Modern Nutrition in
Health and Disease

Modern Nutrition in Health and Disease

Sixth Edition

Edited by

ROBERT S. GOODHART, M.D., D.M.S.

Consultant to the New York Academy of Medicine
on Medical Education and Nutrition
New York, New York

MAURICE E. SHILS, M.D., Sc.D.

Associate Professor of Medicine
Cornell University Medical College
Attending Physician and Director of Clinical Nutrition
Memorial Sloan-Kettering Cancer Center
New York, New York

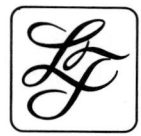

Lea & Febiger
Philadelphia 1980

FIRST EDITION, 1955

SECOND EDITION, 1960

THIRD EDITION, 1964
Reprinted February, 1966

FOURTH EDITION, 1968
Reprinted March, 1970
Reprinted July, 1971

FIFTH EDITION, 1973
Reprinted September, 1974
Reprinted April, 1975
Reprinted July, 1976
Reprinted January, 1978

Library of Congress Cataloging in Publication Data
Main entry under title:

Modern nutrition in health and disease.

  Includes bibliographical references and index.
  Fifth ed. with the same title and the same two editors
is entered under R. S. Goodhart.
  1. Nutrition. 2. Diet in disease. I. Shils,
Maurice Edward. II. Goodhart, Robert Stanley, 1909–
III. Goodhart, Robert Stanley, 1909–   Modern nutri-
tion in health and disease. [DNLM: 1. Diet therapy.
2. Nutrition. WB400.3 M689]
QP141.G63   1980   613.2   79-16842
ISBN 0-8121-0645-8

Published in Great Britain by Henry Kimpton Publishers, London

PRINTED IN THE UNITED STATES OF AMERICA

Print No. 5 4 3 2 1

PREFACE

The sixth edition of *Modern Nutrition in Health and Disease* continues the purposes of previous editions in serving as a textbook on nutrition and as a ready reference book for students and practitioners in the fields of nutrition, medicine, dentistry and public health. The textual arrangement of the fifth edition was well received and this volume continues to group the various aspects of the science of nutrition into major areas which take the reader from basic nutritional science through discussions of the safety and adequacy of the food supply, interrelations of nutrients and metabolism, malnutrition, nutrition during "physiologic" stress and nutrition in the prevention and treatment of diseases.

There have been major revisions and up-dating to keep the reader abreast of the numerous changes which have continued in this vital and expanding field. The contributions to this volume continue to emphasize the fact that the science and practice of nutrition are basic components of clinical medicine. Twenty of the contributors are new with this edition. New chapters have been added on Anatomy and Physiology of the Gastrointestinal Tract, Malnutrition in Hospitalized Patients, Food Fads and Faddism and Effect of Processing on the Nutritional Values of Foods. The chapter on Criteria of an Adequate Diet has been broadened to include discussions of vegetarian diets, dietary fiber and current faddist nonvitamins. The Appendix has expanded information including the composition of numerous defined-formula (elemental) diets.

This book could not have been revised without the support of the contributors: our indebtedness to them is great. We extend appreciation to the staff of Lea & Febiger for their assistance.

New York, New York   Robert S. Goodhart
                         Maurice E. Shils

CONTRIBUTORS

Lilla Aftergood, Ph.D., Associate Research Biochemist, School of Public Health, University of California, Los Angeles, California

Roslyn B. Alfin-Slater, Ph.D., Professor, Environmental and Nutritional Sciences, School of Public Health, Professor of Biological Chemistry, School of Medicine, University of California, Los Angeles, California

Janet A. Appel, Ph.D., Postgraduate Researcher, Department of Nutritional Sciences, University of California, Berkeley, California

Louis V. Avioli, M.D., Shoenberg Professor of Medicine, School of Medicine, Washington University, St. Louis, Missouri

A. E. Axelrod, Ph.D., Professor, Department of Biochemistry, School of Medicine, University of Pittsburgh, Pittsburgh, Pennsylvania

Herman Baker, Ph.D., Professor of Medicine and Preventive Medicine and Community Health, Director, Vitamin Laboratories, College of Medicine and Dentistry, New Jersey Medical School, East Orange, New Jersey

Mark L. Batshaw, M.D., Assistant Professor of Pediatrics and Neurology, The Johns Hopkins University School of Medicine, Baltimore, Maryland

Ernest Beutler, M.D., Chairman, Division of Medicine, City of Hope National Medical Center, Duarte, California

Abby Stolper Bloch, M.S., R.D., Head, Clinical Diet/Nutrition Specialist, Clinical Nutrition Support Kitchen, Memorial Sloan-Kettering Cancer Center, New York, New York

Benjamin Borenstein, Ph.D., Corporate Director, Consumer Research and Development, CPC International Inc., International Plaza, Englewood Cliffs, New Jersey

Jo Anne Brasel, M.D., Associate Professor of Pediatrics, Director, Division of Growth and Development, College of Physicians and Surgeons, Columbia University, New York, New York

Diane L. Bray, Ph.D., Postgraduate Research Nutritionist, Department of Nutritional Sciences, University of California, Berkeley, California

George M. Briggs, Ph.D., Professor of Nutrition, Department of Nutritional Sciences, University of California, Berkeley, California

Selwyn A. Broitman, Ph.D., Professor of Microbiology and Nutrition, Boston University School of Medicine, Boston, Massachusetts

C. E. Butterworth, Jr., M.D., Professor and Chairman, Department of Nutrition Sciences, University of Alabama in Birmingham, Birmingham, Alabama

John E. Canham, M.D., Director, Letterman Army Institute of Research, Presidio of San Francisco, San Francisco, California

Ralph R. Cavalieri, M.D., Professor of Medicine and Radiology, University of California, Chief, Nuclear Medicine Service, Veterans Administration Medical Center, San Francisco, California

Neville Colman, M.B., B.Ch., Ph.D., Assistant Professor of Medicine, State University of New York-Downstate Medical Center, Associate Director, Hematology and Nutrition Laboratory, Veterans Administration Hospital, Bronx, New York

C. L. Comar, Ph.D., Professor Emeritus of Physical Biology, Cornell University, Director, Environmental Assessment Department, Electric Power Research Institute, Palo Alto, California

Marilyn C. Crim, Ph.D., Research Associate, Department of Nutrition and Food Sciences, Massachusetts Institute of Technology, Cambridge, Massachusetts

Charles S. Davidson, M.D., Senior Lecturer in Medicine, Massachusetts Institute of Technology, William Bosworth Castle Professor of Medicine, Emeritus, Harvard Medical School, Boston, Massachusetts

H. F. DeLuca, Ph.D., Professor and Chairman, Department of Biochemistry, University of Wisconsin, Madison, Wisconsin

Phani Dhar, M.D., *Formerly* Research Associate, Mallory Institute of Pathology Foundation, Gastrointestinal Research Group, Boston City Hospital, Boston, Massachusetts

Albert B. Eisenstein, M.D., Professor of Medicine, State University of New York—Downstate Medical Center, Associate Chief of Staff/Research, Veterans Administration Hospital, Brooklyn, New York

Nancy Ernst, M.S., R.D., Chief Nutritionist, Lipid Metabolism Branch, National Heart, Lung and Blood Institute, Bethesda, Maryland

Harry D. Fein, M.D., Associate Professor of Clinical Medicine, New York University School of Medicine, Consultant in Medicine, Former Chief of Gastroenterology, Lenox Hill Hospital, New York, New York

Michael R. Fogel, M.D., Associate Professor of Clinical Medicine, Division of Gastroenterology, Santa Clara Valley Medical Center and Stanford University School of Medicine, Stanford, California

Vincent J. Fontana, M.D., Professor of Clinical Pediatrics, New York University College of Medicine, New York, New York

Oscar Frank, Ph.D., Associate Professor of Medicine, Co-Director, Vitamin Laboratories, College of Medicine and Dentistry, New Jersey Medical School, East Orange, New Jersey

Gerald J. Friedman, M.D., F.A.C.P., Clinical Professor of Medicine, Mt. Sinai School of Medicine, City University of New York, Chief, Section of Diabetes and Metabolism, Beth Israel Medical Center, New York City, New York

C. E. Gibbs, M.D., Professor of Obstetrics and Gynecology, The University of Texas Health Science Center at San Antonio, San Antonio, Texas

Robert S. Goodhart, M.D., D.M.S., Consultant to the New York Academy of Medicine on Medical Education and Nutrition, New York, New York

Francisco Grande, M.D., Professor, Institute of Biochemistry and Nutrition, Fundacion Cuenca Villoro, Zaragoza, Spain

Gary M. Gray, M.D., Professor and Head, Division of Gastroenterology, Stanford University School of Medicine, Stanford, California

Herman Grossman, M.D., Director of Pediatric Radiology, Duke University Medical Center, Durham, North Carolina

Victor Herbert, M.D., J.D., Professor of Medicine, State University of New York—Downstate Medical Center, Chief, Hematology and Nutrition Laboratory, Veterans Administration Hospital, Bronx, New York

Robert E. Hodges, M.D., Professor of Internal Medicine, Chief, Nutrition Section, University of California School of Medicine, Davis, California

Neil A. Holtzman, M.D., Associate Professor of Pediatrics, The Johns Hopkins University School of Medicine, Baltimore, Maryland

M. K. Horwitt, Ph.D., Professor Emeritus, Department of Biochemistry, School of Medicine, St. Louis University, St. Louis, Missouri

Seymour H. Hutner, Ph.D., Professor Emeritus in Residence, Department of Biology and Haskins Laboratories, Pace University, New York, New York

Frank L. Iber, M.D., Chief, Gastroenterology Division, School of Medicine, University of Maryland, Baltimore, Maryland

Elizabeth Jacob, M.B., B.S., M.R.C. Path., Associate Professor of Medicine, University of Manitoba, Winnipeg, Manitoba, Canada

Robert M. Kark, M.D., Professor of Medicine, Rush Medical College, Chicago, Illinois

Ancel Keys, Ph.D., Professor Emeritus of Physiological Hygiene, School of Public Health, University of Minnesota, Minneapolis, Minnesota

Robert I. Levy, M.D., Director, National Heart, Lung and Blood Institute, National Institutes of Health, Bethesda, Maryland

Ting-Kai Li, M.D., Professor of Medicine and Biochemistry, School of Medicine, Indiana University, Indianapolis, Indiana

Charles S. Lieber, M.D., Professor of Medicine and Pathology, Mt. Sinai School of Medicine, City University of New York, Director, Alcoholism Research and Treatment Center, Bronx Veterans Administration Medical Center, Bronx, New York

Nan Sen Tseng Lui, Ph.D., Senior Clinical Research Analyst, Lederle Laboratories, Pearl River, New York

Jean Mayer, Ph.D., Sc.D., President, Tufts University, Boston, Massachusetts

Morton A. Meyers, M.D., Professor and Chairman, Department of Radiology, State University of New York at Stony Brook, Stony Brook, New York

Therese D. Mondeika, R.D., Assistant Director, Department of Foods and Nutrition, American Medical Association, Chicago, Illinois

Fernando Moreno-Pagan, M.D., Chief of Pediatric Allergy, St. Vincent's Hospital and Medical Center, New York, New York

Hamish N. Munro, M.D., Sc.D., Professor of Physiological Chemistry, Department of Nutrition and Food Sciences, Massachusetts Institute of Technology, Cambridge, Massachusetts

Robert A. Neal, Ph.D., Professor, Department of Biochemistry, School of Medicine, Vanderbilt University, Nashville, Tennessee

Paul M. Newberne, D.V.M., Ph.D., Professor of Nutritional Pathology, Massachusetts Institute of Technology, Cambridge, Massachusetts

Robert E. Olson, M.D., Ph.D., Professor and Chairman, Department of Biochemistry, School of Medicine, St. Louis University, St. Louis, Missouri

Bernard L. Oser, Ph.D., President, Bernard L. Oser Associates, Inc., Forest Hills, New York

Joseph H. Oyama, M.D., Assistant Professor of Medicine, Rush Medical College, Chicago, Illinois

H. T. Randall, M.D., Sc.D., Professor and Chairman, Section on Surgery, Brown University Program in Medicine, Surgeon-in-Chief, Rhode Island Hospital, Providence, Rhode Island

Oswald A. Roels, Ph.D., Professor, Department of Marine Studies, University of Texas at Austin, Director, Port Aransas Marine Laboratory, Marine Science Institute, University of Texas, Port Aransas, Texas

Harold H. Sandstead, M.D., Director, Human Nutrition Laboratory, Science and Education Administration, United States Department of Agriculture, North Central Region, Grand Forks, North Dakota

Howerde E. Sauberlich, Ph.D., Chief, Department of Nutrition, Letterman Army Institute of Research, Presidio of San Francisco, San Francisco, California

Joseph Seitchik, M.D., Professor and Chairman, Department of Obstetrics and Gynecology, The University of Texas Health Science Center at San Antonio, San Antonio, Texas

James H. Shaw, Ph.D., Professor of Nutrition, Harvard School of Dental Medicine, Boston, Massachusetts

Spencer Shaw, M.D., Assistant Professor of Medicine, Mt. Sinai School of Medicine, City University of New York, Staff Physician, Section of Liver and Nutrition, Bronx, Veterans Administration Medical Center, New York, New York

Maurice E. Shils, M.D., Sc.D., F.A.C.P., Associate Professor of Medicine, Cornell University Medical College, Attending Physician and Director of Clinical Nutrition, Memorial Sloan-Kettering Cancer Center, New York, New York

Sant P. Singh, M.D., Professor of Medicine, Chicago Medical School, Associate Chief of Staff/Research, Veterans Administration Medical Center, North Chicago, Illinois

Selma E. Snyderman, M.D., Professor of Pediatrics, New York University School of Medicine, Attending Physician, Bellevue Hospital, University Hospital, New York, New York

Edward A. Sweeney, D.M.D., Assistant Dean for Curriculum, Associate Professor of Pediatric Dentistry, Harvard School of Dental Medicine, Senior Associate in Pedodontics, Children's Hospital Medical Center, Boston, Massachusetts

J. C. Thompson, Jr., Ph.D., Director, Department of Physical Biology, New York State College of Veterinary Medicine, Cornell University, Ithaca, New York

Benjamín Torún, M.D., Ph.D., Head, Program of Physiology and Clinical Nutrition, The Institute of Nutrition of Central America and Panama, Guatemala City, Guatemala

David L. Valle, M.D., Assistant Professor of Pediatrics and Medicine, The Johns Hopkins University School of Medicine, Baltimore, Maryland

Bert L. Vallee, M.D., Paul C. Cabot Professor of Biological Chemistry, Harvard Medical School, Boston, Massachusetts

Fernando E. Viteri, M.D., Sc.D., Chief, Division of Human Nutrition and Biology, The Institute of Nutrition of Central America and Panama, Guatemala City, Guatemala

Donald M. Watkin, M.D., M.P.H., F.A.C.P., Research Associate Professor of Medicine, The George Washington University Medical Center, Washington, D.C.

Robin C. Watson, M.D., Professor of Radiology, Cornell University Medical College, Chairman, Department of Diagnostic Radiology, Attending Physician, Memorial Sloan-Kettering Cancer Center, New York, New York

Jean Weininger, Ph.D., Research Fellow, Department of Nutritional Sciences, University of California, Berkeley, California

Roland L. Weinsier, M.D., Dr.P.H., Associate Professor and Director, Division of Clinical Nutrition, Department of Nutrition Sciences, University of Alabama in Birmingham, Birmingham, Alabama

Philip L. White, Sc.D., Director, Department of Foods and Nutrition, American Medical Association, Chicago, Illinois

Myron Winick, M.D., R. R. Williams Professor of Nutrition, Professor of Pediatrics, Director, Institute of Human Nutrition, Director, Center for Nutrition, Genetics and Human Development, College of Physicians and Surgeons, Columbia University, New York, New York

Norman Zamcheck, M.D., Associate Clinical Professor of Medicine, Harvard Medical School, Chief, Gastrointestinal Research Laboratory, Mallory Institute of Pathology Foundation, Boston City Hospital, Boston, Massachusetts

CONTENTS

PART II. SAFETY AND ADEQUACY OF THE FOOD SUPPLY

Contents   xiii

Part I

The Foundations of Nutrition

Chapter *1*

BODY WEIGHT, BODY COMPOSITION AND CALORIE STATUS

Francisco Grande
and
Ancel Keys

The body is, in the most literal sense, the product of its nutrition. Though the transformations are profound, nutrition begins with the foodstuffs and proceeds to the material end-result, the living body and its functions. The most elementary, but certainly not the least important, aspect of nutrition is the gross mass of tissue it produces and maintains. The most obvious, and in many populations perhaps the most common, nutritional defects are those caused by gross calorie imbalance.

Calorie undernutrition is the conspicuous form of malnutrition in underdeveloped countries but, even in the midst of plenty, starvation caused by disease is common because many illnesses interfere with the appetite or the assimilation of food. In the simplest of societies obesity may be rare, either because of chronic food shortages or because physical exercise is an effective preventive, but as society becomes more specialized, more prosperous and more sedentary an excessive accumulation of body fat tends to be the rule unless it is consciously combatted.

Except for changes in hydration, gain of body weight over a period of time is an expression of positive calorie balance, that is, an excess of calorie intake over expenditure, and, conversely, weight loss is an expression of calorie deficit. It must be borne in mind, however, as discussed later, that there is no simple relationship between calorie balance and the rate of weight gain or loss at a given time. Finally, it is possible to maintain constant weight and still be in positive calorie balance; this can happen when muscle is replaced by fat and when body water is lost in the presence of positive calorie balance.

Until recently, in addition to the impressionistic methods of gross inspection and digital feel, gross body weight, sometimes supplemented with a few measurements of external dimensions, had to suffice for studies on living man. Fortunately, new methods are now at hand for analysis of the body mass into metabolically distinct components.[1-3] These, together with the more widespread application of statistical methods and concepts, provide increasingly useful and precise norms for guidance in calorie nutrition.

BODY WEIGHT

The gross body weight per se has some direct metabolic significance. To the extent that it represents the size of the cell mass of the body it determines the basal metabolic rate. The metabolic cost of physical activity is determined by the body weight, since most of the energy cost of physical activity is expended in simply moving the body around. With a fixed amount of activity—number, extent, speed and force of movements—energy expenditure tends to be directly proportional to gross body weight.[4,5]

Actually, grossly overweight persons tend to be relatively inactive; the movements they make are expensive in calories but they make fewer movements than persons of average weight. Many recent studies show that overweight persons are not characterized so much by large food consumption as by physical inactivity.[6-8] However, when a heavyweight has to move quickly there is an excessive demand for energy, and this may mean a strain on one or more vulnerable organs or functions.

Insurance companies report an excessive death rate in overweight persons from a variety of causes, including accidents. A heavy body is an impediment in avoiding many accidents simply because it is harder to move it or to change its direction. Further, the damaging force in a fall increases with increasing body weight.

Nevertheless, the major importance of the body weight is its association with body fatness. The amount of fat in the body may be considered as an expression of the calorie balance status. It is a common error to regard overweight and obesity as identical. Obesity means excessive fatness and it is essential to adhere to this definition.[2,9] Athletes are often overweight but underfat.[10] It is safe to conclude that a middle-aged man who is 30 or more pounds heavier than the average man of the same height is obese, that is, overfat. At lesser degrees of overweight, the relationship between obesity and overweight is not close, particularly at younger ages.[11-13]

Many sedentary persons are excessively fat but not overweight, while the opposite condition, overweight without fat, is common among people doing heavy physical work. The two conditions are, in fact, metabolic opposites, the one tending to result from the lack of activity, the other from excessive activity. Attention to this discrimination discloses differences in characteristics pertinent to circulation and health.[14]

In addition to distinguishing between fat and muscle in the gross body weight, variations in the water content of the body must be considered. In ascites 5 to 10 kg of fluid in the abdominal cavity may be encountered and much larger totals of edema fluid are not rare. One of Simonart's[15] starved patients lost 20 kg in a week while his nutriture was improving. Extreme edema is readily detected, but more moderate variations in hydration are not easily recognizable. Clinical recognition of edema requires an accumulation of the order of 5 to 10 per cent of the total body weight as excess water.[2,16] The variable contribution of water to the total body weight of clinically healthy persons is reflected in the weight fluctuations seen on reducing diets under controlled conditions.[17]

Another contributor to confusion about the meaning of total body weight is the variable weight of the body skeleton. The mineral mass in the adult skeleton averages approximately 6 per cent of the normal body weight of the adult but, in different persons, it may be as low as 4 or as high as 9 per cent.[2]

Perhaps a more important contribution of the skeleton to the body weight is through its form. Overweight and underweight are commonly computed on the basis of weight for height. However, a broad and short skeleton automatically means a large body weight per unit of height and, thus far, no system has been devised to allow for this in a practical manner. The body "frame" types discussed below are theoretical concepts devoid of real utility in the absence of agreed methods of measurement and classification.

The "Constancy" of Body Weight

The literature contains only limited information about daily weight changes. Rapid fluctuations of body weight do, however, occur with no apparent relation to changes in calorie intake, energy expenditure or health status. These short-term fluctuations are difficult to understand but they should be taken into account in metabolic experiments, especially when they involve limited periods of time. In a group of 44 men living under highly controlled conditions, Durnin[18] observed day-to-day changes of body weight up to 1 kg. Similar observations have been reported by Edholm.[19] Elkinton and Danowski[20] measured body weight of a man on 53 out of 56 days and found a standard deviation of ±0.86 pound, equivalent to ±0.51 per cent of his weight. Taggart[21] studied the body weight of a nonpregnant woman for a period of 80 days. The body weight during the period changed from 61.5 to 63.9 kg with daily fluctuations up to 0.8 kg. These changes were not related to the menstrual cycle.

Most of the short-time fluctuations of body weight can be explained by changes in the water content of the body. These fluctuations, however, do not detract from the fact that, over periods of a week or more, food intake and energy intake are closely balanced and the body weight remains relatively constant.[19]

Considerable changes in body weight can be produced by the retention of water associated with deposition of glycogen in muscle and liver. Olsson and Saltin[22] have reported a mean weight gain of 2.4 kg in 19 young men after 4 days of feeding a carbohydrate-rich diet. Muscle glycogen had been previously depleted by intense arm and leg activity while the men were consuming a diet of fat and protein for 3 days just before the diet. Total body water, measured by dilution of tritiated water, rose in the 4 days by an average of 2.2 liters. From determinations of muscle glycogen, it was estimated that the glycogen content of the body increased by some 500 gm, which means that 3 to 5 gm of water are bound with each gram of glycogen deposited. The meal-eating pattern has a marked effect on body weight in the rat, but Swindell et al.[23] found changes of body weight in young women that were unrelated to the frequency of meals.

Body Weight Standards

Until lately almost all statistical evaluations of calorie status, obesity, emaciation and gross nutritional health have been based simply on the gross body weight as related to height. Comparison of a person's actual weight, M, with his *standard* (tabular) *weight*, S, is the most widely used

Table 1–1. Graded Average Weight in Pounds of Men of Different Statures at Various Ages.*

Height, Inches	Age, Years							
	20	25	30	35	40	45	50	55
60	117	122	126	128	131	133	134	135
62	122	126	130	132	135	137	138	139
64	128	133	136	138	141	143	144	145
66	136	141	144	146	149	151	152	153
68	144	149	152	155	158	160	161	163
70	152	157	161	165	168	170	171	173
72	161	167	172	176	180	182	183	184
74	171	179	184	189	193	195	197	198
76	181	189	196	201	206	209	211	212

*From Davenport, C.B.: *Body Build and Its Inheritance.* Publication 329, Carnegie Institute of Washington, 1923.

criterion of leanness/fatness. The degree of over- or underweight may be expressed as the percentage deviation of the actual (M) from the standard weight (S), $\Delta\% = 100$ (M–S)/S, or as *relative body weight*, R = 100 M/S. It should be stressed again that body weight is not a reliable criterion in the diagnosis of obesity. Thus, in a study of 1761 healthy U. S. Army veterans,[24] only a minority of the extreme relative-body-weight categories (120, 125 or more) were frankly obese by skinfold measurements. In the United States, the standard of reference has long been the tables of average weight for height and age originally published by the Association of Life Insurance Medical Directors and the Actuarial Society of America in 1912 under the title "Medico-actuarial Mortality Investigation" (New York). They are summarized in Tables 1–1 and 1–2.

Elsewhere[25,26] we have discussed the limitations of these tables, which merely give the average values for men and women of specified ages who obtained life insurance policies at standard premium rates from 1888 to about 1905, mostly in urban centers on the eastern seaboard. The heights and weights were recorded as for "ordinary clothing;" what this means today is

questionable. However, for men at least, similar values may apply approximately to the undressed state, that is, in socks and shorts, because the heel height (about 1 inch) roughly counteracts the clothing weight customary half a century ago. For women the application is more difficult because of the variability of heel height and the great reduction in female clothing weight over the intervening years.

More recent tables list body weights for the same height under three headings: "light" or "small frame," "medium frame," and "heavy" or "large frame." The medium frame values correspond to the averages in the older tables and the "light" and "heavy frame" weight values are simply some 5 to 8 per cent smaller or larger, respectively. Unfortunately, there is no accepted system for deciding who has a "light frame," and no actual evaluations of frame size were made in developing the tables. Apparently the observed frequency distributions of the weight values used for the original tables of 1912 (where frame was not considered) were merely divided into thirds. The lighter third of men of a given height and age was arbitrarily defined as having a light frame and the mean weight of this group was then considered to be the

Table 1–2. Graded Average Weight in Pounds of Women of Different Statures at Various Ages.*

Height, Inches	Age, Years							
	20	25	30	35	40	45	50	55
56	106	109	112	115	119	122	125	125
58	110	113	116	119	123	126	129	129
60	114	117	120	123	127	130	133	133
62	119	121	124	127	132	135	138	138
64	125	128	131	134	138	141	144	144
66	132	135	138	142	146	149	152	153
68	140	143	146	150	154	157	161	163
70	147	151	154	157	161	164	169	171
72	156	158	161	163	167	171	176	177

*From Davenport, C. B.: *Body Build and Its Inheritance.* Publication 329, Carnegie Institute of Washington, 1923.

average body weight of men of light frame of the given height and age. In other words, these tables have no basis in measurement and are useless and misleading, except to indicate that a single "average" body weight for given height and age is inadequate and that differences in skeletal type may explain some of the variability observed in clinically healthy persons of the same height, age and sex.

Still more recently, the Metropolitan Life Insurance Company has popularized the idea enunciated by Fisher and Fisk[27] that the observed body weights for the average of the population are not necessarily those most conducive to health. In the United States and many other countries it is usual for body weight to increase long after body length growth is finished, but it is possible to argue that the usual gain of weight beyond age 25 or 30 is undesirable or at least unnecessary. Accordingly, tables of "desirable body weight" (at first labeled "ideal") have been provided.[8] Tables 1–3 and 1–4 specify frame size, with no more precise definition than that indicated above, and they indicate a "desirable"

range (of 7 to 8 pounds for different frames and heights) within each height and frame class. Age is not specified, since the theory is that no weight change with advancing age is desirable. The values are, in fact, merely a rearrangement of the 1912 tables but limited to persons of 25 to 30 years of age. The specification of optimal or ideal weight is therefore uncertain. For estimating present averages, without regard to what may be "desirable" values, some data have been obtained from Selective Service records[28] and studies of the Quartermaster Corps.[29,30]

The average white registrant for Selective Service just before World War II was 26 years old, and was, unclothed, 68.5 inches tall and weighed 152.2 pounds. From the old 1912 tables a clothed weight of 152.0 pounds would be predicted for the average 26-year-old man whose height in shoes is 68.5 inches. Unfortunately, the Selective Service data are not analyzed for other ages and heights, and the data for men after several years in the Army differ from those of men first called up for service. An analysis in 1946 and 1949 of

Table 1–3. Weight in Pounds According to Frame (in Indoor Clothing).*

Height with Shoes 1-inch Heels		*Desirable Weights for Men Aged 25 and Over*		
Feet	Inches	Small Frame	Medium Frame	Large Frame
5	2	112-120	118-129	126-141
5	3	115-123	121-133	129-144
5	4	118-126	124-136	132-148
5	5	121-129	127-139	135-152
5	6	124-133	130-143	138-156
5	7	128-137	134-147	142-161
5	8	132-141	138-152	147-166
5	9	136-145	142-156	151-170
5	10	140-150	146-160	155-174
5	11	144-154	150-165	159-179
6	0	148-158	154-170	164-184
6	1	152-162	158-175	168-189
6	2	156-167	162-180	173-194
6	3	160-171	167-185	178-199
6	4	164-175	172-190	182-204

*For nude weight, deduct 5 to 7 lb (male) or 2 to 4 lb (female). Prepared by Metropolitan Life Insurance Company. Derived primarily from data of the Build and Blood Pressure Study, Society of Actuaries, 1959.

Table 1–4.   Weight in Pounds According to Frame (in Indoor Clothing).*

Height with Shoes 2-inch Heels		Desirable Weights for Women Aged 25 and Over		
Feet	Inches	Small Frame	Medium Frame	Large Frame
4	10	92- 98	96-107	104-119
4	11	94-101	98-110	106-122
5	0	96-104	101-113	109-125
5	1	99-107	104-116	112-128
5	2	102-110	107-119	115-131
5	3	105-113	110-122	118-134
5	4	108-116	113-126	121-138
5	5	111-119	116-130	125-142
5	6	114-123	120-135	129-146
5	7	118-127	124-139	133-150
5	8	122-131	128-143	137-154
5	9	126-135	132-147	141-158
5	10	130-140	136-151	145-163
5	11	134-144	140-155	149-168
6	0	138-148	144-159	153-173

*For nude weight, deduct 5 to 7 lb (male) or 2 to 4 lb (female). Prepared by Metropolitan Life Insurance Company. Derived primarily from data of the Build and Blood Pressure Study, Society of Actuaries, 1959.

data on men leaving the Army after several years indicated that, in both white and Negro men, the body weights are higher than would be expected from the 1912 tables.[29] The white separatees averaged 104.4 per cent and the Negro separatees averaged 105.0 per cent of the values listed in the medicoactuarial tables of 1912.

For women the actual averages for the population are still more uncertain. No samples generally representative of the population have ever been studied. A sample of about 8,500 women in the Women's Army Corps and in the Army Nurse Corps averaged 26.9 years old, 63.9 inches tall and 130.9 pounds in body weight; the 1912 tabular weight figure would be 128.5.

A national survey in Canada, covering some 22,000 persons in a carefully selected stratified sample of the entire country, provides more acceptable modern data.[31] The average weights for specified heights found in the Canadian survey are given in abbreviated form in Table 1–5. These weights are for persons in "ordinary" indoor clothing, without shoes.

A 1960-62 health examination survey by the Department of Health, Education and Welfare provides weights for height and age for 6,672 persons, out of a nationwide probability sample of 7,710 persons 18 to 79 years of age selected from the 111 million in the population in that age group in the United States.[32] These data are given in abbreviated form in Table 1–6.

The data of the U.S. health examination survey were compared with those of the 1943 British height/weight survey, the 1953 Canadian survey and the 1959 Society of Actuaries study in this country. Among men 18 to 64 years of age, Britons were found to average 19 pounds less, Canadians 5 pounds less and insured Americans 6 to 7 pounds less than the American men examined in 1960-62. For women of this age, Britons were 14 to 15 pounds less, Canadians 5 to 6 pounds less, and insured Americans 10 to 11 pounds less than the American women examined in 1960-62.

What, then, may be concluded about standard, desirable and "ideal" weights? In the first place, it is obvious that the avail-

Table 1–5. Average Weights (pounds) for Height and Age of Canadians in "Ordinary Indoor Clothing, without Shoes."*

Height in Inches	Age in Years				
	25	35	45	55	65 and over
Men					
60	128	139	136	137	130
62	135	146	144	145	140
64	142	152	152	152	149
66	150	160	161	160	158
68	156	167	169	168	167
70	163	174	177	176	177
72	170	182	186	184	186
74	185	189	194	191	195
Women					
58	113	124	131	137	128
60	118	128	135	142	136
62	123	132	139	146	144
64	128	135	143	151	152
66	133	139	147	156	161
68	138	143	151	160	169
70	143	146	154	165	177

*Abbreviated and adapted from Table 2 of Pett and Ogilvie.[31]

Table 1–6. Average Weight (pounds) for Men and Women, by Age and Height†: United States, 1960-62.*

Height in Inches	Age in Years					
	18–24	25–34	35–44	45–54	55–64	65–74
Men						
62	140	139	150	142	145	161
64	139	147	154	159	158	154
66	160	161	166	164	163	159
68	157	165	170	174	172	164
70	165	180	179	183	173	174
72	169	188	183	183	177	188
74	185	182	204	203	216	
Women						
58	121	121	117	117	136	140
60	122	124	138	137	148	142
62	128	133	143	143	159	154
64	126	140	147	155	156	158
66	142	139	148	157	145	154
68	131	150	160	169	158	200

*From Roberts.[32]
†Height without shoes; weight partially clothed. Clothing weight estimated as averaging 2 pounds.

able data are inadequate to describe the actual weights of "average" members of the population or to specify what weights would be most conducive to health. If anything, the young men of today may be heavier, at the same height, than those of 50 years ago and this may possibly be true of young women as well. The average body weights of older persons are much more uncertain, though there is no doubt that weight, in the United States, tends to change with age in somewhat the same manner as at the turn of the century.

Weights and Heights During Growth

The present discussion is primarily concerned with adults and space does not permit detailed consideration of the situation during growth, that is, in infants and children. Far more data are available on children than on adults. Height/weight data for the United States have been summarized[33] and Garn and Shamir[34] have reviewed anthropometric methods, including fat estimation, in the study of growth. The extensive data on height and weight at different ages have been analyzed by Falkner[35] and are given here in Tables 1–7

and 1–8. During the last 50 years, both sexes in the United States have been getting taller and heavier at any given age through the growing period.[36,37]

Birth-weight-doubling time is usually considered to take place around 5 to 6 months, but current data indicate a trend toward faster weight gain among American babies. Thus, Neumann and Alpaugh[38] have reported average birth-weight-doubling time of 119 days (3.8 months) for American children. Formula-fed babies doubled their birth weight earlier than did breast-fed ones (113 versus 124 days, $p < 0.05$). There is no reason to suppose that a trend to increased rate of weight gain is desirable; on the contrary, faster weight gain in infancy may contribute to later problems with obesity.

Body Weights in Other Countries

Information on average and desirable body weights in many, but not all, other countries is as deficient or worse than that in the United States. Older data, often of doubtful statistical merit, are summarized by Krogman.[39] Useful data are available for Great Britain and Japan. There is no

Table 1–7. Heights and Weights of Boys Aged 4 to 18 Years. Values of the 5th, 50th (median), and 95th Centiles.*

Ages (yrs)	Height (inches)				Weight (pounds)		
	5th	50th	95th		5th	50th	95th
4	38.3	40.8	43.3		30.0	36.1	42.2
5	40.3	43.4	46.4		33.0	40.3	47.6
6	42.8	45.9	49.0		36.0	44.7	53.4
7	44.8	48.1	51.4		40.3	50.9	61.5
8	46.9	50.5	54.1		44.4	57.4	70.1
9	48.8	52.8	56.8		48.0	64.4	80.4
10	50.6	54.9	59.2		51.4	71.4	91.4
11	51.9	56.4	60.9		53.3	78.9	102.5
12	53.5	58.6	63.7		60.0	86.0	113.5
13	55.2	61.3	67.4		65.3	98.6	131.9
14	57.5	64.1	70.7		75.5	118.8	148.1
15	61.0	66.9	72.8		88.0	124.3	160.6
16	63.8	68.9	74.0		97.8	133.8	169.8
17	65.2	69.8	74.4		106.5	139.8	174.0
18	65.9	70.2	74.5		110.3	144.8	179.3

*From Falkner.[35]

Table 1–8.   Heights and Weights of Girls Aged 4 to 18 Years. Values of the 5th, 50th (median), and 95th Centiles.*

Ages (yrs)	Height (inches)				Weight (pounds)		
	5th	50th	95th		5th	50th	95th
4	38.1	40.7	43.3		28.8	36.1	43.4
5	40.6	43.4	46.2		32.2	40.9	49.6
6	42.8	45.9	49.0		35.5	45.7	55.9
7	44.5	47.8	51.1		38.3	51.0	63.7
8	46.4	50.0	53.6		42.0	57.2	72.4
9	48.2	52.2	56.2		45.1	63.6	82.1
10	49.9	54.5	59.1		48.2	71.0	95.0
11	51.9	57.0	62.1		55.4	82.0	108.6
12	54.1	59.5	64.9		63.9	94.4	124.9
13	57.1	62.2	66.8		72.8	105.5	138.2
14	58.5	63.1	67.7		83.0	113.0	144.0
15	59.5	63.8	68.1		89.5	120.0	150.5
16	59.8	64.1	68.4		95.1	123.0	150.1
17	60.1	64.2	68.3		97.9	125.8	153.7
18	60.1	64.4	68.7		96.0	126.2	156.4

*From Falkner.[35]

doubt that, at the same height and age, Britons tend to be lighter than Americans and the age-increment in weight is smaller.[40] In Japan, not only is the relative weight smaller but the age-increment in weight is much smaller than in Americans.[41]

A continuous rise in body weight with age, such as is the situation in the United States, is not inevitable. Among relatively primitive people on islands in the China Sea there is no increase of average body weight after age 25.[42,43] It is interesting that most of the usual age-increment in body weight common among adults in the western world rapidly disappears in populations with short rations who are not actually starving.[2] A relatively moderate reduction in the food supplies available for the entire population tends to produce the greatest loss of body weight in the older, fatter individuals, and the health records of World War II suggest that this may be beneficial.

In recent years we have been able to measure heights and weights of substantially all men aged 40 to 59 in selected areas in Italy, Yugoslavia, Finland, Greece and the Netherlands and have compared these with the findings on statistical samples of railroad employees in the United States. In terms of the medicoactuarial standards (Table 1–1), the medians for relative body weight of different categories of United States railroad employees ranged from 101 to 106 per cent; the corresponding figures for men in the foreign samples were below 100 per cent in all except one group in Italy. It is notable, too, that in all of the foreign samples the relative body weight decreased with age from 40 to 44 and from 55 to 59 years. In other words, these European men tended to gain less weight with age than did the Americans. The inference is that American men tend to excessive fat accumulation with advancing age.

Somatotypes

Human bodies differ in type or shape and recognition of gross differences in the body type is not possible solely from measurements of relative weight or of fatness. The idea that particular body types are dominant among patients with certain diseases is of long standing, but there is lack of agreement on the definition of body type and the distinction between body type and relative obesity is not clear.

Sheldon[44] proposed a scheme of *somatotypes* which is supposed to represent the basic body characteristic, relatively independent of body fatness, and this has been rather widely used. However, it is clear that these types are not, in fact, independent of the state of nutrition.[26,45] Studies on experimental starvation in man have shown that, when starved, the endomorph is so changed that he will be easily classified as an ectomorph. *Endomorphy* and *ectomorphy* appear to be primarily impure expressions of the obesity/emaciation continuum, while the meaning of *mesomorphy* is uncertain. The fact that Sheldon's somatotypes are related to body fatness and to skeletal shape does not confer any special value to somatotyping; better estimates of these items are available by other and less esoteric means.

Optimal Characteristics

All the foregoing discussion leads to the conclusion that the specification of "optimal" or "ideal" weights is hazardous business. For body weight and relative obesity, at least, the only point on which there will be full agreement is that major departures from the population average should be avoided. There is no doubt that there is an excess mortality penalty in later life associated with marked overweight at the time of application for life insurance.

Insurance experience indeed shows increasing mortality rates with increasing degrees of overweight, but there are serious questions about the samples compared and the interpretations thereof. The fact that insurance companies charge extra premiums to overweight persons probably results in biased samples. Moreover, overweight and obesity, though correlated, especially at the extremes, are far from being identical. Obesity, that is, body fatness, has

not been measured in the insurance studies and an excess of weight for given height may reflect bone, muscle or body shape as well as, or instead of, actual obesity.

Physicians and the general public alike are under the pressure of constant propaganda about the health dangers of obesity in general and the development of cardiovascular disease in particular. However, to suggest that the major national health obstacle in the United States is obesity because perhaps a tenth of the population may be 10 per cent or more above the average body weight cannot be sustained from present evidence. Is there actually any serious health hazard necessarily associated with 10 per cent overweight? At what ages? Can we disregard the question of obesity versus overweight? Much more research is needed before scientifically acceptable answers to these questions will be at hand. One thing seems certain. The elimination of gross overweight among Americans cannot, by itself, be expected to bring our adult mortality to a level to compare favorably with that of the Netherlands and the Scandinavian[25] countries, for example. A more penetrating analysis of obesity, rather than mere body weight, might reveal more scope for improvement.

BODY COMPOSITION

The development of methods for estimation of the gross composition of the human body in vivo has provided an important tool for metabolic analysis and the evaluation of nutritional status. The application of these methods makes possible estimation of the main gross components of the human body and, in particular, the measurement of its fat content.[1] Validation of these indirect methods depends on data obtained by the direct analysis of human bodies. The discussion of indirect methods of body composition analysis must start, therefore, with a consideration of the existing data from direct analyses of human bodies.

Direct Analysis of Human Bodies

Technical and legal complications of direct analysis of the main components of whole human bodies are such that few results have been reported in the century since attempts began in this direction. The early work was summarized in the first and subsequent editions of Vierordt's *Tabellen*[46] but the technical methods then available severely limit the utility of the older data.

Table 1–9 summarizes the most reliable modern data on the gross composition of 3 adult male bodies. Two of these can be considered representative of normal bodies, but the body of the 46-year-old man is not free of suspicion of abnormality.

There is a good deal of variability in the total fat content of these selected bodies. Equally significant is the variation in the ratio of ash to protein and in the water content of the fat-free mass. Clearly, the concept of a constant composition of the fat-free portion of the body finds no support from the only direct data we have for man. The data from animals are far more numerous and they also show considerable variation among individuals.

The Compartments of the Body

Metabolically, the most elementary analysis of the body mass begins with the differentation between the parts of the body that are relatively active in energy metabolism and the relatively nonactive parts. In the latter category are the body fat, the extracellular fluid, the mineral portion of the bony skeleton and a negligible part of the horny epidermis, the nails and the hair.[3,26] The body fat tends to be the most variable compartment, though the extracellular fluid mass may increase considerably in cases of edema.

If, from the total mass of the body, the nonactive masses of fat, extracellular fluid and bone mineral are subtracted, the remainder may be termed the *active tissue mass*[47] or *cell residue*. This mass, primarily cells of course, may represent anything from perhaps 30 to 65 per cent of the total body weight, but it accounts for substantially all the energy consumption. The highest values for cell mass, as a percentage of body weight, will be found in lean muscular men in a state of dehydration; the lowest values will occur in sedentary women who are both fat and edematous.

Table 1–9. Body Composition from Direct Chemical Analysis of 3 Male Cadavers*

Reference	Age (years)	Height (cm)	Total weight (kg)	Per cent†				Water % of Fat-free Weight
				Water	Fat	Protein	Ash	
Mitchell et al. 1945	35	183.0	70.6	68.2	12.5	14.5	4.8	77.9
Widdowson et al. 1951	25	179.0	71.8	62.0	15.0	16.6	6.4	72.9
Frobes et al. 1953	46	168.5	53.8	56.0	19.6	18.8	5.6	69.6
Mean	35.3	176.8	65.4	62.6	15.3	16.4	5.7	73.9

*From Brozek, et al.[49] Based on examinations by Mitchell et al.,[144] Widdowson et al.,[145] and Forbes et al.[146]
†Computed as per cent of the body weight accounted for by water, protein and ash, comprising 99.7 per cent of the total body weight.

The foregoing subdivision of the mass of the body into the four compartments—fat, extracellular water, cell residue and bone mineral—is not only metabolically reasonable but it also corresponds to some degree, as we shall see, with the availability of practical methods of measurement in vivo. The distribution of the four main chemical components of the body among the four main compartments is described in Table 1-10.

It will be observed that this system pays little attention to the traditional classifications of the body into kinds of parts—bony skeleton, cartilaginous skeleton, voluntary muscle and so on—or into systems—skeletal system, muscular system, nervous system and so on. Partly this is because the first focus is on gross metabolism; equally important, however, is the fact that no practical methods are available, or even conceivable, to provide reliable measurements of the living human body in these other terms. Furthermore, when the center of interest is nutrition, and especially changes in nutritional state, some questions about organs and organ systems are of only subordinate interest. For example, the mass of the brain and ner-

vous tissue is relatively insensitive to nutritional effects, at least after growth is finished. Mental and nervous functions may be greatly affected, but this is not at all closely related to the mass of the brain and nerves; the mass itself is remarkably constant in the face of starvation or of gross overnutrition of the body as a whole.[2] The degree to which the adult skeletal mass responds to changes in nutrition is unknown, but in any event the change is relatively small and slow. On the other hand the masses of some organs and organ systems seem to respond alike to gross nutritional changes. In starvation, the percentage reductions in the masses of the heart, voluntary muscles, kidneys, testes and many other organs are similar.[2]

In the partition system just described it will be observed that there are no places, as such, for blood, skeleton or adipose tissue. The estimation of total blood volume (and hence its mass) is not difficult and a combination of the dye method (T-1824 dilution) or labeled erythrocyte injection, with a hematocrit, for example, provides estimates of both circulating blood plasma and cells. These measurements are useful and provide additional detail but they are not

Table 1-10. A System of Symbols Used in Describing the Body Compartments and the Main Chemical Components of the Body.*

Body compartments		Chemical Components			
		Water A	Fat F	Protein P	Minerals M
Fat (F)		—	F	—	—
Extracellular water (A_E)		A_E	—	—	—
Cell residue (C)		A_c	—	P	M_c†
Bone (osseous mineral) (M_o)		—	—	—	M_o
Total body weight	$W = A + F + P + M = F + A_E + C + M_o$				
Total body water	$A = A_E + A_c$				
Total body mineral	$M = M_o + M_c$				
Cell residue	$C = A_c + P + M_c + W - (F + A_E + M_o)$				
Total nonfat solids	$S = P + M$				
Cell residue solids	$(M_3) = P + M_c$				

*From Brozek, et al.[49]

†M_c refers to the mineral content of the "cell residue" and represents by definition all mineral that is not osseous ($M_c = M - M_o$) i.e. the mineral in the "cells" and in the extracellular fluid.

essential in the first stage of metabolic analysis. The total mass of the blood is not a large part of the total body mass and it accounts for only an infinitesimal part of the total energy metabolism of the body. The plasma (or rather the plasma water), which normally comprises more than half of the blood volume and makes up about 4 per cent of the body weight, is included in the calculation of extracellular water. The cellular components of the blood account for only about a thirtieth of the total body weight; they are included in the "cell residue" compartment, which also includes the plasma proteins and the plasma minerals in our system of partition.

The skeleton is a large mass and in the living (i.e. fresh, wet) state may average a sixth of the total body mass. In 64 young white men who averaged 70.7 kg of living weight, the dry defatted skeletal weight was 4,259 gm or 6 per cent of the gross body weight.[48] The bone mineral accounts for only a fraction of the total skeletal mass, and the water, protein and fat components are included in the estimates of the total body content of these substances, or in the corresponding compartments (extracellular water, cell residue and fat). From the data of the analyses of the 3 cadavers listed in Table 1–9 we have estimated the mass of bone mineral (after transformation of ash into bone mineral[49]) as 4.8 per cent of the total body weight.

Fat is defined in this chapter as pure fat obtained after ether extraction of the whole body. Adipose tissue is not, as is sometimes supposed, pure fat. From Bozenraad's old studies[50] it often is concluded that human adipose tissue is 80 to 85 per cent pure fat. Actually, he merely reported that when drying samples of adipose tissue in an oven they lost an average of 15 to 20 per cent of their weight. Bozenraad was well aware of the fact that adipose tissue contains connective tissue, blood vessels and cell walls and he did not suggest that this dried adipose tissue was simply fat. He found the water content of adipose tissue in emaciated persons to be considerably greater than in well-nourished persons. In 7 emaciated bodies water averaged 31 per cent of the abdominal "fat," 33 per cent of the heart "fat," and 25 per cent of the kidney "fat." The corresponding averages for 14 well-nourished subjects were 12, 18 and 14 per cent respectively.

Densitometric Determination of Body Fat

The relative proportions of the components of a system consisting of an additive mixture of two substances of different density can be calculated if we know the density of each of the components and that of the mixture. Let W_1 and W_2 be the masses of the components, d_1 and d_2 their densities, and D the density of the mixture. D will be

$$(1) \quad D = \frac{W_1 + W_2}{\left(\frac{W_1}{d_1}\right) + \left(\frac{W_2}{d_2}\right)}$$

If we make $W_1 + W_2 = 1$ and represent the component W_1 as a fraction (w_1) of the total mass we can write

$$(2) \quad D = \frac{1}{(w_1/d_1) + (1 - w_1/d_2)}$$

Solving for w_1

$$(3) \quad w_1 = \frac{1}{D} \cdot \frac{d_1 d_2}{(d_2 - d_1)} - \frac{d_1}{(d_2 - d_1)}$$

$$(4) \quad w_1 = \frac{\left(\frac{d_2}{D} - 1\right)}{\left(\frac{d_2}{d_1} - 1\right)}$$

The application of this equation to the estimation of fat in the living human body requires, then, the measurement of its density, the definition of the two components W_1 and W_2 and assigning values for their densities d_1, d_2.

An early application of densitometry was made by Kohlrausch[51] who used it to demonstrate changes in the body composition of dogs resulting from alterations in nutritional state and in physical exercise. General interest in this method developed later as a result of the pioneer work of Behnke and his colleagues in weighing men under water.[52,53] The development of theory and applications is presented by Keys and Brozek[26] and by Siri.[3] We have published a revision of the constants and assumptions involved in the application of the densitometric method to the determination of body fat in man.[49] The density of the human body is obtained from estimates of the total mass and volume of the body. The measurement of the volume can be made with considerable accuracy by either of two methods. The Archimedean principle of weighing the body under water provides a sensitive measure of body volume, but it requires that an estimate be made of the air in the lungs and respiratory passages at the time of weighing.[26] Measurement of this residual air is not particularly difficult with the nitrogen washout method. In the alternative method, first used by Kohlrausch,[51] the body volume is estimated from the application of the gas laws of Boyle and Gay-Lussac to the body in an air chamber of known capacity. The considerable technical difficulties of the latter method seem to be largely overcome by the use of a foreign gas, such as helium, of which a known amount is injected into the gas chamber; the free space is then estimated from a gas analysis on the dilution principle.[3]

Lean Body Mass versus Fat-free Body. Behnke[52] proposed partition of the body into two parts, (1) fat and (2) "lean body mass." The latter was conceived of as the body with the least amount of fat compatible with health and was considered to include the "essential fat," amounting to 10 per cent of its weight. This definition was later revised so that the lean body mass was held to include 2 per cent of its weight as fat. Since it is impossible to decide how much fat is really essential and since no methods are available to separate body fat into essential and nonessential parts, more recent investigations have either redefined the lean body mass as the body devoid of all fat[54] or, better, have abandoned the term and deal with the fat-free body and the body fat, the latter being the sum of ether-extractable substances in the body.

Pace and Rathbun[55] considered the body to be made up of a nonfat portion and pure fat, and assumed the densities of these two parts to be constant. They then provided a numerical solution for Equation 4 which has been fairly widely used. However, it is now known that their value for fat density is incorrect for living men and that the value for density of the fat-free body is neither a constant nor precisely known for any given situation.[3,26] Moreover, such an equation cannot be accurate because, when the body becomes fatter, it does not do so merely by adding fat to the preexisting mass. Numerous observations in controlled experiments have shown that, in men showing large changes of body weight induced by dietary alterations, the density of the tissue gained or lost is never that of pure fat; in other words, the density of the nonfat part of the body changes with nutritional status.[56]

The Density of Human Fat. Human body fat, as extracted by ether from adipose tissue removed at surgery from the living body, has a density of 0.9000 gm per ml at 37°C.[57] Variations in fat density are small between the sexes and among individuals and locations in the body. This low variability, as well as the low absolute value of the density, provides the basis for estimating the proportion of fat in the body from the density of the living person.[1,3,26,52] It should be noted, however, that the thermal coefficient of expansion of fat is relatively high. Allowance for this must be made in dealing with dead bodies. In human fat the mean change in density is 0.00074 per degree C, over the range of 15 to 37°C, so that, even in the living body, the density will be different in a feverish person than in the same person with hypothermia.[57] Different animal species differ somewhat in the density and thermal expansion of their body fat and in some species, notably the cow and the lamb, subcutaneous and internal fats have different densities. The density of the ether extract from muscle and brain is higher than that of the ether extract from adipose tissue.[58] All these facts must be taken into account in applying the densitometric method for the estimation of total body fat.

The Concepts of "Reference Body" and of "Obesity Tissue." The nonfat portion of the body has an average density something like 1.10 gm per ml at 37°C, but there are individual variations; the value is altered by gross changes of hydration, as in edema, and by changes in the degree of obesity. As a person grows fatter, the bony mineral mass (of high density) tends to remain constant while water, connective tissue and cells, as well as fat, tend to increase.[56,59] This follows from the nature of the adipose tissue and from the fact that many of the soft tissues of the body must make at least slight adjustments to the increase of total body size occasioned by the developing obesity. More muscle is required to carry around the added weight, the blood vessels have to cover more distance, the area of the skin has to increase. These complications, however, do not prevent highly useful estimates of total body fat by densitometry.

Most theoretical and practical needs for the estimation of body fat are satisfied with a relative answer. We have proposed to do this by making comparison with a "standard body," the body of a clinically healthy man aged 25 who corresponds exactly in body weight with the United States average for given height as recorded in standard height/weight tables. By definition such a body is neither obese nor emaciated, neither overweight nor underweight. From measurements on young men selected to correspond with these height/weight requirements such a standard average body is found to have a density of 1.0629 gm per ml at 37°C.[29] The fat content of the standard body was originally estimated as 14 per cent of the total body weight.[26] Bodies with densities less than this are, then, relatively fat and those with densities above this figure are relatively lean.

These differences can be expressed quantitatively in terms of the kind of tissue that the body tends to gain or lose when it is maintained in a state of calorie imbalance for some time. From experiments on under- and overeating to produce body weight changes of the order of 10 to 20 kg in otherwise healthy men in a period of 6 months, it appears that such weight changes involve what we have termed "obesity tissue," that is, the sum of the various substances gained or lost by the body during the process of weight change. As stated, this obesity tissue is not pure fat, nor is it identified with adipose tissue or any other particular tissue of the body. The density of the obesity tissue found in our experiments averaged 0.9478 gm per ml at 37°C.[56] A given individual, then, can be considered as made of two parts, one corresponding in composition to that of the reference body and another corresponding in composition to that of obesity tissue. In other words, a given individual can be considered as equal to the standard body plus or minus a certain amount of obesity tissue.

If g is considered the proportion of the body made up by such obesity tissue and D the observed density of the whole body, we may write, similarly to Equation 4

$$(5) \quad g = \frac{\left(\dfrac{1.0629}{D} - 1 \right)}{\left(\dfrac{1.0629}{0.9478} - 1 \right)}$$

or

$$(6) \quad g = (8.755/D) - 8.237$$

Suppose, for example, we observe a value of D = 1.050 in man. Then we have

(7) g = (8.755/1.050) − 8.237 = 0.101

and we conclude that 10.1 per cent of the body weight of this man is obesity tissue, with 89.9 per cent of his body weight having the composition of our standard young man. A negative value for g would mean deficiency of obesity tissue in comparison with the standard.

The obesity tissue is considered to be made up of fat, extracellular fluid and cell residue. From measurements in experiments on men gaining weight from overeating, it appears that about 14 per cent of the gain is accounted for by extracellular fluid while the remainder is a mixture of fat and cells having an average density of 0.939 gm per ml. From the density of fat, an estimate of the density of the "cells" and the determination of the extracellular fluid, the composition of the obesity tissue was calculated. Our first estimate was that such obesity tissue is composed of 14 per cent extracellular fluid, 62 per cent fat and 24 per cent cell residue.[56]

From the proportions of standard man and of obesity tissue in the body and the proportions of fat in each of these two parts, it is easy to compute the total amount of fat in the body. This will be equal to the sum of the fat in the standard body and in the obesity tissue. In our example we computed that a man with a body density of 1.050 is made up of 10.1 per cent of obesity tissue and 89.9 per cent of standard body. If his weight is 75 kg, his body is made of 7.58 kg (75 × 0.101) of obesity tissue and 67.42 kg (75 × 0.899) of standard body. The amount of fat contributed by the obesity tissue is 7.58 × 0.62 = 4.70 kg, and that contributed by the standard man is 67.42 × 0.14 = 9.44 kg. The total amount of fat, then, is 4.70 + 9.44 = 14.14 kg or 18.85 per cent of the total body weight.

Obviously the validity of these computations depends on the validity of the values assigned to the fat content of the standard body and the obesity tissue. It was originally suggested[29] that the standard body of density 1.0629 contains about 14 per cent fat, a figure accepted as within perhaps 2 per cent of the true value by several later investigators.[3,60] From new experiments in men changing weight, however, in which nitrogen balance as well as body density were determined, it appears that the true value may be near to 16 per cent.

We have proposed the use of a new standard of reference, which we have called the "reference body," based on the analyses of the 3 human cadavers listed in Table 1–9. The density of this reference body was computed from the data of chemical analysis of the cadavers in Table 1–9 as described elsewhere[49] and was found to be 1.064 gm per ml at 37°C. The fat content of the reference body is 15.3 per cent of the total body weight. The composition and density of the reference body are presented in Table 1–11. The differences resulting from the substitution of the new reference body for the previous standard body are small. The important advance consists of replacing an assumed with an empirically determined fat content of the reference body and the corresponding increase in validity of the computation.

Obesity tissue, as defined from the data of the experiment in men gaining weight by overeating,[56] tends to have a quite constant density of 0.9478 gm per ml at 37°C. Other data in the literature,[61,62] as well as new experiments in our laboratory, however, indicate that the density and composition of the obesity tissue gained or lost by the body are not always identical. We have attempted to provide other estimates of the composition and density of the obesity tissue and to correct the data of our previous experiments by using the value of 1.078 as density of the cell residue.[49] This figure was derived, as was the value for the density of the reference body, from the data from the analyses of the 3 male

Table 1–11.   Weights and Volumes of the Components of 1 kg of the Reference Body (Based on the Analysis of 3 Male Cadavers), their Densities, and the Calculated Density (d = 1.064) of the Empirically Defined Reference Body.*

Symbol	Component	Weight gm	Density at 37°C gm/ml	Specific Volume at 37°C ml/gm	Volume at 37°C ml
A	Water	624.3	0.99371	1.0063	628.2
P	Protein	164.4	1.34	0.7463	122.7
F	Fat	153.1	0.9007†	1.1102	170.0
M_o	Bone (osseous) mineral	47.7	2.982	0.3353	16.0
M_c	Non-osseous mineral	10.5	3.317	0.3015	3.2
Total		1000.0	1.064	0.9398	940.1

*From Brozek et al.[49]
†36°C

Table 1–12.   Calculated Percentage Composition of Obesity Tissue Defined on the Basis of Weight Gain, Weight Loss and the Difference Between Low-density and High-density Young Men.*

	Weight Gain	Weight Loss	Static Difference
Sample size	N = 10	N = 10	N = 16 and 21
Extracellular water	14	4	7
Fat	64	64	73
Cell residue	22	32	20
Density	0.948	0.954	0.938

*From Brozek et al.[49]

cadavers listed in Table 1–9. These new estimates of density and composition of obesity tissue cover three different situations: weight gain, weight loss and static weight difference. The last value applies to the difference between two groups of young men of the same age and height but differing markedly in body weight and density. These data are presented in Table 1–12.

Formulas for the Densitometric Estimation of Body Fat. In view of the substantial variations in the composition of the obesity tissue, it seems that no single formula is generally valid for the estimation of body fat. At present it appears that the best estimates will be obtained by using the formula which applies to the particular situation under study. In Table 1–13 we present three formulas based on the three classes of obesity tissue previously discussed. The formulas based on the experiments on gain and loss of weight will be more useful in the evaluation of body composition during periods of rapid dynamic changes of body weight, while the formula based on the static differences between chronically thin and chronically obese individuals will better fit the conditions of slowly changing or stable body weight.

Application of these formulas to our example of a man with a body density of 1.050 gives fat values of 20.63, 20.90 and 21.04 per cent for the formula based on the obesity tissue of weight gain, weight

Table 1–13. Formulas for the Estimation from Body Density (D_B), of the Amount of Obesity Tissue as a Fraction of Total Body Weight, of the Fat Associated with the Obesity Tissue, and of the Total Body Fat as a Fraction of Total Body Weight (Density of Reference Body 1.064; Fat Content 15.3% of Body Weight).*

Item	From Gain	From Loss	From Static Difference
Density (d_G)	0.948	0.954	0.938
Fat content of "obesity tissue" (as fraction, f_G)	0.64	0.64	0.73
"Obesity tissue," g, from body density	$= \dfrac{8.696}{D_B} - 8.172$	$\dfrac{9.228}{D_B} - 8.673$	$\dfrac{7.921}{D_B} - 7.444$
Fat content, f_G, from body density	$= \dfrac{5.565}{D_B} - 5.230$	$\dfrac{5.906}{D_B} - 5.551$	$\dfrac{5.782}{D_B} - 5.434$
Total body fat, f_B, from body density	$= \dfrac{4.235}{D_B} - 3.827$	$\dfrac{4.494}{D_B} - 4.071$	$\dfrac{4.570}{D_B} - 4.142$

*From Brozek et al.[49]

loss and static difference, respectively. These values are not very different from each other, but all of them are higher than the value of 18.85 per cent obtained by the application of the old formula illustrated on pages 17 and 18.

Body Fat from Body Water Measurements

The total amount of water in the body may be estimated on the dilution principle. An intravenous injection is made of an exactly known amount of a substance which penetrates and dissolves in all the water of the body and is not rapidly metabolized. After time is allowed for uniform distribution, a blood sample is drawn and the concentration of the test substance in the water of the blood is measured. Water labeled with isotopic hydrogen, deuterium or tritium[63] is suitable as the test substance, but antipyrine, n-acetyl-4-aminopyrine and urea have also been used.[64-66] Isotopic labeled water can also be orally administered.

Measurement of body water is useful for its own sake but it also has the advantage that it may be used to estimate the other components of the body, at least roughly. The original crude theory was that water

represents a fixed fraction of the mass of the nonfat part of the body.[55] This is not precisely true, even in normally hydrated bodies. In the cadavers listed in Table 1–9, the water represents a range of 69.6 to 77.9 per cent of the fat-free mass. This range may be used to calculate limits for the proportion of fat in the body, when the total body water has been measured. Now, the total body weight (W) must be equal to the sum of the total body water (A), the total body fat (F) and the total body nonfat solids (S).

$$(8) \quad W = A + F + S$$

If we take the total body weight to be unity and represent the fractions of the different components by the corresponding lower-case letters we have

$$(9) \quad 1 = a + f + s$$

and therefore

$$(10) \quad f = 1 - (a + s)$$

In the preceding paragraph it was indicated that we have limits of a = 0.696

(a + s) and a = 0.779 (a + s). The limiting possibilities will then be

(11a) $f = 1 - a/0.696$

(11b) $f = 1 - a/0.779$

The application of Equations 11a and 11b can be illustrated by the case of a man weighing 80 kg who is found to have a total body water mass of 45 kg, i.e. a = 0.56. From Equation 11a we have f = 0.196 and from 11b we have f = 0.281. The conclusion is that the man in question has a body in which from 19.6 to 28.1 per cent of the weight is made up of fat. Such a calculation is not permissible, of course, in the presence of edema or dehydration.

Body fat can also be determined from combined measurements of total body water and extracellular water. The limitations of these systems have been discussed by Keys and Brozek.[26]

Body Fat from Body Water and Densitometry

It may be suggested that a more reliable estimate of body composition would be obtained from a combination of body water and density measurements. We[26] and others have derived equations for this purpose, that of Siri[3] being

(12) $f = (2.057/D) - 0.786a - 1.286$

where D is the density of the whole body and f and a are the proportions of fat and of water in the body. As Siri pointed out, however, this combination really does not eliminate the uncertainty about the fundamental assumptions. The estimate of the body fat by Equation 12 may have a standard deviation around ± 1.7 per cent of the total body weight.[3]

Total Body Potassium in Body Composition Studies

Since potassium is present mainly in the intracellular phase, the measurement of the potassium content of the body offers a possibility for the estimation of the body cell mass. Measurement of the total potassium content of the living body has been achieved by two methods: (1) direct measurement of the gamma radiation emitted by the radioactive ^{40}K which occurs in a constant proportion in natural potassium, (2) measurement of the total exchangeable potassium by isotopic dilution using ^{42}K as a tracer.

Direct measurement of body potassium by means of its natural radioactivity was initiated by Sievert[68,69] and has been developed in this country with the introduction by Anderson et al. of the Los Alamos human counter, which makes it possible to determine the total potassium content of the body in a short period of time.[70] The methods based on the measurement of the exchangeable potassium by isotopic dilution with ^{42}K are widely used at the present.[63,71,72] The available data indicate a reasonable agreement between the results obtained by the two methods,[73-75] although the values found by the dilution method are lower than those found by carcass analysis (Forbes and Lewis[76]). In applying the total potassium content of the body to the determination of body fat, the system is similar to that used in the determination of the fat-free body from the total water content of the body. By dividing the total amount of potassium in the body by the potassium content of 1 kg of fat-free body, the mass of fat-free body in kg can be calculated, and by substracting the fat-free body mass from the total body weight we compute the amount of fat in the body. The problem, then, is to establish the potassium content of the fat-free body. Since the fat-free body is made up of a series of anatomic elements having different compositions, it is clear that the average potassium concentration will depend on the relative proportion of these various components. The high potassium content of muscle is well known, but muscle is only a part of the total fat-free body, and connective tissue and other structural materials, while having a similar degree of hydration, probably have little potassium. Interesting correlations between potassium content and fat-free cell solids (cell-residue solids or Allen's M_3) estimated from total body water have been described and used as a basis for the estimation of body fat.[73] Anderson and Langham[77,78] have used the figure of 73 mEq of potassium per kg for the computation of the lean body mass. Forbes et al.[79,80] have used the figure 68.1 mEq per kg to compute the fat-free body mass. This latter figure is based on data from the analyses of 4 human bodies.[76] The fat-free body mass (in kg) is calculated by these authors by dividing the total body potassium (mEq) by 68.1. Burmeister and Bingert[81] in their extensive studies have calculated "cell mass" from total body potassium determinations, assuming a mean potassium content of 92.5 mEq per kg of cell mass. Fat-free body mass was calculated by these authors as 1.1 × cell mass + extracellular fluid. Extracellular fluid, in turn, was assumed to be 6.1 liters per square meter of body surface. Allen et al.[73] have shown that the total body potassium content measured by the body counter method is proportional to the body mass minus bone mineral, fat and water (this is the compartment M_3 which corresponds with our cell-residue solids). Since the ratio K/M_3 (equivalents of potassium per kg) decreases with age and is lower in the female than in the male, the authors use a correction which takes into account the chronologic age of the subject. M_3 for males beyond age 15 is then given by

(13) $M_3 = K/(0.354 - 0.00082\ \sigma)$

in which M_3 is in kg, K in equivalents, and σ is age in years. Assuming that the ratio of M_3 to total body water and to bone mineral is constant, Allen et al.[73] estimate the amount of fat from M_3 by

(14) $F = M - 4.964\ M_3$

in which F and M represent the masses of fat and of the total body respectively and M_3 the mass of the cell residue solids calculated from Equation 13. More recently Anderson[82] has suggested a system of body partition into muscle, adipose tissue and remaining body mass as being more consistent with their data of total body potassium and total body water.

Isotopic Dilution Methods in Body Composition Studies

The determination of the composition of the human body by isotopic dilution methods has been widely used. Moore and his co-workers[71,83] have published a summary of their extensive and important work.[71] The estimation of the body cell mass depends on the measurement of the exchangeable potassium, assuming a ratio of potassium to nitrogen in the cell mass of 3 mEq of K per gm of N, and an average nitrogen content of 4 per cent (or 25 per cent of protein).

It should be noted that Moore's "body cell mass" does not correspond to the cell residue as defined here. The estimation of the body cell mass assumes uniformity of potassium concentration in all the cells of the body, and the compartment so described excludes such components as connective fibers and plasma proteins included in the cell residue. Final validation of this technique requires more information with direct determination of potassium.

The methods of isotopic dilution have been applied by Haxhe[84] in studies on man and animals under various conditions. The changes observed by Haxhe during undernutrition are in good agreement with the data reported by others. Of particular interest are the data on the constancy of the K/N ratio in undernutrition. This finding tends to support the validity of the measurement of exchangeable potassium in the estimation of the cell mass of the body in the presence of changing nutritional status.

Inert Gas Uptake in the Measurement of Body Fat

The well-known fact that certain gases are highly soluble in fat and little soluble in aqueous media prompted the use of some of these gases in the estimation of the fat content of the body. Nitrogen was originally used by Behnke, but this gas has the practical disadvantage of its extremely slow elimination.

Lesser et al.[85] have measured fat in human subjects using cyclopropane and [85]Kr. Unfortunately, there is no direct comparison with other methods in the same subjects. The results, however, are in general agreement with estimates of body fatness derived from body water measurements, but tend to be somewhat lower than those obtained by the densitometric method. Because of its theoretical simplicity, the inert gas method offers much promise as an independent method for checking the validity of other methods currently used in the estimation of body fat.

Subcutaneous Fat

About half of the total fat in man is in the subcutaneous layer, so measurements of subcutaneous fat may give a good index to the total fat of the body.[12,86,87,88] Unfortunately, the subcutaneous fat layer varies from place to place and the distribution is not the same in different individuals or in the same individual at different ages. For example, in young children the layer of subcutaneous fat over the triceps muscle of the arm is relatively thick, even in thin children, while the layer over the abdomen is much thinner. In adults the proportion is reversed, so data from children[89] do not apply to adults. However, sampling several sites, or even a single site in persons of a given age, may allow a useful rough estimate of the total body fatness.

Equations for the prediction of total body fat or of body density from a combination of measurements of skinfolds at different sites have been developed.[12,13,26,90,91] These show correlations between the values predicted from skinfolds and those obtained from densitometry, with coefficients of r = 0.85 to r = 0.87. This correlation means that almost 20 per cent of the variance is not accounted for by regression.

With experience, a fairly good subjective appraisal of calorie nutritional status can be made simply by digital pinching, but skinfold calipers, used as recommended by a committee of experts,[90,92] allow novice and expert alike to obtain numerical estimates of acceptable reliability.[26,93]

The skinfold should be pinched up to the point where the sides are parallel and the thickness is measured with calipers exerting a pressure of 10 gm per square mm (single jaw face area). Prolonged application of the calipers should be avoided because after the initial deformation of the skinfold under the pressure there is a slowly progressive compression, particularly if edema is present. Advantage may be taken of this slow deformation to evaluate the presence or amount of edema.

The subcutaneous fat thickness in some parts of the body may be accurately estimated from soft-tissue roentgenograms.[26,34,94] Rather good agreement has been found between the skinfold technique and the radiographic method[13] when measuring subcutaneous fat changes. In a group of 52 middle-aged men the correlation between total body fat (from densitometry) and the thickness of the subcutaneous fat measured on roentgenograms was r = 0.75 and r = 0.76 for two sites on the arms, and r = 0.58 for the calf.[95] A better correlation might be expected if the sum of fat thickness at several sites was used.

The topographic distribution of subcutaneous fat tends to be an individual characteristic but *changes in fatness induced by dietary alterations seem to be shared proportionally by all regions of the body.*[86,87,95] When an obese person loses fat on a reducing diet, if the fat thickness over the triceps muscle diminishes by 10 per cent, then approximately a 10 per cent reduction at other sites may be expected. This may be disappointing to reducers who hope to get thinner in some places than in others, but it does mean that simple skinfold measurements are useful for following the changes in the total fat of the body. On the other hand, the process of gaining weight after a period of dietary restriction may proceed at different rates in different places. In experiments in this laboratory it was observed that the abdominal skinfold increased at a disproportionately rapid rate.[86]

Body Composition During Growth

The processes of growth and development require energy and building material over and above the demands of ordinary maintenance and the cost of physical work. The growth of children is retarded by a restriction of food intake[2] and the growth deficit is related to the severity of the undernutrition. The rate of weight increase is more readily affected than is growth in height, but even this latter can be seriously inhibited in extreme calorie deficit.

Growth is not only a change of body size—important changes in body *composition* also take place during the growth period. It has long been known[96] that the concentration of water in the body is high in the fetus and steadily decreases during growth. During intrauterine development total body water as a percentage of total body weight decreases from 94 to about 76 at delivery and continues to fall thereafter, with no difference between the sexes during the growing years.[97]

The change in water content of the developing body was considered by Moulton[98] as one of the basic principles in mammalian development. The other basic principle emphasized by Moulton is that fat is the great variable in the composition of the mammalian body. At a given moment of the development process the proportions of water, protein and minerals in the fat-free portion of the body become stabilized. When this stabilization is achieved the body reaches "chemical maturity." The age at which an animal reaches chemical maturity was considered by Moulton to be a relatively constant fraction of the total life span.

The changes in the total and extracellular water in children have been studied by Friis-Hansen.[97] Total body water was determined by D_2O and extracellular water by thiosulfate. A summary of his results is presented in Table 1–14. Both total body water and extracellular water (as percentages of the total body weight) decrease as age advances, but the proportion of extracellular water decreases more than that of total body water. This is in part an expression of the increase of cell mass at the expense of extracellular fluid, in particular of the development of tissues such as skeletal muscle which have a high pro-

Table 1–14. Average Percentages of the Total Body Weight Represented by Total Body Water and By Extracellular Water and the Ratio of Intracellular Water to Total Body Solids During Infancy and Childhood.*

	0 to 11 Days	11 Days to ½ yr.	½ to 2 Years	2 to 7 Years	7 to 16 Years
Total body water	77.6%	72.2%	59.5%	63.1%	58.4%
Extracellular water	41.6%	33.7%	26.2%	24.7%	19.9%
Intracellular water ÷ total body solids	1.61	1.38	0.82	1.04	0.93

*Data from Friis-Hansen.[97]

portion of intracellular water. In part, the age trend shown in Table 1–14 is also a result of increasing body fatness. That the relative fatness of the body increases during childhood was indicated from densitometric data reported by Zook[99] and Boyd,[100] though the methods used were unsatisfactory. Macy and Kelly[54] estimated averages of 22, 24 and 26 per cent of the body weight represented by fat in boys aged 4 to 6, 7 to 9 and 10 to 12 years, respectively, but their material was small and the calculations were based on many assumptions, including the arbitrary value of 73.2 per cent for the total water in the fat-free body. The densitometric data obtained by Parizkova[101,102] in children 9 to 17 years of age indicate that density increases continuously in the boys, while in the girls it shows a decrease between 14 and 16 years with a slight increase at 17 to 18 years.

Mellits and Cheek[103] have reported a linear relationship between total body water and weight from infancy to young adulthood. Total body water (TW) in liters can be predicted from body weight (WT) in kg by

(15)   TW = 1.065 + 0.603 WT (for males)

(16)   TW = 1.874 + 0.493 WT (for females)

Total body water was found to be a non-linear function of height, represented by a quadratic equation, or by 2 intercepting straight lines.

The increase of cell mass during the period of growth has been well documented by Burmeister and Bingert[81] in studies on 3,143 children using the body counter for the determination of total body potassium.

Many data have been reported in recent years on the changes of subcutaneous tissue thickness during infancy and childhood.[31,101-108] Maximal values are found at the end of the first year and in adolescence with a steady increase during the adult years. The sex differences in subcutaneous tissue thickness are apparent in early childhood.

On the basis of information from a variety of sources, Fomon[109] has estimated the body composition of a hypothetical male reference infant from birth to 3 years (Table 1–15).

The most striking change in body composition during the first 4 months of extrauterine life is the increase in fat content and the parallel decrease in the proportion of water. It is estimated that 41.6 per cent of the 3.5 kg of body weight gained during this period is fat. The percentage of body fat decreases steadily after 4 months of age. There seems to be little change in the percentage of protein during the first 4 months after birth. Thereafter, there is a steady increase in protein percentage, as indicated in Table 1–15.

Body Composition in Old Age

With advancing years there is, in adult age, a progressive decrease of the cell mass of the body. This has been documented by

Table 1–15.   Body Composition of a Reference Body.*

Age (months)	Body Weight (kg)	Whole Body (gm/100 gm)			
		Water	Protein	Lipid	Other
Birth	3.5	75.1	11.4	11.0	2.5
4	7.0	60.2	11.4	26.3	2.1
12	10.5	59.0	14.6	23.9	2.5
24	13.0	61.0	15.7	20.6	2.7
36	15.0	62.0	16.4	18.3	3.3

*From Fomon.[109]

various methods. From densitometric determinations Brozek[110] estimated, in men, an average decrease of 0.11 kg of cell mass per year between ages 25 and 50 years. Total body water (antipyrine space) diminishes with increasing age, without significant change of extracellular water (thiocyanate space), indicating a reduction of the cell mass.[111] Measurements of body potassium, both by analysis of cadavers and by whole body counting, have shown progressive decrease of the total potassium content of the body. The average concentration of potassium per kg of gross body weight decreases steadily with increasing age in adult life,[73,77,112] but the potassium content per kg of fat-free body is lower in the newborn than in the adult.[79]

Recent studies are in agreement that the weight of the cell mass decreases continuously from early adulthood to old age. For example, Burmeister and Bingert[81] found in men an average cell mass of 42.5 kg at 25 to 26 years and of 34.5 kg at 65 to 70 years. There is, therefore, a mean decrease of 8 kg (about 19 per cent of the weight of the cell mass at 25 to 26 years) over 40 to 45 years. This result is in good agreement with the data on total body water reported by Shock et al.[111] These authors found a mean intracellular water volume of 28.2 liters at 20 to 29 years and of 21.9 liters at 60 to 69 years, or a decrease of 6.3 liters. Assuming a water content of 72.7 per cent in the cell mass, this means a reduction in cell mass of 8.6 kg. According to Forbes and Reina,[113] at age 65 to 70 the average man has 12 kg less lean body mass than at age 25. The corresponding figure for females is a decrease of 5 kg.

The results of longitudinal studies reported by Forbes[114] indicate an average reduction of lean body mass during the adult years of the order of 3 kg per decade. The fat content of the body, measured by the inert gas method (Lesser et al.[85]), tends to increase with age in spite of the fact that the relative body weight of the subjects was close to 100 for all the age groups. Fat content of 12 young men (mean age 29.6 years, mean relative weight 99.7) averaged 18.3 per cent, whereas the fat content of 10 older men (mean age 70.1 years, mean relative weight 103.1) averaged 26.3 per cent. The average fat content of 10 young women (23.7 years, 98.9 relative weight) was 23.7 per cent. That of 13 older women (68.8 years, 103.0 relative weight) was 36.0 per cent.

It follows from the preceding data that the average man, maintaining at 65 to 70 years the same body weight that he had at 25 years, must have a higher proportion of body fat at his more advanced age. Because the cell mass represents the metabolically active compartment of the body, the continuous decrease of cell mass through adult life should be taken into consideration in calculating nutrient requirements and drug dosage in older persons.

CALORIE STATUS

The relationship between energy metabolism and body composition will be considered in two main aspects: (1) the relationship between basal metabolism and body composition and (2) the relationship between changes in body composition and changes in calorie balance.

Basal Metabolism and Body Composition

The basal metabolism is the result of energetic processes in the cells which constitute the active mass of the body; fat, extracellular fluid and bone minerals make no direct contribution to this basal metabolism. Though adipose tissue is not metabolically inert, such energy consumption as it exhibits must be attributed to the cells and not to the plain fat in it. Accordingly, it would be reasonable to express the basal metabolic rate in units of the active tissue mass rather than in terms of the gross mass of the body or even of the popular surface area unit. In 1950 we showed that much variation, otherwise unexplained, is eliminated when basal metabolism is expressed in units of fat-free or, better, active tissue mass.[2]

Studies in our laboratory[115] *have also shown that much of the decrease of basal metabolic rate attributed to age seems to be readily explained by changes in the proportion of the body weight made up of fat, changes that have been ignored, for the most part, in cross-sectional surveys.*

For persons of given sex and age the total basal oxygen consumption is correlated to about the same extent with surface area as with fat-free body weight.[61] The utility of the fat-free body weight as a standard of reference is clear when persons of different sex and age are compared.[53,60,110,116] For both males and females over the age range of perhaps 20 to 60 years a single value can be used to indicate the "normal" metabolic rate. The single value of 4.4 ml of oxygen per minute (or about 1.3 calories per hour) per kg of fat-free body weight can be used instead of the customary tables and graphs based on the artificial concept of surface area as the determinant of basal metabolism.

From the foregoing it is an obvious step to suggest the converse, namely, that the fat-free body mass may be estimated simply from the basal metabolism.[53,116,117] With strictly normal, healthy young adults, this estimation is reasonably good, but more general application is questionable because of the susceptibility of the basal oxygen metabolism to hormonal and dietary influences. Obviously this estimation cannot be made if there is any suspicion of abnormality of the basal metabolic rate.

Since it appears that the basal metabolism normally is strictly proportional to the mass of active tissue or cells in the body, it follows that the basal metabolism should be closely correlated with any measure which, in turn, is highly correlated with the active cell mass. In addition to fat-free body weight, such measures are represented by total body water and extracellular fluid mass or volume. Without benefit of the considerations outlined above, it has been found that, indeed,

basal metabolism is highly correlated with the extracellular fluid volume of the body.[118,119] A high correlation ($r = 0.896$) has been found between basal metabolism and total body potassium.[73] While the statistical correlations emphasized above are of great utility, it is essential not to lose sight of the underlying physiology.

Bray et al.,[120] in a study on 18 grossly obese females, reported oxygen consumption to be highly correlated with body weight and surface area, whereas the correlation was much less satisfactory with total body water and exchangeable potassium. The measurements of oxygen consumption reported by these authors do not represent basal oxygen consumption, however. They correspond to the oxygen consumption over a 24-hour period calculated from the average of 6 to 11 samples of expired air taken at various intervals between 8:00 a.m. and 8:00 p.m. The patients rested for 15 to 20 minutes before each collection. The samples taken after meals showed the increase in oxygen consumption corresponding to the specific dynamic action. It is clear that the values of oxygen consumption reported represent neither basal oxygen consumption nor total 24-hour oxygen intake. Most of the data of basal metabolic rate in obese patients indicate that the values tend to be low when referred to actual weight, and high when referred to standard weight.[121]

From the foregoing discussion it might be supposed that all cells or all parts of the active tissue mass of the body have equal rates of metabolism per unit of mass. This is grossly erroneous, as has been emphasized by Brozek and Grande.[122] In man, the brain and liver, together representing only about 4 per cent of the normal body mass, account for over 40 per cent of the total resting oxygen consumption, while the skeletal muscles, amounting to about 40 per cent of the body weight, contribute barely 25 per cent of the basal metabolism. These facts go far toward explaining the otherwise puzzling fact that the basal metabolism early in starvation quickly falls far more than would be predicted from a consideration of the change in total cell mass of the body.[123] Since the active cell mass is made up of tissues with very different metabolic rates, it is obvious that changes in the average metabolic rate of the cell mass can be produced by changes in the proportion among the various components.[117]

On the other hand, it must be considered that the metabolic rate per weight unit of cell mass varies with the partition system adopted, because the various methods used in the determination of the cell mass measure compartments of different size and composition in terms of anatomic structures. In the system of partition which has been described here, the cell residue, by definition, contains not only the active cells of the body but also the plasma proteins, the connective tissue fibers and so on. Consequently, the basal metabolism per weight unit of such a compartment is expected to be lower than that of a compartment defined in a more restricted way and including a higher proportion of metabolically active components. Our measurements[117] in normal young men gave values for the basal metabolism of the cell residue of 1.52 kcal per kg per hour (S.D. = 0.134) for a group of 13 men, and of 1.57 kcal per kg per hour (S.D. = 0.123) for another group of 12 men. The mass of the compartment was estimated by dividing the amount of intracellular water (total body water minus extracellular water) by 0.733. Ryan et al.[124] found in 14 normal men (mean age 34.9 years) a value corresponding to 1.88 kcal per kg of cell mass per hour, when cell mass was determined by dividing intracellular water by 0.70. Bernstein et al.,[36] using the same system to determine the cell mass, found in a group of young women a mean value corresponding to 2.02 kcal per kg per hour. Moore et al.[71] give values between 2.7 and 3.6 kcal per kg per hour for the "body cell mass" estimated from measurements of exchangeable potassium. This seems to indicate that the compartment measured by this method is smaller in terms of mass than the cell residue computed from determinations of total body water and extracellular water. The interpretation of metabolic rates in terms of mass of active tissue compartments requires, then, a precise definition of the nature of the compartment measured and of the methods used. Thus, when the basal caloric production is expressed in terms of lean body mass, the values given in the literature are of the order of 1.00 to 1.17 kcal per kg per hour.[117] It is of interest to compare these basal values with an average of 1.71 kcal per kg per hour reported for the total energy expenditure of young men living in voluntary confinement similar to that in space cabins.[125]

The Calorie Equivalent of Weight Change

Weight loss as a consequence of negative calorie balance has been regarded largely as a reduction of the fat content of the body. Depot fat is the most important storehouse of energy in the body and represents the material preferentially used to compensate for the energy deficit caused by inadequate calorie intake. This fact has been well documented in the classical literature.[126] It must be recognized, however, that the changes in body composition taking place during periods of negative energy balance are more complex than a simple loss of fat.

The most common application of information on body weight and composition is in connection with nutritional correction and control of obesity and emaciation. What is the calorie equivalent of a given amount of weight gain or loss?

The most superficial approach is to estimate that, since 1 kg of animal fat has an energy value of about 9100 kcal, therefore an accumulated nutritional deficit of 9100 kcal would be attended by a weight loss of 1 kg. This value, or the value of 9000 kcal per kg of body weight change, is still quoted from time to time, but disparate values can be found in the medical literature. More commonly, Bozenraad's data on adipose tissue[30] are misconstrued and it is concluded that 1 kg of body weight gain or loss should be the equivalent of 8000 kcal.[127,128] Adipose tissue and obesity tissue, that is, the kind of tissue actually gained or lost when the diet is changed, are not identical in calories, however. Obesity tissue gained or lost in a few months, as in our experiments, would have a value between 6000 and 6500 kcal per kg if it were burned in a calorimeter.

It by no means follows that a dietary deficit of 6000 to 6500 kcal will produce a weight loss of 1 kg. In the first place, the calorie value of the tissue lost is affected by the intensity of the calorie imbalance and the value changes as calorie imbalance continues. During the first few days on a sharply reduced diet the body tends to lose more water than fat and again, after the body has become emaciated, further reductions in body weight represent water and protein loss as well as fat. In both situations the calorie value of the lost tissue is much lower than 6000 kcal per kg. Dole and his colleagues[129] conducted well-controlled experiments on 5 obese women whose diets were alternated between excess and deficiency at 4-day intervals. The observed weight changes corresponded to averages of 2160 to 3610 kcal per kg. We have found similar values with men for the first few days of dietary restriction. Later, however, the calorie value of the weight change rises. In one of our experiments 13 young men subsisted on a carbohydrate diet providing 1000 kcal daily while following a fixed schedule of physical activity to make the energy expenditure at the beginning of the restriction period in the order of 3200 kcal per day. The calorie equivalent of the weight lost during the first 3 days averaged 2596 kcal per kg; that of the weight lost between days 11 and 13 was 7043 kcal per kg.[86] Other data also indicate that the calorie equivalent of

weight loss increases with the duration of the restriction period.[117]

Equally important is the fact that, given time, the body weight tends to reach a steady state and calorie expenditure tends to balance calorie intake, no matter what the level of the latter may be. When we changed the diet of young men from 3500 to 1500 kcal daily the weight loss was rapid at first and decreased exponentially with time until calorie equilibrium was achieved with the body weight being 25 per cent less than it had been.[130]

Much interesting information has been gathered recently in connection with the use of complete starvation as a means of reducing body weight in obese individuals. Under such circumstances the caloric value of the weight loss must be equal to the total energy expenditure, since the only source of energy available is that represented by the body tissue.[126,131] If the energy expenditure is known, the calorie equivalent of the loss can be easily calculated by dividing the total energy deficit (which in this case is equal to the energy expenditure) by the weight loss. Such computation can be made with the data of Consolazio et al.[132] obtained from 6 men who starved for 10 days. The average weight loss was 7.3 kg and the total energy expenditure was estimated as 25,000 kcal, so the calorie equivalent of the loss is of the order of 3400 kcal per kg. This is comparable to some of the data previously reported from short-time experiments, and stresses the fact that much of the weight lost during a limited period of starvation or semistarvation must be water.

By combining measurements of total energy expenditure and nitrogen balance it is possible to calculate the amount of fat lost during periods of starvation or food restriction.[117,133] When the energy expenditure is unknown, useful information about its level can be obtained by computing the energy value of the weight loss from its composition determined by some of the methods already discussed. This, incidentally, offers a means of checking the credibility of some data on body composition changes.[126,131] The results presented in some reports show wild disagreement between the body composition data and elementary considerations of bioenergetics. One of these reports[134] compares the effects of complete starvation and of a ketogenic diet on weight loss and body composition. The mean weight loss for 10 men for 10 days of complete starvation was 9.6 kg, of which 6.2 kg were estimated as lean body mass and 3.4 kg as fat. Simple computation, using commonly accepted constants,[49,126] indicates that such an average daily weight loss would have a caloric value of 3544 kcal. Accordingly, this figure should represent the energy expenditure of the subjects. The figure seems much too high for starving individuals spending no energy for specific dynamic action and who, according to the authors, "had uniform moderate physical activity" in a metabolic ward. Much more incredible are the data on the same individuals when they were given a ketogenic diet (1000 kcal per day) for 10 days. They lost an average of 6.6 kg which was estimated as being made up of 0.2 kg of lean body mass and 6.4 kg of fat. The calorie equivalent of that loss would amount to 5776 kcal per day which, added to the food intake of 1000 kcal per day, would make a total of 6776 kcal per day. The authors offer no explanation for this unbelievable increase of more than 3000 kcal in the daily energy expenditure during the period on the ketogenic diet, when, supposedly, there was no change in the level of physical activity. This example clearly indicates the need for critical examination of body composition data in the light of currently accepted principles of metabolic physiology.

These erroneous data have been interpreted as supporting the view that the composition of the reducing diet influences the rate of weight loss, in apparent violation of basic thermodynamic principles. The findings recently reported by Yang and van Itallie[135] demonstrate that, over a 10-day period, the energy value of the sum of body constituents lost during adherence to a diet of 800 kcal per day was minimally affected by wide variations in the proportion of fat and carbohydrate ingested. Ketosis induced by carbohydrate restriction conferred no advantage regarding nitrogen loss. The authors rightly concluded that the rate of fat loss is a function of the degree of energy deficit.

The energy cost of laying down new tissue has been estimated using various assumptions, but it should be borne in mind that, as stated by Hommes et al.,[136] the energy needed to synthesize specific cell constituents is virtually impossible to determine experimentally.

Fomon[109] used Kielanowski's data, obtained in growing pigs, which indicate that about 7.5 kcal are needed for the synthesis of 1 gm of protein and 11.6 kcal for the synthesis of 1 gm of fat. With these figures, the energy cost of 1 gm of weight gain, including the calorie value of the stored protein and fat, will be of the order of 5.4 kcal per gm for an infant between birth and 4 months. Thus Fomon estimates that the percentage of the calorie intake required for growth, for this period, is 32.8.

Hommes et al.[136] have attempted a more sophisticated approach applying Atkinson's metabolic system of calculating the amounts of ATP and glucose needed for the synthesis of the various compounds deposited. They estimated that the energy cost of growth, including the calorie equivalent of the nutrients deposited in the body, is 13.4 per cent of the total calorie intake. With the data given by the authors this corresponds to about 1.9 kcal per gm of tissue gained. This figure is obviously too low. Assuming that the composition of the weight gained is that given by Fomon for this period of life (41.6 per cent fat, 11.4 per cent protein), the actual caloric value of the gain will be about 4.2 kcal per gm.

Using Kilianowski's data it may be calculated that the energy cost of depositing 1 gm of obesity tissue of weight gain, as described in Table 1–12, is of the order of 7.9 kcal per gm—including the energy equivalent of the stored protein and fat. Since the energy value of the fat and protein stored in this form of obesity tissue is about 6.0 kcal per gm, this means that 76 per cent of the energy needed to deposit obesity tissue appears as stored fat and protein, whereas 24 per cent is used to defray the cost of synthesis of these compounds.

Body Weight in Complete Starvation and Calorie Restriction

The paper by Thomson et al.[137] reports interesting observations about weight loss in obese individuals who fasted for long periods of time. One obese woman fasted for 249 days and lost 34 kg or 28 per cent of her original body weight. With the exception of two patients, who had the lowest initial body weights, all the others lost substantial amounts of weight. In spite of the individual differences, the data clearly show that the average daily loss for the whole period tends to decrease with its duration. Thus the patients who starved for about 40 days showed a mean weight loss of about 0.3 per cent of their original body weights per day. The patient who starved 139 days lost weight at the rate of 0.18 per cent of the initial weight per day and the two women who starved 236 and 249 days had mean daily weight losses of 0.15 and 0.11 per cent respectively. Similar results have been reported by Barnard et al.[138] One of the women studied fasted for 315 days and lost 66.5 kg or nearly 50 per cent of her original body weight. This corresponds to an average weight loss of about 0.15 per cent per day. Another woman starved for 74 days with a loss of about 25 per cent of her original weight and an average weight loss of 0.34 per cent per day.

These data confirm the general idea that the rate of weight loss tends to decrease as the duration of the calorie restriction increases.[2] Even total starvation loses efficiency as a means of weight reduction after a certain time.

No data on body composition or energy exchange were reported by Thomson et al., but some limiting calculations can be made with their data. The mean daily weight loss for 10 women on starvation treatment was 0.219 kg and, assuming that only fat was lost, this would correspond to an energy expenditure of 1970 kcal per day. On the other hand, if we assume that the tissue lost had the composition of what we have defined as "obesity tissue from static difference," the mean energy expenditure would be 1480 kcal per day. These two values give the probable limits of energy expenditure for this group of starving women. Some of them, however, must have had extremely low energy expenditure levels, particularly in the latter part of the starvation period. The values computed from the weight loss would indicate that two of the patients (4 and 6) were not using more than an average of 800 to 1100 kcal per day.

Considerable reduction of body weight can be achieved by prolonged drastic reduction of food intake. Bortz[139] has reported the case of a 35-year-old man who lost 227 kg over a period of 723 days on a diet of 800 kcal per day. The loss corresponds to 72 per cent of his original body weight of 314 kg. The average rate of weight loss was about 0.1 per cent per day and compares with the rates observed in some of the obese women who starved for long periods. The initial maintenance calorie requirement of this patient was estimated to be of the order of 5,000 kcal per day. The estimated protein loss was 13.25 kg or about 5.8 per cent of the total weight loss. This corresponds to an average protein loss of 18 gm per day and is considerably smaller than that observed over shorter periods in starving men and in men on a carbohydrate diet of 400 kcal per day.[132,140]

Allen and Musgrave[141] described the changes of body weight and body composition of obese adult men consuming a diet providing 400 kcal and 45 gm of high-quality protein daily. During a mean of 49 days there was an average weight loss of 12.03 kg. It was assumed that the men were in nitrogen equilibrium and that the loss comprised essentially fat and water. From densitometric determinations it was estimated that the average fat loss was 10 kg or 83 per cent of the total weight loss. The determinations of the specific volume supported the view that the loss was indeed made up of fat and water and the calculations of total energy expenditure from the fat loss gave results in excellent agreement with previous estimates of energy expenditure for subjects with a moderate level of physical activity.[126] This interesting work seems to have achieved the desideratum of weight reduction—loss of fat without loss of protein.

The process of gaining weight, when men shift from a negative to a positive energy balance, likewise does not always give an exact picture of the excess calorie intake. In our experiments[86] it was observed that increase in weight was rapid at the beginning of the refeeding period; later, with the same level of excess calorie intake, no further increase of body weight was detected for some time. Since there was no doubt as to the presence of a positive energy and nitrogen balance, it seems reasonable to assume that the weight change caused by the storage of fat and protein in the body was offset by the loss of some of the water retained in excess during the first few days of refeeding. Similar observations have been reported with respect to nitrogen retention in previously underfed individuals without a corresponding increase of body weight,[9,142] and in constitutionally thin individuals.[143]

There is great variability among outpatients in regard to body weight response to dietary change, partly because of differences in activity habits, partly because the truth about dietary intakes is not always easy to discover. Obese people are not always heavy eaters, and this is true of children as well as of adults.[144] Since physical inactivity is often at least partly responsible, we commonly advise reduction in obesity partly by reducing the diet, partly by increasing exercise. This certainly affects the calorie equivalent of weight loss. Suppose one fat person loses 50 pounds of obesity tissue while another, combining exercise and reduced food, has a net loss of 50 pounds but has gained 10 pounds of muscle tissue? The former has achieved his weight loss at a cost of about 140,000 kcal; the latter has lost 60 pounds of obesity tissue and gained 10 pounds of muscle, making a net equivalent of about 168,000 kcal. We favor the second person's accomplishment.

BIBLIOGRAPHY

1. Grande: In *Obesity in Perspective* (Bray, Ed.). HEW Pub. No. NIH 75-708. Washington, 1975, p. 189.
2. Keys, Brozek, Henschel, Mickelsen and Taylor: *The Biology of Human Starvation*. Minneapolis, University of Minnesota Press, 1950.
3. Siri: *Advances in Biological and Medical Physics*. New York, Academic Press, 1956, p. 239.
4. Food and Agriculture Organization: F.A.O. Nutritional Studies No. 15, Rome, 1957.
5. Keys: J.A.M.A., *142*, 333, 1950.
6. Johnson, Burke and Mayer: Am. J. Clin. Nutr., *4*, 37 and 231, 1956.
7. Mayer: In *Weight Control* (Eppright, Ewanson and Iverson, Eds.). Ames, Iowa State College Press, 1955, p. 199.
8. Metropolitan Life Insurance Co.: Statistical Bulletin, *23*, 6, 23 and 24, 1942.
9. Holmes, Jones and Stanier: Br. J. Nutr., *8*, 173, 1954.
10. Behnke, Feen and Welham: J.A.M.A., *118*, 495, 1942.
11. Brozek and Keys: Science, *112*, 788, 1950.
12. Brozek and Keys: Br. J. Nutr., *5*, 194, 1951.
13. Brozek and Keys: Nutr. Abstr. Rev., *20*, 247, 1951.
14. Taylor, Brozek and Keys: J. Clin. Invest., *31*, 976, 1952.
15. Simonart: *La Dénutrition de Guerre. Etude Clinique, Anatomopathologique et Thérapeutique.* Brussels and Paris, Maloine, 1948.
16. Keys, Taylor, Mickelsen and Henschel: Science, *103*, 669, 1946.
17. Newburgh: Arch. Intern. Med., *70*, 1033, 1942.
18. Durnin: Proc. Nutr. Soc., *20*, 52, 1961.

19. Edholm: Proc. Nutr. Soc., (Brozek and Henschel, Eds.), 20, 71, 1961.
20. Elkinton and Donowski: The Body Fluids. Baltimore, Williams & Wilkins, 1955, p. 26.
21. Taggart: Br. J. Nutr., 16, 223, 1962.
22. Olsson and Saltin: Acta Physiol. Scand., 80, 11, 1970.
23. Swindell, Holmes and Robinson: Br. J. Nutr., 22, 667, 1968.
24. Seltzer, Stoudt, Bell and Mayer: Am. J. Epidemiol., 92, 339, 1970.
25. Keys: Am. J. Public Health, 43, 1399, 1953.
26. Keys and Brozek: Physiol. Rev., 33, 245, 1953.
27. Fisher and Fisk: How to Live. New York, Funk, 1916.
28. Edwards: Medical Statistics Bulletin No. 2, Washington, 1943.
29. Newman and White: Environmental Protection Section Report No. 180. Washington, Office of the Quartermaster General, 1951, p. 1.
30. Randall and Monroe: Environmental Protection Branch Report No. 148. Washington, Office of the Quartermaster General, 1949.
31. Pett and Ogilvie: Hum. Biol., 28, 177, 1956.
32. Roberts: Weight by Height and Age of Adults. U.S. 1960-1962. National Center for Health Statistics, Series 11, No. 14. Washington, HEW, 1966.
33. Hathaway: USDA Home Econ. Res. Rep. No. 2. Washington, Government Printing Office, 1957.
34. Garn and Shamir: Methods for Research in Human Growth. Springfield, Charles C Thomas, 1958.
35. Falkner: Pediatrics, 29, 467, 1962.
36. Bernstein, Johnston, Ryan, Inouye and Hick: J. Appl. Physiol., 9, 241, 1956.
37. Hastings: A Manual for Physical Measurements. 1902. See reference 33.
38. Neumann and Alpaugh: Pediatrics, 57, 469, 1976.
39. Krogman: Tab. Biol., 20, 1, 1941.
40. Kemsley: Ann. Eugen., 16, 18, 23 and 316, 1952.
41. Yanagi, Hayami, Suzuki and Nagamine: Tokyo, Annu. Rep. Nat. Inst. Nutr., 1949–50, p. 1.
42. Fry: J. Clin. Nutr., 1, 453, 1953.
43. Chen, Lee, Ko and Shih: Mem. Fac. Med. Taiwan, 1, 168, 1951.
44. Sheldon: Varieties of Human Physique. New York, Harper, 1940.
45. Lasker: Am. J. Phys. Anthropol., 5, 323, 1947.
46. Vierordt: Daten und Tabellen für Mediciner und Aerzte. Jena, Fischer, 1888.
47. Rubner: Die Gesetze des Energieverbraushs bei der Ernaehrung. Leipzig and Vienna, Deuticke, 1902.
48. Baker and Newman: Am. J. Phys. Anthropol., 15, 601, 1957.
49. Brozek, Grande, Anderson and Keys: Ann. N.Y. Acad. Sci., 110, 113, 1963.
50. Bozenraad: Dtsch. Arch. Klin. Med., 103, 120, 1911.
51. Kohlrausch: Arb. Physiol., 2, 23, 1930.
52. Behnke: Harvey Lect., 37, 198, 1941.
53. Behnke: Ann. N.Y. Acad. Sci., 56, 1095, 1953.
54. Macy and Kelly: Hum. Biol., 28, 289, 1956.
55. Pace and Rathbun: J. Biol. Chem., 159, 685, 1945.
56. Keys, Anderson and Brozek: Metabolism, 4, 427, 1955.
57. Fidanza, Keys and Anderson: J. Appl. Physiol., 6, 252, 1953.
58. Mendez, Keys, Anderson and Grande: Metabolism, 9, 472, 1960.
59. Cheek, Schultz, Parra and Reba: Pediatr. Res., 4, 268, 1970.
60. Döbeln, von: Acta Physiol. Scand., 37, Suppl. 126, 1956.
61. Johnston and Bernstein: J. Lab. Clin. Med., 45, 109, 1955.
62. Ljunggren: Acta Endocrinol., Suppl. 33, 1957.
63. Sagild: Scand. J. Lab. Clin. Med., 8, 44, 1956.
64. Edelman: In Techniques for Measuring Body Composition (Brozek and Henschel, Eds.). Washington, National Academy of Sciences, 1961, p. 140.
65. McCance and Widdowson: Proc. R. Soc. B., 138, 115, 1950.
66. Soberman, Brodie, Levy, Axelrod, Hollander and Steele: J. Biol. Chem., 179, 31, 1949.
67. Faller, Petty, Last, Pascale and Bond: J. Lab. Clin. Med., 45, 748, 1955.
68. Sievert: Ark. Fysik., 3, 337, 1951.
69. Sievert: Strahlentherapie, 99, 185, 1956.
70. Anderson, Schuch, Perrings and Langham: Nucleonics, 14, 26, 1956.
71. Moore, Olesen, McMurray, Parker, Ball and Boyden: The Body Cell Mass and Its Environment. Philadelphia, W.B. Saunders, 1963.
72. Talso, Miller, Cargallo and Vasquez: Metabolism, 9, 456, 1960.
73. Allen, Anderson, and Langham: Gerontology, 15, 348, 1960.
74. Corsa, Olney, Steenburg, Ball and Moore: J. Clin. Invest., 29, 1280, 1950.
75. Rundo and Sagild: Nature, 175, 774, 1955.
76. Forbes and Lewis: J. Clin. Invest., 35, 596, 1956.
77. Anderson and Langham: Science, 130, 713, 1959.
78. Anderson and Langham: Science, 133, 1917, 1961.
79. Forbes: Pediatrics, 29, 477, 1962.
80. Forbes, Gallup and Hursh: Science, 133, 101, 1961.
81. Burmeister and Bingert: Klin. Wochenschr., 45, 409, 1967.
82. Anderson: Ann. N.Y. Acad. Sci., 110, 189, 1963.
83. McMurray, Boling, Davis, Parker, Magnus, Ball and Moore: Metabolism, 7, 651, 1958.
84. Haxhe: La Composition Corporelle Normale ses Variations au Cours de la Sous-alimentation et l'Hyperthyroidie. Bruxelles, Arscia, 1963.
85. Lesser, Deutsch and Markofski: Metabolism, 20, 792, 1971.
86. Brozek, Grande, Taylor, Anderson, Buskirk and Keys: J. Appl. Physiol., 10, 412, 1957.
87. Edwards: Clin. Sci., 10, 305, 1951.
88. Terhederbrügge: Arch. Pathol. Anat. Physiol., 298, 640, 1937.

89. Reynolds: Monogr. Soc. Res. Child Dev., *15*, No. 2, 1951.
90. Brozek (Ed.): *Body Measurements and Human Nutrition*. Detroit, Wayne University Press, 1956.
91. Pascale, Grossman, Sloane and Frank: In *Body Measurements and Human Nutrition* (Brozek, Ed.). Detroit, Wayne University Press, 1956, p. 55.
92. Keys et al.: In *Body Measurement and Human Nutrition* (Brozek, Ed.). Detroit, Wayne University Press, 1956. Hum. Biol., *28*, 1, 1956.
93. Edwards: Voeding (Amsterdam), *16*, 57, 1955.
94. Stuart, Hill and Shaw: Monogr. Soc. Res. Child Dev., *5*, No. 3, 1940.
95. Brozek, Mori and Keys: Science, *128*, 901, 1958.
96. Bezold, von: Z. Wiss. Zool., *8*, 487, 1857.
97. Friis-Hansen: Acta Pediatr., *46*, Suppl. 110, 1957.
98. Moulton: J. Biol. Chem., *57*, 79, 1923.
99. Zook: Am. J. Dis. Child., *43*, 1347, 1932.
100. Boyd: Hum. Biol., *5*, 646, 1953.
101. Parizkova: Nutrition, *14*, 275, 1960.
102. Parizkova: J. Appl. Physiol., *16*, 173, 1961.
103. Mellits and Cheek: Monogr. Soc. Res. Child Dev., *35*, 12, 1970.
103. Garn: In *Body Measurements and Human Nutrition* (Brozek, Ed.). Detroit, Wayne University Press, 1956.
104. Garn: Hum. Biol., *29*, 337, 1957.
105. Novak: Ann. N.Y. Acad. Sci., *110*, 545, 1963.
106. Reynolds and Grote: Anat. Rec., *102*, 45, 1948.
107. Stuart and Meredith: Am. J. Public Health, *36*, 1365 and 1373, 1946.
108. Stuart and Sobel: J. Pediatr., *28*, 637, 1946.
109. Fomon: *Infant Nutrition*, 2nd ed. Philadelphia, W.B. Saunders, 1974.
110. Brozek: Fed. Proc., *11*, 784, 1952.
111. Shock, Watkin, Yiengst, Norris, Gaffney, Gregerman and Falzone: J. Gerontol., *18*, 1, 1963.
112. Myhre and Kessler: J. Appl. Physiol., *21*, 1251, 1966.
113. Forbes and Reina: Metabolism, *19*, 653, 1970.
114. Forbes: Hum. Biol., *48*, 161, 1976.
115. Keys, Taylor and Grande: Metabolism, *22*, 579, 1973.
116. Miller and Blyth: J. Appl. Physiol., *5*, 73 and 311, 1952.
117. Grande: In *Techniques for Measuring Body Composition* (Brozek and Henschel, Eds.). Washington, National Academy of Sciences, 1961, p. 168.
118. Dahlstrom: Acta Physiol. Scand., *21*, Suppl. 71, 1950.
119. Steele, Brodie, Messinger, Soberman, Berger and Galdston: Trans. Assoc. Am. Physicians, *57*, 214, 1949.

120. Bray, Schwartz, Rozin and Lister: Metabolism, *19*, 418, 1970
121. Drenick and Dennin: J. Lab. Clin. Med., *81*, 421, 1973.
122. Brozek and Grande: Hum. Biol., *27*, 22, 1955.
123. Grande, Anderson and Keys: J. Appl. Physiol., *12*, 230, 1958.
124. Ryan, Williams, Ansell and Bernstein: Metabolism, *6*, 365, 1957.
125. Vanderveen: In *Fourth International Symposium of Bioastronautics and the Exploration of Space.* (Roodman, Strughold and Mitchell, Eds.). Brooks AFB Aerospace Medical Division (AFSC), 1968, p. 421.
126. Grande: Ann. Intern. Med., *68*, 467, 1968.
127. Evans: *Diseases of Metabolism*, 3rd ed. Philadelphia, W.B. Saunders, 1936.
128. Wishnofsky: Metabolism, *1*, 554, 1952.
129. Dole, Schwartz, Thorn and Silver: J. Clin. Invest., *34*, 590, 1955.
130. Taylor and Keys: Science, *112*, 215, 1950.
131. Grande: Am. J. Clin. Nutr., *21*, 305, 1968.
132. Consolazio, Mataush, Johnson, Nelson and Krzywicki: Am. J. Clin. Nutr., *20*, 672, 1967.
133. Gilder, Cornell, Grafe, Macfarlane, Asaph, Stubenbord, Watkins, Rees and Thorbjanarson: J. Appl. Physiol., *23*, 304, 1967.
134. Benoit, Martin and Watten: Ann. Intern. Med., *63*, 604, 1965.
135. Yang and van Itallie: J. Clin. Invest., *58*, 722, 1976.
136. Hommes, Drost, Geraets and Reijenga: Pediatr. Res., *9*, 51, 1975.
137. Thomson, Runcie and Miller: Lancet, *2*, 992, 1966.
138. Barnard, Ford, Garnett, Mardell and Whyman: Metabolism, *18*, 564, 1969.
139. Bortz: Am. J. Med., *47*, 325, 1969.
140. Consolazio, Mataush, Johnson, Krzywicki, Isaac and Witt: Am. J. Clin. Nutr., *21*, 803, 1968.
141. Allen and Musgrave: Am. J. Clin. Nutr., *24*, 14, 1971
142. Cook and Auken: Ann. Intern. Med., *34*, 1404, 1951.
143. Passmore, Meiklejohn, Dewar and Thow: Br. J. Nutr., *9*, 27, 1955.
144. Mitchell, Hamilton, Steggerda and Bean: J. Biol. Chem., *158*, 625, 1945.
144. Hunt, Peckos and Fry: *Overeating, Overweight, and Obesity*. New York, National Vitamin Foundation, 1953, p. 73.
145. Widdowson, McCance and Spray: Clin. Sci., *10*, 113, 1951.
146. Forbes, Cooper and Mitchell: J. Biol. Chem., *203*, 359, 1953.

Chapter *2*

THE GASTROINTESTINAL TRACT: AN OVERVIEW OF FUNCTION

Frank L. Iber

The major function of the gastrointestinal (GI) tract is the transfer of nutrients from the lumen of the intestine into the body itself. The gastrointestinal tract must be able to change the many varied physical and chemical forms of food that are eaten, and to process these forms into simple molecules which can be utilized by the body.[1,2]

A second substantial function of the GI tract is the protection of the body from a variety of noxious materials.[3] Along with the foods necessary for the body's maintenance and health, many substances are ingested which have the potential to cause great harm. Thus parasites, bacteria and viruses which are eaten with food, along with the many chemical poisons which are naturally occurring, must be detoxified.

A normal person daily ingests about 3000 gm of liquid and food, the GI tract adds 8000 to 14,000 ml of digestive juices and nearly all is absorbed, so that only 200 gm of solid is evacuated from the GI tract. The GI tract is a muscular tube with a functional lining passing from the mouth to the anus. The major portions are the mouth and pharynx, the esophagus, the stomach, the small intestine (divided into duodenum, jejunum and ileum) and the colon. At all levels the lining is resistant to abrasion and bacterial invasion, and secretes mucus to lubricate itself and enzymes and antibodies to keep bacteria in check. The lining repairs itself rapidly from an injury and renews itself completely in days or weeks.[4] The lining contains specialized cells that secrete, absorb and regulate. The predominant cells vary to account for different functions at different levels of the tract. Absorption cells have a specialized surface with many tiny projections called microvilli.[5] Secretory cells exist at nearly every level of the digestive tract. In the stomach and small intestine these are part of the lining; in other regions they are so large and specialized that they are separate glands with a duct leading their secretions into the intestinal tract. The salivary glands, the liver and the pancreas are the best known of such secretory glands.

The GI tract in eating and evacuation is controlled by the central nervous system.[6] Thus, voluntary and involuntary controls emanate from the brain and there are rich networks of nerves to all of the muscles about the mouth, tongue and throat, and similarly about the anus. To coordinate this function, sensations flow to the brain from these areas; thus odor, taste and consistency of food and drink reach the brain as well as touch, temperature, fullness of the mouth, etc. Sensations from the rectum and its sphincters also are transmitted to the brain. Sensory and pain representation is much more highly developed in the mouth and in the anus than all other regions; minor sores or ulcers in these areas produce profound pain. In the esophagus or in the rectum a few cm from the anus, the mucosa may be pinched off in taking a biopsy with no pain sensation—a marked contrast to areas nearer the extremes.[7]

The processes of digestion, in which complex food molecules are chemically transformed into simple ones, and absorption, in which simple molecules cross the gut wall and reach the blood, require a

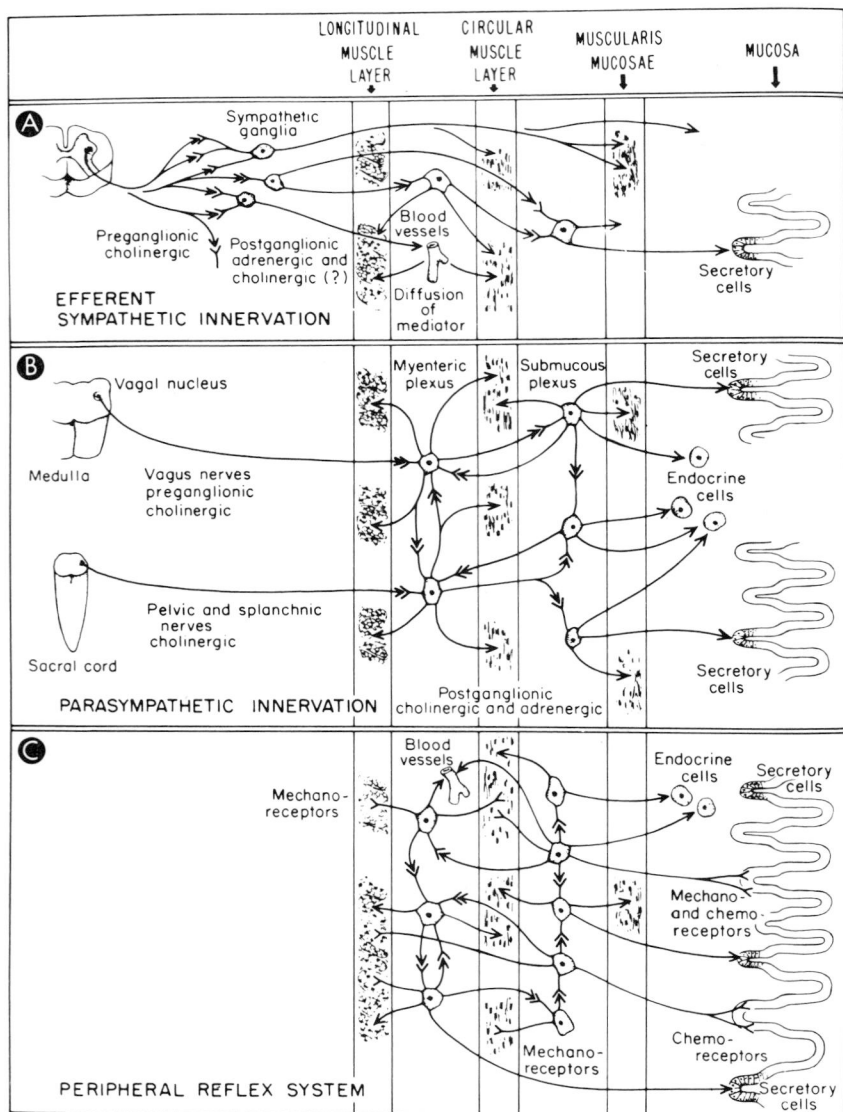

Fig. 2–1. Examples of the autonomic and intrinsic innervation throughout the GI tract. *A:* The interplay of sympathetic nerves from each level of the spinal cord. These go to blood vessels, to secretory cells and to both the longitudinal and circular muscle layers. *B:* The interplay of parasympathetics. *C:* The intrinsic nerves controlling integrative function of peristalsis, emptying and coordinated secretion. (From Davenport.[2] Used by permission.)

highly coordinated sequence of steps. Thus chewing, swallowing, mixing, trituration and movement out of the stomach, adjustment of pH, addition of bile or pancreatic juice and absorption are specific processes that must occur in the proper sequence and at the appropriate level of the gut. Two separate and complementary systems present throughout the GI tract serve to inform the other portions of the tract what is needed and what is happening and to effect this integration: nerves and hormones.

The innervation of the GI tract is almost entirely involuntary, using both the sympathetic and parasympathetic systems; many nerve networks exist confined almost entirely to the GI tract. Thus huge parasympathetic networks arise in the brain stem and pass to the esophagus, the stomach and to a minor degree the pancreas. Sympathetic nerve fibers pass from each spinal cord level to the GI tract. Coordinated muscular activity and spontaneous rhythmic contractions arise from nerve plexuses at each level of the intestinal tract. The normal function of these self-contained nerves is essential for peristalsis.

Figure 2–1[2] illustrates the common type of innervation present within the GI tract. The intrinsic nerves control much of the integrative function, as illustrated in C. A and B illustrate input from the brain and spinal cord. Peristalsis is largely controlled by this form of innervation. Caffeine and many other drugs change the activity of these nerves and thus alter intestine activity and secretion. Severe disease of either the internal lining (mucosa) or the external surface (serosa) such as ulcerative colitis or pancreatitis respectively may make these nerve ganglia edematous and paralyze peristalsis. Actual destruction of the nerves occurs in a few infrequent diseases (such as Chagas disease or amyloid) and in long-standing diabetes.

The second major system of regulation is hormonal.[8] Figure 2–2 illustrates a cell

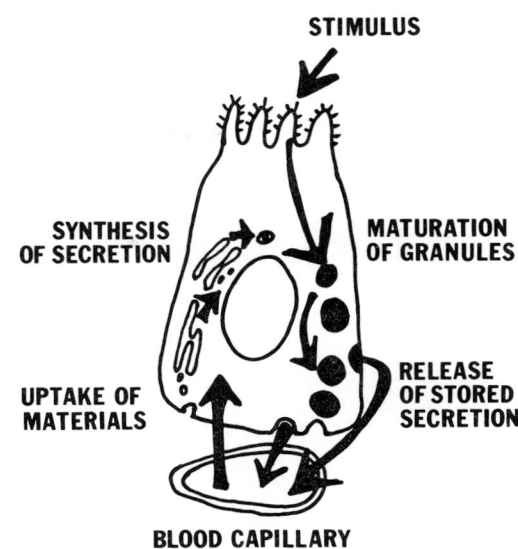

Fig. 2–2. A schematic endocrine cell of the intestinal tract. These cells are of many types, each secreting a hormone and an amine, such as serotonin. The luminal surface of the cell has microvilli that detect signals from the digestants leading to release of granules to the pericapillary space, where they pass into the blood and exert hormonal effects. See Table 2–1 for the more important intestinal hormones.

occurring in both the lining and glandular portions of the GI tract. These cells often have villi on the luminal surface and/or nerve endings, but characteristically contain secretory granules which are released into the pericapillary space by the cell. These granules contain serotonin or histamine and a polypeptide hormone. The cells are more concentrated in the antrum of the stomach, duodenum and upper small intestine and secrete hormones that regulate the GI function. They have many different names depending upon various staining properties (e.g. uptake of silver stains [argentifine] cells or amine precursor uptake and deamination [APUD] cells).

Histochemists and electron micrographers recognize 8 different types of these cells in the lining of the GI tract. The cells of the pancreatic islets are of nearly

Table 2–1. Features of Gastrointestinal Hormones

	Secreting Type*	Cell Location**	Amino Acids	Secretory Activity				Motor Activity		
				Gas	Int	Pan	Bile	Gas	GB	Int
Secretin	S	Int	27	–	–	++++	++	0	0	–
PZM-CCK	I	Int	33	–	+	0	0	–	+++	++
Gastrin	G	Gas Int	17	++++	0	++	+	+	+	0
Entero-glucagon†	EG	Int	29	– – – –						– – –
GIP†	K	Int	43							
Motilin	EC	Int	22					++++	0	++++
VIP	H	Int Pan	28	– –	++	++++	++	– – –		++++

PZM-CCK = pancreozymin-cholecystokinin   **Int = intestine   GB = gallbladder   – inhibits

GIP = gastric inhibitory peptide   Gas = gastric   + promotes

VIP = vasoactive intestinal peptide   Pan = pancreas

*After the Weisbaden classification. See Pearse, Polak and Bloom.[19]

†Both hormones stimulate insulin release from the pancreas.

identical embryologic origin. These cells discharge into the pericellular space the granules containing both the amine and the hormone, in response to a signal, either gained from the absorptive surface of the cell, such as hypertonicity, amino acids or sugars, or from a nerve ending. The amine enhances capillary permeability and permits the rapid entry of the high-molecular-weight hormone into the circulation. Table 2–1 lists some of the accepted hormones. All are now made synthetically. All have multiple actions; thus secretin predominantly stimulates an alkaline secretion of the pancreas, but also increases flow in the bile, retards gastric emptying and increases intestinal secretion. A small fragment of the hormone (4 to 10 amino acid fragments of the parent hormone of 10 to 30 amino acids) will often reproduce all of the actions of the parent hormone.

FUNCTIONS OF THE GI TRACT

Motility and Sphincters

Orderly peristalsis is essential to GI function.[9] If a 6- or 7-cm segment of small intestine is cut free, reversed end for end and replaced in the regular stream, the animal so treated will die because this small reversed segment is sufficient to completely interfere with peristalsis and produce obstruction of the intestine.[9a] Each of the major areas of the GI tract is under separate control for its motility. Swallowing forces a bolus of food or drink into the esophagus and, in smooth continuity with swallowing, peristaltic waves propel the ingested material into the stomach. Simple distention of the esophagus will also initiate peristalsis. The stomach has a "pacemaker" (i.e. specialized nervous tissue in the wall that initiates conducted peristaltic waves) located on the greater curvature; these contractions cease at the pylorus. The small intestine has many pacemakers throughout its length, but the high ones (in the duodenum) set a faster pace than those lower down, and therefore

are usually dominant. The colon has separate peristaltic pacemakers.

Many regions of the GI tract have specialized circular muscles called sphincters, usually located between organs.[10] These muscular regions are usually tightly constricted and thus retard movement of luminal contents and prevent backward flow. The sphincters are innervated so that they relax before a peristaltic wave reaches them. Thus, in the esophagus the lower esophageal sphincter (between the esophagus and stomach) is constricted at a pressure of about 10 mm Hg. When peristalsis moves through the esophagus, this sphincter relaxes *before* the food bolus reaches the sphincter area, thus permitting unimpeded passage. Such sphincters are located at both ends of the esophagus, at the lower end of the stomach (the pylorus), at the lower end of the small bowel (the ileocecal valve) and in the rectum. All of these are influenced by intestinal hormones and by the nerves in the wall and thus control the rate of movement of materials from one section to another.

Disorders of motility produce two different nutritional problems. Disorders of motility of the esophagus produce painful swallowing or sticking of food so that smaller and smaller meals are progressively ingested and weight loss follows.[11] A second form is loss of motility of the stomach and small intestine, most commonly seen in long-standing diabetics and resulting in impaired stomach and intestinal emptying. The ineffective total emptying of both organs allows excessive growth of bacteria. These bacteria may interfere with the orderly digestion of fats or vitamins or may actually injure the surface of the intestine. Intestinal scleroderma, a rare collagen disease, often has severe malnutrition as its principal manifestation.[12]

Secretion[13]

The process of secretion couples the energy-yielding metabolism within a cell to transport systems possessing the properties of enzymes. Secretory processes are known and identified for hydrogen, chloride, bicarbonate, sodium and potassium; for bile salts and uric acid and other organic molecules; and for enzymes and antibodies. Membrane-bound enzymes on the surface of the secreting cell are responsible for transport for the water-soluble smaller molecules (up to 600 to 1000 daltons) but the larger molecules are formed within the cell in membrane-bound packets that are secreted through a process in which the packets fuse with the membrane of the cell and discharge the contents. In nearly every instance both nerve stimuli and hormones act on the membrane of the cell to stimulate or inhibit secretion; this is accomplished in its final pathway either through enhancement or diminution of the rate-limiting enzyme in the transport system. In many of these systems cyclic adenosine monophosphate, cyclic guanosine monophosphate or prostaglandins are the intracellular mediators of this increased enzyme formation.[14,14a] These mediated changes are of such a magnitude that in the stomach acid secretion may be stimulated one millionfold and the fluid secretion in the small intestine can be increased twentyfold.

The salivary glands, the stomach, the pancreas and the liver produce complex secretions containing water, electrolytes, organic molecules, antibodies and enzymes. Only the salivary glands and stomach can produce a hypotonic or hypertonic secretion; all of the other digestive glands and organs produce nearly isotonic secretion. The salivary glands have exclusively autonomic nervous control, the stomach has both nerve and hormone control in approximately equal balance, but the liver and pancreas are largely controlled by hormones. All of these glands alter the composition of their secretion with variations in diet, secretory rate and stimuli.[15] In normal digestion about one fourth to one half of the maximal rate of secretion is utilized. Table 2–2 indicates some of the important properties of these secretions. Figure 2–3 illustrates secreting cells in the pancreas.

The small intestine is an important secretory organ. Enzyme-secreting glands exist in the duodenum but the crypts of Lieberkuhn throughout the small intestine

Table 2–2. Secretion and Absorption in Normal Subjects

Site	Vol Added ml/24 hr	Tonicity	Other* Components	Volume Absorbed ml/24 hr	Net Exit Traffic ml/24 hr
Ingestion	3000	Hi, Lo, Iso	–	0	3000
Salivary	350	Lo, Iso	Amylase	0	3350
Stomach	1000	Hi, Lo, Iso	Acid Pepsin Intrinsic factor	100	4250
Duodenum	1000	Iso	Alkali	100	5150
Pancreas	500	Iso	Amylase Peptidase Trypsin	0	5650
Liver	1500	Iso	Bile salts	0	7150
Jejunum	6000	Iso	Peptidases	8000	5150
Ileum	4000	Iso	Alkali	7000	2150
Colon	1000	Iso	–	2950	200

Hi = hypertonic, Lo = hypotonic, Iso = isotonic
*Immunoglobulin gamma A
 Lysozyme   } in all secretion
 Most plasma electrolytes

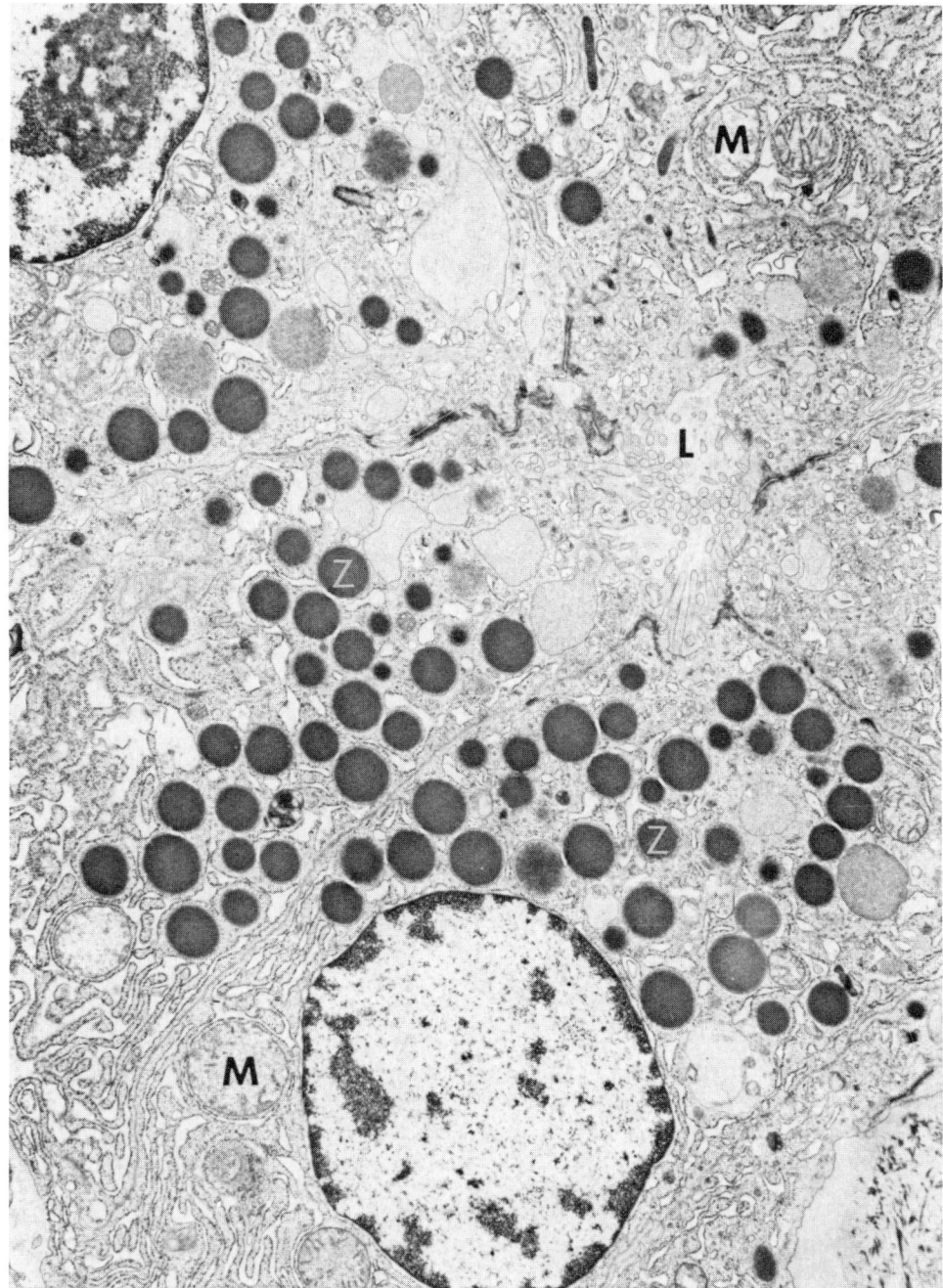

Fig. 2–3. Electron micrograph of a portion of the exocrine pancreas. This specimen was obtained at autopsy from a 65-year-old male who died as a result of a ruptured aortic aneurysm. Note the acinar cells with their distinctive zymogen granules (Z). These cells surround the acinar lumen (L). The swollen mitochondria (M) are the result of anoxia. The zymogen granules discharge into the lumen. The duct cells in the larger cells add watery alkaline secretion (not illustrated) as the major contributors to the volume. (Electron micrograph courtesy of Dr. Ray Jones, Department of Pathology, University of Maryland.)

produce a watery secretion varying in composition to increase the bicarbonate content progressively from duodenum to ileum.[16] The small intestine and colon normally absorb substantially faster than they excrete to produce little or no fluid in the lumen.[17] Under unusual circumstances (in obstruction or stimulation with V. cholerae or E. coli endotoxins) intestinal secretion may increase to as much as 40 liters per 24 hours.[18] Although cholera is the most widely known example of such watery and depleting diarrhea, other infections, certain slow-growing malignancies of the colon (villous adenomas) and certain hormone-secreting tumors of the pancreas (vasoactive intestinal peptide)[19] produce similar depletions.

Absorption

Although there is little absorption in the mouth, esophagus and stomach, all subsequent portions of the GI tract and the gallbladder are highly specialized to accomplish this function. Figure 2–4 indicates the basic structure of absorptive cells. The absorptive surface is highly specialized in having microvilli to increase the membrane surface area; there are high concentrations of enzymes in the microvilli that function to produce absorption, or to complete the final digestive steps before absorption occurs.

Absorption is of several types:[20] (1) active transport in which materials are moved against an electrochemical gradient and therefore require energy, (2) passive transport in which materials flow along an electrochemical gradient and (3) facilitated transport in which the material moves along an electrochemical gradient, but combination with an intermediate or membrane molecule is a necessary step to make absorption possible. "Bulk flow" is a common variant of facilitated transport. When rapid absorption of an osmotically active molecule occurs, the water carried along to preserve isotonicity is not pure water, but contains dissolved molecules of substances present in the lumen. The dissolved molecules transported with the water appear to have been actively transported. Most absorption of major nutrients is not energy requiring, but active transport systems exist for nearly all major and minor components.[21]

The lipid membrane surrounding the intestinal cell must be traversed if absorption is to occur. It is impermeable to most ionized molecules and to water-soluble molecules larger than those with molecular weights of 800 to 1200. Somewhat larger lipid-soluble molecules can pass through the cell wall but larger or charged molecules must usually be absorbed by facilitated transport of one form or another. Many important nutrients require this latter category of transport. Thus, bile salts and cholesterol, many vitamins and most minerals require special absorptive systems, often individually evolved for each type of molecule.

Figure 2–4 illustrates several adjacent intestinal absorptive cells. There is the luminal surface with the microvilli, the cell wall adjacent to another cell in the epithelium, and the cell surface adjacent to the capillaries and lymph space. Processes for active transport are usually located in the microvilli or in the membranes facing the spaces between cells.[22] A few active transport systems are localized on the inner cell surface, depending upon the free diffusion of molecules into the cell from where it is pumped against a concentration gradient into the interstitial space.[23] Cells are connected to one another by tight junctions (Fig. 2–4) which both provide structural stability between cells in the mucosa and prevent diffusion beyond this point.[24] The enzymes of the transport system are often closely related to digestive enzymes bound to membranes, and facilitate absorption. Thus, sucrose and polypeptides of 2 and 3 amino acid fragments are often taken up by the cell faster than their single-molecule components.

Figure 2–5 illustrates an impediment to

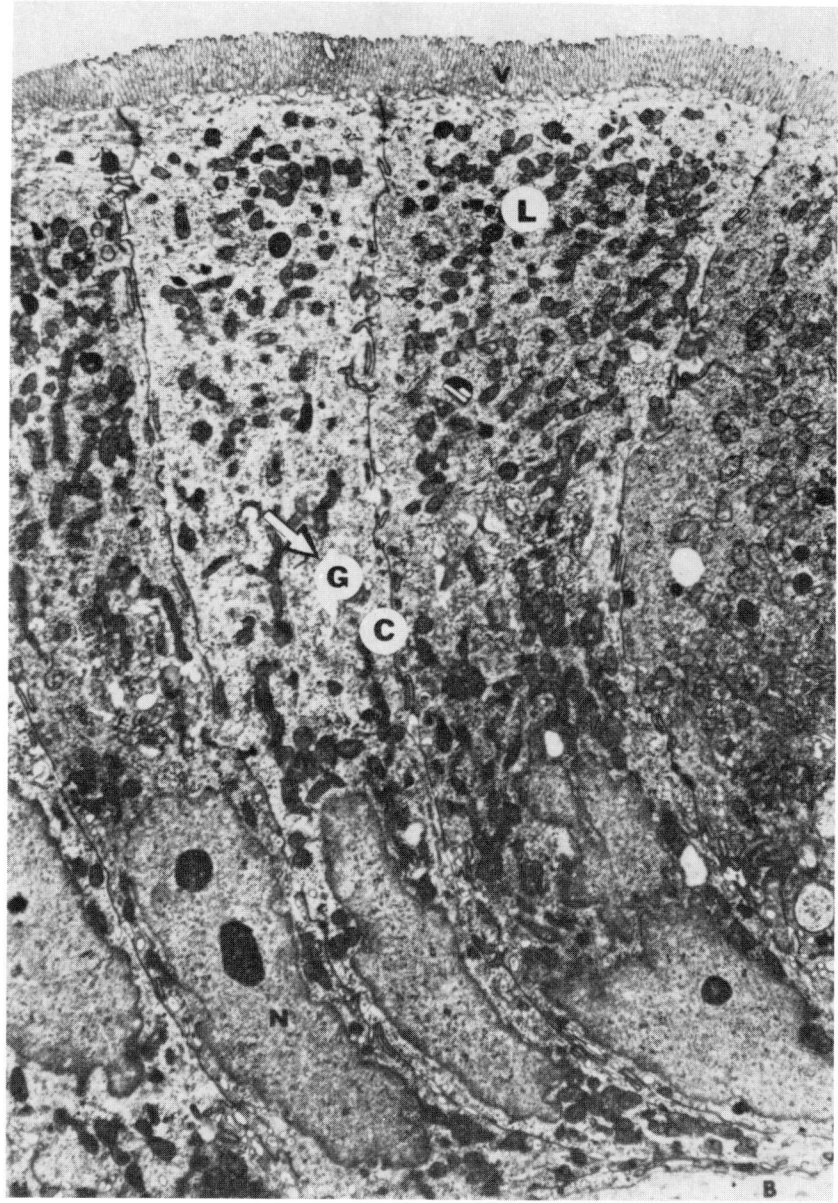

Fig. 2–4. Low-magnification electron micrograph of intestinal absorptive cells from the middle third of a jejunal villus from a normal man. Portions of five cells are shown. V = microvilli, N = nucleus, G = Golgi material, L = lysosomes, M = mitochondria, C = lateral cell membrane (the dark areas above and below this are tight junctions) B = basal lamina. (From Trier: *Handbook of Physiology*, Alimentary Canal (Code, Ed.). Washington, American Physiological Society, 1968. Used by permission.)

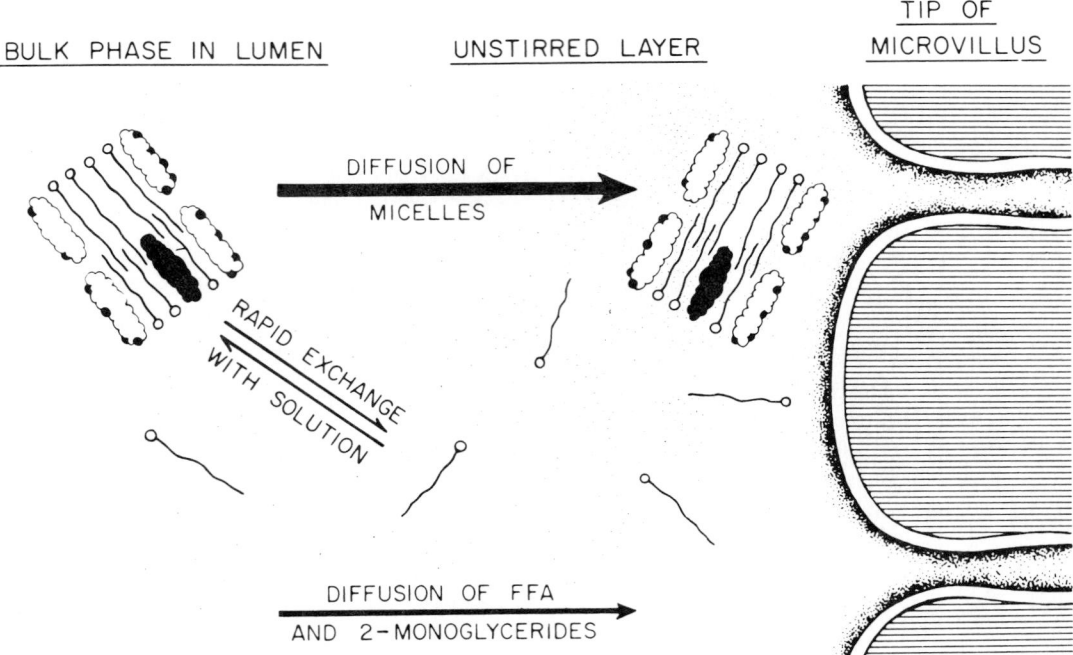

BULK PHASE IN LUMEN   UNSTIRRED LAYER   TIP OF MICROVILLUS

DIFFUSION OF MICELLES

RAPID EXCHANGE WITH SOLUTION

DIFFUSION OF FFA AND 2-MONOGLYCERIDES

Fig. 2–5. The unstirred water layer. The final passage through this layer depends upon diffusion, which is slow for water-insoluble materials such as the illustrated free fatty acids. Formation of micelles substantially overcomes this diffusion block and accelerates absorption. (From Davenport.[2] Used by permission.)

all absorption called the "unstirred water layer." For absorption to occur the nutrient must reach the surface of the intestinal cell. However, peristaltic action and the circular muscular contractions of the intestines do not mix a thin layer of fluid (unstirred water layer), ranging in thickness from 0.01 to 1.0 mm, entrapped by the microvilli. Diffusion of all substances must occur through this layer. Large molecules diffuse more slowly than small ones so that the amount diffused is directly related to the concentration and reciprocally related to the square or cube root of the molecular weight. For large molecules or highly water-insoluble molecules (fatty acids, some vitamins, cholesterol and some drugs) diffusion almost completely determines the rate of absorption and this process per se is slow.[26]

Most higher animals have evolved an absorptive mechanism to overcome this problem which involves bile salts. All naturally occurring bile salts are flat crocodile-shaped molecules in which highly polar and water-soluble groups stick out on one side like the legs of a crocodile, but the remainder is highly lipid soluble. These molecules aggregate in water solution, forming micelles. Figure 2–6 illustrates such a conglomerate. Micelles have a molecular weight of about 100,000 and therefore diffuse slowly through the unstirred water layer. However, the interior of the micelle is lipid and, therefore, lipid-soluble materials are highly soluble there. Thus, for oleic acid, a common food constituent, the micellar concentration is 100 times that in water. This increased concentration transported to the surface of the

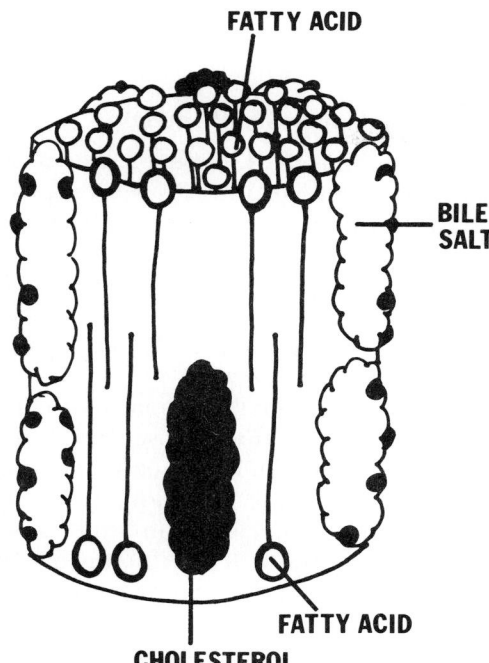

FATTY ACID

BILE SALT

FATTY ACID

CHOLESTEROL

Fig. 2–6. Schematic illustration of a micelle. The bile salts line the outside of the cylinder with the polar groups external and the lipid soluble material internal. Fat-soluble materials fill up the center; in the illustration fatty acid and cholesterol molecules are shown.

cell more than overcomes the slower diffusion of the large micelle and absorption is strikingly facilitated.[27]

PATHOPHYSIOLOGY

Mouth and Pharynx

The processes in the mouth of chewing, salivation, tasting and swallowing contribute in a major fashion to the enjoyment of eating and have some small role in the regulation of choices of food of these oral processes. Although certain cancers, liver disease and zinc deficiency alter taste threshold[28] and influence appetite, only abnormalities of swallowing profoundly affect nutrition. Surface erosions due to trauma, broken teeth, cancers or viral infections may be so painful as to interfere with the intake of food, but the most serious interference is produced with neurologic or muscular disorders influencing swallowing or with obstruction which prevents passage.

Thus, paralytic strokes common in septuagenarians and hypertensives often involve nuclei or tracts in the brain stem which are essential to swallowing. Multiple sclerosis or amyotrophic lateral sclerosis may involve these vital areas. Muscle diseases such as dermatomyositis may on rare occasions interfere seriously with swallowing.

Esophagus

The active conveyance of food from the mouth to the stomach and the exclusion of stomach contents from returning to the esophagus seem the only functions of this organ. Cancers or swallowed hard objects such as bones or pins may obstruct the passage of food and prevent the person from eating, but loss of peristaltic function is a more common problem.

Thus, many persons over age 60, particularly diabetics, lose peristaltic function and swallowing becomes difficult and often painful; weight loss follows.[29] Some collagen diseases injure the smooth muscle of the lower third, still other diseases (Chagas, achalasia) destroy the ganglion cells in the muscular layer and cause similar problems. If the sphincter between the stomach and the esophagus refuses to relax with swallowing obstruction may be profound, but the more common abnormality is that it does not properly exclude a reflux of stomach contents into the esophagus and a consequent partial destruction of its lining, which is not resistant to stomach digestants. This common problem, often associated with hiatus hernia and heartburn, produces major discomfort with the ingestion of food but rarely produces nutritional problems.

Stomach

The secretory and digestive functions of the stomach are well-defined but the organ

can be removed partially or in its entirety
with only modest effects on nutrition except for vitamin B_{12} absorption, which is
totally abolished by removal. The stomach
secretes acid (pH 1.0 is common) which is
promptly neutralized in the first 15 inches
of the duodenum, probably not as a diges-
tant of food but as a destroyer of infectious
agents, for few organisms can survive both
an extreme acid and a slightly alkaline pH.
The emptying of the stomach is exquisitely
controlled by hormones released from the
duodenal wall and by this delicately balanced regulation serves a major digestive
function in releasing complex food to the
upper portions of the small intestine at a
rate that permits efficient absorption. Loss
of the stomach, or even part of it, as the
result of surgery or disease moderately
interferes with this integrative function
and foods, particularly fats, are released to
the small intestine more rapidly, with a
resultant loss of efficiency and increased
losses of food into the feces.

The stomach actively adds fluid to its
lumen so that solutions approach isotonicity.[30] Thus, ingestion of water results in a
concentrated ionic secretion being added
in the stomach, whereas ingestion of a
sugar-containing soft drink (twice the concentration of body fluids) results in a dilute
solution being added. All subsequent portions of the GI tract are freely permeable
to water in both directions so that a hypertonic solution added to the duodenum or
colon results in a rapid entry of water from
the body. Addition of water leads to rapid
absorption.

Sudden distention of any portion of the
intestine stimulates peristalsis so that addition of a hypertonic solution to the
duodenum produces not only swelling of
the contents but hormonal discharge and
rapid evacuation. This discomfort, from
the swelling and its sequelae, is a common
occurrence following removal of major
portions of the stomach and is termed
"dumping."[31] The essential role of the
stomach in intrinsic factor production and

vitamin B_{12} metabolism is separately emphasized in later chapters.

The Upper Small Intestine

Normally, this is the site of the most
important digestive and absorptive processes. The duodenum and first part of the
jejunum may be looked upon as the principal sites of digestion of complex food
substances, initial absorption of simple
molecules and regulation of gastric, pancreatic and biliary function.

Entry of food from the stomach into the
duodenum causes the release from the
duodenum of an alkaline secretion into the
lumen and hormone secretion, secretin,
pancreozymin-cholecystokinin and gastric inhibitory peptide (GIP) into the blood
stream. The hormones stimulate alkaline
and enzyme-rich secretions by the pancreas, produce emptying of the gallbladder, retard stomach emptying and stimulate insulin secretion. Absorption in the
duodenum is limited; only simple
molecules requiring no digestion are absorbed. Iron, calcium and magnesium are
especially well absorbed at this location.

A little further along the small intestine
sufficient digestion occurs so that substantial amounts of simple molecules are available for absorption. In normal individuals,
90 to 95 per cent of all absorption occurs in
the first half of the small intestine,[32] but
many of the functions of the upper small
intestine can be assumed by the lower
bowel or small intestine with the exception
of providing an alkaline secretion (limited
to the duodenum), absorption of iron, calcium and other bivalent metals (probably
necessary before free fatty acids are released) and production of the regulatory
hormones.

Diseases of the upper small intestine are
those of obstructions such as tumors or
injuries to the lining. Peristaltic changes
due to muscular or nerve disease (diabetes,
scleroderma) often result in a major increase in bacterial growth which injures
the lining. Bacterial overgrowth, protein

malnutrition, parasite infestations, gluten sensitivity and lymphatic blockage all produce similar injury to the luminal surface of intestinal cells and are described in more detail in Chapter 31 B. Under these circumstances all active transport processes are impaired, release of regulatory hormones is inappropriate, digestive enzymes attached to the microvilli (lactase, etc.) largely disappear[33] and all of the absorptive processes are rendered inefficient. Because the digestion and absorption of fats are the most complex, impairment of lipid absorption is most profound.

The lining cells of the human small intestine are replaced every 3 to 5 days, requiring active mitosis and available nutrients to carry out this process.[4] Protein deficiency or folic acid deficiency retard the cell replacement.[34] Impaired replacement leads to an older population of cells on the villi with some limit in function. Absorptive defects of vitamins, amino acids, fats and sugars have been demonstrated.

The Lower Small Intestine

This is primarily a pure absorptive area, specialized for the absorption not only of foodstuffs but of water and electrolytes. The final fifth of the small intestine has well-developed and localized active transport systems for absorption of conjugated bile salts and for the B_{12} intrinsic factor combination.[35] The diseases of this region are similar to those of the upper small intestine but the impairment from disease or absence of the distal ileum assumes uniqueness in interfering with both bile salt absorption and B_{12} absorption. Uric acid is actively secreted by the lower small intestine.

The Pancreas

This organ, like the liver, develops in the embryo from an outpouching of the gut. The pancreas is at least three different functional organs combined into one. The digestive enzymes, potent for fat, protein and carbohydrate digestion, are produced by the acinar cells in small granules which are evacuated into the duct. The ducts produce an alkaline secretion responsible for the neutralization of the stomach acid; the release of these secretions is under separate hormone regulation by secretin. Islands of APUD cells secrete insulin, glucagon and possibly other hormones that influence the liver and the entire body.

The pancreatic juice is possibly the most important single digestive juice. The normal pancreas releases into the intestine about 20 to 30 gm of digestants daily, which are used and then destroyed. The manufacture of these 20 to 30 gm of protein depends upon the availability of suitable nutrients, and the pancreatic function is impaired in all forms of protein malnutrition or even voluntary starvation. The alkalinizing function is essential for pancreatic juices to act, for all of the enzymes are active only above pH 6 or even higher; acid pH rapidly inactivates them.[36,36a]

The pancreatic duct may become obstructed with a tumor so the secretion does not reach the intestine or the gland, which may become destroyed with inflammation. Both processes result in inadequate juices and maldigestion with subsequent malabsorption.

The Liver and Biliary Passages

The liver has two substantial roles in nutrition. It produces an important digestive juice—the bile—and it processes, stores and redistributes many nutrients. The digestive function of bile depends upon its content of conjugated bile salts. These materials are essential for micelle formation which in turn is a necessary step in the absorption of fats and fat-soluble vitamins. The entire body contains about 3 or 3.5 gm of bile salts. After a 5- or 6-hour fast these are entirely contained in the gallbladder which empties in response to a meal with the duodenal release of cholecystokinin-pancreozymin (CCK-PZ). These bile salts facilitate digestion through micelle formation (Fig. 2–6) but remain in the lumen of the gut largely until they reach the terminal ileum where they are actively and almost totally reabsorbed. They are absorbed via the portal vein and are rapidly reexcreted by the liver into the gallbladder. If the meal is not completely digested further emptying of these same bile salts is accomplished. In an average day the bile salt pool is reutilized 7 to 9 times; thus 20 to 25 gm of bile salts reach the intestine for use through the *enterohepatic circulation.*[37] In the normal individual, it is so efficient that only 5 per cent is lost per day, and this is replaced by liver synthesis.

Many disease processes occur which impair the enterohepatic circulation. Blocked biliary passages with stone or tumor completely prevent entry of bile acids. Any process producing increased numbers of bacteria in the small intestine results in splitting of the bile salts (deconjugation); this destroys the active transport link in the terminal ileum which is specific for the conjugated form and necessary for absorption. This, in turn, produces increased intestinal losses, depleting the bile salt pool. If the terminal ileum is lost through surgery or disease, the process is impaired. Liver disease such as hepatitis or cirrhosis prevents the rapid reexcretion of bile salts into the biliary passages and therefore the rapid reutilization is interrupted. All of these processes curtail the rapid availability of bile salts and interfere with efficient fat and fat-soluble substance absorption.

The bile also is a convenient excretory pathway for the liver; bilirubin and many other substances utilize this route to get out of the body.

All water-soluble materials absorbed by the intestine are carried from the intestine via the portal vein, which passes directly to the liver and breaks into a capillary bed bringing these materials into intimate contact with the liver cells. Nearly every nutrient passes into the liver cells and may be stored (such as glucose converted to the storage form of glycogen), utilized for energy or converted into other often more complex molecules (ketones, proteins, creatinine and most of the serum proteins are synthesized here).[38] Many vitamins are stored in the liver or are biotransformed into a physiologically active form. Even fat-soluble materials, primarily absorbed via the lymphatics, eventually reach the liver for some storage or processing. Many fatty acids are utilized by the liver; fat-soluble vitamins are stored there or are transformed to more active materials. Carrier proteins for the fat-soluble vitamins and for hormones are often manufactured by the liver.[39]

In liver disease an inefficiency and wastefulness of these myriads of metabolic processes develop. The normal liver can store about 1 year's supply of vitamin B_{12} or vitamin A but the diseased liver probably only a few weeks' or months' supply. Protein synthesis throughout the body is dependent upon a supply of all of the amino acids in proper proportions; in severe liver disease the release of the appropriate concentrations does not occur.

Gallbladder disease without obstruction has little effect upon digestion because the gallbladder per se is not essential to efficient digestion. This is probably because the biliary passages can assume most of its function.

The Colon and Rectum

The colon absorbs relatively large quantities of water and electrolytes; it receives about 1500 ml from the ileum each day and discharges between 100 and 200 ml from the rectum. Movement through the colon is much slower than in all other portions of the GI tract and is dependent upon volume of nonabsorbable materials, often called bulk or fiber.[40] Movement from stomach to the end of the ileum may require 30 to 90 minutes while passage through the colon may require 1 to 7 days.

Bacterial concentration and variety are more intense than in all other parts of the GI tract. Anaerobic and aerobic bacteria are present with counts in excess of 10^8 bacteria per ml of intestinal content.

Many food components not digestible by the intestinal tract are metabolized by this intense combination of bacteria and decreased motility. Thus many complex polysaccharides and a few simple ones (stachyose, lactulose) are digested by the colonic bacteria to hydrogen and carbon dioxide and short-chain fatty acids are produced that usually maintain the stool pH at about 5.5 or 6. Nondigestible protein residues are altered by bacteria to unpleasant odorous molecules (skatole from tryptophan, mercaptans from sulfur-containing amino acids) and nondigested fatty acids are oxidized to agents chemically similar to castor oil, a stimulant of colon secretion.[41]

Water is absorbed from the first two thirds of the colon; the contents become more and more plastic in consistency and the muscular activity necessary to produce propulsion increases. The last portion of the colon is mainly a reservoir requiring marked muscle activity to produce propulsion. Highly purified diets (and therefore with less fiber and bulk in the colon) result in diminished luminal content and make propulsion more difficult. Thickening of the muscle and bulging out of the intestinal lining through defects in the wall where blood vessels penetrate (called diverticulae) are common consequences.

Many normal materials in the diet when properly digested and absorbed have no influence on the colon. However, dysfunction of one type or another in the small intestine may lead to sequelae which profoundly influence colon function. Thus bile salts, normally at least 97 per cent absorbed in the terminal ileum, produce profuse diarrhea when abnormally large amounts enter the colon because of stimulation of secretion. Fatty acids of greater than 10-carbon-chain length stimulate co-

lonic secretion and, if oxidized by bacteria, produce even more diarrhea. Lactose or other simple disaccharides, normally split and completely absorbed in the small intestine, readily produce diarrhea if they reach the colon in quantity, because of both the osmotic effect and the mild secretory and irritant effects of the small-chain acids (lactate) that result from their fermentation.

If the lining of the colon becomes inflamed as it does in colitis, absorption is impossible and increased colonic secretion adds to the fecal stream with resulting copious diarrhea. Many bacterial and parasitic diseases (typhoid fever, shigellosis, salmonellosis, amebiasis) acutely and reversibly injure the lining of the colon. Other similar diseases merely stimulate the secretory cells without injuring the lining where the volume of secretion simply overwhelms the colon's ability to absorb.

BIBLIOGRAPHY

1. Sleisenger and Fordtran: *Gastrointestinal Disease.* Philadelphia, W.B. Saunders, 1973.
2. Davenport: *Physiology of the Digestive Tract.* Chicago, Year Book Medical Publishers, 1977.
3. Schanker: J. Med. Pharmacol. Chem., *2*, 43, 1960.
4. Eastwood: Gastroenterology, *72*, 962, 1977.
5. Almy: In *Gastrointestinal Disease* (Sleisenger and Fordtran, Eds.). Philadelphia, W.B. Saunders, 1973, pp. 3–12.
6. Doty: In *Handbook of Physiology*: Sec 6, Alimentary Canal, Vol IV (Code, Ed.). Washington, American Physiological Society, 1968, pp. 1861–1902.
7. Brooks: *Gastrointestinal Pathophysiology.* New York, Oxford University Press, 1974, pp. 7–52.
8. Bloom: In *Gastrointestinal Physiology II,* International Review of Physiology, Vol. 12 (Crane, Ed.). Baltimore, University Park Press, 1977, pp. 71–103.
9. Code, et al.: In *Handbook of Physiology*: Sec. 6. Alimentary Canal, Vol. V (Code, Ed.). Washington, American Physiological Society, 1968, pp. 2881–2896.
9a. Bortoff: Annu. Rev. Physiol., *34*, 261, 1972.
10. Pope: In *Gastrointestinal Disease* (Sleisenger and Fordtran, Eds.). Philadelphia, W.B. Saunders, 1973, pp. 86–89.
11. Treacy, et al.: Ann. Intern. Med., *59*, 351, 1963.
12. Bluestone, et al.: Gut, *10*, 185, 1969.
13. Binder: In *Gastrointestinal Physiology II,* Vol 12 (Crane, Ed.). Baltimore, University Park Press, 1977, pp. 285–304.
14. Davenport: *Physiology of the Digestive Tract.* Chicago, Year Book Medical Publishers, 1977, pp. 166–184.

14a.Kimberg: Gastroenterology, *67*, 1023, 1974.
15. Sachs, Heinz and Ullrich: *Gastric Secretion*. New York, Academic Press, 1972.
16. Field: Gastroenterology, *66*, 1063, 1974.
17a.Turnberg, et al.: J. Clin. Invest., *49*, 548, 1970.
17b.Turnberg, et al.: J. Clin. Invest., *49*, 557, 1970.
18. Banwell and Sheer: Gastroenterology, *65*, 467, 1973.
19. Pearse, Polak and Bloom: Gastroenterology, *72*, 746, 1977.
20. Sleisenger and Brandborg: *Malabsorption*. Philadelphia, W.B. Saunders, 1977, p. 1.
21. Mathews: In *Biomembranes*, Vol. 4B (Smyth, Ed.). New York, Plenum Press, 1974, p. 647.
22. Crane: In *Gastrointestinal Physiology II*, Vol 12. Baltimore, University Park Press, 1977, pp. 305–365.
23. Diamond and Bossert: J. Gen. Physiol., *50*, 2061, 1967.
24. Trier: In *Gastrointestinal Disease* (Sleisenger and Fordtran, Eds.). Philadelphia, W.B. Saunders, 1973, pp. 840–863.
25. Parson and Prichard: J. Physiol., *212*, 299, 1971.
26. Wilson and Dietschy: J. Clin. Invest., *51*, 3015, 1972.
27. Hofmann: In *Handbook of Physiology:* Sec. 6, Alimentary Canal, Vol. V (Code, Ed.). Washington, American Physiological Society, 1968, pp. 2507–2533.
28. DeWys and Walters: Cancer, *36*, 1888, 1975.
28a.Hambridge and Walravens: In *Trace Elements in Human Health and Disease*. Vol 1 (Pradad, Ed.). New York, Academic Press, 1976, pp 21–32.
29. Katz and Spiro: N Engl J Med *275*, 1350, 1966.
30. Hunt, and Wan: In *Handbook of Physiology*: Sec 6, Alimentary Canal, Vol II (Code, Ed.). Washington, American Physiological Society, 1967, pp. 781–804.
31. Sawyers and Herrington: Surgery, *69*, 263, 1971.
32. Weser: Am. J. Clin. Nutr., *24*, 133, 1971.
33. Winawer and Zamcheck: In *Progress in Gastroenterology*, Vol I (Glass, Ed.). New York, Grune and Stratton, 1968, pp. 339–356.
34. Hermos, et al.: Ann. Intern. Med., *76*, 957, 1972.
35. Garbutt, Lack and Tyor: Am. J. Med., *51*, 627, 1971.
36. Graham: N. Engl. J. Med., *296*, 1314, 1977.
36a.DiMagno, et al.: N. Engl. J. Med. *296*, 1318, 1977.
37. Javitt: In *Diseases of the Liver,* 4th ed. (Schiff, Ed.). Philadelphia, J.B. Lippincott, 1975, pp. 111–145.
38. Combs and Schenker: In *Diseases of the Liver,* 4th ed. (Schiff, Ed.). Philadelphia, J.B. Lippincott, 1975, pp. 204–246.
39. Mallia, Smith and Goodman: J. Lipid Res., *16*, 180, 1975.
40. Spiller and Amen: *Fiber in Human Nutrition.* New York, Plenum Press, 1976.
41. Bright-Asare and Binder: Gastroenterology, *64*, 81, 1973.

Chapter *3*

THE PROTEINS AND AMINO ACIDS

Hamish N. Munro
and
Marilyn C. Crim

Proteins are associated with all forms of life, an observation which dates back to the original identification of proteins as a class by Mulder in 1838, although earlier investigators had evidence of a less precise character for a similar group of compounds associated with living matter.[1] The proteins of living matter act as organic catalysts (enzymes), as structural features of the cell, as messengers (peptide hormones), as antibodies, etc. The accumulation of proteins during growth and development, and the maintenance of tissue proteins in the adult, represent important objectives in ensuring nutritional well-being. A knowledge of how dietary protein is optimally utilized by the body is important in determining how much protein is needed for health and for the restoration of body tissue in disease. For this reason, the chapter begins with the metabolism of amino acids, including their uses as a source of nitrogen for the biosynthesis of other major constituents of the body. The next section describes the roles of individual organs in the utilization of dietary protein, providing an integrated picture of protein metabolism and its responses to food intake. Estimates of the requirements of human subjects for protein and for individual amino acids are then discussed, and changes in such needs as a result of disease are evaluated. Finally this is followed by an account of the sources of protein in the diet, and the patterns of intake.

The importance of protein in the diet is primarily to act as a source of amino acids, some of which are *essential* (indispensable) dietary constituents because their carbon skeletons are not synthesized in the bodies of animals; others are *nonessential* (dispensable) since they can be made within the animal from carbon and nitrogen precursors. A survey[2] of species ranging from single-celled animals (protozoa) to man shows that all animal species from single-celled organisms onward need some preformed amino acids in their diets; furthermore, the list of these essential amino acids is remarkably similar[2] for all animal species. For man, the essential amino acids are histidine, isoleucine, leucine, lysine, methionine, phenylalanine, threonine, tryptophan and valine; in addition, cysteine and tyrosine are synthesized in the body from methionine and phenylalanine respectively. All of these 11 amino acids occur in proteins in the cells of the body. An additional nine amino acids (alanine, arginine, aspartic acid, asparagine, glutamic acid, glutamine, glycine, proline and serine) are present in most proteins. These can, however, be deleted from the diet, since the body has the capacity to synthesize them from simple precursors. They are thus nonessential in the diet. Other amino acids occur in proteins, but these are made by modifying the side chains of one of the above after the protein has been synthesized. For example, hydroxyproline occurs in collagen by hydroxylation of certain proline residues in the collagen peptides as they are being made.[3] Similarly, the contractile proteins actin and myosin of muscle contain 3-methylhistidine, made by methylation of certain histidine residues in these proteins.

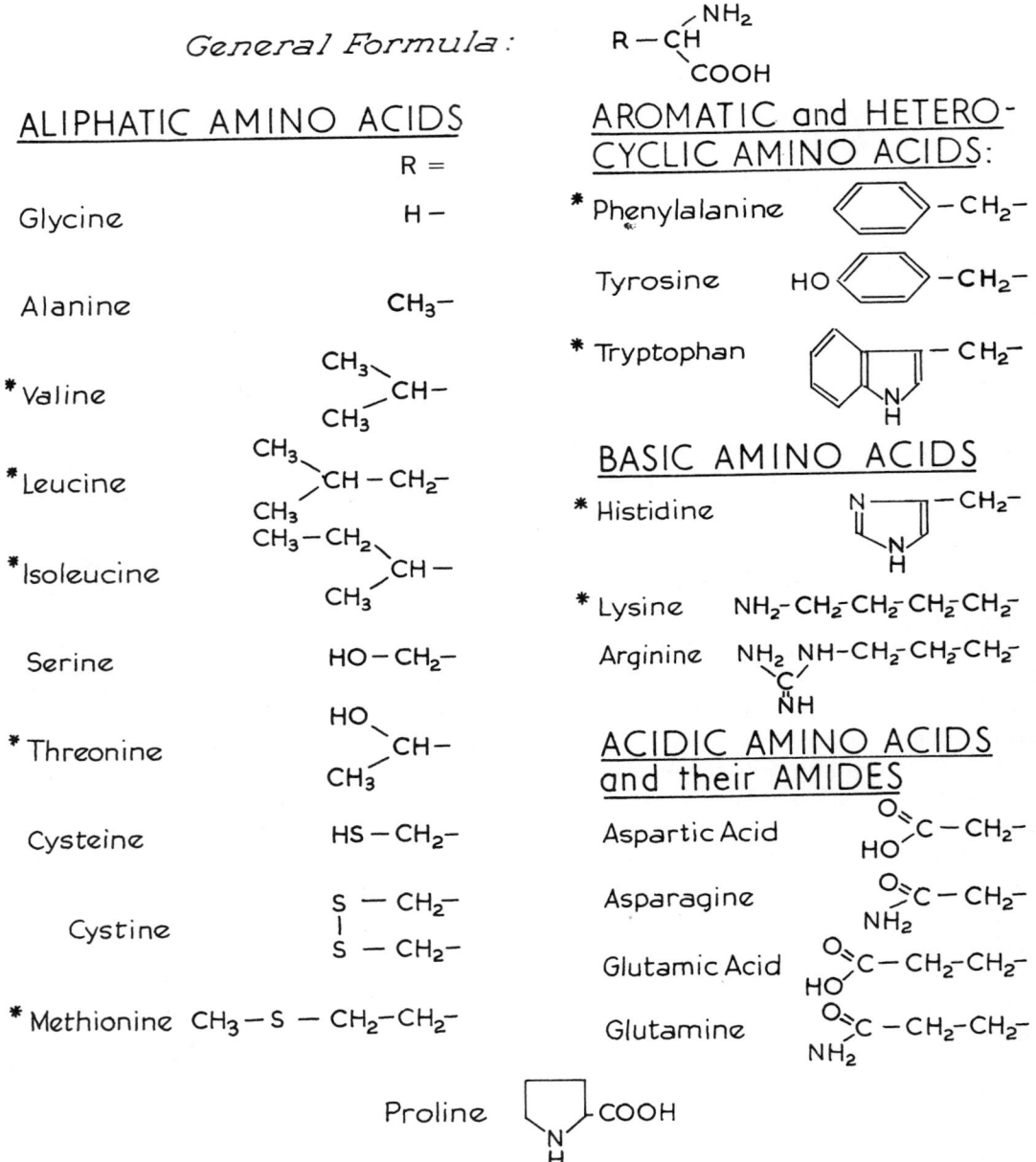

Fig. 3-1. Formulas of the 20 common amino acids found in proteins. Essential amino acids are marked with an asterisk(*).

These derived amino acids are not used again for de novo protein synthesis. When proteins containing them are broken down within the body, they are either metabolized (hydroxyproline) or excreted quantitatively (3-methylhistidine).

Figure 3–1 shows the structural formulas of the 20 amino acids used for protein synthesis. It will be seen that all except glycine have an asymmetrical carbon atom, and thus can exist as optically active isomers that rotate the plane of polarized lights to the left (levorotatory) or to the right (dextrorotatory). Only one out of each amino acid isomer pair is used by the body for constructing its proteins. The amino acid isomers used for protein synthesis all have similar structural conformations around the asymmetric carbon atom, the amino group and the carboxyl group occupying the same relative spatial relationship to one another. These amino acids are therefore designated as the L-series, while those not commonly found in proteins are called the D-series, regardless of how they rotate the plane of polarized light. Many metabolic reactions, including those of protein synthesis and transport across cell walls, distinguish L- from D-forms. However, certain reactions (transaminations) can transform the D-form into the L-form and thus make it available to the body. The capacity to use dietary D-amino acids is limited to certain amino acids which vary from species to species.[2] In man, these are D-methionine and D-phenylalanine.[2] Recent studies with intravenous infusion of D-methionine indicate that it is utilized less efficiently than the L-form.

The structural features of the 20 amino acids show (Fig. 3–1) that some are dibasic (arginine, lysine, histidine) and some diacidic (aspartic acid, glutamic acid). These characteristics are important in determining the properties of proteins containing an abundance of dibasic or diacidic amino acids (e.g. diacidic amino acids are especially abundant in proteins forming parts of membranes). Most amino acids are, however, neutral with an aliphatic or aromatic side chain. The classification of amino acids into neutral, basic and acidic has particular relevance to amino acid transport across membranes, since each amino acid class appears to be carried by a separate carrier mechanism.

METABOLISM OF AMINO ACIDS: INTRACELLULAR EVENTS

Free Amino Acid Pools and Their Metabolic Fates

Protein consumed in the diet is enzymatically hydrolyzed in the alimentary tract and passes into the blood stream as free amino acids which mingle with amino acids coming from the tissues. Amino acids occur in the body in the free form and in the form of body proteins. The concentration of protein-bound amino acids in the tissues averages 2 M, whereas the free amino acids pools are about 0.01 M,[4] that is, 0.5 per cent of the concentration of protein-bound amino acids. Table 3–1 shows the distribution of individual amino acids between the body proteins and the free amino acid pools in the tissues of the young rat. The tissue concentrations of the free essential amino acids are very low, whereas the concentrations of four of the nonessential amino acids (alanine, glutamic acid, glutamine and glycine) are somewhat higher. On the other hand, the concentrations of free amino acids in rat plasma (Table 3–1) all fall within a similar range. This occurs because the four nonessential amino acids present in most abundance in the tissues are extensively synthesized and retained within the cells.

Comparison of the concentrations of free essential amino acids in the body with the essential amino acid requirements for the growing rat (Table 3–1) demonstrates that the free amino acid pool must turn over several times daily through the flux from dietary sources. The magnitude of the flux of amino acids in the body is

Table 3–1.   Amounts of Protein-Bound and Free Amino Acids in the Body of a 50-gm Rat, and the Concentrations of Free Amino Acids in Rat Plasma*

Amino Acid	Total Body Content of Amino Acids (μmoles/100 gm rat)		Free Amino Acids in Rat Plasma (μmoles/ 100 ml)	Daily Amino Acid Requirement (μmoles/100 gm rat)
	Protein-bound	Free		
Essential				
Arginine	8400	7	16	—
Histidine	3600	24	11	140
Isoleucine	8400	10	8	400
Leucine	16500	14	16	500
Lysine	8900	15	41	600
Methionine	4050	6	9	350
Phenylalanine	5800	9	9	450
Threonine	7550	20	24	400
Tryptophan	980	2	—	55
Valine	9400	12	18	500
Nonessential				
Alanine	13500	100	32	—
Aspartic acid	11300	19	1	—
Glutamic acid	17700	132	15	—
Glutamine	—	223	55	—
Glycine	24700	323	45	—
Serine	12400	20	23	—
Tyrosine	3550	8	9	—

*Adapted from Munro[5] and Herbert et al.[6]

increased even further by recycling of amino acids coming from breakdown of proteins in the tissues.

Transport of free amino acids across cell membranes has been extensively studied, and has been found to occur by several carrier mechanisms, each common to a number of amino acids.[4] In general, basic, acidic and neutral amino acids each enter the tissues by different transport mediators. In each category, a degree of competition for the carrier can be demonstrated between any two amino acids of that class. Within the neutral class, Christensen[4] describes two groups of transport mechanisms. One has high affinity for alanine and for α-aminoisobutyric acid, a synthetic nonprotein amino acid. This carrier is sensitive to respiratory inhibitors. On the other hand, the branched-chain neutral amino acids are taken up by a different mechanism which is relatively insensitive to respiratory inhibitors. This second form of uptake appears to depend for its driving force on exchange of intracellular neutral amino acids for extracellular amino acids. Finally, Meister[7] has proposed a transport mechanism located in the cell membrane and involving glutathione for the actual movement of amino acids into cells.

There has been considerable dispute about whether free intracellular amino acids are the ultimate source for protein synthesis within cells, or whether extracellular amino acids charge transfer RNA (tRNA) for protein synthesis without entering the cell fluid.[8,9] This problem is of considerable importance in studies of protein synthesis in whole animals, since breakdown of tissue protein within cells contributes amino acids that dilute the intracellular free amino acid pool more than the plasma pool. In consequence, isotopically labeled amino acids undergo a greater reduction in specific activity within cells than in the blood stream,[10] so that the rate of synthesis of intracellular proteins computed from the specific activity of the free amino acids in each precursor pool can be quite different. Khairallah[11] has measured the specific activity of liver amino-acyl-tRNA after giving labeled leucine to rats, and found that the tRNA had an activity midway between free leucine in the plasma and in the liver cells. He concluded that tRNA is charged with amino acids by a pool closely associated with the cell membrane and receiving amino acids from both external and intracellular sources.

Amino acids are subjected within the body to the series of metabolic reactions outlined in Figure 3–2. Although this represents a complex series of pathways, we can group these reactions into three categories:

1. Part of the free amino acid pool is incorporated into tissue proteins. Because of tissue protein catabolism, these amino acids re-

turn to the free pool after a variable length of time and thus become available for reutilization.

2. Part of the free amino acid pool undergoes catabolic reactions. This leads to loss of the carbon skeleton as CO_2 or its deposition as glycogen and fat, while the nitrogen is eliminated as urea.

3. Some free amino acids are used for synthesis of new N-containing compounds, such as purine bases, creatine and epinephrine. These are subsequently generally degraded without return of end-products to the free amino acid pool (e.g. purines are degraded to uric acid, creatine to creatinine, epinephrine to vanillylmandelic acid). In addition, the nonessential amino acids are made in the body using amino groups derived from other amino acids.

The relative magnitudes of these three pathways in the whole animal is represented by studies in which rats were fed by stomach-tube with 1-mg doses of uniformly labeled L-tyrosine, L-phenylalanine or L-tryptophan.[13] The investigators measured the proportion of absorbed radioactivity excreted during the first 4 hours in the form of CO_2 or recovered from the liver, gut and total skeletal musculature in

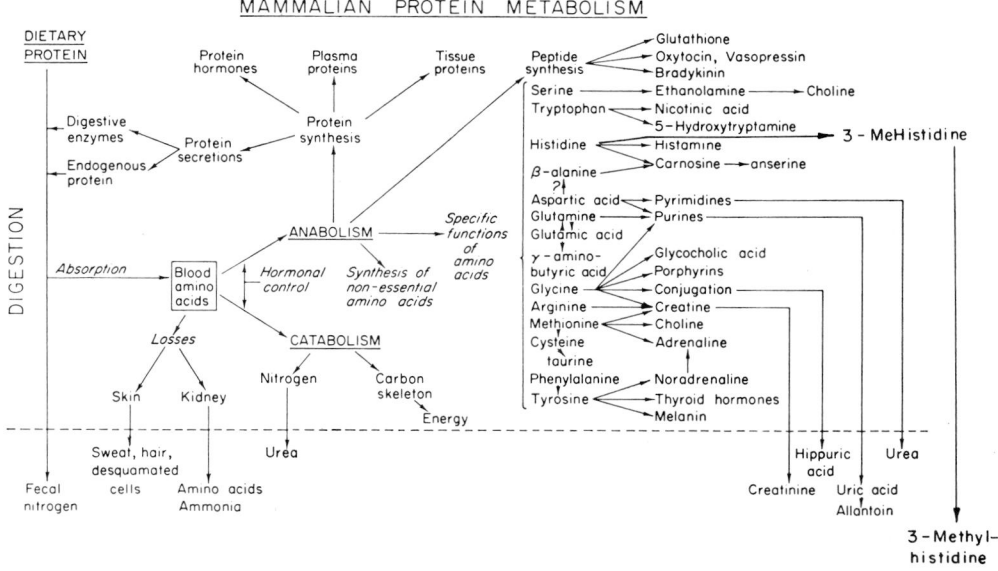

Fig. 3–2. General features of mammalian protein metabolism. (From Munro.[12])

the form of protein-bound activity or as nonprotein compounds. At 15 minutes after feeding, 20 to 40 per cent of the absorbed radioactivity of the three amino acids was recovered as acid-soluble compounds in liver, gut and muscle, most being in muscle. Considerable amounts of nonaromatic radioactive compounds were present at this time, indicating rapid breakdown of the free amino acids. Thereafter, acid-soluble ^{14}C activity decreased whereas output as CO_2 rose and eventually accounted for 19 to 40 per cent of the absorbed dose. Protein-bound activity in the three tissues represented 34 to 51 per cent of the absorbed activity at 4 hours after feeding. The relative magnitudes of these pathways will, of course, depend on the nutritional state of the animal. In a later section, we shall see that the proportion of lysine degraded to CO_2 increases progressively as intake of lysine exceeds requirement, and that this is regulated by the liver.

Protein Synthesis and Degradation

The amount of a protein in a cell can be altered by changes in the rate of either its synthesis or its breakdown or both. The combination of synthesis and breakdown is known as turnover, and in the steady state both synthesis and breakdown are equal. As Figure 3–3 shows, protein synthesis consists of two phases: *transcription*, in which messenger RNA (mRNA) is made on a template of DNA in the nucleus, and *translation*, in which the mRNA is used in the cytoplasm by the ribosomes to synthesize protein. In many cases this is followed by further (post-translational) modification of the newly synthesized peptides.

Transcription and Its Control. The first step is to make the information in chromosomes available by transcribing specific parts of the chromosomal DNA into messenger RNA. It is generally accepted that the histones and acidic proteins of chromosomes regulate the pieces of the encoded information which are made

available, although the details of the mechanism remain uncertain.

As shown in Figure 3–3, the nucleus contains several forms of RNA, separable on sucrose gradients. Ribosomal RNA is formed in the nucleolus, first as a single strand of 45S RNA, which then breaks into shorter lengths resulting in the 28S and 18S RNAs of the two ribosomal subunits (rRNA). In the nuclear sap, RNA of large size (heterogeneous nuclear RNA; HnRNA) is transcribed from the DNA and from this mRNAs are made. The transfer of mRNA from the nucleus to the cytoplasm first acquires polyadenylic acid formed by poly A polymerase except for some messengers (e.g. for histones) which do not include poly A. Finally, the mRNA becomes associated with protein to produce ribonucleoprotein particles (mRNP) which pass to the cytoplasm.[15]

The formation of RNA using a template of eukaryotic DNA involves the action of DNA-dependent RNA polymerase, which can be resolved on DEAE-Sephadex into several species.[16-18] Polymerase I is found in the nucleolus and transcribes ribosomal RNA. Polymerase II occurs in the nucleoplasm and transcribes HnRNA and thus mRNA. Polymerase III synthesizes tRNA and 5S RNA.

Inhibitors of these processes are important for exploring control of protein synthesis. Low doses of actinomycin D inhibit ribosomal RNA synthesis; inhibition of HnRna synthesis requires larger amounts. Formation of mRNA is inhibited by amanitin, which binds specifically to polymerase II,[16,17] while poly A polymerase is inhibited by cordycepin.[19] Consequently these inhibitors can be used to block induction of cell proteins requiring additional mRNA synthesis and transport.

The response of the RNA-synthesizing system to hormones and other factors is an important means for altering protein synthesis. For example, liver RNA content increases following administration of corticosteroid hormones to animals,[20] mainly

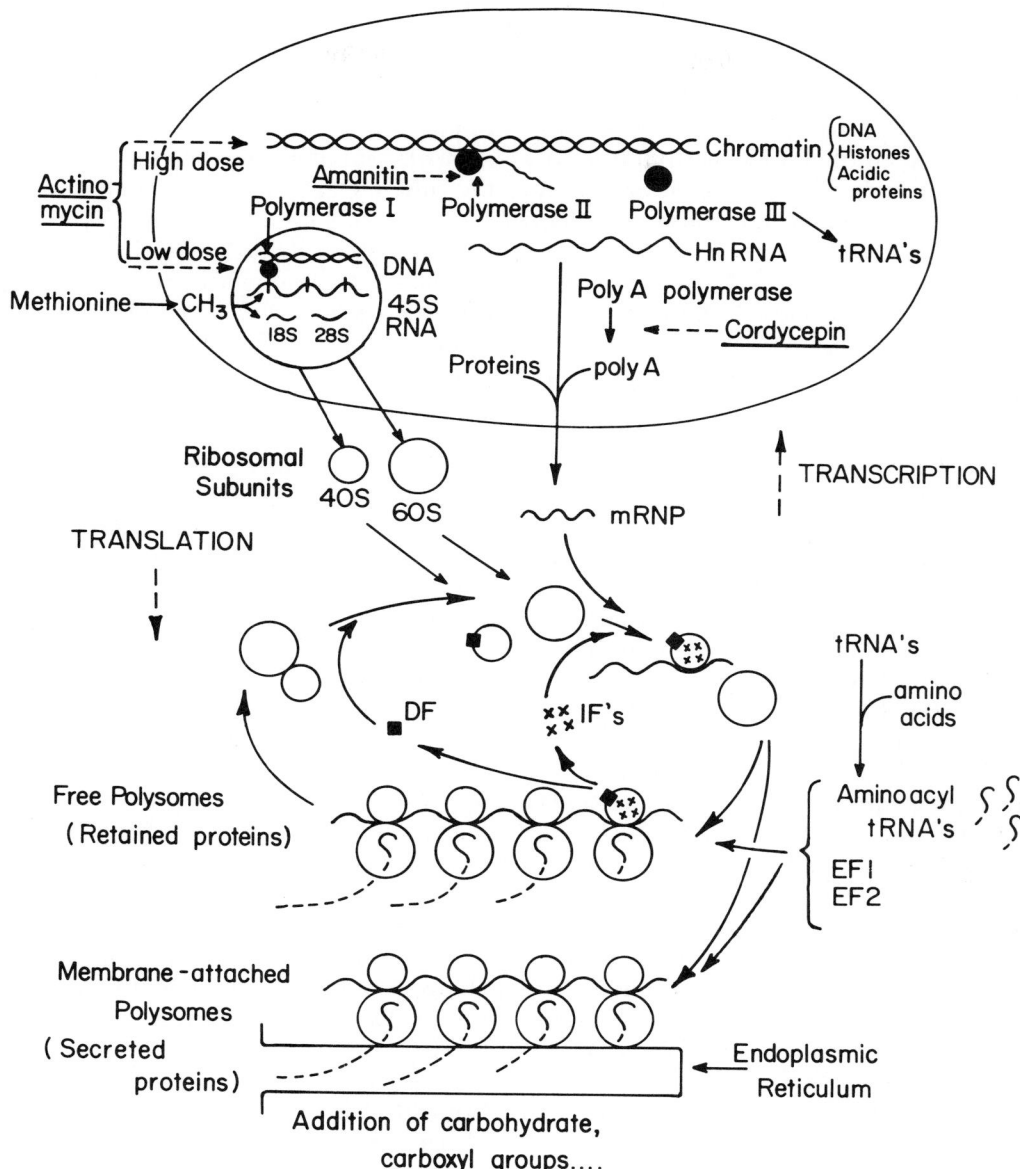

Fig. 3–3. Mechanism of eukaryote protein synthesis. The diagram shows chromatin, RNA polymerases I, II and III and their inhibitors actinomycin D and α-amanitin, poly-A polymerase and its inhibitor cordycepin, mRNA precursor (HnRNA), the transport of the messenger RNA (mRNA) into the cytoplasm as messenger ribonucleoprotein (mRNP), free ribosomes and polyribosome aggregates both free in the cytosol and attached to the endoplasmic reticulum membrane for secretion of proteins. (From Nowak and Munro.[14])

because of increased rRNA synthesis. After a single injection of hydrocortisone into rats, there is an increase in the amount of 45S RNA produced in liver nucleoli which could be the result of exposure of more template DNA to nucleolar polymerase or of an increase in the activity of the nucleolar polymerase I. Sajdel and Jacob[21] have shown that there is a sharp increase in polymerase I (nucleolar enzyme). Some specific mRNAs are also induced. Corticosteroid administration transiently increases tyrosine aminotransferase and tryptophan oxygenase levels in rat liver by a process inhibited by prior administration of actinomycin D.[22] In general, changes in protein synthesis produced by hormones involve specific receptors in the cells of the target organ.[23,24] The hormone enters the target cell and binds to a specific cytoplasmic receptor which then enters the nucleus and binds to the chromatin at a specific site. This is followed by transcription of the DNA at that site, so that new messenger RNA species are made. The mRNAs are then transported into the cytoplasm where they are translated, producing new proteins in the cell or increasing the amounts of existing proteins.

Translation and Its Control. The process of mRNA translation has been reviewed elsewhere.[25] The synthesis of peptide chains on ribosomes occurs in three phases, namely, initiation, elongation and termination (Fig. 3–3). Several protein initiation factors have been identified in eukaryote cells; in addition, initiation requires free ribosomal subunits, mRNA and initiator methionyl tRNA. Initiation is followed by peptide chain elongation, with the addition of successive amino acids to the peptide chain. Some 60 aminoacyl-tRNA species charged with the 20 amino acids of proteins form complexes with elongation factor 1 (EF 1) and GTP, and insert the correct amino acid indicated by the codons of the mRNA into the growing peptide chain. Binding of aminoacyl-tRNA is followed by translocation of the growing

protein chain across the ribosome surface under the influence of elongation factor 2 (EF 2) and GTP, during which the ribosome undergoes conformational changes. Finally termination of the peptide chain requires additional protein factors (not shown). The ribosome then separates from the mRNA (runoff ribosome) and dissociates into subunits by a mechanism requiring a dissociation factor. Repeated initiation of the same mRNA strand results in the mRNA carrying a number of ribosomes bound to the message, that is, a polyribosome (Fig. 3–3). The proportion of the total ribosome population in the forms of polysomes and of runoff ribosomes and subunits is determined by the balance between initiation and elongation. If initiation is reduced, the ribosomes still pass along the mRNA strand and accumulate as runoff ribosomes. Thus polysomes diminish and runoff monosomes and subunits increase. The effects of reduced rate of chain elongation depends on the cause. Thus the antibiotic cycloheximide prevents translocation by altering EF 2 and GTP binding[26] so that the polysome pattern is not disrupted, although movement slows down. On the other hand, puromycin causes premature chain termination and often disrupts the polysomes. If tRNA carrying a single amino acid is not available in adequate amounts, the rate of chain elongation is retarded only at those points where that amino acid must be inserted in the growing peptide chain.[27]

Post-translational Events and Their Control. After the peptide chain has been synthesized, many proteins undergo further change before becoming active cell components. Such post-translational modifications can be useful for identifying the fate of the peptide chain. Thus in the case of actin and myosin, in which some of the histidine residues become methylated after translation, the 3-methylhistidine so formed is released during intracellular turnover of these proteins and is quantitatively excreted in the urine.[28] The amount excreted thus served as an index of muscle protein catabolism (see later).

Some proteins are secreted by cells; many of these are modified by addition of carbohydrates (glycoproteins) after translation.[3] Such secreted proteins are made on ribosomes attached to the membranes of the endoplasmic reticulum, which act as conducting channels for their secretion and also as sites where sugars are added to the peptide chain (Fig. 3–3).

Pathways of Amino Acid Degradation

Each amino acid is degraded by undergoing a special sequence of chemical reactions.[29,30] The details of these are not relevant in this volume, and can be obtained from texts on biochemistry. In Figure 3–4 the routes of degradation of the essential and nonessential amino acids are outlined

to show how NH_3 and glutamic acid are made available by these degradative reactions for eventual excretion as urea. The figure also shows that 7 of the 10 amino acids essential to the rat are primarily degraded in the liver, whereas the other 3 (the branched-chain amino acids isoleucine, leucine and valine) are mostly catabolized in muscle, and also in kidney and brain. Much of the amino group made available by transamination of the branched-chain amino acids in muscle is transferred to pyruvate and glutamate to produce respectively alanine and glutamine, forms in which they go by way of the blood stream to the liver (alanine) and the gut (glutamine). In the gut wall alanine and glutamic acid are formed and the alanine passes by way of the portal system to the liver (Fig. 3–5). This facilitates the

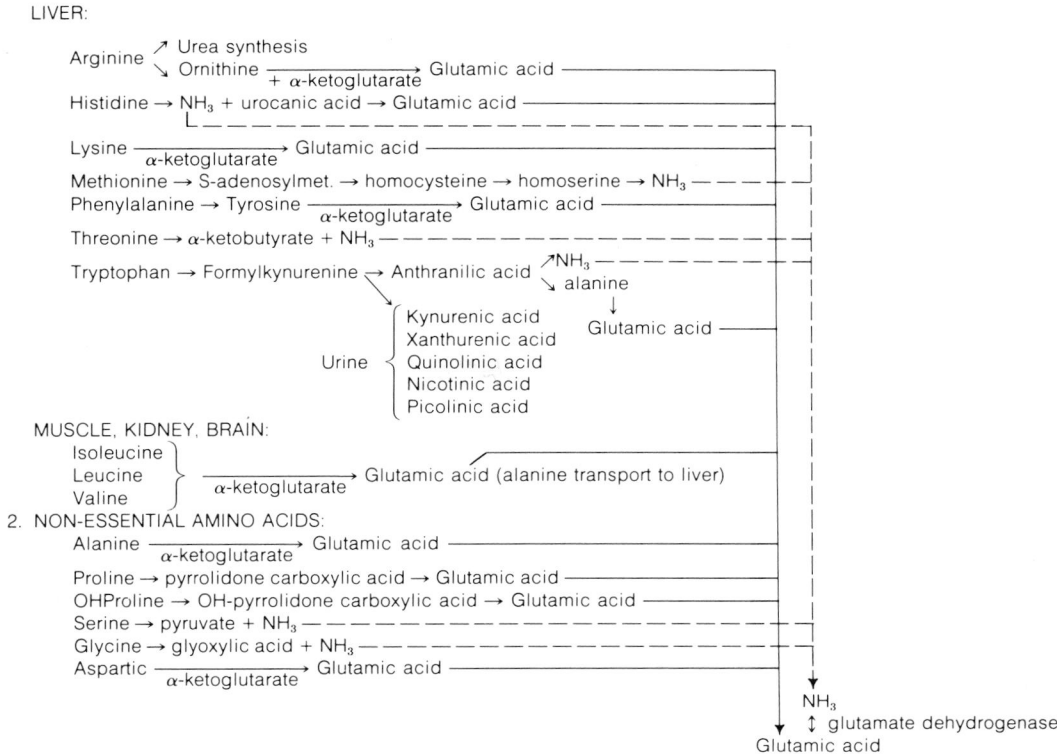

Fig. 3–4. Degradative pathways of amino acid metabolism.

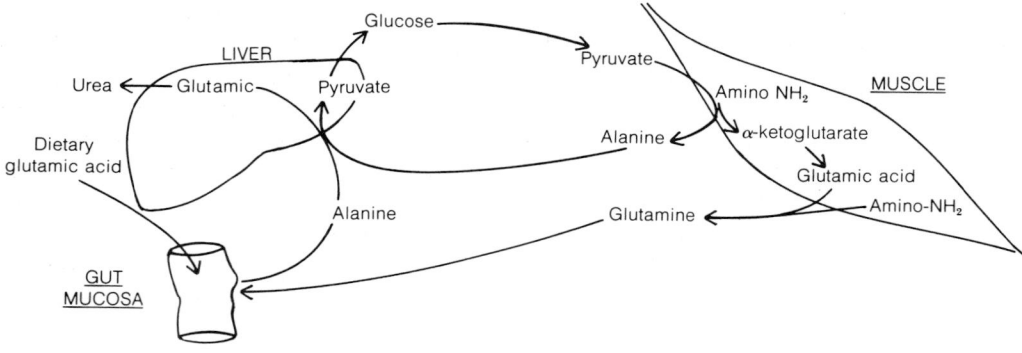

Fig. 3–5. Exchange of nitrogen and carbon between muscle, gut mucosa, and liver.

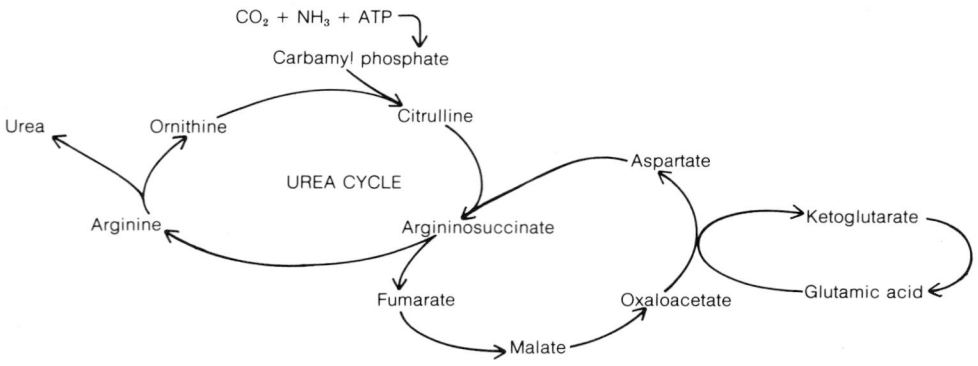

Fig. 3–6. Mechanism of urea synthesis.

transport of amino-N to the liver for urea formation, while the carbon of alanine becomes available for gluconeogenesis.

Urea synthesis is performed in the liver.[30] The process is summarized in Figure 3-6. Ammonia and CO_2 first form carbamyl phosphate. This reacts in turn with ornithine to give citrulline, which then acquires another N from aspartic acid to form argininosuccinate. This splits into arginine and fumarate, the latter going back to the tricarboxylic acid cycle while the arginine is finally split by arginase into urea and ornithine. Ornithine is thus released to participate in another cycle.

Other Pathways Utilizing Amino Acids

Synthesis of Nonessential Amino Acids. The division of amino acids into essential and nonessential was originally made by Rose[31] on the basis of whether they were necessary in the diet for optimal growth of rats. Nonessential amino acids could be deleted from the diet without impairing optimal growth. In the case of adults beyond the stage of growth, it was shown that N balance was impaired by withdrawal of essential amino acids. It has since been shown with isotopic labels that the nonessential amino acids are made from precursors such as glucose whereas

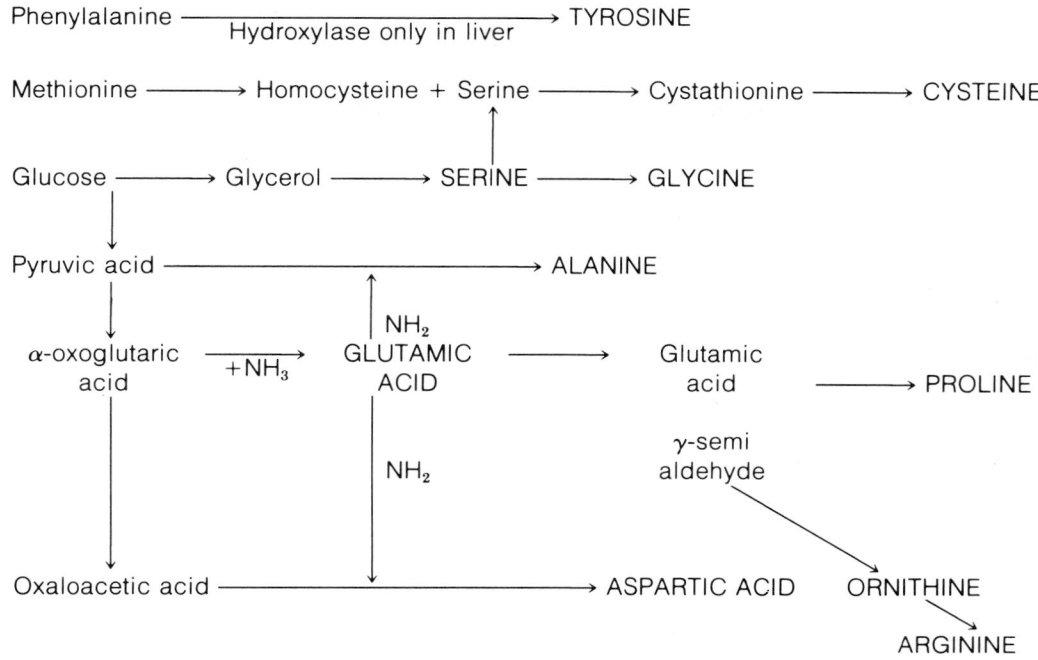

Fig. 3–7. Pathways of synthesis of nonessential amino acid. (From Munro.[2])

the carbon skeletons of the essential amino acids do not take up the labeled precursor.[2] The pathways of synthesis of the nonessential amino acids are well established and are shown in Figure 3–7. These pathways are not always present in all tissues (e.g. tyrosine is formed by hydroxylation of phenylalanine only in the liver) and there can be more than one biosynthetic route (e.g. for serine).

Purine and Pyrimidine Biosynthesis. Purine and pyrimidine bases are synthesized in most cells of the body from simpler carbon and nitrogen precursors.[32] The major reactions are shown in Figures 3–8 and 3–9. These permit the formation of the ribonucleotides of adenine, guanine, uracil and cytosine, which provide high-energy phosphate compounds (di- and triphosphates) in the cell, and also become polymerized to form RNA (see Fig. 3–3). The deoxyribonucleotides found in DNA

are made by reduction of the ribose in the ribonucleotides.

Biosynthesis of purine nucleotides can occur by two routes, namely, de novo and salvage pathways. In de novo synthesis (Fig. 3–8), glycine and phosphoribosylpyrophosphate (PRPP) initially react to form a series of products eventually providing the nucleotide inosine monophosphate (IMP) containing the base hypoxanthine. Adenylic acid (AMP) and guanylic acid (GMP) are then made from this nucleotide by altering substituents on certain carbon atoms of the purine ring (Fig. 3–8). These mononucleotides can be phosphorylated to form the high-energy compounds ADP, ATP, GDP and GTP. They can also undergo degradation to adenosine and adenine or guanosine and guanine. In turn, the free bases adenine and guanine can be deaminated to hypoxanthine and xanthine respectively. Finally, the hypo-

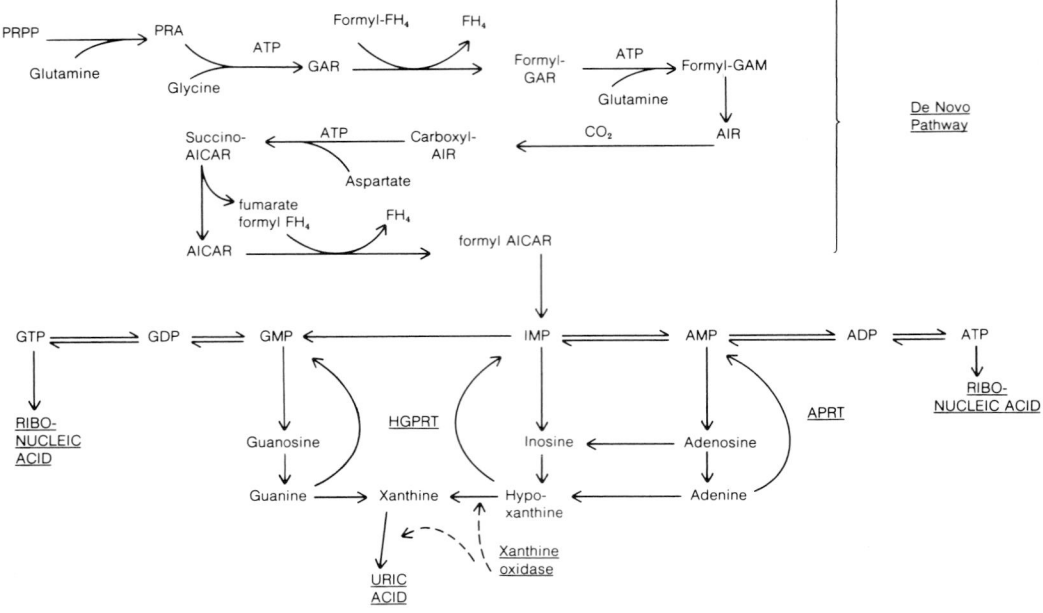

Fig. 3–8. De novo synthesis of purine nucleotides, nucleotide interchange, the salvage pathways and purine degradation routes. *De novo pathway*: PRPP = phosphoribosylpyrophosphate; PRA = phosphoribosylamine; GAR = glycinamide ribonucleotide; formylGAM = N-formylglycinamidine ribonucleotide; AIR = amino-iminazole ribonucleotide; AICAR = amino-iminazole-carboxyamide ribonucleotide. *Nucleotide interchange*: IMP = inosinic acid (hypoxanthine ribonucleotide); AMP = adenylic acid; GMP = guanylic acid. *Salvage pathways*: APRT = adenine phosphoribosyltransferase; HGPRT = hypoxanthine-guanine phosphoribosyltransferase.

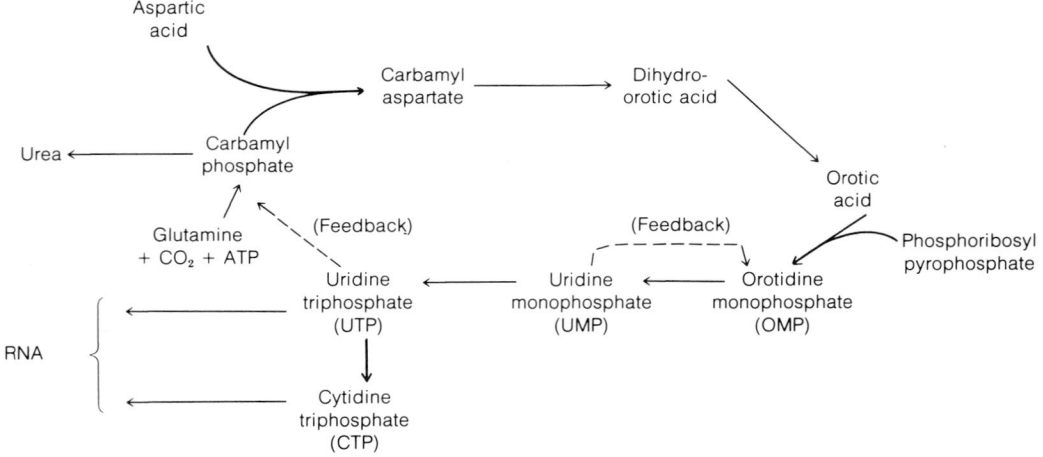

Fig. 3–9. Pyrimidine nucleotide synthesis.

xanthine forms xanthine and the xanthine is irreversibly made into uric acid, the last two reactions being catalyzed by xanthine oxidase.

It will be recognized from Figure 3–8 that de novo synthesis of AMP and GMP requires a considerable number of high-energy phosphate bonds. However, purine nucleotides can also be synthesized by means of the salvage pathways, in which the free purine bases react with phosphoriboxyl pyrophosphate to form the mononucleotides by a route involving only one ATP (Fig. 3–8). Two enzymes, adenine-phosphoribosyl-transferase (APRT) and hypoxanthine-guanine phosphoribosyl-transferase (HGPRT), catalyze the reaction. The latter enzyme is defective in the Lesch-Nyhan syndrome,[33] leading to loss of salvage and consequent increased activity in the de novo pathway to compensate. The failure to salvage guanine leads to excessive formation of uric acid and is thus one cause of gout.

Finally, synthesis of the pyrimidine bases utilizes amino acid N, the initial reaction in the pathway requiring aspartic acid (Fig. 3–9). In addition, the first step in this biosynthetic pathway requires carbamyl phosphate, which is also a substrate for urea synthesis. It has recently been shown[34] that lack of adequate amounts of dietary arginine to prime the urea synthesis cycle can result in diversion of carbamyl phosphate to the pyrimidine biosynthetic pathway. Overload of the latter pathway results in accumulation of orotic acid which is excreted in the urine, thus becoming an indicator of arginine insufficiency.

Creatine and Creatinine. Most of the creatine of the body is found in skeletal muscle where it exists both as creatine and as creatine phosphate. In resting muscle the creatine is present largely in the high-energy phosphate form, whereas in fatigued muscle the concentration of creatine phosphate is insignificant.[34a] This depletion is the result of the biochemical coupling of the conversion of creatine phosphate to creatine with synthesis of ATP, a reversible reaction mediated by the enzyme ATP-creatine transphosphorylase (also known as creatine phosphokinase). This reaction allows the muscle to generate an additional but limited amount of ATP from creatine phosphate under anaerobic conditions.

Creatine is synthesized extramuscularly in a 2-reaction sequence, each step of which is enzymatically mediated. The first is the transamidination reaction between the amino acids arginine and glycine, resulting in the formation of guanidoacetic acid and ornithine. This is followed by the methylation of the guanidoacetic acid by S-adenosyl-methionine to form creatine. The creatine is then transported to the muscle and actively taken up by it. Both creatine phosphate and creatine undergo a nonenzymatic irreversible dehydration to form creatinine, the rate of reaction being twice as fast for creatine phosphate as for creatine. Unlike creatine, creatinine is not bound by muscle but distributes in total body water and is cleared from the body by the kidney. The daily rate of creatinine formation from its creatine precursors is remarkably constant and is estimated to be about 1.7 per cent of the total creatine pool per day.

Recent studies by Crim et al.[35,36] indicate that the body creatine pool can be increased by intake of dietary creatine. This increase in creatine appears to occur without an increase in muscle mass, and thus implies a higher concentration of creatine in muscle. Daily 24-hour urinary creatinine output has been used clinically as a measure of lean body mass. In fact, population studies[36a] have indicated a highly significant correlation between these two parameters. However, since it is clear that the creatine pool in the body of an individual is a composite of dietary intake and synthesis of creatine, this use of urinary creatinine to assess muscle mass is subject to an approximately twofold error related to the variability of muscle creatine concentration, namely from 0.3 to 0.5 per cent.

Clinically, urinary creatinine is also used to estimate the adequacy of a 24-hour collection of urine. On a short-term basis, such as 1 to 2 weeks, this is generally reasonably accurate, since the rate of degradation of creatine to creatinine is so small that large changes in the body pool of creatine would need to occur over a long period before a significant change in the 24-hour output of creatinine would occur. It should, however, be emphasized that this use of creatinine output assumes that, during the collection period, there are no significant sources of dietary *creatinine* since, unlike creatine, it is rapidly excreted in the urine.

Ammonia Synthesis in the Kidney. An important end-product of protein metabolism is urinary ammonia, which increases in amount with acidosis, occurring in conditions such as starvation or uncontrolled diabetes mellitus.[37] Urinary ammonia is derived from plasma glutamine (Fig. 3–10). In the cells of the proximal convoluted tubule of the kidney, glutaminase causes the amide N of glutamine to form ammonia and glutamate; the latter then yields another NH_3, leaving α-ketoglutarate as the other product of the reaction.

This latter is now available for gluconeogenesis, so that in acidosis the kidney becomes a source of glucose in tandem with NH_3 excretion. It has been suggested[39] that the first response to acidosis is the production of glucose by the kidney, to which NH_3 formation is secondary. Ammonia formation allows the body to conserve sodium ion, which would otherwise have to be used to neutralize the acid being excreted. Ammonia formation also permits additional acid secretion through bicarbonate production.

UTILIZATION OF DIETARY PROTEIN: AN INTEGRATED PICTURE

In the preceding section, the pathways of amino acid metabolism were examined individually. Proteins are intimately related to life processes, so that regulation of protein metabolism with its 20 amino acids in an integrated fashion is necessary to maintain bodily function. This concept will now be explored in a description of overall protein metabolism, especially as it responds to intake of a meal.

Digestion and Absorption of Protein

Digestion of the protein of the diet begins with attack by pepsin secreted in the

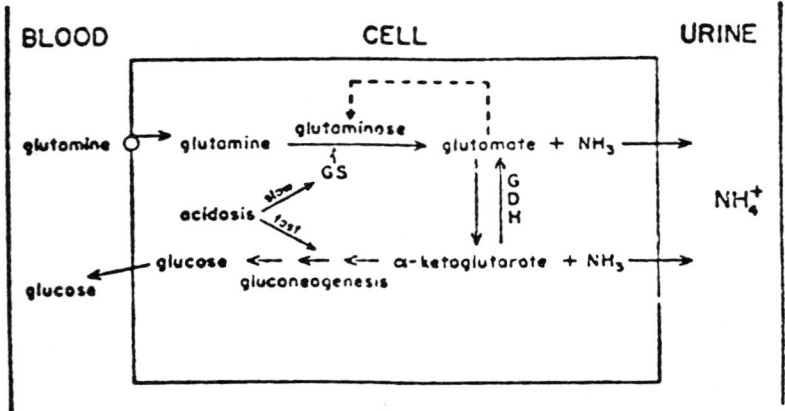

Fig. 3–10. Mechanism for control of ammonia production and gluconeogenesis by the kidney. GS = glutaminase synthesis; GDH = glutamate dehydrogenase. (From Goldstein and Schooler.[38])

gastric juice, followed by proteolytic enzymes from the pancreas and the mucosa of the small intestine.[40] These enzymes are mostly made in precursor (zymogen or proenzyme) form and becomes activated by loss of a small part of their peptide chains through "limited proteolysis." The pancreatic proenzymes become activated on meeting the intestinal juice where enterokinase is present and activates trypsinogen. This is followed by a cascade of activation of the other pancreatic proenzymes, again through selective proteolysis by the active trypsin (Fig. 3–11). Premature activation can occur within the pancreas in association with acute pancreatitis and results in autolysis of the pancreas.

Secretion of proteolytic enzymes by the pancreas appears to be regulated by the presence of dietary protein in the gut contents. In the case of trypsin, it has been shown[42,43] that this enzyme binds to protein in the gut lumen until an excess is present. This excess of free enzyme then operates a feedback regulation system to the pancreatic acinar cells which causes inhibition of synthesis of the precursor trypsinogen (Fig. 3–12). Some plants contain inhibitors of proteolytic enzymes, the best-known being the trypsin inhibitor of the soybean. Feeding of unheated soybean or its trypsin inhibitor to rats results in hypertrophy of the pancreas,[44] presumably because of tenacious binding of the free trypsin and the consequent overstimulation of enzyme formation in the pancreas. This new understanding of control mechanisms in pancreatic secretory activity does not appear as yet to have found an application in cases of acute and recurrent pancreatitis, where the giving of small peptides and free amino acid would be expected to reduce the secretory stimulus caused by whole protein. For example, Lavau et al.[45] have shown experimentally with rats that feeding a meal in which an amino acid mixture replaced casein resulted in a diminution in secretion of trypsinogen.

The events occurring in the course of protein digestion are described in detail by Gitler.[40] Successive proteolytic enzymes attack peptide bonds selected on the basis of

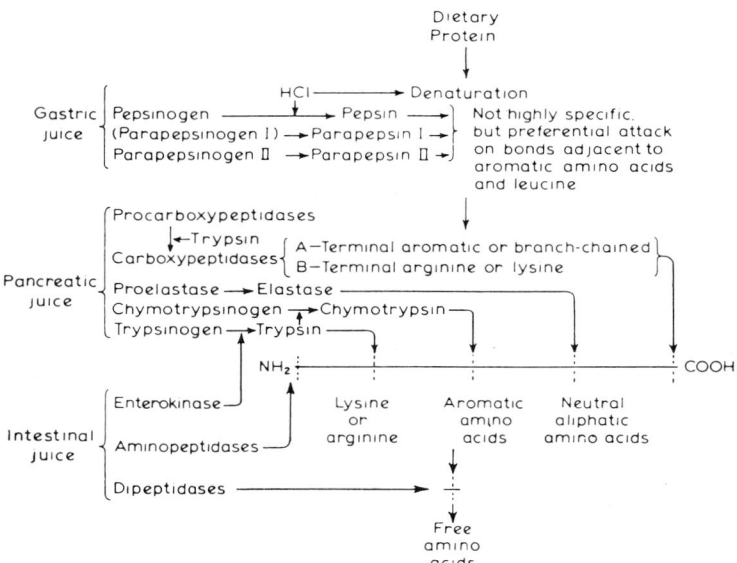

Fig. 3–11. Digestion of protein in the alimentary tract. (From Gitler.[40])

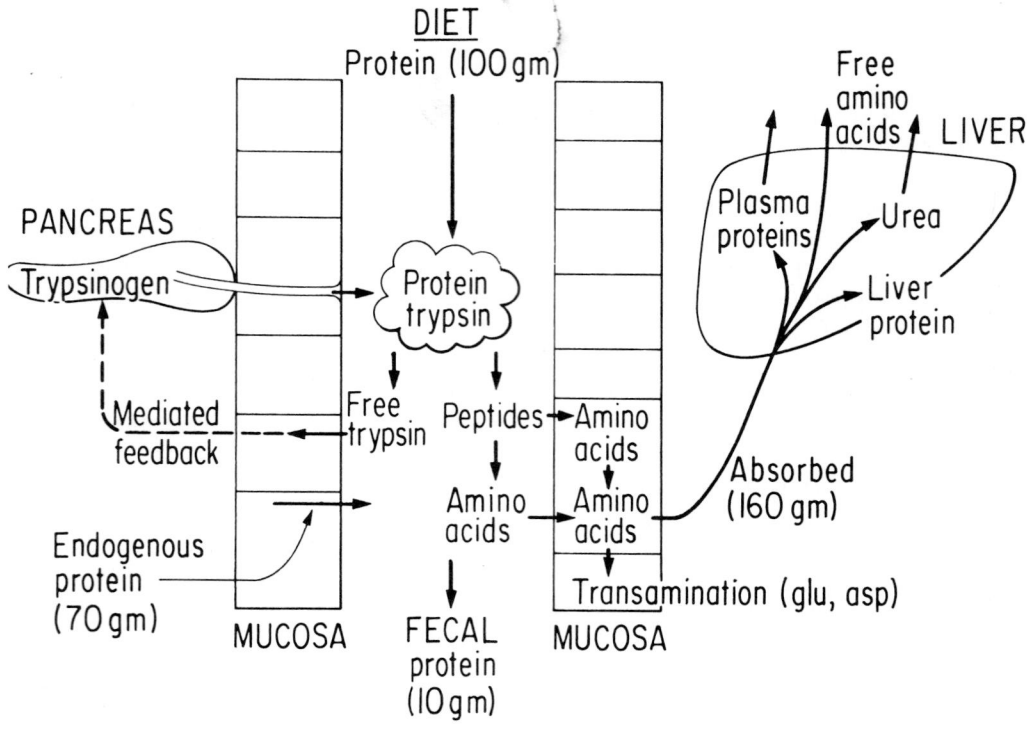

Fig. 3–12. Fate of dietary protein, secretion of endogenous protein, feedback control of pancreatic enzyme secretion and absorption through the mucosa. (From Crim & Munro.[41] Reprinted with permission from the American Medical Association.)

one of the amino acid residues adjacent to the bond (Fig. 3–11). Thus pepsin, which has a relatively low specificity, nevertheless preferentially hydrolyzes bonds adjacent to leucine or the aromatic amino acids, while the enzymes of the pancreatic juice show a greater specificity toward bonds adjacent to lysine or arginine (trypsin), to aromatic amino acids (chymotrypsin) or neutral aliphatic amino acids (elastase). In addition, exopeptidases attack the free ends of the peptide chain. Thus the carboxyl terminal end loses one amino acid at a time through the action of two carboxypeptidases from the pancreas, while the intestinal juice contributes aminopeptidases which perform a similar action at the N terminal end of the peptide.

The end-products of digestion of protein are absorbed through the mucosal cells of the small intestine. Until recently, it was believed that only free amino acids were absorbed. Indeed, some of the protein in the gut lumen is finally hydrolyzed to free amino acids prior to absorption, and numerous studies reviewed by Schultz and Curran[46] confirm that transport of free amino acids into the mucosa involves energy-dependent carriers with some specificity for neutral, basic and acidic classes of amino acids. However, the absorption of small peptides, notably dipeptides, has recently been shown to play a significant role in assimilation of dietary protein.[47,48] Because of the presence of peptide hydrolases in the brush border and cytosol of the mucosal cells, these peptides undergo resolution to free amino acids on entering the mucosal cells, so that only free amino acids pass into the portal vein and to the liver (Fig. 3–12). The transport mechanism for uptake of peptides by mucosal cells differs from the mechanism for free amino acid uptake, notably by absence of competition for absorption between the two. The absorption of peptides is likely to be a major route of amino acid uptake. Thus, although subjects with Hartnup's disease cannot transport free tryptophan into the mucosal cells, they nevertheless grow almost normally,[49] and it must be assumed that their need for the essential amino acid tryptophan is adequately met by its absorption in peptide form. A similar comment can be made about the growth of children with cystinuria, a metabolic defect in which transport of lysine as well as cystine across the intestinal mucosa is defective,[50] yet growth continues.

It is significant to note that the mucosal cells can metabolize some incoming amino acids.[51] A notable pathway is the transamination of glutamic acid to yield alanine (Fig. 3–15). Aspartic acid is also transaminated to alanine by mucosal cells and arginine gives rise to ornithine. The capacity of mucosal cells to transaminate these dicarboxylic amino acids could play an important role in reducing the toxicity of excessive intakes of the acids, which in enormous doses have been shown to cause damage to the hypothalamic regions of the brains of rats and mice[52] but not of primates.[53]

An area of gastrointestinal metabolism now receiving increasing attention is the secretion of protein into the gut. Digestive enzymes represent protein added to the gut contents from endogenous sources, and the epithelial cells of the mucosa are continuously replaced by cell division in the crypts; this is followed by passage of each cohort of cells up the villus and sloughing from the tip of the villus. The extent of endogenous protein secretion is a controversial question. In particular, widely divergent estimates of the contribution of protein from mucosal sloughing have been made. One intermediate estimate is that 70 gm of protein (17 gm present in secreted juices and 50 gm as sloughed mucosal cells) are added to the intestinal contents daily.[54] When added to the 100 gm of protein consumed by the average person eating a western type of diet, this gives a total of 170 gm in the gut lumen available for absorption (Fig. 3–12). Fecal nitrogen output is equivalent to about 10 gm protein daily, so that the efficiency of digestion and absorption of both dietary and endogenous protein must be high. This turnover of protein in the gut wall is sensitive to dietary change. Protein deficiency[55] and starvation[56] both reduce the rate of cell division in the mucosa, without altering cell size or composition.[55] These observations can be correlated with evidence on rats that protein deficiency leads to reduced secretion of endogenous protein into the gut.[57]

Role of the Liver

The absorbed amino acids pass to the liver by way of the portal vein. After a meal of protein, there are changes in the amount and pattern of amino acids in the portal vein, but a less dramatic increase in amino acids levels in the general circulation. This occurs because the liver is the main or only site of catabolism for 7 of the essential amino acids, the remaining 3, the branched-chain amino acids, being degraded mainly in muscle and kidney.[58] The liver monitors the absorbed amino acids and adjusts the rate of their metabolism according to bodily needs. Using dogs fed excessive amounts of meat, Elwyn[58] has shown that much of this incoming amino acid load is immediately degraded to urea, a small proportion is temporarily retained as liver protein presumably mostly as additional enzyme protein, another small portion is secreted as plasma protein, while only about a quarter of the absorbed amino acids pass into the general circulation (Fig. 3–13).

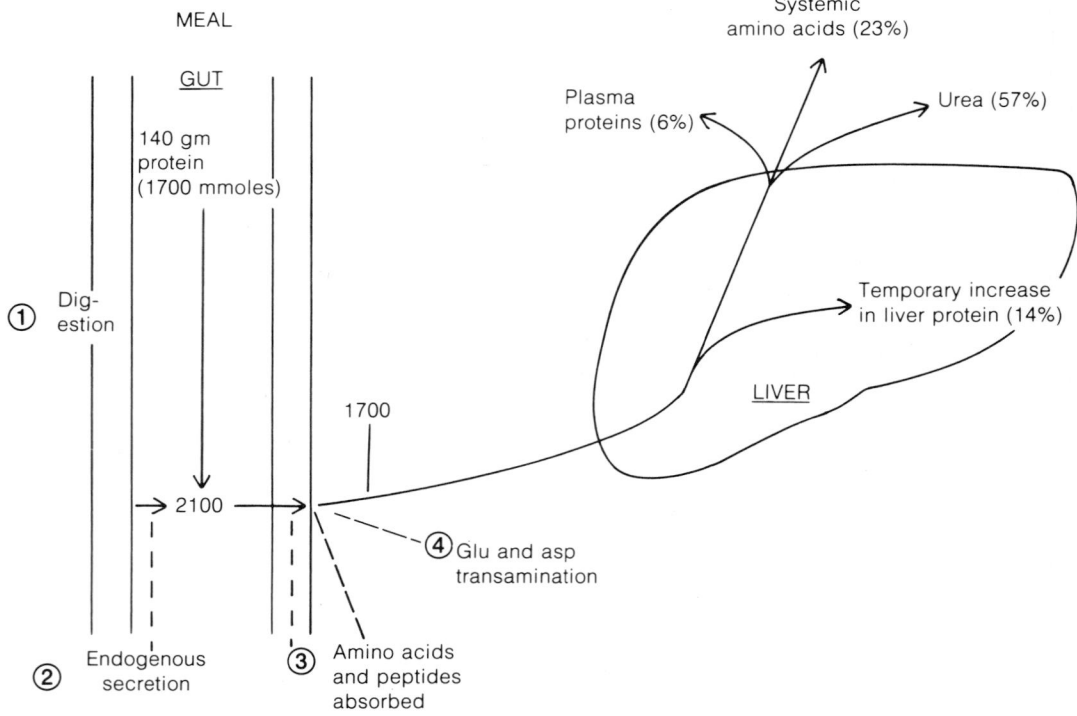

Fig. 3–13. Fate of a meal of meat fed to a dog: role of liver in monitoring incoming amino acids. The data are based on Elwyn's studies.[58]

The process of monitoring of amino acid intake by the liver regulates the amounts of individual essential amino acids available to the body from the diet. When the dietary intake of an essential amino acid is progressively increased, induction of liver enzyme activity usually occurs when intake exceeds requirement. This induction (e.g. threonine dehydratase in Figure 3–14) often shows a sudden increase at levels of intake beyond the needs of the body, indicating that the liver accurately monitors intake in relation to the needs of the body and destroys only essential amino acids extensively above that critical level in the diet. In the case of nonessential amino acids, the levels of enzymes (e.g. glutamic aminotransferase) responsible for their metabolism do not show this inflection but increase progressively with rising intake

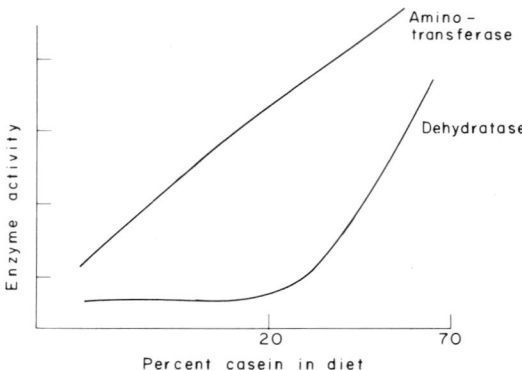

Fig. 3–14. Effect on liver enzymes of increasing the protein content of a diet fed to growing rats. The upper line shows the response of a liver enzyme metabolizing a nonessential amino acid (glutamic acid), while the lower line indicates the response of an enzyme for degradation of an essential amino acid (threonine). (Data from Harper.[59])

(Fig. 3–14). This conservation of essential amino acids is indicated also by studies in which different amounts of lysine were given to young growing rats.[60] At an intake of 100 mg of lysine, gain in body weight was maximal. At intakes beyond 100 mg daily, ^{14}C-carbon dioxide production from injected ^{14}C-lysine showed a rapid increase, indicating that the intake which gave maximal growth corresponded to the point at which the liver began to destroy excess lysine. In rats, the plasma levels of lysine show a response curve similar to that seen with CO_2 production,[61] the level of lysine rising steeply when there is more lysine in the diet than is necessary for maximal growth. This suggests that increases in the peripheral blood levels of essential amino acids provide the signal for enzyme induction in the liver.

Finally, synthesis by the liver of degradative enzymes of amino acid metabolism and probably of other proteins is reflected in increased aggregation of polyribosomes during the absorptive period after a meal containing protein. In the case of the rat, this gives rise to diurnal variations in polyribosome aggregation related to the time of food intake.[62] There is also reduced breakdown of these proteins,[63] presumably resulting from stabilization by their substrates derived from the incoming amino acids. Thus we find that degradative enzymes such as tyrosine aminotransferase[62] and tryptophan pyrrolase[64] show diurnal variations related to meal consumption. In addition, other metabolic events in the liver cell are subject to diurnal variations related to protein intake from the diet. Synthesis of RNA accelerates while RNA breakdown decreases.[65] This latter leads to changes in purine nucleotide pools and there is consequent stimulation of de novo purine biosynthesis after meals containing protein.[66] A scheme coordinating these various metabolic responses with changes in amino acid supply has been presented elsewhere.[67] Some secreted proteins, such as albumin,[68] do not appear to

undergo diurnal rhythms in synthesis in normal animals, but their rate of synthesis increases when protein is given to protein-depleted animals.[69] Elsewhere, it has been suggested[67] that synthesis of albumin by the normal animal is regulated in relation to the plasma level, and responds to protein intake in the depleted animal because the serum albumin level has fallen below this critical control level and is now regulated in relation to amino acid supply. Some secreted proteins, such as the α_{2u}-globulin (molecular weight 20,000) made by the liver of the mature male rat and excreted in the urine, show diurnal responses to protein intake even in well-nourished animals.[70]

Regulation of Blood Amino Acid Levels

As indicated above, the liver monitors the passage of amino acids into the peripheral circulation. However, this process does not completely eliminate excess amino acids beyond what the peripheral tissues are able to use or metabolize. Consequently, plasma levels of many essential amino acids increase when dietary supply exceeds the requirements of the tissues, as previously discussed for lysine. In some cases this increase in the level of an essential amino acid in the peripheral blood occurs quite abruptly when requirement is exceeded. For example, we[71] examined the influence of the age of the rat on the response of its plasma tryptophan concentration to different levels of dietary tryptophan (Fig. 3–15). The rats used were either weanlings or mature adults. As the amount of tryptophan in the diet was increased from less than adequate to more than sufficient for maximal growth, the tryptophan content of the plasma rose sharply beyond the point of requirement at each age. For the rapidly growing weanlings, the point of inflection was 0.1 per cent tryptophan in the diet, above which growth was not stimulated and plasma tryptophan started to rise. For the mature rats, 0.03 per cent dietary tryptophan was

just sufficient to satisfy weight maintenance and above this level plasma tryptophan concentration rose. The findings
are thus interesting in showing that the
method is sensitive to age-related changes
in requirements. This method has been
used to determine the requirements of
human subjects for essential amino acids,
and indeed the point of inflection of tryptophan (3 mg per kg body weight) agrees
with the amount required for N balance of
young adults.[72] However, other essential

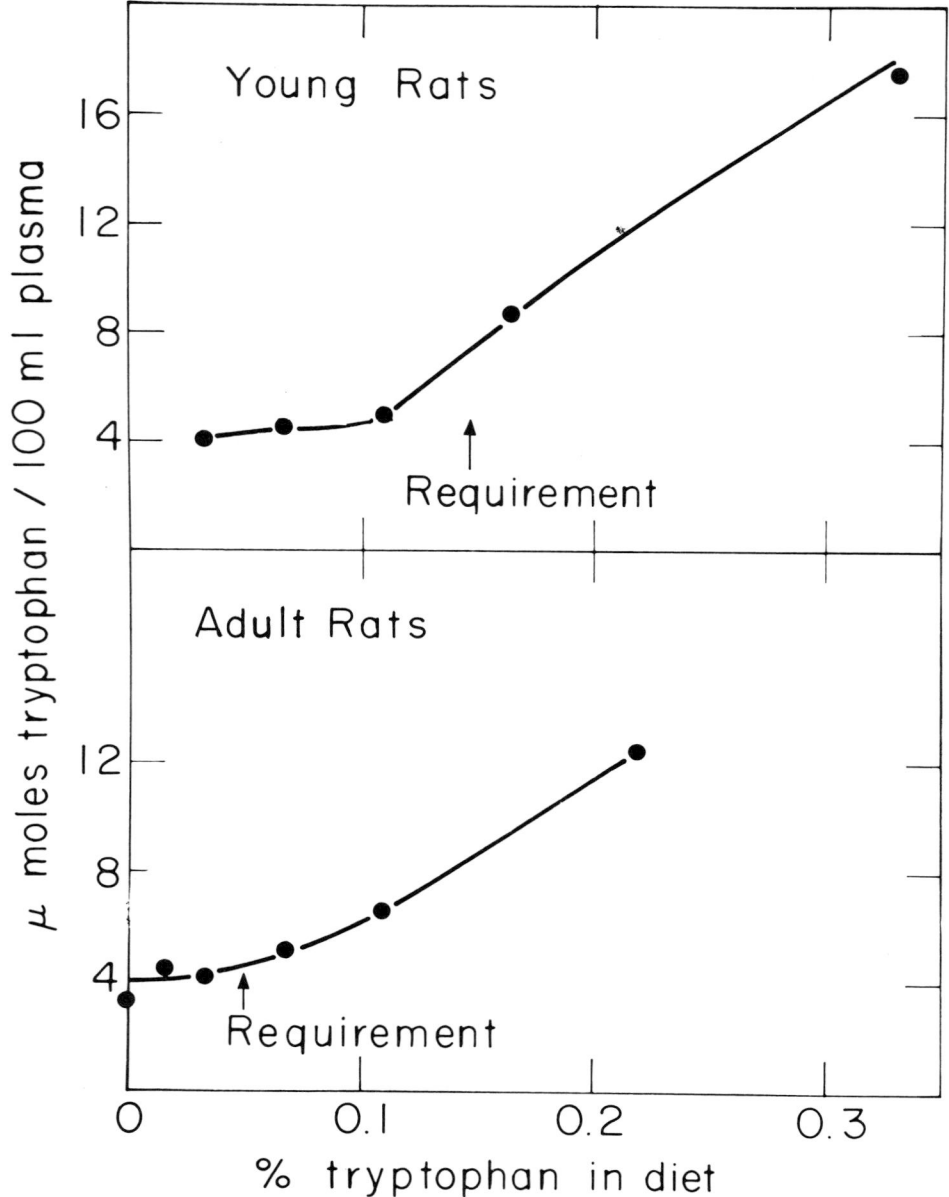

Fig. 3–15.   Plasma levels of young and mature rats fed diets containing various levels of tryptophan in an otherwise adequate diet. (Adapted from Young and Munro.[71])

amino acids such as lysine have given less clear-cut points of inflection and there has also been some dispute about the use of the inflection as a measure of optimal requirements.[73]

The plasma levels of amino acids are also affected by dietary carbohydrate through a mechanism involving insulin secretion. Shortly after consuming carbohydrate, the concentrations of most plasma amino acids decrease because of deposition in muscle through insulin-mediated transport[74] (Fig. 3-16). The effect is maximal for branched-chain amino acids, which can fall as much as 40 per cent after a dose of glucose, whereas some amino acids (e.g. tryptophan) are affected only minimally.[75] The same mechanism is also the basis of a metabolic interaction between dietary protein or amino acids and carbohydrate consumed in the same meal.[74]

The alterations in plasma-free amino acid patterns caused by the protein and carbohydrate components of a meal have significance for the availability of amino acids to the peripheral tissues. In particular, it has been shown that the free tryptophan content of the brain of the rat can be elevated by tryptophan administration, and that this maneuver increases the serotonin content of the brain.[76] Entry of tryptophan into the cells of the brain is also determined by the plasma levels of other competing neutral amino acids, notably the branched-chain amino acids.[77] Following a meal of carbohydrate, the extensive reduction in plasma levels of branched-chain amino acids results in greater passage of tryptophan into the brain and more serotonin is synthesized.

This mechanism is not only significant in regulating serotonin metabolism, it is also critical to brain function under pathologic conditions. As shown in Figure 3-17, the loss of normal liver function associated with hepatic cirrhosis results in a series of metabolic alterations relating to protein metabolism.[78] Amines and ammonia formed by bacterial action in the gut are no longer trapped by the liver but pass freely into the systemic blood and thence to the brain cells. For example, bacterial action produces phenethylamine from phenylalanine; this is transformed to octopamine in the brain where it serves as a false neurotransmitter competing with the catecholamines. Amino acids with metabolism normally regulated in the liver (e.g. tryptophan and phenylalanine) are no longer subject to control, so that their plasma levels rise and are more available to the brain. Finally, the liver normally inactivates a large part of the insulin. In individuals with cirrhosis this no longer occurs and plasma insulin levels rise. This enhances transport of branched-chain amino acids into muscle, resulting in the low plasma levels of branched-chain amino acids observed in cases of cirrhosis. This reduction in the plasma levels of the branched-chain amino acids allows a larger proportion of the already elevated tryptophan content of the plasma to pass into the brain. Excessive levels of serotonin are generated and contribute to hepatic coma. This concept of the role of excess serotonin formation in hepatic coma has received some confirmation from studies showing reversal of the comatose state following administration of branched-chain amino

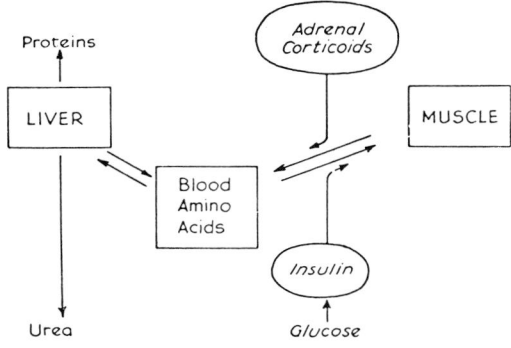

Fig. 3–16. Scheme showing the action of dietary carbohydrate on levels of blood amino acids. Adrenocortical hormones have the opposite action. (From Munro.[74])

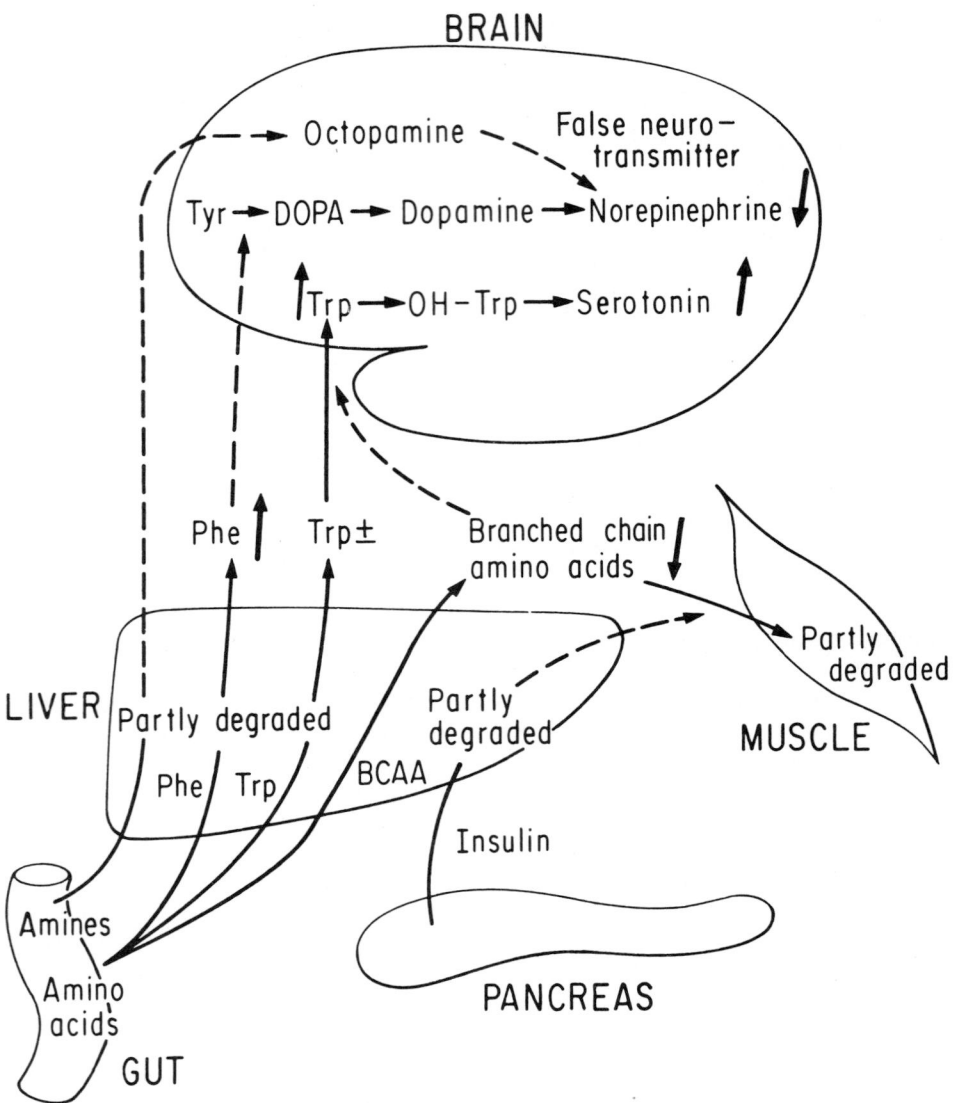

Fig. 3–17. Role of branched-chain amino acids in hepatic coma. Owing to unrestricted passage of insulin into the general circulation in hepatic cirrhosis, branched-chain amino acids are removed excessively by muscle. In consequence of this lowering of plasma branched-chain amino acids, there is less competition with tryptophan and phenylalanine for entry into the brain and thus more serotonin and less norepinephrine are made. (From Crim and Munro.[41] Reprinted with permission from the American Medical Association.)

acids to laboratory animals and patients with hepatic coma.[79]

Role of Skeletal Muscle in Protein Metabolism

Skeletal muscle is the largest tissue in the body.[2] Consequently, metabolism of amino acids in this tissue is of considerable significance for general protein metabolism. Muscle is also the main site of metabolism of the branched-chain amino acids (leucine, isoleucine, and valine). As described above, muscle is a major target for the action of insulin, which promotes entry of amino acids (especially the branched-chain amino acids). Insulin also promotes synthesis of muscle protein and reduces muscle protein breakdown. Corticosteroids have opposite effects (Fig. 3–16).

The effects of hormones and of nutrient intake on muscle protein metabolism have been examined by a variety of techniques, including use of radioactive amino acids. In man two main procedures have been used, namely, measurement of the differences in amino acid levels of blood entering and leaving muscle (arteriovenous differences) and measurement of 3-methylhistidine as a urinary compound proportional to the rate of myofibrillar protein breakdown. The measurement of uptake and release of amino acids indicates that fasting human subjects release large amounts of alanine and glutamine into the blood (Fig. 3–5), equivalent to a loss of 75 gm of protein daily from the muscles of a 70-kg man.[80] The alanine is formed by transamination between pyruvate derived from glucose and amino groups transferred from amino acids present in muscle. In consequence alanine becomes a carrier of nitrogen from muscle to liver, where its carbon skeleton enters the gluconeogenic pathway while its amino group is converted into urea. The other carrier of nitrogen from muscle is glutamine, formed when glutamic acid accepts nitrogen as its amide group (Fig. 3–5). This glutamine passes to the intestine where the amino group is transaminated to alanine which now goes to the liver. By means of these reactions, muscle has a special mechanism which allows transport of nitrogen and carbon to the liver. Following gluconeogenesis in the liver, some of the carbon comes back to muscle as glucose, giving the glucose-alanine cycle between liver and muscle. Measurement of the arteriovenous differences across the forearm have demonstrated that, if insulin or carbohydrate is administered, the output of alanine diminishes, and after a meal is completely reversed so that muscle actually gains protein; thus fluctuations in the A-V loss occur throughout the day.[81] This mechanism implies that, from the body mass of muscle (45 per cent of body weight on the average), a considerable amount of carbon is available for metabolism during fasting or other emergency.

Interpretation of arteriovenous difference data is difficult, however, because of amino acid recycling within the muscle cell. For example, the diminution of arteriovenous difference after insulin administration[80] could be the result of retardation of muscle protein breakdown or increased synthesis of protein through the known stimulant action of insulin on muscle protein synthesis. In order to monitor muscle protein breakdown without reutilization, 3-methylhistidine output in urine has been exploited. Methylation of histidine in actin and myosin occurs only after these proteins have been synthesized in muscle. When the protein of the myofibril is eventually catabolized, 3-methylhistidine is not reused but is excreted quantitatively in the urine and thus provides an index of muscle protein breakdown (Fig. 3–18). Several lines of evidence confirm that 3-methylhistidine in fact fulfills this purpose. First, tRNA and its charging enzymes were prepared from rat muscle and shown not to charge with 3-methylhistidine.[83] This implies that it is not recycled for muscle protein synthesis. Second, analysis of various major tissues and organs of the

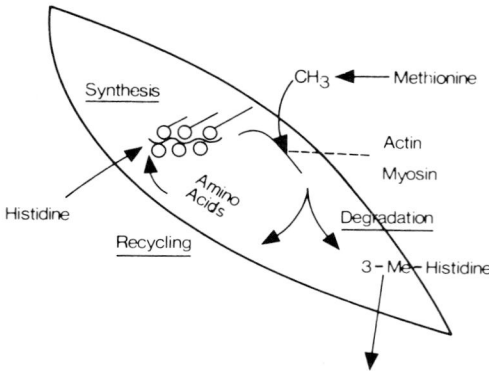

Fig. 3–18. Synthesis of 3-methylhistidine in muscle actin and myosin, and its release and quantitative excretion in the urine following breakdown of these muscle proteins. (From Munro.[82])

rat for their content of 3-methylhistidine shows that skeletal muscle is the overwhelming reservoir of this methylhistidine in the body. Third, by administering [14]CH[3]-labeled 3-methylhistidine to rats[83] and to human subjects[84] it was shown that essentially all was excreted in the urine over a short period.

The output of 3-methylhistidine has been used to study dietary effects on muscle protein breakdown rate. Changes in methylhistidine excretion have been examined in young growing rats receiving either a normal diet or diets deficient in either protein alone or protein and calories.[85] Protein depletion caused a rapid reduction in output of 3-methylhistidine, which declined steadily to 20 per cent of initial output, while on repletion output again rose. In the case of protein-calorie deficiency, however, an initial rise was followed by a gradual fall in 3-methylhistidine output. Thus muscle responds to protein depletion by shutting off breakdown. However, with semistarvation, breakdown at first increases and then diminishes. In similar fashion malnourished children in India showed a low output of methylhistidine for weight, which rose during repletion.[86] We[87] have also observed that grossly obese subjects undergo-

ing prolonged fasting show a progressive reduction in 3-methylhistidine output.

Finally, 3-methylhistidine output is affected by age and by hormonal status. In the newborn, output per kg body weight is higher than in the mature adult, and declines further in old age.[88] Unpublished data of Munro and Young show that output is increased by thyroxine secretion within the normal range of thyroid activity but by corticosterone only at plasma levels of this hormone equivalent to severe stress.

Integration of Body Protein Metabolism

From the preceding information, a composite picture of the daily flux of amino acids in various compartments of the body of an adult man can be assembled; these estimates for a 70-kg man are shown in Figure 3–19. The customary daily protein intake in western countries is about 100 gm, augmented by addition of an estimated 70 gm of protein secreted into the gastrointestinal tract; consequently, the total load for absorption is estimated to be 170 gm protein. Experiments involving ^{15}N suggest that some 300 gm of protein are synthesized daily in the body of the adult.[54] The difference between the intake of 100 gm protein and the daily turnover of 300 gm indicates the

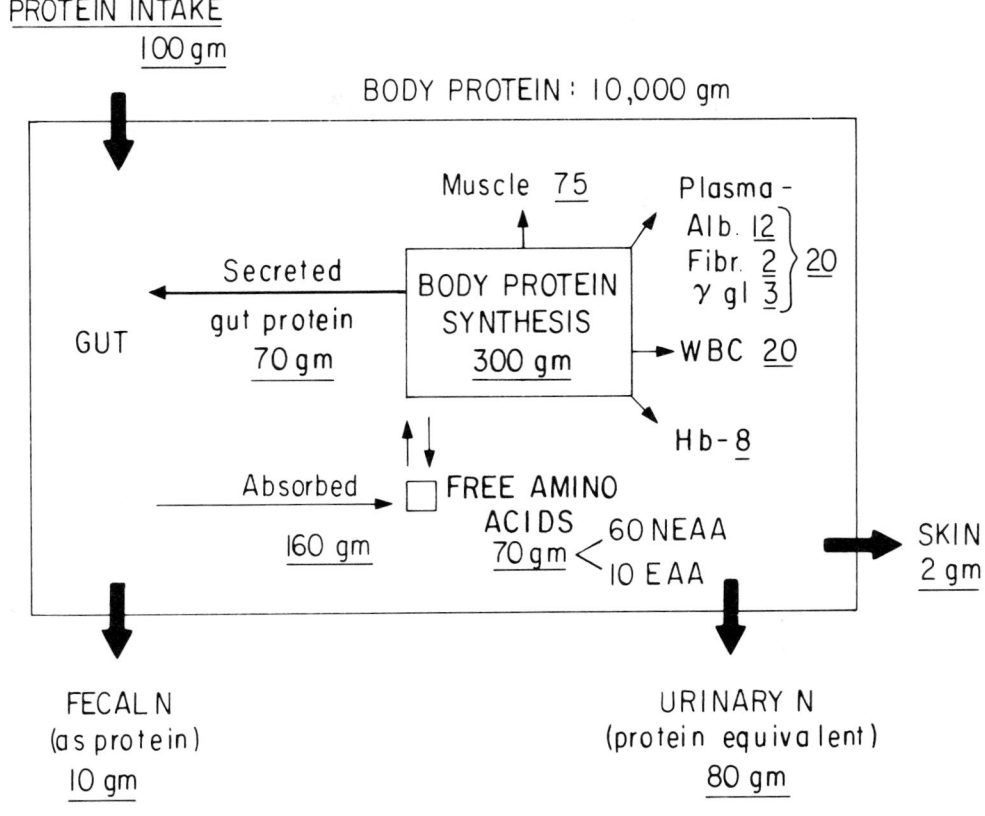

Fig. 3–19. Daily intake and turnover of protein by a 70-kg man. (From Munro.[89])

extensive reutilization of amino acids involved in protein metabolism. Some major components in this daily protein turnover are identified: gut, muscle, plasma proteins, white blood cells, hemoglobin. Note that the free amino acid pool of the body, estimated at 70 gm, is primarily made up of nonessential amino acids, as shown earlier for the rat (Table 3–1).

Metabolic Body Size and Protein Metabolism

It has long been known that among mammals intensity of energy metabolism decreases as mature body size increases. This applies as a general principle to metabolism and affects the relative sizes of some organs intimately concerned with

metabolic regulation, such as the liver.[2] Table 3–2 is based on regression analysis of data from a wide range of mammals of varying mature size. It shows the results as organ weights or metabolic components per kg body weight for animals weighing 200 gm (rat) and 70 kg (man), as predicted by these regression analyses. The proportion of skeletal muscle is constant at 45 per cent of body weight, blood and heart weight are also of the same weight per kg body weight, but liver and kidney, two organs intimately concerned with metabolism of food, are relatively smaller in man than in the rat. The endocrine organs (pituitary, adrenal and thyroid glands) are also smaller. In addition, most metabolic parameters (basal energy

Table 3–2.   The Influence of Body Size on the Relative Weights of Individual Organs and on Several Parameters of Metabolism*

Measurement	Amount of Metabolic or Body Component per kg of Body Weight		
	At 200 gm (rat)	At 70 kg (man)	Ratio $\frac{rat}{man}$
Organ sizes:			
Skeletal muscle weight (gm)	450	450	1.0
Blood weight (gm)	52	48	1.1
Heart weight (gm)	6.0	5.5	1.1
Liver weight (gm)	41	19	2.1
Kidney weight (gm)	9.4	3.8	2.5
Pituitary weight (mg)	360	80	4.5
Adrenal weight (mg)	380	120	3.2
Thyroid weight (mg)	150	90	1.7
Metabolic Parameters:			
Basal energy metabolism (kcal/day)	108	23	4.7
Endogenous urinary N (mg N/day)	230	45	5.1
Threonine requirement (mg/day)	28	7	4.2
Methionine requirement (mg/day)	56	16	3.5
Total body protein synthesis (mg N/day)	1010	218	4.6
Creatinine in urine (mg N/day)	14	8	1.8
Total body albumin (gm)	4.0	4.6	0.9
Albumin turnover (days^{-1})	0.24	0.04	6.0
Ceruloplasmin turnover (days^{-1})	0.49	0.11	4.4

*Data abstracted from Munro.[2]

metabolism, endogenous urinary N output, requirements for the essential amino acids, total body protein synthesis and turnover of albumin and ceruloplasmin) are about five times more intense per kg body weight in the rat than in man. However, the daily excretion of creatinine per kg body weight is less affected by body size of the species, reflecting its relationship to the amount of muscle in the bodies of rat and man.

Nitrogen Excretion and Nitrogen Balance

The end-products of nitrogen metabolism within the body are excreted in the urine (Fig. 3–2), while unabsorbed protein coming from the diet or protein secreted into the lumen of the intestines is voided in the feces. In addition, some nitrogenous materials are lost from the skin as both soluble N (e.g. urea) and as shed epithelials cells. Finally minor routes of N loss are represented by nasal secretions, hair cuttings, menstrual fluid and semen.

The major N compounds in the urine are urea, ammonia, uric acid and creatinine. These respond differently to changes in protein intake (Table 3–3). On a diet of normal protein content, urea accounts for more than 80 per cent of urinary N, but this proportion falls when a diet low in protein is consumed. During fasting, the absolute amount and percentage of ammonia N rise in response to the acidosis. On the other hand, creatinine output tends to be independent of diet since it reflects the pool of creatine in muscle when a creatine-free diet is taken.

The overall metabolism of protein in the body can be summarized by nitrogen bal-

Table 3-3. Partition of Urinary N Output Under Different Nutritional Conditions by Adult Human Subjects*

	High-protein Diet	Low-protein Diet	During Fasting Day 1	During Fasting Day 2
Urinary N Source	Total daily output (gm N)			
Total N	16.80	3.60	10.51	8.77
Urea N	14.70	2.20	8.96	6.62
Ammonia N	0.49	0.42	0.40	1.05
Uric acid N	0.18	0.09	0.12	0.17
Creatinine N	0.58	0.60	0.44	0.39
Undetermined N	0.85	0.27	0.59	0.54
	Percentage of total N output			
Urea N	87.5	61.7	85.1	75.4
Ammonia N	3.0	11.3	3.8	12.0
Uric acid N	1.1	2.5	1.1	1.9
Creatinine N	3.6	17.2	4.2	4.4
Undetermined N	4.9	7.3	5.6	6.1

*From Allison and Bird.[90]

ance. This represents the difference between N intake and N output, the difference being either positive (N retention, as in active growth), negative (N loss) or zero (N equilibrium). The determination of N balance (B) thus requires a careful estimate of intake (I) and of all routes of N loss, namely urine (U), feces (F) and dermal losses (S):

$$B = I - (U + F + S)$$

Thus the balance is obtained by a usually small difference (10 to 15 per cent) between two larger numbers and is thus subject to the combined errors of these estimates. Furthermore, Wallace[91] has pointed out that N intake tends to be overestimated through unconsumed diet while output tends to be underestimated because of losses. There is thus a built-in bias toward a positive balance. In addition, it is unusual to make direct measurements of dermal losses, the custom being to accept a constant (estimated) correction for dermal N, or to ignore this N loss. The contribution of such dermal N losses is discussed in the next section.

Nitrogen balance is also affected by energy intake.[74] Not only does N balance become progressively more negative as energy intake is reduced below the needs of the body but it becomes more favorable when energy intake is increased above the subject's requirements for energy. There is accordingly a continuous relationship between energy intake and N balance from negative at low-energy levels to positive at excessive intakes of energy, as shown by the upper line of Figure 3-20. The lower line in this diagram shows the consequence of limiting the amount of protein in the diet. Restriction of dietary protein prevents further improvement in N balance beyond a certain point. Note that the difference between the two lines results from increase in protein intake. The conclusions to be drawn from this figure are that N balance is the result of both protein intake and energy intake and that studies of factors affecting N balance, such as dietary protein, must be carried out under conditions where the subject's energy intake is carefully defined in relation to his requirements.

Finally, N balance is influenced by hor-

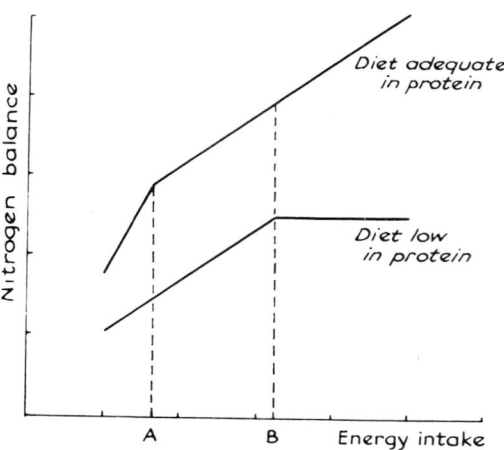

Fig. 3–20. Diagram showing the relationship of N balance and energy intake on diets of different protein content. *Upper line*: Diet adequate in protein; *lower line*: diet deficient in protein. An increase in energy intake evokes an improvement in N balance at both levels of protein intake, but at the lower protein intake increments in energy intake are not effective beyond point B. (From Munro.[74])

mones.[74] These can be divided into anabolic (growth hormone, testosterone) and catabolic (corticosteroids, thyroxine). These hormones are especially effective on protein metabolism in muscle. Because skeletal muscle is such a large tissue, anabolic and catabolic changes in muscle tend to determine alterations in N balance. This can obscure effects of these hormones on protein metabolism in other tissues, such as liver.[74]

REQUIREMENTS OF MAN FOR PROTEIN AND AMINO ACIDS

Unlike that of molecular biology, our knowledge of nutritional principles continues to pursue a slow evolution.[92] In the field of protein requirements, a major advance was achieved in 1946 by Block and Mitchell[93] who showed that various biologic measures of the quality of dietary proteins could be correlated with their content of essential amino acids expressed as a "chemical score," i.e. the concentration

of the essential amino acid in least abundance relative to requirements. The emphasis on essential amino acids as an explanation for the need for dietary protein was further underlined in the period 1950 to 1960 by a series of quantitative estimates of human requirements for individual amino acids. The protein and amino acid requirements of man have been frequently reviewed and recommendations have been made in the publications of expert committees of the World Health Organization and of the Food and Agricultural Organization[94-96] and also in recommended dietary allowances for the United States.[97] The requirement for protein and the requirement for individual essential amino acids will initially be considered separately.

Protein Needs and Allowances

The requirement for protein in the diet can be estimated in two ways. One is to measure all losses of nitrogenous compounds from the body when the diet is devoid of protein and then assume that sufficient nitrogen from high-quality dietary protein to replace these obligatory nitrogen losses will provide the adult human subject with his requirement. This is the so-called factorial method, since it is based on adding up a series of factors that represent obligatory nitrogen losses from the body. Enough protein to replace these should meet requirements. The second procedure for estimating protein requirements is to determine directly the minimum amount of dietary protein needed to keep the subject in nitrogen equilibrium. Ideally, the two methods should arrive at similar estimates of protein requirements. For infants and children, optimal growth and not nitrogen equilibrium is the criterion used, and the special needs in pregnancy and lactation are also considered separately.

The factorial method of measuring dietary protein needs depends on adding all the losses of organic nitrogen by a subject on a nitrogen-free diet. Two major ques-

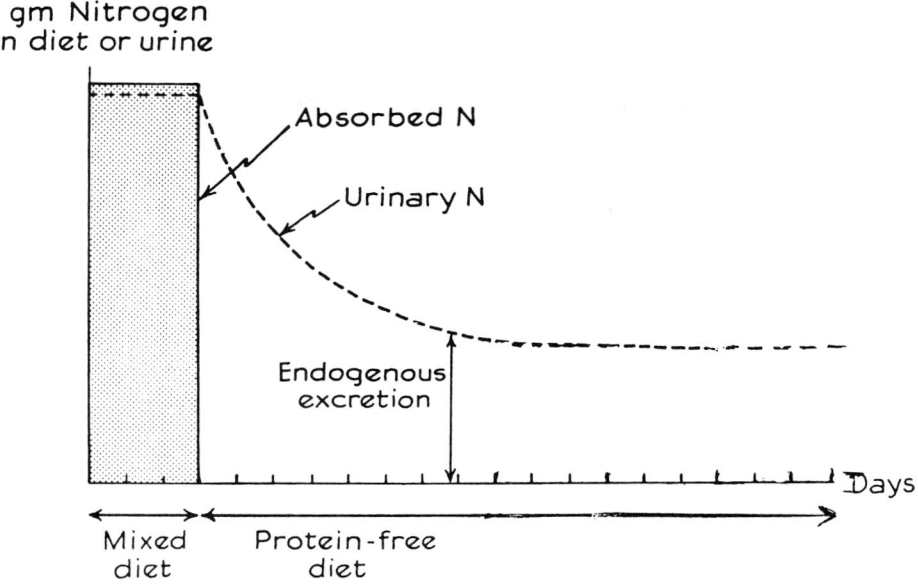

Fig. 3–21.   Effect of a protein-free diet on urinary N output.

tions thus arise: What are the routes of obligatory nitrogen loss, and what is the magnitude of N loss by each channel under these basal conditions on a protein-free diet? A survey of all such experiments has been assembled by Irwin and Hegsted.[98] When a protein-free diet is fed to a human subject or to an animal such as a rat, there is a rapid decrease in urinary N output for a few days, followed by a plateau (Fig. 3–21). Based on two sets of studies,[99,100] this minimum output has been estimated to be 37 mg N per kg body weight. Even on a diet without protein, there is also a loss of N in the feces, representing enzymes and desquamated intestinal cells that have not been fully digested and reabsorbed. This obligatory fecal N output of adults is about 12 mg N per kg body weight. Organic nitrogen is also lost from the skin in the form of desquamated cells, hair and nail clippings and sweat. On the basis of recent direct studies of skin losses conducted under rigorous collection conditions involving minimal sweating,[101] the cutaneous N loss by adult men eating a normal diet in a temperate environment is about 5 mg per kg body weight; this decreases to 3 mg when a protein-free diet is consumed.

In addition to these major routes of N loss, there are a series of minor routes of N excretion, such as ammonia in the breath, nasal secretions, menstrual flow in the female and seminal fluid in the male.[101] For all these minor routes, an estimate of 2 mg N per kg body weight for men and 3 mg N per kg for women approximates the average daily loss.

The factorial approach predicts that protein requirements are the amounts needed in the diet to replace obligatory losses of nitrogen. Table 3–4 shows that the sum of urinary, fecal, cutaneous and minor routes of N loss is 54 mg N per kg body weight. These estimates of obligatory N loss can be expressed as amounts of body protein that have to be replaced daily from dietary sources, using the conversion factor of N × 6.25 to give the weight of protein. Thus, the obligatory N losses would represent a net daily loss of 0.34 gm

Table 3–4. Obligatory Nitrogen Losses by Adult Men on Protein-Free Diets and the Equivalent Loss of Body Protein

	Daily N Loss (mg/kg b wt)	Equivalent Amount of Protein (gm/kg b wt)
Obligatory Losses:		
Urine	37	0.23
Feces	12	0.08
Cutaneous	3	0.02
Minor Routes	2	0.01
Total (Mean)	54	0.34
2 S.D. above mean*	70	0.45
Amount of whole egg protein needed for equilibrium†		0.59

*Additional 30 per cent to cover upper level of individual requirements extending 2 S.D. above the mean.
†Loss of efficiency 30 per cent.

of body protein per kg body weight, if not replaced from the diet. By this method the daily protein requirement of the average adult would be 0.34 gm per kg of a dietary protein that is fully utilized. The data of Scrimshaw et al.[99] and of Calloway et al.[100] show a coefficient of variation of 15 per cent for the obligatory N losses in the urine and feces. Consequently, Table 3–4 also includes a value reflecting the addition of 30 per cent (twice the coefficient of variation of 15 per cent) to cover the range of individual losses for 97.5 per cent of the population. The upper limit of the amount of body protein to be replaced thus becomes 0.45 gm per kg body weight.

It should be possible to test these predictions by feeding different amounts of protein and finding the minimum amount needed to restore N equilibrium. This approach suffers from some general defects. As mentioned above, N balance studies tend to overestimate true protein intake and underestimate N output, thus leading to a more positive apparent balance than really exists.[91] A second problem is that, in calculating N balance, an allowance has to be made for cutaneous and other minor routes of N excretion that are usually not measured. Corrections for these depend on the same published observations as those used in the factorial computations.

Several authors have added different levels of protein to a protein-free diet and have measured the improvement in N balance. In general, addition of increasing amounts of high-quality protein such as whole egg protein[100] has produced a nonlinear response (Fig. 3–22). At lower intakes, the improvement in N balance is proportional to the amount of protein added to the diet, but as intake is further increased the efficiency of utilization falls off so that the amount needed to achieve N equilibrium (i.e. output = intake) is much greater than predicted from the earlier part of the curve. This loss of efficiency as equilibrium is approached has been estimated to add 30 per cent to the amount of whole egg protein needed for N equilibrium and therefore the requirement for dietary protein is increased by this percentage, namely, from 0.45 to 0.59 gm protein per kg body weight (Table 3–4). If the protein of the diet is used less efficiently than egg protein, the amount needed to replace body protein will be correspondingly increased. Thus if the average dietary protein has only 75 per cent of the biologic quality of egg protein, the requirement should be increased to 0.8 gm per kg body weight (0.59 × 100/75), that is, 56 gm protein daily are needed to meet the requirements of a 70-kg man.

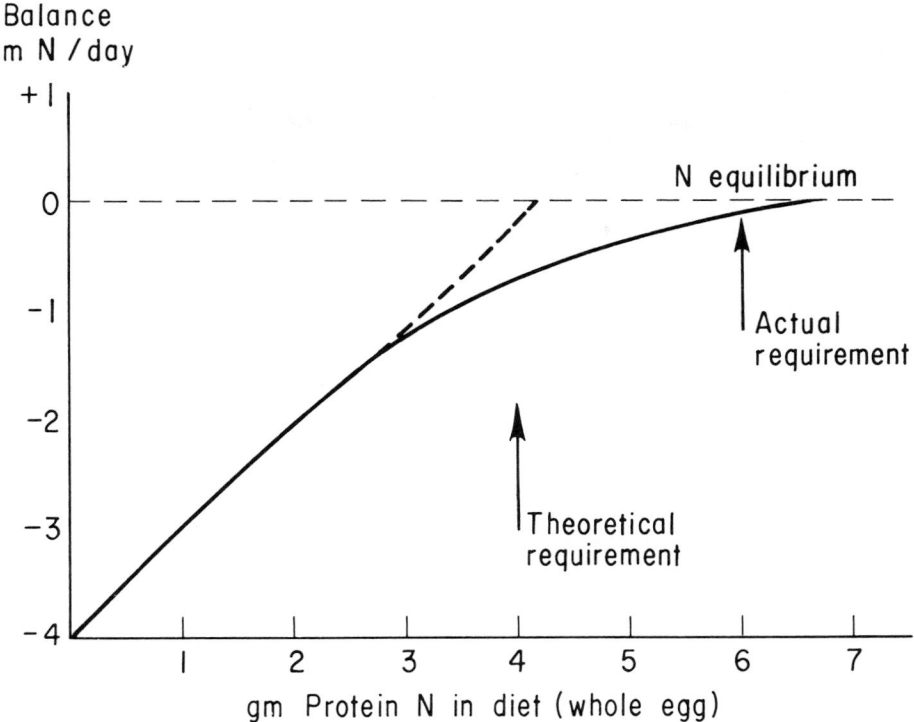

Fig. 3–22. Response of N balance to increasing amounts of whole egg protein added to a protein-free diet.

These conclusions are less secure than such precise calculations would lead one to believe. Nitrogen balance is influenced by energy intake.[74] In the past not enough attention has been given to ensuring energy equilibrium during N balance experiments; in general, there has been a tendency to increase energy intake beyond requirements in order to prevent weight losses on low-protein diets. This confounds the N balance data by improving N retention from the surfeit of calories (see later). This has been well illustrated by Inoue,[102] who showed that the apparent requirement of young men for protein could be altered significantly by changing energy intake. At an intake of energy just sufficient for maintenance (45 cal per kg), the average requirement of egg protein for N equilibrium was 0.65 gm per kg body weight, whereas, at a higher energy intake (57 cal per kg), the requirement fell to 0.45 gm per kg. Similarly, the requirement for rice protein as the sole dietary protein changed from 0.87 gm per kg at the lower caloric intake to 0.58 gm per kg at the higher level of energy. Furthermore, it has been found that the use of a correction factor of 30 per cent for loss of efficiency of utilization of egg protein (Fig. 3–22) may not describe the reduction in utilization of other proteins such as wheat gluten. Finally, it has been found by Garza et al.[103] that 0.57 gm egg protein per kg body weight per day is insufficent to maintain the N balance of young adult men receiving adequate but not excessive energy intakes. At this level of intake serum levels of certain liver enzymes (e.g. transaminases) rose, an effect that disappeared when protein intake was increased. In a more recent study, Garza et al.[104] found that addition of nonessential amino acids to increase protein intake from 0.57 to 0.8 gm per kg allowed young adults to achieve N equilibrium, thus pointing to a major requirement for more nonspecific nitrogen by the adult. This conclusion will also emerge in later comments on the essential amino requirements of adults.

The needs of other age groups for protein have also been explored to various extents. During its first year, the infant increases in weight by about 7 kg. The daily increment in body protein over this period is about 3.3 gm. The estimates of daily protein requirements of infants are based on the amount of milk protein needed to sustain maximal growth, namely, 2.4 gm per kg during the first months declining to 1.5 gm per kg by six months. After the first year, requirements are less well established but are believed to fall progressively from 1.1 gm per kg at 1 year of age to the adult level of 0.8 gm per kg.

During pregnancy, about 1 kg of protein is deposited in the fetus and the maternal body, much of it during the later stages of pregnancy.[97] To meet this need, it is recommended that the pregnant woman should receive an additional 30 gm of protein daily from the second month of gestation onward, i.e. a total of 1.3 gm protein per kg body weight.[97] For a pregnant adolescent, the level of dietary protein should be raised to 1.5 to 1.7 gm per kg to allow the mother's body to grow. During lactation, an additional 20 gm of protein should be added to the diet to offset the secretion of protein in the milk.

Studies of the protein requirements of elderly men and women[105,105a] show that the needs per unit of body weight are similar to those of young adults both regarding output on a protein-free diet[105] and amount of dietary protein needed to achieve N equilibrium.[105a]

Factors Influencing Protein Requirements

While severe psychologic stress has been found to increase N output,[106] the ordinary stresses of living are allowed for in the estimates of protein allowances. Although high environmental temperatures cause excessive N loss through sweat, this is eventually compensated for by a reduction in urinary N output. Heavy work is also not thought to be a significant factor in protein requirements. However, athletes in training may temporarily need more protein during the period of increase in muscle mass.[107] The effect of the energy content of the diet on protein utilization has been well established and the necessity for ensuring an adequate but not surfeit calorie level during determinations of protein needs has already been emphasized.

Essential Amino Acids and Their Needs by Man

For adult man, the essential amino acids are isoleucine, leucine, lysine, methionine, phenylalanine, threonine, tryptophan and valine. Infants also require histidine and small amounts are probably needed by adults. Our ideas on the amino acid needs of adults are based primarily on N balance studies, whereas requirements for infants and children are predicated on the least amounts compatible with maximal growth. Irwin and Hegsted[108] have reviewed all studies of human amino acid needs published before 1971. The conditions used for assaying amino acid requirements are discussed elsewhere in detail.[108a] Published estimates obtained by nitrogen balance measurements show a wide range of estimated needs even within a single study.

In order to extract useful figures from this literature, the middle of the range of values obtained by Rose and his colleagues has been accepted for men on the grounds that requirements for all of the essential amino acids were studied by a single investigator under constant conditions. These

Table 3–5. Essential Amino Acid (EAA) Requirements in mg/kg Body Weight of Human Subjects of Various Ages*

Requirement	Infant (Holt)	Child, 10–12 yr. (Nakagawa)	Adult Man (Rose)	Adult Man (Inoue)	Adult Woman (Hegsted)
Histidine	(25)	—	—	—	—
Isoleucine	111	28	10	11	10
Leucine	153	49	11	14	13
Lysine	96	59	9	12	10
Met. & Cys.	50	27	14	11	13
Phe. & Tyr.	90	27	14	14	13
Threonine	66	34	6	6	7
Tryptophan	19	4	3	3	3
Valine	95	33	14	14	11
Total EAA (excl. histidine)	680	261	81	87	80

*Adapted from Munro.[108a]

midrange values are shown in Table 3–5 expressed per kg body weight for adult men. They agree closely with data on Japanese men obtained by Inoue et al.,[109] who examined the requirement for each amino acid by plotting N balances at several levels of intake and interpolating to zero balance. They also agree with the requirements of women for essential amino acids per kg body weight estimated by Hegsted[110] from regression equations obtained by recalculating all available published data on women. It should be noted that these are *average* needs; in order to compare them with the allowances for protein, it would be necessary to increase the estimates by 30 per cent in order to cover all but the top 2.5 per cent of the population according to normal distribution. Even so, this adjustment would be based on the assumption that the variability of needs for individual essential amino acids follows that of protein.

Regarding amino acid requirements of infants and children, Table 3–5 gives the estimates by Holt and Snyderman[111] of the essential requirements of infants up to 6 months of age growing maximally. Although the data were expressed as ranges,

we have taken the midpoint of the range of values as the average need. Values of the same order have been obtained by Fomon and Filer[112] from amino acid intakes of infants growing optimally on milk-formula diets. The requirements of older children (10 to 12 years of age) have been estimated by Nakagawa et al.[113]

When expressed per kg body weight, the needs for protein and for each essential amino acid decline progressively with increasing age from infancy (Fig. 3–23). However, the requirements for essential amino acids decrease much more extensively than do those for total protein. Consequently, the proportion of total protein needs represented by essential amino acids falls from 43 per cent in the case of infants to 36 per cent for older children and to 19 to 20 per cent for adults. On the basis of this information, it should be possible to dilute egg and other good-quality protein having an overabundance of essential amino acids with nonessential amino acids or with ammonium salts and still maintain N equilibrium. Indeed, various authors[114,115] were able to achieve N equilibrium with adult subjects receiving only 13 to 15 per cent of dietary N in the form of

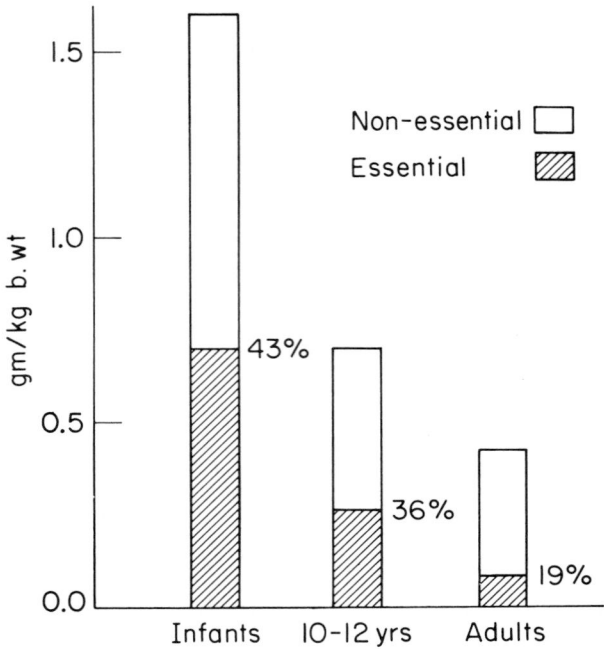

Fig. 3–23. Average requirement for protein and for the sum of eight essential amino acids at 6 months, 10 to 12 years and in adulthood. (From Munro.[108a])

essential amino acids. Similarly, Scrimshaw and co-workers[116] have been able to replace a small part of the nitrogen of egg, beef and milk with nonessential nitrogen from glycine and diammonium citrate without impairing nutritive value. At a level of 0.4 gm protein per kg body weight, N equilibrium could be maintained with dilution of these proteins up to 25 to 30 per cent. The source of nonessential nitrogen may also be important. In contrast to the above positive findings, Daniel et al.[117] found that replacement of milk protein with nonessential nitrogen significantly reduces the biologic value of the protein for 10- to 11-year-old girls, suggesting that their essential amino acid needs are proportionately higher than those of adults. Finally, Snyderman et al.[118] observed that nonessential nitrogen added to cow's milk protein to the extent of about 20 per cent stimulated the growth of young infants. The published data on dilution studies are

thus too variable to indicate whether proteins can be diluted to a greater extent for adult use than for feeding infants.

Protein and Essential Amino Acid Needs in Disease

There are two difficulties in deciding on protein requirements in disease: (1) Individual diseases affect protein needs to different extents and (2) each disease process varies in intensity. Some tentative estimates of protein needs in a variety of major diseases are shown in Table 3–6. In a number of these conditions (fever, fracture, burns and surgical trauma), body protein is lost extensively during the acute phase of the disease and should be regained during convalescence. Hence, we have two problems, the nutritional requirements during the acute phase and the requirements during recovery. Opinion about the desirability of high protein and energy intakes during the height of the

Table 3–6. Protein Requirements in Specific Diseases*

Normal adult
    For N equilibrium: 0.55 gm/kg, raised to 0.8 gm/kg by protein quality correction.
    Customary intake: 1–2 gm/kg.

Metabolic response to severe injury and burning
    Acute phase: 2–4 gm/kg. + increased calories
    Convalescence: 2+ gm/kg.

Malabsorption and gastrointestinal diseases
    Malabsorption syndrome: 1 gm/kg.
    Ulcerative colitis: 1–1.4 gm/kg.†
    Ileocecostomy: 1–1.4 gm/kg.†

Liver disease
    Acute hepatic encephalopathy: very low.‡
    Recovered encephalopathy: 1–1.5 gm/kg.
    Chronic encephalopathy: 0.5 gm/kg.‡

Renal disease
    Uremia: 0.5 gm/kg‡ (? ketoanalogs)
    Nephrosis: 1–1.4 gm/kg.†

Malignant disease
    Increased protein and energy

*From Munro.[119]
†In each condition, losses of protein can double minimal requirement.
‡Intake restricted on clinical grounds.

metabolic response to a severe injury or illness varies. The loss of protein during such illnesses can be appreciable.[120] For example, simple disuse atrophy during bed rest can cause a loss of 0.3 kg body protein. To this can be added 0.4 kg body protein after a gastrectomy, 0.7 kg after fracture of a femur and 1.2 kg after a 35 per cent burn. There is no division of opinion about the need to replace such losses during convalescence. There is evidence from studies on depleted adult rats[121] that during repletion the needs for essential amino acids increase two- to threefold those for maintenance of the adult. The repleting adult animal has the requirements of the growing rat. This is reflected in the recommendation of an essential amino acid pattern for the protein-depleted patient based on that of the rapidly growing child.[122]

In some diseases, protein intake must be restricted, e.g. acute liver failure, where intake has to be restricted in order to avoid hepatic coma, and in uremia, in which capacity to excrete nitrogenous end-products is limited. The problem is to provide sufficient protein to avoid depletion of tissue protein without exceeding the capacity of the patient to deal with the amino acid load. Thus, in the dietary management of uremia, there is clinical evidence[123] that an intake of 0.5 gm protein per kg body weight allows the patient to resist intercurrent infections better than the earlier recommendation of 0.25 gm per kg. In order to reduce the amount of N to be excreted by uremic patients, there have been recent attempts[124] to use nitrogen-free analogs of essential amino acids ("keto-analogs") to provide some of the dietary amino acid supply. Finally, there is evidence that wasting (cachexia) associated with the anorexia of malignant disease reduces the capacity of the patient to withstand vigorous treatment. Nutritional rehabilitation allows the cancer patient to better withstand surgery, chemotherapy and radiation therapy[125] (Chapter 38). In judging the effectiveness of nutritional support, a useful observation is that many patients with cancer cachexia have lost the normal responses of cellular immunity. Responsiveness can often be restored by vigorous nutritional rehabilitation, and becomes an index of the repletion of the depleted body.

Assessment of Protein Depletion and Repletion

Specific criteria of protein depletion and repletion are under continuing exploration. Various indices have been suggested.[41] Loss of weight and other general signs have long been in use, but more specific signs are less satisfactory. The plasma essential-to-nonessential amino acid ratio declines in protein deficiency but this responds too readily to transient alterations in intake, and thus does not represent the degree of depletion. Plasma albumin level does not decline until there is significant depletion. Plasma enzymes mainly indicate liver damage and have fallen into disuse. As indicated above, the competence of antibody-forming processes is of growing importance in indicating depletion and repletion. Leukocyte metabolism undergoes changes in malnutrition but these are technically difficult to establish. Finally, changes in methylhistidine excretion may be helpful, as our rat studies[85] suggest. In addition, changes in

plasma hormone levels occur in protein-calorie malnutrition.[126] As Table 3–7 shows, there are increments in growth hormone levels in kwashiorkor (protein deficiency) but not in marasmus (protein-calorie deficiency). A reduction in somatomedin level has been noted in kwashiorkor and might also prove to be a useful index of changes in the liver in response to diet. A reduction in plasma insulin level might also be helpful. Cortisol is elevated in marasmus but not usually in kwashiorkor, whereas thyroid-stimulating hormone is a sensitive index of calorie deficiency. These alterations occur under extreme conditions of dietary deficiency; however, patterns of endocrine change deserve more attention in less severe malnutrition.

DIETARY SOURCES OF PROTEIN AND AMINO ACIDS

In performing nitrogen balance studies and similar nutritional experiments using normal diets, it is usually assumed that almost all dietary nitrogen takes the form of protein, so that dietary N × 6.25 is accepted as a reasonable approximation of the amount of protein in the diet. This practice is based on two assumptions, first that almost all the N in the diet is protein, and second that the factor 6.25 represents the ratio of total weight to N for most proteins and protein mixtures. These propositions will now be examined.

Table 3–7. Protein-Energy Malnutrition and Endocrine Function*

Hormone	Kwashiorkor (Protein deficiency)	Marasmus (protein-calorie deficiency)
Growth hormone	Elevated	Sometimes raised
Somatomedin	Reduced	—
Insulin	Reduced	Normal
Cortisol	No change	Often elevated
TSH	No change	Much reduced
Thyroxine	Reduced (protein carrier less)	Normal or raised

*From Munro.[127]

Forms of Dietary Nitrogen

Natural foods consist mostly of the tissues of plants and animals, so that the diet will reflect tissue constituents. Analysis of animal tissues such as liver and muscle confirms that indeed almost all the N is present in the form of protein with only a small amount (1 to 2 per cent) as free amino acids or peptides, and an equally small amount as nucleic acids and phospholipid N,[128] and, in the case of muscle, as creatine and the dipeptides carnosine and anserine. However the muscle of fishes is richer in nonprotein N (20 per cent or more), and contains a greater variety of N compounds.[129] Similarly, about 20 per cent of the N in human milk is nonprotein N, most of which is *not* free amino acids (e.g. urea).[130]

In plant tissues, the proportion of nonprotein N is very variable. Seeds contain mostly (95 per cent) protein N. In roots, such as the potato and carrot, less than half the total N is protein,[131] most of the N being present in the form of peptides and free amino acids with glutamine and asparagine especially abundant in the potato.[132] In addition, plant tissues contain an abundance of amino acids that do not occur in proteins. Over 100 such have been identified, some of which can be metabolized in the animal body whereas many are excreted unchanged in the urine, and a few (e.g. hypoglycin A in the fruit of the West Indian Blighia and cyanoalanine in the grain of the East Indian Lathyrus) produce serious toxic effects. In addition, new protein sources, such as single-cell protein, can contain high levels of purine nitrogen.[133]

In view of these findings, it is reasonable to accept the assumption that the N of western mixed diets is essentially protein in nature. However, in the case of some root crops such as cassava, the N content seriously overestimates the true protein content as obtained by hydrolysis followed by analysis of individual amino acids.[134]

The use of the conversion factor N × 6.25 also requires comment. This implies that the average protein contains 16 per cent N. However, Jones[135] has shown that the proteins of individual foods can vary from 15.7 per cent N in the case of milk to 19 per cent in the case of nuts. The use of varying conversion factors from N to protein has in fact been employed in calculating the protein content of foods assembled in some tables of food composition.[136]

The Protein Content of Foods and Diets

The protein content of foodstuffs is usually expressed per 100 gm of the food. As Table 3–8 shows, this varies from 0.5 to 40 per cent or more in some processed foods (e.g. dehydrated egg). However, the value of a foodstuff as a protein source also depends on its energy content, since the caloric needs of the individual determine the amount of food he will consume. Thus, an adult man with a daily protein allowance of 56 gm (244 kcal) and a daily energy requirement of 2,800 kcal would require about 8 per cent of his energy intake in the form of dietary protein of average quality to provide for his protein needs. Table 3–8 therefore also expresses the protein content of foodstuffs as the percentage of calories of the food provided by protein. Any food with less than 8 per cent kcal as protein is presumably inadequate to assure the protein needs of a population if it is the only protein source. Thus some major tropical foods, cassava, plantain and yam flour, all have a low protein content combined with a high content of starch and thus fall below the required percentage of protein calories. On the other hand, Irish potatoes also are low in protein content per 100 gm but have much less starch, so that their protein content per 100 kcal is much more favorable.

In practice, diets in most parts of the world provide 9 to 14 per cent of the calories as protein,[92] and average total intakes range from 50 to 100 gm protein daily. Table 3–9 shows that in 1972 the estimated average intake per head of the

U.S. population was 101 gm, of which more than two-thirds was in the form of animal protein. This average protein intake has not changed much over the 65 years that records of food consumption have been kept by the Department of Agriculture. However, the source of protein has varied considerably during this period; around 1910, half the protein came from vegetable sources.[139] The shift since then has been brought about by a progressive increase in consumption of beef and poultry and a reduction in that of cereals and potatoes.[140] It will also be noted in this table

Table 3–8. Protein Content of Some Foods*

| | Protein | |
| | gm per 100 gm of food | kcal per 100 kcal. of food |
Foodstuff		
Cassava flour	1.5	1.8
Plantain	1.0	3.1
Sweet potato	1.5	5.3
Irish potato	2.0	10.7
Yam flour	3.5	4.4
Milk	3.3	20.6
Rice	7.0	8.0
Maize meal	9.5	10.5
Wheat flour (70% extraction)	10.0	11.4
Eggs	13.0	33.0
Pork, medium fat	14.9	13.9
Beef, medium fat	17.5	27.4
Fish, nonfatty	17.0	93.0
Lean beef	19.0	37.6
Kidney beans	24.0	27.3
Dried eggs	47.0	33.9

*From Platt[136a] and Albanese.[136b]

Table 3–9. Average Daily Consumption of Protein and Essential Amino Acids in the United States Compared with the Estimated Allowances for a 70-kg Adult

Dietary Constituent	U.S. Intake* (gm/day)	Adult Allowance† (gm/day)
Protein	101	56
Animal	71	—
Vegetable	30	—
Essential amino acids		
Isoleucine	5.3	0.7
Leucine	8.2	1.0
Lysine	6.7	0.8
Methionine	2.1	0.9
Phenylalanine	4.7	1.0
Threonine	4.1	0.5
Tryptophan	1.2	0.25
Valine	5.7	0.7

*Mean protein intake in U.S. in 1972 taken from Clark.[137] Mean amino acid intakes in U.S. computed by Consumer and Food Economics Research Division, ARS, USDA, 1970.[138]
†From WHO/FAO Report on Energy and Protein Requirements.[96]

that the protein sources of the average U.S. diet provide an abundance of essential amino acids in comparison with the estimated needs of an adult for these amino acids.

Evaluation of Protein Quality

In a preceding section it was pointed out that proteins differ in their capacity to provide amino acids for utilization in the body. These differences in protein quality are important in computing the amount of protein needed to meet the needs of people, as illustrated in an earlier section. It is therefore important to have reliable procedures for such measures of protein quality. This field has recently been surveyed in a publication[141] which can be consulted for details. Basically, the evaluation of a protein source begins with nitrogen and amino acid analysis and proceeds to biologic tests. Thus we have to consider first the evidence obtained from amino acid analysis and then from evaluation based on biologic assays.

In 1946, Block and Mitchell[93] introduced the concept of assessing the nutritional quality of a protein on the basis of its constituent amino acids. They pointed out that all amino acids must be provided simultaneously at the sites of protein synthesis in the body and that intracellular deficits of any one could result in limitation of the rate of protein synthesis. Accordingly, they proposed that the biologic value of a dietary protein would be determined by the essential amino acid present in least concentration relative to the needs of the animal or human. This is therefore the "most limiting amino acid" from which a "chemical score" of protein quality could be calculated.

In practice, a protein with an ideal amino acid pattern is first established so that it provides all essential amino acids in optimal concentrations to meet requirements when it is fed at adequate levels. Then the concentrations of essential amino acids in 1 gm of the dietary protein source are expressed as percentages of the amounts of each essential amino acid in 1 gm of the ideal standard protein. The amino acid showing the lowest percentage is the "limiting amino acid," and its percentage determines the "chemical score" ("amino acid score") of the protein. A provisional amino acid pattern for scoring has been provided in the FAO/WHO Report on Energy and Protein Requirements.[96] This pattern is based on the essen-

Table 3–10. Essential Amino Acid Composition of Ideal Reference Protein and of Cereal, Legume and Milk Powder Proteins and of a Mixture of All Three*

Protein Source	Amino Acid Content of Protein				Amino Acid Score (limiting amino acid)
	Lysine	Sulfur amino acids	Threonine	Tryptophan	
	%	%	%	%	
Ideal pattern	5.5	3.5	4.0	1.0	100
Cereal	2.4	3.8	3.0	1.1	44 (lysine)
Legume	7.2	2.4	4.2	1.4	68 (SAA)†
Milk powder	8.0	2.9	3.7	1.3	83 (SAA)†
Mixture: cereal-legume-milk (67:22:11)	5.1	3.2	3.5	1.2	88 (threonine)

*Data recalculated from Nutritional Evaluation of Protein Foods.[141]

†SAA = sulfur amino acids.

tial amino acid needs of the preschool child. The percentages of essential amino acids in this ideal pattern are: isoleucine 4 per cent, leucine 7 per cent, lysine 5.5 per cent, methionine + cystine 3.5 per cent, phenylalanine + tyrosine 6 per cent, threonine 4 per cent, tryptophan 1 per cent, valine 5 per cent. Thus, as shown in Table 3–10, cereal protein in which lysine is the limiting amino acid at a concentration of 2.4 per cent would have an amino acid score of

$$\frac{2.4}{5.5} \times 100 = 44$$

Amino acid scoring of protein quality has a number of advantages. As shown in Table 3–10, the most limiting amino acid can be identified and other essential amino acid deficits can be recognized. This allows the protein or diet to be supplemented not only with the least abundant essential amino acids but also with others present in suboptimal concentrations. In addition, the amino acid patterns of several dietary proteins can be compared and then mixed to give a diet in which the excesses of essential amino acids in one protein complement the deficiencies in the other and thus provide a better quality of dietary protein than any of the individual protein sources (Table 3–10).

Although amino acid analysis is thus a powerful tool in establishing the nutritional potential of a dietary protein, there are some limitations to its use, including the finding that proteins totally lacking one essential amino acid can still have some biologic value in supporting slow growth.[142] There is also a problem related to nonavailability of some essential amino acids present in the protein, as discussed below.

Further information about protein quality can be obtained from biologic tests most commonly carried out on the rat and on man. Many biologic assays of quality are based on growth of rats in which weight gain or nitrogen retention is the criterion of efficiency. In man, growth and N retention have been used for infants and N balance for adults. Relationships among various assays based on growth are illustrated diagrammatically in Figure 3–24.

The earliest assay to measure protein quality was the *protein efficiency ratio* (PER). In this, young animals (usually rats) are fed the protein source at a standard level (e.g. 9 per cent) for 10 or more days and the weight gain per gm protein eaten over this period provides the PER. For example, in one series of tests[143] the standard (casein) had a PER of 2.8, soy protein 2.4 and wheat gluten 0.4. This means that the young rat gained 2.8 gm for every gm of casein eaten, but only 0.4 gm for every gm of gluten eaten. However, this makes gluten appear to be of less value than it really is. If a protein-free diet is fed to young rats for 10 days, they will lose several gm in weight. In most of the alternative assays described below, this is recognized by including a control group on zero intake of protein.

The classic procedure for measuring protein quality by changes in body protein is *biologic value* (BV) (Fig. 3–24). It can be applied to growing or adult animals and to man. As originally described,[144] it involves measurement of N intake from the dietary protein and the output of N in the feces and in the urine. A group is also run on a protein-free diet to obtain values for excretion of N at zero protein intake. If the output of N in the feces is increased about this basal level, it indicates less than 100 per cent absorption of the dietary protein. It is thus possible to calculate the amount of dietary N absorbed. The extent of utilization of this absorbed N is indicated by the proportion excreted in the urine above the basal N output observed with animals or humans fed a protein-free diet. Biologic value thus is the fraction of absorbed N retained in the body for growth or maintenance.

A simpler procedure than measurement of BV by N balance is to assay the amount

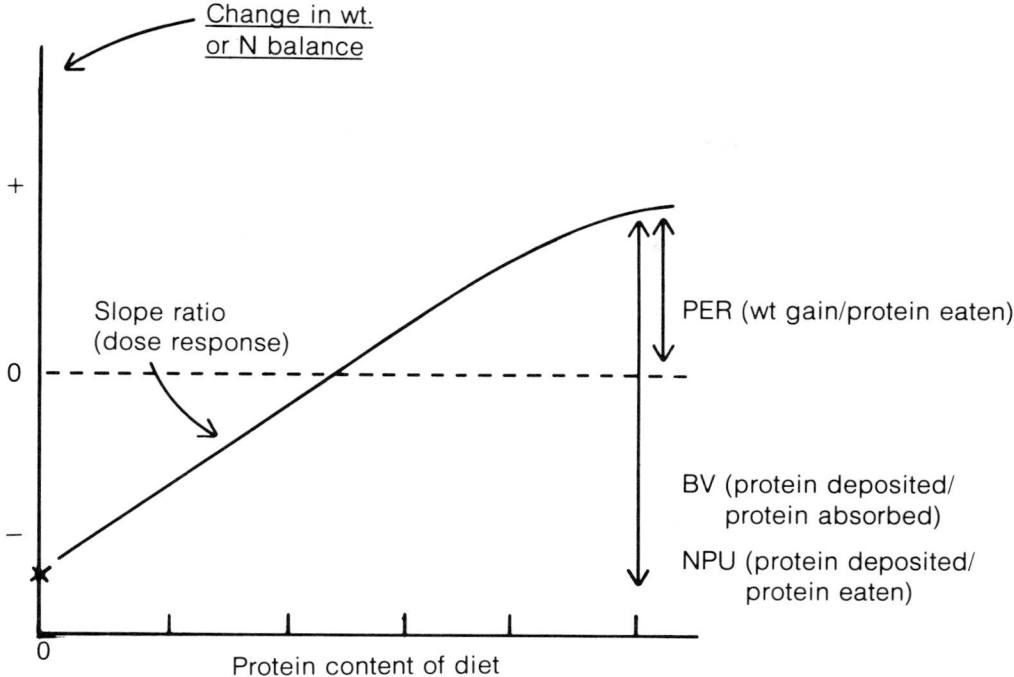

Fig. 3–24. Comparison of different indices of protein quality.

of protein N in the body of the animal at the end of the experiment. This is compared with the carcass N of a group fed a protein-free diet for the same length of time. The gain in N of the group receiving dietary protein is compared with their N intake and the proportion retained in their bodies is computed. This gives *net protein utilization (NPU)* (Fig. 3–24). It will be seen that this index takes no account of digestibility, so that a poorly digested protein would be recorded as having a low value. The NPU procedure appeals because of its relative simplicity and has been widely used with modifications in which the analysis of the carcass N content has been simplified by measuring dry weight or carcass water content.[145,146] Hegsted[146] has modified the procedure by measuring carcass N content at various levels of intake of dietary protein. He then constructs a dose-response line, the slope of which is determined by the biologic quality of the dietary protein. This procedure is representative of *slope ratio assay* methods. A problem associated with such dose-response assays is that the line relating protein consumed to growth rate may not be straight.[146]

Other procedures have been used to evaluate the quality of dietary proteins. These include the growth of microorganisms such as Streptococcus zymogenes[147] and Tetrahymena pyriformis[148] which have amino acid requirements somewhat similar to those of mammals. Assays of quality have also been based on the capacity of dietary protein to replete depleted animals and to cause changes in the protein and nucleic acid content of various organs.[149]

Amino Acid Availability from the Diet

In general, the amino acid composition of the protein in a foodstuff is useful in predicting its nutritive value for animals and man, using the chemical score as an index of quality (see above). However, there are circumstances under which amino acid availability can be less than that indicated by chemical analysis. Some raw plants contain inhibitors of proteolytic digestion, the best known being the trypsin inhibitor of the soya bean which is inactivated by cooking.[150] Reduced biologic availability can also occur as a result of heat treatment or of storage under adverse conditions. This second type of under-availability has been extensively studied because of its relevance to food processing procedures.[151,152]

Four types of damage to amino acids can occur as a result of food processing:

1. Loss of available lysine can occur from mild heat treatment in the presence of reducing sugars, e.g. during milk processing; in this instance, the sugar reacts with free side-chains of lysine residues to render them unavailable.
2. Under severe heating conditions, in the presence of either sugars or oxidized lipids or even without either of these, food proteins can become resistant to digestion so that availability of all amino acids is reduced.
3. When protein is exposed to severe treatment with alkali, lysine and cysteine residues can be eliminated, with formation of lysinoalanine which may be toxic.
4. Conditions of oxidation such as the use of SO_2 give rise to a loss of methionine in the protein.

Heat damage of the first kind occurs when a reducing sugar such as lactose or glucose is heated with a protein, or the protein and sugar are stored together at lower temperatures under moist conditions. As shown in Figure 3–25, the free NH_2 groups on the lysine side chains of the protein form an addition product with the reducing group of the sugar, and this product then undergoes a rearrangement to form fructosolysine. On hydrolysis with strong acid, most of the lysine is released again but about 30 per cent forms furosine and pyridosine during hydrolysis. These two cyclized derivatives can be observed on column chromatography of the hydroly-

sate for amino acids using the ninhydrin reaction, and signal the occurrence of nonavailable forms. In order to quantitate the amount of lysine made unavailable as a result of reaction with reducing sugars, it is desirable to have a reagent that reacts only with unmodified lysine side chains to form a compound which resists acid hydrolysis. The most widely used reagent is fluorodinitrobenzene (FDNB), which reacts with the free NH_2 groups of lysine residues but not with those blocked by sugar adducts.[151] The product formed between FDNB and lysine (DNP-lysine) resists the hydrolysis in strong acid used to liberate amino acids. Consequently, the difference between total lysine in the protein hydrolysate and DNP-lysine represents unavailable lysine in the original protein.

The second type of reduced availability of amino acids is more general and occurs when proteins are heated strongly in the absence of sugars, causing them to undergo peptide bond formation between the side chains of lysine and dicarboxylic acids. On acid hydrolysis, these peptide bonds rupture so that lysine is fully recovered.[152] However, the production of these new cross-linkages between the chains of the intact protein results in resistance to enzymic digestion. If a small amount of sugar is present during heat treatment, it promotes much more extensive cross-linkage with a corresponding increase in resistance to digestion in the gastrointestinal tract.

The third type of damage to proteins as a result of treatment with alkali is detectable by the appearance of a peak of lysinoalanine on conventional column analysis of the protein hydrolysate for amino acids. This is accompanied by a loss of cystine and lysine because of the reaction shown in Figure 3–26. The reaction in alkali begins with cleavage of cystine to form thiocysteine and dehydroalanine. The thiocysteine is unstable and resolves into a series of derivatives, while the de-

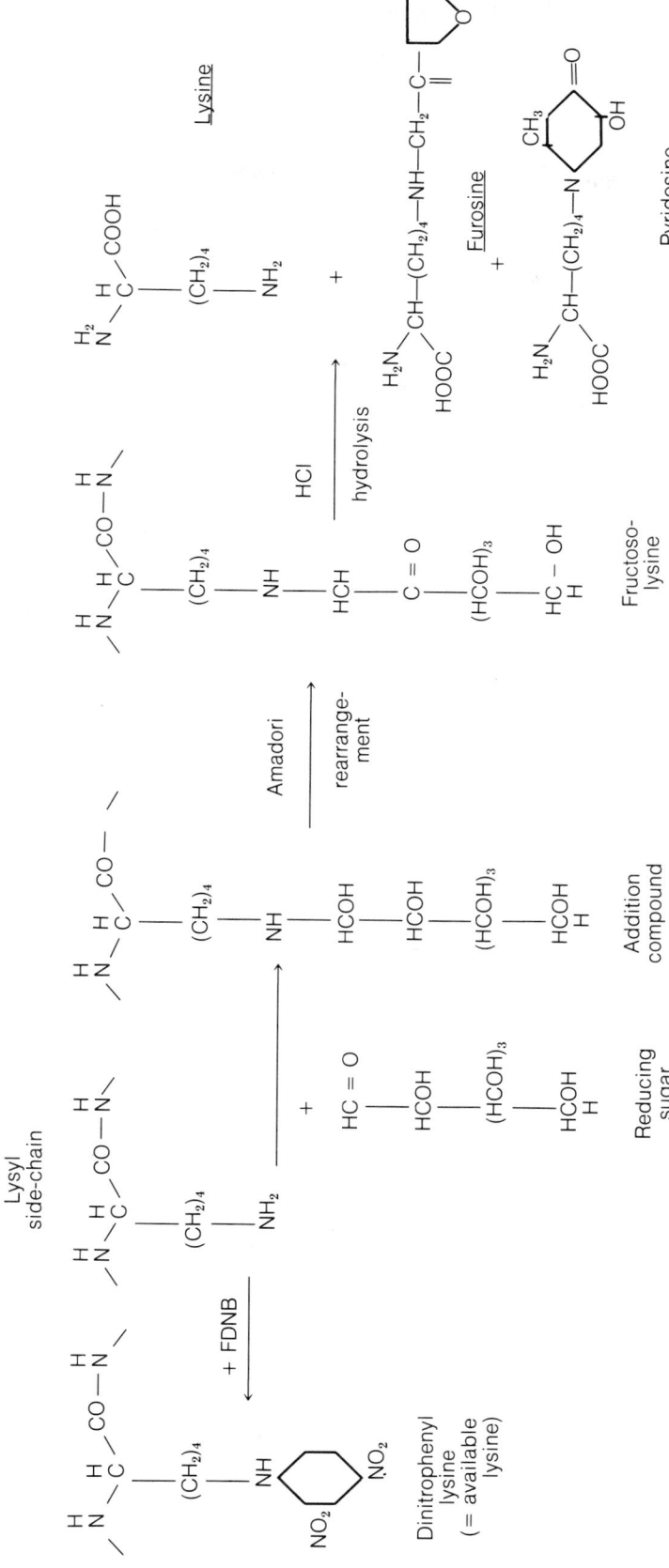

Fig. 3-25. Reactions of lysine side chains in dietary protein with reducing sugars in the diet, and the assay of available lysine with fluorodinitrobenzene (FDNB).

93

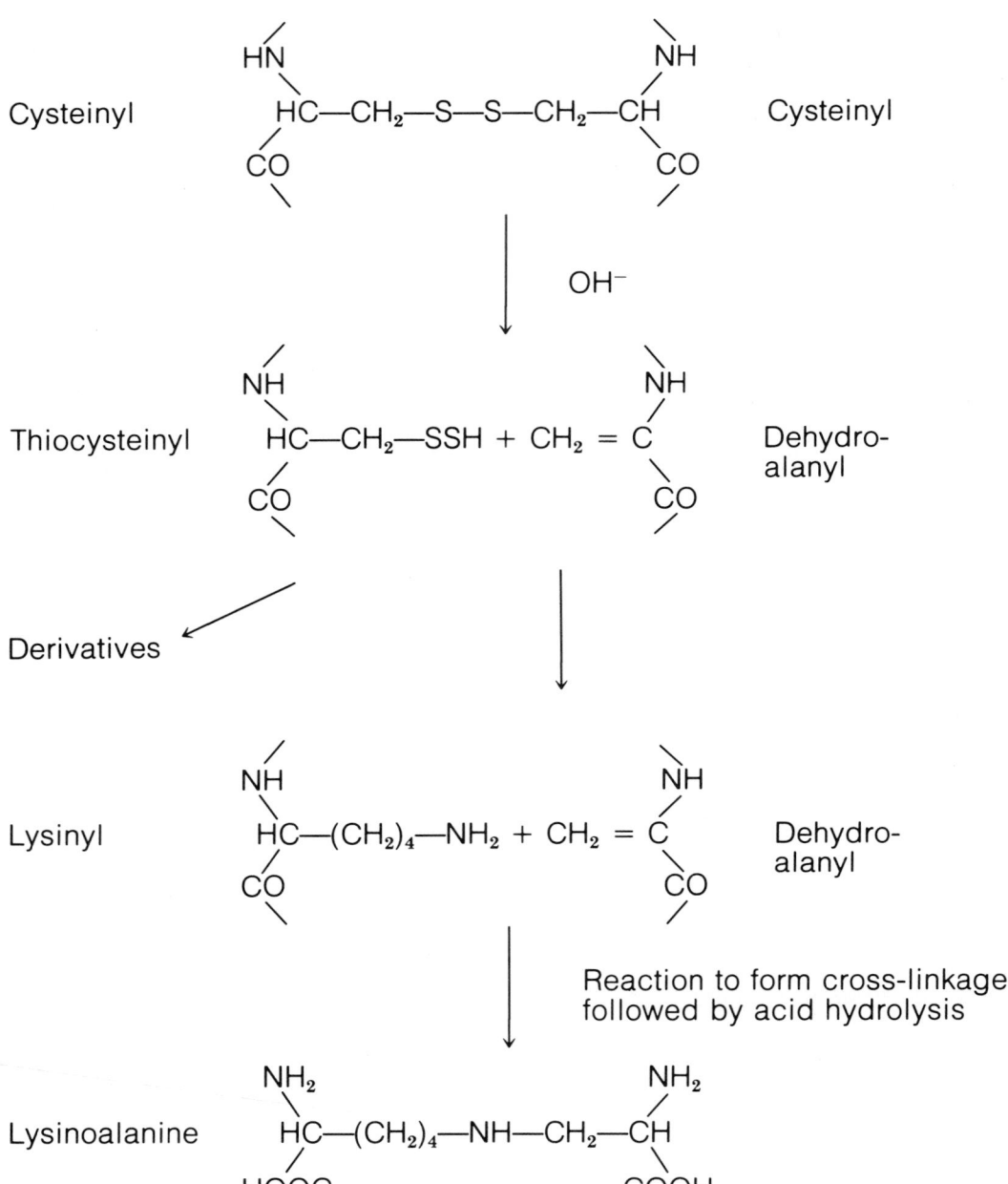

Fig. 3–26. Production of lysinoalanine as a result of treatment of proteins with alkali.

hydroalanine cross-reacts with peptide chains having exposed lysyl, ornithyl or amide side chains. On acid hydrolysis, the products so formed are released as lysinoalanine (Fig. 3–26), ornithinoalanine and β-aminoalanine respectively. Lysino-alanine is of importance not only as a mechanism by which lysine becomes un-available but also because after absorption it becomes concentrated in the cortex of the kidney[153] where it produces cell en-largement and multinucleation.[154,155] The toxicologic implications of these changes in the kidney have not been resolved.

Finally, oxidizing agents used in the treatment of proteins can transform methionine to methionine sulfoxide, with consequent loss of available methionine.

In addition to the loss of essential amino acids from the diet by chemical reactions, their utilization by the recipient can be affected by the presence of excess of other essential or nonessential amino acids.[156] Such disproportionate amounts of amino acids can produce effects on the animal that are classified into toxicities, antagonisms and imbalances. These have been demonstrated primarily with growing animals which respond with a reduction in growth rate and sometimes other changes. The term *amino acid toxicity* describes ad-verse effects from intake of large amounts of individual amino acids. Amino acids differ in the level at which such toxic effects occur; the most toxic are methio-nine and tyrosine, whereas threonine in large excess causes only a moderate reduc-tion in growth rate. *Amino acid antagonism* is the term used when excess of one amino acid in the diet causes depression in growth rate that can be alleviated by the addition of a structurally similar amino acid. The best established example is the antagonism between the branched-chain amino acids leucine, isoleucine and valine. Finally, the term *amino acid imbalance* is used when a change in the proportion of amino acids causes a depression in growth rate that is alleviated by adding more of

the most limiting essential amino acid in the diet. For example, when a mixture of amino acids lacking histidine is added to a diet containing 6 per cent fibrin as the protein, young rats cease to grow.[157] The addition of the amino acid mixture depre-sses growth, even although all the amino acids of the fibrin are still present. The most limiting amino acid in the diet is histi-dine, and growth can be restored by adding histidine to the diet imbalanced by the mix-ture of amino acids lacking it. Thus utiliza-tion of the histidine in fibrin has been im-paired by imbalancing the proportions of the essential amino acids through addition of the mixture lacking histidine. When the imbalanced mixture is fed to rats, the level of histidine in the plasma falls sharply and the animal reduces its food intake, pre-sumably because of an effect of the low plasma amino acid level on appetite con-trol by the brain.[158] The extent to which the normal diet of man can be imbalanced without impairing utilization of essential amino acids is not known. The effects of imbalances are observed in growing ani-mals under special circumstances in which suboptimal intakes of protein are fed, and are unlikely to occur in human subjects at normal levels of dietary protein.[159]

CONCLUSION

Protein metabolism is part of the mech-anism developed by animals to extract nu-trients from their environment and use them for the maintenance of biochemical reactions within the body. An important aspect of tissue function affected by amino acid supply is the capacity for growth and differentiation of the tissues. Of equal im-portance is the functional maintenance of the tissues of the adult. In adult man, there is a progressive loss of function from early adulthood to old age.[160] An important as-pect of nutritional science is to discover nutrient intakes that promote optimal function of the tissues during growth and development and to preserve tissue func-tion during aging. An understanding of the mechanisms of protein and amino acid metabolism is a prerequisite for improving our knowledge of the role of protein in attaining these desirable objectives.

BIBLIOGRAPHY

1. Munro: In *Mammalian Protein Metabolism*, Vol. 1 (Munro and Allison, Eds.). New York, Academic Press, 1964, pp. 1–29.
2. Munro: In *Mammalian Protein Metabolism*, Vol. 3 (Munro, Ed.). New York, Academic Press, 1969, pp. 133–182.
3. Munro and Steinert: Int. Rev. Sci., *7*, 359, 1975.
4. Christensen: In *Mammalian Protein Metabolism*, Vol. 1 (Munro and Allison Eds.). New York, Academic Press, 1964, pp. 105–124.
5. Munro: In *Mammalian Protein Metabolism*, Vol. 4 (Munro, Ed.). New York, Academic Press, 1970, pp. 299–386.
6. Herbert, Coulson and Hernandez: Comp. Biochem. Physiol., *17*, 583, 1966.
7. Meister: Science, *180*, 33, 1973.
8. Hider, Fern and London: Biochem. J., *114*, 171, 1969.
9. Mortimore, Woodside and Henry: J. Biol. Chem., *247*, 2776, 1972.
10. Gan and Jeffay: Biochim. Biophys. Acta, *148*, 448, 1967.
11. Airhart, Vidrich and Khairallah: Biochem. J., *140*, 539, 1974.
12. Munro: In *Mammalian Protein Metabolism*, Vol. 1 (Munro and Allison, Eds.). New York, Academic Press, 1964, pp. 31–34.
13. Dalgleish and Tabechian: Biochem. J., *62*, 625, 1956.
14. Nowak and Munro: In *Nutrition and the Brain*, Vol. II (Wurtman and Wurtman, Eds.). New York, Raven Press, 1977, pp. 193–260.
15. Schumm and Webb: Biochem. Biophys. Res. Commun., *48*, 1259, 1972.
16. Jacob, Sajdel and Munro: Biochem. Biophys. Res. Commun., *38*, 765, 1970.
17. Kedinger, et al.: Biochem. Biophys. Res. Commun., *38*, 165, 1970.
18. Roeder and Rutter: Nature, *224*, 234, 1969.
19. Darnell, Philipson, Wall and Adesnik: Science, *174*, 507, 1971.
20. Goodlad and Munro: Biochem. J., *73*, 343, 1959.
21. Sajdel and Jacob: Biochem. Biophys. Res. Commun., *45*, 707, 1971.
22. Kenney: In *Mammalian Protein Metabolism*, Vol. 4 (Munro, Ed.). New York, Academic Press, 1970, pp. 131–176.
23. Jensen and DeSombre: Science, *182*, 126, 1973.
24. O'Malley and Means: Science, *183*, 610, 1974.
25. Lodish: Annu. Rev. Biochem., *45*, 39, 1976.
26. Baliga and Munro: Nature, *23*, 257, 1971.
27. Fleck, Shepherd and Munro: Science, *150*, 628, 1965.
28. Young, et al.: J. Biol. Chem., *247*, 3592, 1972.
29. Kaplan and Pitot: In *Mammalian Protein Metabolism*, Vol. 4 (Munro, Ed.). New York, Academic Press, 1970, pp. 387–443.
30. Krebs: In *Mammalian Protein Metabolism*, Vol. 1 (Munro and Allison, Eds.). New York, Academic Press, 1964, pp. 125–176.
31. Rose: Physiol. Rev., *18*, 109, 1938.
32. Davidson: *The Biochemistry of the Nucleic Acids*, 7th ed. New York, Academic Press, 1972.
33. Seegmiller: Harvey Lect., *65*, 175, 1971.
34. Prior, Milner and Visek: J. Nutr., *105*, 141, 1975.
34a. Hultman, Bergstrom and Nilsson: Acta Anaesthesiol. Scand., *55*, 28, 1974.
35. Crim, Calloway and Margen: J. Nutr., *105*, 428, 1975.
36. Crim, Calloway and Margen: J. Nutr., *106*, 371, 1976.
36a. Forbes and Bruining: Am. J. Clin. Nutr., *29*, 1359, 1976.
37. Pitts: Fed. Proc., 7, 418, 1948.
38. Goldstein and Schooler: Adv. Enzyme Regul., *5*, 71, 1967.
39. Cahill and Owen: In *Mammalian Protein Metabolism*, Vol. 4 (Munro, Ed.). New York, Academic Press, 1970, pp. 559–584.
40. Gitler: In *Mammalian Protein Metabolism*, Vol. 1 (Munro and Allison, Eds.). New York, Academic Press, 1964, pp. 35–69.
41. Crim and Munro: In *Defined Formula Diets for Medical Purposes* (Shils, Ed.). Chicago, American Medical Association, 1977.
42. Ochoa-Solano and Gitler: J. Nutr., *94*, 249, 1968.
43. Snook: J. Nutr., *97*, 286, 1969.
44. Green, et al.: Proc. Soc. Exp. Biol. Med., *142*, 1162, 1973.
45. Lavau, Bazin and Herzog: J. Nutr., *104*, 1432, 1974.
46. Schultz and Curran: Physiol. Rev., *50*, 637, 1970.
47. Adibi and Soleimanpour: J. Clin. Invest., *53*, 1368, 1974.
48. Kim, et al.: J. Clin. Invest., *51*, 1419, 1972.
49. Asatoor, et al.: Clin. Sci., *39*, 1, 1970 (abstract).
50. Milne: In *Transport across the Intestine* (Burland and Samuel, Eds.). London, Churchill-Livingstone, 1972, p. 95.
51. Fauconneau and Michel: In *Mammalian Protein Metabolism*, Vol. 4 (Munro, Ed.). New York, Academic Press, 1970, pp. 481–522.
52. Olney and Ho: Nature, *227*, 609, 1970.
53. Stegink, et al.: Am. J. Physiol., *229*, 246, 1976.
54. Munro: In *Mammalian Protein Metabolism*, Vol. 3 (Munro, Ed.). New York, Academic Press, 1969, pp. 237–262.
55. Munro and Goldberg: In *The Role of the Gastro Intestinal Tract in Protein Metabolism* (Munro, Ed.). Oxford, Blackwell, 1964, p. 189.
56. Ju and Nasset: J. Nutr., *68*, 633, 1959.
57. Twombley and Meyer: J. Nutr., *74*, 453, 1961.
58. Elwyn: In *Mammalian Protein Metabolism*, Vol. 4 (Munro, Ed.). New York, Academic Press, 1970, p. 523.
59. Harper: Am. J. Clin. Nutr., *21*, 358, 1968.
60. Brookes, Owens and Garrigus: J. Nutr., *102*, 27, 1972.
61. Pawlak and Pion: Ann. Biol. Anim. Biochim. Biophys., *8*, 517, 1968.

62. Fishman, Wurtman and Munro: Proc. Natl. Acad. Sci., 64, 677, 1969.
63. Schimke: In *Mammalian Protein Metabolism*, Vol. 4 (Munro, Ed.). New York, Academic Press, 1970, pp. 177–228.
64. Wurtman: In *Mammalian Protein Metabolism*, Vol. 4 (Munro, Ed.). New York, Academic Press, 1970, pp. 445–479.
65. Enwonwu and Munro: Arch. Biochem. Biophys., 138, 532, 1970.
66. Clifford, et al.: Biochim. Biophys. Acta, 277, 443, 1972.
67. Munro, Hubert and Baliga: In *Alcohol, Nutrition and Protein Synthesis*, Vol. 1 (Rothschild, Oratz and Schreiber, Eds.). New York, Pergamon Press, 1975, p. 33.
68. Peters and Peters: J. Biol. Chem., 247, 3858, 1972.
69. Morgan and Peters: J. Biol. Chem., 246, 3500, 1971.
70. Driscoll, Crim, Zahringer and Munro: J. Nutr., 108, 1691, 1978.
71. Young and Munro: J. Nutr., 103, 1756, 1973.
72. Young, Hussein, Murray and Scrimshaw: J. Nutr., 101, 45, 1971.
73. Young, et al.: J. Nutr., 102, 1159, 1972.
74. Munro: In *Mammalian Protein Metabolism*, Vol. 1 (Munro and Allison, Eds.). New York, Academic Press, 1964, pp. 381–481.
75. Munro and Thomson: Metabolism, 2, 354, 1953.
76. Moir and Eccleston: J. Neurochem., 15, 1093, 1968.
77. Fernstrom and Wurtman: Science, 178, 414, 1972.
78. Munro, Fernstrom and Wurtman: Lancet, 1, 722, 1975.
79. Fischer, et al: Surgery, 78, 276, 1975; 80, 77, 1976.
80. Pozefsky, et al.: J. Clin. Invest., 48, 2273, 1969.
81. Wahren, Felig and Hagenfeldt: J. Clin. Invest., 57, 987, 1976.
82. Munro: In *Aromatic Amino Acids in the Brain* (Ciba Foundation Symposium 22). New York, Elsevier, 1974, pp. 5–24.
83. Young, et al.: J. Biol. Chem., 247, 3592, 1972.
84. Long, et al.: Metabolism, 24, 929, 1975.
85. Haverberg, et al.: Biochem. J., 152, 503, 1975.
86. Narasinga, Rao and Nagabhushan: Life Sci., 12, 205, 1973.
87. Young, Haverberg, Bilmazes and Munro: Metabolism, 22, 1429, 1973.
88. Munro and Young: Am. J. Clin. Nutr., 31, 1608, 1978.
89. Munro: In *Clinical Nutrition Update Amino Acids* (Greene, Holliday and Munro, Eds.). Chicago, American Medical Association, 1977, pp. 141–146.
90. Allison and Bird: In *Mammalian Protein Metabolism*, Vol. 1 (Munro and Allison, Eds.).New York, Academic Press, 1964, pp. 483–512.
91. Wallace: Fed. Proc., 18, 1, 1959.
92. Munro: In *Mammalian Protein Metabolism*, Vol. 2 (Munro and Allison, Eds.). New York, Academic Press, 1964, pp. 3–39.
93. Block and Mitchell: Nutr. Abstr. Rev., 16, 249, 1946.
94. FAO Report: *Protein Requirements*, Nutrition Studies No. 16. Rome, FAO, 1957.
95. WHO/FAO Report: *Protein Requirements*, WHO Technical Report Series No. 301, Geneva, WHO, 1965.
96. WHO/FAO Report: *Energy and Protein Requirements*, WHO Technical Report Series No. 522. Geneva, WHO, 1973.
97. Food and Nutrition Board N.A.S.: Recommended Dietary Allowances, 8th rev. ed. Washington, 1974.
98. Irwin and Hegsted: J. Nutr., 101, 385, 1971.
99. Scrimshaw, et al.: J. Nutr., 102, 1595, 1972.
100. Calloway and Margen: J. Nutr., 101, 205, 1971.
101. Calloway, Odell and Margen: J. Nutr., 101, 775, 1971.
102. Inoue, Fujita and Niiyama: J. Nutr., 103, 1673, 1973.
103. Garza, Scrimshaw and Young: J. Nutr., 107, 335, 1977.
104. Garza, Scrimshaw and Young: J. Nutr., 108, 90, 1978.
105. Uauy, Scrimshaw, Rand and Young: J. Nutr., 108, 97, 1978.
105a. Cheng, et al.: Am. J. Clin. Nutr., 31, 12, 1978.
106. Scrimshaw, et al.: Am. J. Clin. Nutr., 18, 321, 1966.
107. Torun, Scrimshaw, and Young: Am. J. Clin. Nutr., 30, 1983, 1977.
108. Irwin and Hegsted: J. Nutr., 101, 539, 1971.
108a. Munro: In *Parenteral Nutrition* (Wilkinson, Ed.). London, Churchill-Livingstone, 1972, pp. 34–67.
109. Inoue, Fujita and Niiyama: Unpublished results, 1971.
110. Hegsted: Fed. Proc., 22, 1424, 1963.
111. Holt and Snyderman: In *Amino Acid Metabolism and Genetic Variation* (Nyhan, Ed.). New York, McGraw-Hill, 1967, p. 381.
112. Fomon and Filer: In *Amino Acid Metabolism and Genetic Variation* (Nyhan, Ed.). New York, McGraw-Hill, 1967, p. 391.
113. Nakagawa, Takahashi, Suzuki and Kobayashi: J. Nutr., 80, 305, 1964.
114. Kofranyi and Jekat: Hoppe Seylers Z. Physiol. Chem., 338, 154, 1964.
115. Swenseid, Feeley, Harris and Tuttle: J. Nutr., 68, 203, 1959.
116. Scrimshaw, et al.: J. Nutr., 98, 9, 1969.
117. Daniel, Doraiswamy, Swaminathan and Rajalakshmi: Br. J. Nutr., 24, 741, 1970.
118. Snyderman, et al.: J. Nutr., 78, 57, 1962.
119. Munro: Acta Anaesthesiol. Scand., 55 (Suppl.), 81, 1974.
120. Cuthbertson: In *Parenteral Nutrition* (Wilkinson, Ed.). London, Churchill-Livingstone, 1972, pp. 4–23.
121. Steffee, et al.: J. Nutr., 40, 483, 1950.
122. Winters and Hasselmeyer (Eds.): *Intravenous Nutrition in the High Risk Infant*. New York, Wiley, 1975.
123. Ford, et al.: Br. Med. J., 1, 735, 1969.
124. Walser, Coulter, Dighe and Crantz: J. Clin. Invest., 52, 678, 1973.

125. Munro: J. Am. Diet. Assoc., *71*, 380, 1977.
126. Crim and Munro: In *Metabolic Basis of Endocrinology* (De Groot, et al., Eds.). In press.
127. Munro: In *Current Concepts in Parenteral Nutrition* (Greep, Soeters, Wesdorp, Phaf and Fischer, Eds.). The Netherlands, Martinus Niijhoff-Medical Division, 1977, pp. 55–68.
128. Harrison: Biochem. J., *55*, 204, 1953.
129. Tarr: Annu. Rev. Biochem., *27*, 223, 1958.
130. American Academy of Pediatrics: Committee on Nutrition. Pediatrics, *26*, 1039, 1960.
131. Kulkarnie and Sohonie: Indian J. Med. Res., *44*, 511, 1956.
132. Neuberger and Sanger: Biochem. J., *36*, 662, 1942.
133. Protein Advisory Group Bulletin, *5*, 19, 1975.
134. Close, Adriaens, Moore and Bigwood: Bull. Soc. Chim. Biol., *35*, 985, 1953.
135. Jones: U.S. Department of Agriculture, Circular 183 (revised), 1941.
136. McCance and Widdowson: Med. Res. Counc. Spec. Rep. Ser., *297*, 1960.
136a. Platt: Med. Res. Counc. Spec. Rep. Ser. *302*, 1962.
136b. Albanese and Orto: In *Modern Nutrition in Health and Disease*, 5th ed. (Goodhart and Shils, Eds.). Philadelphia, Lea & Febiger, 1970, pp. 28–88.
137. Clark: National Studies of Food Consumption and Dietary Levels. Washington, U.S. Department of Agriculture, 1975.
138. Consumer and Food Economics Research Division, Agricultural Research Service, United States Department of Agriculture, 1970.
139. Weir: In *Fat Content and Composition of Animal Products.* Washington, National Academy of Sciences, 1976, pp. 5–23.
140. Munro: In *Fat Content and Composition of Animal Products.* Washington, National Academy of Sciences, 1976, pp. 24–44.
141. Nutritional Evaluation of Protein Foods. Washington, National Academy of Sciences, 1978.
142. Bender: In *National Academy of Sciences – National Research Council* Pub. 843. Washington, 1961, p. 407.
143. Derse: J. Assoc. Off. Agric. Chem., *43*, 38, 1960.
144. Mitchell: J. Biol. Chem., *58*, 873, 1923.
145. Miller and Bender: Br. J. Nutr., *9*, 382, 1955.
146. Said and Hegsted: J. Nutr., *99*, 474, 1969.
147. Ford: Br. J. Nutr., *16*, 409, 1962.
148. Stott and Smith: Br. J. Nutr., *20*, 663, 1966.
149. Allison: In *Mammalian Protein Metabolism*, Vol. 2 (Munro and Allison, Eds.). New York, Academic Press, 1964, pp. 41–86.
150. Klose, Hill and Fevold: Proc. Soc. Exp. Biol. Med., *62*, 10, 1946.
151. Carpenter: Nutr. Abstr. Rev., *43*, 424, 1973.
152. Mauron: Proceedings IV Congress Food Science and Technology, Vol. 1, 1974, p. 564.
153. Finot, Bujard and Arnaud: In *Protein Crosslinking-B* (Friedman, Ed.). New York, Plenum Publishing, 1977, pp. 51–71.
154. Woodard: Fed. Proc., *32*, 884, 1973.
155. Woodard and Short: J. Nutr., *103*, 569, 1973.
156. Harper: In *Mammalian Protein Metabolism*, Vol. 2 (Munro and Allison, Eds.). New York, Academic Press, 1964, pp. 87–134.
157. Kumta and Harper: Proc. Soc. Exp. Biol. Med., *110*, 512, 1962.
158. Leung and Rogers: Am. J. Physiol., *221*, 929, 1971.
159. Harper: In *Improvement of Protein Nutriture.* Washington, National Academy of Sciences, 1974, pp. 138–166.
160. Shock: J. Am. Diet. Assoc., *56*, 491, 1970.

Chapter *4*

NUTRITIONAL ASPECTS OF DIETARY CARBOHYDRATES

Gary M. Gray
and
Michael R. Fogel

Carbohydrates continue to be the most important worldwide source of calories because of their ready accessibility and relatively low cost. In addition to lactose, which makes up 10 per cent of milk, and refined sucrose, polysaccharides are available in cereals or grains such as rice, potato, rye, yams and corn. Sucrose is found in many fruits and berries, particularly in dates, figs, and bananas, as well as in roots and tubers. In Africa nearly 80 per cent of total calories are taken in as carbohydrate, and in the Caribbean at least 65 per cent.[1] In the United States carbohydrates constitute about 50 per cent of the total caloric intake. The most important source of carbohydrate in the western world is starch, accounting for 50 per cent of saccharide calories; this is followed by sucrose (30 per cent) and lactose (10 per cent). Indigestible saccharides such as raffinose and stachyose are present in legumes but are not hydrolyzed to a significant extent in the small intestine, and hence are not assimilated. They have significant intraluminal metabolic effects, however, as will be discussed in the section concerning fiber in the diet. Because of the importance of carbohydrates as a dietary source, the mechanisms of their assimilation will be considered in some detail.

DIETARY STARCH

Intraluminal Nonrate-limiting Process in Digestion

Starch is comprised of a linear chain of glucose residues connected by an α-type of linkage between carbon 1 and carbon 6 of the adjacent glucose units. Digestion of this linear type of starch, amylose, begins under the influence of salivary α-amylase in the mouth but this occurs only to a minor extent because of the short time that food is in the oral cavity. Salivary α-amylase is inhibited by the acid pH present in the stomach. Significant intraluminal digestion of starch does not occur until the polysaccharide reaches the duodenum, where pancreatic α-amylase acts intraluminally to cleave it to oligosaccharide products. α-Amylase acts at the interior links of the amylose molecule but has little specificity for the linkages at the ends of the molecule, so that the final products possessing only exterior linkages are a disaccharide (maltose) and a trisaccharide (maltotriose).

The bulk of starch contains not only α-1,4 linear chains but also α-1,6 linkages which account for about 6 per cent of the polysaccharide linkages. These linkages constitute a branching point from which

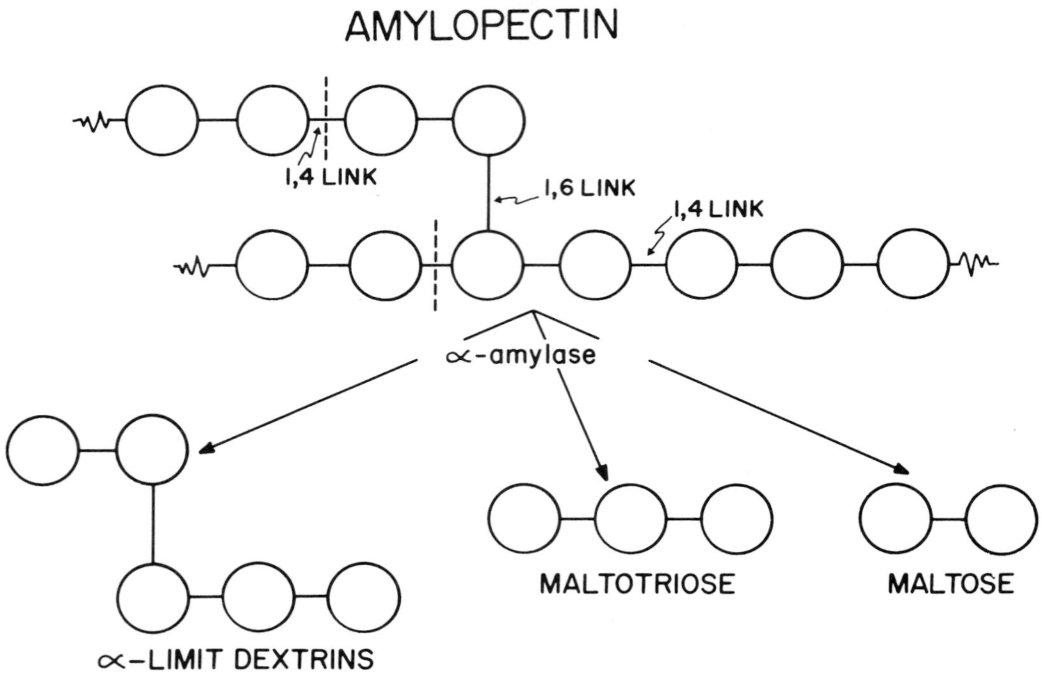

Fig. 4–1. The action of pancreatic α-amylase on the branched starch amylopectin. A portion of the polysaccharide molecule is shown. Because of the resistance to hydrolysis around the α 1,6 branch point, α-limit dextrins (average molecular weight 1500) are formed together with maltose and maltotriose as the final products within the intestinal lumen. (From Gray.[3])

additional α-1,4 straight chains can emanate. α-1,6 Branching points are important nutritionally because α-amylase has very poor specificity for these linkages. Hence, the final oligosaccharide products are not only maltose and maltotriose but also branched oligosaccharides, the α-limit dextrins, which have an average molecular weight of 1500 (Fig. 4–1). No more than a trace of free glucose is released from the hydrolysis of starch because the outer glucose-glucose linkages are not hydrolyzed by α-amylase. The overall action of α-amylase on the starches is highly efficient, so that the starch in a meal can be expected to be completely digested to the final oligosaccharide products by the time the meal reaches the distal duodenum.

In states of disease and malnutrition the secretion of pancreatic α-amylase is usually maintained at levels adequate to hydrolyze the amount of starch ingested. Hence, in patients with severe pancreatic exocrine insufficiency, intraluminal digestion proceeds at nearly the same rate as in normal individuals.[2] As shown in Figure 4–2, the luminal digestion products after a starch meal taken by patients with severe pancreatic exocrine insufficiency consist of oligosaccharides only slightly larger than those found in normal persons. Although total digestion of the starch is not complete by the time the substrate reaches the duodenal-jejunal junction, the average degree of polymerization of the molecule is only 8, and subsequent action of intraluminal α-amylase can be expected to quickly produce the final oligosaccharide products shown in Figure 4–1. Hence starch maldigestion must be rare even in patients

EXTENT OF HYDROLYSIS AT THE
LIGAMENT OF TREITZ

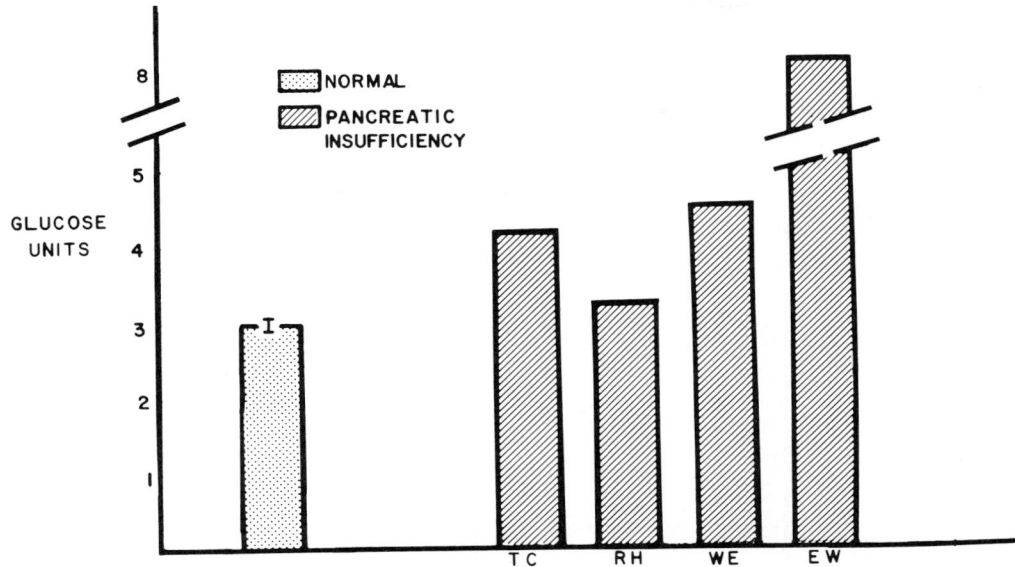

Fig. 4–2. Digestion of starch in normal human subjects (mean ± SE) and in 4 patients with pancreatic exocrine insufficiency (PI). The 50-gm starch meal was ingested and samples collected at the duodenal-jejunal junction. Even though PI patients secreted α-amylase at only 10 per cent of normal rates (data not shown), the starch was nearly completely hydrolyzed; residual hydrolytic products contained an average of only 4.5 glucose units per molecule. (From Fogel and Gray.[2])

with severe pancreatic disease. Starch, being efficiently digested in pancreatic disease, is an important source of calories.

Intestinal Surface Digestion of Oligo- and Disaccharides

The final products of starch digestion, with the disaccharides sucrose and lactose, are presented to the intestinal surface membrane where constitutive brush-border surface enzymes act on them at the lumen-cell interface.[3] The active hydrolytic sites of these enzymes are functionally located at the exterior surface of the membrane; hence, the oligosaccharides do not penetrate the intestinal cell but instead are hydrolyzed at the outer brush-border membrane. This surface hydrolysis is extremely rapid and provides sufficient

monosaccharide substrate for the final transport across the intestinal cell. In general, surface digestion of oligosaccharides is not rate limiting for the overall assimilation of dietary carbohydrate. There is one exception to this, however. As shown in Figure 4–3, the overall assimilation of glucose and galactose from lactose is only about half that which occurs from the equivalent mixture of the two monosaccharides.[4] Thus the hydrolysis of lactose is relatively slow and does not provide sufficient amounts of free glucose and galactose to assure maximal transport of these monosaccharides. The hydrolytic step is rate limiting for lactose. For all other oligosaccharides, however, there appears to be no difference in the rate of assimilation whether the oligosaccharides

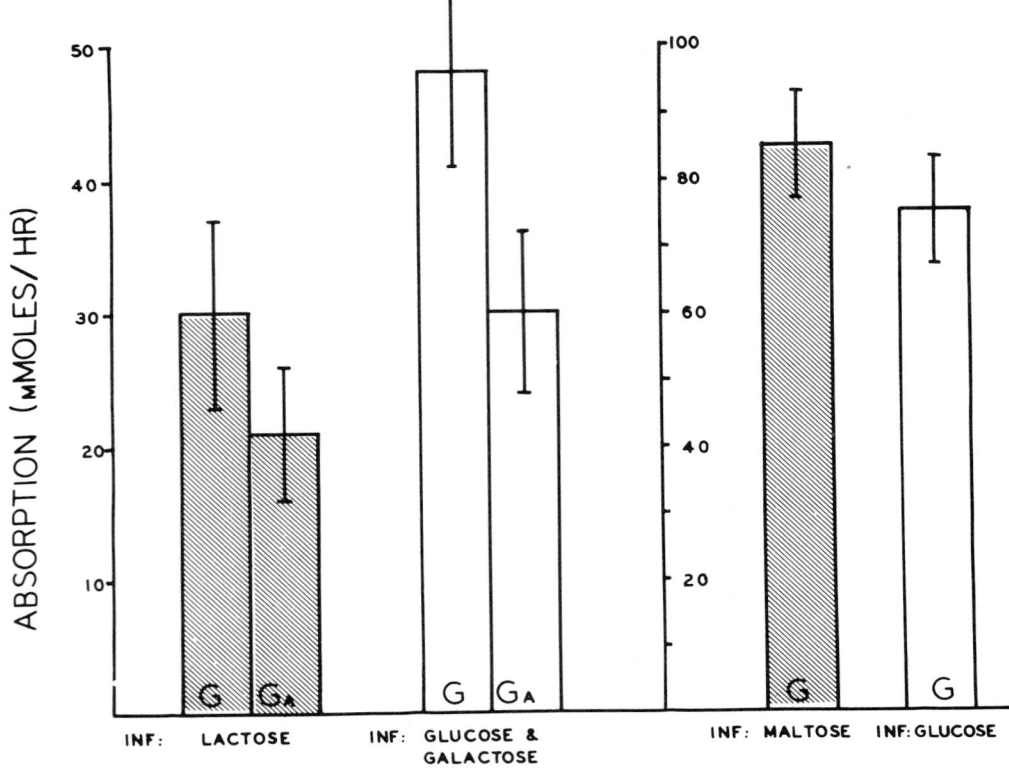

Fig. 4–3. Comparison of disaccharide and monosaccharide assimilation in normal human subjects (mean ± SE, n = 10). A 30-cm segment of jejunum was perfused at 15 ml per hr with 80 mM disaccharide or the equivalent monosaccharide mixture. Assimilation from maltose was comparable to that from the equivalent glucose (right panel). In contrast (left panel), as compared to the equivalent monosaccharide mixture, absorption of both glucose and galactose was appreciably slower from the lactose solution ($p < 0.05$). (From Gray and Santiago.[4])

Table 4–1.   Assimilation of Dietary Carbohydrate

Food Source	% in Diet	Luminal Hydrolysis	Intestinal Surface Hydrolysis	Rate limiting Step
Starch (Amylopectin Amylose)	60	→ Maltose Maltotriose α-Limit Dextrins	→ Glucose	Glucose Transport
Lactose	10	None	→ Glucose and Galactose	Surface Hydrolysis
Sucrose	30	None	→ Glucose and Fructose	Glucose and Fructose Transport

themselves are presented to the intestinal surface or whether an equivalent amount of the final hexose products is provided.

Table 4–1 summarizes the stages and apparent rate-limiting steps in the overall assimilation of dietary carbohydrate.

The Intestinal Oligosaccharidases and Their Control Mechanisms

The characteristics of the human intestinal oligosaccharidases are shown in Table 4–2. Notably all of these enzymes are large glycoproteins of 200,000 to 300,000 daltons, consisting of two general types: (1) the α-glucosidases hydrolyze the α-glucosyl linkages and (2) the β-galactosidase digests the lactose in milk. Man is born with a full complement of these oligosaccharidases, which are constituents of the surface membrane of the intestinal villus cells.[5-7] Crypt cells do not have active forms of these proteins, but precursor enzymes appear to be in the intestinal crypt cells. Although the life of the small intestinal cell is only 2 to 3 days, there is evidence from animal studies that the intestinal disaccharidases probably have a half-life only a fraction of the cell life, and hence that the oligosaccharidases are synthesized and degraded several times during the life of the cell.[8] This suggests that intestinal car-

bohydrases are controlled by mechanisms other than the rate of cell turnover.

The level of intestinal sucrase activity in man appears to be regulated at least in part by the amount of carbohydrate in the diet. Hence, individuals on a low-carbohydrate diet show a significant decrease in sucrase in a matter of only 2 to 5 days.[9] On the other hand, ingestion of large amounts of sucrose and probably also of its monosaccharide products, glucose and fructose, causes an appreciable increase in sucrase levels above those found in individuals maintained on a diet containing only modest amounts of these carbohydrates. Since the oligosaccharidases are known to be synthesized and degraded several times during the intestinal cell life cycle, it appears likely that there is either an increase in the rate of synthesis of this enzyme with feeding of its substrate or that the enzyme already synthesized becomes stabilized and is not subject to degradation. The degradation of intestinal disaccharidases may occur under the influence of pancreatic proteases which cleave them off of the intestinal surface membrane. The mechanism whereby substrates such as sucrose might prevent this degradation is unknown.

The monosaccharide products released at the intestinal surface appear to play an

Table 4–2. Human Brush-border Oligosaccharidases

Enzyme-Type Name	Principal Substrate	Products	% Total Maltase	Km (mM)	Mol Wt
β-Galactosidase: lactase[5]	Lactose	Glucose and galactose		18	280,000
α-Glucosidase: glycoamylase[6]	Malto-oligosaccharides (G_2† → G_9)	Glucose	25	3.8 → 1.1 (G_2) (G_9)	210,000
Sucrase-α-dextrinase*[7]	Sucrose	Glucose and fructose	25	20	280,000
	α-Dextrins	Glucose	50	1.1	
Trehalase	Trehalose	Glucose		3	

*Commonly called sucrase-isomaltase although isomaltose is not a physiologic substrate in the intestine.
†G indicates glucose and the subscript the number of α-(1→4) linked glucose units.

important and immediate role in the regulation of oligosaccharidase action. Since, for most dietary carbohydrates, the rate of hydrolysis at the intestinal surface exceeds the subsequent transport capacity for the released monosaccharides, monosaccharides accumulate at the intestinal surface and are known to have an inhibitor action on the oligosaccharidase when the concentrations are as low as 10 mM.[10] Surface hydrolysis is not allowed to continue wantonly but instead is regulated at a certain finite rate by virtue of the feedback inhibition of these enzymes by their monosaccharide products. This in effect constitutes a coupling of surface hydrolysis and subsequent transport of the products and probably is important to ensure efficient assimilation while still avoiding the release of a marked excess of monosaccharide which might have a deleterious osmotic effect. This will be considered further in the section on oligosaccharidase deficiency syndromes.

Mechanism of Monosaccharide Transport[3]

The principal monosaccharide released at the intestinal surface is glucose which is the hexose component accounting for 80 per cent of digested carbohydrate. Other monosaccharides are galactose, which is almost identical in structure to glucose and utilizes the same transport mechanism, and fructose. These hexoses, being too large to move across the intestinal surface membrane by simple diffusion, require specific transport mechanisms. Two principal mechanisms accommodate these saccharides. The glucose-galactose transport mechanism has a precise structural requirement for a 5-carbon pyranose ring with the location of the hydroxyl group at carbon 2 below the horizontal plane of the molecule. In addition, the presence of a sixth carbon greatly facilitates transport. D-Xylose, a pentose, is the smallest molecule that can be transported, although it is handled poorly. Glucose and galactose have high affinity and are transported

most efficiently. The transport of glucose and galactose occurs by a saturable process that probably involves a protein carrier in the brush-border membrane that somehow facilitates binding and movement of the hexose into the interior of the intestinal cell. This process is aided by sodium ion, which appears to bind at a different site on the carrier. The energy for the system is derived from the sodium pump that facilitates movement of interiorized sodium into the intercellular spaces between cells under the influence of ATPase. The carrier from intestinal mammalian cells has not yet been isolated, but similar carrier proteins have been identified in bacterial systems.

Fructose has a structure considerably different from glucose, and this monosaccharide utilizes a separate transport mechanism that appears to be independent of sodium and does not transport the saccharide against a concentration gradient. This process is about half as efficient as the glucose transport process but it supports uptake of fructose at adequate rates to promote its total assimilation in the small intestine.

Deficiency of the Oligosaccharidases

Pathogenesis of Oligosaccharide Intolerance. As outlined above, essentially all dietary carbohydrate must be hydrolyzed at the intestinal luminal-cell interface since there are no mechanisms for translocation of intact oligosaccharide across the intestinal membrane. Any saccharide that cannot be hydrolyzed by the action of a membrane surface enzyme will remain in the intraluminal fluid. The intestinal luminal fluid is kept isotonic with plasma, and small particles such as oligosaccharides have an osmotic effect that will increase intraluminal fluid to maintain its isotonicity. Furthermore, in the lower ileum and colon, undigested carbohydrates are metabolized by bacteria to 2- and 3-carbon fragments that increase the osmotic effect two- to fourfold. Hence, if 50 gm of a carbohydrate cannot be hydrolyzed on the intestinal surface it may eventually retain anywhere from 150 ml to 1 L of water, resulting in a watery, frothy diarrhea. Secondary malabsorption of other nutrients may occur because of the rapid transit time and the acid pH established by the volatile fatty acid products of the carbohydrate when it is thus metabolized.

Patients typically complain of abdominal fullness, nausea and abdominal cramps up to 60 minutes after ingesting a meal containing the carbohydrate that cannot be digested. Diarrhea may persist as long as 5 hours after ingestion of the offending sugar.

Disaccharidase Deficiency Syndromes. Congenital deficiency of disaccharidases is rare but the most common type in early childhood is sucrase-α-dextrinase deficiency; this may occur in as high as 0.2 per cent of the white western population.[11] Most patients with this deficiency syndrome have several family members with intolerance to sucrose, and these families usually eliminate table sugar from the diet. A small but significant percentage of patients with the irritable-colon syndrome may actually be suffering from sucrase-isomaltase deficiency. Although congenital deficiency of intestinal lactase occurs in the childhood years, it is uncommon.

The most widely recognized disaccharide deficiency is that of acquired lactase, which occurs in childhood or adolescence in a large percentage of the world's population.[12] Typically symptoms develop sometime between 4 and 16 years of age, and the prevalence in the world's population is extremely high. About 10 per cent of healthy North American whites and 70 per cent of American blacks appear to be deficient in intestinal lactase. Other population groups showing a high rate of lactase deficiency are Asians (90 per cent), Israeli Jews (60 per cent), Arabs (80 per cent) and Mexicans (75 per cent). The extremely high prevalence of lactase deficiency in most of the world's population groups has prompted the suggestion that an inherited defect is responsible. This has not yet been established by population analysis, however.

Disaccharidase deficiency in gastrointestinal disorders is common, particularly if the small intestine is involved with the disease process. Hence, essentially all patients with celiac sprue (gluten-sensitive enteropathy, nontropical sprue, and tropical sprue) are deficient in intestinal lactase, the disaccharidase that appears to be most sensitive to injury. Two-thirds to three-fourths of such patients are also deficient in intestinal sucrase and maltase. After treatment, deficiency of lactase persists in only 30 to 60 per cent. Other diseases associated with disaccharidase deficiency include cholera, gastroenteritis, pellagra, the irritable-colon syndrome and postgastrectomy syndromes.[13]

The clinical diagnosis of disaccharidase deficiency is usually relatively easy because of the relationship of symptoms to the offending carbohydrate. Patients usually develop symptoms when a 50-gm load of the offending disaccharide is administered, and a specific diagnosis can be made from enzymatic analysis of the peroral intestinal biopsy. Presumptive diagnosis of disaccharidase deficiency can be made from the oral disaccharide tolerance test or a breath test utilizing ^{14}C-lactose.[14] Another breath test, based on analysis of expired air for hydrogen produced from intestinal bacterial action on lactose, avoids the exposure to radioactive carbohydrate.

Treatment of disaccharide deficiencies consists of elimination of the offending carbohydrate and substitution of another nutrient to which the individual is tolerant. Fortunately, starch can be given as an inexpensive source of carbohydrate calories in patients with deficiency of the intestinal membrane disaccharidases.

DIETARY FIBER

The recent epidemiologic studies of Burkitt, Trowell and others have ushered in a new era of interest in the unabsorbed portion of ingested carbohydrates known as dietary fiber.[16,17] The fact that the western urban diet contains only 20 per cent of the dietary fiber present in the diets of 100 years ago has led to claims that colonic cancer, constipation, diverticulosis, gallstones and even coronary artery disease (disorders not generally well recognized until this century) are caused by a deficient intake of fiber. The nature of dietary fiber, its function, and its relation to the above disorders will be considered.

The Nature of Dietary Fiber

Current analytic methods have determined that dietary fiber is composed of at least six general components listed in Table 4–3.[18] Formerly, fiber was measured by simply weighing the amount of vegetable fiber resistant to acid hydrolysis and alkaline hydrolysis. This crude analysis actually measures mainly the cellulose and lignin fractions. Recently, more accurate methodology[19] has been developed for the measurement of all the components listed in Table 4–3. Fiber can now be measured with sufficient accuracy to conform to Trowell's definition as "the remnant of plant cells resistant to hydrolysis by the alimentary enzymes of man." Thus, lignin, a noncarbohydrate, can be included in his definition.

Bran, the most concentrated form of fiber (Table 4–4), is often used synonymously, but incorrectly, with the term dietary fiber.[20,21] Consisting of the outer layers of wheat grain, bran forms approximately 15 per cent of whole wheat. The composition of bran is variable and depends upon the fineness of the milling process. In addition to the fiber components (cellulose and pentosan), wheat protein, starch, fat and sugar are included in processed bran. Wheat also contains some fiber in its inner core. Commercial flour may contain residual fiber from the wheat core, but most of the bran is removed by the steel rollers that have replaced stone in modern mills.

The Effect of Fiber in the Diet

As shown in Table 4–4, the total quantity of dietary fiber varies markedly in different foods.[20,21] Furthermore, each type of food fiber is composed of different proportions of the six basic components listed in Table 4–3. The properties of fiber most important for human intestinal function are a hydrophilic nature, gel-forming ability and a binding capacity for ions or salts. Although the exact effects of dietary fiber depend on the type and amount of fiber ingested, most of its actions are limited to the large intestine.

Table 4–3. Dietary Fiber

Type	Chemical Characteristics	Representative Molecular Size (daltons)	Plant Cell Function	Special Physical Properties
Cellulose	Unbranched 1-4 β-D-glucose polymers	6×10^5	Cell wall structure	Hydrophyllic
Hemicellulose	Pentose or hexose polymers often branched; soluble in cold alkali	3×10^4	Wall stability	Ion binding
Pectins	β-1,4-D-galacturonic acid polymers usually associated with other polysaccharides	$6–9 \times 10^4$	Wall stability	Gel-forming ability Ion binding
Algal polysaccharides	Some similar to plants, others have sulfated polymers such as agar and carrageenan	2×10^5	Algal cell wall structure	Gel-forming ability
Lignin	Noncarbohydrate substituted phenylpropanes	$1–5 \times 10^3$	Cell wall strength	Possible bile salt binding ability

Table 4–4. Dietary Fiber in Selected Foods*

Food	Total Dietary Fiber	Noncellulose Polysaccharides gm/100 gm	Cellulose	Lignin
White bread	2.7	2	0.7	Trace
Whole meal bread	8.5	6.0	1.3	1.2
All-Bran	27	18	6.0	2.9
Puffed wheat	15	10	2.6	2.5
Beans, baked (canned)	7.3	5.7	1.4	0.2
Peas, frozen (raw)	7.8	5.5	2.1	0.2
Carrot, young (boiled)	3.7	2.0	1.5	Trace
Potato, main crop (raw)	3.5	2.5	1.0	Trace
Peanut butter	7.5	5.6	1.9	Trace
Peaches (whole)	2.3	1.5	0.2	0.6

*Selected from Southgate, et al.[21] Values rounded off to two significant figures.

Theoretically, a diet high in cellulose, hemicellulose and pectin produces a bulky, gel-like stool. In fact, studies going back nearly 50 years show that the addition of high fiber substances to the human diet consistently results in a bulkier stool.[22–24] Such a diet facilitates easy passage of stool and normal distention of the colon. A reduction of fiber elements in the diet results in a firm, small stool and contracted colon. In western urbanized society, the average stool weight is under 150 gm per day. With the addition of 50 gm of fiber, the wet weight of stool increases to over 250 gm per day.[20]

The addition of pectin, certain gums and mucilages might be expected to lower serum calcium, iron and magnesium levels; lipid levels might also be reduced because of binding of bile salts (Table 4–3). In fact, lowered ion levels have been shown with high-fiber diets, but generally these changes are minimal and probably not biologically significant. Although the cholesterol-reducing effect of most dietary fiber is minimal, certain gums, especially guar, are still actively being studied.[25]

Dietary Fiber and Disease Processes

The Irritable-bowel Syndrome and Diverticulosis. The irritable-bowel syndrome, characterized by abdominal aching or cramping pain associated with diarrhea or alternating diarrhea and constipation, is a common affliction of western man. Clearly, it is a leading cause of industrial absenteeism in the United States and the most common entity encountered by the gastroenterologist. Although important psychologic and sociologic factors are related to the prevalence of this syndrome, one major pathophysiologic mechanism is disordered colonic motility. Studies of rural Africans have shown that the disorder does not occur in a rural setting where people eat an unrefined high-fiber diet. This finding has been extrapolated to provide a rational basis for treatment.

Studies on patients with the irritable-bowel syndrome have shown increased pressure in the colonic lumen. LaPlace's law of fluid and pressure relationships in a cylinder (pressure × radius = K × wall tension) may be rearranged:

$$\text{intraluminal pressure} \sim \frac{\text{wall tension (circular muscle)}}{\text{radius}}$$

As shown in this formula, a narrowed colon (decreased radius) results in higher intraluminal pressure if the wall tension is constant. Thus, a low-fiber diet will cause the colon to partially contract, a situation which may be responsible for the localized areas of tonic contraction (hypersegmentation) and circular muscle hypertrophy noted in the irritable-bowel syndrome.

Constipation is the logical result of delayed transit caused by this alteration of colonic function. Abdominal pain may also be related to the localized colonic dilatation produced by the temporary obstructive hypersegmentation.

A further extension of this line of reasoning may explain the low incidence of colonic diverticulosis in rural Africa and the increasing incidence of this disorder in industrialized communities. A lifelong fiber-deficient diet with its resultant hypersegmentation, muscular hypertrophy and increased colonic intraluminal pressure may eventually produce herniation of colonic mucosa at regions of low resistance, e.g. at the sites where nutrient arteries penetrate the muscularis.[26] These mucosal herniations, called diverticula, may be clinically silent but are occasionally associated with diverticulitis and massive colonic bleeding. Because of the vast numbers of patients with colonic diverticula, these complications are common causes of serious morbidity and mortality in our aging population.

The rational treatment of diverticulosis and the irritable-bowel syndrome starts with a high-fiber diet.[27-29] The added bulk increases the radius of the colon and prevents the colonic musculature from being chronically contracted. With a high-fiber diet, colonic pressure should eventually diminish. Although there are no long-term studies demonstrating beneficial colonic pressure changes in patients fed high-fiber diets, short-term studies have demonstrated improved colonic function in patients with diverticulosis and the irritable-bowel syndrome.

Colonic Neoplasia. Colonic cancer and polyps are rare in rural Africa. However, in the United States colonic cancer is a leading cause of cancer deaths. The western diet, perhaps because of the increased ingestion of animal protein, may be associated with the presence of substances in the bowel lumen which may have the capacity to produce neoplasia in animals. These potential carcinogens are postulated to be produced by colonic bacteria which ferment the nutrient products remaining in the colon. Colonic bacteria act upon nitrogenous waste material and bile salts to produce carcinogens such as nitrosamines and phenols. Dietary fiber itself is degraded into volatile fatty acids, hydrogen, carbon dioxide and methane. Although the ingestion of fiber does not seem to change the bacterial flora, the unwanted by-products of bacterial metabolism are diluted by the fluid-retaining properties of the remaining intact dietary fiber; this may decrease the exposure time of the colon mucosa to putative carcinogens.[22] Furthermore, the transit time of colonic contents is related in a curvilinear fashion to the stool weight (Fig. 4–4); transit time decreases with increasing amounts of stool.[30] Thus, dietary fiber may dilute potentially noxious substances produced by colonic bacteria and promotes the more rapid elimination of these substances[31] (see also Chapter 38).

Dietary Fiber and Heart Disease. The epidemiologic studies of Burkitt and Trowell demonstrated in the rural African population not only a lower incidence of colonic disorders but also a diminished rate of coronary artery disease.[16,17] These findings have been confirmed in vegetarian populations of the western world, such as the Seventh Day Adventists. However, the diet of this group, as well as being high in fiber, is low in animal fat. The possibility that high-fiber diets lower the risk of coronary artery disease has been considered by several investigators. The most commonly studied risk factor is the plasma cholesterol level. After early studies yielded conflicting results, a recent, thorough study of normal subjects fed 60 gm of mixed dietary fiber daily or a regular American diet containing approximately 12 gm of dietary fiber[32] for 4 weeks revealed no difference in the serum cholesterol levels of the two groups, despite the fact that stool bulk was increased and transit time was decreased in the

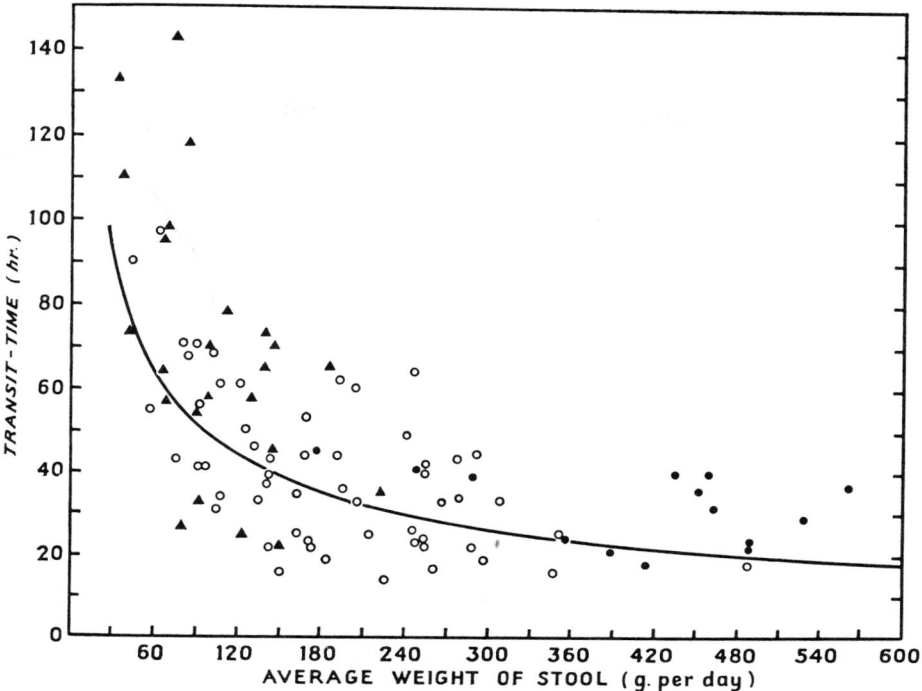

Fig. 4–4. Relationship between stool weight and oral-to-anal transit time for individuals on diets of varying fiber content. O = vegetarians, vegans and African boarding-school (mixed) diet; o = African villagers (high-residue) diet; ▲ = English boarding-school and British Navy (low-residue) diet. Transit time of radioactive plastic pellets included with the meal was detected by exposure of stools to x-ray film. (From Burkitt, Walker and Painter.[30])

high-fiber group. Thus, the colonic effects of the high-fiber diet occurred but were not accompanied by lowering of cholesterol levels. This lack of effect was found whether the subjects ate high-cholesterol or cholesterol-free diets. Although the serum cholesterol may be reduced by a single type of dietary fiber such as pectin or guar, further experiments on the effect of high quantities of specific fiber on cholesterol lowering are indicated. It is unlikely, however, that the ingestion of these substances would be as beneficial as the ion exchange resin, cholestyramine, presently used to reduce cholesterol. The decrease in coronary artery disease and the lower cholesterol levels in the rural African population is more probably caused by the low animal-fat diet and high physical activity than by a high-fiber diet.

Dietary Fiber and Diabetes. In recent years, pectin has been shown to slow the gastric release of ingested food, especially sugars. Thus, postprandial blood sugar might rise more slowly with a resultant lower insulin response. In fact, recent studies have confirmed that fiber-free substances such as apple juice produce higher postprandial insulin levels than do equicaloric quantities of intact apples.[33] Other studies in diabetics have demonstrated lower blood sugar levels after meals containing pectin.[34] Theoretically, pectin may improve diabetic control by reducing the absorption rate of sugar. It is not clear, however, whether this pharmacologic effect is of therapeutic significance. Further studies to determine the therapeutic effectiveness of pectin in diabetic management are warranted.

Dietary Fiber and Gallbladder Disease. Cholelithiasis is another disorder that has been shown epidemiologically to be more prevalent in the western world than in rural Africa. Since cholelithiasis results from chronic supersaturation of bile with cholesterol, reduction of cholesterol synthesis and enhancement of bile salt absorption may allow the biliary cholesterol to become desaturated and to remain in the micellar (soluble) phase. Indeed, some experiments with high-fiber diets have shown a slight decrease in cholesterol synthesis. Also a high-fiber diet could, by shortening transit time, decrease the production of secondary bile salts. The resultant higher levels of primary bile acids would then increase the bile acid pool and improve biliary cholesterol solubility. Although this action is theoretically possible, the most recent data on normal subjects suggest that no prolonged change occurs.[35] Thus, a favorable effect of dietary fiber on cholesterol saturation, and hence cholelithiasis, has not yet been established.

METABOLISM OF MONOSACCHARIDES AFTER ABSORPTION

Because of the rapid assimilation of dietary carbohydrates, plasma glucose rises approximately 25 mg per dl after the ingestion of a carbohydrate load. These plasma levels return rapidly to normal, and the normal fasting level is again achieved by 2 to 3 hours after the meal. Insulin is secreted promptly in response to the carbohydrate load, preventing plasma glucose from reaching high concentrations that would produce hyperosmolality. The delicate glucose-insulin homeostasis is maintained by regulation of insulin and glucose interactions by a finely tuned mechanism. Insulin has two distinct actions. It facilitates the transport of glucose from the plasma to the cells by acting directly on the cell membranes of the adipocyte and muscle cell. Its second action, in liver, is distinctly different, since it does not seem to modify or facilitate membrane transport of glucose but instead activates a series of enzymes that promote glucose metabolism after entry to favor production of α-glycerol phosphate and acetyl CoA fatty acids. In addition, it tends to facilitate synthesis of glycogen and accelerates metabolism through the Krebs cycle to yield energy and carbon dioxide.

The plasma glucose and insulin response depends to a significant extent upon the amount of dietary carbohydrate ingested at the time of a meal. As shown in Table 4–5, both the glucose and insulin response in plasma vary depending upon the amount of carbohydrate in the meal. A moderate increase (12 per cent) in carbohydrate content of the meal results in a slight but significant increase in the plasma glucose and a marked increase in plasma insulin, indicating that the homeostatic mechanism of increased insulin re-

Table 4–5. Carbohydrate Load and Plasma Glucose and Insulin*

Carbohydrate (% in Diet)	Glucose† mg/dl	Insulin† μU/ml
43	115	120
55	132	175

*Adapted from Reaven and Olefsky.[36]
†One-hour postprandial values where significantly higher for the 55 per cent carbohydrate diet for both glucose (p < 0.005) and insulin (p < 0.0001).

Table 4–6.   Effect of Carbohydrate Type on Plasma Glucose and Insulin*

Carbohydrate Source	Glucose† (mg/dl) 30 min	Insulin† (μU/ml) 30 min
Glucose	130	60
Sucrose	135	70
Starch	105	20

*Adapted from Crapo, Reaven and Olefsky.[37]
†Values at 30 minutes after ingestion of 100 gm of glucose equivalent; both glucose and insulin responses were significantly higher after glucose or sucrose than after starch.

Table 4–7.   Maintenance of Normal Plasma Glucose in Mild Diabetes Mellitus*

	Glucose		Insulin	
	(mg/dl)	% Increase	(μU/ml)	% Increase
Normal	115	↓	85	↓
Diabetic	130	14	155	82

*Adapted from Reaven, Olefsky and Farquhar.[38] Glucose (40 gm/cm² body surface) was given orally and venous samples taken 1 hour later.

lease restricts the rise in plasma glucose concentration even among individuals on a high-carbohydrate diet.[36] The glucose and insulin response also varies depending upon the type of carbohydrate in the meal, as shown in Table 4–6.[37] The maximal glucose and insulin response is highest with glucose or sucrose as the source of the final monosaccharide and is much lower when given in the form of starch polysaccharide. This is at first somewhat surprising since starch is rapidly hydrolyzed intraluminally to oligosaccharides which are in turn hydrolyzed to glucose at the intestinal surface. However, the starch meal may retard gastric emptying so that the actual quantity of glucose equivalent available for assimilation per unit time may be lower than with the other saccharides. Indeed, this concept is supported by the fact that the starch meal produces a more prolonged rise in the plasma glucose level than the sucrose or glucose meal.[37]

Patients with mild diabetes mellitus maintain a normal glucose tolerance curve even though their serum insulin levels increase by 80 per cent (about 15 per cent is a normal increase) (Table 4–7). The metabolic response to dietary carbohydrates is precise, and there is only a slight increase in plasma glucose followed by a prompt decline toward fasting levels.[38]

BIBLIOGRAPHY

1. Jerome: In *Carbohydrates in Health* (Hood, Ed.). Avi Publishing Company, Westport, 1977.
2. Fogel and Gray: J. Appl. Physiol., *35*, 263, 1973.
3. Gray: N. Engl. J. Med., *292*, 1225, 1975.
4. Gray and Santiago: Gastroenterology, *51*, 489, 1966.
5. Gray and Santiago: J. Clin. Invest., *48*, 716, 1969.
6. Kelly and Alpers: Biochim. Biophys. Acta, *315*, 113, 1973.
7. Conklin, Yamashiro and Gray: J. Biol. Chem., *250*, 5735, 1975.
8. Olsen and Korsmo: J. Clin. Invest., *60*, 181, 1977.
9. Rosensweig and Herman: J. Clin. Invest., *47*, 2253, 1968.
10. Alpers and Cote: Am. J. Physiol., *221*, 865, 1971.
11. Gray, Townley and Conklin: N. Engl. J. Med., *294*, 750, 1976.
12. Gray: In *The Metabolic Basis of Inherited Disease*, 4th ed. (Stanbury, Wyngaarden and Fredrickson, Eds.). New York, McGraw-Hill Book Company, 1978.
13. Gray: In *Human Health and Disease* (Altman and Katz, Eds.). Bethesda, Fed. Am. Soc. Exp. Biol., 1977.
14. Sasaki, et al.: J. Lab. Clin. Med., *76*, 824, 1970.

15. Newcomer, et al.: N. Engl. J. Med., *293*, 1232, 1975.
16. Burkitt, Walker and Painter: J.A.M.A., *299*, 1068, 1974.
17. Trowell, Painter and Burkitt: Am. J. Dig. Dis., *19*, 864, 1974.
18. Spiller and Amen: *Fiber in Human Nutrition.* New York, Plenum Press, 1976.
19. Southgate: In *Fiber in Human Nutrition* (Spiller and Amen, Eds.). New York, Plenum Press, 1976.
20. Mendeloff: N. Engl. J. Med., *297*, 811, 1977.
21. Southgate, et al.: J. Hum. Nutr., *30*, 303, 1976.
22. Mitchell and Eastwood: In *Fiber in Human Nutrition* (Spiller and Amen, Eds.). New York, Plenum Press, 1976.
23. Kelsay: Am. J. Clin. Nutr., *31*, 142, 1978.
24. Almy: Curr. Concepts Nutr., *4*, 155, 1976.
25. Story and Kritchevsky: In *Fiber in Human Nutrition* (Spiller and Amen, Eds.). New York, Plenum Press, 1976.
26. Fleischner: Gastroenterology, *60*, 316, 1971.
27. Brodribb: Lancet, *1*, 664, 1977.
28. Søltoft, et al.: Lancet, *1*, 270, 1976.
29. Brodribb and Groves: Gut, *19*, 60, 1977.
30. Burkitt, Walker and Painter: Lancet, *2*, 1408, 1972.
31. International Agency for Research on Cancer; Intestinal Microecology Group: Lancet, *2*, 207, 1977.
32. Raymond, et al.: J. Clin. Invest., *60*, 1429, 1977.
33. Harber, Heaton, Murphy and Burroughs: Lancet, *2*, 679, 1977.
34. Jenkins , et al.: Lancet, *2*, 172, 1976.
35. Tarpila, Miettinen and Metsaranta: Gut, *19*, 137, 1978.
36. Reaven and Olefsky: J. Clin. Endocrinol. Metab., *38*, 151, 1974.
37. Crapo, Reaven and Olefsky. Diabetes, *25*, 741, 1976.
38. Reaven, Olefsky and Farquhar: Lancet, *1*, 1247, 1972.

Chapter **5**

LIPIDS

Roslyn B. Alfin-Slater
and
Lilla Aftergood

Lipids are a heterogeneous group of biologically important compounds which are classified together because of their similar solubility in organic solvents, e.g. acetone, ethyl ether, petroleum ether and chloroform. Also, usually in their molecular structure there is a fatty acid or fatty acid derivative. Fats are the most concentrated form of energy available to the body, providing approximately 9 kcal per gm fat. All tissues of the body are able to utilize fatty acids as a source of energy.

LIPID CLASSIFICATION

Fats are of both animal and vegetable origin and, in foods, consist primarily of triglycerides (or triacylglycerols). Triglycerides are composed of 1 molecule of glycerol and 3 fatty acid molecules, which can be the same or different. The physical state of triglycerides depends on the chain length and degree of unsaturation of their fatty acid components—the more unsaturated the fatty acids and the shorter the chain length, the lower the melting point of the fat. In edible fats or oils the fatty acids are usually of either 16 or 18 carbon atoms and may be saturated, unsaturated or polyunsaturated. Animal fats also contain cholesterol, either free or combined with a fatty acid as a cholesteryl ester. Cholesterol is a compound of physiologic importance, which acts as a structural element in the cell wall and is an intermediary

in the synthesis of many physiologically active steroids and hormones in the body. Vegetable oils have no cholesterol but contain plant sterols which are poorly absorbed by the animal body and, in fact, interfere with the absorption of cholesterol. Edible fats also contain small amounts of phospholipids which are important emulsifying agents and are essential for the proper digestion of fats, in general.

Lipids may be classified according to the following abbreviated scheme:

1. Triglycerides (neutral fats) are glycerol esters of fatty acids.
2. Phosphatides (phospholipids) contain phosphate, fatty acids, glycerol and a nitrogenous compound. There are various classes of phospholipids, depending on the particular nitrogen-containing compound and fatty acid residues. For example, lecithin is composed of glycerol, 2 fatty acids (usually one unsaturated), phosphate and choline.
3. Sphingolipids contain a fatty acid, phosphate, choline and an amino alcohol, sphingosine.
4. Glycolipids are composed of a carbohydrate, a fatty acid and an amino alcohol. Cerebrosides, which occur largely in the brain, may also be classified as glycolipids.
5. Steroids and sterols are high-molecular-weight compounds with a characteristic cyclopentanophenanthrene nucleus. The sterols contain a free hydroxyl group and can be considered as high-molecular-weight alcohols. These would include cholesterol and the plant sterols, e.g. sitosterol.

6. Waxes are esters of fatty acids with alcohols other than glycerol.
7. The fat-soluble vitamins A, D, E, and K are also classified as lipids but these will be discussed in separate chapters.

In this chapter we shall review: (1) digestion and absorption of the three major lipid classes, triglycerides, phospholipids and cholesterol and its esters, and factors which affect or interfere with absorption, (2) transport of lipids between lymph and tissues, (3) lipid composition of various organs, (4) biosynthesis of lipids, (5) metabolism of cholesterol and the essential fatty acids and (6) the importance of fat in the diet.

PROPERTIES OF FATS

Fats will combine with iodine and with other halogens in proportion to the number of double bonds. The so-called iodine number or iodine value (I.V.) is a constant which gives information as to the degree of unsaturation of fats. Thus, coconut oil, composed largely of saturated fatty acids, has an iodine number of only 8 to 10. Butter fat has an I.V. ranging from 26 to 38, while linseed oil has the exceedingly high I.V. of 177 to 209. Iodine values for common vegetable fats are: corn oil, 115 to 124; cottonseed oil, 105 to 115; olive oil, 79 to 90; peanut oil, 85 to 100; soybean oil, 130 to 138. In contrast with these values, typical animal fats have the following iodine numbers: lard, 50 to 65; beef tallow, 35 to 45; mutton tallow, 32 to 45.

The unsaturated bonds can be saturated with hydrogen when the fats are subjected to a fairly high temperature in the presence of hydrogen gas together with finely divided nickel, which acts as a catalyst in bringing about the combination of hydrogen with the unsaturated linkages. By means of this process, called hydrogenation, oils, liquid at ordinary temperatures, can be converted to fats, which are ordinarily solid. The extent to which the melting point may be increased depends upon the completeness of hydrogenation. On complete hydrogenation, most of the common animal and vegetable fats reach a maximum melting point of 65°C (194°F), which approximates the melting point of tristearin.

Hydrogenation is widely employed for converting liquid oils into solid fats in the manufacture of shortenings and margarines. Two processes are available for the preparation of these hydrogenated fats, i.e. either the partial hydrogenation of the total fat to the desired melting point (35° to 48°C) resulting in the formation of trans isomers of the naturally occurring cis fatty acids,[1] or the complete hydrogenation of a portion of the fat, which is then mixed with a sufficient amount of the unhydrogenated oil to give a blended fat with an appropriate melting point.[2]

The double bonds of fats are especially vulnerable to oxidation. The addition of oxygen may take place at such linkages, with the formation of oxides, peroxides and hydroperoxides, which eventually give rise to shorter-chain acids and aldehydes. These peroxides are powerful oxidizing agents, and they may destroy important vitamins present in the fats. This is probably one of the reasons for the harmful nutritional effect of rancid fats. However, the spontaneous auto-oxidation of unsaturated fats is markedly inhibited by the presence of natural antioxidants in the fat. The most important of these, which are widely distributed in vegetable oils, are the tocopherols (vitamin E). δ-Tocopherol is the most powerful antioxidant, while γ-, β-, and α-tocopherol have decreasing potencies as antioxidants. The vitamin E activity is exactly opposite, α-tocopherol being the most active and δ-tocopherol the least active form of the vitamin.

In addition to the tocopherols, a number of other compounds have been found to possess antioxidant properties; these are now widely employed in prolonging the shelf life of foods. The commonest of these are NDGA (nor-dihydroguaiaretic acid), gum guaiac, propylgallate and gallic acid, butylhydroxyanisole (BHA), butylhydroxytoluene (BHT) and ascorbic acid.

A second location at which all fats and oils are vulnerable is at the ester linkages where the fatty acids are combined with the alcohol groups of glycerol. The fat molecules may be readily ruptured at these ester linkages by heating with sodium hydroxide or potassium hydroxide. Under such conditions, glycerol is released and the fatty acids are transformed to water-soluble soaps. The saponification of fats, when performed under standardized conditions, can be used as an index of the average molecular weight of the fatty acids present in the fat. The saponification number is defined as milligrams of potassium hydroxide required to saponify 1 gm of fat.

Ordinarily saponification requires heat and strong alkali, but it can also be effected at body temperature under physiologic conditions by enzymes present in the secretions of the gastrointestinal tract. The hydrolysis of fats is an important phenomenon, not only in the digestion and absorption of fats and oils but also in their preservation. One of the common reactions which leads to the spoilage of fats is so-called *hydrolytic rancidity*. This is particularly well recognized in the case of rancid butter, in which the presence of free butyric acid produced in this manner is responsible for the development of the unpleasant odor and flavor.

Dietary fatty acids may exhibit two important types of isomerism (compounds with the same composition but different molecular structure), i.e. positional and geometric. The former involves a difference in location of the double bond, viz. vaccenic acid (a minor fatty acid occurring in tallow and butterfat) is 11-octadecenoic acid and a positional isomer of oleic acid, 9-octadecenoic acid. This shift in double-bond position may result from processing, e.g. hydrogenation. The melting point of the fatty acid is affected to a limited extent by the position of the double bond.

Geometric isomerism (or cis-trans isomerism) is dependent on the configuration of the H atoms attached to the carbons joined by the double bonds. If the H atoms are on the same side of the carbon chain the arrangement is called *cis*, whereas if the H atoms are on the opposite sides of the C chain the arrangement is *trans*. For instance, the octadecamonoenoic acids, elaidic (trans) and oleic (cis), are geometric isomers. The trans isomers have higher melting points than their cis counterparts. In general, cis isomers occur naturally in food fats and oils. Small amounts of trans isomers occur in ruminant fat, although most trans isomers result from industrial hydrogenation processes.

DIGESTION AND ABSORPTION OF TRIGLYCERIDES

Most dietary fat is in the form of triglycerides. Food also contains some phospholipid, cholesterol and its esters and the fat-soluble vitamins. The total fat intake is approximately 150 gm per day, or about 40 per cent of the total daily caloric intake for many Americans. Since 1945 there has been a shift toward the ingestion of a greater proportion of fats of vegetable rather than animal origin,[3] with a present ratio of animal to vegetable fat of approximately 1.6 and a ratio of saturated to unsaturated fatty acids (oleic and linoleic) of 0.6.[4]

Although the glycerol component is constant in structure, the fatty acids may be long or short chain, and saturated or unsaturated. Unsaturated fatty acids may contain 1, 2, 3 or even more double bonds and may be attached to the different carbon atoms of the glycerol molecule. The fatty acids comprising the triglycerides may be all the same or may be mixtures of 2 or 3 different fatty acids. All these variables exert an influence on the extent of digestibility, on the efficiency of absorption and, in general, on the subsequent fate of the molecule.

The mechanism of fat absorption has

been recently reviewed by Westergaard and Dietschy,[5] Ockner and Isselbacher[6] and Masoro.[7]

The digestion and absorption of fat occur in the small intestine where lipids are initially converted to more polar compounds. No digestive changes take place in the mouth. However, the process of chewing yields a certain amount of separation of nutrients by virtue of the action of salivary amylase on the carbohydrate moiety of the ingested food mixture. Further mechanical separation of the fatty material from the other nutrients occurs in the stomach. In addition, in the stomach proteolytic enzymes act on proteins and the amylases continue to catalyze hydrolysis of carbohydrates. As a result, most of the fat is freed from the food mixture as a coarse emulsion. There is some evidence that a limited amount of lipolysis occurs in the stomach. Some hydrolysis of medium-chain triglycerides (i.e. those with fatty acids with 6 to 12 carbon atoms) has been observed in rat stomach, even though pancreatic enzymes were excluded by prolonged diversion of the pancreatic flow.[8] Also, it has been shown recently that glands near the pharynx secrete lipase that acts in the stomach to hydrolyze long-chain triglycerides,[9] forming compounds which may contribute to further emulsification of fats.

The fat emulsion then enters the duodenum in small regulated portions. The time at which this occurs depends on the amount of fat present in the food mixture; the more fat, the longer the food stays in the stomach. In the duodenum the fat emulsion is mixed with bile and pancreatic lipase. Pancreatic lipase is the principle concerned with fat lipolysis in the intestine. Pancreatic lipase attacks the triglyceride molecules specifically and sequentially at the 1 and 3 positions, forming first the 1,2-diglycerides and liberating one fatty acid molecule and, thereafter, forming the 2-monoglyceride and another fatty acid molecule.[10] The rate of hydrolysis of triglycerides by pancreatic lipase is dependent on chain length. Unsaturated fatty acids are hydrolyzed more rapidly than are saturated fatty acids.[11]

In some instances, as much as 80 per cent of dietary triglyceride is absorbed as the 2-monoglyceride.[12] In man, under normal conditions the 2-monoglyceride is the major compound absorbed.[13]

The activity of pancreatic lipase is inhibited by an excess of bile salts. However, another enzyme provided by the pancreas, co-lipase, binds bile salts and thus prevents the inhibition of lipase. Apparently a complex of co-lipase–bile salts–lipase is the enzymatic unit reacting with the lipid emulsion.[14] This microemulsion, consisting of the free fatty acids and the 2 monoglycerides combined with conjugated bile salts, facilitates the entrance of the fat into the mucosa. Partial isomerization of the 2-monoglyceride may take place at this time, as may some further hydrolysis to glycerol and fatty acid, catalyzed by a monoglyceride lipase present in the microsomal fraction of the mucosa.[15] The water-soluble glycerol is quickly absorbed by passive transport.

The conjugated bile salts essential for microemulsion or micelle formation are not absorbed through the mucosa with the fatty acids and monoglycerides; they reenter the lumen in the distal small bowel and are recirculated through the liver and bile back to the intestine (enterohepatic circulation). The bile acid pool is cycled several times daily through the intestine and liver and a relatively small amount of bile acid is synthesized de novo each day to replace that which escapes absorption and is excreted as acidic steroids.[16] Bile acid synthesis is enhanced during feeding and suppressed in fasting.[17] Each individual bile salt molecule synthesized in the liver undergoes 15 to 20 enterohepatic circulations before it is lost via the feces;[18] 97 to 98 per cent of bile salts are reabsorbed.[19] In the colon, bacterial degradation of the bile salt molecule results in a large number of different metabolites, some of which may be potentially carcinogenic.[20]

The most significant role of bile salts in fat absorption is the solubilization of lipids. Solubilization is necessary for optimal rates of transfer of fatty acids and monoglycerides from the lumen to the absorptive cell. Bile salts aid in the absorption process by the stimulation of water secretion from the small and large intestine.[21]

As the longer-chain fatty acids are absorbed they are reesterified. The first step in this process is activation of the fatty acids to form the acyl-CoA derivatives in the presence of the energy supplier, ATP, and with the help of a very active, long-chain fatty acid, thiokinase, in the mucosa, which requires CoA, ATP and Mg^{++} as cofactors. A similar enzyme occurs in liver and in adipose tissue. The fatty acyl-CoA then reacts with L-α-glycerophosphate, formed from glycerol via glycerokinase and ATP, to yield monoglyceride phosphate or lysophosphatidic acid. Lysophosphatidic acid then adds another fatty acyl-CoA to form diglyceride phosphate or phosphatidic acid. The phosphate group is removed by the action of a phosphatidic acid phosphatase, which is quite active in the intestinal mucosa, to form the diglyceride. The diglyceride adds a third fatty acyl-CoA, forming the triglyceride molecule. The generation of triglycerides and phosphoglycerides from the free fatty acids, monoglycerides and lysophosphoglycerides which takes place in the endoplasmic reticulum has been reviewed by Brindley.[22]

Glucose is a good precursor of L-α-glycerophosphate. Both the glycolytic and oxidative pathways of glucose metabolism are active in the gut mucosa and it is probable that both pathways are involved in the conversion of glucose to L-α-glycerophosphate. It has been shown, however, that monoglycerides actually inhibit the α-glycerophosphate pathway of triglyceride synthesis.[23]

The enzymes which rebuild the long-chain triglyceride molecule exhibit a low specificity toward the medium-length fatty acids. As a result, the fatty acids with chain lengths shorter than 12 carbon atoms are transported bound to albumin, without reesterification, directly to the liver via the portal vein.[24] A fatty acid-binding protein is present in the cytoplasm of the intestinal mucosa.[6] Its presence, together with its greater affinity for unsaturated fatty acids, has been suggested by the observation that, despite the equal rates of uptake, unsaturated fatty acids lead to more rapid intestinal lipoprotein formation.[25]

One of the now disproved theories of fat absorption involved the engulfing by mucosal cells of minute, unhydrolyzed fat particles by a process called pinocytosis. Electron microscope studies have ruled out the absorption of triglycerides through pinocytosis as a major pathway.[26]

DIGESTION AND ABSORPTION OF OTHER LIPIDS

Although most fats contain triglycerides as their major component, other lipid substances are present in small amounts. These comprise chiefly phospholipids and the nonsaponifiable fraction—the sterols, the tocopherols, the carotenoids and, in some cases, vitamins A and D.

Phospholipids

Crude fats contain phospholipids but these are largely removed in the refining processes. However, other foods contain a phospholipid component.

Within the lumen of the intestine, the ester bond at the 2 position of dietary lecithin (and possibly other phosphoglycerides) is hydrolyzed. This reaction, yielding free fatty acids and highly polar lysophosphoglycerides, is catalyzed by a phospholipase A of pancreatic origin.[27] Some unhydrolyzed phosphatides may be absorbed by the mucosal cells, although usually there is extensive hydrolysis of the phospholipids. At least one-third of the dietary lecithin is incorporated into the chylomicron lecithin.[28] In the mucosal cell, the lysolecithin is acylated to form lecithin. It has been proposed that phospholipids provide a link between the glyceride and outer protein layer in the formation of the chylomicrons.[29]

Cholesterol

The daily ingestion of cholesterol in western society varies from 0.2 to 2 gm.[30] Cholesterol occurs in foods in the unesterified form as well as esterified to fatty acids. Esterified cholesterol is hydrolyzed in the intestinal lumen by means of a pancreatic cholesterol esterase to free cholesterol and fatty acids; it appears that only free cholesterol is absorbed by the intestine.[31,32] In the mucosa cholesterol mixes with a pool of free cholesterol of endogenous origin. The endoplasmic reticulum utilizes the triglyceride, phospholipid, cholesterol (30 per cent) and cholesteryl ester (70 per cent) along with a specific protein to generate chylomicrons.[33,34]

Cholesterol absorption is enhanced by the presence of dietary fat. Sylven and Borgström[35] reported that the amount of cholesterol absorbed was directly proportional to that which appeared in the lymph; with increasing chain length the amount of cholesterol which appeared in the lymph was also increased. It has been suggested that dietary fat improves cholesterol absorption by stimulating the flow of bile and by increasing solubilization of cholesterol in the intestinal lumen. Also the increased rate of cholesterol absorption may reflect an increased rate of chylomicron formation after fat feeding. Both cholesterol esterases and bile salts are important in cholesterol absorption. Bile is essential for the passage of cholesterol from the intestinal lumen to the lymph.[36]

The peak of cholesterol absorption takes place in approximately 6 to 9 hours. The absorption of cholesterol from food is not complete. There are striking differences among species in capacity for absorption. On the basis of amount per kilogram of body weight, absorption in the dog, cat and rabbit is 35 to 100 times higher than that observed in man, which averages 140 to 260 mg a day.[33,37] The absorption of cholesterol depends on the size of the dose; with increasing amounts fed, the percentage absorbed decreases although the actual amount absorbed is increased. At a high level of intake man absorbs less than 10 per cent of that fed, whereas in other species 30 to 70 per cent of the fed amount is absorbed. The serum concentration of cholesterol in man is essentially unaffected by cholesterol feeding.[38]

With increased absorption of cholesterol two compensatory mechanisms usually occur: an increased excretion and a variable decrease in the total body synthesis.[39]

Borgström,[40] using nonsteady state conditions, reported that the total amount of cholesterol absorbed was proportional to the amount fed; in his experiments as much as 1.8 gm cholesterol per day was absorbed. Bloomfield[41] found that cholesterol was better absorbed when fed with safflower oil than with butter. Unsaturated fatty acid esters of cholesterol seem to be better absorbed than are the medium- and long-chain fatty acid esters. Undoubtedly many factors affect the absorption of cholesterol: amount of cholesterol fed at one time, frequency of ingestion, type of dietary fat fed concomitantly, age of the subject, previous dietary history and genetic factors. There is substantial evidence to indicate a marked variation in the individual responses of plasma cholesterol when man is challenged by increased dietary cholesterol, with a significant number of subjects showing no change at all.[42]

Sterols other than cholesterol are not well absorbed. In fact certain plant sterols, e.g. β-sitosterol, are not only poorly absorbed themselves but also interfere with the absorption of cholesterol.[43] This may be because of competition for the enzyme cholesterol esterase. This property has led to use of plant sterol emulsions as therapeutic tools in reducing hypercholesterolemia.

Undoubtedly foods contain many other

lipids present in minor amounts which may play important metabolic and

cent digestibility) is calculated by the general formula:

$$\frac{\text{Fat ingested—fat excreted (corrected for metabolic fat)}}{\text{Fat ingested}} \times 100 = \% \text{ Digestibility}$$

physiologic roles. For instance cyclopropenoid fatty acids, e.g. sterculic and malvalic acids, occur in small amounts in cottonseed oil.[44]

Thus, through a process of hydrolysis and subsequent resynthesis, dietary lipids, insoluble in water, are being transferred from food via an aqueous medium through the intestine into the blood. In addition, resynthesized lipids are of a composition and configuration suitable for the next step in their metabolism.

FACTORS AFFECTING FAT ABSORPTION

Digestibility

Although all edible fats are practically completely digested and utilized, the rates at which they are utilized may differ considerably. Fats which are absorbed slowly seem to be as well utilized when they are given in small quantities, as are fats which are rapidly absorbed. When a slowly absorbed fat is fed in large doses, a considerable amount may be lost to the feces. As far as its nutritional value is concerned, it does not seem to matter whether the fat is absorbed slowly or rapidly. Fat which is more quickly absorbed is more rapidly available to the tissues and is less likely to produce digestive upsets; fats which are more slowly absorbed and remain in the gastrointestinal tract for a longer period of time extend the period of satiety after a meal and are less of a "burden" on the fat transport systems. They produce a sustained but lower lipemia over a long period of time rather than sudden large hyperlipemias such as occur when rapidly absorbed fats are ingested.

In general, both animal and vegetable fats are practically completely utilized. Their coefficient of digestibility (or per

Ordinarily fats are digested to at least 95 per cent. Calloway and Kurtz[45] studied the digestibility of a number of natural edible fats (coconut oil, butter fat, soybean oil, corn oil, lard and cottonseed oil) and found that they were all practically completely digested. In studies with butter fat, butter oil, cod liver oil, corn oil, lard and two shortenings, Steenbock et al.[46] showed that these lipid substances were all absorbed to the same extent, with the maximum absorption occurring after 6 to 8 hours. The per cent fat absorbed after 2 hours varied from 24 to 41 per cent; after 4 hours, 53 to 71 per cent; after 6 hours, 68 to 86 per cent; after 12 hours, 97 to 99 per cent.

The rate of absorption of hydrogenated fats is comparable to that of natural fats of the same melting point and approximate fatty acid composition. Since the rate of absorption is influenced primarily by melting point, fats having a high content of stearic acid (e.g. completely hydrogenated fats such as hydrogenated lard and hydrogenated cottonseed oil with melting points of 54° and 55°C) have a lower digestibility and a slow rate of absorption. However, digestibility is not impaired in fats containing mixed triglycerides into which stearic acid is incorporated with unsaturated fatty acids. Also, it has been reported that the absorption of tristearin by the rat is improved by the concomitant feeding of triolein, which possibly increases its solubility in the bile.[47]

Amount of Fat Consumed

The rate at which fat leaves the intestine is at first increased when large amounts are present; the percentage of fat absorbed is decreased since some is lost to the feces before it can be absorbed by the intestinal mucosa.

Age of Subject

It has been shown that infants under 1 year of age absorb fat inefficiently.[48] Also, fat is more slowly absorbed and metabolized in aged individuals than in young adults.[49]

Emulsifying Agents

Emulsifying agents such as lecithin and Tween 80 can increase the digestibility of a poorly absorbed fat and can also increase the rate of absorption of fats which are well digested and absorbed.[50] For example, Tween 80 (polyoxyethylene-sorbitan-mono-oleate) was able to increase fat absorption in patients with sprue (a disease in which fat is poorly absorbed) and in those suffering from certain pancreatic disorders.[51]

Fatty Acid Composition of Triglyceride Molecule

In general, short-chain fatty acid triglycerides are absorbed faster than longer-chain fatty acid triglycerides, with triacetin and tributyrin absorbed more rapidly than tricaproin and tricaprylin.[52] Triglycerides with odd-chain fatty acids are absorbed more slowly than those with even chains. It has been shown that triglycerides with palmitic acid on position 2 are better absorbed than are fats with palmitic acid on other positions, or with other fatty acids on position 2. Tomarelli and associates[53] and Filer and co-workers[54] have reported that the absorption of fats is affected adversely when palmitic and/or stearic acids appear in the 1,3 positions of the triglyceride molecule.

Overheating and Auto-oxidation of Fats

Although the heating of fats to temperatures ordinarily employed for frying and cooking (205° to 210°C) neither changes the digestibility of the fat nor produces toxic substances,[55,56] when fats are heated in air at high temperatures (over 250°C) changes in many physical and chemical characteristics are observed. Viscosity is increased, iodine value is decreased and digestibility is reduced.

Auto-oxidation of fats is often induced by air at room temperature. It is a slow process with peroxides formed at double bonds, followed by their breakdown into ketones and aldehydes. The rate of oxidation is usually greatly accelerated at higher temperatures. Linolenic acid (C_{18} with 3 double bonds) is particularly susceptible to oxidation. To minimize the content of such polyunsaturated fatty acids in edible oils and thereby increase stability, some hydrogenation is frequently employed in processing. In addition, the naturally occurring antioxidants, such as tocopherols, are beneficial in improving stability of vegetable oils.

Calcium

The relationship between calcium and fat metabolism has been recognized for many years. It has been reported by Harkins et al.[57] that, in conditions of lipid malabsorption due to a deficiency of bile salts, calcium absorption was decreased. Further interrelationships between calcium and fat, as concerns the absorption of these two nutrients, have been shown with experiments on animals; the absorption of calcium requires the presence of fat in the diet, although at very high levels of fat, especially those with the higher melting points, the absorption of calcium is depressed.[58] Similarly, for optimal absorption of fat, some calcium is required, although at high calcium levels there is a decreased absorption of fats,[59] especially those with high melting points, e.g. those containing lauric, myristic, palmitic and stearic acids in their triglycerides. The digestibility of fats with a high concentration of unsaturated fatty acids, e.g. oleic and linoleic acids, is not affected by the presence of calcium.[60] In fact, triglycerides containing oleic acid enhance calcium absorption.[61]

The mechanism by which calcium interferes with the absorption of saturated fats seems to be the formation of poorly absorbed calcium salts of saturated fatty acids. The proportion of calcium lost in the feces, or the amount of fatty acid not absorbed because it is excreted as the calcium soap, depends on the type of fat in the diet. In rats, fecal fatty acids become progressively more saturated as the calcium content of the diet is increased.[62] In infants ingesting fat other than human milk fat, both calcium and saturated fatty acids of long-chain length are lost in the stool.[63] On the other hand, Gorman et al.[64] reported that the apparent digestibility of fat and the amount of fecal fat were not influenced by low to moderate levels of calcium and protein.

MALABSORPTION OF FATS

Bile Salts and Pancreatic Lipase

Lipid malabsorption may occur for a variety of reasons. As noted above, the process of converting the triglycerides in foods to the triglycerides in chylomicrons involves many steps. It is not surprising to learn that interference with the supply of any of the participating factors may adversely affect fat absorption.[65] The two major compounds involved in digestion and absorption of fats are bile salts and pancreatic lipase.

Bile salts are essential, not only for the absorption of neutral fat but also for the absorption of other lipids from the intestinal tract. They act as detergents, aiding in the emulsification of fat within the lumen of the intestine. They form micellar particles with fat and/or with the digestion products of fat and transport these micelles to the intestinal mucosa where the products of fat digestion are absorbed. Bile salts are synthesized by the liver from cholesterol; the most common bile salts found in mammals are the glycine and taurine derivatives of cholic acid and chenodeoxycholic acid. Bile salts are secreted in rather large quantities. In man, approximately 30 gm are excreted each day; this is approximately 6 times the amount in the body pool and is much larger than can be accounted for by normal biosynthesis. This large amount of available bile salts is made possible by absorption from the intestine, transport to the liver and resecretion by the liver into the ileum of the intestine. This process is called enterohepatic circulation.

It is obvious that any interference with bile salt production, transport, absorption and storage will interfere with the absorption of fat. A decreased supply of bile salts in the intestine may be a result of the inability of the liver to synthesize bile salts or to effect the conjugation of bile salts with glycine or taurine. When unconjugated bile products are secreted they can interfere with micellar formation and, therefore, also with the uptake of lipids by the mucosa. An obstruction in the bile duct can prevent the bile from flowing into the intestine. Also, an impairment in the enterohepatic circulation due to poor absorption of bile salts from the ileum and subsequent losses in the feces may account for an insufficient supply of bile salts and hence decreased fat absorption.

Pancreatic lipase, which is the most important enzyme for fat lipolysis, may be in short supply if there is an inflammation or tumor of the pancreas. The disease cystic fibrosis[66] also results in a deficiency of pancreatic enzymes, causing impaired fat lipolysis and absorption and a subsequent excessive loss of fat through the feces.

Intestinal Mucosa

Any defects in the structure or metabolism of the cells of the intestinal mucosa may have an inhibitory effect on fat absorption[67,68] as well as on the absorption of other nutrients.

Protein and Lipoprotein Formation

Since protein is a necessary component of lipoproteins and chylomicrons, inhibition of protein and lipoprotein synthesis would interfere with chylomicron formation and would therefore prevent the movement of triglyceride into the lymphatics. Isselbacher and Budz have shown that the normal intestinal mucosa can synthesize protein and lipoprotein.[69] It has also been demonstrated that substances which inhibit protein synthesis, e.g. puromycin, acetoxycycloheximide, ethionine and carbon tetrachloride, cause a postprandial accumulation of triglyceride in the intestinal mucosa and a depressed serum triglyceride level.[70]

Fat malabsorption also occurs in rats deficient in essential fatty acids (EFA). This apparently is not caused by the alteration of intraluminal digestive function or by changes in the uptake of fat by the mucosal membrane but rather by the delay in the removal of newly synthesized triglyceride from the mucosa. Either the formation or the removal of chylomicrons is impaired, possibly because of shortage of appropriate phospholipids.[71] Also, saturated fatty acids are absorbed less readily than unsaturated ones.[72] A genetic disease in which there is a deficiency of β-lipoproteins (abetalipoproteinemia) is also associated with impaired fat metabolism; here, also, there is interference with the movement of lipid from the intestinal mucosa into the lymph.[73] In many disorders of fat absorption, triglycerides of medium-chain fatty acids are better absorbed than are the fats composed of long-chain fatty acids,[74] since the shorter-chain fatty acids are absorbed directly into the portal circulation.

Certain physicochemical characteristics such as smaller molecular size and greater water solubility of both medium-chain triglycerides and their associated fatty acids result in differences in physiologic behavior, such as more rapid hydrolysis, no requirement for bile acid, minimal reesterification, no chylomicron formation and subsequently a different route of transport. In turn these compounds have potential therapeutic applications in pancreatic insufficiency, cystic fibrosis, sprue and other cases of lipid malabsorption.[75]

FAT TRANSPORT FROM LYMPH TO TISSUES

Chylomicron Formation

The major portion of the dietary lipid is delivered to the venous blood in the form of chylomicrons which are transported in the thoracic lymph. These chylomicrons are composed by weight of approximately 88 per cent triglyceride, 9 per cent phospholipid, 1.5 per cent cholesterol, 1.5 per cent cholesteryl ester and 1 per cent protein.[76]

Chylomicrons are formed in the smooth endoplasmic reticulum of the mucosal cell. Although the amount of protein in the chylomicron particle is small, it is essential for chylomicron formation. The presence of large amounts of chylomicrons in blood makes the plasma milky (lipemic) in appearance. The half-life of the circulating chylomicron constituents is of the order of a few minutes in rat, and less than 1 hour in man.[76]

Nature of Fatty Acids in Lymph Triglycerides

It is now believed that practically all of the triglycerides (with the exception of the small amount of fatty acids of short- and medium-chain glycerides which may be present in food and which are absorbed directly into the portal circulation), and other lipids as well, enter the lymph from the intestine on their way to the liver and to other tissues. Although most of the fatty acids in chylomicron triglycerides are derived from the diet,[77] endogenous fatty acids may be incorporated in significant amounts, since the mucosal cell cannot distinguish fatty acids from dietary fat from circulating free fatty acids or from lipogenesis. The fatty acid composition of the dietary fat also influences to some degree the fatty acid composition of the chylomicron cholesterol ester and to a lesser degree the composition of the chylomicron phospholipids.[29] Medium-chain triglycerides have been found to induce the highest cholesterol content in chylomicrons.[78]

Lipoproteins

Lipids are ubiquitous components of cells and tissues. Since they are not sufficiently polar to circulate freely in an aqueous medium such as plasma, they are dependent for mobility on combination with a carrier protein to form lipoproteins; this confers the solubility necessary to allow distribution in body fluids.[79] The classification of lipoproteins is based on the method of isolation, i.e. ultracentrifugal separation or electrophoresis. The differentiation, based on density versus electrophoretic mobility, is comparable in most instances, and often these classifications are used interchangeably. Thus very-low-density lipoproteins (VLDL) are identical with the pre-β fraction (density range 0.95 to 1.006 gm per ml), the low-density lipoproteins (LDL) correspond to the β-fraction (1.006 to 1.063 gm per ml) and the high-density lipoproteins (HDL) correspond to the α-fraction identified by paper or gel electrophoresis (1.063 to 1.21 gm per ml).[77] Chylomicrons, which contain a small amount of protein and large amounts of triglyceride (TG) may be considered a borderline group of lipoproteins of a particularly low density. Information concerning the functional significance of lipoproteins has accumulated in recent years.[80-83]

Recent advances in the understanding of the metabolism of lipoprotein emphasize that they are closely interrelated. VLDL are generally regarded as of hepatic origin. However, a significant fraction of endogenous plasma VLDL may be of intestinal origin.[84] They transport the dietary and endogenous TG to muscle and adipose tissue. VLDL appear to be the major, if not the sole, source of plasma LDL through the formation of a transient intermediate LDL form. Conversion of VLDL to LDL involves the loss of core triglycerides and surface apoproteins. LDL is probably removed by the liver.[85]

The major classes of human plasma lipoproteins, their lipid composition, pathologic disorders and treatment are considered in Chapter 34.

Lipoprotein Lipase (LPL) and Chylomicron Hydrolysis

Adipose tissue and muscle remove the triglyceride component of the chylomicrons whereas the cholesteryl esters are removed by the liver.[86] Lipoprotein lipase is involved in the hydrolysis and subsequent transport of triglycerides. It is located on the endothelial surface of the capillary.[87] After extensive hydrolysis of triglycerides, a chylomicron remnant particle is released to the blood from the endothelial surface. The apolipoprotein component becomes a part of HDL. The remnant particle, which is now rich in cholesterol, is transported to the liver and following interaction with the plasma membrane of the hepatocyte a new apolipoprotein and some cholesteryl ester are released into the circulation in the form of LDL. The remaining components of the remnants are hydrolyzed to free fatty acids, glycerol and cholesterol and further utilized by the liver.[88]

Lipoprotein lipase is more or less specific for intact chylomicrons and VLDL; free cholesterol exerts an inhibitory action.[89] No lipoprotein lipase activity has been found in the liver, but it is present in the extracts of heart and adipose tissue.

Lipoprotein lipase activity is modified by the nutritional status of the organism. High-carbohydrate diet increases the activity of LPL in adipose tissue and decreases it in skeletal muscle and heart; in fasted animals the opposite situation obtains.[90] Less lipoprotein lipase activity has been found in the adipose tissue of rats fed saturated fats than in those fed polyunsaturated fatty acids.[91] The lipoprotein lipase activity increases in muscle during starvation, thus enhancing the release of lipids for energy purposes.[92]

It has been established that the lipoprotein lipase that functions at the endothelial cell surface in adipose tissue in vivo is derived from a precursor that exists in the fat cell. Two forms of the enzyme (a and b) differing in molecular weight have been identified. The proportion of the total activity contributed by the form of higher molecular weight is greater in rats in a fed state, suggesting that this is the form functioning at the surface.[93,94]

PLASMA LIPIDS

Triglycerides are the most variable component of the plasma lipids. They range between 10 to 200 mg per ml plasma, depending on individual variation and time elapsed after ingestion of a fat-containing meal. The peak of absorption of lipid and, therefore, the time of maximum lipemia is usually 4 to 6 hours following a meal. Most of the triglyceride is carried in the LDL and VLDL fractions (after entering the circulation in the form of chylomicrons).

Plasma free fatty acids (FFA) are derived from adipose tissue, are bound to albumin and lipoproteins and are characterized by a rapid turnover. Depending on the nutritional status of the animal, their concentration ranges between 0.3 to 0.5 mEq per liter; the higher values occur in the fasting or malnourished animal.

Phospholipids are less variable, although they are present at a rather high level, i.e. 50 per cent of plasma lipids. Most of the phospholipids occurs as lecithin and is carried primarily in the HDL and LDL fractions.

Cholesterol is carried primarily by the LDL and HDL. Total serum cholesterol in the average adult man ranges from 140 to 260 mg per 100 ml plasma. About 70 per cent occurs as cholesterol esterified with fatty acids. The serum cholesterol level varies with race, age, sex and diet and, probably, is under genetic control. Serum cholesterol levels have been thoroughly investigated because of their probable association with atherosclerosis. Recently evidence has been accumulating that HDL facilitates the uptake of cholesterol from peripheral tissues and helps in its transport to liver for subsequent catabolism and excretion. Thus high plasma HDL concentrations are thought to exert a protective effect against atherosclerosis.[95]

TISSUE LIPIDS AND METABOLISM

Erythrocytes

The erythrocytes differ markedly in composition from the blood plasma. Erythrocyte lipids are composed mainly of free cholesterol and phospholipids. Less than 3 per cent of total erythrocyte fatty acids occurs in defined lipids other than phospholipids. The concentration of phospholipids in red cells is approximately double that in plasma and the proportions of the various phospholipids which occur in red cells are also different from those in plasma. For example, 35 per cent of the total phosphatides in erythrocytes is lecithin, whereas lecithin comprises 75 per cent of the plasma phospholipids; ethanolamine phosphoglycerides comprise 30 per cent of total phosphatides in erythrocytes and 5 per cent in plasma; serine phosphoglycerides comprise 10 per cent of erythrocyte phosphatides and are absent from plasma. Plasmalogens make up 20 per cent of the total red cell phosphatides but only 3 to 5 per cent of plasma phosphatides. Of the fatty acids in the erythrocyte phospholipids, about 50 per cent are unsaturated, whereas in plasma neutral lipids, the unsaturated fatty acids constitute 65 to 75 per cent of the total.[96] It has been shown that the fatty acid pattern of human erythrocyte phospholipids can be altered by diet.[97] In the case of cholesterol, the quantity is somewhat lower in the cells than in the plasma. The free cholesterol of plasma lipoproteins readily exchanges with cholesterol in the red cell membrane.[98]

Cell Membranes

Lipids and proteins are the major components of membranes; the relative amounts differ depending on the type of membranes involved. The ratio of lipid to protein in the rat ranges from 0.202 in liver mitochondria to 1.320 in kidney plasma membranes. It is possible that the membranes that act mainly as barriers control the highest lipid:protein mass ratios.[99] The lipid:protein ratio of myelin is 3, whereas most other membranes have ratios of about 0.5. Myelin has large amounts of glycosyl ceramides, the erythrocyte plasma membrane and myelin contain large quantities of sphingolipid, whereas microsomal and mitochondrial membranes have almost none; at the same time these are rich in phosphoglycerides. Cardiolipin is present exclusively in mitochondrial membranes.

In addition to these subcellular differences in lipid composition, studies of a variety of tissues indicate that many of the mammalian organs have characteristic lipid profiles.

Liver

The liver is the major site of lipid metabolism. Most of the triglyceride circulating in the blood is initially removed by the liver.[100] Here it undergoes a variety of energy-producing and energy-consuming processes, the two most important being fatty acid oxidation and fatty acid synthesis. Fatty acids become available for oxidation in the liver through three sources: (1) synthesis in the liver from dietary carbohydrate when provided in excess of need, (2) hydrolysis of the chylomicron triglyceride derived from dietary fat and (3) mobilization of free fatty acids from adipose tissue via an albumin complex in the blood.

The usual disposition of free fatty acids is conversion to triglyceride. There are various factors which regulate the amount of triglyceride which is stored in the liver. One of the processes by which excess triglyceride is removed is through the oxidation of the triglyceride fatty acids to CO_2 and H_2O preceded by lipolysis of the triglyceride to free fatty acids + glycerol.

Fatty Acid Oxidation. Fatty acid oxidation is an energy-producing process which proceeds in a stepwise fashion through successive β-oxidations. The enzymes required for the oxidative reactions are contained in the mitochondria of the cell and the energy which is produced is stored as high-energy compounds such as ATP. The reaction sequence by which fatty acids are oxidized is such that 2-carbon units are successively split off. In this way the complete oxidation of palmitic acid ultimately releases 2500 kcal with approximately 40 per cent of the standard free energy of oxidation being recovered as phosphate bond energy.[101]

The first step in the sequence is the activation of palmitic acid with the formation of the CoA-thioester:

$$\text{Fatty acid} + \text{CoASH} + \text{ATP} \xrightarrow[\text{Mg}^{++}]{\text{thiokinase}} \text{fatty acyl-CoA} + \text{AMP} + \text{PP}$$

There are three different thiokinases which are specific for fatty acids of varying chain lengths. The second step is an α,β-dehydrogenation of the fatty acyl-CoA catalyzed by acyldehydrogenases. Here, too, three enzymes with chain-length specificity have been isolated. The resulting compounds are trans $R \cdot CH = CH \cdot CO \cdot SCoA$ and a reduced acceptor, $FADH_2$ (flavin adenine dinucleotide), which transfers the electrons through another flavoprotein to the cytochrome b of the mitochondrial electron transport system. The third step is the hydration of the α,β-unsaturated fatty acyl-CoA by the enzyme enoyl-CoA hydrase with the production of the L-(+)-hydroxyacyl-CoA derivative. This compound is then oxidized in the fourth step by a β-hydroxyacyl dehydrogenase to beta-ketoacyl-CoA. The electrons are transferred to nicotinamide adenine dinucleotide (NAD^+). The last step is the thiolytic cleavage of the β-ketoacyl-CoA by a thiolase to form a fatty acyl-CoA with two less carbon atoms than the original and one molecule of acetyl-CoA. The equilibrium constant for this reaction favors acetyl-CoA formation:

$$R \cdot CO \cdot CH_2 \cdot CO \cdot SCoA \; + \; CoASH \longrightarrow$$
$$R \cdot CO \cdot SCoA + CH_3 \cdot CO \cdot SCoA$$

The resulting fatty acyl-CoA is now ready for another passage through the oxidation cycle[102] until it is completely degraded to acetyl-CoAs.[102]

Acetyl-CoA is normally oxidized to CO_2 and H_2O via the citric acid cycle. In starvation or in uncorrected diabetes, considerable amounts of acetyl-CoA accumulate because of impaired carbohydrate metabolism. These acetyl-CoAs condense to form ketone bodies, i.e. acetoacetate, β-hydroxybutyrate and acetone. An excessive amount of these compounds produces the condition called ketosis. The condensation of two acetyl-CoAs releases coenzyme A which is then available for activation of fatty acids for further oxidation. Ketone bodies either may be further oxidized to CO_2 and H_2O by extrahepatic tissues or may be excreted in the urine.

For the oxidation of unsaturated fatty acids two additional enzymes, an isomerase and an epimerase, are necessary; these also are located in the mitochondria. The rates of oxidation for both saturated and polyunsaturated fatty acids have been found to be the same.[103]

Fatty acids with odd numbers of carbon atoms undergo the same type of β-oxidation; however, in addition to acetyl-CoA the 3-carbon propionyl CoA is also formed which, following the addition of CO_2 and rearrangement, enters the citric acid cycle.

Fatty acids can also undergo other types of oxidative processes. Mead and Levis,[104] on the basis of analysis of the radioactivity in C_{23} acids of brain cerebrosides, have proposed a theory of α-oxidation of long-chain fatty acids in brain. α-Hydroxy acids are formed by direct hydroxylation of preformed, unsubstituted long-chain fatty acids. Alpha-oxidation is catalyzed by enzymes located in the microsomes.[105] This process involves a series of reactions whereby long-chain fatty acids are oxidatively degraded with the simultaneous release of carbon dioxide from the carboxyl atom and the formation of a free acid containing one less carbon. The required cofactor is NAD^+ and the intermediate is an α-hydroxy-fatty acid:

$$R \cdot CH_2 \cdot COOH \longrightarrow R \cdot CHOH \cdot COOH \longrightarrow$$
$$R \cdot COOH$$

Carnitine (β-hydroxy-γ-trimethyl-aminobutyric acid) which is widely distributed in mammalian tissues[106] plays an important role in lipid catabolism and energy production. It is part of the shuttle mechanism whereby long-chain fatty acids are transformed into acyl carnitine derivatives and transported across the mitochondrial membrane, which is impermeable to long-chain fatty acids per se and to their CoA esters. In this manner it allows β-oxidation to occur with the liberation of energy.

Fatty Acid Synthesis. When the mechanism of the β-oxidation of fatty acids became elucidated it was assumed that fatty acid synthesis occurred by the reversal of the β-oxidation pathway. However, as a result of extensive studies involving a variety of plant and animal tissues[107,108] it has been established that there are three systems responsible for synthesis. These are (1) the cytoplasmic, the de novo or palmitate-synthesizing system, (2) the mitochondrial, concerned with the elongation of available fatty acids and (3) the microsomal, also concerned with elongation, but particularly involved in the synthesis of the unsaturated fatty acids.

In the cytoplasm, fatty acids of C_{16} or C_{18}

are built sequentially from two carbon fragments. The first step is the carboxylation of acetyl-CoA to malonyl-CoA by acetyl-CoA carboxylase which has biotin as its prosthetic group:

$$ATP + HCO_3^- + CH_3 \cdot CO \cdot SCoA \longrightarrow {}^-O \cdot CO \cdot CH_2 \cdot CO \cdot SCoA + ADP + PP$$

The second step is the conversion of malonyl-CoA to palmitate. This is catalyzed by a group of enzymes, the fatty acid synthetases. Protein-bound acyl derivatives have been postulated as intermediates. The following reaction sequence has been established. During the condensation of acetyl-CoA and malonyl-CoA, a simultaneous decarboxylation takes place forming acetoacetyl-S-enzymes. The intermediates remain bound covalently to the protein by thioester linkages. Then acetoacetyl-S-enzyme is reduced by NADPH to D-($-$)-β-hydroxy-butyryl-S-enzyme and dehydrated to trans-2-butenoyl-S-enzyme. The resulting α,β-unsaturated fatty acyl-S-enzyme is reduced by a second NADPH. Electron transfer is mediated by $FMNH_2$ (reduced flavin mononucleotide). Seven passages through this reaction yield palmitic acid according to the following equation:

fatty acids being elongated at a faster rate than their saturated homologs. This is essentially the reverse of the β-oxidation pathway except that the acyl dehydrogenase is replaced by an enzyme which catalyzes the reduction of trans-α,β-unsaturated acyl-CoA by NADPH.

Microsomes contain an enzyme system which catalyzes the elongation of fatty acyl-CoA to longer-chain acids in the presence of malonyl-CoA and NADPH. Acetyl-CoA is inactive in this system and NADPH is the preferred electron donor. Saturated fatty acids of C_{10} to C_{16} are elongated at faster rates than are other saturated acids; however, the more unsaturated the fatty acid the faster is its rate of elongation. In all probability this system is the one responsible for the synthesis of arachidonic acid from linoleic acid.

The desaturation of fatty acids, e.g. production of oleic acid from stearic acid, is catalyzed by an enzyme system found in the microsomal fraction of the cell. NADH is the preferred electron donor. Microsomal enzymes also catalyze the desat-

$$\text{Acetyl-CoA} + 7 \text{ malonyl-CoA} + 14 \text{ NADPH} + 14 \text{ H}^+ \longrightarrow \text{palmitic acid} + 7CO_2 + 8 \text{ CoASH} + 14 \text{ NADP}^+ + 6H_2O$$

Many tissues other than liver, including adipose tissue itself, are capable of fatty acid biosynthesis.[109]

The cytoplasmic system is efficient in producing palmitic and stearic acids. However, since the organism apparently needs longer-chain fatty acids as well, two other systems are operative to elongate these endogenously synthesized fatty acids and fatty acids derived from the diet. In the mitochondria, acetyl-CoA is the carbon donor and both NADH and NADPH (reduced nicotinamide adenine dinucleotide phosphate) are required. The system elongates fatty acids of chain lengths C_{10} to C_{22} at different rates, with unsaturated

uration of monoenoic to dienoic acids but not to the essential dienoic acid, linoleic acid. Since animals have lost the ability to synthesize linoleic acid they have to depend on dietary sources for an adequate supply. However, linoleic acid can be metabolized through sequences of desaturation and elongation yielding arachidonic acid and the longer-chain polyunsaturated fatty acids (PUFA).

Lipid Accumulation. Because of its activity in all aspects of lipid metabolism, a multiplicity of conditions can contribute to an accumulation of triglycerides in the liver. The general mechanisms responsible may be an increased synthesis of triglycerides, a decreased oxidation of triglyceride fatty acids, an increased uptake of triglycerides or fatty acids from the blood, a decreased secretion of triglycerides by the liver or a combination of these factors.[110] Fatty livers resulting from starvation or diabetes are due to an increased mobilization of fatty acids from adipose tissue; a decreased phospholipid synthesis resulting from choline deficiency may also be involved in the impaired lipid removal from the liver.[111] The administration of ethionine, which interferes with lipoprotein synthesis, also may be responsible for neutral fat accumulation.[112] Poisons, such as CCl_4,[113] and drugs, such as puromycin, produce fatty livers together with a decreased plasma lipoprotein level.[114] Orotic acid, which interferes with the normal formation of hepatic nucleotides, causes fatty livers accompanied by low plasma lipoproteins.[115] A fatty liver can result in man from acute or chronic ethanol ingestion.[116] Liver injury is commonly produced when ethanol is ingested in conjunction with deficient, low-fat diets. A diet with 25 per cent of calories as fat appears to be optimal for minimizing the steatogenic effects of ethanol.[117] Hepatic lipid deposition after ethanol administration is accompanied by an increased release of lipoproteins into the blood. However, this adaptive mechanism is generally insufficient to prevent hepatic steatosis. Administration of dietary triglycerides containing medium-chain rather than long-chain fatty acids reduces the ability of alcohol to produce fatty liver in rats.[118] Fatty livers may also be attributable to a deficiency of essential fatty acids, probably in part because of a depressed phospholipid synthesis. An abnormal accumulation of cholesterol also occurs in essential fatty acid deficiency.[119]

Adipose Tissue

Approximately 85 per cent of the fuel reserves of an average adult man is as lipids, 98 per cent of which is stored as triglycerides in adipose tissue.[120,121] This is the final site of deposition of dietary fatty acids in excess of caloric requirement.

Adipose tissue is important as a source of energy in the newborn and in infancy.[122] The lipid content accounts for 40 per cent by weight of the adipose tissue of the newborn and increases with increasing age.[123] Age also has a major influence on the fatty acid composition of the superficial depot fat of children.[124] Linoleic acid appears to be high in the infant, and thereafter decreases.

No sex differences were found at the early stages of development; however, some differences in fatty acids, i.e. lower oleic and higher stearic acid content, have been reported in normal adult males as compared with normal adult females.[125] Inhabitants of the United States have higher levels of myristic, palmitic, stearic and oleic acids and lower levels of palmitoleic, linoleic and linolenic acids in adipose tissue than their Japanese counterparts. In addition, linoleic acid seems to decrease with age in the United States, whereas the Japanese have a higher content of polyunsaturated acids and no correlation with age.[126]

The composition of fat in the fat depots is sensitive to dietary unsaturated fatty acids. The proportions of linoleic and linolenic acids present are functions of their content in the diet. Changes in fatty acid patterns in adipose tissue induced by the diet appear slowly over a period of months.[127] In men fed an unsaturated fat diet for prolonged periods, the linoleic acid content of adipose tissue rose from 11 per cent of the total fatty acids to 32 per cent after 5 years.[128] When animals are exposed to a cold temperature they deposit more liquid fats with a lower melting point and a higher iodine number than in warmer climates.[129]

The process of fat deposition starts at the endothelial surface of the capillaries supplying the adipose tissue depots. Lipoprotein lipase catalyzes the hydrolysis of the triglyceride components of the chylomicrons (and VLDL) to yield free fatty acids and glycerol.[130] Much of this free fatty acid is taken up by the adipocyte and, with L-α-glycerophosphate, which originates from glucose, is converted to triglyceride and deposited in the lipid vacuole of the adipocyte. The glycerol produced is released by adipose tissue and is not utilized for resynthesis of triglycerides, since the enzyme glycerokinase is not usually present in adipose tissue.[131] The correlation between fat-induced hyperlipemia and the tissue level of lipoprotein lipase provides supportive evidence for the functioning of lipoprotein lipase in the uptake of chylomicron triglyceride by the tissues. However, the exchange of plasma triglyceride fatty acids with those of the liver is much more rapid than any net uptake by adipose tissue.[132] Thus, most of the triglycerides appearing in adipose tissue have previously gone through resynthesis in the liver and have lost most of their original identity.

Insulin is intimately involved in the mechanism of fat deposition, since increased secretion following a meal promotes the generation of α-glycerophosphate needed for triglyceride formation and stimulates glycerokinase activity of adipocytes.[133] Lipoprotein lipase activity is also increased under these conditions.

A reciprocal regulation of lipoprotein lipase activity has been established in rat adipocytes.[134] Cyclic AMP (adenosine-3′,5′-monophosphate) activates hormone-sensitive lipase, resulting in the production of free fatty acids. In the presence of glucose and insulin, some of the free fatty acids are reesterified to triglycerides, leading to an increased consumption of ATP and, hence, to a decrease in protein synthesis and consequent reduction in lipase activity.

A normal adult human is estimated to have about 25 billion adipocytes which constitute the actual reservoir of lipids.[135] Hirsch and Han[136] have investigated the effects of age, food restriction and hyperphagia on adipose cellularity in rats. They have established that the number of adipose tissue cells in the normal rat increases up to 15 weeks of age. Subsequently, however, the increase in adipose depot size occurs solely through an increase in cell size, i.e. the amount of lipid per cell. While food deprivation during the first 3 weeks of life leads to a reduction in cell number, as well as in cell size, at a later age starvation has no effect on cell number.[137] This concept, however, has been challenged by Stiles et al.,[138] who found that the number of adipocytes increased in the epididymal depot of rats between 26 and 52 weeks of age. Also feeding high-fat diets to adult mice and rats has resulted in increased numbers of adipocytes in certain depots.[139]

Obesity has been defined as that bodily state in which there is excessive accumulation of fat in both the relative and the absolute sense. It occurs as the result of substrate excess, when food intake exceeds the rate at which foodstuffs are combusted, and also when there is enhanced insulin activity.[140] In a limited survey of obese children, it has been shown that the degree of hyperinsulinemia was a function of duration of obesity and thus correlated with excess fat.[141]

On the other hand, the decrease of basal calorie requirement with age is such that obesity can develop even if food intake is reduced to some extent.[142]

Adipose tissue triglycerides are released as their hydrolyzed products, i.e. fatty acids and glycerol. The rate of fatty acid release from stored adipose tissue triglycerides during periods of caloric deficiency and stress is determined by the relative rates of hydrolysis of these triglycerides, of reesterification of fatty acids and of transport of fatty acids from the cell into blood where they can combine with albumin.[143] Free fatty acids from adipose tissue are utilized in many organs and supply a considerable portion of the metabolic energy of heart and skeletal muscle. The liver utilizes large quantities, which it removes from the circulation.

In fasting mammals there is a high rate of hormone-sensitive triglyceride lipase activity and a low rate of triglyceride biosynthesis in the adipose tissue. Therefore fat mobilization occurs at high rates; very little fat mobilization occurs in fed animals. Catecholamines play a well-defined role in fat mobilization from adipose tissue.[144] They activate lipases by increasing the concentration of cyclic AMP in adipose tissue cells. Tissues of mammals contain compounds called prostaglandins which can modify fat mobilization. These are biosynthesized from the essential fatty acids. In metabolic obesity there may be a biochemical error leading to overproduction of prostaglandins with resultant impaired lipolysis. In addition, prostaglandins may affect lipogenesis.[145]

Gonadal Lipids

The importance of lipids in gonadal function became apparent when male and female rats placed on diets deficient in essential fatty acids exhibited impaired reproductive performance. Analyses of rat testes reveal that 80 per cent of the lipid occurs as phospholipid,[146] predominantly phosphatidylcholine. The major saturated fatty acid of the phospholipid fraction is palmitic, whereas arachidonic acid is the major polyenoic acid. The highly unsaturated docosapentaenoic fatty acid is also present in considerable quantity. The high concentration of this 22-carbon polyenoic fatty acid with 5 double bonds is characteristic of testis tissue in a variety of mammals[147] and seems to be correlated with spermatogenesis and maturation of sperm. A decrease in essential fatty acid content of testes with age corresponds with the involution of the active tissue.[148] Polyenoic fatty acids appear to be functionally important in gonadal tissue, in general, since it has been reported that a high content of PUFA derived from linoleic acid is a characteristic component of Graafian follicle in beef and pork.[149]

Rat testes also contain small quantities of triglycerides and cholesterol; most of the cholesterol is unesterified (96 per cent).[146] However, in ovaries approximately 70 per cent of the cholesterol is esterified.[150] The cholesterol content of the ovary has been shown in the rat to fluctuate with the estrous cycle. Cholesteryl ester depletion occurs simultaneously with steroid hormone secretion in both adrenal and ovarian tissue,[151] resulting apparently from the conversion of cholesterol to pregnenolone. In general, ovarian cholesterol turns over rapidly.[152] Ovaries also contain rather high levels of PUFA, e.g. arachidonic and docosatetraenoic acids.[153]

Adrenal Lipids

The adrenal cortex contains a significant proportion of cholesteryl esters. The cholesterol concentration, particularly cholesteryl arachidonate, is easily decreased by stresses, such as infection, and by hormone treatment.[154] Cholesterol is an obligatory precursor in the biosynthetic pathway of adrenocortical steroids.[155] The apparent selectivity in depletion of cholesteryl esters is probably caused by differences in their rates of hydrolysis.[156] Adrenals are among the most active of the tissues capable of removing cholesteryl esters from plasma.[157]

Takayasu et al.[158] compared the fatty acid composition of human and rat adrenal lipids. The adrenal phospholipid contained about 20 per cent arachidonate in man and about 40 per cent in rats. The docosatetraenoic acid content was also particularly high in the rat and was a major component in human adrenal cholesterol esters. The type of fatty acids incorporated into the cholesteryl ester fraction can be influenced by the fatty acid composition of dietary lipids.[159]

Brain

Brain tissue is particularly rich in lipids. Brain lipids are formed to a large extent before, or immediately after, birth and are then considered to be relatively stable from a metabolic point of view. However, a reduced deposition of brain lipids, as well as an alteration in the fatty acid portion of the phospholipid molecules, was reported when essential fatty acid deficiency was induced early in experimental animals.[160]

Myelination and elongation of fatty acid chains are closely related.[161] Myelin contains high levels of galactolipids, plasmalogens and cholesterol.[162] Seventy per cent of total rat brain cholesterol is contained in myelin, as is practically all of the cerebroside, most of the phosphatidylethanolamine, and 70 per cent of total sulfatides and sphingomyelin.[163] A reduced rate of growth (from malnutrition) causes a delay in the accumulation of lipids in myelin. Myelin composition is fixed and a deficiency of one of the lipid components limits the assembly of the whole lipid portion of the membrane.[164]

Apparently, dietary fatty acids can influence the composition of brain fatty acids.[165] Free fatty acids seem to be the preferred form of transport into the brain.[166] Dhopeshwarkar and Mead[167,168] have shown that palmitate and oleate (as well as linoleate and linolenate) can penetrate the brain tissue lipids without prior degradation by β-oxidation to acetate. These workers[169] have also observed that elongation of fatty acids is more pronounced in the adult brain than in weanling rats. It has been postulated that rat brain may require different amounts of essential fatty acids during aging.[170] The rate of incorporation of arachidonate into the brain glycerolipids was found to be faster than that of the stearate.[171] A large group of even- and odd-numbered α-hydroxy fatty acids with 20 to 26 carbon atoms occurs in brain cerebrosides.[172]

Ketone bodies have been shown to be utilized for fatty acid and sterol synthesis by the brain. The capacity of the brain of developing rats to synthesize complex lipids and produce energy is higher with ketone bodies than with glucose.[173]

Cholesterol in brain is primarily unesterified. During myelination the concentration of esterified cholesterol never exceeds 2 per cent[174] and later it constitutes only 0.1 to 0.2 per cent of the total. After completion of the myelination process, cholesteryl arachidonate is the major ester. During early development large amounts of desmosterol are found in rat brain but they later disappear.[175] Possibly both cholesterol esters and desmosterol may have important roles in sterol synthesis and metabolism during development, differentiation and myelination. In the adult brain, the turnover of brain cholesterol is considerably slower than it is in other tissues.

CHOLESTEROL METABOLISM

Cholesterol is an integral part of cell structure and is synthesized in most tissues, with the possible exception of adult brain. Liver is probably the most active site of cholesterol genesis, although, in man, the extrahepatic tissues biosynthesize more cholesterol than does the liver.[176] In man no more than 40 per cent of circulating cholesterol is derived from the diet even when high-cholesterol diets are consumed.[177] There is a difference in the dietary regulation of cholesterol synthesis between the liver and extrahepatic tissues and between animals and man. In rats and other animals, a negative feedback mechanism operates and, therefore, feeding cholesterol to animals produces a marked suppression of hepatic cholesterol synthesis; however, no significant changes are induced in the gastrointestinal tract. In man, exogenous cholesterol does not suppress cholesterol genesis in extrahepatic tissues and there is still some controversy as to the effect on liver; the existence of a negative feedback control is indeed questionable.[176,178] The rate of cholesterol synthesis in the human intestine may approximate that of cholesterol genesis in the human liver.[33] The concentration of bile may be involved in controlling cholesterol synthesis in the intestine.

The entire cholesterol molecule is biosynthesized from acetyl groups. The complete chemical synthesis of cholesterol and squalene from labeled precursors followed by complete chemical degradation [179,180] made it possible to identify the origin of each carbon atom of the molecule.

Cholesterol biosynthesis may be considered as a sequence of reactions: (1) the conversion of acetyl-CoA to mevalonic acid, (2) the conversion of mevalonic acid through geraniol and farnesol to squalene, (3) the cyclization of squalene to lanosterol and (4) the conversion of lanosterol to cholesterol. One of the important metabolic sites at which cholesterol synthesis is regulated has been demonstrated by Gould and Popják[181] to be the reduction of β-hydroxy-β-methyl-glutaryl-CoA to mevalonate. Other studies[182] have suggested that additional sites beyond the mevalonate stage might also be inhibited by starvation, by high cholesterol diets and by drugs. Also the sterol carrier protein which can be altered by dietary manipulations may play a role in modulating sterol synthesis.[183]

Plasma cholesteryl esters originate in both the liver and plasma.[184] Whereas cholesteryl arachidonate is the major ester in rat plasma, cholesteryl oleate predominates in the liver unless the diet contains high proportions of other fatty acids.[185] Presumably, only some types of cholesteryl esters are secreted into plasma in the rat, but the nature of this selective process is unknown.

The metabolism of cholesteryl esters is considerably different in man than in the rat. The cholesteryl esters of LDL and HDL are similar,[186] with cholesteryl linoleate the most abundant of the esters. Human liver, however, contains mostly saturated esters.

About two-thirds of the cholesteryl esters are carried in the LDL where the greatest turnover occurs. The turnover of the cholesteryl esters in the different lipoproteins is similar in normocholesterolemic and hypercholesterolemic subjects and is not altered by dietary changes, despite marked changes in the composition of the cholesteryl esters.[187] The possible mechanisms that regulate plasma cholesteryl ester turnover have been reviewed by Dietschy and Wilson.[33] Cholesterol in plasma lipoproteins is fairly rapidly equilibrated with cholesterol in blood, liver and intestine and more slowly with cholesterol in muscle, adipose and connective tissues and atheromas.[188,189]

In man most of the cholesteryl esters in plasma are formed as a result of the activity of the lecithin-cholesterol-acyl transferase (LCAT) enzyme.[190,191] This enzyme is responsible primarily for the formation of cholesteryl esters in the HDL fraction.[176,192] It shows some specificity for certain fatty acids, acting primarily in the transfer of linoleic acid in human plasma from the 2-position of lecithin to free cholesterol to form the cholesteryl ester. This esterification is followed by a transfer of esterified cholesterol from HDL to VLDL in exchange for triglycerides.[193] In the rat the activity of the cholesterol-esterifying system in plasma has been shown to be increased during starvation,[194] in diabetes, after the ingestion of ethanol[195] and after treatment with female sex hormones.[147] The composition and distribution of plasma lipoproteins may influence the activity of the LCAT enzyme. High-density lipoprotein promotes this transesterification reaction by acting as an acceptor of the lysolecithin produced during the reaction.[196] Cholesteryl ester turnover is related to the transport of cholesterol from tissues which synthesize cholesterol to the liver, which is the major site of cholesterol catabolism. A hereditary deficiency of LCAT has been reported[197] with interesting biochemical manifestations, e.g. hypercholesterolemia with less than 10 per cent of esterified cholesterol (normal is approximately 30 per cent), high lecithin and low lysolecithin concentration in plasma and a cholesteryl ester composition resembling neither normal hepatic cholesteryl esters nor plasma cholesteryl esters and, therefore, probably derived from the intestine.

Plasma cholesterol levels can be influenced by diet. Alfin-Slater et al.[119] described the relationship between essential fatty acids and plasma cholesterol in rats, and, as early as 1952, Kinsell et al.[198] described the cholesterol-lowering effect of PUFA in humans. The mechanisms by which this is effected are still not clear. Some studies demonstrate a concomitant increase in fecal sterol excretion or turnover with PUFA diets,[199,200] whereas other studies are not in agreement with these results.[201,202] Plant sterols, which are poorly absorbed, also decrease the absorption of dietary and endogenous cholesterol.[43] Saturated and unsaturated fatty acids are incorporated into plasma cholesteryl esters more readily when they are derived from endogenous synthesis rather than from the diet.[186]

A major pathway for the degradation of cholesterol in mammals is the conversion of cholesterol to bile salts, about 33 per cent of cholesterol (350 mg) synthesized daily.[203] This process occurs exclusively in the liver.[204] The chemical changes taking place involve the conversion of the isooctyl side chain of cholesterol to a 5-carbon monocarboxylic acid side chain, the inversion of β-oriented OH at C_3 to α-orientation, the reduction of unsaturation at C_5 and the addition of one or more OH groups at C_7 or C_{12}.[205] The enzymes required for bile acid formation have been found in both the mitchondrial and microsomal regions of liver cell. The microsomes contain enzymes that catalyze the conjugation of bile acids with either glycine or taurine to form conjugated bile salts. It is estimated that about 0.8 gm of cholesterol is degraded to bile acids daily. In human bile the principal bile acids are cholic, chenodeoxycholic and deoxycholic acids.[206]

The formation of bile acids by the liver is under negative feedback control, i.e. the bile acids returning to the liver following absorption from the intestine inhibit the synthesis by liver of new bile acids. On the other hand, when the cholesterol content of the lymph is decreased, as in the case of biliary obstruction, the rate of cholesterol synthesis in the liver is increased.[207] There is, apparently, an active exchange of cholesteryl esters between the liver and plasma lipoproteins, possibly the "remnant" portions of lipoproteins formed through a previous removal of triglycerides by lipoprotein lipase.[208] The plasma contains cholesteryl ester molecules synthesized by the liver, as well as cholesteryl esters formed by the LCAT enzyme. To maintain a constant concentration of cholesteryl esters in plasma some are removed from the circulation as the precursors of bile acids.

Another important aspect of the metabolism of cholesterol is its conversion to steroid hormones. In the adrenals, cholesterol is the precursor of pregnenolone[209] which is the precursor for progesterone, testosterone and estrogens. Cholesterol is also the precursor of adrenocortical steroids, such as aldosterone and cortisol, and of vitamin D formed through the irradiation of 7-dehydrocholesterol in the skin.

It is obvious that the overall regulation of cholesterol metabolism is quite complicated, primarily because of the interlocking nature of various feedback systems. In the liver, synthesis is influenced by the amount of dietary cholesterol, the absorption of which is dependent on the availability of bile acids which, themselves, originate from liver cholesterol. Controls of cholesterol biosynthesis in the intestine are less clear but there also is a strong dependence on bile acid availability. These features of cholesterol metabolism obviously contribute to the difficulty in manipulating serum cholesterol by simple dietary or even pharmacologic means which often produce only temporary effects.[33]

Finally it is important to remember that cholesterol is physiologically important. It plays a structural role as a component of the plasma membranes, particularly those in skin and intestinal mucosa.

ESSENTIAL FATTY ACIDS (EFA)

In the last decade several rather comprehensive reviews on EFA have appeared.[210-212] Research in this area has been quite extensive and rewarding, but much still remains to be elucidated.

EFA are those fatty acids that either cannot be biosynthesized or are synthesized in inadequate amounts by animals that require the nutrients for growth, maintenance and the proper functioning of many physiologic processes. It has been recognized that many fatty acids have essential fatty acid activity but the three most important are linoleic (18:2, cis-9,12-octadecadienoic), linolenic (18:3, cis-9,12,15-octadecatrienoic) and arachidonic acids (20:4, cis-5,8,11,14-eicosatetraenoic); these vary in activity in alleviating symptoms of EFA deficiency. Various deficiency symptoms have been observed in many animal species in response to feeding diets low in or free from EFA: in chickens, low fertility and hatchability; in rabbits, diminished growth and loss of hair; in fish, changes in dermal pigmentation; in rats, loss of weight, eczematous dermatitis, impairment of reproduction, changes in cell membrane function, and changes in enzymatic activity, with characteristic changes in FA composition of tissue lipids. In general, EFA deficiency is associated with decreased concentrations of dienoic, tetraenoic, pentaenoic and hexaenoic acids and increased concentrations of monoenoic and trienoic acids. A diagnostic approach for the assessment of EFA deficiency has been suggested using the ratio of the concentrations of triene to tetraene fatty acids in plasma and tissues; values over 0.4 indicate an EFA deficiency.[213] Some of the deficiency symptoms, such as dry and scaly skin and poor weight gain, have been observed in human infants fed diets low in polyunsaturated fatty acids.[214]

In the rat, feeding cholesterol in the absence of fat causes EFA deficiency symptoms to appear earlier.[215] Cholesterol possibly inhibits the formation of arachidonic acid (which is probably the active form of the essential fatty acids) from linoleic acid.[216] On the other hand, the rate of conversion of linoleate to arachidonate and the synthesis of phospholipids is greater in livers of EFA-deficient rats than in controls.[217] Feeding adequate amounts of arachidonate to EFA-deficient rats cures all deficiency symptoms although the linoleic acid tissue content remains at a level similar to that in EFA-deficient animals.[218]

EFA may be necessary for the efficient transport and metabolism of cholesterol, since it has been reported that, in the absence of fat in the diet, abnormally large amounts of cholesterol, triglycerides and phospholipids[119,217] accumulate in the liver. EFAs undergo chain lengthening and desaturation in the body; linoleate forms arachidonate, and linolenate yields the more highly polyunsaturated fatty acids. It has been suggested[219] that linoleate and linolenate compete for a common system of enzymes for elongation and for conversion to their more highly unsaturated derivatives. For any given chain length, the more unsaturated fatty acid has the greater affinity for the enzyme system. Oleate and linoleate also compete as substrates for the enzymes involved in the transformation of linoleic to arachidonic acid.[220] According to Nervi and Brenner[221] this competitive inhibition may occur at all stages, i.e. at desaturation, elongation and esterification. Saturated fatty acids also interfere with the metabolism of EFA, since, in some instances, an enhanced utilization of residual EFA occurs in animals receiving the essential fatty acid-deficient diet together with saturated fatty acids.[222]

There appears to be a sex difference in EFA requirement. Female rats have 1.3 to 1.6 times more polyenoic acid in tissues than do males.[223] Estrogenic hormones seem to exert a sparing effect on PUFA in the plasma and liver of rats.[224] Although the optimum requirement of EFA for the male rat is approximately 1.3 per cent of calories, that for female rats is approximately 0.5 per cent.[223] Similar differences in EFA requirement have been observed in other animal species as well.[225,226]

EFA deficiency results in alterations in cell membranes. It is probable that the change in the fatty acid composition of phospholipids of the membrane is the primary lesion of EFA deficiency.[227] One of the biochemical criteria for EFA deficiency is the effect on mitochondrial permeability;[228] liver mitochondria prepared from EFA-deficient rats evidently have altered permeability, since they swell rapidly in vitro and possibly in vivo as well, under conditions that preserve the shape and size of normal mitochondria.[229] It has been shown that mitochondria prepared from livers of EFA-deficient rats oxidize substrates of the citric acid cycle more rapidly than do normal mitochondria. At the same time less high-energy phosphate is formed.[230] This uncoupled phosphorylation might explain the increased metabolic rate, the high endogenous respiration and the elevated cytochrome oxidase activity[212] in the EFA-deficient animal.

It is difficult to deplete adult animals of essential fatty acids because of their large reservoir of linoleate in adipose tissue. Even prolonged feeding of a deficient diet may not produce deficiency symptoms, although Collins and Sinclair[230] have produced an EFA deficiency in patients through parenteral feeding of saturated fat. In infants receiving fat-free total parenteral nutrition (TPN) for many weeks, scaly skin lesions, thrombocytopenia and poor wound healing were accompanied by low levels of linoleic and arachidonic acid in plasma and a high concentration of 5,8,11-eicosatrienoic acid (the trienoic acid characteristic of EFA deficiency).[231] More recently, reports of an EFA deficiency syndrome in adult patients during TPN, oral

fat-free feeding or in those with lesions of the GI tract have appeared.[232-235] Essential fatty acid deficiency symptoms have been produced in adult rats by feeding a fat-free diet in restricted amounts until they weighed one-half of their original weight, and then by feeding the fat-free diet ad libitum.[236] It is in young growing animals that essential fatty acid deficiency is produced in the shortest length of time.[237] It is now established that essential fatty acids are required by the human infant. The requirement appears to be 0.5 per cent of calories.[238] Collins et al.[239] concluded that the adult man requires at least 7.5 gm per day of linoleic acid, an amount equal to approximately 2 per cent of the total caloric intake of an adult man consuming a 3000-cal diet. There are some indications that atherosclerosis is accompanied by some derangements of EFA metabolism.[240]

Even though EFA deficiency symptoms have been corrected in some cases by topical application of EFA-rich oils,[241,242] a recent report has shown that this method is not universally effective.[243]

An excessive intake of EFA (and polyunsaturated fatty acids in general) may have some adverse effects. First of all, the antioxidant capability of the body is challenged. Cholesteryl linoleate hydroperoxides have been isolated from atheromatous plaques and they appeared to be similar to those produced by autooxidation.[244] However, most of the natural dietary sources of PUFA are also excellent sources of active forms of vitamin E. The need for vitamin E is related to the amount of PUFA in the diet and in tissues, and this must be considered when the nutritive adequacy of diets high in PUFA is being evaluated.[212] It has been reported[245] that a high PUFA diet did not cause a decrease in serum vitamin E levels in humans. However, supplemental vitamin E may be advisable for an extended period if a high PUFA intake is discontinued.

It has been suggested that a high polyunsaturated to saturated (P/S) fatty acid ratio promotes gallstone formation.[246] Hofman et al.[247] pointed out that this may be due in part to a stimulation of cholesterol biosynthesis. Also, cholesterol secretion into the bile may be increased, causing elevated lithogenicity of the bile.[248]

Similarly there have been suggestions that high PUFA intakes may result in the formation of more bile salts, which can be degraded by carcinogen-producing bacteria, thus increasing the risk of colon cancer.[249]

Further recognition of the importance of essential fatty acids in nutrition has recently been demonstrated by the fact that EFA are precursors for the hormone-like substances called prostaglandins.[250,251]

PROSTAGLANDINS (PG)

About 40 years ago, Goldblatt[252] and von Euler[253] independently discovered that seminal fluid and extracts of vesicular glands contained a lipid fraction with potent vasodepressor activity and able to stimulate smooth muscle. In 1960 Bergström and Sjövall[254] crystallized from many kilograms of sheep vesicular glands an active principle which they named prostaglandin E_1 (PGE$_1$). Three years later, Bergström and co-workers[255] established the structure of PGE$_1$ and also of a series of structurally related compounds.

To date, dozens of different, naturally occurring prostaglandins have been isolated, all of which are derivatives of prostanoic acid (C20-cyclopentanoic acid) and which appear to be widely distributed in animal tissues.[256] Four series of natural prostaglandins have been described, designated by the letters E, F, A and B, corresponding to differences in the ring structure and variations in degree of unsaturation of the side chain.

In 1964, two groups of investigators, Van Dorp et al.[257] and Bergström et al.,[258] reported that prostaglandins could be synthesized from polyunsaturated fatty acids. The conversion involved a ring closure (Fig. 5–1). In the synthesis of prostaglandins from dihomo-γ-linolenic acid and arachidonic acid, prostaglandin endoperoxides and tromboxanes are among the intermediates and metabolites.[259,260] A competition between unsaturated fatty acids was observed in PG formation, i.e. linolenic acid was found to compete irreversibly with arachidonic acid for PG synthetase.[261] Although prostaglandins can be formed from a variety of polyunsaturated fatty acids, Van Dorp and co-workers[273,278] found that biologically active prostaglandins are formed only from those unsaturated fatty acids which have appreciable EFA activity; therefore, these workers postulated that the sole essential function of the EFA was as precursors for prostaglandin formation. However, attempts to cure EFA deficiency in rats by oral or intravenous administration of prostaglandins have been unsuccessful. It is possible, of course, that the administered prostaglandins did not reach the location where they were needed, and it is also possible that there is a difference between administered prostaglandins and prostaglandins formed in situ. However, this is the first time since the discovery of essential fatty acids that the role of EFA as precursors for other physiologically active metabolites has been studied. Recent reports indicate that an increase in dietary linoleic acid intake directly influences prostaglandin biosynthesis.[262] Such findings give support to the hypothesis postulated by Thomasson[263] that the beneficial effects of dietary linoleic acid can be explained by an increased prostaglandin synthesis.

The functions of prostaglandins in animal metabolism are many and varied. Since the highest concentrations of prostaglandin activity are found in accessory reproductive tissues and in semen, it was originally proposed that prostaglandins played a role in reproduction by causing vasodilation, by facilitating ejaculation or by contributing to sperm viability and transport.[264] It has been proposed that, in

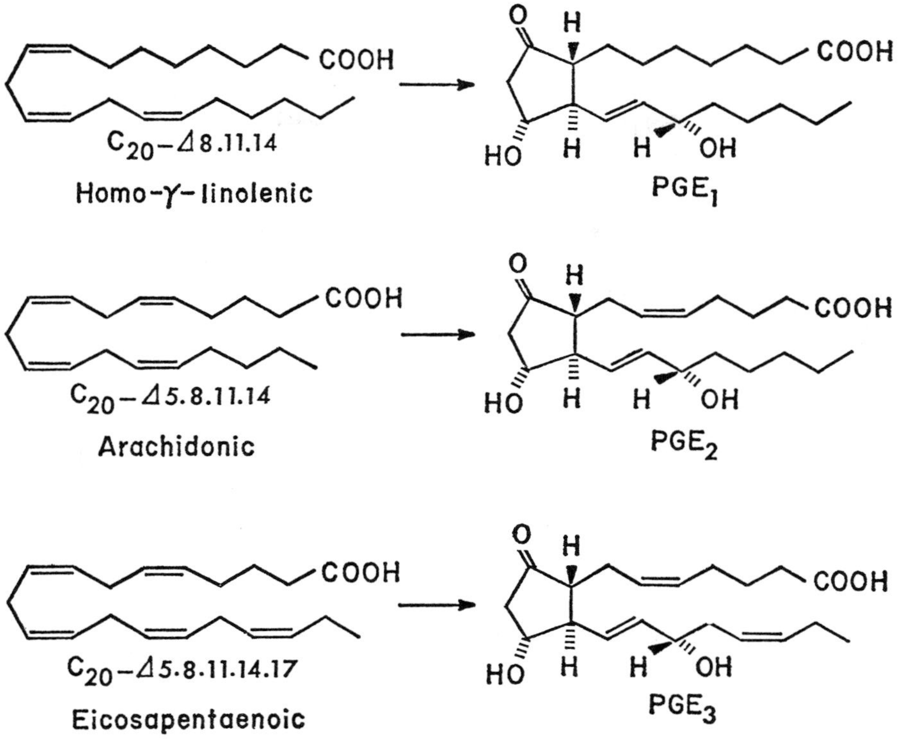

Fig. 5-1. Formation of prostaglandins from unsaturated fatty acids.

man, the seminal prostaglandins inhibit uterine motility, thus facilitating the meeting of sperm and ovum. Although prostaglandins aid in conception, they can also be used in inducing labor and promoting abortion.[265]

Prostaglandins are extremely potent. A few nanograms (1×10^{-9} gm) cause contraction of smooth muscle. In vivo, 1 μg per kg causes a significant drop in blood pressure. Prostaglandins affect heart rate. They are normal constituents of the brain in many species of animals and probably act as transmitters at central nervous synapses.

The prostaglandins are not equally potent nor do they all act in a similar fashion. For example, while PGE_1 and PGE_2 are powerful vasodilators, $PGF_{2\alpha}$ is a vasopressor in dogs and rats.[266] Qualitative differences have been noted among PGE, $PGF_{2\alpha}$

and PGA_1 and quantitative differences between PGE_1 and PGE_2. PGE_1 is a potent inhibitor of lipolysis. In some respects it behaves as a competitive inhibitor of hormones that increase lipolysis.[267] The hormones activate the enzyme system adenyl cyclase, which catalyzes the formation of cyclic AMP from ATP. The antilipolytic action of PGE_1 probably results from the inhibition of adenyl cyclase.[268] Usually less lipolysis takes place in adipose tissue of PUFA-fed rats than in the adipose tissue of rats fed saturated fats, probably because of the conversion of PUFA to PG.[269]

Even low concentrations of PG inhibit lipolysis efficiently. In adipose tissue of EFA-deficient animals, however, there is a decreased release of PGE_2, resulting in an increase in lipolysis and also a pronounced inhibition of lipolysis by administered PGE_2.[270]

Prostaglandins may play a role in metabolic obesity, since it is possible that, in the equilibrium reaction in adipose tissue, whereby triglycerides form free fatty acids and glycerol, prostaglandins favor the formation of triglycerides. If there is a biochemical error leading to an overproduction of prostaglandins, lipolysis will not take place.[145] Prostaglandins may also affect lipogenesis since they have an insulin-like action in enhancing reesterification and de novo synthesis of fat in adipose tissue.

It has been established that PGE_1 prevents the development of, as well as aids in the disappearance of, aggregates of platelets.[271] The endoperoxides of prostaglandins are the compounds which induce platelet aggregation.[272,273] This fact, together with the known effects of prostaglandins on blood pressure and vasodilation, may indicate a possible therapeutic use in cardiovascular disease.

BIBLIOGRAPHY

1. Kummerow: J. Am. Oil Chem. Soc., 51, 255, 1974.
2. Melnick and Luckman: U.S. Patent 2 955 039, 1960.
3. Rizek, Friend and Page: J. Am. Oil Chem. Soc., 51, 244, 1974.
4. Kritchevsky: Lipids, 12, 49, 1977.
5. Westergaard and Dietschy: Med. Clin. North Am., 58, 1413, 1974.
6. Ockner and Isselbacher: Rev. Physiol. Biochem. Pharmacol., 71, 107, 1974.
7. Masoro: Ann. Rev. Physiol. 39, 301, 1977.
8. Clark, Brause and Holt: Gastroenterology, 56, 214, 1969.
9. Hamosh, Klaeveman, Wolf and Scow: J. Clin. Invest., 55, 908, 1975.
10. Desnuelle and Savary: J. Lipid Res., 4, 369, 1963.
11. Hoffmann and Borgström: Biochim. Biophys. Acta, 70, 317, 1965.
12. Raghavan and Ganguly: Biochem. J., 113, 81, 1969.
13. Kayden, Senior and Mattson: J. Clin. Invest., 46, 1695, 1967.
14. Borgström and Donner: J. Lipid Res., 16, 287, 1975.
15. Senior and Isselbacher: Biochem. Biophys. Res. Commun., 6, 274, 1961.
16. Dietschy: J. Lipid Res., 9, 297, 1968.
17. Grundy: J. Clin. Invest., 53, 115, 1974.
18. Tyor, Garbitt and Lack: Am. J. Med., 51, 614, 1971.
19. Grundy, Metzger and Adler: J. Clin. Invest., 51, 3026, 1972.
20. Borgström: Acta Med. Scand., 196, 1,1974.
21. Simmonds: Am. J. Clin. Nutr., 22, 266, 1969.
22. Brindley: Biomembranes, 4B, 621, 1974.
23. Polheim, David, Schultz, Wylie and Johnston: J. Lipid Res., 14, 415, 1973.
24. Jackson: Biomembranes, 4B, 673, 1974.
25. Ockner and Manning: J. Clin. Invest., 54, 326, 1974.
26. McKay, Kaunitz, Csavassy and Johnson: Metabolism, 16, 111, 1967.
27. Borgström: Acta Med. Scand., 196, 1, 1974.
28. Stein and Stein: Biochim. Biophys. Acta, 116, 95, 1966.
29. Schlierf, Falor, Wood, Lee and Kinsell: Am. J. Clin. Nutr., 22, 79, 1969.
30. Keys: In World Trends in Cardiology: Cardiovascular Epidemiology, Vol. 1 (Keys and White, Eds.), New York, Harper & Row, 1965.
31. Goodman: Physiol. Rev., 45, 747, 1965.
32. Borgström: Biomembranes, 4B, 555, 1974.
33. Dietschy and Wilson: N. Engl. J. Med., 282, 1179, 1970.
34. Hamilton: Adv. Exp. Med. Biol., 26, 7, 1972.
35. Sylven and Borgström: J. Lipid Res., 10, 351, 1969.
36. Watt and Simmonds: Biochim. Biophys. Acta, 225, 347, 1971.
37. Kaplan, Cox and Taylor: Arch. Pathol., 76, 359, 1963.
38. Wilson and Lindsey: J. Clin. Invest., 44, 1805, 1965.
39. Quintao, Grundy and Ahrens: J. Lipid Res., 12, 233, 1971.
40. Borgström: In Proceedings 1967 Deuel Conference on Lipids (Cowgill and Kinsell, Eds.). Washington, Government Printing Office, 1967.
41. Bloomfield: J. Lab. Clin. Med., 64, 613, 1964.
42. Sodhi and Mason: Am. J. Med., 63, 325, 1977.
43. Grundy, Ahrens and Davignon: J. Lipid Res., 10, 304, 1969.
44. Carter and Frampton: Chem. Rev., 64, 497, 1964.
45. Calloway and Kurtz: Food Res., 21, 621, 1956.
46. Steenbock, Irwin and Weber: J. Nutr., 12, 103, 1936.
47. Hamilton, Webb and Dawson: Biochim. Biophys. Acta, 176, 27, 1969.
48. Sobel, Besman and Kramer: Am. J. Dis. Child., 77, 576, 1949.
49. Becker, Meyer and Necheles: Gastroenterology, 14, 80, 1950.
50. Augur, Rollman and Deuel: J. Nutr., 33, 177, 1947.
51. Jones, Culver, Drummey and Ryan: Ann. Intern. Med., 29, 1, 1948.
52. Deuel and Hallman: J. Nutr., 20, 227, 1940.
53. Tomarelli, Meyer, Waeber and Bernhart: J. Nutr., 95, 583, 1968.
54. Filer, Mattson and Fomon: J. Nutr., 99,293, 1969.
55. Nolen, Alexander and Artman: J. Nutr., 93, 337, 1967.

56. Alfin-Slater, Morris, Aftergood and Melnick: J. Am. Oil Chem. Soc., *46*, 657, 1969.
57. Harkins, Hagerman and Sarett: J. Nutr., *87*, 85, 1965.
58. Nicolaysen, Eeg-Larsen and Malm: Physiol. Rev., *33*, 424, 1953.
59. Werner and Lutwak: Fed. Proc., *22*, 553, 1963.
60. Cheng, Morehouse and Deuel: J. Nutr., *37*, 237, 1949.
61. Young and Garrett: J. Nutr., *81*, 321, 1963.
62. Fleischman, Yacowitz, Hayton and Bierenbaum: J. Nutr., *88*, 255, 1966.
63. Williams, Rose, Morrow, Sloan and Barnes: Am. J. Clin. Nutr., *23*, 1322, 1970.
64. Gorman, Ritchey, Abernathy and Korslund: J. Am. Diet. Assoc., *57*, 513, 1970.
65. Isselbacher: Fed. Proc., *26*, 1420, 1967.
66. Fernandez, van de Kamer and Weijers: J. Clin. Invest., *41*, 488, 1962.
67. Holt and Clark: Am. J. Clin. Nutr., *22*, 279, 1969.
68. Brice, Owen and Tyor: Gastroenterology, *48*, 584, 1965.
69. Isselbacher and Budz: Nature, *200*, 364, 1963.
70. Hyams, Sabesin, Greenberger and Isselbacher: Biochim. Biophys. Acta, *125*, 166, 1966.
71. Clark, Ekkers, Singh, Balint, Holt and Rodgers: J. Lipid Res., *14*, 581, 1973.
72. Ockner, Pittman and Yager: Gastroenterology, *62*, 981, 1972.
73. Levy, Fredrickson and Laster: J. Clin. Invest., *45*, 531, 1966.
74. Holt, Hashim and Van Itallie: Am. J. Gastroenterol., *43*, 549, 1965.
75. Wiley and Leveille: J. Nutr., *103*, 829, 1973.
76. Eisenberg and Levy: Adv. Lipid Res., *13*, 1, 1975.
77. Seidel: Nutr. Metab., *15*, 9, 1973.
78. Sylven: Acta Physiol. Scand., *79*, 516, 1970.
79. Fredrickson, Levy and Lees: N. Engl. J. Med., *276*, 34, 1967.
80. Bilheimer and Levy: Adv. Exp. Med. Biol., *38*, 39, 1973.
81. Dioguardi and Vergani: Adv. Exp. Med. Biol., *38*, 3, 1973.
82. Smith, Pownall and Gotto: Annu. Rev. Biochem., *47*, 751, 1978.
83. Levy and Eisenberg: Ann. Biol. Clin. *32*: 1, 1974.
84. Mistilis and Ockner: J. Lab. Clin. Med., *80*, 34, 1962.
85. Levy, Morganroth and Rifkind: N. Engl. J. Med., *290*, 1295, 1974.
86. Stein, Stein, Fidge and Goodman: J. Cell Biol., *43*, 410, 1969.
87. Borensztajn, Itone and Sandros: Biochim. Biophys. Acta, *398*, 394, 1975.
88. Eisenberg, Bilheimer, Levy and Lindgren: Biochim. Biophys. Acta, *326*, 361, 1973.
89. Fielding: Biochim. Biophys. Acta, *218*, 221, 1970.
90. Delorme and Harris: J. Nutr., *105*, 447, 1975.
91. Nestle, Carroll and Havenstein: Metabolism, *9*, 1, 1970.
92. Austin and Nestel: Biochim. Biophys. Acta, *164*, 59, 1968.
93. Robinson, Cryer and Davies: Proc. Nutr. Soc., *34*, 211, 1975.
94. Schotz and Garfinkel: Biochim. Biophys. Acta, *270*, 472, 1972.
95. Mjøs: Scand. J. Clin. Lab. Invest., *37*, 191, 1977.
96. Farquhar: Biochim. Biophys. Acta, *60*, 80, 1962.
97. Farquhar and Ahrens: J. Clin. Invest., *42*, 675, 1963.
98. Quarfordt and Hilderman: J. Lipid Res., *11*, 528, 1970.
99. Lucy: FEBS Lett., *40*, S105, 1974.
100. Stein and Shapiro: J. Lipid Res., *1*, 326, 1960.
101. Krebs and Lowenstein: In *Metabolic Pathways. I* (Greenberg, Ed.). New York, Academic Press, 1960.
102. Wakil: In *Lipid Metabolism* (Wakil, Ed.). New York, Academic Press, 1970.
103. Stoffel and Schiefer: Z. Physiol. Chem., *341*, 84, 1965.
104. Mead and Levis: Biochem. Biophys. Res. Commun., *9*, 231, 1962.
105. Fulco: J. Biol. Chem., *242*, 3608, 1967.
106. Mitchell: Am. J. Clin. Nutr., *31*, 293, 1978.
107. Lynen: Prog. Biochem. Pharmacol., *3*, 1, 1967.
108. Wakil, Pugh and Sauer: Proc. Natl. Acad. Sci., *52*, 106, 1964.
109. Patel, Owen, Goldman and Hanson: Metabolism, *24*, 161, 1975.
110. Shapiro: In *Lipids and Lipidoses* (Schettler, Ed.). New York, Springer-Verlag, 1967.
111. Day and Levy: Biochem. Med., *3*, 177, 1969.
112. Olivecrona: Acta Physiol. Scand., *54*, 287, 1962.
113. Aiyar, Fatterpaker and Sreenivasan: Biochem. J., *90*, 558, 1964.
114. Robinson and Seakins: Biochim. Biophys. Acta, *62*, 163, 1962.
115. Creasey, Hankins and Handschumaker: J. Biol. Chem., *236*, 2064, 1961.
116. Lieber and Rubin: Am. J. Med., *44*, 200, 1968.
117. Leiber and DeCarli: Am. J. Clin. Nutr., *23*, 474, 1970.
118. Lieber: Lipid Pharmacol., *2*, 183, 1976.
119. Alfin-Slater, Aftergood, Wells and Deuel: Arch. Biochem. Biophys., *52*, 180, 1954.
120. Cahill: N.Engl. J. Med., *282*, 668, 1970.
121. Havel: N.Engl. J. Med., *287*, 1186, 1972.
122. Shiff, Stern and Leduc: Pediatrics, *37*, 577, 1966.
123. Baker: Am. J. Clin. Nutr. *22*, 829, 1969.
124. Birkbeck: Acta Paediatr. Scand., *59*, 505, 1970.
125. Heffernan: Am. J. Clin. Nutr., *15*, 5, 1964.
126. Insull, Lang, Hsi and Yoshimura: J. Clin. Invest., *48*, 1313, 1969.
127. Hirsch, Farquhar, Ahrens, Peterson and Stoffel: Am. J. Clin. Nutr., *8*, 499, 1960.
128. Dayton, Hashimoto, Dixon and Pearce: J. Lipid Res., *7*, 103, 1966.
129. Williams and Platner: Am. J. Physiol., *212*, 167, 1967.
130. Masoro: In *International Encyclopedia of Pharmacology and Therapeutics*. Pharmacology of Lipid Transport and Atherosclerotic Processes (Masoro, Ed.). Oxford, Pergamon Press, 1975.
131. Ball: Ann. N.Y. Acad. Sci., *131*, 225, 1965.
132. Carlson and Ekeland: J. Clin. Invest., *42*, 714, 1963.

133. Persico, Cerchio and Jeffay: Am. J. Physiol., *228*, 1868, 1975.
134. Patten: J. Biol. Chem., *245*, 5577, 1970.
135. Hirsch and Knittle: Fed. Proc., *29*, 1516, 1970.
136. Hirsch and Han: J. Lipid Res., *10*, 77, 1969.
137. Knittle and Hirsch: J. Clin. Invest., *47*, 2091, 1968.
138. Stiles, Francendese and Masoro: Ann. J. Physiol., *229*, 1561, 1975.
139. Lemonnier: J. Clin. Invest., *51*, 2907, 1972.
140. Rabinovitz: Annu. Rev. Med., *21*, 241, 1970.
141. Schultz: Metabolism, *22*, 359, 1973.
142. Nelson, Anderson, Gastineau, Hayles and Stamnes: J.A.M.A., *223*, 627, 1973.
143. Baldwin: Fed. Proc., *29*, 1277, 1970.
144. Sdrobici, Bonaparte, Pieptea and Sapatino: Nutr. Dieta, *9*, 271, 1967.
145. Curtis-Prior: Lancet, *1*, 897, 1975.
146. Oshima and Carpenter: Biochim. Biophys. Acta, *152*, 479, 1968.
147. Bieri and Prival: Comp. Biochem. Physiol., *15*, 275, 1965.
148. Turchetto, Martinelli and Weiss: Life Sci., *8*, 271, 1969.
149. Holman and Hofstetter: J. Am. Oil. Chem. Soc., *42*, 540, 1965.
150. Aftergood, Hernandez and Alfin-Slater: J. Lipid Res., *9*, 447, 1968.
151. Behrman and Armstrong: Endocrinology, *85*, 474, 1969.
152. Behrman, Armstrong and Greep: Can. J. Biochem., *48*, 881, 1970.
153. Arai and Rennels: Tex. Rep. Biol. Med., *25*, 509, 1967.
154. Aftergood and Alfin-Slater: J. Lipid Res., *12*, 306, 1971.
155. Krum, Morris and Bennett: Endocrinology, *74*, 543, 1967.
156. Gidez and Feller: J. Lipid Res., *10*, 656, 1969.
157. Borkowski, Levin, Delcroix and Klastersky: J. Appl. Physiol., *28*, 42, 1970.
158. Takayasu, Okuda and Yoshikawa: Lipids, *5*, 743, 1970.
159. Egwim and Sgoutas: J. Nutr., *101*, 315, 1971.
160. Galli, White and Paoletti: J. Neurochem., *17*, 347, 1970.
161. Aeberhard, Grippo and Menkes: Pediatr. Res., *3*, 590, 1969.
162. Geison and Weisman: J. Nutr., *100*, 315, 1970.
163. Winick: J. Pediatr., *74*, 667, 1969.
164. Smith, Hasinoff and Fumagalli: Lipids, *5*, 665, 1969.
165. Rathbone: Biochem. J., *97*, 620, 1965.
166. Dhopeshwarkar and Mead: Adv. Lipid Res., *11*, 109, 1973.
167. Dhopeshwarkar and Mead: Biochim. Biophys. Acta, *187*, 461, 1969.
168. Dhopeshwarkar and Mead: Biochim. Biophys. Acta, *210*, 250, 1970.
169. Dhopeshwarkar, Maier and Mead: Biochim. Biophys. Acta, *187*, 6, 1969.
170. Turchetto and Barri: Nutr. Dieta, *11*, 34, 1968.
171. Sun: Lipids, *12*, 661, 1977.
172. Fulco and Mead: J. Biol. Chem., *236*, 2416, 1961.
173. Yeh, Streuli and Zee: Lipids, *12*, 957, 1977.
174. Alling and Svennerholm: J. Neurochem., *16*, 751, 1969.
175. Banik and Davison: J. Neurochem., *14*, 594, 1967.
176. Nestel: Adv. Lipid Res., *8*, 1, 1970.
177. Kudchodkar, Sodhi and Horlick: Metabolism, *22*, 155, 1973.
178. Miettinen: Ann. Clin. Res., *2*, 300, 1970.
179. Cornforth, Gore and Popják: Biochem. J., *65*, 94, 1957.
180. Bloch: Science, *150*, 19, 1965.
181. Gould and Popják: Biochem. J., *66*, 51p, 1957.
182. Gould and Swyryd: J. Lipid Res., *7*, 698, 1966.
183. Frnka and Dempsey: Circulation, *51*, (Suppl. II), 82, 1975.
184. Gidez, Roheim and Eder: J. Lipid Res., *8*, 7, 1967.
185. Morin, Bernick, Mead and Alfin-Slater: J. Lipid Res., *3*, 432, 1962.
186. Nestel and Couzens: J. Lipid Res., *7*, 487, 1966.
187. Nestel, Couzens and Hirsch: J. Lab. Clin. Med., *66*, 582, 1965.
188. Goodman, Noble and Dell: J. Lipid Res., *14*, 178, 1973.
189. Samuel and Lieberman: J. Lipid Res., *14*, 189, 1973.
190. Glomset: J. Lipid Res., *9*, 155, 1968.
191. Gjone and Norum: Scand. J. Clin. Lab. Invest., *33*, Suppl. 137, 1974.
192. Glomset, Janssen, Kennedy and Dobbins: J. Lipid Res., *7*, 69, 1966.
193. Nichols and Smith: J. Lipid Res., *6*, 206, 1965.
194. Swell and Law: Proc. Soc. Exp. Biol. Med., *129*, 363, 1968.
195. Wells: Fed. Proc., *28*, 447, 1969.
196. Glomset: Biochim. Biophys. Acta, *65*, 128, 1962.
197. Gjone and Norum: Acta Med. Scand., *183*, 107, 1968.
198. Kinsell, Partridge, Boling, Margen and Michaels: J. Clin. Endocrinol., *12*, 909, 1952.
199. Connor, Witiak, Stone and Armstrong: J. Clin. Invest., *48*, 1363, 1969.
200. Wood, Shioda and Kinsell: Lancet, *2*, 604, 1966.
201. Hellstrom and Lindstedt: Am. J. Clin. Nutr., *18*, 46, 1966.
202. Avigan and Steinberg: J. Clin. Invest., *44*, 1845, 1965.
203. Grundy and Ahrens: J. Lipid Res., *10*, 91, 1969.
204. Harold, Felts and Chaikoff: Am. J. Physiol., *183*, 459, 1955.
205. Holloway: In *Lipid Metabolism* (Wakil, Ed.). New York, Academic Press, 1970, p. 371.
206. Kritchevsky: In *Lipids and Lipidoses* (Schettler, Ed.). New York, Springer-Verlag, 1967, p. 66.
207. Eastwood: Digestion, *8*, 368, 1973.
208. Goodman and Leguire: Biochim. Biophys. Acta, *398*, 325, 1975.
209. Constantopoulos and Tchen: J. Biol. Chem., *236*, 65, 1961.
210. Alfin-Slater and Aftergood: Lipid Pharmacol., *2*, 43, 1976.
211. Guarnieri and Johnson: Adv. Lipid Res., *8*, 115, 1970.
212. Holman: Prog. Chem. Fats Other Lipids, *9*, 275, 1968.
213. Holman: J. Nutr., *70*, 405, 1960.

214. Hansen, Wiese, Boelsche, Haggard, Adam and Davis: Pediatrics, *31*, 171, 1963.
215. Takasugi and Imai: J. Biochem., *60*, 191, 1966.
216. Aftergood and Alfin-Slater: J. Lipid Res., *8*, 126, 1967.
217. Fukazawa, Privett and Takahashi: Lipids, *6*, 388, 1971.
218. Rahm and Holman: J. Nutr. *84*, 149, 1964.
219. Holman and Mohrhauer: Acta Chem. Scand., *17*, S84, 1963.
220. Dhopeshwarkar and Mead: J. Am. Oil Chem. Soc., *38*, 297, 1961.
221. Nervi and Brenner: Acta Physiol. Lat. Am., *15*, 308, 1965.
222. Alfin-Slater, Morris, Hansen and Proctor: J. Nutr., *87*, 168, 1965.
223. Pudelkiewicz, Seufert and Holman: J. Nutr., *94*, 138, 1968.
224. Aftergood and Alfin-Slater: J. Lipid Res., *6*, 287, 1965.
225. Sewell and McDowell: J. Nutr., *89*, 64, 1966.
226. Reid, Bieri, Plock and Andrews: J. Nutr., *82*, 401, 1964.
227. Sinclair: In *Lipid Pharmacology* (Paoletti, Ed.). New York, Academic Press, 1964.
228. Decker and Mertz: J. Nutr., *91*, 324, 1967.
229. Smithson: Anat. Rec., *157*, 324, 1967.
230. Collins and Sinclair: Aust. Biochem. Soc. Proc., *2*, 19, 1969.
231. White, Turner, Turner and Miller: J. Pediatr., *83*, 305, 1973.
232. Richardson and Sgoutas: Am. J. Clin. Nutr., *28*, 258, 1975.
233. Wene, Connor and Denbesten: J. Clin. Invest., *56*, 127, 1975.
234. Wapnick, Norden and Venturas: Gut, *15*, 367, 1974.
235. Fleming, Smith, Hodges: Am. J. Clin. Nutr., *29*, 976, 1976.
236. Barki, Nath, Hart and Elvehjem: Proc. Soc. Exp. Biol. Med., *66*, 474, 1947.
237. Nørby: Br. J. Nutr., *19*, 209, 1965.
238. Cuthbertson: Am. J. Clin. Nutr., *29*, 559, 1976.
239. Collins, Sinclair, Royle, Coots, Maynard and Leonard: Nutr. Metab., *13*, 150, 1971.
240. Kingsbury and Brett: Postgrad. Med., *50*, 425, 1974.
241. Press, Hartop and Prottey: Lancet, *1*, 597, 1974.
242. Friedman, Shochat, Maisels, Marks and Lamberth: Pediatrics, *58*, 650, 1976.
243. Hunt, Engel, Modler, Hamilton, Bissen and Holman: J. Pediatr., *92*, 603, 1978.
244. Harland, Gilbert and Books: Biochim. Biophys. Acta, *316*, 378, 1973.
245. Christiansen and Wilcox: J. Am. Diet Assoc., *63*, 138, 1973.
246. Sturdevant, Pearce and Dayton: N. Engl. J. Med., *288*, 24, 1973.
247. Hofman, Northfield and Thistle: N. Engl. J. Med., *288*, 46, 1973.
248. Grundy: J. Clin. Invest., *55*, 269, 1975.
249. Rose, Blackburn, Keys, Taylor, Kannel, Paul, Reid and Stamler: Lancet, *1*, 181, 1974.
250. Kupiecki and Weeks: Fed. Proc., *25*, 719, 1966.
251. Hwang, Mathias, Dupont and Meyer: J. Nutr. *105*, 995, 1975.
252. Goldblatt: J. Physiol., *84*, 208, 1935.
253. von Euler: Arch. Exp. Pathol. Pharmakol., *175*, 78, 1934.
254. Bergström and Sjövall: Acta Chem. Scand., *14*, 1701, 1960.
255. Bergström, Ryhage, Samuelsson and Sjövall: J. Biol. Chem., *238*, 3555, 1963.
256. Horton: Physiol. Rev., *49*, 133, 1969.
257. Van Dorp, Beerthuis, Nugteren and Vonkeman: Biochim. Biophys. Acta, *90*, 204, 1964.
258. Bergström, Danielsson and Samuelsson: Biochim. Biophys. Acta, *90*, 207, 1964.
259. Hamberg, Svensson, Wakabayashi and Samuelson: Proc. Natl. Acad. Sci., *71*, 345, 1974.
260. Moncada, Gryglewski, Bunting and Vane: Nature, *263*, —
261. Pace-Asciak and Wolfe: Biochim. Biophys. Acta, *152*, 784, 1968.
262. Hwang, Mathias, Dupont and Meyer: J. Nutr., *105*, 995, 1975.
263. Thomasson: Nutr. Rev., *27*, 67, 1969.
264. Patel: Ann. Intern. Med., *73*, 483, 1970.
265. Kaufman, Freeman and Mishell: Contraception, *3*, 121, 1971.
266. Weeks: Circ. Res., *24*, Suppl. 1, 1969.
267. Stock and Westermann: Life Sci., *5*, 1667, 1966.
268. Bergström and Samuelsson: Endeavour, *27*, 109, 1968.
269. Pawar and Tidwell: Biochim. Biophys. Acta, *164*, 167, 1968.
270. Christ and Nugteren: Biochim. Biophys. Acta, *218*, 296, 1970.
271. Thomasson: Nutr. Dieta, *11*, 228, 1969.
272. Lands and Samuelsson: Biochim. Biophys. Acta, *164*, 426, 1968.
273. Vonkeman and Van Dorp: Biochim. Biophys. Acta, *164*, 430, 1968.

Chapter 6

THE VITAMINS

A. Vitamin A and Carotene

Nan Sen Tseng Lui
and
Oswald A. Roels

Man's earliest knowledge of vitamin A resulted from disease symptoms caused by its absence. One of the first symptoms of vitamin A deficiency is night blindness. Its nutritional cure has been known for thousands of years. Eber's Papyrus, an Egyptian medical treatise of about 1500 B.C., recommends eating roast ox liver, or the liver of black cocks, to cure it. The famous Greek philosopher Hippocrates prescribed raw ox liver for the cure of night blindness. One of us found in 1955 that medicine men in Ruanda-Urundi (central Africa) prescribed chicken liver to cure night blindness.

In the early part of the 20th century, McCollum and his colleagues at the University of Wisconsin and Osborne and Mendel at Yale University were interested in the mysterious ingredients present in natural foods, which were essential to supplement diets of purified proteins, carbohydrates, fats and minerals to support life and growth. In 1915, McCollum and Davis[1] described "fat-soluble A," a growth-promoting factor isolated from animal fats and fish oils. Animals fed a diet consisting mainly of polished rice, casein and minerals did not develop normally unless this factor was added. Drummond[2] suggested later that the "fat-soluble factor

A" should be named vitamin A. Vitamin A deficiency was also shown to be responsible for xerophthalmia[3] and certain forms of night blindness.[4] In the meantime, vitamin A activity had also been found in plant material. Steenbock et al.[5,6] found that vitamin A activity was associated with the yellow carotenes present in plants.

In a now classical paper, Bloch[7] demonstrated clearly that the widespread occurrence of xerophthalmia among children in Denmark could be prevented by feeding them butter fat or cod liver oil. He also proved that the disease could not be attributed to the absence of fat, as such, because children receiving margarine or pork fat suffered severely from xerophthalmia. He had earlier stressed the inhibition of growth and the increased susceptibility to infection in children suffering from xerophthalmia and its accompanying night blindness. Bloch terminated the paper which he read before the World Dairy Congress, Washington, D.C., October 3, 1923, with the following statement:

> What I have said here and proved to you, testifies to the enormous importance of milk as food for the child. No other article can replace milk. Absence of milk from the diet or the inclusion of unfavorably modified milk is the

origin of most serious diseases. By ordering milk, and especially cream and butter, not only is this terrible eye disease cured—which I believe will be discovered in every country when it is looked for—but these dairy products are of the greatest importance for growth and development and for the cure of our greatest infectious diseases.

Moore[8] demonstrated that the carotenes were structurally related to vitamin A and were converted in vivo to the vitamin. Thus, the provitamin status of β-carotene and certain other carotenoids was established.

The structural formulas of vitamin A and β-carotene were first proposed by Karrer et al. in 1930–1931.[9,10] Isler and his colleagues synthesized the first pure vitamin A in 1947.[11] Three years later, Karrer et al.[12] and Inhoffen et al.[13] reported the synthesis of β-carotene. Both retinol and β-carotene are now synthesized by the ton in the pharmaceutical industry.

STRUCTURE OF COMPOUNDS WITH VITAMIN A ACTIVITY

The term *vitamin A* is now used to designate several biologically active compounds.

Retinol, 3-Dehydroretinol and Their Esters

Retinol (vitamin A_1) and 3-dehydroretinol (vitamin A_2) are alcohols with the structures[9,10] shown in Figure 6A–1.

Vitamin A exists naturally in several isomeric forms. This is a cis-trans isomerism resulting from configurational differences at the double bonds in the side chain, illustrated in Figure 6A–2.

The major naturally occurring form of vitamin A is the all-trans isomer. Neovitamin A (13-cis) has about 85 per cent of the potency of the all-trans form, and the 11-cis isomer (neo-b) has 75 per cent of the biologic activity of the all-trans isomer.[14] 3-Dehydroretinol has only about half the

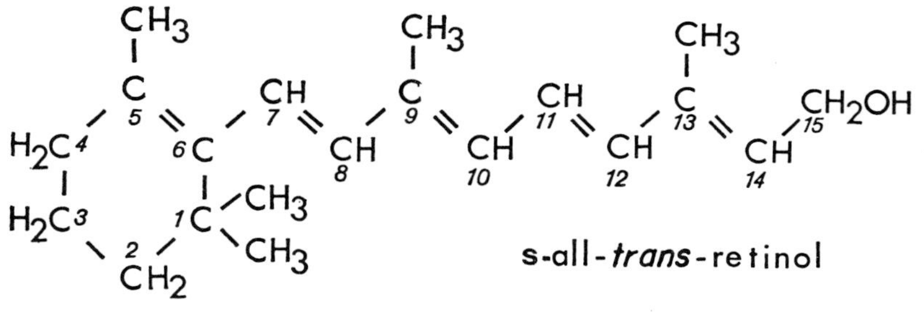

s-all-*trans*-retinol

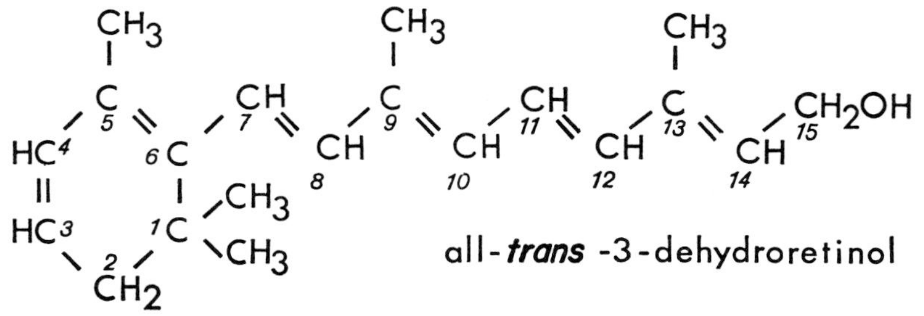

all-*trans*-3-dehydroretinol

Fig. 6A–1. Structures of retinol and 3-dehydroretinol.

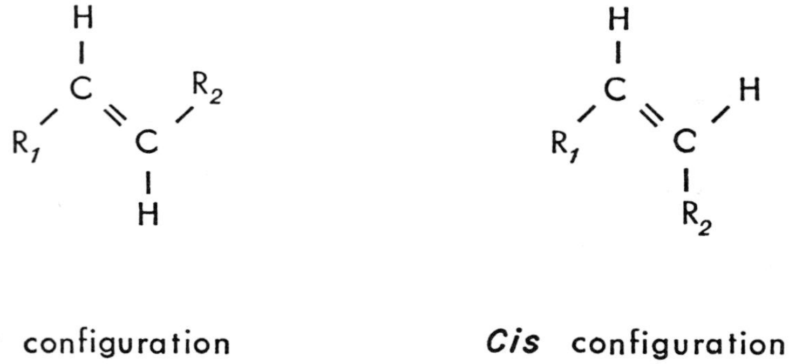

Trans configuration   **Cis** configuration

Fig. 6A–2. Cis-trans isomerism.

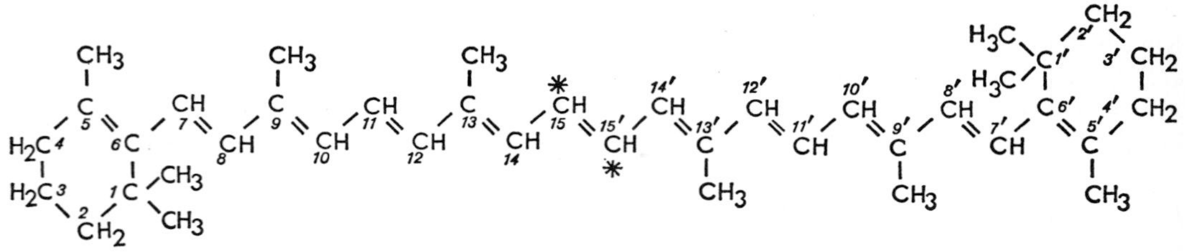

Fig. 6A–3. β-Carotene.

biologic activity of retinol[15] and also exists in various isomeric forms.

$$\overset{O}{\overset{\|}{}}$$

Vitamin A esters (R-CH$_2$O–C–R', where R' is the hydrocarbon chain of the esterifying fatty acid) appear to be the storage form of vitamin A in animal tissues. Reti[16] found that vitamin A was present mainly in the ester form in the livers of various fish, birds and mammals. In mammals, the stored retinyl ester is hydrolyzed by a liver enzyme; free retinol then travels via the blood stream to the tissue where a metabolic requirement exists.[17]

Retinal and Retinoic Acid

Retinal (R—C $\overset{O}{\underset{H}{}}$) is the aldehyde corresponding to retinol. It is the active form of vitamin A in vision[18] and also fulfills certain other functions of vitamin A.[19] Retinoic acid (RCOOH) is the acid corresponding to retinol. It can support growth of vitamin A-deficient animals, but cannot prevent blindness.[20] Retinal and retinoic acid also exist in cis-trans isomeric forms. The structural formulas of retinal and retinoic acid differ only from that of retinol, shown in Figure 6A–1, by having another functional group on carbon atom 15.

Carotenoids with Provitamin A Activity

Among the commonly occurring carotenoids such as α-carotene, β-carotene, γ-carotene and lycopene, β-carotene is the most important provitamin A. β-Carotene is a symmetrical molecule containing two β-ionone rings connected by a conjugated chain. It has the structure shown in Figure 6A–3.

In α-carotene and γ-carotene, one of the β-ionone rings is replaced by the struc-

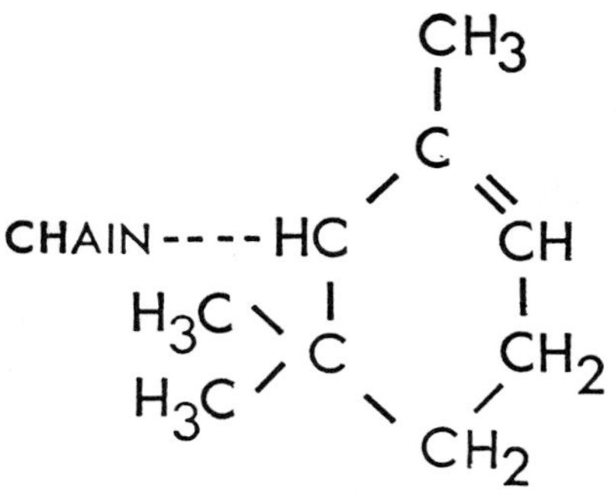

Fig. 6A–4. Replacement of a β-ionone ring in structure shown in Figure 6A–3.

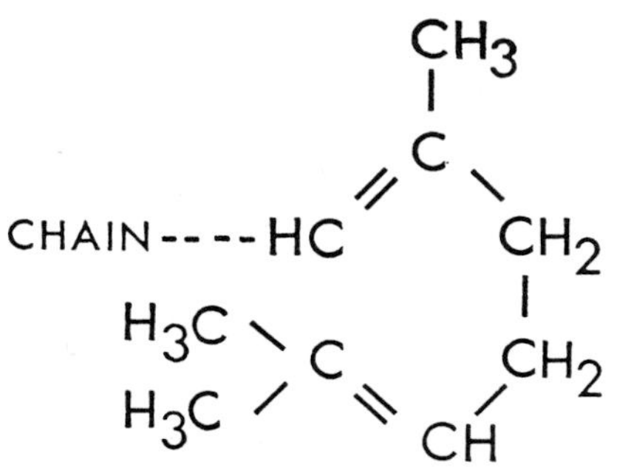

tures shown in Figure 6A–4. The remainder of the molecules are identical.[21,22] The biopotency of α- and γ-carotene is about half that of β-carotene.[23,24] The biologic activity of these carotenoids with provitamin A activity results from their conversion to vitamin A by the organism.[8] The mechanism of this reaction is oxygenation at carbon atoms 15 and 15′ (marked * in Figure 6A–3) and subsequent splitting of the molecule at that point.[25]

GENERAL CHEMICAL PROPERTIES OF VITAMIN A AND THE PROVITAMINS A

Vitamin A

Retinol melts at 63° to 64°C and has an absorption maximum in ethanol at 324 to 325 nm with an $E_{1cm}^{1\%} = 1832$.[26] The vitamin is soluble in fats and in all the usual organic solvents. It is insoluble in water, but may be dispersed in the aqueous phase by emulsification or by attachment to proteins.[26,27] Retinol and its esters have a yellowish-green fluorescence. The fluorescence of retinyl esters in alcoholic solution increases rapidly, then is followed by destruction.[28] In the absence of antioxi-

dants, vitamin A is unstable in oxygen: the oxidation products are ill defined.[29]

Oxidation. Potassium permanganate oxidation of retinol yields retinal.[30] This has led to the use of manganese dioxide as an oxidant to convert allylic alcohols into the corresponding aldehydes.[31] A petroleum ether solution of retinol, left in the dark at room temperature in the presence of manganese dioxide, yields retinal.

Reduction. Lithium aluminum hydride reduces vitamin A aldehydes, acids and acid esters to the corresponding retinol homolog.[32] Sodium or potassium borohydride has the same effect.[33]

Isomerization. Retinal is isomerized by exposure to light. Each isomer gives a steady-state mixture of all possible isomers with the all-trans retinal always dominant.[33,34]

Instability Toward Acids. Vitamin A is extremely sensitive toward acids, which can cause rearrangements of the double bonds and dehydration.[35,36]

Color Reactions. Acidic reagents give transient blue color reactions with vitamin A. These tests are useful for qualitative or comparative measurements. The purple color obtained with sulfuric acid was one of the first methods used to identify vitamin A in liver oils.[27] Later, arsenic trichloride and the Carr-Price reagent (antimony trichloride in chloroform) were used.[37] More recently, other Lewis acids, such as trifluoracetic acid, have been used for the quantitative determination of the vitamin.[38]

Provitamins A

β-Carotene melts at 181° to 182°C. In petroleum ether, all-trans β-carotene has absorption maxima at 453, 481 and 273 nm.[39] Pure synthetic, crystalline all-trans β-carotene, after drying in a high-vacuum pistol, should give an $E_{1cm}^{1\%}$ value of 2,518 at 451 nm in n-hexane. It should have absorption maxima in the same solvent at 451 nm and 479 nm and an absorption minimum at 468 nm.[40] β-Carotene is readily soluble in carbon disulfide, chloroform and benzene. It is almost insoluble in ethanol and methanol. The carotenes take up oxygen rapidly when exposed to air, giving colorless products. This destruction by oxygen is accelerated by light.[41] As do most other carotenoids, carotene produces colors with various reagents, including sulfuric and nitric acids.[42] With antimony trichloride, carotene yields a blue color, as does vitamin A. The reaction is less rapid, however, and two absorption maxima occur at 490 nm[42] and 1020 nm,[43] against 620 nm for vitamin A. Cis-trans isomerism occurs in carotenoids.[44] It may be induced by refluxing the pigment in a solvent, by illumination, by treatment with acids or iodine or by melting the crystals.

THE DETERMINATION OF VITAMIN A AND ITS PROVITAMINS

Vitamin A and its related compounds can be measured by biologic, physical and chemical methods.

Physical Methods

The principal physical assays of vitamin A are based on the characteristic light absorption of vitamin A and of the pro-

vitamin A compounds. Retinol and its related compounds show maximum absorption in the near-ultraviolet.[26] The provitamins show maximum absorption near 460 nm.[39,44] The extinction coefficients of various vitamin A and provitamin A compounds have been carefully determined by different laboratories. Thus, by measuring the extinction at the absorption maximum, the quantity of vitamin A or provitamin A compound in a solution can be calculated. Irrelevant absorption, caused by contaminants, often results in high extinction values for vitamin A at its maximum absorption. To obviate this, Morton and Stubbs[45] introduced a correction procedure which assumes that the absorption curve of the substances responsible for the irrelevant absorption is approximately linear at wavelengths near and on either side of the absorption maximum of vitamin A. Cama et al.[46] have investigated this for retinol and retinyl acetate and arrived at different "fixative points" in different solvents and have given the correction formula in each case. According to these authors, the fixative points for retinol in cyclohexane are E_1 (312.5 nm), E_2 (326.5 mm) and E_3 (336.7 nm). The suggested correction formula is E (corr.) = 7 $(E_2 - 0.442E_1 - 0.578 E_3)$. The Vitamin Division of the International Union of Pure and Applied Chemistry[47] has recommended precise procedures for standard assays of vitamin A oils which would be acceptable in international trade.

The fluorescence of vitamin A has been most successfully exploited by Popper and his associates to detect the vitamin in tissue sections and to study the distribution of the vitamin in the animal body.[48] Fujita and Aoyama[49] described a quantitative fluorimetric assay of total vitamin A (retinyl ester plus retinol) in the unsaponifiable matter of various oils; however, carotene and vitamin D interfered with the assay under the experimental conditions described.

Dunagin and Olson[50] have succeeded in

quantitatively separating retinol and some of its derivatives by gas/liquid chromatography.

Other methods such as infrared spectrophotometry,[51] nuclear magnetic resonance[52] and mass spectroscopy[53] have been used for the identification of stereoisomers of retinol.

Chemical Methods

A number of colorimetric assays are based on color reactions produced by retinol and related compounds with a variety of reagents. Several Lewis acids (trifluoroacetic acid, perchloric acid, stannic chloride, boron trifluoride, antimony trichloride) and glycerol dichlorohydrin produce colored products with vitamin A.[54] These color reactions have been used for quantitative and qualitative determinations. The Carr-Price test[37,55] is one of the most widely used for vitamin A determination. In the test, vitamin A reacts with antimony trichloride in chloroform, giving rise to a blue color with its absorption maximum at 620 nm, $E_{1cm}^{1\%} = 4800$. Neeld and Pearson[38] have introduced a far superior new colorimetric procedure, based on the blue color produced by trifluoroacetic acid with vitamin A. This procedure can also be used to determine retinyl esters, retinal and retinoic acid.[54] The concentration of these forms of vitamin A can be determined by comparing the molar absorptions to those of vitamin A at the appropriate wavelengths. The major advantage of the trifluoroacetic acid method is that the color is more stable and less susceptible to interference by traces of moisture than the Carr-Price method.

Bioassay Procedures

The various forms of vitamin A and provitamin A have a number of common physiologic effects in the animal body. The various vitamin A compounds differ chemically, however, and there are marked differences in their biologic potencies. The definitive assay for vitamin A activity is based upon its biologic activity. The three bioassays generally used are discussed below and are described in great detail by Bliss and Roels.[55a]

The Growth Assay. Young rats are depleted of vitamin A stores until they no longer grow on the vitamin A-free test diet. Different individuals are then fed graded doses of vitamin A or of the compound in which vitamin A is to be determined under standardized conditions, and the gain in weight during the test period is related to the logarithm of the dose. Generally males are used since there is a sexual difference in response to vitamin A deficiency. Because litter mates grow at more nearly the same rate than do rats from different litters, the segregation of litter differences in setting up an assay can increase its precision materially. Coward[56] has used statistical methods to calculate the vitamin A activity of the unknown in International Units. One International Unit of vitamin A corresponds to 0.6 μg of β-carotene and to 0.3 μg of retinol. Most workers agree that, under the conditions most commonly pertaining in biologic testing, these two units have virtually the same activity.

The Vaginal Smear Assay. This method is based on an early symptom of vitamin A deficiency in the female rat, i.e. the interruption of the normal estrous cycle with the persistence of cornified cells in vaginal smears. Administration of vitamin A or of vitamin A-containing compounds leads to quick return of the normal smear. Pugsley and collaborators[57] have developed a quantitative method from this relationship which has several advantages over growth assay in both precision and efficiency. Ovariectomized rats are used to ensure against misinterpreting the response, which is then highly specific for vitamin A. In the range of about 25 to 150 I.U. (the total amount of vitamin A administered over a period of 2 to 3 successive days), the response can be plotted linearly against the log dose of vitamin A.

The Liver Storage Assay. This method, originally devised by Guggenheim and Koch,[58] is based on the assimilation and liver storage of vitamin A by the depleted rat. The vitamin A content of the liver is directly proportional to the ingested dose over a range of 500 to 10,000 I.U. (total amount of vitamin A administered over a period of 2 to 3 days).

THE OCCURRENCE OF VITAMIN A IN FOODS

The carotenoid pigments are widely distributed in plant tissues. They are characterized by their typical red, yellow and orange colors. Since many of them have no vitamin A activity, the occurrence of a pigmented carotenoid in food should not necessarily be taken as an indication of its value as a source of provitamin A.

Xanthophyll and lycopene are among the most frequently occurring carotenoid pigments and have no vitamin A activity whatsoever. Thus, chromatographic separation of different carotenoid pigments, identification of each compound with provitamin A activity and determination of its biologic activity are necessary to correctly establish the provitamin A content of foodstuffs.[59]

Fruits contain varying, but generally low, amounts of carotenoids. Cereals and cereal foods, in general, do not contain carotenoids or preformed vitamin A. The only exception to this is the soybean, which contains traces of carotene. Among the vegetable oils, the richest source of provitamin A is palm oil (the oil extracted from the fruit coat of Elaeis guineensis). The provitamin A activity of the red palm oil from ripe fruits varies from 65,000 to 113,000 I.U. per 100 gm oil.[60]

Preformed vitamin A is found almost exclusively in animals. Human and animal organisms tend to concentrate most of the vitamin A in the liver where it appears to be stored. Other significant pools of vitamin A are found in the kidney, milk and blood plasma. Milk products and eggs are usually rich sources of vitamin A. From skim milk and skim-milk products practically all carotenoids and preformed vitamin A have been removed with the fat. Among the meats, pork, beef, chicken, lamb, rabbit, turkey and veal contain only traces of vitamin A. Fish liver oils are generally extremely rich sources of the vitamin, although the content varies over a wide range. The highest value of vitamin A was found in red steenbras, which contained up to 1,130,000 I.U. per gm of oil.[61]

Extensive data on vitamin A activity of raw, processed and prepared foods were published in 1950 and 1966 by Watt and Merrill of the Bureau of Human Nutrition and Home Economics of the United States Department of Agriculture.[62] In these handbooks, vitamin A values, expressed as International Units, are listed for 751 different foodstuffs.

GENERAL METABOLISM OF VITAMIN A AND THE PROVITAMINS A

Absorption

Carotenoids. In most mammals, most of the ingested provitamin A is converted to vitamin A in the intestinal wall. There is, however, a great deal of species specificity in the ability of different mammals to absorb dietary carotenoids. Man and the bovine can absorb both vitamin A and the carotenoids, and convert carotenoids with provitamin A activity to the vitamin. In contrast, the rat and the pig do not absorb significant amounts of carotenoid pigments. However, they can convert provitamin A to the vitamin in the gut.[63] The small intestine is the most important organ involved in the conversion of provitamin to vitamin, although other tissues are also capable of carrying out this process.[64,65] The carotene cleavage enzyme β-carotene-15, 15'-dioxygenase has been demonstrated in rat intestine, liver and kidney. The reaction catalyzed by the enzyme requires oxygen. The initial and sole product which has been identified is retinal.[66] Two moles of retinal can be formed from each mole of β-carotene.[67] The retinal so formed is subsequently reduced to retinol by a nonspecific aldehyde reductase with NADH or NADPH as cofactor.[68] A number of factors affect the absorption of carotenoids from the intestine. Absorption is significantly hampered when the diet is unusually low in fat.[69] The quality of the fat also influences absorption. The amount of carotene absorbed from raw carrots is highest when low-molecular-weight fatty acids are given, and the percentage of absorbed carotenoids falls as the chain length of the fatty acids increases.[70] Conjugated bile acids with one free hydroxyl group have a stimulating effect on carotene absorption and on cleavage of the carotene molecule in the intestines of the chick, the hamster, the rat and the rabbit.[71]

Vitamin A. The major dietary form of vitamin A is all-trans retinyl ester. In the upper intestine the ester is hydrolyzed by the pancreatic retinyl ester hydrolase and a hydrolase associated with the outer surface of the brush border of the absorptive cells.[72,73] The free retinol is then absorbed into the intestinal mucosal cells in micellar form. Retinol derived from the hydrolysis of dietary retinyl esters or from β-carotene cleavage passes the mucosal cell wall and is mainly esterified and incorporated into chylomicrons,[73,74] but a small portion may be oxidized to retinal and further to retinoic acid.[75,76] Other derivatives of retinol are also readily absorbed: retinal is absorbed as such and is mainly reduced and converted to retinyl ester within the mucosa,[77] although a portion is converted to retinoic acid.[76] Retinoic acid, when administered as its sodium salt in the diet, is absorbed as such.[78]

Transport

Retinyl esters in chylomicrons formed in the intestinal mucosal cells travel through the lymphatic system, via the thoracic duct, to the blood stream, and are stored in the liver. Stored retinyl ester is hydrolyzed there by a liver enzyme,[79] and free retinol then travels via the blood stream to the tissue where a metabolic requirement exists. Only 10 to 17 per cent of the vitamin A content of the blood in normal human subjects in the fasting state is in the ester form. However, in the postabsorptive state, after vitamin A intake, the percentage of the ester in the circulating blood increases rapidly as a result of the vitamin A ester arriving in the blood stream from the gut via the lymphatic system.[80] The blood level of vitamin A is independent of the liver reserves: as long as there are small reserves of vitamin A present in the liver, the blood level remains normal. As soon as the liver is depleted of its vitamin A reserves, the vitamin A level of the blood falls rapidly.[81] In human blood, the newly absorbed vitamin A ester occurs mainly in the Sf 10 to 100 lipoprotein fraction of the blood stream. Twenty per cent of the free retinol present in serum is associated with the Sf 3 to 9 serum lipoprotein fraction, which also carries about 80 per cent of the β-carotene and lycopene in human serum. The major portion of retinol is transported by the high-density plasma protein fraction.[82] Retinol is transported in the plasma in association with a complex consisting of one molecule of a specific transport protein, retinol-binding protein (RBP), and one molecule of prealbumin.[84,85] Free retinol is unstable in aqueous dispersion, whereas the retinol bound to the RBP complex is quite stable.

In normal human subjects, the plasma levels of both vitamin A and prealbumin are proportional to the levels of RBP.[84] Decreased serum vitamin A concentrations have been described in children with protein-calorie malnutrition.[86,87] It has been suggested that the low serum vitamin A levels in kwashiorkor largely reflect a functional impairment in the hepatic release of the vitamin rather than deficiency per se. Hepatic release of vitamin A is impaired because of defective hepatic production of plasma proteins, including the proteins for retinol transport. When dietary proteins and calories are provided, plasma RBP and prealbumin concentrations rise and hence plasma vitamin A increases.[88] Muto et al.[89] have observed a rapid increase in the level of serum RBP when vitamin A was given orally to rats deficient in it.[89] The large pool of RBP which accumulates in the liver of vitamin A-deficient rats can be released rapidly into the serum after the injection of chylomicrons containing the vitamin.[90] The amount of RBP released from the liver is directly related to the dose given.

Storage

In 1931 Moore did the first quantitative determinations of vitamin A in rat tissues using the Carr-Price reaction.[91] He found that the liver contained large amounts of the vitamin, whereas traces were found in the intraperitoneal fat, kidney and lung. When rats are given very large doses of vitamin A, the vitamin can be found in appreciable amounts in the adrenals, and traces are found in the pancreas, thymus and spleen. This distribution throughout the body is typical for many mammals. In birds and fish, the liver is usually also the most important site of storage. However, certain sea birds have stomach oils which are rich in vitamin A and some fish have extraordinarily high amounts in the intestinal wall. In some types of shrimp, the eyes contain practically the entire body reserve of the vitamin.[92] Vitamin A in cod liver oil is present mainly in the ester form.[93] Generally speaking, carotenoids are more evenly distributed throughout the body of those animal species which have carotenoids. Frequently, carotenoids are concentrated in depot fat. The ovaries of animals with yellow body fat sometimes contain high quantities of carotenoids concentrated in the corpora lutea and in the corpora rubra.[94] In rat liver, small amounts of vitamin A alcohol are always present but retinyl palmitate is the dominant storage form.[95] Vitamin A alcohol is stored in the

parenchymal cells of the liver, whereas vitamin A ester is stored in the Kupffer cells.[96]

Catabolism

Within the liver, retinol may be conjugated with uridine diphosphoglucuronic acid to form its O-glucosiduronate, or it may be oxidized to retinal and then to retinoic acid.[97,98] Retinoic acid also forms a glucuronide in the liver, and these glucuronides, together with a small amount of free retinoic acid, are excreted efficiently into the bile.[97,99,100] Retinoic acid may also be decarboxylated in the liver to a series of yet-undefined products, or might possibly lose a 2-carbon fragment from the terminal portion of the side chain, which is subsequently oxidized to CO_2.[101] In the eye, retinol derived from the blood is oxidized to retinal before its isomerization and combination with opsin (described below).[102] The oxidation of retinol to retinal and then to retinoic acid also occurs in the kidney[103] and in the intestine.[75]

Excretion

The vitamin A glucuronides in the bile are partially reabsorbed in the gut and transported back to the liver, in an enterohepatic circulation.[104] Most of the biliary glucuronides of vitamin A, however, seem to be hydrolyzed in the gut, apparently by β-glucuronidase of enteric bacteria. They are then excreted in the feces as a mixture of free retinoic acid, possibly free retinal, the intact glucuronides and some other unidentified products.[101,105]

The existence of a multiplicity of urinary vitamin A metabolites has been published repeatedly.[106-108] Recently Rietz et al.[109] detected several vitamin A metabolites in the lipid extract of human and rat urine after the ingestion of high doses of retinyl esters or retinoic acid. Further characterization of these metabolites after methylation showed four metabolites. The following structures were proposed for the methylated metabolites (I, II, III, and IV).

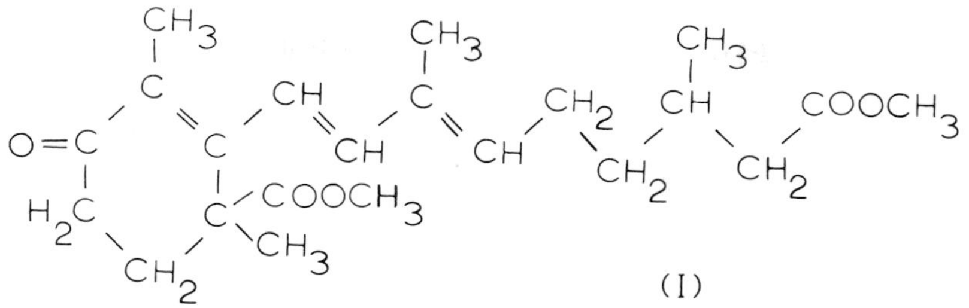

(I)

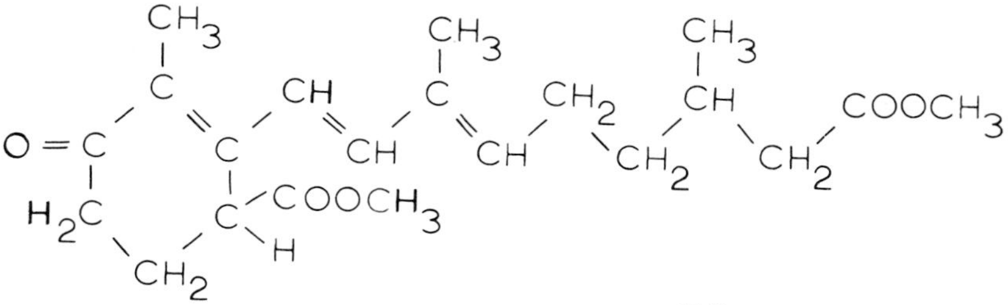

(II)

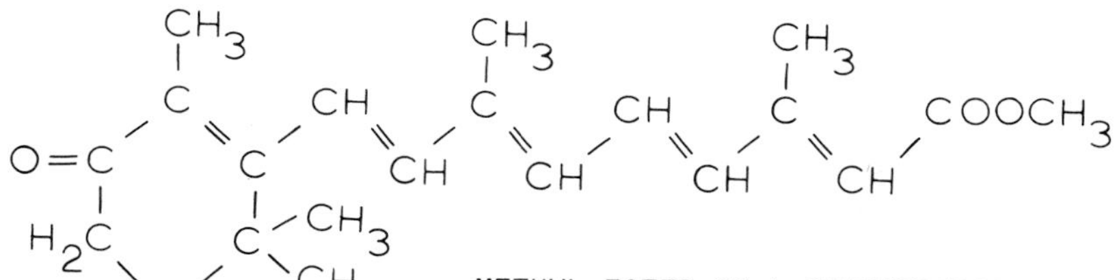

METHYL ESTER OF 4-OXORETINOIC ACID
(III)

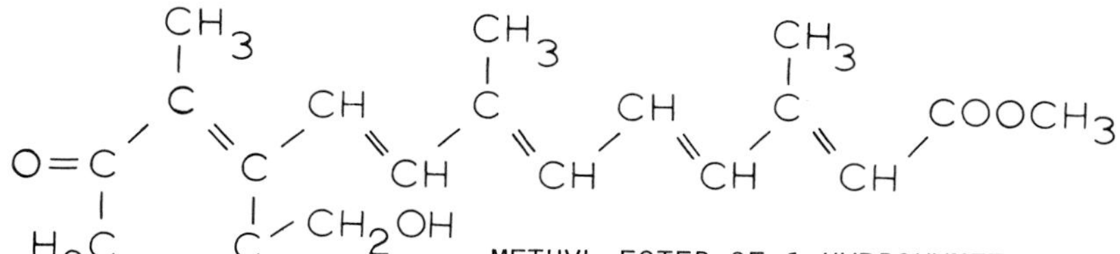

METHYL ESTER OF 1-HYDROXYMETHYL-4-OXORETINOIC ACID
(IV)

Fig. 6A–5. Metabolite structures I, II, III and IV.

Metabolite II is probably derived from metabolite I by loss of one methyl group. Metabolites III and IV seem to be catabolic intermediates between retinoic acid and metabolites I and II.

ROLE OF VITAMIN A IN BIOCHEMICAL SYSTEMS

Function of Vitamin A in Vision

George Wald was awarded the Nobel Prize for Medicine in 1967 for his discovery of the role of vitamin A in the visual system.

The retina of the eye of most vertebrates contains two distinct photoreceptor systems: the cones are concerned with acute perception and the rods are involved with vision in dim light. The photosensitive pigment of the rods is called rhodopsin and is a combination of retinal and a protein, opsin. The photoreceptor of cones contains the same chromophore (retinal) but the protein moiety is different from that in rods and is called iodopsin. The chromophore of the visual pigments in rods and cones of most vertebrates is retinal. 3-Dehydroretinal fulfills the same function in fresh-water fish and certain amphibians.[110,111] In the eye, retinol can be oxidized to retinal. The reaction is catalyzed by an alcohol dehydrogenase with nicotinamide-adenine-dinucleotide as coenzyme.[112] In rhodopsin, retinal is in the 11-cis form. After absorbing quanta of light, the 11-cis retinal of rhodopsin is isomerized, and the pigment is subsequently hydrolyzed to the protein (opsin) and all-trans retinal. The energy exchange in this process causes potential differences, producing a nervous excitation transmitted via the optic nerves to the brain, resulting in visual sensations. In the dark, some of the all-trans retinal is isomerized by retinal isomerase of the eye tissue to the 11-cis isomer, which then combines with opsin to regenerate rhodopsin.[113] Brown and Wald have shown that a similar mechanism operates at high light intensities and enables us to see different colors.[114]

The binding between retinal and opsin is believed to be a Schiff-base type of linkage formed by the condensation of the aldehyde group of retinal with the ϵ-amino group of lysine in opsin.[115] Other studies suggest that retinal may link to lysine or cysteine of opsin by a substituted aldiminic linkage.[116] Kimble and collaborators reported that retinal may be bound to phosphatidylethanolamine of the lipid-opsin complex prior to photolysis; it is transferred from there to a lysine ϵ-amino group of opsin in the process of photolysis.[117]

Function of Vitamin A Outside the Visual Cycle

Effect on Major Metabolic Pathways. Vitamin A deficiency does not disturb the tricarboxylic acid cycle[118] in carbohydrate metabolism. However, glycogen biosynthesis from acetate, lactate and glycerol appears to be slowed down and can be reversed by cortisone administration.[119]

Interaction between vitamin A compounds and other members of the lipid class has also been studied extensively. Vitamin A metabolism is linked with that of coenzyme Q, vitamin E, vitamin D, the sterols and the biosynthesis of squalene. Interaction of vitamin A and E seems to be important in regulating the stability of biologic membranes.[120] Ubiquinone (coenzyme Q) increases in the liver of vitamin A-deficient rats.[121] Vitamin A deficiency increases the biosynthesis of squalene and of ubiquinone in rat liver and reduces cholesterol formation.[122]

The utilization of vitamin A stores in the liver is directly proportional to protein intake when animals are fed a diet low in the vitamin. Low-protein diets retard the onset of deficiency symptoms. Conversely, increased protein intake will rapidly deplete liver reserves of vitamin A.[123] Vitamin A also influences synthesis of both serum and muscle proteins.[124,125] Glycoprotein synthesis in the intestinal mucosa is impaired in vitamin A deficiency: by using a cell-free protein synthesis system, it was found that this lesion was located in the pH 5 fraction. In studying the role of vitamin A in the biosynthesis of glycopeptides, it was found that vitamin A was needed for carrying mono- or oligosaccharide units to an acceptor site for the biosynthesis of glycoproteins situated in the cell membrane.[126]

Effect on Cell Membranes. Vitamin A-deficient animals do not only become blind but die. Many physiologic functions are affected and a large number of pathologic lesions appear in vitamin A-deficient animals.[127] Vitamin A must, therefore, perform an essential metabolic function common to many biochemical systems and to diverse tissues in living animals. In the past few years, an increasing amount of evidence has pointed toward a probable function of vitamin A in regulating membrane structure and function. Liver lysosomes of vitamin A-deficient rats are labilized.[128,129] Normal vitamin A concentration ensures optimum stability of these lysosomes. Large doses of the vitamin labilize the lysosomal membrane in vivo as well as in vitro.[130] The structure and stability of erythrocyte membranes are also markedly altered.[131,132] It has also been demonstrated that vitamin A is associated with several purified biologic membranes. In rat kidney endoplasmic reticulum, the major forms of vitamin A compounds appear to be retinol and retinoic acid.[133]

Active Form of Vitamin A

The active form of vitamin A appears to differ depending on the target organ. Thus, in the photoreceptor in the eye, it is the aldehyde. For reproductive activity, it appears to be retinol itself,[134-136] but for all other tissue activities the form is almost certainly retinoic acid. Retinoic acid supports growth[137] but not vision or reproduction. Whereas retinol and retinal are metabolically interconvertible in the body,

the further oxidation to retinoic acid is irreversible and retinoic acid cannot be stored in the body.

THE PATHOLOGY OF VITAMIN A DEFICIENCY AND EXCESS

Hypovitaminosis A

Vitamin A deficiency causes many lesions; its earliest symptom is a failure of the retina to obtain adequate supplies of retinal for the formation of rhodopsin, resulting in night blindness. This lesion is fully reversible, but may rapidly be followed by structural changes in the retina as a secondary complication.[138] Thus, the first symptoms of vitamin A deficiency are night blindness and xerosis (drying) of the conjunctiva. If deficiency continues, xerosis of the cornea appears, followed by corneal distortion. The loss of continuity of the surface epithelium, with formation of a noninflammatory "ulcer" and infiltration of the stroma, leads to softening of the cornea, perforation and iris prolapse. In untreated cases, the corneal structure melts rapidly into a gelatinous mass. Endophthalmitis frequently supervenes. These advanced changes are known as keratomalacia. Keratomalacia, particularly in infants and young children, is an acute process and may occur rapidly, before the more chronic changes of xerosis occur. The severity of the lesions and the rapidity with which they occur are, in general, inversely proportional to age.[139,140] Blindness caused by vitamin A deficiency is most frequently the result of loss of the lens through perforation of the cornea. It is, therefore, not directly related to the biochemical function of vitamin A in the visual cycle but to the function of the vitamin in general metabolism, which is not clearly understood to date.

Xerosis also occurs throughout the body and can be a prolific source of secondary lesions, such as infections and pathologic calcification. The general tendency of xerosis is to replace columnar epithelia in many sites by thick layers of horny, stratified epithelium. This change is often described as a metaplasia, implying that the tissues have changed in form. The term *keratinization*, implying that the membrane becomes horny, is also used.[141,142] Nerve lesions and increased pressure in the cerebrospinal fluid may accompany bony changes or may develop independently.[143,144] Numerous anatomic deformities can occur in the fetus from vitamin A deficiency in the maternal diet.[134]

Since vitamin A is transported in association with protein, protein deficiency states accentuate retinol deficiency. It is not clear whether the effect is entirely due to poor transport, for it has been shown that, in protein-calorie malnourished children, the administration of high-protein diets leads to improved retinol absorption from the intestinal tract.[145] A special word of caution is necessary here. Patients with kwashiorkor usually have extremely low reserves of vitamin A. When dietary protein supplements are given to these patients, their vitamin A requirement increases and the last reserves of the vitamin are mobilized from the liver, thus precipitating vitamin A deficiency. It is therefore necessary to administer vitamin A as well as protein to protein-deficient patients.[88,146] In developed countries, hypovitaminosis A can occur in association with fat absorption diseases: celiac disease,[147] obstructive jaundice,[148] infective hepatitis[149] and cystic fibrosis of the pancreas.[150] It has been confirmed recently that vitamin A absorption is dependent on the presence of bile acids in the intestinal tract,[151] and this probably explains the vitamin A deficiency associated with certain of the biliary obstruction disorders. Such cases cannot be treated readily by oral dosage of vitamin A because of the poor absorption of the vitamin in oil; in general, water-miscible forms have not produced much elevation of the plasma level either. Consequently, parenteral treatment is necessary.

Hypervitaminosis A

Vitamin A is highly toxic when given in excess. There are several reports in the literature of acute hypervitaminosis A in infants caused by single, massive doses. The main manifestations of toxicity are transient hydrocephalus and vomiting.[152] Outbreaks of acute vitamin A intoxication have been noted in Arctic explorers who ingested large quantities of polar bear liver, a rich source of the vitamin.

Chronic hypervitaminosis A in adults has occurred most frequently in patients who received large doses (20 to 30 times the recommended daily allowance [RDA]) of this vitamin as treatment for dermatologic conditions, and who continued subsequent intake without medical supervision. It has also been reported in food faddists[153] who included large doses of vitamin preparations in their daily dietary regimens. In patients with chronic hypervitaminosis A, fatigue, malaise and lethargy are common complaints, usually accompanied by abdominal discomfort, bone or joint pain or both, severe, throbbing headaches, insomnia and restlessness, night sweats, loss of body hair or brittle nails or both. Constipation, irregular menses and emotional lability have been reported. Physical examination usually reveals dry, scaly, rough skin, peripheral edema and mouth fissures. Exophthalmus is also common.[154,155]

Hypercarotenosis

Massive doses of carotene are not converted to vitamin A rapidly enough to induce vitamin A toxicity, but excess carotene accumulates in the body. Isolated cases of hypercarotenosis have been reported, resulting from grossly excessive intakes of vegetables with high carotenoid content, especially carrots. Unlike vitamin A, excessive intakes of carotenoids do not produce clinical symptoms other than yellow skin, which disappears when excessive ingestion of carotenoids is discontinued.[155]

VITAMIN A REQUIREMENTS OF MAN AND ANIMALS

The vitamin A requirements may be modified by age, growth, caloric intake, physical expenditure and special needs during pregnancy and lactation. The Recommended Daily Allowances (RDA), revised in 1974,[156] of vitamin A are: for infants and children up to age 10 years, from 1,400 to 3,300 I.U.; for adult females, 4,000 I.U.; for adult males, 5,000 I.U.; for pregnant women, 5,000 I.U.; for lactating women, 6,000 I.U. A recent study in the United States[157] has indicated that the adult human male requires at least 600 μg per day of retinol to prevent or cure eye changes and perhaps more to reverse cutaneous lesions. The requirement for β-carotene is approximately 1,200 μg per day. These levels of retinol and β-carotene would not necessarily support optimal levels of plasma vitamin A. Intakes of 1,200 μg per day of retinol or of 2,400 μg per day of β-carotene appear necessary to ensure plasma vitamin A levels above 30 μg per 100 ml, which are judged desirable.

Extensive studies of the vitamin A requirements of rats and farm animals have been undertaken. About 2 I.U. of either vitamin A or β-carotene are required to restore growth in young rats deficient in the vitamin. Much larger doses, however, are necessary to allow maximum longevity (100 I.U. per rat daily) or storage of the vitamin in the liver (30 I.U. per rat daily).[158] For beef cattle, the National Research Council recommended a daily allowance of 22 I.U. of vitamin A (alcohol) per kg body weight or 220 I.U. of carotene per kg body weight. For growing pigs, an allowance of 150 I.U. of carotene per kg body weight is recommended; this dose should be increased to 200 I.U. in pregnancy and to 330 I.U. during lactation.[159]

NORMAL SERUM LEVELS AND LIVER RESERVES OF VITAMIN A IN MAN

Liver is the storage organ for vitamin A. Recent analyses of human tissues obtained at autopsy showed that the vitamin A concentration in kidney, heart, muscle, lung, pancreas, fat, adrenal, prostate, spleen, testes and thyroid was approximately 1 μg per gm, whereas concentration in the liver varied from 17 to 281 μg per gm.[160]

Moore[161] has discussed the vitamin A status in normal health and in experimental deficiency in man at great length in his standard work. He reports that liver reserves were determined in accidentally killed humans in Britain, Holland, South Africa, China, Norway, Sweden and Scotland. He has also reviewed a wide variety of serum vitamin A and serum carotene levels in humans studied in the United States, Great Britain, South Africa and Norway. The grand average of these studies indicates a serum vitamin A level of approximately 40 μg per 100 ml for these human populations. The corresponding serum carotenoid level was 137 μg per 100 ml. Much wider ranges for liver reserves, determined on victims of accidental death, are reported, with the averages from different countries ranging from 24 μg per gm liver for China to 191 μg per gm liver for Scotland.

It was found, in a recent study on Canadians,[162,163] that the liver vitamin A stores of 15 to 32 per cent of subjects examined on autopsy were less than 40 μg per gm; however, many of these specimens were obtained from diseased subjects. A study on autopsy material from Canadians who died in accidents revealed that one group of accidental death victims had higher liver vitamin A reserves than those who died from diseases, whereas another group of accidental death victims had values similar to those who died from disease.

In a study of the vitamin A liver stores of accident victims in New York City,[164] the mean vitamin A content of 101 human livers was 126 μg per gm wet tissue with a range of 7 to 668 μg and a median of 66 μg. Postmortem blood samples were obtained from 50 of the subjects and the serum vitamin A level was 49 ± 16 μg per 100 ml of serum.

The average serum vitamin A content of a well-fed population in West Germany was found to be 52.7 ± 13.2 μg per 100 ml for 165 males and 50.5 ± 12.7 μg vitamin A per 100 ml serum for 216 females. The corresponding carotene concentrations were 85.6 ± 28.6 μg per 100 ml for the males and 94.0 ± 34.3 for the females; some age trends were noticeable.[165]

It should be stressed here that serum levels do not reflect liver reserves of vitamin A in experimental animals, except after almost complete exhaustion of the liver reserves. At that stage, serum vitamin A levels fall rapidly. Low serum levels of vitamin A are, therefore, often, but not always, an indication of vitamin A deficiency: dangerously low liver reserves may occur simultaneously with near normal blood levels of the vitamin.

Levels below 20 μg per 100 ml serum are certainly on the low side and levels below 10 μg per 100 ml are low indeed and more than likely to be indicative of serious vitamin A deficiency.

Serum carotene levels are much more variable than those of vitamin A: they directly reflect dietary intake of carotenoids. Extremely high levels of carotene can be found in populations consuming carotene-rich diets such as red palm oil.

Studies of the liver reserves of patients who died from various diseases have indicated ranges lower than those found in cases of accidental death. Moreover, the loss of vitamin A reserves is greater in some diseases than in others. For example, the loss in appendicitis appears to be about 50 per cent, in pneumonia 70 per cent, and in chronic nephritis 89 per cent. In the last two diseases these losses are due, at least partially, to excretion of the vitamin in the urine. In chronic and incurable diseases the situation may be complicated by failure in the absorption or metabolism of the vitamin. Usually this abnormality may have little effect on the course of the disease, but the possibility of aggravation of the main lesion by superimposed hypovitaminosis A should be borne in mind. The administration of the vitamin seems advisable, provided it causes no digestive disturbance.[166]

VITAMIN A THERAPY

The only unequivocal therapeutic use for vitamin A is for the treatment of hypovitaminosis A. Night blindness and the milder conjunctival changes respond well to 30,000 I.U. of vitamin A daily for a few days, given as cod or halibut liver oil.[167] Corneal damage must be treated as an emergency; a dose causing a rapid increase in the level of vitamin A in the blood plasma seems to be necessary. Since the adult liver can absorb at least 500,000 I.U., doses of the vitamin should be so adjusted as to make this amount available during the first few days of treatment. Children should be given smaller doses.[168]

The materials available for the prevention and cure of vitamin A deficiency include vitamin A-containing foods, fish liver oils, concentrates derived from them, preparations of carotene in oil and synthetic forms of vitamin A, which are available as the palmitate, stearate or acetate ester or in the alcohol form.

In most patients, oral treatment is decidedly more effective than parenteral. When lesions of the gastrointestinal tract are involved, however, the administration of the vitamin by injection may be necessary. If so, an aqueous dispersion of the vitamin should be used.[167]

There is extensive literature on the use of vitamin A in the treatment of skin diseases. The main diseases in which therapeutic benefit has been claimed are pityriasis rubra pilaris (Devergie's disease), psoriasis, keratosis follicularis (Darier's disease) and certain ichthyoses.[169] It has been reported that benefit may be seen in certain patients with these disorders when retinoic acid is applied topically.[170,171] Topical retinoic acid may also help some cases of acne vulgaris.

Over many years, several publications have appeared discussing the possible effect of vitamin A and its analogs on the risk of development of cancer, squamous carcinoma in particular. Direct evidence of the value of vitamin A in protection against cancer has come from experiments in which tissues in organ culture or in intact animals were exposed to carcinogenic polycyclic aromatic hydrocarbons in such a way that they developed squamous cancers.[172-174] Cone and Nettesheim[175] showed that vitamin A protected rats against the early development of squamous neoplasms caused by the carcinogen 3-methylcholanthrene, given by endotracheal instillation. Their observations were particularly important because these workers measured the amount of vitamin A stores in the liver to make sure that rats, which were supposedly vitamin A deficient, really were so. The association of lung cancer and low intake of vitamin A has also been reported.[176] All these findings suggest that it may be possible to protect certain high-risk individuals—perhaps everyone—against the development of certain forms of cancer of epithelial origin by maintaining them in a state of good nutrition in respect to vitamin A.[177]

BIBLIOGRAPHY

1. McCollum and Davis: J. Biol. Chem., *23*, 181, 1915.
2. Drummond: Biochem. J., *14*, 660, 1920.
3. McCollum and Simmonds: J. Biol. Chem., *32*, 181, 1917.
4. Fridericia and Holm: Am. J. Physiol., *73*, 63, 1925.
5. Steenbock and Boutwell: J. Biol. Chem., *41*, 163, 1920.
6. Steenbock and Sell: J. Biol. Chem., *51*, 63, 1922.
7. Bloch: J. Dairy Sci., 7, 1, 1924.
8. Moore: Biochem. J., *24*, 692, 1930.
9. Karrer, Helfenstein, Wehrli and Wettstein: Helv. Chim. Acta, *13*, 1084, 1930.
10. Karrer, Morf and Schopp: Helv. Chim. Acta, *14*, 1036 and 1431, 1931.
11. Isler, Huber, Ronco and Kofler: Helv. Chim. Acta, *30*, 1911, 1947.
12. Karrer and Eugster: Helv. Chim. Acta, *33*, 1172, 1950.
13. Inhoffen, Bohlmann, Bartram, Rummert and Pommer: Ann. Chem., *570*, 54, 1950.
14. Harris, Ames and Brinkman: J. Am. Chem. Soc., *73*, 1252, 1951.
15. Shantz: Science, *108*, 417, 1948.
16. Reti: C. R. Soc. Biol., *120*, 577, 1935.
17. Ganguly: Vitam. Horm., *18*, 387, 1960.
18. Wald: Vitam. Horm., *18*, 417, 1960.
19. Ames: Ann. Rev. Biochem., *27*, 371, 1958.
20. Dowling and Wald: Vitam. Horm., *18*, 387, 1960.
21. Karrer, Morf and Walker: Helv. Chim. Acta, *16*, 975, 1933.
22. Winterstein: Z. Physiol. Chem., *215*, 51, 1933.
23. Deuel, Sumner, Johnston, Polgar and Zechmeister: Arch. Biochem., *6*, 157, 1945.
24. Zechmeister, Pinckard, Greenberg, Straub, Fukui and Deuel, Jr.: Arch. Biochem., *23*, 242, 1949.
25. Olson: J. Biol. Chem., *236*, 349, 1961.
26. Boldingh, Cama, Collins, Morton, Gridgeman, Isler, Kofler, Taylor, Wieland and Bradbury: Nature, *168*, 598, 1951.
27. Drummond and Watson: Analyst, *47*, 341, 1922.
28. Sobotka, Kann and Loewenstein: J. Am. Chem. Soc., *65*, 1959, 1943.
29. Embree and Shantz: J. Am. Chem. Soc., *65*, 906, 1943.
30. Morton: Nature, *153*, 69, 1944.
31. Ball, Goodwin and Morton: Biochem. J., *42*, 516, 1948.
32. Robeson, Cawley, Weisler, Stern, Eddinger and Chechak: J. Am. Chem. Soc., *77*, 4111, 1955.
33. Brown and Wald: J. Biol. Chem., *222*, 865, 1956.
34. Wald, Brown, Hubbard and Oroshnik: Proc. Natl. Acad. Sci., *41*, 438, 1955.
35. Beutel, Hinkley and Pollak: J. Am. Chem. Soc., *77*, 5166, 1955.
36. Barnholdt: Acta Chem. Scand., *11*, 909, 1957.
37. Carr and Price: Biochem. J., *20*, 497, 1926.
38. Neeld and Pearson: J. Nutr., *79*, 454, 1963.
39. Zechmeister and Polgar: J. Am. Chem. Soc., *65*, 1522, 1943.
40. Bickoff, White, Bevenue and Williams: J. Assoc. Off. Agr. Chem., *31*, 633, 1948.
41. Baur: Helv. Chim. Acta, *19*, 1210, 1936.
42. Karrer and Jucker: *Carotenoids.* Amsterdam, Elsevier, 1950.
43. Collins: Nature, *165*, 817, 1950.
44. Zechmeister: *Cis-trans Isomeric Carotenoids, Vitamin A and Arylpolyenes.* Vienna, Springer-Verlag, 1962.
45. Morton and Stubbs: Analyst, *71*, 348, 1946.
46. Cama, Collis and Morton: Biochem. J., *50*, 48, 1951.
47. Brunius: Nature, *181*, 395, 1958.
48. Popper: Physiol. Rev., *24*, 205, 1944.
49. Fujita and Aoyama: J. Biochem., *38*, 271, 1951.

50. Dunagin and Olson: Anal. Chem., *36*, 756, 1964.
51. Brown, Blum and Stern: Nature, *184*, 1377, 1959.
52. Von Planta: Unpublished data, quoted in Kofler and Rubin: Vitam. Horm., *18*, 315, 1960.
53. Bliss and György: *Vitamin Methods*, Vol. 2 (Gyögy, Ed.). New York, Academic Press, 1951.
54. Dugan, Frigerio and Siebert: Anal. Chem., *36*, 114, 1964.
55. Roels and Trout: Am. J. Clin. Nutr., *1*, 197, 1959.
55a.Bliss and Roels: *The Vitamins*, Vol. VI, 2nd ed. (György and Pearson, Eds.). New York, Academic Press, 1967.
56. Coward: *The Biological Standardisation of Vitamins*, 2nd ed. London, Baillière, Tindall & Cox, 1947.
57. Pugsley, Wills and Crandall: J. Nutr., *28*, 365, 1944.
58. Guggenheim and Koch: Biochem. J., *38*, 256, 1944.
59. Booth: *Carotene, Its Determination in Biological Materials*. Cambridge, Heffer, 1957.
60. Hunter and Scott: Biochem. J., *38*, 211, 1944.
61. Rapsan, Schwartz and Van Rensburg: J. Soc. Chem. Ind., *65*, 61, 1945.
62. Watt and Merrill: Agriculture Handbook 8. Washington, U.S. Department of Agriculture, 1950, 1966.
63. Thompson, Brande, Coates, Cowie, Ganguly and Kon: Br. J. Nutr., *4*, 398, 1950.
64. Bieri and Pollard: Br. J. Nutr., *8*, 32, 1954.
65. Zachman and Olson: J. Biol. Chem., *238*, 541, 1963.
66. Olson and Hayaishi: Proc. Natl. Acad. Sci., *54*, 1364, 1965.
67. Goodman, Huang, Kanai and Shiratori: J. Biol. Chem., *242*, 3543, 1967.
68. Fidge and Goodman: J. Biol. Chem., *243*, 4372, 1968.
69. Roels, Trout and Dujacquier: J. Nutr., *65*, 115, 1958.
70. Brown and Bloor: J. Nutr., *29*, 349, 1945.
71. Olson: Fed. Proc., *21*, 473, 1962.
72. David and Ganguly: Indian J. Biochem., *4*, 14, 1967.
73. Mahadevan, Seshadri-Sastry and Ganguly: Biochem. J., *88*, 531, 1963.
74. Mahadevan, Seshadri-Sastry and Ganguly: Biochem. J., *88*, 534, 1963.
75. Huang and Goodman: J. Biol. Chem., *240*, 2839, 1965.
76. Fidge, Shiratori, Ganguly and Goodman: J. Lipid Res., *9*, 103, 1968.
77. Deshmuk, Murthy, Mahadevan and Ganguly: Biochem. J., *96*, 377, 1965.
78. Deshmuk, Malathi, Subba-Rao and Ganguly: Indian J. Biochem., *1*, 164, 1964.
79. Mahadevan, Ayyoub and Roels: J. Biol. Chem., *241*, 57, 1966.
80. Hoch and Hoch: Br. J. Exp. Pathol., *27*, 316, 1946.
81. Dowling and Wald: Proc. Natl. Acad. Sci., *44*, 648, 1958.
82. Krinsky, Cornwell and Oncley: Arch. Biochem. Biophys., *73*, 233, 1958.
83. Kanai, Raz and Goodman: J. Clin. Invest., *47*, 2025, 1968.
84. Smith, Roy and Goodman: J. Clin. Invest., *49*, 1754, 1970.
85. Smith and Goodman: J. Clin. Invest., *50*, 2426, 1971.
86. McLaren, Shirajian, Loshkajian and Shadarevian: Am. J. Clin. Nutr., *22*, 863, 1969.
87. Pereira, Begum and Dumm: Am. J. Clin. Nutr., *19*, 182, 1966.
88. Arroyave, Wilson, Mendez, Behar and Scrimshaw: Am. J. Clin. Nutr., *9*, 180, 1961.
89. Muto, Smith, Milch and Goodman: J. Biol. Chem., *247*, 2452, 1972.
90. Smith, Muto, Milch and Goodman: J. Biol. Chem., *248*, 1544, 1973.
91. Moore: Biochem. J., *25*, 275, 1931.
92. Moore: *Vitamin A*. Amsterdam, Elsevier, 1957.
93. Bacharach and Smith: Q. J. Pharmacol., *1*, 539, 1928.
94. Kuhn and Brockmann: Z. Physiol. Chem., *206*, 41, 1932.
95. Gray and Cawley: J. Nutr., *23*, 301, 1942.
96. Krishnamurthy and Ganguly: Nature, *177*, 575, 1956.
97. Lippel and Olson: J. Lipid Res., *9*, 168, 1968.
98. Mahadevan, Murthy and Ganguly: Biochem. J., *85*, 326, 1962.
99. Dunagin, Meadows and Olson: Science, *148*, 86, 1965.
100. Dunagin, Zachman and Olson: Biochim. Biophys. Acta, *124*:1966.
101. De Luca and Roberts: Am. J. Clin. Nutr., *22*, 945, 1969.
102. Wald: Vitam. Horm., *18*, 417, 1960.
103. Kleiner-Bossaler and De Luca: Arch. Biochem. Biophys., *142*, 371, 1971.
104. Zachman, Dunagin and Olson: J. Lipid Res., *2*, 3, 1966.
105. Natu and Olson: J. Nutr., *93*, 461, 1967.
106. Varma and Beaton: Can. J. Physiol. Pharmacol., *50*, 1026, 1972.
107. Wolf, Kahn and Johnson: J. Am. Chem. Soc., *79*, 1208, 1957.
108. Rietz: Acta Vitaminol. Enzymol., *25*, 123, 1971.
109. Rietz, Wiss and Weber: Vitam. Horm., *32*, 237, 1974.
110. Wald: Vitam. Horm., *1*, 195, 1943.
111. Wald, Brown and Smith: Science, *118*, 505, 1953.
112. Wald and Hubbard: Proc. Natl. Acad. Sci., *36*, 92, 1950.
113. Hubbard and Colman: Science, *130*, 977, 1959.
114. Brown and Wald: Nature, *200*, 37, 1963.
115. Ball, Collins, Dabi and Morton: Biochem. J., *45*, 304, 1949.
116. Heller: Biochemistry, *7*, 2914, 1968.
117. Kimble, Poincelot and Abrahamson: Biochemistry, *9*, 1817, 1970.
118. Wolf, Lane and Johnson: J. Biol. Chem., *225*, 995, 1957.
119. Johnson and Wolf: Vitam. Horm., *18*, 465, 1960.

120. Roels, Trout and Guha: Biochem. J., *97*, 353, 1965.
121. Lowe, Morton and Harrison: Nature, *172*, 716, 1953.
122. Wiss and Gloor: Vitam. Horm., *18* 485, 1960.
123. McLaren: Br. J. Ophthalmol., *43*, 234, 1959.
124. Vakil, Roels and Trout: Br. J. Nutr., *18*, 217, 1964.
125. Moore: Vitam. Horm., *18*, 431, 1960.
126. De Luca and Wolf: Int. J. Vitam. Nutr. Res., *40*, 284, 1970.
127. Moore: *Vitamin A*. New York, Elsevier, 1957.
128. Roxas, Sessa, Trout, Guha and Roels: Fed. Proc., *23*, 293, 1964.
129. Roels, Trout and Guha: Biochem. J., *93*, 23, 1964.
130. Roels: *The Vitamins*. Vol. 1, 2nd ed. (Sebrell and Harris, Eds.). New York, Academic Press, 1967.
131. Anderson, Pfister and Roels: Nature, *213*, 47, 1967.
132. Roels, Anderson, Lui, Shah and Trout: Am. J. Clin. Nutr., *22*, 1020, 1969.
133. Mack, Lui, Roels and Anderson: Biochim. Biophys. Acta, *228*, 203, 1972.
134. Mason: Am. J. Anat., *57*, 303, 1935.
135. Howell, Thomson and Pitt: J. Reprod. Fertil., *7*, 251, 1964.
136. Juneja, Mondgal and Ganguly: Biochem. J., *111*, 97, 1969.
137. Dowling and Wald: Proc. Natl. Acad. Sci., *46*, 587, 1960.
138. Dowling and Wald: Proc. Natl. Acad. Sci., *44*, 648, 1958.
139. McLaren, Oomen, and Escapini: Bull. WHO, *34*, 357, 1966.
140. Paton and McLaren: Am. J. Ophthalmol., *50*, 568, 1960.
141. Wolbach: Vitamins, *1*, 106, 1954.
142. Pillat: Arch. Ophthalmol., *2*, 256, 1929.
143. Coetzer: Biochem. J., *45*, 628, 1949.
144. Mellanby: Proc. R. Soc. B, *132*, 28, 1944.
145. Viteri, Flores, Alvarado and Behar: Am. J. Dig. Dis., *18*, 201, 1973.
146. Oomen, McLaren and Escapini: Trop. Geogr. Med., *16*, 271, 1964.
147. Barnes, Wollaeger and Mason: J. Clin. Invest., *29*, 982, 1950.
148. Blegvad: Acta Ophthalmol., *1*, 172, 1924.
149. Harris and Moore: Br. Med. J., *1*, 553, 1947.
150. Blackfan and May: J. Pediatr., *13*, 627, 1938.
151. Barnard and Heaton: Gut, *14*, 316, 1973.
152. Lindhard: Medd. Groenland, *41*, 461, 1913.
153. Bergen and Roels: Am. J. Clin. Nutr., *16*, 265, 1965.
154. Gerber, Raeb and Sobel: Am. J. Med., *16*, 729, 1954.
155. Josephs: Am. J. Dis. Child., *67*, 33, 1944.
156. Food and Nutrition Board: *Recommended Dietary Allowances*. Washington, National Academy of Sciences—National Research Council, 1974.
157. Sauberlich, Hodges, Wallace, Kolder, Canham, Hood, Raica and Lowry: Vitam. Horm., *32*, 251, 1974.
158. Moore: *Vitamin A*. Amsterdam, Elsevier, 1957, p. 228.
159. *Recommended Nutrient Allowances for Farm Animals*. Washington, National Academy of Sciences—National Research Council, 1944, 1949, 1950.
160. Raica, Scott, Lowry and Sauberlich: Am. J. Clin. Nutr., *25*, 291, 1972.
161. Moore: *Vitamin A*. Amsterdam, Elsevier, 1957.
162. Hoppner, Phillips, Erdsdy, Murray and Perrin: Can. Med. Assoc. J., *101*, 84, 1969.
163. Hoppner, Phillips, Murray and Campbell: Can. Med. Assoc. J., *99*, 983, 1968.
164. Underwood, Siegel, Weisell and Dolinski: Am. J. Clin. Nutr., *23*, 1037, 1970.
165. Kasper: Int. Z. Vitam. Forschung, *38*, 142, 1968.
166. Moore: Biochem. J., *31*, 155, 1937.
167. McLaren: Trans. R. Soc. Trop. Med. Hyg., *60*, 436, 1966.
168. Moore: In *The Vitamins*, Vol. 1, 2nd ed. (Sebrell and Harris, Eds.). New York, Academic Press, 1967.
169. Logan: Arch. Dermatol., *105*, 748, 1972.
170. Frost and Weinstein: J.A.M.A., *207*, 1863, 1969.
171. Fry, MacDonald and McMinn: Br. J. Dermatol., *83*, 391, 1970.
172. Lasmitzki and Goodman: Cancer Res., *34*, 1564, 1974.
173. Chu and Malmgren: Cancer Res., *25*, 884, 1965.
174. Saffiotti et al.: Cancer, *20*, 857, 1967.
175. Cone and Nettesheim: J. Natl. Cancer Inst., *50*, 1599, 1973.
176. Bjelke: Int. J. Cancer, *15*, 561, 1975.
177. Sporn, Dunlop, Newton and Smith: Fed. Proc., *35*, 1332, 1976.

B. VITAMIN D*

H. F. DeLuca

The disease rickets appears to have been evident even in ancient times, possibly resulting indirectly from advances in urbanization.[1] Bardsley, in 1807, wrote about the effective use of cod liver oil in the treatment of osteomalacia,[2] while Palm,[3] in 1890, suggested that sunlight possessed antirachitic action. In 1919 Sir Edward Mellanby succeeded in producing rickets in experimental animals and found it could be prevented by the administration of cod liver oil.[4] McCollum and associates[5] demonstrated that the antirachitic factor in cod liver oil is relatively stable to heat and aeration, thereby differing from the previously discovered vitamin A. McCollum named the factor vitamin D.[6] Also in 1919 Huldshinsky demonstrated clearly that ultraviolet light from either sunlight or ultraviolet lamps could cure rickets.[7] The elegant work of Steenbock and associates[8,9] established that antirachitic activity could be produced in food and other biologic materials by ultraviolet irradiation. This discovery provided the basic information needed for the isolation and identification of vitamin D_2[10,11] and the elimination of rickets as a major medical problem because food could be easily fortified with the antirachitic vitamin.

A distinct time lag exists between administration of vitamin D to deficient animals and detection of a physiologic response[12] (e.g. enhanced intestinal calcium absorption). It is now known that the conversion of vitamin D to active metabolites and the stimulation of protein synthesis and/or assembly constitute the main events occurring during this time period.

By current definitions vitamin D can be considered both a vitamin and a hormone. Vitamin D is an organic compound which acts as a micronutrient; its ingestion is required by most urban populations (i.e. it acts as a vitamin). However, there is no need for vitamin D supplementation in people who are able to meet their vitamin D need through the sunlight activation of 7-dehydrocholesterol in the skin. The vitamin D thus produced is metabolized to an active form(s) which then acts on distinct target tissue with feedback control occurring at the site of active metabolite synthesis. Thus the active metabolite 1,25-dihydroxyvitamin D_3 (1,25-$(OH)_2D_3$), which is produced exclusively in the kidney and functions in intestine and bone, is considered a hormone and vitamin D a prohormone.[12,13]

VITAMIN D CHEMISTRY

The D vitamins are characteristically found in the sterol fraction of biologic extracts. Vitamins D_2 and D_3, the more common forms of the vitamin, are derived from ergosterol and 7-dehydrocholesterol, respectively, and are, therefore, named ergocalciferol and cholecalciferol (Fig. 6B–1).

The triene structure of vitamin D gives a characteristic absorption band at 265 nm with an absorption minimum at 228 nm and a molar extinction coefficient of 18,200 at 365 nm. Vitamin D is fairly stable and is soluble in a wide range of organic solvents, although care should be taken to store solutions of the vitamin under nitrogen in the absence of light, acid and at cold temperatures if possible. The main problem is the ease of oxidation of the triene system, its sensitivity to acid and light-

*Supported by grants from the USPHS (No. AM-14881) and the Harry Steenbock Research Fund.

160

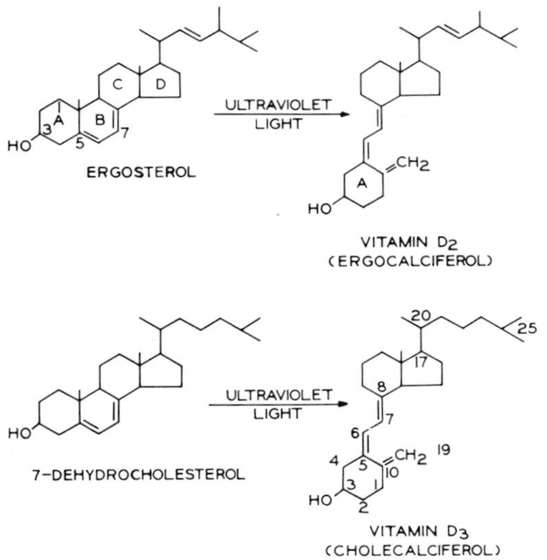

Fig. 6B-1. The conversion of the vitamin D provitamins to their corresponding vitamin D compounds by ultraviolet light.

catalyzed isomerization. Often an antioxidant such as α-tocopherol or butylated hydroxytoluene can be used to help prevent oxidation. Aqueous suspensions are particularly unstable because of dissolved oxygen. Oil or propylene glycol solutions of the vitamin with an antioxidant, however, are quite stable.

Chemical alteration of existing functional groups or double bonds results in a product with decreased antirachitic activity. Vitamin D_4 is produced by the reduction of the 22, 23 double bond in vitamin D_2 and is only one half to three fourths as active as vitamin D_2 in rats. Substitution of a Cl, Br[14] or a mercaptan[15] group for the 3-OH function results in loss of activity. Reduction of the methylene group on ring A and rotation of the ring 180 degrees results in dihydrotachysterol (present in solutions of AT-10), a compound which is less active than the vitamin at low doses but of therapeutic value when given at a pharmacologic level[16] because it acts as an analog of 1,25-$(OH)_2D_3$.[17]

MEASUREMENT OF VITAMIN D

Only a small amount of vitamin D is required (e.g. 1 I.U. in the rat, where 1 mg = 40,000 I.U.) to elicit a physiologic response. Thus the amounts of vitamin D which must be measured in biologic materials are extremely small. Recently high-pressure liquid chromatography (HPLC) coupled to a sensitive ultraviolet absorbance detector has been used for measurement, and will largely replace the biologic assays; however, biologic assays represent the only methods available until wide acceptance of the HPLC is realized.[18]

The rat-line test or calcification test[19] remains the method of choice. A single dose of standard vitamin D will promote calcification in the epiphyseal plate of the rachitic rat. Silver nitrate (1.5 per cent w/v) staining of sectioned bone is used for visual detection of new calcification which increases as a function of the dose of vitamin D.

Per cent bone ash is also used in chicks and rats as an assay for vitamin D. The bone ash content of tibia is determined after feeding chicks a rachitogenic diet and standard doses of vitamin D for 21 days.[20] Increase in per cent bone ash is correlated to the dose of vitamin D. The chick bone ash method is the primary method used for vitamin D_3. To differentiate between vitamins D_2 and D_3 an efficacy ratio of rat to chick response is used. Chicks give a response to vitamin D_3 tenfold greater than to vitamin D_2, while rats respond equally well to both compounds.

VITAMIN D ABSORPTION AND EXCRETION

Vitamin D is generally absorbed with food fats; therefore, inhibition of normal fat absorption (steatorrhea) results in a diminished absorption of ingested vitamin D. Patients with chronic pancreatitis, celiac disease and biliary obstruction were found to malabsorb ^{3}H-vitamin D_3.[21] Absorption occurs in the jejunum and/or ileum. Bile is essential,[22,23] with most of an absorbed dose of vitamin D present in the chylomicrons of the lymphatic system.[21] Vitamin D concentrates rapidly in the liver where it is hydroxylated to 25-hydroxyvitamin D_3 (25-OH-D$_3$).[24,25] The movement of vitamin D from the plasma chylomicrons and lipoproteins appears to occur in the liver by transfer to an α_1-globulin with a molecular weight of 52,000 which acts as a carrier for the vitamin and its metabolites.[26-28]

Bile appears to be the major pathway of vitamin D metabolite excretion. Patients having biliary fistulas excrete little radioactivity from a dose of ^{3}H-vitamin D_3.[29] A significant amount (i.e. 3 per cent) of ^{3}H-vitamin D_3 is also detectable in the urine during the 48 to 72-hour period following an intravenous dosage.[29]

DIETARY IMPLICATIONS

Because of food fortification with vitamin D, the daily vitamin requirement (200 to 400 I.U. or 5 to 10 μg vitamin D_3) can be achieved without vitamin supplementation.[30] However, rickets can occur in breast-fed infants and those fed unfortified milk,[31] in which case a vitamin D supplement is recommended (e.g. 400 I.U. daily). It is currently suggested that prophylactic doses of vitamin D in excess of 1,000 I.U. daily are inadvisable.[32] However, Fomon and associates have shown that moderate overdoses of vitamin D (i.e. 1,380 to 2,370 I.U. daily), common in a substantial number of children in the United States, had no detrimental effect on growth.[33] A high frequency of a mild form of idiopathic hypercalcemia in Great Britain has been associated with a vitamin intake of 4,000 I.U. daily, mainly from fortified infant foods.[34] Of course, an excessive intake of vitamin D (i.e. 50,000 to 100,000 I.U. daily) is potentially dangerous to both normal children[35] and adults[36] and must be avoided. As a precaution, intakes of vitamin D in excess of 1,000 I.U. per day should be taken only if prescribed by a physician and provided that serum calcium concentration or fasting 24-hour

urinary calcium levels are routinely monitored once every month.

There should also be an awareness that improper dietary intake of calcium and/or phosphorus can impair growth and cause bone disease. Infants require 400 to 600 mg of calcium daily, children (1 to 10 years) and adults (over 18 years) require 800 mg daily, while growing children (10 to 18 years) and women during pregnancy need 1,300 mg daily.[31] Phosphorus should be consumed at a level equivalent to calcium with the dietary ratio of the two ions approximately 1:1. A high-phosphorus diet, as afforded by cow's milk, may result in hypocalcemic tetany during early infancy.[37] The high phosphate intake in the United States afforded through soft drinks and meat is also of interest concerning possible long-term effects in children and adults alike. High-phosphate diets decrease the absorption of calcium by the formation of an insoluble calcium complex. Phytate in bread and certain cereals forms insoluble calcium phytate which also interferes with intestinal calcium absorption.[38]

One resultant effect of low blood calcium and phosphorus is the softening and deformity of the maxillary bones. Mellanby and Mellanby reported that, in London between 1945 and 1947, children (i.e. up to 5 years) who had increased availability of calcium and vitamin D possessed markedly improved dental status.[39]

METABOLITES OF VITAMIN D
(Fig. 6B–2)

Column chromatography of chloroform tissue extracts from rats and chicks injected with ^{3}H-vitamin D_3 results in the separation of several vitamin D metabolites. A sulfated vitamin D[40] and a long-chain fatty acid ester of the vitamin[41] have been identified. Recently, interest has developed in polar metabolites which possess additional hydroxy groupings. The major circulating form of the vitamin in vivo has been identified as 25-OH-D$_3$ by DeLuca

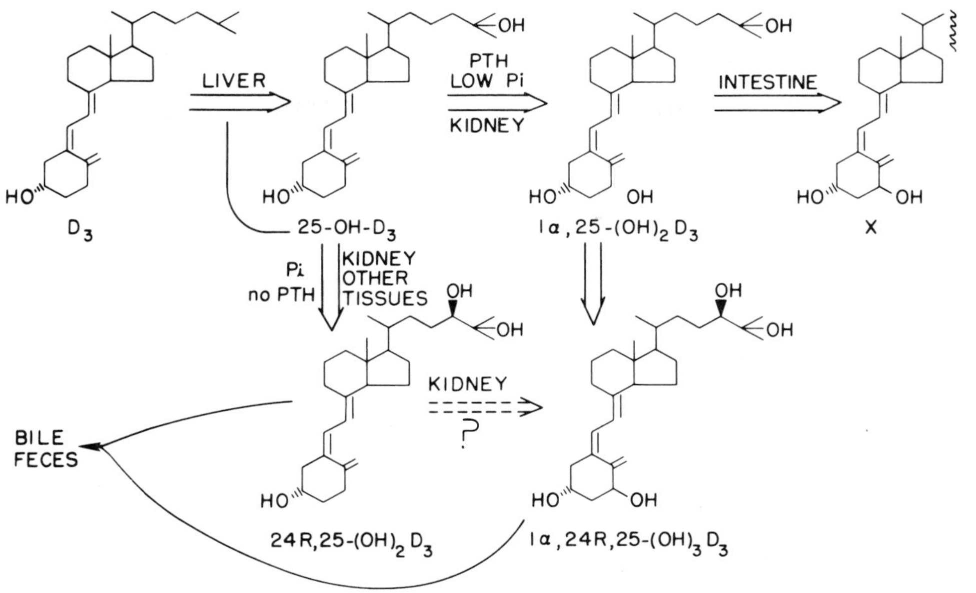

Fig. 6B–2. The known pathways of vitamin D metabolism. Note that $1\alpha,25$-$(OH)_2D_3$ is considered the active hormone in regulating calcium and phosphorus metabolism while 25-OH-D_3 is the major circulating form of the vitamin.

and associates.[42] This polar compound appears to be hydroxylated further wherein 24R,25-dihydroxyvitamin D_3 (24R,25-$(OH)_2D_3$)[43] and 25,26-dihydroxyvitamin D_3 (25,26-$(OH)_2D_3$)[44] have been isolated from hog plasma. Of great importance is the identification of 1,25-$(OH)_2D_3$.[45-47] This metabolite is present in intestine at a concentration of only 0.5 to 1 ng per gm tissue and is extremely active in stimulating intestinal calcium and phosphate transport.

The biologic activity of the metabolites can be summarized with respect to vitamin D_3 as follows:

25-OH-D_3 is 2 to 5 times more active than vitamin D_3 in calcification of bone, intestinal calcium transport and the mobilization of calcium from bone.[48] It acts more rapidly than vitamin D_3, eliciting a response within 12 hours. It is the major circulating form of vitamin D at 20 to 30 ng per ml plasma.

$1\alpha,25$-$(OH)_2D_3$ is the most potent form of vitamin D known, giving an activity of 10 times vitamin D_3 in all systems known to be responsive.[48] It is formed exclusively in the kidney[49] and circulates at a level of 30 to 40 pg per ml in normal adults. It is considered the final active form or hormonal form of vitamin D_3.[50] It is the fastest acting, giving responses within 3 hours.[51]

24R,25-$(OH)_2D_3$ is a major metabolite of vitamin D in terms of quantity, being present at about 1 ng per ml of human plasma. Its function, if any, is unknown and, in rats, it is somewhat less active than 25-OH-D_3.[52] It is apparently formed in the kidney from 25-OH-D_3.

1α,24R,25-Trihydroxyvitamin D_3 (1α,-24R,25-$(OH)_3D_3$) is formed by 24-hydroxylation of $1\alpha,25$-$(OH)_2D_3$, but can also be formed by 1α-hydroxylation of 24R,25-$(OH)_2D_3$.[53] It is 60 per cent as active as $1\alpha,25$-$(OH)_2D_3$.[54] Its function is also unknown, although the best assumption is that 24-hydroxylation is probably an inactivation mechanism.

25,26-$(OH)_2D_3$ is the least active of the

known metabolites, being one tenth as active as 25-OH-D$_3$ on intestine, and its function is unknown.[44]

In all cases, the corresponding vitamin D$_2$ metabolites have been isolated and identified.[55,56] The pathway of vitamin D$_2$ metabolism is identical to the vitamin D$_3$ pathway. In birds, the vitamin D$_2$ metabolites are one tenth as active as the vitamin D$_3$ metabolites but they are equal in activity in the rat.[57] So far as is presently known, $1\alpha,25$-(OH)$_2$D$_3$ carries out all the known functions of vitamin D.

FUNCTIONS OF VITAMIN D

Vitamin D brings about normal mineralization of bone and endochondral calcification, preventing the disease rickets in the young and osteomalacia in the adult. It also plays an important role in the prevention of hypocalcemic tetany, a function it shares with the parathyroid hormone. Because the vitamin is essential for calcium absorption, it may also function in the prevention of osteoporosis by ensuring adequate calcium from the environment, thus preventing reliance on the skeleton to support normal serum calcium concentration. To prevent hypocalcemic tetany and to provide for normal mineralization of bone and cartilage, vitamin D is responsible for the elevation of plasma calcium and phosphorus concentration to supersaturation.[12,13] Although it may function at the calcification sites, there is no clear evidence of this. To elevate plasma calcium and phosphorus, vitamin D activates active transport of calcium[58] and phosphorus[59] in the intestine, improves renal reabsorption of calcium[60] and stimulates the mobilization of calcium from the bone fluid compartment.[61] All of these mechanisms then result in the elevation of plasma calcium and phosphorus concentrations to normal levels.

There is evidence that vitamin D functions to improve muscle strength, but the nature of this function is not known.

1,25-(OH)$_2$D$_3$ As a Hormone

Vitamin D is converted in the liver to 25-OH-D$_3$ and subsequently in the kidney to 1,25-(OH)$_2$D$_3$ before it functions. Nephrectomized animals do not synthesize 1,25-(OH)$_2$D$_3$[62] and the target organs of intestine[63] and bone[64] thus do not respond to physiologic doses of 25-OH-D$_3$ and vitamin D$_3$ but do respond normally to 1,25-(OH)$_2$D$_3$. Since 1,25-(OH)$_2$D$_3$ is made exclusively in kidney and functions in bone and intestine, it is considered a hormone.[12,13] As a hormone, its biosynthesis is stimulated by hypocalcemia, hypophosphatemia and certain hormones. It is the major calcium-regulating hormone and serves as an important phosphate-regulating hormone.

Calcium Homeostasis

A fall in serum calcium concentration stimulates secretion of the parathyroid hormone. This peptide hormone stimulates biosynthesis of 1,25-(OH)$_2$D$_3$.[65] The 1,25-(OH)$_2$D$_3$ stimulates intestinal calcium absorption and, together with the parathyroid hormone, stimulates renal reabsorption of calcium and mobilization of calcium from bone.[66] The resultant rise in serum calcium suppresses parathyroid hormone secretion, thus shutting down 1,25-(OH)$_2$D$_3$ biosynthesis and calcium mobilization. When calcium rises above normal, the C cells of the thyroid secrete another hormone called calcitonin which blocks mobilization of calcium from bone and perhaps stimulates calcium and phosphorus excretion in the kidney, thus restoring calcium to normal.

It is important to note that parathyroid hormone does not bind to intestine and thus does not directly influence calcium absorption.[67] Rather it stimulates calcium absorption by stimulating 1,25-(OH)$_2$D$_3$ synthesis.[68] In the bone and kidney, however, both parathyroid hormone and 1,25-(OH)$_2$D$_3$ must be present to stimulate the mobilization and retention of calcium.[66] The parathyroid hormone is rapid acting and its actions are spent in minutes. On the other hand, the stimulation of 1,25-$(OH)_2D_3$ and its actions require many hours.[51] Thus short-term control of serum calcium is by parathyroid hormone acting on kidney and bone with existing 1,25-$(OH)_2D_3$ while longer hypocalcemic stimulation causes 1,25-$(OH)_2D_3$ to increase, thus stimulating the intestine to absorb calcium. Thus the ability to adjust calcium absorption to the needs of the organism is by parathyroid hormone–1,25-$(OH)_2D_3$ stimulation. Exogenous parathyroid hormone or 1,25-$(OH)_2D_3$ eliminates the ability of the intestine to adapt.[68,69] Thus Nicolaysen's "endogenous factor" is the parathyroid hormone–vitamin D endocrine complex.[70]

MECHANISM OF ACTION OF 1,25-$(OH)_2D_3$

1,25-$(OH)_2D_3$ is believed to bind to a 3.2–3.7 cytosol receptor[71,72] which is transferred to the nucleus[73] and to initiate transcription of genes[74] which code for calcium and phosphate transport proteins. Indeed, 1,25-$(OH)_2D_3$ is located in the nucleus in the functioning intestine consistent with the steroid hormone receptor mechanism.[75] Further, receptor proteins have been identified and shown to bind to nuclei.

The nature of the calcium–phosphorus transport proteins remains unknown. Wasserman and co-workers identified a calcium-binding protein in chick and mammalian species which was once believed to be the transport protein.[76] There is uniform agreement that the site of the intestinal epithelial cell affected by 1,25-$(OH)_2D_3$ ultimately is the brush border surface, presumably by an induced transport protein. The calcium is shuttled to the basal-lateral membrane by either membrane vesicles or mitochondria. Calcium is released into the serosal fluid by a sodium-dependent reaction.[77]

Little is known concerning the phosphate transport system of intestine except that it requires sodium and is active.[78]

In the bone, 1,25-$(OH)_2D_3$ binds to a 3.2S receptor[79] and ultimately appears in the nuclei of osteoclasts and/or osteoblasts.[80] It initiates calcium mobilization by a transcriptive event since this action is blocked by actinomycin D.[51]

VITAMIN D DEFICIENCY AND DISEASE STATES

Many biochemical and physiologic imbalances occur in the deficient state, which, if not corrected, result in rickets in growing children and osteomalacia in adults. Characteristic biochemical changes include low plasma calcium and inorganic phosphorus levels with a concomitant high plasma alkaline phosphatase. Early in deficiency a defect in calcium absorption occurs. This often leads to secondary hyperparathyroidism, in which parathyroid hormone is secreted in response to a low plasma calcium concentration. With remaining 1,25-$(OH)_2D_3$, bone calcium is mobilized, restoring serum calcium to normal, but parathyroid hormone also causes a phosphaturia, giving a hypophosphatemia which results in a failure of mineralization and bone disease.[81] Rickets occurs when the newly synthesized organic matrix fails to mineralize, resulting in soft bones. Most striking is the failure of endochondral calcification, resulting in widening of the epiphyseal plate and the buildup of osteoid tissue.

Vitamin D affects citrate metabolism, as evidenced by the fact that the serum citrate from 10 rachitic infants was 1.5 mg per 100 ml compared to 2.5 mg per 100 ml in normal infants.[82] Vitamin D treatment (i.e. 600,000 I.U.) resulted in elevation of the serum citrate; however, it is now clear that the citrate response is a consequence of, rather than a participant in, the vitamin-induced changes in mineral metabolism.[83]

Diagnosis of rickets is usually made from the characteristic bony deformities seen on radiographs and from the plasma calcium, phosphorus and alkaline phosphatase values. The noncalcified epiphyseal plate becomes more apparent and there are broadening and irregularity in the adjacent regions of the epiphysis and metaphysis.

Although vitamin D-deficiency rickets is now rare in the western world, several disorders still exist in which there is an apparent lack of the vitamin's action within the calcium homeostatic system. It is now clear that vitamin D is converted to an active hormone which acts on the target tissue, resulting in appropriate responses. Thus some diseases of bone are probably the result of a defective vitamin D metabolism, regulation or target organ response.

Refractory or Vitamin D-Resistant Rickets (Familial Hypophosphatemia)

This disease is usually manifest in early childhood and is characterized by hypophosphatemia and an X-linked dominant inheritance.[84] Although the exact resulting molecular defect which causes the disease is not known, the most characteristic dysfunction is a renal loss of phosphate. In addition, intestinal calcium absorption is below normal. Abnormal vitamin D metabolism has been reported in this disease,[85] but the phosphate defect is not corrected by the administration of 1,25-$(OH)_2D_3$ or 25-OH-D_3.[86] It is likely that there is a generalized defect in phosphate transport mechanisms which may or may not be related to abnormal vitamin D metabolism. However, the defective absorption of calcium in the disease is corrected by 1,25-$(OH)_2D_2$ or 1 α-OH-D_3.

Treatment with massive doses of vitamin D (e.g. 50,000 to 100,000 I.U. daily) gives variable results.[87] Some investigators have reported better success by using lower amounts of vitamin D (e.g. 15,000 to 50,000 I.U. daily) in conjunction with oral phosphate supplements.[88]

Recently 1,25-$(OH)_2D_3$ has been used in the treatment of the disease, together with oral phosphate, with good success. The oral phosphate provides a replacement for the renal loss of phosphate while the 1,25-$(OH)_2D_3$ is used to repair the calcium transport mechanism and to prevent secondary hyperparathyroidism.

Hypoparathyroidism

Hypoparathyroidism usually occurs as a result of surgical removal of the parathyroid glands. Idiopathic hypoparathyroidism is uncommon. This rare disease frequently persists with major convulsive seizures in addition to tetanic spasms. Such patients have often had years of anticonvulsant therapy before the underlying pathologic condition is detected. In this context it is interesting that the long-term use of anticonvulsant drugs apparently accelerates the metabolic breakdown of vitamin D.[89,90]

Hypoparathyroidism has been treated with high doses of dihydrotachysterol or vitamin D_2. Dihydrotachysterol is reported to be the more active compound on a weight basis.[90] Occasionally hypoparathyroid patients develop a resistance to treatment with vitamin D and dihydrotachysterol, necessitating the search for derivatives which may be more active. 25-OH-D_3 is more effective than vitamin D_3 or dihydrotachysterol.[91] Of great importance is the fact that parathyroid hormone stimulates 1,25-$(OH)_2D_3$ synthesis; thus, hypoparathyroid patients produce inadequate 1,25-$(OH)_2D_3$ in response to hypocalcemia. Exogenous 1,25-$(OH)_2D_3$ and its analog 1α-OH-D_3 are effective at physiologic doses in management of this disease, provided dietary calcium is adequate.[92,33]

Vitamin D-Dependency Rickets

Prader and his associates have described a vitamin D-resistant rickets in children which is completely curable with doses of vitamin D ranging from 50,000 to 100,000 I.U. daily.[94] Vitamin D-dependency rickets differs from familial hypophosphatemia in that the latter does not respond completely to vitamin D, and the former is an autosomal recessive trait. Several children suffering from this disease have responded to 30 to 500 μg 25-OH-D$_3$ daily.[95] The disease is not the result of a block in 25-hydroxylation of vitamin D, since pharmacologic amounts of this form of the vitamin are required. However, it is probably a specific genetic block in 1-hydroxylation of 25-OH-D$_3$, since physiologic amounts (0.05 μg per kg) of 1,25-(OH)$_2$D$_3$ will cure the disease[95] and low blood levels of 1,25-(OH)$_2$D$_3$ have been found (DeLuca and Fraser, unpublished results). Cure with 25-OH-D$_3$ probably results from excess 25-OH-D$_3$ substituting for small amounts of 1,25-(OH)$_2$D$_3$ in the receptor mechanisms.

Azotemic Chronic Renal Failure

Patients suffering from chronic renal failure often exhibit abnormally low intestinal calcium absorption, low plasma calcium, secondary hyperparathyroidism and osteodystrophy.[96,97] Such patients have features of both osteitis fibrosa and/or osteomalacia. They are resistant to vitamin D and show abnormal vitamin D metabolism.[98] These patients respond satisfactorily to 50 to 100 μg per day of 25-OH-D$_3$ as compared to much larger doses of vitamin D.[99] Recently it has been shown that renal tissue is responsible for the metabolism of 25-OH-D$_3$ to 1,25-(OH)$_2$D$_3$, the metabolically active form of vitamin D. It is likely that, in chronic renal disease, 1,25-(OH)$_2$D$_3$ is not made in sufficient amounts and thus a "vitamin D"-deficient intestine and ultimately bone result. The resulting hypocalcemia brings about secondary hyperparathyroidism and osteitis fibrosa; the total lack of 1,25-(OH)$_2$D$_3$ gives rise to osteomalacia. The 1,25-(OH)$_2$D$_3$ satisfactorily restores calcium absorption to normal in nephrectomized rats.[63] Furthermore, 1,25-(OH)$_2$D$_3$ and 1α-OH-D$_3$ are used in the successful treatment of a high proportion of renal osteodystrophy patients.[100-103] Pharmacologic amounts of 25-OH-D$_3$ are also successfully employed in the treatment.[99]

Other bone diseases may also be of interest in regard to vitamin D metabolism. The vitamin D resistance of such diseases as hepatic rickets and Fanconi syndrome makes the investigation into the use of vitamin D metabolites for the treatment of such illnesses an exciting area of clinical investigation.

Hypervitaminosis D (Vitamin D Toxicity)

Care should be taken to detect any hypercalcemia or hypercalciuria, when using large doses of vitamin D, which could be indicative of intoxication. Irreversible renal, heart and aortic damage is known to result from prolonged hypercalcemia. Serum calcium should not be permitted to rise above 12 mg per 100 ml.[104]

Treatment in mild cases consists of withdrawing vitamin D until serum calcium falls; this necessitates the readministration of vitamin D, usually at a reduced level. More severe cases may require the use of glucocorticoids to reduce serum calcium concentration.[105] Calcitonin may also occasionally be used in the treatment of hypervitaminosis D.[106] Toxicity of vitamin D is believed to be the result of high circulating 25-OH-D levels which substitute for 1,25-(OH)$_2$D$_3$ on the receptors when at excessive concentrations. Thus calcium transport and bone resorption goes on at high and unchecked rates, giving hypercalcemia and nephrocalcinosis.

IMPORTANT ANALOGS OF 1,25-(OH)$_2$D$_3$

A synthetic analog of great importance is 1α-OH-D$_3$, which is not naturally occurring.[107] It has been shown to be converted in the liver to the active hormone 1,25-(OH)$_2$D$_3$ before it acts.[108] It is relatively easy to synthesize and is used therapeutically as a substitute for 1,25-(OH)$_2$D$_3$.

Dihydrotachysterol$_2$ is a reduction

product of vitamin D_2 or the photoisomer tachysterol$_2$. The 9,10 double bond is reduced and the A ring is rotated about the 5,6 double bond.[17] Thus the 3-OH group is in the spatial position of the 1-OH of 1,25-(OH)$_2$D$_3$. It, therefore, acts without undergoing 1-hydroxylation. Similarly, the 5,6-trans vitamin Ds act without 1-hydroxylation. They are, however, poor substitutes for 1,25-(OH)$_2$D$_3$.[108]

SUMMARY

In summary, the mode of action for vitamin D is becoming increasingly clear; witness the recent discovery of the kidney-based vitamin D endocrine system and the hydroxylated vitamin D metabolites, especially 1,25-(OH)$_2$D$_3$. Vitamin D is first hydroxylated in the liver to 25-OH-D$_3$, which represents the major circulating form of the vitamin in blood. Further hydroxylation of 25-OH-D$_3$ to 1,25-(OH)$_2$D$_3$ occurs in the kidney. It is the latter compound which acts directly to carry out the functions of vitamin D.

The realization that vitamin D serves only as a precursor for the synthesis of a hormone suggests that some vitamin D-related diseases may involve a block in the production of the active form of the vitamin. It is already apparent that such diseases as renal osteodystrophy, vitamin D dependency and hypoparathyroidism are such diseases. These and several other diseases are managed with the active metabolites of vitamin D.

BIBLIOGRAPHY

1. Griffenhagen: Bull. Natl. Inst. Nutr., 2, No. 9, 1952.
2. Bennett: Treatise on the Oleum Jecoris Aselli or Cod-liver Oil, Edinburgh, 1848.
3. Palm: Practitioner, 45, 270, 1890.
4. Mellanby: J. Physiol., 52, Liii, 1919.
5. McCollum, Simonds, Becker and Shipley: J. Biol. Chem., 53, 293, 1922.
6. McCollum, Simonds, Becker and Shipley: Bull. Johns Hopkins Hosp., 33, 229, 1922.
7. Huldshinsky: Dtsch. Med. Wochenschr., 45, 712, 1919.
8. Steenbock and Black: J. Biol. Chem., 61, 405, 1924.
9. Steenbock: Science, 60, 224, 1924.
10. Askew, Bourdillon, Bruce, Jenkins and Webster: Proc. R. Soc., B107, 76, 1931.
11. Windaus, Schenck and von Werder: Hoppe-Seylers Z. Physiol. Chem., 241, 100, 1936.
12. DeLuca: Vitam. Horm., 25, 315, 1967.
13. DeLuca: Fed. Proc., 33, 2211, 1974.
14. Bernstein, Oleson, Ritter and Sax: J. Am. Chem. Soc., 71, 2576, 1949.
15. Bernstein and Sax: J. Org. Chem., 16, 685, 1951.
16. Parfitt: Aust. Ann. Med., 16, 114, 1967.
17. Hallick and DeLuca: J. Biol. Chem., 246, 5733, 1971.
18. Jones: In Vitamin D: Biochemical, Chemical and Clinical Aspects Related to Calcium Metabolism (Norman, Schaefer, Coburn, DeLuca, Fraser, Grigoleit and von Herrath, Eds.). Berlin, Walter de Gruyter, Inc., 1977.
19. U. S. Pharmacopoeia, 15th Revision, U.S.P. XV. Easton, Mack Publishing, 1955.
20. Association of Official Analytical Chemists, Horwitz (Ed.). Box 540, Benjamin Franklin Station, Washington.
21. Thompson, Lewis and Booth: J. Clin. Invest., 45, 94, 1966.
22. Schachter, Finkelstein and Kowarski: J. Clin. Invest., 43, 787, 1964.
23. Greaves and Schmidt: J. Biol. Chem., 102, 101, 1933.
24. Ponchon and DeLuca: J. Clin. Invest., 48, 1273, 1969.
25. Bhattacharyya and DeLuca: Arch. Biochem. Biophys., 160, 58, 1974.
26. Botham, Ghazarian, Kream and DeLuca: Biochemistry, 15, 2130, 1976.
27. Imawari and Goodman: J. Clin. Invest., 59, 432, 1977.
28. Haddad and Walgate: J. Biol. Chem., 251, 4803, 1976.
29. Avioli, Williams, Lund and DeLuca: J. Clin. Invest., 46, 1907, 1967.
30. Recommended Dietary Allowances, 8th rev. ed. Washington, National Academy of Sciences, National Research Council, 1974.
31. Maternal Nutrition and Child Health, Bull. 123. Washington, National Research Council, Food and Nutrition Board, 1950 (reprinted 1957).
32. Fraser and Salter: Pediatr. Clin. North Am., May, 417, 1958.
33. Fomon, Younozai and Thomas: J. Nutr., 89, 345, 1966.
34. Fellers and Schwartz: N. Engl. J. Med., 259, 1050, 1958.
35. Anning, Dawson, Dolby and Ingram: Q. J. Med., 17, 203, 1948.
36. Hess and Lewis: J.A.M.A., 91, 783, 1928.
37. Gardner: Pediatrics, 9, 534, 1952.
38. Bruce and Callow: Biochem. J., 28, 517, 1934.
39. Mellanby and Mellanby: Br. Med. J., 2, 409, 1948.
40. Higaki, Takahashi, Suzuki and Sahashi: J. Vitaminol., 11, 261, 1956.
41. Lund, DeLuca and Horsting: Arch. Biochem. Biophys., 120, 513, 1967.
42. Blunt, DeLuca and Schnoes: Biochemistry, 7, 3317, 1968.

43. Suda, DeLuca, Schnoes, Ponchon, Tanaka and Holick: Biochemistry, 9, 2917, 1970.
44. Suda, DeLuca, Schnoes, Tanaka and Holick: Biochemistry 9, 4776, 1970.
45. Holick, DeLuca and Schnoes: Proc. Nat. Acad. Sci., 68, 803, 1971.
46. Holick, Schnoes, DeLuca, Suda and Cousins: Biochemistry, 10, 2799, 1971.
47. Semmler, Holick, Schnoes and DeLuca: Tetrahedron Letters, 40, 4147, 1972.
48. Tanaka, Frank and DeLuca: Endocrinology, 92, 417, 1973.
49. Fraser and Kodicek: Nature, 228, 764, 1970.
50. DeLuca and Schnoes: Annu. Rev. Biochem., 45, 631, 1976.
51. Tanaka and DeLuca: Arch. Biochem. Biophys., 146, 574, 1971.
52. Tanaka, DeLuca, Ikekawa, Morisaki and Koizumi: Arch. Biochem. Biophys., 170, 620, 1975.
53. Tanaka, Castillo, DeLuca and Ikekawa: J. Biol. Chem., 252, 1421, 1977.
54. Holick, Kleiner-Bossaller, Schnoes, Kasten, Boyle and DeLuca: J. Biol. Chem., 248, 6691, 1973.
55. Suda, DeLuca, Schnoes and Blunt: Biochemistry, 8, 3515, 1969.
56. Jones, Schnoes and DeLuca: Biochemistry, 14, 1250, 1975.
57. Jones, Baxter, DeLuca and Schnoes: Biochemistry, 15, 713, 1976.
58. Schachter: In The Transfer of Calcium and Strontium Across Biological Membranes (Wasserman, Ed.). New York, Academic Press, 1963.
59. Chen, Castillo, Korycka-Dahl and DeLuca: J. Nutr., 104, 1056, 1974.
60. Steele, Engle, Tanaka, Lorenc, Dudgeon and DeLuca: Am. J. Physiol., 229, 489, 1975.
61. Carlsson: Acta Physiol. Scand., 26, 212, 1952.
62. Gray, Boyle and DeLuca: Science, 172, 1232, 1971.
63. Boyle, Miravet, Gray, Holick and DeLuca: Endocrinology, 90, 605, 1972.
64. Holick, Garabedian and DeLuca: Science, 176, 1146, 1972.
65. Garabedian, Holick, DeLuca and Boyle: Proc. Natl. Acad. Sci., 69, 1673, 1972.
66. Garabedian, Tanaka, Holick and DeLuca: Endocrinology, 94, 1022, 1974.
67. Zull and Repke: J. Biol. Chem., 247, 2195, 1972.
68. Ribovich and DeLuca: Arch. Biochem. Biophys., 175, 256, 1976.
69. Ribovich and DeLuca: Arch. Biochem. Biophys., 170,, 529, 1975.
70. Boyle, Gray, Omdahl and DeLuca: In Endocrinology 1971 (Taylor, Ed.). London, Wm. Heinemann Medical Books, 1972.
71. Kream, Reynolds, Knutson, Eisman and DeLuca: Arch. Biochem. Biophys., 176, 779, 1976.
72. Brumbaugh and Haussler: Life Sci., 16, 353, 1975.
73. Brumbaugh and Haussler: J. Biol. Chem., 249, 1258, 1974.
74. Emtage, Lawson and Kodicek: Nature, 246, 100, 1973.
75. Chen and DeLuca: J. Biol. Chem., 248, 4890, 1973.
76. Wasserman and Corradino: Annu. Rev. Biochem., 40, 501, 1971.
77. Martin and DeLuca: Am. J. Physiol., 216, 1351, 1969.
78. Walling: In Vitamin D: Biochemical, Chemical and Clinical Aspects Related to Calcium Metabolism (Norman, Schaefer, Coburn, DeLuca, Fraser, Grigoleit and von Herrath, Eds.). Berlin, Walter de Gruyter, 1977.
79. Kream, Jose, Yamada and Deluca: Science, 197, 1086, 1977.
80. Weber, Pons and Kodicek: Biochem. J., 125, 147, 1971.
81. Fraser, Kooh and Scriver: Pediatr. Res., 1, 425, 1967.
82. Harrison and Harrison: Yale J. Biol. Med., 24, 273, 1952.
83. Harrison and Harrison: Am. J. Physiol., 199, 265, 1960.
84. Williams, Winter and Burnett: In The Metabolic Basis of Inherited Disease (Stanbury, Wyngaarden and Fredrickson, Eds.). New York, McGraw-Hill, 1966.
85. Avioli, Williams, Lund and DeLuca: J. Clin. Invest., 46, 1907, 1967.
86. Glorieux, Scriver, Holick and DeLuca: Lancet, 2, 287, 1973.
87. Harrison: J. Pediatr., 64, 618, 1964.
88. Wilson, York, Jaworski and Yendt: Medicine, 44, 99, 1965.
89. Richens and Rowe: Br. Med. J., 4, 73, 1970.
90. Harrison, Lifshitz and Blizzard: N. Engl. J. Med., 276, 894, 1967.
91. Pak, DeLuca, Chavez de los Rios, Suda, Ruskin and Delea: Arch. Intern. Med., 126, 239, 1970.
92. Kooh, Fraser, DeLuca, Holick, Belsey, Clark and Murray: N. Engl. J. Med., 293, 840, 1975.
93. Neer, Holick, DeLuca and Potts: Metabolism, 24, 1403, 1975.
94. Prader, Illig and Heierli: Helv. Paediatr. Acta, 16, 452, 1961.
95. Fraser, Kooh, Kind, Holick, Tanaka and DeLuca: N. Engl. J. Med., 289, 817, 1973.
96. Stanbury and Lumb: Medicine, 41, 1, 1962.
97. Kimberg, Baerg and Gershon: Arch. Intern. Med., 126, 891, 1970.
98. Avioli, Birge, Lee and Slatopolsky: J. Clin. Invest., 47, 2239, 1968.
99. Teitelbaum, Bone, Stein, Gilden, Bates, Boisseau and Avioli: J.A.M.A., 235, 164, 1976.
100. Silverberg, Bettcher, Dossetor, Overton, Holick and DeLuca: Can. Med. Assoc. J., 112, 190, 1975.
101. Brickman, Sherrard, Jowsey, Singer, Baylink, Maloney, Massry, Norman and Coburn: Arch. Intern. Med., 134, 883, 1974.
102. Pierides, Kerr, Ellis, Peart, O'Riordan and DeLuca: Clin. Nephrol., 5, 189, 1976.
103. Chan, Oldham, Holick and DeLuca: J.A.M.A., 234, 47, 1975.
104. Yendt, DeLuca, Garcia and Cohanim: In The Fat Soluble Vitamins (DeLuca and Suttie, Eds.). Madison, University of Wisconsin Press, 1969.

105. Connor, Hopkins, Thomas, Carey and Howard: J. Clin. Endocrinol., *16*, 945, 1956.
106. Milhaud: In *Parathyroid Hormone and Thyrocalcitonin (Calcitonin)* (Talmage and Belanger, Eds.). New York, Excerpta Medica, 1968.
107. Holick, Semmler, Schnoes and DeLuca: Science, *180*, 190, 1973.
108. Holick, Tavela, Holick, Schnoes, DeLuca and Gallagher: J. Biol. Chem., *251*, 1020, 1976.

C. Vitamin K

Robert E. Olson

While studying cholesterol biosynthesis in chicks fed a fat-extracted diet, Dam in 1929[1] observed an unexpected hemorrhagic disease. He soon demonstrated that it was caused by a deficiency of a previously unrecognized fat-soluble substance in the diet. This factor was not identical with any known lipid or the then known fat-soluble vitamins A, D and E, and was found to be broadly distributed in the plant kingdom, particularly in green leafy vegetables. Dam christened the new substance "vitamin K" for Koagulation vitamin. McFarland et al. in 1931[2] confirmed Dam's finding and reported that fish meal was a source of the new vitamin K.

Efforts were then initiated to attempt to isolate the new factor from both alfalfa and fish meal, the vitamin K content of which was greatly increased by intentional putrefaction.[3] In 1939, Doisy and his colleagues[4] and Dam and his colleagues[5] announced the isolation of vitamin K from alfalfa. In addition, Doisy's group reported the isolation of a related but not identical vitamin K from putrefied fish meal.[6] They named these compounds vitamins K_1 and K_2.

CHEMISTRY OF THE K VITAMINS

Vitamin K_1, now known as phylloquinone, was identified by Doisy's group[7] as 2-methyl-3-phytyl-1,4-naphthoquinone, shown in Figure 6C–1. It is the only homolog of vitamin K synthesized by plants. Vitamin K_2, isolated from fish meal, was originally believed to be 2-methyl-3-di-farnesyl-1,4-naphthoquinone,[8] but has since been shown to have 7 isoprene units in the side chain instead of 6, and is now called menaquinone-7.[9] Traces of MK-6 were also found. The menaquinone family of K_2 homologs is a large series of vitamins containing unsaturated side chains, which differ in the number of isoprenyl units. Menaquinone-4 is synthesized in animals and birds from menadione (2-methyl-1,4-naphthoquinone),[10] formerly known as vitamin K_3, by alkylation with digeranyl pyrophosphate. The enzyme has been partially purified and characterized from chick and rat liver microsomes.[11] The other menaquinones are products of bacterial biosynthesis and range from menaquinone-7 to menaquinone-13.[12,13] Partially saturated menaquinones, menaquinone-9-H[14] and menaquinone-8-H[15], are known.

ESTIMATION OF VITAMIN K

Except for vitamin K-rich foods, vitamin K is present in animal and plant tissues in concentrations less than 1 μg per gm of fresh weight. Such a low concentration makes chemical determinations difficult, particularly since all the vitamin K homologs are labile to alkali and light. Extraction of desiccated tissue with neutral solvents, followed by column and thin-layer chromatography, has resulted in the isolation of a variety of vitamin K homologs from various tissues.[15,16] When purified in sufficient quantity, the vitamin

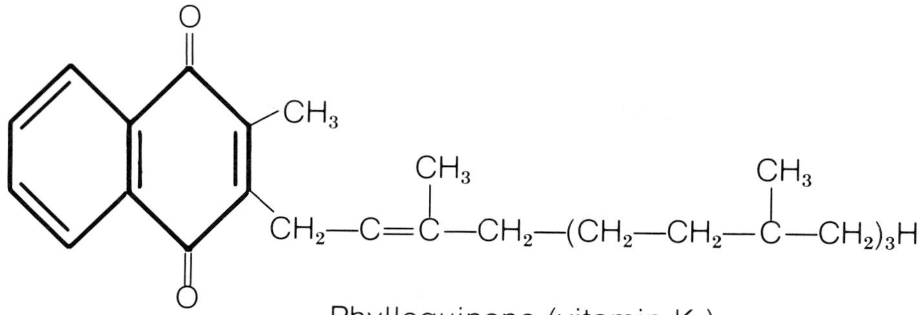

Phylloquinone (vitamin K_1)

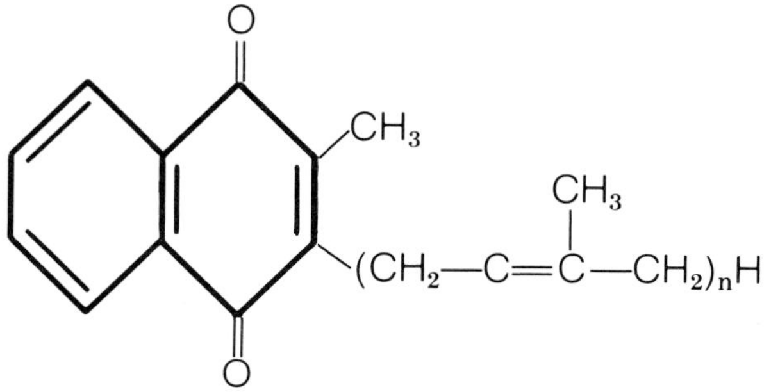

Menaquinone-n (MK-n, vitamin K_2)

Fig. 6C–1. Structures of 2-methyl-3-phytyl-1.4 naphthoquinone and menaquinone.

Ks can be identified by a distinctive absorption spectrum: the molecular extinction coefficient at 248 mμ is 19,000.

The most commonly used technique for measuring the vitamin K content of foods is the chick bioassay, which is sensitive to 0.1 μg phylloquinone per gm of diet. Chicks made deficient in vitamin K by receiving a vitamin K-free diet for 10 days are then fed a supplement containing the assay food. The prothrombin level of the blood is then compared with a standard curve resulting from the feeding of known amounts of phylloquinone.[18,19]

The vitamin K content of common foods as determined by bioassay in chicks is presented in Table 6C–1. In general, green leafy vegetables are high, fruits and cereals are low, and meats and dairy products are intermediate. These bioassays were done on an "as-is" basis, without extraction, which, in the instances of green vegetables, gave less than the actual content of vitamin K_1. In fact, the intestinal absorption of vitamin K from plant sources ranges from 30 to 70 per cent of the actual content determined by extraction. It appears that tobacco is one of the richest sources of phylloquinone known. It contains about 5 mg per 100 gm, a small percentage of which is volatilized in smoking and absorbed through the mucous membranes of the nasopharynx and bronchi.[20]

ABSORPTION, DISTRIBUTION AND METABOLISM OF VITAMIN K

The absorption of phylloquinone and the menaquinones requires bile and pancreatic juice for maximum effectiveness.[21] These alkylated lipid-soluble homologs are incorporated into chylomicrons and appear in the lymph.[22] Efficiency of absorp-

Table 6C–1. Average Vitamin K Content of Some Ordinary Foods*

Food	Vitamin K µg/100 gm	Food	Vitamin K µg/100 gm
Milk & Milk Products		*Vegetables*	
Milk (cows)	3	Asparagus	57
Cheese	35	Beans, green	14
Butter	30	Broccoli	200
		Cabbage	125
Eggs		Lettuce	129
		Peas, green	19
Hens (whole)	11	Spinach	89
		Turnip greens	650
Meat & Meat Products		Potato	3
Ground beef	7	Pumpkin	2
Beef liver	92	Tomato	5
Ham	15	Watercress	57
Pork tenderloin	11		
Chicken liver	7	*Fruits*	
Pork liver	25	Applesauce	2
Bacon	46	Banana	2
		Orange	1
Fats		Peach	8
Corn oil	0	Raisins	6
Safflower oil	0	Strawberries	—
Beef fat	15		
		Beverages	
Cereals & Grain Products		Coffee	38
Rice	—	Cola	2
Maize	5	Tea, green	712
Whole wheat	17	Tea, black	—
Wheat flour	4		
Bread	4		
Oats	20		

*Data taken from the studies of Dam and Glavind,[18] Richardson,[104] Doisy[20] and Matschiner and Doisy.[19]

tion has been measured from 10 to 70 per cent, depending upon the vehicle in which the vitamin is administered and the extent of the enterohepatic circulation generally characteristic of isoprenoid lipids. When isotopically labeled phylloquinone was administered by mouth in doses ranging from the physiologic to the pharmacologic to animals[23] and man,[24] the vitamin appeared in the plasma within 20 minutes and peaked at 2 hours. It then declined exponentially to low values over a period of 48 to 72 hours. During this period, it appeared to be transferred from the chylomicrons to the β-lipoproteins. Between 8 and 30 per cent of the administered radioactivity was recovered in the urine over a 3-day period in both animals and man, whereas total fecal radioactivity accounted for 45 to 60 per cent of the administered dose over a 5-day period. About one third of this was unchanged vitamin K_1. The administration of nonabsorbable lipids, such as mineral oil or squalene, greatly reduced the absorption of vitamin K in animals.[25]

As much as 50 per cent of a parenterally administered dose of vitamin K_1 may appear in the liver within 1 hour. After oral administration, the liver may contain as much as 20 per cent of the administered dose in 2 hours; this then declines to low values after 24 hours. The relative concentration of vitamin K in kidney, heart, skin and muscle increased to maximum values over a 24-hour period, and then declined. The principal sites of uptake, after liver, were skin and muscle. Fractionation of liver tissue, after the administration of phylloquinone-^{3}H to rats, showed the following relative distribution of radioactivity: nuclei, 13 per cent; mitochondria, 9 per cent; microsomes, 63 per cent; cytosol, 14 per cent.[26] In omnivorous animals, such as man, both phylloquinone and the higher-molecular-weight menaquinones (MK-7 to MK-13), of bacterial origin and probably derived from intestinal flora, are found in the liver.[27,28]

Wiss et al.[29] observed that the principal excretory form of vitamin K in rat urine has a metabolite resembling the lactone of vitamin E first described by Simon, Gross and Milhorant.[30] It was identified as a chain-shortened and oxidized derivative of vitamin K, which forms a gamma lactone and is probably excreted as a glucuronide. Vitamin K oxide has also been identified as a metabolite of vitamin K in rats.[31]

When menadione (2-methyl-1,4-naphthoquinone) is administered to animals or man, only a small amount (0.05 to 1.0 per cent) is converted to an active vitamin, menaquinone-4.[32-34] The principal metabolites of menadione are the sulfate and glucuronide of dihydromenadione.[35] Menadione also reacts with free sulfhydryl groups in proteins to form a thioether linkage, first described by Fieser,[36] which may account for some of its reported toxicity.[37]

PHYSIOLOGIC FUNCTION OF VITAMIN K

Shortly after the discovery of vitamin K, Dam et al.[38] demonstrated that the anticoagulant effect of vitamin K deficiency in the chick was caused by a reduction in the content of plasma prothrombin. Subsequently, it was learned that three other coagulation proteins—factor VII,[39] factor IX[40] and factor X[41] —were also regulated by vitamin K. An abbreviated clotting scheme depicting the proteolytic cascade hypothesis proposed by Biggs and McFarlane[42] and by Davie and Ratnoff,[43] and showing the role of the vitamin K-dependent factors, is shown in Figure 6C–2.

The four vitamin K-dependent coagulation factors are distributed in the extrinsic system, which is activated by injury, the intrinsic system, which is activated by platelets, and the final common pathway leading to the conversion of fibrinogen to fibrin. In deficient animals or man, the administration of vitamin K brings about a prompt response and return toward normal of depressed coagulation factors in 4 to 6 hours. In the absence of the liver, this response does not occur.[44]

Since 1935, several hypotheses have been proposed to account for the action of vitamin K in controlling the activity of these factors. Originally it was thought that vitamin K was a component of prothrombin. Other ideas put forward more recently suggested that vitamin K regulated (1) mammalian electron transport,[45] (2) specific mRNA synthesis and uptake by ribosomes[46] and (3) the post-translational modification of a precursor peptide by addition of a prosthetic group.[47] The discovery of γ-carboxyglutamic (Gla) (Fig. 6C–3) in a tetrapeptide (Leu-Gla-Gla-Val) isolated from bovine prothrombin and representing residues 6 to 9 by Stenflo and his colleagues at the University of Lund in Malmo,[48] followed by independent reports of similar findings by Nelsestuen et al.[49] from Minneapolis and Magnusson et al.[50] from Arrhus, was the first specific clue to the action of the vitamin. This new amino acid was absent from the corresponding peptide derived from the abnormal inactive prothrombin present in the plasma of cows which had been fed Dicumarol. These findings strengthened the view that vitamin K was involved in a post-translational carboxylation of an inactive precursor peptide. Magnusson et al.[50] observed that not only were residues 7 and 8 γ-carboxyglutamate, but in fact in the first

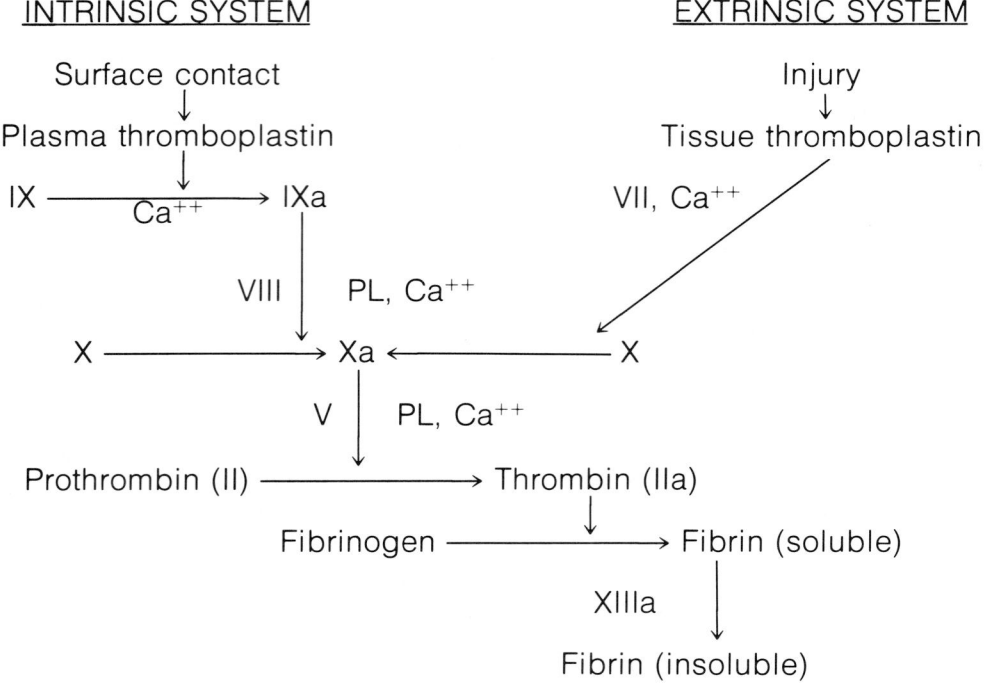

INTRINSIC SYSTEM

Surface contact

Plasma thromboplastin

IX $\xrightarrow{\text{Ca}^{++}}$ IXa

VIII | PL, Ca^{++}

X $\longrightarrow$ Xa $\longleftarrow$ X

V | PL, Ca^{++}

Prothrombin (II) $\longrightarrow$ Thrombin (IIa)

Fibrinogen $\longrightarrow$ Fibrin (soluble)

EXTRINSIC SYSTEM

Injury

Tissue thromboplastin

VII, Ca^{++}

XIIIa |

Fibrin (insoluble)

Fig. 6C–2. Factors II (prothrombin), VII (proconvertin), IX (Christmas factor) and X (Stuart-Prower factor) are vitamin K-dependent and occupy the core of the clotting scheme. Activation of these factors requires calcium ions. Factor V is acceleration globulin: factor VIII is antihemophilic globulin; factor XIII is fibrin-stabilizing factor, a transpeptidase; PL is phospholipid; factor a is active enzyme.

40 amino acids from the N terminus all glutamic acids (at positions 7, 8, 15, 17, 20, 21, 26, 27, 30 and 33) were γ-carboxylated.

The discovery of γ-carboxyglutamate in prothrombin stimulated a flurry of studies of CO_2 fixation into prothrombin under various conditions. In vitamin K-deficient rats given $H^{14}CO_3^-$, Olson[46] found little evidence of additional $^{14}CO_2$ incorporation into prothrombin beyond that seen in albumin from glutamate synthesis. Girardot et al.[51] dosed vitamin K-deficient rats with $H^{14}CO_3^-$ and reported that a ^{14}C-tryptic peptide from plasma prothrombin contained a labeled acidic amino acid which yielded unlabeled glutamate on boiling. These inconclusive experiments were just a beginning and several laboratories took up the study of the function of vitamin K in peptide-bound glutamate carboxylation.

The first vitamin K-dependent system which produced prothrombin in vitro was that described by Shah and Suttie.[52] Postmitochondrial supernatants from vitamin K-deficient rats were shown to respond to

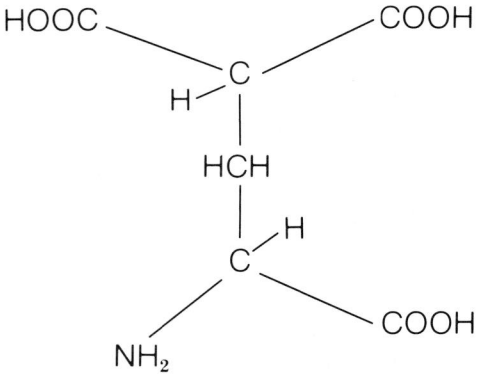

Fig. 6C–3. γ-Carboxyglutamate.

the addition of vitamin K by producing a significant amount of biologically active prothrombin in the presence of cycloheximide. Esmon et al.[53] then demonstrated that the same postmitochondrial supernatant would catalyze a vitamin K-dependent incorporation of $H^{14}CO_3^-$ into the endogenous microsomal precursor protein. Radioactive prothrombin formed in this in vitro system was isolated and essentially all of the radioactivity was shown to be present as γ-carboxyglutamic acid residues in the N-terminal portion of prothrombin. These observations offered final proof that vitamin K was concerned with the post-translational carboxylation of glutamate residues in a prothrombin precursor. The vitamin K-dependent synthesis and modification of precursor prothrombin has also been demonstrated in H-35 hepatoma cells in culture.[54]

The vitamin K-dependent carboxylase system is a membrane-bound component of microsomes. It has been solubilized[55-57] and in the soluble form retains most of the properties of the microsomal system. The system requires a peptide substrate, O_2, $^-HCO_3$ and either vitamin K plus NADH or vitamin K hydroquinone. ATP is not required. The active form of the vitamin is the reduced form and constitutes the electron donor for a microsomal electron transport system involving vitamin K hydroquinone and oxygen. This electron transport system is coupled to a CO_2 fixation reaction converting peptide-bound glutamate to γ-carboxyglutamate. Artificial substrates imitating partial sequences of prothrombin precursor have proven to be active in the system. Suttie[58] has reported that the pentapeptide Phe-Leu-Glu-Glu-Val, analogous to residues 5 to 9 in bovine precursor prothrombin, can be carboxylated in the solubilized rat microsomal system. Houser et al.[57] compared the activity of this pentapeptide with the homologous pentapeptide from the rat, Phe-Leu-Glu-Glu-Ile, and found that the Ile peptide was three times as active as the

Val peptide in the solubilized rat microsomal system.

Jones et al.[60] investigated the active species of "CO_2" utilized by the microsomal system by the low-temperature method of Filmer and Cooper.[59] This was possible only because short-chain homologs of vitamin K such as menaquinone-2 are quite active at 10°C. The reactions were carried out with washed microsomes in the presence of cycloheximide, avidin and acetazolamide to inhibit respectively protein synthesis, biotin-dependent reactions and carbonic anhydrase. By generating $^{14}CO_2$ or $H^{14}CO_3^-$ preferentially and measuring the rate of uptake of isotope from each species into γ-carboxyglutamate residues in microsomal protein at minute intervals, it was concluded that CO_2 and not bicarbonate was the preferred substrate. Physiologists have long believed that CO_2, being uncharged, is a principal form of transport of "CO_2" through membranes. Biotin is clearly not involved in this CO_2 fixation[60,61] because (1) biotin-deficient rats showing marked depression of biotin-dependent enzyme activity show no depression in plasma prothrombin, (2) avidin, a potent inhibitor of biotin-dependent reactions, is ineffective in blocking the vitamin K-dependent carboxylation, even in the detergent-solubilized microsomal system, (3) ATP is not required and (4) CO_2 and not bicarbonate is the active species of "CO_2."

All primary biotin-catalyzed CO_2 fixations involve ATP and $^-HCO_3$.[62] The mechanism by which vitamin K catalyzes the transfer of CO_2 from the membrane to peptide-bound glutamate is not yet elucidated. Reaction mechanisms which have been suggested include formation of a dehydro vitamin K-hemicarbonate, activation of the γ-proton of peptide-bound glutamate by the conjugate base of dehydro vitamin K, formation of the peroxide anion of vitamin K which could also form a hemicarbonate and an indirect action of vitamin K[63] through a regulatory protein upon the carboxylase. Epoxidation of vitamin K is associated with carboxylation of prothrombin precursors in whole microsomes, but whether epoxide formation is required for carboxylation is controversial.[63,64] Additional work will be required to elucidate the molecular action of vitamin K in prothrombin formation.

BONE AND KIDNEY PROTEINS CONTAINING γ-CARBOXYGLUTAMATE

Recent reports have indicated that proteins containing γ-carboxyglutamic acid also occur in mineralized tissue. Hauschka, Lian and Gallop[65] reported such a protein, which they named "osteocalcin." It could be isolated from metatarsal bones of 14-week-old chickens by extraction with 0.5 molar EDTA. It was adsorbable on barium sulfate, and could be chromatographed on hydroxyapatite. Price et al.[66,67] isolated a similar, probably homologous, protein from bovine bones and determined its amino acid sequence; it contained 49 amino acids including 3 γ-carboxyglutamate residues and had a molecular weight of 5,700.

Hauschka[68] observed that the appearance of osteocalcin in embryonic chick bones coincides with the beginning of mineralization. He noted that injection of Dicumarol or warfarin into eggs containing developing embryos reduced the Gla content of osteocalcin by 20 to 50 per cent. Vitamin K-deficient chicks and rats showed comparable reduction in the Gla content of EDTA-extractable bone proteins. Several case reports of the Conradi-Hunermann type of chondrodysplasia punctata in infants born of mothers taking warfarin during the first trimester suggest that warfarin may be a teratogen because of its inhibition of osteocalcin synthesis and perhaps the synthesis of other vitamin K-dependent proteins concerned with the maturation of bony tissue.[61-72] The role of osteocalcin may be to modulate calcium deposition in the bone matrix by interacting with hydroxyapatite crystal nuclei as they form.

Lian and Prien[73] have reported the presence of another Gla containing protein in the matrix of hydroxyapatite [$Ca_{10}(PO_4)_6(OH)_2$] and calcium oxalate renal stones in man. This protein has an apparent molecular weight of 18,000 and contains 3 or 4 residues of Gla. It may prevent crystallization of Ca^{++} stones in normal urine.

COUMARIN ANTICOAGULANT DRUGS

A hemorrhagic disease in cattle which had consumed spoiled clover was described by Schofield[74] in 1922 and attributed to a depressed prothrombin level in 1931.[75] In 1941, Link and his associates[76] demonstrated that the active agent in spoiled clover was dishydroxycoumarin (Dicumarol). A variety of related compounds, either derivatives of 4-hydroxycoumarin or phenindione, have been synthesized and tested for anticoagulant activity in animals and man. One of the more popular ones in the United States is warfarin [3-(α-acetonylbenzyl)-4-hydroxycoumarin], which is more soluble than Dicumarol. Structures are shown in Figure 6C–4.

The oral anticoagulant agents regulate the biosynthesis of prothrombin (factor II) and factors VII, IX and X in the liver. They also induce hypoprothrombinemia at the same rate when given in saturating doses, even though the half-life of various drugs varies from hours to days. As soon as there is an effective concentration of the drug, prothrombin biosynthesis by the liver is shut off and the factors then decay in plasma at their specific half-lives.[77] Hydroxylated products of these drugs, generated by the enzymes in the liver microsomes, are inactive.

There is presently a controversy on the mode of antagonism of the coumarin drugs and vitamin K. Some believe that the interaction is competitive at some common

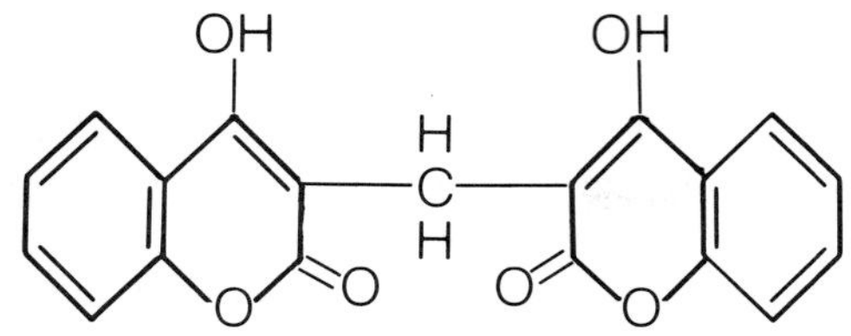

Fig. 6C–4. Structures of Dicumarol and warfarin.

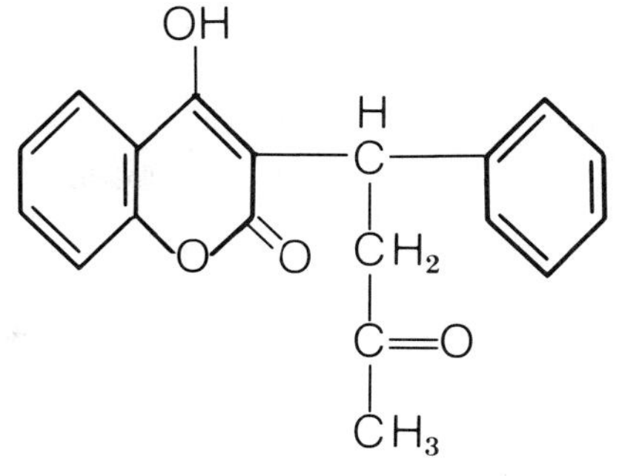

site on a regulatory protein or enzyme involved in prothrombin synthesis,[78,79] and others feel that the kinetics are not competitive[77,80,81] and are probably allosteric.[82]

Warfarin inhibits the in vitro vitamin K-dependent carboxylation of prothrombin precursor in rat liver microsomes, but has little effect on the solubilized carboxylase system.[63] Warfarin inhibits several vitamin K-metabolizing enzymes, including vitamin K reductase and vitamin K epoxide reductase. All of these data support the view that warfarin is not a direct inhibitor of the carboxylase, but acts to inhibit indirectly through an ancillary enzyme or regulatory protein.

O'Reilly et al.[83] have discovered a kindred of genetically determined resistance to the anticoagulant action of coumarin drugs. The genetic defect may be due to a reduced affinity of a regulatory protein for coumarin drugs. Responsiveness to vitamin K in these patients was normal. A related group of coumarin-resistant rats[79,84,85] appears to have a high resistance to coumarin drugs and a slightly increased vitamin K requirement, suggesting that the mutant protein in the rat may have altered sites for both coumarin and vitamin K.

Thierry et al.[86] and Lorusso and Suttie[87] observed that microsomal fractions from warfarin-resistant rats showed less binding of ^{14}C-warfarin than those from normal Sprague-Dawley rats. Searcey et al.[88] have reported the isolation of warfarin-binding proteins from Sprague-Dawley and warfarin-resistant rats which appear to be homologous but differ in their affinities for the 4-hydroxycoumarin drugs. By using differential warfarin binding, these proteins were isolated from 0.2 to 0.4 M KC1 extracts of polysomes derived from the two strains of rats by chromatography on DEAE-cellulose. The warfarin-binding protein isolated from Sprague-Dawley rats was half saturated at 8 μM warfarin and bound 0.7 mole warfarin per mole of protein at saturation. The corresponding protein from warfarin-resistant rats did not saturate at levels of 30 μM warfarin and bound only 0.1 mole warfarin per mole protein. The molecular weights of the binding proteins from normal and warfarin-resistant rats were each 32,000 by SDS gel electrophoresis. The ^{14}C-warfarin binding by these proteins was inhibited by unlabeled warfarin, phylloquinone and tryptic digestion. The S-enantiomer of warfarin was the preferred ligand. On the basis of these data, it is possible that this protein is the warfarin-receptor protein which mediates the effect of the drug on prothrombin synthesis.

When overdosage with coumarin drugs occurs in patients who have received anticoagulant agents to prevent thrombosis (coronary artery disease, pulmonary embolic disease), the intravenous administration of pharmacologic doses of vitamin K_1 in the milligram range reinitiates prothrombin synthesis within minutes, gives protective levels of prothrombin within hours and normal values in 24 hours. Water-soluble derivatives of menadione (e.g. Synkavite) are largely ineffective against the coumarin anticoagulant drugs because, as previously mentioned, the rate of conversion to menaquinone-4 is so slow that pharmacologically effective levels of the alkylated vitamin are not attained.[89,90]

VITAMIN K DEFICIENCY

Primary vitamin K deficiency is uncommon in man. This is because of the widespread distribution of vitamin K in plant and animal tissues and the microbiologic flora of the normal gut, which synthesize the menaquinones in amounts that may supply the bulk of the requirement for vitamin K.

Newborn infants represent a special case of vitamin K nutrition because (1) the placenta is a relatively poor organ for the transmission of lipids and (2) the gut is sterile during the first few days. In normal infants, the plasma prothrombin concentration may decrease to as low as 20 per cent in the second and third days of life, and then gradually climb to normal adult values over a period of weeks. If values fall below 10 per cent, hemorrhagic disease of the newborn may occur.[91] Both water-soluble and lipid-soluble forms of vitamin K are effective in restoring prothrombin levels and controlling hemorrhage in these infants.[92,93] The advisability of giving vitamin K routinely to expectant mothers is controversial.[94,95]

Healthy adult subjects fed diets low in vitamin K (less than 20 μg per day) for periods of several weeks show minimal signs of vitamin K deficiency, i.e. plasma prothrombin values of 60 to 90 per cent, unless they are also given bowel-sterilizing

antibiotics such as neomycin.[20,96,97] In one study, intravenous nutrition of apoplectic patients plus neomycin was required to lower the vitamin K-dependent clotting factors to below 20 per cent of normal[97] in 4 weeks. The intravenous administration of vitamin K in various doses (0.03 to 1.5 μg per kg) to these patients caused a proportional rise in the concentration of these depressed values to normal.

Udall[96] showed that large amounts of vitamin K (of the order of 500 mg per day) instilled into the cecum did not elevate depressed coagulation factors in anticoagulated patients, whereas the same dose given orally produced a prompt response. It appears that the microorganisms synthesizing vitamin K in the gut must reside in the ileum, where absorption of vitamin K is possible. In unusual cases, self-imposed dietary restriction has been observed to induce hypoprothrombinemia with hemorrhage responsive to oral vitamin K.[89,99]

Any disorder that hinders the delivery of bile to the small bowel, such as obstructive jaundice or bile fistula, reduces the absorption of vitamin K from the bowel and causes a reduction in plasma concentration of the vitamin K-dependent factors that can be prevented or relieved by the administration of parenteral vitamin K, or oral vitamin K plus bile salts. Malabsorption syndromes associated with sprue, pellagra, bowel shunts, regional ileitis and ulcerative colitis also cause a secondary vitamin K deficiency.[100]

In chronic liver disease, hypoprothrombinemia with bleeding may occur because of lack of functional hepatic ribosomes to respond to vitamin K.

NUTRITIONAL REQUIREMENTS FOR VITAMIN K

The vitamin K requirement of mammals is met by a combination of dietary intake and microbiologic biosynthesis in the gut. Furthermore, genetic factors no doubt influence the vitamin K requirement in both animals and man. In conventional rats, the vitamin K requirement is about 10 μg per kg per day, whereas, in germ-free rats, the requirement is more than doubled to about 25 μg per kg per day.[101]

In human subjects, the vitamin K homologs stored in the liver suggest that about 40 to 50 per cent of the daily requirement is derived from plant sources, i.e. vitamin K_1, and the remainder from microbiologic biosynthesis. Rietz, Gloor and Wiss[28] reported that 50 per cent of the vitamin K of human liver was vitamin K_1 and the remainder a mixture of menaquinone-7, menaquinone-8, menaquinone-9, menaquinone-10 and menaquinone-11.

If it is assumed that the intravenous dose of vitamin K required to raise depressed vitamin K to normal for 1 day is 1 μg per kg,[97] and that 50 per cent of the vitamin K appearing in the lumen of the gut each day is absorbed, the total daily requirement for the vitamin would be 2 μg per kg per day. If, on the other hand, the assumption is that 50 per cent of the requirement is derived from intestinal microorganisms, then the dietary requirement would be reduced again to 1 μg per kg per day. With the information at hand, this is a rough estimate, particularly since there is controversy on the relative activity of phylloquinone and the menaquinones in stimulating prothrombin synthesis.[102,103] From the dietary information presented in Table 6C–1, it can be calculated that a "normal mixed diet" in the United States will contain from 300 to 500 μg of vitamin K per day, an amount more than adequate to supply the dietary requirement.

BIBLIOGRAPHY

1. Dam: Biochem. Z., 215, 475, 1929.
2. McFarland, Graham and Richardson: Biochem. J., 25, 358, 1931.
3. Almquist and Stokstad: J. Nutr., 12, 329, 1936.
4. Binkley, MacCorquodale, Thayer and Doisy: J. Biol. Chem., 130, 219, 1939.
5. Dam, Geiger, Glavind, Karrer, Karrer, Rothchild and Salomon: Helv. Chim. Acta, 22, 310, 1939.
6. McKee, Binkley, Thayer, MacCorquodale and Doisy: J. Biol. Chem., 131, 327, 1939.
7. Binkley, Cheney, Holcomb, McKee, Thayer, MacCorquodale and Doisy: J. Am. Chem. Soc., 61, 2558, 1939.
8. Binkley, McKee, Thayer and Doisy: J. Biol. Chem., 133, 721, 1940.
9. Isler, Rüegg, Chopard-dit-Jean, Winterstein and Wiss: Helv. Chim. Acta, 41, 786, 1958.
10. Martius and Esser: Biochem. Z., 331, 1, 1958.
11. Dialameh, Yekundi and Olson: Biochim. Biophys. Acta, 223, 332, 1970.
12. Matschiner, Taggart and Amelotti: Biochemistry, 6, 1243, 1967.
13. Pennock: Vitam. Horm., 24, 307, 1966.
14. Gale, Arison, Trenner, Page and Folkers: Biochemistry, 2, 200, 1963.
15. Scholes and King: Biochem. J., 97, 766, 1965.
16. Martius: Am. J. Clin. Nutr., 9, 97, 1961.
17. Matschiner and Taggart: Anal. Biochem., 18, 88, 1967.
18. Dam and Glavind: Biochem. J., 32, 485, 1938.
19. Matschiner and Doisy: J. Nutr., 90, 97, 1966.
20. Doisy: Unpublished work.
21. Mann, Mann and Bollman: Am. J. Physiol., 158, 311, 1949.
22. Blomstrand and Forsgren: Int. J. Vitam. Nutr. Res., 38, 45, 1968.
23. Wiss and Gloor: Vitam. Horm., 24, 575, 1966.
24. Shearer, Barkhan and Webster: Br. J. Haematol., 18, 297, 1970.
25. Matschiner, Hsai and Doisy: J. Nutr., 91, 299, 1967.
26. Bell and Matschiner: Biochim. Biophys. Acta, 184, 597, 1969.
27. Matschiner and Amelotti: J. Lipid Res., 9, 176, 1968.
28. Rietz, Gloor and Wiss: Int. J. Vitam. Res., 40, 351, 1970.
29. Wiss and Gloor: Vitam. Horm., 24, 575, 1966.
30. Simon, Gross and Milhorat: J. Biol. Chem., 221, 797, 1956.
31. Matschiner, Bell, Amelotti and Knauer: Biochim. Biophys. Acta, 201, 309, 1970.
32. Billeter, Bolliger and Martius: Biochem. Z., 340, 290, 1964.
33. Taggart and Matschiner: Biochemistry, 8, 1141, 1969.
34. Dialameh, Taggart, Matschiner and Olson: Int. J. Vitam. Nutr. Res., 41, 391, 1971.
35. Losito, Owen and Flock: Biochemistry, 6, 62, 1967.
36. Fieser and Turner: J. Am. Chem. Soc., 69, 2335, 1947.
37. Mezick and Cornwell: Biochim. Biophys. Acta, 219, 361, 1970.
38. Dam, Schønheyder and Tage-Hansen: Biochem. J., 30, 1075, 1936.
39. Owen: Bull. Am. Coll. Surg., 32, 256, 1947.
40. Naeye: Proc. Soc. Exp. Biol. Med., 91, 101, 1956.
41. Hougie, Barrow and Graham: J. Clin. Invest., 36, 485, 1957.
42. Biggs and McFarlane: *Human Blood Coagulation and Its Disorders*, 3rd Ed. Philadelphia, F.A. Davis, 1962.
43. Davie and Ratnoff: Science, 145, 1310, 1964.

44. Andrus, Lord and Moore: Surgery, 6, 899, 1939.
45. Martius: Vitam. Horm., 24, 441, 1966.
46. Olson: Vitam. Horm., 32, 483, 1974.
47. Suttie: Vitam. Horm., 32, 463, 1974.
48. Stenflo, Fernlund, Egan and Roepstorff: Proc. Natl. Acad. Sci., 71, 2730, 1974.
49. Nelsestuen, Zytkovicz and Howard: J. Biol. Chem., 249, 6347, 1974.
50. Magnusson, Sottrup-Jansen, Petersen, Morris and Dell: FEBS Lett., 44, 189, 1974.
51. Girardot, Delaney and Johnson: Biochem. Biophys. Res. Commun., 59, 1197, 1976.
52. Shah, and Suttie: Biochem. Biophys. Res. Commun., 60, 1397, 1974.
53. Esmon, Sadowski and Suttie: J. Biol. Chem., 250, 4744, 1975.
54. Munns, Johnston, Liszewski and Olson: Proc. Natl. Acad. Sci., 73, 2803, 1976.
55. Esmon and Suttie: J. Biol. Chem., 251, 6238, 1976.
56. Mack, Suen, Girardot, Miller, Delaney and Johnson: J. Biol. Chem., 251, 3269, 1976.
57. Houser, Carey, Dus, Marshall and Olson: FEBS Lett., 75, 226, 1977.
58. Suttie, Hageman, Lehrman and Rich: J. Biol. Chem., 251, 5827, 1976.
59. Filmer and Cooper: J. Theor. Biol., 29, 131, 1970.
60. Jones, Gardner, Cooper and Olson: J. Biol. Chem., 252, 7738, 1977.
61. Friedman and Shia: Biochem. J., 163, 39, 1977.
62. Wood and Utter: Essays in Biochemistry. New York, Academic Press, 1965.
63. Olson and Suttie: Vitam. Horm., 35, 59, 1977.
64. Sadowski, Schnoes and Suttie: Biochemistry, 16, 3856, 1977.
65. Hauschka, Lian and Gallop: Proc. Natl. Acad. Sci., 72, 3925, 1975.
66. Price, Otsuka, Poser, Kirstaponis and Raman: Proc. Natl. Acad. Sci., 73, 1447, 1976.
67. Price, Poser and Raman: Proc. Natl. Acad. Sci., 73, 3374, 1976.
68. Hauschka: Biochem. Biophys. Res. Commun., 71, 1207, 1976.
69. Pettifor and Benson: J. Pediatr., 86, 459, 1975.
70. Warkang: Am. J. Dis. Child., 129, 287, 1975.
71. Fourie and Hay: S. Afr. Med. J., 49, 2081, 1975.
72. Shaul, Emery and Hall: Am. J. Dis. Child., 129, 360, 1975.
73. Lian and Prien, Jr.: Fed. Proc. 35, 1763, 1976.
74. Schofield: Can. Vet. Rec., 3, 74, 1922.
75. Roderick: Am. J. Physiol., 96, 413, 1931.
76. Campbell, Smith, Roberts and Link: J. Biol. Chem., 138, 1, 1941.
77. O'Reilly and Aggeler: Pharmacol. Rev., 22, 35, 1970.
78. Quick and Collentine: J. Lab. Clin. Med., 36, 976, 1950.
79. Hermodson, Suttie and Link: Am. J. Physiol., 217, 1316, 1969.
80. Babson, Malament, Mangun and Phillips: Clin. Chem., 2, 243, 1956.
81. Woolley: Physiol. Rev., 27, 308, 1947.
82. Olson, Philipps and Wang: Adv. Enzyme Regul., 6, 213, 1968.
83. O'Reilly, Aggeler, Hoag, Leong and Kropatkin: N. Engl. J. Med., 271, 809, 1965.
84. Greaves and Ayres: Nature, 215, 877, 1967.
85. Pool, O'Reilly, Schneiderman and Alexander: Am. J. Physiol., 215, 627, 1968.
86. Thierry, Hermodson and Suttie: Am. J. Physiol., 219, 854, 1970.
87. Lorusso and Suttie: Mol. Pharmacol., 8, 197, 1972.
88. Searcey, Graves and Olson: J. Biol. Chem., 252, 6260, 1977.
89. Douglas and Brown: Br. Med. J., 1, 412, 1952.
90. Dam: Vitam. Horm., 24, 295, 1966.
91. Brinkhous, Smith and Warner: Am. J. Med. Sci., 193, 475, 1937.
92. Dam, Tage-Hansen and Plum: Lancet, 237, 1157, 1939.
93. Brinkhous: Medicine, 19, 329, 1940.
94. Potter: Am. J. Obstet. Gynecol., 50, 235, 1945.
95. Webster and Fitzgerald: Surg. Clin. North Am., 23, 85, 1943.
96. Udall: J.A.M.A., 194, 107, 1965.
97. Frick, Riedler and Brogli: J. Appl. Physiol., 23, 387, 1967.
98. Kark and Lozner: Lancet, 2, 1162, 1939.
99. Aggeler, Lucia and Fishbon: Am. J. Dig. Dis., 9, 227, 1942.
100. Clark, Dixon, Butt and Snell: Mayo Clin. Proc., 14, 407, 1939.
101. Gustafsson, Daft, McDaniel, Smith and Fitzgerald: J. Nutr., 78, 461, 1962.
102. Matschiner and Taggart: J. Nutr., 94, 57, 1968.
103. Isler and Wiss: Vitam. Horm., 17, 53, 1959.
104. Richardson, Wilkes and Ritchey: J. Nutr., 73, 363, 1961.

D. Vitamin E

M. K. Horwitt

In 1922, Evans and Bishop[1] noted that a fat-soluble factor prevented fetal resorption in animals that had been fed a rancid lard diet. This was confirmed by Mattill et al.[2] and designated as vitamin E by Sure[3] in 1924. The term "tocopherol" was proposed by Evans from the Greek word *tocos* meaning childbirth or offspring, the Greek noun *phero*, to bring forth, and *ol* for alcohol. The usefulness of the study of fetal resorption as an assay method overwhelmed the significance of the early study of Olcott and Emerson[4] on the antioxidant properties of tocopherol which was amply supported by Moore,[4a] Dam,[5] Filer et al.,[6] and others.[7-9]

In more recent times, the function of α-tocopherol as an antioxidant of the polyunsaturated fatty acids in the tissues has been supported by Tappel,[10] Horwitt,[11] Draper,[12] and Witting.[13] That it can also protect coenzyme Q has been claimed by Folkers.[14] Since coenzyme Q is involved in the transfer of electrons, additional studies on this relationship to vitamin E may serve to resolve a current controversy—whether α-tocopherol is an integral part of an enzyme system[15,16] or whether it protects the integrity of the lipid component of enzyme systems or of the cellular structures that produce or support the enzymes. The possibility that vitamin E is both a biologic antioxidant and a component of some enzyme systems cannot be precluded.

Gilbert[16a] has shown that α-tocopherol can stimulate the growth and reproduction of rotifers, a phenomenon which cannot be related to an antioxidant effect.

CHEMISTRY

Pure vitamin E was first isolated by Evans and the Emersons[17] from the unsa-ponifiable fraction of wheat germ oil in 1936. Its chemical structure[18] and synthesis[19] were reported in 1938. Although α-tocopherol is the active compound most often designated as vitamin E, there are seven other naturally occurring tocopherols. These are designated[20] by the number and position of the methyl groups on either the tocol or tocotrienol complex (Fig. 6D–1) as shown in Table 6D–1. The alpha, beta, zeta and gamma tocopherols have approximately 135, 50, 30 and 10 per cent relative biologic activity,[21] respectively. Not as much is known about the others but their relative biologic activities are quite low, ranging from 5 for epsilon tocopherol to 1 for delta tocopherol.

The most important sources of the tocopherols are the various vegetable oils. Usually, the amount of α-tocopherol present is related to the percentage of linoleic acid in the triglyceride.[8] Thus, safflower

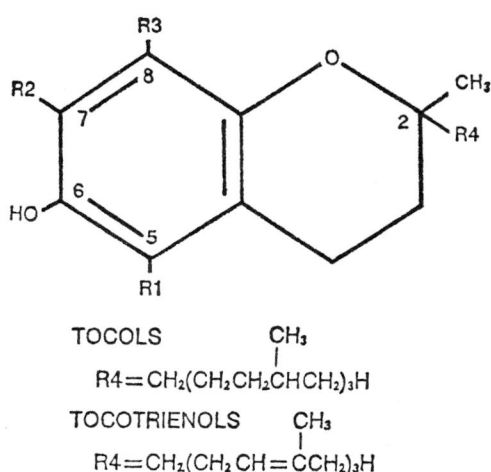

$$TOCOLS$$
$$R4 = CH_2(CH_2CH_2CHCH_2)_3H$$ with CH_3 branch

$$TOCOTRIENOLS$$
$$R4 = CH_2(CH_2 CH = CCH_2)_3H$$ with CH_3 branch

Fig. 6D–1. Structural formulae of vitamin E compounds.

Table 6D–1.   Naturally Occurring Tocopherols

Tocol	Tocotrienol	Methyl Positions
α-(alpha)	ζ-(zeta)	5, 7, 8
β-(beta)	ε-(epsilon)	5, 8
γ-(gamma)	η-(eta)	7, 8
δ-(delta)	8-methyl-tocotrienol	8

oil, which is about 80 per cent linoleate, has one of the highest contents of α-tocopherol. An exception to this rule is corn oil, which, although containing about 50 per cent linoleic acid, has about 90 per cent of the total tocopherol in the gamma tocopherol form. The amounts of total tocopherol present in commercial oils vary greatly with the refining process used.

Differences in activity among the tocopherols are probably a function of the ability of cellular components to distinguish between the compounds and to remove them at different rates. There seems to be no significant difference in the rate at which the individual tocopherols are absorbed from the intestine. Tocopheryl acetate, which has no antioxidant activity before the acetate is removed by cellular esterases, is partially hydrolyzed in the intestine and partially absorbed as the intact ester.[22] Maximum liver storage also occurs more quickly with the free tocopherol than with the acetate derivatives. However, there may be some theoretical advantage to the slower utilization of the acetates. Not only are they less likely to be oxidized before absorption but it has been demonstrated in rats and in chicks fed tocopherol-deficient diets containing different levels of polyunsaturated fatty acids that dividing a tocopherol supplement into smaller, more frequent doses protects better than giving the same total amount once a week.

Various metabolites of α-tocopherol have been investigated for biologic activity: among these are α-tocopherylquinone, the hydroquinone and tocopheronolactone. Both the quinone and hydroquinone derivatives are active in restoring the fertility of rats on E-deficient diets[22,23] and can prevent or cure nutritional muscular dystrophy induced by vitamin E deficiency in the rat and rabbit.[24] Tocopheronolactone has no effect on the fertility of deficient rats as measured by the gestation-resorption test. Like the former derivatives however, it maintains tissue levels of coenzyme Q.[25]

Knowledge of the chemistry of α-tocopherol and its oxidation products is still far from complete. Similarly, the metabolic fate of tocopherol in man is largely unknown, although two conjugated urinary metabolites have been described following the ingestion of large quantities of vitamin E.[26] These may represent final degradation products or intermediates in the formation of other metabolites. However, the possibility exists that some of the presumed metabolites described recently may be formed in vitro, post mortem or during isolation.[27]

UNITS OF MEASUREMENT

One mg of dl-α-tocopheryl acetate has been designated as having 1 International Unit. On the basis of relative biologic activity, which in the past has been a function of efficacy in the prevention of fetal resorption in rats, dl-α-tocopherol, d-α-tocopheryl acetate and d-α-tocopherol have been assigned International Units of 1.1, 1.36 and 1.49, respectively. An approximate confirmation of this relationship between d- and dl-α-tocopheryl acetate was obtained during resupplementation of adult men whose stores of α-tocopherol had been depleted[28] under controlled experimental conditions.

EFFECTS OF DEFICIENCY ON PHYSIOLOGIC FUNCTION

Experimental deprivation of vitamin E in animals is followed by a more baffling array of diverse physiologic abnormalities than has been encountered with any other vitamin. For the sake of discussion, although all of the syndromes have proven to be related, as least in part, to the levels of polyunsaturated fats in the diet and the tissues affected, the pathologic changes studied in mammals may be divided into effects upon the reproductive system, the musculature, the nervous system and the vascular system, respectively. These changes have been described in detail by Mason.[29]

Reproductive System

The seminiferous epithelium of vitamin E-deficient male rats shows no injury until active spermatogenesis begins during the third month of life, when there is a relatively rapid degeneration of the epithelium. To prevent these changes, tocopherol must be given about 2 weeks prior to the appearance of histologic injury. The degeneration is characterized by the following sequence of events: (1) inhibition of spermatogenesis with abnormal swelling and fusion of mature sperm, (2) marked diminution of sperm and nuclear chromatolysis in spermatids and secondary spermatocytes, (3) sloughing of germ cells, and fusion of many into large multinucleate cells, (4) nuclear fragmentation and hydropic degeneration of remaining germ cells, (5) eventual lining of the shrunken tubules by a vacuolated, fibrous Sertoli syncytium. The testes are grossly atrophied, brownish, flabby and watery when cut. The rabbit, dog and monkey show testes damage resembling the early phases of injury in the rat but the mouse is remarkably resistant, taking many more months before marked atrophy of the germinal epithelium occurs.

In the female rat, all reproductive events are apparently normal up to the time of implantation, which occurs at about the seventh day after insemination. Impaired vascular relationships between fetal and maternal components of the placenta appear to be responsible for asphyxia, starvation and death of the fetus. Fetal resorption can be prevented if sufficient tocopherol is given during the first week of pregnancy. In rats given doses that are less than adequate, death may be delayed but pronounced changes may appear in the vascular system prior to death. Changes in the ovaries of young rats have not been demonstrated; the pathologic condition noted seems to be due to uterine dysfunction. Similar intrauterine effects of vitamin E deficiency have been noted in the mouse, hamster and guinea pig. There is no good evidence to relate malfunction of the reproduction process in man with an increased need for vitamin E.

Muscular System

The term "nutritional muscular dystrophy" refers to a form of myopathy which is noted in animals on vitamin E-deficient diets and should not be confused with human "muscular dystrophy." Although it may be proper to consider that nutritional muscular dystrophy can be produced in man[30] under specially defined conditions, the distinction between the disorder that can be produced by nutritional means and the hereditary human disease termed "muscular dystrophy" should be emphasized.

In animals, it is possible to produce a form of muscle paralysis, usually preceded by a pronounced creatinuria,[31] by decreasing the ratio of tocopherol to polyunsaturated fats fed or by inhibiting the optimum utilization of tocopherol by feeding diets which are deficient in either selenium and/or sulfur amino acids.[32] Grossly, the skeletal muscle may be pale, ischemic and gritty owing to calcium deposition. Microscopically there may be edema, leukocyte infiltration and segmental fragmentation of the muscle fibers. The amount of such changes may depend on the severity of the disorder, which is a function of the degree of deficiency, the level of polyunsaturated lipids in the tissues, the time of onset and many related stresses and other nutritional imbalances which can alter the picture.

Herbivorous animals appear to be particularly susceptible to such nutritional myopathies, but how much of this increased susceptibility may be related to the higher levels of polyunsaturated fat in the usual diets of these animals is not certain.[33] The cardiac muscles of herbivorous animals (rabbit, sheep and cattle) are particularly sensitive to low tocopherol regimens;[34] sudden death through myocardial failure may appear before the development of the acid-fast pigment that is characteristic of deficiency in other animals.

The accumulations of the acid-fast pigments have been studied most intensively in the smooth muscle of rats. The changes in the uterus constitute a prototype for those observed elsewhere.

Pigment granules, which give the uterus a chestnut-brown fluorescent color, appear first at the pole of the nucleus and gradually push the myofibrils peripherally, eventually distorting the muscle cells. A similar pigment referred to as lipofuscin or ceroid pigment has been found in the smooth muscle of the stomach, intestine, bronchial wall and bladder of children dying with cystic fibrosis of the pancreas,[35] especially those over 2 years of age. It has also been described in adults with chronic pancreatitis.[36] It is noteworthy that the children with cystic fibrosis of the pancreas showed an excessive creatinuria which could be diminished by administering α-tocopherol.[37] In addition, one adult male patient with pronounced muscular weakness and high creatinuria showed marked improvement after tocopherol therapy. A

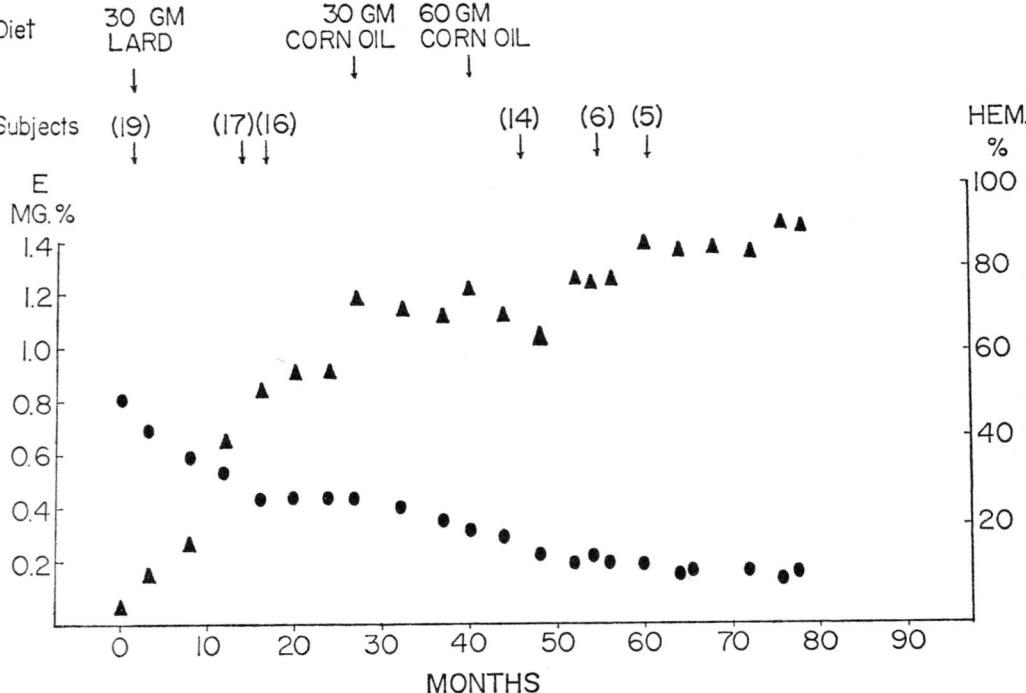

Fig. 6D–2. Decrease in average plasma total tocopherols (•) and increase of peroxide hemolysis test results (▲) with time and with progressive increase in dietary content of polyunsaturated fatty acids. Figures in parentheses indicate number of adult male subjects remaining on controlled depletion regimen at times indicated. (This figure is an extension of one previously reported.[28])

thorough study of the latter patient,[30] in which remission and exacerbation of the symptoms could be controlled by providing or withholding tocopherol, indicated that the basic difficulty might be secondary to the malabsorption of lipids resulting from a deficiency of pancreatic lipase.

Nervous System

Although extensive lesions in the vestibular nuclei and pyramidal tracts and changes in the motor horn cells of the spinal tract have been reported in experimental animals,[38] interpretations as to whether these are the causes or effects of muscular degeneration have been controversial. Pigment accumulation in vitamin E-deficient rats has been confirmed in the anterior horn cells, glial cells and macrophages; however, sclerotic motor cells in the spinal cord have been noted only occasionally in more recent work.[39] In another study, the claim is made that the metabolic derangements may affect the muscles and nervous system independently.[40]

Nutritional encephalomalacia in the chick is apparently also a function of the relative ratio of tocopherol to polyunsaturated fats in the diet.[41] It is characterized by motor incoordination, ataxia and head retraction, followed by prostration and death. Two cases of human cerebellar encephalomalacia[42] related to tocopherol deficiency have been reported, but in only one of these was there a satisfactory dietary history. In that one,[43] an infant had been given, intravenously, a lipid preparation which provided a high proportion of linoleic acid without compensatory high levels of tocopherol. Necropsy did not reveal abnormalities in the cerebral hemispheres, but the cerebellum was the site of widespread hemorrhages, proliferation of capillaries and absence of Purkinje cells. The histopathology could be differentiated from that found in Wernicke's encephalopathy.

Vascular System

Hemorrhages are common manifestations in vitamin E deficiency. Those in the brain have already been noted. The syndrome called exudative diathesis in chicks is usually manifested by the appearance of large patches of subcutaneous edema on the breast and abdomen. There is increased permeability of the capillaries with interfascial accumulations of a fluid colored greenish by decomposed hemoglobin.

The decreased ability of the erythrocyte to withstand peroxidative deterioration by hydrogen peroxide when the level of tocopherol in the blood is low has become the basis for the so-called peroxide hemolysis test.[44] The erythrocytes of premature and newborn infants are particularly susceptible to peroxide hemolysis. It may be generalized that when the plasma tocopherol level is below 0.5 mg per 100 ml such hemolysis tests are positive.

An evaluation of the peroxide hemolysis test in adult men was made in a study sponsored by the Food and Nutrition Board of the National Research Council in which the diet was limited to approximately 3 mg of α-tocopherol per day for over 6 years.[45] The erythrocytes of the men on this diet showed a gradual increase in peroxide hemolysis which was almost maximal within 2 years in most of the subjects. When the fat in the diet, which had been "stripped" lard, was changed to "stripped" corn oil, in order to increase the amounts of polyunsaturated fat consumed, there was a further increase in the degree of peroxide hemolysis, along with a decrease in levels of tocopherol in the plasma, although there was appreciably more tocopherol remaining in the stripped corn oil than in the stripped lard.[28] Figure 6D–2 gives the trend of the average data obtained in the depleted subjects and further shows that when the stripped corn oil intake was doubled from 30 to 60 gm per day there was a further decrease in the plasma tocopherol levels.

After over 6 years on the diet, when the plasma tocopherol had reached a plateau approximating 0.2 mg of tocopherol per 100 ml of plasma, there was a small but significant decrease in erythrocyte survival time[46] as measured by ^{51}Cr erythrocyte-life techniques. It should be emphasized that these subjects were not anemic, possibly because special controls were built into the experiment to supply protein, ascorbic acid and iron in amounts considered adequate to forestall anemia. Nevertheless, when they were supplemented with 300 mg d-α-tocopherol acetate per day, 4 out of 5 depleted subjects showed a small but significant increase in reticulocytes, which was not obtained in any patients in the control groups who were similarly supplemented.[47] These small changes in reticulocyte response would not have been convincing but for the studies of Dinning[48] and Fitch,[49] who obtained marked erythropoietic responses when α-tocopherol was administered to vitamin E-deficient monkeys. The beneficial effect of α-tocopherol administration on red cell survival in patients with proven malabsorption and low serum tocopherols has recently been confirmed by Leonard and Losowsky.[50]

A direct relationship between erythrocyte stability in vivo and the in vitro peroxide hemolysis test cannot be made since the sensitivity of the erythrocyte to dilute peroxide is far greater than to anything that it normally encounters. It has been shown in man[51] and more recently confirmed and elaborated by Bieri and Poukka[52] in studies of rat erythrocytes that the peroxide hemolysis test is primarily related to the level of tocopherols in the plasma and only secondarily a function of the level of polyunsaturated fatty acids in the erythrocyte. The phospholipids in the erythrocyte membrane are peroxidized[53] at a rate related to the amount of tocopherols present.

Currently, there is a debate on whether vitamin E has a hemopoietic effect in children with protein-calorie malnutrition. Since such children usually have low levels of lipoproteins in their blood and the serum tocopherol levels are related to the level of blood lipids, it is possible that many children with low levels of serum tocopherol have adequate levels of vitamin E in their tissues. Thus, different workers may have been treating patients who were not equivalent in their states of vitamin E deficiency. The direct relationship between total blood lipid levels and serum tocopherol levels, which has been studied by Horwitt et al.,[54] may make it necessary to report levels of serum tocopherols as a function of the level of blood lipids rather than as mg per 100 ml as has been done in the past.

MODE OF ACTION

The disagreement among investigators with respect to the function of vitamin E has not been resolved despite many years of work in this field. There is relative harmony regarding the following:

1. When polyunsaturated fatty acid (PUFA) intake is sufficient only to supply the minimal needs for health, relatively little vitamin E seems to be required. Increasing the levels of the more unsaturated lipids in the diet, which, in turn, increases the levels of PUFA in the various tissues at different rates, increases the requirement for vitamin E. This is true for chicks,[41] rats,[31] cattle[55] and man.[11] It is noteworthy that tissues such as the testes, which accumulate the more unsaturated fatty acids to a higher degree, are among the first to break down during vitamin E deficiency.[56]

2. The amount of lipofuscin pigment found in the tissues is a function of time, increased ingestion of PUFA and decreased ingestion of vitamin E.[57,58]

3. The substitution of other lipid antioxidants for α-tocopherol can prevent or diminish the incidence of vitamin E deficiency in animals fed diets containing no detectable amount of tocopherols.[59] The efficacy of such antioxidants is limited by their different absorbabilities, transport and the fact that they are foreign to the body.

The opponents of the antioxidant theory contend that so vital a compound as vitamin E must be a component of an enzyme or transport system in an action unrelated to its antioxidant function. In consequence, since a vitamin E-deficient animal presents a staggering list of apparently unrelated histopathologic sequelae, many deficient enzyme systems have been reported to be present in vitamin E deficiency. Arguments that the breakdown by peroxidation or free radical reactions of membrane phospholipids, coenzyme Q, vitamin A and other compounds could cause such enzyme dysfunctions are not considered conclusive. Arguments that other antioxidants can prevent abnormality are countered with the belief that only minute amounts of tocopherol are needed when other antioxidants are present.

It is hoped that future research will prove that both the "antioxidant" and "enzyme" proponents for vitamin E function will prove to be correct.

DISTRIBUTION, FOOD SOURCES AND STORAGE

The vegetable and seed oils are the largest contributors of the tocopherols to the diet. It is interesting that in nature there is a rough proportionality between the level of the tocopherols in a seed oil and the concentration of linoleic acid in the oil,[8] as though the antioxidant were placed there to protect the PUFA from auto-oxidation. Unfortunately, the different tocopherols are not uniformly distributed so that the amounts of α-tocopherol available to the consumer may not always be optimal. Thus, in corn oil, which has approximately 50 per cent linoleic acid, there are 100 mg of total tocopherol per 100 gm, of which only about 10 per cent is α-tocopherol. In cottonseed oil, approximately 60 per cent of the total tocopherols is α-tocopherol; in safflower oil, approximately 90 per cent.

Animal products are relatively poor sources of α-tocopherol but variations are quite large, depending upon the source of fat in the animal's diet.

The losses of natural concentrations of α-tocopherol[60] during cooking procedures and commercial processes are substantial. In the preparation of wheat flour, in addition to the large losses incurred during the separation of the bran and the sperm, nearly all of the remaining tocopherol may be lost if chlorine dioxide is used in the bleaching process.[61] Much tocopherol is removed from oils by purification processes before they reach the market; in fact, the by-products of such processes serve as important sources for the production of tocopherol concentrates sold for human and animal supplementation.

The depot fats and the liver may be the chief repositories of tocopherol and serve as convenient indices of previous intake in animal studies. The pituitary and the adrenals become very rich in tocopherol[62]

Table 6D–2. Fat and d-α-Tocopherols in Various Food Groups Available for Consumption in the United States in 1960

	Fat (gm/day)	d-α-Tocopherols Content (mg/100 gm fat)	Amount (mg/day)
Visible fats			
Butter	7.19	1.6	0.115
Lard	9.55	2.3	0.220
Margarine	9.42	10.2	0.961
Shortening	15.62	10.0	1.562
Other fats and oils	14.14	50.0	7.063
Total	55.92	..	9.921
Other food fats			
Dairy products	23.31	1.6	0.378
Eggs	5.33	10.7	0.572
Meats, etc.	52.08	1.7	0.893
Beans, peas, nuts, etc.	5.33	9.3	0.496
Fruits and vegetables	1.74	91.7	1.597
Grain products	2.23	48.9	1.092
Total	90.02	..	5.028
Totals	145.94	..	14.949

(From Harris and Embree.[64])

soon after tocopherol is fed. However, these observations become less spectacular if the level of tocopherol is expressed in terms of mg tocopherol per gm of fat, after which the relative levels in blood and in the tissues with the more unsaturated lipids—the adrenals, pituitary and tests—become quite similar. Thus, the ratio of approximately 1 mg tocopherols per gm lipid, a ratio which is in the same range noted in vegetable oils, is found in some animal tissue fats.

The amounts of α-tocopherol found in the ordinary components of human diets differ much more than is usually appreciated, depending upon source, preparation and age of the food. Dicks[63] has surveyed the literature to show that the tocopherol content of most foods may vary severalfold. Accordingly, the data given in Table 6D–2, which show an average consumption of 15 mg of α-tocopherols per day, should be interpreted as only an approximation of average consumption in the United States.

NUTRITIONAL REQUIREMENTS

The average intake of α-tocopherols by adults is 15 mg per day but the range of intake must be considered to be quite large, since individuals fed diets high in protein and low in plant fat would consume less than 10 mg per day, whereas those fed diets high in polyunsaturated oils could be ingesting over 60 mg per day. Since, in both cases, the amount of tocopherol consumed is probably close to the requirement, the question of what to recommend as a universal requirement is not easy to resolve. Harris and Embree,[64] using the Elgin studies[28] as a basis, suggested that the E:PUFA ratio should be 0.6. Thus, a man consuming 60 gm of PUFA, which is 50 per cent polyunsaturated, would require 21.6 mg of α-tocopherol or 32 I.U. Extrapolation of studies of various animals of different sizes tends to confirm the estimate of 30 I.U. for a 70-kg man.[65] A similar calculation for infants gives 3 to 6

I.U. of vitamin E, which is in good agreement with the range suggested by clinical studies[66] and is readily supplied by their normal diets.

Some certification of the tocopherol requirement when the diet contained approximately 38 gm of linoleic acid a day is supplied by data from the Elgin studies, in which adult male patients were maintained on 3 mg of α-tocopherol for over 6 years (Fig. 6D–2). Control subjects on the same diet, who were supplemented with 15 mg of α-tocopherol acetate (a total of approximately 24 I.U. per day), showed no signs of vitamin E deficiency but they also had no reserves, since examination of their erythrocytes showed a rapid increase in "peroxide hemolysis" soon after the supplement was removed.[28] Supplementation of 9 depleted subjects at 54 months with various levels of vitamin E indicated that the addition of 20 I.U. to the 4.5 I.U. in the diet was not sufficient to maintain blood levels even after 138 days of supplementation.

It should be understood that an adult does not require 30 I.U. per day unless he is consuming the equivalent of 60 gm of an unsaturated oil per day—and, if he is, he is probably obtaining the required amounts of tocopherols from the oil being consumed. The need for a stated requirement is not so much for normal individuals fed normal diets as for those who have absorptive difficulties or who for various reasons are consuming oxidized fats or large amounts of fish oils. Fish oils have a high peroxidative potential[47] and relatively low levels of tocopherols. In other words, the need for supplementation of normal diets which happen to have low levels of PUFA and corresponding low levels of vitamin E is not indicated in normal individuals on the basis of current evidence.

DEFICIENCY IN MAN

Although mammals on prescribed diets that are deficient in vitamin E can show a bewildering spectrum of pathologic symptoms, there is no good evidence to indicate that the healthy man is susceptible to vitamin E deficiency when he consumes and absorbs the constituents of the average American diet. What happens when his absorption of lipids is deficient is another matter, as has been noted in the above section on effects of deficiency on physiologic function. As early as 1908, a peculiar lesion of muscle was reported in a patient with sprue.[67] Many children with cystic fibrosis of the pancreas who have steatorrhea had excessive creatinuria while fed a low-creatine diet;[68-70] this was decreased after supplementation with vitamin E. More recently, a study of adult patients with proven malabsorption was reported in which impaired red cell survival was demonstrated.[50]

The anemia of prematurity and its relationship to inadequate absorption of α-tocopherol by the premature infant has been studied extensively.[70a-70c] Some pediatricians have concluded that it is advisable to supplement vitamin E from the tenth day onward in premature infants who are artificially fed. In one well-controlled study,[70d] immature infants have been shown to have a lower incidence of retrolental fibroplasia when supplemented with vitamin E.

A syndrome consisting of edema, skin lesions, an elevated platelet count and morphologic changes in erythrocytes has been described in premature infants receiving formula mixtures that contained relatively high levels of PUFA.[71] The abnormalities disappeared rapidly after the administration of vitamin E and were not observed in infants fed identical diets supplemented with vitamin E. Ehrenkranz et al., in a preliminary report, provide evidence that vitamin E administration during the acute phase of therapy for the respiratory-distress syndrome in premature neonates may favorably modify the development of bronchopulmonary dysplasia.[71a]

Although the requirement for vitamin E for what is considered normal health is relatively noncontroversial, the possible need for antioxidants to promote improved function and decreased rate of aging is another matter.[72] The hypothesis supporting the belief that aging is, at least in part, a progressive accumulation of cellular deteriorations that come from free-radical damage, either from cosmic rays, pollution or peroxidative sequelae, has found many proponents. The story of free radical pathologic condition and the possibility that antioxidants can inhibit such a condition has been reviewed by Pryor.[73] The most that can be said for this theory is that it is attractive, that the clues of prolonged survival of small animals given antioxidants are most interesting but that concrete evidence to support it has not yet been published. It is possible that the accumulated effects of small changes over a 60-year period cannot be demonstrated in the cells of small animals with relatively short life spans.

So much α-tocopherol acetate has been ingested by so many that it may be concluded, in the absence of any apparent physiologic signs, that this is one of the least toxic of all the vitamins. It has been consumed by many at levels of more than a gram per day for many months, despite the fact that the benefits claimed remain to be proved.

PHARMACOLOGIC EFFECTS

Any discussion of the biologic usefulness of vitamin E should distinguish between its requirement as an essential nutrient and its possible pharmacologic action when ingested in amounts many times the generally recognized nutritional requirement. For example, there have been claims for many years by numerous clinicians that vitamin E can prevent thrombus formation by an effect on blood clotting. Because these claims were not based upon controlled experiments, they were properly discounted by most nutritional scientists. Recently[74] attention has been directed to the possibility that an oxidation product of α-tocopherol, α-tocopheryl quinone, which had been shown to be an inhibitor of vitamin K more than 20 years ago,[75] was responsible for this prolongation of blood clotting time. This may explain the observation made by Corrigan and Marcus[76] that large doses of vitamin E potentiated the effect of warfarin on a patient. The latter effect was confirmed by Schrogie.[77]

Although the in vitro production of the quinone by $FeCl_3$ or other oxidative agents is a simple procedure, only small amounts are found in the tissues.[78] There has been a report that there is a marked increase of the quinone in the livers of mice after intraperitoneal administration of large amounts of tocopherol acetate.[79] However, most of the tocopheryl quinone would probably not have to be absorbed to have its effect upon intestinal sources of vitamin K produced by normal bacterial synthesis. In view of the large amounts of vitamin E consumed by food faddists for many years without any apparent harm, this effect on blood clotting would not be expected to be deleterious. Nevertheless, while the effect on blood clotting may turn out to be a useful clinical tool, care should be taken that patients receiving anticoagulants are not taking large amounts of vitamin E. Whether earlier discounted claims that vitamin E may inhibit the incidence of cardiovascular accidents should be reinvestigated remains to be determined.

A study conducted at the National Institutes of Health, of individuals who had been ingesting up to 800 I.U. of vitamin E for more than 3 years, did not find any evidence of toxicity.[80]

BIBLIOGRAPHY

1. Evans and Bishop: Science, 56, 650, 1922.
2. Mattill, Carman and Clayton: J. Biol. Chem., 61, 729, 1924.
3. Sure: J. Biol. Chem., 58, 693, 1924.
4. Olcott and Emerson: J. Am. Chem. Soc., 59, 1008, 1937.
4a. Moore: Biochem. J., 34, 1321, 1940.
5. Dam: Pharmacol. Rev., 9, 1, 1957.
6. Filer, Rumery and Mason: Transactions First Conference on Biological Antioxidants. New York, Josiah Macy Foundation, 1946.
7. Hickman: Rec. Chem. Prog., 9, 104, 1948.
8. Hove and Harris: J. Am. Oil Chem. Soc., 28, 405, 1951.
9. Hove: Am. J. Clin. Nutr., 3, 328, 1955.
10. Tappel: Vitam. Horm., 20, 493, 1962.
11. Horwitt: Borden's Rev. Nutr. Res., 22, 1, 1961.
12. Draper: In International Encyclopedia of Food and Nutrition, Vol. 9 (Morton, Ed.). New York, Pergamon Press, 1970.
13. Witting: Lipids, 2, 109, 1967.
14. Folkers: Int. J. Vitam. Res., 39, 334, 1969.
15. Boguth: Vitam. Horm., 27, 1, 1969.
16. Green and Bunyan: Nutr. Abstr. Rev., 39, 321, 1969.
16a. Gilbert: Am. J. Clin. Nutr., 27, 1005, 1974.
17. Evans, Emerson and Emerson: J. Biol. Chem., 113, 319, 1936.
18. Fernholz: J. Am. Chem. Soc., 60, 700, 1938.
19. Karrer, Fritzsche, Ringier and Salomon: Helv. Chim. Acta, 21, 520, 1938.
20. Pennock, Hemming and Kerr: Biochem. Biophys. Res. Commun., 17, 542, 1964.
21. Century and Horwitt: Fed. Proc., 24, 906, 1965.
22. Wiss, Bunnell and Gloor: Vitam. Horm., 20, 441, 1962.
23. Green, Edwin, Diplock and Bunyan: Biochim. Biophys. Acta, 49, 417, 1961.
24. MacKensie and MacKensie: J. Nutr., 72, 322, 1960.
25. Green, Diplock, Bunyan, Edwin and McHale: Nature, 189, 747, 1961.
26. Simon, Eisengart, Sundhein and Milhorat: J. Biol. Chem., 221, 807, 1956.
27. Plack and Bieri: Biochim. Biophys. Acta, 84, 729, 1963.
28. Horwitt: Am. J. Clin. Nutr., 8, 451, 1960.
29. Mason: In The Vitamins, Vol. 3 (Sebrell and Harris, Eds.). New York, Academic Press, 1972.
30. Vester and Williams: Clin. Res., 11, 180, 1963.
31. Witting and Horwitt: J. Nutr., 82, 19, 1964.
32. Witting and Horwitt: J. Nutr., 84, 351, 1964.
33. Blaxter: Vitam. Horm., 20, 633, 1962.
34. Swahn and Thafvelin: Vitam. Horm., 20, 645, 1962.
35. Kerner and Goldbloom: J. Dis. Child., 99, 597, 1960.
36. Braunstein: Gastroenterology, 40, 224, 1961.
37. Nitowsky, Hsu and Gordon: Vitam. Horm., 20, 559, 1962.
38. Einarson: J. Neurol. Neurosurg. Psychiatry, 16, 98, 1953.
39. Mason: In Pharmacology and Disease (Bourne, Ed.). New York, Academic Press, 1960.
40. West: In Muscular Dystrophy in Man and Animals (Bourne and Golarz, Eds.). New York, Hafner Publishing Co., 1963.
41. Century, Horwitt and Bailey: Arch. Gen. Psychiatry, 1, 420, 1959.
42. Bailey: Am. J. Clin. Nutr., 12, 275, 1963.
43. Horwitt and Bailey: Arch. Neurol., 1, 312, 1959.
44. György, Cogan and Rose: Proc. Soc. Exp. Biol. Med., 81, 536, 1952.
45. Horwitt, Harvey, Duncan and Wilson: Am. J. Clin. Nutr., 4, 408, 1956.
46. Horwitt, Century and Zeman: Am. J. Clin. Nutr., 12, 99, 1963.

47. Horwitt: Vitam. Horm., *20*, 541, 1962.
48. Dinning: Nutr. Rev., *21*, 289, 1963.
49. Fitch: Vitam. Horm., *26*, 501, 1968.
50. Leonard and Losowsky: Am. J. Clin. Nutr., *24*, 388, 1971.
51. Horwitt, Harvey and Harmon: Vitam. Horm., *26*, 487, 1968.
52. Bieri and Poukka: J. Nutr., *100*, 557, 1970.
53. Heikkila, Mezick and Cornwell: Physiol. Chem. Phys., *3*, 93, 1971.
54. Horwitt, Harvey, Dahm and Searcey: Ann. N.Y. Acad. Sci., *203*, 223, 1972.
55. Blaxter: In "Vitamin E." Atti del terzo Congresso Internationale Venezia, Edizioni Valdonega Verona, 1956.
56. Witting, Likhite and Horwitt: Lipids, *2*, 103, 1967.
57. Sulkin and Srivanij: J. Gerontol., *15*, 2, 1960.
58. Witting, Theron and Horwitt: Lipids, *2*, 97, 1967.
59. Draper, Bergan, Chiu, Csallany and Boaro: J. Nutr., *84*, 395, 1964.
60. Harris: Vitam. Horm., *20*, 603, 1962.
61. Moore: Br. Med. Bull., *12*, 44, 1956.
62. Quaife, Swanson, Dju and Harris: Ann. N.Y. Acad. Sci., *52*, 300, 1949.
63. Dicks: Vitamin E Content of Foods and Feeds for Human and Animal Consumption. Agric. Exp. Station Bull., 435. Laramie, University of Wyoming, 1965.
64. Harris and Embree: Am. J. Clin. Nutr., *13*, 385, 1963.
65. Harris: Ann. N.Y. Acad. Sci., *52*, 240, 1949.
66. MacKensie: Pediatrics, *13*, 346, 1954.
67. Bramwell and Muir: Q. J. Med., *1*, 1, 1907-8.
68. Gordon, Nitowsky and Cornblath: Am. J. Dis. Child., *90*, 669, 1955.
69. Nitowsky, Cornblath and Gordon: Am. J. Dis. Child., *92*, 164, 1956.
70. Nitowsky, Tildon, Levin and Gordon: Am. J. Clin. Nutr., *10*, 368, 1962.
70a. Oski and Barness: J. Pediatr., *70*, 211, 1967.
70b. Gross and Melhorn: J. Pediatr., *85*, 753, 1974.
70c. Lo, Frank and Hitzig: Arch. Dis. Child., *48*, 360, 1973.
70d. Johnson, Schaffer and Boggs: Am. J. Clin. Nutr., *19*, 147, 1974.
71. Hassan, Hashim, Van Itallie and Sebrell: Am. J. Clin. Nutr., *19*, 147, 1966.
71a. Ehrenkranz, Bonta, Ablow and Warshaw: N. Engl. J. Med., *299*: 564, 1978.
72. Tappel: Geriatrics, *23*, 97, 1968.
73. Pryor: Chem. Eng. News, June 7, 1971, pp. 34–51.
74. Horwitt: Am. J. Clin. Nutr., *29*, 569, 1976.
75. Woolley: J. Biol. Chem., *159*, 59, 1945.
76. Corrigan and Marcus: J.A.M.A., *230*, 1300, 1974.
77. Schrogie: J.A.M.A., *232*, 19, 1975.
78. Csallany, Draper and Shah: Arch. Biochem. Biophys., *98*, 142, 1962.
79. Aristarkova, Burlakova and Khrapova: Biofizika, *19*, 703, 1974 (English translation).
80. Farrell and Bieri: Am. J. Clin. Nutr., *28*, 1381, 1975.

E. Thiamin

Robert A. Neal
and
Howerde E. Sauberlich

Recognition of vitamin B_1 activity dates back to 1890 when the Dutch physician Eijkman observed that chickens fed a diet which consisted mainly of polished rice developed polyneuritic symptoms similar to those common to beriberi patients. Additional studies showed that the paralysis resulting from feeding polished rice could be cured by adding rice polishings to the diet. As a result of these studies Eikjman suggested the toxic principle was contained in polished rice but could be neutralized by some protective factor in rice polishings.

Takaki of Japan was the first to advance an explanation that beriberi was actually a nutritional deficiency. In 1884 he began experiments in which he modified the diet fed sailors aboard ships of the Japanese Navy in an attempt to decrease the disastrous incidence of beriberi. The major modification was the inclusion of dry milk and additional meat in the diet. The modified diet resulted in a dramatic decrease in the incidence of beriberi.[1] He concluded from these experiments that beriberi was caused by a lack of nitrogenous food components in association with excessive intake of non-nitrogenous food.

The correct explanation for the etiology

of beriberi was proposed in 1901 by Grijns.[2] Grijns found that in addition to rice polishings, Katjang idjo (a small green pea), a green bean and meat could also prevent beriberi in fowl fed a diet consisting mainly of starch. As a result of these studies he postulated that natural foodstuffs contained an unknown factor, absent in polished rice, which prevented the development of polyneuritis.

Funk[3] reported the isolation of a substance from rice polishings which cured beriberi, and named it vitamine. However, the active product he isolated still contained little of the active principle.

Jansen and Donath,[4] employing adsorption onto fuller's earth, were able to isolate crystalline material which cured polyneuritis in rice birds. The trivial name aneurine was suggested by Jansen. This name was commonly used throughout Europe for a considerable time. However, this nomenclature was not accepted in the United States because of its therapeutic implications. The name aneurine was eventually replaced by thiamin (thiamine).

In 1934 R. R. Williams and his colleagues,[5,50] using an improved process, isolated a sufficient quantity of the vitamin to make structure elucidation possible.

STRUCTURE, CHEMICAL SYNTHESIS, CHEMICAL AND PHYSICAL PROPERTIES

Work by R. R. Williams and his colleagues made it clear that thiamin was composed of a pyrimidine and a thiazole moiety and in 1936 established its structure as 3-(2′-methyl-4′-amino-5′-pyrimidylmethyl)-5-(2-hydroxyethyl)-4-methylthiazole.[6]

Thiamin

Thiamin has been synthesized by the formation of the pyrimidine and thiazole moieties separately followed by a coupling of the two moieties or by synthesizing the pyrimidine with a suitable side chain which can react with a second compound to form the thiazole ring.

Williams and Cline[7] used the first method in their original synthesis of thiamin. The 4-hydroxypyrimidine was synthesized in a reaction between acetamidine and the sodio derivative of ethyl-2-ethoxy-1-formylpropionate. The 4-hydroxypyrimidine was converted in a series of steps to 2-methyl-4-amino-5-bromomethylpyrimidine. The thiazole moiety was synthesized by reacting 3-acetyl-3-chloropropanol with thioformamide. The coupling of the two moieties gave thiamin bromide hydrobromide.

An example of the second type of synthesis is that of Todd and Bergel.[8] These workers condensed ethyl-1-ethoxymethylene-1-cyanoacetate with acetamidine to form 5-cyano-4-hydroxy-2-methylpyrimidine. This compound was converted in a series of steps to 2-methyl-4-amino-5-aminomethylpyrimidine. Reaction of this latter compound with potassium dithioformate yielded 2-methyl-4-amino-5-thioformamidomethylpyrimidine. Condensation of this compound with 3-acetyl-3-chloropropanol yielded thiamin.

One gram of thiamin chloride hydrochloride can dissolve in 1 ml of water. It is soluble to about 1 per cent in ethanol but rather insoluble in other common organic solvents. The hemihydrate of thiamin melts at 248 to 250°C. Thiamin has a characteristic odor very much like that of yeast.

The vitamin exhibits absorption bands in the ultraviolet region of the spectrum. At pH 7 in aqueous solution the absorption maxima are at 235 and 267 nm, corresponding to the pyrimidine and thiazole moieties respectively. At pH 1 there is one maximum at 247 and a shoulder at 260 nm, again corresponding to the pyrimidine and thiazole moieties respectively.

Thiamin is destroyed at elevated temperature unless the pH is below 5. At pH values above 7 thiamin rapidly loses its biologic activity. In alkaline solution under oxidizing conditions (e.g. potassium ferricyanide) thiamin is oxidized to the fluorescent compound thiochrome, a reaction widely used for the detection and quantitation of thiamin.

Thiochrome

Sulfite ion at room temperature attacks the methylene bridge between the two ring systems of thiamin to yield the separate pyrimidine and thiazole moiety.[6] The products of this reaction are 2-methyl-4-amino-5-pyrimidylmethylsulfonic acid and 5-(2-hydroxyethyl)-4-methylthiazole.

BIOLOGIC FUNCTIONS OF THIAMIN

Thiamin in the form of pyrophosphate participates as a coenzyme in the oxidative

alpha ketoglutarate to lipoic acid. This transfer may take place either by an electrophilic attack by oxidized lipoic acid on the number 1 carbon of the fragment displacing thiamin pyrophosphate or by a preliminary oxidation of the "active aldehyde" intermediate to yield an acyl thiamin pyrophosphate followed by nucleophilic attack of reduced lipoic acid to displace thiamin pyrophosphate. There is some evidence to indicate the latter route may be the correct one.

The final step in the oxidative decarboxylation of pyruvate and alpha ketoglutarate is the transfer of acetate and succinate respectively from lipoic acid to coenzyme A. The oxidative decarboxylation reactions of pyruvate and alpha ketoglutarate are important from the standpoint of energy production in plants and in animal organisms.

An additional important thiamin pyrophosphate requiring enzyme in plants and animals is transketolase. The enzyme catalyzes the reaction

xylulose-5-phosphate + ribose-5-phosphate $\longrightarrow$ sedoheptulose-7-phosphate + glyceraldehyde-3-phosphate

decarboxylation of alpha keto acids to aldehydes. The most important substrates for this type of reaction are pyruvate which is metabolized to acetyl coenzyme A and alpha ketoglutarate which is metabolized to acetyl coenzyme A and alpha ketoglutarate which is metabolized to succinyl coenzyme A. Both these reactions require the participation of lipoic acid, NAD and coenzyme A. The mechanism of these reactions involves first the formation of an "active aldehyde" intermediate between the substrate (pyruvate or alpha ketoglutarate) and enzyme-bound thiamin pyrophosphate. The intermediate in the decarboxylation of pyruvate is 2-(1-hydroxyethyl)-thiamin pyrophosphate. In the decarboxylation of alpha ketoglutarate the intermediate is 2-(1-hydroxy-3-carboxypropyl)-thiamin pyrophosphate.

The next step is the transfer of the 2-carbon fragment in the case of pyruvate and the 4-carbon fragment in the case of

In this reaction xylulose-5-phosphate is cleaved between carbons 2 and 3 to form a 2-(1,2-dihydroxyethyl)-thiamin pyrophosphate intermediate and glyceraldehyde-3-phosphate. The 1,2-dihydroxyethyl group is then transferred from thiamin to the number 1 carbon of ribose-5-phosphate to yield sedoheptulose-7-phosphate. This reaction is important in the phosphogluconate pathway, a reaction sequence which carries out the interconversion of 3-, 4-, 5-, 6- and 7-carbon sugars. This pathway is also an important source of reduced NADP.

Other enzyme-catalyzed reactions requiring thiamin as a coenzyme are the nonoxidative decarboxylation of alpha keto acids and the phosphoketolase reaction, both of which are important only in microorganisms.[32] The latter reaction involves the cleavage of a ketopentose phosphate to triose phosphate and acetyl phosphate.

METHODS OF ASSAY

There are various methods for assay for thiamin in biologic materials. These include animal assays as well as chemical and microbiological assays.

The thiochrome procedure[9] is the most widely used chemical method for assay of thiamin in biologic materials. It depends on the alkaline oxidation of thiamin to thiochrome. Thiochrome exhibits an intense blue fluorescence and can be measured fluorimetrically. In this procedure thiamin is isolated from biologic materials by passing a solution containing the vitamin over a column of the synthetic zeolite Decalso. The thiamin absorbed to the Decalso is eluted and oxidized to thiochrome using an alkaline solution of ferricyanide. The thiochrome is extracted into isobutanol and quantitated by measuring the fluorescence of the isobutanol solution. Since thiamin pyrophosphate forms a thiochrome derivative poorly soluble in isobutanol, the thiochrome procedure can be used to distinguish between free thiamin and its pyrophosphate forms by assaying an extract before and after incubation with a phosphatase enzyme.

Other chemical tests for thiamin are the formaldehyde-diazotized sulphanilic acid method,[10] the diazotized p-aminoacetophenone method[11,12] and the bromthymol blue method.[13]

The microbiologic method which is most widely used currently is assay with Lactobacillus viridescens.[14] This organism requires the intact thiamin molecule for growth; neither the thiazole nor pyrimidine moieties nor their phosphorylated forms are active. Thiamin monophosphate and diphosphate are as active as thiamin while the hydroxyethyl derivative of thiamin is only 80 per cent as active.

Other useful but less widely used microorganisms for thiamin assay include Phycomyces blakesleeanus,[15] Kloeckera brevis (Kloeckera apiculata),[16] Lactobacillus fermentum,[17] and Ochromonas danica.[18]

With the development of chemical and microbiologic assays for thiamin the applicability of animal assays decreased. Animal assays are still useful, however, for determining the availability of thiamin in a food source or a new form or preparation of the vitamin. The response may be measured in various animals including pigeons and chicks, but the rat is the animal of choice. The rat assay measures the curative effect of the food source or new preparation containing thiamin on rats which have been made thiamin deficient. The response is compared to the curative effect of pure synthetic thiamin hydrochloride. The response most commonly measured is growth, although the length of cure of bradycardia or of polyneuritis is sometimes used.

Numerous methods have been used to assess the state of thiamin nutrition in man.[32] The most important of these are the measurement of the activity of erythrocyte transketolase, a thiamin pyrophosphate-requiring enzyme, the measurement of blood or urinary levels of thiamin using various chemical and microbiologic techniques and measurement of blood levels of pyruvate and alpha ketoglutarate. The best methods currently in use appear to be the erythrocyte transketolase method of Brin[19,61,62,74] as modified by others,[20-22, 66,71-73] and the measurement of thiamin in urine using the modified thiochrome procedure of Hennessy and Cerecedo.[9,63-65]

DEFICIENCY IN EXPERIMENTAL ANIMALS AND MAN

One of the first recorded signs of thiamin deficiency in experimental animals was the characteristic head retraction in the pigeon.[23] Thiamin-deficient pigeons also show ataxia and leg weakness, cardiac failure with tachycardia, abnormalities of the electrocardiogram and necrosis of the heart muscle. Chicks repond to thiamin deficiency in a manner similar to pigeons.

The major symptoms of thiamin deficiency in rats are loss of appetite (anorexia), weight loss, convulsions, slowing of the heart rate (bradycardia) and lowering of the body temperature. Loss of muscular tone and lesions of the nervous system may also develop. The urine of deficient rats contains a higher pyruvate/lactate ratio than that of normal animals. Thiamin-deficient rats also exhibit a reduced erythrocyte transketolase activity. The administration of thiamin brings about a remarkable reversal of the deficiency in 24 hours.

The classical pathologic condition arising from thiamin deficiency in man is called beriberi.[50,55,56] The symptoms and treatment of beriberi are discussed in detail in Chapter 23.

NUTRITIONAL REQUIREMENT

The requirements for thiamin in human nutrition are usually based on caloric intake. Various investigators have indicated the daily adult requirement for thiamin is from 0.23 to 0.5 mg per 1,000 calories.[21,24-26]

The Food and Nutrition Board recommends 0.5 mg of thiamin for each 1,000 calories in the diet. Older persons may use thiamin less efficiently;[57,58] therefore, a daily intake of 1 mg of thiamin is recommended even if they consume less than 2,000 calories daily. The recommended average intake of thiamin for men is 1.2 to 1.5 mg and for women, 1.0 to 1.1 mg. In women during pregnancy and lactation, an increased daily allowance of 0.3 mg is recommended to meet increased needs.[67-69]

The recommended daily intakes of thiamin for infants and children are: 0 to 6 mo, 0.3 mg; 6 mo to 1 yr, 0.5 mg; 1 to 3 yr, 0.7 mg; 4 to 6 yr, 0.9 gm; 7 to 10 yr, 1.2 mg; boys 11 to 14 yr, 1.4 mg; and girls 11 to 14 yr, 1.2 mg.

Good sources of thiamin are pork, beef, organ meats, wheat or other whole or enriched grains and fresh vegetables, especially peas and beans (see Table 61–1).

Thiamin requirements and metabolism may be altered by various thiaminases[43] and thiamin antagonists such as caffeic acid (3,4-dihydroxycinnamic acid)[39,40] and compounds present in tea,[44,60,70] coffee,[41] rice bran[42] and other sources.[46-48] Approximately 80 per cent of the thiamin in the body is present as thiamin pyrophosphate. The remainder is present in decreasing order of amount as thiamin triphosphate, thiamin monophosphate and thiamin. The adult human body contains about 30 mg of thiamin.

Thiamin is absorbed from the small intestine by both a passive diffusion process and active transport that involves Na^+ and ATPase.[51] In alcoholics, thiamin absorption is often depressed; this may be related to a folic acid deficiency.[52-54,59]

TOXICITY

Thiamin produces a variety of pharmacologic effects when administered in large amounts. However, these effects are seen only in doses which are thousands of times larger than those required for optimum nutrition.

Death in animals after intravenous injection of thiamin is caused by depression of the respiratory center.[27] The lethal dose of thiamin administered by intravenous injection is 125 mg per kg in mice, 250 mg per kg in rats, 300 mg per kg in rabbits and 350 mg per kg in dogs.[28] The ratios of the lethal doses on intravenous injection to those on subcutaneous and oral administration were found to be 1:6:40. In monkeys, intravenous administration of 200 mg per kg failed to elicit any symptoms[28] and only 600 mg per kg caused any toxic effects.

Rats have been maintained for three generations on a daily intake of 0.08 to 1.0 mg of thiamin without harmful effects.[6] These are doses up to 100 times the daily requirement for the vitamin.

No toxic effects of thiamin administered by mouth have been reported in man. Generally toxic effects have not been reported on subcutaneous, intramuscular, intraspinal or intravenous injection of doses 1 to 200 times larger than the daily maintenance doses. In rare cases, however, thiamin has caused reactions resembling anaphylactic shock in man. Most of these reactions are in patients who had previously received large doses of thiamin by injection. Thus, they apparently developed a hypersensitivity to thiamin.

THIAMIN METABOLISM

Over two dozen metabolites of thiamin have been noted to occur in the urine of rats[29,30] and of men[31-33] given the vitamin labeled in either the pyrimidine or thiazole moieties. Only 6 of these have thus far been identified: 2-methyl-4-amino-5-pyrimidine carboxylic acid,[31] 4-methylthiazole-5-acetic acid,[33,34,35] 2-methyl-4-amino-5-hydroxymethylpyrimidine,[36] 5-(2-hydroxyethyl)-4-methylthiazole,[37] [3-(2'-methyl-4'-amino-5'-pyrimidylmethyl)-4-methylthiazole-5 acetic acid] (thiamin acetic acid)[37] and 2-methyl-4-amino-5-formylaminomethylpyrimidine.[37]

Thiamin and its thiazole moiety are metabolized to their corresponding acids in the rat by liver alcohol dehydrogenase.[49] Although thiamin itself was a poor substrate for the enzyme, its thiazole moiety was oxidized at a faster rate than ethanol.

BIBLIOGRAPHY

1. Takaki: Lancet, 2, 189, 1887.
2. Grijns: Research on Vitamins 1900–1911, J. Noorduyn. Gorinchem., 37, 38, 1935.
3. Funk: J. State Med., 20, 341, 1912.
4. Jansen and Donath: Koninkl. Ned. Akad. Wetenschap. Proc., 29, 1390, 1926.
5. Williams, Waterman and Keresztesy: J. Am. Chem. Soc., 56, 1187, 1934.
6. Williams and Spies: Vitamin B₁. New York, Macmillan, 1938.
7. Williams and Cline: J. Am. Chem. Soc., 58, 1504, 1936.
8. Todd and Bergel: J. Chem. Soc., 364, 1937.
9. Hennessy and Cerecedo: J. Am. Chem. Soc., 61, 179, 1939.
10. Kinnersley and Peters: Biochem. J., 32, 1516, 1938.
11. Prebluda and McCollum: J. Biol. Chem., 127, 495, 1939.
12. Melnick and Field: J. Biol. Chem., 130, 97, 1939.
13. Gupta and Cadwallader: J. Pharm. Sci., 57, 112, 1968.
14. Deibel, Evans and Niven: J. Bacteriol., 74, 818, 1957.
15. Schopfer and Jung: C. R. 5th Congr. Int. Tech. Chem. Ind. Agr. Scheveningen 1, 22, 1937.
16. Hoff-Jorgensen and Hansen: Acta Chem. Scand., 9, 552, 1955.
17. Sarett and Cheldelin: J. Biol. Chem., 155, 153, 1944.
18. Baker, Pasher, Frank, Hutner, Aaronson and Sobotka: Clin. Chem., 5, 13, 1959.
19. Brin: Ann. N.Y. Acad. Sci., 98, 528, 1962.
20. Warnock: J. Nutr., 100, 1057, 1970.
21. Ziporin, Nunes, Powell, Waring and Sauberlich: J. Nutr., 85, 297, 1965.
22. Stevens, Sauberlich and Long: In Automation in Analytical Chemistry. New York, Mediad Incorporated, 1968.
23. Suzuki, Shamimura and Okade: Biochem. Z., 43, 89, 1912.
24. Nat. Acad. Sci.–Natl. Res. Council Pub., 8th ed. Washington, 1974.
25. Ziporin, Nunes, Powell, Waring and Sauberlich: J. Nutr., 85, 287, 1965.
26. Sauberlich, Herman and Stevens: Am. J. Clin. Nutr., 23, 671, 1970.
27. Haley: Proc. Soc. Exp. Biol. Med., 68, 153, 1948.
28. Mouriquand and Coisnard: Presse Med., 53, 369, 1945.
29. Neal and Pearson: J. Nutr., 83, 343, 1964.
30. Balaghi and Pearson: J. Nutr., 89, 265, 1966.
31. Neal and Pearson: J. Nutr., 83, 351, 1964.
32. Sauberlich: Am. J. Clin. Nutr., 20, 528, 1967.
33. Ariaey-Nejad, Balaghi, Baker and Sauberlich: Am. J. Clin. Nutr., 23, 764, 1970.
34. Ariaey-Nejad and Pearson: J. Nutr., 96, 445, 1968.
35. Suzuoki, Tominaga, Matsuo, Sumi and Miyakawa: J. Nutr., 96, 433, 1968.
36. White, Amos and Neal: J. Nutr., 100, 1053, 1970.
37. Amos and Neal: J. Biol. Chem., 245, 5643, 1970.
38. Sauberlich, Dowdy and Skala: Laboratory Tests for the Assessment of Nutritional Status. Cleveland, CRC Press, 1974.
39. Berüter and Somogyi: Int. J. Vitam. Nutr. Res., 37, 169, 1967.
40. Schaller and Höller: Int. J. Vitam. Nutr. Res., 46, 143, 1976.
41. Somogyi and Nägeli: Int. J. Vitam. Nutr. Res., 46, 148, 1976.
42. Kumar De and Chaudhuri: Int. J. Vitam. Nutr. Res., 46, 154, 1976.
43. Evans: Vitam. Horm., 33, 467, 1975.
44. Buhr and Hilker: Fed. Proc., 35, 443, 1976 (abstract).
45. Tang and Hilker: J. Food Sci., 35, 676, 1970.
46. Somogyi: In Toxicants Occurring Naturally In Foods, 2nd ed. Washington, National Academy of Sciences, 1973.
47. Hilker and Peter: Experientia, 24, 1146, 1968.
48. Sreevanich, Phornphiboul and Dunn: J. Med. Assoc. Thail., 51, 666, 1968.
49. Dalvi, Sauberlich and Neal: J. Nutr., 104, 1476, 1974.
50. Williams: In Toward the Conquest of Beriberi. Cambridge, Harvard University Press, 1961.
51. Rindi and Ventura: Physiol. Rev., 52, 821, 1972.
52. Thomson and Leevy: Clin. Sci., 43, 153, 1972.

53. Thomson, Baker and Leevy: Gastroenterology, *60*, 756, 1971.
54. Howard, Wagner and Schenker: J. Nutr., *104*, 1024, 1974.
55. Goldsmith: Prog. Food Nutr. Sci., *1*, 559, 1975.
56. Tanphaichitr, Vimokesant, Dhanamitta and Valyasevi: Am. J. Clin. Nutr., *23*, 1017, 1970.
57. Horwitt, Leibert, Kreisler and Wittman: Investigations of human requirements for B-complex vitamins. National Research Council Bull. 116. Washington, National Academy of Sciences, 1948.
58. Oldham: Ann. N.Y. Acad. Sci., *98*, 542, 1962.
59. Tomasulo, Kater and Iber: Am. J. Clin. Nutr., *21*, 1341, 1968.
60. Hilker, Chan, Chen and Smith: Nutr. Rep. Int., *4*, 223, 1971.
61. Brin: Methods Enzymol., *19*, 125, 1970.
62. Brin: Newer Methods Nutr. Biochem., *3*, 407, 1967.
63. Manual for Nutrition Surveys. Interdepartmental Committee on Nutrition for National Defense. Washington, Superintendent of Documents, 1962.
64. Muiruri, Romsos and Kirk: Am. J. Clin. Nutr., *27*, 837, 1974.
65. Edwin, Jackman and Hebert: Analyst, *100*, 689, 1975.
66. Warnock, Frattali and Preston: Clin. Chem., *21*, 432, 1975.
67. Heller, Salkeld and Körner: Am. J. Clin. Nutr., *27*, 1221, 1974.
68. Kaminetzky, Langer, Baker, Frank, Thomson, Munves, Opper, Behre and Glista: Am. J. Obstet. Gynecol., *115*, 639, 1973.
69. Lockhart, Kirkwood and Harris: Am. J. Obstet. Gynecol., *46*, 358, 1943.
70. Vimokesant, Nakornchai, Rungruangsak, Dhanamitta and Hilker: J. Nutr. Sci. Vitaminol., *22* (Suppl.), 1, 1976.
71. Bayoumi and Rosalki: Clin. Chem., *22*, 327, 1976.
72. Warnock: Clin. Chem., *21*, 432, 1975.
73. Smeets, Miller and DeWael: Clin. Chim. Acta, *33*, 379, 1971.
74. Brin and Danon: J. Sci. Ind. Res., *29*, S39, 1970.

F. Riboflavin

M. K. Horwitt

The food fraction termed "water-soluble B" reported by McCollum and Kennedy[1] in 1916, with the suggestion that it might be identical with the antiberberi substance, was first shown to be dual in nature in 1920 by Emmett and Luros.[2] This was further studied by Smith and Hendrick[3] who, in 1926, divided the complex into a beriberi preventative material which was destroyed by heat and an antipellagric substance which was more heat stable. About the same time Goldberger and Lillie[4] were making their classical demonstrations that pellagra could be cured by dietary means, and the term "vitamin B_1" began to represent the water-soluble, heat-labile, antineuritic fraction, and vitamin B_2 or G the heat-stable antipellagric fraction. Soon after Warburg and Christian[5] discovered the first flavoprotein in 1932, the close correlation between the vitamins and biologic oxidations was recognized from the combined observations of Ellinger and Koschara,[6] Booher,[7] and Kuhn et al.[8] and riboflavin deficiency was proved responsible for some of the abnormalities formerly associated with pellagra.

ISOLATION AND CHEMICAL NATURE

Although the water-soluble, yellow-green fluorescent compound in whey was known to chemists in the 19th century,[9] it was not isolated from milk and shown to be a part of the B complex until 1933 by Kuhn, György and Wagner-Jauregg.[8] In the meantime Warburg and Christian,[5] while studying yellow fluorescent tissue extracts as parts of various enzyme systems in tissues, had reported sufficient revealing chemical data to uncover the close relationship of their yellow enzyme to the vitamin-like yellow-fluorescent compound in milk. The identification of the colored component of the "yellow oxidation enzyme" with the vitamin made the recognition of riboflavin as the prosthetic group of the active flavoprotein enzymes possible. At about the same time Booher[7] confirmed the fact that the growth-promoting property of whey was associated with its water-soluble yellow fluorescent pigment.

The synthesis of riboflavin was accomplished by Kuhn[10] and Karrer[11] and associates in 1935; they showed that the compound was 6,7-dimethyl-9-(dl'-ribityl) isoalloxazine.

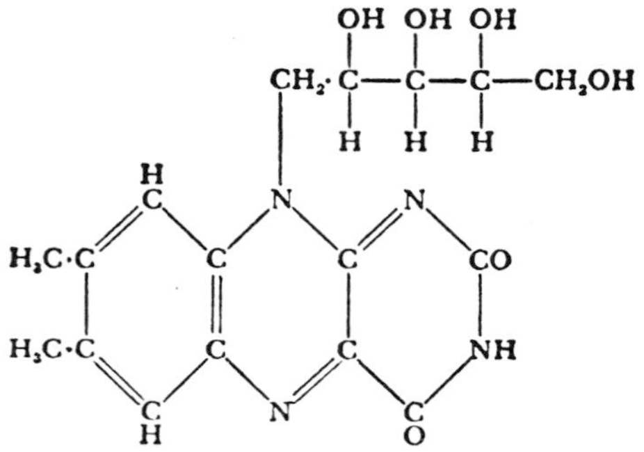

Fig. 6F–1. Riboflavin (6,7-dimethyl-9-(dl'-ribityl) isoalloxazine).

The methods of isolation varied somewhat with the source of the material but nearly all the early workers used adsorption on fuller's earth for slightly acid extracts. The resulting adsorbate was extracted with pyridine solutions or dilute ammonia, and the eluate, after concentration, was precipitated with a heavy metal to form a salt of flavine. Until it was recognized that all were dealing with the same substance, the pigments were given specific names such as ovoflavin, lactoflavin, hepatoflavin and uroflavin.

Riboflavin crystallizes in yellowish brown needles. Solubility is relatively slight, being only 12 mg per 100 ml at 27.5°C. Riboflavin-5-phosphate, the "flavin mononucleotide," is much more soluble. Both riboflavin and its phosphate are decomposed by exposure to light and in strongly alkaline solutions. The typical fluorescence of riboflavin is dependent upon the presence of a free 3-imino group, and neither 3-substitute riboflavin nor the enzyme systems will fluoresce.

THE ESTIMATION OF RIBOFLAVIN

Although the growth of rats[12] and chicks[13] may occasionally be used to assay riboflavin in mixed diets, the biologic method of assay has been generally superseded by microbiologic methods.[14,14a]

The chemical assay of riboflavin relies upon the fact that the fluorescence of riboflavin is proportional to its concentration under controlled conditions of salt concentration, pH and temperature. Interfering substances may be removed by potassium permanganate[15] or by adsorption on Florisil.[16] More recently, procedures which make use of paper chromatography, column chromatography and radioisotopic methods have been described.[16a]

The present U.S.P. Reference Standard is a recrystallized sample of riboflavin obtainable from the U.S.P. Reference Standard Committee. Comparisons of purified riboflavin with biologic units have shown that one Bourguin-Sherman rat growth unit,[17] which upon daily addition will produce an average gain of 3 gm per rat per week, is equal to about 2.5 μg of riboflavin. Von Euler[18] proposed a unit of 5 μg of riboflavin, an amount which produced an increase in weight of 0.8 to 1.0 gm per day in young rats. A Cornell unit[19] is defined as the growth effect on chicks equivalent to that produced by 1 μg of riboflavin.

The need for biologic standards of activity continues to exist especially in the study of derivatives of riboflavin. For example, in the assay of a water-soluble derivative prepared by Stone,[20] fluorometric assay yielded a value of 57.2 per cent riboflavin, a microbiologic assay by U.S.P. XIII revision method gave a value of 33 per cent riboflavin, whereas the biologic assay by rat growth method showed that the riboflavin potency was negligible.

DEFICIENCY IN EXPERIMENTAL ANIMALS

The effects of riboflavin deficiency in rats, dogs, foxes, pigs, young ruminants, other mammals and birds have been reviewed by Horwitt.[21] The primary effect of riboflavin restriction is the cessation of growth. When less than the minimum requirement is provided rats show severe ophthalmia and a bilateral, symmetrical alopecia which almost completely denudes the head, neck and trunk. An eczematous condition of the skin affects especially the nostrils and eyes. The eyelids become denuded of hair and may be stuck together with a serous exudate. Conjunctivitis, blepharitis, corneal opacities and vascularization of the cornea are common manifestations of rat ariboflavinosis.

The importance of riboflavin in the reproductive cycle is often overlooked. Its absence from the diet of rats may produce anestrus, and the damage is irreparable[22] if riboflavin is not restored in 10 weeks. Riboflavin-deficient female rats gave birth to litters with congenital malformations.[23]

The deficiency of riboflavin in dogs was evaluated by Sebrell[24,25] who noted a characteristic fatty liver followed by collapse, coma and death in about 3 months. Patek et al.[26] characterized riboflavin deficiency in the pig as a syndrome which included retarded growth, corneal opacities, dermatitis, changes in the hair and hoofs and terminal collapse associated with hypoglycemia. Mitchell et al.[27] considered the absolute and relative neutrophilic granulocyte concentrations in the blood as the most sensitive indices of riboflavin deficiency in the pig. Rhesus monkeys[28] develop a freckled type of dermatitis on the face, hands, legs and groin. Foy and Kondi[29] have studied ariboflavinosis in the baboon which, after 10 weeks, developed swollen and edematous bleeding gums and ulcerated seborrheic keratitis of the face, nose, eyebrows, armpits and scrotum.

BIOCHEMICAL AND PHYSIOLOGIC FUNCTIONS OF RIBOFLAVIN

Knowledge of the close relationship between the vitamins and biologic oxidations may be said to date from 1932, the year in which the first flavoprotein was discovered. This compound, often referred to as the "old yellow enzyme," was soon separated into a protein and a yellow prosthetic group.[5] Stern and Holiday[30] found that the prosthetic group of Warburg's yellow enzyme was a derivative of alloxazine. This fact, when combined with the observations of correlations between vitamin B_2 requirements and concentrations of the yellow-green fluorescence, was soon corroborated by the synthesis of riboflavin. Theorell's[31] demonstration that Warburg's enzyme contained 1 molecule of phosphate and the proof of constitution of riboflavin-5'-phosphate were the concluding steps in the first separation, identification and synthesis of the prosthetic group of an enzyme.

Riboflavin is a constituent of 2 coenzymes, riboflavin-5'-phosphate, erroneously called flavin mononucleotide (FMN) since ribitol is an alcohol, and flavin adenine dinucleotide (FAD). The formulas are on page 200.

The riboflavin coenzymes are essential parts of a number of oxidative enzyme systems involved in electron transport. These include the amino acid oxidases, xanthine oxidase, the succinic dehydrogenase complex, glutathione reductase and many others. Some of the relationships of deficiencies in such enzyme systems to endocrine imbalances have been reviewed by Rivlin.[31a]

It is axiomatic that cellular growth cannot evolve in the absence of riboflavin. During periods of riboflavin deficiency, negligible amounts of riboflavin are excreted in the urine and it might be sur-

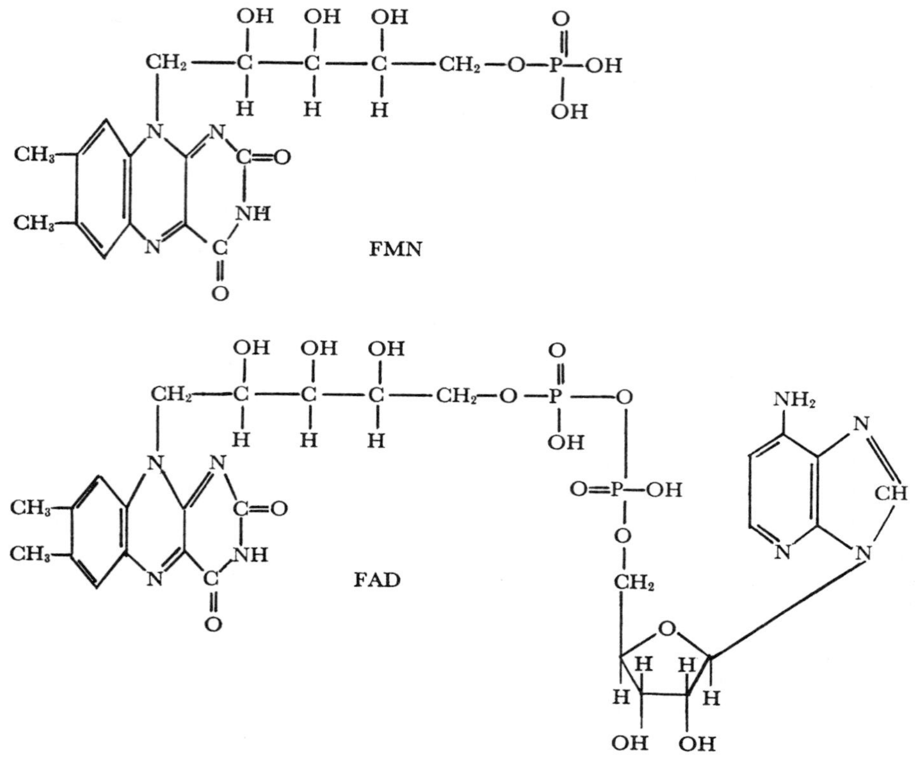

Fig. 6F–2. Structures of FMN and FAD.

mised that the body is capable of utilizing much of the riboflavin released by its own catabolic processes. However, the day-by-day needs of this vitamin for tissue turnover in the adult appear to be greater than 0.5 mg, and the decomposition products of riboflavin must be excreted in forms not recognized at present.

It is reasonable that any local trauma to the skin must be repaired by new growth.[32] Such trauma might range from erosions at the angles of the mouth, an area that is constantly flexed, to surgical intervention. The lesions formed are repaired by local growth only to the extent that riboflavin and protein are available. In the absence of riboflavin, minor injuries become aggravated and the so-called specific manifestations of ariboflavinosis become apparent.

CLINICAL ASPECTS OF RIBOFLAVIN DEFICIENCY

The first description of the clinical findings, which have subsequently become known as ariboflavinosis, was published by Stannus in 1912,[33] 20 years before riboflavin itself was discovered. His findings were confirmed and augmented by Bahr[34] in Ceylon, Scott[35] in Jamaica, Moore[36] in West Africa, Landor and Pallister[37] in Singapore, Aykroyd and Krishnan[38] in South India and Goldberger and Wheeler[39] and Tanner[40] in the United States. It was generally recognized that the lesions were on the basis of some dietary deficiency and that they could be cured by administration of vitamin B complex.

Lesions of the eye, in particular corneal vascularization, were described in the rat by Bessey and Wolbach[41] and by Spies,[42] Sydenstriker[43] and Kruse[44] in the human being. Extensive corneal vascularization among members of the Royal Canadian Air Force which seemed to respond to riboflavin administration was observed by Tisdall, McCreary and Pearce.[45]

The concept of riboflavin deficiency in man as a syndrome characterized by angular stomatitis, glossitis, seborrheic dermatitis about the nose and scrotum and vascularization of the cornea has been generally accepted since the publication of the findings of Sebrell and Butler.[46] This was confirmed and extended by the controlled experiment of Horwitt, Hills et al.[32] In the latter study,[32,47] although scrotal dermatitis was observed frequently, no evidence of circumcorneal injection or unusual vascularization of the cornea was observed. The tendency of small vascular twigs in the margins of the cornea to disappear and reappear months later was frequently noted, but no proliferation of the vessels of the limbic plexus was seen. No other ocular abnormalities were noted except for a tendency on the part of 3 subjects in the deficient group whose flicker fusion thresholds were increased. None of the subjects had any evidence of glossitis. There was nothing to suggest "magenta" tongue, "red" tongue or loss of the normal papillae. Studies of the capillary bed mentioned earlier failed to reveal any evidence of a "capillary dyskinesia," suggested by Stannus[48] to be the fundamental pathologic change of hyporiboflavinosis.

None of the results of these tests in themselves is entirely satisfactory, but taken as a group they are suggestive that no significant changes took place in the general capillary bed. There were no neurologic abnormalities, and no change of attitude, activity or appetite, such as appears in thiamin deficiency, was noted. Biochemically there was a sharp contrast between the behavior of these subjects and that of those exposed to deficiency of

thiamin as previous reported,[49,50] in that the "double metabolic load" of glucose plus exercise failed to reveal any abnormality of the levels of lactic and pyruvic acids in the blood. This was surprising because of the intimate role played by both these vitamins in the enzyme systems involved in the metabolism of carbohydrate.

Erythrocyte glutathione reductase, which is decreased when the consumption of riboflavin is deficient, has been used to evaluate population groups.[50a]

RIBOFLAVIN REQUIREMENTS OF MAN

Evidence of ariboflavinosis has not been confirmed on experimental diets which provided 0.8 to 0.9 mg per day[49,51] for over 2 years. Interpretation of the results of urinary excretions at different levels of riboflavin intake[52] has indicated that a tissue reserve of riboflavin may not be maintained in adult men at levels of intake below 1.2 mg per day. When intake was restricted to levels between 0.55 and 1.1 mg per day, less than 10 per cent of the ingested riboflavin was excreted in the urine. At levels of 1.3 mg per day or higher, over 20 per cent was excreted. Similar results have been obtained in female adults.[53,54]

The requirement for riboflavin does not appear to be related to calorie requirement or to muscular activity. However, the urinary excretion is markedly affected by alterations in nitrogen balance.[55-57] Less is excreted in the urine, on a given intake, when tissue growth is rapid, as during convalescence after severe trauma,[58] during lactation[59] or after administration of testosterone propionate;[60] more is excreted after severe burns or surgical procedures where protein losses indicate cellular decomposition.[61]

As a consequence of these observations, and the knowledge that in animal growth studies the amounts of riboflavin and protein in the diet are proportionately limiting, this reviewer has suggested that the daily mg riboflavin allowances be computed from the daily gm protein allowances, because protein utilized has been related to changes in the lean body mass[62] by those responsible for estimating protein requirements. This correlates similar conditions which increase the need for riboflavin and protein simultaneously, such as growth, pregnancy, lactation and wound healing. One advantage of relating the riboflavin and protein allowances is in facilitating a simple calculation of the needs of individuals who are growing faster than the average, or for those who, for a time, need more protein and riboflavin for tissue repair as a consequence of surgery, burns or other trauma.

In recent years there has been a tendency to relate riboflavin requirements to metabolic body size. Thus the Food and Nutrition Board has recommended that the allowance be calculated as a function of kg of body weight to the 0.75 power. The assumption is made that infants require 0.1, children 0.08, and adults 0.07 mg per kg.[75] In effect, this somewhat relates the riboflavin requirement to the protein requirement and curbs recommendations that would make it necessary to drink large amounts of milk when expending large amounts of energy. Included in current Recommended Dietary Allowances are increased riboflavin intakes of 0.3 mg per day during pregnancy and 0.5 mg per day during lactation. On this basis, infants need 0.4 to 0.6 mg, children 0.6 to 1.2 mg, adults 1.3 to 1.7 mg and pregnant and lactating women 1.8 and 2.0 mg per day, respectively.

SOURCES OF RIBOFLAVIN

It is not difficult to conceive a riboflavin-deficient diet if dairy foods and other animal protein sources are omitted.[63] Conversely, a mixed diet that contains a pint of milk and the usual portions of meat products is not likely to be deficient in riboflavin. Fortunately, the relative heat stability of riboflavin in the absence of light favors its preservation in ordinary cooking procedures.[64] The major losses which may occur are probably attributable to the extraction of the vitamin by the water used in cooking or blanching.[65-67] Loss due to exposure to light during cooking[68] may be important.

The relative insolubility of riboflavin makes it logical to give divided doses during therapeutic administration of the vitamin. However, a single daily oral administration of 6 mg appears to be assimilated as satisfactorily as 3 2-mg doses at 4-hour intervals.[52] Where more rapid saturation is desired, a single dose of 25 mg of the sodium salt of riboflavin phosphate may be administered[69] intramuscularly. The intramuscular administration is preferred, since the intravenous injection of 50 gm in 1 minute produced evidence of a slight decrease in pulse rate in all of 5 adult subjects tested.

TOXICITY

The low solubility of riboflavin may be responsible for its low toxicity. The oral administration of 10 gm per kg to rats and 2 gm per kg to dogs produced no ill effects.[70] Mice receiving 340 gm per kg intraperitoneally, which is 5,000 times the therapeutic dose, or an equivalent of 20 gm per day for a man, showed no apparent effect. The rat LD_{50} following intraperitoneal administration was 560 gm per kg.[70]

BIBLIOGRAPHY

1. McCollum and Kennedy: J. Biol. Chem., 24, 491, 1916.
2. Emmett and Luros: J. Biol. Chem., 43, 265, 1920.
3. Smith and Hendrick: Public Health Rep., 41, 201, 1926.
4. Goldberger and Lillie: Public Health Rep., 41, 1025, 1926.
5. Warburg and Christian: Biochem. Z., 266, 377, 1933.
6. Ellinger and Koschara: Chem. Ber., 66, 315, 808, 1933.
7. Booher: J. Biol. Chem., 102, 39, 1933.
8. Kuhn, György and Wagner-Jauregg: Chem. Ber., 66, 317, 576, 1034, 1933.
9. Blyth: J. Chem. Soc., 35, 530, 1879.

10. Kuhn, Reinemund, Weygand and Strobele: Chem. Ber., *68*, 1765, 1935.
11. Karrer, Salomon, Schopp and Benz: Helv. Chim. Acta, *18*, 1143, 1935.
12. von Euler and Malmberg: Z. Physiol. Chem., *250*, 158, 1937.
13. Jukes: J. Nutr., *14*, 223, 1937.
14. Snell and Strong: Ind. Eng. Chem., Anal. Ed., *11*, 346, 1939.
14a. Baker and Frank: In *Riboflavin* (Rivlin, Ed.). New York, Plenum Press, 1975.
15. van Eekelen and Emmerie: Acta Brev. Ned., *5*, 77, 1935.
16. Andrews: Cereal Chem., *21*, 398, 1944.
16a. Fazekas: In *Riboflavin* (Rivlin, Ed.). New York, Plenum Press, 1975.
17. Bourguin and Sherman: J. Am. Chem. Soc., *53*, 3501, 1931.
18. von Euler: Institut International di Chimie Solvay, Sixieme Conseil de Chimie, rapport et discussions Sur les Vitamines et les Hormones. Paris, 1938.
19. Norris, Wilgus, Ringrose, Heiman and Heuser: Cornell Univ. Agr. Exp. Sta. Bull., *660*, 3, 1936.
20. Stone: Science, *111*, 283, 1950.
21. Horwitt: *The Vitamins*, Vol. 5 (Sebrell and Harris, Eds.). New York, Academic Press, 1972.
22. Coward, Morgan and Waller: J. Physiol., *100*, 423, 1942.
23. Warkany: Vitam. Horm., *3*, 73, 1945.
24. Sebrell: Natl. Inst. Health Bull., *162*, Part 3, 23, 1933.
25. Sebrell and Onstatt: Public Health Rep., *53*, 83, 1938.
26. Patek, Post and Victor: Am. J. Physiol., *133*, 47, 1941.
27. Mitchell, Johnson, Hamilton and Haines: J. Nutr., *41*, 317, 1950.
28. Cooperman, Waisman, McCall and Elvehjem: J. Nutr., *30*, 45, 1945.
29. Foy and Kondi: Vitam. Horm., *26*, 653, 1968.
30. Stern and Holiday: Chem. Ber., *67*, 1104, 1442, 1934.
31. Theorell: Biochem. Z., *272*, 155, 1934.
31a. Rivlin: N. Engl. J. Med., *283*, 436, 1970.
32. Horwitt, Hills, Liebert and Steinberg: J. Nutr., *39*, 357, 1949.
33. Stannus: Trans. R. Soc. Trop. Med. Hyg., *5*, 112, 1912.
34. Bahr: *Researches on Sprue in Ceylon*, 1912–1914. London, Cambridge University Press, 1915.
35. Scott: Ann. Trop. Med., *12*, 109, 1918.
36. Moore: West Afr. Med. J., *4*, 46, 1930; J. Trop. Med., *42*, 109, 1939.
37. Landor and Pallister: Trans. R. Soc. Trop. Med. Hyg., *19*, 121, 1935.
38. Aykroyd and Krishnan: Indian J. Med. Res., *24*, 411, 1936.
39. Goldberger and Wheeler: Hygienic Laboratory Bulletin, No. 120. Washington, U.S. Treasury Department, Public Health Service, 1920.
40. Goldberger and Tanner: Public Health Rep., *40*, 54, 1925.
41. Bessey and Wolbach: J. Exp. Med., *69*, 1, 1939.
42. Spies, Vilter and Ashe: J.A.M.A., *113*, 931, 1939; Spies, Bean and Ashe: Ann. Intern. Med., *12*, 1830, 1939.
43. Sydenstricker, Geeslin, Templeton and Weaver: J.A.M.A., *113*, 1697, 1939.
44. Kruse, Sydenstricker, Sebrell and Cleckley: Public Health Rep., *55*, 157, 1940.
45. Tisdall, McCreary and Pearce: Can. Med. Assoc. J., *49*, 5, 1943.
46. Sebrell and Butler: Public Health Rep., *53*, 2282, 1938.
47. Hills, Liebert, Steinberg and Horwitt: Arch. Intern. Med., *87*, 682, 1951.
48. Stannus: Br. Med. J., *2*, 103, 1944.
49. Horwitt, Liebert, Kreisler and Wittman: National Research Council Bull. *116*, Washington, 1948.
50. Horwitt and Kreisler: J. Nutr., *37*, 411, 1949.
50a. Sauberlich, Judd, Nichoalds, Broquist and Darby: Am. J. Clin. Nutr., *25*, 756, 1972.
51. Williams, Mason, Cusick and Wilder: J. Nutr., *25*, 361, 1943.
52. Horwitt, Harvey, Hills and Liebert: J. Nutr., *41*, 247, 1950.
53. Davis, Oldham and Roberts: J. Nutr., *32*, 143, 1946.
54. Brewer, Porter, Ingalls and Ohlson: J. Nutr., *32*, 583, 1946.
55. Sarett and Perlzweig: J. Nutr., *25*, 173, 1943.
56. Sarett, Klein and Perlzweig: J. Nutr., *24*, 295, 1942.
57. Pollack and Bookman: J. Lab. Clin. Med., *38*, 561, 1951.
58. Andrea, Schenker and Browne: Fed. Proc., *5*, 3, 1946.
59. Roderick, Coryell, Williams and Macy: J. Nutr., *32*, 267, 1946.
60. Beher and Gaebler: J. Nutr., *41*, 447, 1950.
61. Pollack and Halpern: Therapeutic Nutrition. Washington, National Research Council, 1951.
62. Horwitt: Am. J. Clin. Nutr., *18*, 458, 1966.
63. Horwitt, Sampson, Hills and Steinberg: J. Am. Diet. Assoc., *25*, 591, 1949.
64. Levine and Remington: J. Nutr., *13*, 525, 1937.
65. Mayfield and Hedrick: J. Am. Diet. Assoc., *25*, 1024, 1949.
66. Wagner, Strong and Elvehjem: Ind. Eng. Chem., *39*, 985, 1947.
67. Krehl and Winters: J. Am. Diet. Assoc., *26*, 966, 1950.
68. Cheldelin, Wood and Williams: J. Nutr., *26*, 477, 1943.
69. Horwitt and Wilson: Unpublished.
70. Unna and Greslin: J. Pharmacol. Exp. Ther., *76*, 75, 1942.
71. Kuhn and Boulanger: Z. Physiol. Chem., *241*, 233, 1936.
72. Kuhn: Klin. Wochenschr., *17*, 122, 1938.
73. Demole: Z. Vitaminforsch., *7*, 138, 1938.

G. Niacin

M. K. Horwitt

Pellagra first appeared in Europe about 1720, coincident with the introduction of corn (maize) planting. The first recorded description of symptoms of pellagra as an individual disease was by Casal, a Spanish physician, in 1735. The term *pellagra*, or rough skin, which had been used by the peasantry in Italy to describe the symptoms, was not published until 1771 by Frapolli. Despite its antiquity, the recognition that this was a dietary deficiency disease did not evolve until after Goldberger's classical studies which began in 1913, when the U.S. Public Health Service undertook an investigation of an epidemic in the south where about 200,000 cases a year were being recorded. As early as 1913, Sandwith had suggested that pellagra was due to a deficiency of tryptophan in maize.[1] Wilson,[2] working in Egypt, had claimed in 1920 that pellagra was due to the poor biologic value of the protein in corn, a point with which Goldberger[3] concurred. In fact, Tanner, an associate of Goldberger (quoted by Sebrell[4]), in a letter written in 1921 describes the rapid cure of a pellagrous patient by the administration of tryptophan. However, the discovery that a yeast extract devoid of amino nitrogen was effective in curing pellagra delayed the recognition of the significance of these observations. It was not until 1937, when Elvehjem et al.[5] demonstrated that nicotinic acid could cure the animal analogs of pellagra, that the direct correlation between human pellagra and nicotinic acid became apparent.[6-10] Almost 8 more years were to pass before the biologic transformation of tryptophan to niacin was fully appreciated.[11] Even today some tables in textbooks in use report the niacin content of foods without reference to the tryptophan content.

DISCOVERY AND CHEMICAL NATURE

Although nicotinic acid was prepared as a pure chemical substance in 1867[12] and isolated from rice polishings by Funk in 1911,[13] its recognition as a vitamin was not fully established until 1937 when Elvehjem, Madden, Strong and Woolley[5] showed that the deficiency disease black tongue in dogs was cured by this substance. The recognition that nicotinic acid (niacin) was the human antipellagra vitamin was

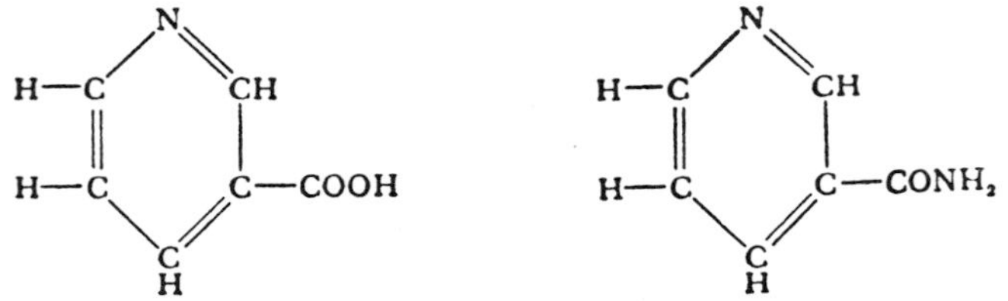

Nicotinic acid (Niacin)
pyridine-3-carboxylic acid

Nicotinamide (Nicotinic Acid Amide; Niacinamide)
pyridine-3-carboxylic acid amide

Fig. 6G–1. *Left*: Nicotinic acid (niacin) (pyridine-3-carboxylic acid). *Right*: Nicotinamide (nicotinic acid amide; niacinamide) (pyridine-3-carboxylic acid amide).

soon confirmed by numerous investigators.

Niacin is β-pyridine carboxylic acid. This is easily converted to the physiologically active nicotinic acid amide (niacinamide). Niacin is a nonhygroscopic, stable, white crystalline solid which sublimes without decomposition at about 230°C. It is soluble in water (1 gm to 60 ml at 25°C) and in alcohol (1 gm in 80 ml at 25°C) and insoluble in ether. Niacinamide is much more soluble in water (1 gm in 1 ml) and in alcohol (1 gm in 1.5 ml) and is also soluble in ether.

THE ESTIMATION OF NICOTINIC ACID

Although animals have never been completely satisfactory subjects for the assay of the pellagra-preventive factor, dogs have been used to produce uncomplicated niacin deficiency.[14,15] The chemical technique most often used depends upon the König reaction[16] in which the pyridine compound reacts with cyanogen bromide and an organic base to form a yellow color.[17,18] In recent years the microbiologic methods (as illustrated by that of Snell and Wright[19]) have been more popular. These depend upon the amount of lactic acid produced by L. arabinosus on a synthetic medium containing all known growth factors except niacin.

THE BIOLOGIC FUNCTION OF NICOTINIC ACID

The physiologic significance of nicotinic acid was understood in 1935 by Warburg and Christian[20] before its importance in nutrition was recognized. The isolation by these investigators of coenzyme II, a compound of adenine, nicotinamide, 2 molecules of ribose and 3 molecules of phosphoric acid, was followed by the recognition that this coenzyme, triphosphopyridine nucleotide (TPN), was a specific codehydrogenase for a series of dehydrogenases which included, among other enzymes, those involved in changing glucose-6-monophosphate to phosphogluconic acid and citric acid to α-ketoglutaric acid. Coenzyme I (cozymase) or diphosphopyridine nucleotide (DPN) is similar in general action and in structure except that it contains 2 molecules of phosphoric acid. It is a specific codehydrogenase for enzymes responsible for converting lactic acid to pyruvic acid, alcohol to acetaldehyde, β-hydroxybutyric acid to acetaldehyde, and many other reactions. The modern terms for DPN and TPN are NAD and NADP, the currently accepted abbreviations for nicotinamide adenine dinucleotide and nicotinamide adenine dinucleotide phosphate, respectively.

NAD and NADP serve as parts of the intracellular respiratory mechanism of all cells. They assist in the stepwise transfer of hydrogen from a product of glycolysis to flavin mononucleotide which in turn, with the help of specific enzymes, transfers this hydrogen to the cytochromes which in turn transfer the hydrogen to oxygen to form water. NAD and NADP can accept electrons from many biologic substrates. Reduced NAD (NADH) usually donates its hydrogens to flavin adenine dinucleotide (FAD) in the cell respiratory chain responsible for energy release. NADPH gives up its hydrogens most often to cellular biosynthetic processes such as the synthesis of fatty acids.

CLINICAL ASPECTS OF NICOTINIC ACID DEFICIENCY

Although the disease has been endemic in corn-eating areas of the world for over 200 years, it was not until about 1908 that the diagnostic symptoms of pellagra were clearly recognized.[21] Usually, the early symptoms are weakness, lassitude, anorexia and indigestion. These are followed by the classic "three Ds," dermatitis, diarrhea and dementia.

The dermatitis has a characteristic appearance on those parts of the body exposed to sunlight, heat or mild trauma. The lesions are distributed on the face, neck and surfaces of the hands, feet, elbows and other parts of the body which may be subject to mechanical irritations or to contact with body secretions. Usually the lesions of pellagra are bilaterally symmetrical. In a study by Goldsmith et al.[22] of experimentally produced pellagra, the importance of oral lesions as diagnostic signs was confirmed.

Although diarrhea is a prominent feature in the pellagrous patient, it may not develop in all cases.[23] The diarrhea may be severe and accompanied by vomiting and a dysphagia, a mouth inflammation which may be so painful that the patient refuses food and becomes emaciated.

The mental symptoms develop in untreated cases.[24] Irritability, headaches, sleeplessness, loss of memory and other signs of emotional instability often accompany the early signs of pellagra. In advanced cases, toxic confusional psychosis with symptoms of acute delirium and catatonia has been observed.

Lesions of the nervous system are nonspecific. Scattered degeneration of the axis cylinders of the pyramidal cells of the cortex and a myelin degeneration of fibers of the spinal column have been found.[25] Peripheral lesions are uncommon.

Recognition of the deficiency of dietary intake of nicotinic acid, or tryptophan-containing proteins, can be obtained by analyzing the urine for its N^1-methylnicotinamide content. Whereas the normal daily excretion is usually over 3 mg, subjects on a restricted diet providing 4.7 mg of niacin and 190 mg of tryptophan for 60 days had excretions of approximately 0.5 mg per day.[22] Slightly higher excretions of N^1-methylnicotinamide were obtained in another study in which a diet providing 5.8 mg niacin and 265 mg of tryptophan daily was fed for more than a year.[26] The latter study also showed that the pyridone of N^1-methylnicotinamide was not excreted unless the excretion of N^1-methylnicotinamide approached satisfactory levels. In effect, if the pyridone is found in the urine

at minimal levels the diet is generally found to be adequate in niacin/tryptophan.

NICOTINIC ACID REQUIREMENTS OF MAN

Dietary levels of less than 7.5 mg a day have been associated with the production of pellagra[22,27,28] but it is not correct to speak about nicotinic acid needs without considering the amount of tryptophan in the diet. Not only can tryptophan alone heal the lesions of pellagra[29-31] but it may be more nearly correct to think of pellagra as a tryptophan deficiency, since corn products are relatively more deficient in tryptophan than in nicotinic acid.[32,33]

The term *niacin-equivalent*[32] was introduced to facilitate the calculation of the combined effects of nicotinic acid and tryptophan in the diet. The amount of tryptophan chosen to be equivalent to 1 mg of nicotinic acid was 60 mg. This ratio is a compromise based upon studies of the amounts of tryptophan converted to N^1-methylnicotinamide and its metabolites in human subjects.[26,34] Obviously, such a relationship cannot be expected to be inflexible under all conditions of genetic, physiologic and dietary variations, but the fact that some protein foods practically devoid of nicotinic acid can supply all the niacin-equivalents necessary for optimal health makes it practical to have some estimation of the amounts of tryptophan in the diet in order to evaluate nicotinic acid requirements. This is illustrated in Table 6G–1.

It should be emphasized that, although most studies[35-38] have confirmed that an average of 60 mg of tryptophan is converted to 1 mg of niacin, this equivalence will vary from individual to individual. Of special interest are data[39] from women in the third trimester of pregnancy who can convert tryptophan to niacin metabolites 3 times as efficiently as nonpregnant females. It would appear from interpretation of studies on the effect of tryptophan

load tests during pregnancy or after ingestion of contraceptive steroids or steroid
hormones that the estrogens cause stimulation of tryptophan oxygenase which is apparently the rate-limiting enzyme in the
tryptophan-nicotinic acid ribonucleotide
pathway.[40,41]

An interesting point that comes out of
studies of human requirements is the calculation that the requirement for niacin-
equivalents is dependent upon the total
caloric intake as a function of either
metabolism plus work or body size. Accordingly, it may be necessary to think of
niacin/tryptophan requirements, as
thiamin requirements, as being related to
calories consumed. An illustration of this
may be had from comparing the experimental pellagra-producing diet used by
Goldberger[27] with those used by Goldsmith
et al.[22] and in the Elgin studies.[26] The
Goldberger diet provided 6.7 mg
nicotinamide and 330 mg tryptophan in
3,000 calories, or 4.1 niacin-equivalents
per 1,000 calories, whereas diets in the
other studies, which provided 5.2 mg of
nicotinamide plus 235 mg tryptophan in
2,000 calories or 4.4 niacin-equivalents per
1,000 calories, did not produce pellagra.
In the Tulane studies,[22] diets which provided less than 4.4 niacin-equivalents per
1,000 calories at levels of intake of 2,000
calories did produce pellagra.

To put the figure of 4.4 mg of niacin-
equivalent per 1,000 calories in proper
perspective, it should be compared with
levels of intake of thiamin and riboflavin
below which pathologic symptoms appear.
This would be about 0.18 mg of thiamin
per 1,000 calories and about 0.6 mg of
riboflavin per day.

Some nutritional workers have objected
to the use of a niacin-equivalent because of
the absence of easily accessible tables that
present the tryptophan content or niacin-
equivalence of common foods. With the
niacin content of many packaged foods
now presented on the label, it can be
confusing if the niacin amount listed does

Table 6G–1. Niacin-equivalents of Representative Foods[26]

Food	Niacin mg/1000 calories	Trypto- phan mg/1000 calories	Niacin- equivalent per 1000 calories
Cow's milk	1.21	673	12.4
Human milk	2.46	443	9.84
Beef, round	24.7	1280	46.0
Whole eggs	0.60	1150	10.8
Salt pork	1.15	61	2.17
Wheat flour	2.48	297	7.43
Corn grits	1.83	70	3.00
Corn	4.97	106	6.74

not allow for the contribution from protein. It should be noted that a simple
approximation of the tryptophan content
of a protein can be made by assuming that
1 per cent of the protein is tryptophan.
Actually, if more precision is desired the
following approximations may be used:
corn products 0.6 per cent, other grains,
fruits and vegetables 1.0 per cent and
animal protein products 1.5 per cent. Dividing the milligrams of tryptophan by 60
gives an acceptable niacin-equivalent contributed by the protein in the food.

Another possible objection to the use of
a niacin-equivalent may be based on the
fact that pregnant women[39] and those taking oral contraceptives convert niacin to
tryptophan more efficiently. The rate of
conversion seems to be related to the
amount of estrogen produced or ingested[45] and, in the case of pregnancy, is
reduced to a normal level soon after parturition. Since a greater need for niacin by
pregnant women has been postulated, this
increase in conversion may be a safety
factor built in by nature and should not be
considered an objection to the evaluation
and tabulation of niacin-equivalents. Current confusion will continue until workers
are made aware that some of the best
antipellagragenic foods contain very little
niacin per se.

THERAPY

Since the ingestion of large, therapeutic amounts of nicotinic acid usually produces a flushing reaction, niacin prescribed for correction of nutritional deficiency is more often administered as the nicotinamide (niacinamide). The amounts of nicotinamide generally recommended for therapeutic purposes are about 10 times the daily minimum requirement (assuming adequacy of protein) and range from 50 to 250 mg per day. Recommended allowances as defined by the Food and Nutrition Board range from 5 to 8 niacin-equivalents for infants to 20 niacin-equivalents for lactating females. Since 75 gm of good protein will supply about 15 mg niacin-equivalents from its tryptophan content and practically all mixed diets with adequate calories will add more than 5 mg of niacin, this allowance of 20 mg niacin-equivalents is easy to achieve.

Large doses of nicotinic acid, from 3 to 6 gm per day, reduce the levels of cholesterol, beta-lipoproteins and triglycerides in the blood.[42,43] Nicotinamide is ineffective. The flushing reaction and itching resulting from oral ingestion of nicotinic acid disappear after about 3 days of therapy, but prolonged use has raised some problems of gastrointestinal irritation and possible liver damage.[44]

BIBLIOGRAPHY

1. Sandwith: Trans. Soc. Trop. Med. Hyg., 6, 143, 1913.
2. Wilson: J. Hyg., 20, 1, 1921.
3. Goldberger: J.A.M.A., 78, 1676, 1922.
4. Sebrell: J. Nutr., 55, 3, 1955.
5. Elvehjem, Madden, Strong and Woolley: J. Am. Chem. Soc., 59, 1767, 1937; J. Biol. Chem., 123, 137, 1938.
6. Fouts, Helmer, Lepkovsky and Jukes: Proc. Soc. Exp. Biol. Med., 37, 405, 1937.
7. Smith, Ruffin and Smith: J.A.M.A., 109, 2054, 1937.
8. Spies, Cooper and Blankenhorn: J.A.M.A., 110, 622, 1938.
9. Spies, Bean and Stone: J.A.M.A., 111, 584, 1938.
10. Schmidt and Sydenstricker: J.A.M.A., 110, 2065, 1938; Sydenstricker: Arch Intern. Med., 67, 746, 1941; Sydenstricker and Cleckley: Am. J. Psychiatry, 98, 83, 1941.
11. Krehl, Sarma, Teply and Elvehjem: J. Nutr., 31, 85, 1946.
12. Huber: Liebeg's Ann. Chem., 141, 271, 1867.
13. Funk: J. Physiol. 43, 395, 1911; J.A.M.A., 109, 2086, 1937.
14. Waisman, Mickelsen, McKibbin and Elvehjem: J. Nutr., 19, 483, 1940; McKibbin, Waisman, Mickelsen and Elvehjem: Wis. Agr. Exp. Sta. Bull. No. 446.
15. Schaefer, McKibbin and Elvehjem: J. Biol. Chem., 144, 679, 1942.
16. König: J. Prakt. Chem., 69, 105, 1904, 70, 19, 1904.
17. Swaminathan: Nature, 141, 830, 1938.
18. Bandier and Hald: Biochem. J., 33, 264, 1939.
19. Snell and Wright: J. Biol. Chem., 139, 675, 1941.
20. Warburg and Christian: Biochem. Z., 275, 464, 1935.
21. Elvehjem: Physiol. Rev., 20, 249, 1940.
22. Goldsmith, Sarett, Register and Gibbons: J. Clin. Invest., 31, 533, 1952.
23. Bicknell and Prescott: Vitamins in Medicine, 3rd ed. New York, Grune & Stratton, 1953.
24. Frostig and Spies: Am. J. Med. Sci., 199, 268, 1940.
25. Youmans: Nutritional Deficiencies. Philadelphia, J. B. Lippincott, 1943.
26. Horwitt, Harvey, Rothwell, Cutler and Haffron: J. Nutr., 60, Suppl. 1, 1956.
27. Goldberger and Wheeler: Arch. Intern. Med., 25, 451, 1920.
28. Frazier and Friedeman: Q. Bull. Northwest. Med. Sch., 20, 24, 1946.
29. Bean, Franklin and Daum: J. Lab. Clin. Med., 38, 167, 1951.
30. Sarett: J. Biol. Chem., 193, 627, 1951.
31. Vilter, Mueller and Bean: J. Lab. Clin. Med., 34, 409, 1949.
32. Horwitt: Am. J. Clin. Nutr., 3, 244, 1955.
33. Horwitt: J. Am. Diet. Assoc., 34, 914, 1958.
34. Goldsmith: Am. J. Clin. Nutr., 6, 479, 1958.
35. Goldsmith, Miller and Unglaub: J. Nutr., 73, 172, 1961.
36. Moyer, Goldsmith, Miller and Miller: J. Nutr., 79, 423, 1963.
37. deLange and Joubert: Am. J. Clin. Nutr., 15, 169, 1964.
38. Vivian: J. Nutr. 82, 395, 1964.
39. Wertz, Lojkin, Bouchard and Derby: J. Nutr., 64, 339, 1958.
40. Rose and Braidman: Am. J. Clin. Nutr., 24, 673, 1971.
41. Brin: Am. J. Clin. Nutr., 24, 704, 1971.
42. Miller, Hamilton and Goldsmith: Am. J. Clin. Nutr., 8, 480, 1960.
43. Shawver, Scarborough and Tarnowski: Am. J. Psychiatry, 117, 741, 1961.
44. Christensen, Achor, Berge and Mason: Dis. Chest, 46, 411, 1964.
45. Horwitt, Harvey and Dahm: Am. J. Clin. Nutr., 28, 403, 1975.

H. Pantothenic Acid

Howerde E. Sauberlich

Pantothenic acid was recognized in 1933[1] as a growth factor for yeast. Following its isolation[2,3] and synthesis,[4] it was found that the vitamin could prevent or cure chick dermatitis.[5,6] Subsequently it was recognized as an essential nutrient for the rat, mouse, monkey, pig, dog, fox, turkey, fish, hamster and other species. It is widely distributed in nature and has been found in all forms of living things. Liver, meat, cereal, milk, egg yolk, fresh vegetables and many other foods are good sources (Table 6I–1).[7]

CHEMISTRY AND BIOCHEMICAL FUNCTIONS OF PANTOTHENIC ACID

Pantothenic acid has a molecular weight of 219 and consists of α, γ-dihydroxy β, β' dimethyl butyric acid and β-alanine joined by a peptide linkage. Since the vitamin itself is a pale yellow viscous oil, it is commonly available as a synthetic white crystalline calcium salt. The vitamin is stable in neutral solution but is readily destroyed by heat at either alkaline or acid pH.

Pantothenic acid is converted via pantetheine to coenzyme A which is an important catalyst of biologic acetylation reactions,[8-11] or in a broader sense in acyl transfers. Coenzyme A contains β-mercaptoethylamine the terminal sulfhydryl group of which is the reactive site of the molecule in biologic reactions.[12,13] All known acyl derivatives of coenzyme A are thiol esters. These acyl derivatives of coenzyme A may participate in a number of metabolic reactions. Thus coenzyme A is

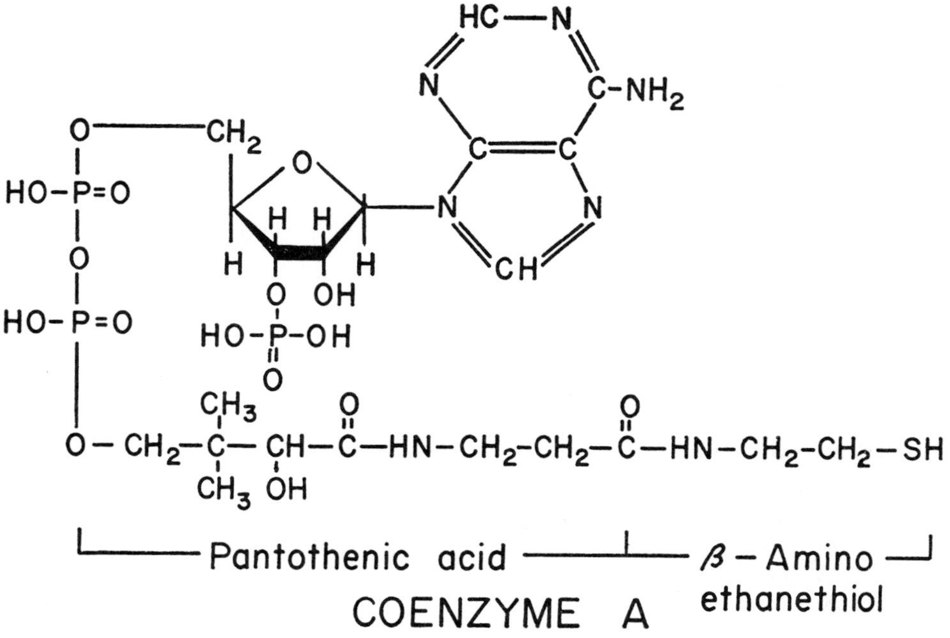

Fig. 6H–1. Structure of coenzyme A.

involved in condensation and addition reactions, acyl group interchanges and nucleophilic attack. In this manner, coenzyme A is enzymatically involved in (1) acetylation of choline and certain aromatic amines such as sulfonamides, (2) oxidation of fatty acids, pyruvate, α-ketoglutarate and acetaldehyde, and (3) synthesis of fatty acids, cholesterol, sphingosine, citrate, acetoacetate, porphyrin and sterols. Thus coenzyme A may serve not only as an acetyl acceptor or acetyl donor but also as an acceptor or donor of acyl groups.[14-17]

Pyruvate and α-ketoglutarate are converted to acetyl coenzyme A and to succinyl coenzyme A, respectively, through the participation of thiamin pyrophosphate, niacin adenine dinucleotide (NAD) and lipoic acid. Additional roles of coenzyme A in carbohydrate metabolism have been noted.[18-20] Acetoacetyl coenzyme A may conjugate in the liver with acetyl coenzyme A to form β-hydroxy-β-methylglutaryl coenzyme A, an important precursor of cholesterol and other sterols. Coenzyme A participates in the biosynthesis of sphingosine and ceramide.[21] Histones of liver nuclei are acetylated by coenzyme A.[22]

Fatty acids are converted into an active state for oxidation in the mitochondria by the formation of fatty acyl/coenzyme A esters by the catalyzed reactions of enzymes such as thiophorases, acetate thiokinase, medium and long-chain fatty acid thiokinases and a guanine triphosphate-specific acid thiokinase.[23,24] Enzymatic β-oxidation of the straight-chain fatty acids with even-number carbon atoms results in the production of acetyl coenzyme A. Quantities of propionyl coenzyme A and methylmalonyl coenzyme A result from the oxidation of odd-carbon or branched-chain fatty acids and unsaturated fatty acids.[25] Propionyl coenzyme A is converted by the biotin-requiring propionyl carboxylase enzyme into methylmalonyl coenzyme A. The vitamin B_{12} containing methylmalonyl mutase enzyme converts methylmalonyl coenzyme A into

succinyl coenzyme A which may then enter the tricarboxylic acid cycle.[26]

The de novo synthesis of long-chain fatty acids proceeds mainly through malonyl coenzyme A as an intermediate.[27-30] Malonyl coenzyme A is formed by carboxylation of acetyl coenzyme A through the action of acetyl coenzyme A carboxylase. This enzyme appears to play an important role in the control of fatty acid synthesis.[28] Through the involvement of a cytoplasmic multienzyme complex, acetyl coenzyme A and malonyl coenzyme A are converted to palmityl coenzyme A and stearyl coenzyme A.[31] Further elongation may occur in the mitochondria with the participation of acetyl coenzyme A or in the microsomes with the participation of malonyl coenzyme A.[32] The metabolism of medium-chain fatty acids likewise involves coenzyme A.[17,33,34]

Fatty acid biosynthesis in the cytoplasm and mitochondria involves an additional role of pantothenic acid in the form of the co-factor, 4'-phosphopantetheine. This factor is bound to a protein commonly referred to as the acyl carrier protein (ACP).[36] This protein, with 4'-phosphopantetheine, appears to be involved in all fatty acid synthesizing

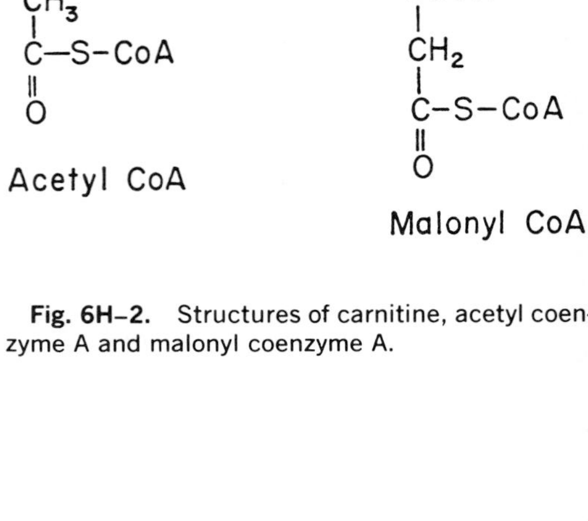

Fig. 6H–2. Structures of carnitine, acetyl coenzyme A and malonyl coenzyme A.

systems.[30,37-39,130] The acyl intermediates formed during fatty acid synthesis are esterified to the sulfhydryl group of the 4'-phosphopantetheine linked to the acyl carrier protein. Phosphopantetheine is a cofactor bound to the guanosine triphosphate-dependent acyl coenzyme A synthetase.[40] Thus, 4'-phosphopantetheine serves in a capacity during fatty acid synthesis analogous to that of coenzyme A during fatty acid oxidation. The fatty acids formed may be converted to triglycerides via the participation of their fatty acyl coenzyme A esters.[41] Coenzyme A also participates in the biosynthesis of ceramides.

Carnitine reacts with fatty acyl coenzyme A esters to form fatty acyl carnitine esters. The acylated carnitines are capable of crossing the mitochondrial membrane which is impermeable to acyl coenzyme A.[27,42-44] Following passage into the mitochondria, the fatty acyl group is transferred from carnitine to coenzyme A again to form fatty acyl coenzyme A. Coenzyme A is synthesized within the cells as blood coenzyme A fails to permeate liver cells.[45]

An additional form of pantothenic acid, present in tomato juice, has been purified and identified as 4'O-(β-D-glucopyranosyl)-D-pantothenic acid.[131] Although the significance of the compound is unclear, it serves as a growth stimulant for a strain of Pediococcus cerevisiae.

METHODS OF ASSAY

Pantothenic acid may be measured with the use of chemical methods, microbiologic procedures and the chick curative bioassay. Although the chick and rat prophylactic and curative bioassays were commonly used in early studies on pantothenic acid, they have been replaced by microbiologic procedures for assaying natural products.[46] Pantothenic acid, pantetheine and coenzyme A are equally active in the animal bioassays. The microbiologic assays use either Saccharomyces uvarum (Saccharomyces carlsbergensis), Lactobacillus casei or L. plantarum (L. arabinosus) as the test organism.[47-49] More recently, some investigators have employed Pediococcus acidilacti[124] and the protozoan Tetrahymena pyriformis[50] for measuring pantothenic acid levels in natural products and biologic fluids. Most of the pantothenic acid in foods and biologic materials exists as coenzyme A and other bound forms. Microbiologic assays for total pantothenic acid content require enzymatic hydrolysis of the samples to provide free pantothenic acid. Pantethine and pantetheine have been estimated in samples with the use of L. helveticus.[47,51] Pharmaceutic preparations of pantothenic acid can be readily assayed with the use of L. plantarum.[52] Pantothenyl alcohol (panthenol), a compound with equivalent pantothenic acid activity for animals and man,[53] can be

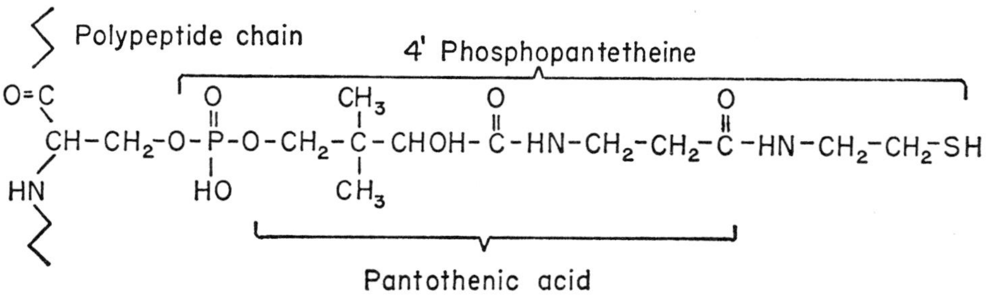

Fig. 6H–3. Acyl carrier protein (ACP).

measured in pharmaceutic products with the use of Leuconostoc mesenteroides.[47,54] Chemical procedures, including gas chromatography[108,125,126] are also available for determining pantothenic acid and pantothenyl alcohol in dry or liquid multivitamin preparations.[47,55-57] Pantoic acid, a metabolite and constituent of pantothenic acid, can be estimated with the use of an Escherichia coli mutant.[58] Procedures for measuring coenzyme A have also been described.[59,60] Recently, the development of a radioimmunoassay for the determination of pantothenic acid has been reported.[140,141]

DEFICIENCIES

Experimental Animals

Although the effects of a pantothenic acid deficiency vary greatly from species to species, certain common denominators exist, particularly that of growth failure.[61] In addition, a deficiency of the vitamin in the rat results in dermatitis, achromotrichia (graying), adrenal necrosis and hemorrhage,[127] "spectacled eyes" (hair loss about the eyes), spastic gait, anemia, leukopenia, impaired antibody production,[109] gonadal atrophy, infertility, duodenal ulcer, altered adrenal synthesis of corticosterone[132] and decreased urinary excretion of the vitamin.[133] Congenital malformations may occur in offspring of pantothenic-deficient rats.[62,63] Increased levels of fat in the diet did not increase the requirement for pantothenic acid in the rat, based upon body weight changes, adrenal weights or onset and incidence of graying of the hair. Pantothenic acid-deficient rats did, however, have lower liver coenzyme A values when fed a high-fat diet.[64] A pantothenic acid deficiency in the mouse resembles that in the rat. The mouse, however, does not develop hemorrhagic and necrotic adrenals but exhibits a partial paralysis of the hind legs with nerve tissue degeneration.

Dogs develop hair changes, decreased appetite, irritability, fatty livers, gastrointestinal tract disturbances, hypoglycemia, convulsions, coma and death. Similar observations have been reported for monkeys. Swine develop dermatitis, spastic gait ("goose-stepping"), hair loss, excessive nasal secretions, diarrhea, ulcerative colitis, degenerative lesions of the spinal cord and peripheral nerves and alterations in sodium, potassium and glucose absorption.[65] The coenzyme A activity of cells from colonic mucosa was markedly reduced in pantothenic acid-deficient swine.[65] These observations suggest a relationship between coenzyme A content of colonic tissue and diarrhea and ulcerative colitis.

A pantothenic acid deficiency in the chick results in the classical dermatitis in the corners of the mouth and on the toes and upper surface of the foot. Other signs of deficiency include poor feathering, spinal cord degeneration, incoordination, paralysis, involution of the thymus, fatty degeneration of the liver and death.[66,128] Symptoms of a pantothenic acid deficiency in turkeys resemble closely those in chickens.[67] In addition, ducks deficient in pantothenic acid develop anemia and show an impaired ability to develop antibodies when stimulated with bacterial, viral or erythrocyte antigens.[68,69] A pantothenic acid deficiency can be induced in other species, including the guinea pig and cat.[70]

Man

Pantothenic acid is of such widespread distribution in foods that an occurrence of a deficiency of the vitamin is probably exceedingly rare. However, significant amounts of pantothenic acid are lost in foods when canned, cooked, frozen or processed.[138] In malnutrition, however, multiple deficiencies frequently exist and a deficiency in pantothenic acid may not be recognized as part of the condition. Means of detecting and evaluating a pantothenic acid deficiency are limited. In studies in which attempts were made to control dietary intakes of pantothenic acid, results indicate that the urinary excretion of the vitamin by man is related to its dietary intake.[71,72,111-115,142] Urinary excretions of less than 1.0 mg per day are considered abnormally low for the human adult. Both serum and erythrocytes contain relatively high levels of pantothenic acid but whether changes in these levels can indicate a pantothenic acid deficiency is uncertain.[50,73,74,114-120,143,144]

Serum contains free pantothenic acid and no coenzyme A, while most of the vitamin is present in the erythrocytes as coenzyme A. Blood levels of the acid are higher in the newborn than in the mother and they appear to be related to the levels in maternal circulation at delivery.[134-136,144] The mean free pantothenic acid levels in pregnant subjects, postpartum subjects, and nonpregnant subjects were observed to be 8, 8, and 6 μg per dl blood, respectively.[115] The total blood pantothenic acid values (free plus bound) for these same subjects were 103, 112 and 183 μg per dl blood, respectively. A total pantothenic acid level of less than 100 μg per dl blood has been considered suggestive of low or inadequate dietary intakes of the vitamin. Various diseases have little or no influence on serum pantothenic acid levels.[137,143] The level of bound pantothenic acid in blood appears to decline with age.[139]

The measurement of changes in the blood and urine levels of the vitamin after test loads of 10 to 50 mg of the vitamin is not very useful in the diagnosis of pantothenic acid deficiency.[75,76] Patients with chronic malnutrition tend to have lower levels of pantothenic acid in blood and urine.[77,78] Poorly nourished alcoholic patients have been observed to have low serum and urinary levels of pantothenic acid.[79,145] The elevated serum copper levels noted in pellagrins were lowered significantly by injections of pantothenic acid.[80] The vitamin has been reported to afford relief in nutritional neuropathy and Korsakoff's psychosis.[81] Pantothenic acid treatment improved the burning or electric foot syndrome (nutritional melalgia)[82,83] which was noted in prisoners of the Japanese during World War II.[84-86] Subjects with this syndrome have been reported to have a reduced ability to acetylate para-aminobenzoic acid.[87] Pantothenic acid has been reported to improve the ability of well-nourished subjects to withstand stress.[88,89] In patients with chronic ulcerative and granulomatous colitis, the coenzyme A activity in the mucosa was considerably lower than that found in normal gut mucosa.[143]

The most well-defined signs and symptoms of a pantothenic acid deficiency have been those observed in human volunteers maintained on a diet deficient in pantothenic acid and on a pantothenic acid antagonist, omega methyl pantothenic acid.[90-94,121] Subjects on the pantothenic-deficient diet developed vomiting, malaise, abdominal distress and burning cramps. Later during the deficiency, tenderness in the heels, fatigue and insomnia occurred. Subjects who received both omega methyl pantothenic acid and the deficient diet developed similar symptoms somewhat earlier. The subjects were observed to have pain and soreness in the abdomen, nausea, some personality changes, insomnia, weakness and cramps in the legs, and paresthesia in the hands and feet. There was an impaired eosinopenic response to ACTH and an elevated sedimentation rate. Adrenocortical function appeared to remain normal. Antibody production against tetanus was impaired by the pantothenic acid deficiency. The combination of pantothenic acid and pyridoxine deficiencies exaggerated the impaired antigenic response when bacterial antigens were used, but not when poliomyelitis virus was employed. Administration of large doses of pantothenic acid reversed most of the signs and symptoms and laboratory changes ascribed to the pantothenic acid deficiency.

NUTRITIONAL REQUIREMENT

Ordinary foods customarily used in American diets provide an intake of approximately 7 mg of pantothenic acid per day, with a range of 5 to 20 mg per day.[71,95,121] Intakes of less than 4 mg per day were observed for low-income women[122] and teenage girls.[115] Diets adequate for children of 7 to 9 years of age provide about 4 to 5 mg of pantothenic acid.[72] The Food and Nutrition Board has not established a recommended dietary allowance for pantothenic acid but states that a daily intake of 5 to 10 mg is probably adequate for children and adults.[96] Pregnancy and lactation may increase the requirement.[115,119] Approximately 2 mg of pantothenic acid is present in a liter of human milk,[144] while cow's milk contains about 3.5 mg per liter. Pantothenic acid is unstable to heat with losses ranging from 15 to 30 per cent in heat-dried, canned and cooked meats.[97]

THERAPEUTIC USE, TOXICITY AND METABOLISM

Although pantothenic acid has been reported as an antigray-hair factor in man and as a means to relieve postoperative paralytic ileus and provide benefit in cases of burn and skin lesions, these effects have not been corroborated.[89,98-102] At present, no clearly defined therapeutic use of pantothenic acid exists, although the vitamin is commonly present in multivitamin preparations and in products employed in intravenous and oral alimentation. Synthetic calcium pantothenate is usually employed for these purposes, although the sodium salt is used in aqueous dispersions where the calcium ion must be avoided. Only the D (+) enantiomorph has biologic activity. Pantothenyl alcohol (panthenol) may also be used in the preparation of injectable and other liquid pharmaceutic preparations.

Pantothenic acid has been administered to human subjects in the amounts of 10 to 20 gm as the calcium salt. The only evidence of toxicity from these high intakes was an occasional diarrhea.[103,104,123]

The metabolism of pantothenic acid has not been studied in depth in man. Although the germ-free rat has been reported not to metabolize and break down pantothenic acid,[105] limited information suggests that man does metabolize daily a quantity of the vitamin.[89] Antagonists of pantothenic acid have been reported to possess antimalarial properties.[106,107]

BIBLIOGRAPHY

1. Williams, Lyman, Goodyear, Truesdail and Holaday: J. Am. Chem. Soc., 55, 2912, 1933.
2. Williams: Science, 89, 486, 1939.
3. Williams, Weinstock, Rohrmann, Truesdail, Mitchell and Meyer: J. Am. Chem. Soc., 61, 454, 1939.
4. Williams and Major: Science, 91, 246, 1940.
5. Jukes: J. Am. Chem. Soc., 61, 975, 1939.
6. Wooley, Waisman and Elvehjem: J. Am. Chem. Soc., 61, 977, 1939.
7. Orr: Pantothenic Acid, Vitamin B_6 and Vitamin B_{12} in Foods. Home Economics Research Report No. 36, U. S. Dept. Agr., 1969.
8. Lipmann, Kaplan, Novelli, Tuttle and Guirard: J. Biol. Chem., 167, 869, 1947.
9. Baddiley: Adv. Enzymol., 16, 1, 1955.
10. Lipmann: Bacteriol. Rev., 17, 1, 1953.
11. Jaenicke and Lynen: In The Enzymes, Vol. 3 (Boyer, Lardy and Myrbäck, Eds.). New York, Academic Press, 1960.
12. Stern and Ochoa: J. Biol. Chem., 179, 491, 1949.
13. Lynen, Reichert and Rueff: Liebigs Ann. Chem., 574, 1, 1951.
14. Clayton: Q. Rev. Chem. Soc. London, 19, 168, 1965.
15. Frantz and Shroepfer: Annu. Rev. Biochem., 36, 691, 1967.
16. Lennarz: Annu. Rev. Biochem., 39, 359, 1970.
17. Shapiro: Annu. Rev. Biochem., 36, 247, 1967.
18. Cooper and Bendict: Biochemistry, 7, 3032, 1968.
19. Nakashima, Pontremoli and Horecker: Proc. Nat. Acad. Sci., 64, 947, 1969.
20. Weber, Lea and Stamm: Lipids, 4, 388, 1969.
21. Morell: J. Biol. Chem., 245, 342, 1970.
22. Gallwitz and Sekeris: Hoppe Seylers Z. Physiol. Chem., 350, 150, 1969.
23. Galigzna, Rossi, Sartorelli and Gibson: J. Biol. Chem., 242, 2111, 1967.
24. Greville and Tubbs: Essays in Biochemistry, New York, Academic Press, 1968.
25. Dupont and Mathias: Lipids, 4, 478, 1969.
26. Hogenkamp: Annu. Rev. Biochem., 37, 225, 1968.
27. Stumpf: Annu. Rev. Biochem., 38, 159, 1969.
28. Numa, Nakanishi, Hashimoto, Iritani and Akazaki: Vitam. Horm., 28, 213, 1970.
29. Vagelos: Annu. Rev. Biochem., 33, 139, 1964.

30. Schweizer, Willecke, Winnewisser and Lynen: Vitam. Horm., 28, 329, 1970.
31. Hansen and Hanser: Acta Chem. Scand., 23, 2180, 1969.
32. Seubert, Lamberts and Kramer: Biochim. Biophys. Acta, 164, 498, 1968.
33. Bar-Tana and Rose: Biochem. J., 109, 283, 1968.
34. Bar-Tana, Rose and Shapiro: Biochem. J., 109, 269, 1968.
35. Mooney and Barron: Biochemistry, 9, 2138, 1970.
36. Majerus and Vagelos: Adv. Lipid Res., 5, 2, 1967.
37. Pugh and Wakil: J. Biol. Chem., 240, 4727, 1965.
38. Larrabee, McDaniel, Bakerman and Vagelos: Proc. Natl. Acad. Sci., 54, 267, 1965.
39. Vanaman, Wakil and Hill: J. Biol. Chem., 243, 6420, 1968.
40. Rossi, Alexandre and Galzigna: J. Biol. Chem., 245, 3110, 1970.
41. Dagley and Nicholson: An Introduction to Metabolic Pathways. New York, John Wiley and Sons, 1970.
42. Fritz and Yue: J. Lipid Res., 4, 279, 1963.
43. Rossi, Alexandre and Sartorelli: Eur. J. Biochem., 4, 31, 1968.
44. Thomitzek: Ergeb. Physiol., 62, 68, 1970.
45. Domschke, Liersch and Decker: Hoppe Seylers Z. Physiol. Chem., 352, 85, 1971.
46. Bliss, Bird and Thompson: The Vitamins, Vol. VII, 2nd ed. (György and Pearson, Ed.). New York, Academic Press, 1967.
47. Bird and Thompson: The Vitamins, Vol. VII, 2nd ed. (György and Pearson, Ed.). New York, Academic Press, 1967.
48. Atkin, Williams, Schultz and Frey: Ind. Eng. Chem., Anal. Ed., 16, 67, 1944.
49. Clarke: Anal. Chem., 29, 135, 1957.
50. Baker and Frank: Clinical Vitaminology. New York, Interscience Publishers, 1968.
51. Snell and Wittle: In Methods in Enzymology, Vol. III (Colowick and Kaplan, Ed.). New York, Academic Press, 1957.
52. U. S. Pharmacopeia, Revision XVI. Easton, Mack Publishing, 1960.
53. Abiko, Tomikawa and Shimizu: J. Vitam., 15, 59, 1969.
54. Bird and McCready: Anal. Chem., 30, 2045, 1958.
55. Panier and Close: J. Pharm. Sci., 53, 108, 1964.
56. Zappala and Simpson: J. Pharm. Sci., 50, 845, 1961.
57. Sheppard and Prosser: In Methods in Enzymology, Vol. XVIII (McCormick and Wright, Ed.). New York, Academic Press, 1970.
58. Rogers and Campbell: Anal. Chem., 32, 1662, 1960.
59. Allred: Anal. Biochem., 29, 293, 1969.
60. Abiko: In Methods in Enzymology, Vol. XVIII (McCormick and Wright, Ed.). New York, Academic Press, 1970.
61. Follis: In Deficiency Disease. Springfield, Charles C Thomas, 1958.
62. Jennings: In Vitamins in Endocrine Metabolism. Springfield, Charles C Thomas, 1970.
63. Nelson, Wright, Baird and Evans: J. Nutr., 62, 395, 1957.
64. Williams, Chu, McIntosh and Hincenbergs: J. Nutr., 94, 377, 1968.
65. Nelson: Am. J. Clin. Nutr., 21, 495, 1968.
66. Milligan and Briggs: Poul. Sci., 28, 202, 1949.
67. Kratzer and Williams: Poul. Sci., 27, 518, 1948.
68. Schulman and Rickert: J. Biol. Chem., 226, 181, 1957.
69. Axelrod and Hopper: J. Nutr., 72, 325, 1960.
70. Gershoff and Gottlieb: J. Nutr., 82, 135, 1964.
71. Fox and Linkwiler: J. Nutr., 75, 451, 1961.
72. Pace, Stier, Taylor and Goodman: J. Nutr., 74, 345, 1961.
73. Stanbery, Snell and Spies: J. Biol. Chem., 135, 353, 1940.
74. Pelezar and Porter: Proc. Soc. Exp. Biol. Med., 47, 3, 1941.
75. Spies, Stanbery, Williams, Jukes and Babcock: J.A.M.A., 115, 523, 1940.
76. Krahnke and Gordon: J.A.M.A., 116, 2431, 1941.
77. Makila: Int. Z. Vitaminforsch., 40, 81, 1970.
78. Kerrey, Crispin and Fox: Am. J. Clin. Nutr., 21, 1274, 1968.
79. Leevy, Baker, ten Houe, Frank and Cherrick: Am. J. Clin. Nutr., 16, 339, 1965.
80. Fidnlay and Venter: J. Invest. Dermatol., 31, 11, 1958.
81. Gordon: Pantothenic Acid in Human Nutrition. University of Chicago Symposium on Biological Action Vitamins, 1942.
82. Harrison: Lancet, 1, 961, 1946.
83. Cruickshank: Lancet, 2, 369, 1946.
84. Gopalan: Indian Med. Gaz., 81, 23, 1946.
85. Glusman: Am. J. Med., 3, 211, 1947.
86. Denny-Brown: Medicine, 26, 41, 1947.
87. Sarma, Menon and Venkatachalam: Curr. Sci., 18, 367, 1949.
88. Ralli: Nutr. Symp. Series, 5, 78, 1952.
89. Ralli: In The Vitamins, Vol. II (Sebrell and Harris, Eds.). New York, Academic Press, 1954.
90. Hodges, Bean, Ohlson and Bleiler: Am. J. Clin. Nutr., 11, 85, 1962.
91. Hodges, Bean, Ohlson and Bleiler: Am. J. Clin. Nutr., 11, 187, 1962.
92. Bean and Hodges: Proc. Soc. Exp. Biol. Med., 86, 693, 1954.
93. Hodges, Ohlson and Bean: J. Clin. Invest., 37, 1642, 1958.
94. Hodges, Bean, Ohlson and Bleiler: J. Clin. Invest., 39, 1421, 1959.
95. Mangay Chung, Pearson, Darby, Miller and Goldsmith: Am. J. Clin. Nutr., 9, 573, 1961.
96. Recommended Dietary Allowances, 8th ed. Washington, Natl. Acad. Sci.–Natl. Res. Council, 1974.
97. Anon.: Nutr. Rev., 20, 257, 1962.
98. Goldman: J. Invest. Dermatol., 11, 95, 1948.
98a. Scichounoff and Naz: Schweiz. Med. Wochenschr., 75, 767, 1945.
99. Combs and Zuckerman: J. Invest. Dermatol., 16, 379, 1951.

100. Frost: Physiol. Rev., *28*, 368, 1948.
101. Jacques: Lancet, *2*, 861, 1951.
102. Watne, Mendoza, Rosen, Nadler and Case: J.A.M.A., *181*, 827, 1962.
103. Gershberg, Rubin and Ralli: J. Nutr., *39*, 107, 1949.
104. Gershberg and Kuhl: J. Clin. Invest., *29*, 1625, 1950.
105. Anon.: Nutr. Rev., *14*, 116, 1956.
106. elslager, Hutt and Werbel: J. Med. Chem., *11*, 1071, 1968.
107. Razdan, Reinsel and Zitko: J. Med. Chem., *13*, 546, 1970.
108. Prosser and Sheppard: J. Pharm. Sci., *58*, 718, 1969.
109. Axelrod: Am. J. Clin. Nutr., *24*, 265, 1971.
110. Sauberlich, Dowdy and Skala: Laboratory Tests for the Assessment of Nutritional Status. Cleveland, CRC Press, 1974.
111. Schmidt: Int. Z. Vitaminforsch., *21*, 257, 1949–51.
112. Schmidt: J. Gerontol., *6*, 132, 1951.
113. Fox, Lee and Chen: Fed. Proc., *23*, 243, 1964 (abstract).
114. Koyanagi, Hareyama, Kiruchi, Takanohaski, Oikawa and Akazawa: Tohoku J. Exp. Med., *98*, 357, 1969.
115. Cohenour and Calloway: Am. J. Clin. Nutr., *25*, 512, 1972.
116. Ishiguro, Kobayashi and Kaneta: Tohoku J. Exp. Med., *74*, 65, 1961.
117. Denko, Grundy and Porter: Arch. Biochem., *13*, 481, 1947.
118. Koyanagi, Hareyama, Kikuchi and Kimura: Tohoku J. Exp. Med., *88*, 93, 1966.
119. Ishiguro: Tohoku J. Exp. Med., *78*, 7, 1962.
120. Ellestad, Nelson, Adson and Palmer: Fed. Proc., *29*, 820, 1970 (abstract).
121. Fry, Fox and Tao: J. Nutr. Sci. Vitaminol. *22*, 339, 1976.
122. Johnson and Nitzke: Home Econ. Res. J., *3*, 241, 1975.
123. Ralli and Dumm: Vitam. Horm., *11*, 133, 1953.

124. Solberg, Hegna and Clausen: J. Appl. Bacteriol., *39*, 119, 1975.
125. Tarli, Benocci and Neri: Anal. Biochem., *42*, 8, 1971.
126. Tesmer and Hötzel: Fresenius Z. Anal. Chem., *277*, 124, 1975.
127. Kazuko, Kubato, Nishigaki and Kikutani: Chem. Pharm. Bull., *23*, 1, 1975.
128. Gries and Scott; J. Nutr., *102*, 1269, 1972.
129. Hellendoorn, de Grott, Mijill Dekker, Slump and Willems: J. Am. Diet. Assoc., *58*, 434, 1971.
130. Qureshi, Lornitzo and Porter: Biochem. Biophys. Res. Commun., *60*, 158, 1974.
131. Eto and Kakagawa: Inst. Brew. London, *81*, 232, 1975.
132. Pietrzik, Hesse and Hötzel: Int. J. Vitam. Nutr. Res., *45*, 251, 1975.
133. Pietrzik, Hesse, Wiesch and Hötzel: Int. J. Vitam. Nutr. Res., *45*, 153, 1975.
134. Kaminetzky, Langer, Baker, Frank, Thomson, Munves, Opper, Behrle and Glista: Am. J. Obstet. Gynecol., *115*, 639, 1973.
135. Kaminetzky, Baker, Frank and Langer: Am. J. Obstet. Gynecol., *120*, 697, 1974.
136. Baker, Thomson, Frank and Leevy: Am. J. Clin. Nutr., *27*, 676, 1974.
137. Markkanen: Int. J. Vitam. Nutr. Res., *43*, 302, 1973.
138. Schroeder: Am. J. Clin. Nutr., *24*, 562, 1971.
139. Ishiguro: Tohoku J. Exp. Med., *107*, 367, 1972.
140. Wyse and Hansen: Fed. Proc., *35*, 660, 1976 (abstract).
141. Wyse and Hansen: Fed. Proc., *36*, 1169, 1977 (abstract).
142. Jellery and Calloway: J. Nutr., *106*, 17, 1976 (abstract).
143. Ellestad-Sayed, Nelson, Adson, Palmer and Soule: Am. J. Clin. Nutr., *29*, 1333, 1976.
144. Srinivasan and Belavady: Int. J. Vitam. Nutr. Res., *46*, 433, 1976.
145. Tao and Fox: J. Nutr. Sci. Vitaminol., *22*, 333, 1976.

I. Vitamin B₆

Howerde E. Sauberlich
and
John E. Canham

In 1934, a factor was recognized that prevented skin lesions in the rat ("rat acrodynia"); the name "vitamin B₆" was proposed by György for this factor.[1-3] The crystalline compound was isolated and reported on by three groups of investigators in 1938.[4-6] Subsequently, the vitamin was characterized[7-9] and synthesized.[10] Following the knowledge of the structure of the molecule, the term *pyridoxine* came into use for the synthesized vitamin. Bacterial studies later revealed the existence of two

Table 6I–1. Vitamin Content of Selected Foods
(per 100 gm of edible portion)

Food Item	Pantothenic Acid [1,3] (mg)	Vitamin B$_6$[1,3] (μg)	Thiamin[2,3] (μg)
Meats			
Beef (raw)			
Liver	7.700	840	250
Round	0.470	330	90
Kidney	3.850	430	360
Heart	2.500	250	530
Pork (raw)			
Ham (cured), lean	0.525	320	890
Loin	0.600	350	980
Liver	6.400	650	300
Veal (raw)			
Loin	0.900	340	140
Frankfurters (all meat)	0.430	140	160
Lamb (raw)			
Leg	0.550	275	180
Fish			
Ocean perch fillet (raw)	0.360	230	100
Halibut, fresh (raw)	0.275	430	70
Tuna, canned	0.320	425	50
Salmon, canned	0.550	300	30
Chicken (raw)			
Dark	1.000	325	80
Light	0.800	683	50
Eggs (raw)			
Whites	0.200	2	Trace
Yolk	4.400	300	220
Whole	1.600	110	110
Cheese			
Cheddar	0.500	80	30
Cottage	0.220	40	30
Milk			
Cow			
Whole	0.314	42	38
Skim	0.330	40	36
Evaporated	0.640	50	46
Condensed	0.730	50	90
Dry, whole	2.270	300	280
Dry, skim	3.570	360	415
Human	0.220	20	10
Cereals and Grain Products			
Bread, white	0.430	40	250
Bread, whole wheat	0.760	180	260
Oatmeal, dry	1.500	140	600
Corn grits, dry (enriched)	—	147	440
Cornmeal (enriched)	0.580	250	440
Corn flakes (cereal)	0.185	65	430
Rice, dry, regular (enriched)	0.550	170	440
Rice, precooked (enriched)	0.285	34	440
Shredded wheat (cereal)	0.706	244	220
Flour, all-purpose (enriched)	0.465	60	440

Table 6I–1. Vitamin Content of Selected Foods (Continued)

Food Item	Pantothenic Acid [1,3] (mg)	Vitamin B₆[1,3] (µg)	Thiamin[1,2] (µg)
Cereals and Grain Products (cont.)			
Soybean flour (defatted)	2.220	724	1090
Macaroni, dry (enriched)	– –	64	880
Noodles, egg, dry (enriched)	– –	88	880
Fruits and Vegetables			
Apples (raw)	0.100	30	30
Bananas (raw)	0.260	510	50
Apricots (canned)	0.092	54	20
Avocados (raw)	1.070	420	110
Blueberries (canned)	0.068	39	10
Cherries, sour (canned)	0.105	44	30
Grapefruit (raw)	0.283	34	40
Grapes (raw)	0.075	80	50
Oranges (raw)	0.250	60	100
Plums (canned)	0.072	27	20
Peaches (canned)	0.050	19	100
Pears (canned)	0.022	14	100
Pineapple (canned)	0.100	74	80
Strawberries (raw)	0.340	55	30
Cantaloupe (raw)	0.250	86	40
Cranberries (raw)	0.219	35	30
Cabbage (raw)	0.205	160	50
Cauliflower (raw)	1.000	210	110
Lettuce (raw)	0.200	55	60
Peas, green (raw)	0.750	160	350
Potatoes, white (raw)	0.380	250	100
Potatoes, sweet (raw)	0.820	218	100
Squash, summer (raw)	0.360	82	50
Turnip greens (frozen)	0.140	100	60
Beans, green snap (fresh)	0.190	80	80
Navy beans (dried)	0.725	560	650
Corn, yellow (canned)	0.220	200	30
Spinach, leaf (frozen)	0.150	150	100
Tomatoes, ripe (raw)	0.330	100	60
Nuts			
Almonds (dry)	0.470	100	240
Peanuts (roasted)	2.100	400	320
Pecans	1.707	183	860
Walnuts (English)	0.900	730	330
Dried Fruits			
Dates	0.780	153	90
Figs	0.435	175	100
Peaches	– –	100	100
Prunes	0.460	240	90
Raisins (seedless)	0.045	240	110
Beverages, alcoholic			
Beer	0.080	60	Trace
Wine	0.030	40	Trace

[1]From Home Economic Research Report No. 36, U.S. Dept. Agr., 1969.
[2]From Agriculture Handbook No. 8, U.S. Dept. Agr., 1963.
[3]From Agriculture Handbook No. 8–1, U.S. Dept. Agr., 1976..

other natural forms of the vitamin—pyridoxal and pyridoxamine.[11,12] Since the three forms are essentially equally effective in animal nutrition, the group of compounds is referred to collectively as vitamin B_6.

The vitamin is essential for man, rat, mouse, chick, pig, dog, turkey and other species, including many microorganisms. Once the rumen has developed, cattle and sheep and other ruminants do not require a dietary source of vitamin B_6. Horses similarly synthesize the vitamin in the cecum. Vitamin B_6 occurs widespread in foods, with meats, cereals, lentils, nuts and some fruits and vegetables rich sources (Table 6I–1). It occurs in animal products largely in its pyridoxal and pyridoxamine forms while in vegetable products pyridoxine is the more prevalent form.[11,13,14] Several comprehensive reviews on vitamin B_6 are available.[15-21,184-186,189,190]

CHEMISTRY AND BIOCHEMICAL FUNCTIONS OF VITAMIN B_6

Pyridoxine hydrochloride, the commonly available synthetic form, has a molecular weight of 205.6 and occurs as white platelets readily soluble in water.[208] Pyridoxine is quite stable in acid solutions, but rapid destruction by light occurs in neutral and alkaline solutions.[207] Pyridoxal and pyridoxamine are also available but less used. The coenzyme activities of vitamin B_6 were recognized with the discovery and identification of pyridoxal-5-phosphate.[22-25] The phosphorylated form of pyridoxamine was subsequently shown to occur naturally.[26] Additional information on the early history of vitamin B_6 may be found in reviews.[27-30]

Pyridoxal-5-phosphate represents the coenzyme form of vitamin B_6, although pyridoxamine can also activate a number of vitamin B_6-dependent enzymes.[28-34]

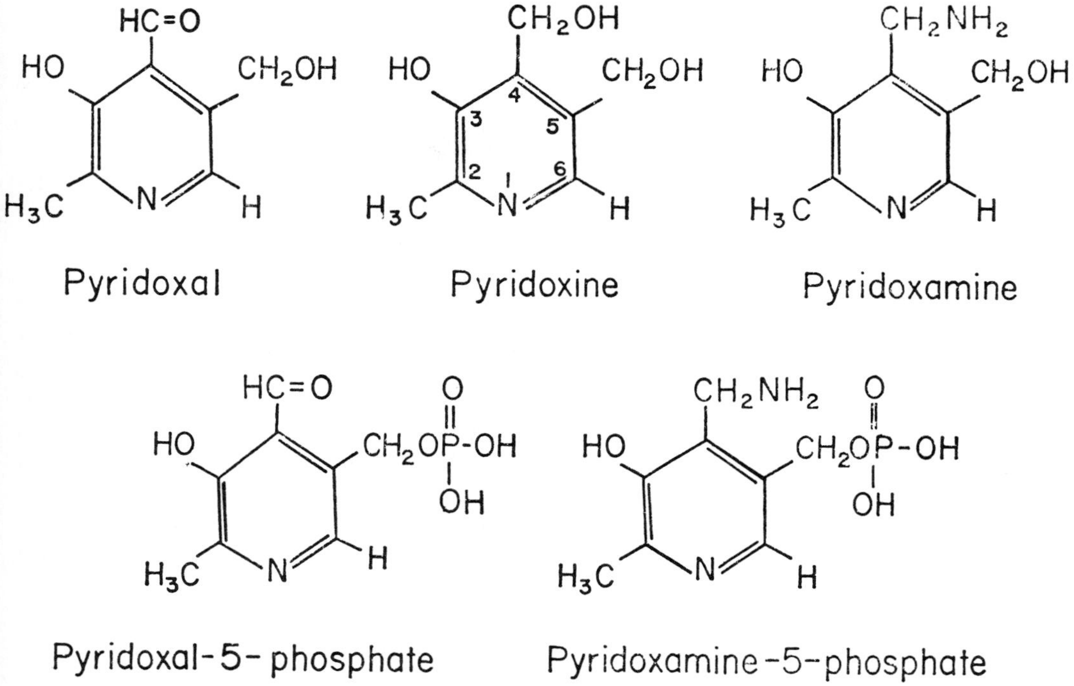

Fig. 6I–1. Structures of the various forms of vitamin B_6.

Pyridoxine, pyridoxamine and pyridoxal are converted through enzymatic pathways to the coenzyme form.[16,20,28,35,36,184,200] A number of compounds structurally related to pyridoxine have been synthesized, with some possessing vitamin B_6 activity.[16,20,28,37] Other analogs possess antivitamin B_6 action.[15,16,19,20,190,207,208] 4-Deoxypyridoxine, for example, has been used to induce vitamin B_6-deficiency symptoms in animals and man.[16,19,37-43] Other antagonists function as binding agents to inactivate the vitamin. Included in this group are isoniazid (INH), penicillamine, semicarbazide and cycloserine.[15,16,19,207,208]

Vitamin B_6, in the coenzyme form, is concerned with a vast number and variety of enzyme systems almost entirely associated with nitrogen metabolism. Well over 60 pyridoxal phosphate-dependent enzymes are known.

Some of the reactions catalyzed by these enzymes involving amino acids include transamination, racemization, decarboxylation, cleavage, synthesis, dehydration and desulfhydration. The transaminases represent a major group of the pyridoxal phosphate-catalyzed enzymes. The α-amino group of amino acids such as alanine, arginine, asparagine, aspartic acid, cysteine, isoleucine, lysine, phenylalanine, tryptophan, tyrosine and valine is removed by transamination. Usually α-ketoglutarate serves as the final acceptor of the amino groups for channeling into reactions whereby the nitrogenous end-products such as urea are formed. Following deamination, the carbon skeletons of the amino acids undergo oxidative degradation to compounds that are metabolized in the tricarboxylic acid cycle. Pyridoxal phosphate functions in transaminases in a Schiff base (ketimine) mechanism.[15-19,45,46] Glutamic oxaloacetic acid transaminase (GOT), glutamic pyruvic acid transaminase (GPT) and other transaminases are located almost entirely within the cell. Elevated levels of serum transaminase activity are commonly employed as diagnostic aids for following cellular involvement in certain disease processes.[51]

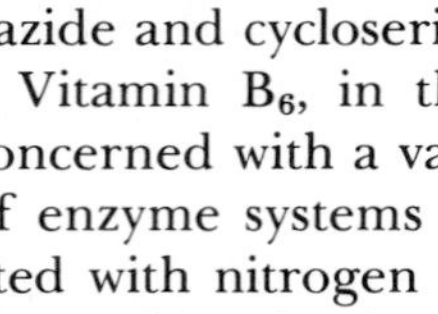

The pyridoxal phosphate-dependent decarboxylases are of considerable importance in mammalian tissues.[15-19,45,46] Thus, aromatic L-amino acid decarboxylase reacts on tyrosine, histidine, dopa and tryptophan to form their respective amines.[189] Serotonin is produced by the action of this enzyme on 5-hydroxytryptophan.[47,185] Glutamic acid decarboxylase catalyzes the formation of γ-aminobutyric acid from glutamic acid in the central nervous system.[48,185] Cysteine sulfinic acid decarboxylase converts cysteine to taurine.[188] Tryptophan metabolism, including its conversion to nicotinic acid, requires a number of pyridoxal phosphate-catalyzed reactions.[15,16,49,50,188] Consequently, when a deficiency in vitamin B_6 occurs tryptophan metabolism is altered, giving rise to excessive urinary excretion of xanthurenic acid, kynurenine, 3-hydroxykynurenine and quinolinic acid, while the excretion of nicotinic acid and N^1-methylnicotinamide may be reduced.[51-61,167,186,187]

The vitamin is also required in the conversion of cysteine to pyruvic acid[62] and oxalate to glycine,[63] and in the synthesis of

4-Deoxypyridoxine

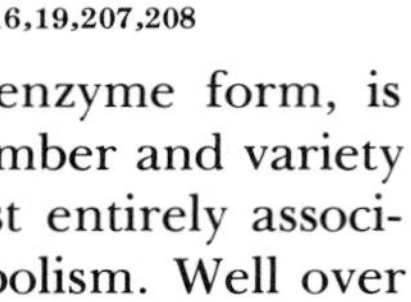

Penicillamine

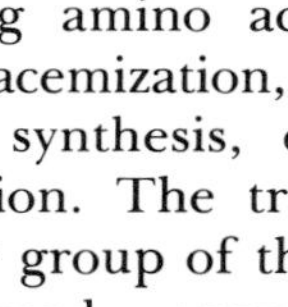

Isoniazid (INH)

Fig. 6I–2. Structures of agents which inactivate vitamin B_6.

δ-aminolevulinic acid,[16,64-66] an intermediate in the formation of porphyrin. Pyridoxal phosphate is a cofactor for a number of dehydratases, racemases, transferases, hydroxylases, synthetases and other classes of enzymes.[16-18,190] Unique of the enzymes requiring pyridoxal phosphate is phosphorylase,[18,67,68] the enzyme that catalyzes the breakdown of glycogen to form glucose-1-phosphate. The coenzyme plays an important conformational or structural role in this enzyme, but whether it also plays an essential catalytic role is unclear. Although vitamin B$_6$ has been implicated in lipid metabolism, the role appears to be mediated through secondary effects.[16,69-72] Additional information on the biochemical roles of vitamin B$_6$ is available in a number of reviews.[15-20,46,73,74]

METHODS OF ASSAY

Microbiologic assay, chemical methods and animal bioassay procedures are available to measure vitamin B$_6$.[193] The animal bioassays, using either the rat or chick,[75,76] are time consuming, expensive and variable and therefore have been generally replaced by microbiologic and chemical methods. Saccharomyces carlsbergensis is the test organism commonly used in the microbiologic method since pyridoxine, pyridoxal and pyridoxamine are equally active on a molar basis for this organism.[21,77] The individual forms may be determined by a differential assay employing Lactobacillus casei to measure pyridoxal, Streptococcus faecalis to measure combined pyridoxal and pyridoxamine, and S. carlsbergensis to measure total vitamin B$_6$ content.[20,21,78-80,191] A more recent procedure involves the chromatographic separation of the three forms of vitamin B$_6$ followed by assay of the eluates with S. carlsbergensis.[20,21,81-85] The protozoan Tetrahymena pyriformis has also been used to measure vitamin B$_6$ in biologic materials as has Kloeckera brevis.[192]

Since the majority of the forms of vitamin B$_6$ occur in natural substances in phosphorylated and bound forms, extraction and hydrolytic procedures are required prior to assay.[21,86] Fluorometric and enzymatic procedures have been described for measuring pyridoxal and pyridoxal phosphate in biologic material.[20,21,87-89,169-171,195-198] Thin-layer chromatography and gas/liquid chromatography methods appear promising for application to pharmaceutic preparations.[20,90-92] The major metabolite of vitamin B$_6$ is 4-pyridoxic acid, for which fluorometric procedures are available.[21,93,94] Measurement of this metabolite has been useful in clinical and research studies on vitamin B$_6$ nutrition and metabolism.[60] Blood or plasma pyridoxal phosphate levels can provide useful information concerning nutritional status.[186,194,201] Simple and sensitive enzymatic assays for pyridoxal phosphate have been described, based on the measurement of $^{14}CO_2$ evolved during the decarboxylation of L-tyrosine-1-^{14}C by pyridoxal phosphate-dependent tyrosine apodecarboxylase from S. faecalis.[169,196-199]

DEFICIENCIES

Experimental Animals

Dermatitis (acrodynia) is the characteristic sign of a vitamin B$_6$ deficiency in the rat. The lesions occur on the paws, ears, nose, chin, submental region and upper thorax.[16,96-97] The acrodynia resembles the dermatologic effects of an essential fatty acid deficiency, but the nature of the relationship is not clear.[69,96,99] A high-fat diet will delay the appearance of pyridoxine-deficiency dermatitis[100] and pyridoxine has a similar effect on the dermatitis of essential fatty acid deficiency.[101] A pyridoxine deficiency in the rat also induces poor growth, muscular weakness, fatty livers, convulsive seizures,[102] anemia,[103] reproductive impairment,[104] edema, nerve degeneration, enlarged adrenal glands, increased excretion of xanthurenic acid, urea and oxalate, decreased transaminase activities, reduced synthesis of ribosomal and messenger ribonucleic acid and deoxyribonucleic acid,[105,106] impaired immune responses[206] and numerous other alterations in biochemical processes.[16] Lesions noted in the pyridoxine-deficient mouse resemble those in the rat.[107] As with the rat, high protein intakes induce more readily the characteristic skin lesions and death in animals fed a vitamin B_6-deficient diet.

Similar alterations have been noted in vitamin B_6-deficient chicks, hamsters, dogs, monkeys, swine, calves, turkeys and rabbits. The most commonly observed effects of a deficiency in these species have been microcytic hypochromic anemia, degeneration of nervous tissues and convulsions.[16,98]

Man

The first evidence of the essentiality of vitamin B_6 for the human was reported in 1939.[110] Patients on poor diets were observed to have an ill-defined syndrome characterized by weakness, irritability and nervousness, insomnia and difficulty in walking. Although the symptoms did not respond to treatment with other members of the B complex, relief was obtained within 24 hours when pyridoxine was administered. Shortly thereafter pyridoxine was reported to be effective in healing cheilosis which did not respond to riboflavin.[111] The reports on the widespread occurrence of convulsive seizures and nervous irritability in infants fed an autoclaved commercial liquid milk formula low in vitamin B_6[112-116] were convincing evidence of its essentiality in human nutrition. Approximately 300 cases with overt symptoms responsive to pyridoxine therapy were noted.[116] The clinical improvement was corroborated by return of the abnormal electroencephalographic patterns to normal.[15,115]

More clearly defined symptoms of a vitamin B_6 deficiency in man have been obtained by placing experimental subjects on diets low in the vitamin and administering certain antivitamin B_6 compounds.[15,16,19,60,61] The earliest such study was conducted in 1948 by administering a purified diet deficient in vitamin B_6 to an adult for 55 days.[117] No clear-cut symptoms of a pyridoxine deficiency appeared although mental depression was noted. Derangement of tryptophan metabolism, manifested by the excretion of xanthurenic acid, was observed within 3 weeks in adult human subjects maintained on a vitamin B_6-deficient diet.[118] In subsequent years, the tryptophan load test has commonly been used in vitamin B_6-deficiency and -requirement studies.[15,16,19,60,61,186,194,202-205,209]

Convincing deficiency symptoms were produced in 2 infants placed on a vitamin B_6-deficient diet.[55] The infants ceased to gain weight after several months. Pyridoxic acid disappeared from the urine and urinary pyridoxine was reduced to very low values. The ability to convert tryptophan to nicotinic acid was lost. Convulsions occurred in one and hypochromic anemia in the other. The administration of pyridoxine readily corrected these abnormalities, except for the ability to convert tryptophan to nicotinic acid, which was slower to respond.

Vitamin B_6 deficiency has been induced in 50 human adults with the associated use of a pyridoxine antagonist, 4-deoxypyridoxine.[38,39] Lesions resembling seborrhea appeared about the eyes, in the nasolabial folds and around the mouth and spread to involve the face, forehead, eyebrows and skin behind the ears. The scrotal and perineal regions were involved occasionally. Intertrigo developed under the breasts and in other moist areas. Hyperpigmented scaly pellagra-like dermatitis also developed occasionally in the collar region and on the forearms, elbows and thighs. Cheilosis, glossitis and stomatitis occurred and were morphologically indistinguishable from the oral lesions of nicotinic acid and riboflavin deficiency. Three patients developed peripheral neuropathy of a sensory type; motor function was impaired later. Weight loss was noted in all subjects, with apathy, somnolence and increased irritability occurring in some. Although there was a strong tendency to develop infections, particularly of the genitourinary tract, production of antibodies to typhoid and erythrocyte antigens was not measurably impaired.[119]

Another group of investigators similarly induced a B_6 deficiency in human subjects with the use of a deficient diet and deoxypyridoxine.[43] In this study there was a slight impairment of the formation of antibodies against tetanus and typhoid. Most of the subjects, including all those who developed clinical signs of deficiency, excreted large amounts of xanthurenic acid in the urine after a test dose of tryptophan, but their ability to convert tryptophan to N^1-methylnicotinamide was not impaired. In a companion study, subjects were given a diet deficient in pantothenic acid and pyridoxine and supplemented with deoxypyridoxine and omega methylpantothenic acid.[120] These subjects became ill and were completely unable to respond to tetanus and to typhoid O antigen.

In more recent years, vitamin B_6 deficiency has been induced in human volunteer subjects without the use of pyridoxine antagonists.[15,16,19,53,54,56,60,61,121-127,201,202,230] Subjects on a vitamin B_6-deficient diet have been observed to develop personality changes manifested by irritability, depression and loss of the sense of responsibility.[61] The subjects also developed filiform hypertrophy of the lingual papilla, aphthous stomatitis, nasolabial seborrhea and an acneiform papular rash of the forehead. Abnormal electroencephalograms were observed.

Tryptophan metabolism was altered, with high urinary excretions of xanthurenic acid after tryptophan loading. Pyridoxine repletion corrected all of the abnormalities noted. Vitamin B_6 in natural foods was as available as crystalline pyridoxine.[15,16] Although there appears to be no apparent effect of increased caloric utilization on vitamin B_6 requirements,[61] high intakes of protein hastened the onset of a deficiency.[15,19,61,121,123,124,209] A tryptophan load induces in the vitamin B_6-deficient subject marked urinary excretions not only of xanthurenic acid but also of kynurenine, hydroxykynurenine, kynurenic acid, acetylkynurenine, and quinolinic acid.[53,56,121,123,194,201,202,230,234] Plasma and blood levels of vitamin B_6 and urinary excretion of vitamin B_6 and 4-pyridoxic acid fall with decreased intakes of the vitamin.[19,121,124,126,133,147,148,230] In pyridoxine deficiency, methionine metabolism is altered;[223,227,228,234] in contrast, cysteine metabolism is only slightly changed.[60,125] Glutamic oxaloacetate transaminase (GOT) and glutamic pyruvate transaminase (GPT) activities in blood and its components are lowered in deficiency.[15,19,60,61,122,126–132,147,230] Changes in plasma and urinary levels of free amino acids may occur in pyridoxine deficiency.[19,127,134,209,230] Certain metabolic defects appear to respond to increased intakes of pyridoxine.[146] Several infants with convulsive seizures dating from shortly after birth have been found to respond to 2 mg of pyridoxine daily.[135-137] A number of patients with pyridoxine-responsive anemia, classified as sideroblastic anemia, have been reported.[15,16,19,138-144,210,211] In these individuals the production of hemoglobin and erythrocytes is dependent upon the administration of 2.5 gm or more of vitamin B_6 daily. Iron, folic acid and vitamin B_{12} are without effect. Other types of vitamin B_6-dependency syndromes have been reported.[146] Oxaluria may occur in persons receiving deoxypyridoxine or isoniazid.[45,145,160] A vitamin B_6 deficiency may occur in uremic patients and in patients with various forms of liver disease.[233] Evidence of vitamin B_6 deficiency in chronic alcoholic patients has been reported.[149,172,212–214] Ingestion of diets high in leucine has been indicated to increase the requirement for vitamin B_6.[225,226]

A metabolic interrelationship between steroid hormones and vitamin B_6 has been observed.[16] Women taking steroid hormones for contraceptive purposes have been observed to excrete grossly increased amounts of tryptophan metabolites following a tryptophan load.[19,61,150-155,167,173,174, 204,231] Vitamin B_6 supplementation corrects this abnormality.[203] Impaired glucose tolerance occurs in some women ingesting oral contraceptive agents.[203,216,217] In addition, the use of oral steroid contraceptives may be accompanied by increases in the stimulation in vitro of erythrocyte glutamic oxalacetic transaminases,[203,218,219] decreased plasma concentration of pyridoxal-phosphate,[229] depression,[203,220] hypertriglyceridemia[221] and malaise.[222] At present, the effects of estrogens on tryptophan and vitamin B_6 metabolism have no satisfactory molecular explanation.[19] Whether the use of oral contraceptive agents produces a true vitamin B_6 deficiency is equivocal.[205] However, 15 to 20 per cent of the users of these agents have direct biochemical evidence of deficiency.[203] Nevertheless, present knowledge does not appear to justify routine supplementation with pyridoxine.[203,205,223] Pregnant women may excrete abnormal amounts of kynurenine, xanthurenic acid and 3-hydroxykynurenine, which may be decreased with pyridoxine supplements.[15,16,156,157,167,224] Supplements of vitamin B_6 failed to change complications of pregnancy.[158] Evidence has been reported indicating the vitamin requirement is increased in patients with hyperthyroidism.[159]

NUTRITIONAL REQUIREMENT

The Food and Nutrition Board[161] has established a recommended daily dietary allowance of 2.0 mg of vitamin B_6 for adult men and women. During pregnancy and lactation, an allowance of 2.5 mg per day is recommended. For younger age groups, lesser amounts have been suggested as being adequate. Requirements for the adult have been reasonably well established from controlled depletion and repletion experimental human investigations.[15,16,19,60,61,121-126,201,202,243] These studies have demonstrated an influence of protein intake on the requirement for vitamin B_6.[16,209] Adult males ingesting 100 gm of protein daily appeared to have a daily B_6 requirement of 1.75 to 2.0 mg, while persons on a low protein intake had a requirement of 1.25 to 1.5 mg per day.[202] An intake of 1.5 mg has been suggested as adequate for young women.[201] Information as to the actual pyridoxine requirement of infants, children and adolescents is exceedingly limited.[15,16,161,235-237] A daily allowance of 0.3 to 0.4 mg appears adequate for infants.[235] For artificially fed infants, an allowance of 0.4 mg per day (0.04 mg per 100 kcal) has been considered ample. A vitamin B_6 intake of approximately 1.25 mg per day appears adequate for boys and girls 7 to 9 years of age.[236]

Abnormalities associated with vitamin B_6 inadequacies in pregnant women have been largely corrected by vitamin B_6 supplements of 2 to 5 mg per day.[198,224,239-242] Human milk provides approximately 0.10 to 0.25 mg per liter.[235,237,238] The vitamin B_6 content of milk appears to reflect the nutritional state of the mother with respect to the vitamin.[237,238] Intakes of 2.5 mg or more per day will provide milk with a B_6 content in excess of 0.20 mg per liter.[237,238]

The average diet in the United States provides the amounts of vitamin B_6 recommended, though certain poor or restricted diets do not.[95] Although meats serve as a good source of vitamin B_6, a considerable loss occurs during cooking.[14,168,232]

THERAPEUTIC USE, TOXICITY AND METABOLISM

Pyridoxine hydrochloride is frequently present in multivitamin preparations.[207]

The compound is used as an adjunct in prophylaxis and treatment of multiple vitamin B-complex deficiencies and is included in preparations designed for intravenous and oral alimentation. It has also been used in the treatment of dermatoses, neuromuscular and neurologic diseases. Such administration has been largely ineffective except in cases with inborn errors of vitamin B_6 metabolism, or in association with the use of a vitamin B_6 antagonist or in a dietary deficiency of the vitamin. Oral doses of 1 to 150 mg per day have been used. Similar levels have been used in treating pyridoxine-responsive anemias. Pyridoxine supplements are commonly employed as a precautionary measure when isoniazid is used in the treatment of tuberculosis.[162,185,207] Where other drugs possessing antivitamin B_6 properties are used for extended periods, such as penicillamine in the treatment of Wilson's disease and other conditions, pyridoxine supplements are recommended.[19,163,185,207] Pyridoxine has been used for a number of years by obstetricians for the control of nausea and vomiting of pregnancy. The effectiveness of this treatment has not been proven by carefully controlled studies. Pyridoxine has been employed in the treatment of hyperoxaluria and recurring oxalate kidney stones,[175,176] chorea,[177] isoniazid toxicity,[178,185] and levodopa-induced dystonia.[179-181,185] Excess pyridoxine, however, can reduce the clinical benefits of levodopa therapy in Parkinson's disease.[182,183,185] Pyridoxal-5-phosphate (as the calcium salt) has also been used for prophylaxis and treatment of deficiency. Pyridoxamine dihydrochloride possesses hypnotic properties.[185]

The toxicity of pyridoxine is extremely low.[207,208] Doses up to 1 gm per kg of body weight were tolerated without ill effects by dogs, rats and rabbits. The pharmacodynamic effects are few and none has been observed in man. The toxicity of pyridoxamine and pyridoxal is also very low, although pyridoxal was about twice as toxic as pyridoxine or pyridoxamine for animals.[16,164]

Vitamin B_6 is extensively metabolized by man. The major metabolite is 4-pyridoxic acid, which accounts for 20 to 40 per cent of the vitamin metabolized daily.[124,165,166,186,194] Isotopic studies indicate the presence in the urine of a number of unknown metabolites derived from pyridoxine. Small amounts of pyridoxal, pyridoxamine and pyridoxine and their phosphorylated analogs are present in the urine.[124,165]

BIBLIOGRAPHY

1. György: Nature, *133*, 498, 1934.
2. Birch, György and Harris: Biochem. J., *29*, 2830, 1935.
3. Birch and György: Biochem. J., *30*, 304, 1936.
4. Lepkovsky: Science, *87*, 169, 1938.
5. Keresztesy and Stevens: Proc. Soc. Exp. Biol. Med., *38*, 64, 1938.
6. György: J. Am. Chem. Soc., *60*, 983, 1938.
7. Stiller, Keresztesy and Stevens: J. Am. Chem. Soc., *61*, 1237, 1939.
8. Kuhn, Wendt and Westphal: Chem. Ber., *72B*, 310, 1939.
9. Harris, Stiller and Folkers: J. Am. Chem. Soc., *61*, 1242, 1939.
10. Harris and Folkers: Science, *89*, 347, 1939.
11. Snell: J. Biol. Chem., *157*, 491, 1945.
12. Snell, Guirard and Williams: J. Biol. Chem., *143*, 519, 1942.
13. Rabinowitz and Snell: J. Biol. Chem., *176*, 1157, 1948.
14. Orr: Pantothenic Acid, Vitamin B-6 and Vitamin B-12 in Foods. Home Economics Research Report No. 36. Washington, U.S. Dept. Agr., 1969.
15. Harris, Wool and Loraine (Eds.): Vitam. Horm., *22*, 361, 1964.
16. Sebrell and Harris (Eds.): *The Vitamins,* Vol. II. New York, Academic Press, 1968.
17. Snell and DiMari: In *The Enzymes,* Vol. III, 3rd ed. (Boyer, Ed.). New York, Academic Press, 1970.
18. Harris, Muson and Diczfalusy. (Eds.): Vitam. Horm., *28*, 265, 1970.
19. Kelsall (Ed.): Ann. N.Y. Acad. Sci., *166*, 1, 1969.
20. McCormick and Wright (Eds.): Methods Enzymol., *18*, 431, 1970.
21. Sauberlich: In *The Vitamins,* Vol. VII, (György and Pearson, Eds.). New York, Academic Press, 1967.
22. Gunsalus, Bellamy and Umbreit: J. Biol. Chem., *155*, 685, 1944.
23. Heyl, Luz, Harris and Folkers: J. Am. Chem. Soc., *73*, 3430, 1951.
24. Baddiley and Mathias: J. Chem. Soc., 2583, 1952.

25. Schlenk and Snell: J. Biol. Chem., *157*, 425, 1945.
26. Rabinowitz and Snell: J. Biol. Chem., *169*, 643, 1947.
27. Robinson: *The Vitamin B Complex.* New York, John Wiley and Sons, 1951.
28. Snell: Vitam. Horm., *16*, 77, 1958.
29. Meister: In *The Enzymes,* Vol. 6 (Boyer, Lardy and Myrbäck, Eds.). New York, Academic Press, 1962.
30. Braunstein: In *The Enzymes,* Vol. 2 (Boyer, Lardy and Myrbäck, Eds.). New York, Academic Press, 1960.
31. Meister: Adv. Enzymol., *16*, 185, 1955.
32. Velick and Vavra: In *The Enzymes,* Vol. 6 (Boyer, Lardy and Myrbäck, Eds.). New York, Academic Press, 1962.
33. Ellis and Davies: Biochem. J., *78*, 615, 1961.
34. Davies and Ellis: Biochem. J., *78*, 623, 1961.
35. Brown and Reynolds: Annu. Rev. Biochem., *32*, 447, 1963.
36. Wada and Snell: J. Biol. Chem., *236*, 2089, 1961.
37. Snell: In *Comprehensive Biochemistry,* Vol. II (Florkin and Stotz, Eds.). Amsterdam, Elsevier, 1963.
38. Mueller and Vilter: J. Clin. Invest., *29*, 193, 1950.
39. Vilter, Mueller, Glazer, Jarrold, Abraham, Thompson and Hawkins: J. Lab. Clin. Med., *42*, 335, 1953.
40. Glazer, Mueller, Thompson, Hawkins and Vilter: Arch. Biochem. Biophys., *33*, 243, 1951.
41. Will, Repasky, Mueller and Glazer: Am. J. Clin. Nutr., *9*, 245, 1961.
42. Muller and Iacono: Am. J. Clin. Nutr., *12*, 358, 1963.
43. Hodges, Bean, Ohlson and Bleiler: Am. J. Clin. Nutr., *11*, 180, 1962.
44. Faber, Feitler, Bleiler, Ohlson and Hodges: Am. J. Clin. Nutr., *12*, 406, 1963.
45. Guirard and Snell: In *Comprehensive Biochemistry,* Vol. 15 (Florkin and Stotz, Eds.). Amsterdam, Elsevier, 1964.
46. Yamada, Katunuma and Wada (Eds.): *Symposium on Pyridoxal Enzymes.* Tokyo, Maruzen, 1968.
47. Weissbach, Bogdanski, Redfield and Udenfriend: J. Biol. Chem., *277*, 617, 1957.
48. Kellam and Bain: J. Pharmacol. Exp. Ther., *119*, 225, 1956.
49. Henderson, Gholson and Dalgliesh: In *Comprehensive Biochemistry,* Vol. 4 (Florkin and Stotz, Eds.). Amsterdam, Elsevier, 1962.
50. Coursin: Am. J. Clin. Nutr., *14*, 56, 1964.
51. Searcy: *Diagnostic Biochemistry.* New York, McGraw-Hill, 1969.
52. Price, Brown and Larson: J. Clin. Invest., *36*, 1600, 1957.
53. Yess, Price, Brown, Swan and Linkswiler: J. Nutr., *84*, 229, 1964.
54. Brown, Yess, Price, Linkswiler, Swan and Hankes: J. Nutr., *87*, 419, 1965.
55. Snyderman, Holt, Carretero and Jacobs: Am. J. Clin. Nutr., *1*, 200, 1953.
56. Kelsay, Miller and Linkswiler: J. Nutr., *94*, 27, 1968.
57. Fouts and Lepkovsky: Proc. Soc. Exp. Biol. Med., *50*, 221, 1942.
58. Greenberg, Bohr, McGrath and Rinehart: Arch. Biochem., *21*, 237, 1945.
59. Lepkovsky and Nielson: J. Biol. Chem., *144*, 135, 1942.
60. Linkswiler: Am. J. Clin. Nutr., *20*, 547, 1967.
61. Sauberlich, Canham, Baker, Raica and Herman: J. Scientif. Ind. Res., *29*, S28, 1970.
62. Binkley, Christensen and Jensen: J. Biol. Chem., *194*, 109, 1952.
63. Pasquarillo and Tenconi: Acta Vitaminol., *15*, 163, 1961.
64. Schulman and Richert: J. Biol. Chem., *226*, 181, 1957.
65. Richert and Schulman: Am. J. Clin. Nutr., *7*, 416, 1959.
66. Burnham and Lascilles: Biochem. J., *87*, 462, 1963.
67. Illingworth, Jansz, Brown and Cori: Proc. Natl. Acad. Sci., *44*, 1180, 1958.
68. Brown and Cori: In *The Enzymes,* Vol. 5 (Boyer, Lardy and Myrbäck, Eds.). New York, Academic Press, 1961.
69. Witten and Holman: Arch. Biochem. Biophys., *41*, 266, 1952.
70. Swell, Law, Schools and Treadwell: J. Nutr., *74*, 148, 1961.
71. Rosen and Nichol: Vitam. Horm., *21*, 135, 1963.
72. Goswami and Coniglio: J. Nutr., *89*, 210, 1966.
73. Dagley and Nicholson: *An Introduction to Metabolic Pathways.* New York, John Wiley and Sons, 1970.
74. Fasella: Annu. Rev. Biochem., *36*, 185, 1967.
75. Bliss and György: In *The Vitamins,* Vol. VII (György and Pearson, Eds.). New York, Academic Press, 1967.
76. Sarma, Snell and Elvehjem: J. Biol. Chem., *165*, 55, 1946.
77. Atkin, Schultz, Williams and Frey: Ind. Eng. Chem., Anal. Ed., *15*, 141, 1943.
78. Rabinowitz and Snell: J. Biol. Chem., *176*, 1157, 1948.
79. Gregory: J. Dairy Res., *26*, 203, 1959.
80. Gregory and Mabbitt: J. Dairy Res., *28*, 293, 1961.
81. MacArthur and Lehmann: Assoc. Off. Agr. Chem. J., *42*, 619, 1959.
82. Polansky and Murphy: Am. Diet. Assoc. J., *48*, 109, 1966.
83. Toepfer and Lehmann: Assoc. Off. Agr. Chem. J., *44*, 426, 1961.
83a. Thiele and Brin: J. Nutr., *90*, 347, 1966.
84. Toepfer, MacArthur and Lehmann: Assoc. Off. Agr. Chem. J., *43*, 57, 1960.
85. Toepfer, Polansky, Richardson and Wilkes: J. Agr. Food Chem., *11*, 523, 1963.
86. Woodring and Storvick: Assoc. Off. Agr. Chem. J., *43*, 63, 1960.
87. Storvick, Benson, Edwards and Woodring: Methods Biochem. Anal., *12*, 183, 1964.
88. Donald and Ferguson: Anal. Biochem., *7*, 335, 1964.

89. Boxer, Pruss and Goodhart: J. Nutr., *63*, 623, 1957.
90. Ahrens and Karytnyk: Anal. Biochem., *30*, 413, 1969.
91. Prosser, Sheppard and Libby: Assoc. Off. Anal. Chem. J., *50*, 1348, 1967.
92. Korytnyk, Fricke and Paul: Anal. Biochem., *17*, 66, 1966.
93. Reddy, Reynolds and Price: J. Biol. Chem., *233*, 691, 1958.
94. Woodring, Fisher and Storvick: Clin. Chem., *10*, 479, 1964.
95. Mangay Chung, Pearson, Darby, Miller and Goldsmith: Am. J. Clin. Nutr., *9*, 573, 1961.
96. Sullivan and Nicholls: J. Invest. Dermatol., *3*, 317, 1940.
97. Antopol and Unna: Arch. Pathol., *33*, 241, 1942.
98. Follis: *Deficiency Disease*. Springfield, Charles C Thomas, 1958.
99. Carter and Phizackerley: Biochem. J., *49*, 227, 1951.
100. Birch: J. Biol. Chem., *124*, 775, 1938.
101. Schneider, Steenback and Platz: J. Biol. Chem., *132*, 539, 1940.
102. Chick, Sadr and Worden: Biochem. J., *34*, 595, 1940.
103. Batchen, Cheesman, Copping and Trusler: Br. J. Nutr., *9*, 49, 1955.
104. Nelson and Evans: J. Nutr., *43*, 281, 1951.
105. Montjar, Axelrod and Trakatellis: J. Nutr., *85*, 45, 1965.
106. Trakatellis and Axelrod: Biochem. J., *95*, 344, 1965.
107. Boutwell, Rusch and Chiang: Proc. Soc. Exp. Biol. Med., *77*, 860, 1951.
108. Baker, Frank, Ning, Gellene, Hutner and Leevy: Am. J. Clin. Nutr., *18*, 123, 1966.
109. Baker and Frank: *Clinical Vitaminology*. New York, Interscience Publishers, 1968.
110. Spies, Bean and Ashe: J.A.M.A., *112*, 2414, 1939.
111. Smith and Martin: Proc. Soc. Exp. Biol. Med., *43*, 660, 1940.
112. Vitamin B-6 in Human Nutrition. M. and R. Conference, Chicago, November 19, 1953.
113. Coursin: Vitam. Horm., *22*, 756, 1964.
114. Malony and Parmelee: J.A.M.A., *154*, 405, 1954.
115. Coursin: J.A.M.A., *154*, 406, 1954.
116. Hawkins: Science, *121*, 880, 1955.
117. Hawkins and Barsky: Science, *108*, 284, 1948.
118. Greenberg, Bohr, McGrath and Rinehart: Arch. Biochem., *21*, 237, 1949.
119. Wayne, Will, Friedman, Becker and Vilter: Arch. Intern. Med., *101*, 143, 1958.
120. Hodges, Bean, Ohlson and Bleiler: Am. J. Clin. Nutr., *11*, 187, 1962.
121. Baker, Canham, Nunes, Sauberlich and McDowell: Am. J. Clin. Nutr., *15*, 59, 1964.
122. Canham, Baker, Raica and Sauberlich: Proc. Seventh Int. Cong. Nutr., *5*, 558, 1966.
123. Miller and Linkswiler: J. Nutr., *93*, 53, 1967.
124. Kelsay, Bysal and Linkswiler: J. Nutr., *94*, 490, 1968.
125. Swan, Wentworth and Linkswiler: J. Nutr., *84*, 220, 1964.
126. Baysal, Johnson and Linkswiler: J. Nutr., *89*, 19, 1966.
127. Aly, Donald and Simpson: Am. J. Clin. Nutr., *24*, 297, 1971.
128. Raica and Sauberlich: Am. J. Clin. Nutr., *15*, 67, 1964.
129. Jacobs, Cavill and Hughes: Am. J. Clin. Nutr., *21*, 502, 1968.
130. Woodring and Storvick: Am. J. Clin. Nutr., *23*, 1385, 1970.
131. Cinnamon and Beaton: Am. J. Clin. Nutr., *23*, 696, 1970.
132. Cheney, Sabry and Beaton: Am. J. Clin. Nutr., *16*, 337, 1965.
133. Baker and Frank: World Rev. Nutr. Diet., *9*, 124, 1968.
134. Harding, Sauberlich and Canham: In *Automation in Analytical Chemistry*—Technicon Symposia (Skeggs, Ed.). New York, Mediad Inc., 1965.
135. Hunt, Stokes, McCrory and Stroud: Pediatrics, *13*, 140, 1954.
136. Bessey, Adam and Hansen: Pediatrics, *20*, 33, 1957.
137. Waldinger and Berg: Pediatrics, *32*, 161, 1963.
138. Harris, Whittington, Wesiman and Horrigan: Proc. Soc. Exp. Biol. Med., *91*, 427, 1956.
139. Bickers, Brown and Sprague: Blood, *19*, 304, 1962.
140. Hines and Harris: Am. J. Clin. Nutr., *14*, 137, 1964.
141. Horrigan and Harris: Vitam. Horm., 22, 722, 1964.
142. Nordio and Massino: Ann. Paediat., *207*, 160, 1966.
143. Weintraub, Conrad and Crosby: N. Engl. J. Med., *275*, 169, 1966.
144. Wohllebe and Paul: Folia Haematol., *86*, 445, 1966.
145. Johnston and Donald: Am. J. Clin. Nutr., *12*, 413, 1963.
146. Frimpter, Andelman and George: Am. J. Clin. Nutr., *22*, 794, 1969.
147. Gailani, Holland, Nussbaum and Olson: Cancer, *21*, 975, 1968.
148. Ziegler, Reinken and Berger: Int. Z. Vitaminforsch., *39*, 192, 1969.
149. Walsh, Howorth and Marks: Am. J. Clin. Nutr., *19*, 379, 1966.
150. Rose: Clin. Sci., *31*, 265, 1966.
151. Rose: Nature, *210*, 196, 1966.
152. Price, Brown and Thornton: Am. J. Clin. Nutr., *18*, 312, 1966.
153. Price, Brown and Yess: Adv. Metab. Disord., *2*, 159, 1965.
154. Wolf, Price, Brown and Kawamura: Eighth Int. Cong. Nutr., Prague, 1969.
155. Brown, Thornton and Price: J. Clin. Invest., *40*, 617, 1961.
156. Wachstein, Moore and Graffeo: Proc. Soc. Exp. Biol. Med., *96*, 326, 1957.
157. Friedman, Becker, Thompson and Vilter: J. Lab. Clin. Med., *46*, 817, 1955.
158. Hillman, Cabaud, Nilsoon, Arpin and Tufano: Am. J. Clin. Nutr., *12*, 427, 1963.

159. Wohl, Levy, Szutka and Maldia: Proc. Soc. Exp. Biol. Med., *105*, 523, 1960.
160. McCoy, Anast and Naylor: J. Pediatr., *65*, 208, 1965.
161. Recommended Dietary Allowances, 8th ed. Washington, National Academy of Sciences— National Research Council, 1974.
162. McKusick and Hsu: Arthritis Rheum., *4*, 426, 1961.
163. Jaffe, Altman and Merryman: Clin. Invest., *43*, 1869, 1964.
164. Kraft, Fiebig and Hotovy: Arzneim. Forsch., *11*, 922, 1961.
165. Tillotson, Sauberlich, Baker and Canham: Proc. Seventh Int. Cong. Nutr., *5*, 554, 1966.
166. Johansson, Lindstedt, Register and Wadström: Am. J. Clin. Nutr., *18*, 185, 1966.
167. Brown: Am. J. Clin. Nutr., *24*, 653, 1971.
168. Schroeder: Am. J. Clin. Nutr., *24*, 562, 1971.
169. Chabner and Livingston: Anal. Biochem., *34*, 413, 1970.
170. Takanashi, Matsunaga and Tamura: J. Vitam., *16*, 132, 1970.
171. Evangelopoulos, Karni-Katsadimas and Kalogerakos: Enzymologia, *40*, 37, 1971.
172. French: N. Engl. J. Med., *283*, 1173, 1970.
173. Baumblatt and Winston: Lancet, *1*, 832, 1970.
174. Luhby, Davis and Murphy: Lancet, *2*, 1083, 1970.
175. Gibbs and Watts: Clin. Sci., *38*, 277, 1970.
176. Gershoff and Prien: Am. J. Clin. Nutr., *20*, 393, 1967.
177. Paulson: Am. J. Psychiatry, *127*, 1091, 1971.
178. Katz and Jobin: Am. Rev. Respir. Dis., *101*, 991, 1970.
179. Jameson: J.A.M.A., *211*, 1700, 1970.
180. Friedman: J.A.M.A., *214*, 1563, 1970.
181. Golden, Mortati and Schroeter: J.A.M.A., *213*, 628, 1970.
182. Du Voison, Yahr and Cote: Trans. Am. Neurol. Assoc., *94*, 81, 1969.
183. Cogzias: J.A.M.A., *210*, 1255, 1969.
184. Snell and Haskell: In *Comprehensive Biochemistry*, Vol. 21 (Florkin and Stotz, Eds.). New York, Academic Press, 1971.
185. Ebadi: In *Proceedings of a Workshop on Vitamin B₆*. Washington, National Academy of Sciences, 1977.
186. Sauberlich, Canham, Baker, Raica and Herman: Am. J. Clin. Nutr., *25*, 629, 1972.
187. Henderson and Hulse: In *Proceedings of Workshop on Vitamin B₆*. Washington, National Academy of Sciences, 1977.
188. Sturman: In *Proceedings of a Workshop on Vitamin B₆*. Washington, National Academy of Sciences, 1977.
189. Ebadi and Costa: Adv. Biochem. Psychopharmacol., *4*, 1, 1972.
190. Sauberlich: Proc. Ninth Int. Cong. Nutr., *1*, 88, 1975.
191. Anderson, Peart and Fulford-Jones: J. Clin. Pathol., *23*, 233, 1970.
192. Barton-Wright: Analyst, *96*, 314, 1971.
193. Haskell: In *Proceedings of a Workshop on Vitamin B₆*. Washington, National Academy of Sciences, 1977.
194. Sauberlich, Skala and Dowdy: Laboratory Tests for the Assessment of Nutritional Status. Cleveland, CRC Press, 1974.
195. Haskell and Snell: Anal. Biochem., *45*, 567, 1972.
196. Shane: In *Proceedings of a Workshop on Vitamin B₆*. Washington, National Academy of Sciences, 1977.
197. Bhagavan, Coleman and Coursin: Biochem. Med., *14*, 201, 1975.
198. Hamfelt and Tuvemo: Clin. Chim. Acta, *41*, 287, 1972.
199. Bhagavan, Koogler and Coursin: Int. J. Vitam. Nutr. Res., *46*, 160, 1976.
200. Johansson, Lindstedt and Tiselius: J. Biol. Chem., *249*, 6040, 1974.
201. Donald: In *Proceedings of a Workshop on Vitamin B₆*. Washington, National Academy of Sciences, 1977.
202. Linkswiler: In *Proceedings of a Workshop on Vitamin B₆*. Washington, National Academy of Sciences, 1977.
203. Rose: In *Proceedings of a Workshop on Vitamin B₆*. Washington, National Academy of Sciences, 1977.
204. Leklem, Rose and Brown: Metabolism, *22*, 1499, 1973.
205. Leklem, Brown, Rose and Linkswiler: Am. J. Clin. Nutr., *28*, 535, 1975.
206. Robson, Schwarz and Perkins: In *Proceedings of a Workshop on Vitamin B₆*. Washington, National Academy of Sciences, 1977.
207. Bauernfeind and Miller: In *Proceedings of a Workshop on Vitamin B₆*. Washington, National Academy of Sciences, 1977.
208. Brin: In *Proceedings of a Workshop on Vitamin B₆*. Washington, National Academy of Sciences, 1977.
209. Canham, Baker, Harding, Sauberlich and Plough: Ann. N.Y. Acad. Sci., *166*, 16, 1969.
210. Horrigan: Blood, *42*, 187, 1973.
211. Mudd: Fed. Proc., *30*, 970, 1971.
212. Li: In *Proceedings of a Workshop on Vitamin B₆*. Washington, National Academy of Sciences, 1977.
213. Pierce, McGuffin and Hillman: Arch. Intern. Med., *136*, 283, 1976.
214. Davis and Smith: Med. J. Aust., *2*, 357, 1974.
215. Driskell, Geders and Urban: J. Lab. Clin. Med., *87*, 813, 1976.
216. Spellancy, Buhi and Birk: Contraceptives, *6*, 265, 1972.
217. Adams, Wynn, Folkard and Seed: Lancet, *1*, 759, 1976.
218. Salkeld, Knorr and Korner: Clin. Chim. Acta, *49*, 195, 1973.
219. Rose, Adams and Strong: Br. J. Obstet. Gynecol., *80*, 82, 1973.
220. Adams, Wynn, Seed and Folkard: Lancet, *2*, 516, 1974.
221. Rose, Leklem, Fardal, Baron and Shargo: Am. J. Clin. Nutr., *30*, 691, 1977.
222. Winston: Am. J. Psychiatry, *130*, 1217, 1973.
223. Leklem, Linkswiler, Brown, Rose and Anand: Am. J. Clin. Nutr., *30*, 1122, 1977.
224. Dempsey: In *Proceedings of a Workshop on Vitamin*

B_6. Washington, National Academy of Sciences, 1977.
225. Rao, Raghuram and Krishnaswamy: Nutr. Metab., *18*, 318, 1975.
226. Krishnaswamy, Rao, Raghuram and Srikantia: Am. J. Clin. Nutr., *29*, 177, 1976.
227. Park and Linkswiler: J. Nutr., *100*, 110, 1970.
228. Krishnaswamy: Int. J. Vitam. Nutr. Res., *42*, 468, 1972.
229. Lumeng, Cleary and Li: Am. J. Clin. Nutr., *27*, 326, 1974.
230. Donald, McBean, Simpson, Sun and Aly: Am. J. Clin. Nutr., *24*, 1028, 1971.
231. Leklem, Brown, Rose, Linkswiler and Arend: Am. J. Clin. Nutr., *28*, 146, 1975.
232. Gregory and Kirk: In *Proceedings of a Workshop on Vitamin B_6*. Washington, National Academy of Sciences, 1977.
233. Spannuth, Mitchell, Stone, Schenker and Wagner: In *Proceedings of a Workshop on Vitamin B_6*. Washington, National Academy of Sciences, 1977.
234. Shin and Linkswiler: J. Nutr., *104*, 1348, 1974.
235. McCoy: In *Proceedings of a Workshop on Vitamin B_6*. Washington, National Academy of Sciences, 1977.
236. Ritchey, Johnson and Korslund: In *Proceedings of a Workshop on Vitamin B_6*. Washington, National Academy of Sciences, 1977.
237. Kirksey and West: In *Proceedings of a Workshop on Vitamin B_6*. Washington, National Academy of Sciences, 1977.
238. West and Kirksey: Am. J. Clin. Nutr., *39*, 961, 1976.
239. Cleary, Lumeng and Li: Am. J. Obstet. Gynecol., *121*, 25, 1975.
240. Shane and Contractor: Am. J. Clin. Nutr., *28*, 739, 1975.
241. Lumeng, Cleary, Wagner, Yee and Li: Am. J. Clin. Nutr., *29*, 1376, 1976.
242. Brophy and Siiteri: Am. J. Obstet. Gynecol., *121*, 1075, 1976.
243. Sauberlich: Vitam. Horm., *22*, 807, 1964.

J. Folic Acid and Vitamin B_{12}*

Victor Herbert
Neville Colman
and
Elizabeth Jacob

The history of vitamin B_{12} and folic acid is rather a long one.[1-3] In 1822, Combe[4] reported to the Royal Medical and Surgical Society of Edinburgh on the "history of a case of anemia" which he surmised was due to "some disorder of the digestive and assimilative organs." Thus was launched the study of pernicious anemia in particular and megaloblastic anemia in general, after restimulation by Addison's description, in 1849 and 1855,[5] of what his contemporaries evidently recognized as pernicious anemia, even though he did not mention glossitis, jaundice or nerve damage. He did mention "the disease having uniformly occurred in fat people," which

would imply deficiency of vitamin B_{12} rather than of folate, since deficiency of the latter tends to be associated with wasting.

The nutritional basis of pernicious anemia was suspected by Flint[6] in 1860, when he stated that "in these cases there exists degenerative disease of the glandular tubuli of the stomach." Another two-thirds of a century had passed when the classic work of Castle[7] and his associates demonstrated that normal human gastric juice contains an "intrinsic factor" that combines with an "extrinsic factor" contained in animal protein to result in absorption of the "antipernicious anemia principle." When vitamin B_{12} was isolated in 1948 almost simultaneously in the United States[8] and England,[9] Berk and his associates[10] showed that this vitamin was

*Supported in part by USPHS Grants #AM 15163 and 20526 and by the Medical Research Service of the Veterans Administration.

both "extrinsic factor" and "antipernicious anemia principle."

Early reports of disease now attributable to probable folate deficiency include those of Channing[11] and Barclay,[12] who reported a severe form of anemia in pregnancy and the puerperium which was often fatal when it resulted from several pregnancies superimposed on a bad diet. Osler[13] postulated that megaloblastic anemia of pregnancy and the puerperium was "caused by an agent which differs from that which causes the anemia of Addison." Evidence for this hypothesis emerged a decade later when Wills and her associates[14] described a macrocytic anemia in Hindu women in Bombay, usually associated with pregnancy, that responded to therapy with a commercial preparation of autolyzed yeast called marmite. By feeding the same type of diet ingested by their patients to monkeys, they produced in them a similar macrocytic anemia, which responded to a "Wills factor" present in crude but not purified liver extracts. We now know that the more purified extract consisted of a fairly pure solution of vitamin B_{12}, and that the Wills factor removed from the crude liver extract in the process of purification is folic acid. This gradually became clear after the purification of pteroylglutamic acid in 1943 by Stokstad,[15] its crystallization from liver in the same year by Pfiffner and associates,[16] its synthesis and structural identification by Angier and his co-workers,[17] and the 1948 isolation of crystalline vitamin B_{12}. The rapid isolation of vitamin B_{12} by the American workers was greatly aided by a microbiologic assay based on Shorb's[18] discovery that "LLD factor," a growth factor required by Lactobacillus lactis Dorner, was not only the "animal protein factor" necessary for proper growth and function in animals fed an all-vegetable diet, but was also present in liver extracts in amounts that closely paralleled their potency in the treatment of pernicious anemia.

Folic acid proved to be not only the Wills factor but also the vitamin M contained in dried brewer's yeast which corrected the deficiency anemia, leukopenia, diarrhea and gingivitis of monkeys studied by Day and associates.[19] It also proved to be the vitamin B_c contained in yeast that corrected the deficiency syndrome in chicks characterized by anemia and growth failure. Furthermore, folic acid proved to be the norite eluate factor (i.e. it could be adsorbed on and eluted from charcoal) of liver, described by Snell and Peterson[20] as essential to the growth of Lactobacillus casei (and therefore also called the "L. casei factor"). The term *folic acid* was coined by Mitchell and co-workers[21] because they found this material in a leafy vegetable (spinach). At that time, it was not recognized that vitamin B_{12}, and not folic acid, was the active ingredient in the oral liver therapy which Minot and Murphy[22] reported in 1926 as successful in treating pernicious anemia (for which work they received the Nobel Prize in Medicine in 1934).

CHEMISTRY[3,23,24]

Neither cyanocobalamin nor pteroylglutamic acid, the common pharmaceutic forms of vitamin B_{12} and folic acid, is present as such in significant quantity in either the human body or the various foods from which these agents were isolated. In the body and in foods, they are present in various reduced metabolically active coenzyme forms, often conjugated (in the case of vitamin B_{12} to peptide and in the case of folate to one or more glutamates) in peptide linkage. During the extraction procedure these labile active forms are either destroyed by oxidation (particularly folates) or oxidized and converted to cyanocobalamin or pteroylglutamic acid, which are the stable forms of the respective vitamins. These stable forms are partially oxidized and not known to be metabolically active; not until they are reduced by metabolic systems present within gut and other tissue cells do they become metabolically active cobalamins or folates.

Vitamin B_{12}[3,23,25,27]

Figure 6J–1 shows the structural formula of vitamin B_{12} (cyanocobalamin); delineation of this structure, using x-ray crystallography, by Hodgkin and her coworkers was partly responsible for her winning the 1964 Nobel Prize in Chemistry. The chemistry of the vitamin has been reviewed by Smith.[23] The two major portions of the molecule are the corrin nucleus (a planar group) and a "nucleotide" lying in a plane nearly at right angles to the corrin nucleus and linked to it by D-1-amino-2-propanol. The "nucleotide" (5-6-dimethyl-benzimidazole) is attached to ribose by an alpha-glycoside linkage. A second bond between the two major parts

of the molecule is the coordinate linkage of the cobalt atom to one of the nitrogen atoms of the "nucleotide."

In cyanocobalamin, the anionic ($-R$) group in coordinate linkage with the cobalt is cyanide. Fortuitously, the original isolation of B_{12} from liver yielded a stable product, cyanocobalamin, because the unstable linkage of the 5'-deoxyadenosyl anionic group to the rest of the molecule in coenzyme B_{12} (the form naturally present in liver) was ruptured and replaced by cyanide which leached from the charcoal columns used in the isolation procedure.

Cyanocobalamin crystals are dark red, the substance absorbs water and the official product in the U.S.P. contains 12 per cent absorbed moisture. The activity is destroyed by heavy metals and strong oxidizing or reducing agents, but not by auto-

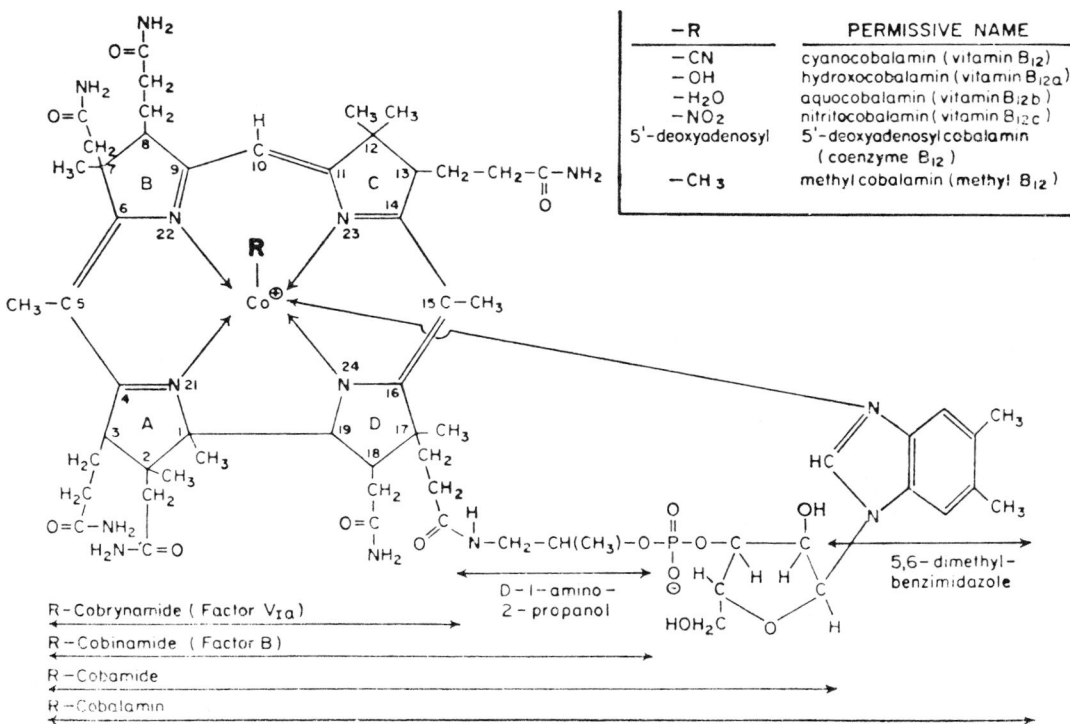

$-R$	PERMISSIVE NAME
$-CN$	cyanocobalamin (vitamin B_{12})
$-OH$	hydroxocobalamin (vitamin B_{12a})
$-H_2O$	aquocobalamin (vitamin B_{12b})
$-NO_2$	nitritocobalamin (vitamin B_{12c})
5'-deoxyadenosyl	5'-deoxyadenosylcobalamin (coenzyme B_{12})
$-CH_3$	methyl cobalamin (methyl B_{12})

Fig. 6J–1. Structural formula of vitamin B_{12} (cyanocobalamin). The numbering system for the corrin nucleus is made to correspond to that of the porphin nucleus by omitting the number 20. (Modified from Brown and Reynolds: Annu. Rev. Biochem., *32*, 419, 1963.)

claving for short periods at 121°C. It is soluble 1:80 in water, and stable in solution. Aqueous solutions are neutral; maximal stability is at pH 4.5 to 5.

Coenzyme B_{12} (5'-deoxyadenosylcobalamin) and methylcobalamin (methyl-B_{12}) are the two vitamin B_{12} coenzymes known to be metabolically active in man, and constitute the dominant forms of B_{12} in mammalian tissues. Both are unstable in light and undergo photolysis with formation of aquocobalamin, or, in the presence of potassium cyanide, cyanocobalamin. Under the rules of the International Union of Pure and Applied Chemistry (IUPAC) Commission on Biochemical Nomenclature,[28] cyanocobalamin is a permissive (semisystematic) name for vitamin B_{12} and the term vitamin B_{12} without qualification means cyanocobalamin exclusively. However, the term is also entrenched in the literature as a generic term for all of the cobalamins active in man. The permissive term cobalamin (or B_{12}) is used to describe the vitamin B_{12} molecule minus the cyanide group, and is prefixed by the designation of the anionic R group (see Figure 6J–1) attached to the cobalt. The terms coenzyme B_{12} and vitamin B_{12} coenzyme are not interchangeable; the former means 5'-deoxyadenosylcobalamin exclusively, and the latter applies to any coenzyme form of B_{12}.

Figure 6J–1 delineates some of the family of natural and semisynthetic cobalamins; others include dicyanocobalamin, thiocyanatocobalamin, chlorocobalamin and sulfitocobalamin. The alphabetic congeners of vitamin B_{12} (B_{12a}, B_{12b}, B_{12c}) listed in Figure 6J–1 are believed equipotent in treatment of vitamin B_{12} deficiency (unless that deficiency is due to a congenital or acquired defect in enzymes involved in converting one B_{12} form to another). However, minimal dose therapy suggests[29] that coenzyme B_{12} is more potent therapeutically than cyanocobalamin; therapy with doses greater than minimal is always used clinically, and all forms of B_{12} appear equipotent when used in greater than minimal doses.

Folic Acid[3,24,30]

Figure 6J–2 presents the structural formula of folic acid (pteroylglutamic acid), the parent compound of the folate vitamin forms. The major subunits of the molecule are the pteridine moiety linked by a methylene bridge to para-aminobenzoic acid, which is joined by peptide linkage to glutamic acid.

Crystalline folic acid is yellow. The free acid is almost insoluble in cold water, but the disodium salt is more soluble (about 1.5 gm per 100 ml). Injectable solutions are prepared by dissolving folic acid in isotonic sodium bicarbonate solution, or by using the disodium salt. Folic acid is destroyed at pH below 4, but is relatively stable above pH 5, with no destruction in 1 hour at 100°C. The molecule usually splits into pteridine and para-aminobenzoyl glutamate.

The rules of the International Union of Pure and Applied Chemistry[28] are that pteroylglutamic acid may be designated generically as folic acid, and that the pure substance hitherto known as folic acid, folacine or vitamin B_c shall be named pteroylglutamic acid. However, the term

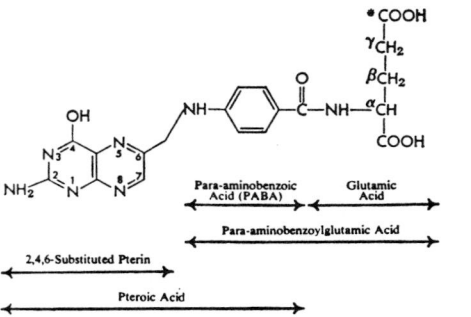

*Site of attachment of extra glutamate residue(s) of pteroyl di-, tri-, or hepta-glutamate.

Folic Acid (Pteroylmonoglutamic Acid)

Fig. 6J–2. Structural formula of folic acid (pteroylglutamic acid). (From Herbert[3] with permission of the Macmillan Co.)

folic acid is entrenched in the literature not only generically but also as a synonym for pteroylglutamic acid. Therefore, when the context does not make the meaning clear, it is preferable to use the term folate for the generic meaning (as done by WHO Scientific Group, 1968,[31] and FAO/WHO Expert Group, 1970).[31]

Pteroylglutamic acid is not normally found in foods or in the human body in significant concentrations. The forms which are found in such sources are indicated in Figure 6J–3. They differ from the parent compound by virtue of 1 to 3 structural modifications. First, all are reduced folates and, except for 7,8-dihydrofolate, all are 5,6,7,8-tetrahydrofolate (THF). Second, as indicated in Figure 6J–3, various 1-carbon adducts may be linked to THF at the N-5, N-10, or 5,10 position, conferring on folates their role as 1-carbon carriers; it has been suggested[30] that there are only 5 natural 1-carbon substitutions on THF and that N^5 formyl THF (folinic acid; citrovorum factor) represents nonenzymatic conversion of folate during processing of natural materials. Third, the number of glutamate residues may vary from 1 to 8, each linked by peptide bonds between its amino group to the gamma-carboxyl group of the preceding glutamate (see Fig. 6J–2).

UNITS OF MEASUREMENT AND METHODS OF ASSAY

Vitamin B_{12}[3,23,32]

Human serum levels of vitamin B_{12} are measured in picograms (pg: 10^{-12} grams, $\mu\mu g$ [micromicrograms]) per ml of serum; normal values range from 200 to 900 pg per ml; values below 80 pg per ml repre-

	R	OXIDATION STATE
N^5 formyl THFA	—CHO	formate
N^{10} formyl THFA	—CHO	formate
N^5 formimino THFA	—CH=NH	formate
$N^{5,10}$ methenyl THFA	>CH	formate
$N^{5,10}$ methylene THFA	>CH$_2$	formaldehyde
N^5 methyl THFA	—CH$_3$	methanol

*Broken lines indicate the N^5 and/or N^{10} site of attachment of various 1-carbon units for which THFA acts as a carrier.

5,6,7,8-Tetrahydrofolic Acid (THFA)(FH$_4$)(R=—H)

Fig. 6J–3. Structures and nomenclature in the folate field. The table above the formula lists some of the possible 1-carbon adducts formed with THFA. (From Herbert[3] with permission of the Macmillan Co.)

sent unequivocal B_{12} deficiency according to the WHO Scientific Group on Nutritional Anemias.[31] This tiny quantity of vitamin B_{12} activity may be measured only microbiologically or by radioassay. Many microorganisms require vitamin B_{12} in order to grow, and therefore there are many microbiologic assays for vitamin B_{12}. Radioassay has the advantage over microbiologic assay in that false low results do not occur if serum contains antibiotic or other substances which inhibit growth of microorganisms, whereas the microbiologic assays do yield false low results in such circumstances. Radioassay for vitamin B_{12} was first described in 1958;[33] the most widely used such assay applies coated charcoal[34,35] to separate free from bound vitamin B_{12}.

Human serum and tissues contain not only biologically active "true B_{12}" but also analogs of varying to no activity. Radioassays which do not use pure intrinsic factor (which binds only "true B_{12}," i.e. "true cobalamins")[35a] measure "total B_{12}" ("total cobinamides") rather than "true B_{12}," and thus may not pick up early B_{12} deficiency, since in early deficiency only that portion of "total B_{12}" which is "true B_{12}" may fall, and analogs may still be in the normal range.[35b,35c,35d] It must also be recognized that heat plus the presence of large amounts of vitamin C will destroy vitamin B_{12} unless the B_{12} is protected by cyanide, $-S$ or another protective mechanism.[35e]

Larger quantities of vitamin B_{12} may be assayed colorimetrically, spectroscopically, fluorometrically or chemically.

The U.S.P. assay for vitamin B_{12} is spectrophotometric. Although liver extract for injection was deleted from the U.S.P. in 1960, such products are still being used, assayed by a microbiologic method for their vitamin B_{12} content.

Folic Acid[3,35]

Normal human serum contains 7 to 16 nanograms (ng: 10^{-9} grams; mμg [milimicrograms]) of folic acid activity per ml of serum. These tiny quantities could be measured only microbiologically, as originally described in 1959,[38-42] until a radioisotopic assay was described in 1970.[43] The dominant folate in serum and red cells is 5-methyltetrahydrofolate, and folate assays must therefore be capable of measuring this derivative. Because L. casei is the only microorganism known to grow well on this folate, the only microbiologic assay which adequately measures serum and red cell folate in man uses L. casei. Similarly, the only radioassays which accurately measure serum folate are those which measure 5-methyltetrahydrofolate; these are mainly done at pH 9.3, where folic acid and serum folate have similar reactivity.[44]

Recently, a technique has been developed for the simultaneous radioisotope determination of serum vitamin B_{12} and folate in the same test tube.[45] This assay correlates well with other radioassays[46] and considerably simplifies the assay of the two vitamins. It may be the method of choice for use in most laboratories.

Since serum folate is labile, false low values for serum folate activity occur if the serum has not been protected against oxidative destruction prior to assay. Such protection is brought about by storing the serum frozen, storing it in the presence of a reducing agent such as ascorbate, or both. It must be remembered that ascorbate may destroy B_{12} in storage.[35e]

Larger quantities of folate activity than those normally present in human serum may be measured chemically, fluorometrically, by paper and thin-layer chromatography, enzymatically or by animal assay.[35]

THE CAUSES OF NUTRITIONAL DEFICIENCY OF VITAMIN B_{12} AND FOLIC ACID

In the final analysis, nutritional deficiency means there is inadequate usage of a nutrient in one or more intracellular systems to sustain normal biochemical

Table 6J-1. Etiologic Classification of Vitamin B_{12} and Folate Deficiency in Man*

I. Vitamin B_{12} Deficiency (normal B_{12} body stores last 3 to 6 years after cessation of B_{12} absorption)
  A. Indequate Ingestion
    1. Poor diet (lacking animal protein and microorganisms, the sole B_{12} sources)
      a. Vegans
      b. Chronic alcoholism (folate deficiency more common)
      c. Poverty, religious tenets, ignorance, dietary faddism
  B. Inadequate Absorption
    1. Lesions of the stomach
      a. Secretion of abnormal intrinsic factor
        1. Hereditary
      b. Inadequate or absent secretion of intrinsic factor
        1. Hereditary failure of intrinsic factor secretion with normal gastric mucosa
        2. Gastric atrophy associated with multiple autoantibodies and polyendocrinopathy, or with hypothyroidism
        3. Hereditary degenerative gastric atrophy (Addisonian pernicious anemia) (i.e. included in Addison's original cases)
        4. Gastric atrophy as the end-result of superficial inflammatory gastritis; superficial gastritis with atrophy (probably also included among Addison's cases)
        5. Lesions which destroy the gastric mucosa (ingested corrosives, linitis plastica, etc.)
      c. Intrinsic factor inhibitor in gastric secretion
        1. Antibody to intrinsic factor (in saliva or gastric juice)
          a. Blocking antibody
          b. Binding antibody
      d. Gastrectomy
        1. Total
        2. Subtotal
          a. Proximal
          b. Distal
    2. Small intestine disorder (affection ileum, which is the main site of B_{12} absorption)
      a. Gluten-induced enteropathy (childhood celiac disease; adult celiac disease) (idiopathic steatorrhea, nontropical sprue)
      b. Tropical sprue
      c. Regional ileitis
      d. Strictures or anastomoses of the small bowel, jejunal diverticulosis, gastrocolic fistulas, other "stagnant bowel" syndromes
      e. Intestinal resection (particularly involving ileum)
      f. Malignancies and granulomatous lesions involving the small intestine
      g. Other conditions characterized by chronically disturbed intestinal function
      h. Drugs
        1. Para-aminosalicylic acid (PAS)
        2. Colchicine
        3. Neomycin
        4. Ethanol
        5. Oral contraceptive agents?
      i. Specific malabsorption for vitamin B_{12}
        1. Due to long-term ingestion of calcium-chelating agents
        2. Due to inadequately alkaline pH in ileum (Zollinger-Ellison syndrome; inadequate pancreatic bicarbonate)
        3. Unknown causes (absence of intestinal receptors for B_{12}-intrinsic factor complex? absence of "releasing factor"?)
          a. Congenital (Imerslund-Gräsbeck syndrome)
          b. Acquired (forme fruste of sprue)
        4. Inadequate pancreatic exocrine secretion (chronic pancreatitis, fibrocystic disease of pancreas, etc.)
    3. Competition for vitamin B_{12} by intestinal parasites or bacteria
      a. Fish tapeworm (Diphyllobothrium latum)
      b. Bacteria: The blind loop syndrome (B_{12}-greedy bacteria) (overlaps "stagnant-bowel" syndrome)

Table 6J–1. Etiologic Classification of Vitamin B_{12} and Folate Deficiency in Man
(Continued)

C. Inadequate Utilization
   1. Vitamin B_{12} antagonists
      a. Substituted B_{12} amides and anilides
      b. Cobaloximes
   2. Protein malnutrition?
   3. Malignancy?
   4. Liver disease?
   5. Renal disease?
   6. Thiocyanate intoxication?
   7. Congenital or acquired enzyme deficiency or deletion
      a. Methylmalonyl-CoA mutase
      b. Methyltetrahydrofolate-homocysteine methyltransferase
      c. B_{12a} reductase
      d. $B_{12\gamma}$ reductase
      e. Deoxyadenosyltransferase
      f. Other enzyme reduction or deletion
   8. Abnormal B_{12}-binding protein in serum, irreversibly binding B_{12} and making it unavailable to tissues
      a. Abnormal cobalophilins (myeloproliferative disorders)
      b. Abnormal cobalophilins and/or TC II (liver disease)
   9. Inadequate serum B_{12}-binding protein
      a. Congenital absence of TC II
  10. Nitrous oxide anesthesia
D. Increased Requirement
   1. Hyperthyroidism
   2. Increased hematopoiesis?
   3. Infancy?
   4. Parasitization
      a. By fetus
      b. By malignant tissue?
E. Increased Excretion
   1. Inadequate B_{12}-binding protein in serum?
   2. Liver disease (inadequate retention of B_{12})
   3. Renal disease?
F. Increased Destruction
   1. Excessive vitamin C intake? (may also reduce B_{12} absorption)
II. Folic Acid Deficiency (normal folate body stores will last only 3 to 6 months after cessation of folate ingestion)
  A. Inadequate Ingestion
   1. Poor diet (lacking unprocessed fresh, uncooked or slightly cooked food) (folates are heat-labile)
      a. Nutritional megaloblastic anemia
         1. Tropical
         2. Nontropical
         3. Scurvy (diets poor in vitamin C are also poor in folate)
      b. Chronic alcoholism with or without cirrhosis
  B. Inadequate Absorption (affecting upper one third of small intestine which has the largest surface and thus is the main site of folate absorption)
   1. Defective folate polyglutamate hydrolysis
      a. Congenital or acquired conjugase deficiency (not described)
      b. Conjugase inhibitors
         1. In foods (yeast and beans)
         2. Drugs?
         3. Low pH
   2. Defective mucosal transport
      a. Specific for folate
         1. Congenital

Table 6J–1. Etiologic Classification of Vitamin B$_{12}$ and Folate Deficiency in Man
(Continued)

    2. Drugs — diphenylhydantoin (Dilantin)

        — ethanol (in presence of prior folate deficiency)— primidone, barbiturates, cycloserine

    3. High pH

  b. As part of malabsorption syndromes (any chronic functional or structural disorder involving the upper small intestine)

    1. Gluten-induced enteropathy (childhood and adult celiac disease)

    2. Tropical sprue

  3. Blind loop syndrome (folate-greedy bacteria) (more commonly bacteria *produce* folate)

C. Inadequate Utilization (metabolic block)

  1. Folic acid antagonists (dihydrofolate reductase inhibitors)

    a. 4-Amino-4-deoxyfolates   (Chemotherapy, immunosuppression,
       (i.e. methotrexate, aminopterin)   psoriasis)

    b. 2,4-Diaminopyrimidine (i.e.
       Pyrimethamine   (Malaria, toxoplasmosis)
       Trimethoprim   (Antibacterial)

    c. Triamterene   (Diuretic)

    d. Diamidine compounds (i.e.   (Pneumocystis carinii,
       pentamidine isethionate)   protozoacidal)

  2. Anticonvulsants?

  3. Enzyme deficiency

    a. Congenital

      1. Formiminotransferase

      2. Dihydrofolate reductase?

      3. Methyltetrahydrofolate transmethylase?

      4. Cyclohydrolase?

      5. Other enzymes, including those secondarily affecting folate (e.g. cystathione synthase)

    b. Acquired

      1. Liver disease

        a. Formiminotransferase

        b. Other enzymes

  4. Vitamin B$_{12}$ deficiency ("methyl folate trap")

  5. Alcohol (both specific and nonspecific interference with folate metabolism)

  6. Dietary amino acid excess (glycine, methionine)

  7. Uremia (interferes with folate transport)

  8. Sex steroids (e.g. oral contraceptives)

D. Increased Requirement

  1. Parasitization

    a. By fetus (especially in multiple pregnancies)

    b. By breast-fed infant

    c. By malignant tissue (especially lymphoproliferative disorders; myeloproliferative disorders to a lesser extent; extensive carcinomatosis, etc.)

  2. Infancy (especially prematurity)

  3. Increased hematopoiesis (hemolytic anemias; chronic blood loss [including scurvy])

  4. Increased metabolic activity (e.g. hyperthyroidism)

  5. Lesch-Nyhan syndrome (increased reliance on folate-dependent pathways)

  6. Drugs (L-dopa?)

E. Increased Excretion

  1. Vitamin B$_{12}$ deficiency? (of obligatory excretion of folate in urine and bile?) (due partly to inability to incorporate folate in cells)

  2. Liver disease?

  3. Kidney dialysis.

F. Increased Destruction

  1. Scurvy?

  2. Dietary oxidants?

---

*Compiled mainly from information in Symposium on Vitamin B$_{12}$ and Folate (Herbert, guest ed.). Am. J. Med. *48*, 539, 1970, and from Herbert.[131]

functions. Such inadequate usage falls in one or more of six basic categories:

1. Inadequate ingestion
2. Inadequate absorption
3. Inadequate utilization
4. Increased requirement
5. Increased excretion
6. Increased destruction.

Any one or combination of these 3 inadequacies and 3 excesses may result in nutritional deficiency. Table 6J–1 presents the currently known possible etiologic factors in each of these 6 categories which may produce nutritional deficiency of vitamin B_{12} or folic acid. The ensuing sections will discuss in more detail mechanisms of inadequate absorption and utilization of these two vitamins.

ABSORPTION

Vitamin B_{12}[3,23,47-51]

There are two separate and distinct mechanisms for the absorption of vitamin B_{12}. The *physiologic* mechanism, the derangement of which accounts for much human vitamin B_{12} deficiency, is capable of handling a maximum of 1.5 to 3 μg of free vitamin B_{12} at any one time. This mechanism operates as follows: (1) Ingested vitamin B_{12} is freed from its polypeptide linkages to food by gastric acid and gastric and intestinal enzymes, (2) the free vitamin B_{12} attaches to the gastric intrinsic factor of Castle (a glycoprotein of molecular weight in the range of 50,000, produced by normal gastric parietal cells, which dimerizes on combination with vitamin B_{12} so that a complex is formed consisting of 2 molecules of intrinsic factor and 2 molecules of vitamin B_{12}), (3) the vitamin B_{12}-intrinsic factor complex is carried down to the ileum, where it is plastered onto the brush border of the ileal mucosal cells in the presence of ionic calcium and a pH above 6, (4) via a currently uncertain mechanism, the vitamin B_{12} is released from its complex with intrinsic factor probably at but possibly within the ileal

enterocyte (epithelial cell); (5) the vitamin then finds its way across the enterocyte into the portal venous blood, at which point it is attached to serum vitamin B_{12}-binding proteins (see Fig. 6J–4). Bicarbonate and trypsin from the pancreas facilitate this mechanism, largely probably by selectively destroying nonintrinsic factor B_{12} binders, a phenomenon we were not able to demonstrate, but others subsequently did demonstrate at more alkaline pH.[51a,51b]

The other, or *pharmacologic,* mechanism of vitamin B_{12} absorption appears to be diffusion.[48] It accounts for the absorption along the entire length of the small intestine of approximately 1 per cent of *any* quantity of *free* vitamin B_{12} in the small bowel. This is the mechanism which makes possible oral (rather than parenteral) therapy for vitamin B_{12} deficiency due to vitamin B_{12} malabsorption. However, such therapy is less reliable than parenteral therapy.[3]

Folate[3,24,48,52,53]

Current evidence suggests that food folate is absorbed primarily from the proximal third of the small intestine, although it is capable of being absorbed from the entire length of the small bowel. Folate in food is present primarily in polyglutamate form. Prior to absorption, the "excess" glutamates must be split off the side chain of the vitamin molecule by conjugases. The products of conjugase action are detectable in the intestinal lumen prior to absorption,[54] and preliminary evidence suggests that this may be due to a surface-active brush border conjugase functionally and chromatographically distinguishable from intracellular conjugase.[55] Conjugase action may be specifically inhibited by food factors described in yeast and beans[56] and may be nonspecifically impaired at acid pH.[57]

However, impaired mucosal transport of monoglutamyl folates after deconjugation probably accounts for most instances of folate malabsorption. Active mucosal transport is accelerated by glucose[58] and galactose and impaired by unidentified factors present in many foods.[59,60]

It is probable that a small but relatively unchanging percentage of ingested folate is absorbed by passive diffusion after deconjugation,[61] as is the case with vitamin B_{12}.

TRANSPORT, DISTRIBUTION, STORAGE, FATE AND EXCRETION

Vitamin B_{12} (Fig. 6J–4)[3,25,49,62,63]

Vitamin B_{12} in human serum is bound to 3 different vitamin B_{12}-binding proteins, transcobalamin I, II and III (TCI, TCII, TCIII). The normal total vitamin B_{12}-binding capacity (TBBC) of serum ranges from about 1000 to 1800 pg per ml and the unsaturated vitamin B_{12} binding capacity (UBBC) ranges from 600 to 1400 pg per ml, normally largely (450 to 1000 pg per ml) due to TCII.[64] TCI and TCIII are glycoproteins; are synthesized largely in granulocytes,[63] but possibly also in salivary glands, gastric mucosa and some hepatomas;[65] have a molecular weight of about 60,000 and appear to have largely a storage function, although TCIII may be involved in redelivery of vitamin B_{12} to the liver, to which it may attach via a terminal galactose.[63,65] The amounts of unsaturated TCI and TCIII in serum range from 30 to 110 and 120 to 300 pg per ml respectively.[64] These glycoproteins are referred to by some as cobalophilins (R proteins); they are microheterogeneous mixtures of various isoproteins in different proportions.[65]

TBBC, UBBC and serum vitamin B_{12} levels all tend to be elevated in any situation in which the total body neutrophil pool is increased (as in myeloproliferative disorders). It has been shown that this is due to an increase in the amounts of unsaturated TCI and TCIII.[66] These glycoproteins, however, do not deliver vitamin B_{12} to the bone marrow, as illustrated by the fact that a patient with chronic myelogenous leukemia and pernicious anemia had a normal serum vitamin B_{12} level because of these glycoproteins and yet the tissues were starved of the vitamin to the point where biochemical deficiency was severe.[67]

Further evidence that TCI and TCIII do not participate in transport of the vitamin to bone marrow and nervous tissue is provided by the report[63] of two brothers with congenital lack of these proteins who had low serum vitamin B_{12} levels but no hematologic or other manifestations of tissue B_{12} deficiency.

Unlike the cobalophilins (TCI and TCIII), which are glycoproteins, TCII is a pure protein. It has an apparent molecular weight of 38,000,[65] is synthesized largely in the liver,[68-70] is a beta-globulin and is chiefly responsible for transport and delivery of the vitamin. There is relatively little vitamin B_{12} attached to it in vivo because of the rapidity with which it is degraded as it delivers B_{12} to tissues. When a sample of blood is drawn, only 10 to 20 per cent of plasma vitamin B_{12} (which is mainly methyl-B_{12}) is bound to TCII; the rest is bound to cobalophilin, largely TCI (which is 80 to 100 per cent saturated with B_{12}). The plasma survival time of TCIII is very short (minutes) compared to TCII, which in turn is short (hours) compared to TCI (days) and the cobalophilins in chronic myelogenous leukemia and hepatoma.[65]

Vitamin B_{12}, when it enters the blood stream, is bound by TCs in proportion to their binding capacity and delivered by TCII to liver, bone marrow cells, reticulocytes, lymphoblasts, fibroblasts and tumor cells via a mechanism similar to that by which intrinsic factor delivers the vitamin to ileal mucosal cells. Bone marrow cells, reticulocytes and many other cells contain on their surfaces "receptor sites" for the TCII-B_{12} complex; these sites will take up the complex only in the presence of ionic calcium and a pH greater than 6;[71] liver cells may contain receptor sites for TCIII.[63,65] Thus, delivery of B_{12} to the gut enterocyte and the immature erythrocytes both require (1) a transport protein, (2) pH above 6, (3) ionic calcium and (4) a receptor site for the protein-vitamin B_{12} complex on the surface of the cell.

The importance of TCII in the absorption, transport and delivery of vitamin B_{12} to the tissues is emphasized by the finding of individuals with congenital absence of TCII who have defective vitamin B_{12} delivery and therefore require treatment with large frequent parenteral doses of the vitamin.[72,73] The possible "acute phase reactant" status of TCII may be important,[73a] including elevated TCII in autoimmune disease.[73b]

"Normal" stores of vitamin B_{12} range between 1 and 10 mg,[32,74,75] with the liver containing 50 to 90 per cent of the total stored vitamin (averaging 1 μg B_{12} per gm of liver). Average stores range between 2 and 5 mg. There is no evidence for significant catabolism of vitamin B_{12} by man, and it is probable that loss occurs only by excretion, mainly in the bile. The wholebody turnover of vitamin B_{12} is between 0.1 and 0.2 per cent daily, regardless of whether body stores are normal or reduced. Coenzyme B_{12} appears to be the main storage form, and methyl-B_{12} appears to be the main serum transport form.[23,25]

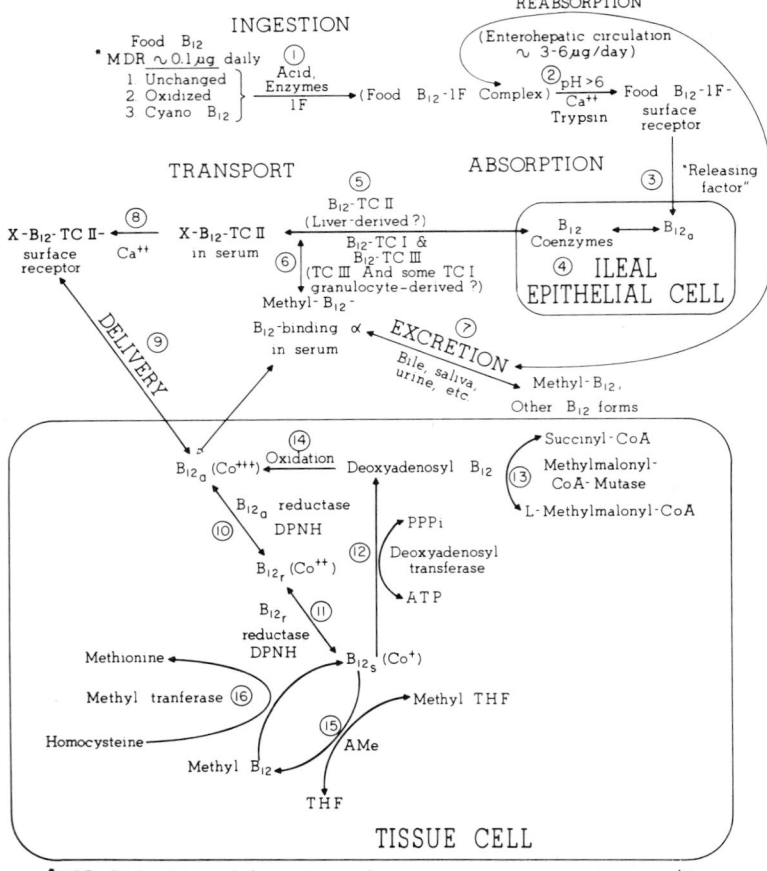

*MDR = Adult minimum daily requirement from exogenous sources to sustain normality

Fig. 6J–4. *A*: Cobalamin (B_{12}) metabolism in man. (From Herbert[149] with permission of W. B. Saunders.)

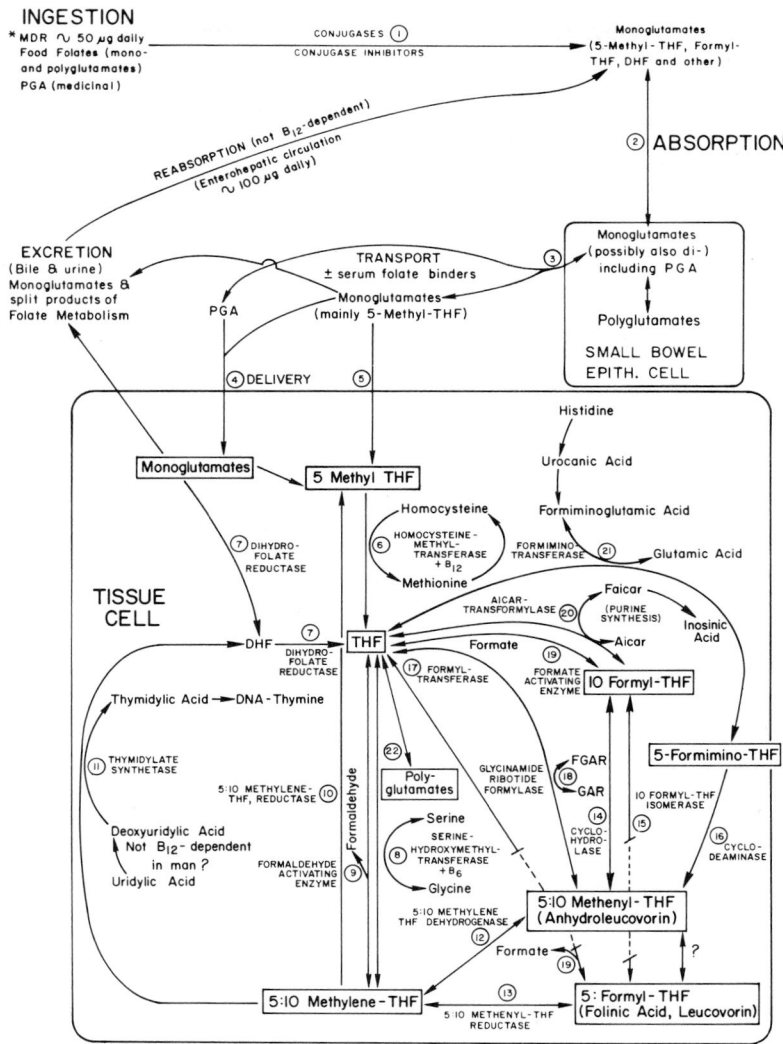

Fig. 6J–4. *B*: Flow chart of folate metabolism in man. Circled numbers identify individual steps in folate metabolism. In mammals, the same enzyme catalyzes reactions 12, 14 and 19,[147] and another single enzyme catalyzes both steps 16 and 21.[148] THF = tetrahydrofolate, DHF = dihydrofolate. (From Herbert[149] with permission of W. B. Saunders.)

There is normally an enterohepatic circulation of vitamin B_{12} which may account for from approximately 0.6 to approximately 6 μg of the vitamin excreted daily in the bile and reabsorbed in the ileum.[3,76-78] This almost total conservation of vitamin B_{12} explains why pure vegetarians, who eat almost no vitamin B_{12}, take decades to develop deficiency of the vitamin. It is only when the reabsorption phase of the enterohepatic circulation of the vitamin is damaged, by damage to the stomach, ileum or pancreas, that vitamin B_{12} deficiency disease develops more rapidly (i.e. in 3 to 6 years).

Folate (Fig. 6J–4)[3,30,79-82]

Plasma transport of folate remains far less clearly elucidated than that of vitamin B_{12}. Folate in plasma appears to be distributed in 3 fractions. Free folate and that loosely bound to low-affinity binders are similar in magnitude, whereas much less is bound to high-affinity binders.

Low-affinity binding is a nonspecific property of many different plasma proteins and is similar to nonspecific binding of bilirubin and various drugs. It was detected many years ago using ultrafiltration (which overestimates the amount bound), equilibrium dialysis and gel filtration. The potential binding capacity is several hundred times greater than the amount of folate in serum. Early data showing failure to half-saturate these binders at very high concentrations of free folate indicate that the affinity constant of the system is less than 10^4 liters per mole, which is less than the 10^6 liters per mole affinity constant of the carrier-mediated cell transport systems for folate.[82]

Study of the high-affinity serum folate binders was initiated by Rothenberg's serendipitous discovery of such binders in chronic myeloid leukemia cells,[83] and subsequently in the serum of the same patients. They are demonstrable in granulocytes of a proportion of nonleukemic subjects, and are released into the serum by

these cells.[84] Although their release has not yet been detected in most normal subjects, it has been shown that all human (and animal) serum contains these binders,[80] which more often than not are largely saturated.

Current data[80] suggest that there is only one class of high-affinity serum folate binders—glycoproteins with a molecular weight of about 40,000, probably granulocyte-derived but modified by liver and perhaps kidney. They have binding constants (K_d) of approximately 10^{-10} M folic acid and of the order of 10^{-8} M 5-methyltetrahydrofolate, the main folate present in serum. Although these affinities indicate that binder would only be half-saturated at usual serum methyltetrahydrofolate concentrations, they normally average 67 per cent saturation. This may be due to the presence of very small quantities of nonmethyl unsubstituted folates on binders. These binders carry less than 5 per cent of serum folate. Their physiologic function has not yet been demonstrated, but at least three lines of inquiry are currently being pursued: (1) The binders may play a role in folate delivery to liver similar to the role of transcobalamin I in vitamin B_{12} transport. (2) They may be important in controlling folate distribution, breakdown and excretion in deficient states. (3) Their presence in cerebrospinal fluid,[85] their increased affinity for oxidized folate and the active transport of oxidized folates out of cerebrospinal fluid[86] all suggest that they may function as carriers important in transporting oxidized folates from cerebrospinal fluid to blood.

Folate is delivered to bone marrow cells, reticulocytes, liver, cerebrospinal fluid, and renal tubular cells against a concentration gradient in a manner which suggests energy-dependent carrier-mediated transport.[82] The transport constant of these systems is about 10^{-6} M. Methyltetrahydrofolate, which accounts for almost all of serum folate, appears to be transported more efficiently than folic acid across the intestinal cell and into the cells of the body.

Normal total-body folate stores are in the range of 5 to 10 mg, of which approximately half is in the liver.[31] It has been suggested that the enterohepatic circulation, which transports about 0.1 mg of biologically active folate daily,[3] is important in the maintenance of serum folate levels.[87]

Most stored folate is present as polyglutamates,[30] which have far greater molecular size and charge than monoglutamates. Transport across cell walls probably requires hydrolysis to monoglutamates, and the enzymes responsible for polyglutamate synthesis and hydrolysis may thus play a major role in folate storage. These enzymes, which have been incompletely characterized, are known respectively as polyglutamate synthetase and conjugase (polyglutamate hydrolase; gamma-glutamylcarboxypeptidase). Conjugase, which has been more fully studied than the synthetase, is present in almost all mammalian tissues and is under partial hormonal control. Some of the folate-dependent reactions shown in Figure 6J-4 are altered by varying glutamyl chain lengths, and it is thus probable that conjugase and polyglutamate synthetase affect the metabolic role of folate as well as its storage.

Folate is excreted in urine and bile in metabolically active and inactive forms. Urinary excretion of the biologically active material occurs after glomerular filtration of the free fraction and reabsorption of some filtered folate by active transport across the tubular cell wall. The principal breakdown product of folate in urine, acetamidobenzoylglutamate, suggests that the principal route of folate catabolism occurs through oxidative cleavage of the folate molecule at the 9–10 bond, with acetylation of the para-aminobenzoyl moiety in the liver prior to excretion.[81] Some workers[88] believe that scorbutic patients may lose large amounts of folate through irreversible oxidation of 10-formyltetra-hydrofolate to 10-formylfolate and excretion of the latter in the urine.

As mentioned above, about 100 μg of biologically active folate is excreted in the bile daily. In addition, studies with radioactive tracer folates[89] indicate that a large proportion of injected radioactivity is excreted in the bile as a biologically inactive compound which is not a product of 9–10 cleavage, but which has not been well characterized. Alcohol interferes with the folate enterohepatic cycle.[87]

NUTRITIONAL REQUIREMENTS AND NATURAL SOURCES

The term *minimal daily requirement* (MDR), as used in this chapter, means the minimal daily requirement *from exogenous sources* required to sustain normality, with normality defined as the absence of any biochemical hypofunction which is correctable by addition of greater quantities of the vitamin. By this definition, the minimal daily requirement for vitamin B_{12} of a normal subject would be only 0.1 μg, since this quantity will sustain normality in a normal subject.[90–91] The minimal daily requirement for vitamin B_{12} of a patient with gastric or ileal structural or functional damage would be greater, since such damage not only eliminates the normal absorption of vitamin B_{12} from exogenous (food) sources, but also eliminates the normal daily reabsorption from the ileum of almost all the vitamin B_{12} normally excreted each day in bile.

The minimal daily requirement can be reduced to a formula[92] applicable generally to essential (i.e. required from exogenous sources) nutrient deficiency, as follows:

$$(1) \quad \text{MDR (units/day)} = \frac{\text{UBS (units)}}{\text{D (days)}}$$

where:

MDR = minimal daily requirement of nutrient from exogenous sources
UBS = utilizable body stores of nutrient
D = number of days required to develop tissue

deficiency after cessation of absorption from exogenous sources of nutrient (with appropriate correction for *incomplete* cessation of absorption).

The above formula may also be written as:

$$(2) \qquad D = \frac{UBS}{MDR}$$

or

$$(3) \qquad UBS = D \times MDR$$

As suggested above, one can predict the time it would take any given nutrient deficiency to develop in any given person after reduction or cessation of absorption of the nutrient if one knows (or can reasonably estimate) the MDR for the nutrient and the utilizable body stores thereof.

The Recommended Dietary Allowances (RDA) "are the levels of intake of essential nutrients considered, in the judgment of the Food and Nutrition Board (of the National Academy of Sciences) on the basis of available scientific knowledge, to be adequate to meet the known nutritional needs of practically all healthy persons."[91] The RDA for each nutrient is intentionally greater than the MDR in order to allow for normal variation in utilization and requirements and because there is a tendency to err on the positive side when information is incomplete: small surpluses of nutrients are rarely detrimental whereas small deficits may cause deficiency over a long period of time.

Vitamin B_{12}

Nutritional Requirements.[3,29,33,74,90,91] Vitamin B_{12} requirements have been estimated from three different types of study:[30] (1) those designed to determine the minimal amount needed to prevent or cure megaloblastic anemia resulting from vitamin B_{12} deficiency, (2) those correlating the relationship between the levels of vitamin B_{12} in serum and in liver in deficient and healthy subjects and (3) those correlating body stores and turnover rates of vitamin B_{12}.

The results of such studies[30] demonstrated that: (1) the minimal quantity of vitamin B_{12} which would produce a hematologic response in patients with uncomplicated vitamin B_{12} deficiency was in the range of 0.1 μg daily, and 0.5 to 1 μg of the vitamin daily produces maximum hematologic responses, with similar amounts maintaining a normal picture. (2) Patients with moderate vitamin B_{12} deficiency resulting from B_{12} malabsorption had an average liver vitamin B_{12} content of 0.16 μg per gm wet weight of liver, associated with serum vitamin B_{12} levels ranging from 80 to 130 pg per ml and an average total body B_{12} of approximately 250 μg. (A second group of individuals who were also suffering from vitamin B_{12} malabsorption, but who had not yet developed morphologic evidence of blood damage due to vitamin B_{12} deficiency, all had serum levels between 130 and 200 pg per ml, associated with approximately 0.28 μg of vitamin B_{12} per gm wet weight of liver and an average total body vitamin B_{12} content of approximately 525 μg). (3) The daily whole body turnover of vitamin B_{12} measured with tracer doses of radioactive vitamin indicates a radioactivity turnover of between 0.1 and 0.2 per cent daily, regardless of whether the body vitamin B_{12} stores are normal or reduced.

Loss of 0.1 to 0.2 per cent of radioactive vitamin B_{12} daily means less than that quantity of vitamin is lost from the body stores daily, since the radioactive B_{12} excreted in the bile mixes with nonradioactive B_{12} in the diet, and some of the radioactive B_{12} that would otherwise be reabsorbed in the ileum is replaced by absorbed nonradioactive vitamin. The net result is a gradual reduction in the radioactivity of the body vitamin B_{12} stores, but a much lesser reduction in the actual vitamin B_{12} content of those stores.

The Food and Nutrition Board of the National Research Council (NRC) set the RDA for vitamin B_{12} at 3 μg per day for adolescents and normal adults "assuming that at least 50 per cent of quantities up to 3 μg of food vitamin B_{12} is absorbed."[91] On the other hand, the Joint FAO/WHO Expert Group[74] recommends a daily intake of 2 μg of vitamin B_{12} for the normal adult. The recommendation of the NRC group is based almost entirely on studies of the body turnover of radioactive vitamin B_{12}, studies that seem to have no relation to minimal daily requirement, since such turnover tends to be a fixed percentage of body stores regardless of the size of body stores. On the other hand, the 2 μg daily intake recommended for adults by the FAO/WHO group is based not only on the same radioactivity turnover studies on which the NRC relied almost exclusively but also on studies of minimal amounts needed to prevent or cure megaloblastic anemia resulting from vitamin B_{12} deficiency, and on studies of the relationship between the levels of vitamin B_{12} in serum and in liver in deficient and healthy subjects. The recommended daily allowance (RDA) of 3 μg of vitamin B_{12} for adults by the NRC group carries a greater margin above normal physiologic requirements than does the FAO/WHO recommendation.

Vitamin B_{12} deficiency does not occur in breast-fed infants unless their mothers are deficient in the vitamin. Infants showing such deficiency respond hematologically to 0.1 μg of vitamin B_{12} orally.[93] In the economically advanced countries, breast milk supplies 0.3 μg of vitamin B_{12} daily, which is clearly adequate as manifested by lack of evidence of any deficiency in the infant. Available evidence suggests that the milk from mothers whose serum contains vitamin B_{12} concentrations close to the lower limit of normality (i.e. 200 pg per ml) is also adequate. The Joint FAO/WHO Expert Group therefore recommends 0.3 μg of vitamin B_{12} daily as the intake for infants on artificial feeding,[74] as does the NRC.

Vitamin B_{12} deficiency does not occur in normal children on adequate calorie and animal protein intakes. Therefore, the Joint FAO/WHO Expert Group[74] calculated desirable intakes of vitamin B_{12} for different ages in relation to the calorie intakes recommended for the respective age groups: 0.9 μg daily for children age 1 to 3 years (1 μg RDA), 1.5 for children age 4 to 9 years, 2 for age 10 years and over (3 μg RDA).

Pregnancy produces an increased requirement for vitamin B_{12} due to the fetal drain on maternal stores. The fetus removes approximately 0.2 μg of vitamin B_{12} daily from the maternal stores in the latter half of pregnancy; the Joint FAO/WHO Expert Group[74] calculated the desirable daily intake of vitamin B_{12} in pregnancy to be 3 μg (4 μg RDA).

Total recommended intake during lactation is 2.5 μg per day (4 μg RDA) based on the recommended daily intake of 2 for the normal adult (3 μg RDA) plus an additional 0.5 μg to accommodate the approximately 0.3 μg lost in the milk of nursing mothers.[74]

Natural Sources.[2,3,23,25–27,32,74,91,94] The sole source of vitamin B_{12} in nature is synthesis by microorganisms. The vitamin is not found in plants except when they are contaminated by microorganisms. Fruits, vegetables and grains and grain products are usually devoid of vitamin B_{12}. However, the root nodules of certain legumes contain microorganisms which make vitamin B_{12} and unwashed vegetable products may also contain vitamin B_{12} because of contamination by soil or fecal matter. These small amounts of vitamin B_{12} in legumes and food contamination may well provide the only dietary source of vitamin B_{12} for strict vegetarians. The usual dietary sources of vitamin B_{12} are meat and meat products (including shellfish, fish and poultry), and, to a lesser extent, milk and milk products. Rich sources of vitamin B_{12} (greater than 10 μg per 100 gm of wet weight) are organ meats such as lamb and beef liver, kidney and heart and bivalves (clams, oysters) which siphon large quantities of vitamin B_{12}-synthesizing microorganisms from the sea. Moderately high amounts (3 to 10 μg per 100 gm of wet weight) are present in nonfat dry milk, some seafood (crabs, rock fish, salmon, sardines) and egg yolk. Moderate amounts (1 to 3 μg per 100 gm wet weight) are found in muscle meats, some seafood (lobster, scallops, flounder, haddock, swordfish, tuna) and fermenting cheeses (Camembert, Limburger). There is less than 1 μg per 100 gm of wet weight in fluid milk products and in cream, cheddar and cottage cheese. Bacteria in the knobby growths of some seaweeds make the vitamin,[94a] and some manufacturers add the vitamin to breakfast cereals.

The vitamin B_{12} molecule is resistant to heat unless exposed in an alkaline medium to temperatures in excess of 100°C; the molecule splits at 250°C. Thus, hamburgers cooked on a hot griddle may lose some of their B_{12} from the surface flat against the hot griddle, but the vitamin B_{12} deep within the patty is preserved. Eight per cent of the vitamin B_{12} in liver is lost by boiling at 100°C for 5 minutes, while boiling muscle meat at 170°C for 45 minutes results in a loss of 30 per cent of the vitamin from the meat. Milk pasteurized for 2 to 3 seconds loses 7 per cent of its available vitamin B_{12}; when boiled for 2 to 5 minutes, it loses 30 per cent. Sterilization in a bottle for 13 minutes at 119 to 120°C causes a loss of 77 per cent; rapid sterilization (3 to 4 seconds) with superheated steam at 143°C destroys only about 10 per cent of the vitamin.[74] It should be noted that, in the presence of ascorbic acid, vitamin B_{12} is less heat stable and that substantial amounts in food may be destroyed by 0.5 gm of ascorbic acid.[35e,95,96,97] In light of this, if ascorbic acid is added to food, as has been suggested in some schemes of iron fortification,[98,99] this may lead to a significant reduction in vitamin B_{12} intake. In some circumstances, large doses of ascorbic acid may reduce vitamin B_{12} absorption.[99a]

The enzymatically active forms of vitamin B_{12} (coenzyme B_{12} and methylcobalamin) are the dominant forms in foodstuffs, in which they are generally attached to polypeptides. Cyanocobalamin per se is probably not present to a significant extent in any natural source. This stable form of vitamin B_{12} results from the action of cyanide on natural vitamin B_{12} coenzymes; thiocyanate ingestion and absorption of cyanide from tobacco smoke may convert a small amount of enzymatically active cobalamins in blood and tissues to cyanocobalamin.

Folic Acid

Nutritional Requirements.[3,32,74,90,91,100] The minimal daily requirement (MDR) for folate is in the range of 50 μg for adults. The FAO/WHO Expert Group recommends[30] a daily dietary intake (allowing for less than 100 per cent absorption) of 200 μg of "free" folate (defined as folate available to the microorganism L. casei without conjugase treatment) for adults, 50 μg for infants, 100 μg for children, 400 μg during pregnancy and 300 μg during lactation. The Nutrition Board's RDA for total folate, as assayed by L. casei from dietary sources after conjugase treatment, is 400 μg for adults and children over 10 years of age; it ranges from 50 μg for infants (under one year) through 100 μg (1 to 3 years), 200 μg (4 to 6 years) and 300 μg (7 to 10 years) to 600 μg for lactating women and 800 μg in pregnancy.[91] Since the daily folate requirement is hinged to the daily metabolic and cell turnover rates, it is increased by anything which increases metabolic rate (such as infection and hyperthyroidism), and anything which increases cell turnover (such as hemolytic anemia and rapid tissue growth in the fetus and malignant tumors). Folate consumption by individual cells is proportional to their rate of 1-carbon-unit transfer. Alcohol interferes with folate utilization, and thereby increases folate requirement.[101]

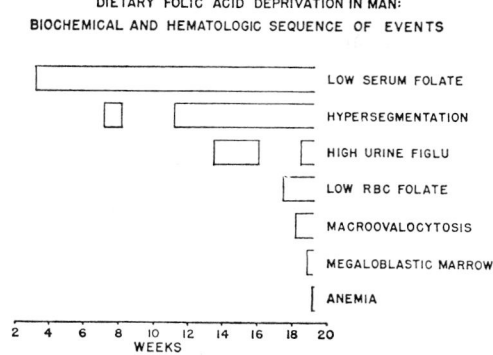

DIETARY FOLIC ACID DEPRIVATION IN MAN:
BIOCHEMICAL AND HEMATOLOGIC SEQUENCE OF EVENTS

LOW SERUM FOLATE
HYPERSEGMENTATION
HIGH URINE FIGLU
LOW RBC FOLATE
MACROOVALOCYTOSIS
MEGALOBLASTIC MARROW
ANEMIA

2   4   6   8   10 12 14 16 18 20
WEEKS

Fig. 6J–5. Biochemical and hematologic sequence of events in developing dietary folate deficiency in man. (From Herbert: Trans. Assoc. Am. Physicians, 75, 307, 1962.)

The sequence of events in developing folate deficiency in man is depicted in Figure 6J–5.

Natural Sources.[24,91,102–105] Unlike vitamin B_{12}, which is present only in animal protein, folates are ubiquitous in nature, being present in nearly all natural foods. Unlike vitamin B_{12}, folate is highly susceptible to oxidative destruction; 50 to 95 per cent of the folate content of foods may be destroyed by protracted cooking or other processing, such as canning, and all folate is lost from refined foods such as hard liquor and hard candies. Foods with the highest folate content per unit of dry weight include yeast, liver and other organ meats, fresh green vegetables and some fresh fruits.

The naturally occurring folates are active metabolic forms, usually in polyglutamate linkage[30] (with pteroylheptaglutamates dominant in yeast). Conjugases present in vegetable and mammalian tissues[106] (including human intestine) liberate pteroyldiglutamates and pteroylmonoglutamates from the conjugates, thereby making the folate available for absorption. About 90 per cent of monoglutamate is absorbed by humans when ingested on its own, but this proportion is markedly de-

creased in the presence of many foods, irrespective of whether the folate was derived from or added to the food.[59,60] Prior data suggesting that polyglutamate was poorly absorbed compared with monoglutamate were probably affected by other factors in the foods from which polyglutamate was derived, since the efficiency of polyglutamate hydrolysis in intestine[53,54] appears to rule it out as a rate-limiting step in folate absorption unless conjugase inhibitors are present.

The pharmaceutic product pteroylglutamic acid (PGA), like the pharmaceutic product cyanocobalamin, is not usually found as such in natural sources. Its isolation from natural sources, like the isolation of cyanocobalamin, was the result of oxidation and deconjugation of the naturally occurring conjugated forms to a stable form.

METABOLIC FUNCTIONS AND INTERRELATIONSHIPS[2,3,25,107–109]

DNA Synthesis

As illustrated in Figure 6J–6, both vitamin B_{12} and folic acid are required for synthesis of thymidylate, and therefore of DNA. A vitamin B_{12}-containing enzyme removes a methyl group from methyl folate and delivers it to homocysteine, thereby converting homocysteine to methionine (methyl-homocysteine) and regenerating THFA, from which the 5,10-methylene THFA involved in thymidylate synthesis is made. Since methyl folate is the dominant form of folate in human serum and liver, and probably also in other body storage depots for folate, and since methyl folate may only return to the body's folate pool via a vitamin B_{12}-dependent step, when a patient suffers from vitamin B_{12} deficiency much of his folate is "trapped" as methyl folate, and thus is metabolically useless. This "folate trap" hypothesis[52,107–110] may provide much of the explanation of why the hematologic damage of vitamin B_{12} de-

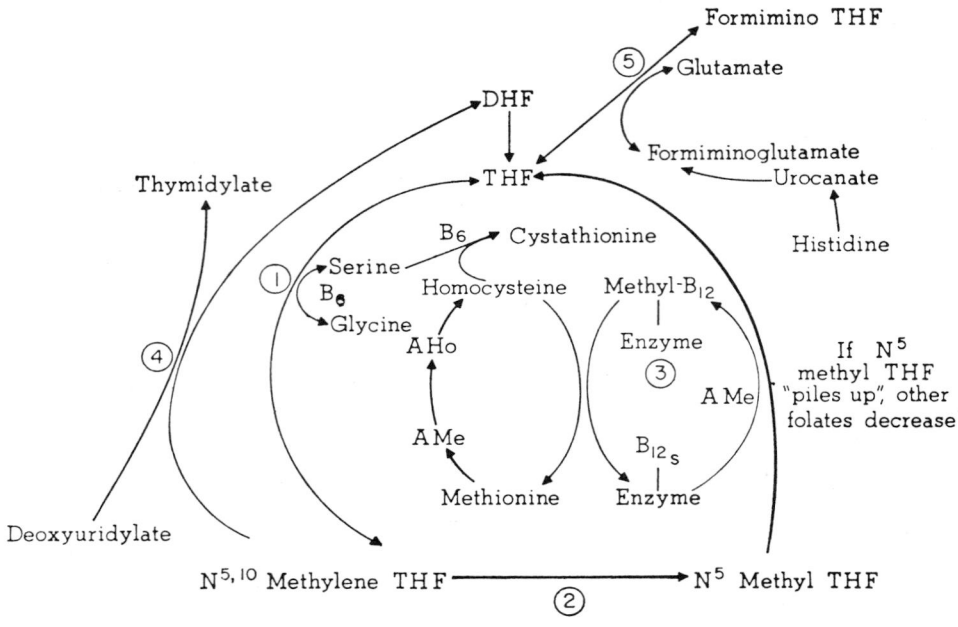

Fig. 6J–6. Interrelationships of vitamin B_{12}, B_6 and folate. (From Herbert [25] with permission of J. & A. Churchill.)

ficiency is not clinically distinguishable from that of folate deficiency. In both instances, the hematologic damage results from lack of adequate 5,10-methylene THFA, which delivers its methyl group to deoxyuridylate to convert that substance to thymidylate, and thus makes DNA during the S phase. In either deficiency lack of adequate DNA synthesis causes many hematopoietic cells to die in the bone marrow, very possibly without ever completing the S phase of cell replication (i.e. a form of "ineffective erythropoiesis").

Megaloblastosis (the presence of giant germ cells) is the end-product of deranged DNA synthesis of any cause. It is most easily understood as an arrest in the S (synthesis) phase of cell replication, usually because of inadequate availability of vitamin B_{12} or folate, with most replicating cells in the body, instead of being in a resting phase, being in the process of attempting (with poor success) to double

their DNA in order to divide. The underlying biochemical defect which translates poor thymidylate synthesis (due to folate and/or vitamin B_{12} deficiency) into morphologic megaloblastosis may be failure to elongate DNA chains in the presence of a relatively normal capacity to initiate DNA synthesis, presumably because the lowered thymidylate concentrations remain adequate to serve as substrate for "initiating" DNA-polymerase but not for "elongating" DNA polymerase.[111]

Morphologic changes are most striking in bone marrow cells, with the "ineffective hematopoiesis" resulting in peripheral blood pancytopenia (anemia, leukopenia and thrombopenia). However, megaloblastosis is also present in all other duplicating cells of the body[3,112] and may be strikingly noted in the epithelial cells of the entire alimentary tract, producing glossitis and variable degrees of megaloblastosis along the entire alimentary tract epithelium. It is not yet clear why gut changes associated with vitamin B_{12} deficiency are often associated with constipation whereas those associated with folate deficiency are more commonly associated with diarrhea; these differences may be related to phenomena other than the nutrient deficiency per se.

Since growth is dependent on cell replication, and cell replication is dependent on DNA synthesis, both vitamin B_{12} and folic acid are required for growth.

"Packaging" Folate in Cells

Another important interrelationship of these two vitamins is the involvement of vitamin B_{12} in the transport and storage of folate in cells.[113-118] In vitamin B_{12} deficiency, there is impaired transport of methyltetrahydrofolate into bone marrow cells[116] and transformed lymphocytes,[115] with correction of the defect after addition of vitamin B_{12}.[116] Similarly, humans and experimental animals with vitamin B_{12} deficiency have low erythrocyte folate and decreased liver folate stores. These defects are probably attributable to failure of vitamin B_{12}-dependent homocysteine: methionine transmethylation. Failure to remove the methyl group from folate, causing an intracellular "methyl trap,"[3,112] may interfere with dissociation of the carrier-folate complex at the inner cell wall and impair transport into the cell,[82] and it does impair folate storage because tetrahydrofolate is preferred over methyltetrahydrofolate as a substrate for polyglutamate synthetase.[117,118]

Inadequate myelin synthesis with resultant neurologic damage results from vitamin B_{12} deficiency but not from folate deficiency.[3,112] The biochemical basis for this defective myelin synthesis is unknown. Since myelin is lipoprotein, vitamin B_{12} must have some as yet undetermined role in synthesis of either the lipid or the protein component of myelin. It has been proposed that the neurologic damage relates to the B_{12} requirement for the propionate-methylmalonate conversion, but this is probably not so because infants born lacking the apoenzyme for this conversion do not have damaged myelin, and the abnormalities reported in fatty acids in myelin of vitamin B_{12}-deficient subjects[119] may well relate to plasmalogen[120] rather than to B_{12} deficiency. The nervous system damage caused by vitamin B_{12} deficiency involves,[112] in addition to myelinated peripheral nerves, the myelinated posterior and lateral cords of the spinal column, and therefore nervous system damage from this deficiency has been variously termed subacute combined degeneration, combined system disease, posterolateral sclerosis and funicular degeneration. However, the disease usually starts insidiously and not subacutely, combined lesions are often absent and lesions of the peripheral nerves occur more frequently and earlier than lesions of the central nervous system. For these reasons, the nervous system changes are more accurately described by direct reference to the actual involvement (i.e. peripheral nerve or spinal cord or cerebral damage).

The various neurologic symptoms and signs resulting from the inadequate myelin synthesis caused by vitamin B_{12} deficiency include paresthesia, especially numbness and tingling in the hands and feet, diminution of vibration sense and/or position sense (usually but not always occurring first in the ankles and feet), unsteadiness, poor muscular coordination with ataxia, moodiness, mental slowness, poor memory, confusion, agitation, depression and central scotomata (sometimes with dim vision due to optic atrophy or tobacco amblyopia); delusions, hallucinations and even overt psychosis (usually with paranoid ideas) may occur. The wide variety of sensory and motor changes tend to be symmetrical, especially if present for a period of weeks or months.

It has been our observation that economically advantaged people with vitamin B_{12} deficiency tend to have relatively severe neurologic damage and relatively mild hematologic damage, whereas poor people with vitamin B_{12} deficiency tend to have relatively equal severity of neurologic and hematologic damage. We believe that a major explanation for the variable degree of hematologic damage with fixed amount of neurologic damage in vitamin B_{12} deficiency is the quantity of folate in the diet. Well-to-do people tend to eat better diets, richer in high-folate-containing foods such as fresh fruits and fresh vegetables as well as fresh meats. The folate retards development of hematologic damage, while allowing neurologic damage to progress.

Folate deficiency does not damage myelin, but it is associated with a high frequency of irritability, forgetfulness and, often, hostility and paranoid behavior. These phenomena often strikingly improve within 24 hours of the start of therapy with folic acid. Other neurologic sequelae attributed by some to folate deficiency have been reviewed elsewhere,[121] but the association has not been convincingly demonstrated.[85]

Cerebration may improve rapidly when vitamin B_{12} deficiency is appropriately treated, but the neurologic damage resulting from inadequate myelin synthesis heals slowly. Since the nerve damage is related to deterioration of the axon underneath the deteriorated myelin, healing is related to the speed of regeneration of damaged axons; this regeneration creeps peripherally from the nerve head at the rate of 0.1 mm per day.

B_{12} in Fat and Carbohydrate Metabolism[3,23,25,27,30,122]

Since coenzyme B_{12} is required for the hydrogen transfer and isomerization whereby methylmalonate is converted to succinate,[23,25] B_{12} is involved in both fat and carbohydrate metabolism. As indicated above, although it is an attractive speculation that one reason for the neurologic damage of patients with vitamin B_{12} deficiency is inability to make the lipid portion of the lipoprotein myelin sheath

(due to inadequate propionic acid utilization related to inadequate interconversion of methylmalonate and succinate), there is not yet evidence to tie this to the neurologic damage of vitamin B_{12} deficiency in man.

More recently, it has been shown that rat glial cells grown in vitamin B_{12}-deficient media produce 2 odd-chain fatty acids which are not found when the cells are grown in the presence of vitamin B_{12}.[123] Further, nerve biopsies from subjects with vitamin B_{12} deficiency incubated in ^{14}C-labeled proprionate produced labeled [15]C and ^{14}C fatty acids, whereas biopsies from normal subjects produced labeled ^{12}C and ^{14}C fatty acids.[124] The explanation for this finding and its relationship to the functional and histologic changes have not yet been elucidated.

B_{12} in Protein and Fat Metabolism[23,25,27,30]

Vitamin B_{12} is involved in protein synthesis through its role in the synthesis of the amino acid methionine, and possibly in other ways as well. Since methionine is involved in making available more of the lipotropic substances choline and betaine, this is another point where cobalamin may play a role in lipid metabolism.

B_{12} as a Reducing Agent[3,23,125]

Vitamin B_{12} appears concerned in maintenance of sulfhydryl groups in the reduced form necessary for function of many SH-activated enzyme systems. Vitamin B_{12} deficiency is characterized by a decrease in reduced glutathione (which is changed from GSH to GSGG) of erythrocytes and liver. This is correctable by administration of vitamin B_{12}. In vitro, vitamin B_{12} derivatives catalyze the nonenzymatic oxidation of sulfhydryl derivatives.

Folates in 1-Carbon-unit Transfers[24,30,126]

Folate coenzymes are concerned with mammalian metabolic systems involving transfer of a 1-carbon unit. These reactions include (1) de novo purine synthesis (formylation of glycinamide ribonucleotide [GAR] and 5-amino-4-imidazole carboxamide ribonucleotide [AICAR]), (2) pyrimidine nucleotide biosynthesis (methylation of deoxyuridylic acid to thymidylic acid), (3) 3 amino acid conversions: (a) the interconversion of serine and glycine (which also requires vitamin B_6), (b) catabolism of histidine to glutamic acid, (c) conversion of homocysteine to methionine (which also requires vitamin B_6), (4) generation of formate into the formate pool (and utilization of formate), (5) methylation of small amounts of transfer RNA. The suggestion that folate may be involved in physiologic methylation of biogenic amines[127] has been refuted.[128]

Role of Ascorbic Acid

It is possible that ascorbate in vivo may aid in the protection against oxidative destruction of reduced folates in the body. There is no evidence that ascorbate plays any role in the reduction of pteroylglutamic acid to tetrahydrofolic acid, a reaction mediated by folate reductases; the original such evidence proved to be protection by ascorbate of the end-product against oxidative destruction.

Selective Nutrient Deficiency

A possibly important new area of nutrition research is selective nutrient deficiency in one cell line and not another in the same patient. Two papers describing selective folate deficiency in white cells but not red cells were recently published.[128a,128b] Those studies delineated the use of lymphocytes (which in their resting form in the human blood stream appear impervious, not only to vitamin B_{12} and folic acid, but also to other nutrients, such as nicotinamide[128c]) to measure past nutrient deficiency up to two months after therapy,[128a] and also to measure covert folate deficiency in iron-deficient patients.[128b] Only when lymphocytes are making DNA do they appear to become pervious to nutrients.[128a,128b,128c]

THERAPY[3]

The only established therapeutic use of vitamin B_{12} or folic acid is in treating deficiency of the respective vitamin. Claims made for nutritional value of either of these vitamins in clinical situations in which deficiency of the vitamin does not exist are without foundation in fact.

When the deficiency is of vitamin B_{12}, only this vitamin should be used for therapy; conversely, when the deficiency is of folate, only that vitamin should be used for therapy. The use of folic acid in the treatment of a patient whose deficiency is of vitamin B_{12} will often produce hematologic improvement of a temporary nature, but will allow the neurologic damage of the underlying vitamin B_{12} deficiency to progress, often to an irreversible state.

Although liver extract for injection was deleted from the U.S.P. in 1960, such products are still being used by some practitioners and appear in the National Formulary. For clinical purposes the injectable unit is approximately the equivalent of 1.33 μg of vitamin B_{12}. It should be noted that since preparations of liver extract contain hematopoietic materials other than vitamin B_{12} (e.g. folic acid, folinic acid), they constitute shotgun therapy, like many other multi-ingredient therapies, and such use is to be avoided.

The signs and symptoms of deficiency of vitamin B_{12} or folate in man[1-3,111,129-131] are listed in Table 6J–2.

Therapy of the Critically Ill Patient

It is rarely necessary to institute immediate therapy prior to determining the cause of megaloblastic anemia. Major indications for emergency therapy include severe thrombocytopenia (platelet count less than 50,000 per cu mm) associated with bleeding, severe leukopenia (white cell count less than 3,000 per cu mm) associated with infection, infection itself, coma, severe disorientation, marked neurologic damage, severe hepatic disease, uremia or

Table 6J–2.   Clinical Picture of the Megaloblastic Anemias

1. Symptoms
    Weakness, tiredness
    Dyspnea
    Sore tongue
    Paresthesia (B_{12} deficiency only)
    Diarrhea (especially folate deficiency)
    Constipation (especially B_{12} deficiency)
    Irritability and forgetfulness (especially folate deficiency)
    Anorexia
    Syncope
    Headache
    Palpitation
2. Signs
    Megaloblastic bone marrow (orthochromatic megaloblasts, giant metamyelocytes)
    Anemia, leukopenia, thrombocytopenia, with macroovalocytes (normal MVC = 87 ± 5 cu μ) and "hyper-segmented polys" (normal Arneth count 2 lobes = 20 to 40 per cent, 3 lobes = 40 to 50 per cent, 4 lobes = 15 to 25 per cent, 5 lobes = 0 to 5 per cent, 6 lobes = 0 to 0.1 per cent, more than 6 lobes = 0) (normal "lobe average" = 3.17 ± 0.25). (Rule of fives: When 100 neutrophils counted, the presence of 5 or more with 5 or more lobes means hypersegmentation.)
    Morphologic red herrings: congenital hypersegmentation (approximately 1 per cent of population), hypersegmentation with renal disease; twinning deformities; macrocytes of pyruvate kinase deficiency, aplastic anemia, reticulocytosis, hypothyroidism, neoplasia.
    Fever
    Icterus plus pallor (lemon-yellow skin)
    Glossitis
        Acute
        Chronic atrophic
    Neurologic damage (only proven in B_{12} deficiency, which damages myelin)
        Vibration sense diminished
        Position sense diminished, ataxia, "combined systems disease"
        Impaired mentation, paranoid ideation (seen in both deficiencies)
    Malabsorption
    Achylia gastrica (primary with B_{12} deficiency, secondary with folate deficiency) (reduced intrinsic factor)
    Splenomegaly (in approximately one third of cases, if looked for radiologically)
    Weight loss (especially folate deficiency)
    Pigmentation; vitiligo
    Postural hypotension (especially B_{12} deficiency)
    Low serum vitamin B_{12} or folate level
    Elevated serum lactic dehydrogenase (LDH)
    Elevated urine formiminoglutamate
    Methylmalonic aciduria (B_{12} deficiency only)
    High serum iron, increased saturation of iron-binding capacity of serum, increased bone marrow iron stores, normal free erythrocyte protoporphyrin
    Low red cell folate is present in either deficiency
    Circulating antibody to intrinsic factor in two-thirds of pernicious anemia patients
    Circulating antibody to gastric parietal cells in most patients with gastric damage, regardless of cause
    Abnormal "dU suppression test"
    Abnormal liver function tests
    Subnormal intestinal absorption
    Low red cell B_{12} or folate level; low lymphocyte B_{12} or folate

other debilitating illness complicating the anemia. The anemia itself is not a problem since the dyspnea and occasional angina which may accompany a hematocrit of less than 15 volumes per cent are relieved by a transfusion of 1 to 2 units of packed erythrocytes. Transfusion is unwarranted in the absence of symptoms of anemia. When venous pressure is elevated, transfusion of packed erythrocytes should be accompanied by withdrawal of equivalent or slightly smaller quantities of whole blood. This will reduce rather than raise the venous pressure; transfusion of whole blood without withdrawal of blood has been responsible for acute rises in venous pressure with resultant irreversible congestive failure in elderly patients with megaloblastic anemia and unrecognized elevated venous pressure. Ideally, venous pressure should be determined prior to transfusion, and monitored during both the transfusion of packed cells and the simultaneous withdrawal of whole blood. This may easily be done by use of a 3-way stopcock, injecting the packed cells in units of 50 ml, followed by determination of venous pressure change and withdrawal of 30 to 50 ml of whole blood, prior to repeating the whole procedure with injection of another 50 ml of erythrocytes. An alternate to exchange transfusion is to precede the administration of blood by the parenteral injection of a diuretic.

When, for one or more of the reasons discussed above, immediate vitamin therapy is necessary before etiologic diagnosis, 100 μg of cyanocobalamin and 15 mg of folic acid are given intramuscularly, followed by 5 mg of folic acid by mouth and 100 μg of vitamin B_{12} intramuscularly daily, for a week. Such treatment will produce excellent hematologic response except in cases in which hematopoiesis is suppressed by infection, uremia, chloramphenicol administration or some other factor.

Vitamin B_{12} Therapy

Vitamin B_{12} deficiency in man is nearly always due to inadequate ingestion and/or inadequate absorption, and therapy is guided by adequate etiologic diagnosis (Table 6J–1).

Inadequate ingestion of vitamin B_{12} is corrected by adding to the daily diet any food containing vitamin B_{12} (i.e. meat or meat products, including fish, shellfish or poultry). If the patient, because of poverty, cannot afford meat or meat products, or, for religious or other reasons, is a strict vegetarian, adequate treatment consists of 1 μg of vitamin B_{12} orally daily supplied as liquid or tablet.

When the vitamin B_{12} deficiency is due to inadequate absorption, 1 μg of vitamin B_{12} parenterally (subcutaneously or intramuscularly) daily constitutes adequate therapy. A single injection of 100 μg or more of vitamin B_{12} will produce a complete therapeutic remission in any patient whose deficiency is not complicated by unrelated systemic disease or other factors. The remission is sustained for life by monthly injections of 100 μg of vitamin B_{12}. It is important to point out to the patient who has permanent gastric or ileal damage that he must receive monthly injections of vitamin B_{12} for life.

For simultaneous differential diagnosis and therapy, patients should be treated with an injection of 1 μg of vitamin B_{12} daily for 10 days, after a control period of a few days to establish the constancy of the reticulocyte level, elimination of dietary sources of vitamin B_{12} and folic acid (by provision of a diet consisting exclusively of well-cooked finely particulate grains or vegetables, such as rice and beans, and beverages devoid of vitamin B_{12} and folate, such as tea, coffee and soft drinks). Such a therapeutic trial is illustrated in Figure 6J–7, from Herbert.[129] Not shown in the figure is the leukopenia or thrombopenia often seen in untreated megaloblastic

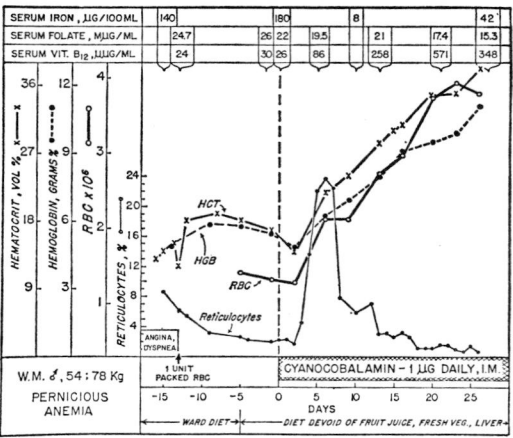

Fig. 6J–7. Response of a patient with uncomplicated vitamin B_{12} deficiency to therapy with 1 μg daily of parenteral vitamin B_{12}. (From Herbert[129] with permission of the New England Journal of Medicine.)

Folic Acid Therapy

For combined differential diagnosis and therapy, the patient is treated with 100 μg of folic acid orally daily (if the suspected diagnosis is dietary inadequacy), or parenterally (if the suspected diagnosis is folate malabsorption). This dosage will produce a maximal hematologic response in patients with folate deficiency, but will not produce hematologic response in patients with vitamin B_{12} deficiency. Therapeutic trial with a parenteral dose of 50 μg of pteroylglutamic acid daily in a patient with folate deficiency is shown in Figure 6J–8, again from Herbert.[129] Note in the figure that ascorbic acid per se has no hematopoietic effect in folate deficiency. The expected sharp fall in plasma iron level does not occur when ascorbate therapy is used, because vitamin C produces a rise in serum iron which cancels out the early fall that otherwise develops when folate deficiency is treated with folate (or vitamin B_{12} deficiency is treated with

anemia; granulocytes and platelets return to normal levels within 1 week after the start of therapy, at approximately the time reticulocytes reach their peak level.

Initial therapy with doses of vitamin B_{12} greater than 1 μg daily is desirable when the vitamin B_{12} deficiency is complicated with other debilitating illness such as infection, hepatic disease, uremia, coma, severe disorientation or marked neurologic damage. In such cases, 30 μg or more of vitamin B_{12} is given daily parenterally for 5 to 10 days. Daily parenteral doses larger than 30 μg have no proven therapeutic advantage, and much of the excess is rapidly excreted in the urine.

Hydroxocobalamin and other depot preparations of vitamin B_{12} may be retained longer at the site of injection and in serum, but this possible slight therapeutic advantage over cyanocobalamin does not warrant their greater cost; they also may have undesirable side effects. More detailed discussion of vitamin B_{12} preparations, routes of administration, dosage and therapeutic responses may be found in *The Pharmacological Basis of Therapeutics.*[3]

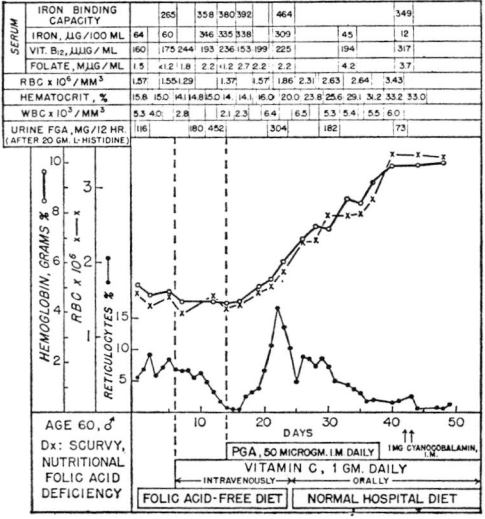

Fig. 6J–8. Hematologic response to parenteral administration of 50 μg of folic (pteroylglutamic) acid daily, in a patient with nutritional folate deficiency and treated scurvy. (From Herbert[129] with permission of the New England Journal of Medicine.)

vitamin B_{12}).[132] As in treated vitamin B_{12} deficiency, treatment of folate deficiency returns subnormal leukocyte and platelet levels to normal within a week after the start of therapy, at approximately the time of the reticulocyte peak.

Therapy with doses of folic acid larger than 0.1 mg daily is desirable when the folate deficiency state is complicated by conditions which may suppress hematopoiesis (such as unrelated systemic disease), conditions that increase folate requirement (pregnancy, hypermetabolic states, alcoholism, hemolytic anemia) and conditions that reduce folate absorption. Therapy should then be with 0.5 to 1 mg daily. There is no evidence that doses greater than 1 mg daily have any greater efficacy; additionally, loss of folate in the urine becomes roughly logarithmic as the amount administered exceeds 1 mg.

Maintenance therapy is normally 0.1 mg of folic acid daily for 1 to 4 months, and then should be stopped only if the diet contains at least one fresh fruit or fresh vegetable daily. If the daily folate requirement is increased due to an increased metabolic or cell-turnover rate the maintenance dose should be 0.2 to 0.5 mg daily.

Ideal nutritional therapy for dietary folate deficiency is the ingestion of one fresh fruit or one fresh vegetable daily; such a diet would probably wipe nutritional folate deficiency from the face of the earth.[130] As it is, nutritional folate deficiency probably encompasses approximately a third of all the pregnant women in the world.[74]

The Prevention of Folate Deficiency

It is the consensus that pregnant women should receive folate supplements,[3] and they have been recommended in clinical disorders which increase the risk of folate deficiency. Major problems have been encountered in the delivery of such supplements to patients. It has been shown that significant numbers of pregnant women do not ingest iron tablets given to them,[133] but this problem may not be as severe when tablets containing both iron and folate are given, since a separate report[134] suggests that the adverse gastrointestinal effects of iron ingestion may be decreased when folic acid is simultaneously ingested. The largest component of the problem is that antenatal care is not available to, or taken advantage of by, large numbers of pregnant women, particularly in populations where folate deficiency is common.[135] This phenomenon has again been highlighted by the observation that of 110 consecutive women seeking prenatal care in New York City, 61 were in the second trimester and 26 already in the third trimester of pregnancy.[136]

As an alternative approach to the alleviation of the problem, a series of studies was devised to determine the feasibility of fortifying staple foods with folic acid.[60,135,137-140] When the data generated in these studies are judged against criteria delineated by an Expert Committee of the World Health Organization (WHO) and Food and Agricultural Organization (FAO),[141] such fortification appears feasible, inexpensive, effective and safe in populations with a demonstrable need for increased dietary levels of folic acid. It has been suggested that such elevations may increase the incidence and/or severity of neurologic damage in subjects with pernicious anemia, but the literature contains little data to support this view. This reservation thus seems minor when weighed against the primary object of food fortifications, namely, the elevation of dietary folate levels in large undernourished populations to amounts present in the diet of more affluent people who rarely suffer folate deficiency, i.e. to levels approaching the RDA. A joint meeting of the WHO and other bodies has recommended that authorities concerned with populations in which folate deficiency is common should initiate trials to determine the feasibility and effectiveness of food fortification with folate in those populations.[142]

TOXICITY[3]

It is hard to accept that either vitamin B_{12} or folic acid, being necessary for life, could, in quantities close to minimal daily requirements, be toxic in man. In fact, these substances are nontoxic in man not only in small doses but also in doses which exceed the minimal daily adult human requirement by 10,000-fold for vitamin B_{12} and several hundred-fold for folic acid. Being water-soluble, excesses of these vitamins tend to be excreted in the urine rather than, like the fat-soluble vitamins, being stored in tissues. Vitamin B_{12} and folic acid both appear to require binding to polypeptides as a precondition of storage; excesses above the limited serum- and tissue-available-binding capacity tend to be excreted rather than retained.

A rare allergic reaction has been reported, possibly due to impurities in a rare preparation of crystalline cyanocobalamin.[25] Hydroxocobalamin injections and injections of various depot preparations of cyanocobalamin have been associated with the appearance of antibody to plasma vitamin B_{12}-binding protein.[127] While the significance of this antibody is not yet clear, such preparations offer no clear advantage over cyanocobalamin to warrant their use, especially in view of their greater cost and the pain on injection of some of the depot preparations.

One questionable instance of an allergic reaction to folic acid has been reported in man.[2] Daily doses of up to 15 mg in man are without toxic effects; this daily dose is well below that which could lead to precipitation of crystalline folic acid in the kidneys (precipitation produces renal toxicity in rats given massive doses of folic acid). Folic acid has been reported to partially reverse the antiepileptic effects of phenobarbital, diphenylhydantoin, and primidone, and thereby increases seizure frequency in patients getting anticonvulsant therapy.[121,144]

Although no such effect has been observed in many controlled studies using an oral dose of 15 mg folic acid daily, there is now firm experimental and clinical evidence that very high concentrations of folic acid can have a convulsant effect.[121] Most of the data were obtained in experimental studies in animals and indicated that the convulsant dose of folic acid in normal rats was 45 to 125 mg if administered intravenously and 15 to 30 mg if preceded by the induction of a focal cortical lesion.[145] Convulsions have been reported in one of 8 epileptics given parenteral folic acid under electrocephalographic monitoring;[146] this occurred after the rapid intravenous infusion of 14.4 mg folic acid, which presumably elevated serum folate concentration in the cerebral vessels several times higher than would be the case after folic acid ingestion.[85,121]

BIBLIOGRAPHY

1. Castle: Trans. Am. Clin. Climatol. Assoc., *73*, 53, 1961; Kass: *Pernicious Anemia*. Philadelphia, W.B. Saunders, 1976.
2. Chanarin: *The Megaloblastic Anemias*. Philadelphia, F. A. Davis, 1969.
3. Herbert: In *The Pharmacological Basis of Therapeutics*, 5th ed. (Goodman and Gilman, Eds.). New York, The Macmillan Co., 1975.
4. Combe: Trans R. Med. Chir. Soc. Edinb., *7*, 194, 1822.
5. Addison: *On the Constitutional and Local Effects of Disease of the Suprarenal Capsules*. London, S. Highley, 1855.
6. Flint: Am. Med. Times, *7*, 181, 1860.
7. Castle: Am. J. Med. Sci., *178*, 748, 1929.
8. Rickes, Brink, Koniuszy, Wood and Folkers: Science, *107*, 396, 1948.
9. Smith and Parker: Biochem. J., *43*, viii, 1948.
10. Berk, Castle, Welch, Heinie, Anker and Epstein: N. Engl. J. Med., *239*, 911, 1948.
11. Channing: N. Engl. Q. J. Med. Surg., *1*:157, 1842.
12. Barclay: Quoted by Castle.[1]
13. Osler: Br. Med. J., *1*, 1, 1919.
14. Wills, Clutterbuck and Evans: Biochem. J., *31*, 2136, 1937.
15. Stokstad: J. Biol. Chem., *149*, 573, 1943.
16. Pfiffer, Binkley, Bloom, Brown, Bird and Emmett: Science, *86*, 404, 1943.
17. Angier, Boothe, Hutchings, Mowat, Semb, Stokstad, Subba Row, Walter, Cosulich, Farrenbach, Hultquist, Kuh, Northey, Seeger, Sickels and Smith: J. Am. Chem. Soc., *103*, 667, 1946.
18. Shorb: Science, *107*, 397, 1948.
19. Day, Mims, Totter, Stockstad, Hutchings and Sloane: J. Biol. Chem., *157*, 423, 1945.
20. Snell and Peterson: J. Bacteriol., *39*, 273, 1940.

21. Mitchell, Snell and Williams: J. Am. Chem. Soc., 63, 2284, 1941.
22. Minot and Murphy: J.A.M.A., 87, 470, 1926.
23. Smith: *Vitamin B₁₂*, 3rd ed. London, Methuen & Co.: New York, John Wiley & Sons, 1965. Babior (Ed.): *Cobalamin*. New York, John Wiley & Sons, 1975. Pratt: *Inorganic Chemistry of Vitamin B₁₂*. New York, Academic Press, 1972.
24. Blakley: *The Biochemistry of Folic Acid and Related Pteridines*. New York, John Wiley & Sons, 1969; Food and Nutrition Board: *Folic Acid*. Washington, National Academy of Sciences, 1977.
25. Arnstein and Wrighton (Eds.): *The Cobalamins*, London, J. & A. Churchill, 1971.
26. Heinrich (Ed.): *Vitamin B₁₂ and Intrinsic Factor*, Second European Symposium. Stuttgart, Ferdinand Enke Verlag, 1962.
27. Perlman (Ed.): Vitamin B₁₂ Coenzymes, a Symposium. Ann. N.Y. Acad. Sci., 112, 547, 1964.
28. IUPAC-IUB Commission on Biochemical Nomenclature: Nomenclature of vitamins, coenzymes and related compounds. Tentative rules. J. Biol. Chem., 241, 2991, 1966.
29. Sullivan and Herbert: N. Engl. J. Med., 272, 340, 1965.
30. Scott and Weir: Clin. Haematol., 5, 547, 1976.
31. WHO Scientific Group: Nutritional anemias. WHO Tech. Rep. Ser. #450, 1968; FAO/WHO Expert Group: Requirements of ascorbic acid, vitamin B₁₂, folate, and iron. WHO Tech. Rep. Ser. #452, 1970.
32. Skeggs: *Vitamin B₁₂* in *The Vitamins: Chemistry, Physiology, Pathology, Methods*, Vol. VII, 2nd ed. (Gyorgy and Pearson, Eds). New York, Academic Press, 1967.
33. Herbert: Am. J. Clin. Nutr., 7, 433, 1959.
34. Lau, Gottlieb, Wasserman and Herbert: Blood, 26, 202, 1965.
35. Herbert: In *B₁₂ and Folate Analysis with Radionuclides in Hematopoietic and Gastrointestinal Investigations with Radionuclides* (Gilson and Smoak, Eds.). Springfield, Charles C Thomas, 1972.
35a. Gottlieb, Retief, and Herbert: Biochim. Biophys. Acta, 141, 560, 1967.
35b. Kolhouse, Kondo, Allen, Podell and Allen: N. Engl. J. Med., 299, 785, 1978.
35c. Cooper and Whitehead: N. Engl. J. Med., 299, 816, 1978.
35d. Donaldson: N. Engl. J. Med., 299, 827, 1978.
35e. Herbert, Jacob, Wong, Scott and Pfeffer: Am. J. Clin. Nutr., 31, 253, 1978.
36. Herbert and Bertino: In *The Vitamins: Chemistry, Physiology, Pathology, Methods*, Vol. VII, 2nd ed. (Gyorgy and Perarson, Eds.). New York, Academic Press, 1967.
37. Herbert: In *Clinical Biochemistry* (Curtius and Roth, Eds.). Berlin and New York, Verlag Walter de Gruyter, 1974.
38. Herbert, Wasserman, Frank, Pasher and Baker: Fed. Proc., 18, 246, 1959.
39. Baker, Herbert, Frank, Pasher, Hutner, Wasserman and Sobotka: Clin. Chem., 5, 275, 1959.
40. Herbert, Baker, Frank, Pasher, Sobotka and Wasserman: Blood, 15, 228, 1960.
41. Herbert: J. Clin. Invest., 40, 81, 1961.
42. Herbert: J. Clin. Pathol., 19, 12, 1966.
43. Waxman, Schreiber and Herbert: Blood, 36, 858, 1970; 38, 219, 1971. Rothenberg, da Costa and Rosenberg: N. Engl. J. Med., 286, 1335, 1972.
44. Longo and Herbert: J. Lab. Clin. Med., 87, 138, 1976.
45. Gutcho and Mansbach: Clin. Chem., 23, 1609, 1977.
46. Jacob, Colman and Herbert: Clin. Res., 25, 537A, 1977.
47. Glass: Physiol. Rev., 43, 529, 1963.
48. Herbert: Gastroenterology, 54, 110, 1968. Herbert: Semin. Nucl. Med., 2, 220, 1972.
49. Grasbeck: In *Intrinsic Factor and Other Vitamin B₁₂ Transport Proteins* in *Progress in Hematology*, Vol. VI (Brown and Moore, Eds.). New York, Grune & Stratton, 1969.
50. Carmel, Rosenberg, Lau, Streiff and Herbert: Gastroenterology, 56, 548, 1969.
51. Corcino, Waxman and Herbert: Am. J. Med., 48, 562, 1970. Chanarin: J. Clin. Pathol., 24 (Suppl.) (R. Coll. Pathol.), 5, 60, 1971.
51a. Bernstein and Herbert: Am. J. Clin. Nutr., 26, 340, 1973.
51b. Allen, Beetharam, Allen, and Podell: J. Clin. Invest., 61, 1628, 1978.
52. Butterworth and Krumdieck: Br. J. Hematol. 31 (Suppl.), 111, 1975.
53. Rosenberg: Clin. Haematol., 5, 589, 1976.
54. Halsted, Baugh and Butterworth: Gastroenterology, 68, 261, 1975.
55. Reisenauer, Krumdieck and Halsted: Fed. Proc., 36, 1120, 1977.
56. Butterworth, Newman and Krumdieck: Trans. Am. Clin. Climatol. Assoc., 86, 11, 1974.
57. Tamura, Shin, Buehring and Stokstad: Br. J. Haematol., 32, 123, 1976.
58. Gerson, Cohen, Hepner, Brown, Herbert and Janowitz: Gastroenterology, 61, 224, 1971.
59. Tamura and Stokstad: Br. J. Haematol., 25, 513, 1973.
60. Colman, Green and Metz: Am. J. Clin. Nutr., 28, 459, 1975.
61. Smith, Matty and Blair: Biochim. Biophys. Acta, 219, 37, 1970.
62. Hall: Ann. Intern. Med., 75, 297, 1971. Stenman: Scand. J. Haematol., 14, 91, 1975. Allen: Br. J. Haematol., 33, 161, 1976.
63. Herbert: Am. J. Clin. Nutr., 7, 433, 1959. Castro, Herbert, and Wasserman: J. Clin. Invest., 40, 66, 1961. Herbert: Blood, 32, 305, 1968. Carmel and Herbert: Blood, 40, 542, 1972.
64. Jacob, Wong and Herbert: J. Lab. Clin. Med., 89, 1145, 1977.
65. Allen: Prog. Hematol., 9, 57, 1975. Stenman: Scand.J. Clin. Lab. Invest., 35, 157, 1975. Gräsbeck: Br. J. Haematol., 31 (Suppl.), 103, 1975.
66. Begley and Hall: Blood, 45, 287, 1975.
67. Corcino, Zalusky, Greenberg and Herbert: Br. J. Haematol., 20, 511, 1971.
68. Tan and Hansen: Proc. Soc. Exp. Biol. Med., 127, 740, 1968.
69. Cooksley, England, Louis, Down and Tavill: Clin. Sci. Mol. Med., 47, 531, 1974.

70. Savage and Green: Fed. Proc., *34*, 905, 1975.
71. Retief, Gottlieb and Herbert: J. Clin. Invest.,*45*, 1907, 1966.
72. Hakami, Neiman, Cannellos and Lazerson: N. Engl. J. Med., *285*, 1163, 1971.
73. Scott, Hakami, Teng and Sagerson: J. Pediatr., *81*, 1106, 1972.
73a. Fleming, Ogunfunmilade and Carmel: Am. J. Clin. Nutr., *31*, 1732, 1978.
73b. Frater-Schroder, Hitzig, Grob and Kenney: Lancet, *2*, 238, 1978.
74. FAO-WHO Expert group: Requirements of ascorbic acid, vitamin D, vitamin B_{12}, folate, and iron. WHO Tech. Rep. Ser., #452, 1970.
75. Rappazzo, Salmi and Hall: Br. J. Haematol., *18*, 427, 1970.
76. Okuda, Grasbeck and Chow: J. Lab. Clin. Med., *51*, 17, 1958.
77. Grasbeck, Nyberg and Reizenstein: Proc. Soc. Exp. Biol. Med., *97*, 780, 1958.
78. Heinrich: Semin. Hematol., *1*, 199, 1964.
79. Colman and Herbert: In *Topics in Hematology* (Seno, Takaku and Irino, Eds.). Amsterdam, Excerpta Medica, 1977.
80. Colman and Herbert: Blood, *48*, 911, 1976.
81. Murphy, Keating, Boyle, Weir and Scott: Biochem. Biophys. Res. Commun., *71*, 1017, 1976.
82. Goldman: Ann. N.Y. Acad. Sci., *186*, 400, 1971.
83. Rothenberg: Proc. Soc. Exp. Biol. Med., *133*, 428, 1970.
84. Colman and Herbert: Program, 17th Annual Meeting of American Society of Hematology, 1974.
85. Colman and Herbert: Clin. Res., *25*, 336A, 1977. Herbert and Colman: In *Folic Acid and the Nervous System* (Botez and Reynolds, Eds.). New York, Raven Press, 1979.
86. Spector and Lorenzo: Am. J. Physiol.,*229*, 777, 1975.
87. Hillman, McGuffin and Campbell: Trans. Assoc. Am. Physicians, *90*, 145, 1977.
88. Stokes, Melikian, Leeming, Portman-Graham, Blair and Cooke: Am. J. Clin. Nutr., *28*, 126, 1975.
89. Lavoie and Cooper: Clin. Sci. Mol. Med., *46*, 729, 1974.
90. Herbert: Am. J. Clin. Nutr., *27*, 743, 1968.
91. Food and Nutrition Board, National Research Council: *Recommended Dietary Allowances*, 8th ed. Washington, National Academy of Sciences, 1974.
92. Herbert: N. Engl. J. Med., *284*, 976, 1971.
93. Jadhav, Webb, Vaishava and Baker: Lancet, *2*, 903, 1962.
94. Lichtenstein, Beloian and Murphy: *Vitamin B_{12}: Microbiological Assay Methods and Distribution in Selected Foods*. Home Econ. Res. Rep. #13. Washington, U.S. Department of Agriculture, 1961.
94a. Ericson and Banhidi: Acta Chem. Scand., *7*, 167, 1953. Lindenbaum: Personal communication.
95. Herbert and Jacob: J.A.M.A., *230*, 241, 1974.
96. Newmark, Scheiner, Marcus and Prabhudesai: Am. J. Clin. Nutr., *29*, 645, 1976.
97. Herbert, Jacob and Wong: Am. J. Clin. Nutr., *30*, 297, 1977.
98. Sayers, Lynch, Jacobs, Charlton, Bothwell, Walker and Mayet: Br. J. Haematol., *24*, 209, 1973.
99. Sayers, Lynch, Charlton, Bothwell, Walker and Mayet: Br. J. Haematol., *28*, 483, 1974.
99a. Herbert, Landau, Shang, Chayes and Colman: Blood, *52* (Suppl. 1), November 1978.
100. Colman: In *Advances in Nutritional Research* (Draper, Ed.). New York, Plenum Press, 1977.
101. Sullivan and Herbert: J. Clin. Invest., *43*, 2048, 1964.
102. Herbert: Am. J. Clin. Nutr., *12*, 17, 1963.
103. Hurdle, Barton and Searles: Am. J. Clin. Nutr., *21*, 1202, 1968.
104. Hoppner, Lampi and Perrin: J. Inst. Cancer Sci. Tech. Aliment., *5*, 60, 1972.
105. Perloff and Butrum: J. Am. Diet. Assoc., *70*, 161, 1977.
106. Reed, Weir and Scott: Am. J. Clin. Nutr., *29*, 1393, 1976.
107. Herbert and Zalusky: J. Clin. Invest., *41*, 1263, 1962.
108. Metz, Kelly, Swett, Waxman and Herbert: Br. J. Haematol., 4, 575, 1968.
109. Das and Herbert: Clin. Haematol., *5*, 697, 1976.
110. Noronha and Silverman: *On Folic Acid, Vitamin B_{12}, Methionine and Formiminoglutamic Acid Metabolism in Vitamin B_{12} and Intrinsic Factor*, 2nd European Symposium. Stuttgart, Enke Verlag, 1962.
111. Hoffbrand, Ganeshaguru, Hooton and Tripp: Clin. Haematol., *5*, 727, 1976.
112. Herbert: *The Megaloblastic Anemias*. New York, Grune & Stratton, 1959.
113. Herbert: Proc. R. Soc. Med., *57*, 377, 1964.
114. Cooper and Lowenstein: Blood, *24*, 502, 1964.
115. Das and Hoffbrand: Br. J. Haematol., *19*, 203, 1970.
116. Tisman and Herbert: Blood, *41*, 465, 1973.
117. Spronk: Fed. Proc., *32*, 471A, 1973.
118. Shane, Brody and Stokstad: Fed. Proc., *36*, 1120, 1977.
119. Frenkel: J. Clin. Invest., *50*, 33a, 1971.
120. Marcus, Ullman, Safier and Ballard: J. Clin. Invest., *41*, 2198, 1962.
121. Colman and Herbert: In *Biochemistry of Brain* (Kunar, Ed.). Oxford, Pergamon Press, 1979.
122. Weissbach and Taylor: Vitam. Horm. 28, 395, 1968.
123. Barley, Sato and Abeles: J. Biol. Chem., *247*, 4270, 1972.
124. Frenkel: J. Clin. Invest., *52*, 1237, 1973.
125. Ellenbogen: In *Newer Methods of Nutritional Biochemistry*, Vol. 1 (Albanese, Ed.). New York, Academic Press, 1963.
126. Herbert and Das: Vitam. Horm., *34*, 1, 1976.
127. Pearson and Turner: Nature, *258*, 173, 1975.
128. Meller, Rosengarten, Friedhoff, Stebbins and Silber: Science, *187*, 171, 1975.
128a. Das and Herbert: Br. J. Haematol., *38*, 219, 1978.
128b. Das, Herbert, Colman and Longo: Br. J. Haematol., *39*, 357, 1978.

128c.Colman and Herbert: Blood, 52 (Suppl. 1), November 1978.

129. Herbert: N. Engl. J. Med., 268, 201 and 368, 1963.

130. Herbert: Semin. Hematol., 7, 2, 1970.

131. Herbert: In *Disease-A-Month*. Chicago, Year Book Medical Publishers, 1965.

132. Zalusky and Herbert: N. Engl. J. Med., 265, 1033, 1961.

133. Bonnar, Goldberg and Smith: Lancet, 1, 451, 1969.

134. Sood, Ramachandran, Mathur, Gupta, Ramalingaswamy, Swarnabai, Ponniah, Mathan and Baker: Q. J. Med., 44, 241, 1975.

135. Colman, Barker, Green and Metz: Am. J. Clin. Nutr., 27, 339, 1974.

136. Herbert, Colman, Spivack, Ocasio, Ghanta, Kimmel, Brenner, Freundlich and Scott: Am. J. Obstet. Gynecol., 123, 175, 1975. Herbert: In *Nutritional Disorders of American Women* (Winick, Ed.). New York, John Wiley & Sons, 1977.

137. Colman, Larsen, Barker, Barker, Green and Metz: Am. J. Clin. Nutr., 28, 465, 1975.

138. Colman, Barker, Barker, Green and Metz: Am. J. Clin. Nutr., 28, 471, 1975.

139. Colman, Larsen, Barker, Barker, Green and Metz: S. Afr. Med. J., 48, 1763, 1974.

140. Colman, Green, Stevens and Metz: S. Afr. Med. J., 48, 1795, 1974.

141. FAO/WHO: Food fortification and protein-calorie malnutrition. WHO Tech. Rep. Ser., #477, 1971.

142. WHO: Control of nutritional anaemia with special reference to iron deficiency, Report of IAEA/USAID/WHO Joint Meeting. WHO Tech. Rep. Ser., #580, 1975.

143. Hom, Olesen and Schwartz: Scand. J. Haematol., 5, 107, 1968.

144. Reynolds: Brain, 91, 197, 1968. Herbert and Tisman: In *Biology of Brain Dysfunction* (Gaul, Ed.). New York, Plenum Press, 1973.

145. Hommes, Or, Obbens Eamt and Wijffels: J. Neurol. Sci., 19, 63, 1973.

146. Chi'en, Krumdieck, Scott and Butterworth: Am. J. Clin. Nutr., 28, 51, 1975.

147. Paukert, Straus, and Rabinowitz: J. Biol. Chem., 251, 5104, 1976.

148. Drury, Bazar, and MacKenzie: Arch. Biochem. Biophys., 169, 662, 1975.

149. Herbert: In *Textbook of Medicine*, 14th ed. (Beeson and McDermott, Eds.). Philadelphia, W.B. Saunders, 1975.

K. *Ascorbic Acid*

Robert E. Hodges

Perhaps the earliest account of the ancient disease now known as scurvy was written by the Egyptians in the Papyrus Ebers about 1550 B.C.[1] Later the Greeks and Romans referred to a plague that was almost certainly scurvy.[2] This disease is remarkable in that it reshaped the course of history, since military rations seldom contained adequate amounts of vitamin C.[3] Vivid accounts of scurvy appear in the writings of explorers and military leaders who lived in the 16th, 17th and 18th centuries A.D.[4,5]

Very little is known about scurvy during the early centuries of the Christian era, but in 1536 Jacques Cartier, then in Newfoundland, was gravely concerned when most of his crew fell ill with the disease.[6] He was advised by friendly Indians to give them an extract of the arborvitae tree (a white cedar),* which promptly cured the survivors. In that same century Sir Richard Hawkins described the use of oranges and lemons in treating British sailors who had scurvy,[7] and in Sweden, Urban Hiaerne reported that cloudberries were effective treatment.[8] Thus it is now apparent that many authors have erroneously credited the Scottish naval surgeon James Lind with the original discovery that oranges and lemons can cure scurvy.[9,10]

The first edition of the *Encyclopedia Britannica—1771*[7] gives a fascinating though disjointed discussion of scurvy. Obviously some of the suggested forms of therapy were useless but many were undoubtedly helpful for they described foods

---

*Other sources refer to Ameda or Hanneda (thought to be a sassafras) tree.

or potions containing varying amounts of ascorbic acid. For example, one author recommended "plenty of fresh greens or vegetables . . . particularly sallads of garden cresses." In referring to James Lind's treatise, the encyclopedia reported "the oranges and lemons had the best effect" . . . and later—"but as oranges and lemons are apt to spoil, let the juice of these fruits be well cleared from the pulp, and depurated by standing some time; after which it may be poured off from the gross sediment. Let it then be poured into any clean open vessel of china or stoneware . . . that it may evaporate more readily. Put this into a pan of water over a clear fire; let the water come almost to a boil, and continue nearly in that state with the bowl full of juice in the middle of it, till the juice is found of the consistence of a thick syrup when cold. When it is cold, it is to be corked up in a bottle for use. Two dozen of good oranges weighing five pounds, when evaporated . . . will be equal to less than three ounces . . . and the virtues of this extract, thus made, . . . will serve one man at sea several years. . . ." One wonders how much ascorbic acid was preserved in this way.

The *Encyclopedia Britannica* goes on to say "it will likewise be of great use to seamen to have gooseberries . . . preserved in bottles . . . also small onions pickled in vinegar; cabbage, french beans, etc. may be preserved by putting them in clean dry stone jars, with a layer of salt at the bottom, then a thin layer of the vegetable covered with salt, and so alternately till the jar is full." Also, ". . . this is the manner in which they preserve that never-failing remedy, Greenland scurvy-grass."

"Poor people that winter in Greenland . . . preserved themselves from the scurvy by spruce-beer, which is their common drink." "Likewise, the simple decoction of fir-tops has done wonders." "The shrub black spruce of America makes this most wholesome drink. . . ." "A simple decoction of the tops, cones, leaves, or even of the green bark or wood of these is an excellent

antiscorbutic; but perhaps it is much more so when fermented. By carrying a few bags of spruce to sea, this wholesome drink may be made at any time. . . ." Patients with scurvy were treated . . . "with raisins or currants . . . but more particularly pickled cabbage and small onions boiled. Most of their food ought to be well-acidulated with orange or lemon juice . . . and salads of all kinds are beneficial, but more particularly dandelion, sorrell, endive, lettuce, sumitory, and purslane; to which may be added scurvy-grass, cresses, and the like." "Summer fruits are all good, as [are] oranges, lemons, citrons, apples, etc. In the wintertime, genuine spruce-beer, with lemons and orange juice is proper; or antiscorbutic ale made of an infusion of wormwood, horseradish, mustard-seed, and the like.

"Van Swieten says, he has often seen whole families cured of the scurvy in Holland, by the use of a cask of ale in which were put heads of a red cabbage cut small, twelve handfuls of scurvy-grass, and a pound of fresh horseradish, freshly infused."

Obviously, some of these foods must have contained substantial amounts of ascorbic acid whereas others probably had little or none, for we know that fermentation to make beer or wine destroys most if not all of the ascorbic acid content of fruit or vegetable juices.

The Lords of the British Admiralty, confronted with this background of information and misinformation, undoubtedly were sorely vexed when their admiral, George A. Anson, undertook a voyage around the world in the ship *Centurion* between 1740 and 1744.[3] He started with 6 ships and 1,955 men, yet only the flagship returned. One thousand fifty-one died, most of scurvy. These losses inspired James Lind (or perhaps he was ordered) to seek the cure of scurvy. No doubt he was aware of at least some of the aforementioned forms of treatment when, on the ship *Salisbury*, he performed his classical experiment on May 20, 1747.[10] Yet he did not publish his treatise until 7 years later, and it was not until 1795 (48 years after Lind's experiment) that the Admiralty prescribed lemon juice for all British sailors, hence the nickname "limey." But Lind's studies had neither a prompt nor a profound effect upon a close friend, the enthusiastic Captain James Cook,[11,12] who was not content with his recommendations but insisted upon other measures, including unprecedented cleanliness and personal hygiene aboard ship. He sent men ashore at every opportunity to gather all manner of greens, even grasses, which were prepared, served and eaten. He employed the ingenious technique of insisting that his officers eat this strange food in front of the men, whereupon they deemed it more than suitable and ate their share. By these methods Captain Cook was the first British commander to demonstrate that prolonged ocean voyages did not necessarily result in scurvy among the crew. His first voyage from 1768 to 1771 and his second from 1772 to 1775 conclusively demonstrated that scurvy could be prevented. His third and final voyage began in 1776 and unfortunately 3 years later he was killed by natives in Hawaii.

Yet the efforts of many early explorers and later of James Lind and Captain James Cook were insufficient to impress upon a civilized world the lesson they sought to teach. Indeed, as recently as 1912, when Captain Robert Falcon Scott explored the South Pole, he and his team met with tragic death as a result of scurvy,[13] and, in the middle of the 19th century during the American Civil War,[14] scurvy was rampant among the troops of both the north and the south. Only in the past half century has scurvy become rare among military personnel.

CHEMISTRY AND BIOCHEMISTRY

Once investigators had found that certain foods contained a factor capable of preventing or curing scurvy in both guinea pigs and man, it remained to identify this elusive substance. Zilva and his associates worked at isolation and synthesis of vitamin C between 1910 and 1920. They demonstrated that this substance was necessary not only for prevention of scurvy but for development of teeth in susceptible species of animals.[15] By this time an astonishing fact had become apparent; only a few species of animals need to consume ascorbic acid in their diet, whereas most other species are able to synthesize their own.[16] Herein lies one of the great genetic mysteries, which is still incompletely solved.[17]

The actual isolation of ascorbic acid was accomplished independently in 1928 by two different teams of investigators, one of which was headed by Szent-Györgyi, who was later to receive a Nobel prize for his work. In 1928 Svirbely and Szent-Györgyi isolated "hexuronic acid" from orange juice, cabbage juice and adrenal glands.[18] Meanwhile, King and his associates, working independently, isolated vitamin C from lemon juice and demonstrated that the substance named hexuronic acid by Szent-Györgyi was identical with vitamin C.[19] Both of these discoveries were published in 1932 and, subsequently, it was only a short step to the synthesis of ascorbic acid by two men: Hayworth,[20] who determined its structure, and Reichstein,[21] who finally synthesized it in 1933.

Chemically, L-ascorbic acid, or vitamin C, is a rather simple compound with the empiric formula $C_6H_8O_6$. It has a molecular weight of 176, is very soluble in water, less so in ethyl alcohol and quite insoluble in most lipid solvents. L-Ascorbic acid has been considered to be the active form of vitamin C, but dehydro-L-ascorbic acid also has antiscorbutic activity. Recently, a urinary metabolite of ascorbic acid, ascorbate-3-sulfate,* has been studied for its antiscorbutic activity and other metabolic functions. Although it will cure scurvy in certain species of fish and in guinea pigs, it does not prevent or cure

---

*This may be ascorbate-2-sulfate.

scurvy in nonhuman primates and, presumably, would not be active in humans.[22-25]

Ascorbic acid is derived primarily from plant foods, especially fresh, rapidly growing fruits or vegetables, but even those species of animals that can synthesize vitamin C have relatively low concentrations of this substance in their tissues. Burns[26] described the mechanisms of synthesis of L-ascorbic acid by animals and plants. In rats, and presumably in other mammals that do not require a dietary source of ascorbic acid, glucose is converted through a series of steps to D-glucuronic acid, then to L-gulonic acid, to L-gulonolactone, which is converted to 2-keto L-gulonolactone, then to L-ascorbic acid. According to Burns, the basic defect in man, monkeys and guinea pigs, all of which require vitamin C in the diet, is an inability to convert L-gulonolactone to L-ascorbic acid. Burns found no detectable conversion of L-gulonolactone-1-^{14}C to labeled L-ascorbic acid in human, monkey and guinea pig liver homogenates.

L-Gulonolactone, L-galactonolactone, D-glucuronolactone and methyl-D-galacturonate can be converted to L-ascorbic acid by cress seedlings. Obviously the major pathway for biosynthesis of L-ascorbic acid from D-glucose in plants is completely different from that found in animals.

Vitamin C is widely distributed throughout plant foods, especially those that are fresh and rapidly growing. Plant foods that are dormant, such as nuts, seeds and grains, contain little or no vitamin C. Ascorbic acid is easily destroyed by oxidation, but its perishability has been somewhat exaggerated. Heat, exposure to air and alkaline medium and contact with metallic copper or iron hasten the oxidation of ascorbic acid to dehydro-L-ascorbic acid, then to diketogulonic acid, oxalic acid and other derivatives. Fortunately, many foods rich in ascorbic acid also contain factors, such as other organic acids and antioxidants, that help to protect and preserve the vitamin C contained therein. Prolonged cooking, especially if the cooking water is discarded, will result in heavy losses of vitamin C.

Foods supplying ascorbic acid can be conveniently divided into three categories: excellent, good and fair. The "excellent" category includes foods containing 100 or more mg per 100 gm. Broccoli, Brussels sprouts, collards, black currants, guava, horseradish, kale, turnip greens, parsley and sweet peppers are included in this group. The second or "good" category of foods contains 50 to 99 mg per 100 gm, and includes cabbage, cauliflower, chives, kohlrabi, orange pulp, lemon pulp, mustard greens, beet greens, papaya, spinach, strawberries and watercress. The third or "fair" category contains 30 to 49 mg per 100 gm, and includes asparagus, lima beans, Swiss chard, gooseberries, red currants, grapefruit, limes, loganberries, melons (cantaloupe), okra, tangerines, potatoes and turnips. Note that potatoes and cabbage, which may be consumed in large quantities by low-economic groups, can provide generous intakes of ascorbic acid.

Despite the high level of interest and the prolonged period of study relating to the functions of vitamin C, we know surprising little about it. Its most important function, obviously, is to prevent scurvy, but even though we can describe scurvy in minute detail (Table 6K–1) we have yet to understand most of the mechanisms involved.

At the biochemical level, ascorbic acid may function in hydrogen ion transfer systems and aid in regulation of intracellular oxidation-reduction potentials. It is a powerful water-soluble antioxidant, and is thought to protect other antioxidants, even some that are lipid-soluble, such as vitamin E, vitamin A and the essential fatty acids. It facilitates gastrointestinal absorption of iron and is believed to play a role in conversion of folic acid to its active form, folinic acid. Ascorbic acid may also play a

Table 6K–1. Manifestations of Ascorbic Acid Deficiency in Man

1. Systemic
    Fatigability
    Lassitude
2. Hemorrhagic
    Petechiae
    Perifollicular hemorrhages
    Ecchymoses
    Bleeding gums
3. Psychologic
    Depression
    Hypochondriasis
    Hysteria
4. Secretory
    Dry skin
    Xerophthalmia } Sjögren's syndrome
    Xerostomia
    Follicular hyperkeratosis
5. Vasomotor instability
    Altered metabolism of neurotrophic amines
6. Hematologic
    Impaired iron absorption
    Impaired folate metabolism
7. Connective tissues
    Scorbutic arthritis
    Impaired wound healing

role in detoxification of poisonous substances by virtue of its cofactorial role in hydroxylation reactions. L-Ascorbic acid functions as a coenzyme in some situations where the rate of reaction is important. For example, in hydroxylation reactions which depend upon maintenance of either copper or iron in a reduced state, ascorbic acid has been found to be critical.[40,41] It also is necessary for hydroxylation of proline in the synthesis of collagen,[42] for hydroxylation of tryptophan to 5-hydroxytryptophan[43] and for metabolism of 3,4-dihydroxyphenylethylamine to norepinephrine.[44,45] It is quite certain that ascorbic acid is essential for conversion of hydroxyphenylpyruvate to homogentisic acid in the formation of tyrosine.[46,47] Perhaps these activities explain some of the physiologic abnormalities of vascular reactivity and some of the psychologic changes that have been observed in patients with scurvy.[35,39,48]

PHYSIOLOGY

In this chapter, reference is made to three different levels of ascorbic acid administration. The first is the *minimal daily requirement*, which represents the least amount of vitamin C that can prevent clinical signs or symptoms of scurvy. The second or *physiologic dose* represents the recommended level of intake designed to ensure that practically everyone ingesting this amount of vitamin C not only will avoid developing scurvy but will have a sufficient surplus to maintain a normal metabolic pool of ascorbic acid and to meet emergency demands. The third level of vitamin C intake is referred to as the *pharmacologic dose*, which may exert effects entirely alien to vitamin C, and which will be regarded as medicinal therapy for conditions entirely unrelated to scurvy.

Deficiency of vitamin C results in a specific syndrome known as scurvy. The characteristics of this syndrome vary somewhat from one susceptible species to another, but many of the manifestations listed in Table 6K–1 will be found in subhuman species that require a dietary source of ascorbic acid. Certainly one of the major manifestations of scurvy is interference with metabolism of mesenchymal tissues,[27–29] accompanied by interference with blood-clotting mechanisms.[30] In young animals impairment of bone formation and disruption of dentition occur, presumably as a result of impaired synthesis of collagen.[31,36] In studies of scurvy in human volunteers, both the British Medical Research Council study[33] and the Iowa City studies[34,35] failed to demonstrate impairment of wound healing. If one reviews the original report by Crandon,[32] one finds that a surgical wound *appeared* to be healing adequately because there was normal proliferation of epithelial cells, but subcutaneous tissues were not repaired, presumably because of failure to synthesize collagen properly and failure to form new blood vessels in the wounded area. There are, however, other reports of both experimental and spontaneous scurvy wherein there has been unequivocal impairment of wound healing and faulty healing of bony fractures.[49,50]

Hemorrhagic manifestations of scurvy[51] include subperiosteal bleeding, petechial hemorrhages, ecchymoses, bleeding into joints, into the peritoneal cavity and into the pericardial sac. Massive hemorrhage into the adrenals has been observed in scorbutic guinea pigs and may be the major cause of death. The explanation for these hemorrhagic phenomena is no longer self-evident. For many years, the theory of Wolbach and Howe[36] that lack of intercellular cement permitted disruption of the endothelial cells that comprised the membrane and resulted in capillary hemorrhages was an attractive explanation. This was particularly so in view of the many negative results of attempts to detect impairment of any of the blood-clotting factors in either animal or human scurvy. Recent electron microscopic studies of tissues taken from patients with scurvy at a time when they had abundant evidence of hemorrhagic phenomena failed to demonstrate any capillary disruption or loss of the hypothetical intercellular cement.[34] Perhaps another explanation will be found for the bleeding that characterizes scurvy.

Infectious diseases have consistently been much more common among people with scurvy.[52] Although numerous animal experiments support these observations,[53] both the leukocyte count and the immune response to antigenic challenge remain normal in scorbutic animals[54,55] and in man.[35] Perhaps disruption of epithelial surfaces and impairment of mucus secretions play a role.

The finding of a high concentration of ascorbic acid in the adrenal cortex suggests that deficiency of vitamin C might result in impairment of adrenal cortical function.[56] In most carefully controlled animal studies, however, adrenal cortical activity does not seem to be diminished by a reduction in ascorbic acid intake, and may even be increased during experimental scurvy.[56,57]

Studies in both experimental animals and man[37–39,58] have demonstrated that vascular reactivity is seriously impaired during scurvy. There is suggestive evidence that this results from faulty metabolism of sympathetic amines, another phenomenon that could explain sudden death in scurvy.

Apparently, ascorbic acid is essential for normal protein metabolism, both in experimental animals[59] and in humans.[60] Deficiency of ascorbic acid was found to result in lowering of the albumin fraction of the serum and in raising of the globulin fraction. This was accompanied by an excessive rate of urinary loss of nitrogen.[35]

Lipid metabolism also may be influenced by ascorbic acid.[61] For many years Russian physicians prescribed large doses of ascorbic acid as a means of avoiding hypercholesterolemia in the hope of preventing atherosclerosis.[62] Although other investigators failed to confirm these observations, it is of interest that Fox and Dangerfield in South Africa[63] and Hodges et al. in the United States[35] observed a significant *rise* in serum cholesterol of scorbutic subjects given repleting doses of vitamin C. These changes occurred without any other modifications of the diet. Reports by Mumma et al.[22,25] suggested that ascorbate-3-sulfate might mobilize tissue stores of cholesterol. Somewhat more convincing is the report by Ginter et al.[64] that ascorbic acid is involved in hepatic hydroxylation of cholesterol and in the formation of bile acids. Ginter felt that his observations would support the theory of Spittle[65] that large doses of vitamin C lower the plasma cholesterol concentration of adults. Not only have numerous studies failed to confirm this observation but Davies and Newson[66] found a *positive* correlation between levels of cholesterol and levels of ascorbate in the plasma of pastoral Africans.

Other aspects of the physiology of ascorbic acid metabolism in man deserve attention. The American public has been exposed to an unprecedented level of publicity relating the potential benefits that may derive from taking large doses of vitamin C. Although the 1974 (8th ed.) report of the Committee on Dietary Allowances of the Food and Nutrition Board, National Research Council[66] recommends 45 mg per day as a generous allowance for adult men and women (nonpregnant, nonlactating), the American public has been advised that much larger amounts could lead to better health. Two thousand to 3,000 mg per day have been suggested and, in some instances, much larger amounts have been advocated for specific illnesses. In the opinion of the author, these suggestions are probably ill advised, for there are several natural biologic characteristics that help mankind avoid high levels of ascorbic acid in plasma: (1) There are limited concentrations of ascorbic acid in our regular food supplies. The average American diet contains between 50 and 150 mg of ascorbic acid in a day's ration. It is possible by increasing the amount of fresh fruits and vegetables to increase the intake of ascorbic acid, but it is virtually impossible to devise attractive diets that supply the 2,000- to 2,500-mg level recommended by some. (2) The human kidney handles ascorbic acid in much the same way as it handles glucose. The renal tubules actively reabsorb ascorbic acid so long as a plasma concentration is within normal limits. When the plasma concentration rises above a certain point known as the renal threshold, the tubules reach their maximum reabsorptive capacity known as tubular maximum, or Tm, and the result is that ascorbic acid is excreted in the urine. The rise in urinary excretion is directly proportional to further increases in the plasma concentration of ascorbic acid. This serves to prevent or minimize hyperascorbemia.[68] (3) Absorption of ascorbic acid from the human digestive tract is highly efficient at low levels of intake but becomes progressively less efficient with greater levels of intake.[69] More than 70 per cent of doses up to 180 mg are absorbed, but with doses of 1,500 mg the absorption is about 50 per cent and with doses of 12,000 mg absorption is only 16 per cent. Unabsorbed ascorbic acid exerts an osmotic effect which accounts for the diarrhea that commonly occurs in persons who take massive doses. (4) Ingestion of very large amounts of ascorbic acid for a prolonged period of time results in metabolic changes that can be explained by postulating induction of a catabolic enzyme that destroys ascorbic acid at an accelerated rate.[70] Individuals given large doses for a prolonged period manifest a fall in the concentration of ascorbic acid in the white blood cells. After the large doses are stopped, the concentration of ascorbate in serum and in white blood cells falls rapidly. This phenomenon can also be demonstrated in guinea pigs given excessively large amounts of ascorbic acid followed by an abrupt decrease to low levels of intake.

The question of an optimal level of intake for ascorbic acid persists despite an enormous body of evidence. The World Health Organization Expert Committee has recommended 30 mg per day for men and nonpregnant, nonlactating women throughout the world. A similar recommendation has been made in Great Britain. In the United States the recommendation is 45 mg daily, and in some other countries it is substantially higher. If one compares the level of health in countries having a low intake with that of those having a high intake, it is impossible to detect any difference in the types or prevalence of illness that may have been influenced by the amount of vitamin C ingested. No one denies that an intake of 10 mg daily can and will prevent scurvy, but the implication has been that lack of sufficiently large doses of vitamin C may contribute to the ravages of a number of illnesses the causes of which remain in doubt. These include atherosclerotic diseases, malignant diseases, susceptibility to infectious diseases and certain forms of mental illness, to mention a few. Enormous sums of money have been invested in studies designed to evaluate extravagant claims that ascorbic acid may prevent or cure certain disease processes for which current therapy is less than optimal. The work of Srikantia et al. in India[69] strongly supports the concept that modest doses of ascorbic acid not only prevent scurvy but also maintain "tissue saturation" at or near optimal levels. Recent studies conducted by the author and associates[34,35,60,72] demonstrated (Fig. 6K–1) that the body pool of healthy adult men averages about 1,500 mg and that the rate of metabolism of ascorbic acid is about 3 per cent per day of the existing body pool. When a diet devoid of ascorbic acid is fed for a prolonged period of time, the size of this ascorbate pool diminishes steadily and reaches a point within approximately 2 months where the amount of vitamin C available for catabolism is barely adequate to prevent scurvy. Below this point, signs and symptoms of scurvy begin to develop in a progressive fashion.

Replenishment with labeled ascorbic acid has been shown to result in prompt reversal of all of the signs and symptoms of scurvy and, at the same time, to result in gradual restoration of body stores of ascorbic acid. The metabolic machinery is remarkably parsimonious in handling small quantities of ascorbic acid and, indeed, no L-ascorbic acid can be excreted in the urine until the body pool has been substantially replenished.

UNITS OF MEASUREMENT

Unlike most other vitamins, ascorbic acid is measured in milligrams rather than arbitrary International Units. Quantitative

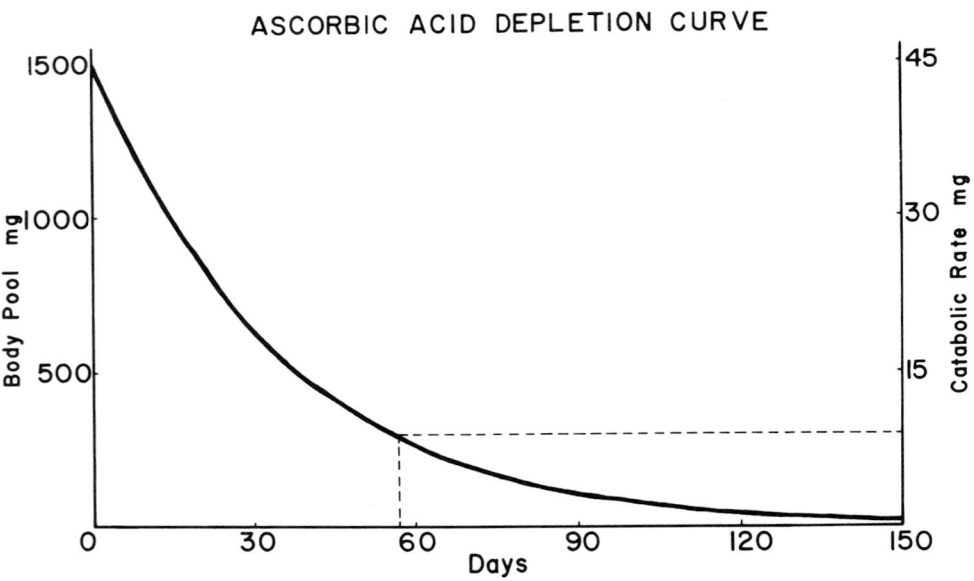

Fig. 6K–1. Curve of ascorbate pool derived from data of 9 men whose body pool of ascorbate was labeled with [14]C L-ascorbic acid. They were then fed a diet devoid of vitamin C. Initially the body pool averaged 1500 mg. The average daily rate of catabolism was 3 per cent of the existing body pool. Thus, the maximal rate of catabolism approximated 45 mg per day. When the body pool fell below 300 mg total and the catabolic rate below 9 mg per day, signs of scurvy began to appear (about 55 days). From this curve the approximate body pool size can be estimated from the dose. Thus, with a daily intake of 30 mg, the pool size should be about 1,000 mg.

estimation of L-ascorbic acid is generally accomplished by taking advantage of its reducing properties. An example of this is the 2,6,dichlorophenolindophenol method of Bessey.[73] This technique, however, is time consuming and measures principally reduced L-ascorbic acid. The more popular method is that of Schaffert and Kingsley,[74] which measures total ascorbic acid using 2,4,dinitrophenylhydrazine.

Different investigators have employed a variety of chemical and physiologic techniques for estimating the state of ascorbic acid nutrition of animals or of man. The simplest of these is measurement of the vitamin C content of serum or plasma: another method employs whole blood, whereas still another measures the ascorbic acid content of the buffy coat of centrifuged blood.[71] This layer is composed chiefly of leukocytes and platelets. A variety of values can be found in the literature. Table 6K–2 gives a composite approximation of values suggested by leading investigators. It should be emphasized that neither serum, whole blood nor buffy coat concentrations of ascorbic acid can provide a valid estimate of nutritional stores. These can be measured only by isotopic techniques which are not practical for routine clinical use. For purposes of comparison, however, Table 6K–2 includes estimates of the metabolic body pool size in milligrams.

Throughout the years physicians have attempted to ascertain the ascorbic acid status of patients by utilizing a variety of load tests. These are based upon the principle of *tissue saturation*, a term that actually implies a finite body pool that can be saturated by giving a specified amount of ascorbic acid. The methods employed generally consist of administering, either orally or parenterally, one or several doses of ascorbic acid and collecting, at intervals, samples of blood or urine, or both. By measuring the rate of increase in the concentration of ascorbic acid in these biologic pools, one can then get some estimate of the ascorbic acid status of a given patient.

The most precise and specific technique employs L-ascorbic acid that has been radioactively labeled with either ^{14}C or ^{3}H. After a sufficient period of equilibration, the specific radioactivity of L-ascorbic acid in plasma or blood can be estimated, and from this the approximate body pool size can be calculated. Since excretion of radioactive materials occurs largely in the urine, with only negligible amounts lost in feces, sweat and expired CO_2,[60] the daily rate of excretion of radioactivity in the urine gives an estimate of the daily rate of catabolism of ascorbic acid. Hornig performed metabolic studies in guinea pigs labeled with radioactive L-ascorbic acid and found that the distribution of this nutrient is highest in the adrenals, pancreas, spleen, salivary glands and testes, with gradual accumulation in brain tissue and in the eyes.[75] Other investigators, using slightly different techniques, have found high concentrations of ascorbic acid in the eyes, the pituitary gland and the brain.[76]

Table 6K–2. L-Ascorbic Acid Nutritional Status of Man

	Serum or Plasma Concentration (mg/100 ml)	Whole Blood Concentration (mg/100 ml)	Buffy Coat Concentration (μg/10⁸ cells)	Body Pool Size (mg)
Well nourished*	> 0.60	> 1.0	> 16	1500
Adequate*	0.40–0.59	0.60–0.99	11–15	600–1499
Low	0.10–0.39	0.30–0.59	2–10	300–599
Deficient	< 0.10	< 0.30	< 2	0–299

*These represent approximate ranges, not absolute values. This table is offered chiefly as a guide to interpretation of current publications.

The demonstration of ascorbate-3-sulfate* in human urine, as well as in the urine of guinea pigs, rats and trout, suggests that this compound is a common metabolite of ascorbic acid, but the question of whether it is an active metabolite or a metabolic end-product has not yet been answered. It could act as a sulfate donor, as suggested by Chu and Slaunwhite[77] as well as by Mumma. It could serve a function in transport across cellular membranes, inasmuch as ascorbate-3-sulfate is a dinegative ion at physiologic pH and appears to interact strongly with metallic ions. It is possible that ascorbate sulfate plays a role in the transfer of L-ascorbic acid across the blood-brain barrier, although this is speculation based on the observations by Hammerström and others that free L-ascorbic acid does not rapidly cross this barrier.[78]

NUTRITIONAL REQUIREMENTS VERSUS RECOMMENDED ALLOWANCES

As mentioned above, the recommended level of intake for ascorbic acid has varied greatly from time to time and from country to country. For example, in 1968, a tabulation of the recommended allowances by country showed that 30 mg daily was proposed for the United Kingdom, 75 mg for West Germany and 60 mg for the United States. At the present time the recommended level is 45 mg in the United States.

No one pretends that mere avoidance of deficiency disease represents an optimal nutrient intake for man. But the term *tissue saturation*, when referring to vitamin C allowances, suggests that there is something healthful about "full saturation" with this nutrient. The same philosophy has never been used with regard to any other nutrient, with the possible exception of dietary protein. For example, we make no effort to try to attain the highest possible tissue concentration of thiamin or of

riboflavin or of pantothenic acid or, indeed, even of iron.

Efforts to estimate the human requirement from the amount of ascorbic acid apparently synthesized by those mammalian species that do not require a dietary source of this vitamin are fraught with considerable hazard. Perhaps the most reliable information on this subject comes from reports of the plasma concentrations of ascorbic acid found in ordinary farm animals. Sheahan observed that cows had an average plasma ascorbic acid concentration of 0.38 mg per dl, bulls 0.40, sheep 0.34 and pigs 0.33.[79] These values are closely similar to the values of healthy adult men and women who consume a diet containing between 40 and 50 mg of ascorbic acid per day.

DEFICIENCY IN MAN

Only a brief description of scurvy is given here but the reader is referred to the chapter concerning clinical manifestations of certain vitamin deficiencies. The onset of scurvy can be detected between 60 and 90 days after beginning a diet that contains no ascorbic acid. The earliest manifestations consist of a few petechial spots and small ecchymoses. These fade within a few days but are soon replaced by others. Somewhat later, larger ecchymoses appear and may be accompanied by petechiae which become perifollicular in location. At the same time follicular hyperkeratosis develops, especially on the buttocks, thighs and calves. Many hyperkeratotic lesions contain fragmented or coiled hairs and some demonstrate the classical lesion of scurvy; *the hyperkeratotic follicle with a red hemorrhagic halo* (Fig. 6K–2). A little later the gums become swollen and bleed easily. It is noteworthy that the gums do not become involved if the patient has no teeth and gum lesions are seldom severe in subjects who practice good dental hygiene. A unique characteristic of scurvy is the development of Sjögren's (sicca) syndrome:[80] dryness of the mouth and eyes, loss of hair,

---

*or ascorbate-2-sulfate

dry itchy skin and loosening of teeth and dental fillings. Scurvy may be characterized by weakness and lethargy, followed by aching of the legs, arthralgia and joint effusions. A peculiar form of vasomotor instability has been observed and may be accompanied by pitting edema of the feet and ankles. Oliguria has also been observed in severe scurvy. Psychologic changes are common and have been characterized as the "neurotic triad,"[48] which consists of hysteria, depression and hypochondriasis. Peripheral neuropathy was observed in one scorbutic subject who developed hemorrhages into the femoral nerve sheaths of both legs.[81] In infants, scurvy is most apt to occur shortly after the child is removed from the breast unless ascorbic acid supplements are fed. Subperiosteal hemorrhages result in pain in the legs and arms. The lower end of the femur and the upper end of the humerus are most likely to be tender. Epiphyseal separations occur, resulting in typical chest deformities.

Therapy

Although a great deal has been written about therapy of scurvy, much of this has been conjectural and arbitrary. As we have seen from accounts of scurvy in ancient times, even small quantities of ascorbic acid have proven to be sufficient to alleviate the symptoms and signs quickly. This was the experience of the British Medical Research Council and it was our experience in treating 9 subjects who participated in the Iowa City studies. Doses of vitamin C ranging from 6.5 to 60 mg daily caused prompt and sustained improvement in the signs and symptoms of severely scorbutic subjects. Accordingly, we feel it is reasonable

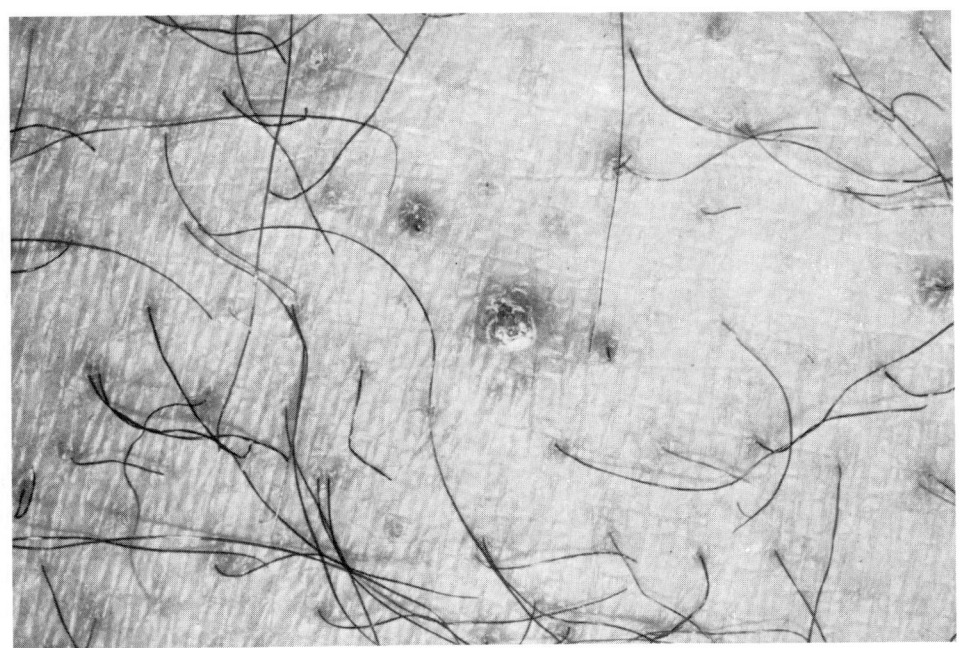

Fig. 6K–2. Follicular hyperkeratosis with perifollicular hemorrhage. Scurvy interferes with protein synthesis and with lubricating secretions. The results are swan-neck deformities of hairs and, in some hair canals, extrusion of irregular hyperkeratotic materials. Perifollicular hemorrhages can be seen around several hairs.

to recommend that scurvy be treated with modest doses of vitamin C, starting with 100 mg of ascorbic acid 3 times daily, by mouth if tolerated or parenterally if not. Massive doses of ascorbic acid can cause gastrointestinal distress, electrolyte disturbances and even hemolysis when given parenterally. A total intake of 300 mg daily should result in replenishment of body pools in a little more than 5 days, since the vitamin is almost completely absorbed at this dose level and, in the deficient state, almost none is lost in the urine. One word of caution should be given however—scurvy can result in sudden death, so treatment must not be delayed.

PHARMACOLOGIC DOSES AND TOXIC EFFECTS

Thus far we have dealt with a discussion of the manifestations of ascorbic acid deficiency and the daily dose of this vitamin necessary to prevent or cure scurvy. We have shown that an allowance of 45 mg daily should be sufficient to maintain the metabolic body pool at or near maximum and that much smaller amounts will prevent or cure scurvy. Any discussion of the hypothetical protective or curative effects of huge doses of vitamin C (in the neighborhood of 100 to 1,000 times the physiologic dose) is based more on conjecture than on well-documented evidence.

Many articles have been published since 1939 attesting to or denying the virtues of giving large doses of ascorbic acid, in the hope of preventing or ameliorating the common cold. The author has not been convinced that any of these articles has provided conclusive evidence either that ascorbic acid prevents upper respiratory infections or that it significantly shortens the duration of symptoms. Indeed, one of the studies that reportedly showed the strongest effect in lessening the number of days of illness was that of Coulehan et al. in 1974.[82] Coulehan et al. repeated this study, and 2 years later reported that there was

no difference in the number of schoolchildren who became ill, in the number of episodes or in the mean duration of illness. Furthermore, children with the higher ascorbate levels had a longer duration of illness.[83] Similarly, Anderson et al.[84] studied the effects of large doses of vitamin C in preventing or treating colds. The differences in the number and duration of colds were not significant, but the number of subjects who remained well and the total number of days of disability were significantly different, thus suggesting a small beneficial effect from vitamin C. Anderson et al. then repeated these studies[85] using different daily doses of vitamin C (250, 1,000, or 2,000 mg) for prophylaxis and 4,000 or 8,000 mg for therapy. There were no differences in the numbers of illnesses, and only small and questionable prophylactic and therapeutic effects. Of even greater interest, however, was the fact that the smallest dose was as effective as the largest dose. Consequently, Anderson and his group did a third study[86] in which they administered either 500 mg of vitamin C or a placebo once a week and, if a subject caught cold, he or she was advised to take 1,500 mg on the first day and then 1,000 mg daily for 4 additional days. Vitamin C was given as either sustained-release or regular tablets. There were no significant differences in the results of these two preparations. Both vitamin groups, however, had less severe illnesses than those receiving the placebo, and the vitamin-treated subjects had 25 per cent fewer days indoors. It is interesting to note that these results were achieved with an *average* daily intake of about 70 mg of ascorbic acid.

Perhaps the best summary of this topic was presented by Chalmers,[87] who reviewed the "best" 14 clinical trials published throughout the world and concluded that 8 were creditable. In these, the differences in the mean numbers of colds per year averaged 0.09, and the differences in the mean duration of colds averaged 0.11 days. He concluded that these minor benefits were not worth the potential risk, however small.

A well-established principle of pharmacologic therapy is that *all* substances are potentially toxic if the dose is large enough—including oxygen, water and, of course, vitamin C. We have established that 10 mg or a little less will prevent or cure scurvy and we have compared the recommended daily allowances of various countries. In the United States this amount is 45 mg.

Administration of 50 to 100 times this amount may or may not have measurable effects. We can conjecture that harmful or undesirable consequences may follow prolonged ingestion of massive doses of ascorbic acid, doses in the range of 5,000 to 15,000 mg daily. The earliest effect may be nausea, followed by diarrhea. A large amount of ascorbic acid will be excreted in the urine where it may interfere with simple tests for glycosuria, giving a false-positive reaction with the copper-containing reagents and a false-negative reaction with the glucose-oxidase methods used in the popular (glucose oxidase-horseradish peroxidase) dipstick tests.[88,89]

The osmotic diarrhea that results from taking more vitamin C than can be absorbed has another important meaning for the medical practitioner. Ascorbic acid in large concentrations in the feces can and will interfere with most of the popular tests for occult blood in the stool (Jaffe et al.[110]). This, of course, could result in failure to diagnose gastrointestinal bleeding, and might have serious consequences.

Ascorbate is well known for its ability to enhance iron absorption, a result far from desirable in men who are not anemic.[90,91] It can also "mobilize" the minerals of the bony skeleton, but the consequences of this action are not yet known.[92–94] Some ascorbate is converted to oxalate[95,96] and fear has been expressed that this may lead to stones in the urinary tract. Although a low pH should protect against calcium oxalate stones, it would favor formation of uric acid stones and cystine stones.[97]

Animal studies have demonstrated that large doses of ascorbic acid may cause infertility or abortion[98,99] or adverse effects on the fetus.[100] In one clinical study human pregnancies were interrupted by giving large amounts of ascorbic acid orally.[101] Of even more concern, however, is the recent report by Stich et al., indicating that large doses of ascorbic acid may have a mutagenic effect.[102]

In rats, huge doses of an analog of vitamin C, dehydroascorbic acid, can, like alloxan, produce permanent diabetes,[103] and L-ascorbic acid itself can potentiate the diabetogenic effect of alloxan in rats.[104] There is as yet no clear-cut evidence that massive doses of vitamin C damage the islet cells of the human pancreas, but definitive tests have not yet been reported and there may be concern about individuals who maintain an excessive intake of ascorbic acid for a number of years.

Ascorbic acid in massive doses may interfere with anticoagulant therapy, both with heparin and with coumadin drugs,[105–107] and large amounts of ascorbic acid have been shown by Klevay to raise the cholesterol level of human volunteers.[108]

Excessive amounts of ascorbic acid given to chicks may interfere with intestinal absorption of certain trace minerals, especially copper.[109] Herbert and Jacob have shown[111] that large doses of vitamin C taken orally may inactivate or destroy dietary vitamin B_{12}. This has been disputed, but Herbert has evidence that cannot be dismissed lightly.

Vitamin C is an essential nutrient. In proper doses it prevents scurvy. At the present time there is no convincing evidence that larger doses are beneficial. Overdoses of an essential nutrient may result in a "conditioned deficiency," i.e. a relative lack of responsiveness to normal doses.[97] Accordingly, it seems to the author that patients should be advised against self-medication with abnormally large doses of ascorbic acid.

BIBLIOGRAPHY

1. Papyrus Ebers: Medical Writings, ca 1550 B.C. Quoted in Encyclopedia Britannica, Chicago, 1964.
2. Hippocrates: *The Genuine Works of Hippocrates,* ca 600 B.C., (Adams, Ed.). Lond. Sydenham Soc., *1*, 196, 267, 1849. Pliny: Compages in Genubers Solverentur, ca 63 A.D. In Major: *Classic Descriptions of Disease with Biographical Sketches of the Authors.* Springfield, Charles C Thomas, 1945.
3. Anson: *A Voyage Around the World in the Years 1740, 1, 2, 3, 4.* 3rd ed. (Compiled by Richard Walter, M.A., Chaplain of H.M.S. Centurion, London, 1748.)
4. Hess: *Scurvy, Past and Present.* Philadelphia, J. B. Lippincott, 1920.
5. Thomas: Experiment versus authority. James Lind and Benjamin Rush. N. Engl. J. Med., *281*, 932, 1969.
6. Cartier: La Grosse Maladie. Reproduction photographique de son 'Brief Recit et Succincte Narration, 1545, suive d'une traduction en langue anglaise du chapitre traitant des aventures de Cartier aux prises avec le scorbut et d'une nouvelle analyse du Mystère de l'Anneda' (Frank, et al.). Montreal, XIX Congrès International de Physiologie, The Ronald Printing Co., 1953.
7. *Encyclopedia Britannica,* Vol. III, 1st ed., 1771.
8. Åberg: Urban Hiaerne—The first Swedish chemist. J. Chem. Educ., *27*, 334, 1950.
9. *Encyclopedia Britannica*: Admiral George A. Anson, 1:1027, James Lind, 14:150, 15:204, Captain James Cook, 10:148, 1964.
10. Lind: *A Treatise on the Scurvy.* London, A. Millar, 1753. (Republished Edinburgh, Edinburgh University Press, 1953.)
11. Villiers: Nutr. Today, *4*, 8, 1969.
12. Kodicek and Young: Notes and Records of the Royal Society of London. *24*, 43, 1969.
13. Priestley: Nutr. Today, *4*, 18, 1969.
14. Hunt: In *Contributions Relating to the Causation and Prevention of Disease* (Flint, Ed.). New York, published for the U.S. Sanitary Commission by Hurd and Houghton, 1867.
15. Zilva and Wells: Proc. R. Soc. Lond. Series *B, 90*, 505, 1917–19.
16. Stone: Acta Genet. Med. Gemellol., *XV*, 345, 1966.
17. Chadhuri and Chatterjee: Science, *164*, 435, 1969.
18. Svirbely and Szent-Györgyi: Biochem. J., *26*, 865, 1932.
19. King and Waugh: Science, *75*, 357, 1932.
20. Haworth and Hirst: J. Soc. Chem. Ind., *52*, 645, 1933.
21. Reichstein, Grüssner and Oppenhauer: Helv. Chim. Acta, *16*, 561, 1933.
22. Mumma: Biochim. Biophys. Acta, *165*, 571, 1968.
23. Mead and Finamore: Biochemistry, *8*, 2652, 1969.
24. Baker, Hammer, March, Tolbert and Canham: Science, *173*, 826, 1971.
25. Mumma and Verlangieri: Fed. Proc., *30*, 370, 1971 (abstract).
26. Burns: Am. J. Med., *26*, 740, 1959.
27. Antonowicz and Kodicek: Biochem. J., *110*, 609, 1968.
28. Mussini, Hutton and Udenfriend: Science, *157*, 927, 1967.
29. Barnes, Constable and Kodicek: Biochim. Biophys. Acta, *184*, 358, 1969.
30. Pirani, Bly and Sutherland: Arch. Pathol., *49*, 710, 1950.
31. Kodicek: In *Structure and Function of Connective and Skeletal Tissue.* Proceedings of an Advanced Study Institute Organized under the Auspices of N.A.T.O. held at the University of St. Andrews, Scotland. (Jackson et al. Eds.). London, Butterworths, 1965.
32. Crandon, Lund and Dill: N. Engl. J. Med., *223*, 353, 1940.
33. Bartley, Krebs and O'Brien: Medical Research Council Special Report Series 280. London, Her Majesty's Stationery Office, 1953.
34. Hodges, Baker, Hood, Sauberlich and March: Am. J. Clin. Nutr., *22*, 535, 1969.
35. Hodges, Hood, Canham, Sauberlich and Baker: Am. J. Clin. Nutr., *24*, 432, 1971.
36. Wolbach and Howe: Arch. Pathol., *1*, 1, 1926.
37. Lee and Lee: Am. J. Physiol., *149*, 465, 1947.
38. Lee: Ann. N.Y. Acad. Sci., *92*, 295, 1961.
39. Abboud, Hood, Hodges and Mayer: J. Clin. Invest., *49*, 298, 1970.
40. Goldberg: Br. J. Haematol., *5*, 150, 1959.
41. Staudinger, Krisch and Leonhäuser: Ann. N.Y. Acad. Sci., *92*, 195, 1961.
42. Peterkofsky and Udenfriend: Proc. Natl. Acad. Sci., *53*, 335, 1965.
43. Cooper: Ann. N.Y. Acad. Sci., *92*, 208, 1961.
44. Levin, Levenberg and Kaufman: J. Biol. Chem., *235*, 2080, 1960.
45. Friedman and Kaufman: J. Biol. Chem., *240*, PC552, 1965.
46. Avery, Clow, Menkes, Ramos, Scriver, Stern and Wasserman: Pediatrics, *39*, 378, 1967.
47. Sealock and Silberstein: Science, *90*, 517, 1939.
48. Kinsman and Hood: Am. J. Clin. Nutr., *24*, 455, 1971.
49. Bourne: Proc. Nutr. Soc., *4*, 204, 1946.
50. Edwards and Dunphy: N. Engl. J. Med., *259*, 224, 1958.
51. Hess: *Scurvy, Past and Present.* Philadelphia, J. B. Lippincott, 1920.
52. Scrimshaw, Taylor and Gordon: Interactions of Nutrition and Infection. Geneva, World Health Organization, 1965.
53. Honjo, Takasaka, Fujiwara, Imaizumi and Ogawa: Jpn. J. Med. Sci. Biol., *22*, 149, 1969.
54. Kumar and Axelrod: J. Nutr., *98*, 41, 1969.
55. Stepto, Pirani, Consolazio and Bell: Endrocrinology, *49*, 755, 1951.

56. Banerjee and Singh: Am. J. Physiol., *190*, 265, 1957.
57. Morgan: Vitam. Horm., *9*, 161, 1951.
58. Beyer: J. Pharmacol. Exp. Ther., *76*, 149, 1942.
59. Torre and Green: J. Nutr., *97*, 61, 1969.
60. Baker, Hodges, Hood, Sauberlich, March and Canham: Am. J. Clin. Nutr., *24*, 444, 1971.
61. Bronte-Stewart, Roberts and Wells: Br. J. Nutr., *17*, 61, 1963.
62. Simonson and Keys: Circulation, *24*, 1239, 1961.
63. Fox and Dangerfield: Proc. Transvaal Mine Medical Officer's Assoc., *19*, 267, 1940.
64. Ginter, Nemec and Bobek: Br. J. Nutr., *28*, 205, 1972.
65. Spittle: Lancet, *2*, 1280, 1971.
66. Davies and Newson: Am. J. Clin. Nutr., *27*, 1039, 1974.
67. Recommended Dietary Allowances, 8th rev. ed. Washington, National Academy of Sciences, 1974.
68. Ahlborg: Acta Physiol. Scand., *12* (Suppl. 36), 78, 1946.
69. Kübler and Gehler: Int. Z. Vitam. Forsch., *40*, 442, 1970.
70. Masek und Hruba: Int. Z. Vitam. Forsch., *34*, 39, 1964.
71. Srikantia, Mohanram and Krishnaswamy: Am. J. Clin. Nutr., *23*, 59, 1970.
72. Baker, Hodges, Hood, Sauberlich and March: Am. J. Clin. Nutr., *22*, 549, 1969.
73. Bessey: J. Biol. Chem., *126*, 771, 1938.
74. Schaffert and Kingsley: J. Biol. Chem., *212*, 59, 1955.
75. Hornig: World Rev. Nutr. Diet., *23*, 225, 1975.
76. Kuether, Telford and Roe: J. Nutr., *28*, 347, 1944.
77. Chu and Slaunwhite: Steroids, *12*, 309, 1968.
78. Hammarström: Acta Physiol. Scand., *70* (Suppl. 289), 1, 1966.
79. Sheahan: J. Comp. Pathol. Ther., *57*, 28, 1947.
80. Hood, Burns and Hodges: N. Engl. J. Med., *282*, 1120, 1970.
81. Hood: N. Engl. J. Med., *281*, 1292, 1969.
82. Coulehan, Reisinger, Rogers and Bradley: N. Engl. J. Med., *290*, 6, 1974.
83. Coulehan, Eberhard, Kapner, Taylor, Rogers and Garry: N. Engl. J. Med., *295*, 973, 1976.
84. Anderson, Reid and Beaton: Can. Med. Assoc. J., *107*, 503, 1972.
85. Anderson, Suranyi and Beaton: Can. Med. Assoc. J., *111*, 31, 1974.
86. Anderson, Beaton, Corey and Spero: Can. Med. Assoc. J., *112*, 823, 1975.
87. Chalmers: Am. J. Med., *58*, 532, 1975.
88. Präuer: N. Engl. J. Med., *284*, 1328, 1971.
89. Glatzel and Rüberg-Sehweer: Med. Klin., *61*, 1249, 1966.
90. Moore: Am. J. Clin. Nutr., *3*, 3, 1955.
91. Pirzio-Biroli, Bothwell and Finch: J. Lab. Clin. Med., *51*, 37, 1958.
92. Thornton: J. Nutr., *100*, 1479, 1970.
93. Thornton and Omdahl: Proc. Soc. Exp. Biol. Med., *132*, 618, 1969.
94. Ramp and Thornton: Proc. Soc. Exp. Biol. Med., *137*, 273, 1971.
95. Lamden and Chrystowski: Proc. Soc. Exp. Biol. Med., *85*, 190, 1954.
96. Lamden: N. Engl. J. Med., *284*, 336, 1971.
97. Med. Lett. Drugs Ther., *12* (No. 26), 105, 1970.
98. Neuwiler: Int. Z. Vitam. Forsch., *22*, 392, 1951.
99. Mouriquand and Edel: C. R. Soc. Biol., *147*, 1432, 1953.
100. Cochrane: Can. Med. Assoc. J., *93*, 893, 1965.
101. Samborsakaya and Ferdman: Bull. Exp. Biol. Med., *8*, 96, 1966.
102. Stich, Karim, Koropatnik and Lo: Nature, *260*, 722, 1976.
103. Patterson: J. Biol. Chem., *183*, 81, 1950.
104. Levy and Suter: Proc. Soc. Exp. Biol. Med., *63*, 341, 1946.
105. Owen, Tyce, Flock and McCall: Mayo Clin. Proc., *45*, 140, 1970.
106. Sigell and Flessa: J.A.M.A., *214*, 2035, 1970.
107. Rosenthal: J.A.M.A., *215*, 1671, 1971.
108. Klevay: Proc. Soc. Exp. Biol. Med., *151*, 579, 1976.
109. Hunt, Landesman and Newberne: Br. J. Nutr., *24*, 607, 1970.
110. Jaffe, Kasten, Young and MacLowry: Ann. Intern. Med., *83*, 824, 1975.
111. Herbert and Jacob: J.A.M.A., *230*, 241, 1974.

L. Biotin

Janet A. Appel
and
George M. Briggs

Biotin, a water-soluble vitamin of the B complex, occurs in a wide variety of foods and is also synthesized by bacteria which inhabit the gastrointestinal tract of human beings and many animal species. Biotin functions in metabolism as a cofactor for several key carboxylating enzymes. In 1977, Balnave reviewed the effects of biotin deficiency in several species of animals,[1] and Bonjour prepared an extensive review of investigations of biotin nutrition in human beings.[2]

CHEMISTRY

In 1942, du Vigneaud[3] described his work and the contributions of others in determining the structure of biotin as a ureido ring containing a sulfur atom and a valeric acid side chain, following the isolation of the vitamin by Kögl.

Microbiologic assay for biotin using Saccharomyces cerevisiae or Lactobacillus plantarum is used routinely. Other test organisms, including Lactobacillus casei, Micrococcus sodonensis, Neurospora crassa, Rhizobium trifolii and Ochromonas danica, have also been used with varying results.[4] Biologic assays, using the rat and chick, have been used and may continue to be of value in determining the bio-availability of biotin from different food sources.[5,6] An isotopic dilution assay for biotin has been recently developed which is sensitive, reproducible and possibly less time consuming than microbiologic assays.[7,8]

OCCURRENCE IN FOODS

Foods containing the greatest concentrations of biotin include yeast (approximately 200 μg of biotin per 100 gm), liver and other organ meats (approximately 100 μg of biotin per 100 gm), soybeans and rice bran (approximately 60 μg of biotin per 100 gm) and egg yolk (approximately 50 μg of biotin per 100 gm).[9] Most muscle meats, dairy products, grains, fruits and vegetables contain lower quantities of biotin, often 10 μg per 100 gm or less. Exceptions in this group of foods include mackerel, sardines, cauliflower and cowpeas, which all contain roughly 20 μg of biotin per 100 gm. Nuts contain a moderate amount of biotin, approximating 30 μg per 100 gm.[9] It has been estimated that the average American diet contains 100 to 300 μg of biotin per day.[10]

Biotin occurs in free form in fruits and vegetables but is apparently bound by proteins in many food sources,[11] including a recently identified biotin-binding protein in egg yolk.[12] Recent evidence of biotin deficiency in poultry and pigs fed practical rations containing biotin suggests that substances in the feed may decrease availability of biotin.[5–6,13–14] Biotin is bound tightly, and consequently inactivated, by avidin, a heat-labile protein found in egg albumin.[15] This interaction resulted in initial identification of biotin deficiency as "egg-white injury" in rats fed a diet containing raw egg white.[16] It has continued to be of experimental and clinical importance in the development of biotin deficiencies.

BIOSYNTHESIS

Synthesis of biotin by microorganisms which normally inhabit the intestinal tract of animals and human beings occurs in most bacteria via a pathway consisting of several steps from pimelic acid to substituted pelargonic acids and eventually to biotin.[17] Biotin thus formed contributes, along with dietary biotin, to the total amount of the vitamin available for metabolic needs.[1,18-20] The type of carbohydrate in the diet and the presence of other B vitamins have been shown to influence the amount of microbial biotin synthesized in the gut of rats.[20]

ABSORPTION, BLOOD AND URINE LEVELS

Evidence from a study of several animal species indicates that biotin is absorbed from the upper portion of the small intestine, and an active transport mechanism has been suggested in some of these species.[21] In human beings, it has been shown, by increases in urinary output of biotin following direct instillation of the vitamin into the distal colon, that biotin can be absorbed at this site.[22]

Bhagavan and Coursin found average biotin concentrations of 32 mμg per 100 ml of whole blood in infants, and a significantly lower concentration of 26 mμg per 100 ml of whole blood in adults.[23] While these amounts are in agreement with several other workers, Nisenson and Sherwin have reported much higher levels in serum, averaging 120 mμg per 100 ml of serum in infants and 160 mμg per 100 ml of serum in adults.[24] Baker and his co-workers recently measured blood biotin levels in a group of 174 women at parturition and found an average biotin concentration of 42 mμg per 100 ml of whole

blood, which was not significantly different from a level of 59 mμg per 100 ml of whole blood found in nonpregnant controls.[25] These results do not support an earlier report of markedly lower blood biotin levels found in a group of 9 pregnant women.[26] The differences in circulating biotin levels reported in the literature may well be caused by several factors, including differences in methods of analysis and wide individual variability of blood biotin concentration, small sample sizes and differences in nutritional status. It has been suggested that biotin levels below 10 mμg per 100 ml of whole blood may be indicative of biotin deficiency.[23]

Low levels of biotin in the liver have been found in patients suffering from fatty livers as a result of alcoholism, possibly indicating a decreased storage capacity for biotin in the fat-infiltrated liver.[27]

In human urine, the principal biotin excretory product found is intact free biotin, in amounts which vary according to assay conditions, individual differences and possibly dietary biotin intake.[18,19,28] Oppel reported an average urinary biotin excretion of 46 μg per 24 hours (range 14 to 111 μg) in 20 adults.[18] Gardner, Parsons and Peterson found values within this range and also showed greater excretions when biotin intake was increased by including liver in the diet, but not when comparable amounts of biotin were fed in yeast.[28] Swendseid and her colleagues showed that, under starvation conditions, urinary biotin excretion did not decrease in all human subjects studied, indicating considerable intestinal synthesis under these conditions.[19] Fecal biotin excretion usually equaled or exceeded urinary biotin output in these studies, and the total amount of biotin excreted in urine and feces was greater than dietary intake because of the contribution of bacterial synthesis.[2,18,19,28] It has been reported that achlorhydria may be accompanied by decreased biotin absorption, as reflected by decreased urinary biotin excretion.[2]

ROLE IN METABOLISM

Biotin is an essential cofactor for the enzymes acetyl CoA carboxylase, propionyl CoA carboxylase, pyruvate carboxylase, β-methylcrotonyl carboxylase, geranoyl CoA carboxylase and methylmalonyl CoA transcarboxylase.[29] Decreased activity of some of these enzymes has been demonstrated in tissues of biotin-deficient rats and chicks.[30] It has been shown that biotin also activates urea amidolyase in microorganisms.[29] In each of these enzyme systems, ATP and magnesium, in addition to biotin, are required for activity. The mechanism of biotin action involves a two-step process initiated by the binding of carbon dioxide to the ureido-1'-nitrogen of biotin, in combination with the apoenzyme. The reaction is completed by the release of the carbon dioxide moiety to another substrate.[31]

Direct and indirect effects of biotin on fatty acid synthesis, carbohydrate metabolism and protein and nucleic acid synthesis have been partially elucidated.[29,30,32]

Lipid Metabolism

Alterations in lipid metabolism in biotin-deficient rats indicative of decreased lipid synthesis include a decreased incorporation of ^{14}C-labeled acetate into phospholipids of liver tissue.[33] Decreased amounts of C_{18} fatty acids and relatively greater amounts of C_{16} fatty acids have also been found in biotin-deficient rats and chicks, although the total amount of fat in the liver may remain unchanged.[34,35] Biotin deficiency may interfere with cholesterol metabolism, as indicated by hypercholesteremia and possible impairment of cholesterol storage seen in some biotin-deficient species, including human beings.[36]

Carbohydrate Metabolism

Interference with carbohydrate metabolism in biotin-deficient rats includes decreased gluconeogenesis, probably resulting from inhibition of pyruvate metabolism and lack of sufficient reducing equivalents.[37,38] Biotin-responsive fasting hypoglycemia has been reported in some cases of biotin deficiency in rats, and a hypoglycemic response to shock stress has also been found.[39,40] On the other hand, Dakshinamurti and his co-workers found an impaired glucose tolerance in biotin-deficient rats which was alleviated by insulin or biotin, possibly acting through stimulation of glucokinase enzyme in the deficient liver.[41] In pharmacologic doses, biotin has been shown to bring about results similar to insulin in the activation of the glucokinase enzyme in the liver of diabetic rats,[42] an effect which may be caused by a stimulation of insulin synthesis or secretion. Glycogen synthesis has been reported to decrease in biotin deficiency in some studies of rats[43] but not under all conditions.[44] While Wagle found no change in carbon dioxide production from glucose during biotin deficiency in rats,[45] Bhagavan, Coursin and Dakshinamurti reported an enhancement of glucose oxidation.[43] In contrast, Dakshinamurti, Modi and Mistry reported a decrease in oxidative phosphorylation in biotin-deficient rat liver.[41] Some of these discrepancies may be due to differences in the stage of deficiency studied, to the effect of decreased food intake of deficient animals or to other differences in experimental conditions.[39,41,44] An increased rate of glycolysis in rats during biotin deficiency has been attributed to interference with normal pyruvate metabolism.[46]

Protein Metabolism

Decreased utilization of glucose for protein synthesis has been found, and interference with protein synthesis, at the level of RNA metabolism has also been suggested in biotin-deficient rats.[32,38]

Vitamin Interrelationships

A recent report shows that biotin increases the rate of conversion of conjugated folacin to unconjugated forms, but does not support previous evidence that biotin increases the rate of folate biosynthesis.[47] A possible interrelationship in rats between the metabolism of biotin and vitamin B_{12} has been found by Marchetti and his co-workers. Administration of pharmacologic doses of ascorbic acid and other reducing agents appears to alleviate biotin-deficiency symptoms in rats[36] but not in turkey poults,[49] suggesting species differences in mechanisms of ascorbic acid synthesis or an effect on gut microflora.

BIOTIN DEFICIENCY

Animals

Since the early reports of "egg-white injury" in 1927,[16] biotin deficiency has been produced in rats, mice, guinea pigs, pigs, dogs, monkeys, rabbits and several species of poultry and fish.[50–55] In most of these species except poultry, it has been necessary to include avidin from raw egg white, antibiotics or sulfa drugs in the diet to bring about biotin-deficiency symptoms in conventional animals. Germ-free rats have also been used successfully in studies of biotin deficiency. Common signs of deficiency include alopecia, especially around the eyes, a scaly dermatitis, depigmentation, anorexia, decreased growth rate, spastic gait or paralysis, perosis in poultry, fatty infiltration of the liver and reproductive abnormalities.[1,36,50–55]

Human Beings

Sydenstricker and his colleagues produced an experimental biotin deficiency in human subjects by feeding raw egg-white diets in 1942. A scaly dermatitis, atrophy of lingual papillae, graying of mucous membranes, increasing skin dryness, depression, lassitude, muscle pains, paresthesia, anorexia, nausea, hypercholesteremia and, finally, electrocardiogram abnormalities were found during a 10-week course of deficiency.[56] Signs and symptoms were completely alleviated by the injection of

150 to 300 μg of biotin daily for a period of 3 to 5 days.

Spontaneous biotin deficiency has occurred on rare occasions when individuals have subsisted on diets rich in raw eggs and little else for periods of several months. Signs of biotin deficiency similar to those found by Sydenstricker, but less severe in nature, disappeared following biotin therapy.[57,58]

Establishment of a precise quantitative dietary requirement for biotin is precluded because of the contribution of intestinal biotin synthesis in unknown and apparently changeable amounts. However, any dietary need for the vitamin would probably be less than the injected doses of 150 to 300 μg found necessary by Sydenstricker to relieve deficiency symptoms under conditions of avidin ingestion.[56] The amount of biotin found effective by Sydenstricker is in the same range as the estimate of average dietary biotin intake in the United States (100 to 300 μg per day[10]). Thus, the amount of the vitamin usually ingested, in addition to biotin available from intestinal synthesis, is likely to be well in excess of minimal biotin requirements under normal dietary conditions.

Administration of large doses of antibiotics or sulfa drugs has been used routinely to decrease intestinal biotin synthesis and bring about biotin deficiency in experimental animals.[20] From limited evidence available in human beings, it appears that commonly used doses would have relatively little effect on biotin synthesis, when given for short periods of time.[59] However, large doses (6 gm of streptomycin daily for 10 to 20 days) resulted in notable reduction of urinary biotin levels in 3 human subjects.[60]

Administration of biotin has been beneficial in alleviating symptoms of seborrheic dermatitis and Leiner's disease in some infants. Therapy has usually involved administration of oral or injected doses of 5 to 10 mg of biotin daily for several days, or as a single treatment.[61–63]

Factors in addition to a dietary biotin deficiency may play prominent roles in this syndrome, since a complicating circumstance of diarrhea is common and use of other treatments, including administration of antibiotics or other B vitamins, has also been found to be beneficial.[61-63] In addition, while some infants suffering from the disease have low blood and urine levels of biotin, others afflicted with similar symptoms have normal concentrations.[53] Treatment of the mothers of breast-fed infants with seborrheic dermatitis by the injection of pharmacologic doses of biotin has also been reported to be of benefit.[61,62]

In human beings, rare inborn errors of metabolism affecting the activity of propionyl CoA carboxylase and β-methylcrotonyl carboxylase have been sometimes found to respond to pharmacologic doses of biotin.[64-66]

Evidence exists of a relationship between biotin deficiency and the occurrence of sudden death following liver and kidney damage in young chickens.[1,2,13] The hypoglycemic response to stress described in biotin-deficient rats[40] has been proposed as the ultimate cause of death in these cases.[1,13,67]

TOXICITY

Although no studies of biotin toxicity in human beings have been conducted, toxicity appears to be low, since the injection of 5 to 10 mg daily to infants less than 6 months of age for treatment of seborrheic dermatitis has shown no adverse effects. Contradictory findings concerning a toxic effect of biotin on reproduction in the female rat have been reported. Paul, Duttagupta and Agarwal found that rats injected with 5 to 50 mg biotin per kg body weight prior to pregnancy had increased numbers of resorptions, ovarian atrophy and estrus irregularities.[68] On the other hand, Mittelholzer repeated the experiments reported by Paul and his co-workers and found none of the abnormalities attributed to biotin excess by the earlier authors.[69] A more recent report by Paul and Duttagupta claiming decreased placental and fetal weights in offsprings of rats injected during pregnancy with 100 mg biotin per kg body weight has not been confirmed.[70]

BIBLIOGRAPHY

1. Balnave: Am. J. Clin. Nutr., *30*, 1408, 1977.
2. Bonjour: Int. J. Vitam. Nutr. Res., *47*, 107, 1977.
3. du Vigneaud: Science, *96*, 455, 1942.
4. Baker, Frank, Matovitch, Pasher, Aaronson, Hutner and Sobotka: Anal. Biochem., *3*, 31, 1962.
5. Wagstaff, Dobson and Anderson: Poult. Sci., *40*, 503, 1961.
6. Scheiner and De Ritter: J. Agr. Food Chem., *23*, 1157, 1975.
7. Dakshinamurti, Landman, Ramamurti and Constable: Anal. Biochem., *61*, 225, 1974.
8. Hood: J. Sci. Food Agr., *26*, 1847, 1975.
9. Hardinge and Crooks: J. Am. Diet. Assoc., *38*, 240, 1961.
10. Food and Nutrition Board: Recommended Dietary Allowances, 8th ed. Washington, National Academy of Sciences, 1974.
11. Lampen, Bahler and Peterson: J. Nutr., *23*, 11, 1942.
12. White, Dennison, Fera, Whitney, McGuire, Meslar and Sammelwitz: Biochem. J., *157*, 395, 1976.
13. Anon: Nutr. Rev., *34*, 217, 1976.
14. Brooks, Smith and Irwin: Vet. Rec., *101*, 46, 1977.
15. Eakin, Snell and Williams: J. Biol. Chem., *140*, 535, 1941.
16. Boas: Biochem. J., *21*, 712, 1927.
17. McCormick: Nutr. Rev., *33*, 97, 1975.
18. Oppel: Am. J. Med. Sci., *204*, 856, 1942.
19. Swendseid, Schick, Vinyard and Drenick: Am. J. Clin. Nutr., *17*, 272, 1965.
20. Ham and Scott: J. Nutr., *51*, 423, 1953.
21. Spencer and Brody: Am. J. Physiol., *206*, 653, 1964.
22. Sorrell, Frank, Thomson, Aquino and Baker: Nutr. Rep. Int., *3*, 143, 1971.
23. Bhagavan and Coursin: Am. J. Clin. Nutr., *20*, 903, 1967.
24. Nisenson and Sherwin: J. Pediatr., *69*, 134, 1966.
25. Baker, Frank, Thomson, Langer, Munves, De Angelis and Kaminetzky: Am. J. Clin. Nutr., *28*, 56, 1975.
26. Bhagavan: Int. J. Vitam. Res., *39*, 235, 1969.
27. Baker, Zitter, Goldfarb, Leevy and Sobotka: Am. J. Clin. Nutr., *14*, 1, 1964.
28. Gardner, Parsons and Peterson: Am. J. Med. Sci., *211*, 198, 1946.
29. Lynen: Biochem. J., *102*, 381, 1967.
30. Arinze and Mistry: Comp. Biochem. Physiol., *38B*, 285, 1971.
31. Knappe: Annu. Rev. Biochem., *39*, 757, 1970.
32. Boeckx and Dakshinamurti: Biochem. J., *140*, 549, 1974.

33. Dakshinamurti and Desjardins: Can. J. Biochem. *46*, 1261, 1968.
34. Puddu, Zanetti, Turchetto and Marchetti: J. Nutr., *91*, 509, 1967.
35. Donaldson: Proc. Soc. Exp. Biol. Med., *116*, 662, 1964.
36. Terroine: Vitam. Horm., *18*, 1, 1960.
37. Arinze, Deodhar, Chiang and Mistry: Int. J. Biochem., *5*, 715, 1974.
38. Bhagavan and Coursin: J. Nutr. Sci. Vitaminol., *22*, 79, 1976.
39. Bhagavan, Coursin and Stewart: Life Sci., *8*, 299, 1969.
40. Bhagavan, Coursin and Stewart: Life Sci., *8*, 1117, 1969.
41. Dakshinamurti, Modi and Mistry: Proc. Soc. Exp. Biol. Med., *127*, 396, 1968.
42. Anon: Nutr. Rev., *28*, 242, 1970.
43. Bhagavan, Coursin and Dakshinamurti: Arch. Biochem. Biophys., *110*, 422, 1965.
44. Patel and Mistry: Proc. Soc. Exp. Biol. Med., *134*, 264, 1970.
45. Wagle: Arch. Biochem. Biophys., *103*, 267, 1963.
46. Deodhar and Mistry: Life Sci., *9*, 581, 1970.
47. Nair and Noronha: J. Nutr. Sci. Vitaminol., *20*, 243, 1974.
48. Marchetti and Testoni: J. Nutr., *84*, 249, 1964.
49. Arends and Kienholz: J. Nutr., *102*, 1667, 1972.
50. Sebrell and Harris (Eds.): *The Vitamins*, Vol. 1, New York, Academic Press, 1954.
51. Coots, Harper and Elvehjem: J. Nutr., *67*, 525, 1959.
52. Smith: Am. J. Physiol., *144*, 175, 1945.
53. Waisman, McCall and Elvehjem: J. Nutr., *29*, 1, 1945.
54. Hegsted, Mills, Briggs, Elvehjem and Hart: J. Nutr., *23*, 175, 1942.
55. Poston and McCartney: J. Nutr., *104*, 315, 1974.
56. Sydenstricker, Singal, Briggs and DeVaughn: Science, *95*, 176, 1942.
57. Baugh, Malone and Butterworth: Am. J. Clin. Nutr., *21*, 173, 1968.
58. Williams: N. Engl. J. Med., *228*, 247, 1943.
59. Oppel: Am. J. Med. Sci., *215*, 76, 1948.
60. Sarett: J. Nutr., *47*, 275, 1952.
61. Nisenson: J. Pediatr., *51*, 537, 1957.
62. Nisenson: Pediatrics, *44*, 1014, 1969.
63. Messaritakis, Kattamis, Karabula and Matsaniotis: Arch. Dis. Child., *50*, 871, 1975.
64. Barnes, Hull, Balgobin and Gompertz: Lancet, *2*, 244, 1970.
65. Gompertz, Draffan, Watts and Hull: Lancet, *2*, 22, 1971.
66. Bartlett and Gompertz; Lancet, *2*, 804, 1976.
67. Wight, Siller, Evans, Bannister, Whitehead and Blair: Lancet, *1*, 1339, 1975.
68. Paul, Duttagupta and Agarwal: Curr. Sci., *42*, 623, 1973.
69. Mittelholzer: Int. J. Vitam. Nutr. Res., *46*, 33, 1976.
70. Paul and Duttagupta: J. Nutr. Sci. Vitaminol., *22*, 181, 1976.

M. *Bioflavonoids*

Jean Weininger
and
George M. Briggs

The first clinical use of flavonoids was reported in 1936 by Szent-Györgyi and his co-workers.[1] They claimed that extracts of red pepper or lemon juice were effective, while ascorbic acid was ineffective, in the treatment of patients with certain pathologic conditions characterized by increased permeability or fragility of the capillary wall. The crystalline flavone fraction of lemon — called citrin—was also reported to decrease tissue hemorrhages and prolong the life of scorbutic guinea pigs.[2] The name vitamin P was proposed for these flavone substances because of their presumed action on vascular permeability.[1,2]

When subsequent work, by the same and other authors, failed to establish that these substances were true vitamins, the Joint Committee on Biochemical Nomenclature of the American Society of Biological Chemists and the American Institute of Nutrition recommended in 1950 that the term vitamin P be discontinued.[3] The word *bioflavonoids*—designating flavonoids having biologic activity—was introduced to replace vitamin P,[4] although the latter term continues to appear in the medical literature.

CHEMISTRY AND OCCURRENCE IN FOODS

The flavonoids are a large group of generally insoluble phenolic compounds widely distributed in plants.[5] The basic flavone structure consists of a 1,4-benzopyrone with a phenyl substitution at the 2 position (Fig. 6M–1). Hydroxyl group substitutions enable naturally occurring flavonoids to combine with sugars to form glycosides. Flavonoids can also form che-

lates with metals. The chemistry and biochemistry of the major classes are discussed systematically in the comprehensive text *The Flavonoids*.[6] The structures of some common bioflavonoids are given in Figure 6M–2.

Flavonoids have been shown to act as antioxidants, protecting ascorbic acid and other plant components from oxidation.[5,7] As pigments in fruits and vegetables, flavonoid compounds range from the pale yellow and colorless flavanones in citrus fruit to the red and blue anthocyanins in berries.[5,7,8] Most flavonoids are concentrated in the skin, peel and outer layers of fruits and vegetables—the areas most accessible to light.

The amounts of different flavonoids in various foodstuffs are presented in two recent reviews.[5,7] Although onions with colored skins have an exceptionally high content, most root vegetables have low concentrations; leafy vegetables have higher concentrations. Citrus fruits contain about 50 to 100 mg per 100 gm of

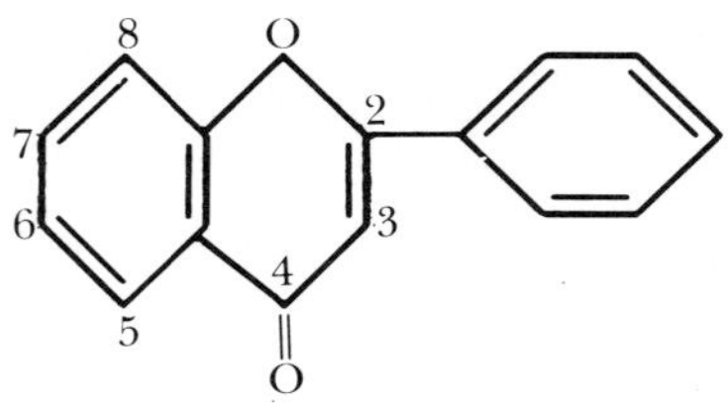

Fig. 6M–1.   Basic flavone structure.

Quercetin

Hesperidin

Rutin

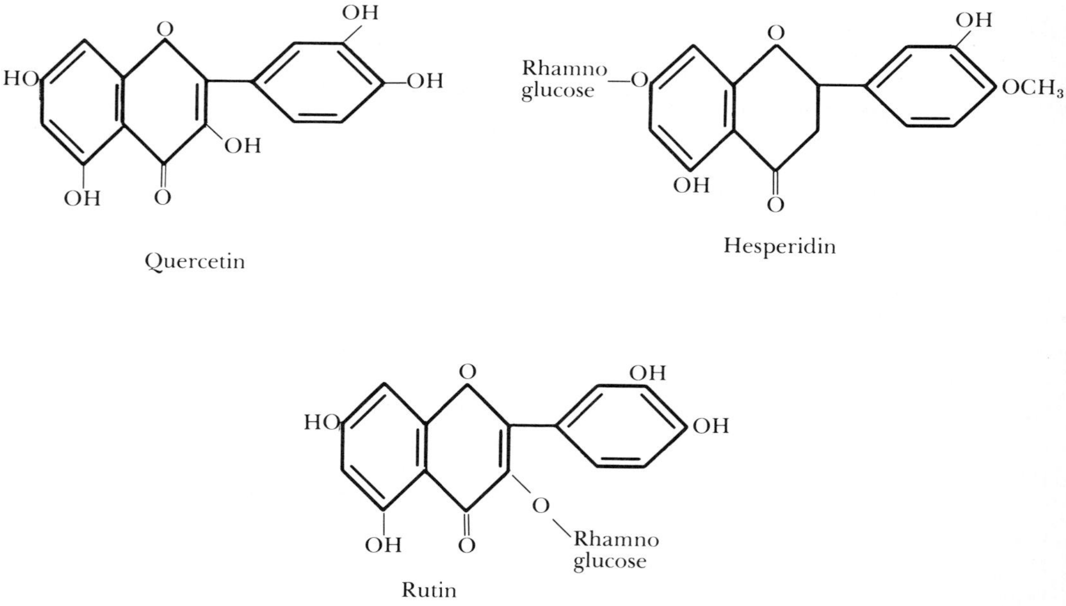

Fig. 6M–2.   Structures of some common bioflavonoids.

fresh material. Beverages, such as tea, coffee, wine, and beer also contain significant amounts of flavonoids. An average daily intake of about 1 gm of flavonoids might be expected in a typical mixed diet.[5] About one-half of the amount ingested is thought to be absorbed in a physiologically active form, the rest being degraded by intestinal bacteria.[5]

NUTRITIONAL AND CLINICAL SIGNIFICANCE

Aside from one unconfirmed report of "vitamin P" deficiency in two people,[9] there is no known bioflavonoid deficiency condition. Bioflavonoids cannot be considered vitamins because they have not been demonstrated to be essential in the diet of humans or of any other species. However, they are among the many food substances that have definite biologic activity.

Some recent work indicates that certain bioflavonoids inhibit aldose reductase, an enzyme involved in the formation of cataracts in diabetes mellitus and galactosemia, though there is no evidence that they actually interfere with cataract formation in humans.[10,11] If bioflavonoids do reduce red blood cell aggregation,[12] or decrease bleeding associated with capillary fragility,[4] as reported, it is probably because of a weak pharmacologic effect rather than a normal structural or functional physiologic role.[13]

Some of the observed effects may be explained by the ability of bioflavonoids to chelate metals or by their antioxidant effects, which may spare ascorbic acid.[5] Some of the inconsistent findings may be results of the variable actions of the different flavonoids under investigation as well as of different study designs.

Despite claims of usefulness,[5,13,14] there is no accepted therapeutic role of bioflavonoids in vascular purpura, hypertension, degenerative vascular disease, rheumatic fever, arthritis, cancer or any other condition.

At this time, no conclusive evidence exists that bioflavonoids serve any *unique* role in human nutrition or in the prevention or treatment of disease in humans.

BIBLIOGRAPHY

1. Rusznyák and Szent-Györgyi: Nature, *138*, 27, 1936.
2. Bentsáth, Rusznyák and Szent-Györgyi: Nature, *138*, 798, 1936.
3. Joint Committee on Nomenclature: Science, *112*, 628, 1950.
4. Miner (Ed.): Bioflavonoids and the capillary. Ann. N.Y. Acad. Sci., *61*, 637, 1955.
5. Kühnau: World Rev. Nutr. Diet., *24*, 117, 1976.
6. Harborne, Mabry and Mabry (Eds.): *The Flavonoids*, Part 1 and Part 2. New York, Academic Press, 1975.
7. Herrmann: J. Food Technol., *11*, 433, 1976.
8. Hughes: J. Hum. Nutr., *32*, 47, 1978.
9. Scarborough: Lancet, *2*, 644, 1940.
10. Varma, Mikuni and Kinoshita: Science, *188*, 1215, 1975.
11. Varma and Kinoshita: Biochem. Pharmacol., *25*, 2505, 1976.
12. Robbins: Int. J. Vitam. Nutr. Res., *47*, 373, 1977.
13. Pearson: J.A.M.A., *164*, 1675, 1957.
14. Shils and Goodhart: *The Flavonoids in Biology and Medicine,* Nutrition Monograph Series No. 2. New York, The National Vitamin Foundation, Inc., 1956.

N. Choline

Janet A. Appel
and
George M. Briggs

Choline is a key part of the phospholipid lecithin and is present in certain sphingomyelins. It also acts as a source of a labile methyl group for the synthesis of other methylated products, and is the precursor of acetylcholine.

While choline is a component of many foods common to the diets of animals and human beings, it can also be synthesized by many animal species.[1,2] However, the rate of choline synthesis has been shown to be insufficient to meet physiologic needs in some animal species, especially in the young.[1,2] In addition, dietary choline deficiency, resulting in liver and kidney damage, has been produced experimentally in several species by exclusion from the diet of choline and nutrients essential for its synthesis.[1-4] Hence, choline is generally classified as a vitamin by comparative nutritionists who work with experimental animals.

The synthesis of choline probably also occurs in human beings. We know, however, of no experimental efforts to develop a choline deficiency in human subjects, so proof of its need in the diet and knowledge of the amount of choline normally synthesized by human beings are lacking. Clinical evidence of a dietary choline deficiency has not been found and, thus, it is not possible to state that choline is an essential vitamin for man.

CHEMISTRY

Choline, known chemically as (β-hydroxyethyl)trimethylammonium hydroxide and depicted by the formula

$$(CH_3)_3\overset{\displaystyle OH}{\overset{\displaystyle |}{N}}CH_2CH_2OH,$$

can be measured by a colorimetric reaction with ammonium reineckate and subsequent light absorbance of choline reineckate in acetone or acetonitrile solution.[5,6] Microbiologic assay for choline using a mutant strain of Neurospora crassa has also been used routinely.[3] Recently, more sensitive or more specific methods have been developed: fluorometric enzyme assay, enzymatic radioisotopic assay and gas chromatography.[7,8]

OCCURRENCE IN FOODS

Choline is widespread in our food supply. It is found in muscle meats and grains in amounts approximating 100 mg choline per 100 gm. Egg yolks and organ meats such as liver have considerably greater choline concentrations (approximately 1,700 mg and 600 mg per 100 gm, respectively).[3,9,10] Legumes are also good sources, containing approximately 200 to 300 mg choline per 100 gm.[9,11] Fruits and vegetables are generally poor choline sources, but they may contain appreciable amounts of betaine, which has been shown to decrease the need for dietary choline in experimental animals.[4] It has been estimated that an average American diet contains between 400 and 900 mg of choline per day.[12]

The need for preformed choline has been shown, in animal studies, to depend to some extent on methionine availability and the vitamin B_{12} and folacin content of the diet. Also choline metabolism can be altered by other diet constituents (see later section), which may then affect the amount of choline needed.[3,13] Therefore it is not possible to assess the adequacy of choline intake from diets of experimental animals without considering the amounts of these other nutrients available from the diet. The practical significance of such interrelationships on the need for choline by human beings is unknown.

Because of its widespread occurrence in foods, it would be virtually impossible to eat a conventional diet low in choline that is not also lacking in several other nutrients.[4] An exception to this probability exists in formula diets, based on a limited number of foods low in choline or its precursors. Such a situation is presented in infant formulas based on milk substitutes. The potential harm of choline deficiency and lack of toxic symptoms from choline ingested by infants fed milk-based formulas or breast milk has prompted the Committee on Nutrition of the American Academy of Pediatrics to recommend the inclusion of choline in infant formulas to the level found in milk-based formulas (i.e. at least 7 mg per 100 kcal).[14]

DEFICIENCIES IN ANIMALS

The importance of choline in animal nutrition was discovered in 1931, when it was found that feeding choline in the form of lecithin caused reduction of fat accumulated in the livers of insulin-supported depancreatized dogs.[15] C.H. Best and his colleagues later showed that rats fed a low choline diet developed fatty livers which could be prevented by choline supplementation.[16] The term *lipotropic* was coined in 1935 by Best, Huntsman and Ridout to describe the effect of ". . . substances which decrease the rate of deposition and accelerate the rate of removal of liver fat."[17] Since the 1930s, a syndrome of dietary choline deficiency has also been established in mice, pigs, calves, rabbits, guinea pigs, monkeys, baboons, trout and

poultry.[3,18] The most common signs of choline deficiency in mammals are fatty infiltration of the liver and hemorrhagic kidney damage. Choline-deficient poultry suffer primarily from perosis, a tendon defect resulting in permanently deformed legs.[3,4]

METABOLISM

Analysis of liver and plasma lipids in choline-deficient animals and isotopic tracer studies have shown that the lipotropic effect of choline on choline-deficient fatty livers is probably effected through the manufacture of lecithin, thus influencing the synthesis or secretion of lipoproteins with their role in the removal of triglycerides from the liver.[19-21] It is possible that the kidney lesions associated with choline deficiency are caused by decreased amounts of acetylcholine and interference with the blood-clotting mechanism at Factor V, but a causal relationship has not been conclusively established.[22]

Transmethylation

Participation of choline in transmethylation reactions was first revealed by Tucker and Eckstein in 1937, when they showed that methionine, but not other sulfur-containing amino acids lacking a labile methyl group, could decrease liver fat in choline-deficient rats.[23] Work that followed by du Vigneaud and his colleagues elucidated the transmethylation reactions which allow choline synthesis from ethanolamines and from excess methionine in the diet.[24] Subsequently, reactions were recognized in which choline donates a labile methyl group to homocystine to form methionine, which in turn reacts with guanidoacetic acid to form creatine.[3,24,25] Such transmethylation reactions allow the replacement of choline with methionine or homocystine, betaine and certain ethanolamines in the diets of rats and some other species studied, without incurring a specific choline deficiency.[3,24,26]

Biosynthesis of Choline and Lecithin

Two mechanisms of lecithin synthesis have been demonstrated in vivo in rats. In a reaction scheme similar to choline synthesis from preformed ethanolamine and the labile methyl group of methionine, lecithin can be synthesized by three trans-methylations from methionine to phosphatidylethanolamine.[27] The second pathway of lecithin synthesis consists of the reaction of cytidine diphosphate choline with a D,1-2 diglyceride.[28] While evidence of enzyme systems essential to carry out these reactions has been found in species other than the rat, differences in activity of methyltransferase enzymes involved in the reactions have been reported.[3,29]

Such species differences include a very limited ability of the guinea pig and some species of poultry to methylate ethanolamine and phosphatidylethanolamine directly when fed low-choline diets containing these substances as the only precursors for choline biosynthesis.[3,29] Monomethylethanolamine, not usually a constituent of foods, and labile methyl sources such as methionine or betaine can be used by these species for choline and lecithin synthesis, however.[2,3]

A recent, unconfirmed report provides indirect evidence that the rate of trans-methylation reactions leading to choline or methionine synthesis may be increased in human beings when dietary intake of both of these nutrients is low for several days.[30] Whether such adaptation can continue for extended periods of time, or is at the expense of other essential metabolic products, is unknown. Kushwaha and Jensen found, in a study of Japanese quail which appear to have an absolute dietary requirement for preformed choline, that no adaptation of the rate of choline synthesis occurred during restriction of dietary intake.[29] These authors also reported finding contradictory results concerning the rate of choline synthesis during choline deficiency in studies of rats.[29]

It has been shown in rats that vitamin B_{12} and folacin are involved in the biosynthesis de novo of methyl groups, which can be used to synthesize choline and methionine.[31,32] Adequate intakes of vitamin B_{12} and folacin will, therefore, decrease the need for preformed choline in the diet, a point which was unrecognized in early studies of choline deficiency, when diets often lacking these two vitamins were commonly used.

Factors which Affect the Need for Choline in Animals

Choline metabolism is affected by several dietary and physiologic factors in addition to the precursors and accessory factors directly involved in choline synthesis. Under experimental conditions, the amount and type of fat in the diet,[33] energy intake, type of carbohydrate eaten,[34] total amount of protein in the diet[4] and possibly the amount of dietary cholesterol[35] influence the quantity of choline required.[2,4] Excessive ethanol in the diet may cause an increased rate of choline metabolism in some species[36,37] or may have a nonspecific effect on choline need through its caloric contribution to the diet.[38] It has been reported that methotrexate interferes with choline synthesis from de novo methyl groups, in rats, and that the administration of choline or methionine overcomes that effect.[39]

Young animals, which may have an increased need for choline and/or methionine as well as a less efficient synthetic system for choline, appear to be more susceptible to choline deficiency.[2,3] Environmental temperature also affects choline metabolism: rats raised in cold temperatures did not have the signs of choline deficiency seen in rats grown at room temperature and fed the same diet.[40]

USE OF CHOLINE IN HUMAN BEINGS

In human beings, the use of choline in the treatment of the fatty liver of alcoholism and of kwashiorkor has been investigated by several workers, prompted by the apparent similarity of these human symptoms with fatty livers seen in choline-deficient animals. However, administration of choline by itself has generally proved to be ineffective in these cases.[4,41]

Administration of pharmacologic doses of choline may alleviate symptoms of tardive dyskinesia and Huntington's disease in human beings.[42-44] This effect appears to be beyond specific dietary needs for choline in normal persons.

TOXICITY

No studies have been reported which evaluate the toxicity of choline in healthy human beings. However, oral pharmacologic doses of up to 20 gm per day of choline chloride have been used for periods of several weeks in the treatment of the above neurologic disorders.[42] In some patients, ingestion of these high levels of choline chloride have resulted in dizziness, nausea, diarrhea or possibly a slightly longer P-R interval in electrocardiograms.[42] A fishy odor, apparently caused by bacterial degradation of choline to trimethylamines in the intestine, is common in patients treated with high oral doses of choline.[42,43] These levels of intake are more than 20 times that estimated for an average mixed diet.

IMPORTANCE OF DIETARY VERSUS ENDOGENOUS CHOLINE

Attempts to determine the relative importance of exogenous versus endogenous choline supplies are confused because of the number of factors which affect choline metabolism. Species differences in enzyme activities governing choline synthesis and degradation exist[1,3,29] and physiologic and dietary factors can influence the total amount of choline needed in metabolism.[2,3] Amounts of dietary methionine and betaine and the presence of folacin and vitamin B_{12} will directly affect rates of choline synthesis. For these reasons a quantitative dietary requirement for choline cannot be stated.

A perpetual negative balance between endogenous supply and metabolic need for choline exists for some species such as the guinea pig, quail and chicken, suggesting that choline is a vitamin for these animals. It has been shown in numerous studies of rats that these animals are able to meet their choline needs through biosynthesis, when they are provided with essential precursors and accessory factors in the diet. Nevertheless, choline can function as an important nutrient for rats in its contribution to the total amount of choline available for synthesis of phospholipids, acetylcholine and other methylated products essential to metabolism. Whether a dietary source of choline is necessary to prevent signs of deficiency in the animal species studied appears to depend on the balance between the dietary and physiologic factors which determine the rate of choline synthesis and the total amount of choline needed for metabolism.

Little is known about either the magnitude of choline synthesis in human beings or the effect of dietary and physiologic factors on the synthesis and metabolism of choline. For these reasons, we must await further studies before determining whether choline is a vitamin for man.

BIBLIOGRAPHY

1. Stekol: Am. J. Clin. Nutr., 6, 200, 1958.
2. Griffith and Dyer: Nutr. Rev., 26, 1, 1968.
3. Sebrell and Harris (Eds.): The Vitamins, Vol. III. New York, Academic Press, 1971.
4. Lucas: Am. J. Clin. Nutr., 6, 504, 1958.
5. Engel: J. Biol. Chem., 144, 701, 1942.
6. Argoudelis and Tobias: Anal. Biochem., 64, 276, 1975.
7. Hanin: Choline and Acetylcholine: Handbook of Chemical Assay Methods. New York, Raven Press, 1974.
8. Wang and Haubrich: Anal. Biochem., 63, 195, 1975.
9. Engel: J. Nutr., 25, 441, 1943.
10. McIntire, Schweigert and Elvehjem: J. Nutr., 28, 219, 1944.
11. Glick: Cereal Chem., 22, 95, 1945.

12. Food and Nutrition Board: Recommended Dietary Allowances, 8th ed. Washington, National Academy of Sciences, 1974.
13. Lombardi: Fed. Proc., *30*, 139, 1971.
14. Committee on Nutrition: Pediatrics, *57*, 278, 1976.
15. Hershey and Soskin: Am. J. Physiol., *98*, 74, 1931.
16. Best and Huntsman: J. Physiol., *75*, 405, 1932.
17. Best, Huntsman and Ridout: Nature, *135*, 821, 1935.
18. Hoffbauer and Zaki: Arch. Pathol., *79*, 364, 1965.
19. Chalvardjian: Can. J. Biochem., *47*, 207, 1969.
20. Mookerjea: Fed. Proc., *30*, 143, 1971.
21. Mookerjea, Park and Kuksis: Lipids, *10*, 374, 1975.
22. Wells: Fed. Proc., *30*, 151, 1971.
23. Tucker and Eckstein: J. Biol. Chem., *121*, 479, 1937.
24. du Vigneaud, Cohn, Chandler, Schenck and Simmonds: J. Biol. Chem., *140*, 625, 1941.
25. Simmonds, Cohn, Chandler and du Vigneaud: J. Biol. Chem., *149*, 519, 1943.
26. Best, Ridout and Lucas: Can. J. Biochem. Pharmacol., *47*, 73, 1968.
27. Gibson, Wilson and Udenfriend: J. Biol. Chem., *236*, 673, 1961.
28. Kennedy: Fed. Proc., *30*, 216, 1958.
29. Kushwaha and Jensen: J. Nutr., *105*, 226, 1975.
30. Mudd and Poole: Metabolism, *24*, 721, 1975.
31. du Vigneaud, Ressler and Rachele: Science, *112*, 267, 1950.
32. Stekol and Weiss: J. Biol. Chem., *186*, 343, 1950.
33. Carroll and Williams: J. Nutr., *107*, 1263, 1977.
34. Furuno, Shimakawa and Suzucki: J. Nutr., *105*, 1263, 1975.
35. Patek, Bowry and Hayes: Proc. Soc. Exp. Biol. Med., *148*, 370, 1975.
36. Uthus, Skurdel and Cornatzer: Lipids, *11*, 641, 1976.
37. Klatskin and Krehl: J. Exp. Med., *100*, 615, 1954.
38. Koch, Roatta, De Conti and Monserrat: Nutr. Rep. Intl., *15*, 9, 1977.
39. Tuma, Barak and Sorrell: Biochem. Pharmacol., *24*, 1327, 1975.
40. Radomski and Orme: J. Nutr., *92*, 19, 1967.
41. Gabuzda: Am. J. Clin. Nutr., *6*, 280, 1958.
42. Davis, Hollister, Barchas and Berger: Life Sci., *19*, 1507, 1976.
43. Growden, Hirsch, Wurtman and Wiener: N. Engl. J. Med., *297*, 524, 1977.
44. Fernstrom: Metabolism, *26*, 207, 1977.

O. *Inositol*

Janet A. Appel
and
George M. Briggs

While the presence of inositol in biologic tissues was discovered over 150 years ago by Scherrer,[1] remarkably little is known today concerning its nutritional significance. Biosynthesis of inositol appears to be a relatively widespread phenomenon in microorganisms and in higher plants and animals. Nevertheless, a dietary requirement for the substance has been demonstrated in some species of animals under certain dietary conditions. Recent advances in research concerning the possible biologic roles of inositol, primarily in cell membrane functions and in lipoprotein synthesis, have prompted several reviews of inositol metabolism.[2-4]

CHEMISTRY
Structure

Only 1 of the 9 isomers of inositol which exist is of metabolic importance. This form, properly called *myo*-inositol (meso-inositol, i-inositol, bios I and inosite are obsolete terms for the substance), is chemically known as 1,2,3,5/4,6 cyclohexanehexol and has a structure which closely resembles that of glucose:

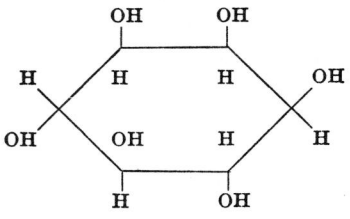

Occurrence

In pure form, this is a remarkably stable, white, crystalline substance which is water soluble and has a sweet taste.[2] *Myo*-inositol is found in virtually all living cells, where it often occurs in combined forms of ethers, phosphates or as a component of phospholipids.[2] The most common form of *myo*-inositol found in plants is the hexaphosphate known as phytic acid. This substance readily binds divalent cations, often forming insoluble salts. Studies of animals and of human subjects have shown that dietary phytate can decrease gastrointestinal absorption of minerals such as calcium, zinc and iron.[5] Phytase enzymes capable of hydrolyzing these salts have been identified in some plant and animal tissues.[6]

In animal tissues, *myo*-inositol most frequently occurs either in the free form (in amounts ranging from 0.43 to 0.46 mg per 100 ml human plasma[7] to as much as 500 mg per 100 gm human lens tissue[8]) or in phospholipids.[2] Phosphatidylinositol, diphosphoinositide (phosphatidylinositol 4-phosphate) and triphosphoinositide (phosphatidylinositol 4,5 biphosphate) have been found in various amounts in virtually all animal tissues.[3] Highest concentrations of phosphatidylinositols have been found in kidney (1.23 mg per gm rat kidney) and neural tissue (0.67 mg per gm rat brain) with lesser amounts in liver, muscle tissues, erythrocytes, body fluids and other organs.[2,3] Phytic acid, in association with calcium ions (phytin), has been found in nucleated erythrocytes of fowl and turtles[9] and an inositol-containing disaccharide has recently been identified in rat mammary gland and milk.[10]

Relatively high levels of phosphatidylinositol have also been found in yeast and other microorganisms, primarily in cell membranes and cell wall polysaccharides.[3] As would be expected from its widespread occurrence in plant and animal tissues, food sources of *myo*-inositol are plentiful and varied.[2] Estimates of average

daily inositol intake of humans in the United States range from 300 mg[11] to 1000 mg[2] per day.

Analysis

The traditional microbiologic method for *myo*-inositol analysis makes use of the inositol requirement for growth of the yeast Saccharomyces carlsbergensis.[2] A similar assay using Saccharomyces cerevisiae as the test organism has also been described.[12] While both of these methods involve turbidometric measurements of growth, a cup-plate method using Kloeckera apiculatus has recently been developed.[13] A time-consuming chemical method involving reaction with periodate is also available.[2]

Microbiologic assays and chemical methods appear to be giving way to more rapid chromatographic methods (paper and thin-layer)[2,3] and more extensive development of gas-liquid chromatography.[2,14,15] Enzyme assays[2] and ion-exchange chromatography[16] have also been developed for inositol analysis. Extensive treatment may be necessary to free inositol from bound forms prior to analysis, depending on the method used and the nature of combined forms present in the samples to be analyzed.[2,17]

BIOLOGIC SIGNIFICANCE

Deficiency Signs in Animals

In 1941, Woolley described a dietary inositol deficiency in mice characterized by decreased rate of growth and occurrence of alopecia.[18] Signs of deficiency occurred in about 50 per cent of the animals studied and spontaneous recoveries were noted on occasion.[2] Subsequently, Hegsted and his co-workers found that inositol increased the growth rate of chicks fed semipurified diets.[19] Pavcek and Baum found inositol effective in alleviating the "spectacle eye" condition in rats;[20] however, the diet used in this experiment was lacking in biotin also. Other workers have shown a response of spectacle eye to biotin, indicating that the effect of inositol may have been an indirect one resulting from increased biotin synthesis by gut bacteria.[2] A more recent study has shown a growth response in rats fed semipurified diets supplemented with inositol; however, no other deficiency signs were found during the 3-month period of the feeding trials.[21]

Since 1973, Hegsted and his co-workers have reported several studies of inositol deficiency in female gerbils.[22,23] Female animals (and castrated males) fed semipurified diets lacking inositol showed signs of hypocholesteremia, excessive fat deposition in the intestinal mucosa (lipodystrophy) and eventually dermatitis, weight loss and death.[23] Intact male animals were apparently protected from dietary deficiency by adequate inositol synthesis in the testes. When male animals were fed inositol-deficient, semipurified diets containing highly saturated fat as the fat source, they also developed intestinal lipodystrophy, but to a lesser extent than the females.[22]

In 1957, Eagle and his colleagues reported their studies of inositol requirements of a number of different cell types, using tissue culture techniques.[24] They found that many normal and malignant human cells required an exogenous source of inositol. As emphasized by these workers and others, there are several critical differences between the tissue culture environment and the internal environment of the intact animal. Therefore, extrapolation of these results to the in vivo situation of the whole animal is limited.[4,24] Furuya and co-workers used similar techniques and found that monkey kidney cells, some cultures of rat liver cells, and rat thymus cells did not require exogenous inositol to achieve maximal growth rates.[25]

Several investigations of rats, mice and hamsters fed semipurified diets have failed to demonstrate a dietary need for inositol.[26-28] Notable in this group of papers is that of Burton et al., who found de-

creased free inositol levels in some tissues of neonatal rats fed inositol-deficient diets from 6 days to 72 days of age, but found no signs of abnormal development or of lipid deposition in any tissues.[28]

Metabolism

Gavin and McHenry provided the initial evidence for a metabolic role of *myo*-inositol as a lipotropic factor, when they found it alleviated fatty livers in rats fed a particular semipurified diet.[29] Many studies have been conducted since this discovery in attempts to further clarify this point. These investigations have revealed a number of dietary and physiologic factors which appear to influence the amount of inositol required for metabolism. Because of these effects, a dietary need for inositol may be demonstrated in some species under certain dietary and environmental conditions, while such a need may not be found in other species or under different conditions.

Some dietary influences which appear to affect inositol metabolism include dietary choline content, the amount of fat in the diet, its degree of saturation, and its specific fatty acid composition.[4,30-32] Physiologic and environmental stress may also affect inositol utilization, as pointed out in studies by Wright[33] and by Burton and Wells.[34] Wright found that the fatty liver syndrome in commercial laying chickens responded to supplementary inositol.[33] It was hypothesized that genetic factors maximizing egg production and decreasing body size, as well as modern feeding and housing practices, may have led to increased inositol need by the layers. Transient development of fatty livers in lactating rats fed inositol-deficient diets throughout pregnancy and lactation was found by Burton and Wells.[34] *Myo*-inositol content of milk and mammary tissue declined in the dams, and tissue levels of *myo*-inositol in offspring were below normal. However, no clinical abnormalities were found in the offspring which were followed through their own reproduction cycles. Liver lipid content of the inositol-deprived dams spontaneously returned to normal when lactation ceased. In these special cases it seems that inositol needs exceeded the biosynthetic capabilities of the organisms studied.

The mechanism for the lipotropic action of inositol found in some of these studies remains unknown. However, evidence is accumulating which points to its role in phospholipid synthesis and a consequent effect on the synthesis and secretion of lipoproteins involved in lipid transport.[2-4]

A number of studies have revealed aspects of inositol metabolism other than its lipotropic action. Wiebelhaus, Betheil and Lardy showed that absorption of myo-inositol in rats is virtually complete within 24 to 48 hours after ingestion. This group also provided evidence that inositol ingested under fasting conditions could be catabolized similarly to glucose, as less than 1 per cent of the dose was excreted in the urine, and it was effective in reducing ketosis in the rats studied.[35] Conflicting reports appear in the literature concerning a possible role of inositol in amylase secretion[36] and an unconfirmed report describes an increase in calcium uptake in bones of rats given supplemental inositol.[37] Some evidence also exists for a role of inositol in esterification of cholesterol in gerbils, hens and rats.[4,23,38,39] Early claims of a metabolic interrelationship between inositol and para-aminobenzoic acid and between inositol and ascorbic acid have not been upheld.[40-42]

Considerable interest has been generated recently in the role of myo-inositol in cell membrane functions. Studies have provided as yet inconclusive evidence for possible functions of inositol in mitochondrial contraction,[43] sperm motility[44] and regulation of cell membrane permeability, affecting ionic transport and neural transmission.[3,45,46] Evidence for these roles of inositol through its function

as a cell surface receptor has been reviewed by Michell.[47]

The kidney appears to be a primary site of myo-inositol catabolism. In studies with rats, the pathway from inositol to glucuronic acid to xylulose and the pentose phosphate cycle has been identified as the major route of inositol breakdown. Inositol oxidase, capable of catalyzing the first step in the reaction sequence, has been isolated from rat kidney tissue.[2]

Synthesis

Proof of myo-inositol biosynthesis from glucose is available, in most part from tracer studies of germ-free rats,[48] conventional rats,[49] microorganisms[50] and tissue cultures of different cell types.[51-53] Characterization of catalyzing enzymes and of intermediates in the reaction sequence has been accomplished to some extent.[2,3,54] In addition, the major pathway for incorporation of myo-inositol into phosphatidylinositols, involving reaction with cytidin diphosphate diglycerides, has been established.[2,3] Enzymes have also been identified in several tissues which are involved in transfer of phosphate groups during synthesis of polyphosphoinositides.[3]

Significance in Human Beings

Signs of inositol deficiency have not been found in human populations and we are not aware of any experimental efforts to study effects of inositol deprivation in human subjects. Because of the widespread occurrence of inositol in the food supply, low intakes would not be expected in diets normally consumed. Concern has focused on some infant formulas based on nonmilk protein sources, and on some of the chemically defined diets designed for therapeutic purposes which are low or lacking in inositol.[55,56] While it is unknown whether use of these products constitutes risk of inositol deficiency, the Committee on Nutrition of the American Academy of Pediatrics has recommended that inositol be included in infant formulas at levels at or above those found in milk-based formulas[55] as a precautionary measure.

Toxicity

Few studies of inositol toxicity are available, but from evidence in rats and other animals it appears to be relatively nontoxic.[2,57] Human subjects fed 3 gm of *myo*-inositol per day for a short period of time showed no toxic signs, and others given single intravenous doses up to 1 gm showed no effects.[2]

Relevant Clinical Conditions

Patients with renal diseases and nephrectomized rats have shown excessively high levels of *myo*-inositol in the blood.[11,58] In addition, diabetic patients and rats with experimentally induced diabetes show high *myo*-inositol levels in blood and urine.[59–62] It is not clear whether these high levels are the results of hyperglycemia and competition with glucose for renal excretion, a possible dependence of *myo*-inositol on insulin for cell entry,[60] or decreased catabolism of inositol by the kidney.[58–60] Recent evidence supports the theory of decreased inositol catabolism as a primary cause, however.[63]

The changes in *myo*-inositol metabolism in diabetes and renal disease have been implicated in decreased motor nerve conduction velocity in experimental animals and in human subjects.[59,61,62] Attempts have further been made to explain peripheral neuropathies associated with diabetes and renal diseases on the basis of changes in *myo*-inositol metabolism. However, causal relationships between motor nerve conduction velocity and occurrence of neuropathies have not been consistently found.[58,61,62] As Anderson pointed out, changes in *myo*-inositol levels in body fluids are only one of many metabolic changes occurring in these diseases which have been shown to affect neurologic function.[61]

In conclusion, research investigations to date have provided clues to the functions of *myo*-inositol in metabolism and have brought to light physiologic and environmental factors which may affect its utilization. The studies available have failed to provide any evidence, however, that *myo*-inositol is an essential nutrient for human beings.

BIBLIOGRAPHY

1. Neukomm: *Ueber das Vorkommen von Leucin, Tyrosin und Andered Umsatzstoffe in Menschlichen Korper bei Krankheiten.* Zurich, Orell, Fussli u. Comp., 1859.
2. Anderson, et al.: Inositols. In *The Vitamins,* Vol. 3, 2nd ed. (Sebrell and Harris, Eds.). New York, Academic Press, 1971.
3. Hawthorne and White: Vitamin. Horm., *33,* 529, 1975.
4. Kuksis and Mookerjea: Nutr. Rev., *36,* 233, 1978.
5. Reinhold, Ismail-Beigi and Faradji: Nutr. Rep. Int., *12,* 75, 1975.
6. Rapoport, Leva and Guest: J. Biol. Chem., *139,* 621, 1941.
7. Freinkel, Dawson, Ingbar and White: Proc. Soc. Exp. Biol. Med., *100,* 549, 1959.
8. Heyningen: Biochem. J., *65,* 24, 1957.
9. Rapoport: J. Biol. Chem., *135,* 403, 1940.
10. Naccarato, Ray and Wells: J. Biol. Chem., *250,* 1872, 1975.
11. Clements, DeJesus and Winegrad: Lancet, *1,* 7813, 1973.
12. Woolley: J. Biol. Chem., *140,* 453, 1941.
13. Yamada and Tsukahara: J. Nutr. Sci. Vitaminol., *19,* 205, 1973.
14. Seifert: J. Assoc. Off. Anal. Chem., *55,* 1194, 1972.
15. Clements and Starnes: Biochem. Med., *12,* 200, 1975.
16. Cosgrove: Ann. N.Y. Acad. Sci., *165,* 677, 1969.
17. Taylor and McKibbin: J. Biol. Chem., *201,* 609, 1953.
18. Woolley: J. Biol. Chem., *139,* 29, 1941.
19. Hegsted, Briggs, Mills, Elvehjem and Hart: Proc. Soc. Exp. Biol. Med., *47,* 376, 1941.
20. Pavcek and Baum: Science, *93,* 502, 1941.
21. Yagi, Kotaki and Yamamoto: J. Vitaminol., *11,* 14, 1965.
22. Hegsted, Gallagher and Hanford: J. Nutr., *104,* 588, 1974.
23. Anonymous: Nutr. Rev., *32,* 210, 1974.
24. Eagle, Oyama, Levy and Freeman: J. Biol. Chem., *226,* 191, 1957.
25. Furuya, Takaoka, Nagai and Katsuta: Jpn. J. Exp. Med., *41,* 471, 1971.
26. McCormick, Harris and Anderson: J. Nutr., *52,* 337, 1954.
27. Shepherd and Taylor: Proc. Nutr. Soc., *33,* 63A, 1974.
28. Burton, Ray, Bradford, Orr, Nickerson and Wells: J. Nutr., *106,* 1610, 1976.
29. Gavin and McHenry: J. Biol. Chem., *139,* 485, 1941.

30. Best, Lucas, Patterson and Ridout: Science, *103*, 12, 1946.
31. Best, Lucas, Patterson and Ridout: Biochem. J., *48*, 448, 1951.
32. Anderson and Holub: J. Nutr., *106*, 529, 1976.
33. Wright: Nutr. Rep. Int., *2*, 209, 1970.
34. Burton and Wells: J. Nutr. *106*, 1617, 1976.
35. Weibelhaus, Betheil and Lardy: Arch. Biochem., *13*, 379, 1947.
36. Slaby and Bryan: J. Biol. Chem.,*251*, 5078, 1976.
37. Angeloff, Skoryna and Henderson: Acta Pharmacol. Toxicol., *40*, 209, 1977.
38. Herrmann: Proc. Soc. Exp. Biol. Med., *63*, 436, 1946.
39. Kotaki, Sakurai, Kobayashi and Yagi: J. Vitaminol., *14*, 87, 1968.
40. Martin: Am. J. Physiol., *136*, 124, 1942.
41. Ershoff: Proc. Soc. Exp. Biol. Med., *56*, 190, 1944.
42. Anderson, Coots and Halliday: J. Nutr., *64*, 167, 1958.
43. Vignais, Vignais and Lehninger: J. Biol. Chem., *239*, 2011, 1964.
44. Voglmayr: Biol. Reprod., *11*, 593, 1974.
45. Koch and Diringer: Biochem. Biophys. Res. Commun., *58,* 361, 1974.
46. Charalampous: J. Biol. Chem., *246*, 456, 1971.
47. Michell: Biochim. Biophys. Acta, *415*, 81, 1975.
48. Halliday and Anderson: J. Biol. Chem.,*217*, 797, 1955.
49. Imai: J. Biochem., *53*, 50, 1963.
50. Chen and Charalampous: J. Biol. Chem., *240*, 3507, 1965.
51. Hauser and Finelli: J. Biol. Chem., *238*, 3224, 1963.
52. Imai: J. Biochem., *55*, 126, 1964.
53. Naccarato, Ray and Wells: Arch. Biochem. Biophys., *164*, 194, 1974.
54. Chen and Eisenberg: J. Biol. Chem., *250*, 2963, 1975.
55. Committee on Nutrition: Pediatrics, *57*, 278, 1976.
56. Young, Heuler, Russell and Weser: Gastroenterology, *69*, 1338, 1975.
57. Hasan, Nishigaki, Tsutsui and Yagi: J. Nutr. Sci. Vitaminol., *20*, 55, 1974.
58. Melmed, Bank and Lewin: Isr. J. Med. Sci., *10*, 1518, 1974.
59. Palmano, Whiting and Hawthorne: Biochem. J., *167*, 229, 1977.
60. Clements and Reynertson: Diabetes, *26*, 215, 1977.
61. Anderson: Am. J. Clin. Nutr., *29*, 402, 1976.
62. Winegrad and Greene: N. Engl. J. Med., *295*, 1416, 1976.
63. Melmed, Lewin and Bank. Am. J. Med. Sci.,*274*, 55, 1977.

P.   *Carnitine*

Diane L. Bray
and
George M. Briggs

In 1947, Fraenkel, while investigating the role of folic acid in the nutrition of insects, found that the meal worm (Tenebrio molitor) required a growth factor, present in the charcoal filtrate of yeast, which had not previously been recognized.[1] To this factor he gave the name "vitamin B_T," though it is not recognized as a vitamin today since there is no absolute dietary need in any higher animal.

If the meal worms were fed a synthetic diet deficient only in vitamin B_T, they died in 4 to 5 weeks. So constant was this finding that Fraenkel was able to develop a technique for bioassay of vitamin B_T based on the rate of growth of larvae of Tenebrio molitor.[2] Using this technique, he found there was a wide distribution of vitamin B_T in yeast, milk, liver and whey, with particularly large quantities in muscle and meat extracts.[3] These have been proven to be the most potent natural sources of this substance. Although some other insects could not synthesize vitamin B_T, Fraenkel and his co-workers found that most insects they studied, as well as higher animals, synthesized the compound in their tissues.

Fraenkel concentrated large amounts of crystalline vitamin B_T in 1948. In studies with Carter,[4-7] he proved that this compound was identical with carnitine, a quaternary ammonium compound, which had been discovered in muscle by Gulewitsch and Krimberg[8] in 1905. Carnitine is beta-hydroxygamma-trimethylaminobutyrate; its formula is

$$\underset{(CH_3)_3N \cdot CH_2 \cdot \overset{\displaystyle OH}{\overset{\displaystyle |}{CH}} \cdot CH_2 \cdot COOH}{}$$

With the molecular structure established, and its role as a vitamin for certain insects described, the search for the metabolic function of carnitine was intensified. Fritz[9] noted in 1955 that carnitine, when added to a rat liver homogenate containing fatty acids of 8 or more carbons, increased the rate of fatty acid oxidation. Concurrently, Friedman and Fraenkel[10] isolated an enzyme, acetyl carnitine transferase, from pigeon liver which reversibly acetylated carnitine according to the reaction

acetyl CoA + carnitine $\longrightarrow$ acetyl acylcarnitine + CoA

These two observations inspired much research into the role of carnitine in fatty acid metabolism and led to the suggestion that a primary function of carnitine may be as a carrier molecule translocating long-chain fatty acids across the inner mitochondrial membrane to the matrix where they are accessible to oxidative enzymes. There is some speculation that carnitine may also function as a methyl donor,[11] but most of the evidence to date supports the hypothesis that carnitine plays its major role in lipid metabolism.[12,13]

The role of carnitine in human metabolism continues to be explored through its determination in blood and tissues of healthy humans, and through studying disease states in which the observed levels deviate from the normal. Unfortunately the establishment of normal levels has been hampered by a lack of uniformity of assay methods among laboratories. The only method available to early

workers was the biologic assay mentioned above. Since then, enzymatic techniques, with radiometric modifications, have been developed,[14,15] based upon the ability of the enzyme acetyl carnitine transferase to transfer acyl groups to carnitine, as in the reaction shown. The free CoA is then measured colorimetrically. Much of the recent work has relied upon these latter methods, and there has been little utilization of the two approaches on the same samples, making the comparison of data extracted from the literature difficult. Moreover, variables which probably affect these levels—e.g. age, sex, race and diet history of the subjects—have not been controlled. The plasma or serum values of carnitine using the biologic assay range from 860 to 2870 μg per dl.[16] When the enzymatic method or one of its variations is used, the range found for carnitine is 378 to 1196 μg per dl.[16] Most of the determinations of muscle carnitine have been based on the enzymatic method, and the range reported is 457 to 2479 μg per gm dry weight.[16]

The diseases in which carnitine levels have been most extensively studied have been lipid storage myopathies, the most common symptoms of which are muscle weakness and lipid accumulation between muscle fibers.[17,18] Since carnitine had been implicated in lipid metabolism, the search for the cause of the disease included determinations of carnitine levels, which were found, in general, to be lower than normal. This functional deficiency of carnitine may result from one of three metabolic disorders. (1) A genetic defect affecting the synthesis of one or more of the enzymes required for the synthesis of carnitine would depress levels of carnitine in the blood and tissues. (2) Even if synthesis were normal, the use of the endogenous carnitine might still be impaired by its presence in plasma in an unavailable form, by a lack of acyl carnitine transferase, or by a defect in the sarcolemma rendering it less permeable to carnitine. (3) Abnormally rapid degradation of carnitine could cause symptoms of deficiency to appear.[19] When the metabolic disorder involved is either decreased synthesis or increased catabolism, treatment with dietary carnitine has been reported to relieve symptoms.[17] However, in those cases where the defect lies in the body's ability to use the available carnitine, the administration of carnitine is not the answer. In one case improvement was seen on a diet low in fat and, in another, clinical improvement occurred with prednisone therapy.[20,21]

Low fluid and tissue carnitine levels have also been noted in diseases such as diabetes, dystrophy and hyperthyroidism, as well as in such normal physiologic states as fasting, pregnancy and physical exertion.[19] These states are also generally characterized by alterations in lipid metabolism, the area in which in vitro work has suggested that carnitine has its major function.

Under normal conditions, there is no dietary requirement for carnitine; therefore, it cannot be considered to be a vitamin for humans. However, where a metabolic abnormality exists which inhibits synthesis, interferes with use or increases catabolism of carnitine, symptoms appear which are sometimes relieved by dietary supplement. Future research focusing on the metabolic function of this compound should further delineate the dietary role of carnitine in human health and disease. Braunwald suggests that, through augmenting anaerobic metabolism, carnitine might possibly help reduce myocardial injury following coronary artery occlusion.[22]

BIBLIOGRAPHY

1. Fraenkel: Nature, *161*, 891, 1948.
2. Fraenkel: Fed. Proc., *10*, 183, 1951.
3. Fraenkel: Arch. Biochem., *34*, 457, 1951.
4. Fraenkel: Arch. Biochem., *34*, 468, 1951.
5. Carter, Bhattacharyya and Fraenkel: Fed. Proc., *10*, 170, 1951.
6. Carter, Bhattacharyya and Fraenkel: Arch. Biochem. Biophys., *35*, 241, 1952.
7. Carter, Bhattacharyya, Weidman and Fraenkel: Arch. Biochem. Biophys., *38*, 405, 1952.
8. Gulewitsch and Krimberg: Z. Physiol. Chem., *45*, 326, 1905.
9. Fritz: Acta Physiol. Scand., *34*, 364, 1955.
10. Friedman and Fraenkel: Arch. Biochem. Biophys., *59*, 491, 1955.
11. Fraenkel and Friedman: Vitam. Horm., *15*, 73, 1957.
12. Mitchell: Am. J. Clin. Nutr., *31*, 293, 1978.
13. Friedman and Fraenkel: In *The Vitamins*, Vol. 5 (Sebrell and Harris, Eds.). New York, Academic Press, 1972.
14. Marquis and Fritz: J. Lipid Res., *5*, 184, 1964.
15. Cederblad and Lindstedt: Clin. Chim. Acta, *37*, 235, 1972.
16. Mitchell: Am. J. Clin. Nutr., *31*, 481, 1978.
17. Karpati, et al.: Neurology, *25*, 16, 1975.
18. Angelini: J. Neurol., *214*, 1, 1976.
19. Mitchell: Am. J. Clin. Nutr., *31*, 645, 1978.
20. Smyth, Lake, MacDermot and Wilson: Lancet, *1*, 1198, 1975.
21. Vandyke, Griggs, Markesberg and Dimauro: Neurology, *25*, 154, 1975.
22. Braunwald: Harvey Lect., *71*, 247, 1975–1976.

Chapter 7

MAJOR MINERALS

A. *Calcium and Phosphorus*

Louis V. Avioli

Calcium and phosphorus are considered together since they constitute the major part of the mineral content of the skeleton. Over 99 per cent of the total-body calcium and approximately 85 per cent of the phosphorus are in the bones. The ratio of calcium to phosphorus in the bone is a little over 2/1 and is approximately constant. Thus, marked changes in the body content of one of these minerals will be reflected in changes in the other.

Many phosphorus compounds are present in the body, and phosphorylated compounds are involved in a number of metabolic pathways. No attempt is made in this chapter to discuss these functions of phosphorus, since they are considered in standard textbooks of biochemistry. Attention is directed primarily toward the nutritional requirement of calcium and phosphorus and, since phosphorus is ordinarily considered to occur in adequate amounts in most diets consumed by man, primary discussion is given to calcium requirements. It is remarkable that, in spite of the prominence given to calcium in the nutrition literature, there is much argument as to its nutritional significance in most diets. Increasing knowledge has served primarily to emphasize how little is known of calcium requirements and the need for additional criteria to estimate requirements and adequacy of calcium intake.

CALCIUM

Calcium is the most abundant cation and the fifth most common inorganic element of the human body. It not only serves as the principal component of skeletal tissue, imparting to it the structural integrity essential to support the increasing body size of the individual during growth, but also plays a vital role in a variety of essential physiologic and biochemical processes. The functions of the calcium ion include its influence on blood coagulation, neuromuscular excitability, cellular adhesiveness, transmission of nerve impulses, maintenance and function of cell membranes and activation of enzyme reactions and hormone secretion. The skeleton, a huge reservoir of insoluble complexes of calcium, is in dynamic equilibrium with physicochemically soluble forms of circulating calcium. These are maintained at a remarkably constant level, with a diurnal plasma variation of ± 3 per cent. This fluctuation in circulating calcium is comparable to that of plasma sodium (± 3 per cent) and is lower than the range of variation for the potassium (± 12 per cent) or the hydrogen ion (± 10 per cent). Although the primary homeostatic mechanism that controls the plasma calcium concentration is a function of the parathyroid glands and biologically active vitamin D metabolites, a variety of other hormones, vitamins, inhibitors of biologic calcification, such as inorganic pyrophosphate, and other less well-understood factors prevent the fluctuation of calcium over a wide range, despite the enormous insoluble skeletal reservoir and wide variations in intake and output.[1] Disruption of this exquisite control system leads ultimately to derangements in skeletal and extraosseous calcium metabolism. These, in turn, often result in characteristic clinical manifestations and alterations in both chemical and roentgenographic findings, which serve to define the pathologic state.

Calcium in Bone

The average adult human contains 1,000 to 1,200 gm of calcium or 20.7 to 24.8 gm per kg of fat-free body tissue. Whereas, quantitatively, 30 per cent of body sodium and 50 per cent of body magnesium are stored in bone, over 99 per cent of the body calcium resides in the skeleton. Calcium in the solid mineral phase of bone is usually considered to be a variant of poorly crystalline hydroxyapatite, $Ca_{10}(PO_4)_6(OH)_2$, the unit cell of the crystal lattice containing all 18 ions of the formula. It has been suggested, from studies on synthetic and biologic hydroxyapatites, that the apatite portion of bone mineral does *not* have the ideal stoichiometry $Ca_{10}(PO_4)_6(OH)_2$, but is approximately 10 per cent deficient in calcium, with the structure remaining generally intact.[2] A noncrystalline amorphous phase combined with phosphate, $Ca_3(PO_4)$, has also been identified in osseous tissue.[3]

The hydroxyapatite crystals are tubular hexagons with average dimensions of $40 \times 50 \times 600$ Å. Although calcium and phosphate are the principal ions in hydroxyapatite, the crystal contains significant amounts of Na^+, Mg^{++}, CO_3^{2-} and citrate^{3-} ions[4] which, with the exception of Mg^{++}, can substitute for either calcium or phosphate in the apatite lattice and can be adsorbed on its surface or incorporated into its hydration shell.

Trace elements[5] and so-called bone-seeking ions, such as strontium (Sr), radium (Ra), plutonium (Pu), lead (Pb) and fluorine (F), are also incorporated into or adsorbed onto the crystal. This assumes importance when their radioactive isotopes (e.g. ^{90}Sr from fallout or Ra from luminous paints) are ingested, since their accumulation may lead to radiation damage and malignant degeneration of bone cells. The release of mineral from bone during resorption buffers hydrogen ions, whereas the formation of bone mineral generates hydrogen ions, 8 H^+ released per unit cell of the crystalline lattice. This may assume significant proportions in the growing skeleton wherein, during the process of skeletal mineralization and hydroxyapatite synthesis, approximately 20 mEq of H^+ are released by the deposition of 1 gm of calcium.[6] Bone, therefore, not only represents a calcium depot for the miscible calcium pool but also assumes an important role as a reservoir for electrolytes and buffers. The presence of the amorphous calcium phase accounts for a Ca/P ratio in bone (1/5) which is lower than that found in synthetic hydroxyapatite. This metastable noncrystalline calcium phase is characteristic of newly deposited bone mineral and spontaneously changes to the poorly crystallized hydroxyapatite after it is deposited. The relative concentration of the amorphous phase in bone decreases with the increasing biologic age of the skeleton.[7,8]

Bone affords an enormous depot of calcium which, when appropriately stimulated by a variety of hormones and metabolic agents, serves as the guardian of the circulating calcium pool. Unlike the mineral of tooth enamel, which is relatively inert, bone undergoes constant remodeling and turnover. The dynamic process of bone turnover normally releases into blood and then reaccumulates from 250 mg to 1 gm of calcium per day. Little calcium is deposited in the fetus during the first trimester of pregnancy, but the concentration rises rapidly subsequently until a body weight of 0.5 kg is attained.[9] Gradual increments are observed thereafter until term. During the final trimester, when maternal levels of circulating parathyroid hormone[10] and intestinal calcium absorption[11] are increased, the human fetus acquires approximately 20 gm of calcium from maternal sources. The total calcium content of a full-term neonate weighing 3,500 gm approaches 30 gm, or about 1 per cent of the body weight.

The turnover of skeletal calcium varies with age. It has been estimated to be 100 per cent per annum in infants up to 1 year and decreases with age to a turnover rate of 10 per cent in older children. The skeleton weighs approximately 100 gm at birth and actually doubles in weight during the first year of life. Skeletal growth during childhood involves calcium retention of not more than 150 mg per day until after the first decade. During peak adolescent growth, bone development is at its maximum and calcium retained as bone may range between 275 to 500 mg per day. The rate of turnover is higher in cancellous or trabecular bones (e.g. vertebrae and ribs) than in compact bones, such as the skull and mandible. In adults, after epiphyseal closure and longitudinal growth have ceased, the turnover rate is approximately 2 to 4 per cent per annum.

During adult life skeletal growth does not entirely cease, since both subperiosteal bone formation and the later adolescent shift to endosteal bone formation or apposition continue to some extent. At this time, skeletal maintenance requires the deposition of approximately 180 gm of calcium per annum, or 18 per cent of the total skeletal content. The skeleton is in a relative steady state, since bone formation equals bone resorption, with no net change in skeletal mass.

Between the fourth and fifth decades, there is a shift in this equilibrium and bone resorption dominates. Skeletal mass then begins to decline with advancing age at a

rate approximating 0.7 per cent of the total mass per annum (Fig. 7A–1).[12] This inevitable decrease in bone mass with advancing years obtains independent of wide variations in calcium intake and dietary habits. The significant features are: (1) Among young adults, the skeletal mass is greater in males than females and greater in blacks than whites. (2) The loss begins earlier in females than in males. (3) Taller subjects of both sexes lose bone less rapidly. (4) Although the onset of loss in the females antedates the menopause, the rate of skeletal loss in some females is distinctly accelerated after the menopause.[12] Thus, since the maximum skeletal mass at maturity is less for the white female than for the male or Negro of either sex, and because the loss begins earlier in the female and proceeds at a more rapid rate

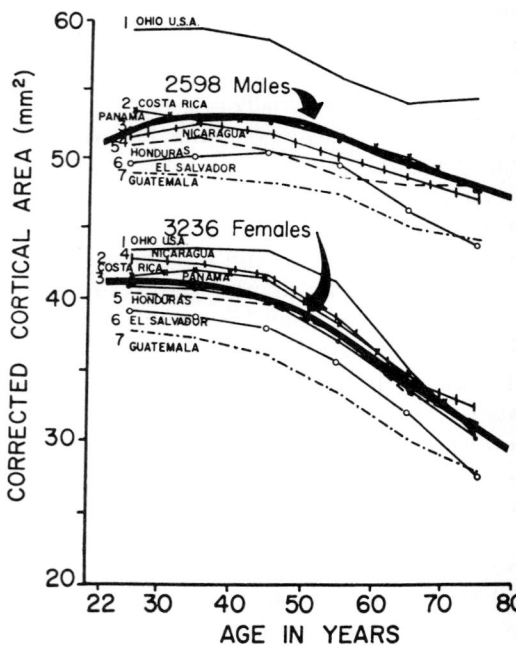

Fig. 7A–1. Age-associated decrease in the metacarpal cortical area of males and females from 7 countries. The overall trend of bone loss for all subjects is depicted by the heavy black lines that represent pooled weighted mean values. (From Garn et al.: Clin. Orthop., 65, 51, 1969. Used with permission of authors and publisher.)

after the menopause, net skeletal mass is lowest in the menopausal white female.

The exchange of calcium between bone and circulating fluids is still ill defined and poorly understood. It appears to be divisible into the slow processes of bone formation and resorption and the far more rapid processes of ion exchange with accessible crystal surfaces. The osteon surfaces, or Haversian units, of compact bone plus the surfaces afforded by trabecular bone provide an enormous surface area for interchange between extracellular fluids and bone mineral. Normally, less than 1 per cent of the skeletal calcium is available for free ionic exchange with the extracellular fluid.[13] The calcium in blood, extracellular fluid and extraosseous cellular compartments accounts for 1 per cent of whole-body calcium and, together with the exchangeable calcium of bone, comprises the miscible, or readily exchangeable, calcium pool. Since most of the skeletal calcium is not in a form that is readily diffusible to combat hypocalcemia and maintain homeostasis, calcium must be mobilized by active resorptive processes.

Bone lability is maintained by the concurrent activities of bone formation and resorption. Osseous tissue is continually being deposited and resorbed, primarily as a result of the activity of the connective tissue cells covering its surfaces. Changes in bone resorption are not simply consequent to changes in the activity of existing cell machinery but depend on the continuous transformation of resting undifferentiated cells to osteocytic cells, osteoblasts and osteoclasts. Osteoclastic and osteocytic responses to parathyroid hormone represent one of the most singularly effective control mechanisms available to facilitate the resorption of bone. The regulating action of parathyroid hormone is normally accomplished through continuous secretion, which is inversely related to the extracellular fluid calcium ion concentration.

In contrast to the action of parathyroid hormone on bone, the inhibition of bone resorption is the principal, if not sole, function of the hormone calcitonin.[1,14,15] It is noteworthy that the resorptive activity of osteoclasts decreases in response to calcitonin, the action of which is rapid and short lived, relative to parathyroid hormone. Calcitonin is elaborated by the parafollicular cells of the thyroid in response to *elevations* in circulating ionized calcium concentration. Together with parathyroid hormone, calcitonin constitutes the dual proportional control system which effectively maintains a constant extracellular calcium concentration.[1,14,15] In addition, vitamin D, through its biologically active metabolites, alters the responsiveness of bone to both parathyroid hormone and calcitonin, so that alterations in bone resorption serve the needs of skeletal growth and remodeling as well as calcium homeostasis.[1,14,15]

Although the roles of parathyroid hormone, calcitonin and vitamin D metabolites in maintaining calcium homeostasis are of paramount importance, insulin, growth hormone, thyroxine, androgens, estrogens, adrenal corticosteroids and inorganic phosphate are also contributory in this regard.[1]

Calcium in Plasma

The total calcium concentration of blood plasma or serum of man is remarkably constant, ranging between 2.25 and 2.75 mM, with 2.5 mM (10 mg per 100 ml or 5.0 mEq/L) the average value.[16] In men, the serum calcium decreases with age, paralleling a decrease in both total serum protein and albumin, whereas in women, despite similar decrements in total serum protein, serum calcium remains rather constant with advancing years. Serum total calcium also decreases 5 to 10 per cent during pregnancy until the end of the third trimester, when it tends to rise. The values begin to fall in the second or third month, attaining the lowest values in the seventh or eighth months. The "free" ionized calcium concentration is not significantly altered during pregnancy, so the reduction in total calcium can best be explained by the lower amount of protein-bound calcium. The latter may reflect the 20 to 30 per cent fall in circulatory albumin which normally obtains during the third trimester.

Calcium exists in three forms in the blood and body fluids: (1) protein-bound calcium, (2) ionized calcium and (3) diffusible calcium complexed with organic acids such as citrate or inorganic acids such as sulfate or phosphate.[16] The free and complexed calciums are often referred to as the nonprotein-bound or ultrafilterable fraction. The physiologic properties of calcium are all functions of the free ionic calcium. Because of the compartmentalization of plasma calcium, total calcium may often fail to reflect the free ionic calcium levels, particularly in subjects with acidosis, alkalosis or abnormal plasma protein concentrations. In normal plasma the protein-bound calcium accounts for about 46 per cent of the total[16] (Fig. 7A-2). Albumins and globulins are the principal plasma proteins to which calcium is bound, with the prealbumin fraction accounting for the highest degree of binding affinity. About 81 per cent of the protein-bound calcium is bound to albumin, the globulins accounting for the remainder. For the protein-poor fluids of the body, such as the cerebrospinal and extracellular fluids, the calcium concentration is generally about 1.25 mM/L (5 mg per 100 ml) and is virtually all in the ultrafilterable form. A small fraction of this is also in the form of nonionized diffusible complexes. The ionized calcium fraction is the physiologically active form; alterations in its concentration are critical for the regulation of neuromuscular excitability. Plasma ionized calcium concentrations normally range between 0.94 to 1.33 mM/L (mean 1.14 mM/L). When this plasma concentration is reduced, increased neuromuscular irritability results.

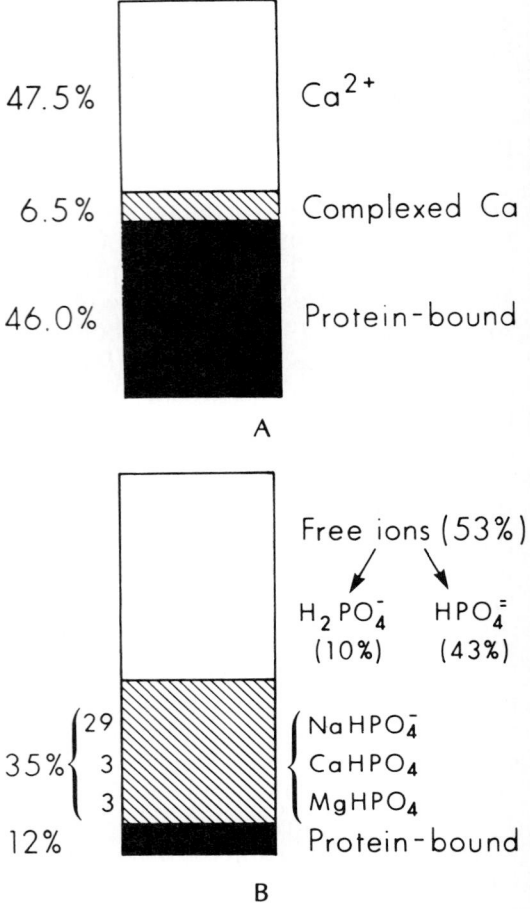

Fig. 7A-2. *A*, State of calcium in normal human plasma. *B*, State of phosphorus in normal human plasma. (Modified from Walser.[16])

Although increases in total serum calcium are occasionally associated with the increases in the level of ionized calcium, there is no apparent correlation between serum-ionized and total calcium concentrations. Thus, neither serum total calcium nor ultrafilterable calcium provides a reliable index of serum-ionized calcium. The protective effect of acidosis against hypocalcemic tetany may not result entirely from an increased concentration of ionized calcium, since the hydrogen (or hydroxyl) ion exerts a depressive effect on neuromuscular irritability, even though it does not affect the inotropic response of the heart to calcium ions.

In normal subjects, a relation exists between plasma calcium and inorganic phosphate. When expressed in terms of total calcium (mg per 100 ml) and inorganic phosphate (mg per 100 ml), the "ion product" or Ca × P solubility product normally averages 35. This calculated circulating ion product has no theoretical significance and its values are extremely variable in normal man. In molar units, the ion product calculated by this method is 0.2 to 0.3 times the actual plasma ion product, $(Ca^{+2}) \times (HPO_4{}^{2-})$, which in human plasma averages $0.72 \times 10^{-6}M$. A "solubility product constant" can be defined as the ion product at concentrations of the ions at which the rates of solution and precipitation of the salt are equal. A solubility product constant thus physicochemically defines conditions present at equilibrium.

Despite many uncertainties concerning the mineralizing propensity of plasma and the exact chemical nature of either the earliest form of bone mineral or of the fluids in direct contact with bone mineral in vivo, it has been suggested that ionic interchange between bone and tissue fluids exhibits a solubility relationship. The ion product of hydroxyapatite ($1 \times 10^{-25}M$) is considerably lower than that of $(Ca^{+2}) \times (HPO_4{}^{2-})$ in extracellular fluid. At normal plasma pH the body fluids are, in effect, supersaturated with respect to the final mineral bone phase. This has been interpreted as meaning that mineral can be extracted from the surrounding fluids with great efficiency during bone formation. Moreover, it has been suggested further that a fall in the Ca × P ion product in the extracellular fluid leads to a dissolution of the exchangeable bone mineral and, conversely, an increase leads to increased deposition of these elements into bone.

It seems more than likely that the formation of inorganic crystals in bone occurs by a process of heterogeneous phase transformation, which does not occur within the lumen of blood vessels and in soft tissue. This implies that calcium and phosphate from the fluids bathing bone are rendered "mineralizable" by the interaction of ions in the bathing fluids with a unique "nucleating center" in bone (most probably collagen fibrils). In order for heterogeneous nucleation to occur, the tissue fluid in contact with the nucleation center in bone must be in metastable equilibrium. To date, this hypothesis has not been verified, since it cannot be determined a priori from the chemical composition and properties of the fluids bathing bone whether they are in metastable equilibrium with the mineral phase of bone. Therefore, until the determination of the plasma Ca × P ion product can be correlated in vivo with the mineralizing propensity of plasma, and the effective ion product which governs mineralization in vivo is known, it appears unwise to consider the plasma Ca × P ion product a precise physiologic determinant of new bone formation and skeletal turnover.

Calcium Absorption

The homeostasis of calcium in blood and extracellular fluid represents an exquisite biologic control system in man. The level of circulating calcium depends on a balance between the amount added by the resorption of bone, intestinal absorption and renal tubular reabsorption on one hand and the calcium lost by skeletal formation, or "accretion," and renal and intestinal excretion on the other.

It should be stressed that measurements of "calcium balance" in man are likely to be poor estimates of actual calcium absorption or retention.[17] Since the "balance" is, in essence, the calculated difference between a large intake and a large excretion, the difference between these is inherently inaccurate. The usual errors, namely, failure of the subject to consume all of the diet and failure to collect all of the excreta, often lead to false-positive balances. The extent to which such errors have influenced prevailing concepts of calcium homeostasis in health and disease is unknown. The absorptive efficiency of the intestine for calcium is dependent on amount of exposure to ultraviolet light[18] and vitamin D intake, the sex and age of the individual, the food source and total calcium content of the source. Whereas during periods of active skeletal growth children may absorb up to 75 per cent of ingested calcium, normal adults, with daily intakes of 400 to 1,000 mg, absorb 30 to 60 per cent.[19] Dietary factors which increase calcium absorption include certain amino acids, such as lysine and arginine, vitamin D and lactose. Cocoa, soybeans, kale, spinach (or other high oxalate-containing foods) and foods with high phosphate content, such as unpolished rice, hexaphos-phoinositol in bran or wheat meal,[20-22] decrease the intestinal absorptive efficiency for calcium. Other factors which decrease calcium absorption include the ingestion of alkali, increased gastrointestinal transit time, stress, immobilization, thyroid hormone and cortisol or any of its synthetic analogs. Antibiotics such as penicillin, neomycin and chloramphenicol may actually enhance the absorption of calcium.[23,24]

The effect of inorganic phosphorus on calcium absorption is controversial. Earlier reports of an inhibition of calcium absorption induced by supplemental phosphate feeding[25] conflict with later studies demonstrating no effect of dietary phosphorus increments on calcium absorption.[26] Calcium absorption is more efficient in males than in females. This may be related to

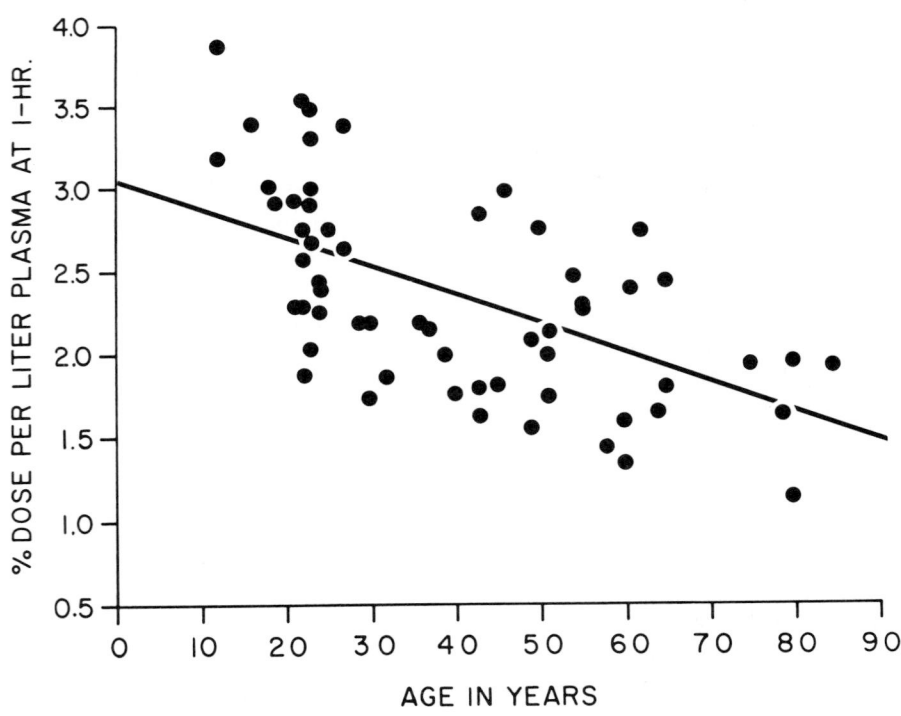

Fig. 7A–3. Regression slope as determined by the method of least squares and scattergram of plasma [47]Ca values (ordinate) 1 hour after the administration of [47]CaCl in 20 mg of calcium as $CaCl_2$. Patients fasted overnight before the study and had been adapted to weighed calcium intakes of 170 to 380 mg per day for 14 to 21 days before the test. (From Avioli et al.[28] Used with permission of authors and publisher.)

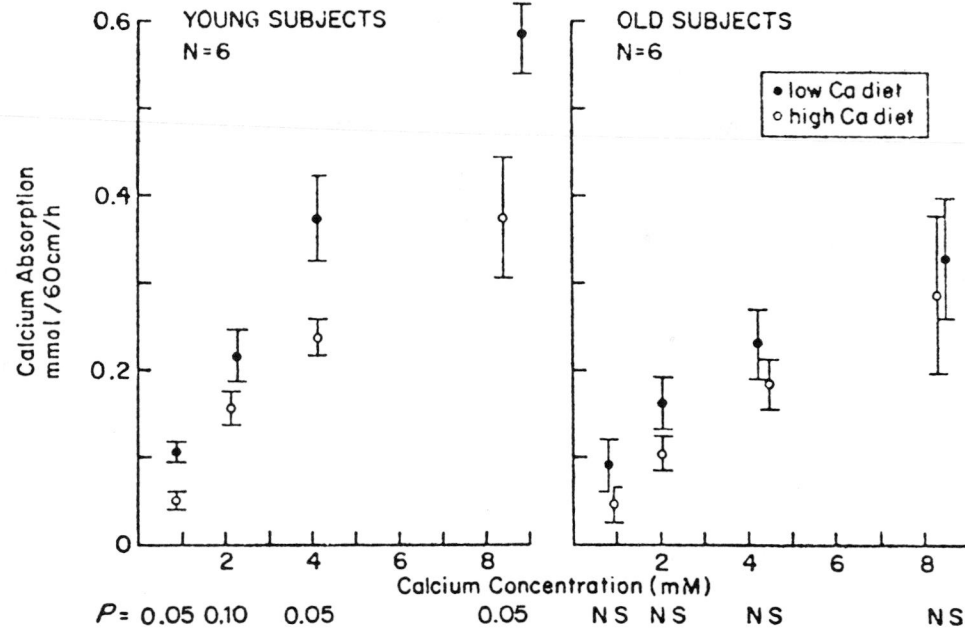

Fig. 7A–4. Effect of calcium intake on calcium absorption rates in young and old subjects. Each subject was studied on a high- and low-calcium diet. The rate of calcium absorption in the old subjects was significantly less than that observed in younger individuals, and the intestinal response of old individuals to calcium deprivation blunted. NS = no significant difference. In this study, urinary calcium was higher in the older subjects despite the fact that they absorbed less calcium (From Ireland and Fordtran.[29] Used with permission of authors and publishers.)

reports of stimulated calcium absorption when androgens are administered to females.[27] Absorption decreases as individuals age[28,29] (Fig. 7A–3); the adaptive efficiency of the intestine to fluctuations in calcium intake is one whereby, with decreasing calcium intake, the per cent absorbed increases.[29,30] This intestinal adaptive efficiency appears to be also blunted by the aging process[29] (Fig. 7A–4). Despite the recognized inverse relation between calcium absorption and intake, prolonged fasting paradoxically results in decreased absorption[31] and absorption may actually increase as calcium intake rises, with absorptive capacities of more than 1.0 gm per day documented at intakes of 7.5 gm.[32] Although it has been reported that calcium is significantly better absorbed when given to human subjects as the lactate than as the

gluconate salt,[33] it has also been observed that no difference exists in the utilization of calcium from milk, gluconate, lactate, carbonate or sulfate salts.[34,35]

Fecal calcium consists not only of unabsorbed ingested calcium but also the endogenous calcium secreted into the gastrointestinal tract and not absorbed. About 85 per cent of the calcium entering the intestine in this manner is secreted proximal to the site of absorption and thus is presented to the absorptive sites and is assumed to be handled with the same efficiency as the calcium of dietary origin. Approximately 15 per cent of the total intestinal calcium secretion is assumed to be nonabsorbable, even under conditions when dietary calcium is completely absorbed. Total intestinal calcium excretion in man averages 0.194 ± 0.073 gm per day, whereas the secreted calcium that is not absorbed, *endogenous fecal calcium,* averages 130 mg per day.

These values are based on the assumption that dietary calcium mixes homogeneously with endogenously secreted calcium, that the absorptive efficiencies for both are identical and that a portion of the endogenous calcium is unabsorbed because it enters the gut distal to the absorptive site(s). There is general agreement that this endogenous fecal fraction, like the daily losses of calcium in sweat, exerts little effect on the day-to-day regulation of calcium balance. It should be noted, however, that in certain clinical situations, such as overt hyperthyroidism, the calcium losses in sweat, which normally range between 20 and 350 mg per day,[17] may be considerable because of the increased concentrations of calcium in the sweat, as well as the increased volume of sweat. Also, calcium losses in sweat may approximate 1 gm per day in individuals working at high temperatures.

Calcium Excretion

Once absorbed, calcium enters the extracellular fluid and rapidly exchanges with the calcium in the exchangeable moiety of bone mineral and that in the glomerular filtrate. The daily urinary excretion of calcium in normal human subjects on diets containing 600 to 1,000 mg of calcium per day ranges between 80 to 250 gm.[36] An exponential relationship exists between dietary and urinary calcium, so that wide variations in intake are accompanied by parallel but only slight alterations in excretion. The urinary excretion of calcium is determined more by the absorption of calcium from the intestine than by the dietary intake. The more efficient the intestinal absorption of calcium, the greater will be the absolute change in urinary calcium for a given change in calcium intake. Since the efficiency of absorption decreases in man with advancing age,[28,29] the variation of

urine calcium with calcium intake is greater in young than in older individuals. Variations in urinary calcium excretion normally play an insignificant role in modifying the effect of wide swings in calcium intake on calcium homeostasis. There is a diurnal variation in the rate of calcium excretion, with the greatest excretion occurring during the day and a nadir observed during the evening hours.[36]

The amount of nonprotein-bound calcium filtered by the glomeruli in man averages 10,000 mg per 24 hours. Normally, approximately 99 per cent of the filtered load is reabsorbed by the renal tubules, so that, *on the average,* 100 mg of calcium are excreted per day. In hypocalcemic states (i.e. serum calcium concentration below 7.5 mg per 100 ml) renal tubular reabsorption of calcium is so complete that calcium virtually disappears from the urine. The major part of calcium reabsorption, like that of sodium, occurs in the proximal convoluted tubule and in the ascending limb of Henle's loop; presumably the remainder is absorbed in more distal parts of the nephron. Whereas the distal tubular reabsorption of calcium appears independent of sodium, calcium and sodium ions appear to share a common pathway of active transport in the proximal tubule. To this extent, excretion is dependent upon simultaneous sodium excretion, the latter governing the excretion of the free calcium ion. Calcium excretion is increased not only by saline diuresis but also by carbohydrate ingestion, phosphate deprivation,[37] metabolic acidosis, cortisol or any of the synthetic glucocorticoids, thyroid and growth hormones[36] and diets rich in protein[38] and magnesium. Hypercalciuria is often seen in bone diseases characterized by rapid bone destruction, with or without simultaneously occurring hypercalcemia. The renal tubular reabsorption of calcium is increased by parathyroid hormone, a fall in plasma calcium, metabolic alkalosis and benzothiazine diuretics.[36]

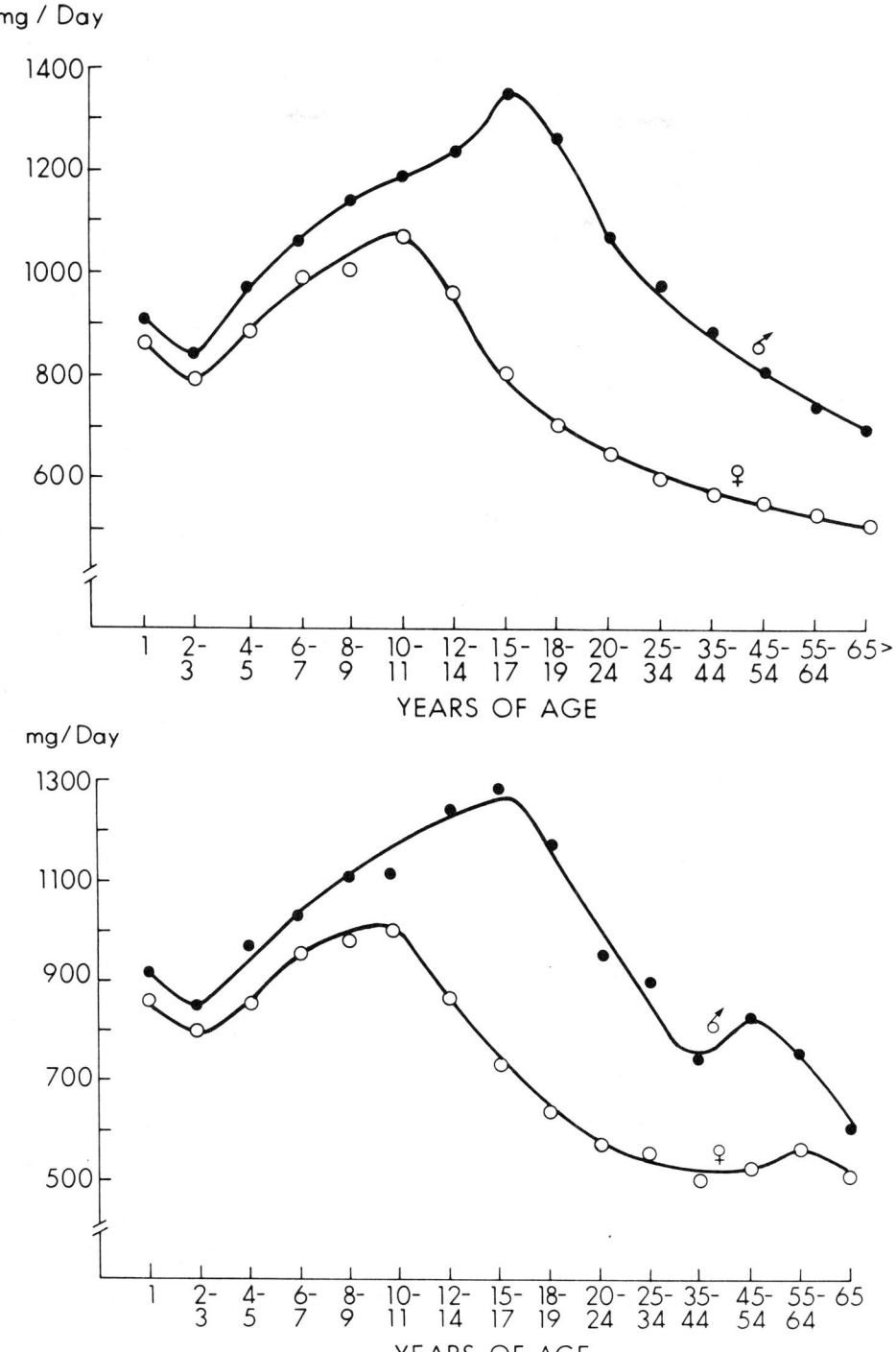

Fig. 7A–5. Mean *(top)* and median *(bottom)* calcium intakes of men and women in the United States for the years 1971–1974. (Adopted from DHEW Publication No. (HRA)77–1647, July 1977.)

Calcium Requirements

A number of dietary surveys reveal that among western populations the mean adult calcium intake ranges between 400 to 1300 mg calcium per day.[39] At all ages, men consume more calcium than women (Fig. 7A–5), and at all ages there are individual men and women who ingest 2 to 4 times the recommended allowances of calcium.[39]

The full-term infant contains about 25 gm of calcium, about half of which is deposited during the last lunar month of pregnancy at a rate of approximately 300 mg per day. It has been demonstrated that the reproductive process is not impaired when the diets of pregnant women range between 700 mg to 1.2 gm per day.[40,41] More recent estimates place the calcium requirement of pregnant women at 2.0 gm per day,[42] although this has been contested.[43]

A young baby receives about 200 mg calcium per day while ingesting 650 ml of breast milk during early lactation, and by 8 months of age the infant's daily calcium intake has increased to 350 mg.[44] Assuming a maintenance calcium requirement of 3 mg per kg body weight and an efficiency of utilization of 30 per cent, it has been estimated that a lactating mother will require from 1 to 2 gm of calcium per day in order to ensure adequate calcium supply in breast feedings and skeletal balance.[45] The needs for the third trimester of pregnancy and normal lactation, as recommended by the Joint FAO/WHO Expert Group on Calcium Requirements, has been set at 1,200 mg per day,[46] although it is recognized that many women have lactated adequately on lower intakes.

A premature infant needs about 90 to 120 gm calcium per kg body weight and 60 to 90 mg phosphorus per kg daily, amounts which are easily provided by 100 gm of whole cow's milk per kg of body weight.[47] An average 1-month-old infant, weighing 4 kg, will obtain 235 mg of calcium daily from breast milk, and at 3 months approximately 300 gm calcium per day, amounts sufficient to meet his skeletal demands.[48] Formula-fed children up to 1 year of age require no more than 600 mg of calcium per day for adequate skeletal development and growth.[20] For children from 1 to 10 years with adequate vitamin D intakes, 800 mg per day appears sufficient to ensure normal skeletal growth.[20]

Preadolescent growing children, however, may need 2 to 4 times as much calcium as does an adult.[20] Higher intakes of calcium, on the order of 1 to 1.5 gm daily, are recommended during preadolescence and puberty because of the demands of rapid skeletal growth. Intakes greater than this need not be advocated, since maximal calcium retention obtains in children and young adults at this level of intake.

Although the majority of young and middle-aged adults are capable of maintaining a positive calcium balance on an average daily intake of 600 to 1,000 mg per day, higher intakes may be essential to maintain mineral and skeletal homeostasis in middle-aged and elderly individuals.[48–52] The age-related needs for additional dietary calcium may result in part from the fact that absorption, as well as the adaptive efficiency of the intestine to fluctuations in calcium intake, decreases with age.[28,29] The negative calcium balances observed in osteoporotic patients on low but seemingly adequate calcium intakes have variously been ascribed to slow and noncompensatory adaptation to low calcium intakes, defective renal adaptation with relative hypercalciuria and lactose intolerance resulting from intestinal lactase deficiency.[12]

Evidence that calcium deprivation leads to "osteoporosis" in man stems primarily from controversial retrospective and epidemiologic studies.[12] Some reports reveal no significant difference in the incidence of "osteoporosis" between patients who historically ingested less than 500 mg calcium per day and those with intakes greater than 1,500 mg per day;[53–55] others demonstrate a lower calcium intake in symptomatic "osteoporotic" individuals than in age-matched normal control subjects.[56-63] Epidemiologic and dietary survey studies may ultimately prove misleading, regardless of the conclusions derived, unless more specific emphasis is placed on dietary habits, the degree of mobilization, the daily intake of minerals other than calcium, the dietary intake of protein and vitamin D and the extent of sunlight exposure.

Modern diets, which are characteristically rich in animal proteins and phosphorus with low Ca/P ratios, may prove deleterious to bone, since they may promote hypercalciuria and stimulate the release of parathyroid hormone with a resultant progressive decrease in bone mass.[12,64-67] Immobilization, or the relative inactivity which often attends the infirmities of age, promotes skeletal demineralization; peculiar dietary habits may also lead to increased urinary calcium loss and a negative calcium balance, despite an adequate intake. Not only may calcium intakes be inadequate in geriatric populations[39] but vitamin D deficiency and inadequate sunlight exposure[18] may also prevent maximal absorption of ingested calcium. There is also accumulating evidence that it may be possible to prevent the normal bone loss which attends senescence and the pathologic fractures seen in the severely "osteoporotic" postmenopausal female by calcium supplementation.[12]

Calcium intakes ranging from 1,000 to 2,500 mg per day do not result in hypercalcemia in normal individuals. Ingestion of larger amounts, as may occur with ulcer patients consuming large amounts of milk and antacid (alkali) products (chiefly products containing calcium carbonate), may result in hypercalcemia and in rapid deterioration of renal function.[68-70] An acquired or inherited vitamin D-sensitive hyperabsorption of calcium occurs in patients with sarcoidosis and in certain hypercalciuric individuals with renal calculi; in these subjects hypercalcemia and/or hypercalciuria result from only modest increments in dietary vitamin D supplementation of diets containing 800 to 1,500 mg calcium per day.[71-73]

PHOSPHORUS

Of the 11 to 14 gm of phosphorus per kg fat-free tissue in the normal adult, 85 per cent is in the skeleton. The remainder is distributed between tissue and membrane components of skeletal muscle, skin, nervous tissue and other organs. Whereas most of the phosphorus in soft tissue and cell membranes is in the form of organic esters, almost all of the phosphorus in bone is contained in the mineral phase as inorganic orthophosphate and small amounts of inorganic phosphate. The regulation of plasma phosphate is not as readily explained as that of plasma calcium since the circulating phosphate is in equilibrium not only with skeletal and cellular inorganic phosphate but also with a large number of organic compounds resulting from cellular metabolism. The phosphate ion is essential for the metabolism of carbohydrate, lipids and protein, functioning as a cofactor in a multitude of enzyme systems and contributing to the metabolic potential in the form of "high-energy-phosphate" compounds. Phosphate functions to modify acid-base equilibrium in plasma and within cells and plays fundamental roles in modifying the development and maturation of bone, in the renal excretion of hydrogen ions and in modifying the effects of the B vitamins.

Although the sequence of events which obtains during the nucleation of bone collagen is still imperfectly understood, collagen fibrils exhibit a remarkable faculty to form covalent bonds with phosphate. The phosphorylation of collagen has been considered the initiating event in the nucleation of bone. Phosphate, in addition to its conditioning role in the formation of the apatitic structure, also affects bone resorption, mineralization and collagen synthesis and thus plays an integral role in calcium homeostasis. The available evidence is consistent with the interpretation that these effects are direct effects of phosphate upon the metabolic functions of bone cells.[1]

Plasma Phosphate

In the human adult, plasma inorganic phosphate ranges between 2.5 to 4.4 mg per dl, with a mean of 3.5 mg per dl. Dietary phosphate, stage of growth and age, time of day, hormonal interplay and renal function all contribute to the variability of the fasting serum phosphate concentration. Eighty-eight per cent of the plasma phosphate is unfilterable (Fig. 7A–2); some of this is complexed with mono- or divalent cations such as Na^+, Ca^{++} and Mg^{++}. At normal blood pH, 85 per cent of the ultrafilterable phosphate is in the form of HPO_4^{-2}, the remainder existing mainly as $H_2PO_4^-$.[16]

As noted earlier for calcium, the concentration of plasma phosphate varies with age. In prepubertal children the mean value for circulating phosphate approximates 5 mg per 100 ml with an upper normal limit approaching 6 mg per 100 ml. Normal adult values are gradually approached by the third decade, after which, in men, plasma phosphate decreased progressively with advancing age.[74] The trend of values for plasma phosphate in females represents a unique circumstance: they decline gradually between ages 20 and 35 and rise after age 40.[74] The higher levels of phosphate in the female over 40 years of age seem to be related to the menopause. This assumes more significance since not only are postmenopausal females deficient in estrogen (a phosphaturic substance) but a positive correlation reportedly exists between serum inorganic phosphate and the extent of bone resorption in middle-aged and elderly women.[75]

Total serum phosphate may also normally fluctuate by as much as 1 to 2 mg per 100 ml. These variations generally reflect abrupt shifts of inorganic phosphate between extracellular fluid and intracellular compartments, rather than a net gain or loss of phosphate from the body. The administration of hexoses or hormones such as insulin, glucagon or epinephrine results in a reduction in serum phosphate, presumably by simulating the cellular utilization of glucose and accelerating the formation of intracellular phosphate esters. A systemic alkalosis has been associated with a fall in circulating phosphate and attributed to a shift of phosphate out of the extracellular fluid compartment. The fall in plasma phosphate concentration is apparently greater in respiratory than in comparable levels of metabolic alkalosis. Thus, the evaluation of hypophosphatemia should always include measurements of the pH and total CO_2 content of plasma.

Whereas starvation is occasionally associated with a decrease in plasma inorganic phosphate, acidosis and excessive catabolism of body tissue associated with starvation or lysis of neoplastic lymphoid cells during therapy[76] may lead to cellular release of phosphorus, hyperphosphatemia and reciprocal hypocalcemia. Severe hypophosphatemia has also been reported in hypokalemia states, independent of the attendant metabolic alkalosis. Variations in the plasma level of inorganic phosphate most probably contribute to the regulation of bone turnover[77] and to bioactivation of the vitamin D metabolite 25-hydroxycholecalciferol to 1,25-dihydroxycholecalciferol.[78,79] It is noteworthy in this regard that severe dietary phosphate deprivation results in hypophosphatemia and increased circulating 1,25-dihydroxycholecalciferol in women, whereas insignificant changes in the plasma levels of either substance obtain in phosphate-depleted males.[37]

Phosphate Absorption

Most if not all of the dietary phosphorus is absorbed as free phosphate. The efficiency of phosphate absorption is a function of both the dietary intake and the food source.[80] Sixty to 70 per cent is absorbed on a normal intake and maximal absorption (up to 90 per cent) is achieved on very low intakes.[81] Various dietary forms of organic phosphate esters, such as the phytic acid of cereals and seeds, are not readily available to man, since the human intestine is relatively deficient in the enzyme phytase, essential for hydrolysis of the organic esters. Organic phosphate ester compounds may also interfere with calcium absorption, since they form insoluble calcium salts within the intestinal lumen. In animals, unsaturated fatty acids, iron and aluminum interfere with intestinal phosphate absorption.[82-84] Vitamin D increases intestinal phosphate absorption in certain animal species;[78] however a direct effect of vitamin D (or its biologically active metabolites) on phosphate absorption in man is still to be adequately demonstrated. There is no known effective physiologic mechanism regulating the intestinal absorption of phosphate in man, the control of the phosphate economy being achieved primarily by variations in dietary intake and renal excretion.[36] Fecal phosphorus represents both unabsorbed phosphate and that secreted into the gastrointestinal tract.[81] In man with phosphorus intakes approximately 1 to 1.50 gm per day, the secretion of endogenous phosphate into the intestinal lumen averages 3 mg per kg per day.[81] Dietary phosphorus is absorbed to a greater extent than is calcium and, consequently, the renal excretion of phosphorus is much greater than that of calcium.[36]

Phosphate Excretion

Urinary phosphorus is largely inorganic phosphate, the amount depending primarily upon how much is absorbed from the intestinal tract. Phosphate exists in the forms of $HPO_4^{2-}/H_2PO_4^-$ in the glomerular filtrate in a ratio of 4 to 1. With normal renal function, urinary phosphorus usu-

ally amounts to approximately two-thirds of the dietary phosphorus. Normally, a diurnal variation in phosphate clearance occurs with the usual pattern, that of a matitudinal increase in urinary phosphorus/creatinine ratios. This circadian rhythm is related to physical activity, with the nadir appearing a few hours after the end of sleep. The loss of diurnal variation in adrenal-insufficient states and the documented inverse correlation between phosphate excretion and plasma cortisol levels suggest that this rhythm is controlled by the adrenal glands.[36]

In man, the tubular reabsorption of phosphate cleared by the glomeruli is normally 85 to 95 per cent.[36] This is an age-related and rate-limited process, with a maximum tubular reabsorptive capacity in adults of 4 to 8 mg per min. The tubular reabsorption of phosphate is increased by short-term cortisol therapy and growth hormone, and is decreased by digoxin, estrogen, thyroid hormone, parathyroid hormone, long-term cortisol therapy and elevations in circulating calcium.[36]

Phosphorus Requirements

The average daily phosphorus requirement of adults in the United States is estimated at 0.8 to 1.5 gm per day.[25,80,85] Whereas the primary source of calcium in the American diet is milk, major sources of phosphorus are milk, poultry, fish and meat. Non-nutritious soft drinks containing excess phosphorus in the form of phosphoric acid also serve as sources for children and adults alike. The relative greater availability of phosphate-containing foodstuffs has resulted in a calcium/phosphate dietary ratio in western diets much lower than that recommended to maintain the integrity of skeletal tissue. This matter is of some concern, since diets with a low Ca/P ratio have led to progressive bone loss in rats,[86] dogs[86,87] and horses,[89] and may stimulate secondary hyperparathyroidism in man.[90]

With the exception of young infants, the

recommended allowance of phosphorus per day is the same as that of calcium, although the Ca/P ratio of diets ingested throughout the world today is reported less than 0.75.[91,92] The Ca/P ratio of cow's milk of 1.3/1, compared with a Ca/P ratio of 2/1 in breast milk,[91] may contribute to the syndrome of "idiopathic hypocalcemia" and tetany of infants on formula feedings. Phosphorus depletion in man, a syndrome characterized by weakness, anorexia, malaise and skeletal aches, can obtain during prolonged and excessive intake of nonabsorbable antacids.[95] Specific abnormalities, such as hemolytic anemia, granulocyte dysfunction, erythrocyte glycolysis, hypercalciuria and renal calculi may also result from phosphate depletion.[93,94] The syndrome has been experimentally produced in man and is readily reversed when the medication is discontinued and sufficient amounts of dietary phosphorus are consumed.[95] Its frequency in the very large population of individuals ingesting antacids is unknown, but it is probably rare, based on the infrequency of published reports of this complication.[95] Recognition and appropriate therapy require medical supervision, particularly when adjustments in drug therapy for peptic ulcer are involved.

Since the kidney is capable of excreting 600 to 900 mg of phosphorus daily, hyperphosphatemia is rare in the absence of chronic renal disease and then only when the glomerular filtration rate falls below 20 mg per min.[36] Hyperphosphatemia is also characteristic of disorders of parathyroid secretion and metabolism, such as hypoparathyroidism[96-98] and pseudohypoparathyroidism,[99,100] and can be accentuated by phosphate feeding. There are no specific signs or symptoms of hyperphosphatemia per se, although the hypocalcemia often associated with hyperphosphatemia (and exacerbated by phosphate feeding) can result in enhanced neuroexcitability, tetany and convulsions.

BIBLIOGRAPHY

1. Raisz: In Metabolic Bone Disease, Vol. 1 (Avioli and Krane, Eds.). New York, Academic Press, 1977.
2. Robinson: Clin. Orthop., 112, 263, 1975.
3. Termine and Eanes: Calcif. Tissue Res., 10, 171, 1972.
4. Termine: Clin. Orthop., 85, 207, 1972.
5. Becker, Spadaro and Berg: J. Bone Joint Surg., 50A, 326, 1968.
6. Kildeberg, Engel and Winters: Acta Paediatr. Scand., 58, 321, 1969.
7. Termine and Posner: Science, 153, 1523, 1966.
8. Harper and Posner: Proc. Soc. Exp. Biol. Med., 122, 137, 1966.
9. Pitkin: Am. J. Obstet. Gynecol., 121, 724, 1975.
10. Cushard, Creditor, Canterbury and Reiss: J. Clin. Endocrinol. Metab., 34, 767, 1972.
11. Heaney and Shillman: J. Clin. Endocrinol. Metab., 53, 661, 1971.
12. Avioli: In Metabolic Bone Disease, Vol. 1 (Avioli and Krane, Eds.). New York, Academic Press, 1977.
13. Heaney: Clin. Orthop., 31, 153, 1963.
14. Root and Harrison: J. Pediatr., 88, 1, 1976.
15. Harrison and Harrison: Biomembranes, 4B, 793, 1974.
16. Walser: J. Clin. Invest., 40, 723, 1961.
17. Isaksson, Lindholm and Sjogren: Metabolism, 16, 303, 1967.
18. Neer, et al.: Nature, 229, 255, 1971.
19. Mautalen, Cabrejas and Soto: Metabolism, 18, 395, 1969.
20. Irwin and Kienholz: J. Nutr., 103, 1021, 1973.
21. McCance and Widdowson: J. Physiol., 101, 44, 1942.
22. Reinhold, Faradji, Abadi and Ismail-Beigi: J. Nutr., 106, 493, 1976.
23. Heggeness: J. Nutr., 68, 573, 1959.
24. Migicovsky, Nielson, Gluck and Burgess: Arch. Biochem., 34, 479, 1951.
25. Leichsenring, Norris, Lamison, Wilson and Patton: Br. J. Nutr., 45, 407, 1951.
26. Spencer, Menczel, Lewin and Samachson: J. Nutr., 86, 125, 1965.
27. Jaworski, Brown, Fedoruk and Seitz: N. Engl. J. Med., 269, 1103, 1963.
28. Avioli, McDonald and Lee: J. Clin. Invest., 44, 1960, 1965.
29. Ireland and Fordtran: J. Clin. Invest., 52, 2672, 1973.
30. Spencer, Lewin, Fowler and Samachson: Am. J. Med., 46, 197, 1969.
31. Fromm, Litvak and Degrossi: Lancet, 1, 616, 1970.
32. Heaney, Saville and Recker: J. Lab. Clin. Med., 85, 881, 1975.
33. Spencer, Scheck, Lewin and Samachson: J. Nutr., 89, 283, 1966.
34. Bronner, Harris, Moor and Benda: MIT Report A-81C, 1960.
35. Patton and Sutton: J. Nutr., 48, 443, 1952.
36. Massry, Friedler and Coburn: Arch Intern. Med., 131, 828, 1973.

37. Gray, Wilz, Caldas and Lemann: J. Clin. Endocrinol. Metab., *45*, 299, 1977.
38. Linkswiler, Joyce and Anand: Trans. N.Y. Acad. Sci., *36*, 333, 1974.
39. Vital and Health Statistics: Series 11-Number 202, 1977.
40. Thomson: Br. J. Nutr., *13,* 190, 1959.
41. Thomson: Br. J. Nutr., *13*, 509, 1959.
42. Duggin, et al.: Lancet, *2*, 926, 1974.
43. Walker: Lancet, *1*, 107, 1975.
44. Sterns: Physiol. Rev., *19*, 415, 1939.
45. Mitchell and Curzon: *Actualities Scientifiques et Industrilles*, No. 771. Paris, Hermann and Co., 1968.
46. Food and Agriculture Organization: Rome, Series No. 30, 1962.
47. Hovels and Stephan: Ernahrung, *2*, 178, 1961.
48. Leitch and Aitken: Nutr. Abstr. Rev., *29*, 393, 1959.
49. Ohlson and Stearns: Fed. Proc., *18,* 1076, 1959.
50. Heaney, Recker and Saville: Am. J. Clin. Nutr., *30*, 1603, 1977.
51. Whedon: Fed. Proc., *4,* 1112, 1959.
52. Calcium Requirements. FAO Nutr. Meet. Rep. Series, No. 30, 1962.
53. Smith and Frame: N. Engl. J. Med., *273*, 73, 1965.
54. Garn, Rohmann and Wagner: Fed. Proc., *26*, 1729, 1967.
55. Garn: Am. J. Clin. Nutr., *23*, 1149, 1970.
56. Riggs, et al.: J. Bone Joint Surg., *29*, 915, 1967.
57. Hurxthal and Vose: Calcif. Tissue Res., *4*, 245, 1969.
58. Owen, Irving and Luall: Acta Med. Scand., *103*, 235, 1940.
59. Vinther-Paulsen: Geriatrics, *8*, 76, 1953.
60. Smith and Nordin: Proc. R. Soc. Med., *57*, 868, 1964.
61. Harrison, Fraser and Mullan: Lancet, *1*, 1015, 1961.
62. Lutwak and Whedon: DM, 1, 1963.
63. Krook, Lutwak, Whalen, Henrikson, Lesser and Uris: Cornell Vet., *62*, 32, 1972.
64. Schwartz, Woodcock, Blakely and MacKellar: Am. J. Clin. Nutr., *26*, 519, 1973.
65. Lutwak: Nutr. Rev., *37*, 1, 1974.
66. Beal: J. Am. Diet. Assoc., *53*, 450, 1968.
67. Nordin, Young, Bulusu and Horsman: In *Osteoporosis* (Barzel, Ed.). New York, Grune and Stratton, 1970.
68. Ivanovich, Fellows and Rich: Ann. Intern. Med., *66*, 917, 1967.
69. Henneman: Fed. Proc., *18*, 1093, 1959.
70. E.J.H. (editorial): Ann. Intern. Med., *66*, 1021, 1967.
71. Jackson and Dancaster: J. Clin. Endocrinol. Metab., *19*, 658, 1959.
72. Bell, Gill and Bartter: Am. J. Med., *36*, 500, 1964.
73. Henneman, Dempsey, Carroll and Albright: J. Clin. Invest., *35*, 1229, 1956.
74. Keating, Jones, Elveback and Randall: J. Lab. Clin. Med., *73*, 825, 1969.
75. Kelly, Jowsey, Riggs and Elveback: J. Lab. Clin. Med., *69*, 110, 1967.
76. Clarkson, Blondin and Cryer: Metabolism, *22*, 611, 1973.
77. Haddad and Avioli: Endocrinology, *87*, 1245, 1970.
78. DeLuca: Fed. Proc., *32*, 2211, 1974.
79. Hughes, Haussler, Wergedal and Baylink: Science, *190*, 578, 1975.
80. Moon, Malzer and Clark: J. Am. Diet. Assoc., *64*, 386, 1974.
81. Nordin and Smith: In *Diagnostic Procedures in Disorders of Calcium Metabolism*. Boston, Little Brown, and Co., 1965.
82. Sewell, Trout, Field and Treadwell: Proc. Soc. Exp. Biol., *92*, 613, 1956.
83. Street: J. Nutr., *24*, 111, 1942.
84. Cox, Dodds, Wigman and Murphy: J. Biol. Chem., *92*, 11, 1931.
85. Recommended Dietary Allowances: Washington, National Academy of Sciences, 1958.
86. Draper, Lie and Bergan: J. Nutr., *102*, 1133, 1972.
87. Krook, Lutwak, Henrikson, Kallfelz, Hirsch, Romanus, Belanger, Marier and Sheffy; J. Nutr., *101*, 233, 1971.
88. LaFlamme and Jowsey: J. Clin. Invest., *51*, 2834, 1972.
89. Argenzio, Lowe, Hintz and Schryver: J. Nutr., *104*, 18, 1974.
90. Reiss, Canterbury, Bercovitz and Kaplan: J. Clin. Invest., *49*, 2146, 1970.
91. Beal: J. Am. Diet. Assoc., *53*, 450, 1968.
92. Lorenz and Burr: J. Pediatr., *85*, 522, 1974.
93. Knochel: Arch. Intern. Med., *137*, 203, 1977.
94. Kreisberg: Hosp. Prac., *12*, 121, 1977.
95. Cooke, Teitelbaum and Avioli: Arch. Intern. Med., *138*, 1007, 1978.
96. Avioli: Am. J. Med., *57*, 34, 1974.
97. Peden: Am. J. Hum. Genet., *12*, 323, 1960.
98. Parfitt: J. Clin. Endocrinol. Metab., *34*, 152, 1972.
99. Potts: In *The Metabolic Basis of Inherited Disease* (Stanbury, Wyngaarden and Fredrickson, Eds.). New York, McGraw-Hill, 1970.
100. Farriaux: Am. J. Dis. Child., *130*, 180, 1976.

B. Magnesium

Maurice E. Shils

Human magnesium deficiency was first described in a small number of patients in 1934.[1] Understanding of the prevalence of this deficiency, its symptomatology, relationships to other electrolytes and association with various disease states has come slowly. The observations of Flink and co-workers indicating depletion of this ion in alcoholics[2] were an important step forward. Beginning 5 years later, a series of clinical case reports began to focus attention on hypomagnesemia in malabsorptive states. Endocrine disorders, abnormalities in the newborn, renal tubular defects and iatrogenic influences have been added to the list. With increasing ease and frequency of measurement of magnesium in body fluids[3] it has become obvious that human depletion occurs much more commonly than had been assumed previously.

BODY PARTITION

Magnesium shares some of the attributes of calcium in its characteristics of absorption and storage in bone, a similarity to potassium in being an important intracellular constituent and a resemblance to sodium in the efficiency with which the normal kidney retains the ion when serum levels fall. This eclectic state is of additional interest, since it is now apparent that a deficiency of magnesium affects the metabolism of each of the other three ions in some manner.

The adult human weighing 70 kg contains approximately 20 to 28 gm of magnesium,[4-6] equaling 1,667 to 2,400 mEq of this ion (1 mEq = 0.5 mM = 12 mg). About 55 per cent is present in bone and about 27 per cent in muscle. Muscle, liver, heart and pancreas contain about the same amount (approximately 16 mEq per kg wet weight).[6,7] Erythrocyte content varies from 4.3 to 6.2 mEq/L depending on method.[7] Normal serum levels also vary depending on method but, with atomic absorption methods, the range is usually 1.5 to 2.1 mEq/L.[8] Magnesium ion in erythrocytes and plasma exists in free, complexed and protein-bound forms; in plasma the approximate percentages are 55, 13 and 32, respectively.[7] Cerebrospinal fluid magnesium is greater than that of plasma (approximately 2.5 mEq/L) despite the absence of protein; about 55 per cent is free and the remainder is complexed.[7] Magnesium in sweat averages 0.6 mEq/L in man in a hot environment.[9]

Thirty per cent of bone magnesium is in a surface-limited pool present either within the hydration shell or on the crystal surface. In adult man, the larger fraction of bone magnesium does not appear to be associated with bone matrix but is an integral part of the bone crystal. Both magnesium pools are increased in patients with chronic renal failure.[9a] In vitro studies suggest that surface magnesium rapidly reflects changes in serum magnesium levels, whereas the deeper pool is probably deposited at the time of bone formation with mobilization being dependent upon the resorptive processes.[9a]

INTAKE, EXCRETION AND HOMEOSTASIS

Magnesium intake varies greatly because of the widely variable content of different foods.[6] Fifteen to 40 mEq per day is probably an average range for healthy individuals in the United States and western Europe.[10] Of this intake approximately 60 to 70 per cent is excreted in the stools by most individuals.[7,10] The remainder (other than that retained in new tissue or lost in sweat or desquamated skin) is excreted in the urine. A number of physiologic factors influence normal absorption. These include total magnesium intake, intestinal transit time, rate of water absorption and resultant luminal magnesium concentration, and the amounts of calcium, phosphate and lactose in the diet.[7] When radioactive magnesium (^{28}Mg) was given intravenously only 2 per cent[11] or less[12] was excreted in the stool. With a high magnesium intake (47 mEq per day) absorption of the ingested radioisotope (used as a tracer) was 23.7 per cent; at the more usual intake of 20 mEq per day, absorption was 44.3 per cent; with a very low intake (1.9 mEq per day), it was 75.8 per cent.[12] Water influx ("solvent drag") through the intestinal epithelium appears to play a significant role in absorption of this ion.

When magnesium intake is severely restricted, output becomes very small. On intakes of less than 1 mEq per day, daily urinary and fecal losses each averaged less than 1 mEq after an initial adjustment period.[13,14] As magnesium intake increases after a period of deficiency urinary excretion increases markedly as serum levels approach the lower normal range.[13] Supplementing a normal intake increases urinary excretion without altering normal serum levels.[15] The intestinal and renal conservation and excretory mechanisms in normal individuals permit homeostasis over a wide intake of dietary magnesium, just as they do for sodium. However, contrary to the case of sodium, there does not appear to be an efficient hormonal homeostatic mechanism for regulating serum magnesium. The normal range is the result of a balance between gastrointestinal absorption and renal excretion. Since gastrointestinal mechanisms of magnesium transport are not very efficient, the renal threshold is presumably the critical factor in determining that level. Summaries of data on renal handling of magnesium have been published recently.[7,15] Reabsorption probably occurs in a manner similar to that for calcium and sodium and there is interdependence in the clearance of these three ions.[7]

The major site of tubular absorption of magnesium, at least in the rat, appears to be in the ascending loop of Henle, with lesser but significant amounts in the proximal tubule.[15a] Heaton has suggested that, in the rat at least, magnesium filtered from serum with concentrations below the lower limit of normal is reabsorbed, and the magnesium appearing in the urine at higher serum concentrations is derived from tubular secretion.[15]

Since parathyroid hormone (PTH) mobilizes bone salts, its administration to normal animals may be expected to affect serum and urinary magnesium. The hormone in moderate doses caused little or no rise in plasma magnesium in normal rats,[16] dogs[17,18] or man.[19,20] In hypoparathyroid subjects[20] an early fall in urinary magnesium excretion occurs following administration of PTH; this is followed by an increased excretion of magnesium and calcium. The magnesium excretory response in normal subjects is variable.[7,20,21a,21b] Calcitonin derived from pig causes hypocalcemia but no significant change in serum magnesium in the dog,[22,23] monkey[24] or normal man.[24,25] Urinary magnesium in the dog may be decreased[22] or unchanged[23] under various experimental conditions.

Administration of magnesium to normal pigs[25a] or addition to in vitro systems with porcine thyroid glands[25b] or perfusion of porcine thyroid glands stimulated the release of calcitonin.[25c] Acute infusion of magnesium salts to patients with metastatic medullary carcinoma of the thyroid produced a striking fall in circulating calcitonin.[25d] Acute administration of mineralocorticoids had no significant effect on calcium and magnesium excretion in the dog[25e] or man.[25f] Prolonged administration of aldosterone to sheep caused an increase in magnesium excretion.[25g] In primary aldosteronism, hypomagnesemia and high renal clearance of magnesium have been reported.[25h] DOCA administered daily for a 6-day period to dogs caused no change in urinary calcium and magnesium for the first 2 days but thereafter there was an average 8-fold increase in calcium and 2-fold increase in magnesium.[25i] There was no significant change in serum magnesium. The more potent diuretics, furosemide and ethacrynic acid, significantly increase excretion of magnesium.[25j,25k] Thiazides have less effect, while spironolactone does not affect renal loss. Triamterene conserves magnesium as well as potassium.[25k]

BIOCHEMISTRY

Magnesium plays a key role as a prosthetic group in many essential enzymatic reactions. The enzymes include those that hydrolyze and transfer phosphate groups (phosphokinases). Thus, magnesium is involved in reactions involving ATP and in those, at almost every step, in the phosphorylation of glucose in its anaerobic metabolism and in its oxidative decarboxylations in the citric acid cycle requiring thiamin pyrophosphate, in the activities of alkaline phosphatase and of pyrophosphatase and in the activation of amino acids. It is further involved in protein synthesis through its action on ribosomal aggregation, its roles in binding messenger RNA to 70S ribosomes and in the synthesis and degradation of DNA. Magnesium is required for the conversion of ATP to cyclic AMP by the enzyme adenylate cyclase, the substrate of which is magnesium ATP. Cyclic AMP appears to play a role in the regulation of parathyroid hormone secretion.[25l] Documentation of these and other enzymatic functions is given elsewhere.[7,8,26,27] Magnesium plays an important role in neuromuscular transmission and activity: it acts at some points synergistically with calcium, while at others it is antagonistic. This complex area has been reviewed elsewhere.[7,8,28,29]

MAGNESIUM DEFICIENCY

Experimental Animals

Acute and near-total deprivation of this cation in diets fed to growing animals produces one of the most rapidly developing and, in the rat, one of the most dramatic of all deficiencies. After 3 to 5 days of acute deficiency young rats develop peripheral vasodilatation which increases for approximately 1 week and then gradually subsides; concomitantly the animals become progressively hyperkinetic when disturbed and then develop tonic-clonic convulsions which are often fatal.[30] This study established the association between magnesium depletion and neuromuscular changes. Other signs of deficiency in rats include reduced growth, alopecia, skin lesions and edema and hypertrophic gums. Calcification and degenerative changes in various organs, especially the kidney, have been prominent on the usual diets, which tend to be fairly high in calcium. Calcification begins in the kidney as luminal concretions in the ascending loop of Henle. Studies in the kidney[31] and heart[32] permit understanding of the sequence of changes

Table 7B–1. Effect of Experimental Magnesium Depletion: Serum Calcium Levels in Various Species*

| Species | Calcium Levels | | |
	Increased	Unchanged	Decreased
Rat	+ φ	+ φ	+
Mouse		+	+
Guinea pig		+	+
Chick			+ (2)
Dog		+ (4)	+ (4)
Pig			+
Sheep			+ (2)
Cow		+	+ (3)
Monkey			+ (2)
Man		+	+

*Modified from Shils,[45f] where the detailed references are given.

φNumerous references. There has been only one report of decreased serum Ca in the rat.

()Numbers in parentheses indicate number of reports from different investigators.

from subcellular organelles to gross alterations. Although the rat has been by far the most widely used animal, many other species have been studied, including various fowl,[33] guinea pig,[34] mouse,[35] pigs,[36] sheep and cattle,[37-39] dogs,[40-43] monkeys[44,45] and man.

It is apparent that the rat is not a representative species either with respect to certain symptomatology or to serum calcium changes (Table 7B–1). Other species do not develop the peripheral vasodilation. The deficient mouse does not develop the repetitive tonic-clonic convulsions but usually dies in a sudden brief convulsion.[45a] Deficient monkeys develop spasticity, tremors and convulsion when hypocalcemia develops; increasing the oral calcium does not raise serum calcium or prevent the symptomatology.[45b]

Magnesium deficiency depresses immunoglobulin concentrations in rats[45c] and mice.[45d] The number of antibody-synthesizing cells is decreased.[45d]

The availability of the rich store of magnesium from bone during a period of deficient intake depends upon the age of the animal.[45e,45f] A large percentage is exchangeable in young animals, e.g. 30 to 40 per cent in the rat, and very little in older animals, e.g. 4 to 6 per cent in the rat.[45f]

Human Deficiency

The symptomatology and biochemical abnormalities ascribable to this deficiency are still not completely defined and areas of disagreement exist despite (or because of) numerous clinical case reports. This situation is attributable to two major factors: (1) Experimentally induced symptomatic human deficiency has been induced to date in only one study,[13,46,47] and (2) symptomatic human deficiency observed in patients has always developed in a setting of predisposing and complicating disease states. The latter have included severe malabsorption of various etiologies,[48-58] chronic alcoholism with malnutrition,[2,48,49,59-62] prolonged magnesium-free

parenteral feeding, usually in association with prolonged losses of gastrointestinal secretions,[2,48,49,55,63] burns,[64] acute or chronic renal disease involving tubular dysfunction,[1,65,65a] lactation losses,[66] childhood malnutrition,[67,68] postnatal tetany syndromes,[69-71,79,80,86] familial disorders of renal[72] or intestinal conservation,[80,86] congestive heart failure in conjunction with the use of diuretics,[25k] diabetic acidosis[80a] and parathyroid disorders, especially in the immediate postparathyroidectomy period.[73-75] In such clinical circumstances, associated complex and uncontrolled variables—multiple dietary inadequacies, changes in oral and parenteral nutrients and medications, metabolic abnormalities, manifestations of basic disease and severe

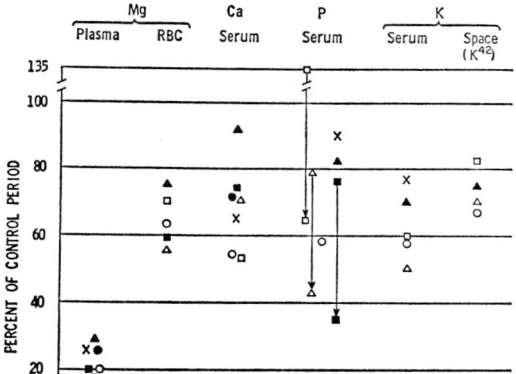

Fig. 7B–1. Biochemical changes observed in the course of experimental human magnesium depletion. The maximum deviation observed in the course of the depletion is indicated as a percentage of the average control levels for each subject for magnesium, calcium, inorganic phosphate and potassium. K[42] space indicates the estimate of exchangeable body potassium using [42]K. The transient decrease in serum inorganic phosphate noted in 3 individuals immediately following magnesium repletion is indicated by a line connecting values observed in the late depletion period with those observed in early repletion. (From Shils.[13] Used by permission of Williams and Wilkins.)

infection occurring in close proximity to the magnesium therapy—often make it difficult and potentially misleading to ascribe certain clinical manifestations specifically to magnesium deficiency.

There are four recorded efforts to induce magnesium deficiency experimentally in human volunteers.[13,76-78] In the study in which symptomatic depletion occurred,[13,46,47] plasma magnesium fell progressively on the magnesium-deficient diet (< 0.8 mEq per day) to levels which were 10 to 30 per cent those of control periods (Fig. 7B–1). Erythrocyte magnesium declined more slowly and to a lesser degree. Urine and fecal magnesium decreased to extremely low levels within 7 days. Hypocalcemia occurred in 6 of the 7 subjects, despite adequate calcium intake and absorption and no prior evidence of gastrointestinal or parathyroid abnormalities. Hypocalciuria was noted early in the depletion in all cases. Serum phosphate was normal or slightly low in all but one subject and urinary excretion was usually unaffected. Most deficient subjects developed hypokalemia and negative potassium balance; serum sodium remained normal and the subjects were in positive sodium balance.

Neurologic signs occurred in 5 of the 7 after deficiency periods ranging from 25 to 110 days. Hypomagnesemia, hypocalcemia and hypokalemia were present in all consistently symptomatic patients (Figs. 7B–1 and 7B–2). Despite the hypocalcemia,

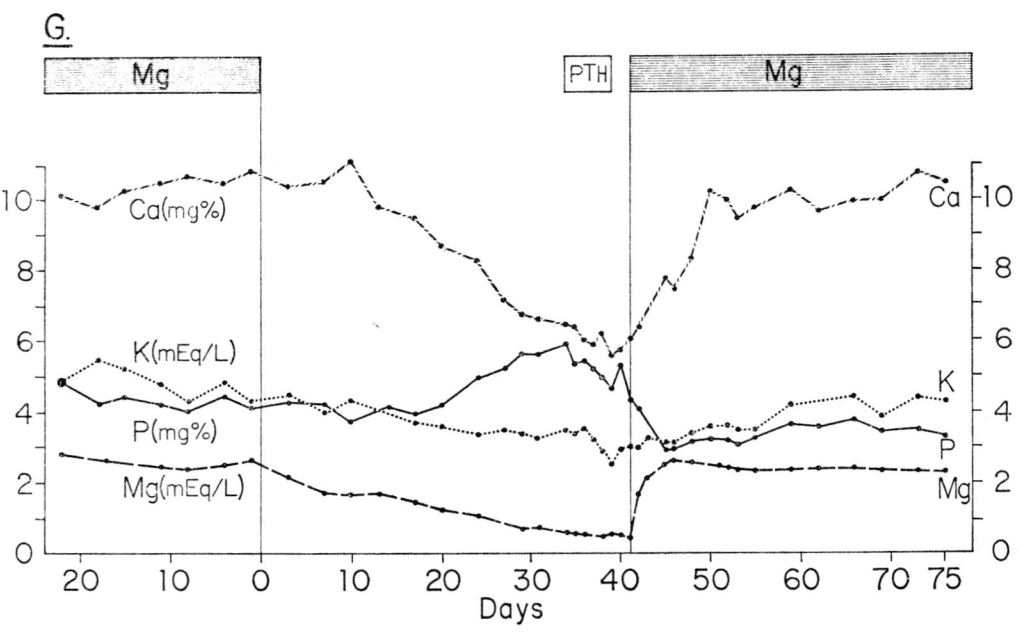

Fig. 7B–2. Blood chemistries in subject on experimental magnesium (Mg) depletion. Mg was omitted after a month on the control diet. The rise in serum inorganic phosphate (P) with Mg depletion in this patient was unique among the depleted subjects. On depletion day 25 Trousseau and Chvostek signs first occurred and the former became progressively stronger as plasma calcium (Ca), Mg and potassium (K) continued to decline. On depletion day 35, parathyroid hormone (PTH) was given i.m. at 50 units t.i.d. for 5 days; this had no effect on plasma Ca but appeared to decrease P. On day 41, anorexia, nausea, paresthesias and generalized muscle spasticity developed; 17 mEq of Mg IV was then given with rapid improvement. This was followed by similar amounts of Mg IM 12 and 15 hours later. Dietary Mg (40 mEq daily) was resumed on the third repletion day. (From Shils.[13] Used by permission of Williams and Wilkins.)

deep tendon reflexes were either normal or decreased. The electromyogram revealed rapid-firing high-pitched potentials during the deficiency period in the 5 patients tested. The electroencephalogram showed no changes related to the deficiency. Anorexia, nausea and apathy occurred frequently and heralded exacerbation of the neurologic changes. When electrocardiographic changes occurred, they were compatible with coexisting hypocalcemia or hypokalemia. All abnormalities reverted to normal with reinstitution of magnesium. Strongly positive potassium balances associated with negative sodium balances occurred as magnesium was retained, electrolytes returned to normal and urine magnesium and calcium rose.

√ It is concluded from this study that magnesium is essential for the normal metabolism of potassium and calcium in adult man, that magnesium is essential for the mobilization of calcium from bone, that the signs and symptoms are associated with complex electrolyte changes occurring secondarily to magnesium deficiency, that the alterations in various electrolytes in blood and tissues and their relative intakes influence the development and manifestation of clinical and biochemical changes and that the occurrence in clinical situations of otherwise unexplained hypokalemia and hypocalcemia should suggest the possibility of significant magnesium depletion.

In another study, hypomagnesemia occurred with hypocalciuria, but without hypocalcemia or symptoms of deficiency, in 2 subjects ingesting 2 to 5 mEq of magnesium per day.[78] The 4 subjects in the remaining two experimental studies did not become hypomagnesemic within the 20 to 38 days of deficiency.[76,77] The numerous differences in types of subjects and diet composition in these experiemental studies have been discussed.[13]

The signs and symptoms noted in the experimental depletion[13,46,47] covered a wide spectrum, including personality change, spontaneous generalized muscle spasm, tremor, fasciculations and Trousseau and Chvostek signs. These have been described separately or in various combinations in clinical cases of hypomagnesemia.[2,49,51,55,57,58,65,66,70] The subjects in the experimental study[13] had no coma, convulsions, significant myoclonic jerks or athetoid movements, which have been reported to occur in certain cases.[2,49,55,58,67,69-71,79,80] Convulsions with or without coma seem to occur much more frequently in acutely deficient infants than in adults. Normoreflexia or hyporeflexia was noted in association with hypocalcemia and positive Trousseau signs in the experimental depletion; hyperreflexia was never seen.[13] The clinical literature on this point is contradictory: hyperreflexia has been reported frequently in symptomatic cases with hypomagnesemia, while others have noted normal or depressed reflexes.[2,50,51,54] Our experience and that of others are not in accord with statements that the Chvostek sign, but not the Trousseau sign, is elicited in magnesium deficiency.[55,81] The development of anorexia, nausea and vomiting, heralding exacerbation of neurologic symptoms, has been one of the more striking observations in experimental depletion.[13,46]

A striking change in the hypomagnesemic subjects becoming symptomatic in the experimental study was the development of hypocalcemia and hypokalemia.[13,46] The clinical literature is also in disagreement about the relationship of magnesium deficiency to hypocalcemia and to latent or overt tetany (defined here as a positive Trousseau sign or spontaneous carpopedal spasm). Some investigators have expressed the opinion that tetany is not a manifestation of magnesium deficiency per se.[2,50,55,82-84] However, there is increasing evidence that the hypocalcemia developing with marked magnesium deficiency cannot be effectively treated with calcium administration alone; it does improve with magnesium administration.[48,]

[51,52,54,56–58,70,80,85–87] It is worth emphasizing that continued parenteral administration of large amounts of calcium is potentially dangerous in the magnesium-depleted individual because of the predisposition toward soft tissue calcification in this deficiency.

Another type of clinical picture has been noted in which hyperirritability, tetany and other neuromuscular abnormalities occurred in a setting of hypomagnesemia and *normocalcemia*; these responded to magnesium but not to calcium salts.[49,67, 68,71,88] This author has not observed this syndrome in any one of numerous cases of clinical magnesium depletion or in his experimental studies in man.

There is increasing support for the view that hypokalemia and total-body depletion of this ion occur in serious magnesium depletion in adults.[13,45,58,78] However, the majority of cases of neonatal tetany associated with hypomagnesemia and hypocalcemia showed normal serum potassium; no data are given on potassium balance or body stores. In malnourished children with magnesium depletion hypokalemia is often present.[67,68]

In experimental human magnesium depletion serum magnesium began to decline early and before changes occurred in red cell concentration;[13] normal muscle magnesium content was found in the presence of reduced serum levels.[78] Reports of the relation among serum, muscle and bone levels of this ion in the clinical literature on magnesium deficiency are conflicting. They include findings of decreased serum and muscle magnesium with normal bone level,[83] normal serum and erythrocyte levels with decreased muscle magnesium and potassium,[89] reduced serum level with normal muscle content,[57] reduced muscle levels in association with normal serum, erythrocyte and bone magnesium levels[90] and consistently reduced serum concentrations with variable muscle levels.[91] Alfrey et al.[92] measured muscle, erythrocyte and bone magnesium in patients with reduced, normal and increased serum magnesium levels. Muscle magnesium content was shown to vary directly with muscle potassium levels and independently of other body magnesium stores. While serum magnesium did not consistently reflect muscle magnesium concentration, there was a highly significant correlation between serum and bone magnesium levels. Bone and extracellular fluid magnesium are the major magnesium pools in man which are decreased during magnesium depletion and increased during magnesium excess.

Hypomagnesemia has been described in chronic heart failure.[25k] Decreased food intake and/or impaired absorption, use of certain diuretics and digitalis toxicity may be contributing factors. The deficiency may predispose to the occurrence of cardiac arrhythmias and may aggravate digitalis toxicity. Administration of magnesium may be useful in hypomagnesemic or digitalis-toxic tachyarrhythmias.[25k]

Associations have been made between hardness of drinking water and mortality from cardiovascular disease in areas of England, Wales, Scotland, the United States and Sweden, with softer water being associated with a higher mortality rate.[93] Preliminary data indicating lower magnesium levels in the coronary arteries in men in soft water areas are insufficient at present to allow more than speculation; even if corroborated, the lower magnesium levels may be related to pathologic changes unrelated to magnesium intake or metabolism.

Thirty-seven per cent of infants born to diabetic mothers have been found to be hypomagnesemic during the first 3 days of life, and this was related to the severity of maternal diabetes and prematurity.[94]

TREATMENT OF MAGNESIUM DEPLETION

The amount and route of magnesium administration will depend upon the severity of depletion and its etiology. Symptomatic deficiency is best treated by the intravenous or intramuscular route. It is our practice to initiate treatment in older children and adults with relatively small amounts of magnesium sulfate intravenously (i.e. 2 gm [17 mEq]) over 1 or 2 hours in saline or dextrose solutions, with other nutrients as required. In the presence of cardiac arrhythmias and electrolyte abnormalities, the patient is monitored during the initial infusion. Another 2 to 4 gm are then given by continuous infusion over the remaining 24 hours or by periodic intramuscular injections. This administration is given daily for 2 or more days and the situation reassessed. An estimate of the degree of depletion may be obtained by measuring daily urinary magnesium levels during repletion. When a sudden increase in urine levels occurs, serum magnesium levels usually have become persistently normal and immediate repletion has been achieved.[13]

A program of longer-term oral or, if necessary, periodic intravenous or intramuscular administration should then be established to maintain normal serum levels. Supplementary magnesium may be given as tablets of milk of magnesia or as gelatin capsules packed with powdered magnesium sulfate (Epsom salts), magnesium chloride or magnesium oxide; one is given 3 to 6 times per day. Improvement of existing steatorrhea will decrease fecal magnesium losses. Treatment of other underlying disease, replacement of potassium deficits and avoidance of alcohol are essential where indicated. Calcium administration in the treatment of hypocalcemia secondary to magnesium deficiency is unnecessary unless tetany—overt or latent (i.e. positive Trousseau sign)—is apparent. Serum calcium usually will return to normal levels within a week of initiating magnesium repletion.

Alternative programs of magnesium replacement in adults have been utilized, usually with higher doses than advocated here.[95] Asymptomatic hypomagnesemia may be treated with smaller or less frequent doses. Reported experience in the treatment of symptomatic magnesium depletion in infants is unanimous concerning the rapid efficacy of relatively small amounts of intravenous or intramuscular magnesium in controlling neurologic signs and restoring serum levels.[69-71,79,80,120] Administration of 0.5 to 1.0 ml of 50 per cent magnesium sulfate solution (2 to 4 mEq of magnesium ion) 2 or 3 times per day appears adequate. The duration and follow-up of treatment will depend upon the etiology of the depletion.

INTERRELATIONSHIPS AMONG MAGNESIUM, CALCIUM, PARATHYROID HORMONE, VITAMIN D AND BONE METABOLISM

Rat Studies. Studies have shown that magnesium-deficient rats often developed hypercalcemia, hypophosphatemia, hypocalciuria and hyperphosphaturia suggestive of a hyperparathyroid state.[16,96-98] Parathyroidectomy eliminated the relative hypercalcemia,[16,98-100] further strengthening the relationship between magnesium deficiency and increased activity of the parathyroid gland in this species. However, despite the hypercalcemia, histologic studies in intact magnesium-deficient rats have indicated that the parathyroid gland was not enlarged.[101] Furthermore, restriction of dietary calcium in the magnesium-deficient rat results in hypocalcemia,[102,103] revealing an important and complicated role of dietary calcium intake in the rat that does not appear to hold for other species, particularly during periods of active growth.

In Vitro Studies. In studying the formation of parathyroid hormone in cultured explants of normal bovine parathyroid glands, Targovnik et al.[104] found that there is a first-order relationship between hormone release from the glands and the total concentration of the divalent cations calcium and magnesium. These ions were equivalent in affecting the release of hormone; as one was decreased and the other increased so that the total divalent ion concentration was constant, parathyroid hormone secretion remained unchanged. However, when magnesium concentration was very low, the hormone was diminished regardless of the total cation concentration. On the other hand, Hamilton and colleagues[105] found increased incorporation of amino acids in the parathyroid hormone isolated from the tissue or from the medium when the concentration of calcium was lowered in the medium. However, changes in the magnesium concentration had no effect on the biosynthesis of parathyroid hormone. These authors suggested that calcium ions affect directly and indirectly both the synthesis and secretion of parathyroid hormone while magnesium ions affect only secretion. These apparent discrepancies remain to be resolved. Perfusion studies of goat or sheep parathyroid glands in vivo have suggested also that the parathyroid gland is sensitive to low magnesium concentrations with resultant increased output of the hormone.[106] When parathyroid extract (PTE) was added to rat bones in vitro, less calcium was released from the bone when the medium was low in magnesium[107] or when the bone was derived from magnesium-deficient rats.[99] These studies suggest that magnesium deficiency induces a degree of refractoriness of bone to the action of parathyroid hormone. If this observation holds for the intact animal it creates an apparent contradiction, since serum calcium is higher in the deficient rat.

In Vivo Studies. Further insight into the relative effects of calcium and magnesium on PTH secretion has been obtained in recent studies with calves.[107a] PTH was assayed in parathyroid venous blood collected at timed intervals as solutions of sodium EDTA and/or $MgCl_2$ were infused into the jugular vein in order to alter plasma calcium and magnesium levels. The effect of magnesium on PTH secretion rate was found to be similar to that of calcium but the effect of variations in plasma magnesium concentration was approximately one-third to one-half as great as that observed with changes in plasma calcium concentration.

Effect of Parathyroid Extract In Vivo

Experimental Animals. Because of the evidence suggesting that a hyperparathyroid state exists in the magnesium-depleted rat, various investigators have tested the effects of PTE given to parathyroidectomized or thyroparathyroidectomized rats and other species. The results of individual studies are listed in Table 7B–2. With the exception of the chick, the species tested—including the rat, dog and monkey—appear to be capable of responding to PTE with respect to elevation of serum calcium levels during magnesium deficiency, although one study with dogs suggests that there may be a relative refractoriness of bone. The abnormality occurring in these magnesium-deficient mammals appears to reside primarily in the inability of the parathyroid gland to secrete an amount of hormone appropriate to the serum calcium level. However, direct evidence for this belief has been obtained only in the

Table 7B–2. Effect of Parathyroid Extract Injection on Serum Calcium in Magnesium-deficient Animals Versus Controls*

| | Surgical State | | |
Species	Intact	PTX	T-PTX
Rat	S	S	R
Chick	R		
Dog	PR		S
Monkey	S		

*Abbreviations: PTX = parathyroidectomized, T-PTX = thyroparathyroidectomized, S = similar response, PR = partially refractory, R = refractory. From Shils,[45b] where the original references may be found.

study of Levi et al.,[108] where the immuno-crossreactivity between canine and bovine PTH was utilized to detect circulating PTH in canine serum.

Human Response. Observations have been made in a relatively small number of deficient adults and children and these have been reviewed recently.[45b,109] Responses in terms of rise in serum calcium and renal excretion of phosphate and cyclic AMP have been variable in deficient adults, but, in general, the expected rise was depressed. In those in whom the PTE response was retested following institution of magnesium, the rise in calcium was appreciably greater than that during the deficiency period in most subjects. Certain methodologic problems are associated with a number of these studies, particularly in relation to variable degrees of deficiency and treatments and to the calcium rise attributed to PTE when the calcemic effect of magnesium repletion was also occurring. A calcemic response was observed in the majority of deficient children; these had primary hypomagnesemia—a clinical state very different from the more complex situation occurring with malnourished adults with magnesium depletion. However, in many of the children the degree of deficiency and previous treatment varied. Despite these variations and unresolved differences, a significant percentage of deficient patients appear to have an end-organ resistance to PTE.

Vitamin D "Resistance" in Magnesium Deficiency

Lack of calcemic response to vitamin D in hypocalcemic states has been reported in the presence of magnesium deficiency in rats[110] and in patients with hypoparathyroidism[111] and rickets.[112] Pharmacologic doses of vitamin D have been reported to cause no or only partial calcemic effect[113] or a good response[114] in magnesium-deficient hypocalcemic patients with malabsorption or alcoholism. 1:25 Dihydroxy-cholecalciferol appears to have a direct

stimulatory effect similar to that of PTH on osteoclast-like cells from rat bone in culture and an inhibitory effect on osteoblastic-like cells. Unlike PTH, the vitamin D metabolite did not increase cellular cyclic AMP.[115]

PTH Levels in Magnesium-Deficient Patients

A resolution to the inter- and intra-species differences and discrepancies in these interrelations appeared to be at hand with the advent of immunoassays for circulating parathyroid hormone. At this time data from at least 8 different laboratories on a total of 36 hypomagnesemic patients are available and have been reviewed in some detail.[45b,109] Ten of these

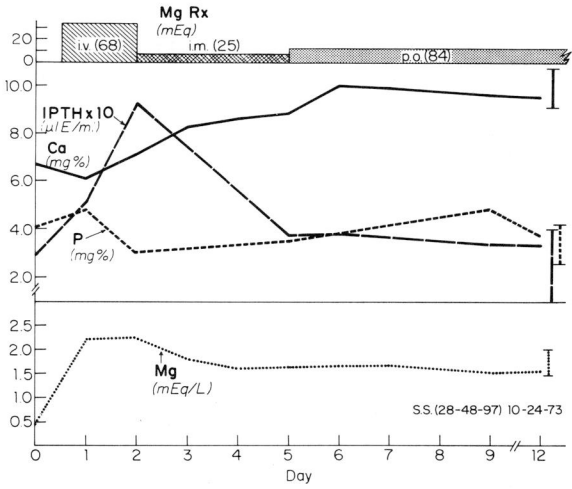

Fig. 7B–3. The effect of magnesium deficiency and repletion on plasma levels of magnesium, calcium, phosphate and immunoreactive parathyroid hormone (IPTH) in an adult woman with malabsorption. The normal range for each is indicated by the vertical lines at the right. The dosage and route of administration of magnesium (as sulfate) are indicated at the top. Note that magnesium levels rose in association with increases in IPTH and with a lag in elevation of calcium; as calcium increased IPTH returned to the normal range. Clinical symptoms disappeared within 12 hours after instituting magnesium in this patient but full recovery may be delayed for 2 or more days when deficiency has been prolonged. (From Shils.[45b])

individuals had levels so low as to be undetectable, 18 had values in the "normal"
range which were, however, inappropriately low for the degree of hypocalcemia
present and 8 had elevated levels. Many of
the patients with the very low or normal
IPTH concentrations had significant increases in hormone levels following magnesium administration. The rise in IPTH
occurred before the serum calcium rose.
Patients with high levels during deficiency
returned toward or to normal when repletion occurred. An example of the serum
IPTH, calcium and magnesium values before and during magnesium therapy is
shown in Figure 7B–3. When IPTH measurements were done serially hourly or
daily when moderate amounts of magnesium were given intramuscularly or
slowly intravenously, there appeared to be
a lag of hours or days before IPTH was
maximal. However, when 12 or 25 mEq of
magnesium were given rapidly by intravenous injection serum IPTH rose in 1
minute to very high levels in association
with elevations of serum magnesium but
without any detectable rise in serum calcium over the next 30 to 60 minutes.[109]
The various reports suggest that the deficiency leads to impaired secretion of
PTH as well as to an impaired end-organ
responsiveness to PTH.

With adequate magnesium repletion
serum calcium usually begins to rise in 2 or
more days and continues until normal
levels are attained. With this rise there is a
decline in serum PTH.

Sequence of Effects of Magnesium Deficiency and Response to Repletion

The following sequences of magnesium
deficiency are postulated to explain most
of the observations mentioned above:

**Sequence I—The Initiation of Hypo-
calcemia.** When there is an adequate intake of calcium, negative calcium balance
does not occur; consequently calcium depletion can be ruled out as the etiology of
hypocalcemia occurring as the result of

magnesium deficiency. There must develop, as a primary factor, a failure of
calcium to leave the metabolically labile
bone mineral. This defect is associated
with a deposition in bone mineral or in soft
tissues of absorbed dietary calcium with a
resultant progressive fall in serum calcium.
In the deficient rat and older animals of
certain species fed relatively large amounts
of calcium who do not become hypocalcemic, the failure to mobilize calcium from
bone may be counterbalanced by increased
absorption of calcium from the intestine
with a resultant maintenance of serum
calcium. There are at least two major
mechanisms responsible for the failure of
calcium release from bone: (1) a decreased
heteroionic exchange of magnesium for
calcium at the bone surface and (2) impairment by magnesium deficiency of the
normal metabolic activity of osteocytes in
maintaining mineral homeostasis by active
bone resorption. This cellular change may
be related in whole or in part to the development of resistance to PTH (which may
operate through impaired cyclic AMP
generation) and possibly to 1:25 dihydroxycholecalciferol.

**Sequence II—The Perpetuation of
Hypocalcemia.** With the development of
hypocalcemia, one would expect PTH
production and secretion to increase. At
this stage of magnesium depletion some
individuals do have elevated levels of the
hormone; nevertheless their serum calcium levels remain depressed, indicating a
resistance to the hormone. Other subjects
have low levels of hormone or "normal"
levels which are inappropriate to the circulating calcium level; this situation indicates an inadequacy of PTH production
and/or secretion. Thus, there is a failure at
two levels in the PTH mechanism designed
to maintain calcium homeostasis. It is
tempting to speculate that these two stages
are related to the degree of deficiency with
bone resistance occurring first and then
being followed by a PTH production or
secretion failure as the deficiency becomes

severe. Excessive calcitonin does not appear to be involved. At present there is no evidence for or against involvement of a failure of formation or function of the metabolically active form(s) of vitamin D, although resistance to vitamin D has been reported to occur in magnesium deficiency.

Sequence III—The Regression of Hypocalcemia. Following administration of magnesium an increase in PTH occurs, its rapidity depending upon the route and amount of magnesium given. There is an associated lag period before serum calcium begins to rise. Presumably in this interval the administered magnesium ions are entering the hydration shell of bone, permitting calcium exchange to begin; this exchange may occur early in repletion and may explain the rapid improvement that occurs in some of the neuromuscular abnormalities with little or no detectable change in circulating calcium. When failure of calcium release is associated with end-organ insensitivity, magnesium repletion leads to entry of magnesium into bone mineral and results in heterionic exchange; the availability of magnesium ion at critical sites on the osteocytes induces responsiveness to hormones with resultant bone resorption. With or without end-organ resistance, elevated PTH levels would be expected to occur following repletion until serum calcium has risen, at which time the hormone levels will decline.

REQUIREMENTS

Establishment of firm data for adequate intake of magnesium for individuals of different ages and physiologic status is difficult because of the complex dietary and physiologic interrelationships of magnesium with calories, calcium, phosphate, protein, lactose, potassium and probably other nutritional factors. A large number of balance studies have been performed on adults to obtain data on magnesium requirements (reviewed by Seelig[10]). However, some reservations about much of these data are indicated, either because of the short duration of the study or the inadequacy of the analytical procedures.

The Recommended Dietary Allowances for magnesium of the National Research Council suggest 40 to 70 mg per day for infants rising to 250 mg as children increase in age up to 10 years. Adult males and nonpregnant and nonlactating females have recommended values of 300 to 400 mg with 450 mg for pregnancy and lactation.[116] Seelig recommends 6 mg per kg especially for adult males.[10] These amounts appear to be more than adequate for normal individuals; they may be grossly inadequate for those with serious intestinal and renal absorptive defects.

HYPERMAGNESEMIA AND MAGNESIUM TOXICITY

The normal kidney is capable of excreting absorbed or injected magnesium ion so rapidly that serum levels do not rise to clinically significant levels. In the treatment of preeclampsia and eclampsia with magnesium, relatively massive doses have been given with the objective of maintaining the serum level at 5 to 8 mEq/L and patients with normal kidneys were able to excrete 40 to 60 gm of magnesium sulfate per day.[95] Hypermagnesemia may develop in other clinical situations where magnesium-containing drugs, usually antacids, are given to individuals with renal insufficiency.[1,117,118] The pharmacology of magnesium has been reviewed by Walser.[7] It has been reported that central depression begins to appear at levels about 8 mEq/L and pronounced anesthesia occurs at about 20 mEq/L. Infusion of magnesium sulfate, raising plasma concentrations of magnesium to approximately 15 mEq/L, induced profound paralysis of skeletal muscle (with the exception of the diaphragm and a few other muscles) in 2 human subjects; there was no evidence of anesthesia and the authors question the previous literature suggesting this.[119] In addition to paralysis, very high blood levels are associated with respiratory depression, coma and death in experimental animals. Calcium infusion counteracts magnesium toxicity. While such dangerously high serum levels are unlikely in the usual clinical situations, avoidance of magnesium-containing medications in patients with significant renal disease is recommended unless otherwise indicated and monitored.

BIBLIOGRAPHY

1. Hirschfelder: J.A.M.A., *102*, 1138, 1934.
2. Flink, et al.: J. Lab. Clin. Med., *43*, 169, 1954.
3. Alcock: Ann. N.Y. Acad. Sci., *162*, 707, 1969.
4. Duckworth and Warnock: Nutr. Abstr. Rev., *12*, 167, 1942–43.
5. Widdowson, McCance and Spray: Clin. Sci., *10*, 113, 1951.
6. Schroeder, Nason and Tipton: J. Chronic. Dis., *21*, 815, 1969.
7. Walser: Ergeb. Physiol., *59*, 185, 1967.
8. Wacker and Parisi: N. Engl. J. Med., *278*, 658, 1968.
9. Consolazio, et al.: J. Nutr., *79*, 407, 1963.
9a. Alfrey and Miller: J. Clin. Invest., *52*, 3019, 1973.
10. Seelig: Am. J. Clin. Nutr., *14*, 342, 1964.
11. Avioli, Lynch and Blastomsky: Clin. Res., *11*, 40, 1963.
12. Graham, Caesar and Burgen: Metabolism, *9*, 646, 1960.
13. Shils: Medicine, *48*, 61, 1969.
14. Barnes, Cope and Gordon: Ann. Surg., *152*, 518, 1960.
15. Heaton: Ann. N.Y. Acad. Sci., *162*, 775, 1969.
15a. Brunnette, Vigneault and Carriere: Am. J. Physiol., *227*, 891, 1974.
16. Heaton: Clin. Sci., *28*, 543, 1965.
17. Greenberg and Mackey: J. Biol. Chem., *98*, 765, 1932.
18. Roberts, Murphy, Miller and Rosenthal: Surg. Forum, *5*, 509, 1954.
19. Gill, Bell and Bartter: Clin. Res., *10*, 405, 1962.
20. Bethune, Turpin and Inoue: J. Clin. Endocrinol. Metab., *28*, 673, 1968.
21a. Shelp, Steele and Rieselbach: Metabolism, *18*, 63, 1969.
21b. Paunier, Ray and Wyss: Helv. Med. Acta, *35*, 504, 1969–70.
22. Cramer, Parkes and Copp: Can. J. Physiol. Pharmacol., *47*, 181, 1969.
23. Clark and Kenny: Endocrinology, *84*, 1199, 1969.
24. Bell, Barrett and Patterson: Proc. Soc. Exp. Biol. Med., *123*, 114, 1966.
25. Foster, et al.: Lancet, *1*, 107, 1966.
25a. Littledike and Arnaud: Proc. Soc. Exp. Biol. Med., *136*, 100, 1971.
25b. Bell: J. Clin. Invest., *49*, 1368, 1970.
25c. Care, Bell and Bates: J. Endocrinol., *57*, 381, 1971.
25d. Anast, et al.: J. Clin. Invest., *56*, 1615, 1975.
25e. Massry, et al.: J. Lab. Clin. Med., *70*, 563, 1967.
25f. Lemann, Piering and Lennon: Clin. Res., *15*, 362, 1967.
25g. Scott and Dobson: Q. J. Exp. Physiol., *50*, 42, 1965.
25h. Horton and Biglieri: J. Clin. Endocrinol., *22*, 1187, 1962.
25i. Massry, et al.: J. Lab Clin. Med., *71*, 212, 1968.
25j. Editorial Comment: Br. Med. J., *1*, 170, 1975.
25k. Iseri, Freed and Bures: Am. J. Med., *58*, 837, 1975.
25l. Abe and Sherwood: Biochem. Biophys. Res. Commun., *48*, 396, 1972.
26. Sutherland: J.A.M.A., *214*, 1281, 1970.
27. Wacker and Vallee: In *Mineral Metabolism* Vol. 2. (Comar and Bronner, Eds.). New York, Academic Press, 1964.
28. Thesleff and Quastel: Annu. Rev. Pharmacol., *5*, 263, 1965.
29. Hubbard, Llinas, and Quastel: *Electrophysiologic Analysis of Synaptic Transmission*, Monog. 19, Physiol. Soc., London. London, Edward Arnold, 1969.
30. Kruse, Orent and McCollum: J. Biol. Chem., *96*, 519, 1932.
31. Schneeberger and Morrison: Lab. Invest., *14*, 674, 1965.
32. Heggtveit: Ann. N.Y. Acad. Sci., *162*, 758, 1969.
33. Van Reen and Pearson: J. Nutr., 51, 191, 1953.
34. Grace and O'Dell: J. Nutr., *100*, 37, 1970.
35. Hamuro: J. Nutr., *101*, 635, 1971.
36. Miller, et al.: J. Nutr., *85*, 13, 1965.
37. Rook and Storey: Nutr. Abstr. Rev., *32*, 1055, 1962.
38. Girard, Brochart, Parodi and Sevestre: Ann. Biol. Anim. Biochim. Biophys., *4*, 345, 1964.
39. Rook: Ann. N.Y. Acad. Sci., *162*, 727, 1969.
40. Syllm-Rapoport and Strassburger: Acta Biol. Med. Ger., *1*, 141, 1958.
41. Vitale, Hellerstein, Nakamura and Lown: Circ. Res., *9*, 387, 1961.
42. Bunce, Jenkins and Phillips: J. Nutr., *76*, 17, 1962.
43. Wener, et al.: Am. Heart J., *67*, 221, 1964.
44. Vitale, Velez, Guzman and Correa: Circ. Res., *12*, 642, 1963.
45. Shils: Unpublished data.
45a. Alcock and Shils: Proc. Soc. Exp. Biol. Med., *146*, 137, 1974.
45b. Shils: In *Trace Elements in Human Health and Disease*, Vol. 2 (Prasad, Ed.). New York, Academic Press, 1976.
45c. Alcock and Shils: Proc. Soc. Exp. Biol. Med., *145*, 885, 1974.
45d. Elin: Proc. Soc. Exp. Biol. Med., *148*, 620, 1975.
45e. Blaxter: In *Bone Structure and Metabolism* (Wolstenholme and O'Conner, Eds.). Boston, Little, Brown and Co., 1956.
45f. Breibart, Lee, McCoord and Forbes: Proc. Soc. Exp. Biol. Med., *105*, 361, 1960.
46. Shils: Am. J. Clin. Nutr., *15*, 133, 1964.
47. Shils: Ann. N.Y. Acad. Sci., *162*, 847, 1969.
48. Randall, Rossmeisl and Bleifer: Ann. Intern. Med., *50*, 257, 1959.
49. Vallee, Wacker and Ulmer: N. Engl. J. Med., *262*, 155, 1960.

50. Hanna, Harrison, MacIntyre and Fraser: Lancet, *2*, 172, 1960.
51. Fletcher, Henly, Sammons and Squire: Lancet, *1*, 522, 1960.
52. Balint and Hirschowitz: N. Engl. J. Med., *265*, 631, 1961.
53. Booth, Babouris, Hanna and MacIntyre: Br. J. Med., *2*, 141, 1963.
54. Petersen: Acta Med. Scand., *173*, 285, 1963.
55. Gerst, Porter and Fishman: Ann. Surg., *159*, 402, 1964.
56. Heaton and Fourman: Lancet, *2*, 50, 1965.
57. Muldowney et al.: N. Engl. J. Med., *281*, 61, 1970.
58. Gerlach, Morowitz and Kirsner: Gastroenterology, *59*, 567, 1970.
59. Mendelson, Ogato and Mello: Ann. N.Y. Acad. Sci., *162*, 918, 1969.
60. Jones, Shane, Jacobs and Flink: Ann. N.Y. Acad. Sci., *162*, 934, 1969.
61. Sullivan, Wolpert, Williams and Egan: Ann. N.Y. Acad. Sci., *162*, 947, 1969.
62. Wolfe and Victor: Ann. N.Y. Acad. Sci., *162*, 973, 1969.
63. Baron: Br. J. Surg., *48*, 344, 1960–61.
64. Broughton, Anderson and Bowden: Lancet, *2*, 1156, 1968.
65. Randall: Ann. N.Y. Acad. Sci., *162*, 831, 1969.
65a. Bar, Wilson and Mazzaferri: Ann. Intern. Med., *82*, 646, 1975.
66. Greenwald, Dubin and Cardon: Am. J. Med., *35*, 854, 1963.
67. Back, Montgomery and Ward: Arch. Dis. Child., *37*, 106, 1962.
68. Cadell: N. Engl. J. Med., *276*, 535, 1967.
69. Davis, Harvey and Yu: Arch. Dis. Child., *40*, 289, 1965.
70. Dooling and Stern: Can. Med. Assoc. J., *97*, 827, 1967.
71. Wong and Teh: Lancet, *2*, 18, 1968.
72. Gitelman, Graham and Welt: Ann. N.Y. Acad. Sci., *162*, 856, 1969.
73. Agna and Goldsmith: N. Engl. J. Med., *259*, 222, 1958.
74. Potts and Roberts: Am. J. Med. Sci., *235*, 206, 1958.
75. Hanna, North, MacIntyre and Fraser: Br. Med. J., *2*, 1253, 1961.
76. Fitzgerald and Fourman: Clin. Sci., *15*, 635, 1956.
77. Barnes, Cope and Gordon: Ann. Surg., *152*, 518, 1960.
78. Dunn and Walser: Metabolism, *15*, 884, 1966.
79. Clarke and Carre: J. Pediatr., *70*, 806, 1967.
80. Paunier et al.: Pediatrics, *41*, 385, 1968.
80a. Martin and Wertman: J. Clin. Invest., *26*, 217, 1947.
81. Fishman: Arch. Neurol., *12*, 562, 1965.
82. Booth, Babouris, Hanna and MacIntyre: Br. Med. J., *2*, 141, 1963.
83. MacIntyre, Hanna, Booth and Read: Clin. Sci., *20*, 297, 1961.
84. Smith, Hammarsten and Eliel: J.A.M.A., *174*, 77, 1960.

85. Fourman and Morgan: Proc. Nutr. Soc., *21*, 34, 1962.
86. Friedman, Hatcher and Watson: Lancet, *1*, 703, 1967.
87. George and Chambers: Tex. Med., *58*, 812, 1962.
88. Miller: Am. J. Dis. Child., *67*, 117, 1944.
89. Montgomery: Lancet, *2*, 74, 1960.
90. Lim and Jacobs: Nephron, *9*, 300, 1972; Q. J. Med., *41*, 291, 1972; J. Lab. Clin. Med., *80*, 313, 1972.
91. Stendig-Lindberg, Bergström and Hultman: Acta Med. Scand., *201*, 273, 1977.
92. Alfrey, Miller and Butkus: J. Lab. Clin. Med., *84*, 153, 1974.
93. Crawford and Crawford: Lancet, *1*, 229, 1967.
94. Tsang, et al.: J. Pediatr., *89*, 115, 1976.
95. Flink: Ann. N.Y. Acad. Sci., *162*, 901, 1969.
96. MacIntyre, Boss and Troughton: Nature, *198*, 1058, 1963.
97. Lifshitz, Harrison, Bull and Harrison: Metabolism, *16*, 345, 1967.
98. Gitelman, Kukolj and Welt: J. Clin. Invest., *47*, 118, 1968.
99. MacManus, Heaton and Lucas: J. Endocrinol., *49*, 253, 1971.
100. Hahn, Chase and Avioli: J. Clin. Invest., *51*, 886, 1972.
101. Mirra, Alcock, Shils and Tennenbaum: Fed. Proc., *31*, 707, 1973.
102. MacManus and Heaton: Clin. Sci., *36*, 297, 1969.
103. Suh, Csima and Fraser: J. Clin. Invest., *50*, 2668, 1971.
104. Targovnik, Rodman and Sherwood: Endocrinology, *88*, 1477, 1971.
105. Hamilton, Spierto, MacGregor and Cohn: J. Biol. Chem., *246*, 3224, 1971.
106. Buckle, Care, Cooper and Gitelman: J. Endocrinol., *42*, 529, 1968.
107. Raisz and Niemann: Endocrinology, *85*, 446, 1969.
107a. Mayer and Hurst: Endocrinology. *102*, 1803, 1978.
108. Levi et al.: Metabolism, *23*, 323, 1974.
109. Rude, Oldham and Singer: Clin. Endocrinol., *5*, 209, 1976.
110. Lifshitz, Harrison and Harrison: Proc. Soc. Exp. Biol. Med., *125*, 472, 1967.
111. Rösler and Rabinowitz: Lancet, *1*, 803, 1973.
112. Reddy and Sivakumar: Lancet, *1*, 963, 1974.
113. Medalle, Waterhouse and Hahn: Am. J. Clin. Nutr., *29*, 854, 1976.
114. Petersen: Acta Med. Scand., *173*, 285, 1963.
115. Wong, Luben and Cohn: Science, *197*, 663, 1977.
116. National Academy of Sciences: Recommended Dietary Allowances, 8th ed. Washington, 1974.
117. Randall, Cohen, Spray and Rossmeisl: Ann. Intern. Med., *61*, 73, 1964.
118. Freeman, Lawton and Chamberlain: N. Engl. J. Med., *276*, 113, 1967.
119. Somjen, Hilmy and Stephens: J. Pharmacol. Exp. Ther., *154*, 652, 1966.

C. Iron*†

Ernest Beutler

Iron is essential to higher forms of life because its central role in the heme molecule permits oxygen and electron transport. The total quantity of body iron varies with weight, hemoglobin concentration, sex and size of the storage compartment. A broad range of individual values exists (Table 7C–1), with an average level of about 50 mg per kg of body weight in adult men and 35 mg per kg in adult women.[1,2]

The amount of iron that must be absorbed from food in order to maintain body iron levels is determined by the amount excreted, the loss in menstrual flow or from hemorrhage, the demands of pregnancy and, in children, the needs related to growth.

Two functional compartments of body iron are recognized: (1) an essential component, comprising about 70 per cent of the total, which is contained in hemoglobin, myoglobin, heme enzymes, cofactor and transport iron and (2) the remainder, nonessential storage iron, found predominantly in liver, spleen and bone marrow as ferritin and hemosiderin. Quantitative distribution of the essential fraction is approximately as follows: 85 per cent in hemoglobin, 5 per cent in myoglobin, 10 per cent in the ubiquitous intracellular heme enzymes (cytochromes, cytochrome oxidase, peroxidase, catalase, etc.) or serving as a cofactor in other enzyme systems, and 4 mg as transport iron bound to transferrin in the plasma.[1-3]

When iron deficiency is well developed, insufficient iron is available to sustain normal hemoglobin production and an anemia characterized, in its severe form, by hypochromic microcytic red blood cells results; defective synthesis of the other heme complexes and iron-containing metalloenzymes may be responsible for the fatigue, epithelial changes and other associated clinical manifestations. Iron-deficiency anemia is a medical and public health problem of prime importance, causing few deaths but contributing seriously to the weakness, ill health and substandard performance of millions of people. Iron deficiency too mild to produce anemia can now be detected with reasonable accuracy, and appears to have a relatively high incidence among children and young women; whether it impairs performance or causes symptoms is still uncertain. Iron excess or overload is of increasing clinical concern. It occurs in patients with certain types of refractory anemia and thalassemia, particularly when multiple transfusions are given, and in patients with idiopathic hemochromatosis.

The main metabolic pathways of iron[4,5] are summarized in Figure 7C–1.

INTAKE

Information concerning dietary iron intake is still fragmentary. Most published figures have been obtained from dietary surveys rather than from actual analysis and indicate that the average daily intake is between 10 and 30 mg.[6] The diets of people who live in western countries contain about 5 to 7 mg of iron per 1,000

*This chapter is a revision of one previously contributed by the late Carl Moore. Dr. Moore was a giant in the field of medicine, and particularly in the area of iron and nutrition. This chapter is dedicated to his memory in recognition of his valuable contributions to science and as a token of my personal esteem and a warm friendship. I am grateful to Mrs. Bonnie Beutler for her valuable editorial assistance.

†This work was supported, in part, by NIH Grant HL07449.

324

Table 7C–1. Estimates of Total Body Iron in Adults to Emphasize the Wide Variations Produced by Body Size and Normal Range of Hemoglobin Values

	Male, 70 kg Hb 16 gm/100 ml	Male, 100 kg Hb 18 gm/100 ml	Female, 45 kg Hb 12 gm/100 ml
"Essential" iron			
Hb Fe	2.67 gm	4.2 gm	1.26 gm
Functional tissue iron*	~.45	~.64	~.29
Transport iron	~.005	~.007	~.003
Storage iron	0.5 – 1.5	0.5 – 1.5	0.3 – 1.0
Total: as low as			<2 gm
as high as		>6 gm	

*Myoglobin, metalloenzymes.

calories.[1] A weight-conscious young woman who limits her intake to between 1,000 and 1,500 calories per day will therefore consume only 6 to 9 mg of food iron. These estimates, however, ignore the iron content of beverages and that added or lost during food preparation. Exogenous iron is of particular significance in the iron-rich diet of the Bantu; the iron is derived largely from the iron pots used for cooking and for the preparation of fermented beverages.[4]

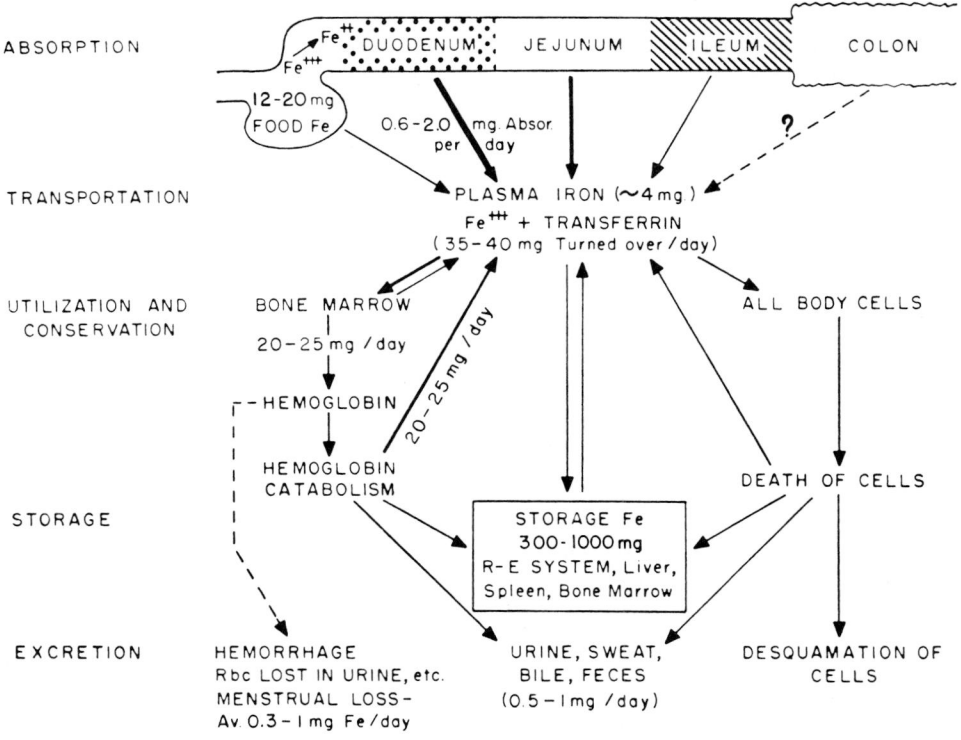

Fig. 7C–1. Schematic outline of iron metabolism in adults.

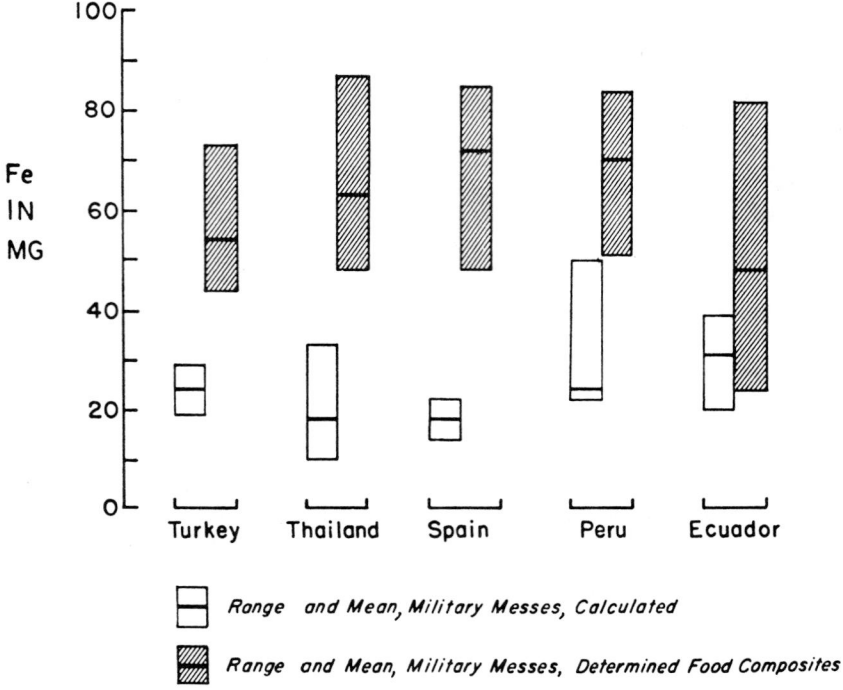

Fig. 7C–2. Iron intake (mg) per man per day in military messes. Note that in each case the values are much higher when determined on food composite than when calculated from food composition tables.

The United States Committee on Nutrition for National Defense has published a series of studies[7] of the iron content of meals served to military personnel in a number of countries. Some of the results are illustrated in Figure 7C–2 and contain two surprises: (1) the *calculated* mean iron intake was comparatively high (20 to 30 mg per day), and (2) in every instance the values *determined* by analysis of the food served were even higher. The food had been prepared in iron cooking utensils. Studies of the effect of cooking in cast-iron skillets or Dutch ovens, utensils commonly found in American kitchens, revealed that iron utensils contribute significantly to the iron content of cooked foods. The gradual substitution of aluminum and stainless steel in the manufacture of cooking equipment has almost certainly had an adverse effect on dietary iron intake. The iron content of canned food may increase significantly when the cans are stored for a matter of months.

Failure to consider the iron content of drinking fluids introduces into dietary surveys another source of error which is of varying significance in different areas. Cider and wine may contain as much as 2 to 16 mg of iron or more per liter.[8] The iron content of city water supplies is usually low, but amounts greater than 5 mg per liter may be found in the water from some deep wells or bore holes.[9]

ABSORPTION

Mechanism and Regulating Factors

Since iron loss is very limited, normal iron balance is maintained largely by regulation of the iron absorbed. Ingested iron is solubilized and ionized largely by the acid gastric juice, reduced to the ferrous state and chelated; substances which form low-molecular chelates such as ascorbic acid, sugars and amino acids tend to promote absorption (Fig. 7C–1). The concept that only ferrous forms of iron traverse the brush border of intestinal mucosal cells may be an oversimplification. The much greater solubility of ferrous than of ferric hydroxide at the neutral to alkaline pH of the duodenum may be of great importance. Normal gastric secretions contain a chemically unidentified stabilizing factor, probably an endogenous chelate, which helps slow the precipitation of ingested iron at the alkaline pH of the small intestine.[10] Impaired absorption in achlorhydria and in gastrectomized subjects is presumably related to decreased solubilization and chelation of the ferric iron in food.[11]

Absorption may occur at any level of the small intestine, but it is most efficient in the upper portion. The chemical form of iron that enters mucosal cells, the nature of receptor sites and the transmucosal transport system are unknown. Iron-binding compounds which have been purified may play a role in iron transport by the gastrointestinal system.[12] Ferritin was once believed to impede iron transport across the mucosa, but it seems doubtful that it plays such a role.[2,5] Most of the iron absorbed into the blood stream passes rapidly through the mucosal cells in the form of small molecules; that portion exceeding the rapid transport capacity combines with apoferritin to form ferritin. Some of the ferritin iron may later be released for uptake into the blood stream, but most of it seems to remain in the mucosal cells until they are desquamated at the end of their 2- to 3-day life span. Direct entry into lymphatic channels is insignificant.

Intraluminal Factors

Intraluminal influences that decrease absorption include: rapid transit time, achylia, malabsorption syndromes, precipitation by alkalinization, phosphates, phytates, and ingested alkaline clays[13] or antacid preparations. A gastric chelate of high molecular weight (gastroferrin) which reputedly binds iron and prevents absorption has also been described.[14] Low levels of this factor in hemochromatosis and iron deficiency were postulated to partially explain augmented absorption in these conditions. The existence of gastroferrin has been disputed.[5] As the intraluminal concentration of iron is increased, the percentage absorbed decreases but the total amount retained by the body rises steadily. When the logarithm of iron dosage is plotted against the logarithm of iron absorbed a straight line is obtained.[15] The following equation describes the relationship between the amount of iron absorbed (A) and iron dosage (D):[16]

$$A = .022 \times D^{0.676} \text{ for males and}$$
$$A = .025 \times D^{0.668} \text{ for females}$$

This relationship indicates that for each 2-fold increment in iron dosage a 1.6-fold increment in absorption can be anticipated. Uptake is increased by ascorbic acid, certain weak chelating agents (e.g. ascorbic acid, succinic acid, sugars, sulfur-containing amino acids) and possibly by the stabilizing gastric factor previously mentioned.[10] Alcohol and deficiency of pancreatic exocrine secretions have been reported to stimulate absorption, but there is not general agreement about these findings.

Systemic Regulation

The systemic regulatory mechanisms which influence iron absorption have never been identified in spite of intensive search.[2,4,5] They operate to: (1) increase absorption in iron deficiency and in hemochromatosis, during the latter half of pregnancy and when erythropoiesis is stimulated (including ineffective erythropoiesis) and (2) decrease absorption in iron overload, and when erythropoiesis is depressed.

Various possible mechanisms have been

investigated, including decreased saturation of plasma transferrin, local hypoxia, humoral factors and mucosal iron concentration. For several decades the concept of a "mucosal block" of iron absorption dominated the literature. Ferritin was regarded as the mediator of absorption; uptake was thought to continue until the intracellular concentration of ferritin blocked further assimilation. Compelling reasons for rejecting the theory have been documented.[2,5] More recently, it has been suggested that the signal which determines whether or not iron is to be absorbed is built into the mucosal cells. It was postulated that: (1) The columnar mucosal cells formed in crypts at the base of villi contain a variable amount of transferrin-derived iron, (2) the size of this intracellular deposit regulates, within limits, the quantity of intraluminal iron which enters cells, (3) the cellular iron may enter the body according to need or remain within the cells to limit absorption and be lost when the cells are sloughed from the tips of villi at the end of their brief life spans. According to this concept, little iron is incorporated from transferrin into mucosal cells of iron-deficient subjects, and absorption is enhanced. Conversely, in iron-loaded subjects, the mucosal cells formed are well endowed with iron, absorption is limited and the cellular iron is excreted when desquamation occurs.

Heme iron, an important dietary form of iron, is absorbed by a mechanism different from that described above for inorganic and nonheme forms of food iron. Some investigators believe that heme is taken up by mucosal cells after it has been released from its globin combination by proteolytic duodenal enzymes, while others believe that the protein portion is removed largely within the mucosal epithelium.[11,17] In either case, iron is liberated by a heme-splitting substance, probably the enzyme heme-oxygenase,[18] and is transferred to plasma in a form that can be bound by transferrin. Only a small portion of the heme absorbed by mucosal cells is delivered to the portal blood as the iron-porphyrin complex.[19] Absorption of heme iron is increased in iron deficiency, but less than that of inorganic ferrous salts. Unlike nonheme forms of iron, absorption of heme is not increased by ascorbic acid nor is it depressed by such substances as phytates and desferrioxamine. Its absorption is inhibited less by simultaneous administration of inorganic iron than is that of nonheme forms,[20-22] and it has a slower rate of appearance in plasma.

Absorption from Foods

Information about the absorption of iron from foods is difficult to obtain and thus is meager.[6,22,23] It is estimated that healthy subjects absorb 5 to 10 per cent of dietary iron, and iron-deficient subjects 10 to 20 per cent. The maximum amount of iron absorption expected from an average diet in the United States is about 1 to 2 mg in normal adults and 3 to 6 mg in iron-deficient patients.

The earliest measurements were made with nonisotopic balance techniques.[24] Several of these studies were done with meticulous care, yet the small difference between oral intake and fecal loss was difficult to measure with precision, and differentiation between excreted and unabsorbed iron was not possible. The studies have the merit of having been done on mixed diets fed over a period of several weeks, so that the effect of daily variation on results was minimized. Absorption, calculated on the basis of positive balance, ranged from 7.3 to 21 per cent.[2,22]

Most data have been obtained by measuring the absorption of iron from single foods prepared or grown so as to contain radioactive iron. Isotopic methods can be used to measure absorption from these foods after they were prepared and fed as would be a normal diet. Figure 7C–3 presents some results obtained using this technique.[22] The overall average absorption in 219 normal subjects approximated

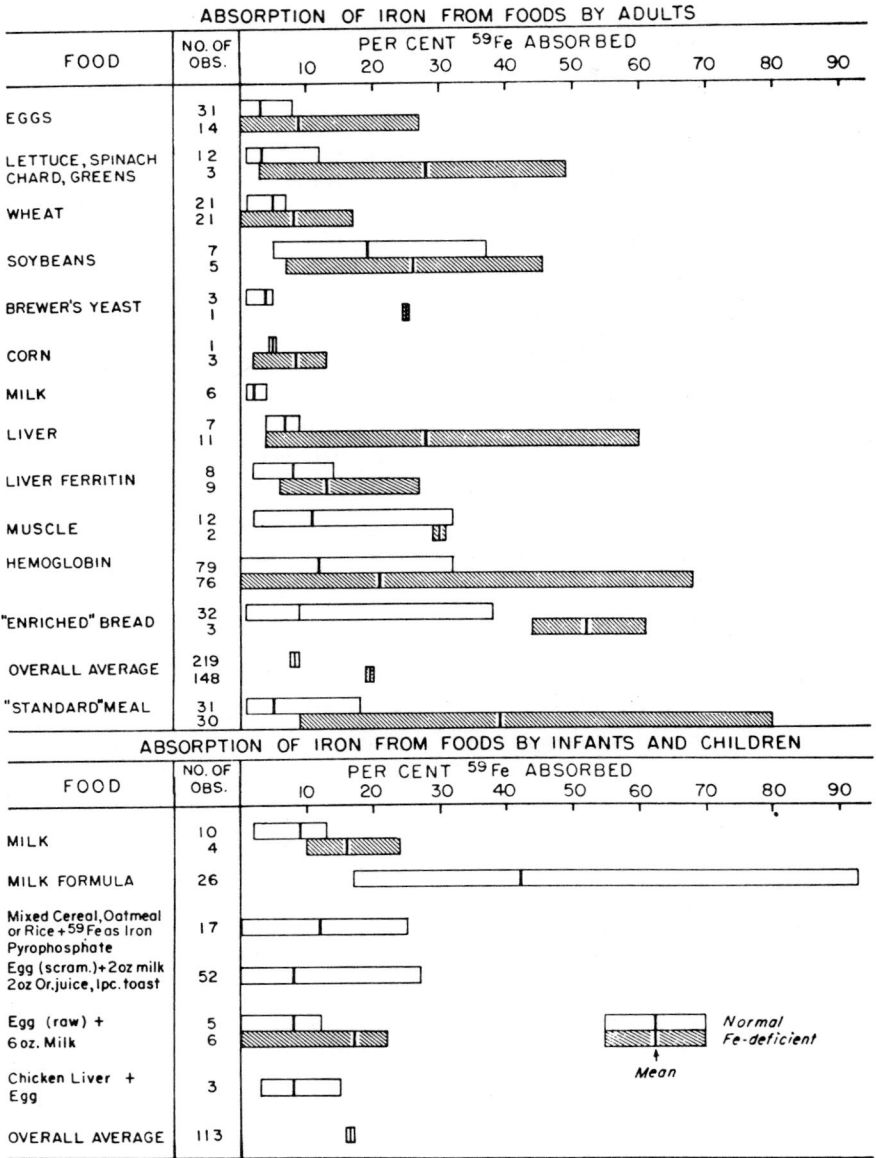

Fig. 7C–3. Radioiron measurements of the absorption of iron from foods by adults, infants and children. The length of the bars indicates the variation among different subjects for each food; the heavy vertical line across each bar indicates the average value. The amount of iron in each feeding varied from 1 to 17 mg. Clear bars = normal subjects; cross-hatched bars = iron-deficient patients.

10 per cent and that in 148 iron-deficient patients 20 per cent. Absorption from any given food varies widely, and is greater from liver, muscle, hemoglobin and soybeans than from eggs, milk and cereals. It is generally greater in children than in adults.

These data have been extensively augmented as the result of a collaborative effort between investigators in Venezuela and Seattle.[23] Figure 7C–4 summarizes results obtained on 520 subjects using 7 foods of vegetable origin and 5 of animal origin. Absorption exceeded 10 per cent from animal foods, was poor from rice and spinach and somewhat better from soybeans than from other vegetable sources. Since radioiron-tagged foods were given as a single test dose, daily variations in absorption were not measured, nor was the effect of possible interaction of foods on iron absorption determined. Ascorbic acid, for instance, will increase[2] while eggs have been reported to decrease[25] the uptake of iron from some foods.

The effect on absorption of certain foods has also been investigated. [26–28] One vegetable (maize or black beans) and one animal food (fish or veal muscle) tagged with different isotopes (^{55}Fe and ^{59}Fe) were fed to the same subjects separately and mixed in the same meal. Veal iron absorption was diminished about 20 per cent when veal was combined with vegetable foods; iron absorption from either corn or black beans was almost doubled when these foods were mixed with animal food. It was further demonstrated that the enhancing effect could be duplicated by substituting amino acids in the same composition as those found in fish muscle, and that cysteine seemed to be the amino acid

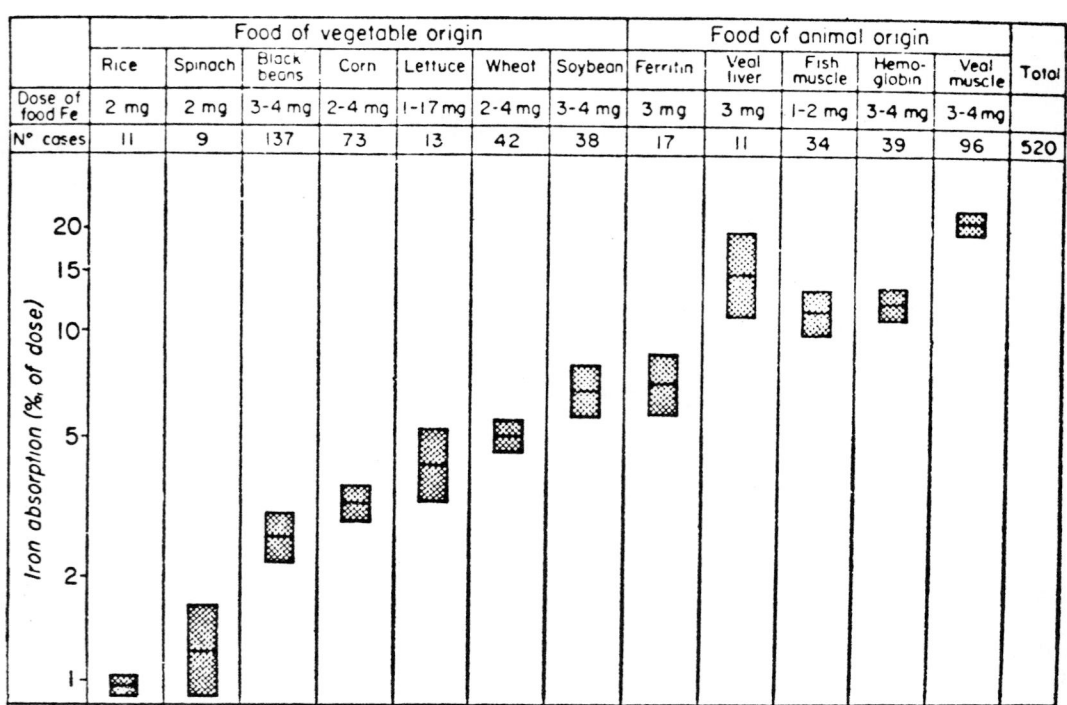

Fig. 7C–4. Absorption of iron from foods. (From Layrisse and Martinez-Torres.[23] Used with permission of Grune and Stratton.)

primarily responsible for the enhancing effect.

These results emphasize the difficulty of obtaining composite data on absorption of iron from a complete diet, and have re-stimulated interest in the use of "standard" or mixed meals[22,29] to which a tracer dose of inorganic radioiron is added as an external tag. Nonheme iron in food appears to be converted into a common pool during cooking and digestion, and absorption of the external tag provides a measure of the iron absorbed from this pool.[28,30] The laborious and difficult isotopic labeling of individual foods can be circumvented in this way and the effect of interaction of different foods on absorption can more easily be studied. It appears that radioiron-tagged hemoglobin will similarly serve as an external tag for measuring the absorption of heme iron in food. Absorption from a complete diet, therefore, can be determined by using both an inorganic and a hemoglobin external tag.

TRANSPORT

Iron is transported in plasma bound to transferrin, a beta$_1$ globulin carrier protein with a molecular weight of 86,000 and a biologic half-life of 8 to 10.5 days.[31] Formed in the liver, the 7 to 15 gm of transferrin present in the normal adult are equally distributed in the intra- and extra-vascular space. It serves a dual function in the transport process. It must *accept* iron from the intestinal tract or from sites of storage or hemoglobin destruction. It must then *deliver* this iron to the bone marrow for hemoglobin synthesis, to reticuloendothelial cells for storage, to the placenta for fetal needs and to all cells for iron-containing enzymes.

Transferrin has two separate binding sites each capable of binding one atom of ferric iron.[32,33] There are conflicting data regarding the identity of the two binding sites. Fletcher and Huehns[33] suggested that the sites were different, one having a greater affinity for iron than the other. Evidence for nonequivalence of the two iron-binding sites, designated A and B, is also provided in vivo in the rat by Awai and Brown[34] and in vitro by Princiotto and Zapolski,[35] but recent data of Harris and Aisen[36] suggest that the two binding sites of human and rabbit transferrin are equivalent with respect to their ability to donate iron to reticulocytes. The metal is tightly bound at physiologic pH, particularly in the presence of bicarbonate and certain other anions;[37] exchange occurs at specific cellular receptor sites. The best-studied are

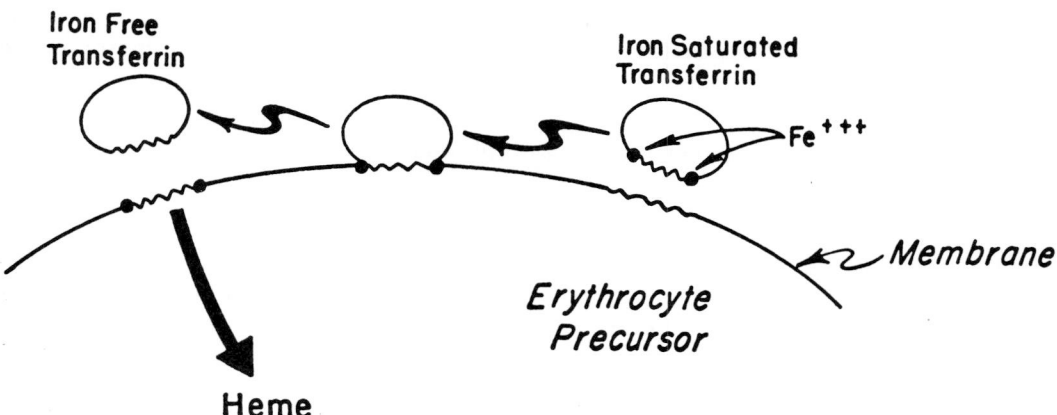

Fig. 7C–5. Schematic representation of the transfer of iron from transferrin to an erythrocyte precursor.

the receptor sites on developing red blood cells; they gradually diminish in number as the cells mature.[38] Transferrin apparently attaches itself to the receptors on the erythroblast or reticulocyte, gives up one or both atoms of iron and then recirculates as a carrier protein (Fig. 7C–5).

Little attention has been paid to iron transport to cells other than erythrocytes, probably because of technical difficulties. Cultured skin fibroblasts represent a suitable system for such studies, however, and transferrin may also play a role in iron delivery to these cells. When cultured fibroblasts are incubated with increasing concentrations of iron tagged with ^{59}Fe, rapid incorporation of iron occurs. The amount of iron incorporated into fibroblasts increases much more rapidly than the concentrations of iron itself. This finding is the opposite of that which would be expected if a carrier mechanism were involved, and is compatible with the concept of membrane damage by ionized iron. On the other hand, if the iron is first complexed to transferrin, the relationship between the concentration of iron and the amount of iron incorporated into fibroblasts follows saturation kinetics. These findings strongly suggest that fibroblasts, like reticulocytes, contain specific binding sites for transferrin.

At least 19 genetic variants of transferrin have been recognized;[39] all seem to function in the same way. The average trans-

binding sites. The remaining two-thirds represent a latent or unsaturated iron-binding capacity (UIBC). The plasma iron level undergoes diurnal variation, with morning values being about 30 per cent higher than those in the evening; it is not influenced by season, exercise or normal meals.

Although only 3 or 4 mg of iron circulates bound to transferrin, the iron turnover rate is rapid.[3,40] About 70 to 90 per cent of the total is transported to the bone marrow where it is transferred to developing red blood cells to support hemoglobin synthesis. Except for a small fraction, which is used for myoglobin and cellular metalloenzymes, the remainder is exchanged largely with reticuloendothelial and hepatic parenchymal cells. The plasma iron turnover rate (PITR) can be determined with reasonable accuracy. After the intravenous injection of trace amounts of radioiron (as ^{59}Fe-citrate or ^{59}FeCl$_3$), the disappearance of radioactivity is followed for 2 or 3 hours and plotted semilogarithmically (Fig. 7C–6). The time required for the activity to reach half that initially present (T½) varies in normal subjects from 60 to 120 minutes. More rapid clearance rates are found in patients with iron deficiency or accelerated erythropoiesis; slower rates occur in those with erythroid hypoplasia. Using the T½ and plasma iron values, the PITR can be calculated from the following formula:

$$\text{PITR (mg/day)} = \frac{0.693 \times \text{Fe (mg/ml plasma)} \times \text{plasma vol (ml)} \times 24}{^{59}\text{Fe T½ (hr)}}$$

ferrin content of normal plasma varies from 215 to 350 mg per 100 ml, but concentration is ordinarily expressed in physiologic terms as total iron-binding capacity (TIBC): roughly 300 to 450 μg per 100 ml. The amount of iron in plasma (90 to 180 μg per 100 ml in males and 70 to 150 μg in women) is sufficient to saturate only about one-third of the available iron-

Normal PITR values range from 25 to 40 gm per day. The PITR is increased when erythropoiesis is stimulated and decreased when erythropoiesis is depressed. In iron deficiency, where the T½ is rapid and the plasma iron value is low, the PITR is usually normal. If the disappearance of plasma iron is followed for a period of many hours a second and even a third

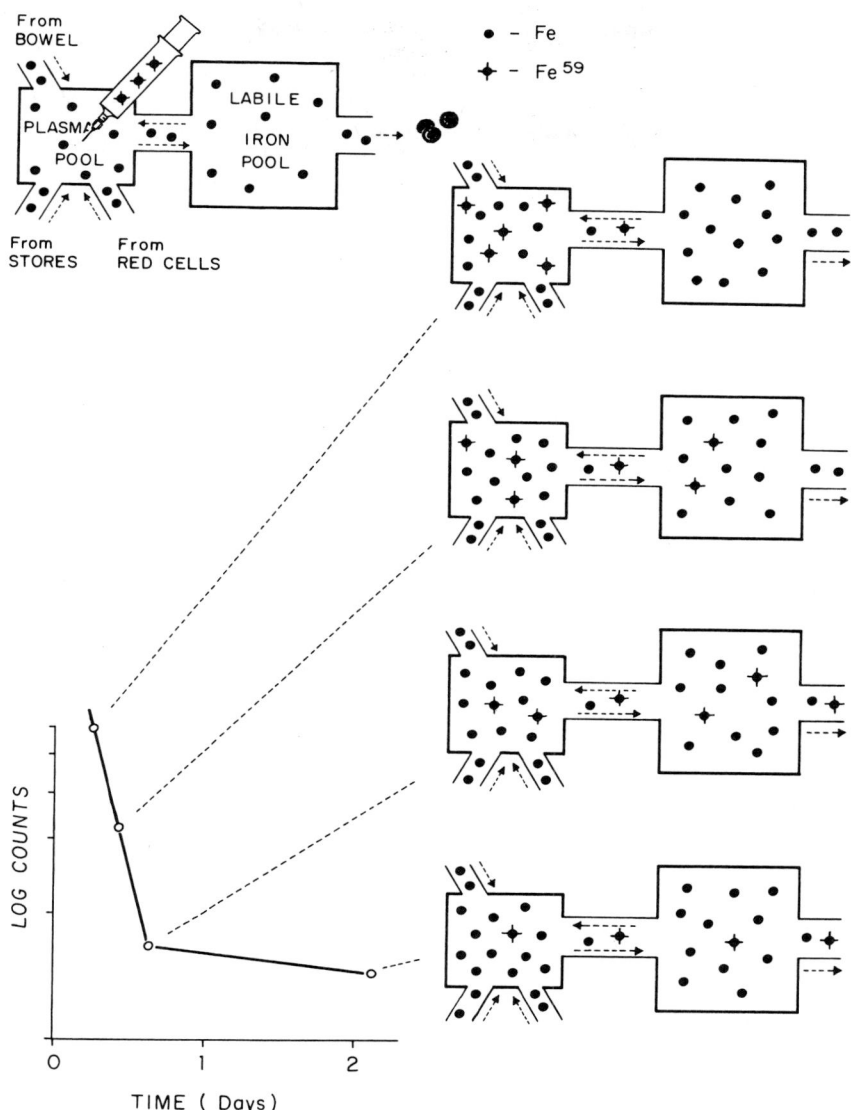

Fig. 7C–6. The mechanism by which two component iron clearance curves may be produced. [59]Fe is injected into the plasma iron pool and the first, rapid, clearance component represents dilution of the radioactive iron by nonradioactive iron coming from iron stores, bowel, red cells and a labile iron pool. However, the radioactive iron mixes with the iron in the labile iron pool until the specific activity of both pools has become equal. The second, slower slope now results from the dilution of the larger, combined pool by iron from the stores, bowel and red cells. The fractional loss from this much larger pool is less, and therefore the slope is not as steep. (Modified from Fairbanks, Fahey and Beutler.[5])

component of the clearance curve can be measured. This finding suggests that the iron which is cleared from the plasma is not simply being incorporated into stable iron compounds but that some is entering other compartments, e.g. "the labile iron pool" from which iron is fed back into the plasma. Complex mathematical models have been constructed to describe the movement of iron among different compartments in the body.[41] Such models are of little clinical value.

Changes in the iron-binding capacity and plasma iron levels are useful diagnostic indicators of various diseases (Fig. 7C–7). Increased total iron-binding capacity is found in iron deficiency, in the third trimester of pregnancy and in response to hypoxia. Decreased levels occur in infection, in protein malnutrition, in many types of iron overload and in conditions in which protein is lost, such as nephrosis or

protein-losing enteropathies. The level of plasma iron represents the balance between iron extracted from the blood by organs of utilization or storage and that delivered to the blood by absorption, hemolysis or release from storage sites. Consequently, it is low in patients with iron deficiency, accelerated erythropoiesis or inflammatory states in which release from reticuloendothelial cells is impaired. It is generally high in those with iron overload, hemolysis or depressed rates of red blood cell formation.

Trace amounts of the iron storage compound ferritin (see below) have also been detected in the plasma using a sensitive radioimmunoassay technique.[42–44] The normal serum ferritin level is in the range of 2 to 20 μg per 100 ml, representing some 0.4 to 4 μg per 100 ml of iron. Ferritin iron does not appear to be a transport form of iron but rather the result of

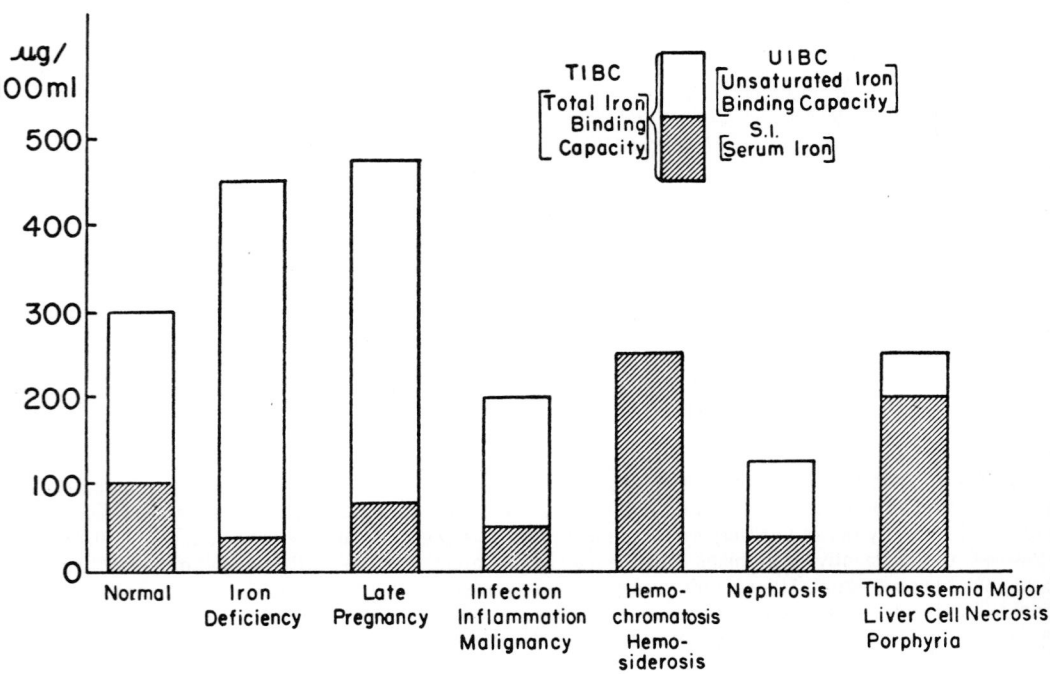

Fig. 7C–7. Relationships of serum iron, unsaturated iron-binding capacity and total iron-binding capacity in various clinical conditions.

"leakage" from various body cells. The measurement of the serum ferritin levels has been advocated as a useful means for the estimation of total body iron stores (see below).

UTILIZATION

The amount of iron utilized for hemoglobin synthesis in a normal adult is approximately 20 to 25 mg per day. These values can be calculated as follows:

A man with a blood volume of 5,000 ml and a hemoglobin level of 15 gm per 100 ml has 750 gm of circulating hemoglobin or 2.55 gm of circulating hemoglobin iron (Hb multiplied by 0.34 per cent). Since the normal life span of the red cell is about 120 days, 2.55 gm ÷ 120 or 21 mg of iron would be required daily to replace the catabolized hemoglobin. Iron utilization can also be determined after a tracer dose of radioiron is given intravenously. The amount of injected radioactive iron which is utilized for hemoglobin synthesis and delivered to the peripheral blood in newly formed erythrocytes is then measured. Normally, red cell radioactivity rises for 7 to 14 days and then levels off at 75 to 90 per cent of the injected amount. The PITR in mg per 24 hr is multiplied by the maximum percentage of radioactivity in circulating hemoglobin to give the amount of iron used daily for hemoglobin formation. For example,

> if the PITR is 35 mg/day, *and* if 80 per cent of the injected dose appears in circulating hemoglobin, then 35 × 80% = 24 mg Fe used for hemoglobin synthesis/day

For a detailed discussion of these ferrokinetic considerations, see Bothwell and Finch[4] and Finch et al.[41]

A normally functioning marrow can effect a 6-fold increase in its production of red blood cells and of hemoglobin; under maximal stimulation, therefore, as much as 100 to 125 mg of iron could be used for hemoglobin synthesis per day.

STORAGE AND TISSUE IRON

Iron in excess of need is stored intracellularly as ferritin and as hemosiderin. Ferritin consists of a shell of 24 chemically identical protein subunits surrounding a micelle of ferric hydroxyphosphate.[45] Ferritin has a characteristic "tetrad" appearance on electron microscopy. The amount of iron varies, but those molecules that are completely filled with iron have a molecular weight of 900,000 and contain approximately 5,000 ferric atoms per molecule—enough to form 1,250 hemoglobin molecules. Recent work has established at least a limited organ specificity for ferritin: liver and spleen ferritins have different electrophoretic mobilities and some differences in the amino acid structure of the protein subunits. Hemosiderin has a higher iron content than does ferritin, and may represent partially denatured ferritin. The major sites of storage are the hepatic parenchymal cells and reticuloendothelial cells of the bone marrow, liver and spleen.

The immediate source of most reticuloendothelial iron stores is hemoglobin iron released from erythrocytes phagocytosed at the end of their life spans. Hepatic parenchymal iron probably comes primarily from plasma transferrin. In the liver and spleen of normal animals, there is a slight preponderance of ferritin over hemosiderin iron. With increasing concentrations of tissue iron, this ratio is reversed and at high levels the additional storage iron is deposited as hemosiderin. Both forms are capable of being mobilized for hemoglobin synthesis when the need for iron exists. The mechanism by which ferritin iron is released to the plasma is obscure.[45] Recently the existence of an enzyme system which may reduce iron and remove it from ferritin has been demonstrated.[46,47]

Quantitative measurement of normal iron stores has proved difficult, but reasonable estimates derived from available data are 300 to 1,000 mg for adult women and 500 to 1,500 mg for adult men. More individuals appear to fall into the lower half of these ranges than into the upper half. For instance, Scott and Pritchard[48] measured the iron actually available for hemoglobin synthesis in 11 healthy college women with normal hemoglobin values who had never bled abnormally nor been pregnant. Systematic phlebotomy was carried out over a period of weeks to determine how much hemoglobin their iron stores could regenerate. In 3 subjects, the iron converted into hemoglobin was less than 100 mg, in 5 it ranged from 112 to 348 mg and in only 3 did it amount to more than 500 mg (606 to 743 mg).

An increase in the amount of stored iron may occur as a result of a shift of iron from the red cell mass to the stores. This occurs in all anemias except those due to iron deficiency. A true increase in total body iron is found in patients with hemochromatosis, transfusion hemosiderosis or, rarely, after excessive and prolonged iron therapy. The amount in tissues may exceed 30 gm. An estimation as to whether iron stores are deficient or excessive may be made from the serum iron, total iron-binding capacity, serum ferritin[42,43,49,50] and stainable iron in bone marrow aspirates.[4,5,51–55]

At one time it was believed that iron enzymes were "inviolate" in iron-deficiency anemia.[56] Extensive studies in experimental animals have shown that iron enzymes are, in point of fact, quite sensitive to depletion in iron deficiency. The degree of loss varies from enzyme to enzyme and from tissue to tissue. Cytochrome c[57] and aconitase[58] are quite readily depleted, while cytochrome oxidase appears to be less susceptible[59] and catalase[60] most resistant of all to depletion. It has been relatively difficult to extend such studies to human subjects, since most of the iron-containing enzymes are not readily accessible. However, investigations of human leukocytes[61] and buccal mucosa[62] have shown depletion of cytochrome oxidase, even in relatively mild iron deficiency.

Conservation

The avid manner in which the body conserves and reutilizes iron is an important characteristic of iron metabolism. Mention has already been made of the fact that a normal adult catabolizes enough hemoglobin each day to release 20 to 25 mg of iron. If this amount were excreted, the iron requirement would be enormously increased and would far exceed the dietary iron absorbed. Actually, more than 90 per cent is conserved so that it can be reutilized repeatedly. Iron released from cells that die anywhere in the body is presumably conserved in a similar manner.

Iron Transfer to the Fetus

The fetus has a highly effective acceptor system for assimilating iron. Iron from the maternal transferrin is transferred to the placental tissue, to the fetal transferrin and then to the fetal tissues. This seems to be a unidirectional pathway, capable of operating effectively against increased maternal requirements for iron and functioning even in the face of maternal iron deficiency. During the last trimester of pregnancy it may account for a transfer of 3 to 4 mg of iron per day to the fetus.[63,64]

EXCRETION

The body has a limited capacity to excrete iron. The best estimates of daily iron turnover in adult men have been calculated to average between 0.90 and 1.05 mg or approximately 13 μg per kg of body weight in subjects studied in Seattle, Venezuela and South Africa.[65] The external loss is distributed roughly as follows:

	mg
Gastrointestinal	
Blood	0.35
Mucosal	0.10
Biliary	0.20
Urinary	0.08
Skin	0.20

However, the classical concept that no compensatory iron loss occurs from the body of individuals with increased iron stores does not hold up to scrutiny of the experimental evidence. A few estimates of iron loss in individuals with increased iron burdens have been made and show that the loss of iron exceeds that of normal persons. The available data are presented in Figure 7C–8. Urinary iron excretion may be increased significantly in patients with proteinuria, hematuria, hemoglobinuria and hemosiderinuria; the etiologic role of hemosiderinuria in the iron deficiency associated with cardiac anemia (e.g. implanted artificial heart valves, calcific aortic stenosis) is of considerable clinical importance. The iron excreted in feces is derived from blood lost into the alimentary canal (1.2 ± 0.5 ml whole blood per day),[69] from unabsorbed biliary iron and from desquamated intestinal mucosal cells. Disagreement has existed about the magnitude of dermal loss, with some workers claiming that it

may be particularly high among people living in hot, moist climates. The computed daily losses of Durban Indians who worked in a laundry where both temperature and humidity were very high were not significantly greater than those in sedentary, white office workers who lived in a temperate climate.[65,70]

It is difficult to quantitate the "normal" iron loss due to menstruation or pregnancy, because of the wide variation which is encountered. While the menstrual blood loss for any individual normal woman tends to be quite constant from month to month, the difference among women is considerable.[71] In an extensive study[72,73] among Swedish women, the mean menstrual loss was found to be 43 ± 2.3 ml, equivalent to an average of about 0.6 to 0.7 mg of iron per day. No great difference was found among the several age groups except the smallest mean value occurred among the 15-year-old girls and

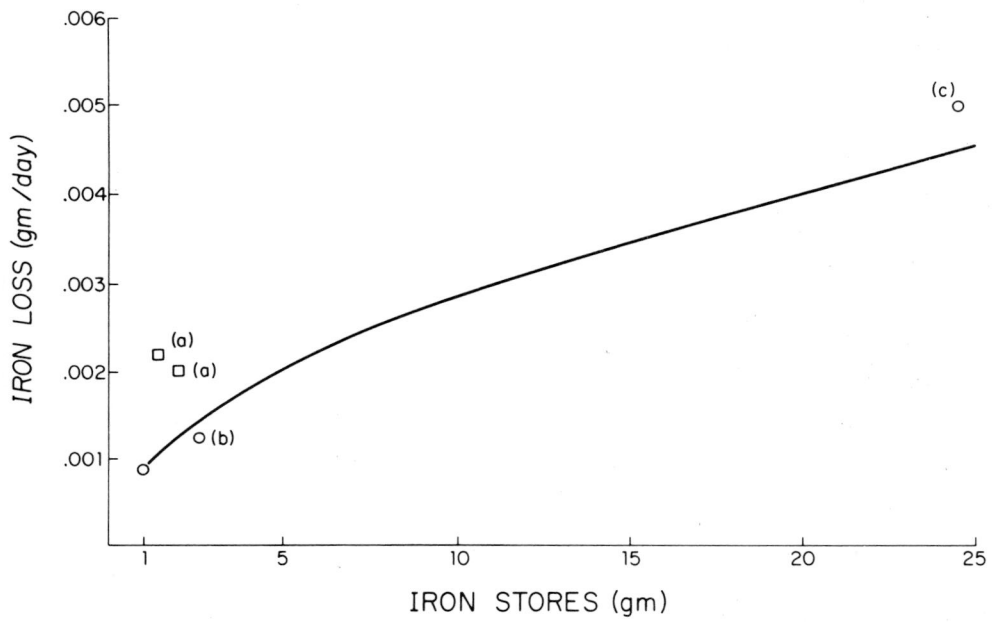

Fig. 7C–8. The relationship between iron stores and iron loss. The curve fits the equation L = .0009 $\sqrt{F}$, where L is the iron loss in gm per day and F represents the iron stores in gm. The points designated (a) are based on the data of Bothwell et al.,[63,66] the point labeled (b) is from the data of Finch,[67] while point (c) is from Crosby et al.[68]

the largest among women in the 50-year group. The upper normal limit of menstrual loss was somewhere between 60 to 80 ml per period. In 95 per cent of women, loss was found to average less than 1.4 mg Fe per day. Women who consider their menses normal may lose more than 100 ml and occasionally more than 200 ml per period. Menstrual blood losses are influenced by intrauterine devices, which increase menstrual bleeding,[74] and by birth control pills, which decrease it.[75]

The iron "cost" of pregnancy is high.[1,76] The external loss in urine, feces and sweat continues and amounts to about 170 mg for the gestational period. About 270 mg (200 to 370 mg) are contributed to the fetus, and another 90 mg (30 to 170 mg) are contained in the placenta and cord. The amount of iron lost in hemorrhage at delivery has been underestimated in the past, and is now believed to average about 150 mg (90 to 300 mg). Iron is required for the expansion of the red blood cell mass that occurs during the last half of pregnancy, but this amount is largely recovered when the circulating red blood cell volume is returned to normal after delivery. Lacta-

tion causes an additional drain of approximately 0.5 to 1 mg of iron per day. If one ignores the external loss, since it represents an amount roughly equal to a year's menstrual loss, plus the iron needed for the expanded blood volume and the enlarging uterus, since it is largely conserved, then the total iron "cost" of a normal pregnancy can be estimated to vary from about 420 to 1030 mg (Table 7C–2), or 1 to 2.5 mg per day spread over the 15-month period of pregnancy and lactation.

Pathologic bleeding from any site constitutes an important form of iron loss: 1 ml of blood with a hemoglobin concentration of 15 gm per 100 ml contains 0.5 mg of iron. A rough but useful rule-of-thumb is that 1 ml of packed red cells contains 1 mg of iron. The chronic loss of only a small volume of blood, therefore, may significantly increase iron requirements. Recognition must also be given to the fact that each 500 ml of blood removed for transfusion purposes removes from the donor between 200 and 250 mg of iron. Spread equally over a year, that amounts to roughly 0.6 to 0.7 mg per day. The effect of multiple donations is obvious.

Table 7C–2. Iron "Cost" of a Normal Pregnancy

Iron contributed to fetus	200–370 mg
In placenta and cord	30–170
In blood loss at delivery	90–310
In milk, lactation 6 months	100–180
	420–1030 mg
Average per day (pregnancy 9 mo, lactation 6 mo)	1–2.5

IRON REQUIREMENTS

Growth

The iron required for growth and its attendant increase in circulating hemoglobin mass is obviously influenced by the rate of growth, i.e. the rapid growth during infancy and the growth spurt of adolescent males. The calculations in Table 7C–3 provide a rough estimate of an average

Table 7C–3. Estimates of Average Daily Iron Requirements for Growth

	Boys	Girls
Adult wt greater than birth wt by	50–100 kg	45–70 kg
Normal body iron per kg	50 mg	35 mg
Iron in total wt gained	2,500–5,000 mg	1,575–2,450 mg
Years of growth	20 yr	15 yr
Estimated iron required for growth: Av per year	125–250 mg	100–163 mg
Av per day	0.35–0.70 mg	0.3–0.45 mg

iron requirement of 0.35 to 0.7 mg per day for boys and 0.3 to 0.45 mg for girls.

Nutritional Allowances

The foregoing discussion has emphasized the limitations of our information about iron loss, the dietary intake of iron and the efficiency of iron absorption from the gastrointestinal tract. In addition, the variations from person to person are relatively large. Enough data are available, however, to permit reasonable estimates of the amount of iron required to maintain a positive balance at various age levels of the population. These approximations suffice to serve as a guide to physicians and health organizations in their attempts to decrease the high incidence of iron deficiency. They are summarized in Table 7C–4. Calculations of the daily food iron requirement are based on an average absorption of 10 per cent—an assumption that seems reasonable since assimilation tends to become more efficient as need increases. It is evident that men and nonmenstruating women, in the absence of pathologic bleeding, should have little difficulty obtaining the iron they need from diets prevalent in the United States (12 to 18 mg Fe per day). The balance may be precarious, however, in many menstruating women and adolescent girls who, because of concern about weight, restrict their diets and frequently have a low iron intake of 10 mg or less per day. The requirements during pregnancy are frequently so large that they are greater than the amount available from diet alone. Particularly in women with depleted stores supplemental iron therapy is necessary during the latter half of pregnancy if iron deficiency is to be prevented.

IRON DEFICIENCY AND IRON-DEFICIENCY ANEMIA

Iron deficiency is without a doubt the most common deficiency of a nutrient. Indeed, it seems likely that it is the most common organic disease of man, excluding, of course, such nearly universal maladies as chickenpox, dental caries, constipation and acne vulgaris.

Iron deficiency is common in infants, and is nearly universal in the premature unless iron supplements are administered.[77] In children over the age of 4, anemia has been reported to occur in 0.6 to 7.7 per cent.[78] Relatively advanced iron-deficiency anemia was found in 5.5 per cent of poor children aged 5 to 8.[79] Thirty-five to 58 per cent of young, healthy women have been found to have some degree of iron deficiency;[80-82] during

Table 7C–4. Estimated Iron Requirements in Mg/Day

	External Loss*	Menses	Pregnancy "Cost"	Growth	Fe Requirement	Daily Food Intake Requirement‡
Adult males (50–100 kg)	0.65–1.3				0.65–1.3	6.5–13
Nonmenstruating women (45–70 kg)	0.6 –0.9				0.6 –0.9	6–9
Menstruating women (45–70 kg)	0.6 –0.9	0.1–1.4			0.7 –2.3	7–23
Pregnancy (50–80 kg)	0.65–1.0		1.0–2.5		1.65–3.5	16.5–35
Adolescent boys (50–100 kg)	0.65–1.3			0.35–0.7	1–2	10–20
Adolescent girls (45–70 kg)	0.6 –0.9	0.1–1.4		0.3–0.45	1–2.7	10–27
Children†					0.4 –1.0	4–10
Infants†					0.5 –1.5	5–15

*0.013 mg/kg.
†Estimates taken from Finch et al.[1]
‡Assuming 10 per cent absorption.

pregnancy, the incidence is even higher.[71,83] In areas in which intestinal helminthiasis exists in a large proportion of the population, iron deficiency anemia is nearly universal.

Pathogenesis

Iron deficiency results from one or a combination of the following: inadequate diet, impaired absorption, blood loss or repeated pregnancies. If an individual reaches adult weight with normal body stores of iron, deficiency caused solely by poor diet or poor absorption takes years to develop, in the absence of blood loss or pregnancy, because iron excretion is limited; these factors are more frequently contributory rather than primary causes. In temperate zones, the two most common causes of iron deficiency among adults are increased menstrual bleeding and hemorrhage from the alimentary canal.[84] The development of iron deficiency in an adult man or a postmenopausal woman should be assumed to be due to blood loss until proved otherwise.

Defective absorption can be caused by diets that are grossly iron deficient or high in cereal content and low in animal protein. Geophagia interferes with the absorption of iron, probably because the ingested clay chelates or precipitates iron as insoluble compounds in the lumen of the gut.[13] Clay-eating is practiced particularly by children and adult women. Among the poor its prevalence is probably much greater than is generally realized. Inadequate uptake of iron occurs in malabsorption syndromes and in chronic diarrhea from any cause. After partial or total gastrectomy two defects in iron absorption are observed: absorption of food iron is subnormal[85] and the increase in absorption that usually accompanies iron deficiency does not take place.[86,87] When patients with atrophic gastritis and achlorhydria become iron deficient they also are not able to increase the uptake of

iron as much as are comparable individuals with normal gastric function.

Except for pregnancy, large losses of iron are most commonly caused by bleeding. Hemorrhage from wounds, from the nose or mouth, genitourinary tract, and from hemorrhoids is obvious. Bleeding from the gastrointestinal canal is often occult and amounts up to 30 ml, if lost by adults high in the tract, may not cause guaiac-positive stools. Hiatus hernia, peptic ulcers, varices, salicylate ingestion, diverticuli, benign or malignant tumors, intestinal parasitic infestation (particularly hookworm disease) and regional enteritis or ulcerative colitis are the most common causes of occult hemorrhage. Occult gastrointestinal blood loss may be detected in nearly 50 per cent of affected infants;[88] usually no discrete lesions can be identified. The effect of normal menstrual loss on iron requirements has been discussed. Women frequently, however, fail to recognize an abnormal flow. Menstrual volume may be excessive if: double pads must be worn because one soaks through, duration of periods is greater than 5 days, large clots are passed and more than 12 pads per period are needed. The use of intrauterine devices increases menstrual bleeding. The admirable and necessary donation of blood for transfusions and the collection of large amounts of blood for diagnostic study must be regarded as forms of hemorrhage. Iron deficiency as a result of transferrin loss through a nephrotic kidney has been reported[89] but must be rare.

Sometimes the cause for iron deficiency is not found during the course of careful clinical evaluation: the diet seems adequate, no absorptive defect can be recognized, no blood loss can be detected. In the careful clinical study of patients seen at the Radcliffe Infirmary at Oxford, 17 per cent of 371 patients fell into this category.[84] No distinctive features could be found. In all probability, blood loss in such patients goes unrecognized because it is intermittent or very small in amount.

Under four conditions, iron-deficient erythropoiesis may be found even though body iron is normal or greater than normal: (1) hereditary absence of transferrin, (2) idiopathic pulmonary hemosiderosis, (3) paroxysmal nocturnal hemoglobinuria and (4) inflammation with the inability to mobilize iron from reticuloendothelial cell depots. Increased amounts of iron are found in these conditions in the liver, lungs, kidneys and reticuloendothelial systems, respectively, but not enough is made available to the bone marrow to support normal hemoglobin synthesis.

Diagnosis

In most disorders, the fully developed disease state is easy to detect, but the milder disorder may be difficult to diagnose. Iron deficiency is no exception to this rule. *Severe iron-deficiency anemia* is characterized by hypochromia and microcytosis of the red blood cells.[90] Erythrocytes are not only small and pale when observed on the blood smear but they vary greatly in size and shape. The serum iron concentration is diminished, and the iron-binding capacity is greatly augmented.[51,52] As a consequence, the saturation of the iron-binding protein is reduced; generally, less than 16 per cent of the available iron-binding sites are saturated. The free protoporphyrin level of the erythrocytes is increased[91-93] and the ferritin content of the serum is diminished.[42,43,49,50,94,95] Examination of the bone marrow generally reveals a decrease in the amount of storage iron in reticuloendothelial cells.[5,48,55,96] An exception to this rule is encountered in individuals who have been transfused within the previous few months or who have been given parenteral iron preparations; in such persons, reticuloendothelial storage iron may be present in the face of well-developed iron-deficiency anemia.[5,97] The number of sideroblasts, red cell precursors containing stainable iron, is also diminished in the bone marrows of patients with iron-deficiency anemia.[52,53]

The diagnosis of *mild iron-deficiency anemia*, or iron deficiency in the absence of anemia, is much more difficult to establish than that of the severe form. Mildly anemic patients do not manifest the microcytic hypochromic cells which are characteristic of the severe iron-deficiency state.[90] Neither is the plasma iron level invariably diminished nor the iron-binding capacity increased. The transferrin may be normally saturated with iron.[52] The serum ferritin levels are usually diminished even in mild iron deficiency,[42,43,49,50,94,98] however, and free erythrocyte protoporphyrin levels are increased.[91-93] With the exception of patients who have been given blood transfusions or parenteral iron therapy, the bone marrow iron stores are depleted, even in the mildest degree of iron deficiency.[5,48,55,96]

It is important to differentiate iron-deficiency anemia from other anemias, particularly hypochromic anemias which may simulate it. Patients with thalassemia minor are frequently misdiagnosed as iron deficient. Such persons generally have normal plasma iron levels and bone marrow iron stores. The diagnosis of β-thalassemia minor is established by demonstrating the increased levels of hemoglobin A_2 which are characteristic of this disorder. α-Thalassemia is characterized by the presence of hemoglobin H.[99] Sometimes iron-deficiency anemia may be confused with the hypochromic anemia which may result from the inheritance of an unstable hemoglobin or with hereditary or acquired sideroblastic anemia. Patients with these anemias have ample bone marrow iron stores, the level of plasma iron is normal or increased and that of the iron-binding capacity is usually normal or diminished. Differentiation of iron-deficiency anemia from the sideroblastic anemias is particularly important, since patients with sideroblastic anemia tend to accumulate excess amounts of iron in the tissues. As a result, they frequently develop iron storage disease. In such circumstances, iron therapy not only fails to benefit the patient but, instead, may hasten the appearance of complications of iron storage disease.

Study of patients with iron-deficiency anemia is never complete until the cause for the deficiency is recognized. The source of any blood loss which may underlie the deficiency state must be identified. Carcinomas of the gastrointestinal tract may occasionally be detected in this search long before other manifestations would have appeared. At times it is helpful to tag a sample of the patient's red blood cells with radioactive chromium, readminister the blood and then measure the radioactivity that will be found in the feces if blood is oozing from a gastrointestinal lesion.[69] The same technique may be used to provide a quantitative measure of menstrual loss.

Clinical Manifestations

It is often assumed that the manifestations of iron-deficiency anemia result from the lowering of the hemoglobin concentration of the blood. A number of clinical observations suggest that this is not the case: (1) The severity of symptoms is not closely correlated with the degree of anemia. (2) Response to treatment often seems to precede rise in the hemoglobin concentration of the blood. (3) Certain clinical manifestations such as koilonychia and esophageal webs cannot be accounted for on the basis of anemia alone.

For these reasons, it was suggested long ago that symptoms in iron-deficient individuals may arise from alterations in tissue metabolism.[10,100,101] Indeed, it was proposed that iron deficiency might produce symptoms in the absence of any anemia at all; a double-blind study in nonanemic, chronically fatigued women suggested that those who were iron depleted responded better symptomatically to iron than to placebo.[102] The concept that iron deficiency might produce symptoms through

mechanisms distinct from its effect on the hemoglobin of the blood should not be surprising. In pernicious anemia, it is quite clear that the neurologic symptoms are related to the metabolic effects of vitamin B_{12} deficiency on nonhematopoietic tissues; there is no reason why iron deficiency could not produce symptoms through an analogous mechanism.

Nonetheless, the concept that iron deficiency is a systemic disorder in which symptoms do not arise from the anemia alone has received increasing support only in the past few years. It has been suggested that iron deficiency may produce scholastic underachievement and behavioral disturbances[103,104] in children, possibly through defects in the metabolism of monamines involved in neural transmission.[104-106] Iron-deficient rats are unable to exercise normally even if transfused to a normal hemoglobin level, apparently because of an iron-deficiency-induced abnormality in muscle metabolism, particularly in α-glycerophosphate dehydrogenase activity.[107] Much attention has been paid to the possible relationship between iron deficiency and immunity to infectious diseases.[108-112] The effect of iron deficiency on tissue metabolism requires further study, and it is likely that a variety of iron-deficiency-induced defects will emerge.

Some patients with iron-deficiency anemia are unaware of being in ill health. Even these individuals, however, often experience an unaccustomed feeling of well-being once iron therapy is initiated.[100] Apparently they considered their reduced level of function as normal, since it had been present for a long period of time. Often the vague symptoms of iron-deficient women have been ascribed to tension, boredom, psychoneurosis or some other form of complex psychopathology. In symptomatic patients with moderately severe to severe degrees of anemia, most of the complaints are common to all anemias: weakness, fatigability, pallor, dyspnea on exertion, palpitation and a sense of being dead tired. When standardized exercise is carried out on a bicycle ergometer, it can be shown that the time needed to restore cardiorespiratory functions to preexercise resting values is markedly prolonged.[113] Coldness and paresthesia of the hands and feet are not infrequent. Only a minority of iron-deficient patients complain of the abnormality causing the anemia, e.g. hiatus hernia, peptic ulcer, hemorrhoids. Symptoms are usually so insidious in onset that their duration cannot be dated with accuracy.

Manifestations related to the oral cavity and the gastrointestinal tract have attracted attention both because of their frequency and because of uncertainty as to their pathogenesis. Vague gastrointestinal complaints—capricious appetite, flatulence, epigastric distress with eructation, constipation or diarrhea and nausea—are fairly common. Pica is practiced by some patients with iron deficiency: geophagia, starch-eating and pagophagia.[114] Geophagia is often but not always corrected by iron therapy.[115] The suggestion has been made that severe degrees of iron deficiency may cause secondary malabsorption phenomena, possibly related to a decrease in iron-containing or iron-dependent enzymes in intestinal mucosal cells.[116] Glossitis characterized by varying degrees of papillary atrophy and soreness is found more often in patients over the age of 40 years and with greater frequency in women than in men. Angular stomatitis occurs in 10 to 15 per cent of patients, particularly among those who are edentulous. Dysphagia, hypochromic anemia and postcricoid esophageal stricture, often accompanied by a web at this site, constitute an interesting triad (the Paterson-Kelly or Plummer-Vinson syndrome) found particularly but not exclusively in middle-aged women. It has been regarded as a precancerous lesion, but that relationship has been doubted.[117] Gastroscopic examination with gastric biopsy done on northern

Europeans has demonstrated gastritis with varying degrees of glandular damage in about 80 per cent of cases and atrophic gastritis in a few.

It is by no means certain that these oral and gastrointestinal manifestations are direct results of iron deficiency. For instance, the incidence of glossitis, angular stomatitis and dysphagia varies greatly among patients in different population groups and seems to be decreasing in communities where iron deficiency remains prevalent. The varying incidence of these epithelial changes plus the fact that they seem to occur more frequently in "low-input" than in "high-output" (blood loss) iron deficiency suggest that they may be caused by associated deficiencies. Hypochlorhydria and achlorhydria occur more commonly than in comparable population groups that are not iron deficient; their incidence varies with the methods used for stimulating gastric secretion, with the age of the patient and with the cause of iron deficiency. For instance, achlorhydria is unusual in chronic iron deficiency and hookworm disease.[118] In the Oxford series, the incidence was about 40 per cent of the single-dose histamine test, but only 16 per cent with the augmented histamine test.[84] In patients with achlorhydria the secretion of acid may return after treatment with iron, particularly in younger patients, but usually it does not.[119] The histologic appearance of the gastric mucosa has only rarely been observed to improve.[84] The suggestion that impairment of iron absorption itself might be the *result* of iron deficiency as well as its *cause* was first made many years ago.[120] More recent data also show flattening of postabsorptive curves after iron loading[121] but such data cannot be interpreted as unequivocally indicating impaired absorption.[54,121]

The fingernails, and sometimes the toenails as well, may become lusterless, thin, brittle, flattened and then spoon-shaped (koilonychia). When the hemoglobin falls below 6 gm per 100 ml the heart may become dilated and hemic murmurs may be heard. The spleen is occasionally sufficiently enlarged to be palpable at the costal margin. Mild degrees of vitiligo and of dependent edema are not infrequent. Neurologic examination is normal in spite of paresthesias. Rarely, papilledema, visual disturbances and elevated cerebral spinal fluid pressure, simulating intracranial tumors, may be found in iron-deficient patients; these unusual manifestations are corrected by iron therapy.[5] Another interesting syndrome occurs among young males in Iran: dwarfism, iron-deficiency anemia, hepatosplenomegaly, hypogonadism and geophagia.[122] A similar syndrome without geophagia has been observed in Egypt; coexistent zinc deficiency may be responsible.

The leukocyte count in severely iron-deficient patients is normal or may be slightly low. Platelet counts may be elevated, but thrombocytopenia also occurs[123-125] and may be quite severe.[126]

Treatment

Adequate therapy must not only correct the deficiency but also treat its cause. Increased menstrual flow, occult loss of blood from the urinary or gastrointestinal tracts or defective absorption must be detected and corrected if possible. Appropriate selection of a therapeutic agent requires understanding of the maximum expected hematologic response, the amount of iron required to produce this maximum effect and the absorption that can be expected from a given iron compound. The physician should observe the patient to make certain that a response is obtained: a satisfactory rise in the hemoglobin level attributable to the iron therapy constitutes final proof of the correctness of the diagnosis.

Hematologic Response and Amount of Iron Required for Maximum Effect. About 7 to 10 days after therapy is initiated, the reticulocyte level begins to rise, reaches a peak between 12 and 16 days and then falls to normal levels during the next 2 weeks; the height of the reticulocyte peak is inversely proportional to the original hemoglobin value and may exceed 20 per cent in severely anemic patients. The hemoglobin begins to increase after about 10 to 14 days; it rises at a rate of 0.2 to 0.3 gm per 100 ml per day when the anemia is severe and at 0.1 to 0.2 gm per 100 ml when the initial hemoglobin level is greater than 7.5 gm per 100 ml. As the hemoglobin concentration approaches normal, the rate of increase slows; from 4 to 8 weeks are required before normal values are attained. Return of the plasma iron to normal may take another 1 or 2 months. The response in children is somewhat more rapid than that of adults, and some data suggest that after intravenous infusion of iron dextran a substantial change in the hemoglobin concentration may be observed even after 1 week.[127]

The *daily* dose of iron ideally should be sufficient to support a maximum hemoglobin increase: 0.3 gm per 100 ml per day or 15 gm of new circulating hemoglobin in a patient with a blood volume of 5 liters. This requires absorption of 50 mg of iron. The exact amount obviously varies with the blood volume and with other factors, but 50 mg of absorbed iron is a reasonable average quantity to provide for adults. The comparable figure for children varies with body weight and can be calculated by estimating the blood volume to be 70 ml per kg body weight.

The *total* amount of iron that must be absorbed or injected to correct the deficiency can also be estimated. If, for example, a woman with severe iron-deficiency anemia has a hematocrit of only 15 per cent, each 1,000 ml of blood is deficient approximately 300 ml of packed red cells. If the patient's blood volume is 4 liters, enough iron must be supplied to provide 4 times as many red cells, i.e. 1,200 ml. Since each ml of red cells contains about 1 mg of iron, 1.2 gm of iron are needed to restore the red cell mass to normal. In addition, 0.5 to 1 gm of iron should be provided to replete the stores. The total amount needed to correct the deficiency in this instance, therefore, would be 1.7 to 2.2 gm.

Oral Therapy. The ideal iron preparation for oral therapy should be well absorbed, well tolerated by the gastrointestinal tract in therapeutic doses and inexpensive. Since ferrous iron is so much more efficiently absorbed than the ferric form, simple highly soluble ferrous salts come closest to approaching the ideal. Ferrous sulfate is generally recognized as the standard against which all other compounds must be evaluated. The most elegant com-

parison of absorption from different iron compounds has been made by Brise and Hallberg with a double isotope technique.[128] Thirty mg of iron as ferrous sulfate and 30 mg as the preparation under study were given on alternate days for a total of 10 days. The two preparations were labeled with two different isotopes of iron so that absorption from the preparation under study could be compared with that from ferrous sulfate (Fig. 7C–9). A number of compounds were absorbed about as well as ferrous sulfate: ferrous succinate, ferrous lactate, ferrous fumarate, ferrous glycine sulfate, ferrous glutamate and ferrous gluconate; none

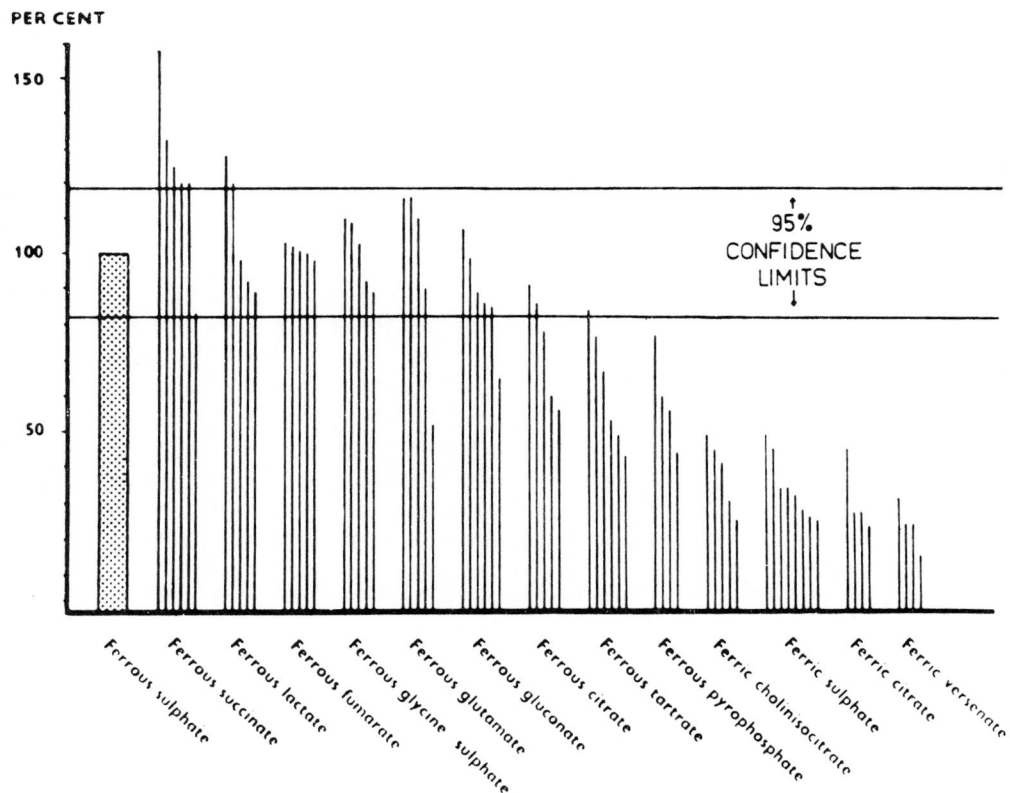

Fig. 7C–9. Comparison of the absorption of iron from ferrous sulfate and from various iron compounds. Daily dose equivalent to 30 mg elemental iron. Ferrous sulfate and the other compounds under study were tagged with different isotopes of iron and given on alternate days for 10 days. (From Brise and Hallberg.[128])

was clearly superior. Relatively large amounts of ascorbic acid given with ferrous sulfate increased absorption of iron.

Each of the preparations listed in Table 7C–5 is entirely acceptable. An iron-deficient patient will absorb approximately 20 per cent of the iron in these tablets. Since the recommended daily dose provides roughly 200 to 240 mg of iron, the desired 40 or 50 mg should be absorbed. Much has been made of the putative gastrointestinal irritating qualities of medicinal iron salts. In point of fact, iron preparations are much better tolerated by patients than is generally believed. In a double-blind study in which iron was given at a slightly lower dosage than that usually employed, no difference could be observed between the effects of placebo and iron (Fig. 7C–10). On the other hand, there is little doubt that a few patients encountered difficulty in tolerating iron medication given in full therapeutic dosage. In those patients who complain of severe epigastric distress, tolerance can frequently be induced by reducing the dose to 1 tablet per day and then gradually adding 1 tablet per day until the full therapeutic dose is reached. Alternatively, other preparations may be tried until one is found that can be tolerated. Children tend to have less gastrointestinal distress from iron therapy than do adults. A satisfactory schedule is to give half the adult dose to children who weigh from 15 to 35 kg, and the full dose to those heavier than

35 kg. For smaller children, and those unable to take tablets, liquid preparations are available.

A common error is to discontinue iron therapy after the 2 or 3 months required for correction of the anemia. Replenishment of iron stores occurs slowly when iron is given orally because absorption falls off as the hemoglobin rises toward normal; consequently, oral therapy must be continued for 6 to 12 months if stores are to be repleted. If the chronic bleeding responsible for iron deficiency cannot be corrected or controlled, continuous iron therapy is required.

Preparations which, in addition to iron, contain molybdenum, copper, cobalt, ascorbic acid, the various vitamins including folic acid and B_{12}, liver or bone marrow extracts, etc. are more expensive, no more effective in correcting iron deficiency and, in some instances, have distinct disadvantages. Fortunately, most are being withdrawn in the United States by order of the Food and Drug Administration. Injections of folic acid and of vitamin B_{12} do not increase the response to iron. Also to be deplored is the prevalent practice of packaging ferrous sulfate in enteric-coated tablets or in capsules containing delayed-release granules. The fraction of iron absorbed from some of these preparations is distinctly less because iron is released more distally in the small intestine where absorption is less efficient. As a result, the expected response to treatment does not

Table 7C–5. Recommended Oral Iron Preparations

Preparation	gm/tablet	Iron Content %	Iron Content mg Fe/tablet	Acceptable Adult Dose tablets/day
Ferrous sulfate·7H$_2$O	0.32	20	60	4
Ferrous sulfate, exsiccated	0.2	29	60	4
Ferrous gluconate	0.32	12	40	4 or 5
Ferrous fumarate	0.2	33	66	4
	0.32	33	105	2 or 3
Ferroglycine sulfate	0.25	16	40	5

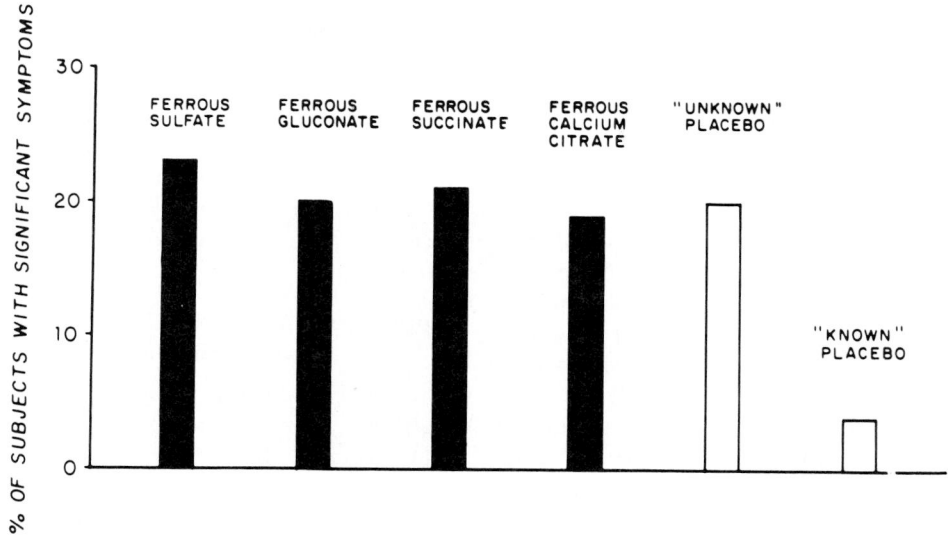

INCIDENCE OF INTOLERANCE TO
FOUR IRON PREPARATIONS (35 mg Fe ++, t.i.d.)
AND TWO PLACEBOS

Fig. 7C–10. The production of symptoms by iron and placebo in a group of women receiving 35 mg of iron in the form of various commonly used iron preparations. When a placebo was included which the subjects thought was an iron preparation ("unknown placebo"), the reaction rate was the same as for all of the iron preparations. When they were told that a control pill was being given ("known placebo"), the reaction rate was very low. (Based on the data of Kerr and Davidson.[129])

occur or is suboptimal.[131] While adequate responses may be observed with some so-called delayed-release iron preparations, such capsules presumably actually release iron quite rapidly.[132] However, the most widely used preparation of this type, Feosol Spansule capsules, is quite ineffective.[131,133]

Oral iron therapy may fail in patients with malabsorption syndromes or with diarrhea, or in those who have had a gastrectomy. In the latter two instances, iron tablets may move so quickly through the small intestine that they reach the cecum before disintegrating; x-ray films of the abdomen may demonstrate the radiopaque pellets in the large bowel.

Parenteral Therapy. Parenteral administration of iron should be reserved for those subjects who are unable to tolerate or absorb orally administered iron: (1) patients with ulcerative colitis, regional enteritis, intestinal shunts, colostomy or ileostomy, (2) patients with malabsorption syndromes, (3) the rare person who is unable or unwilling to cooperate or who has severe intolerance to oral therapy, (4) patients in whom the rate of blood loss is so rapid that it is desirable both to introduce large amounts of iron into the body quickly and to reestablish iron stores.

The most widely used and most satisfactory parenteral iron preparation is iron dextran (Imferon). This preparation may be given either intramuscularly or intravenously. The possibility of an anaphylactoid response may be slightly greater when iron dextran is given by the intravenous route, but intravenous administration also has certain advantages. First of all, it is possible to infuse a large dose, even the total dose required, at one time. Intramuscular administration of iron produces staining of the skin and may also result in local discomfort. Because iron dextran in very large doses has the capacity to induce sarcomas in experimental animals, there has been some concern about its possible carcinogenesis in man. However, after over 25 years of extensive use, there are only scattered reports of the appearance of such tumors.[134] Indeed, so few cases of sarcomas at or near the site of iron dextran injection have been observed that a cause-and-effect relationship cannot be considered to be established in man. The total dose should be calculated to correct the hemoglobin deficit and to provide at least an additional 1,000 mg for storage. Intramuscular injections should be given via a zigzag needle tract to minimize unsightly staining of the skin. Systemic reactions are unusual but may be severe: headache, fever, arthralgia, back pain and, rarely, peripheral vascular collapse. Rates of hemoglobin increase do not differ significantly from those produced by proper oral therapy.

Blood transfusions are rarely necessary in the treatment of iron-deficiency anemia and should generally be reserved for patients who have serious complications demanding immediate correction of the anemia: angina, congestive heart failure or severe pneumonia. Healthy young adults are able to tolerate levels of hemoglobin as low as 2.5 or 3 gm per 100 ml with remarkably little discomfort or danger. The patient's clinical status, not the numerical value of the hemoglobin, should be given primary consideration in reaching a decision regarding the advisability of blood transfusion. Patients with active bleeding who are iron deficient must sometimes be transfused. In these instances, however, the purpose of the transfusion is not primarily to correct the anemia but rather to restore a falling blood volume to normal, thus avoiding the development of hemorrhagic shock.

Prognosis

Recurrence of iron-deficiency anemia is common because the precipitating cause is not recognized, continues or recurs.[84] Patients with chronic severe epithelial changes in the oral cavity have a somewhat higher attack rate of carcinoma of the upper gastrointestinal tract. In affected children whose growth and development are retarded, iron therapy frequently produces at least partial correction of the defect.

Supplements to Prevent Development of Iron Deficiency

In the United States and several other countries, the cereal most commonly eaten, usually wheat flour or rice, is being fortified with iron. Flour in the United States is enriched with 12 mg iron per pound (460 gm): bread baked under commercial conditions contains about 0.022 to 0.037 mg Fe per gm of wet weight. That the iron can be absorbed was proved in experiments in which bread fortified with radioactive iron was fed: normal subjects absorbed from 1 to 12 per cent, while iron-deficient subjects assimilated several times as much.[135] Soluble inorganic iron added to food is absorbed to the same extent as is the intrinsic iron in that food.[30] Since iron in rice and corn is poorly absorbed,[23] these cereals are poor vehicles for fortification. Approximately 10 per cent of the iron is absorbed from iron-fortified cereals prepared for infants.[136] The exact amounts may differ considerably, however, varying not only with the iron compound used but also with the particle size and presumably with method of preparation of the food. Although wheat flour has received the most emphasis as a vehicle for iron supplementation, other foodstuffs may be equally or more suitable, particularly in certain countries. Thus, sugar,[137] fish sauce[138] and salt[139] have recently been found to be suitable vehicles for iron supplementation. Their effectiveness, however, has been vigorously challenged by Elwood in a series of publications,[25,140] and is currently being reevaluated in several countries.

There are two times in life when iron supplementation is recommended: during infancy and pregnancy. A daily dietary allowance of 1.0 to 1.5 mg dietary iron per kg per day achieves optimal iron nutrition for a substantial majority of the infant population.[77,93,141] In an infant of average weight, an intake of 6 to 9 mg per day at 3 months of age, gradually increased to 8 to 12 mg per day at 6 months of age and to 10 to 15 mg per day by 12 months of age will satisfy this allowance, according to Sturgeon's data. He believes that no further increase is necessary in later infancy. Supplementation by iron-enriched cereals or by iron salts is usually required if an intake of 15 mg is to be achieved. In a careful study from Montreal, de Leeuw and her associates found that 78 mg (but not 39 mg) of elemental ferrous iron daily for 24 weeks to normal pregnant women in the McGill University Clinic were adequate to achieve optimal hemoglobin mass and to maintain iron stores.[142]

IRON OVERLOAD

An excessive body burden of iron can be produced by greater-than-normal absorption from the alimentary canal, by parenteral injection, or by a combination of both mechanisms. The excess iron is deposited largely as hemosiderin in reticuloendothelial cells, or in the parenchymal cells of certain tissues. The site of deposition is in part dependent on the portal of entry. When excess iron is derived from intestinal absorption, it is carried to tissues bound by plasma transferrin and transferred to parenchymal and reticuloendothelial cells as well as to developing erythroblasts. On the other hand, parenterally administered iron, given usually as transfused blood, accumulates largely in reticuloendothelial cells where the transfused erythrocytes are eventually destroyed and their hemoglobin degraded. In iron overload the plasma iron and transferrin saturation are usually in-

creased, the total iron-binding capacity somewhat depressed (Fig. 7C–7). A simple classification based on mechanism of production is:

1. Excessive absorption of iron
   A. "Idiopathic" hemochromatosis
   B. Excessive intake (siderosis in the Bantu; prolonged therapeutic administration of iron to subjects not iron deficient)
   C. Chronic alcoholism, chronic liver disease (usually portal cirrhosis) and possibly pancreatic insufficiency
   D. Certain types of refractory anemia, usually associated with ineffective erythropoiesis, and increased hemolysis
2. Transfusional hemosiderosis.

The term *hemosiderosis* has been used to designate an increase in iron storage without associated tissue damage. Hemochromatosis indicates that such damage is present, particularly in the liver, that the iron is widely dispersed and that the amount of iron is greatly increased (usually 20 to 40 gm).[4,143] The "classical triad" of hemochromatosis—cirrhosis, diabetes and hyperpigmentation of the skin—summarizes the most prevalent clinical features of this disorder. The fourth major clinical feature of hemochromatosis is cardiac failure, often preceded by atrial arrhythmias. Hypofunction of endocrine glands is also common. Patients with idiopathic hemochromatosis manifest increased susceptibility to infection. Particularly before the days of antibiotics, the sudden onset of overwhelming sepsis and shock was a common cause of death in patients with this disorder. Idiopathic hemochromatosis appears to be a rare inborn error of metabolism, in which increased intestinal absorption of iron results in slow accumulation of the metal throughout life. It has been suggested that it is caused by a single gene which may affect the transferrin acceptors on tissue cells.[144] However, we have been unable to demonstrate a defect in iron uptake from transferrin by fibroblasts, and the precise pathogenesis of hemochromatosis must be considered to be unknown.

It is not clear whether the high concentrations of iron which accumulate in various tissues are responsible, per se, for tissue injury, or whether an additional nutritional or toxic insult is required for clinical manifestations to appear. Indeed, putative environmental causes of hemochromatosis have been championed by MacDonald, who questions the validity of evidence favoring the existence of a genetic defect.[145] The failure of animal experiments to provide a definitive solution may be related to the fact that iron overload has usually been induced by injecting forms of iron which are taken up primarily by reticuloendothelial cells and are not readily redistributed to parenchymal sites; furthermore, induction of tissue damage may take longer than the animals can usually be kept alive.[146] Those who do believe that iron has a noxious effect point out that cirrhosis, fibrosis and disturbance of organ function are particularly likely to occur when excessive amounts of iron are absorbed from the alimentary canal and deposited primarily in parenchymal rather than (or in addition to) reticuloendothelial cells.

In the Bantu, a positive correlation exists between the concentration of iron in the liver and the incidence of portal cirrhosis: with concentrations greater than 2 gm per 100 gm dry weight, most of the patients have portal cirrhosis.[147] The large amount of intracellular iron may cause progressive destruction of parenchymal cells and replacement by fibrous tissue.[148] The relationship between diabetes mellitus and cardiomyopathies on the one hand and deposition of hemosiderin in the pancreas and myocardium on the other has also been cited as evidence favoring toxicity of the iron. The improvement reported in patients with idiopathic hemochromatosis after removal of a large fraction of their

excess iron by therapeutic phlebotomy would seem to argue strongly for a noxious effect of iron overload.

Of greatest nutritional interest are the forms of secondary iron overload caused by increased alimentary uptake.

Siderosis in the Bantu[4,149,150]

Iron overload in the Bantu results from long-continued exposure to diets containing too much iron, derived largely from cooking pots and from the drums used in the preparation of fermented alcoholic beverages. In adult males, the intake may exceed 100 mg iron per day. The condition frequently becomes manifest in late adolescence, reaches its greatest severity between the ages of 40 and 60 years and is usually more severe in males whose alcoholic consumption tends to be greater. The pathologic pattern of the iron overload is one of hepatic and reticuloendothelial involvement. Portal cirrhosis becomes evident in the majority of patients (but not in all) when the hepatic concentration of iron reaches 2 gm or more per 100 gm of dry weight.[147] Redistribution of iron takes place so that parenchymal deposits of hemosiderin are found in the epithelial cells of many organs, particularly the pancreas and the myocardium. Approximately 20 per cent of these subjects develop clinical diabetes, but myocardial failure has not been described. To what extent these changes are caused by iron alone, by chronic alcoholism or by the associated nutritional disturbances is unknown.

Portal Cirrhosis, Chronic Alcoholism and Pancreatic Insufficiency

Patients with alcoholic or nutritional portal cirrhosis of the liver frequently have increased amounts of stainable iron in their livers, although the total amount present is rarely greater than 1 gm.[151] With the larger amounts, hemosiderin deposits are found in parenchymal cells of the liver, pancreas, heart and adrenal glands. Clinical similarity to hemochromatosis is accentuated by the occurrence in portal cirrhosis of increased skin pigmentation, a greater-than-normal incidence of diabetes mellitus and testicular atrophy. Cardiac failure, when it occurs, can usually be accounted for on other grounds. More males than females are affected and clinical manifestations are most prominent in late middle life.

A number of possible explanations for the iron overload have been cited. Patients with portal cirrhosis are frequently wine drinkers, consuming several liters daily: American and European wines contain significant quantities of iron and several milligrams per day may be derived from that source alone.[8] Alcohol increases the absorption of ferric iron.[152] Patients with chronic liver disease or chronic pancreatitis absorb iron excessively from the gut.[153,154] Whether these patients should be regarded as having hemochromatosis or portal cirrhosis with hemosiderosis is difficult to determine. The body load of excess iron is usually distinctly less than that reported for hemochromatosis. Some workers, however, contend that no sharp distinction is possible; they believe that hemosiderosis may progress, with increasing and more widespread distribution of iron, to the complete picture of hemochromatosis without any sharp dividing line.

Prolonged Iron Therapy

In rare instances, the prolonged administration of iron to patients who did not need it has been responsible for iron overload;[155–158] manifestations indistinguishable from hemochromatosis may have been secondary to increased iron intake, although the possibility that these individuals had the hereditary defect of idiopathic hemochromatosis cannot be ruled out. Since iron preparations are advertised widely in the United States, are available without prescription and are consumed in large quantities, it is of interest that more examples have not been reported. For this reason, the potential of

iron preparations for the production of iron storage disease deserves special attention. On the basis of present-day knowledge of iron metabolism, it is possible to make some rough estimates of the amount of iron which might accumulate in the body of normal persons when different amounts of medicinal iron are administered over long periods of time. The rate of increase, ΔF, is obviously the difference between the amount of iron absorbed, (A) and the amount of iron lost from the body (L): $\Delta F = A - L$. Both of these functions depend upon the amount of stored iron already present in the body; storage iron decreases iron absorption and increases iron loss.

Scant data are present to define either of these parameters, but on the basis of those data which are available[66–68,159] L may be approximated as $.0009 \sqrt{F}$ for males or $.0009 \sqrt{F + .0005}$ for menstruating

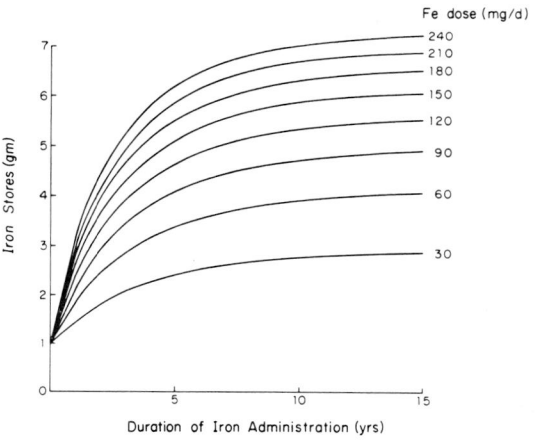

ACCUMULATION OF IRON STORES AT DIFFERENT SINGLE DAILY DOSAGES IN WOMEN

Fig. 7C–11. The expected accumulation of iron in menstruating women receiving single daily doses of 30 mg of iron per day. These data are based on the assumptions that iron absorption in females is $.025 \times D^{0.668}$, where D is the dose of iron in gm, that iron absorption is modified by stores to the extent of $e^{-0.196(F-1)}$ and that excretion is $.0009 \times \sqrt{F} + .0005$, where F is the iron stores in gm.

females, where F is the body iron store in gm (Fig. 7C–8). We have already pointed out that the amount of iron absorbed from a given dose is:

$$A = 0.022 \ D^{0.676} \text{ for males and}$$
$$A = 0.025 \ D^{0.668} \text{ for females}$$

This seems to be modified by the amount of storage iron by a factor of approximately $e^{-0.196(F-1)}$, based on modification of iron absorption in man with different levels of iron burden.[65,66,160] As the fraction of iron absorbed decreases and the amount excreted increases, an equilibrium is established at a level of body iron which depends upon the dose given. The results of calculations of the expected body iron burden at different doses of medicinal iron taken over long periods of time are shown in Figure 7C–11.

Refractory Anemia[4,5]

The amount of iron found in the tissues of patients with refractory anemia, particularly those with a hypercellular marrow and ineffective erythropoiesis, is occasionally greater than can be accounted for by the transfusions they have received. In some cases, little blood was given during the course of the illness yet excess iron was present. Not all of these subjects have erroneously been treated with iron, although that has happened in some instances. Excessive absorption of dietary iron must have occurred, supposedly because of the accelerated but ineffective erythropoiesis. Bothwell and Finch found 31 such patients reported in the literature: the anemias included refractory anemia, what would now be called sideroblastic anemia, thalassemia major and paroxysmal nocturnal hemoglobinuria; all had a cellular erythroid marrow.[4] Twenty-six had portal cirrhosis and an additional 4 had increased portal tract fibrosis; 5 had diabetes and 6 more had impaired glucose tolerance; at least 15 showed increased pigmentation of the skin. In patients such as these, large amounts of hemosiderin are found in parenchymal as well as in reticuloendothelial cells. Why they develop the changes of hemochromatosis, whereas transfusional hemosiderosis is found in most multitransfused subjects with similar loads of body iron, remains a mystery. Nutritional differences between the two groups cannot clearly be identified. Factors of possible significance include cirrhosis resulting from serum hepatitis and the possibility that parenchymal distribution of iron may be related to the gastrointestinal portal of entry of a significant portion of the excess body iron.

BIBLIOGRAPHY

1. Finch, Beutler, Brown, Crosby, Hegsted, Moore, Pritchard, Sturgeon and Wintrobe: J.A.M.A., 203, 407, 1968.
2. Moore: Harvey Lect., 55, 67, 1960.
3. Moore and Moore: Mineral Metabolism, Vol. 2. New York, Academic Press, 1962.
4. Bothwell and Finch: Iron Metabolism. Boston, Little, Brown, & Co., 1962.
5. Fairbanks, Fahey and Beutler: Clinical Disorders of Iron Metabolism, 2nd ed. New York, Grune and Stratton, 1971.
6. Moore: Ser. Haematol., 6, 1, 1965.
7. U.S. Interdepartmental Committee for National Defense Nutrition Survey of the Armed Forces: Iran, 1956. Turkey, 1958. Spain, 1958. Ethiopia, 1959. Peru, 1959. Ecuador, 1960. The Kingdom of Thailand, 1961.
8. MacDonald: Arch. Intern. Med., 112, 82, 1963.
9. Taylor: In The Examination of Water and Water Supplies, 7th ed. (Tresh, Beale and Suckling, Eds.). Boston, Little, Brown & Co., 1970.
10. Beutler, Fairbanks and Fahey: Clinical Disorders of Iron Metabolism. New York, Grune and Stratton, 1963.
11. Conrad: In Iron Deficiency (Hallberg, Harwerth and Vannotti, Eds.). New York, Academic Press, 1970.
12. Pollock and Lasky: J. Lab. Clin. Med., 87, 670, 1976.
13. Minnich, Okcuoglu, Tarcon, Abcasoy, Cin, Yoeruekoglu, Benda and Demirag: Am. J. Clin. Nutr., 21, 78, 1968.
14. Luke, Adel, Davis and Deller: Lancet, 2, 844, 1968.
15. Beutler, Kelly and Beutler: Am. J. Clin. Nutr., 11, 559, 1962.
16. Heinrich: In Iron Deficiency (Hallberg, Harwerth and Vannotti, Eds.). New York, Academic Press, 1970.
17. Weintraub, Weinstein, Huser and Rafal: J. Clin. Invest., 47, 531, 1968.
18. Raffin, Woo, Roost, Price and Schmid: J. Clin. Invest., 54, 1344, 1974.

19. Brown, Hwang, Nicol and Ternberg: J. Lab. Clin. Med., 72, 58, 1968.
20. Turnbull, Cleton and Finch: J. Clin. Invest., 41, 1897, 1962.
21. Hallberg and Solvell: Acta Med. Scand., 181, 335, 1967.
22. Moore: In Symposia of the Swedish Nutrition Foundation VI (Blix, Ed.). Stockholm, Alquist and Wiksell, 1968.
23. Layrisse and Martinez-Torres: Prog. Hematol., 7, 137, 1971.
24. Josephs: Blood, 13, 1, 1958.
25. Elwood: Lancet, 2, 516, 1968.
26. Layrisse, Cook, Martinez, Roche, Kuhn, Walker and Finch: Blood, 33, 430, 1969.
27. Martinez-Torres and Layrisse: Blood. 35, 669, 1970.
28. Layrisse, Martinez-Torres, Cook, Walker and Finch: Blood, 41, 333, 1973.
29. Pirzio-Biroli, Bothwell and Finch: J. Lab. Clin. Med., 51, 37, 1958.
30. Cook, Layrisse, Martinez-Torres, Walker, Monsen and Finch: J. Clin. Invest., 51, 805, 1972.
31. Awai and Brown: J. Lab. Clin. Med., 61, 363, 1963.
32. Laurell: Pharmacol. Rev., 4, 371, 1952.
33. Fletcher and Huehns: Nature, 218, 1211, 1968.
34. Awai, Chipman and Brown: J. Lab. Clin. Med., 85, 769, 1975.
35. Princiotto and Zapolski: Nature, 255, 87, 1975.
36. Harris and Aisen: Nature, 257, 821, 1975.
37. Schlabach and Bates: J. Biol. Chem., 250, 2181, 1975.
38. Jandl and Katz: J. Clin. Invest., 42, 314, 1963.
39. Giblett: Genetic Markers in Human Blood. Philadelphia, F.A. Davis, 1969.
40. Conrad and Crosby: Blood, 22, 406, 1963.
41. Finch, Deubelbeiss, Cook, Eschbach, Harker, Funk, Marsaglia, Hillman, Slichter, Adamson, Ganzoni and Giblett: Medicine, 49, 17, 1970.
42. Jacobs, Miller, Worwood, Beamish and Wardrop: Br. Med. J., 4, 206, 1972.
43. Lipschitz, Cook and Finch: N. Engl. J. Med., 290, 1213, 1974.
44. Halliday, Gera and Powell: Clin. Chim. Acta. 58, 207, 1975.
45. Crichton: N. Engl. J. Med., 284, 1413, 1971.
46. Sirivech, Frieden and Osaki: Biochem. J., 143, 311, 1974.
47. Frieden and Osaki: Adv. Exp. Med. Biol., 48, 235, 1975.
48. Rath and Finch: J. Lab. Clin. Med., 33, 81, 1948.
49. Siimes, Addiego and Dallman: Blood, 43, 581, 1974.
50. Jacobs and Worwood: Br. J. Haematol., 31, 1, 1975 (annotation).
51. Bainton and Finch: Am. J. Med., 37, 62, 1964.
52. Beutler, Robson and Buttenwieser: Ann. Intern. Med., 48, 60, 1958.
53. Weinfeld: Acta Med. Scand., 427 (Suppl.), 1, 1964.
54. Beutler: N. Engl. J. Med., 256, 692, 1957.
55. Beutler, Drennan and Block: J. Lab. Clin. Med., 43, 427, 1954.
56. Hahn and Whipple: Am. J. Med. Sci., 191, 24, 1936.
57. Beutler: Am. J. Med. Sci., 234, 517, 1957.
58. Beutler: J. Clin. Invest., 38, 1605, 1959.
59. Beutler: Acta Haematol., 21, 371, 1959.
60. Beutler and Blaisdell: J. Clin. Invest., 37, 833, 1958.
61. Beutler: Ill. Med. J., 116, 16, 1959.
62. Jacobs: Lancet, 2, 1331, 1961.
63. Bothwell, Pribilla, Mebust and Finch: Am. J. Physiol., 193, 615, 1958.
64. Davies, Brown, Stewart, Terry and Sisson: Am. J. Physiol., 197, 87, 1959.
65. Green, Charlton, Seftel, Bothwell, Mayet, Adams, Finch and Layrisse: Am. J. Med., 45, 336, 1968.
66. Bothwell, Seftel, Jacobs, Torrance and Baumslag: Am. J. Clin. Nutr., 14, 47, 1964.
67. Finch: In Iron Metabolism. An International Symposium (Gross, Ed.). Berlin, Springer-Verlag, 1964.
68. Crosby, Conrad and Wheby: Blood, 22, 429, 1963.
69. Ebaugh, Clemens, Rodnan and Peterson: Am. J. Med., 25, 169, 1958.
70. Bothwell: In Iron Deficiency (Hallberg, Harwerth and Vannotti, Eds.). New York, Academic Press, 1970.
71. Hallberg and Nilsson: Acta Obstet. Gynecol. Scand., 43, 352, 1964.
72. Hallberg, Hoegdahl, Nilsson and Rybo: Acta Obstet. Gynecol. Scand., 45, 320, 1966.
73. Rybo: In Iron Deficiency (Hallberg, Harwerth and Vannotti, Eds.). New York, Academic Press, 1970.
74. Guillebaud, Bonnar, Morehead and Matthews: Lancet, 1, 387, 1976.
75. Mears and Grant: Br. Med. J., 2, 75, 1962.
76. Moore: In Iron Metabolism. An International Symposium (Gross, Ed.). Berlin, Springer-Verlag, 1964.
77. Sturgeon: In Iron in Clinical Medicine (Wallerstein and Mettier, Eds.). Berkeley, University of California Press, 1958.
78. Pearson, Abrams, Fernbach, Gyland and Hahn: Pediatr. Res., 1, 169, 1967.
79. Karp, Haaz, Starko and Gorman: Am. J. Dis. Child., 128, 18, 1974.
80. Fielding, Haughnessy and Brunstroem: Lancet, 2, 9, 1965.
81. Monsen, Kuhn and Finch: Am. J. Clin. Nutr., 20, 842, 1967.
82. Scott and Pritchard: J.A.M.A., 199, 897, 1967.
83. Pritchard and Hunt: Surg. Gynecol. Obstet., 106, 516, 1958.
84. Beveridge, Bannerman, Evanson and Witts: Q. J. Med., 34, 145, 1965.
85. Magnusson: Scand. J. Haematol., 26 (Suppl), 7, 1976.
86. Baird and Wilson: Q. J. Med., 28, 35, 1959.
87. Stevens, Pirzio-Biroli, Harkins, Nyhus and Finch: Ann. Surg., 149, 534, 1959.
88. Hoag, Wallerstein and Pollycove: Pediatrics, 27, 199, 1961.
89. Hancock, Onstad and Wolf: Am. J. Clin. Pathol., 65, 73, 1976.
90. Beutler: Ann. Intern. Med., 50, 313, 1959.
91. Lund: Am. J. Obstet. Gynecol., 62, 947, 1951.

92. Piomelli, Brickman and Carlos: Pediatrics, *57*, 136, 1976.
93. Sturgeon: J. Pediatr., *17*, 341, 1956.
94. Burks, Siimes, Mentzer and Dallman: J. Pediatr., *88*, 224, 1976.
95. Rios, Lipschitz, Cook and Smith: Pediatrics, *55*, 694, 1975.
96. Hutchison: Blood. *8*, 236, 1953.
97. Beutler: J. Lab. Clin. Med., *51*, 415, 1958.
98. Sies and Grosskofp: Eur. J. Biochem., *57*, 513, 1975.
99. Comings: In *Hematology* (Williams, Beutler, Erslev and Rundles, Eds.). New York, McGraw-Hill, 1972.
100. Heilmeyer and Ploetner: *Das Serumeisen und Die Eisenmangelkrankheit.* Jena, Gustav Fischer, 1937.
101. Jasinski and Roth: *Larvierte Eisenmangelkrankheit.* Basel, Benno Schwabe, 1954.
102. Beutler, Larsh and Gurney: Ann. Intern. Med., *52*, 378, 1960.
103. Webb and Oski: J. Pediatr., *82*, 827, 1973.
104. Pollitt and Leibel: J. Pediatr., *88*, 372, 1976.
105. Symes, Sourkes, Youdim, Gregoriadis and Birnbaum: Can. J. Biochem., *47*, 999, 1969.
106. Voorhess, Stuart, Stockman and Oski: J. Pediatr., *86*, 542, 1975.
107. Finch and Mackler: Clin. Res., *24*:480A, 1976 (abstract).
108. Buckley: J. Pediatr., *86*, 993, 1975.
109. Chandra and Saraya: J. Pediatr., *86*, 899, 1975.
110. MacDougall, Anderson, McNab and Katz: J. Pediatr., *86*, 833, 1975.
111. Masawe and Swai: Lancet, *1*, 1241, 1975 (letter).
112. Chandra: Nutr. Rev., *34*, 129, 1976.
113. Andersen and Barkve: Scand. J. Clin. Lab. Invest., *25* (Suppl. 114), 9, 1970.
114. Coltman: J.A.M.A., *207*, 513, 1969.
115. Lanzkowsky: Arch. Dis. Child., *34*, 140, 1959.
116. Kimber and Weintraub: N. Engl. J. Med., *279*, 453, 1968.
117. Jacobs: Br. J. Cancer, *15*, 736, 1961.
118. Foy and Kondi: Trans. R. Soc. Trop. Med. Hyg., *54*, 419, 1960.
119. Lees and Rosenthal: Q.J. Med., *27*, 19, 1958.
120. Jasinski: Schweiz. Med. Wochenschr., *79*, 291, 1949.
121. Gross, Stuart, Swender and Oski: J. Pediatr., *88*, 795, 1976.
122. Halsted, Prasad and Nadimi: Arch. Intern. Med., *116*, 253, 1965.
123. Nutr. Rev., *34*, 25, 1976.
124. Kasper, Whissell and Wallerstein: J.A.M.A., *191*, 359, 1965.
125. Sahud, Olsen and Pedemont: Ann. Intern. Med., *81*, 132, 1974 (letter).
126. Scher and Silber: Ann. Intern. Med., *84*, 571, 1976 (letter).
127. Mehta, Lotliker and Patel: Indian J. Med. Res., *61*, 1818, 1973.
128. Brise and Hallberg: Acta Med. Scand., *376* (Suppl.), 23, 1962.
129. Kerr and Davidson: Lancet, *2*, 489, 1958.
130. Beutler: Clin. Med., *71*, 1889, 1964.
131. Beutler and Meerkreebs: N. Engl. J. Med., *274*, 1152, 1966.
132. Baird, Walters and Sutton: Br. Med. J., *4*, 505, 1974.
133. Beutler: Blood, *15*, 288, 1960.
134. MacKinnon and Bancewicz: Br. Med. J., *2*, 277, 1973.
135. Steinkamp, Dubach and Moore: Arch. Intern. Med., *95*, 181, 1955.
136. Schulz and Smith: Am. J. Dis. Child., *93*, 30, 1957.
137. Layrisse, Martinez-Torres, Renzi, Velez and Gonzalez: Am. J. Clin. Nutr., *29*, 8, 1976.
138. Garby: Unpublished data, 1976.
139. Sayers, Lynch, Charlton, Bothwell, Walker and Mayet: Br. J. Haematol., *28*, 483, 1974.
140. Elwood, Benjamin, Fry, Eakins, Brown, De Kock and Shah: Am. J. Clin. Nutr., *23*, 1267, 1970.
141. Moe: Acta Paediatr. Scand., *150* (Suppl.), 1, 1963.
142. DeLeeuw, Lowenstein and Hsieh: Medicine, *45*, 291, 1966.
143. Finch and Finch: Medicine, *34*, 381, 1955.
144. Brown and Goldstein: Prog. Med. Genet., *1*, 103, 1976.
145. MacDonald: Prog. Hematol., *5*, 324, 1966.
146. Brown, Durbach, Smith, Reynafarje and Moore: J. Lab. Clin. Med., *50*, 862, 1957.
147. Isaacson, Seftel, Keeley and Bothwell: J. Lab. Clin. Med., *58*, 845, 1961.
148. Block, Moore, Wasi and Haiby: Am. J. Pathol., *47*, 89, 1965.
149. Charlton and Bothwell: Prog. Hematol., *5*, 298, 1966.
150. Bothwell: Ser. Haematol., *6*, 56, 1965.
151. MacDonald and Pechet: Arch. Intern. Med., *116*, 381, 1965.
152. Charlton, Jacobs, Seftel and Bothwell: Br. Med. J., *2*,1427, 1964.
153. Callender and Malpas: Br. Med. J., *2*, 1511, 1963.
154. Davis and Badenoch: Lancet, *2*, 6, 1962.
155. Castleman and Towne: N. Engl. J. Med., *247*, 992, 1952.
156. Castleman and Kibbee: N. Engl. J. Med., *258*, 652, 1958.
157. Wallerstein and Robbins: Am. J. Med., *14*, 256, 1953.
158. Turnberg: Br. Med. J., *1*, 1360, 1965.
159. Pollycove: In *Iron Metabolism. An International Symposium* (Gross, Ed.). Berlin, Springer-Verlag, 1964.
160. Prizio-Biroli, Finch and Loden: J. Lab. Clin. Med., *55*, 216, 1960.

Chapter *8*

WATER, ELECTROLYTES AND ACID-BASE BALANCE

H. T. Randall

Water is an essential and major component of all life on earth. Not just a passive solvent in which inorganic salts, organic compounds and dissolved gases interact, water participates actively in forming the building blocks for cells and is a component of most of them, as well as being the environment in which cells live and from which they obtain their nutrition.

Electrolytes comprise a wide variety of compounds, from simple inorganic salts of sodium, potassium and magnesium to complex organic molecules often synthesized by and unique to the individual. Electrolytes share the phenomenon with water itself of dissociating into positively and negatively charged ions, and have the additional property of variably affecting the concentration of hydrogen ion in solution; this effect depends both on individual ion characteristics and on interaction with other ionized and partially ionized substances in the solution. Major differences in specific ion concentrations exist between cell fluid and extracellular fluid; these differences are maintained by a substantial expenditure of energy by cells and are critical to cell metabolism and survival.

The hydrogen ion concentration of intracellular fluid and extracellular fluid differs. Both are held within narrow ranges by a complex series of reactions within the organism and by the ability selectively to excrete excessive acid or base loads by the kidneys. Diets vary in the effective amount of acid and base they contain. Metabolic processes of the body create an additional acid load which must be excreted to maintain optimum concentration.

The term *balance* implies a state of equilibrium which is dynamic for intakes of water, electrolytes and other nutrients, the conversion and utilization of metabolizable nutrients and the excretion of ingested substances or their end-products of metabolism. The net result is that the stable individual remains in energy balance, and in equilibrium of water, electrolyte and hydrogen ion concentration. Growth requires a positive balance. However, fluid, electrolyte and acid-base balance constitutes far more than just a consideration of intake and output of water and electrolytes and of the differences between them. This discussion considers body composition including body cell mass and supporting and protecting tissues, fluid compartments and their size, composition and function, metabolism of water and electrolytes and the regulatory mechanisms that defend the volume, content and acid-base balance of the body. With these as background, alterations in water balance, in electrolyte composition and distribution, and acidosis and alkalosis are analyzed. Parenteral fluid and electrolyte therapies are discussed as alternative and often necessary means of maintaining or correcting abnormalities in fluid, electrolyte and acid-base balances.

NORMAL BODY COMPOSITION

Knowledge of what constitutes normal body composition is essential to an understanding of the requirements of normal man for water and electrolytes as a part of nutrition. The reader is referred to Chapter 1 of this book for a detailed description of body composition, variations with age and by sex and body habitus and the methods used for analysis.

For purposes of this chapter, the studies and terminology of Moore and his associates[1] are used. By isotopic dilutional techniques and chemical analysis they have determined not only the major chemical composition of the body but, more importantly, its functional compartments. The range of normal body composition in both males and females over a wide span of age has been established, and abnormal changes in body composition resulting from disease or injury have been evaluated.

Total Body Water

The largest single component of the body is water. Body water is distributed throughout the cells, the extracellular fluids and the solid supporting structures. The highest concentration of water is present in metabolically active cells of muscle and viscera, the lowest in relatively inert and inactive supporting structures such as the skeleton. Isotope dilution studies using either heavy water (^2H_2O, or D_2O) or tritiated water (^3H_2O) have shown that, in the normal adult male under the age of 40, approximately 60 per cent of body weight is water. In young women the exchangeable body water averages about 50 per cent of body weight, chiefly because the percentage of fat is higher than in men and the percentage of skeletal muscle is lower. In both sexes there is considerable normal variation of total body water content which makes accurate prediction of total body water difficult in a given individual. In the studies of Moore and his associates,[1] total body water is expressed as regression equations based on total body weight. Table 8–1 presents data from studies of 132 normal males and 88 normal females. Each series is divided to show differences due to age. Significant differences in regression equations exist for each group. There is a gradual and significant decline with age in total body water as a percentage of body weight.

Hume and Weyers[2] have suggested that total body water is closely correlated with body surface area. Table 8–2 presents a summary of their data; the regression equations and correlation coefficients are based on data from analysis of body water composition of 30 male and 30 female hospitalized patients using ^3H_2O isotope dilution measured at 2 and 3 hours after injection. Figures for 11 obese and 19

Table 8–1.　Total Body Water (TBW) by Sex and Age[1]

Sex	Age Group (years)	Subjects	Mean Body Wt (kg)	Mean TBW (liters)	95% Confidence Limits of Mean as % of Mean	Ratio (%) TBW(L) to Weight (kg)
Male	16–30	63	71.75	42.26	±16	58.9
Male	31–60	56	73.57	40.24	±17	54.7
Male	61–90	13	69.42	35.82	±16	51.6
Female	16–30	54	60.89	30.99	±13	50.9
Female	31–90	34	62.62	28.36	±21	45.2

Predicted normal:

Males: $\dfrac{\text{TBW in L}}{\text{body wt in kg}} \times 100 = 79.45 - 0.24 \,(\text{wt}) - 0.15 \,(\text{age})$

Females: $\dfrac{\text{TBW in L}}{\text{body wt in kg}} \times 100 = 69.81 - 0.2 \,(\text{wt}) - 0.12 \,(\text{age})$

Table 8–2. Relationship Between Measured Total Body Water and Height, Weight and Predicted Body Surface Area in Adults*

Sex	Number	Age Group	Regression Equation: TBW on H and W**	Multiple Correlation Coefficient TBW, and H and W	95% Confidence Limit—1 Patient H and W Known
M	30	35–71, x̄ 54.5	TBW = 0.194781 H + 0.296785W − 14.012934; r,H and W = 0.547(P<0.01); r,H + TBW = 0.711(P<0.001); r,W + TBW = 0.920(P<0.001)	r = 0.953	±27.5%
F	30	33–84, x̄ 53.7	TBW + 0.344547H + 0.183809W − 35.270121; r,H and W = 0.589(P<0.001); r,H and TBW = 0.770(P<0.001); r,W and TBW = 0.913(P<0.001)	r = 0.957	±27.5%

Sex	Number	Age Group	Regression Equation on Surface Area Predicted on TBW Measured***	Correlation Coefficient	
M Nonobese	25	40–71, x̄ 57.2	Y = 0.5244 + 0.03193X	r = 0.916 P < 0.001	Although not stated, 95% confidence limits for predicting TBW in one individual would be of the order of ± 25%.
F Nonobese	19	41–84, x̄ 56.4	Y = 0.4172 + 0.03831X	r = 0.826 P < 0.001	
F Obese >10% over x̄ for adults	11	33–63, x̄ 50.2	Y = 0.9013 + 0.02811X	r = 0.813 P < 0.001	

* Data taken from Hume and Weyers[2] showing regression equations for total body water based on height, weight and predicted body surface area. Figures are based on a hospitalized patient population.

** Where TBW is in liters, H (height) in cm and W (weight) in kg.

*** Y = body surface area in meters^2, X = TBW in liters.

nonobese females are expressed as regressions of predicted surface area on measured body water using the DuBois formula for prediction of surface area (Fig. 8–1). A high correlation is noted between predicted body surface and predicted total body water in their male and female populations, as might be expected when linear regression of body water is based on height and weight. They suggest that estimates of surface area and of total body water are essentially interchangeable in defining predicted normal lean body mass, total body potassium, normal red cell volume and cardiac output.

A comparison of predicted total body water between Moore's data[1] and those of Hume and Weyers[2] indicates a somewhat higher percentage of total body water by the Hume and Weyers' method for both males and females of middle age. For example, an average-height, average-weight 55-year-old male (177 cm, 79 kg) would have a predicted body surface area of 1.97 square meters (see Fig. 8–1) and a total body water of 45.3 liters, while the expected total body water of males in this age group from Moore's data is 54.7 per cent of body weight or 43.2 liters, and 41.3 liters from the prediction formula in Table 8–1. Similarly, a 162-cm, 67.3-kg 55-year-old female with a body surface area of 1.72 square meters would have a total body water of 34.0 liters, compared to 47.2 per cent of body weight or 31.8 liters from Moore's group average and 30.7 liters from the prediction formula. Individual variation is so great, with 95 per cent confidence limits for total body water of the order of ± 16 per cent of the mean in Moore's series and ± 25 per cent of the calculated individual value in Hume and Weyers' series, that such differences have no statistical significance. The differences might be predicted, however, on the basis that Hume and Weyers' patients were recovering in the hospital, many from such stressful states as myocardial infarction, cardiovascular accident, acute bronchitis and peptic ulcer, and they might be expected to have a somewhat expanded total body water under these circumstances.

Because of the relative simplicity of determining body surface area using the graph devised by DuBois[3] and the close correlation between predicted surface area

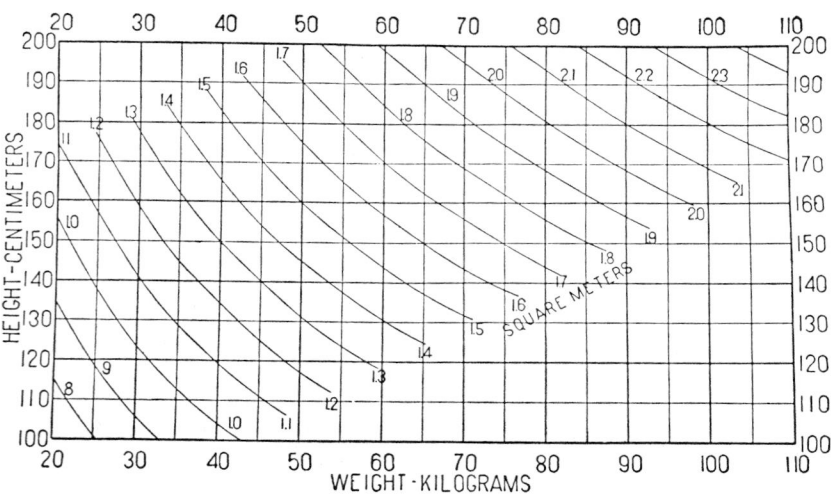

Fig. 8–1. Graph showing the relationship of height in centimeters and weight in kilograms to body surface area in square meters. (From DuBois.[3])

and predicted total body water shown by Hume and Weyers,[2] Figures 8–1, 8–2, and 8–3 are provided for guidance in making estimates of predicted total body water. Wide normal individual variation must be expected.

Total body water, as a percentage of body weight, is higher in children and in adults who are lean or who have larger than normal skeletal muscle mass. It tends to decrease as body weight increases with obesity. Body water as a percentage of

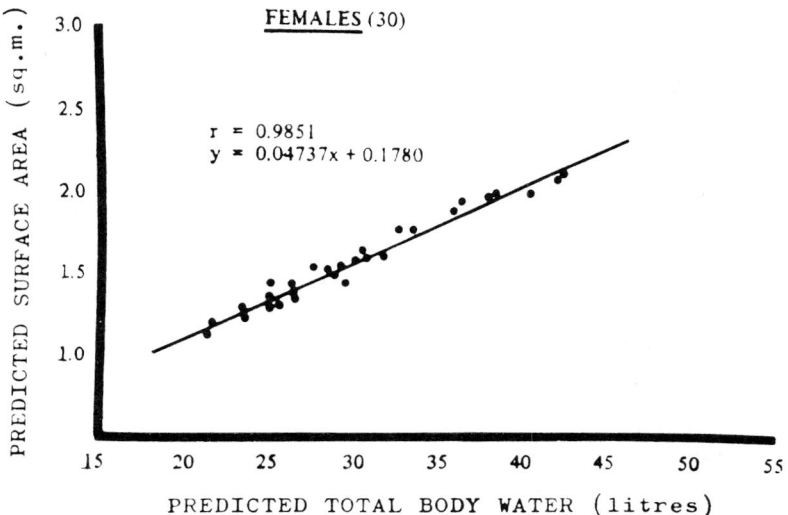

Fig. 8–2. Relationship between predicted body surface and predicted body water for women of middle age. (From Hume and Weyers.[2])

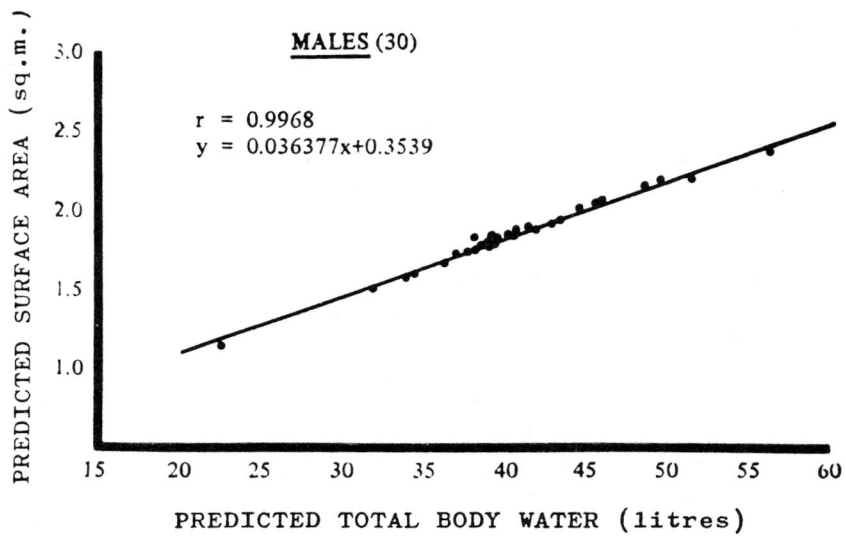

Fig. 8–3. Relationship between predicted body surface area and predicted body water for men of middle age. (From Hume and Weyers.[2])

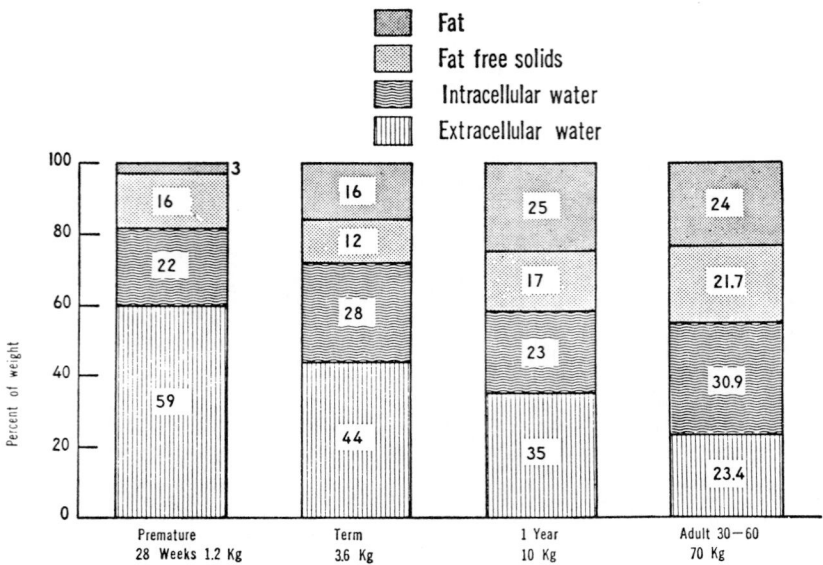

Fig. 8–4. Comparison of water content as per cent of total weight of premature and term infants, a child of 1 year and normal adult 70-kg male. Total water decreases progressively as does extracellular water, while intracellular water increases with increase in body cell mass. (Data from Widdowson[4] and Moore et al.[1])

body weight also declines slowly with age in both sexes. Figure 8–4, utilizing Widdowson's data on growth and composition of the fetus and newborn[4] and Moore's studies of adults,[1] illustrates the extremely high total body water content of the fetus and newborn infant, with progressive decreases in both total body water and the relative proportion of extracellular fluid to body weight and to total water with growth and maturation.

Body water constitutes a higher percentage of body weight in athletes than in nonathletes. Novak, Hyatt and Alexander[5] found an average of 70 per cent of body weight as water in 21 college gymnasts, track men and swimmers; these men had remarkably lean bodies (95 to 96 per cent of body weight was estimated to be fat free). Sixteen football and 10 baseball players of the same age group (19 to 22

years) averaged 14 per cent of body weight as fat and 63 per cent of weight as water.

Brill et al.[6] have measured total body water in markedly obese patients (260 to 440 pounds) in preparation for small bowel bypass operation. Such patients had a 21.3 ± 12.4 per cent greater total body water content than was anticipated on the basis of ^{40}K estimates of lean body mass, and exhibited a relatively expanded extracellular fluid space. They were also noted to have a much increased insensible water loss, averaging a daily evaporative loss of 2.4 to 2.9 liters as compared to a normal value of 0.9 liters.

Total body water may be considered as being distributed in two major compartments or spaces, based on differential concentration of the two major cations sodium and potassium, and by the volume represented by dilution of radioactive isotopes or other substances which appear to reach equilibrium in a portion of the total water pool.[1] The two major compartments are intracellular water (ICW) and extracellular water (ECW). *Intracellular water* is that portion of TBW within cells. Body composition studies indicate that from 50 to 58 per cent (average 55 per cent) of TBW is intracellular in normal healthy adults. Lean individuals with a relatively large skeletal muscle mass, such as trained young male athletes, have a higher percentage of TBW within cells, while females tend to have a more nearly equal distribution of TBW between ICW and ECW. *Extracellular water* consists of the water component of the extracellular fluids, plasma, interstitial fluid and the water component of extracellular solids including tendon, fascia, dermis, collagen, elastin and skeleton. Since there is no way of distinguishing in vivo among the various areas of distribution of ECW, except for measurement of plasma volume and total ECW, ECW is usually considered as a two-subcompartmental distribution of interstitial fluid and plasma.

The size of the ECW compartment as a volume or space depends upon methods used for measurements, and varies from 15 to 16 per cent of body weight when inulin, sucrose or mannitol is the indicator; it is as high as 27 per cent of body weight if ^{24}Na is assumed to be distributed entirely extracellularly, which it is not. Measurement of other small ions, such as $^{35}SO_4^=$ and $^{82}Br^-$, gives equilibration values of distribution of from 21 to 26 per cent of body weight for ECW; these data suffer from the fact that these ions enter into cells to some degree with time. As a practical matter, ECW can be considered as 23 per cent of body weight in normal adults, or even as 20 per cent of body weight as is commonly used clinically for extracellular fluid estimation in water and electrolyte balance problems.

Figure 8–5 illustrates the proportions of body weight as total body water in normal adult men and women, and its distribution as ICW, interstitial fluid and plasma. Comparison of this figure with Figure 8–4 indicates the major differences in water content and distribution that exist between

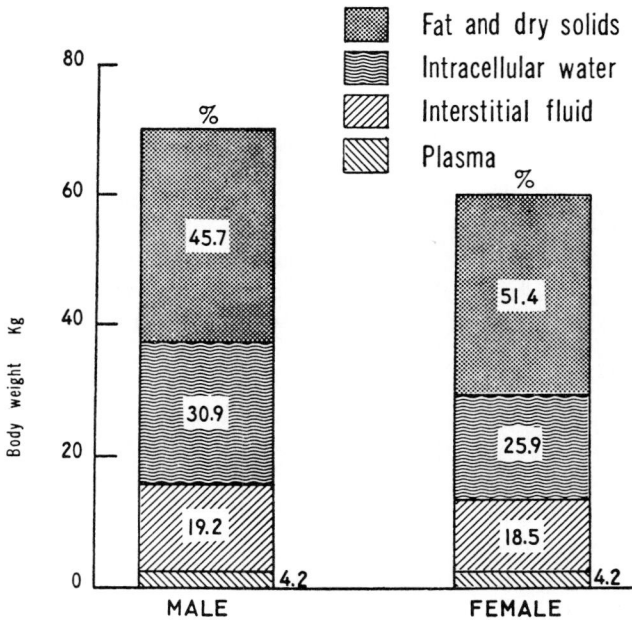

Fig. 8–5. Body water as percentage of body weight, with approximate distribution as intracellular water, interstitial water and plasma water, for adult men and adult women. (Data from Moore et al.[1])

adults and infants and emphasizes a reason for the special problem of water and electrolyte balance in infants.

Total Body Solids:
Fat and Fat-free Solids

Total body solids (TBS) are the remainder of body weight when total body water is subtracted:

$$\text{TBS (kg)} = \text{Body wt (kg)} - \text{TBW (L)}$$

Total body solids are divided into body fat and fat-free solids.

Total body fat (TBF) is a derived figure in body composition analysis and is discussed in more detail in Chapter 1. In normal individuals, the assumptions are made that body fat is anhydrous and that the fat-free body is 73.2 per cent water, as determined by simultaneous multiple isotope dilution:

$$\% \text{ Body fat} = 100 - \frac{\% \text{ Body water}}{0.732}$$

$$\text{Body fat (kg)} = \% \text{ Body fat} \times \frac{\text{Body wt (kg)}}{100}$$

This estimate depends heavily on the state of hydration of the fat-free body,

which may vary from 0.67 to 0.85 or so. Moore has prepared a nomogram based on the ratio intracellular water/total body water which should be consulted for greater accuracy in predicting or estimating TBF.[1]

Fat-free solids (FFS) is another derived value, obtained by subtracting total body fat from total body solids:

$$\text{FFS (kg)} = \text{TBS}_{kg} - \text{TBF}_{kg}$$

The relative proportion of total body solids to body weight in men and women is shown in Figure 8–5.

The Major Electrolytes of Body Water: Sodium, Chloride and Potassium

Total Body Sodium. The sodium ion content of the normal human body is stated to be from 52 to 60 mEq per kg in the adult male, and 48 to 55 mEq per kg in the female. A 70-kg man would therefore have from 3,600 to 4,200 mEq (83 to 97 gm) of sodium. From 35 to 40 per cent of the total body sodium is in the skeleton, and 65 to 75 per cent of skeletal sodium is unexchangeable or very slowly exchanged with that in body fluids and isotope tracers.[1,7]

Total Exchangeable Sodium (Na$_e$). Na$_e$ is the pool of sodium within the body with which ^{24}Na$^+$ or ^{22}Na$^+$ comes into equilibrium, as usually measured at 24 hours after administration of the isotope. It is about 65 per cent of total body sodium and does not change significantly with age or sex in normal adults. Na$_e$ per kg is lower in females than in males since the former have a higher percentage of body fat. Individual variation in Na$_e$ is considerable and is a function of body composition. Average Na$_e$ in normal adult males and females is given by Moore et al.[1] as:

	Age Group (yrs)	Number	Na$_e$ (mEq/kg)	95% C.L.* (% of mean)
Males	16–84	149	40.5	±21%
Females	16–90	78	37.1	±17%
	* Confidence limits			

Table 8–3 gives prediction values for Na$_e$.

Residual Sodium. The portion of exchangeable sodium not accounted for by the product of extracellular water volume (ECW) and extracellular water sodium concentration in mEq/L is residual sodium. This averages 10 to 15 per cent of Na$_e$.

Total Body Chloride. This averages about 33 mEq per kg in a normal adult male;[8] a 70-kg man contains about 2,300 mEq or 81.7 gm. Predominantly an extracellular ion, chloride is found in low concentration in bone and is probably loosely

Table 8–3. Formulas for Predicting Normal Values in Body Composition For the Adult[1]

1. *Total Body Water (TBW)*

   Males
   $$\frac{\text{TBW (L)}}{\text{Body wt (kg)}} \times 100 = 79.45 - 0.24 \text{ (body wt)} - 0.15 \text{ age}$$

   Females
   $$\frac{\text{TBW (L)}}{\text{Body wt (kg)}} \times 100 = 69.81 - 0.26 \text{ (body wt)} - 0.12 \text{ age}$$

2. *Intracellular Water (ICW)*

   Males
   $$\frac{\text{ICW}}{\text{TBW}} \times 100 = 62.3 - 0.16 \text{ age}$$

   Females
   $$\frac{\text{ICW}}{\text{TBW}} \times 100 = 52.3 - 0.07 \text{ age}$$

3. *Exchangeable Potassium (K_e)*

   Using ICW for males or females as appropriate
   $$K_e(\text{mEq}) = 150 \text{ (ICW}_L) + 4(\text{TBW} - \text{ICW})$$

4. *Exchangeable Sodium (Na_e)*
   $$Na_e(\text{mEq}) = 163.2(\text{TBW}_L) - 69 - K_e(\text{mEq})$$

5. *Exchangeable Chloride (Cl_e)*
   $$Cl_e(\text{mEq}) = 0.7315(Na_e) - 16$$

6. *Regression Equation for $Na_e + K_e$ on TBW*
   $$Na_e(\text{mEq}) + K_e(\text{mEq}) = 163.19(\text{TBW}_L) - 69$$

7. *Extracellular Water (ECW)*
   $$ECW = TBW - ICW$$
   $$ECW = \text{Plasma volume} \times 0.93 + \text{Interstitial fluid volume} \times 0.98$$

8. *Extracellular Fluid (ECF)*
   $$ECF = \text{Plasma volume} + \text{Interstitial fluid}$$
   $$ECF = ECW \times 1.03$$

9. *Osmolar Balance*
   $$\frac{Na_e(\text{mEq}) + K_e(\text{mEq})}{\text{TBW (L)}} = 150$$

bound, but exchangeable, in connective tissue. Chloride is in part intracellular; the erythrocytes have the highest cellular concentration with gastric mucosa, gonads and skin containing lesser amounts.

Exchangeable Chloride (Cl_e). This is usually determined by equilibration with $^{82}Br-$, although $^{36}Cl^-$ has been reported recently as a useful tracer.[9] Data for exchangeable chloride are as follows[1]:

	Age Group (yrs)	Number	Cl_e (mEq/kg)	95% C.L.* (% of mean)
Males	16–90	67	29.4	±23%
Females	16–90	60	26.4	±21%
	* Confidence limits			

Cl_e bears a specific relationship to Na_e such that $Cl_e = 0.7315 (Na_e) - 16$.

Total Body Potassium. This value in the healthy young adult male is stated to be from 42 to 48 mEq per kg body weight.[1] A 70-kg man would contain from 2,940 to 3,360 mEq (115 to 131 gm) of potassium. In trained athletes with larger-than-normal muscle mass, total body counting of ^{40}K gives values of 60 and 65 mEq per kg body weight.[5] Virtually all of body potassium appears to be exchangeable with ^{42}K in the normal adult in 24 hours. The only exceptions are potassium in the erythrocytes, which is slowly exchanging, and in the skeleton, where the small amount present may not exchange fully. For practical use total body potassium and exchangeable potassium (K_e) are the same.

Total Exchangeable Potassium (K_e). This is the pool of potassium within the body which comes into equilibrium with ^{42}K in 24 hours. Approximately 98 per cent of K_e is considered to be intracellular. Since the potassium concentration of extracellular fluids averages 3.5 to 5.0 mEq/L, the total extracellular potassium in a 70-kg adult male is about 60 mEq.

Exchangeable potassium differs in males and females and declines in both sexes as a function of age as indicated below[1]:

	Age Group (yrs)	Number	K_e (mEq/kg)	95% C.L.* (% of mean)
Males	16–30	97	48.1	±23%
	31–60	34	45.1	±20%
	61–90	20	37.3	±16%
Females	16–30	59	38.3	±20%
	31–60	28	34.2	±23%
	61–90	21	29.7	±29%

* Confidence limits

Total Body Potassium by ^{40}K Counting. Brill et al.[6] and Novak et al.[5] have determined total body potassium by whole body counting of naturally occurring ^{40}K, which emits gamma rays of 1.46 Mev maximal energy, and occurs as a small fraction (0.0119 per cent) of the stable potassium pool of ^{39}K (93.08 per cent) and ^{41}K (6.91 per cent). When calibrated with known amounts of ^{40}K in properly distributed geometry, body counts can be directly interpreted in terms of mEq potassium. Normal values for K_e can be predicted from body weight, sex and age (Table 8–3).

Na_e, K_e and TBW. The sum of K_e and Na_e, called "total base" by Moore et al.,[1] has a very high correlation with TBW when each of the three variables is measured independently by isotope dilution techniques. The regression equation for this relationship is:

$$Na_e \text{ (mEq)} + K_e \text{ (mEq)} = 163.19 \text{ TBW(L)} - 69$$
$$r = 0.99 \ (P<0.001)$$

Unaffected by age groups or sex, this relationship permits close estimation of the third factor, when any two are known. Na_e bears a close relationship to extracellular water in both males and females, as does Cl_e. K_e bears an even closer relationship to intracellular water, since the concentrations of K are very low in all extracellular fluids (4 mEq/L) as compared to the intracellular value (150 mEq/L).

In healthy individuals, Na_e/K_e ratios approximate 0.85 in males and 1.0 in females. In a wide variety of illness, such as trauma, sepsis, cardiac or renal insufficiency, and prolonged inadequate nutrition whether due to failure of intake or to malabsorption, the Na_e/K_e ratio rises; values of 1.5 or higher are not unusual in debilitated edematous individuals.

Body Cell Mass and Extracellular Tissues

A functional consideration of normal body composition involves division of the body into its living cells and their fluid and solid extracellular supporting structures (Fig. 8–6).

Body cell mass (BCM), a concept defined and developed by Moore et al.,[1] consists of all of the cells of the body, regardless of their location. All have a high intracellular potassium concentration, and all utilize chemical energy from food, or tissue catabolism, to perform thermal, chemical and sometimes mechanical work. The body cell mass is not uniform in metabolic rate, in chemical, mechanical or thermal work done, or in fuel requirements, since these vary from one cell type and location

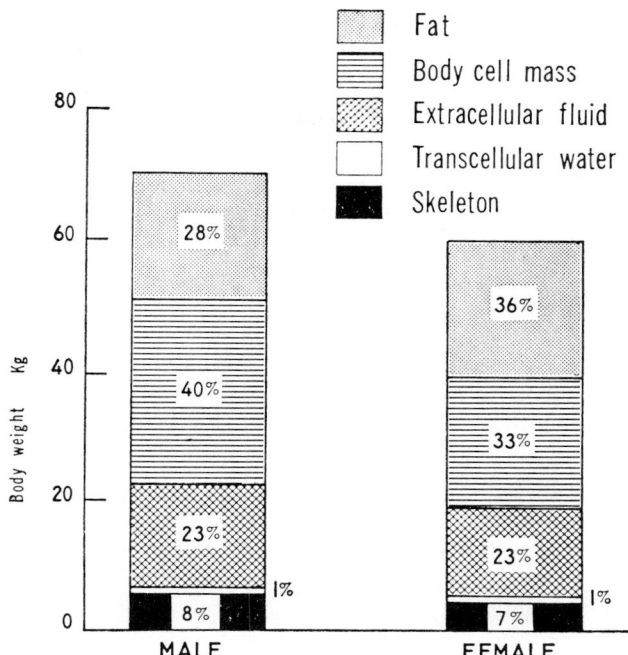

Fig. 8–6. Body cell mass and its proportional relationship to supporting structures. Extracellular fluid includes noncellular elements of connective tissue and tendons, as well as interstitial fluid and plasma. Transcellular fluid is fluid of joints, cerebrospinal fluid and the content of the resting gastrointestinal tract. (Based on data from Moore et al.[1])

to another and with the activity of the body.

Chemical analysis of representative samples of cellular tissues from man indicate a K/N ratio of very close to 3 mEq of potassium for each gram of nitrogen. Virtually all the potassium and a high percentage of protein are intracellular. Assuming an average K/N ratio of 3 mEq per gm N, and a total net weight of average cells (excluding extracellular fluid) of N × 25,[1] body cell mass can then be calculated:

$$BCM = \frac{(K_e - ECK) \times 25}{3}$$

Since extracellular potassium (ECK) is relatively small it can be ignored and

$$BCM_{gm} = K_e(mEq) \times 8.33$$

Intracellular water (ICW) can be calculated from K_e on the basis of $\frac{K_e(mEq)}{150} = ICW (L)$ in normals, since potassium concentration intracellularly is approximately 150 mEq/L (149.7 ± 7.2). Intracellular K concentration can be adjusted for changes in extra-

cellular fluid tonicity by adjustment of the equation

$$\frac{Na_e + K_e}{TBW} = 150$$

a ratio which is an expression of the osmolar equilibrium between cells and extracellular fluids. As noted previously, ICW is normally 50 to 58 per cent of TBW, with males tending to have a higher percentage of TBW as ICW. The ratio ICW/TBW is altered in a variety of diseases, almost all of which result in a decreased ratio by expansion of both TBW and ECW as a percentage of body weight, with or without loss of BCM as well.

Oxygen consumption and caloric expenditure are closely correlated with BCM. Kinney et al.[10] have measured oxygen consumption as 8 to 10 ml per min per kg BCM, and caloric expenditure as 2.7 to 3.6 calories per hr per kg BCM. Novak et al.[5] measured basal oxygen consumption of young athletes as 6.6 to 7.58 ml O_2 per min per kg BCM.

Creatinine excretions have been reported of 60 to 80 mg per kg BCM per day[10] and of 47 to 51 mg per kg BCM per day.[5] This author has become doubtful of the value of daily creatinine excretion as a measure of skeletal muscle mass in seriously ill patients, having observed in many patients a striking fall in total creatinine excretion and in plasma creatinine levels following introduction of a high-caloric amino acid nutritional regimen. This occurred whether the high-caloric material was given intravenously or as chemically defined diets. Plasma creatinine levels of 0.4 mg per 100 ml and total creatine excretion in the urine of less than 0.5 gm a day in adults accompanied a positive nitrogen balance. These data suggest that some part of creatinine production is related to muscle catabolism.

Extracellular tissues (ECT) are those fluids and solids of the body that are wholly outside of cells. Even though some of these have extremely small cell components, only the extracellular part of such tissues is considered as ECT. *Extracellular fluid (ECF)* has been discussed. The extracellular solids include the skeleton, tendons, fascia, dermis, collagen and elastin. *Interstitial fluid* comprises about three-fourths of total extracellular fluid and 15 to 18 per cent of body weight. Interstitial fluid is in intimate communication with plasma, being separated only by capillary walls which permit easy diffusion of all but large protein molecules. Its protein content is much lower and therefore its water content is higher than that of plasma, as are concentrations of chloride and bicarbonate as required by the Gibbs-Donnan distribution equilibrium. The plasma component of extracellular fluid varies between 3.5 and 5 per cent of body weight and averages 4.2 per cent. Normal protein concentration is approximately 7 gm per 100 ml, and therefore plasma is about 93 per cent water. Because of the lower water content of plasma and the presence of protein molecules which behave as nondiffusible anions, the concentration of cations in plasma water is higher than that in interstitial fluid, and the concentration of inorganic anions is somewhat lower.

No measurement of extracellular water takes accurately into account the *extracellular solids,* of which the skeleton is the largest component. The skeleton is estimated to be 10.5 per cent of the normally hydrated fat-free body weight in health, which makes it of the order of 8 per cent of total body weight in males and 7 per cent total body weight in females of normal body composition (Fig. 8–6). Skeletal bone contains about 30 per cent water. It also contains a substantial amount of sodium, 230 to 288 mEq per kg in fat-free dry cortical bone, of which 65 to 75 per cent is unexchangeable, and as much as 85 per cent not associated with chloride. Potassium content of bone is low.[1] A nomogram of skeletal weight based on K_e and K_e/FFS has been prepared by Moore and associates and is useful for more precisely estimating skeletal weight.[1] In wasting diseases, in which there is substantial loss of both BCM and fat, the skeleton assumes a much larger percentage of body weight.

Dense connective tissue of fascial sheaths and tendons together with other collagen in the body has been estimated to comprise 6 per cent of body weight in dogs and 2 to 3 per cent in man. Subcutaneously equilibrated, fat-free collagen of fascia in the dog has been shown by Fulton to contain 70 per cent water and 57 mEq Na^+ per kg, suggesting that 45 per cent of the water content is bound in a way to exclude sodium.[11]

Extracellular solids are, therefore, not chemically homogeneous with extracellular fluids. Equilibria for water, sodium, chloride and probably hydrogen ion within extracellular solids appear to be rather specific for the solid tissue considered. These observations are of importance when considering the behavior of ECF, particularly interstitial fluid, in the derangements of acid-base balance and, particularly, with hypoxic hypoperfusion.

Electrolyte Concentration of Body Fluids

Figure 8–7, modified from the famous diagrams of Gamble,[12] illustrates the approximate composition of interstitial fluid and intracellular water in comparison with that of plasma with its more precisely known values. Table 8–4 gives the range of normal and the analytic error of laboratory determinations for the major electrolytes of plasma as usually determined in serum. Values in this table are from the literature and from our laboratories.[13-15] It should be remembered that there are both a range of values present in normal individuals and an error present in any laboratory determination. The ranges shown take into consideration both the normal variation and the 95 per cent confidence limits of the

laboratory procedure in a well-run clinical laboratory. Repeating any laboratory test will reduce the probability of error due to the test. When laboratory reports do not help to confirm the clinical diagnosis or course, it is wise both to repeat the test and to reexamine and reevaluate the patient.

An approximation of the accuracy of determination of the sodium, chloride and bicarbonate concentrations of the plasma or serum or the determination of the existence of a major electrolyte abnormality in the patient can be made by equating the serum sodium concentration (in mEq) with the sum of the chloride and bicarbonate concentrations (in mEq) plus 10 mEq:

$$mEq\ Na = mEq\ HCO_3 + mEq\ Cl + 10$$

Since the sum of the cations and the anions in any biologic system must be equal, and since sodium ion is the major

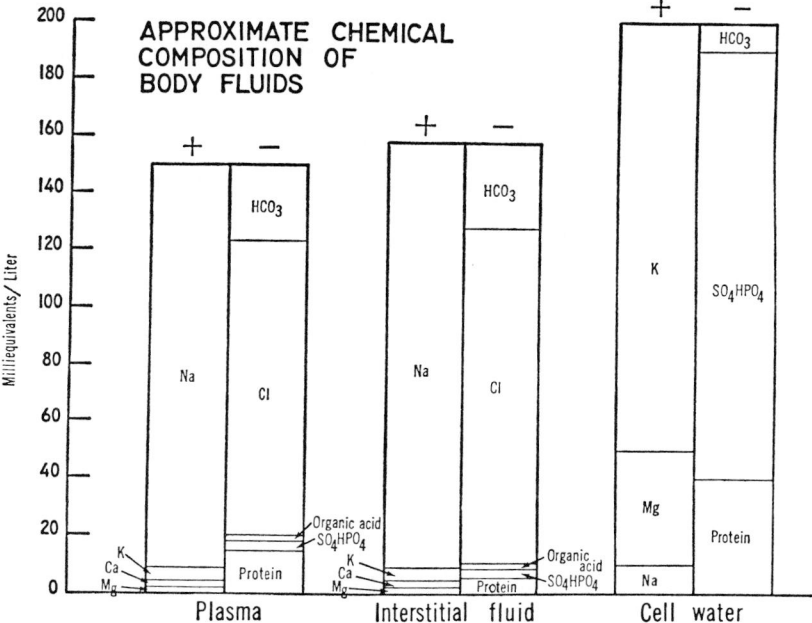

Fig. 8–7. The electrolyte concentrations of plasma and interstitial fluid are compared with an approximation of the electrolytes in cell water. Cell membranes separate and maintain striking concentration and electrolyte differences between intracellular and extracellular fluids. (Modified from Gamble.[12])

Table 8–4. Normal Electrolyte Concentration of Serum

Electrolytes	Range of Normal including Laboratory-method Variance	Reliability of Laboratory Test- 95% Confidence Limits
Cations		
Sodium	136–145mEq/L	± 3 mEq
Potassium	3.5–5.0 mEq/L	± 0.2 mEq
Calcium	4.5–5.5 mEq/L	± 0.1 mEq
	(9.0–11.0 mg/100 ml)	
Magnesium	1.5–2.5 mEq/L	± 0.04 mEq
	(1.8–3.0 mg/100 ml)	
Anions		
Chloride	96–106 mEq/L	± 2.0 mEq
CO_2(content)TCO_2	24–28.8 mEq/L	± 0.2 mEq
Phosphorus (inorganic)	3.0–4.5 mg/100 ml	Considerable variance due
	(1.9 to 2.85 mEq/L as $H PO_4 =$)	to analytic problem
Sulfate (as S)	0.8–1.2 mg/100 ml	Method dependent
	(0.5–0.75 mEq/L as $SO_4 =$)	
Lactate	0.7–1.8 mEq/L	Method dependent
	(6 to 16 mg/100 ml)	
Protein	6.0–7.6 mg/100 ml	Method dependent
	(14–18 mEq/L)	
	Depends on albumin	

cation of extracellular fluid and of serum or plasma, most of the anions balance sodium. The anionic structure of serum or plasma is somewhat more complex than that of the cations, because of the presence of a substantial amount of plasma protein, the molecules of which behave primarily as anions at the pH of plasma. The sum of bicarbonate (27 mEq) and chloride (105 mEq) equals all but 10 mEq of the normal sodium concentration. The relationship between the sum of the two anions and the serum sodium concentration normally remains constant. If the sum of bicarbonate plus chloride plus 10 mEq is *less* than ± 5 mEq of the sodium concentration on repeated determinations, one of two conditions exist; either there has been the addition of substantial amounts of another anion or there is a major error in the laboratory determination of one or more of the three components. Conversely, if HCO_3 + Cl + 10 is greater than sodium by more than 3 to 5 mEq, hypoproteinemia is

the likely cause if laboratory error is ruled out.

Much less is known about intracellular fluid (ICF) than about plasma and interstitial fluid. Muscle cells, liver cells and erythrocytes obviously contain different functional proteins within them, and their electrolyte content is different as well. However, the body cell mass has certain characteristics which all its cells share in common and many of these are different from extracellular fluid. The major intracellular cations are potassium and magnesium; there is relatively little sodium. Bicarbonate ion is present within cells in less than one-half the concentration in ECF. The predominating intracellular anions are organic phosphates and protein in substantial amounts (Fig. 8–7). Approximately 23 per cent of BCM is protein.

The osmolality of intracellular fluid is generally considered to be about the same as ECF, since water diffuses freely into and out of cells as shown by isotope dilution.

The only exception in man would appear to be the medullary area of the kidney, where an osmotic gradient nearly 4 times that of ECF, and presumably of renal tubular cells, is maintained.

FORCES CONTROLLING THE WATER AND ELECTROLYTE BALANCE BETWEEN CELLS AND EXTRACELLULAR FLUID

Osmolality and Osmotic Pressure

A substance in solution in water on one side of a semipermeable membrane which is freely permeable to water but through which the solute cannot pass exerts an effect such that water molecules tend to diffuse in larger numbers *toward* the solution side where the water molecule concentration (or activity) is less. Osmotic pressure is the physical force necessary on the solution side of the membrane to *prevent* the net movement of water across the membrane toward the solution and to maintain equilibrium. One gram molecular weight (GMW) of a substance which does not dissociate into ions, such as glucose or urea, contains 6.06×10^{23} molecules and is termed 1 osmole; dissolved in 1 liter of water 1 osmole will require a pressure equal to 17,004 mm Hg on the solution side to maintain equilibrium across a membrane permeable only to water. One milliosmole (mOsm or mO) is 1/1000th of an osmole and when dissolved in 1 liter of water has an osmotic pressure of 17 mm Hg.

Since the number of particles determines osmotic pressure, substances which ionize affect osmotic pressure according to the degree of dissociation. For example, sodium chloride dissociates into Na^+ and Cl^- in such fashion that at 0.154 molar concentration (that of body fluid) there are about 1.85 particles for each original molecule. A pressure of 286 mO, rather than 308 mO, is exerted.[16]

Osmolality of a solution can be determined on the basis that 1 osmole dissolved in 1 liter of water will depress the freezing point of water by 1.86° C. Normal plasma or serum (fibrogen molecules are very large so their absence makes virtually no difference) freezes at—0.533° C and osmolality is therefore 0.553/1.86 or 297 mO. Freezing point depression osmometers are widely available in clinical laboratories today and are of great value in determining not only plasma osmolality but that of urine and other biologic fluids, thereby assisting the clinician in evaluation of fluid and electrolyte balance in his patient.

With such large forces present even with small differences in osmolality, and the fact that cell membranes, with very limited exceptions such as the distal nephron of the kidney, are quite freely permeable to water, osmolality must be nearly if not exactly equal within cells and their surrounding extracellular fluids. Such is almost certainly the case despite substantial differences in individual ion content and protein concentration between cells and ECF (Fig. 8–7). In order to permit such ionic discrepancies to exist, other forces must be at work and energy must be expended. *The Gibbs-Donnan equilibrium rule* provides that under equilibrium conditions the *product* of concentration of any pair of diffusible cations and anions on one side of a membrane will equal the *product* of the same pair of ions on the other side. When a nondiffusible ion is present on one side of a membrane, the situation is altered so that, while the products of the concentration of the pairs of diffusible ions are equal, the concentrations on the two sides are unequal, and remain so. Within cells, organic phosphates and protein are nondiffusible and hold an excess of the cations K and Mg (Fig. 8–7). These forces are balanced by the remarkable property of living cells of keeping sodium out of the cell by continuous pumping. This counter-osmotic gradient, together with the probability that not all the ions and protein molecules are active (some being "bound" in large protein aggregates), provides the best current explanation of the ability of the body cell mass to maintain the transmembrane differences that are essential to life.

Osmotic Pressure, Diffusion and Reabsorption in Tissue Nutrition

Starling[17] observed that 1 per cent saline solution was rapidly absorbed from subcutaneous tissue and measured the protein oncotic pressure (colloid osmotic pressure) of dog serum against 1.03 per cent saline as 30 to 41 mm Hg. His hypothesis of filtration of plasma against this gradient at the high-pressure end of a capillary and the return of the filtrate at the low-pressure end is well known, but accounts for a very small fraction of the total extracellular circulation according to Pitts.[16]

The major exchanges of water, electrolytes, nutrient substances, oxygen, carbon dioxide and other end-products of metabolism occur by diffusion. Water and plasma electrolytes, which are very small ions, diffuse rapidly back and forth across capillary membranes. Capillary water exchanges with intersitital water several times a second. Sodium, chloride, glucose and urea diffuse at different rates exchanging at rates of 2 times a second to 40 times a minute. *Net* transfer by diffusion depends on diffusion down a gradient with glucose and oxygen moving toward cells and carbon dioxide, organic acids and new water toward the capillary. Oxygen and carbon dioxide, because of their lipid solubility, are free to diffuse across all of the capillary membrane while water and electrolytes are believed to pass through minute pores in the endothelial membrane.[18]

The electrolyte diffusion mechanism across capillary membranes is in contrast with cell membranes where the sequence of cation selectivity resembles narrow-pore fixed-site systems, as described by Eisenman et al.,[19] including active transport mechanisms, such as that associated with Na-K activated ATPase for sodium and potassium.

The distribution of fluid volume between plasma and the interstitial fluid compartments is controlled by a balance of hydrostatic forces. Capillary hydrostatic pressure, including both blood pressure and gravity, and high capillary flow rates result in net flow from capillaries to the interstitial fluid. Colloid osmotic pressure of plasma protein, tissue elasticity and slow capillary flow rates result in a new return flow into capillaries. Anything which alters capillary permeability, such as injury due to heat, toxins or prolonged hypoxia with acidosis, results in varying degrees of loss of plasma protein into the interstitial fluid. Loss of colloid osmotic pressure reduces return flow to the capillary, with resulting local expansion of the intracellular fluid space. Edema becomes clinically evident when the interstitial fluid volume increases above approximately 50 per cent.

Cells are compound structures, with organelles that in complexion appear to be related to cell metabolism and function. As pointed out by Leaf,[20] the regulation of intracellular volume and ionic concentration is a function *primarily of each individual cell*, with some assistance from neighboring cells in organ systems. The concentration of water, ions, protein, nucleic acids and even hydrogen ion probably varies from site to site within cells. Gross averages do not reflect these important gradients.

Regulation of cell volume and concentration of ions within cells is an energy-requiring process involving active transport of sodium and potassium across cell membranes. The source of energy for this active transport system, as it is for practically every kind of energy expenditure by cells, is the metabolism of adenosine triphosphate. Katz and Epstein[21] have reviewed the substantial evidence developed in the last few years that, in addition to ATP, an enzyme, sodium-potassium activated ATPase, is always present in cells that pump sodium and potassium. This enzyme has an absolute requirement for magnesium, but also requires that both sodium and potassium be present together for maximal activity. It has one site with a high affinity for K^+, and another quite separate for Na^+. The enzyme is present on cell membranes and their extensions. It is inhibited by the presence of cardiac glycosides on the outside of the cell membrane, as is active transmembrane transport of sodium. Changes in Na-K activated ATPase in the kidney appear to be correlated with work of Na and K transport, adding further evidence that the enzyme has something to do with the "sodium pump" that enables cells to maintain their intracellular ionic integrity.

One of the effects of differing concentrations of potassium and other ions on opposite sides of a cell membrane is the development of an electrical potential across the membrane. A potential of −90 mV exists within muscle cells when compared to the ECF surrounding them. This negative potential may help to explain the rejection of Cl^- ion by most cells not involved in chloride transport.

Leaf[20] has postulated that a balance of solutes stabilizes cell volume; extracellular sodium balances the effects of intracellular colloids, and a dynamic steady state results. As much as one-third of the total resting energy of skeletal muscle cells may be directed to the sodium pump. When metabolism of cells is interfered with by hypoxia or any other metabolic inhibitor, cells swell. The mechanism appears to be the entrance of Na^+ and Cl^- ions into the cell, producing increased intracellular osmolality, and results in increased water content as water follows solute. At the same time, K^+ is lost, but not equivalently to sodium, so that the result is a net gain in water. Figure 8–8 illustrates schematically the processes involved. If the cell survives, a new equilibrium appears to be established with time in which the intracellular Na^+ concentration, and probably Cl^-, is higher than normal while the total water content of the tissue returns approximately to control levels. Analysis of the potassium, sodium, chloride, water and magnesium content by wet weight of fascia and gross fat-free abdominal rectus muscle of rats has been made, following a standard surgical incision through the muscle and its repair as compared to untraumatized muscle.[22] The injured muscle shows a rapid and significant increase in water, sodium and chloride content by the time of completion of the operation. Water content reaches its peak by day 2 and decreases slowly thereafter, reaching control level by day 20. Sodium content, how-

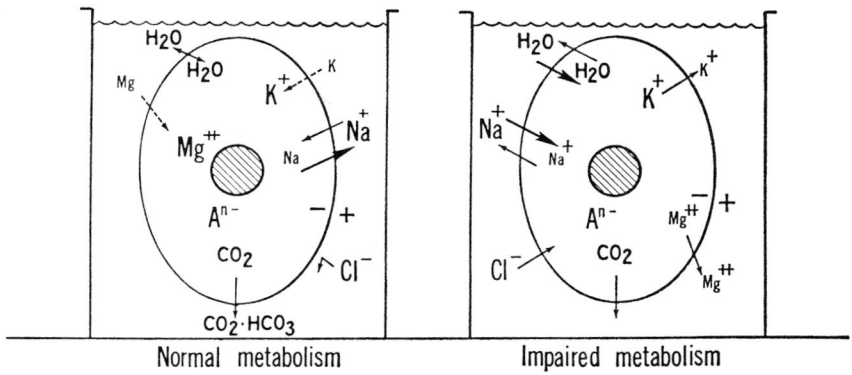

Normal metabolism   Impaired metabolism

Fig. 8–8. The effect of injury, including hypoxia, on the electrolyte and water content of cells. Inhibition of normal metabolism results in depression of the cell membrane sodium pump. Sodium, chloride and water enter the cell, while potassium and magnesium are lost. Water influx results in swelling of the cell. (Modified from Leaf.[20])

ever, continues to rise and potassium content to fall independent of change in total water content until day 10, following which there is a slow fall in sodium and chloride content of muscle matched by a progressive rise in potassium content over the next 50 days to the end of the experiment. These observations suggest that there is a range of dynamic equilibria in skeletal muscle, with different ratios of intracellular and extracellular ions, that is compatible with survival. Repair by replacement of sodium by potassium and magnesium within the cells proceeds slowly and is relatively independent of changes in water content.

Similar processes may occur in severe debilitating illness as well as with the hypoxia of hypoperfusion and acidosis of shock. Intracellular sodium may be higher than normal and intracellular potassium lower per unit of intracellular water in severe illness; in addition, a substantial expansion of the ECF and an increase in TBW with Na_e/K_e ratios substantially greater than 1.0 have been demonstrated.[1]

THE METABOLISM OF WATER AND ELECTROLYTES

Water Balance

Man requires free water to maintain water balance. Even with maximum concentration of urine solutes, the water contained in the foods of a normal diet and the water produced by oxidation of food are inadequate to provide for urinary excretion of the end-products of metabolism, for losses of water from the bowel and, through vaporization, from the respiratory tract and skin. The amount of water and dilute liquids ingested daily varies widely with habit and climate, but in temperate climates averages 1,000 to 2,500 ml a day. Water in semisolid and solid foods averages 1,000 to 1,500 ml. Water of oxidation adds 200 to 400 ml a day. The average adult therefore adds a total of 2,500 to 4,500 ml of water daily to a body pool of 30 to 50 liters.

Loss takes place by four different routes: urinary output and the water content of stool, both of which are measurable, and by evaporation from the respiratory tract and from the skin, measured only with great difficulty and termed "insensible losses." In the normal individual water intake and loss balance very closely, and daily body weight fluctuates less than 2 per cent and usually less than 1 per cent if determined at the same time of day. Insensible losses depend on body size, physical exertion, and environmental temperature and humidity. In an environment of moderate temperature and humidity losses are substantially less than in a warm humid environment where sweat loss becomes large. Respiratory insensible loss averages 300 to 500 ml per day in females and up to 750 ml per day in males. Surface evaporation and sweat together average 400 to 600 ml a day. Total insensible water loss is between 300 and 500 ml per M^2 of body surface area per day with minimal activity in a temperate environment.[13,14,23] Sweat volume is small in a temperate climate except with vigorous activity, but may reach several liters a day, with serious losses of both water and sodium chloride, in warm humid environments with exposure to the sun.

Daily or more frequent *weighing* is the only reliable method of keeping track of insensible losses. Combined with a record of measured intake and of urinary volume and bowel output, body weight permits reasonably accurate accounting of water balance on a day-to-day basis.

Urinary volume represents the difference between total water intake plus water of oxidation and the sum of insensible losses plus the water in stool (normally 100 to 200 ml per day). Normal adults excrete from 1,000 to 2,500 ml of urine a day. Minimal urine volume with normal kidney function in a young adult is 400 to 600 ml per day. This requires the ability to concentrate the urine to a specific gravity of above 1.030 and with an osmolality of 1,000 to 1,400 mO. Urea represents more than one-half the total solutes from a normal diet. Urea excretion is increased by high protein intake and by trauma or sepsis which produces increased catabolism of body cell mass. A large protein intake or illness may substantially increase minimal urine volume. Renal disease increases the minimal volume required to clear a given solute load, since the ability to concentrate the urine is diminished or lost.

Thirst. Physiologic stimuli produce a sensation of dryness of the mouth and hypopharynx and the desire to drink, thereby stimulating ingestion of water. These stimuli result from a decrease in volume of body fluids without change in osmolality or an increase in osmolality without change in volume and are usually a combination of both. A 1 to 2 per cent decrease in total body water is the usual stimulus, and represents a change of 350 to 700 ml in the normal adult. A decrease in intravascular volume, as seen with acute hemorrhage, and the infusion or ingestion of hypertonic solutions are also effective stimuli to the sensation of thirst. The centers for control of thirst are located in the ventromedial and anterior hypothalamus, and are in close relationship to or overlap the centers of the neurohypophysis which regulate antidiuretic hormone (ADH).[16,24]

Thirst may occur in spite of a normal or even overexpanded total body water if intracellular fluid is decreased by infusion of hypertonic extracellular fluids, or if effective interstitial and intravascular fluid volumes are decreased by rapid sequestration of a part of the volumes into an area of injury, such as a burn or an infection, or by rapid accumulation of ascitic fluid or peripheral edema. Thirst is inhibited by expansion of total body water, by reduction of osmolality, or by isotonic expansion of body fluids. Experimental and accidental traumatic lesions of the ventromedial and anterior hypothalamus and tumors of this region may affect both thirst mechanism and ADH secretion.[24]

Antidiuretic Hormone (ADH). As thirst is the regulator of input of water in man, so antidiuretic hormone has a fundamental role in the regulation of water balance and the control of water excretion. By altering the permeability to water of the cells of distal renal tubules and collecting ducts, ADH controls the amount of water reabsorbed and the volume of urine excreted. When ADH level is high in the plasma, the epithelium of the distal tubules and collecting ducts is more permeable to water which diffuses from the tubules into the hypertonic medullary interstitium of the kidney and is thus returned to the circulation. When ADH levels are low, the distal nephron is relatively impermeable to water and a larger volume of urine of a lower osmolality is excreted. With severe reduction in plasma ADH, as occurs with injury to the neurohypophysis, very large volumes of very dilute urine are excreted, necessitating ingestion of many liters of water a day to prevent dehydration from this state of diabetes insipidus.

The tracts responsible for the synthesis, storage and release of ADH consist of paraventricular hypothalamic and supraoptic nuclei and the neurohypophyseal tract of axons arising from cells in these nuclei which pass down the stalk of the pituitary into the posterior lobe of the gland. The hormone must be stored within the hypothalamic course of these axons as well as in the neurohypophysis, since, following hypophysectomy or pituitary stalk section for such conditions as metastatic breast cancer, only a minor fraction of the patients have permanent diabetes insipidus.

Table 8–5 summarizes the factors which are known to stimulate or inhibit ADH secretion. The normal half-life of ADH in the circulation is about 15 to 20 minutes. The length of time necessary for a water load to shut off ADH is 90 to 120 minutes. Most of the ADH in the circulation is

Table 8–5.   Factors Which Stimulate or Inhibit Release of ADH[24]

	Stimulate	*Inhibit*
Osmotic	Hyperosmolar extracellular fluid	Hypoosmolar extracellular fluid
Nonosmotic	Decreased carotid artery and aortic blood pressure via baroreceptors	Elevated blood pressure
	Decreased tension in left atrial wall and pulmonary veins	Increased left auricular pressure
	Emotional stress or pain	
	Quiet standing	Supine position
	Elevated temperature of blood	Cold, ↓ blood temperature
	Drugs: Acetylcholine, morphine, meperidine, barbiturates, nicotine	Alcohol, diphenyl-hydantoin, epinephrine? atropine?
	? Low oxygen saturation via carotid body	
	Low plasma volume or ECF	

deactivated by the liver and kidneys, while about 10 per cent is excreted in the urine.[24,25]

Inappropriate secretion of ADH results in major alteration of body fluid balance through water retention. The clinical findings, as discussed by Bartter and Schwartz,[25] are: (1) hyponatremia with hypoosmolality of the plasma, (2) continued renal excretion of Na^+ despite hyponatremia, (3) absence of clinical evidence of volume depletion, (4) urine less than maximally dilute, (5) normal renal and adrenal function.

The primary causes of the syndrome of inappropriate secretion of ADH include tumors (particularly cancer of the lung or pancreas which synthesizes ectopic ADH); injury, infection, trauma or tumors of the brain or its meninges; pulmonary infection of severe degree, often with cavity formation; the postoperative state with anesthesia and sepsis; and, most commonly, injudicious overloading of patients with parenteral dextrose and water.

Symptoms appear to be related to the rate of change of the sodium concentration and osmolality of the plasma. If these fall slowly, over several days or weeks, there are essentially no complaints until the sodium concentration falls to approxi-

mately 120 mEq/L. With a rapid dilution by water ingestion or infusion or when the serum sodium is below 120 mEq/L, loss of appetite, nausea, vomiting and weakness are the chief complaints. Patients become drowsy, irritable, confused and sometimes hostile. Muscle weakness is pronounced, deep tendon reflexes are diminished or absent, and neurologic signs resembling bulbar palsy may be seen. Coma, convulsions and death may occur. Edema is rare, except with water overloading in excess of 3 to 4 liters.

Plasma sodium and chloride concentrations tend to fall together in patients with inappropriate ADH release. Bicarbonate concentration of the plasma remains nearly normal, as does blood pH. The urine volume is not increased, and a relative oliguria may exist. The finding of substantial amounts of sodium in the urine (30 to 50 mEq/L or more) in the face of hyponatremia is characteristic, and is seen only with inappropriate ADH, adrenal insufficiency or severe renal disease.

Treatment consists of water restriction. A maximum intake of 500 to 700 ml a day in the adult, with 150 gm of carbohydrate either orally or as 25 per cent dextrose in the limited volume of water given slowly intravenously into the superior vena cava will result in a progressive rise in plasma sodium and osmolality. Urine volume tends to rise. If water intoxication from excessive water by infusion is the cause, a brisk diuresis may occur, while urine sodium excretion diminishes. Unless sodium depletion is known to exist concurrently, sodium salts usually should not be administered.

The inappropriate ADH syndrome may persist for a long period of time. Nolph's study of such a case[26] suggests that water retention is independent of sodium intake. With an expanding volume on a constant sodium intake, sodium loss in the urine increased while potassium was retained. The sodium loss, however, was insufficient to explain the resulting hyponatremia without substantial water retention. Neither an increase in glomerular filtration rate nor a decrease in aldosterone secretion explained the sodium loss which accompanied volume expansion. Nolph postulated a decrease in proximal renal tubular sodium reabsorption, possibly triggered by the expansion of ECF volume to explain the phenomenon. Water restriction resulted in a markedly positive sodium balance in his patient, while increasing sodium intake merely resulted in isotonic expansion.

An excellent review of regulation of body fluids by Shore and Claybaugh[27] is recommended as a resource for greater detail.

Electrolyte Metabolism

In this section consideration is given to the metabolism of sodium, potassium and chloride. Calcium, magnesium, phosphate, iron, iodine and other trace elements have been considered in other chapters.

Sodium Balance. *Sodium Intake.* The value of salt, sodium chloride in relatively pure state, has been recognized since early recorded history as not only a pleasurable but also essential component of man's diet. In most of the world today intake of sodium salts is regulated more by taste, custom and habit than by need. Careful planning of diets is necessary to reduce sodium intake below 1 gm a day, which is approximately the minimal requirement for an active normal adult in a temperate climate. Diets containing less than 0.3 gm of sodium are unpalatable and not well tolerated by most patients.

Normal sodium intake varies from 2 gm to as much as 10 gm a day. A group of 28 adults who volunteered to undergo metabolic balance studies for 2 weeks prior to elective surgery for gallbladder disease or inguinal hernia were permitted to select their own diets and seasoning, the only limitation being moderate fat restriction for those with gallstones and a total caloric intake of 30 to 40 calories per kg body weight a day. Thirty-five diet weeks yielded an average sodium intake in food and added salt of 98.9 mEq (2.28 gm) a day, with two-thirds of the group selecting an intake of from 76 to 120 mEq (1.75 to 2.75 gm). Potassium intake ranged from 65 to 88 mEq (2.5 to 3.4 gm) and chloride from 85 to 145 mEq (2.4 to 4.1 gm).[23] All but 6 to 10 mEq of the ingested sodium and 4 to 6 mEq of potassium were recovered from urine and stool in these patients. Since the patients neither gained nor lost significant weight and were in nitrogen balance, the missing sodium and potassium were interpreted as "insensible loss," probably losses from the skin cells. Streeten, Rapaport and Conn[7] found a mean surface loss of 3.3 mEq of sodium a day in normal volunteers bathed in distilled water whose clothes were also analyzed for sodium loss, so our estimates may be somewhat high.

Renal Regulation of Electrolyte Balance. With an adequate intake of sodium, regulation of sodium concentration of body fluids and of sodium balance is renal. However, sodium balance is not merely a matter of glomerular filtration and of the secretion of sufficient aldosterone to control distal renal tubular reabsorption of sodium. Sodium salts are the primary determinant of the volume and composition of extracellular fluid, and indirectly of the osmolality and composition of cells as well. Extrarenal factors are important in renal regulation of sodium balance.

In a normal adult of average size, approximately 125 ml of plasma are filtered through glomerular membranes each minute. This filtrate contains not only the electrolytes of plasma in their normal concentration in plasma water but also glucose, urea, uric acid, amino acids and creatinine. In 180 liters of glomerular filtrate, taking the Donnan factor of 0.95 for univalent cations and 1.05 for univalent anions into consideration, almost 24,000 mEq of sodium (552 gm), along with nearly 20,000 mEq of chloride, 5,100 mEq of bicarbonate and 684 mEq of potassium, are filtered each day![16] This represents more than 8 times the total body sodium content and 250 times the average daily intake. In order to maintain balance, about 99.5 per cent of the filtered sodium and chloride, virtually all of the bicarbonate and 92 per cent of the potassium must be reabsorbed, along with all of the glucose, most of the amino acids and a substantial portion of urea and uric acid. Only creatinine is excreted without reabsorption. It is obvious, therefore, that regulation of sodium balance by the kidneys depends upon perception of small changes in extracellular fluid and plasma volume. Regulation is both intrarenal and extrarenal.[28,29]

Intrarenal Factors Controlling Sodium Balance. When the *glomerular filtration rate* falls, the fall in sodium excretion is proportionately much larger than the decrease in the glomerular filtration rate. Since 99.5 per cent of filtered sodium is normally reabsorbed, a small change in filtration rate represents a substantial reduction in the total amount of sodium filtered. With a rise in GFR there is relatively little increase in sodium excreted.

The proximal renal tubule is probably responsible for much of the "balance" changes in proximal *tubular absorption* which occur very rapidly with change in GFR and are probably not humorally controlled. Aldosterone controls distal tubular sodium reabsorption and potassium secretion. Changes in dietary sodium intake induce reciprocal levels of aldosterone secretion by the adrenals, and by this mechanism balance is maintained under normal conditions.

However, patients adrenalectomized for advanced breast cancer, or adrenal hyperplasia, can maintain sodium balance on varied intakes of sodium and a constant intake of cortisone, provided sodium intake is not extremely low. Also, escape from administered aldosterone occurs by excretion of sodium in the urine after excessive (300 mEq) sodium loading by saline infusion. While aldosterone takes about one hour to produce an effect, decrease in blood volume produces an almost immediate effect on renal sodium excretion. These facts have led to postulation of the existence of a "third factor" in renal control of sodium which is released by volume expansion and which decreases sodium reabsorption by the proximal nephron.[28]

Extrarenal Factors Controlling Sodium Balance. A decrease in left auricular pressure results in increased renal sodium retention, as does a decrease in blood volume. Conversely, an increase in left auricular pressure results in increased sodium output, as does isotonic volume loading unless cardiac output is decreased.

Salt depletion enhances renin output, activating aldosterone through angiotensin mediators and resulting in sodium retention. Salt loading increases renal blood flow and decreases renin output with a resultant increase in sodium excretion.

Edema, whether due to right-sided heart failure, liver disease, the nephrotic syndrome or hypovolemia and hypoproteinemia on a nutritional basis, results in decreased renal excretion of sodium and in an expansion of the ECF. Because of decreased GFR and renal blood flow, the kidneys behave as if the blood volume were decreased. Renal control of sodium balance is based on "effective" or "functional" blood volume and ECF, rather than absolute values of either.

The common causes of hyponatremia and of hypernatremia are listed in Table 8–6. Absolute deficiency or excess of sodium, which determines treatment, depends not only on *concentration,* but also on total *volume* of plasma and ECF, which must be assessed on the basis of history and physical examination of the patient.

Potassium Balance. Daily potassium intake in food usually varies from 60 to 100 mEq; almost all of this is excreted in the urine with a small component in feces in the absence of diarrhea. Intracellular potassium is lost with debilitating diseases entailing loss of body cell mass, in substantial amounts with diuretics and as the result of steroid administration. Immediately following surgical operations or other trauma, potassium is lost in excess of that expected from nitrogen loss, and appears in high concentration in the urine. There is often a transient rise in plasma potassium concentration during and immediately after surgical treatment, a rise that is accentuated in the debilitated, hyponatremic patient with an expanded extracellular fluid. Potassium is retained, and a positive balance is achieved in 1 or 2 days before nitrogen balance becomes positive in early convalescence following illness.

Plasma or Serum Potassium Concentration. This is *not* a reliable index of total body potassium, nor is it per se an indication for the administration or withholding of potassium. Only the extremes of high and low concentration are of themselves important. Potassium concentration in excess of 6 mEq/L with no hemolysis in the specimen requires an explanation and ap-

Table 8–6. Causes of Hyponatremia and Hypernatremia

1. Hyponatremia = plasma sodium concentration less than 135 mEq/L:
    A. In patients with chronic wasting illnesses, e.g. cancer, chronic infection, liver disease, semistarvation, ulcerative colitis, congestive heart failure, ascites and edema.
    B. Following major surgical treatment or extensive trauma, e.g. extensive soft tissue injury, burns, major fractures, severe infection, fluid sequestration in a third space of tissue injury, transcellular pooling, anesthesia, morphine, and meperidine.
    C. With excessive water intake, usually iatrogenic, e.g. antidiuresis of trauma or chronic debility, excessive intravenous glucose and water, retained water from irrigations or hypotonic wet dressings, excessive oral intake, acute renal insufficiency without adequate water restriction, inappropriate ADH syndrome.
    D. As the result of abnormal external loss of sodium with inadequate replacement, e.g. gastrointestinal losses through diarrhea or vomiting or intestinal intubation, bowel, biliary or pancreatic fistulas, decompression of incompletely obstructed distal urinary tract, osmotic diuresis from glucose, mannitol or urea, excessive sweating, adrenal insufficiency.
    E. As the result of dietary restriction or drugs, e.g. chlorothiazide, mercurial diuretcs, ethacrynic acid or furosemide diuresis, low sodium diets for prolonged periods, particularly in chronic heart, liver or kidney disease and for hypertension.
    F. Factitious, e.g. laboratory error or sampling error with dilution by glucose infusion or other sodium-free sources of water.
2. Hypernatremia = plasma sodium more than 150 mEq/L:
    A. Dehydration by loss of hypotonic fluid (desiccation) without adequate water replacement, e.g. respiratory loss with fever, dry oxygen, tracheotomy, hyperventilation of dyspnea and metabolic acidosis, skin losses with burns, fever of various etiologies, prolonged exposure to dry heat.
    B. Excessive solute loading: Concentrated tube feedings of all types high in protein and salts without adequate supplemental water intake, electrolyte solutions as the total source of water intake.
    C. Large volume of dilute urine, e.g. ineffective antidiuretic hormone level, diabetes insipidus, brain stem injury, and posthypophysectomy state.

propriate treatment. Levels of potassium of 7 mEq/L or higher constitute an emergency requiring immediate action for the patient who is threatened with cardiac arrest.

Respiratory or metabolic acidosis, hypoxia, dehydration, renal insufficiency and extensive trauma all tend to raise the plasma potassium concentration by transfer of potassium from cells to extracellular fluid. Patients with chronic debilitating illnesses are likely to have an exaggerated rise in potassium concentration in the immediate postoperative period, and particular attention should be paid to the risk of hyperkalemia in such patients despite the fact that their total body potassium may be diminished by as much as 50 per cent.

Significantly low potassium concentrations begin with values below 3.5 mEq/L. Values of 2.5 mEq or lower are serious, particularly if accompanied by a metabolic alkalosis, as is usually the case. Infusions of dextrose in water will lower the plasma potassium in a fasting patient by about 0.5 mEq/L below resting levels, since potassium is withdrawn from the plasma in the process of glycogen synthesis. Alkalosis, both metabolic and respiratory, lowers plasma potasssium concentration as the result of an intracellular shift and increased renal excretion of potassium.

Hypokalemia. A plasma potassium level of less than 3.5 mEq/L is often accompanied by disordered smooth muscle function, with production or prolongation of paralytic ileus. Sensitivity to digitalis is one of the most important hazards of hypokalemia, with digitalis toxicity appearing with otherwise normal doses. The electrocardiogram in hypokalemia is frequently associated with depressed R-ST, flattened or inverted T waves, prolonged Q-T interval and U waves; various arrhythmias may develop. Marked weakness and lethargy are common. Occasionally the usual hyporeflexia progresses to ascending skeletal muscle paralysis and interference with function of the muscles of respiration; swallowing becomes a serious and sometimes fatal event. Common causes of hypokalemia are listed in Table 8–7.

Hypokalemic alkalosis is commonly seen in patients who have lost chloride, hydrogen ion and potassium from the gastrointestinal tract by vomiting or gastric suction. In the early phases a fall in potassium concentration is related to alkalosis as bicarbonate rises to compensate for

Table 8–7. Common Causes of Hypokalemia

Hypokalemia = plasma potassium levels less than 3.5 mEq/L:

1. Loss of chloride as acid gastric juice leading to metabolic alkalosis and potassium loss by vomiting or aspiration of the stomach.
2. Administration of diuretics, particularly the chlorothiazide types, with a metabolic alkalosis and marked renal potassium loss.
3. Following trauma, surgical treatment or anesthesia, with antidiuresis and sodium conservation, and major urinary loss of potassium in excess of nitrogen; usually potassium intake is markedly reduced in these situations. (Often a transient hyperkalemia precedes postoperative hypokalemia.)
4. Administration of adrenal steroids or the presence of Cushing's disease.
5. In the rehydration phase, following dehydration, particularly in patients with dehydration due to diabetic acidosis, where severe hypokalemia may occur during rehydration, insulin therapy and treatment of acidosis.
6. In chronic renal disease where there is tubular wastage of potassium.
7. With prolonged acidosis or alkalosis, of whatever cause, due to renal wastage of potassium.
8. In patients on prolonged parenteral fluid therapy with inadequate potassium replacement, particularly those with small bowel fistulas or prolonged suction drainage of the gastrointestinal tract.

N.B. All of the above are enhanced by a preexisting deficit of total body potassium due to wasting diseases with loss of body cell mass and expansion of extracellular fluid.

chloride loss. Laboratory values show a plasma chloride below 95 mEq/L and total carbon dioxide in excess of 30 mEq/L. Plasma sodium concentration may be low, particularly with inadequate replacement. Plasma potassium will be in the range of 2.5 to 3.2 mEq/L and pH will be 7.45 to 7.52 if P_{CO_2} is normal. Urine pH is initially alkaline but becomes acid, despite elevated plasma total carbon dioxide, bicarbonate and pH levels. Recent work has shown that both chloride ion and potassium must be administered to correct the alkalosis, which begins with loss of chloride and hydrogen ion, is increased in severity by renal wastage of potassium in the presence of an alkalosis, and is perpetuated by an increased renal tubular reabsorption of bicarbonate, which continues the alkalosis and results in the paradoxical aciduria.

The treatment of hypokalemia is the administration of potassium chloride. Intravenous solutions should not exceed 40 mEq/L of potassium ion per liter, and the salt must therefore be given in 5 per cent glucose in water or other isotonic solutions. The rate of intravenous administration of potassium salts should not normally exceed 30 mEq per hour in the average-sized adult, except in emergency situations such as digitalis toxicity or skeletal muscle paralysis when constant electrocardiogram monitoring is essential. Therapeutic doses of potassium chloride are 50 to 150 mEq per day, and 40 mEq per day is indicated in baseline parenteral fluids. Potassium can be given by mouth either in the form of high-potassium fluids such as orange or grapefruit juice or as solutions of KCl (7.5 to 10 per cent). High concentrations of potassium salts are irritating to the stomach, and should be diluted before administration.

Hyperkalemia. Plasma levels of potassium above 6 mEq/L must be considered abnormally elevated and potentially dangerous, and levels of 7 mEq/L or higher are emergencies. The biochemistry laboratory should notify the floor staff and the responsible physician at once when plasma potassium levels of 6.5 mEq/L or more are found. The electrocardiogram changes include peaking of T waves and widening of the QRS complex, and various arrhythmias may develop. The chief danger is death from cardiac arrest. Causes of this condition are listed in Table 8–8. The most common cause is renal insufficiency, and some degree of renal insufficiency exists with hypovolemia in most patients with hyperkalemia, except that caused by acute hypoxia.

Immediate treatment of hyperkalemia consists of measures to decrease the plasma concentration rapidly, including:

1. The administration of sodium bicarbonate intravenously to combat acidosis and shift potassium intracellularly; 44 mEq in 200 ml of 5 per cent glucose in water can be used as a test dose, with electrocardiogram monitoring. Decreases in the amplitude and spiking of T waves are favorable signs.

Table 8–8.   Common Causes of Hyperkalemia

Hyperkalemia = plasma potassium 6.0 mEq/L or more; emergency level 7.0 mEq/L or more.
1. Acute or chronic renal failure, whether due to parenchymal disease, perfusion, deficiency or obstruction.
2. Acute dehydration, adrenal insufficiency, diabetic acidosis.
3. Immediately following massive injury, burns, major operations. Potentiated by preexisting body cell wasting disease and increased by the presence of devitalized tissue and extravascular blood.
4. Severe metabolic or respiratory acidosis and with prolonged inadequate perfusion of tissues (shock).
5. Major infection, hemorrhage into the gastrointestinal tract or other causes of rapid and massive catabolic use of protein, in the presence of some degree of renal insufficiency.
6. Overly rapid infusion of high concentrations of potassium salts.
7. Factitious factors, e.g. hemolysis of blood specimen or laboratory error in measurement.

2. The administration of glucose with insulin intravenously to utilize potassium for glycogen synthesis. One unit of regular insulin for each 5 gm of glucose is usually safe. If mixed with the glucose, thorough initial mixing and frequent agitation of the flask to assure uniform distribution of the insulin are important.

3. The intravenous use of calcium gluconate for temporary alleviation by calcium of the effects of hyperkalemia on the heart.

Further treatment includes the elimination of potassium intake in food and parenterally and the use of sodium-charged polystyrene sulfonate resins (Kayexalate) either orally or by enema. In patients with renal failure, peritoneal dialysis or hemodialysis is often necessary. Such measures are essential when plasma potassium levels of 7 mEq/L persist or recur after the emergency treatment outlined.

Chloride. Normal plasma chloride concentration is 100 to 106 mEq/L, a value which, like that of plasma sodium, is subject to very little normal variation. Dietary intake is usually in excess of sodium and virtually all of the intake is excreted in the urine, the excess constituting, with phosphate, sulfate and uric acid, a titratable acidity of 40 to 60 mEq of hydrogen ion a day. Changes in chloride ion concentration in the plasma follow those of sodium in dilutional hypotonicity and in desiccation dehydration. Deviation from the normal plasma sodium/chloride ratio of slightly less than 3:2 is usually due to excessive chloride loss from the gastrointestinal tract or kidneys or to chloride retention with renal disease or ureterointestinal anastomoses (Table 8–9).

ACID-BASE BALANCE

L. J. Henderson in 1909 pointed out the significance of bicarbonate as a reserve of alkali in excess of acids other than carbonic, and developed the "Henderson equation." Hasselbalch devised a hydrogen electrode which would function in the presence of carbon dioxide, demonstrated the influence of respiration on blood pH and suggested the logarithmic form of Henderson-Hasselbalch equation (vide infra). D. D. Van Slyke, who recounted these facts in *Summary of Acid Base History in Physiology and Medicine*,[30] developed volumetric apparatus for measuring the total CO_2 content of plasma and demonstrated that the Gibbs-Donnan theory, as applied

---

Table 8–9. Common Causes of Hypochloremia and Hyperchloremia

Hypochloremia = plasma chloride level less than 98 mEq/L.
1. Dilutional, with hyponatremia, in an expanded extracellular fluid following trauma, with wasting diseases, in water retention with overloading, with sequestration of extracellular fluid in a third space of injury.
2. Chloride loss from the gastrointestinal tract, particularly from vomiting or gastric suction but common with salt loss from all levels without adequate replacement.
3. Diuretics, with a loss of chloride in excess of sodium and with high loss of potassium in urine.
4. Adrenal steroids, with sodium retention and potassium and chloride loss in urine.
5. Compensating mechanism in chronic respiratory acidosis, with high plasma carbon dioxide level and normal or low pH.
6. Combined with an elevated plasma carbon dioxide level and pH and a low plasma potassium level in hypokalemic hypochloremic alkalosis.
7. Chronic renal disease and acute renal failure.
Hyperchloremia = plasma chloride above 110 mEq/L.
1. Combined with hypernatremia in desiccation dehydration, with excess solute loading, or in diabetes insipidus or brain stem injury.
2. Ureterointestinal anastomoses due to reabsorption of chloride by the bowel, potentiated by renal insufficiency and by prolonged exposure of bowel mucosa to urine.
3. Iatrogenic—with excessive administration of ammonium chloride or hydrochloric acid.

to the distribution of electrolytes across membranes, fitted chloride and bicarbonate distribution with oxidation and reduction of hemoglobin in the erythrocyte-plasma system. He also defined buffers as ". . . substances which by their presence in a solution increase the amount of acid or alkali that must be added to cause a unit change in pH." Peters and Van Slyke in 1931 introduced the terms *metabolic acidosis and alkalosis* and *respiratory acidosis and alkalosis,* referring to those conditions in the body which produced changes primarily in the plasma bicarbonate concentration as metabolic and to those primarily affecting CO_2 tension as respiratory.[31]

This physiologic language has persisted in clinical medical practice where acidosis and alkalosis are defined as abnormal conditions caused by the accumulation or loss of acid or base.

With rapidly increasing use of pH determination of the blood by clinicians and clinical laboratories in recent years, greater emphasis is being placed on the state of the blood in which pH deviates from normal. In this laboratory language, acidosis and alkalosis are defined in terms of change in pH of the blood and as changes in whole-blood buffering systems in terms of base excess or negative base excess, depending upon the amount of strong acid or strong alkali necessary to return a sample of blood to normal pH under standard conditions of temperature, O_2 saturation and P_{CO_2}.

Definitions of Acid-base

Because of the differences in physiologic (clinical) and laboratory terminology in definition of acidosis and alkalosis and the confusion that resulted, an International Conference was held in 1966 to attempt to develop common definitions. The following definitions are those agreed upon by an ad hoc committee of the Conference[32] and are used in the clinical discussion which follows.

The Brønsted-Lowery System. An *acid* is a substance which is a proton donor. A *base* is a substance which is a proton recipient. The general form for acid-base relationship is given as:

$$A_1 + B_2 \rightleftarrows A_2 + B_1$$

where A_1, B_1 represent one conjugate acid-base pair and A_2, B_2 represent a second conjugate acid-base pair. This takes into consideration the active role of water in solutions.

$$A_1 + B_2 \rightleftarrows A_2 + B_1$$
$$CH_3COOH + H_2O \rightleftarrows [H_3O^+] + [CH_3COO^-]$$
$$H_2CO_3 + H_2O \rightleftarrows [H_3O^+] + [HCO_3^-]$$

Water and H_3O^+ represent one conjugate pair in both systems, acetic acid and the acetate ion and carbonic acid and bicarbonate ion the second conjugate pairs, respectively.

Under Van Slyke's definition of buffers, carbonic, phosphoric, organic acids and the acidic portions of protein molecules (proton donor sites) together with their conjugate bases are *buffers.* Sodium, potassium, magnesium, calcium and chloride *ions* as such do not function as buffers and are neither acids nor bases. They are "aprotes" since they neither donate nor receive protons.

pH is the logarithm of the reciprocal of the hydrogen ion concentration:

$$pH = \log \frac{1}{[H^+]}$$

In thermodynamic terms, pH defines the *hydrogen ion activity:*

$$pH = \log \frac{1}{a_{H^+}} = -\log {}^aH^+$$

Since the activity coefficient for hydrogen ion is not precisely known, it is assumed to be 1, therefore:

$$aH^+ = cH^+$$

where cH is *hydrogen ion concentration* expressed as nanomoles (nM) per liter (10^{-9}

moles). At pH values of whole blood compatible with survival, the concentration of hydrogen ion at 37° C is:

pH	$cH(nM/L)$
7.0	100
7.1	80
7.2	63
7.3	50
7.4	40
7.5	32
7.6	25
7.7	20

It is essential that the temperature and whether whole blood or plasma is examined be stated in reporting both pH and hydrogen ion content or activity.

The Carbon Dioxide System. *Total carbon dioxide concentration* (TCO_2) is the total carbon dioxide extractable from a biologic fluid with strong acid. This includes dissolved carbon dioxide, carbonic acid, bicarbonate ion and carbamino compounds. This is the usual value reported by clinical laboratories as total CO_2 or CO_2 content of plasma.

The *partial pressure of carbon dioxide* (Pco_2) in gas phase in equilibrium with a biologic fluid is usually reported in mm Hg. While Pco_2 can be directly measured by diffusion through a specially prepared Teflon membrane standardized with gas of known CO_2 concentration, the value is often calculated from pH and TCO_2 by use of a nomogram based on the Henderson-Hasselbalch equation.

Carbonic acid concentration (H_2CO_3), in biologic fluids, is very small in comparison to dissolved carbon dioxide concentration. The usual units are mM/L or mEq/L.

Dissolved carbon dioxide concentration, strictly speaking, is the quantity of dissolved carbon dioxide gas in a specified volume; usually H_2CO_3 is included. The sum of the two is designated as S × Pco_2 where S is the solubility coefficient relating the sum of the concentrations of dissolved CO_2 and H_2CO_3 in mM/L to Pco_2 in mm Hg. This value is temperature dependent; at 37° C for blood or plasma, S = 0.0306.

Bicarbonate ion concentration (HCO_3^-) is chemically defined as the concentration of HCO_3^- in biologic fluids. However, in physiologic studies and clinical use, it is calculated as total CO_2 − S × Pco_2. This value includes carbamino compounds and carbonate ion in addition to bicarbonate ion, which makes very little difference in plasma or interstitial fluid but introduces large errors for intracellular fluid:

$$[HCO_3^-] = TCO_2 - S \times P_{CO_2}$$

Standard bicarbonate concentration is the plasma bicarbonate ion concentration of plasma equilibrated at Pco_2 of 40 mm Hg and 37° C. Units are mEq/L.

Bicarbonate concentration at standard pH is similar to standard bicarbonate concentration except that pH is set at 7.40 and Pco_2 is the variable. Units are mEq/L.

Carbon dioxide combining power refers to the total carbon dioxide concentration of plasma, anaerobically drawn and separated from blood, and equilibrated to Pco_2 of 40 mm Hg at room temperature. Units are mM/L. This value is rarely used because of dependence on conditions in the blood when the plasma is separated, and because it is dependent on uncontrolled room temperature.

Buffer Base. The sum of the concentration of buffer ions of whole blood bicarbonate, plasma proteins, and hemoglobin is considered the buffer base. Units are mEq/L. This value and base excess, which is derived from it, are determined on whole blood, and are hemoglobin dependent.

Base Excess. As defined by Astrup and Siggard-Anderson:[32,33] "The base concentration (*of whole blood*) as measured by titration with strong acid to pH 7.40 at a Pco_2 of 40 mm Hg at 37° C. For negative base excess, the titration must be carried out with strong base." Units are mEq/L. Negative base excess is sometimes termed *base deficit.*

Henderson-Hasselbalch Equation.

$$pH = pK_i + \log \frac{[\text{total } CO_2 - S \times P_{CO_2}]}{[S \times P_{CO_2}]}$$

$$pH = pK_i + \log \frac{[HCO_3^-]}{[S \times P_{CO_2}]} \text{ where } pK_i = 6.11$$

The Henderson-Hasselbalch equation is for serum or plasma. Calculation of one value (usually P_{CO_2}) from the other two is frequently done in clinical laboratories.

Acid-base Status of the Blood

Two methods of reporting and evaluating the acid-base status of whole blood and plasma are in current use. Both have strong advocates and each method has both advantages and disadvantages.

The CO_2-bicarbonate Buffer System Method. The older and more commonly used method in the United States characterizes the acid-base status of the *blood* (and by inference of the patient) in terms of the CO_2-bicarbonate buffer system of the plasma. Clinically the most useful measurements are: plasma bicarbonate, $[HCO_3^-]$, blood or plasma P_{CO_2} and plasma pH. Plasma bicarbonate is determined from total CO_2 content of plasma and the pH from the Henderson-Hasselbalch equation. P_{CO_2} is either directly measured with one of several instruments that depend on diffusion of CO_2 through a special CO_2 membrane or it is calculated from total CO_2 and pH. Plasma pH is measured directly from plasma protected against CO_2 loss to air, using a glass electrode pH meter which is standardized against precisely prepared buffer solutions of known pH. The measurement is made at 37° C.

Plasma bicarbonate concentration is used as a measure of the *metabolic* component of acid-base abnormalities, recognizing that alternations in plasma bicarbonate concentration may be manifestations of a primary metabolic derangement or may reflect compensatory changes secondary to a respiratory P_{CO_2} derangement. Similarly, P_{CO_2} is regarded as a measure of the *re-spiratory component* of acid-base disequilibria, recognizing that such changes may either represent the primary derangement or result from secondary compensatory changes.

The Whole Blood Base Excess, or Δ Buffer Base Method. Proponents of this system, based on the work of Siggard-Anderson and Astrup,[33] hold that the metabolic component of acid-base equilibrium can be most precisely determined by titrating to pH 7.40 with strong acid the base excess of *whole blood* which is equilibrated at P_{CO_2} at 40 mm Hg at 37° C. The determination of the number of mEq of base lost or gained by 1 liter of whole blood under these circumstances is independent of respiratory function and represents nonvolatile acid or base accumulation. It is stated that the two most valuable parameters for clinical evaluation of acid-base metabolism are P_{CO_2} and the accumulation of nonvolatile acids or bases.

Values that are determined include: whole blood base excess or ΔBb, blood or plasma P_{CO_2}, plasma pH.

Base excess is not independent of P_{CO_2} in vivo. The titration curve of blood in vivo is slightly different than in vitro. As with any system of analysis of acid-base status, a careful assessment of the patient is essential for clinical interpretation and for determination of therapy.

In the discussion which follows, the first of the two methods will be used. Interconversion is possible with a graph if both oxygen saturation and hemoglobin concentration of whole blood are known, as is often the case with seriously ill patients. Regardless of which method of acid-base terminology and analysis is used, it must be remembered that there are very few independent acid-base variables in blood and that pH, total CO_2, $[HCO_3^-]$, $[H^+]$, $[OH^-]$ and $[\text{hemoglobin}^-]$ are *dependent* variables. Stewart[34] has shown that independent variables constitute only three groups: (1) the partial pressure of CO_2, P_{CO_2}, which is under respiratory control, (2) the difference between the sum of the inorganic cations (excluding H^+) and the anions of strong acids; this component is under renal control through renal regulation of both cation and anion concentrations, and (3) the total buffer present per liter, including protein, and hemoglobin in the case of blood. With knowledge of these three independent variables, the concentration of all the dependent variables, including pH and $[HCO_3^-]$, can be calculated from computer-derived nomograms.

There are two main causes of acid-base disturbance: *respiratory,* due to abnormalities of CO_2 excretion, and *metabolic,* due to abnormalities of production, ingestion or excretion of hydrogen ion.[31,35] Disturbances in one of the two categories usually provoke compensation by the other system. Most patients have a primary defect in one system, with a secondary compensating change in the other. However, 41 per cent of 139 patients studied in detail had mixed primary types of derangements resulting from a wide variety of diseases.

Acidosis and alkalosis should be referred to as conditions which would result in alteration of the pH of blood and plasma *if there were no secondary compensating changes,* and may result in pH changes even with compensation. Acidosis or alkalosis can be further defined as respiratory, metabolic or mixed as the laboratory findings and the clinical pattern indicate. More specific descriptive adjectives, such as renal, diabetic, lactic or respiratory, can be used, without necessarily indicating a change in pH per se.

The Ad Hoc Committee on Acid Base Terminology[32] strongly advised that secondary compensatory mechanisms *are not* and *should not* be considered as acidosis or alkalosis. Rather the primary etiologic factor should be described and compensation indicated, such as "metabolic acidosis with compensatory fall inPco_2" or, better still, simply the laboratory numbers as observed.

Mixed disturbances exist when there are two or more distinct etiologic factors present. These should be described clearly to differentiate them from a single factor with compensation, e.g. "mixed disturbance—metabolic acidosis and respiratory alkalosis," or "mixed disturbance—diabetic and renal acidosis."

Table 8–10 gives the range of normal values found for the set of determinations commonly used in acid-base evaluation. A Siggard-Anderson curve nomogram (Radiometer A/S, Copenhagen, Denmark) is used in determining buffer base and base excess after equilibrating arterial blood (90 per cent saturated with oxygen or more) at 37° C at two standard Pco_2 values, one higher and one lower than Pco_2 40 mm Hg.

A wide variety of nomograms relating pH, total CO_2 amd Pco_2 are in use today. One variant developed by R. V. Stephens in our laboratory from the nomogram devised by Poppell[36] has proved useful clini-

Table 8–10. Whole Blood and Plasma Values for Acid-Base Evaluation

	Range of Normal	95% Confidence Limits of Laboratory Method
Hemoglobin	12.5–16.0 gm/100 ml	± 5% of value
pH (arterial)	7.35–7.45	± 0.02 pH units
Pco₂ (arterial)	35–45 mm Hg	± 3% of value
Plasma total CO₂	24–28.8 mM/L	± 0.2 mM/L
[HCO₃⁻] plasma	22.85–27.45 mEq/L	Calculated value, see text.
Buffer base	43–47 mEq/L whole blood	See text
Base excess	−3 to +3 mEq/L	See text

cally because it relates the two most commonly measured factors in acid-base determination, pH and total CO_2, to acidosis and alkalosis of both metabolic and respiratory origin. The pH is plotted in such a fashion that P_{CO_2} values are straight lines, thus making the determination simpler.[37] Its use is demonstrated in later figures.

Metabolic Acidosis

Metabolic acidosis is a set of conditions that without compensatory changes would tend toward a decrease in the pH of blood. *Usually compensation is incomplete.* The pH of arterial blood is less than 7.38, total CO_2 less than 24 mEq and P_{CO_2} less than 35 mm Hg. The common causes of metabolic acidosis may be divided into four major groups.

1. Increased production of organic acids.
   A. Ketosis with increased fat metabolism, occurring in diabetes mellitus; starvation; hypermetabolism of thyrotoxicosis, fever and sepsis; high-fat low-carbohydrate diets; following trauma and major operations, often combined with relative starvation and acute dehydration, particularly in infants.
   B. Cellular hypoxia including lactic acidosis resulting from prolonged inadequate oxygenation of tissues; pulmonary insufficiency, acute or chronic; hypermetabolism, due to exertion, seizures, fever; congestive heart failure; shock, whether due to hemorrhage or sepsis; anesthesia, cardiopulmonary bypass and acute adrenal insufficiency.
2. Decreased excretion of hydrogen ion due to renal dysfunction, with retention of $[SO_4^=]$ and $[HPO_4^=]$ ions, occurring with decreased renal blood flow in shock, cardiac failure, hypovolemia and vascular disease, intrinsic renal disease, acute or chronic; ob-

structive uropathy; renal disease plus a high-protein diet, $MgSO_4$, NH_4Cl or methionine and ureterosigmoidostomy with renal disease.
3. Loss of base in excess of chloride and sulfate ions resulting from dehydration with sodium loss from diarrhea, biliary or pancreatic fistulas, long tube drainage or small bowel fistula and diuretics that inhibit carbonic anhydrase.
4. Increased intake of acid, e.g. acidifying salts such as NH_4Cl and $CaCl_2$; amino acid solutions given parenterally or in elemental diets, particularly if the amino acids are present as hydrochlorides or sodium chloride in the presence of reduced renal function.

Compensation for metabolic acidosis is both respiratory and renal. Respiration is increased in rate and particularly in depth with a lowering of P_{CO_2} and a partial return of pH toward normal. Renal adjustment, if renal function permits, is a slower process involving an increase in both ammonium ion production and titratable acidity with increased hydrogen ion excretion and conservation of base to restore plasma bicarbonate toward normal. High correlation exists between plasma P_{CO_2} and plasma $[HCO_3^-]$ (r = .97) and between blood pH and plasma P_{CO_2} (r = .83) in a series of 60 children with uncomplicated metabolic acidosis.[38] Respiratory compensation by marked and sustained hyperventilation is characteristic of metabolic acidosis and a useful clinical sign of its presence.

Treatment is directed toward the cause of acidosis. In addition, therapy must be planned to reinforce the diminished bicarbonate reserve and combat the hyperkalemia, which may become a serious threat. Efforts should be made to keep the CO_2 content of the plasma at or above 15 mEq/L, and the best drug for this purpose is sodium bicarbonate, which provides sodium without the anion of a strong acid. Experience has demonstrated that it takes

STATE	ΔpH	ΔPCO$_2$	ΔTCO$_2$	EARLY SECONDARY COMPENSATION
Metabolic Alkalosis	↑	± TO ↑	↑ *	Variable ΔPCO$_2$ within O$_2$ limits, Renal excretion [HCO$_3$]$^-$
Respiratory Alkalosis	↑	↓ *	± TO ↓	Renal? [HCO$_3$]$^-$ excretion ↑Organic acid c̄ Hypoxia
Metabolic Acidosis	↓	↓	↓ *	Hyperventilation, Renal [H]$^+$ excretion
Respiratory Acidosis	↓	↑ *	↑	Renal excretion of Cl$^-$ and [H]$^-$

* INITIAL AND PRIMARY CHANGE

Fig. 8–9. Primary changes in pH, PCO$_2$ and total CO$_2$ resulting from metabolic or respiratory alkalosis and acidosis. Compensatory changes are also indicated.

2 mEq of NaHCO$_3$ per liter of extracellular fluid to raise the plasma CO$_2$ by 1mEq/L. Thus, a patient who has a CO$_2$ content of 10 mEq/L and who weighs 70 kg will require 140 mEq of NaHCO$_3$ to restore the CO$_2$ to 15 mEq/L ($70 \times 0.2 \times 5 \times 2 = 140$). This may be administered as an isotonic solution (1.2 per cent) or in critically ill patients as a 5 per cent solution given slowly intravenously. Serum potassium level may fall markedly and, hence, must be carefully monitored. Potassium must be administered if this occurs. It is not necessary to give enough NaHCO$_3$ to bring the plasma CO$_2$ to normal levels, and the amount of sodium required to do so may be excessive. Titration to maintain a CO$_2$ somewhere above 15 mEq/L is usually adequate in the short-term management of metabolic acidosis.

Figure 8–9 summarizes the primary changes that occur in pH, PCO$_2$ and total CO$_2$ in metabolic and respiratory acidosis and alkalosis, together with the early compensatory changes induced by the primary condition.

Respiratory Acidosis

Retention of carbon dioxide is a condition which, if compensating mechanisms were not available, would produce a fall in the pH of blood. Although complete compensation is seen in mild cases, compensation is usually incomplete, with a fall in pH of the blood, accompanied by a compensatory increase in total CO$_2$ of the plasma. There is an increase of hydrogen ion and a decrease in pH of the blood caused by an increase in PCO$_2$ and in H$_2$CO$_3$. The pH of blood is usually less than 7.38, and the PCO$_2$ is more than 47 and usually more than 50 mm Hg. The CO$_2$ content of the plasma is not altered in the acute phase but rises with compensation and is elevated in chronic form. Arterial blood gas and pH determinations are diagnostic.

Common causes of respiratory acidosis are: (1) hypoventilation, which may be due to airway obstruction, pneumothorax, pleural effusion, atelectasis, pneumonitis, thoracotomy, upper abdominal incisions or skeletal muscle weakness (carbon dioxide retention often occurs acutely as the result of medications which depress respiration, e.g. anesthesia, narcotics, barbiturates and other sedatives or muscle relaxants), (2) arteriovenous shunting in poorly ventilated segments of the lungs due to atelectasis or pneumonitis or interstitial edema, resulting in elevation of systemic arterial P_{CO_2}, (3) inadequate ventilation with respirators.

Compensation for respiratory acidosis is renal with increased tubular reabsorption of sodium and bicarbonate and increased secretion of chloride and hydrogen ion. The result is a rise in plasma bicarbonate which partially or completely restores pH to normal.

Acute respiratory acidosis requires emergency treatment, the success of which rests on recognition of inadequate ventilation long prior to the development of cyanosis. Restlessness and a rise in blood pressure and pulse rate may be the first signs of hypercapnea and hypoxia. Hypotension follows. The use of narcotics only increases the problem through suppression of the respiratory center. Making certain of the airway, administering oxygen cautiously, and assisting respiration are indicated.

Figure 8–10 demonstrates on the Stephens nomogram the changes that occur with respiratory acidosis and with metabolic acidosis. Line A-A, from Elkinton,[35] represents the effect of inhalation of 7.5 per cent CO_2 on normal individuals with resultant acute respiratory acidosis. There is no change in total CO_2 beyond that due to dissolved CO_2 with the increased P_{CO_2}. Lines B-B and C-C represent two different groups of patients with respiratory acidosis from the study of Eichenholz et al.[40] Group I (line B-B) were patients not treated with factors likely to produce metabolic alkalosis, while group II patients (line C-C) had received diuretics or steroid therapy, or had vomited or been on gastric suction, all factors known to produce metabolic alkalosis. The increased levels of bicarbonate at several levels of P_{CO_2} in the second group of patients are evident. This group constitutes a

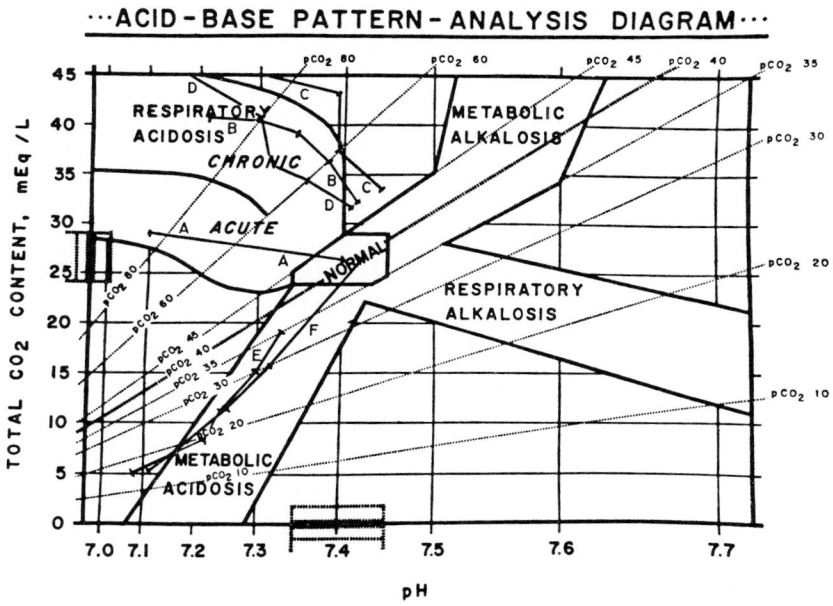

Fig. 8–10. Patient data from the literature showing acute and chronic respiratory acidosis and metabolic acidosis. These data are plotted on the Stephens nomogram relating pH and total CO_2 of plasma to P_{CO_2} and indicating the zone of values usually seen in primary disturbances.[37] A-A: Acute respiratory acidosis,[35] B-B: chronic respiratory acidosis,[40] C-C: mixed disturbance, chronic respiratory acidosis and metabolic alkalosis,[40] D-D: linear regression, respiratory acidosis,[35] E-E: metabolic acidosis, adults,[35] F-F: metabolic acidosis, children.[38] Plots are corrected to reflect total CO_2.

mixed disturbance of respiratory acidosis with compensation by an increase in total CO_2 and in bicarbonate. Line D-D, also from Elkinton,[35] is a plot of the regression $[HCO_3^-] = 20.6 + 0.20 \ P_{CO_2}$. Elkinton points out that the relationship of the rising bicarbonate to rising P_{CO_2} is curvilinear and would better fit a curvilinear regression as is suggested by the curves of B-B and C-C.

Metabolic acidosis with compensation by hyperventilation with reduction of P_{CO_2} is illustrated by lines E-E and F-F. E-E is a plot of data on 27 patients with metabolic acidosis.[35] The regression equation for this series is $P_{CO_2} = 8.8 + 1.51 \ [HCO_3^-] \pm 4.0$. Data on 60 children with uncomplicated metabolic acidosis observed by Albert et al.[38] (F-F) have the regression equation of $P_{CO_2} = 1.54 \ [HCO_3^-] + 8.36$. The similarity of response of the adults and the children is striking and would appear to indicate an essentially normal response.

Metabolic Alkalosis

Metabolic alkalosis is a condition which would tend to elevate the pH of blood or plasma in the absence of compensatory changes and which does so when compensation is incomplete. The common causes of metabolic alkalosis are a loss of body acid, particularly loss of chloride ion, and excess of base, usually sodium, and the loss of significant amounts of potassium.

1. Loss of acid results from vomiting; gastric intubation with loss of acid gastric secretion; gastrocolic fistula or aciduria with potassium and chloride depletion.
2. Excess of base results from absorbable antiacids—particularly $NaHCO_3$; sodium salts of weak acids, particularly lactate, citrate, blood transfusions with ACD anticoagulant; Ringer's lactate solution to replace acid or neutral losses from the gastrointestinal tract; or with vegetable diets.
3. Potassium depletion results from the use of diuretics, particularly thiazides

and furosamide; gastrointestinal losses, particularly lower GI tract, diarrhea; prolonged unreplaced loss of chloride ion with alkalosis and enhanced renal secretion of potassium; lack of potassium intake, particularly in intravenous fluids and with vomiting; adrenal steroid administration, or Cushing's disease or potassium-losing renal tubular disease.

Compensation for metabolic alkalosis is also respiratory and renal. In some patients there is diminished ventilation with some increase in P_{CO_2}, particularly when the CO_2 content of the plasma rises above 35 mEq/L. However, respiratory compensation is small and cannot be detected in the majority of patients.

Goldring et al.[39] studied normal volunteers made alkalotic under controlled conditions by administration of buffers, diuretics and aldosterone. Alkalosis induced by sodium bicarbonate, THAM, and ethacrynic acid was associated with high values of arterial P_{CO_2} (P_{CO_2} values of 46 to 48 mm Hg) while alkalosis induced by thiazide diuretics and aldosterone was associated with normal arterial blood P_{CO_2} values despite comparable increase in HCO_3^- values to a range of 30 to 34 mEq/L.

Figure 8-10 indicates that some patients have an increase in P_{CO_2} values at 35 mEq total CO_2 to compensate in this range. However, Figure 8-11, plotted from Elkinton's data[35] on patients with simple metabolic alkalosis (line G-G), suggests relatively little compensation for rising HCO_3^- by inhibition of CO_2 loss through hypoventilation.

Initial renal compensation following the loss of chloride ion occurs by excretion of sodium bicarbonate resulting in an alkaline urine. Unless adequate amounts of sodium, potassium, chloride and water are made available, this soon leads to dehydration. Metabolic alkalosis increases renal excretion of potassium, and as depletion of this ion develops renal tubular reabsorption of bicarbonate increases, leading to

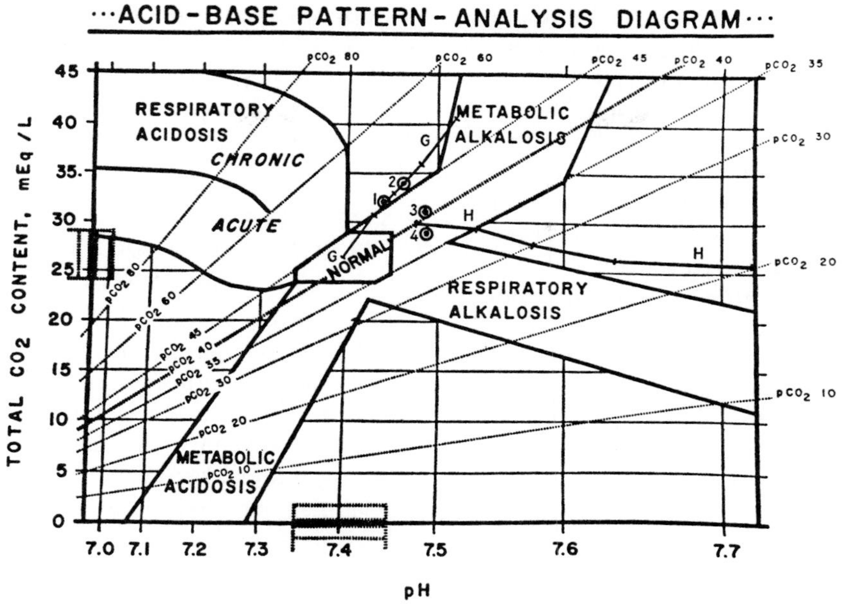

···ACID–BASE PATTERN–ANALYSIS DIAGRAM···

Fig. 8–11. Patient data from the literature showing metabolic alkalosis and respiratory alkalosis. G-G: Regression of P_{CO_2} on $[HCO_3^-]$, $P_{CO_2} = 42.1 + .18\,[HCO_3^-]$, suggesting only slight respiratory compensation,[35] H-H: respiratory alkalosis, $[HCO_3^-] = 20.6 + 0.20\,P_{CO_2}$.[35] Points 1 and 2 and 3 and 4 from Goldring et al.[39] Plots corrected to reflect total CO_2.

the paradox of an acid urine in an alkalotic patient and helping to perpetuate the alkalosis.

Treatment is directed to correction of the cause. Alkalosis caused by sodium retention (steroids or exogenous administration) will correct itself on cessation of therapy. Alkalosis caused by chloride and potassium loss responds to the administration of chloride and potassium. Both ions are required, and potassium chloride is the drug of choice. Isotonic saline solution also provides additional chloride.

Respiratory Alkalosis

Respiratory alkalosis is a primary decrease in P_{CO_2} and H_2CO_3 and is reflected in an increase in pH of the blood. The cause is increased ventilation, in both rate and depth with a reduction of the normal alveolar P_{CO_2} below 35 mm Hg. Initially there is no change in the CO_2 content of the plasma.

The causes of hyperventilation and respiratory alkalosis are multiple and include: (1) apprehension and pain, (2) fever, particularly if associated with some lung infection or atelectasis, (3) hepatic failure with elevated blood ammonia, (4) central nervous system injury, (5) respirators with hyperventilation, (6) septicemia, particularly gram-negative sepsis, (7) salicylate intoxication.

A mild degree of respiratory alkalosis is a common finding in a high percentage of postoperative patients and is often associated with some degree of metabolic alkalosis as well.[41]

The adult respiratory distress syndrome occurs in patients who have undergone major operative procedures, have suffered extensive skeletal trauma or have serious sepsis. Patients develop progressive dyspnea associated with marked hyperventilation, and initially demonstrate a respiratory alkalosis together with a fall in Pa_{O_2}

and in oxygen saturation of hemoglobin. The work of breathing is markedly increased as the result of hyperventilation and decreased compliance of the lungs. Prompt and vigorous action by controlled volume ventilation often with positive end-expiratory pressure (PEEP), and by treatment of fluid overload, if present, is essential for survival in severe cases.[42,43]

Severe respiratory alkalosis produces hypocapneic vasoconstriction (which reduces cerebral circulation) and hypoxia by decreasing the release of oxygen from hemoglobin and decreasing arterial P_{O_2}, with the production of excess lactic acid. In addition, depression of the ionization of calcium may lead to tetany, and the fall in plasma potassium leads to cardiac arrhythmias and digitalis intoxication. With circulatory failure, there is rapid conversion to a severe and often lethal metabolic acidosis.

The *compensation for respiratory alkalosis* is renal with the excretion of sodium bicarbonate in the urine. However, sodium retention and antidiuresis following trauma substantially or completely block this compensation and, as a result, an alkaline urine is seldom seen.

Treatment of respiratory alkalosis depends on its severity. A mild degree of alkalosis, partially respiratory in origin, is seen in a large percentage of postoperative patients upon whom blood-gas analysis is performed. In general, these patients have good cardiac, pulmonary and renal function and will recover without treatment. The development of respiratory alkalosis may be an early clinical indication of the presence of septicemia and should lead the observant physician to institute vigorous antibiotic therapy if signs of infection exist. It may also herald the onset of the adult respiratory distress syndrome. Severe respiratory alkalosis has a poor prognosis owing to the underlying causes of the hyperventilation. Within the limits imposed by oxygen demand, narcotics have proved effective in reducing ventilation.

Theoretically, the inhalation of an oxygen–carbon dioxide mixture, with sufficient CO_2 to raise the P_{CO_2} to normal, should be effective. In the few instances tried, patients have tolerated this procedure poorly.

THE EFFECT OF DIET ON WATER, ELECTROLYTE AND ACID-BASE BALANCE

In relating water, electrolyte and acid-base balance to nutrition, this chapter is not complete without examining the results of normal body metabolism and the effects of variations in dietary intake, including total starvation.

Cellular metabolism of neutral dietary or tissue content results in the production of hydrogen ion and of fixed acid anions, both of which require excretion if acid-base balance is to be preserved. For example, a neutral substance such as glucose in the process of metabolism is converted into lactic and pyruvic acids, with the production of hydrogen ion. Unless there is interference with the normal metabolic sequence, however, these intermediary products of metabolism are then promptly oxidized to neutral end-products, CO_2 and water. Other organic anions, such as citrate and acetoacetate, are metabolized to CO_2. When P_{CO_2} is constant, as is the case with normal respiratory function, the amount of CO_2 lost by respiration is equal to the amount produced. Of the order of 15 to 20,000 mM of CO_2 are produced by the average adult per day.

Nonvolatile acids are also produced as the result of digestion of dietary intake and normal cellular metabolism. Strong inorganic acid anions include Cl^- and $SO_4^=$, the latter resulting from the metabolism of the sulfur-containing amino acids cysteine and methionine as well as from ingested sulfate. In addition, phosphate ($HPO_4^=$) is produced from the metabolism of proteins and phospholipids. While phosphate behaves as a buffer salt, it cannot be excreted in the form H_3PO_4 in the urine because the pH required is too low; in effect, it too behaves as a strong acid anion. Uric acid, the end-product of metabolism of purine bases in man and other·primates, is also excreted in the urine, representing about 5 per cent of the normal acid load.

The average North American diet contains an excess of cations of approximately 1 mEq per kg of body weight per day.[44] This excess is paritally balanced by the excretion in stool of an average excess of cations over inorganic anions of 35 mEq per day, so that in healthy individuals nonvolatile acid production is equal to renal acid excretion plus 25 to 35 mEq neutralized by the dietary cation excess. However, dietary intake is highly variable. Fruit, vegetables, milk and coffee contain more inorganic cation than anion, while meat and eggs contain more inorganic anion than cation.

Renal mechanisms for disposal of nonvolatile acid anions involve two processes. Buffer salts which enter the renal tubule in the glomerular filtrate are transformed by exchange of hydrogen ion for sodium or potassium into acid salts, and inorganic cation is also preserved by combining inorganic anions with ammonium ions derived from amino acids. These processes are schematically illustrated by Pitts[16] as follows:

$$Na_2HPO_4 + H_2CO_3 \longrightarrow NaH_2PO_4 \text{ (excreted)} + NaHCO_3 \text{ (reabsorbed)}$$
$$Na_2SO_4 + 2 H_2CO_3 + 2 NH_3 \longrightarrow (NH_4)_2SO_4 \text{ (excreted)} + 2 NaHCO_3 \text{ (reabsorbed)}$$

Titratable acidity of the urine is defined as the amount of strong base necessary to return urine to the pH of plasma. The total acid load excreted in the urine is the sum of the titratable acidity (buffer effect) plus the strong acid anions combined with ammonium ion. According to Pitts,[16] titratable acid in the urine is 10 to 30 mEq per day in normal man, while acid combined with ammonia is 30 to 50 mEq per day. Thus, 40 to 80 mEq of strong acid anions in excess of fixed base—in effect 40 to 80 mEq (H$^+$)—are excreted daily in the urine.

Both of the above mechanisms are utilized in renal compensation for respiratory and nonrenal metabolic acidosis as previously discussed. When organic acid anions such as lactate and the keto-acid ions, acetoacetate and beta-hydroxybutyrate are presented to the kidneys in very large amounts and require excretion, fixed base, largely sodium, and water are both excreted in abnormal amounts, resulting in dehydration and loss of plasma bicarbonate. When an excess of sodium is filtered in the presence of an elevated plasma bicarbonate, sodium and bicarbonate ions are excreted in an alkaline urine; this is a situation often seen in persons who are strict vegetarians.

Starvation

Starvation induces major changes in both water and electrolyte balance. Initially, weight loss is substantially greater than can be accounted for on the basis of endogenous protein and fat metabolism. While weight loss in starvation is to some extent conditioned by the prefasting diet, and particularly by previous levels of sodium intake in obese patients, Weinsier[45] reported that an initial weight loss of 800 to 1,500 gm occurs in the first 24 hours, followed by an average loss of 1 kg a day for about 10 days. There is then a progressive fall in weight loss to 300 gm a day in the second month of fasting.

Initial weight loss is largely water and salt. The sodium loss exceeds that produced by simple dietary sodium restriction. Initially it is about 150 to 250 mEq a day and slowly declines to 1 to 15 mEq a day with prolonged fasting. Even if the patient is on a sodium-restricted diet before fasting, sodium excretion is still elevated by fasting. Administration of a sodium supplement with water[45,46] or a balanced salt solution containing sodium and potassium[47] fails to prevent sodium and water loss. Since sodium is the major extracellular cation, reduction in extracellular fluid volume as the result of water and sodium loss may be reflected in a decrease in blood volume. An average reduction in 10 days of 14 per cent was observed by Maagøe[48] in a series of patients who were 51 to 61 per cent overweight. The decrease in blood volume was significantly reduced to 5 per cent or less when fasting patients were given 90 mEq of sodium as sodium chloride a day. Bloom[49] has shown that the sodium loss in starvation is not due to ketosis but, rather, to an abrupt decrease in available carbohydrate. This confirms the observations of Gamble[12] that the mild ketoacidosis of starvation does not in itself produce loss of fixed base and that ketones in the urine in starvation can be substantially reduced by the administration of small amounts of carbohydrate.

Potassium is also lost in starvation. Initial losses of 40 to 45 mEq a day gradually diminishing to a level of 10 to 15 mEq a day after the tenth day were reported by Cahill.[50] The plasma potassium concentration usually remains at a low normal level. The potassium and nitrogen losses in starvation are the result of mobilization of body protein for gluconeogenesis from the glucogenic amino acids.[50] About 75 gm of protein (representing 12 gm of nitrogen and 35 to 40 mEq of potassium) are required, together with 16 gm of glycerol and 36 gm of lactate and pyruvate recycled through the Cori cycle, to provide about 150 gm of glucose a day—which appear to be essential in early starvation as substrate for energy requirements of the central nervous system and bone marrow. Some glucose is regularly required by red blood cells for their metabolism.

Amino acid metabolism in starvation has also been studied. Felig et al. have shown that if amino acids are determined as a group there is a slight but significant fall in serum levels; individual amino acids behave differently, however.[51] Some, including glycine, increase in starvation; valine, leucine and isoleucine increase transiently and then fall while arginine levels decrease progressively. Alanine behaves uniquely; it is extracted by the splanchnic circulation to a greater extent than all other amino acids combined, and it appears to be the regulatory mechanism which controls hepatic gluconeogenesis. Infusion of small amounts of alanine results in a rapid increase in blood glucose concentration, offering further confirmation of the hypothesis.[50,51]

The Effects of Carbohydrate

Bloom[49] observed that placing obese starving patients on a 600-kcal diet promptly prevented excessive loss of sodium and water in the urine. Individual tests with salt, protein, fat and carbohydrate showed that only carbohydrate produced sodium retention and associated water retention in the fasted then refed patient. Diet mixtures containing 1,500 and 2,000 kcal composed of protein and fat, with or without salt, failed to prevent a starvation type of sodium and water excretion. The addition of as little as 50 gm of glucose, isocalorically in exchange for fat in these diets, resulted in prompt sodium and water retention. Subsequent studies[45-47] have shown that sodium retention associated with carbohydrate feeding is not related to significant changes in aldosterone excretion, nor is it blocked by spironolactone. It does not appear to be a result of or influenced by glucocorticoids or by changes in catecholamine excretion. It is of interest that glucose administration inhibits furosamide induction of natriuresis and that insulin appears to be necessary for the sodium retention effect of glucose to be apparent in diabetics.[46,47]

The exact nature of the mechanism by which carbohydrate affects sodium and water balance remains unknown. However, this effect must be kept in mind whenever seriously ill patients are being treated. We have observed that a weight gain of 2 to 4 per cent of body weight occurs promptly (within 1 to 2 days) when patients are placed either on high caloric parenteral nutrition or on purified diets which consist largely of amino acids and either glucose or sucrose. A prompt loss of 2 to 4 per cent of body weight occurs when either the parenteral regimen or the "elemental" diet is stopped, even if the patient is immediately able to tolerate a diet of reasonably normal composition. This suggests that the effect of carbohydrate on sodium and water balance is not confined to starvation and refeeding; it may occur with substantial carbohydrate loading. The role of insulin in this phenomenon merits further investigation.

Prolonged Meat and Fat Diets

McClellan and DuBois[52,53] more than 40 years ago studied the effects of a diet of meat and animal fat on two Arctic explorers who lived in New York City for 1 year on a diet composed exclusively of beef, veal, lamb, pork and chicken. The carbohydrate intake was very small, consisting solely of the glycogen of the meat. Protein content of the diet ranged from 100 to 140 gm, the fat from 200 to 300 gm and carbohydrate from 7 to 12 gm a day. Both explorers, and DuBois himself who tried the diet for 10 days, lost weight during the first week. Weight loss ranged from 1.8 to 3.6 per cent of body weight, and this loss was explained as a "shift in the water content of the body while adjusting itself to the low-carbohydrate diet."

The two explorers remained mentally alert, physically active and showed no specific changes in any body system. While on the diet both men consistently excreted "acetone bodies" in the urine. Urine volume was higher when carbohydrate was first omitted, and was at its lowest level when carbohydrate was first added. A persistently negative calcium balance was the only potentially serious abnormality, amounting to about 0.3 gm per day.[52]

High urine specific gravity, 1.020 to 1.030 in urine volumes of 1,500 ml or more a day, was observed and reflects the 40 to 50 gm of urea excreted together with substantial amounts of phosphate, sulfate and potassium. Modern high-protein, low-carbohydrate diets sometimes used for weight reduction require a substantial fluid intake to provide sufficient urine volume to avoid prerenal azotemia.

BIBLIOGRAPHY

1. Moore, Olsen, McMurray, Parker, Ball, and Boyden: *Body Cell Mass and its Supporting Environment: Body Composition in Health and Disease.* Philadelphia, W. B. Saunders, 1963.
2. Hume and Weyers: J. Clin. Pathol., *24*:234, 1971.
3. DuBois: *Basal Metabolism in Health and Disease,* 3rd ed. Philadelphia, Lea & Febiger, 1936.
4. Widdowson: In *Biology of Gestation,* Vol. II (Assali, Ed.). New York, Academic Press, 1968.
5. Novak, Hyatt and Alexander: J.A.M.A., *205*, 764, 1968.
6. Brill, et al.: Am. J. Surg., *123*, 49, 1972.
7. Streeten, Rapaport, Abraham and Conn: J. Clin. Endocrinol. Metab., *23*, 928, 1963.
8. Boling, Taylor, Entenman and Behnke: J. Clin. Invest., *41*, 1840, 1962.
9. Swan, Nelson and Hankes: Ann. Surg., *174*, 287, 1971.
10. Kinney, Lister and Moore: Ann. N.Y. Acad. Sci., *110*, 711, 1963.
11. Fulton: Ann. Surg., *172*, 861, 1970.
12. Gamble: *Chemical Anatomy, Physiology, and Pathology of Extracellular Fluid: A Lecture Syllabus,* 5th ed. Cambridge, Harvard University Press, 1947.
13. Bland: *Clinical Metabolism of Body Water and Electrolytes.* Philadelphia, W. B. Saunders, 1963.
14. Randall: Surg. Clin. North Am., *56*, 1019, 1976.
15. Kinney, J. M. (Ed.): *Manual of Preoperative and Postoperative Care,* 2nd ed. Committee on Preoperative and Postoperative Care, American College of Surgery. Philadelphia, W. B. Saunders, 1971.
16. Pitts: *Physiology of the Kidney and Body Fluids.* Chicago, Year Book Medical Publishers, 1963.
17. Starling: J. Physiol., *19*, 312, 1895–96.
18. Pappenheimer: Physiol. Rev., *33*, 387, 1963.
19. Eisenman, Sandblom and Walker: Science, *155*, 965, 1967.
20. Leaf: Am. J. Med., *49*, 291, 1970.
21. Katz and Epstein: N. Engl. J. Med., *278*, 253, 1968.
22. Rocchio and Randall: Am. J. Surg., *121*, 460, 1971.
23. Randall: Surg. Clin. North Am., *32*, 3, 1952.
24. Kleeman and Fichman: N. Engl. J. Med., *277*, 1300, 1967.
25. Bartter and Schwartz: Am. J. Med., *42*, 790, 1967.
26. Nolph: Am. J. Med., *49*, 534, 1970.
27. Shore and Claybaugh: Annu. Rev. Physiol., *34*, 235, 1972.

28. Earley and Daugharty: N. Engl. J. Med., *281*, 72, 1969.
29. Ulbrich and Marsh: Annu. Rev. Physiol., *25*, 91, 1963.
30. Van Slyke: Ann. N.Y. Acad. Med., *133*, 5, 1966.
31. Peters and Van Slyke: *Quantitative Clinical Chemistry—Interpretations.* Baltimore, Williams and Wilkins, 1931.
32. Siggard-Anderson: Scand. J. Clin. Lab., Invest., *12*, 311, 1960.
33. Ad Hoc Committee on Acid-Base Terminology: In *Current Concepts of Acid-Base Measurement* (Weyer, Ed.). Ann. N.Y. Acad. Sci., *133*, 1, 1966.
34. Stewart: Personal communication.
35. Elkinton: Med. Clin. North Am., *50*, 1325, 1966.
36. Poppell, Vanamee, Roberts and Randall: J. Lab. Clin. Med., *47*, 885, 1956.
37. Randall: In *Critical Surgical Illness* (Hardy, Ed.). Philadelphia, W. B. Saunders, 1971.
38. Albert, Dell and Winters: Ann. Intern. Med., *66*, 312, 1967.
39. Goldring, Cannon, Heinemann and Fishman: J. Clin. Invest., *47*, 188, 1968.
40. Eichenholz, Blumentals and Walker: J. Lab. Clin. Med., *68*, 265, 1966.
41. Lyons and Moore: Surgery, *60*, 93, 1966.
42. Blaisdell: Surgery, *74*, 251, 1973.
43. Burrows: *Respiratory Insufficiency.* Chicago, Year Book Medical Publishers, 1975.
44. Harrington and Lemann: Med. Clin. North Am., *54*, 1543, 1970.
45. Weinsier: Am. J. Med., *50*, 233, 1971.
46. Gozansky and Herman: Am. J. Clin. Nutr., *24*, 869, 1971.
47. Vervebrants and Arky: J. Clin. Endocrinol., *29*, 55, 1969.
48. Maagøe: Metabolism, *17*, 133, 1968.
49. Bloom: Am. J. Clin. Nutr., *20*, 157, 1967.
50. Cahill: N. Engl. J. Med., *282*, 668, 1970.
51. Felig, Owen, Wahren and Cahill: J. Clin. Invest., *48*, 584, 1969.
52. McClellan and DuBois: J. Biol. Chem., *87*, 651, 1930.
53. McClellan, Rupp and Toscani: J. Biol. Chem., *87*, 669, 1930.

Chapter *9*

TRACE ELEMENTS

A. *Iodine*

Ralph R. Cavalieri

Although scientific knowledge of the role of iodine in human nutrition has been accumulated entirely within the past 150 years, the use of iodine-containing medicaments for the treatment of goiter goes back into antiquity. This disorder was certainly known to the ancients. Seaweed and burnt sponge, which we now know to be rich in iodine, were employed in the treatment of goiter by the ancient Chinese, the Egyptians and the Incas of South America.

The first true milestone of modern times was the discovery of elemental iodine by Courtois in 1811. During the processing of Chilean saltpeter in the manufacture of gunpowder for Napoleon's army, Courtois was annoyed by the corrosion of his copper vats. He traced the corrosive agent to the mother liquor of the saltpeter, from which he isolated a violet crystalline substance. Within 3 years, Gay-Lussac named the substance *Iode* (from the Greek for violet-colored) and Davey proved its elemental nature. Credit for the introduction of iodine into medical use and its popularization is usually given to two Geneva physicians, Coindet and Straub (1820). However, the first recorded therapeutic use of the newly discovered element was by Prout, an English physician, who prescribed solution of potassium iodate for simple goiter (1816). By 1819, iodine was on the formulary of London's St. Thomas' Hospital.

The first suggestions that endemic goiter might be due to iodine deficiency were made in 1830–31 by Prevost in Switzerland and Baussingault in France. Prevost and Maffoni in 1846 actually stated that the cause of endemic goiter and cretinism is the absence of iodine in the drinking water and air of those regions affected. Between 1859 and 1876, the French chemist Chatin undertook the ambitious task of measuring the iodine content of samples of soil, water and air from various regions. He concluded from his studies that iodine lack caused goiter and that iodine is a specific in the treatment of the disorder. Unfortunately, Chatin's chemical methods were not adequate, and his conclusions came under criticism. In addition, the widespread, indiscriminate use of iodine for the treatment of all sorts of thyroid disorders with uneven success led to a reaction against his views.[2]

It was not until 1896 that iodine was identified in the thyroid gland by Baumann, although Kocher, the famous Swiss pioneer in the surgery of goiter, had suggested years earlier that iodine might be a physiologically important constituent of the gland. The chemical studies of Baumann and Oswald led to the next important milestone, the isolation by Kendall in 1914–15 of the first of the two active principles of the thyroid, thyroxine. Harington, in the 1920s, characterized the structure of thyroxine and proved it definitively by synthesizing the hormone.[3] When radioactive iodine became available as a tracer, further advances in the field followed rapidly. Gross and Pitt-Rivers (1952) identified the second thyroid hormone, triiodothyronine.[4]

In parallel with early chemical studies, investigation was proceeding at the clinical level. Although cretinism had been known since ancient times, it remained for Gull (1874) to describe adult hypothyroidism and Ord (1878) to give it the name *myxedema*. Within a decade, mainly through the experimental work of Schiff, Hofmeester and Horseley and the astute clinical observations of Kocher and the Reverdins on patients who had undergone total thyroidectomy, it became apparent that myxedema is the result of thyroid failure. In what now seems a logical next step, patients suffering from spontaneous myxedema were given thyroid replacement therapy (Murray, 1891). The results were dramatic and rewarding. The modern era of clinical thyroidology had begun.[3]

The credit for awakening interest in the importance of iodine in the prevention of simple goiter must go to David Marine and his co-workers in the United States.[5] Their classical studies among schoolchildren of Ohio in 1917–18 demonstrated conclusively that iodine supplementation greatly reduced the incidence of goiter in that region. The importance of adequate dietary iodine is now well accepted by the health-science community. Effective public health measures have finally been instituted in most of the regions of the world affected.

METABOLISM OF IODINE IN MAN

Dietary iodine is converted largely to iodide in the gastrointestinal tract. Absorption of iodide is rapid and complete. Once it enters the circulation, iodide ion is distributed throughout the extracellular fluid.[6] There is no significant binding of iodide ion in plasma. Certain tissues possess the ability to concentrate iodide: salivary glands, gastric mucosa, lactating mammary glands, the choroid plexus and, most importantly, the thyroid gland. Of these tissues, only the thyroid is capable of utilizing iodine in the synthesis of the thyroid hormones (Fig. 9A–1).

The kidneys are responsible for nearly all of the excretion of iodide from the body.[7] The urinary clearance rate of iodide in man is about 30 ml plasma per minute; there is no renal mechanism for conserving iodide in the face of dietary deficiency of the element. Normally, little organic iodine is excreted in the feces. Impairment of renal function, if severe, will diminish urinary excretion of iodide and thereby cause an elevation in the plasma iodide level (if dietary intake is unchanged). On the other hand, an osmotic diuresis will increase urinary iodide loss and thereby lower the plasma level.

The initial step in the biosynthesis of the thyroid hormones is the transport of iodide from the blood into the follicular cells of the thyroid gland by the concentrating mechanism already mentioned. This thyroidal iodide "trap" is dependent upon metabolic energy generated within the thyroid cells by aerobic processes. Certain monovalent anions, e.g. perchlorate, thiocyanate and nitrate, inhibit the trap by competing with iodide. Perchlorate is the most potent of these inhibitors.

Once within the thyroid gland, iodide is rapidly oxidized to a higher oxidation state, perhaps $I°$ or I^+, by a specific enzyme, iodide peroxidase, which is located within the follicular cells. This active form of iodine reacts with tyrosine residues within thyroglobulin to form mono- and diiodotyrosine residues. The latter iodotyrosines then react in a coupling process to yield the active hormones thyroxine (T_4) and triiodothyronine (T_3). All of these

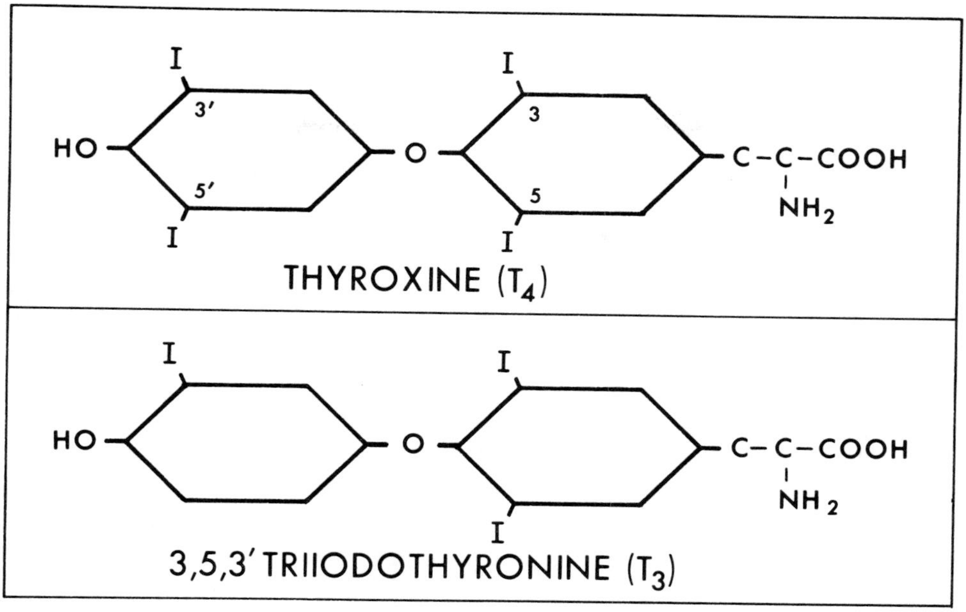

Fig. 9A–1. Structural chemical formulas of the thyroid hormones, thyroxine (T_4) and 3,5,3'-triiodothyronine (T_3). The numerals within the aromatic rings are used to designate the position of the iodine-substituents. When not occupied by an iodine atom, the "corners" of each aromatic ring are occupied by a hydrogen atom (not shown). The alanine side chain of each hormone is the L-isomer.

reactions, from the initial organic binding of iodine to the coupling reaction, are believed to occur within the thyroglobulin molecule. This protein is a large (MW = 670,000) glycoprotein synthesized only in the thyroid gland and stored in the colloid. It contains 120 tyrosine residues, about two thirds of which are available for iodination. The iodine content of thyroglobulin from normal human glands varies widely, depending in part on the iodine supply, though many factors influence the degree to which thyroglobulin is iodinated.[8]

Secretion of Hormones

In order for the hormones to be released from the thyroid into the blood, thyroglobulin must be broken down by proteolytic enzymes into its constituent amino acids. In the process, free hormones T_4 and T_3 and free iodotyrosines are released inside the follicular cells. The iodotyrosines are normally stripped of iodine by a specific iodotyrosine deiodinase: the iodide which is released is available for reutilization by the gland. This intrathyroidal mechanism for recycling iodine serves the important function of conserving iodine in the face of a low dietary supply.[8]

The release of T_4 and T_3 into the blood probably occurs by passive diffusion, although the thyroid hormone-binding protein in plasma may facilitate the process of release from the gland. About 20 molecules of T_4 are secreted for every molecule of T_3, but the ratio of the two hormones varies with conditions (see below).

Distribution and Metabolism of the Hormones

In normal humans, approximately one-third of the total quantity of T_4 in the body (excluding that within the thyroid) is in the plasma, one-third is in the liver, and the remainder is distributed among other tissues.[9] Both the circulating pool and the hepatic pool of T_4 probably serve as reservoirs of the hormone and as buffers to modulate abrupt changes in the level of T_4 at sensitive sites in the body, e.g. the heart.

Both T_4 and T_3 are reversibly bound to a specific plasma "carrier," thyroxine-binding globulin (TBG). Because of the strong binding between T_4 and TBG, the level of free T_4 is only a small fraction (about 1/2000) of the level of total T_4 in plasma. It is this free (unbound) fraction of

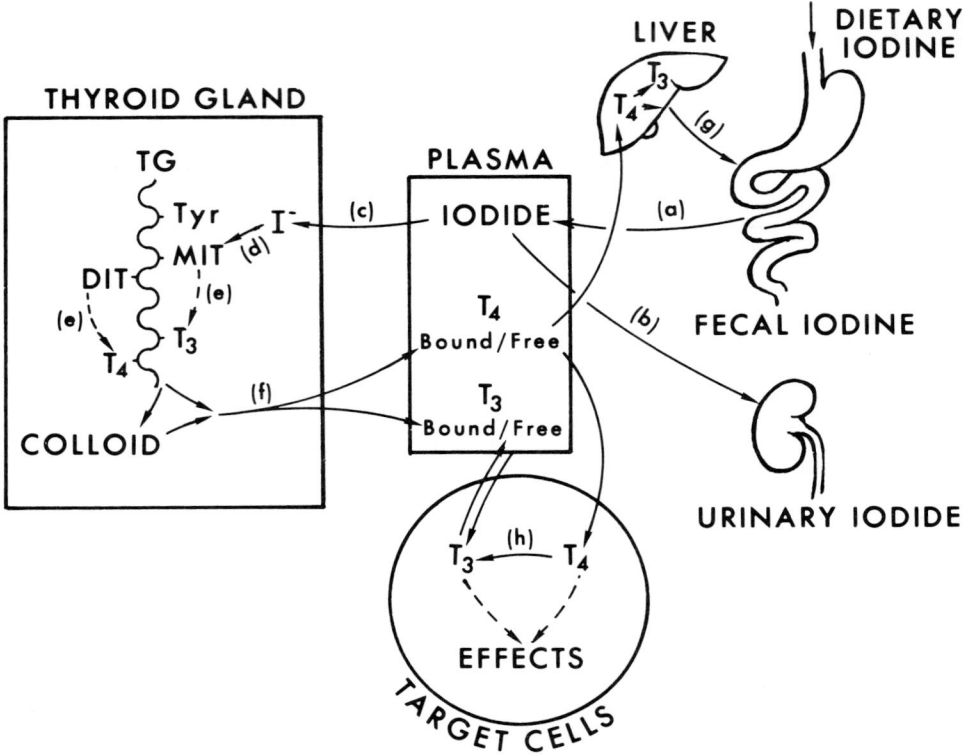

Fig. 9A–2. Schematic outline of iodine metabolism. Dietary iodine is converted to inorganic form (iodide) and rapidly absorbed from the gastrointestinal tract (a). Circulating iodide is either excreted into the urine (b) or taken up by the thyroid gland (c), wherein it enters the biosynthetic pathway toward thyroid hormone synthesis (d and e) initially incorporated into monoiodotyrosine (MIT) and diiodotyrosine (DIT), finally into the hormones triiodothyronine (T_3) and thyroxine (T_4), all within the large protein, thyroglobulin (TG). Secretion of T_4 and T_3 into the blood involves proteolysis of TG (f), usually after a period of temporary storage within the lumen of the follicle, still as TG (colloid). All of the intrathyroidal processes (c–f) are regulated by thyroid-stimulating hormone (TSH) a product of the anterior pituitary (not shown here). Within the plasma, T_4 and T_3 each exists in free and bound forms. Although they are in rapid equilibrium with the protein-bound form, only free T_4 and free T_3 are available to tissues such as the liver, kidneys, heart, skeletal muscle, etc. Cells of the liver contain a considerable amount of T_4, some of which is converted to T_3 and some excreted into the bile (g), ultimately to be reabsorbed into the blood or excreted in the feces. Tissues other than the liver also convert T_4 to T_3 by an enzymatic deiodination (h). Some of the T_3 so produced is returned to the circulation. In many tissues, including the liver, both thyroid hormones are degraded by deiodination to inactive products (not depicted in this figure), the iodide being recirculated through the plasma. The liver is both a target of hormone action and an organ of metabolism and excretion of thyroid hormones.

circulating T_4 which is believed to be the form available for entry into most tissues (particularly the liver) and which ultimately exerts the multiple effects of the hormone.

The distribution of T_3 in man is quite different from that of T_4. Most of the extrathyroidal pool of T_3 is in tissues, predominantly skeletal muscle, and relatively little is in the circulation.[11] T_3 is bound much less strongly to TBG than is T_4, which explains the more rapid onset and shorter duration of action of the former hormone. The intrinsic biologic potency of T_3 is about 3 times greater than that of T_4, a difference which is not due to differences in binding to plasma proteins. In normal humans, about one-third of the T_4 that is turned over each day is converted into T_3 by 5'-monodeiodination in various tissues, including the liver and kidney. This conversion of T_4 in extrathyroidal sites accounts for approximately 80 per cent of the total production of T_3, the remainder being secreted as T_3 by the thyroid.[12]

There is good evidence that the peripheral production of T_3 from T_4 is an enzymatic process under physiologic regulation; any stress or severe systemic illness is associated with a reversible inhibition of the process.[13] In addition, starvation and even short-term caloric restriction, especially of carbohydrate, cause a prompt decrease in T_4-to-T_3 conversion. This phenomenon, which seems to involve the liver to a large degree, may be an appropriate physiologic response in the face of limited dietary intake. (The fall in T_3 seems to correlate with a diminished metabolic rate, as measured by O_2 consumption.) Although the conversion of T_4 to T_3 results in an augmentation of the hormonal activity of thyroid hormone, it is believed that T_4 has intrinsic biologic potency.

An alternative pathway of T_4 deiodination has been identified recently, i.e. 5-monodeiodination which yields the isomer of T_3, 3,3',5'-triiodothyronine (reverse-T_3), which is virtually inactive as a hormone.[14] The production of reverse-T_3 from T_4 has been shown to be augmented in some of those conditions in which T_4-to-T_3 conversion is diminished. The production of T_3 by 5'-deiodination and of reverse-T_3 by 5-deiodination, together, account for about three-quarters of the total amount of T_4 turned over in man.[15]

Further deiodination of these products yields diiodothyronines and monoiodothyronines, none of which appears to have biologic activity.[16] The iodine removed in the sequential deiodination of T_4 and its products is returned to the plasma iodide pool. Other routes of metabolism of T_4 (and T_3) include: Oxidative deamination of the alanine side chain to the acetic acid derivatives (weakly active as hormones) and metabolism in the liver to the glucurono- and sulfoconjugates, which enter the intestinal tract via the bile. A portion of these products is recovered by deconjugation in the gut and reabsorbed, and the remainder is excreted in the feces.

The effects of thyroid hormones on the body are complex and far reaching. Their profound influences on growth and development, protein synthesis, differentiation and energy metabolism have been studied extensively.[17] Still, it is not known whether all of these effects are mediated via a single mechanism. In regard to the intracellular mechanism of action of thyroid hormones, much attention has been given recently to specific "receptors" which bind T_3 and T_4 in the nucleus and which appear to be closely linked to the processes of genetic control over the protein-synthetic machinery of the cell.[18] However, specific binding sites have also been found in mitochondria, supporting the idea that there is not a single locus but many sites within the cell where thyroid hormones initiate their multitudinous effects.

Regulation of Iodine Metabolism

The most important single regulator of the activity of the thyroid gland is thyrotropic hormone (TSH), a protein secreted by the anterior pituitary. TSH stimulates every step in the biosynthesis and secretion of the thyroid hormones, from the initial "trapping" of iodide ion to the proteolysis of thyroglobulin. In the absence of TSH, for example, in hypopituitarism, thyroid gland activity slows to a small fraction of the normal level. Administration of TSH in this situation restores full activity to normal. TSH also stimulates growth of the thyroid by increasing the size and number of follicular cells.

There is a sensitive feedback mechanism between the pituitary and the thyroid which serves to maintain an adequate level of thyroid hormone. A fall in output of hormone from the thyroid, for example, evokes an increase in TSH secretion. Contrariwise, an increase in the circulating level of thyroid hormone causes a lowering in TSH.[19]

The pituitary-thyroid axis is influenced in turn by centers in the hypothalamus (a portion of the midbrain). A potent hypothalamic hormone has been identified which causes the secretion of TSH from the pituitary. This thyrotropin-releasing hormone (TRH), a tripeptide, has been synthesized and is available for diagnostic testing of pituitary function. Considerable research is being conducted on the physiologic relationships involving the central nervous system, the pituitary and the thyroid.

The supply of iodine influences thyroid activity in several ways. Under conditions of iodine lack the iodide transport process is stimulated, with the result that an increased proportion of the circulating iodide pool becomes available to the gland. The individual follicular cells increase in size (hypertrophy) and number (hyperplasia). Thyroglobulin is synthesized more rapidly. More T_3 and less T_4 are formed and secreted proportionately. These alterations in function induced by iodine lack are for the most part mediated by an increase in TSH, but the thyroid gland seems to be capable also of self-regulation independent of changes in the circulating level of TSH. The effect of these changes is to enable the normal individual to maintain a normal metabolic state (euthyroidism) in the face of a limited supply of iodine.[20]

PHARMACOLOGIC EFFECTS OF EXCESS IODIDE

An excellent review of the diverse effects of excessive amounts of iodide in humans has appeared.[21] Small to moderate increments in iodide intake, i.e. up to 10 times the "normal" requirement of about 100 μg per day, lead to little or no chemical effects in individuals with normal thyroids. The gland for a time takes up more iodine than it releases (positive iodine balance), but, within a few weeks, the absolute amount of I^- taken up by the thyroid is reduced toward normal. During the entire period of excess iodide ingestion, the rate of hormonal secretion remains normal. In patients with hyperthyroidism, in contrast, the effects are quite different. Small doses of iodide, as little as 1 mg per day, cause a prompt inhibition of hormone release and marked amelioration of the symptoms of thyrotoxicosis.[22] This effect appears to be a direct one on the hyperactive gland itself and not an effect on the pituitary, as it occurs both in cases of toxic nodular goiter and in untreated Graves' disease, in which disorders blood levels of TSH are low.[23]

Administration of exogenous TSH has been shown to reverse the iodide-induced inhibition of hormone release. This particular effect of iodide has been used with advantage in the treatment of hyperthyroidism, especially in the period before the advent of the thionamide class of antithyroid drugs. The actual mechanism is not well understood, but the results of treatment with iodides ("Lugolization") are diminution in the vascularity of the gland, increase in colloid deposits and decrease in the size of the follicular cells. Unfortunately, the inhibitory effect is often short-lived; many cases "escape" after a period of a few weeks, and thyroid hyperfunction returns full-blown in spite of continuation of iodide therapy. Once they have escaped, such cases are resistant to attempts at reinduction of iodide inhibition.

The acute effects of large doses of iodide in experimental animals and in humans without hyperthyroidism include an inhibition of thyroid hormone synthesis. This phenomenon was discovered in rats by Wolff and Chaikoff.[24] Elevation of the plasma level of iodide about 20 to 35 μg per 100 ml caused a prompt cessation of thyroxine synthesis. However, the animals escaped from this acute inhibition within a day or two. This escape has been termed *adaptation* and apparently is due to a diminution of the iodide-transport process. The biochemical mechanism of the Wolff-Chaikoff effect is not well understood. The effect also occurs in humans, but most individuals appear to "adapt" to excessive doses of iodide and thyroid hormone synthesis proceeds unimpaired. Some are unable to adapt, however.[25] In such cases, most of whom have a history of some preexisting thyroid disorder, prolonged ingestion of iodide (200 mg or more daily for weeks to months) leads eventually to hypothyroidism and usually some degree of thyroid enlargement (iodide goiter). Such iodide-induced hypothyroidism is usually rapidly reversed on withdrawal of the iodide. Either iodide itself (e.g. KI) or any drug which contains iodine (e.g. iodopyrine, an antiasthmatic medication) has been shown to cause iodide myxedema and/or goiter.

In addition to the sporadic cases of iodide goiter, an interesting endemic form has been studied.[21] Along the coast of the Northern Island of Japan, a relatively common form of simple goiter affecting nearly 10 per cent of the population has been traced to an extremely high dietary intake of iodine in the form of seaweed ("kombu"). Studies of iodine metabolism in such cases show evidence of the Wolff-Chaikoff type of block in thyroid hormone synthesis, an effect which can be reversed on withdrawal of seaweed from the diet and reestablished with administration of potassium iodide. Typically, the goitrous individuals in this endemic area are euthyroid, perhaps because ingestion of the seaweed is intermittent throughout the year. The fact that only a minority of all persons exposed develop obvious goiters suggests a preexisting partial biochemical defect in the thyroids of those individuals.

Still another effect of excess iodine was noted almost as soon as the element came into widespread use in the treatment of goiter in iodine-deficient areas. A few euthyroid patients with long-standing goiter developed hyperthyroidism on iodine therapy. This phenomenon, termed *jodbasedow* (literally, Basedow's disease secondary to iodine), occurred often enough to lead to a reaction against the use of the treatment for goiter. Jodbasedow has been reported to occur in modern times in places as far apart as Tasmania[26] and Belgium.[27] It can occur even in localities with a sufficient dietary supply of iodine, when individuals with preexisting nontoxic multinodular or colloid goiter are given large daily doses (100 mg or more) of iodine.[28] The most likely explanation for jodbasedow is that such goitrous thyroids contain autonomous areas which are functioning only poorly until supplied with a sufficient supply of iodine, at which point hyperthyroidism ensues.

ESTIMATION OF DIETARY IODINE

Table 9A–1 lists the iodine content of each of several categories of food determined by direct chemical analysis of samples of diets employed at the Clinical Center, National Institutes of Health.[29] The authors of this study emphasize that these data apply to this institution and are not necessarily applicable to foods available elsewhere and prepared under other conditions. The iodine content of a given food varies widely, depending on the types of

Table 9A–1. Iodine Content of Composites of Food Categories*

Food Categories	No. of Samples	Iodine (µg/wet kg) Mean ± S.E.	Median
Seafoods	7	660 ± 180	540
Vegetables	13	320 ± 100	280
Meat products	12	260 ± 70	175
Eggs	11	260 ± 80	145
Dairy products	18	130 ± 10	139
Bread and cereal	18	100 ± 20	105
Fruits	18	40 ± 20	18

*From Vought and London.[29]

soil, fertilizers, animal feed and method of processing. For example, in some regions of the United States bread may account for a large proportion of iodine intake (150 µg per slice) because certain bakeries add iodate to dough as a stabilizing agent.[30,31] The consumption of iodized salt is another important variable. An individual may add as much as 8 gm of table salt to his food per day. If iodized, this would provide up to 600 µg iodine. The average is about 2 gm salt (150 µg I).

In view of the difficulties in estimating dietary iodine, many workers have employed total daily urinary excretion of iodine to estimate iodine intake. This assumes, of course, that the subject is in iodine balance, i.e. intake equals excretion, during the period of the study. It has been demonstrated, however, that normal and goitrous individuals may be in positive or negative balance for prolonged periods of time.[32,33] It follows, then, that the only certain method of determining iodine intake, short of using formula diets, is to perform analyses on samples of the actual diet consumed or of food categories.

TESTS OF THYROID FUNCTION IN MAN

A variety of techniques have been developed for the quantitative assessment of normal and abnormal thyroid function in humans.[34] Each type of procedure tests a specific aspect of thyroid physiology. The radioiodine uptake determination, although less often employed now than in former years, is useful in evaluating overall activity of the thyroid gland, particularly in suspected hyperthyroidism.[35] In this procedure, a tracer dose of labeled iodine (^{131}I or preferably ^{123}I) is administered orally and the percentage of the dose taken up by the thyroid gland is determined by external gamma counting at standard times, usually between 2 and 6 hours and again at 24 hours postdose. Normal thyroid uptake values vary widely in different areas of the world, depending upon the local dietary iodine intake.[31] In most areas in the United States, the normal 24-hour uptake ranges from 10 to 30 per cent. Most patients with untreated hyperthyroidism show values greater than 30 per cent. (The test is not useful in the diagnosis of hypothyroidism because of considerable overlap into the normal range.)

Determination of the thyroid uptake of radioiodine is also done to test for thyroid gland autonomy in patients suspected of having Graves' disease (diffuse toxic goiter or exophthalmic goiter). In this procedure (thyroid suppression test), the thyroid uptake is measured (at 24 hours after a dose of radioiodine) before and again after an 8-day course of T_3 administration, 75 to 100 µg per day. Patients with active Graves' disease typically show no decline in the thyroid uptake (thyroid autonomy), whereas those without this disorder and those whose disease is in remission exhibit a decrease in uptake to one-half or less of the original value, as a result of the suppression of TSH secretion by the administered T_3.[23]

Thyroid scanning is often performed in conjunction with the thyroid uptake test. The scan shows the distribution of radioiodine taken up in the gland, thereby providing an estimate of gland size, permitting detection of focal areas of hyperfunction ("hot" nodules) and areas of hypofunction ("cold" nodules). Fluorescent thyroid scanning is a new technique which permits the determination of the distribution and total content of stable iodine (^{127}I) in the gland by detecting characteristic x rays emitted from ^{127}I atoms during excitation by gamma radiation from an external source (Americium-241). This procedure, which does not require the administration of radioiodine to the patient, is useful in the diagnosis of some forms of thyroiditis (low ^{127}I content) and in assessing thyroid gland anatomy in patients whose thyroid uptake of radioiodine is too low to permit conventional scanning.

The concentration of free thyroxine (T_4) in the blood is the most reliable indicator of thyroid status, i.e. whether an individual is hyperthyroid or hypothyroid. A rapidly reversible equilibrium exists in plasma between the bound and free forms of T_4 and T_3. In normal individuals, the free T_4 fraction is only about 0.03 per cent of the total, i.e. 2 to 3 ng per 100 ml, a concentration too low to measure conveniently for routine purposes. Various combinations of in vitro tests have been devised to estimate indirectly the concentration of free T_4 in plasma. In the usual procedure, the total T_4 is measured by a specific, sensitive radioassay (competitive-binding assay or radioimmunoassay). An additional test is performed to assess the overall thyroid hormone-binding power of the plasma proteins, e.g. T_4 or T_3 resin uptake test. From the results of these two tests on the patient's plasma, the total T_4 concentration and the resin uptake test, the free T_4 level can be estimated.[10] Methods have been devised which provide an index proportional to the free T_4 concentration in a single procedure suitable for rapid, routine testing of large numbers of plasma samples.[37] The free T_4 concentration (or index) is elevated in nearly all patients with untreated hyperthyroidism and is decreased in hypothyroidism.[38]

One of the reasons why the free thyroxine index has become so widely used as a diagnostic screening test of thyroid status is that the plasma protein (TBG) which binds T_4 (and T_3) is altered in a large number of nonthyroidal disorders and by various medications. Among the latter, the most common are oral contraceptives containing estrogens. Euthyroid women taking such birth-control agents show elevated serum T_4 levels due to high TBG but a normal free T_4 index. (The same combination of results is seen during normal pregnancy.) Thus, the free T_4 index is presently the most reliable indicator of thyroid status.

In a small proportion of patients with hyperthyroidism (less than 5 per cent) the hypermetabolic state is maintained solely by an elevated circulating level of T_3.[39] In such rare cases, since the concentrations of total and free T_4 are within the normal range, the diagnosis of "T_3 thyrotoxicosis" is established by finding an elevated plasma T_3 concentration by means of a specific radioimmunoassay for T_3.[40] It is in the diagnosis of hyperthyroidism, in fact, that the T_3 radioimmunoassay is most useful. Virtually every untreated patient with this disorder exhibits an elevation in plasma T_3, often more than 5 times the normal level (approximately 1.2 ng per ml). In contrast, the plasma T_3 concentration is much less helpful in evaluating patients with suspected hypothyroidism. As discussed above, a wide variety of systemic illnesses, not directly involving the thyroid, as well as alterations in caloric intake, depress the circulating T_3 level without affecting the T_4 concentration. For this reason, the total, and especially the free T_4 level, is more reliable in the diagnosis of hypothyroid conditions than the T_3 concentration.[13]

Hypothyroidism is, in most cases, the result of failure or destruction of the thyroid gland. In a small percentage of patients, however, the hypothyroid state is secondary to a lack of TSH secretion from the pituitary gland. This condition is usually caused by a lesion within the pituitary but, in rare instances, may be a consequence of disease in the hypothalamus with lack of TRH secretion. Determination of the serum level of TSH by radioimmunoassay distinguishes cases of hypothyroidism due to thyroid gland failure or from those due to pituitary or hypothalamic disease. In the former TSH is elevated, while in the latter TSH is depressed. Hypothyroid patients whose serum TSH is *not* increased can be tested using TRH in order to determine whether the pituitary or the hypothalamic center is at fault. If, in such cases, the serum TSH does not rise after TRH administration, it may be concluded that the pituitary is diseased.[41]

SIMPLE GOITER

Simple goiter may be defined as an enlargement of the thyroid gland with hypertrophy and/or hyperplasia of the follicular epithelial cells not primarily caused by inflammatory or neoplastic processes. There may be excessive accumulation of colloid as well. The goiter is usually diffuse and, in its early stages, at least partially reversible with the administration of thyroid hormone. In long-standing cases, the goiter may become multinodular and fail to completely regress with hormone replacement. The pathogenesis of simple goiter is not completely understood. However, most authorities regard the condition as a compensatory response, at least in part involving the TSH mechanism, to inadequate secretion of thyroid hormones by the thyroid gland.

Iodine Deficiency

The once widely accepted view that iodine deficiency is *the* cause of all cases of goiter in endemic areas has been modified. Administration of iodine in large-scale prophylactic programs in endemic goiter areas, such as the Congo, New Guinea and the Andean regions of South America, have markedly reduced the formerly high incidence of goiter. This response supports the thesis that iodine deficiency was one causative factor in these areas.[42] On the other hand, there are several reasons to implicate other factors: Before iodine administration, the incidence of goiter, although high in certain iodine-deficient localities, never reached 100 per cent: some individuals in these areas escaped goiter even though they were exposed to severely iodine-deficient diets. Iodine replacement does not prevent goiter completely.[43]

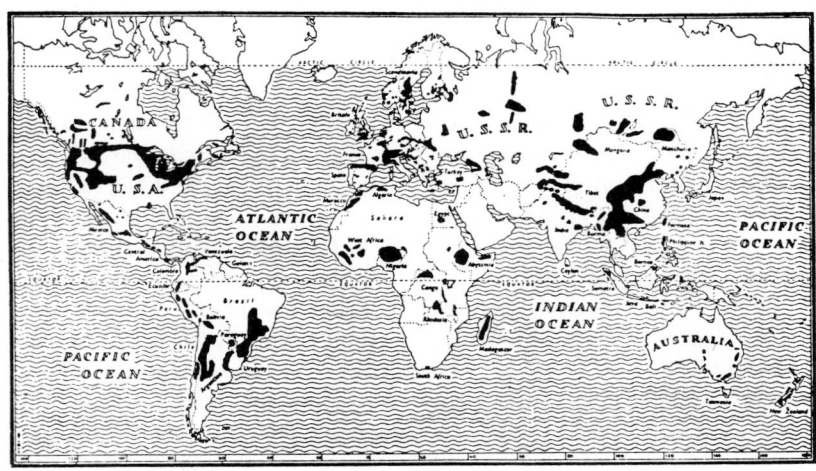

Fig. 9A–3. Goiter areas of the world. (From World Goiter Survey.[2])

Within a given endemic area, the incidence of goiter does not correlate with the iodine intake (as estimated from daily urinary excretion of iodine). For example, on the Idjwi Island (Lake Kivu) in the Congo, the incidence of goiter is 54 per cent in the north and only 5 per cent in the south, yet the average urinary excretion of iodine was found to be similar in both locales (less than 20 μg I per 24 hours).[44] These and other considerations have led workers to conclude that factors other than iodine deficiency may be important, at least in some endemic areas.[45,46] Such factors might include genetically determined defects in the enzymes responsible for thyroid hormone biosynthesis, dietary goitrogens and infectious agents. Bacterial goitrogens have been detected in the water supply of certain districts.[47]

According to this view, iodine deficiency plays a permissive role by "uncovering" borderline or subtle biochemical defects (genetic or acquired) in hormone synthesis.[44] One may imagine that, in a given population, a continuum of varying degrees of susceptibility to goiter exists. In areas where plenty of iodine is available, the incidence of "iodine-deficiency" goiter is relatively low since only those individuals with severe biochemical defects are affected. Under conditions of more limited iodine supply, an increasing proportion of the susceptible group develops goiter until, in extreme iodine deficiency, an endemic situation prevails.

Antithyroid Drugs

Many types of external agents are capable of inducing simple goiter in man.[48] Common to all of these is their ability to inhibit the synthesis, the secretion or the effectiveness of thyroid hormones. The most common antithyroid drugs are the thiocarbamides, or thionamides. Propylthiouracil and methimazole, the most potent of this class, block hormone synthesis within the thyroid by inhibiting coupling of iodotyrosines and, to a lesser extent, by inhibiting formation of iodotyrosines. A number of agents used in medicine for other purposes possess incidental antithyroid activity. For example, para-aminosalicylic acid, used in the treatment of tuberculosis, can induce goiter by virtue of its propylthiouracil-like action. Other drugs with similar effects, but less potent, include sulfonamides, tolbutamide, resorcinol and iodide itself (see above).

A second class of agents induce goiter (and hypothyroidism) by interfering with the thyroidal iodide transport mechanism. Thiocyanate and perchlorate are of this type. Lithium, which has been used for years in the treatment of certain mental disorders, exerts antithyroid activity both by inhibiting the secretion of hormone from the thyroid gland and by altering the peripheral metabolism of thyroxine.[49]

Fig. 9A–4. Chemical formulas of some antithyroid compounds. Propylthiouracil and methimazole are used in the treatment of hyperthyroidism. Goitrin is a potent antithyroid substance present in rutabaga and other members of the cabbage family.

Dietary Goitrogens

Certain foods have been shown to contain substances which induce goiter in experimental animals. In a series of painstaking studies, Greer and his associates isolated from rutabagas and turnips a substance which has antithyroid activity similar in potency to thiouracil.[50] They named the material *goitrin*. Subsequently, goitrin was detected in other vegetables of the cabbage family. Certain other foods also exhibit some degree of antithyroid activity, but the active substance in them has not been identified. Goiter caused solely by dietary goitrogens is probably uncommon. However, if such foods are consumed in large quantities, especially in an iodine-deficient environment, goiter might develop.

Biochemical Defects in Thyroid Hormone Synthesis

In areas of the world outside of recognized "goiter belts," simple goiter sometimes occurs in certain families. There may or may not be coexisting hypothyroidism or cretinism. When such familial cases have been investigated, selective defects in one or another of the steps in thyroid iodine metabolism have usually been found, presumably on a genetic basis.[42] The most common form of defect involves the process by which iodide is oxidized and incorporated into tyrosyl residues, probably as the result of deficient thyroidal iodide peroxidase activity. Another defect consists of a lack of the iodotyrosine deiodinase enzyme. It is interesting that patients with the latter defect are successfully treated by daily administration of a few mg of iodine. The latter observation supports the idea that some cases of iodine-deficiency goiter may represent instances of a partial thyroid enzyme defect which has been brought out by a relative iodine lack.

The dietary requirement for iodine must, therefore, be different for different regions, depending upon the presence or absence of goitrogens in the diet, and for different individuals within each region, depending upon genetic and acquired factors which influence the ability to adapt to limited iodine supply. Nevertheless, as a general guide, a daily intake of 100 μg iodine is considered adequate for most adults, assuming there is no exposure to goitrogenic agents. The iodine requirement is probably somewhat greater in childhood, during the growth spurt of adolescence and during pregnancy and lactation.

Treatment of Simple Goiter

There is no question that wide-scale supplementation of the diet with iodine has significantly reduced the incidence of goiter in areas where it was once highly prevalent. In the United States, iodized salt contains 76 μg iodine per gm. On a reasonably varied diet and with an average consumption of added iodized salt (2 to 6 gm per day), the typical American takes in somewhat more than 500 μg iodine per day.[29] In most countries of Europe, salt is iodized to approximately one-tenth the American level. In those areas of the world where iodine deficiency continues to be a problem and where socioeconomic conditions preclude widespread use of dietary supplementation, administration of iodized oil by intramuscular injection in mass-inoculation programs promises to be an effective means of preventing endemic goiter.[51]

Simple goiters often regress somewhat in size under treatment with iodides, to the degree that iodine deficiency contributes to their causation. The response of large, long-standing goiters to iodides is often disappointing. The preferred treatment in such cases is thyroid hormone. In fact, the most effective means of obtaining regression of almost any type of nontoxic goiter, regardless of the cause, is to administer thyroid hormone. Thyroxine, 0.1 to 0.3 mg daily, is the form most commonly used.

BIBLIOGRAPHY

1. Iason: *The Thyroid Gland in Medical History*. New York, Forben Press, 1946.
2. World Goiter Survey: Iodine Facts. Facts 271–380. London, Iodine Educational Bureau, 1946.
3. Harington: *The Thyroid Gland: Its Chemistry and Physiology*. London, Oxford University Press, 1933.
4. Gross and Pitt-Rivers: Lancet, *1*, 439, 1952.
5. Kimball and Marine: Arch. Intern. Med., *22*, 41, 1918.
6. Berson: Am. J. Med., *20*, 653, 1956.
7. Wayne, Koutras and Alexander: *Clinical Aspects of Iodine Metabolism*. Philadelphia, F.A. Davis, 1964.
8. Pitt-Rivers and Cavalieri: In *The Thyroid Gland*, Vol. 1 (Pitt-Rivers and Trotter, Eds.). Washington, Butterworth, 1964.
9. Cavalieri and Searle: J. Clin. Invest., *45*, 939, 1966.
10. Robbins and Rall: In *Hormones in Blood*, Vol. 1, 2nd ed. (Gray and Bacharach, Eds.). London, Academic Press, 1967.
11. Cavalieri, Steinberg and Searle: J. Clin. Invest., *49*, 1041, 1970.
12. Braverman, Ingbar and Sterling: J. Clin. Invest., *49*, 855, 1970.
13. Cavalieri and Rapoport: Ann. Rev. Med., *28*, 57, 1977.
14. Chopra: J. Clin. Invest. *58*, 32, 1976.
15. Gavin, Castle, McMahon, Martin, Hammond and Cavalieri: J. Clin. Endocrinol. Metab., *44*:733, 1977.
16. Pittman and Pittman: Handbook Physiol., *3*, 233, 1974.
17. Tata: In *Actions of Hormones on Molecular Processes* (Litwack and Kritchevsky, Eds.). John Wiley & Sons, 1964.
18. Oppenheimer: N. Engl. J. Med., *292*, 1063, 1975.
19. Hershman and Pittman: N. Engl. J. Med., *285*, 997, 1971.
20. Studer and Greer: *The Regulation of Thyroid Function in Iodine Deficiency*. Berne, Hans Huber, 1968.
21. Wolff: Am. J. Med., *47*, 101, 1969.
22. Volpe and Johnston: Ann. Intern. Med., *56*, 577, 1962.
23. Ingbar and Woeber: In *Textbook of Endocrinology*, 5th ed. (Williams, Ed.). Philadelphia, W.B. Saunders, 1973.
24. Wolff and Chaikoff: J. Biol. Chem., *172*, 855, 1948.
25. Braverman, Woeber and Ingbar: N. Engl. J. Med., *281*, 816, 1969.
26. Vidor, et al.: J. Clin. Endocrinol. Metab., *37*, 901, 1973.
27. Ermans and Camus: Acta Endocrinol., *70*, 463, 1972.
28. Vagenakis, et al.: N. Engl. J. Med., *287*, 523, 1972.
29. Vought and London: Am. J. Clin. Nutr., *14*, 186, 1964.
30. London, Vought and Brown: N. Engl. J. Med., *273*, 381, 1965.
31. Pittman, Dailey and Beschi: N. Engl. J. Med., *280*, 1431, 1969.
32. Malamos, et al.: J. Clin. Endocrinol. Metab., *27*, 1372, 1967.
33. Vought, Maisterrana, Tovar and London: J. Clin. Endocrinol. Metab., *25*, 551, 1965.
34. Rosenberg: N. Engl. J. Med., *286*, 924, 1972.
35. Cavalieri: In *The Thyroid*, 4th ed. (Werner and Ingbar, Eds.). New York, Harper & Row, 1978.
36. Hoffer, Berstein and Gottschalk: Semin. Nucl. Med., *1*, 379, 1971.
37. Abreau, et al.: J. Nucl. Med., *14*, 740, 1973.
38. Cavalieri: In *Atomic Medicine*, 5th ed. (Behrens, King and Carpender, Eds.). Baltimore, Williams and Wilkins, 1969
39. Sterling, Refetoff and Selenkow: J.A.M.A., *213*, 571, 1970.
40. Gharib, et al.: J. Clin. Endocrinol. Metab., *33*, 509, 1971.
41. Hershman and Pittman: N. Engl. J. Med., *290*, 886, 1974.
42. Stanbury: In *Metabolic Basis of Inherited Disease*, 3rd ed. (Stanbury, Wyngaarden and Fredrickson, Eds.). New York, McGraw-Hill, 1971.
43. Gaitan, Wahner, Correa, Bernal, Jubiz, Gaitan and Llanos: J. Clin. Endocrinol. Metab., *28*, 1730, 1968.
44. Beckers: In *Endemic Goiter*. Pan-American Health Organization, Scientific Publication No. 193, 1968.
45. Roche and Lissitzky: In *Endemic Goiter*. Basel, World Health Organization Monograph No. 44, 1960.
46. Wahner, Mayberry, Gaitan and Gaitan: J. Clin. Endocrinol. Metab., *32*, 491, 1971.
47. Gaitan, Island and Liddle: Trans. Assoc. Am. Physicians, *82*, 141, 1969.
48. Greer: Recent Prog. Horm. Res., *18*, 187, 1962.
49. Temple, Berman, Carlson, Robbins and Wolff: Mayo Clin. Proc., *47*, 872, 1972.
50. Greer: J. Clin. Endocrinol. Metab., *12*, 1259, 1952.
51. Kevany, Fierro-Benitez, Pretell and Stanbury: Am. J. Clin. Nutr., *22*, 1597, 1969.

B. The Biochemical and Nutritional Roles of Other Trace Elements

Ting-Kai Li
and
Bert L. Vallee

The importance of inorganic elements in biochemical and physiologic processes is now well established at all levels of cellular complexity. Although more than 60 elements have been discovered in bacteria, fungi, higher plants, animals and man, few of them have been studied intensively. Investigations have necessarily been restricted to those occurring in amounts large enough to be measurable, even if not always precisely, by available techniques. Calcium, carbon, chlorine, hydrogen, iodine, iron, nitrogen, magnesium, oxygen, phosphorus, potassium, sodium and sulfur comprise this group.

Trace elements, micronutrient elements or *minor elements* are terms applied to the remaining elements occurring constantly in biologic systems. The following are generally included among the trace elements: aluminum, antimony, arsenic, barium, boron, bromine, cadmium, chromium, cobalt, copper, gallium, lead, lithium, manganese, mercury, molybdenum, nickel, rubidium, selenium, silicon, silver, strontium, tin, titanium, vanadium and zinc. They have been grouped together quite arbitrarily but have in common the uncertainty of assigning to them definite physiologic functions and the difficulty in measuring their concentration in biologic fluids; this varies from 1×10^{-6} to less than 1×10^{-12} gm per gm wet weight of tissue. Thus, these designations often have implied reference both to the total amounts and to the problems in qualitative and quantitative detection of the elements, but they are also sometimes inferred to denote uncertainty as to biologic significance.

Perhaps for the latter reason iron, iodine and fluorine, though occurring in these concentration ranges, are generally considered as distinct from the trace element group because their established importance to health and their medical significance are no longer questioned. The roles of these elements are discussed in separate chapters.

Criteria for the essentiality of any element in nutrition have been stated:[1] In the absence of a specific element, a deficiency state develops on diets otherwise adequate and satisfactory, i.e. containing all other dietary essentials in adequate amounts and proportions and free from toxic properties. Dietary supplementation of this specific element and this element alone reverses the deficiency state, resulting in repeated and significant responses in growth and health.

With some elements, the deficiency state has been correlated further with the findings of subnormal concentrations of the element in the blood, tissues and organs of the deficient animals and of altered metabolism. At the present time, chromium, copper, cobalt, manganese, molybdenum, selenium and zinc are classified as *essential* trace elements in animal nutrition. There are recent reports that nickel, tin, vanadium and silicon[2] may be essential nutrient elements for chicks and rats. The essentiality of bromine, barium and strontium is less certain, and other elements, such as cadmium, have suspected functions of significance because of their consistent presence in tissues and cellular components and association with specific macromolecules. No doubt, many of the elements of currently unknown physiologic activity will be found to participate in vital processes and, as analytic techniques improve, the exact loci of these trace elements and their metabolic functions will be identified.

Trace elements and the many avenues of approach to medical problems which they seem to offer have generated much speculation and many hypotheses in regard to their roles in human diseases. The obvious experimental difficulties in appraising the functional significance of trace elements in normal and disease states (vide infra) have often led to confusion as to their true roles and to skepticism among serious investigators. As a consequence, much debate has been occasioned by the observation of the decrease or increase of a given metal ion concentration in the blood of patients with a given disease, and efforts to relate such data to the etiology of the disease have not been uniformly successful. Trace metals have been invoked as mechanistic factors in disease states as diverse as cancer, arteriosclerosis, hypertension, arthritis, porphyria, lupus erythematosus, multiple sclerosis and amyotrophic lateral sclerosis, but the evidence has often not stood the test of time. Even though variations in metal ion concentrations of tissues and body fluids are commonly observed in many disease states, such findings do not necessarily have etiologic significance.

HISTORICAL DEVELOPMENT AND PRESENT PERSPECTIVE

Awareness of the presence and functional significance of trace elements in living systems began about a century ago when iron, copper and zinc were found to be essential to the growth of plants and microorganisms and to be constituents of certain respiratory and blood pigments in snails and molluscs. Later, vanadium was discovered to function in the respiration of tunicates. Investigations of cellular respiration and the involvement of iron in oxida-

tive processes first suggested that metals may be an essential part of enzymatic reactions and pointed the way to the eventual discovery of metalloenzymes. However, the idea of a generalized function for the trace elements was slow to emerge, and most of the experimental work leading to the presently more secure basis of understanding has been performed within the last 45 years.

Knowledge of the essentiality of trace metals to animal nutrition emerged principally through two approaches: basic studies of the effects on animals of highly purified or specially constituted diets designed to be low or high in the trace elements in question, and applied studies of a number of naturally occurring endemic diseases of man or animals that were found to be due to deficiency or excess of one or more trace elements. During the last 30 years, there have been intensive investigations of the metabolic dynamics of metals within the body and their modes of action within the tissues. This development was greatly assisted and stimulated by the advent of isotopes and other concurrent developments in analytic chemistry and enzymology. Radioactive isotopes permitted studies of the absorption, retention and excretion of various elements. It became possible to measure the ranges of normal concentrations of a variety of trace elements in plant and animal tissues and to relate such data to age, sex, geography and disease.[3-5] The discovery of *metalloenzymes* and *metal-enzyme complexes* demonstrated conclusively that trace metals served critical roles in enzymatic processes. These advances have directed particular attention in recent years to the basic biochemical lesions associated with the diverse manifestations of trace element deficiencies and excesses in the animal body.

Classically, the appearance of specific lesions or abnormalities in the animal was used to define the limiting factors in diseases of nutritional origin. Clinical and pathologic studies have served as essential diagnostic tools in the investigation of all trace element deficiencies and toxicities. It is important, nevertheless, to recognize their limitations. Not all trace element disorders result in specific and characteristic clinical signs or pathologic changes which are recognized readily, especially if the disorder is mild. Symptomatology and histopathology may vary depending upon a variety of factors: species, sex and age, the timing, duration and severity of deprivation, the nature of the element itself and its relation to other elements or constituents of the diet. Bone deformities, anemia, reproductive failure, neurologic dysfunction and defective development of the integument and its appendages are common. Mild micronutrient imbalances are often indistinguishable from primary dietary deficiency due to starvation or simply the loss of appetite. Moreover, the clinically or pathologically obvious functional or structural abnormality may be merely the final expression of a defect arising earlier in a chain of metabolic events and may bear no simple relationship to the limiting element.

Because trace elements are biologically active at very low concentrations, rigidly controlled experimental conditions are essential. Failure to observe appropriate precautionary measures has often led to erroneous conclusions. Moreover, a given nutrient element may have multiple modes of action and the specific biologic response to this element may occur within a relatively narrow concentration range. At concentrations above this range, the element may actually become inhibitory or deleterious to the organism, a toxic or pharmacologic manifestation resulting from interaction of the element at other sites.

A further difficulty in the interpretation of many studies results from the frequent occurrence of abnormalities in metal metabolism brought about by *metal ion antagonism* or *conditioned deficiencies* occurring when the normal intake of a nutrient does not meet the needs of an organism because of unusual secondary circumstances or factors. Failure to absorb a metabolite, the inability to synthesize it into a biologically active intermediate and excessive excretion are among the simplest examples of such conditioning factors. The antagonistic action of zinc and molybdenum with copper may serve to illustrate the type of problem encountered frequently: The anemia, subnormal growth and reproductive failure in rats induced by excess zinc in diets and the severe diarrhea and loss of condition in cattle attributed to molybdenum intoxication in a disease known as *teart* were both later found to be caused by conditioned copper deficiency.

Another problem in assessing the function of trace metals in biologic processes arises from the fact that their roles are frequently indirect. Thus, cobalt alone is completely ineffective in the treatment of patients with pernicious anemia; it is therapeutically significant only as a constituent of the vitamin B_{12} molecule. These and similar problems underlie the difficulties encountered in establishing meaningful relationships between disease and alterations in trace metal metabolism.

For these reasons and because the determination of concentrations of trace elements, like that of concentrations of other metabolites, in tissues, cells, subcellular components and body fluids is a corollary to the elucidation of their role in health and disease, the attention of present-day investigators has centered upon the *distribution* and *function* of metals at the subcellular, enzymatic and molecular levels. Moreover, advances in analytic chemistry, biochemistry and molecular biology have permitted the formulation of new hypotheses and their experimental evaluation by means previously unavailable.

Presently, reliable measurements of small concentrations of trace elements present in tissues, cells, subcellular particles, body fluids, proteins and nucleic acids can be performed by colorimetry, fluorimetry, polarography, emission spectrography, flame spectrophotometry, neutron activation analysis, x-ray fluorescence, atomic absorption spectrometry and microwave excitation emission spectrometry. The last method, recently developed, is particularly sensitive for the measurement of certain metals. Thus it is possible, for example, to detect zinc, cadmium, manganese, copper, cobalt and lead in picogram amounts.[6]

Such studies are becoming indispensable in detecting and defining trace element disorders and in delineating the environmental limits under which they are likely to occur. As understanding of the sites and modes of action of micronutrient elements grows, it seems likely that chemical analyses or enzyme assays of particular parts of tissues or cell components will become even more effective diagnostic aids. When these criteria are used jointly and the combined evidence is assessed by the discerning investigator, rapid and revealing data for the recognition and prediction of both deficiency and toxicity states may be obtained even when these are mild.

SOIL-PLANT-ANIMAL RELATIONS

The natural occurrence of deficiency or intoxication of a trace element in animals and man depends ultimately upon the plant, soil and water supply of mineral nutrients. Deficiency and intoxication states in plants and farm animals, which depend upon a limited area for grazing and upon fodder or regulated feedings, usually are recognized readily and the responsible element can be identified. Trace element deficiencies, toxicities and imbalances in man are usually milder, more restricted and more difficult to diagnose and trace to their natural sources, for a variety of reasons.[1] Human mineral requirements are low compared with those of modern breeds of animals, because of a slower growth rate and lower rate of reproduction. The sources of human foods and beverages usually comprise minerals derived from a range of soil types. Modern human dietaries contain a great variety of types of foods, so that trace element abnormalities which may be present in particular parts of plants, animal tissues or fluids can be offset by the consumption of other types of food not affected by deficiencies. The industrial treatment of various foods provides the opportunity both for gains and for losses of trace elements during storage, transport, preservation and processing. Thus, the impact of these influences upon the qualitative adequacy of human diets combines to render the nutritional abnormalities in man far more likely to be associated with poor choice of foods rather than with their sources, and, more commonly, the deficiency or intoxication states occur as *conditioned imbalances* brought about by other factors, e.g. poor absorption. However, when the choice and quality of foods are poor and the dependence on locally grown foods is high, local soil deficiencies or excesses may accentuate the dietary abnormalities and adversely affect human health and nutrition.

BIOCHEMISTRY AND PHYSICAL CHEMISTRY

The search for an explanation of the physiologic role of trace elements has emphasized their association with enzyme systems in living cells. For operational purposes, the enzymes which are affected by metals can be considered in two groups: metalloenzymes and metal-enzyme complexes.[7]

A *metalloenzyme* contains a metal as an integral part of the molecule in a fixed amount per molecule of protein. The small numbers of metal atoms are bound firmly to a limited number of apparently specific sites and are not removed from the protein by mild procedures. When the element is dissociated from the protein moiety by more vigorous manipulation, all measurable biologic activity is lost and is not readily restored by the readdition of this or any other metal. The specific and unique chemical nature of the metal-protein interactions apparently confers both stability and reactivity on the molecule. In some metalloenzymes, the metal atom serves primarily as a component of the active site and participates directly in the catalytic process. In other instances, the metal may serve to maintain the tertiary and quaternary structures of the protein, and its loss affects catalytic function indirectly by causing structural changes. In some enzymes, the metals appear to play both catalytic and structural roles. The elucidation of the physical and chemical basis of metal-protein interactions and their relationship to biologic function constitutes a rapidly advancing and widening area of modern biochemistry.

A large number of metalloproteins, with and without known enzymatic function, have now been isolated from a variety of sources ranging from bacteria to man and are characterized sufficiently to be considered "pure." Copper, cadmium, cobalt, manganese, molybdenum, selenium and zinc may be mentioned in this group. Although relatively few of these metalloproteins have been obtained from human sources, their significance with respect to the biochemistry, physiology and pathology of man is becoming increasingly clear, since their function in different phyla constitutes a common biologic denominator. Structurally, chemically and catalytically similar metalloenzymes are found in species of widely diverse evolutionary histories, thereby indicating their general metabolic importance.

Metalloenzymes may be contrasted with *metal-enzyme complexes*, which compose a far larger group of enzymes that are more loosely associated with metals, the criterion of association being the *activation* of catalysis. In this group, the specificity of association cited above is lacking. The metals may be removed quite readily and different ones may substitute for one another in many instances. The metals which have

been found to activate metal-enzyme complexes include magnesium, manganese, cobalt, zinc, cadmium, chromium, nickel, calcium and other alkaline earths, iron, copper and mercury. Some of the rare earths have also been found to activate a few enzymes. The metal ion is not an integral part of the molecule and, in many instances, the enzymes may be active in the absence of the metal ion. These circumstances increase the difficulties of assessing the biologic significance of these in vitro findings.

Some investigators have considered the differences between these two groups of metal-enzyme systems to be a matter only of degree rather than of kind. A continuous spectrum of the firmness of association between metal and protein has been postulated, with metalloenzymes at one end and metal-enzyme complexes at the other, both having similar biochemical function. Other workers have emphasized the dissimilarities. Whatever the viewpoint, metalloenzymes operationally lend themselves more readily to a definitive assessment of the physiologic role of a metal in enzyme systems at this time, since the element and the enzyme may be studied jointly in vitro and in vivo, the inherent specificity of their association lending biologic significance to the results and providing a chemical basis for the biologic manifestations. While metal-enzyme complexes have been of great theoretical importance in the understanding of catalytic phenomena and general mechanisms of metalloenzyme function, the nature of the underlying chemistry has been more difficult to establish.

Delineation of the role of trace metals in the function and structure of enzymes represents a significant advance in our understanding of the manner in which metals participate in biologic processes and provides a fundamental basis in relating trace elements to health and disease. The discovery of substantial quantities of firmly bound metals, including nickel, chromium, cobalt and manganese, in ribonucleic acids[8] constitutes another potentially important new avenue for the investigation of the role of metals in biology. These metals apparently stabilize the secondary and tertiary structure of RNA[9] and may play an important role in protein synthesis.

The following sections deal with the individual trace elements currently thought to be important for the health and nutrition of man. With a few exceptions, most of the references point to authoritative reviews and pertinent studies published in recent years.

COPPER

Copper is a constituent and essential nutrient of most if not all animals and plants, and its deficiency can lead to severe derangement of growth and metabolism. It has been known to be an essential component of respiratory pigments for over a century and is being detected in an increasing number of proteins and enzymes. It serves as an oxygen carrier in the hemolymph of molluscs and arthropods. In plants, cuproenzymes serve as oxidoreductants of phenols and, in animals, they additionally participate in melanin formation. In animals, copper is involved in activities as diverse as hemoglobin synthesis, bone and elastic tissue development and the normal function of the central nervous system.[10,11]

Physiology and Metabolism

The average copper concentration of an adult vertebrate is of the order of 1.5 to 2.5 μg per gm fat-free tissue. A total of 100 to 150 mg of copper is found in normal man. In general, the liver (10 to 15 mg), kidney, heart, hair and brain (10 mg) contain the highest concentrations of copper. Spleen, lung, muscle and bone contain intermediate, while pituitary, thyroid and thymus have the lowest concentrations. There are about 45 μg of copper per gm dry weight of adult human liver, while there may be 5 to 10 times as much in fetal liver. During growth, the highest concentrations of copper appear in the rapidly developing structures.

Over 90 per cent of the copper in mammalian plasma is associated with the α_2-globulin ceruloplasmin, while over 60 per cent of the copper in erythrocytes is presumed to be associated with erythrocuprein, now known to be the enzyme superoxide dismutase. A small amount of plasma copper is bound to amino acids, i.e. histidine, threonine and glutamine, apparently in equilibrium with that bound to albumin.[12] In other tissues and fluids the biochemical substances with which the major part of the copper is associated are largely undefined.

On a normal diet copper is not accumulated preferentially by any tissue. About 25 per cent of the ingested copper is absorbed from the upper alimentary tract, enhanced by acid and prevented by calcium. Copper complexed with neutral or anionic organic substances may be absorbed more readily than the free ion. A mechanism for the regulation of the absorption of copper from the gastrointestinal tract according to demand, similar to that for iron, has not been established. The bile is the major pathway of copper excretion and a small amount, usually less than 30 μg per 24 hour volume, is excreted in the urine independent of the intake. Less than 5 per cent of ingested copper is retained.

Human whole blood contains about 100 μg of copper per 100 ml volume, distributed about equally between erythrocytes and plasma. The concentration of serum copper in normal individuals is constant and is independent of age, sex, menstrual cycle, food intake, diurnal or seasonal influences and tissue stores. Compared with that of adults, serum copper concentration in newborn infants is low, primarily because of the low concentration of ceruloplasmin. The transport of copper, absorbed either gastrointestinally or administered intravenously, has been studied with radioactive copper, [64]Cu. There is a transient initial rise in serum copper associated with the albumin fraction, followed by a slower secondary rise associated with the α_2-globulin fraction, ceruloplasmin. Ingested copper, loosely bound to serum albumin, is transported rapidly to the liver, bone marrow and other organs where it is stored and becomes incorporated into cuproproteins. The slow secondary rise of serum radioactivity associated with ceruloplasmin can be taken to represent the incorporation of copper into this protein by synthesis and, perhaps, by exchange. The amino acid bound fraction in serum may be involved with the transport of copper across cell membranes.[13] Administration of estrogens markedly increases both serum copper and ceruloplasmin concentrations. Increased serum copper concentrations are found in pregnancy and in hepatic cirrhosis due to hyperestrogenism.

The subcellular distribution of copper in rat liver has been studied: ^{64}Cu distributes differentially between the nucleus and cytoplasm, the uptake in the cytoplasm being much greater than that in the nucleus. The supernatant fractions contain the highest concentrations and about 65 per cent of the total liver copper, as compared to 27 per cent of the total liver nitrogen. A protein having characteristics similar to metallothionein has recently been isolated from rat liver but was thought actually to be a different protein and was termed copper chelatin.[14] The function or significance remains to be resolved.

Factors which influence the concentrations in the liver include diet, age, hormones and pregnancy. Diets abnormally high or low in copper content generally cause corresponding changes in the concentrations of the liver and, frequently, of the blood. Sheep and cattle are extremely sensitive to the copper content of the diet, and in these species the copper concentration of the liver varies directly as a function of the intake.

Table 9B–1. Representative Cuproenzymes and Cuproproteins

Enzyme or Protein	Source
Ceruloplasmin	Blood plasma
Tyrosinase	Skin and melanomas, mushrooms
Uricase	Liver and kidney
Dopamine β-hydroxylase	Adrenal glands
Lysyl oxidase	Connective tissue
Spermine oxidase	Bovine plasma
Benzylamine oxidase	Pig plasma
Diamine oxidase	Kidney
Ascorbic acid oxidase	Squash, cucumber
Laccase	Latex of lacquer tree
D-Galactose oxidase	Doctylium dendroides
Copper chelatin	Liver, kidney, yeast
Mitochondrocuprein	Neonatal liver
Hemocyanin	Molluscs, arthropods
Enzymes Containing Copper and Heme	
Cytochrome c oxidase	Mitochondria
Tryptophan-2,3-dioxygenase	Liver
Enzymes Containing Copper and Zinc	
Superoxide dismutase (cytocuprein, erythrocuprein, hepatocuprein)	Brain, erythrocytes, liver
Enzymes Containing Copper and Manganese	
Diamine oxidase	Human placenta

Biochemistry

The growing number of biochemical systems with which copper is specifically associated suggest its involvement in a broad range of biologic functions.[15] Some of the purified cuproenzymes and copper-containing proteins are shown in Table 9B–1. Importantly, copper is a constituent of cytochrome oxidase, the terminal oxidase of the electron transport chain from which ATP is synthesized oxidatively. This enzyme also contains heme as a prosthetic group. Cuproenzymes catalyze oxidation reactions, including phenolic substrates such as the catecholamines. Ceruloplasmin, the copper-transport protein in plasma, also exhibits phenol oxidase activity, and there is a good correlation between the copper content of the serum and its capacity to oxidize substances such as paraphenylenediamine, benzidine and other phenols, including catecholamine. Furthermore, it exhibits ferro-oxidase activity, i.e. it oxidizes ferrous iron to ferric iron.[16] Ceruloplasmin has a molecular weight of 132,000 and each molecule contains 6 atoms of copper which can be removed in the presence of ascorbic acid.[17] The copper-free, colorless, apoceruloplasmin can be recombined with cuprous ions to form ceruloplasmin. The copper atoms of ascorbate oxidase can also be reversibly restored and appear to serve both catalytic and structural roles in the molecule. Dopamine β-hydroxylase from adrenal medulla converts dopamine to norepinephrine.[18] Tyrosinase or phenoloxidase activity, present in plants such as potatoes and mushrooms, is also found in melanocytes and melanoma tissue of animals and man. The enzymatic activity is associated with the mitochondrial fractions of cells and is responsible for melanin formation. The skin of human albinos has no detectable tyrosinase activity, indicating a deficiency of this enzyme as the basis for the absence of pigment in the skin and uveal tract. Enzymes involved in the oxidation of mono- and diamines, uric acid and galactose are all copper proteins. Amine oxidase activity is also involved in the oxidative deamination of ϵ-amino groups of lysyl residues forming desmosine, the cross-linking group of elastin.[19] Cross-linking of collagen is similarly dependent upon this cuproenzyme. In addition to these cuproenzymes, a number of enzymes such as ureidosuccinase, lecithinase and oxaloacetic decarboxylase are activated by copper, i.e. they form metal-enzyme complexes.

Cerebrocuprein, erythrocuprein and hepatocuprein, collectively called cytocuprein, are identical bluish-green soluble proteins containing about 0.35 per cent copper.[20] They contain 2 atoms each of copper and zinc per molecule of protein.[21] These proteins exhibit superoxide dismutase activity, and are now called superoxide dismutases, i.e. they catalyze the breakdown of superoxide radicals to oxygen and hydrogen peroxide and function to protect living cells against the toxic effects of oxygen.[22] Extracts of brain from patients with hepatolenticular degeneration (Wilson's disease) contain an abnormal copper protein which is isolated together with cerebrocuprein. A protein with high copper affinity has also been demonstrated in the liver of such patients. This protein is similar to mitochondrocuprein isolated from the mitochondria of neonatal liver which contains 3 per cent copper and is insoluble.[20] The amino acid composition of mitochondrocuprein is remarkably similar to that of metallothionein, a cadmium- and zinc-containing protein from kidney (see below). It has been suggested that mitochondrocuprein is a polymeric form of metallothionein.

Low-molecular-weight proteins, in many respects similar to metallothionein or copper-chelatin, have been identified in the cytosol of bovine duodenum and rat intestine.[23] Transport functions for these proteins have been postulated.

Ribonucleic acid isolated from a number of biologic sources contains significant amounts of firmly bound copper in addition to other metals. Significant concentrations of copper have also been found in isolated and purified viruses, perhaps through association with nucleic acid.

Copper influences erythropoiesis; its deficiency impairs iron absorption and transport and decreases hemoglobin synthesis. Concomitant with the decrease in plasma ceruloplasmin concentration, there is reduced transport of iron from the intestine and from the iron stores in tissues and liver to the plasma. The oxidation of ferrous iron to ferric iron catalyzed by ceruloplasmin is apparently important for the formation of transferrin.[24] In copper deficiency the utilization of iron for hemoglobin synthesis is also impaired and abnormal erythrocytes with shortened life span are produced.

Nutrition

The necessity of copper for animal nutrition has now been recognized for more than 30 years, although chemical and clinical evidence of copper deficiency in man did not emerge until recently. Because copper is widely distributed in foods and cooking utensils, it seems improbable that copper deficiency would occur in man except under extreme conditions. Dietary sources of copper are similar to those of iron. Milk products are relatively poor sources. The normal copper intake of man is estimated to be 2.5 to 5 mg per day, an amount adequate for the maintenance of positive copper balance.[25] Children require about 0.05 to 0.1 mg per kg body weight daily.

Copper deprivation leading to hypochromic anemia has been demonstrated in rats, rabbits, chickens, pigs, dogs, sheep, goats and cattle. The absorption of iron from the gastrointestinal tract is decreased and there is a reduction in the survival time of red blood cells. Total-body iron stores are reduced, and the capacity of bone marrow to produce erythrocytes is limited. Malnourished prisoners of war and mentally defective infants placed on diets identical to those producing copper deficiency in swine do not develop hypocupremia or any other evidence of copper deficiency. However, anemia responding to the administration of copper has been reported to occur in infants fed a milk diet for several months following recovery from kwashiorkor,[26] in very premature infants,[27] and in infants[28] and adults[29] receiving total parenteral nutrition.

Copper is essential for the normal development of bone, the central nervous system and connective tissue. Lambs born of copper-deficient ewes develop *enzootic ataxia,* or swayback, characterized by an incoordination of gait. A similar disease has been observed in calves and piglets. Histologic examination shows diffuse symmetric cerebral demyelinization with secondary degeneration of the motor tracts in the spinal cord. Cerebellar folia are absent or deformed. Deficiencies in sheep and cattle lead to osteoporosis and spontaneous fractures. Growing animals develop a rickets-like disease and osteoblastic activity is impaired. Bone collagen from copper-deficient animals shows increased solubility and decreased cross-linking. Bone amine oxidase and cytochrome oxidase activities are decreased. Abnormalities in pigmentation and crimp of hair, and wool, the former presumably related to decreased activity of the phenol oxidases, have also been found in a number of species. Alopecia and dermatoses as well as alterations in the texture and quality of hair and wool have been observed.

Severe copper deprivation in cows leads to myocardial fibrosis and a seasonal incidence of sudden death known as "falling disease." Cardiac hypertrophy has been observed in pigs. It has been suggested that the reduction of cytochrome oxidase activity in copper deprivation may lead to the observed cardiac hypertrophy in an effort to compensate for the reduction in respiratory activity. Cardiac and aortic aneurysms and rupture have also been observed in copper-deficient pigs and chicks. Studies of the aorta have shown decreased tensile strength and elastin content and striking pathologic change of the elastic fibers. There is an increased amount of a soluble protein which appears to be an elastin precursor. The lysine content of elastin is markedly increased by the failure of conversion of lysine to desmosine, the cross-linking residues of elastin.[30] This reaction is catalyzed by amine oxidase, which is decreased in activity in the serum, aorta, heart and kidney of copper-deficient animals.[31] The close similarity of these findings to those observed in lathyrism produced by β-aminopropionitrile, a chelating agent and inhibitor of amine oxidase, suggests that they share common mechanisms in generating the observed abnormalities of bone and connective tissue. The manifestations of copper de-

Table 9B–2.   Manifestations of Copper Deficiency and their Enzymatic Basis

Pathology	Metabolic Derangement	Enzyme Defect
Anemia	Iron transport and heme synthesis	Ceruloplasmin ? Cytochrome oxidase
Skeletal, dermal and vascular defects	Cross-linking of collagen and elastin	Lysyl oxidase
Achromotrichia	Melanin formation	Tyrosinase
CNS disorders	Myelination Catecholamine content	Cytochrome oxidase Dopamine β-hydroxylase
Kinky (steely) hair	Keratinization	? Sulfhydryl oxidase

ficiency and their enzymatic basis are summarized in Table 9B–2.

Several *conditioned* copper intoxication or deficiency diseases in animals have been observed. In cattle, a disease known as *teart*, characterized by severe diarrhea and loss of condition, was initially attributed to molybdenum intoxication. The resemblance of this disease to that exhibited by cattle in certain copper-deficient areas led to the empirical and successful use of copper sulfate in treatment. It soon became apparent that molybdenum in the diet of ruminants could exert a profound effect on copper metabolism. Conversely, sheep grazing on pastures with low molybdenum content rapidly accumulated toxic quantities of copper, whereas a surfeit of molybdenum led to signs of copper deficiency and depletion of tissue copper stores. Furthermore, the "toxicity" of molybdenum is greatly enhanced by an increased intake of inorganic sulfate and perhaps reduced by an increased intake of manganese. Neither molybdenum nor sulfate alone interferes with copper retention, and the effectiveness of either increases to a maximum as the intake of the other is increased. Apparently molybdenum plus sulfate interferes with the availability of copper by blocking tissue utilization or promoting copper excretion or both.

The copper deficiency caused by excess dietary zinc in rats, resulting in anemia, subnormal growth and reproductive failure, is another example of a conditioned copper deficiency. Feeding of excess dietary zinc reduces the liver cytochrome oxidase and catalase activities of rats markedly, and the administration of small amounts of copper sulfate restores the enzymatic activities to normal. In addition, excess zinc in the diet suppresses liver copper concentrations if the copper intake is marginal. On the other hand, an excess intake of copper reduces the zinc concentration of the liver.

Other biochemical studies have shown that copper deprivation leads to decreased tyrosinase, polyphenol oxidase and ascorbic acid oxidase activities in plants. In copper-deficient rats, cytochrome oxidase, amine oxidase and superoxide dismutase activities and ceruloplasmin and hemoglobin concentrations are reduced. Extreme copper deficiency leads to the loss of oxidative capacity in mitochondria because of a decrease of cytochrome oxidase activity. ATP synthesis is decreased and phospholipid synthesis is depressed.[32] Mitochondria become fragile and more susceptible to aging. A reduction in NAD cytochrome c reductase and increased isocitric dehydrogenase activities have also been observed.

Copper Metabolism and Human Disease

Serum copper concentrations are increased in a number of acute and chronic pathologic conditions.[11] Viral and microbial infections, rheumatoid arthritis, rheumatic fever, lupus erythematosus, myocardial infarction, severe thyrotoxicosis, acute and chronic leukemia, a variety of malignant neoplasms, hemochromatosis, portal and biliary cirrhosis may be listed. In general the concentration in red blood cells is unaffected. In infections and myocardial infarction, ceruloplasmin concentration rises concomitant with the increase in copper concentration. A parallel increase in serum oxidase activity is observed. These increases in copper and ceruloplasmin content are unexplained and are not correlated with the change in sedimentation rate. In patients with portal and biliary cirrhosis the copper content of liver is increased.

Hypocupremia has been observed in a variety of states. In the nephrotic syndrome the urinary excretion of copper is increased in direct proportion to the amount of protein lost in the urine. Ceruloplasmin, not normally detected in the urine, is excreted and serum ceruloplasmin concentrations are decreased. Low serum copper concentrations have been observed also in kwashiorkor, sprue, celiac disease and idiopathic hypoproteinemia, presumably a result of an imbalance in the rate of synthesis and breakdown of ceruloplasmin.

An uncommon malady of infants is characterized by edema, hypoproteinemia, anemia, hypoferremia and hypocupremia and decreased serum ceruloplasmin concentrations. These manifestations are similar to the combined copper- and iron-deficiency anemias produced in swine on milk diets, and are corrected by administration of iron and copper. A pure syndrome of copper deficiency in premature infants with gastrointestinal dysfunction and fed diets deficient in copper has recently been described.[33] Features include a refractory sideroblastic anemia, neutropenia, osteopenia by x-ray examination, depigmentation of skin and hair, hypotonia and psychomotor retardation. Serum copper and ceruloplasmin concentrations, plasma iron clearance and erythrocyte iron uptake are decreased. The ad-

ministration of copper alone reverses all abnormalities of this syndrome.

Hepatolenticular degeneration or Wilson's disease is a rare, genetic disease transmitted as a recessive autosomal trait and is the condition best known to be associated with hypocupremia.[34] The cardinal manifestations are the neurologic abnormalities arising from dysfunction of the lenticular region of the brain, signs of hepatic cirrhosis and the demonstration of a brown or gray-green (Kayser-Fleischer) ring at the limbus of the cornea. Renal abnormalities characterized by aminoaciduria, glucosuria, phosphaturia, uricosuria, proteinuria and polypeptiduria may be present along with hypophosphatemia and hypouricemia. The serum copper concentration is usually depressed while urinary excretion is markedly increased. Ceruloplasmin concentration is generally decreased, and leukocyte cytochrome oxidase activity is decreased. The liver, basal ganglia, cerebral cortex, kidney and Kayser-Fleischer corneal rings of patients with Wilson's disease contain excessive quantities of copper. In liver the largest amount of copper is present in a subfraction of liver cells corresponding to neonatal hepatic mitochondrocuprein. Variations in serum copper concentration are due to a high and variable content of the loosely bound copper associated with albumin. Studies with radioactive copper indicate that absorption is increased in individuals with hepatolenticular degeneration: up to 0.56 mg per day per mg of ingested copper or 20 to 50 times normal is retained. Although the incorporation of copper into ceruloplasmin is deranged, the plasma concentration of free or loosely bound (to albumin) copper is increased. The pathogenesis of the disease remains unknown. It has been suggested that patients with this disease may synthesize abnormal proteins having an increased affinity for copper. However, the hypothesis favored by many is that a combination of factors, including decreased incorporation of copper by ceruloplasmin because of abnormalities of its synthesis and impaired binary excretion of copper, may jointly determine the increased deposition of copper in liver. When the copper-binding capacity of liver is exceeded, deposition in other tissues and organs (brain, kidneys, cornea) then occurs, leading to damage.

Attempts to eliminate excessive copper in body tissues and to prevent reaccumulation are the most promising modes of therapy. Various copper chelating agents which are excreted in the urine have been employed, including 2,3-dimercaptopropanol (BAL), ethylenediaminetetraacetate (Versene) and β,β-dimethylcysteine (penicillamine). The latter, when given orally, has given the most encouraging clinical results.[35]

Menkes' kinky (steely) hair syndrome[36] is another disease of abnormal copper metabolism in man. It is inherited as an X-linked recessive trait and is characterized by pili torti, developmental regression, seizures, temperature instability, intimal abnormalities of arteries and scorbutic bone changes. Cerebral degeneration is progressive, usually leading to death before 3 years of age. The copper content of blood, liver and perhaps brain is diminished in patients with the syndrome and decreased activity of cuproenzymes, such as cytochrome oxidase, connective tissue amine oxidase, dopamine β-hydroxylase and tyrosinase, is presumed to underlie many of these abnormalities. The fundamental defect in this disease appears to be a derangement in the transport of copper out of the intestinal mucosal cells into the blood stream, because the uptake of copper by intestinal cells is normal and the copper content of the intestinal cells is increased but blood and liver content of copper is decreased. Recently, cultured skin fibroblasts from patients with Menkes' disease have been shown to exhibit increased copper content.[37] Thus, the abnormality of cellular transport does not appear to be limited to the cells of the intestinal mucosa.

Several inbred strains of mice exhibit abnormalities of copper metabolism or of cuproenzyme function. One of these is the result of a mutation at the X-linked *mottled* locus. Its phenotypic expressions are very similar to those observed in Menkes' syndrome, thus constituting an excellent animal model of the disease.[36] Other mutants are the crinkled and quaking mice which exhibit connective tissue and pigment abnormalities and axial tremors, respectively. In crinkled mice the copper content of hair is decreased and in quaking mice that of brain is diminished. Interestingly, copper supplementation during the prenatal and neonatal periods of growth can ameliorate or prevent the phenotypic expressions of these mutant genes. The precise abnormality in copper metabolism in these mutants remains to be elucidated.[38,39]

Copper Intoxication

Chronic ingestion of excess copper in fodder of sheep leads to accumulations 10 to 20 times the normal concentration of copper in the liver. The animals suffer no apparent ill effects until suddenly a large amount of excess copper is liberated into the blood stream, producing hemolytic anemia, hemoglobinuria and jaundice. Over 60 per cent of the circulating red cells may be destroyed during the crisis and atrophy of the liver may occur. A similar type of hemolytic jaundice has been observed in cattle. Acute copper intoxication in man due to ingestion of copper produces nausea, vomiting, epigastric pain, diarrhea, ptyalism, headache, dizziness, weakness and a metallic taste. In more severe cases tachycardia, hypertension and coma may ensue, followed by jaundice and hemolytic anemia, hemoglobinuria, uremia and death. Serum ceruloplasmin concentrations are increased, as is loosely bound serum copper.[40]

ZINC

The presence of zinc in living organisms and its role as an essential nutrient have been recognized for almost a century, but difficulties in analysis limited early investigations to qualitative efforts. It was not until 1934 that conclusive evidence was adduced that zinc is essential to the normal growth and development of animals. The isolation and purification by Keilin and Mann in 1940 of carbonic anhydrase, found to contain zinc as a component of the molecule and essential for enzymatic function, offered the first concrete basis for an explanation of a mode of action of this element. Since then zinc has been found in many highly purified enzymes, revealing the diversity of its function in protein, nucleic acid, lipid, mucopolysaccharide and carbohydrate metabolism. Zinc-deficiency states in mammals as well as in man have been described.[41,42]

Physiology and Metabolism

The total amount of zinc in the human body has been estimated to be between 2 and 3 gm. Zinc is found in all human tissues, varying from 10 to 200 μg per gm wet weight. Most organs, including the pancreas, contain 20 to 30 μg, while liver, voluntary muscle and bone contain 60 to 180 μg per gm. Larger quantities of zinc are found in the tissues of the eye, particularly the iris, retina and choroid. Zinc is not accumulated preferentially by any tissue although the prostate, prostatic secretions and spermatozoa are remarkably high in zinc content (860 μg per gm for normal human prostate) which is not accounted for by the content of either carbonic anhydrase or alkaline phosphatase. There is no functional explanation for the high concentration of zinc in the male reproductive tract. Differences in organ content from species to species are not remarkable in most instances.

Human whole blood contains about 900 μg of zinc per 100 ml. Normal serum zinc concentrations average 121 ± 19 μg per 100 ml.[43] Normal erythrocytes contain 1.4 mg per 100 ml of packed red blood cells. Three per cent of all blood zinc is found in leukocytes which contain 3.2×10^{-2} μg zinc per million cells, about 25 times more than is found in a comparable number of erythrocytes. Blood zinc concentrations do not exhibit seasonal or diurnal variations and there is no difference in concentration between the sexes. Practically all zinc in serum is protein bound and is distributed in at least two and possibly more fractions.[44] Globulins bind zinc most firmly and an α_2-macroglobulin has been isolated and shown to be a zinc metalloprotein.[45] Most of the remainder, 80 per cent, is probably bound loosely to albumin which appears to be concerned primarily with transport. A large percentage of the erythrocyte zinc appears to be associated with carbonic anhydrase and that in leukocytes with alkaline phosphatase. Serum zinc decreases during pregnancy and with estrogen administration.

The distribution of ^{65}Zn injected in the mouse and the dog indicates that the liver accumulates the largest fraction of the total dose, and the most rapid turnover of ^{65}Zn was observed to occur in liver, pancreas, kidney and pituitary. About 10 per cent of the total ^{65}Zn given was excreted in the pancreatic juice within the first few days. Bone and red blood cells accumulated ^{65}Zn.

Zinc is widely distributed in a variety of foods. Foodstuffs from animal sources, particularly shellfish, are rich in this element. The average human dietary intake is about 10 to 15 mg per day, of which about 5 mg are retained. The site and mechanism of absorption of zinc from the intestine are not known with certainty. The availability of zinc for absorption is decreased by phytic acid, a phosphorus storage compound of plant seeds, which forms insoluble zinc-phytate complexes. Calcium can further decrease its availability by forming the more insoluble mixed zinc-calcium-phytate complex.[46] Once absorbed, zinc is excreted primarily in gastrointestinal and pancreatic secretions. Urine contains about 0.5 mg per day, an amount apparently independent of intake and urinary volume. Studies in the rat indicate that, in contrast to iron, the body stores of zinc are not readily mobilized and, hence, there is an unusual dependence upon a regular, exogenous supply of the element, particularly during periods of growth.

Biochemistry

Zinc is closely associated with a large variety of proteins and enzymes. As a result, the total zinc content of tissues is an inadequate guide to the manifold functions of the metal. The large number of zinc metalloenzymes which have now been isolated point to the wide importance of this metal in metabolism. More than 80 zinc-containing enzymes and proteins have now been discovered from diverse sources throughout all phyla and at least one zinc metalloenzyme has been identified in each of the 6 major enzyme categories classified according to function, i.e. oxidoreductase, transferase, hydrolase, lyase, isomerase and ligase. A representative list is shown in Table 9B–3. Alcohol dehydrogenase, alkaline phosphatase, carboxypeptidase and carbonic anhydrase have been isolated from human tissues and erythrocytes. In these and other zinc metalloenzymes, the metal is essential for the catalytic function and/or the structural integrity of the molecule.

Alcohol dehydrogenase, which is present in liver as well as other organs, oxidizes ethanol and other primary and secondary alcohols, as well as vitamin A alcohol, and reduces retinene. Retinene reductase of the retina is apparently identical or very

Table 9B–3.   Representative Zinc Metalloenzymes and -proteins

Enzyme	Source
Alcohol dehydrogenase	Horse and human liver yeast
d-Lactate cytochrome c reductase	Yeast
Aspartate transcarbamylase	E. coli
RNA polymerase	E. coli, yeast, E. gracilis
DNA polymerase	E. coli, sea urchin
Reverse transcriptase [RNA-dependent DNA polymerase]	Mammalian viruses
Alkaline phosphatase	Mammalian livers, kidneys, placenta and leukocytes, E. coli
Phospholipase C	B. cereus
α-D-Mannosidase	Jack bean
AMP-aminohydrolase	Rabbit muscle
Leucine aminopeptidase	Mammalian kidney, bovine lens, porcine kidney
Carboxypeptidase C	Orange peel
Carboxypeptidase A	Beef, human pancreas
Carboxypeptidase B	Beef, pig pancreas
Dipeptidase	Pig kidney, mouse ascites tumor cells, E. coli
Aldolase	Yeast, Aspergillus niger
Carbonic anhydrase	Mammalian erythrocytes
δ-Aminolevulinate dehydratase	Beef and rat liver, erythrocytes
Phosphomannose isomerase	Yeast
Pyruvate carboxylase	Pig liver, yeast
Protein synthesis elongation factor	Rat liver
Methionyl t-RNA synthetase	E. coli
Enzyme Containing Zinc and Copper	
Superoxide dismutase	Bovine liver, erythrocytes
Enzyme Containing Zinc and Cobalt	
Oxaloacetate Transcarboxylase	Propionibacterium shermanii
Enzyme Containing Zinc and Calcium	
Thermolysin	B. thermolyticus

similar to this enzyme from liver. Horse liver alcohol dehydrogenase contains 4 atoms of zinc per molecule of protein and zinc is essential not only to the catalytic function of the enzyme but also to maintain the subunit structure.[47,48] In addition to ethanol, alcohol dehydrogenase from *human* liver also oxidizes methanol and ethylene glycol, serving as the primary mechanism of detoxification of these and other similar compounds.[49]

Carbonic anhydrase, which catalyzes the reaction $CO_2 + H_2O = H_2CO_3$, is present in erythrocytes in high concentrations and many tissues exhibit this enzymatic activity. Without this enzyme carbon dioxide elimination cannot take place with sufficient rapidity to sustain life and, hence, this enzyme is as important to carbon dioxide transport as is hemoglobin to oxygen transport. Carbonic anhydrases from ox, monkey and human erythrocytes all contain 1 gm atom of zinc per mole of enzyme and correlations have been obtained between the zinc content and enzyme activity in red blood cells under both normal and pathologic conditions. Substitution of cobalt for zinc results in an enzymatically active carbonic anhydrase.[50]

Both carboxypeptidase A and B from pancreatic juice contain 1 atom of zinc per molecule of protein. The single zinc atom is indispensable for the catalytic activities of these enzymes which hydrolyze peptide bonds to liberate the amino acids from the carboxy terminals of proteins and peptides. The zinc in carboxypeptidase A can be replaced in vitro by other metals, e.g. Co, Mn, Ni, Fe, Cd, Hg and Pb, with consequent dramatic alterations in catalytic activity and substrate specificity.[51] Both carboxypeptidase A and B are excreted into the gastrointestinal tract and are implicated in proteolysis and digestive processes.

The zinc atoms of alkaline phosphatase from E. coli appear to be essential for both catalytic function and subunit structure of the enzyme. A decrease in alkaline phosphatase activity has long been noted in zinc-deficient experimental animals, a change which may now be attributed to a failure of synthesis of the active holoenzyme. The alkaline phosphatase of leukocytes may well be identical with the zinc-containing protein of human leukocytes, which contains 0.3 per cent of zinc per gm dry weight of protein, and is responsible for 80 per cent of all zinc found in human leukocytes.

One of the important recent advances is the discovery that DNA and RNA polymerases from both procaryotic and eucaryotic microorganisms are zinc metalloenzymes.[52] Although these enzymes from mammalian sources have yet to be similarly identified, they are likely to be zinc metalloenzymes, since impaired growth, protein synthesis and DNA and RNA metabolism are prominent features in zinc-deficient animals. Even tumor growth has been shown to be inhibited by dietary zinc deficiency in rats. The relationship of zinc to cellular growth has recently been investigated in Euglena gracilis, and a number of striking morphologic and chemical changes accompany zinc deficiency-induced growth arrest:[53,54] Cell volume and size increase while osmophilic granules and paramylon accumulate; cellular DNA content doubles while RNA and protein content decrease; peptides, amino and other organic acids, nucleotides and polyphosphates accumulate.

Further studies have shown that zinc is present in subnuclear structures and is translocated to and from the nucleolus, the mitotic spindle apparatus and chromosomes at each stage of mitosis. In zinc deficiency, the progression of the cell through the various phases of mitosis (G_1, G_1, s, G_2) is impaired. These findings indicate that zinc is essential not only for protein and nucleic acid synthesis but also for the processes of cellular development, division and differentiation (Fig. 9B–1). Zinc has also been shown to be essential for polyribosome formation[55] and to be a component of protein synthesis elongation factor 1 from rat liver, which catalyzes the binding of amino acyl-tRNA to ribosomes.[56]

A further important advance in zinc biochemistry is the recent demonstration of its involvement in neoplastic processes. Studies of normal and leukemic leukocytes more than 25 years ago revealed a strikingly lowered zinc content in leukemic cells, generating the postulate that alterations of a zinc-dependent enzyme or enzymes might be critical to the pathophysiology of leukemias.[57] This hypothesis has recently found support in studies of the metal content of the RNA-dependent DNA polymerases (reverse transcriptases) from type C oncogenic viruses. Thus the enzymes from avian myeloblastosis, murine, simian, feline and RO-114 RNA tumor virus have now been shown to be zinc metalloenzymes. These viruses are associated with the induction of leukemia in these species. Moreover, studies of CCRF-CEM lymphoblasts, which are human lymphoid cells grown in culture from the blood of leukemic patients, have

shown that low concentrations of the chelating agent, 1,10-phenanthroline, inhibit the growth of both normal and leukemic CEM lymphoblasts. Interestingly, however, the chelating agent is cytotoxic to the leukemic cells at concentrations which cause only growth arrest of normal cells.[58] This unusual sensitivity may perhaps relate to the known difference in the zinc content between normal and leukemic leukocytes, and may lead to novel therapeutic approaches.

In addition to its critical role in the mechanism of action of zinc metalloenzymes, zinc increases the activities of many other enzymes. This effect may not be specific since other metal ions also activate most of these systems. The zinc-activated metal-enzyme complexes include carnosinase, histidine deaminase, enolase, dinucleotide pyrophosphatase, phosphoenolpyruvate carboxylase, pyridoxal kinase and others.[59] Among other metals, zinc has also been found to be present in RNA and DNA where it is likely to serve a role in maintaining structure. It has also been claimed that zinc stabilizes cell mem-

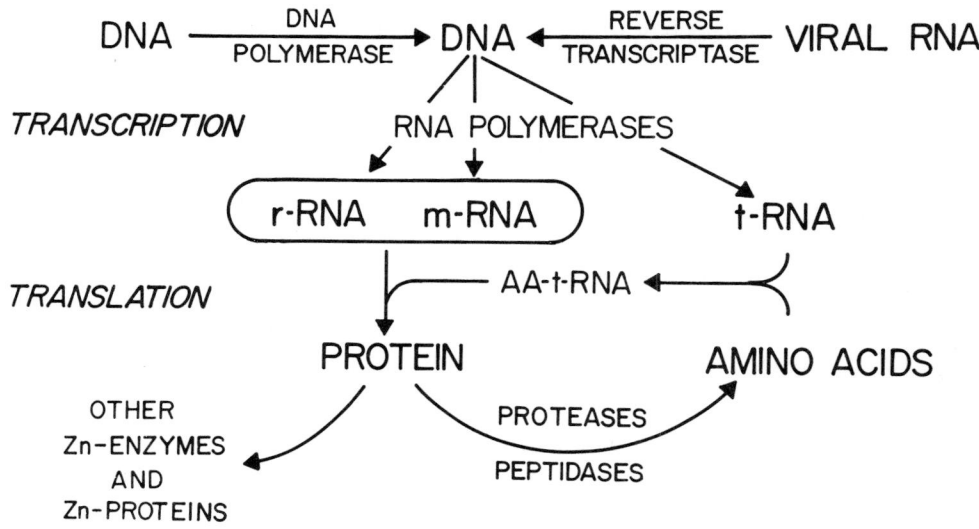

Fig. 9B–1. Zinc in nucleic acid and protein metabolism. The dependent steps are indicated by script over the arrows or breaking them.

branes and protects them against peroxidative damage.

A relationship between zinc and porphyrins has long been known and the excretion of zinc complexes of uroporphyrin and coproporphyrin in urine has been described in human diseases such as porphyria. However, the significance of these compounds is uncertain, since zinc porphyrins are known to form nonenzymatically. The enzymatic incorporation of zinc into porphyrins by an enzyme, zinc chelatase, present in chromatophores of Rhodopseudomonas spheroides[60] and also found in mammalian organs, has been demonstrated. At present, however, there is no known biologically active zinc porphyrin.

A relationship of zinc to the action of insulin, glucagon, corticotropin and other hormones has been postulated. Despite much study and circumstantial evidence, a role for zinc in hormonal function has not been established with certainty. However, it now appears that zinc is required for the ACTH-stimulated steroidogenesis by adrenal glands. The crystallization of insulin at pH values near 6 may be accomplished only in the presence of zinc ions or other metals such as cadmium, cobalt or nickel. Two atoms of zinc associate with 6 molecules of insulin to form a hexamer of MW 36,000. Porcine proinsulin also reacts with zinc.[61] However, physiologically active insulin can be prepared in both amorphous and crystalline form, entirely free of zinc and other metals. Thus the association of zinc with insulin in vitro has not been shown to be a compositional or structural feature essential for function. It cannot be judged from available evidence whether an insulin-zinc complex forms in vivo and is necessary for biologic activity.

Nutrition

Zinc deficiency has been observed or experimentally produced in a large variety of animal species as well as in man. The syndrome is characterized by failure to grow, anorexia, testicular atrophy, decreased size of the accessory sex glands and skin lesions. A decrease in food intake is an early sign of the deficiency state and forced feeding produces signs of ill health. Zinc supplementation promptly restores appetite. Apparently zinc deficiency has adverse effects on the gustatory system and a loss of taste acuity results.[14] In rats hypoplasia of the coagulating and prostate glands and seminal vesicles and hypospermia occur, reversed by the administration of zinc. Testicular degeneration, when it occurs, is not reversible. Notably, cadmium also destroys testicular tissue when administered subcutaneously to rats, but when it is injected together with a large excess of zinc acetate testicular degeneration is prevented. This metal ion antagonism between cadmium and zinc is not limited to the testes, since zinc deficiency in chickens becomes more severe when cadmium is administered simultaneously and higher concentrations of zinc are required to overcome the deficiency state.

Zinc-deficient rats characteristically develop hyperuricemia and the activities of pancreatic enzymes are decreased, as are intestinal and kidney alkaline phosphatase activities. In vitro addition of zinc to homogenates of the intestine and kidney from zinc-deficient animals fully restores alkaline phosphatase activity.[62] Synthesis of the apoenzyme apparently is unimpaired, but enzyme activity is lacking, entirely because concentrations of zinc are inadequate to form the active holoenzyme. Pancreatic carboxypeptidase activity has been shown to decrease quite specifically and rapidly in response to zinc deficiency and return to normal on repletion.[63] Changes in the activities of a number of dehydrogenases in the bone, kidney, intestine, esophagus and testes of zinc-deficient rats and swine have been noted.[64] Apparently these tissues are most sensitive to zinc depletion. Lowering of carbonic anhydrase activity is not usually encountered although there is slight anemia.

The RNA polymerase and thymidine kinase activities of growing tissues are decreased, as is also the incorporation of thymidine.[65] Plasma vitamin A levels are lowered, apparently as a result of a defect in the mobilization of the vitamin from liver into the circulation.[66] However, it is presently not established whether the same enzyme catalyzes this interconversion in retina and liver.

The most striking histologic finding in zinc-deficient rats is hyperkeratinization of the epidermis and parakeratosis of the esophagus, as is found also in other animal species.[67] This may relate in part to the strikingly abnormal sulfur and mucopolysaccharide metabolism which has been found to occur in zinc-deficient animals.[68]

Offspring of rats made zinc deficient for even short periods of time during pregnancy develop major congenital malformations involving the skeleton, brain, heart, eyes, gastrointestinal tract and lungs, emphasizing the importance of zinc to normal growth and development.[69] Fetal mortality is also increased. Interestingly, the deleterious effects of zinc deficiency can be offset by the feeding of a calcium-deficient diet.[70] It appears that the concomitant calcium deficiency, through bone resorption, increases the availability of skeletal zinc stores which are not readily mobilized normally. Abnormalities and decrease in plasma proteins have been reported in zinc-deficient rats, chicks, swine and the Japanese quail. Table 9B–4 summarizes and compares the morphologic, chemical and enzymatic alterations which have been observed in zinc-deficient animals with those in plants and microorganisms.

In hogs, zinc deficiency may occur spontaneously or be induced experimentally and is called porcine parakeratosis. This disease is characterized by dermatitis, diarrhea, vomiting, anorexia, severe weight loss and eventual death. The spontaneous disease has occurred in animals fed specialized diets and has been attributed to the practice of adding bone meal to

Table 9B–4. Zinc Deficiency in Different Phyla

	Morphologic Changes	Chemical Compositions Decrease	Chemical Compositions Increase	Decrease in Enzyme Activity
Micro-organisms	Growth retardation Increase in cell size	Protein RNA (ribosomal) Pyridine nucleotides	DNA Amino acids Polyphosphates Phospholipids ATP Organic acids	Alkaline phosphatase Alcohol dehydro-genase Lactate dehydrogenase Tryptophan desmolase
Plants	Stunted growth Small abnormal leaves Chlorotic mottling Decreased fruit production	Auxin Ethanolamine	Amino acids	Tryptophan desmolase Carbonic anhydrase Aldolase Pyruvate carboxylase
Animals	Growth retardation Fetal wastage Birth anomalies Testicular atrophy Parakeratosis Coarse, sparse hair	Hemoglobin Serum protein	Uric acid	Alkaline phosphatase Alcohol dehydro-genase Pancreatic proteases Leucine amino-peptidase Thymidine kinase RNA polymerase Lactate and malate dehydrogenase NADH diaphorase

the diet to accelerate growth and ossification. The experimental disease is aggravated by large amounts of dietary calcium, and, thus, parkeratosis in hogs is a conditioned zinc deficiency. The mechanism of the Ca-Zn antagonism is unknown. Supplements of zinc carbonate in the diets of hogs with either spontaneous or experimentally induced parakeratosis result in prompt recovery. A similar disease has been reported in cattle.

A syndrome of severe iron deficiency, anemia, hepatosplenomegaly, hypogonadism, hyperpigmentation and dwarfism in Iranian and Egyptian men was described in 1963 and attributed to primary zinc deficiency.[71] Geophagia was common in the Iranian dwarfs, and it was suggested that zinc deficiency may have resulted from excessive consumption of a cereal diet containing large amounts of phytate which inhibits iron and zinc absorption. A similar syndrome in Egyptians studied in greater detail showed, in addition, evidence of primary pituitary hypofunction associated with reduced activities of gonadotropic and growth hormones. The plasma zinc content and that of the red blood cells and hair were decreased, as was the 24-hour exchangeable zinc pool, while plasma turnover of zinc was increased. Sweat and urinary zinc excretion and serum alkaline phosphatase activity were decreased. Upon treatment with supplemental zinc salts a striking response in growth and development and of secondary sex characteristics was observed, exceeding that seen on treatment with a balanced diet alone. Serum zinc concentrations rose to normal. The anemia which was attributed to the concomitant iron deficiency of these patients due to parasitic infestations was not reversed by the administration of zinc. The above findings have recently been confirmed in Iranian women and school children. The deficiency syndrome is now being recognized also in the United States and elsewhere, particularly in young individuals with intestinal malabsorption of

prolonged duration during adolescence,[72,73] or with chronic total parenteral nutrition.[74] Because of marginal or deficient dietary intake, some children in the United States have been reported to exhibit decreased body zinc stores as measured by the content of zinc in hair. These children also exhibit poor growth, anorexia and hypogeusia, manifestations which are consistent with the existence of a mild but clinically significant deficiency state.[75] Serum zinc is consistently decreased during pregnancy. However, much of the decrease appears to be accountable on the basis of diminished binding by albumin and a relationship to marginal zinc nutritional status cannot be drawn.[76]

Zinc in Human Disease States

Serum zinc concentrations are decreased below the range of normal values in acute and chronic infections such as pneumonia, bronchitis, erysipelas and pyelonephritis and are restored upon recovery. The hypozincemia associated with acute inflammatory stresses has been found to be mediated by a protein which is released from leukocytes and stimulates the flux of zinc from plasma to liver.[77] It has been given the name *leukocytic endogenous mediator*. It appears also to have other broad actions in mediating some of the generalized host responses to an inflammatory stimulus, e.g. the synthesis of acute phase reactants by the liver. Serum zinc concentrations are also decreased in myocardial infarction and accompany the well-known changes in a variety of enzyme activities and increase in the copper concentration of serum. Decreased serum zinc values have also been reported in various malignancies, although a uniform pattern is not discernible. Increase in leukocyte zinc has been observed in patients with refractory anemia, while the zinc concentration of leukocytes in acute and chronic lymphatic and myelogenous leukemia is decreased to 10 per cent of the normal value. This phenomenon is apparently independent of the maturity of the cells but may be related to the decreased leukocyte alkaline phosphatase activities in some of these conditions. Excessive zinc excretion has been noted in leukemia and Hodgkin's disease though no cause is immediately apparent. The zinc content and carbonic anhydrase activity of red cells parallel each other and are significantly correlated in normal individuals as well as in those afflicted with anemia, polycythemia vera, secondary polycythemia, leukemia and congestive failure. Both parameters vary directly with the hematocrit level and the hemoglobin concentration. In untreated pernicious anemia, however, the erythrocyte zinc concentration and carbonic anhydrase activity are close to normal, while serum zinc concentrations are decreased. Serum concentrations return to normal with vitamin B_{12} therapy.

Dietary and conditioned zinc deficiency is a potential problem in patients with alcoholism and liver disease, chronic renal disease, rheumatoid arthritis, inflammatory bowel disease and malabsorption syndrome. Patients with chronic hemolytic anemias, such as sickle-cell disease,[78] exhibit zinc deficiency. Plasma and erythrocyte zinc concentrations are decreased and there is zincuria. The growth failure and hypogonadism in these patients may be related to zinc deficiency. Postsurgical patients may also develop zinc deficiency and, in these individuals, wound healing may be impaired.[79] Zinc deficiency can be induced by the administration of zinc chelating agents, such as penicillamine and histidine. In the latter instance, anorexia, taste and smell dysfunction and CNS abnormalities have been reported to be induced and were reversed by the administration of zinc.

Zinc and Postalcoholic Cirrhosis. The discovery of zinc in liver alcohol dehydrogenase stimulated the study of zinc metabolism in human liver disease.

Marked abnormalities in the metabolism of this metal were found to occur in postalcoholic cirrhosis.[43] The concentration of zinc in the serum of patients with a severe degree of this disease was decreased to 66 ± 19 μg per 100 ml as compared to the normal of 121 ± 19 μg per 100 ml. Greatest depressions were noted in patients in hepatic coma and concentrations of less than 30 μg per 100 ml signified an ominous prognosis. Among tests on liver function the zinc data correlated best with BSP retention. Analyses of liver tissue from patients who died of postalcoholic cirrhosis revealed only half the normal content of zinc and iron, while calcium, magnesium, aluminum, manganese and copper concentrations were normal. Significantly, patients with postalcoholic cirrhosis excrete abnormally large quantities of zinc in the urine, 1000 ± 200 μg per 24 hours. The decrease in serum zinc concentration and increased urinary excretion may in part be due to hypoalbuminemia and decreased protein binding of zinc. Administration of zinc sulfate in physiologic quantities to such patients tends to restore the normal excretory pattern in urine. A tendency toward restoration of normal liver function was often noted.[80] Apparently a conditioned zinc deficiency may be a feature of postalcoholic cirrhosis in man. It has been suggested that the low serum zinc concentration in cirrhosis may reflect a change in the synthesis, degradation, metal content, or specific activity of the zinc-containing enzymes which are cardinally involved in intermediary and protein metabolism. It cannot be stated, however, whether these abnormalities of zinc metabolism constitute primary or secondary manifestations of the disease. They do emphasize the significance of the metal to this nosologic entity. Human liver alcohol dehydrogenase has been isolated and identified as a zinc metalloenzyme.[81,82] Studies of this protein in patients with postalcoholic cirrhosis should be of special interest in furthering understanding of the subcellular pathology and etiology of this disease.

The effect of chronic ethanol ingestion has recently been studied in rats. Liver, plasma and muscle zinc content all decreased progressively. The most severe depletion was observed in liver, particularly from the mitochondrial compartment. These effects were seen as early as 2 weeks after the onset of ethanol feeding. The findings clearly indicate that hepatic zinc metabolism is deranged by ethanol long before the onset of cirrhosis.[83]

Acrodermatitis Enteropathica. The first inherited zinc-deficiency disorder was recently described as characterized by alopecia, dermatitis occurring in an acral distribution, diarrhea, photophobia, psychological changes and failure to thrive.[84] The disease is transmitted as an autosomal recessive trait. The patients and their family members exhibit low plasma zinc levels.[85] The primary defect is unknown, though abnormality of zinc absorption has been postulated. Small daily supplements of zinc are curative. This would seem to be the first human disease in which zinc reverses all pathologic lesions and accompanying clinical signs and symptoms. This may justly be thought to be a milestone in the biology and pathology of this hitherto elusive metal.

Toxicity

Compared to copper, lead, mercury and arsenic, zinc is relatively nontoxic. However, *inhalation* of zinc oxide fumes in high concentration, as may occur in industrial settings, produces an acute illness of relatively short duration characterized by chills, fever, cough, salivation, headache, leukocytosis and pulmonary infiltrates. Constant exposure produces tolerance, but intermittent exposure results in recurrence of the illness.

Poisoning due to *ingestion* of zinc may occur when foods have been stored in galvanized containers. Signs and symptoms of toxicity are nausea, vomiting, abdominal cramps, diarrhea and fever. In experimental animals, feeding of massive doses of zinc produces anemia, retarded growth and eventual death.

MANGANESE

A considerable amount of evidence has accumulated that manganese is essential in animal nutrition.[86,87] Although its essentiality for man has never been demonstrated clearly, functions similar to those in other mammals are assumed.

Physiology and Metabolism

Manganese is widely distributed in mammalian tissues, the highest concentrations (about 2 to 3 μg per gm) occurring in bone, pituitary, liver, pineal, and lactating mammary glands and the lowest in lung, connective tissue and muscle. The total manganese content of an adult human has been estimated to be about 20 mg, and the concentrations in individual organs tend to remain relatively constant throughout life. Within cells, manganese is located both in the nucleus and in cytoplasmic organelles. The turnover rate and concentration are relatively high in mitochondria and relatively low in the nucleus. Injected ^{56}Mn tends to localize preferentially in liver and pancreatic tissues and in cytoplasm rather than in nuclei.

As is iron, manganese is absorbed rather poorly from the intestinal tract. High dietary concentrations of calcium and phosphorus decrease absorption but information about the factors that control assimilation from foods is meager. It is presumably transported in plasma by binding to a β-1 globulin designated *transmanganin*. It is not entirely clear, however, that transmanganin differs from transferrin, since the latter protein has been shown to bind manganese and copper as well as iron. In normal persons the plasma concentration is about 2.5 μg per 100 ml, distributed approximately equally between cells and plasma. Manganese is excreted largely via the intestinal tract, much of it in the bile and pancreatic juice. Urinary excretion is very small. It has been reported that estrogen increases the concentration of manganese in serum, and glucocorticoids alter its body distribution.[87]

The average daily intake of manganese in adult man has been estimated to be 3 to 9 mg; about 40 per cent is absorbed. Children presumably require at least 200 μg per kg of body weight. The element is widely distributed in foodstuffs, particularly in wheat germs, seeds, nuts, leafy vegetables and meat. Animal tissues, seafoods, poultry and dairy products are relatively poor sources of manganese.

Biochemistry

Manganese has been shown to activate a large number of metal-enzyme complexes involving transferase, hydrolase, lyase, isomerase and ligase reactions. This effect is not specific since other metals, in particular magnesium, may substitute for manganese in most instances.[59] Arginase, cysteine desulfhydrase, prolinase, thiaminase, dipeptidases, phosphoglucomutase, glucokinase, leucine aminopeptidase, isocitric dehydrogenase, carnosinase, glutamine synthetase, acetyl CoA synthetase and enolase are examples. Fully active arginase binds 4 atoms of manganese per molecule of enzyme. Two of the manganese atoms are bound strongly and cannot be removed without significant protein denaturation. Manganese is required for the enzymatic incorporation of xylose and galactose[88] into glycoproteins. These sugars are present in the mucopolysaccharides, heparin, chondroitin sulfate and dermatan sulfate, which are joined to the protein by a xylosyl-serine bond. Manganese, present in high concentrations in melanocytes, also appears to participate in the final autooxidation of melanin granules.

The biotin-dependent *pyruvate carboxylase* of chicken liver was the first manganese metalloenzyme to have been identified; it contains 4 gm atoms of manganese per mole of protein.[89] More recently,

superoxide dismutases from the mitochondria of chicken liver and from E. coli have been found to be manganese metalloenzymes.[28] Human placental diamine oxidase has been reported to be a metalloenzyme containing both manganese and copper. L-Arabinose isomerase, a manganese-dependent enzyme from Lactobacillus gayonii, may be another manganese metalloenzyme. Avimanganin, a protein previously isolated from chicken liver mitochondria on the basis of its content of manganese, is probably inactivated superoxide dismutase.

Manganese also replaces the native zinc atoms of carboxypeptidase A of bovine pancreas and the neutral protease of B. subtilis, giving rise to enzymatically active products. In addition to chromium, nickel and other metals, manganese has been found to be firmly associated with ribonucleic acids isolated from diverse sources, presumably serving as an important determinant of the native structure.[9] It may also function in protein synthesis by stimulating RNA polymerase activity. A manganese porphyrin in the erythrocytes of man, rabbits and birds has been reported.[90] Manganese ions have been postulated to play a role in oxidative phosphorylation and in the metabolism of fatty acids and cholesterol synthesis. Mitochondria from manganese-deficient animals exhibit marked morphologic abnormalities which may be related to the role of superoxide dismutase. Manganese appears also to be involved in the synthesis of dopamine from L-dopa in brain.[91]

Nutrition

In both mammals and birds, manganese deficiency is characterized by defective growth, bone abnormalities, reproductive dysfunction, central nervous system manifestations, in particular ataxia, and disturbances in lipid metabolism.[1,87] Manganese deficiency has been induced in rats, mice, rabbits, pigs and cattle. Liver arginase activity and manganese concentration are reduced in manganese-deficient rabbits. Manganese-deficient guinea pigs exhibit impaired glucose tolerance and decreased granulation of the beta cells of the pancreatic islets. In rats, manganese is essential for lactation, and maternal manganese deficiency results in abnormal otic labyrinth development in the offspring. In this regard, an interesting relationship between manganese and a genetic disease of rats (pallid strain) exists. Pallid rats have an inherited defect in the formation of otoliths and lack postural orientation when blindfolded or placed in water. Feeding pregnant pallid rats manganese will prevent the phenotypic expression of this disease in their offspring.[92] An analogous recessive mutation, termed *pastel*, has recently been discovered in mink.[93] Birds develop spontaneous manganese deficiency of two forms: *chondrodystrophy*, characterized by defective growth, edema and generalized bone disease occurring in embryonic life and associated with high mortality, and *perosis*, evidenced by shortening and thickening of the bones, accompanied by slipping of the epiphyses and of the Achilles tendon, occurring in postembryonic life.

The biochemical mechanisms in which manganese is involved for proper osteogenesis are unknown but do not appear to relate to calcification. Skeletal maturation is retarded because of a depression or suppression of endochondral bone growth at the epiphyseal cartilages, including matrix formation and cell proliferation. A reduction in mucopolysaccharide and hexosamine content of the epiphyseal cartilage occurs,[94,95] and the galactotransferase enzyme activity of cartilage is decreased.[96] The cartilage of newborn manganese-deficient guinea pigs, which exhibit widespread skeletal defects, has a decreased content of hyaluronic acid, chondroitin sulfate and heparin.[97] Bone and blood phosphatase activities are lowered. In addition to perosis and chondrodystrophy, deficient chicks frequently exhibit neurologic symptoms, particularly ataxia. Susceptibility to manganese deficiency in chickens appears to be genetically controlled and is aggravated by a diet high in calcium, phosphorus or ferrous citrate. In borderline cases the deficiency is improved or prevented entirely by the additional intake of inositol or choline.

Deficiency states attributable specifically to manganese have not been identified in humans and no human diseases have been proved to be causally related. On the basis of the protective effects of manganese against chronic hydralazine poisoning in animals, it has been suggested that lupus erythematosus and the "hydralazine syndrome" in man may be related to manganese deficiency.[98] The possible interrelations between manganese metabolism and aspects of certain diseases and their therapy, in particular the extrapyramidal syndromes, have been considered.[87,90]

Toxicology

Chronic manganese poisoning occurs primarily in miners who inhale large quantities of manganese dust over prolonged periods. The disease is characterized by an encephalitis-like picture with manifestations of extrapyramidal disease. In mild cases, symptoms are reversed by withdrawal from exposure or treatment with disodium dicalcium ethylenediaminetetraacetate.[99] Increased concentrations of the metal are found particularly in the lung. Pulmonary changes similar to pneumoconiosis may occur. Clinical changes begin insidiously with asthenia, anorexia, apathy, headache, impotence, leg cramps and speech disturbances. Eventually the syndrome simulates a progressive hepatolenticular degeneration and in some aspects resembles Parkinson's disease. Facial expression is mask-like, the voice monotonous, and intention tremor, muscle rigidity and spastic gait appear. Tendon reflexes are exaggerated and clonus may develop.

Ingestion of potassium permanganate

results in acute poisoning. A strong oxidizing agent, it causes irritation and necrosis of gastric mucosa, hemolytic jaundice and capillary damage. Protracted ingestion of large amounts of manganese results in elevated concentrations in the liver, but no other ill effects, such as extrapyramidal symptoms, develop.

COBALT

Cobalt serves its paramount, known biologic function as a component of vitamin B_{12}. The biochemistry, physiology, nutrition and metabolism of this vitamin are discussed in Chapter 6, Section J. Hence, this section will concern other aspects of the biochemical and nutritional role of this element, which, however, are still closely related to vitamin B_{12} in most instances. The chemistry and biochemistry of vitamin B_{12} and related corrinoids have been reviewed recently.[100] Cobalt is widely distributed in nature, prompting a search for other biologic functions. The first nonvitamin-B_{12} cobalt enzyme, the biotin-dependent oxaloacetate transcarboxylase containing about 2 atoms of cobalt and 4 of zinc per molecule, has been isolated recently from Proprionbacterium shermanii.[101] Experimentally, cobalt can replace zinc in a number of zinc enzymes, e.g. carboxypeptidase A and B, bovine, human and monkey carbonic anhydrases, the neutral protease of B. subtilis and horse liver alcohol dehydrogenase, resulting in active enzymes with catalytic functions that are modified in characteristic fashion. Cobalt activates a number of enzymes, among them a variety of phosphotransferases and lyases, although these are active in the complete absence of metals or in the presence of other metals.[59] In pharmacologic doses cobalt stimulates erythropoiesis.

Metabolism

The synthesis of vitamin B_{12} by bacteria requires cobalt. In ruminants this occurs in the proximal portion of the intestine from which the vitamin is then absorbed. The total ingestion of 0.07 to 0.08 mg of cobalt per day is sufficient for the bacterial synthesis of the vitamin required by sheep and probably by cattle as well.[1] In other animals and man, however, where bacterial formation of vitamin B_{12} takes place only in the colon, absorption is minimal. Therefore, to be of nutritional value for the human, cobalt must be ingested or injected as vitamin B_{12}. Humans obtain their requirement of this nutrient largely from animal tissues. If man has a need for cobalt other than vitamin B_{12}, the requirement is unknown, although about 0.1 μg of cobalt per day would be sufficient to supply the amount needed to synthesize an adequate amount of vitamin B_{12}. The normal diet supplies about 10 to 200 μg per day.[1]

In view of the small quantities of cobalt present in tissues and body fluids, its quantification has been a major problem and much of the analytic data on record is of dubious value. In animals, orally absorbed or intravenously administered cobalt is excreted primarily in the urine. The greater part of ingested cobalt is not absorbed and is excreted in the stool; the fraction retained is concentrated mostly in the liver and kidneys, which contain about 0.2 parts per million based on the dry weight of the organs. The mode of storage, however, is uncertain. The cobalt concentration of human plasma is about 60 to 80 $\mu\mu g$ per ml and that of whole blood 80 to 300 $\mu\mu g$ per ml. Its estimation by bioassay as part of vitamin B_{12} has become a clinical test, since the determination of cobalt itself at these concentrations is difficult. The whole-body content of cobalt has been estimated to be 1.1 mg for an average-sized adult.

Nutrition

Cobalt deficiency in ruminants, variously called enzootic marasmus, pine or bush sickness, in essence is a vitamin B_{12} deficiency which manifests itself as impaired growth, listlessness, anorexia, progressive emaciation and varying degrees of anemia.[1] The livers of affected animals are deficient in cobalt but contain excessive amounts of iron. Ingestion of cobalt both prevents and cures the condition, but injected cobalt is ineffective. Therapeutic response to liver extract or vitamin B_{12} in amounts comparable to those used for treatment of pernicious anemia in man has been disappointing. About 300 μg of vitamin B_{12} per week is the dose required to alleviate the symptoms. Ruminants apparently have a much higher requirement for the vitamin than do man and other animals. High concentrations of molybdenum in the forage interfere with and may actually arrest the synthesis of vitamin B_{12} in the rumen of cattle, presumably because of the effect on the metabolism of the microorganisms in the rumen.

The Erythropoietic Stimulating Effect of Cobalt

Administration of pharmacologic amounts of cobalt, either orally or parenterally, will induce polycythemia in rats, mice, guinea pigs, rabbits, dogs, pigs, chickens, ducks, hogs and man. The development of polycythemia is apparently independent of other metals but is inhibited or prevented by methionine, cysteine, histidine, choline, nicotinamide and ascorbic acid. Reticulocytosis, elevated erythrocyte and hemoglobin levels, increased total red blood cell mass and normoblastic hyperplasia in the marrow occur. This effect is not mediated through vitamin B_{12}. Cobalt may induce polycythemia by increasing the formation or inhibiting the destruction of erythropoietin, the erythropoietic stimulating hormone secreted primarily by the kidney,[102] but it does so in pharmacologic, not physiologic, doses. There is as yet no evidence that cobalt is a part of erythropoietin, a glycoprotein, or essential to the maintenance of a normal concentration of the hormone under physiologic conditions. Cobalt administration apparently also increases iron absorption as well as globin synthesis. The value

of cobalt therapy of human anemias has been studied extensively.[103]

Toxicity

Congestive heart failure from cardiomyopathy has been reported in individuals who consumed large quantities of beer which had 1.2 ppm of cobalt added during processing as a foam stabilizer. In addition, the afflicted individuals developed polycythemia, pericardial effusion, thyroid hyperplasia and neurologic abnormalities. On autopsy, the heart contained 10 times the normal amount of cobalt, and showed vacuolar degeneration of the muscle and degenerative changes in the myofilaments, mitochondria and sarcoplasmic reticulum. In experimentally induced cobalt cardiomyopathy, the metabolism of pyruvate and fatty acids is impaired. Cobalt is known to bind to lipoic acid and may perhaps interfere with critical decarboxylation reactions in this manner.[104] The anatomic and metabolic changes induced by cobalt in myocardium, however, are not specific, and the toxic effects of cobalt and ethanol may be synergistic in beer-drinkers' cardiomyopathy.

SELENIUM

The physical and chemical properties of selenium closely resemble those of sulfur. However, until recently, little was known about its participation in biochemical reactions.[105] Within the last 15 years, selenium has been recognized to be an essential nutrient element in certain species, and its function in redox reactions as a component of several enzymes has been identified.[106] Selenium prevents dietary liver necrosis in the rat and pig, a fatal exudative diathesis in chicks and turkeys, nutritional muscular dystrophy in lambs, calves and chicks and multiple necrotic degeneration of heart, liver, muscle and kidney in the mouse.[1]

These diseases result from diets multiply deficient in vitamin E and selenium. In other studies selenium by itself has been shown to be required for the optimal growth of chicks. Chicks fed a diet deficient in selenium alone also show poor feathering and atrophy of the pancreas. The latter lesion leads to impaired absorption of fats as well as of vitamin E, and serum vitamin E concentrations of these chicks become abnormally low.[107] In the rat, pure selenium deficiency is manifested by growth retardation, cataract formation, and aspermatogenesis.[108] Various reports have demonstrated that children with kwashiorkor have decreased selenium stores, suggesting that human selenium deficiency may occur with protein-calorie malnutrition.[109] A recent study has shown that selenium is an essential trace nutrient for the growth of diploid human fibroblasts in tissue culture.[110]

The highest concentrations of selenium are found in liver, kidney, heart and spleen. There are about 0.22 μg of selenium per ml of blood in man. It is excreted in the urine. Absorption seems to depend on the solubility of the selenium compound ingested and on the dietary ratio of selenium to sulfur. Once absorbed, selenium is deposited in various amounts in all tissues of the body except fat. In ruminants, a large percentage of the ingested selenium is incorporated by the bacteria of the rumen into seleno-analogs of cysteine and methionine which are absorbed and deposited in tissues as seleno-amino acids and then incorporated into proteins.[111] Selenium has been found in many highly purified proteins, e.g. aldolase, cytochrome c, hemoglobin, myoglobin, myosin and ribonucleoproteins.[112] Even in nonruminants much of the ingested selenium is incorporated in body tissues as selenocysteine and selenomethionine. Although most of the selenium in the body is present as part of various proteins, small-molecular-weight selenium compounds are also present. Thus one of the major selenium compounds excreted in the urine is the trimethylselenonium ion,

and dimethylselenide can be excreted in the breath.

The physiologic role of selenium puzzled workers in the field for many years. The mutually sparing actions of selenium and vitamin E suggested that it may serve an antioxidant role. However, the exact manner in which selenium functioned was not known until 1973 when it was found to be an integral part of the enzyme glutathione peroxidase in rat erythrocytes.[113] Subsequent studies showed that the enzyme from bovine blood contains 4 equivalents of selenium per mole[114] and that most of the selenium in rat liver mitochondria is present in glutathione peroxidase.[115] More than 75 per cent of the selenium in erythrocytes is present in this enzyme. Glutathione peroxidase activity in erythrocytes, plasma, liver, lung and other tissue decreases in direct proportion to decreases in dietary selenium intake, and deficiency of this enzyme is believed to account for many of the manifestations of selenium deficiency. The enzyme catalyzes the transfer of reducing equivalents from reduced glutathione to hydrogen peroxide or to lipid peroxides, thus serving to protect cells and membranes against oxidative damage. Selenium has also been found to be a component of formate dehydrogenase and glycine reductase in microorganisms. The organoselenium component of glycine reductase has been identified as selenocysteine.[116] On the other hand, selenium in glutathione peroxidase is present as a low-molecular-weight organic prosthetic group.[117] A selenoprotein has been isolated from skeletal muscle of sheep but its catalytic function is unknown. Selenium is also incorporated into the protein matrix in teeth. Therefore, it is likely that the element may have additional roles in mammalian metabolism which remain to be identified. Selenium or selenium compounds may serve to protect animals against the toxicity of heavy metals such as cadmium and mercury.[118,119]

Toxic amounts of selenium may act as

antagonists of sulfur metabolism and are known to inhibit certain enzymes, such as succinic dehydrogenase, urease, choline oxidase, tyramine oxidase and proline oxidase. The element also adversely affects embryonic development: it inhibits mitosis at metaphase and bone and cartilage develop abnormally.[1]

Selenium poisoning occurs in animals grazing on alkali (high salt) pastures.[1] The acute toxicity syndrome, blind staggers, is characterized by blindness, abdominal pain, salivation, muscle paralysis and death from respiratory failure. Chronic toxicity, alkali disease, produces dullness and roughness of coat, loss of hair, sore hoofs, erosion of the joints of long bones, cardiac atrophy, cirrhosis of the liver and anemia in cattle. Some of these signs may be attributed to the replacement of cystine by selenocystine in keratin. Poisoning occurs owing to the ingestion of certain plant species which accumulate selenium from the soil. A diet high in protein affords some protection, as does sulfate. Interestingly, arsenic given at low levels of 5 parts per million in the drinking water prevents selenosis. The mechanism of its action is not known. However, there is no evidence that humans living in seleniferous areas develop symptoms attributable to selenium intoxication, although their urinary excretion of the element is above normal levels.

CHROMIUM

In recent years evidence has been adduced that chromium may have an important role in the carbohydrate and lipid metabolism of animals and their utilization of glucose. Thus far its involvement in glucose metabolism and insulin action has been explored most extensively in rats.[120] Deficiency syndromes have also been produced in mice and squirrel monkeys. Presently there is only indirect evidence to support the view that chromium deficiency occurs in man.

The amount of chromium present in animal tissues is not well defined, largely owing to difficulties in analysis. Concentrations ranging between 10 and several hundred parts per billion have been reported. This discrepancy may be partly methodologic and also may reflect geographic variation. The total-body content of chromium is low, less than 6 mg. Highest concentrations are found in skin, fat, adrenal glands, brain and muscle. Geographic variations are large, and a progressive decline in tissue concentrations with age has been reported in the United States.[121] Serum concentrations of chromium are less than 10 ng per ml.

Knowledge of the metabolic movements of chromium is sparse. Only a small percentage of ingested chromium is absorbed. It is excreted mainly by way of the kidney. Trivalent chromium is bound to transferrin in serum, whereas hexavalent chromium has a selective affinity for red blood cells. These properties have permitted the use of radioactive chromium isotopes for the study of mass and turnover of erythrocytes and plasma proteins. Neither the oxidation state nor the physiologic function of chromium in tissues is known.

In vitro chromium has been found to react with biologic macromolecules and enzymes similar to other transition elements. Its use for the tanning of skins is well known. Chromium has been found associated with RNA isolated from many different species, together with Ni, Fe, Mn and other elements. It activates several enzymes, including the succinate-cytochrome dehydrogenase system and phosphoglucomutase and has been noted to stimulate fatty acid and cholesterol synthesis.[122]

The effect of trivalent chromium in reversing a diet-induced mild glucose intolerance in rats was discovered in 1959. Rats raised on a Torula-yeast diet developed a mild impairment of glucose utilization as measured by intravenous glucose tolerance testing. When given trivalent chromium in amounts not much above the estimated daily intake, glucose tolerance returned to the normal range within 24 hours, whereas 40 other elements were ineffective.[123] When great care was taken to minimize extraneous metal contamination, rats eventually developed more severe symptoms of chromium deficiency. Depression of growth rates, severe impairment of glucose metabolism approaching frank diabetes and increased incidence of atheromatous lesions in the aorta were observed.[120] Corneal opacification has been noted to develop in rats fed a diet low in both protein and chromium, but not in protein alone.[121]

The mode of action of trivalent chromium in regulating glucose metabolism has been studied, using chromium-deficient epididymal adipose tissue. Chromium itself does not stimulate the incorporation of glucose into lipids and conversion to CO_2, but it enhances the stimulatory effects of insulin.[124] It has been suggested that, among other factors, chromium facilitates the binding of insulin to cell membranes by forming a "bridge" between the insulin molecule and the membrane.[120] The concentration range within which chromium is stimulatory is narrow and excess amounts of chromium depress insulin activity. Trivalent chromium as part of an organic complex, termed glucose tolerance factor, has been found to be more effective than the inorganic metal alone in potentiating the action of insulin.

The above findings have naturally raised the question of whether chromium metabolism is related to diabetes. To date, the evidence correlating impaired chromium metabolism with glucose intolerance in man is still incomplete. However, in certain instances, chromium supplementation in maturity-onset diabetic patients improves glucose utilization.[125,126] Improvement of glucose tolerance in some children with kwashiorkor has also been reported.[127] Association of chromium deficiency with low-birth-weight infants,

insulin-dependent juvenile-onset diabetes, and gestational diabetes has also been suggested. Chromium nutrition in man and the need to develop more sensitive and reliable techniques for the measurement of this interesting element have been reviewed.[128]

MOLYBDENUM

Molybdenum began to attract attention as a trace element of nutritional importance when it was demonstrated some 30 or 40 years ago that the growth of Azotobacter was increased several times by the addition of minute amounts of molybdate, if gaseous nitrogen served as the only source of nitrogen. Subsequent work showed that traces of molybdenum are present in all plants and animal tissues. The functional significance of molybdenum in normal animal metabolism gained credence when the addition of molybdenum to the diet of rats increased the xanthine oxidase activity of tissues.[129] Subsequently the element was found to be a constituent of various flavin-dependent enzymes, e.g. xanthine and aldehyde oxidases in animal tissues and nitrate reductases in plant tissues. However, an unequivocal requirement of molybdenum for the growth and maintenance of normal life cycles of experimental animals remains to be demonstrated. While great strides in the biochemistry of this element have been made, no syndrome characteristic of molybdenum deficiency has been recognized in animals.[130] Similarly its nutritional role is uncertain. The subsequent discussion will emphasize the rather impressive biochemical evidence for a presumed nutritional role.

Animal tissues contain small amounts of molybdenum, 0.1 to 3 parts per million, based on the dry weight of tissues.[1,130] The largest amounts are found in the liver, kidney, bone and skin. Molybdenum is absorbed readily from the intestinal tract and is excreted rapidly in the urine. A small amount is also excreted in bile. Especially in liver, kidney and bone, the concentrations of tissue molybdenum can be increased or decreased by raising or lowering dietary intake. Diets deficient in molybdenum decrease intestinal and liver xanthine oxidase activities. This can be corrected by additions of small amounts of molybdate to the diet. Increase in dietary sulfate and copper is accompanied by an increase in urinary excretion of molybdenum and its depletion in blood and tissues.

The chemical forms in which molybdenum exists in tissues have not been proven unequivocally, though it seems probable that, during oxidation and reduction, molybdenum cycles between Mo(V) and Mo(VI).[131] At least part is bound to the various molybdoproteins. The protein donor groups which bind molybdenum are also uncertain, though the weight of evidence favors binding to sulfur. Xanthine oxidases from milk and animal tissues catalyze the oxidation of a number of substrates, among which are purines, aldehydes, pteridines, DPNH, certain pyrimidines and other heterocyclic compounds. They contain both molybdenum and iron as well as the flavin coenzyme FAD.[132]

Present evidence indicates the presence of 2 molecules of FAD, 2 atoms of molybdenum and 8 atoms of iron per molecule of highly purified preparations of xanthine oxidase of milk. Xanthine oxidase from mammalian livers also contains 4 gm atoms of iron and 1 gm atom of molybdenum per mole of FAD but that from bird livers contains 8 gm atoms of molybdenum per mole of bound FAD. Aldehyde oxidase from mammalian liver in addition contains 1 to 2 moles of coenzyme Q_{10}. The iron in these enzymes appears to be associated with a stoichiometric quantity of acid-labile sulfur, such as is found in the ferrodoxins. These enzymes therefore are complex metalloflavoproteins containing at least two metals, iron and molybdenum, necessary for their catalytic activity; whether the metals are required solely for electron transport or whether they participate in maintaining the structural integrity of the enzymes as well is poorly understood. It is generally agreed that, in oxidation-reduction, hydrogen from the donor is transferred sequentially to the oxygen acceptor through Mo, FAD and Fe.[131] A molybdohemeprotein, sulfite oxidase, has been isolated from bovine liver.[133] This enzyme catalyzes the oxidation of sulfite to sulfate. Its physiologic importance is emphasized by the recognition in a child of the lack of hepatic sulfite oxidase activity. In this instance, the urine contained sulfite and thiosulfate and severe pathophysiologic sequelae were fatal.[134]

Molybdenum is also essential for nitrogen fixation of leguminous plants and for the biologic conversion of nitrate to ammonia or amino acids by fungi and higher plants, as well as other processes in plant metabolism.[131] Nitrate reductase isolated from plants and bacteria contains FAD, heme and molybdenum, but their stoichiometric relationship has not been defined. Molybdoferredoxins from Azotobacter vinelandii and Clostridium pasteurianum contain Mo, Fe and acid-labile sulfur and are required for the ATP-dependent reductive assimilation of nitrogen.[135] Molybdoferredoxin is a component of the nitrogenase enzyme complex, which also contains ferredoxin.[136] Formate dehydrogenase from E. coli was recently identified as a molybdenum-containing metalloenzyme. A complex molecule of 590,000 daltons, it contains in addition heme, nonheme iron, selenium and acid-labile sulfide.[137]

The nearest approximation to an induced deficiency state has been produced by feeding tungsten, a specific inhibitor of molybdenum, to chickens.[138] This results in depletion of tissue xanthine oxidase, increased excretion of xanthine and hypoxanthine, decreased excretion of uric acid, growth retardation and death. These effects can be overcome by the administration of sufficient amounts of molybdenum. A growth-promoting effect of molybdenum in the growing lamb has been reported. A stimulating effect on cellulose-degrading microorganisms was suggested as the mechanism, with subsequent increase in ruminal cellulose degradation.

Chronic ingestion of excess amounts of molybdenum produces a disease state called "teart" in several animal species. Its interrelationship with copper and sulfate in nutrition has been the subject of intensive investigation (vide supra).

CADMIUM

Minute concentrations of cadmium have been found in tissues and fluids of most animals but no biologic function for this element has as yet been demonstrated.[1] The isolation and characterization of a cadmium-containing protein from horse, rabbit and human kidneys demonstrated that this element can be a normal constituent of biologic matter, rather than a contaminant.[139] These findings have awakened interest in the possible biochemical and physiologic role of the element, since the specific association of an element with a native biologic macromolecule represents an important first step toward the eventual definition of its biologic function.

Metabolism

In most animal tissues cadmium concentrations are of the order of less than 1 μg per gm wet tissue. The total-body concentration of cadmium in man increases with age and varies in different areas of the world.[5] The cadmium content of the liver and the kidney is significantly higher than that of other tissues. Equine and human kidneys may contain amounts varying from 10 to 100 μg per gm wet weight.

Recent studies suggest that both in liver and in kidney cadmium is bound specifically to metallothionein.[140] Cadmium localizes predominantly in the renal cortex, in regions corresponding to the proximal tubules. Deposits in the glomeruli or blood vessels have not been detected.

There is no conclusive evidence for a physiologic regulation of cadmium absorption or excretion. The element is absorbed poorly from the gastrointestinal tract and is excreted slowly. In dogs the total excretion of injected cadmium proceeds at a rate equivalent to a half-life of approximately 1 year and mainly through the intestinal tract. In man the average daily net uptake of cadmium is between 15 and 35 μg and urinary excretion is approximately 10 μg per liter.[140] Epidemiologic data suggest that cigarettes are a major source of cadmium for man.

The physiologic function of cadmium is unknown. It has been suggested that cadmium is a toxic element and an etiologic factor in essential hypertension.[142] Cadmium given orally or parenterally to rats induces hypertension, reversed by chelating agents,[143] but in other animal species the effect may be hypotension.[144] Analyses of kidney cortex containing the major fraction of the renal cadmium content do not reveal large differences between normal material and that obtained from individuals succumbing from hypertension or a variety of renal disorders, but the ratio of cadmium to zinc appears higher in the hypertensive group. However, it is significant to note that there is *no* increased incidence of essential hypertension in patients suffering from chronic cadmium poisoning and no correlation between cadmium accumulation and hypertension or cardiovascular disease in man.[145] Hence, evidence that cadmium exposure may lead to hypertension in man is largely inferential, and experimental proof is lacking.

Biochemistry

Cadmium is specifically associated with a protein of molecular weight 6,700 first isolated from horse kidney cortex and named metallothionein.[146] It represents 1 to 2 per cent of the total weight of soluble proteins in horse renal cortex. Such preparations contain as much as 5.9 per cent cadmium, 2.2 per cent zinc and 9 per cent sulfur. Cadmium and zinc compete for the same binding sites and may be isomorphic in metallothionein. The sulfur is accounted for by cysteine which constitutes 30 per cent of the amino acids in the protein, and 1 atom of cadmium or zinc is apparently bound to 3 sulfhydryl groups.

Further studies have indicated that horse liver and kidney metallothioneins are proteins of 6,600 daltons containing 20 cysteinyl residues and a total of 6 atoms of zinc, cadmium and copper per mole of protein. The protein exhibits microheterogeneity, as evidenced by the presence of 2 or more electrophoretically distinct molecular forms.[147] The amino acid sequence of one of the two principal molecular forms of horse kidney metallothionein has recently been elucidated.[148] Similar proteins have been isolated from human and rabbit kidney and liver,[149,150] and from liver and kidney of zinc- or cadmium-treated pigs, rats, chickens and rabbits. As with metallothionein from horse kidney, the proteins isolated from cadmium-exposed rat and chicken liver exhibit a high content of cysteine, 30 mol%, and contain no aromatic amino acids, but their molecular weights are about 10,000.[152] Induced synthesis of metallothionein by cadmium was recently demonstrated in pig kidney cells grown in tissue culture.[153]

The unique physical and chemical properties of metallothionein have suggested distinctive physiologic and biochemical roles in the homeostatic mechanisms of zinc absorption, cellular transport and storage. Despite numerous efforts,[154,155] however, definite evidence for such functions has not yet been adduced. Alternatively metallothionein may function in detoxification against heavy metals. It is of interest that substantial quantities of mercury have been found in metallothionein, displacing zinc and cadmium, when it was isolated from kidneys of patients who had received mercurial diuretics.

Cadmium activates a considerable number of enzymes, among them carnosinase, arginase, histidase, tryptophan oxygenase and formylglutamic acid deformylase. This action is not specific, since several of these enzymes are also activated by other metals. Cadmium can replace the native zinc atom of carboxypeptidases A and B, resulting in a change of the substrate specificity of these enzymes.

Toxicity

Pulmonary emphysema occurring in workers manufacturing alkaline accumulators and castings of copper-cadmium alloys has been described, a syndrome thought to be due to chronic long-term exposure to cadmium.[156] Proteinuria occurs in about 80 per cent of individuals exposed in this manner for 8 years and more, and aminoaciduria, especially of serine and threonine, is frequent. Renal damage ranges from mild and scattered tubular degeneration to severe tubular and glomerular lesions. Anemia has also been described in some cases of human cadmium toxicity. The livers and kidneys of these patients accumulate 10 to 100 times more cadmium than that found in the organs of healthy unexposed individuals. These high tissue cadmium concentrations remain for many years after cessation of exposure, indicating that excretion is slow. However, death usually results from progressive pulmonary decompensation rather than from kidney damage.

A syndrome of osteomalacia and nephropathy (ouch-ouch disease or itai-itai byo) has been described in Japanese women and is thought to be due to chronic cadmium poisoning.[157] The patients develop extreme bone pain due to osteomalacia and pseudofractures (hence the name of the disease) and have proteinuria, aminoaciduria, glucosuria and hypercalciuria. The syndrome is largely confined to women who have had multiple pregnancies or who are postmenopausal and whose urinary and tissue concentrations of cadmium are increased. The incidence of hypertension may be higher than in the normal population. The epidemiology has been traced to contamination of river water by waste products from a cadmium mine. Cadmium concentrations of crops in that area were increased. Ingestion of water and produce from this region over long periods apparently gave rise to the disease.

Prolonged administration of large amounts of cadmium to rabbits produces tubular lesions similar to those observed in man.[158] However, chronic ingestion of 0.1 to 10 parts per million of cadmium has no discernible adverse effects on rats, as judged by general health, growth rate and pathologic examination, although large amounts of the metal are retained in liver and kidney. Higher doses, however, cause stunted growth, accompanied by hypochromic-microcytic anemia and tubular atrophy and interstitial fibrosis of the kidneys. Both renal and skeletal abnormalities are observed when cadmium is administered to rats fed a calcium-deficient diet.[159]

The parenteral administration of a single dose of cadmium chloride to rats results in necrosis and atrophy of the testis and placental necrosis, without permanent damage to other organs.[160] Cadmium sterilization, apparently brought about through interference with testicular circulation, also occurs in mice, rabbits, guinea pigs and hamsters. Strikingly, the toxic action of cadmium on the testis and placenta is prevented by previous administration of zinc, suggesting these two metals compete for the same binding site of some critical biologic molecule in these tissues. Chronic cadmium intoxication in cattle results in stunted growth, liver and kidney damage, abnormal testicular growth and sperm production. These effects are also partially offset by the concomitant administration of zinc.

Cadmium is known to interact with the sulfhydryl groups of certain enzymes, resulting in inactivation. This circumstance may be pertinent to the effects which have led to its classification as a "toxic" element. Most transition and group IIB metals will exert such toxic effects when administered in excess or by an unusual route.

BIBLIOGRAPHY

1. Underwood: *Trace Elements in Human and Animal Nutrition*, 3rd ed. New York, Academic Press, 1971.
2. Nielsen and Sandstead: Am. J. Clin. Nutr., *27*, 515, 1974.
3. Bowen: *Trace Elements in Biochemistry*. New York, Academic Press, 1966.
4. Tipton and Cook: Health Phys., *9*, 103, 1963.
5. Tipton, Schroeder, Perry and Cook: Health Phys., *11*, 403, 1965.
6. Kawaguchi and Vallee: Anal. Chem., *47*, 1029, 1975.
7. Vallee: In *Enzymes*, Vol. 3B, 2nd ed. (Boyer, Lardy and Myrback, Eds.). New York, Academic Press, 1960.
8. Wacker and Vallee: J. Biol. Chem., *234*, 3257, 1959.
9. Fuwa, Wacker, Druyan, Bartholomay and Vallee: Proc. Natl. Acad. Sci., *46*, 1298, 1960.
10. Scheinberg and Sternlieb: Pharmacol. Rev., *12*, 355, 1960.
11. Adelstein and Vallee: In *Mineral Metabolism*, Vol. 2B (Comar and Bronner, Eds.). New York, Academic Press, 1962.
12. Sarkar and Kruck: In *Biochemistry of Copper* (Peisach, Aisen and Blumberg, Eds.). New York, Academic Press, 1966.
13. Neumann and Suss-Kortsak: J. Clin. Invest., *46*, 646, 1967.
14. Winge, Premakumar, Wiley and Rajagopolan: Arch. Biochem. Biophys., *170*, 253, 1975.
15. Peisach, Aisen and Blumberg: *Biochemistry of Copper*. New York, Academic Press, 1966.
16. Osaki, Johnson and Frieden: J. Biol. Chem., *241*, 2746, 1966.
17. Frieden and Hsieh: Adv. Enzymol., *44*, 187, 1976.
18. Blumberg, Goldstein, Lauber and Peisach: Biochim. Biophys. Acta, *99*, 187, 1965.
19. Hill, Starcher and Kim: Federation Proc., *26*, 129, 1967.
20. Porter: In *Biochemistry of Copper* (Peisach, Aisen and Blumberg, Eds.). New York, Academic Press, 1966.
21. Carrico and Deutsch: J. Biol. Chem., *245*, 723, 1970.
22. Fridovich: Adv. Enzymol., *41*, 35, 1974.
23. Evans, Majors and Cornatzer: Biochem. Biophys. Res. Commun., *40*, 1142, 1970.
24. Roeser, Lee, Nacht and Cartwright: J. Clin. Invest., *49*, 2408, 1970.
25. Gubler: J.A.M.A., *161*, 530, 1956.
26. Cordano, Baertl and Graham: Pediatrics, *34*, 324, 1964.
27. Al Rashid and Spangler: N. Engl. J. Med., *285*, 841, 1971.
28. Karpel and Peden: J. Pediatr., *80*, 32, 1972.

29. Dunlap, James and Hume: Ann. Intern. Med., *80*, 470, 1974.
30. O'Dell, Elsden, Thomas, Partridge, Smith and Palmer: Nature, *209*, 401, 1966.
31. Bird, Savage and O'Dell: Proc. Soc. Exp. Biol. Med., *123*, 250, 1966.
32. Gallagher and Reeve: Aust. J. Exp. Biol. Med. Sci., *49*, 21, 1971.
33. Ashkenazi, Levin, Djaldetti, Fishel and Benvenisti: Pediatrics, *52*, 525, 1973.
34. Bearn: In *The Metabolic Basis of Inherited Disease*, 3rd ed. (Stanbury, Wyngaarden and Fredrickson, Eds.). New York, McGraw-Hill Book Co., 1972.
35. Sternlieb and Feldmann: Gastroenterology, *71*, 457, 1976.
36. Holtzman: Fed. Proc., *35*, 2276, 1976.
37. Goka, Stevenson, Hefferan and Howell: Proc. Natl. Acad. Sci., *73*, 604, 1976.
38. Hurley: Fed. Proc., *35*, 2271, 1976.
39. Keen and Hurley: Science, *193*, 244, 1976.
40. Holtzman, Eliott and Heller: N. Engl. J. Med., *275*, 347, 1966.
41. Vallee: Physiol. Rev., *39*, 443, 1959.
42. Vallee: In *Mineral Metabolism*, Vol. 2B (Comar and Bronner, Eds.). New York, Academic Press, 1962.
43. Vallee, Wacker, Bartholomay and Robin: N. Engl. J. Med., *255*, 403, 1956.
44. Himmelhoch, Sober, Vallee, Peterson and Fuwa: Biochemistry, *5*, 2523, 1966.
45. Parisi and Vallee: Biochemistry, *9*, 2421, 1970.
46. Oberleas, Muhrer and O'Dell: *Zinc Metabolism* (Prasad, Ed.). Springfield, Charles C Thomas, 1966.
47. Li: Adv. Enzymol., *45*, 427, 1977.
48. Drum, Harrison, Li, Bethune and Vallee: Proc. Natl. Acad. Sci., *57*, 1434, 1967.
49. Blair and Vallee: Biochemistry, *5*, 2026, 1966.
50. Lindskog and Malmstrom: J. Biol. Chem., *237*, 1129, 1962.
51. Vallee, Riordan and Coleman: Proc. Natl. Acad. Sci., *49*, 109, 1963.
52. Falchuk, Mazus, Ulpino and Vallee: Biochemistry, *15*, 4468, 1976.
53. Falchuk, Fawcett and Vallee: J. Cell Sci., *17*, 57, 1975.
54. Falchuk, Krishan and Vallee: Biochemistry, *14*, 3439, 1975.
55. Weser, Seeber and Warnecke: Biochim. Biophys. Acta, *179*, 422, 1969.
56. Kotsiopoulos and Mohr: Biochem. Biophys. Res. Commun., *67*, 979, 1975.
57. Vallee, Fluharty, Gibson: Acta Union Int. Contre Cancer, *6*, 869, 1949.
58. Vallee: In *Cancer Enzymology* (Schultz and Ahmad, Eds.). New York, Academic Press, 1976.
59. Vallee and Coleman: *Comprehensive Biochemistry*, Vol. 12 (Florkin and Stotz, Eds.). Amsterdam, Elsevier, 1964.
60. Neuberger and Tait: Biochem. J., *90*, 607, 1964.
61. Grant and Coombs: Essays Biochem., *6*, 69, 1970.
62. Iqbal: Enzymol. Biol. Clin., *11*, 412, 1970.
63. Mills, Quarterman, Williams, Dalgarno and Panic: Biochem. J., *102*, 712, 1967.
64. Prasad, Oberleas, Wolf and Horwitz: J. Clin. Invest., *46*, 549, 1967.
65. Prasad and Oberleas: J. Lab. Clin. Med., *83*, 634, 1974.
66. Smith, McDaniel, Fair and Halsted: Science, *181*, 954, 1973.
67. Follis: *Zinc Metabolism* (Prasad, Ed.). Springfield, Charles C Thomas, 1966.
68. Hsu and Anthony: J. Nutr., *100*, 1189, 1970.
69. Hurley and Mutch: J. Nutr., *103*, 649, 1973.
70. Tao and Hurley: J. Nutr., *105*, 220, 1975.
71. Prasad: Fed. Proc., *26*, 181, 1967.
72. Solomons, Rosenberg and Sandstead: Am. J. Clin. Nutr., *29*, 371, 1976.
73. MacMahon, Parker and McKinnon: Med. J. Aust., *2*, 210, 1968.
74. Tucker, Schroeter, Brown and McCall: J.A.M.A., *235*, 2399, 1976.
75. Hambidge, Hambidge, Jacobs and Baum: Pediatr. Res., *6*, 868, 1972.
76. Giroux, Schechter and Schoun: Clin. Sci. Mol. Med., *51*, 545, 1976.
77. Pekarek, Wannemacher and Beisel: Proc. Soc. Exp. Med., *140*, 685, 1973.
78. Prasad, Schoomaker, Ortega, Brewer, Oberleas and Oelshlegel: Clin. Chem., *21*, 582, 1975.
79. Sandstead, Lanier, Shepard and Gillespie: Am. J. Clin. Nutr., *23*, 514, 1974.
80. Vallee, Wacker, Bartholomay and Hoch: N. Engl. J. Med., *257*, 1055, 1957.
81. Von Wartburg, Bethune and Vallee: Biochemistry, *3*, 1775, 1964.
82. Lange, Sytkowsky and Vallee: Biochemistry, *15*, 4687, 1976.
83. Wang and Pierson: J. Lab. Clin. Med., *85*, 50, 1975.
84. Moynahan and Barnes: Lancet, *2*, 399, 1974.
85. Hirsh, Michel and Strain: Arch. Dermatol., *112*, 475, 1976.
86. Cotzias: Physiol. Rev., *38*, 503, 1958.
87. Cotzias: *Mineral Metabolism*, Vol. 11B (Comar and Bronner, Eds.). New York, Academic Press, 1962.
88. Robinson, Telser and Dorfman: Proc. Natl. Acad. Sci., *56*, 1859, 1966.
89. Scrutton, Utter and Mildvan: J. Biol. Chem., *241*, 3480, 1966.
90. Cotzias: Proceedings Sixth International Congress of Nutrition. Edinburgh, E. & S. Livingstone, 1964.
91. Cotzias, Papavasiliou, Mena, Tang and Miller: Adv. Neurol., *5*, 235, 1974.
92. Hurley: Fed. Proc., *27*, 193, 1968.
93. Erway and Mitchell: J. Hered., *64*, 110, 1973.
94. Leach and Meunster: J. Nutr., *78*, 51, 1962.
95. Leach: Fed. Proc., *26*, 118, 1967.
96. Leach, Muenster and Wein: Arch. Biochem., *133*, 22, 1969.
97. Tsai and Everson: J. Nutr., *91*, 447, 1967.
98. Comens: In *Metal Binding in Medicine* (Seven, Ed.). Philadelphia, J.B. Lippincott, 1960.

99. Penalver: Arch. Ind. Health, *16*, 64, 1957.
100. Hill: In *Inorganic Biochemistry* (Eichhorn, Ed.). Amsterdam, Elsevier, 1973.
101. Northrop and Wood: J. Biol. Chem., *244*, 5801, 1969.
102. Jacobson, Gurney and Goldwasser: Adv. Intern. Med., *10*, 297, 1960.
103. Wintrobe: *Clinical Hematology*, 6th ed. Philadelphia, Lea & Febiger, 1974.
104. Alexander: Ann. Intern. Med., *70*, 411, 1969.
105. Rosenfeld and Beath: *Selenium*. New York, Academic Press, 1964.
106. Stadtman: Science, *183*, 915, 1974.
107. Thompson and Scott: J. Nutr., *100*, 797, 1970.
108. Sprinker, Harr, Newberne, Whanger and Weswig: Nutr. Rep. Int., *4*, 335, 1971.
109. Burk, Pearson, Wood and Viteri: Am. J. Clin. Nutr., *20*, 723, 1967.
110. McKeehan, Hamilton, and Haur: Proc. Natl. Acad. Sci., *73*, 2023, 1976.
111. Shrift and Virupaksha: Biochim. Biophys. Acta, *100*, 65, 1965.
112. McConnell and Roth: Proc. Soc. Exp. Biol. Med., *120*, 88, 1965.
113. Rotruck, Pope, Gauther, Swanson, Hafeman and Hoekstra: Science, *179*, 588, 1973.
114. Hohe, Gunzler and Schock: FEBS Lett., *32*, 132, 1973.
115. Levander, Morris and Higgs: Biochem. Biophys. Res. Commun., *58*, 1047, 1974.
116. Cone, Martin del Rio, Davis and Stadtman: Proc. Natl. Acad. Sci., *73*, 2659, 1976.
117. Oh, Ganther and Hoekstra: Biochemistry, *13*, 1825, 1974.
118. Chen, Whanger and Weswig: Bioinorg. Chem., *4*, 125, 1975.
119. Kosta, Byrne and Zelenko: Nature, *254*, 238, 1975.
120. Mertz, Toepfer, Roginski and Polansky: Fed. Proc., *23*, 2275, 1974.
121. Mertz: Physiol. Rev., *49*, 163, 1969.
122. Curran: J. Biol. Chem., *210*, 765, 1954.
123. Schwarz and Mertz: Arch. Biochem. Biophys., *85*, 292, 1959.
124. Mertz, Roginski and Schwarz: J. Biol. Chem., *236*, 318, 1961.
125. Glinsmann and Mertz: Metabolism, *15*, 510, 1966.
126. Levine, Streeten, and Doisy: Metabolism, *17*, 114, 1968.
127. Hopkins, Ransome-Kuti and Majaj: Am. J. Clin. Nutr., *21*, 203, 1968.
128. Hambidge: Am. J. Clin. Nutr., *27*, 505, 1974.
129. Richert and Westerfeld: J. Biol. Chem., *203*, 915, 1953.
130. de Renzo: In *Mineral Metabolism,* Vol. 2B (Comar and Bronner, Eds.). New York, Academic Press, 1962.
131. Bray, Palmer and Beinert: J. Biol. Chem., *239*, 2667, 1964.
132. Bray: In *Enzymes*, Vol. 7A, 2nd ed. (Boyer, Lardy and Myrback, Eds.). New York, Academic Press, 1963.
133. Cohen and Fridovich: J. Biol. Chem., *246*, 359, 1971.
134. Irreverre, Mudd, Heizer and Laster: Biochem. Med., *1*, 187, 1967.
135. Bui and Mortenson: Proc. Natl. Acad. Sci., *61*, 1021, 1968.
136. Vandecasteele and Burris: J. Bacteriol., *101*, 794, 1970.
137. Enoch and Lester: J. Biol. Chem., *250*, 6693, 1975.
138. Higgins, Richert and Westerfeld: J. Nutr., *59*, 539, 1956.
139. Margoshes and Vallee: J. Am. Chem. Soc., *79*, 4813, 1957.
140. Piscator: Nord. Hyg. Tidskr., *45*, 76, 1964.
141. Pulido, Fuwa and Vallee: Anal. Biochem., *14*, 393, 1966.
142. Schroeder: J. Chronic Dis., *18*, 647, 1965.
143. Schroeder and Buckman: Arch. Environ. Health, *14*, 693, 1967.
144. Dalhamn and Friberg: Acta Pharmacol. Toxicol., *10*, 199, 1954.
145. Syverson, Stray, Syverson and Ofstad: Scand. J. Clin. Lab. Invest., *36*, 251, 1976.
146. Kägi and Vallee: J. Biol. Chem., *235*, 3460, 1960; and *236*, 2435, 1961.
147. Kägi, Himmelhoch, Whanger, Bethune and Vallee: J. Biol. Chem., *249*, 3537, 1974.
148. Kojima, Berger, Vallee and Kägi: Proc. Natl. Acad. Sci., *73*, 3413, 1976.
149. Pulido, Kägi and Vallee: Biochemistry, *5*, 1768, 1966.
150. Piscator: Nord. Hyg. Tidskr., *45*, 76, 1964.
151. Winge and Rajagopalan: Arch. Biochem. Biophys., *153*, 755, 1972.
152. Winge, Premakumar and Rajagopalan: Arch. Biochem. Biophys., *170*, 242, 1975.
153. Webb and Daniel: Chem. Biol. Interact., *10*, 269, 1975.
154. Richards and Cousins: J. Nutr., *106*, 1591, 1976.
155. Chen, Whanger and Weswig: Biochem. Med., *12*, 95, 1975.
156. Friberg: Arch. Ind. Health, *20*, 401, 1959.
157. Emmerson: Ann. Intern. Med., *73*, 854, 1970.
158. Axelsson and Piscator: Arch. Environ. Health, *12*, 360, 1966.
159. Itokawa, Abe, Tabei and Tanaka: Arch. Environ. Health, *28*, 149, 1974.
160. Chiquoine: J. Reprod. Fertil., *10*, 263, 1965.

Part II

Safety and Adequacy of the Food Supply

Chapter *10*

CRITERIA OF AN ADEQUATE DIET

Robert S. Goodhart

Diet patterns and food habits vary not only from one nation to another but also from individual to individual. There is no single pattern of diet which must be followed to ensure good nturition, nor no single food which can be designated essential for life or health. The animal body does require calories, certain fatty acids, amino acids, vitamins and minerals in sufficient amounts and in proper combinations to permit optimum growth and maintenance and repair of tissues under the environmental conditions to which the particular individual is exposed. The essential nutrients are widely dispersed in nature and can be obtained from many combinations of foods with varying ease.

Not only do diet patterns and food values vary but so also do requirements for specific nutrients, depending on genetic and environmental factors, diet patterns, severity and nature of stress situations, age, sex, rate of growth, etc. Largely because of these two factors—differences in nutritional needs of individuals and variation in nutritive value of foods—it is impossible to devise a general food plan that will be just right for everyone.[1] Other influences are of major importance in determining the dietary requirements either of the individual or of groups of persons: the organism's ability to adapt to its diet and to adjust to its environment, and the aspirations of the individual and of the society in which he lives. For example, the nutritional requirements for maximum size, early maturity, active sex life and maximum muscular development are not identical with those for maximum longevity. Diets designed to protect the individual against bacterial infections, e.g. tuberculosis, may lower resistance to certain viral infections and predispose the individual to obesity and coronary artery disease in later years. It is known that both malaria and cerebral malaria tend to spare undernourished persons.[1a]

How these various considerations may influence dietary recommendations is suggested by the various standards of different United States agencies and those of other countries. Table 10–1 gives the recommendations for certain nutrients for the young, healthy, moderately active, adult male made by two American agencies and by Canada and Japan. Although all the committees which formulated these recommendations had access to the same basic information, there are considerable differences among their conclusions. For example, an FAO/WHO Expert Group concluded that calcium intakes of 400 to 500 mg per day represented a practical allowance for adults,[6] a conclusion that appears to be shared by Canada and the I.C.N.N.D. (in evaluating diets in relatively underprivileged areas of the world). The recommendations of the NRC (Table 10–1) appear to be conditioned by our past dietary practices and the results of calcium balance studies. Hegsted[7] points out that "although most of the people of the world do not consume enough calcium to meet dietary recommendations, and thus are

Table 10–1. United States, Canadian and Japanese Recommended Dietary Intakes for Young, Healthy, Normally Active Male Adults§

Standard	Wt. in lb.	Calories	Protein gm	Calcium gm	Vitamin A I.U.	Iron mg	Thiamin mg	Riboflavin mg	Niacin mg	Ascorbic Acid mg	Vitamin D I.U.
National Research Council, United States[2]	154	2700	56	0.8	5000*	10	1.4	1.6	18 (equiv.)	45	0
I.C.N.N.D., United States[3]	154	2900	70	0.4	3500	9	0.96	1.2	10	30	0
Dietary Standard for Canada[4]	158	2850	48	0.5	3700†	6	0.9	1.4	9	30	
Standard Nutritional Requirements for Japanese[5] (light work)	123	2500	70	0.6	2000‡	10	1.3	1.3	13	65	400

* Assuming two-thirds of the total vitamin A activity as carotene and one-third as the preformed vitamin. If the sole source were preformed vitamin A, the allowance would be 3000 I.U.

† Based on the mixed Canadian diet supplying both vitamin A and carotene. As the preformed vitamin A, the suggested intake would be about two-thirds of that indicated.

‡ All as preformed vitamin A.

§ The figures given in this table, and elsewhere in this chapter, for agency-recommended dietary intakes are those which were current at the time of revision of this chapter (August 1977). The Food and Nutrition Board of the National Research Council, in common with the other mentioned agencies, periodically revises its recommendations, a fact which emphasizes, of course, the tentative nature of the recommendations.

often said to be calcium deficient, there is no convincing evidence that this is true." According to the World Health Organization, "since the publication of the report, much new evidence has supported the position taken by the Expert Group, which expressed its recommended intakes as ranges—for example 400 to 500 mg daily for adults. Recent work has justified the use of the low figures in the ranges for assessing the adequacy of diets. . . ."[8]

It should be apparent that the recommendations of national or international bodies on dietary intakes cannot be used, by themselves, as standards for the assessment of nutritional status of either individuals or population groups. Their practical uses are three: (1) in the planning of food production and distribution programs, (2) in the planning of mass feeding or food rationing programs, (3) as a useful starting point for nutrition therapy.

Tables setting forth the recommended dietary allowances of the World Health Organization, Canada and the Food and Nutrition Board of the United States are given in the Appendix to this volume. An additional table (Table 10–2), a concoction of the United States Food and Drug Administration,[9] may interest some readers; it lists the U.S. recommended daily allowances (U.S.RDA) derived by the Food and Drug Administration (FDA) from the recommended dietary allowances published in 1968 by the Food and Nutrition Board of the National Research Council. The FDA has ruled that "dietary supplements shall contain in the specified daily quantity not less than the lower limit nor more than the upper limit of any nutrient specified [in Table 10–2] for the groups for which the supplement is offered." This ruling does not apply to preparations intended for ingestion in tablet, capsule or liquid form or, if intended for ingestion in such a form, does not simulate and is not represented as conventional food, is not represented for use as a sole item of the meal or of the diet, and is not represented for use

in the treatment or management of specific diseases or disorders of children or of pregnant and lactating women. This exemption does not apply to minimum potency requirements. "Whenever a vitamin or mineral for which a U.S.RDA has been established is included in a dietary supplement, the supplement shall provide in the recommended daily quantity at least the lower potency limit for the vitamin or mineral established by [Table 10–2]."[9,10] If the above is confusing, it is more the fault of the Congress than of the FDA.

The table in the Appendix of nutrient intakes recommended by the World Health Organization (WHO) presents the recommendations on energy in terms of both kilocalories and megajoules. The kilocalorie (kcal) is the amount of heat required to raise the temperature of one kilogram of water one degree Celsius, from 14.5° to 15.5°C. The kilojoule (KJ) is equal to 0.239 kcal and the megajoule (MJ) is 1000 times this amount or 239 kcal. In the International System of Units, the unit of work, energy or quantity of heat is the joule, which is the work done in moving a mass a distance of one meter against a force of one newton. A newton is the force which, when acting continuously upon a mass of one kilogram, will impart to it an acceleration of one meter per second per second.[10] The WHO recognizes a trend to increasingly define energy requirements in terms of joules.[8] Personally, I am happy with calories.

Since the requirements for energy and the various nutrients are described in detail in the preceding and following chapters, and are summarized in the tables in the Appendix, they will not be dwelt on to any extent in this chapter, which will be restricted largely to the discussion and illustration of some general principles of dietary management. However, I would first like to correct an oversight in previous editions of this book and revise the definition of "vitamins."

A commonly accepted definition of

Table 10–2. U. S. Recommended Daily Allowances (U.S. RDA) and Permissible Compositional Ranges for Dietary Supplements of Vitamins and Minerals (from Federal Register[9])

	Unit of Measurement	Children under 4 Years of Age[1]			Adults and Children 4 or More Years of Age			Pregnant or Lactating Women		
		Lower limit	RDA	Upper limit	Lower limit	RDA	Upper limit	Lower limit	RDA	Upper limit
Vitamins—Mandatory:										
Vitamin A	International units	1,250	2,500	2,500	2,500	5,000	5,000	5,000	8,000	8,000
Vitamin D[2]	do	200	400	400				400	400	400
Vitamin E	do	5	10	15	15	30	45	30	30	60
Vitamin C	Milligrams	20	40	60	30	60	90	60	60	120
Folic acid[3]	do	.1	.2	.3	.2	.4	.4	.4	.8	.8
Thiamin	do	.35	.70	1.05	.75	1.50	2.25	1.50	1.70	3.00
Riboflavin	do	.4	.8	1.2	.8	1.7	2.6	1.7	2.0	3.4
Niacin	do	4.5	9.0	13.5	10.0	20.0	30.0	20.0	20.0	40.0
Vitamin B$_6$	do	.35	.70	1.05	1.00	2.00	3.00	2.00	2.50	4.00
Vitamin B$_{12}$	Micrograms	1.5	3.0	4.5	3.0	6.0	9.0	6.0	8.0	12.0
Optional:										
Vitamin D	International units				200	400	400			
Biotin	Milligrams	.075	.150	.225	.150	.300	.450	.300	.300	.600
Pantothenic acid	do	2.5	5.0	7.5	5.0	10.0	15.0	10.0	10.0	20.0
Minerals—Mandatory:										
Calcium	Grams	.125	.800	1.200	.125	1.000	1.500	.125	1.300	2.000
Phosphorus[4]	do	.125	.800	1.200	.125	1.000	1.500			
Iodine	Micrograms	35	70	105	75	150	225	150	150	300
Iron	Milligrams	5	10	15	9	18	27	18	18	60
Magnesium	do	40	200	300	100	400	600	100	450	800
Optional:										
Phosphorus[4]	Grams							.125	1.300	2.000
Copper	Milligrams	.5	1.0	1.5	1.0	2.0	3.0	1.0	2.0	4.0
Zinc	do	4.0	8.0	12.0	7.5	15.0	22.5	7.5	15.0	30.0

[1] When labeled for use by infants, a dietary supplement shall contain not less than the lower limit designated for a nutrient in this set of columns, nor more than 100 per cent of the infant U.S. RDA for a nutrient except that the level of biotin, when used, shall be 0.05 mg daily recommended quantity.

[2] Optional for adults and children 4 or more years of age.

[3] Optional for liquid products.

[4] Optional for pregnant or lactating women. When present, the quantity of phosphorus may be not greater than the quantity of calcium.

vitamins is that they are chemically unrelated organic substances that are essential in small amounts for the maintenance of normal metabolic functions but are not synthesized within the body and, therefore, must be furnished from exogenous sources.[12-14]

From a clinical point of view, the agents generally considered to be vitamins are those organic compounds the absence of which can cause specific metabolic defects.[13]

This definition is not quite correct in that a few organic compounds generally recognized to be vitamins for man can be and are synthesized within the human body and, under suitable conditions, in amounts adequate to support normal metabolic processes. Vitamin D is formed by the activation of 7-dehydrocholesterol in the skin by sunlight. Vitamin A is synthesized within the body from a number of carotenoids with varying degrees of efficiency, and niacin can be made within the body from tryptophan. However, deficiencies of vitamins A, D and niacin resulting in serious metabolic defects are known to occur and exogenous sources of the preformed vitamins appear to be essential for most people.

It must also be borne in mind that the exogenous sources referred to are not always foods. Both vitamin K and biotin are normally synthesized by the bacterial flora of the gut. The vitamin B_{12} formed by bacterial action in the colon is, of course, not normally available to the human host living under modern hygienic conditions.

A more accurate definition would be that vitamins are chemically unrelated organic compounds, essential in minute amounts for the maintenance of normal metabolic functions, which are either not synthesized within the body or are generally not synthesized within the body in adequate amounts, so that exogenous sources of supply are usually necessary. This still leaves vitamin D in a somewhat

anomalous position, but perhaps D would be better classified as a hormone than as a vitamin.

One other point on the subject of vitamins: There is no such thing as vitamin B_{17}. Laetrile, amygdalin, a substance derived from pulverized apricot pits,[16] is not essential in any amount for the maintenance of any normal metabolic function, and calling it vitamin B_{17} does not make it so. It has no value in human nutrition and there is "no valid scientific evidence which indicates that Laetrile has any potential value in cancer management."[16] It has no nutrient or therapeutic value whatsoever, and no judge and no act of any legislature can change that. In fact, there is good evidence that laetrile may be poisonous, even lethal, to both men and animals.[16a] Much the same assessment can be made of pangamic acid, another apricot-pit derivative. Pangamic acid has been reported to be a mixture of sodium or calcium gluconate, glycine and diisopropylamine dichloroacetate.[16b] It is not a vitamin nor an essential nutrient of any kind. There is no such thing as vitamin B_{15}.

Dietary Goals for the United States, a report of the Senate Select Committee on Nutrition and Human Needs, emphasizes the importance of cardiovascular disease, hypertension, certain forms of cancer, diabetes and cirrhosis as causes of death and morbidity in the United States and the health bill associated with these diseases, and arrives at the following goals:[15]

1. Increase carbohydrate consumption to account for 55 to 60 per cent of the energy (calorie) intake.
2. Reduce overall fat consumption from approximately 40 to 30 per cent of the energy intake.
3. Reduce saturated fat consumption to account for about 10 per cent of the total energy intake and balance with polyunsaturated and monounsaturated fats which should account for about 10 per cent of energy each.
4. Reduce cholesterol consumption to about 300 mg a day.

5. Reduce sugar consumption by almost 40 per cent to account for about 15 per cent of the energy intake.
6. Reduce salt consumption by about 50 to 85 per cent, to approximately 3 gm a day.

It proposes the following changes in food selection and preparation to achieve these goals:

1. Increase consumption of fruits and vegetables and whole-grain cereals.
2. Decrease consumption of meat and increase consumption of poultry and fish.
3. Decrease consumption of foods high in fat and partially substitute polyunsaturated fat for saturated fat.
4. Substitute nonfat for whole milk.
5. Decrease consumption of butterfat, eggs and other high-cholesterol sources.
6. Decrease consumption of sugar and foods high in sugar content.
7. Decrease consumption of salt and foods high in salt content.

These goals, and the recommended procedures for achieving them, seem sensible enough, but they are unlikely to change much. As the Council on Foods and Nutrition of the AMA has pointed out,[17] "Efforts to improve the nutritional status of populations by introduction of new foods and by attempts to change food habits often have not been effective. Improvement of the nutritive value of widely used foods through enrichment, restoration, or fortification can provide good nutrition to populations at risk, without the necessity of extensive efforts to change food consumption patterns."

Actually, no healthy man with catholic tastes, who regularly eats a variety of cereal products, vegetables and fruits, with little or no sugar, and a small amount of animal protein at each of his three daily meals, is in any danger of developing any nutritional deficiency. By a small amount of animal protein I mean 2 to 3 ounces of fish, meat, poultry or cheese or 1 egg or 2 glasses of milk; this is adequate for any healthy adolescent or adult male provided that caloric requirements are met. Weight should be maintained at or about the level recommended for height (Chap. 1). Serum

cholesterol and triglyceride levels among Americans appear to be more dependent upon degree of adiposity than on frequency of consumption of fat, sugar, starch or alcohol.[18]

Healthy women taking oral contraceptives may require some supplementation of the above diet. Biochemical evidences for deficiencies of vitamin B_6, folacin, vitamin C and vitamin B_{12} have been reported, while the blood levels of vitamin A, iron and copper are said to be elevated. However, according to the 1975 report on oral contraceptives and nutrition of the Committee on Nutrition of the Mother and Preschool Child, Food and Nutrition Board,[19] in spite of the widespread metabolic changes observed relatively few clinical correlations have been identified. Mental depression, which occasionally occurs, may be a manifestation of vitamin B_6 deficiency, which could impair tryptophan-serotonin metabolism in the brain, and, rarely, a megaloblastic anemia responsive to folate therapy has been seen.

More recently, however, Leklem et al., in a controlled study in which urinary cystathionine levels were ascertained before and after methionine loading, came to the conclusion that the use of oral contraceptives has little if any effect on the vitamin B_6 requirement of most women.[45]

Also, the Food and Nutrition Board has expressed concern over the iron intake of women of childbearing age on the "typical American diet"[2] and has recommended that they increase their iron intake "By selecting iron-rich foods whenever possible and by including in the diet foods that are known to increase the absorption of iron present in the diet; for example, meat and citrus fruit." The World Health Organization has expressed concern about the inadequacy of the dietary intake of iron by women of childbearing age who are on diets providing less than 10 per cent of the calories from animal foods,[8] certainly not the typical American diet. The Food and Nutrition Board recommends 18 mg of iron per day for young women, whereas the WHO recommends 14 mg and 28 mg, the higher figure for women on diets very low in animal protein. For a more complete discussion of iron, refer to Chapter 7C. I close my references to the subject with the following quotations and remarks.

> In view of these similarities, it is remarkable that plants and animals have been able to develop, during evolution, methods for keeping many of their tissues and organs free of microbial invaders. In animal systems, the methods involving humoral and cellular immunity are well known. Much less attention has been given to a possible third method: that of nutritional immunity. In this method, the invaded host would attempt to withhold an essential nutrilite from the pathogenic microorganisms. However, because of the qualitative and quantitative similarities between the essential nutrilites of animal hosts and invading microorganisms, such a process appears at first glance to be highly impractical. Nevertheless, hosts go to considerable lengths to deprive invaders of at least one nutrilite (iron), and there exists much evidence that this example of nutritional immunity is an important defense component in our never-ending war with potential pathogens.[20]

> When hosts are rendered hypoferremic by injection of viable bacteria or bacterial products, e.g. BCG vaccine or endotoxin, respectively, their plasma gains antimicrobial activity in direct proportion to the loss of iron and the decrease in iron saturation of transferrin. This antimicrobial action, in in vitro tests, is readily neutralized by addition of iron to the serum. In in vivo tests, animals rendered hypoferremic are more resistant to pathogenic invaders than are controls. Likewise, animals injected with deferoxamine mesylate (the chelator used in hemosiderotic patients to remove iron via renal excretion) were found to have enhanced resistance to listerial bacteria.[20]

> Streptococcus mutans and Vibrio cholerae, but not Escherichia coli, were killed by incubation with purified human apolactoferrin. Concentrations of lactoferrin below that necessary for total inhibition resulted in a marked reduction in viable colony-forming units. This bactericidal effect was contingent upon the metal[iron]-chelating properties of the lactoferrin molecule.[21]

Murray and Murray treated 71 iron-deficient nomads with 900 mg of ferrous sulfate daily for 30 days. Another group of 66 iron-deficient nomads received placebo only. Active infection occurred during or shortly after iron therapy in 27 nomads (38 per cent) and included malaria in 13, brucellosis in 5 and tuberculosis in 3. Five cases of infection occurred in the placebo group (8 per cent) and included 1 malaria, 2 abscesses and 2 schistosomiases.[21a]

Also, a hematocrit value around the generally accepted upper limit of normal may be an important factor in the causation of occlusive vascular disease.[21b] Nicolaides et al.[21c] found that whole-blood viscosity, hematocrit, red-cell flexibility and plasma-fibrinogen concentration were all higher in persons with angina pectoris. They further found that, when the viscosity was corrected to a standard hematocrit (45 per cent), there was no significant difference in viscosity between the group with angina and the group without angina.

Much of the advertising of special dietary products for the aged seems to me to imply an increased metabolic requirement for vitamins and minerals by people beyond a certain age (Have you noticed how early in life old age often begins these days for actors on television programs promoting products for senior citizens?), but this is not so. Nor do they appear to have any more difficult a time, generally, in meeting their requirements than do people in other age groups. The National Nutrition Survey conducted in New York City in the late 1960s found that individuals "over age 60 generally had better results than other age groups with regard to vitamin A and riboflavin; they were not appreciably worse off than other age groups in the case of other biochemical tests. . . ."[22]

Neither the Food and Nutrition Board of the National Research Council-National Academy of Sciences[2] nor the World Health Organization[8] recognizes any need for increasing the vitamin and mineral allowances for healthy, elderly individuals above those levels recommended for the younger healthy adult. Somewhat to the contrary, as a matter of fact, the Food and Nutrition Board decreases slightly the recommended dietary allowances for adult males over the age of 51 years for niacin, riboflavin, thiamin and iodine and, for females over 51 years, decreases the allowances for niacin, riboflavin, iodine and iron. This is consistent with the decreased energy consumption and expenditure of persons in this age group and with the postmenopausal condition of females with respect to iron.

The requirements for sundry vitamins and minerals may be increased by conditions such as those which increase metabolism or cause malabsorption, metabolic blocks or excessive urinary losses, but they are not increased, after reaching adulthood, by age per se. The situations which might demand an intake of some vitamins and/or minerals in amounts greater than normal requirements may present themselves at any age. None of them is unique to old age, however that is defined (also see Chap. 28).

Female vegetarians may have great difficulty in meeting their dietary requirements for iron and both male and female vegetarians may be deficient in calcium and zinc, unless dietary supplementation is resorted to. Also, strict vegetarians (vegans) lack a dietary source of vitamin B_{12}, since man normally obtains this vitamin only from foods of animal origin. Among the better sources of iron available to vegetarians are blackstrap molasses, brewers' yeast, wheat germ, wheat bran, pulses, eggs and enriched flour. (It is necessary to ensure that brewers' yeast is dead. Fungemia and systemic Saccharomyces infections have resulted from the ingestion of live brewers' yeast.[23]) One study of hospital diets found that the ovolactovegetarian diet provided 81 per cent of the adult recommended dietary allowance for zinc, whereas the regular diet provided 97 per cent.[24] The authors postulate that a strict vegetarian diet would furnish even less

zinc, not only because of the high concentration of zinc in animal proteins but also because varying amounts of both calcium and zinc are made unavailable by the phytate found in cereals. A diet depending solely on cereal grains for protein is not to be recommended. Many cereals are deficient in lysine which can be compensated for by adding pulses to the diet. Also, the pulses generally have about twice as much protein as the cereals. Cooked rice provides 1 gm of protein for every 47.6 calories, whereas dried cooked peas provide 1 gm of protein for every 14.4 calories.

Both the whole cereal grains and the pulses are good sources of most of the B vitamins, with the notable exceptions of folacin and vitamin B_{12} and, in the case of maize, niacin and available tryptophan, and the cereal germ oil contains vitamin E. Other vegetables and fruits supply varying amounts of low-calorie bulk, vitamin A, in the form of carotene, ascorbic acid and folacin. Bananas are an exception in regard to calories in that they may supply 85 to 100 calories per 100 gm (plantain = 119 calories per 100 gm). They are a rich source of potassium, of which orange juice is also a good source.[25]

Thus strict vegetarians on diets based largely on cereals may find themselves lacking in calcium, iron and zinc, as well as vitamin B_{12} and lysine. Vegetarian diets based largely on maize may require supplementation with both lysine and tryptophan.[26]

In further regard to lysine, the following quotation from "The Great Protein Fiasco" by Donald S. McLaren is pertinent:

> By about 1966 protein sources which started as a by-product of the dairy industry began to yield some ground to a by-product of the nylon industry. Lysine supplementation of wheat commenced. It has proved extremely difficult to demonstrate any benefit from this to humans, even under very artificial conditions. Human dietaries are usually not especially deficient in lysine; and other foodstuffs—

legumes or milk—tend to make up for the deficiency in bread.[27]

Also, it needs to be mentioned that a new variety of maize, Opague-2 maize, which is higher in lysine and tryptophan and lower in leucine than is common maize, has been developed and has been used successfully in the nutritional rehabilitation of children with severe protein malnutrition.[28]

Vegetarians are likely to get plenty of dietary fiber. Dietary fiber is the residue of plant food resistant to hydrolysis by human alimentary enzymes. It is composed of cellulose, hemicellulose and lignin.[29] It provides bulk to the stool and laxation to the bowels and it has been postulated that dietary fiber is protective against colonic disorders, such as cancer and diverticulosis, and a number of metabolic diseases, such as ischemic heart disease and other vascular disorders, diabetes mellitus and obesity,[29-34a] and may also be protective against certain toxic dietary effects.[35] The pertinent observations on man have been primarily of an epidemiologic nature and it can hardly be said that the evidence in favor of the postulates mentioned above is much more than suggestive, although Brodribb[32] has reported the demonstration, with a double-blind controlled trial, of the relief of symptoms of diverticular disease with a high-fiber diet, and an increase in dietary fiber over the small amount usually found in the diet in industrialized countries can prevent constipation.[36] However, high-fiber diets may also have some adverse effects on some people.

Phytobezoars (gastrointestinal concretions composed of vegetable matter, such as skins, seeds and fibers of fruits and vegetables) are common in Africans who have a high consumption of fruits and other fibrous material. In this respect, persimmons are particularly bad.[37] Phytobezoars are also a not uncommon complication in postoperative peptic ulcer patients;[38,39] in fact, Bucholz[39] has stated that they may be the most common complication found in such patients. He emphasizes the necessity for clear and emphatic instructions to avoid fibrous foods, especially oranges, "unless these foods can be finely chewed or mechanically minced prior to ingestion." He states further that the total elimination of oranges would prevent 80 to 90 per cent of such bezoars following gastric surgery.

Gastric phytobezoars may respond to enzymatic softening or dissolution with or without endoscopic destruction.[40,41] If a bolus results in mechanical obstruction of the small bowel, surgery is mandatory.[39]

Naturally occurring toxicants in foods are discussed elsewhere in this book (Chap. 12), but there are two that bear mention at this point: (1) Lead is ubiquitous in the environment and, when eaten by animals, is concentrated in the bones. Crosby[42] reports a case of a middle-aged actress who suffered severe, crippling lead poisoning as the result of the chronic ingestion of a "health food," powdered bone meal, made from horse bone and prescribed—by a physician—as a calcium supplement. (2) By the Salmonella typhimurium test, extracts of Japanese raw fish, treated in the laboratory with nitrite, showed mutagenic activity which was prevented by the addition of ascorbate. Extracts from similarly treated beef and hot dogs were non-mutagenic.[43] The authors suggest that the mutagenic activity in nitrosated fish might be relevant to the question of the etiology of human gastric cancer. They also refer to reports of an inverse relationship between the consumption of foods rich in ascorbate and gastric cancer.

Among the foods to which unusual health properties are often ascribed must be included yogurt. Perhaps, but yogurt contains no nutrient of any significance which is not in the milk from which it is made. It does, however, contain lactase, derived from the yogurt culture, and, as Kilara and Shahani suggest,[44] cultured yogurt might be beneficial for persons with limited abilities to digest lactose, not only because of its reduced lactose content but also because of the lactase released from the cultures during digestion.

Two rules for nutritional health can perhaps be promulgated as being generally applicable: (1) Eat a variety of foods regularly. (2) Eat and drink in moderation. Further, there is one lesson still to be learned by many institutional food managers and dietitians: No food or meal has any nutritional value unless it is eaten or otherwise internally consumed by the person for whom it is intended. Meals intended to be eaten should be more than just barely edible. They should be palatable.

Agriculture Handbook 456, "Nutritive Value of American Foods in Common Units," by Catherine F. Adams and published in December 1975, can be obtained by sending a check or money order for $5.15 per copy to the Superintendent of Documents, U. S. Government Printing Office, Washington, D. C. 20402.

BIBLIOGRAPHY

1. Page and Phipard: Home Economics Research Report No. 3. Washington, USDA, 1957.
1a. Murray, Murray, Murray and Murray: Am. J. Clin. Nutr., 31, 57, 1978.
2. National Research Council, Food and Nutrition Board: Recommended Dietary Allowances, 1974, Washington.
3. Interdepartmental Committee on Nutrition for National Defense: Manual for Nutrition Surveys, 2nd ed. Washington, Government Printing Office, 1963.
4. Canadian Council on Nutrition: Dietary Standards for Canada 1963: March 1964 (protein revised 1968). Ottawa, Department of Public Printing and Stationery.
5. Ministry of Health and Welfare, Japan: Nutrition in Japan 1960. Tokyo, 1960.
6. World Health Organization: Calcium Requirements, WHO Tech. Rep. Ser. No. 230. Geneva, 1962.
7. Hegsted: J. Am. Diet. Assoc., 50, 105, 1967.
8. World Health Organization: Handbook of Human Nutritional Requirements. Geneva, 1974.
9. Federal Register: 41, 46172, October 19, 1976, Washington, D. C.
10. Federal Register: 42, 20294, April 19, 1977, Washington, D. C.
11. Dorland's Illustrated Medical Dictionary, 24th ed. Philadelphia, W. B. Saunders, 1965.
12. Grollman and Grollman: Pharmacology and Therapeutics, 7th ed. Philadelphia, Lea & Febiger, 1970.
13. Guyton: Textbook of Medical Physiology. W. B. Saunders, Philadelphia, 1976.
14. Goodman and Gilman: The Pharmacological Basis of Therapeutics, 5th ed. New York, Macmillan, 1975.
15. Hegsted: Nutr. Notes, 13, 4, 1977.
16. Food and Drug Administration: FDA Drug Bull., 7, 2, 1977.
16a. Schmidt, Newton, Sanders, Lewis and Conn: J.A.M.A., 239, 943, 1978.
16b. Anon: Med. Lett., 20, 44, 1978.
17. Council on Foods and Nutrition, AMA: J.A.M.A., 225, 1116, 1973.
18. Nichols, Ravenscroft, Lamphiear and Ostrander: J.A.M.A., 236, 1948, 1976.
19. Committee on Nutrition of the Mother and Preschool Child, Food and Nutrition Board: Washington, National Research Council-National Academy of Sciences, 1975.
20. Weinberg: J.A.M.A., 231, 39, 1975.
21. Arnold, Cole and McGhee: Science, 197, 263, 1977.
21a. Murray and Murray: Am. J. Clin. Nutr., 31, 700, 1978.
21b. Thomas, Marshall, Russell, Wetherly-Mein, Boulay, Pearson, Symon and Zilkha: Lancet, 2, 941, 1977.
21c. Nicolaides, Horbourne, Bowers, Kidner and Besterman: Lancet, 2, 943, 1977.
22. Newman and Martin: Ann. N. Y. Acad. Sci., Ser. 11, 33, 316, 1971.
23. Jensen and Smith: Arch. Intern. Med., 136, 332, 1976.
24. Brown, McGuckin, Wilson and Smith: J. Am. Diet. Assoc., 69, 632, 1976.
25. Passmore and Robson (Eds.): A Companion to Medical Studies, Vol. 1. Oxford and Edinburgh, Blackwell Scientific Publications, 1968.
26. Clark, Bailey and Brewer: Am. J. Clin. Nutr., 30, 674, 1977.
27. McLaren: Lancet, 2, 93, 1974.
28. Maffia, Clark and Mertz: Am. J. Clin. Nutr., 29, 817, 1976.
29. Trowell: Am. J. Clin. Nutr., 29, 417, 1976.
30. Kiem, Anderson and Ward: Am. J. Clin. Nutr., 29, 895, 1976.
31. Burkitt: Nutr. Today, 11, 6, 1976.
32. Brodribb: Lancet, 1, 664, 1977.
33. Kritchevsky: Am. J. Clin. Nutr., 30, 979, 1977.
34. MacGregor: J.A.M.A., 227, 911, 1974.
34a. Symposium on role of dietary fiber in health. Am. J. Clin. Nutr., 31(Suppl.), 1, 1978.
35. Kritchevsky: Fed. Proc., 36, 1692, 1977.
36. Medical Letter, 17, 93, 1975.
37. Thomas and Clain: Am. J. Gastroenterol., 64, 392, 1975.
38. Amjad, Kumar and McCaughey: Am. J. Gastroenterol., 64, 327, 1975.
39. Bucholz: Resid. Staff Physician, 61, March 1976

40. Rozen and Gilat: Am. J. Gastroenterol., *64*, 397, 1975.
41. Feffer and Norton: J.A.M.A., *236*, 1578, 1976.
42. Crosby: J.A.M.A., *237*, 2627, 1977.
43. Marquardt, Rufino and Weisburger: Science, *196*, 1000, 1977.
44. Kilara and Shahani: J. Dairy Sci., *59*, 2031, 1976.
45. Leklem, Linkswiler, Brown, Rose and Anand: Am. J. Clin. Nutr., *30*, 1122, 1977.

Chapter *11*

FOOD FADS AND FADDISM

Philip L. White
and
Therese D. Mondeika

Mysticism and food faddism are probably as old as civilization itself. Waxing and waning, constantly changing, man's belief in the curative, protective and magical properties of foods has led to cultism that often becomes a blend of a pseudoscience and a religion.[1-5] Unusual dietary patterns are adopted with the zeal of religious fanaticism by certain segments of our population as a means of creating a spiritual awakening or rebirth. There is no doubt that some of the philosophies provide satisfying emotional experiences for their followers. Many sensible, sincere people are also motivated to seek alternative food styles for ecological reasons. They are worried about environmental pollution through the use of agricultural chemicals and have, thus, turned to "organic" and "health" foods. The pressure of these ecological concerns has increased both the number of people and the emotional intensity involved in this practice. This same concern about the natural environment and the food supply has existed through the generations. Although concern for environmental protection is commendable, a line must be drawn between healthy skepticism and paranoia.[6]

The health food movement produces persuasive leaders who charm their followers with their own brand of proselytism. Examples may be found in the careers of Graham, Kellogg and Post.[5]

Frequently a lucrative business develops from fads and cults, as with the present-day health food enterprise. The power of advertising and communications helps to expand and perpetuate the myths upon which the business was based. The enterprise builds upon the consumer's ignorance, desperation or fear until mere interest evolves into zealotry.

Real or imagined apprehension about the quality and safety of the food supply or specific concern about particular food manufacturing practices and food additives leads many people to seek alternative food practices and nonconventional approaches to personal nutrition. When dealing with alternative food practices that appear to be mere faddism, it is important to distinguish between debatable issues that have a basis in science and issues that represent personal philosophies. For example, people may be convinced that all chemicals used in foods are unsafe and unnecessary. That belief represents personal philosophy—they wish things as God made them, simple and pure. In reality, the issue is based in science relating to the particular chemical and the use it serves. The issue of risk and benefit relative to food chemicals cannot be debated solely on the basis of personal philosophy.

Cultism can emerge as a result of confusion between the significance of uncertain or implied environmental risk and that of unequivocal risk to health. The natural or organic food movement relates to this as people became concerned about modern agricultural practices which rely on chemical sprays and other agricultural chemicals. Apprehension about the safety and quality of processed foods also fans the fires of faddism. Customers patronizing health food stores are led to believe that foods presumably grown without the use of pesticides or artificial fertilizers but with the application to the soil of natural fertilizers (manures) and other organic matter are more nourishing and less likely to be hazardous. "Natural foods" are those that have undergone little or no processing and do not contain additives.[7] In large measure, the movement is based upon distortion of fact and exploitation of the unwary. The movement has also produced an uncompromising situation related to the demand for absolute safety in our environment and our foods. Today, as the result of strong societal pressures, experts are asked to provide evidence of absolute safety rather than evidence of hazard, an unrealistic and unattainable goal.[8]

The natural food concept is also based on the belief that naturalness or "organicness" lends particular health-giving properties to foods and nutrients. The unwary are led to believe that vitamins are not vitamins unless they are derived or extracted directly from plant or animal products. The consumer pays dearly for that bit of myth in the form of exorbitant prices for such products as vitamin C from rose hips or acerola berries. Perpetuation of the myth is absolutely necessary for the continued vitality of the health food movement.

It is unlikely that customers patronizing health food stores and paying for so-called organically grown or natural foods are unaware of the increased prices. Aside from the cost factor, there is more reason to be concerned about the health delusion that may have attracted the consumer initially.

Wolff pointed out that most people who patronize health food stores and restaurants know what they are doing and what they want. They have their own set of beliefs about the cultural significance of food and about the quality and safety of more conventional foods. They do not believe and behave as they do because of the books they read; rather, what they read is determined by their beliefs.[9] Their motivation generally is a desire for a simpler diet not related to the highly processed, convenience foods produced by the American food industry.

> Foods most often bought in health food stores were (reported in descending order of frequency): whole grain products, whole wheat bread, fresh vegetables and fruits, raw nuts, wheat germ, brown rice, honey, yogurt, dried fruits, brewers' yeast, seeds. Foods most frequently avoided in the diet were (in descending order of frequency): refined sugar, processed and canned foods with chemical additives, white flour products and white bread, carbonated drinks, meat from animals raised in the United States, monosodium glutamate, processed meats such as hot dogs and luncheon meats, chocolate, processed cereals, white rice, coffee.[9]

What was once considered to be a fad (a regimen followed with great enthusiasm for a short period of time) may now be thought of as a subculture that is, in reality, only a departure from some conventionally defined norm.[9,10] "What has been called the counterculture can perhaps best be understood as an expression of disaffection, alienation perhaps, or disappointment with an environment that is becoming increasingly man made and yet increasingly foreign, frustrating and incomprehensible."[9] Wolff states that health foodists (his coined word) believe and behave in opposition to the culture in which they were raised and are able to maintain their opposition because they receive strong reinforcements: ". . . a sense of community, a shared (counter) culture, and a feeling of well being." They feel a need to react to what they perceive to be an overly and shortsightedly manipulated environment. Work to improve the diets of this subculture group, should that be necessary, would require a completely different approach than that required to correct dietary faults resulting from ignorance, indifference or poverty.

The willingness of segments of American industry to turn to its own advantage the words of the counterculture, organic and natural, may have produced apparent confirmation of concern. From organic eye shadow to natural breakfast cereals, industry plays both sides of the street by promoting such products. The immediacy of commerce and the ability to tailor-make products to capitalize on consumer interests or concerns may serve at times to confirm a given fear. Thus, the difference between the conventional food industry and the health food industry becomes confused. Perhaps in the confusion the words "organic" and "natural" will lose their significance.

Each generation is visited by what Herbert calls "the health hustlers."[11] These are the proselytes mentioned earlier. Some are self-styled "experts" who know the protection inherent in the First Amendment to the Constitution and use it to further their own careers. Others are simply misguided laymen who have seen the nutritional light—often of a different wavelength than seen by the scientist. Both mislead the public, undermine faith in medicine and nutrition as they promote their own brands of pseudonutrition. Those brands usually include the prescription of vitamins and/or minerals to prevent or cure whatever disease or condition is currently confounding the medical profession. So-called megavitamin therapy, or orthomolecular medicine, is the current panacea for everything from schizophrenia to cancer.[12,13] Because the "health hustlers" are treated with undue respect by the media of mass communications, the public is often incapable of differentiating the "hustler" with inappropriate credentials from the qualified scientist.[14,15] So

long as the health hustlers successfully avoid the infringement of laws and regulations concerned with protecting the public against pretended medical skills or unlawful medical practice, false and misleading food and drug claims on labels, or misuse of the United States mails, they are free to prey on the unsuspecting public.[11]

The publication of books and articles in magazines and newspapers pertaining to nutrition and health abounds in this country. Unfortunately, much of the information is erroneous or misleading. The public is being bombarded with nutrition misinformation at an alarming rate. What is even more unfortunate is that no reliable mechanism exists to help the public evaluate this information and put it into proper perspective. In the absence of such a mechanism, it behooves members of the media and publishers to assume the responsibility for assuring that statements and recommendations made to the public are based on scientific fact rather than on personal opinion.

The chicanery practiced by the health food store "medicine man" who diagnoses ailments and dispenses roots, herbs, teas or nutritional supplements to "cure" disease or relieve its symptoms differs only in degree from that involved in medical quackery.[16] While the latter is more serious because the quack may deprive gravely ill patients of appropriate medical treatment, the rationale for turning to any charlatan is no doubt similar. Bernard[17] succinctly appraised it:

> The need to believe in a therapeutic miracle, when medical science is or seems to be failing, can be so strong that it drives one's intelligence into twisting the facts to fit emotional necessity. Thus, faith in the quack, under such conditions, can be maintained without too much offense to reason by mobilizing such arguments as: the quack may have hit upon something of which medical science is still ignorant; the quack is a genius who is too far ahead of his time to be accorded recognition; the quack is a great healer who is the victim of organized medicine's vindictive jealousy or protection of a professional monopoly, and so on. Clearly,

the psychological situation is very different for those who turn toward quackery in extremis when medicine is impotent than for the majority of those on whose gullibility and weaknesses quackery trades.

The key words are "the need to believe in a therapeutic miracle" and "emotional necessity." It is on these needs that quackery thrives. The recipients are in reality paying for benefits that are not there. They believe, and that very belief may be sufficient justification for action.

It is important to recognize that unconventional or apparently bizarre dietary habits may reflect alternative styles of life or perhaps some long-standing cultural or religious practice that is simply different from the usual pattern. Many people may have a rational argument for nutritional behavior that is based on a cultural or religious viewpoint rather than on misinformation in terms of scientific knowledge of nutrition. Therefore, if attempts are made to change their behavior, it is imperative to understand their way of thinking and start from their point of view. When the resultant nutrient intake is appropriate, there is little reason to be concerned. At the same time, it should be recognized that aberrant diets or exotic regimens derived from a given religious philosophy can be fraught with biologic hazard for the devotee. Such was the case with the so-called Zen Macrobiotic Diet publicized by Georges Oshawa.[18] Several deaths and cases of severe vitamin deficiencies have been reported in individuals who attempted to practice the most extreme aspect of the regimen.[18-20] While the Zen Macrobiotic regimen is an extreme example of a diet derived from a given religious philosophy, it does illustrate that quackery can exist within a mask of culture or religion. By the same token, quacks can slip behind the curtain of religion to avoid persecution and prosecution. The only rational way to bring about behavior modification among followers of a sect or subculture that embraces a hazardous diet or dietary practice is to work within that system of beliefs. Within the value system, changes can be brought about that will improve the nutritional status.

Weight reduction regimens promoted to the public as the answer to the fat person's prayers exemplify the fad diet. They are followed with great excitement for short periods of time. Their popularity is more directly related to the persuasiveness of the promotion and the personality of the "originator" than to the value of the diet. Essentially all reducing diets will help remove weight, especially if the dieter can be swept up with the lure of the regimen. Ultimately, the behavior pattern that precipitated the obesity in the first place takes over and failure begins. The dieter then becomes a candidate for the next highly publicized crash diet.

Most fad diets are based on imbalance, not necessarily calorie imbalance, which is the thermochemical logic of weight reduction, but rather on macronutrient imbalance. Through the years, there have been diets that are excessive in fat, protein or carbohydrates at the expense of one or the other of these nutrients. The ketogenic diets are ketogenic because of the minimal carbohydrate and the excessive fat content. The body water loss, the reduced appetite associated with ketosis and the inability to consume unlimited quantities of high-fat foods apparently explain the weight loss that occurs with such diets. The Council on Foods and Nutrition published a statement criticizing the low-carbohydrate high-protein high-fat reducing diets and warned of the metabolic problems that could develop as a result of these diets, problems related to the excretory demands of the high protein intake, the electrolyte imbalance associated with lean body tissue catabolism and ketosis, and the management of the high-fat diet.[21]

Starvation and semistarvation diets appear, disappear and reappear regularly. While short-term starvation as a means of losing weight has been incorporated into weight reduction programs by some physicians, the exploitation of extended fasting as a popular method of weight reduction is not in the public interest. There are too many hazards associated with unsupervised starvation to justify its popularization. Nevertheless, books and lecturers still extol the virtues of the extended fast for weight control. The protein-sparing modified fast based upon the provision of 1 to 2 gm of protein per kg ideal body weight, with or without a few hundred kcal from carbohydrate, is currently being used in the management of obesity.[22]

Why, in this enlightened age, does the public fall prey to the counterculture of nutrition and medicine? Why is health fraud becoming more lucrative with little probability that public support will diminish? It would seem to relate to a condition of human frailty, the expectation of miracles. Part of the answer can be found in a study of health and opinions sponsored by the federal government.[23]

The study was based on extensive interviews with a national area probability sample of 2,839 adults. Among the findings, the most common misconception reported was that three-fourths of the public believe that extra vitamins provide more pep and energy. Twenty-six per cent, representing about 35 million adults, were found to have used nutritional supplements expecting observable benefits, without the advice of a physician.

Among the more shocking findings was the fact that 42 per cent of the people interviewed, representing 50 million adults, would not be convinced by almost unanimous expert opinion that a hypothetical "cancer cure" was worthless. Only 45 per cent thought such a medicine should be banned by law. The study and interpretive report provide considerable insight into the attitudes about health values in this country: "The study found that informed, systematic thinking about health is rare and that, with certain exceptions, few people have an organized set of health beliefs. While some people act on the basis of specific beliefs, true or false, many more make health decisions believing that 'anything is worth a try.' " This is identified as "rampant empiricism."[23]

In this approach, rational judgment is ruled out since even a total lack of scientific evidence does not eliminate the possibility that a treatment or practice may appear to benefit some users. Psychosomatic effects and unaided recovery, which occur frequently, reinforce faith in the results assumed from this uncritical trial-and-error approach. Further, millions of people appear to be basing important health decisions on the idea that, since there are individual differences in people, there is a chance that almost any treatment may be beneficial. In other words, because it did not work for one does not mean that it might not work for another.

Bruch[24] has discussed the possibility that quackery may be an expression of the relative failure of the scientific approach:

> The great progress of modern medicine during the nineteenth and twentieth centuries, based on the scientific method, has led in its extreme application to a model of medical practice in which the patient is dealt with as a passive object on whom the scientific physician practices his special knowledge. This model overlooks that the doctor-patient interaction rests on a number of shared assumptions and social roles. Talcott Parsons, the sociologist, feels there is need to consider the *function* of medical practice, what is ordinarily called therapy, not simply as the goal of the physical but as the *collectively*-constituted interaction by physician and patient taken together.[25] When a patient is treated 'purely' as an object, his contribution becomes zero, leaving him frustrated and dissatisfied. . . .
>
> Many physicians may give in to the demands from patients for 'special' medications, and at least a few may convince themselves of their effectiveness in the absence of any real data. Thus, in its application, modern medicine may have a magical component called the placebo effect, which on closer and more specific definition should be called magical thinking. . . .

The rampant empiricism mentioned earlier would have as part of its basis the well-known placebo effect mentioned by Bruch. It can be appreciated, if quackery is related to the failure of the scientific approach, that nutrition to the quack is a philosophy, not a science. Unencumbered by science and the truth, the quack knows only those bounds defined by the law.

Rynearson,[26] in an article dealing with the philosophic leaders of food and nutrition faddism, cites many examples of hazardous statements used to fool the public. His article "Americans Love Hogwash" should be required reading for all nutrition students. Rynearson concludes that the American public is sufficiently interested in nutrition to spend vast sums of money in being misled by so-called nutrition experts who have no factual credentials and, further, that a handful of such pseudoauthorities make a fortune out of the business of faddism. He cites the five general origins of food faddism proposed by Mann:[27] (1) philosophical-religious, (2) hucksterism, (3) medical abandonment, (4) the influence of the respected but badly informed or adventurous scientist and (5) fear of the orthodox food industry. "The situation is so complex and people are so confused that the next salesman they meet in the health food store will seem like a nutrition expert."[6]

The more benign fads that come and go are probably nourished by the "fashion followers" who are simply experimenting with the latest in weight reduction regimens or high-fiber diets.

The AMA Conference on Food Faddism and Cultism[6] concluded that food faddism and health quackery probably could not be significantly discouraged by education alone, that there must be a subtle interaction between education and regulation. At the federal level, the Food and Drug Administration, the Federal Trade Commission and the Post Office Department have the major regulatory responsibilities that could act to discourage illicit health practices. Each agency is handicapped by lack of adequate budget and manpower to muster adequate forces to control quackery. Their efforts are further diminished by an amendment to the Food, Drug and Cosmetic Act (PL 94–278, Title V, 4/22/76) that significantly reduces FDA ability to regulate dietary supplements.[28] The composition of dietary supplements can be limited only by the manufacturer's imagination and FDA ability to show toxicity. The government must now evaluate the safety of dietary supplement components.

The amendment is the result of the entry of the health food industry into legislative affairs.[12] This marks a new era in the fight against health fraud that will warrant close scrutiny in the future.

BIBLIOGRAPHY

1. Smith: *The Health Hucksters*. New York, Thomas Y. Crowell, 1960.
2. Young: *The Medical Messiahs*. Princeton, Princeton University Press, 1967.
3. Trager: *The Bellybook*. New York, Grossman Publishers, 1972.
4. Barrett and Knight (Eds.): *The Health Robbers*. Philadelphia, George F. Stickley, 1976.
5. Deutsch: *The New Nuts Among the Berries*. Palo Alto, Bull Publishing Company, 1977.
6. Council on Foods and Nutrition, AMA: *Conference on Food Faddism and Cultism*. Unpublished data, 1971.
7. White: Food Tech., *26*,, 29, 1972.
8. White: Food Drug Cosmetics Law J., *31*, 497, 1976.
9. Wolff: Am. J. Clin. Nutr., *26*, 438, 1973.
10. Erhard: Nutr. Today, *8*, 4, 1973; *9*, 20, 1974.
11. Herbert: In *The Health Robbers* (Barrett and Knight, Eds.). Philadelphia, George F. Stickley, 1976.
12. Jukes: J.A.M.A., *233*, 50, 1975.
13. Herbert: Food Nutr. News, *47*, No. 4, March-April 1976.
14. White: Nutr. News, *36*, No. 3, October 1973.
15. Gunther: In *The Health Robbers* (Barrett and Knight, Eds.). Philadelphia, George F. Stickley, 1976.
16. Frankle and Heussenstamm: Am. J. Public Health, *64*, 11, 1974.
17. Bernard: Am. J. Public Health, *55*, 1143, 1965.
18. Council on Foods and Nutrition, AMA: J.A.M.A., *218*, 397, 1971.
19. New Jersey State Department of Health: Public Health News, June 1966.
20. Sherlock and Rothschild: J.A.M.A., *199*, 130, 1967.
21. Council on Foods and Nutrition, AMA: J.A.M.A., *224*, 415, 1973.
22. Lindner and Blackburn: Obesity/Bariatric Med., *5*, 198, 1976.

23. National Analysts, Inc.: *A Study of Health Practices and Opinions*. Contract No. FDA 66–193. Springfield (Va.), National Technical Information Service, 1972.
24. Bruch: J. Am. Diet. Assoc., *57*, 316, 1970.
25. Parsons: *Social Structure and Personality*. Glencoe, Free Press of Glencoe, 1964.
26. Rynearson: Nutr. Rev., *32* (Suppl. 1), 1, 1974.
27. Mann: Panhandle Magazine, *6*, 18, 1972.
28. White: Postgrad. Med., *6*, 204, 1976.

Chapter 12

NATURALLY OCCURRING FOOD-BORNE TOXICANTS

Paul M. Newberne

In the context of this chapter, diet and nutrition are not synonymous; diet is the total of the various substances consumed while nutrition includes only those substances that serve to nourish the individual, that is, to promote growth, reproduction, maintenance and repair. Toxic foods and non-nutritive substances are usually excluded from nutrition considerations even though they often interact with nutrients and exert enormous effects on the health of the individual.

Inadequate quality or quantity or an imbalance of nutrients as well as the presence of toxins in the diet may contribute to disease. Nutrition should, therefore, be concerned with the entire spectrum of health, including preventive as well as therapeutic medicine. This demands continued study about the metabolism and interactions of nutrients and other dietary components, including toxins, native to foods or residing there as contaminants.

Malnutrition occurs in the United States; it is particularly severe in other areas of the world where it appears at the end of a chain of conditions extending across national borders. Whatever actions may comprise appropriate solutions must include a worldwide increase in the production of food. This implies not only an increase in conventional sources but the introduction of new and novel foods which carry with them the potential for problems of safety.

There are thousands of chemical compounds in the diet of man but only a few of them have nutritional significance. The concept that toxicity may be produced by chemical entities that are normal ingredients of plant and animal foodstuffs is relatively new. Only in recent years has public concern stimulated demands for safer and better food. The increasing complexity of our modern industrial society and the wide-ranging nature of the international food trade have increased the risk of contamination of foods by chemical and biologic agents. However, nature has exceeded man in the introduction of toxic substances into foods. In our broadening search for new sources of food as well as the identification of additional uses for old sources of food, we must be alert to the potential for natural and man-made toxicity occasioned by harmful chemicals in foods eaten as they are grown, or by chemicals entering foods as accidental contaminants or as a result of food processing.

Although food contamination may arise from environmental and industrial pollution (mercury, lead, arsenic), agricultural technology (fertilizers, pesticides) or food processing (nitrosamines, polynuclear hydrocarbons), some of the more dangerous food contaminants occur naturally (natural toxic factors of plant and animal foodstuffs, pathogenic microorganisms, fungal toxins). Thus the primary concern of this chapter is to address those components of the diet, natural or man-made, which have adverse effects on health.

Naturally occurring toxicants have been

generally accorded a lower order of concern in terms of human health than non-nutritive components, including contaminants. Increasing use of plant foodstuffs containing low levels of toxicants to which human populations may be exposed over long periods of time force a reassessment of this area. There is also concern for some of the more obvious additives and contaminants which result from man's activities. Acute disease resulting from exposure to high levels of a specific toxin and overt clinical disease creates one set of problems; long-term exposure to low concentrations creates quite a different set. Different kinds of risks are involved with different toxicants and varying levels of exposure, and different solutions are required. For example, acute allergic reaction to strawberries or toxic reactions to shellfish poisoning (saxitoxin) represent hazards different from long-term, low-level exposure to aflatoxins or nitrosamines. We understand very little about the former and virtually nothing about the latter, even though all of them clearly represent problems in environmental health.

Numerous surveys have identified large numbers of chemicals added to foods by man as well as those which are natural toxicants or contaminants. From this extensive assemblage, only a few have been chosen for examination in this chapter. This brief resume of selected foodstuffs is not meant to imply that other problems do not exist; it reflects our ignorance about many problems and indicates a critical need for continuing surveillance over our food supply and its capacity to properly nourish a growing population.

TOXINS FROM PLANT FOODS

Many toxic components of plant food have been chemically characterized but large numbers of these poisonous plants and their toxic compounds have not been carefully examined either chemically or biologically as to their effects on health. They constitute only a very small fraction of the total food supply and therefore are

considered a low risk to human health. However, no segment of the environment to which humans are exposed is as chemically complex as food, yet knowledge of the intrinsic chemical components of food, except for the nutrients, is poor indeed.[1,2]

While it is generally assumed that the natural components of food, even those known to be toxic, do not constitute a significant or widespread health hazard, there is little definitive information on the toxic effects resulting from ingestion of these compounds by human populations. Even less is known about interactions of toxins and nutrients. We cannot conclude, without appropriate investigation, that these substances are innocuous simply because they have been consumed for many centuries without obvious health effects.

The absence of data on the normal background levels of the non-nutrient components of food makes it impossible to assess the potential health consequences of new plant varieties which may possess radically altered compositions because of genetic manipulation. Such assessments will be necessary since new plant varieties are not generally recognized as safe and must pass certain standards of safety before they can be used as food. Changes in levels of essential nutrients must also be monitored.

When subjected to a variety of stress conditions, most commonly due to fungal invasion, a number of plants undergo metabolic changes which can result in the production and accumulation of abnormal and, in some cases toxic, metabolites. Most notable are those plant "stress" metabolites possessing antifungal activity (the phytoalexins). Genetic manipulation to create new plant varieties may result in the introduction of the stress mechanism.[3] Specific examples of types of substances in food and feed plants considered important in human health are summarized in the following pages.

Protease Inhibitors

Compounds which can inhibit the proteolytic activity of certain enzymes are found throughout the plant kingdom, particularly among legumes. One of the better known inhibitors, trypsin inhibitor, is present in raw soybeans. However, this may contribute very little to an explanation for the poor growth of animals fed unheated soybean meal.[4] The antitryptic factor in soybeans was first described by Read and Haas in 1938[5] and independently discovered by Ham and Sandstedt in 1944.[6] When it was described, it appeared to offer an explanation. However, shortly thereafter, various studies using amino acid rations to which crude soybean trypsin inhibitors were added indicated that some other factor was responsible for the poor growth-promoting properties of raw soybeans.[7]

The effect of heat in improving the nutritional value of soy proteins was recognized as early as 1917 when Osborne and Mendel[8] showed that rats grew better after the soybean meal had been heated. One of the early explanations for the effect of heat involved a change in the protein so that the sulfur amino acids became more available.[7,9] The metabolic explanation for this observation is still not clear. Recent work has shifted from an emphasis on the poor absorption of the sulfur amino acids in raw soybeans to a disturbance in the metabolism of cystine and methionine when raw soybeans are fed to rats. There is an increase in the percentage of labeled carbon dioxide expired by rats given labeled methionine.[10,11]

At present, there is no valid explanation for the growth-inhibiting action of raw soybeans; it is likely that growth inhibition may be due to a number of factors. Most of the harmful biologic effects observed when raw soybeans are fed largely disappear when the meal is properly roasted.

Even properly heated soybean meal as a primary source of protein may produce a zinc deficiency in some species of animals. The explanation for the deficiency appears to be related to the presence of phytic acid in the soybean meal.[12] However, an increased calcium concentration in the diet may enhance zinc deficiency;[13,14] sesame meal also results in zinc deficiency in chicks,[15] but there is now no logical explanation for this effect.

Iodine is another mineral deficiency associated with the ingestion of soybean meal. The work of McCarrison[16] led him to suggest the presence of a goitrogenic substance in soybean meal, since large amounts of iodine in the diet did not prevent the development of this condition. Subsequent work with rats[17,18] and chicks[19] indicated that the iodine requirement is increased when soybeans are included in the ration and that heating the soybeans does not completely eliminate this effect. With the wider use of soybean milk as a liquefied formula for infants, a few reports have appeared describing enlarged thyroids in a few infants fed this formula.[20,21] In all of these cases, the heat treatment used in processing the soybean meal was adequate to destroy its goitrogenic effect.[22] The addition of iodine to the liquid soy formula eliminates the thyroid enlargement.[23]

One of the several trypsin inhibitors in soybeans has been isolated in crystalline form and chemically characterized;[24,25] it is known as a Kunitz inhibitor, after the investigator who first isolated and characterized it.[24] Recently the sequence of amino acids in Kunitz inhibitor has been determined.[25]

A trypsin inhibitor has been isolated and characterized from the lima bean; it has a very high content of cystine but no tryptophan.[26] Another trypsin inhibitor has been purified from the seeds of the mung bean, a staple to some human populations.[27] This inhibitor is stable to heat, particularly under acid conditions, and contains a high cystine content. Since trypsin is essential for adequate digestion and absorption, the presence of inhibitors decreases the utilization of protein. This, in turn, results in reduced growth and generally decreased efficiency of food utilization. Since protein is the most expensive part of the diet, trypsin inhibitors can have economic as well as public health implications. Other plant foodstuffs which contain protease inhibitors are peanut, oat, chickpea, field bean, buckwheat, barley, sweet potato, lentil, rice, lima bean, navy bean, field or garden pea, white potato, wheat, broad bean, fava bean, cowpea, black-eyed pea, and corn. Others could be added to this list, but these examples constitute a major portion of the class of staple foods consumed by a significant segment of population groups around the world and indicate the widespread distribution of inhibitors.

Hemagglutinins

Substances in many plants have the property of agglutinating red blood cells. These compounds have been collectively classified as phytohemagglutinins or lectins; they are present mainly in seeds, but they also exist to a lesser extent in leaves, bark, roots and tubers.[28] Many botanical groups including mono- and dicotyledons, molds and lichens contain them. The highest concentrations are in Leguminosae and Euphorbiaceae and it is in these that the inhibitors most often occur. The first of these compounds to be identified was extracted from castor beans by Stillmark;[29] it agglutinates the red cells from both human and animal blood. The nutritional significance of the phytohemagglutinins is detailed in a number of papers in the literature.[30] Much of the toxic fraction of hemagglutinins is destroyed or neutralized in the digestive tract and only a relatively small amount appears to be absorbed.[31]

In addition to the castor bean, other plant materials contain phytohemagglutinins; these include the soybean, the red kidney bean (phytohemagglutinin A), the black bean (phaseolotoxin A), the yellow wax bean (hemagglutinin) and the jack bean which contains concanavalin A.[31] Since these compounds occur in nature and have profound biologic activity, particularly on mitosis,[32] they may be an important class of environmental toxins.

The hemagglutinating factor in soybeans has been eliminated as a possible factor responsible for growth inhibition. A part of the evidence for its inactivity came from Liener's work showing there was no relation between the hemagglutinating activity of his preparations and their growth-depressing activity.[33]

Some of the hemagglutinins, such as ricin from the castor bean, produce an intense inflammation with destruction of epithelial cells of the GI tract; local hemorrhages may also be observed elsewhere. Liver, kidney and heart damage has also been reported for several of them. The important effect on lymphocytes is the induction of mitosis. This has made some of these compounds (mitogens) useful in biomedical work, particularly in studies related to immunocompetence where exposure in vitro causes lymphocytes to increase DNA synthesis and undergo changes equated with cell division. These proteins are associated in the plant with other protein material and thus are not easily detected by chemical analysis. Instead, they currently must be determined by their activities.

Lathyrism

Lathyrism is a neurologic disease seen in human subjects who have consumed large amounts of Lathyrus sativus (chickling vetch), L. cicera (flat-podded vetch) or L. clymenum (Spanish vetchling).[37] L. sativus is cultivated in India and grows wild in the Tian Shian mountains of western China; L. cicera is used as cattle feed in France, Italy and Algeria and is used in making bread when wheat is in short supply; L. clymenum is grown in Spain, North Africa and the Orient.[38]

The symptoms of lathyrism in human subjects were described by Cantani in 1873 who gave the disease its current name.[38] However, the condition has been recognized for centuries, with one of the earliest descriptions provided by Hippocrates.[39] This disease occurs in countries bordering the Mediterranean; Algeria has more cases than the other countries. It is endemic in India where as many as 7 per cent of the people in certain villages are afflicted.[37,40] The lathyrus plants grow even in severe drought and provide food when the regular food supply is decreased. Under such conditions or during famines these legumes may make up as much as one-third to one-half the total diet.[37] If high consumption of the legumes continues for six months or more, lathyrism frequently follows.[40,41]

Human lathyrism is often referred to as neurolathyrism.[39] This condition usually develops in individuals between the ages of 15 and 30 years and occurs 12 to 20 times more frequently in men than in women.[38,39] The first symptom is a feeling of heaviness of the legs, with weakness setting in shortly thereafter. While standing the leg muscles become tremulous, and when the individual starts to walk he may drag his feet. The leg muscles may become spastic and rigid. The gait becomes jerky; short steps are taken by walking on the balls of the feet. Tingling sensations are felt in various parts of the body. There may be complete loss of sensation to heat and pain.[44] Most of these symptoms are associated with lesions[38] of the lateral pyramidal tracts and funiculi of Goll of the spinal cord.

Although a number of attempts have been made to associate lathyrism with dietary deficiencies,[42,43] there is ample evidence that the consumption of the seeds of various lathyrus plants is responsible for the disease. More recently, many attempts have been made to isolate the toxic factor from lathyrus seeds. In most cases, the relevance of these compounds to human lathyrism remains obscure. Ressler and associates[44] isolated L-α-γ-diaminobutyric acid from seeds of L. latifolius (perennial sweet pea) and L. sylvestris (flat pea) and β-cyano-L-alanine from the seeds of Vicia sativa.[45] When given by stomach tube to rats, both these compounds produce

hyperirritability, tremors, convulsions and, within 2 to 3 days, death. Subcutaneous administration results in less obvious neurologic symptoms. The concentrations of these compounds in the pea and vetch seeds vary but are reported to be from about 0.1 to 1.5 per cent.

The cyanoalanine compound theoretically is related to the aminopropionitriles responsible for the development of osteolathyrism. Decarboxylation of the alanine compound should lead directly to the parent nitrile compound.[44] Whether or not this reaction occurs under natural conditions is unknown. The cyanoalanine and diaminobutyric acid, which were reported to produce neurotoxic symptoms in rats, have not been isolated from L. sativus and, for this reason, the significance of their physiologic reactions has been open to question.[45]

A neurotoxic substance has been isolated from L. sativus. The first suggestion for such a substance came from a report that an alcoholic extract of the seeds, when injected into day-old chicks, produced retraction of the head and twisting and stiffening of the neck.[46] The symptoms disappeared about 12 hours after a single injection. Injection of small doses of the extract each day into chicks maintained the symptoms permanently. One of the compounds isolated from the alcoholic extract and associated with these symptoms was (β - N - oxalyl) - α,β - diaminopropionic acid.[47] Injection of 20 mg of this compound into day-old chicks produced neurologic disturbances with recovery after a few hours. Injection of 48 mg produced death. The susceptibility of different species to this compound varies, as shown by the fact that when mice were injected intraperitoneally with 48 mg they showed no immediate symptoms other than dragging their hind legs. That the oxalic acid present in the compound was not responsible for the symptoms became evident when an equivalent amount was injected into day-old chicks with no untoward results. The essential nature of oxalic acid as an integral part of the molecule was shown when the free diaminopropionic acid proved innocuous after injection into chicks.[48]

Much of the early experimental work with Lathyrus seeds involved osteolathyrism or odoratism.[39] Both these terms are used to describe the condition produced in rats fed rations containing considerable amounts of the legume L. odoratus. When the ration contained 25 per cent ground seeds of this species, weanling rats developed deformities of the spinal cord in 3 to 4 weeks. These abnormalities were readily detected by means of x rays.[49] Similar skeletal abnormalities were seen when the ration contained L. hirsutus (caley pea), or L. tingitanus or L. pusillus (Singletary pea).[42,43,50]

The compound initially isolated from L. odoratus and shown to produce odoratism was β - (N - γ - L - glutamyl) - aminopropionitrile.[50,52] This compound was present in five different varieties of L. odoratus at levels ranging from 58 to 160 mg per 100 gm, whereas in L. pusillus and L. hirsutus its concentration was 62 and 21 mg per 100 gm respectively.[37] Shortly after the announcement of its structure, three different laboratories showed that the gamma glutamyl group was not essential for its action.[37]

The incorporation of the active compound, β-aminopropionitrile, in a ration at a level of 0.1 to 0.2 per cent reproduces all the symptoms including skeletal abnormalities which are otherwise rare in rats (kyphosis, scoliosis, increased shaft diameter, exostoses and rib cage deformities), hernias, reproductive failure and dissecting aneurysms of the aorta.[37,43] All these changes are traceable to alterations in collagen. The collagen of rats with odoratism is abnormal both in form and distribution,[112] resulting in a reduction in its tensile strength. Studies with isotopic sulfur indicate that the primary change is a failure in the formation of chondroitin sulfates A and C and their complexes with proteins resulting in a defect in fibrogenesis.[53] The defect in odoratism involving primarily collagen formation is in sharp contrast to the human disease or lathyrism in which the essential lesion involves the nervous tissue.

Intriguing results have derived from the isolation of toxic compounds from both the L. odoratus and L. sativus groups of peas. However, the substance responsible for the development of human lathyrism still appears to be unknown. The oxalyl diaminopropionic acid which on intraperitoneal injection produces neurologic alterations in chicks, ducklings and pigeons has no visible effect when injected into monkeys.

Favism

Sensitivity to fava or broad beans appears to be an example of an inherited metabolic disturbance. In sensitive individuals, the inhalation of pollen from these plants or ingestion of the bean in either the cooked or raw state produces a hemolytic anemia. Sensitive individuals have a deficiency of glucose-6-phosphate dehydrogenase in their blood and a reduction in glutathione blood levels.[54] The glutathione level in the red blood cells of sensitive individuals is still further reduced following the eating of fava beans; the mechanism of this action is unknown. Hemolysis of the older but not the young red cells follows. Why the younger red cells are resistant is unknown. This explains why, except under peculiar conditions, the individuals recover once the hemolysis ceases.[55]

Most sensitive individuals are children of parents who originated from the Mediterranean area, Asia or Taiwan.[56] Since the enzymatic deficiency in favism appears to be common to a number of other disturbances, it is assumed to be transmitted in the same way, i.e. sex linked. The mother of the affected male carries the genetic defect.[55] Favism may be more complicated than is suggested by the enzymatic deficiency seen in individuals with this disease. This is evident from the fact that not everyone who is deficient in this enzyme develops hemolysis after eating fava or broad beans. The enzymatic defect is common in blacks in the United States, but favism is rarely seen in these individuals. They do, however, exhibit hemolysis when treated with the antimalarial compound primaquine, certain sulfonamides and a number of other compounds.[55]

In some areas of the world, the sensitivity to fava or broad beans affects a significant proportion of the people. In one outbreak along the Caspian Sea 1143 individuals developed hemolysis following the ingestion of broad beans; of these, 16 died.[57] In that geographic area, the hemolytic condition routinely affects a large number of people especially during the spring of the year, with a peak load in June when broad beans are harvested. In Iran, the hemolysis is reported to occur to a greater extent among adults than in children. The incidence of favism in Iran is reported to be almost five times greater among men than women.[57]

The toxic substance in fava beans does not appear to have been isolated although there were reports from Taiwan[58-60] indicating that the toxic substance is vicine (2,4 diamino-6-hydroxypyrimidine-β-D-glycopyranose). This chemical is present in fava beans to the extent of about 0.5 per cent of their dry weight.

Hepatotoxins

Senecio Alkaloids. A number of substances toxic to the liver have been identified in several plant species, including the Senecio genus of plants which occurs across a broad area of the world. At least 25 species of this genus are poisonous to livestock or to human beings, and a large number of alkaloids have been isolated from them. An important characteristic of toxins from these sources is the delayed liver damage which they cause in animals

and man.[61] Senecio disease has been observed in human populations from grains used for breads contaminated with seeds from the poisonous plants.[62] The chemistry of several of these compounds has been worked out.[61]

In some areas of the United States, the seeds of Crotalaria are present in wheat and corn harvested from land where the plants grow interspersed among the grain plants; mechanical harvesters collect both grain and the poisonous seeds of the Crotalaria. The potential for such contaminants in human food requires consideration.[63]

The alkaloids produced by the Senecios are potent liver toxins with a profound effect on mitosis. In low to moderate exposure they produce a delayed effect including veno-occlusive disease and cirrhosis in man: in animals, liver cancer is also induced.[64,65]

The fact that nutritional factors can modify effects of the alkaloids make this a fruitful area for research.[66-70]

Plants of the genus which produce the toxic alkaloids are used to make teas in the southeastern United States and in Curacao. Consumption of these teas has been associated with esophageal and other forms of cancer in man.[70] Only a few publications are available on mechanisms of actions of the toxins and the data are not conclusive.[71,72] The hepatotoxicity appears to be due to the formation of pyrrolic metabolites.[73]

Mycotoxins. There are a large number of fungal toxins in foods but only a few of them appear to be of real or potential danger to the health of man. These include the aflatoxins, patulin, ochratoxin, penicillic acid and trichothecene toxin.[74] The aflatoxins are now known to be hepatotoxic for man[75] and animals and carcinogenic for many animal species.[76]

Aflatoxins. Indications for man's susceptibility to aflatoxin poisoning derive from epidemiologic evidence, an outbreak in India, a childhood disease in Thailand

(Reyes syndrome) and a limited number of experiments designed to define the pattern of aflatoxin metabolism by the liver in vitro. From this data it seems that, compared with some experimental animal species, man is relatively resistant to both the acute and chronic effects.

Interspecies differences and many other factors influence an individual's response.[78] Female animals and castrated males are more resistant to both the acute and chronic effects of aflatoxin. From epidemiologic studies it appears that women are somewhat less susceptible than men to the carcinogenic effects of dietary aflatoxin.[77] Furthermore, in animals, nutrition plays an important role in both acute toxicity and chronic disease.[79-85] High-protein diets are generally protective since they enable the liver's detoxifying enzymes to function optimally. In some cases however they activate other procarcinogens to the active form. Protein deficiency, certain vitamin deficiencies and diets rich in saturated fats render the animal more susceptible to aflatoxin poisoning. Among other environmental factors, excessive exposure to ultraviolet light and other dietary hepatotoxins (e.g. alcohol, plant toxins and other mycotoxins) may have synergistic effects on aflatoxin.[64]

Animal experiments suggest that aflatoxin is immunosuppressive. For this reason, exposure to the toxin is liable to worsen the effects of any concurrent infectious illnesses or to predispose to infectious disease.[86-89]

An assessment of man's likely exposure to aflatoxin can be based on the fact that cow's milk is a more-or-less universal major food and that animal feedstuffs are occasionally contaminated with aflatoxin.[77,90-92] When this happens it can be assumed that cow's milk will almost certainly contain the toxic metabolite aflatoxin M. With a typical analytic detection limit of 0.04 ppb, it follows that up to 0.02 ppb of this toxin could escape detection and yet be ingested by man in his daily half-liter of milk.[81,94]

While definite conclusions regarding the hazards of aflatoxin exposure to man cannot be drawn at this time, there is compelling evidence to suggest that he is quite susceptible to it. Epidemiologic studies suggest a correlation between primary liver cancer and exposure to aflatoxin in parts of Africa, the Philippines and Thailand.[93-97] Sudden deaths from acute encephalopathy and fatty degeneration of the viscera have been ascribed to aflatoxicosis.

The serious outbreak of acute aflatoxin poisoning in man and dogs which recently occurred in India is worthy of further description.[75] In October 1975, the epidemic broke out in several tribal villages of the western states of Gujarat and Rajasthan. The incidence reached a peak in November and December and declined rapidly in January. The presenting features were jaundice, rapidly developing ascites, portal hypertension and a high mortality rate. In most cases death was caused by massive gastrointestinal tract bleeding.

The possibility that the epidemic was the result of an infectious agent was ruled out, since the disease occurred simultaneously in almost 200 villages; it did not involve children, who are generally more susceptible to infections, and it affected only the very poor tribal population whose nutritional status is inadequate. There was no evidence of transmission through contact and the disease failed to respond to antibiotics or other drugs.

Examination of the various items of food collected randomly from the affected households showed that the maize was heavily contaminated with Aspergillus flavus. The aflatoxin load in these samples varied from 6 to 15 ppm, which means that the affected subjects must have consumed 2 to 6 mg of toxin daily for almost a month. Evidence for aflatoxin as the etiologic agent came from the following data.

The disease was confined to the poorest of the people who subsisted mainly on maize during these months because of economic reasons, even though it was obviously shriveled and damaged. The outbreak began with the harvesting and consumption of maize which was affected by excessive rain and badly stored; the incidence subsided as soon as the stock was exhausted. Households located near the fields and away from the villages suffered the most. The inmates of a boys' hostel in the same region, for whom maize was not the staple, did not suffer from the disease.

One liver sample obtained at autopsy and several samples of serum and urine were examined for the presence of aflatoxin or metabolites. Aflatoxin B_1 was not found in either the liver or the samples of urine but 2 out of 7 specimens of serum from affected patients yielded detectable traces. Thin-layer chromatographic analysis of liver extracts exhibited three fluorescent spots. Histopathologic examination of the liver revealed extensive bile duct proliferation with periductal fibrosis and multinucleated giant cells, the latter being peculiar to aflatoxin injury in man.

A disease of children endemic in Thailand has been described by Shank and colleagues.[98] Food consumed by patients and tissues from victims of the encephalopathy and fatty degeneration of the viscera (Reyes syndrome) contained significant concentration of aflatoxins.

These reports provide further evidence of a more direct nature incriminating aflatoxin in toxicologic disease of man. Data accumulated by the International Agency for Research in Cancer strongly suggest that aflatoxin is a human carcinogen.[73]

Fusaria Species. Alimentary toxic aleukia (ATA) in the Soviet Union in 1944 was the cause of a large number of human fatalities; it was traced to consumption of overwintered cereals infected with species of Fusarium.[99]

The clinical features of ATA are usually divided into four stages. The first stage occurs shortly after eating food prepared from toxic grain. The patient feels a burning sensation in the mouth, tongue, throat, palate, esophagus and stomach as a result of the action of the toxin on the mucous membranes. Inflammation of the gastric and intestinal mucosa results in vomiting, diarrhea and abdominal pain. In most cases excessive salivation, headache, dizziness, weakness, fatigue and tachycardia accompany this stage, and there may be fever and sweating as well. The leukocyte count may decrease to levels of 2000 per cu mm with relative lymphocytosis, and there may be an increased erythrocyte sedimentation rate.

The second stage, often called the latent stage because early in this period the patient feels fairly well and is capable of normal activity, is characterized later by disturbances in the hematopoietic system; there is progressive leukopenia, granulopenia, a relative lymphocytosis, anemia and a decrease in platelets. In addition to changes in the hematopoietic system, disturbances also occur in the central and autonomic nervous systems. Weakness, headache, palpitations and mild asthmatic symptoms may occur. The skin and mucous membranes are often icteric, the pupils are dilated, the pulse is soft and feeble and the blood pressure is decreased. The body temperature is usually normal and may even be below normal. This stage may blend almost imperceptibly into the third stage.

The first visible signs of the third stage are petechial hemorrhages on various parts of the body, with slight trauma causing hemorrhages to increase in size. Areas of necrosis may appear on the lips and on the skin of the nose, jaws and eyes. Regional lymph nodes are frequently enlarged. Esophageal lesions may occur and involvement of the epiglottis with laryngeal edema often results in death by strangulation. Some patients suffer from an acute parenchymatous hepatitis accompanied by jaundice. Bronchopneumonia, pulmonary hemorrhages and lung abscesses are frequent complications.

The fourth stage, assuming survival, is convalescence; its course and duration depend on the intensity of the toxicosis. Usually two months or more elapse until the blood-forming capacity of the bone marrow returns to normal.

Although there is no direct information on human exposure, except for inferences from descriptions of alimentary toxic aleukia (ATA) described by Joffe,[99] the ubiquitous nature of Fusaria molds suggest reasons for considering this a potential threat to public health.

Psoralens. The psoralens, phototoxic furocoumarins produced by Sclerotinia sclerotiorum, are responsible for pink rot in celery. Celery pink rot causes a dermatitis characterized by erythema, edema and vesicles with a serous discharge. The skin of the fingers, hands and forearms is affected after exposure to sunlight or ultraviolet light at a wavelength between 320 and 370 nm.[100] The toxins are easily isolated.[101] The 8-methoxy compound has been used with limited success to treat depigmentation of human skin (vitiligo) and to protect against sunburn by increasing skin pigmentation. The extent of human exposure and seriousness of the disease is considered modest.

Ochratoxins. The ochratoxins are dihydroisocoumarins and were first discovered by mycologists of the South African Council for Scientific and Industrial Research in a screening program for toxigenic fungi in foods. The compounds, produced by Aspergillus ochraceus on corn, were identified in 1965.[102,103] It is doubtful that ochratoxins constitute a health problem of significant dimension in man but, in the interest of completeness, they should be mentioned here. They have been associated with renal pathology in swine[104] and with the "Balkan nephropathy" in people of Yugoslavia.[105]

The oral LD_{50} for ochratoxin A in the duckling is approximately 150 mg per animal,[106] in the 1-day-old cockerel 100 to 200 μg per animal,[107] and in the 150-gm rat 20 mg per kg.[106] The duckling develops a fatty infiltration of hepatocytes without necrosis or bile duct proliferation; swelling of

mitochondria and dilation of the endoplasmic reticulum with loss of microsomes are also seen.[108] Low doses in rats produce hyaline degeneration and focal liver necrosis.[108] Higher doses produce renal injury. Chronic ingestion failed to produce tumors.[107] The liver appears to hydrolyze ochratoxin A at the peptide bond to yield phenylalanine and the nontoxic chlorolactone acid, which is excreted in the bile.[109,110] If the association of ochratoxin with the nephropathy of man in Yugoslavia turns out to be a real entity, these toxins will assume a much more important position in human mycotoxic disease.

Trichothecene Toxins. The trichothecene toxins are produced by at least 8 of the 9 species of Fusarium recognized in the Snyder and Hansen system of classification and, at least in the laboratory, by several other genera of fungi.[111] Since before 1900 feed grains heavily invaded by some of these species[112] of Fusarium have been recognized as toxic to animals that consumed them. Recent interpretation of data indicates that ATA as described by Joffe[99] is caused by one or more of the trichothecene toxins (T-2 toxin, neosolaniol, T-2 tetraol).[74]

The incidence and concentration of the trichothecene toxins in foods and crops have been described as more widespread and significant than those of the aflatoxins. Most of the data available are about T-2 toxin; this is the mycotoxin most commonly recognized in foods, because the analysis is relatively easy. More than half of the corn samples examined in the United States in 1973 were positive, making this family of toxins of considerable potential importance.[113]

Zearalenone. Zearalenone, or F-2 toxin, is produced by Fusarium graminearum (Gibberella zeae), Fusarium tricinctum, Fusarium roseum, Fusarium gibbosum, Fusarium roseum equiseti and Fusarium roseum graminearum.[114] Stob[115] and Urry[116] elucidated its structure, 6-(10-hydroxy-6-oxo-*trans*-1-undecenyl) - β - resorcylic acid lactone. Zearalenone has strong uterotrophic activity and has been implicated in estrogenism in pigs fed moldy corn. Feeding the toxin to pigs produces true estrus. These changes are reversible when treatment is halted. Pigs receiving 1 mg zearalenone per day for 8 days develop interstitial edema of mammary tissues and edema and hyperplasia in all uterine layers. In the cervix, the mucosal epithelium undergoes a metaplasia producing an irregular thick layer of stratified squamous cells.[117] Rats given a total of 20 to 650 μg intramuscularly over 7 days developed enlarged uteri.[114] Diets containing 300 mg zearalenone per kg (300 ppm) fed to turkey poults and chicks produce the estrogenic response in 4 days. The compound is an effective growth promoter in lambs, and its use as a supplement to animal feed has been suggested.

Zearalenone is not a toxin in the true sense of the word, i.e. there are no acute effects. There are no reports implicating zearalenone as affecting humans through ingestion of food. However, although zearalenone has not been known to cause any human health problems, it has been found in corn destined for food in the United States, in amounts known to cause vulvovaginitis in swine.[114] Corn may constitute 50 per cent or more of the ration of swine, but it is a major item in the diet of humans only in a few regions, as in portions of Mexico and Africa. Zearalenone has been reported in feeds from the United States, Australia, Ireland, France, Italy, Yugoslavia, Rumania, Hungary, Denmark, Canada, Russia, Japan, Mexico and South Africa, indicating worldwide distribution. The widespread distribution of this potential health hazard in staple foods requires that it be kept under surveillance.

Goitrogens

Goitrogens are natural products in plant foods consumed by man and animals.

They cause hypothyroidism and an enlargement of the thyroid gland. The major cause of goiter is iodine deficiency, and increased iodine consumption is used under most circumstances to prevent or cure the condition. According to folklore, some people believe that simple goiter is caused by eating certain foods.[119] In spite of this belief it appears that there is little to indicate that consumption of goitrogenic plants of the Brassica genus causes goiter. Nevertheless there are factors in some plant foods that can cause enlargement of the thyroid gland with symptoms of iodine deficiency. The Brassica genus includes a number of widely eaten plant foods— cabbage, turnips, rutabagas, mustard greens, horseradish, radish and white mustard. Most of these plants contain small quantities of thioglucosides as goitrogens.

Enlargement of the thyroid gland has been reported in people who eat soybeans and peanuts.[120] Less is known, however, about the goitrogens in these foods compared to the Brassica family. From an economic standpoint, it may also be desirable to conduct research on the rapeseed, one of the six major seeds having commercial value for producing oil. Although oil and proteins from the rapeseed may serve many useful purposes, a technique must be developed to eliminate the toxins from the protein fraction prior to human consumption.

There are about fifty identified natural plant thioglucosides, most of which have been characterized.[121] Although the chemicals occur in many different parts of the plant, the seeds contain the highest concentrations. A number of investigators have observed that goitrogens are transmitted from the milk of cows to man.[120,122] The significance of this remains to be determined; however, since it is potentially important in human health it will be pursued in more detail.

Recent attention to this problem stems largely from the 1954 report of Clements[123] that children in certain parts of Australia and Tasmania developed goiters which were not prevented by potassium iodide administration. These children drank milk from cows fed marrowstem kale (choumoellier, Brassica oleracea var. acephala), a good source of the L-5-vinyl-2-thioxazolidone isolated by Greer and co-workers from a number of goitrogenic plants.[124] This and a number of compounds structurally related to it inhibit the incorporation of iodine into the thyroid hormone.[125]

Peltola[126] initiated a study in Finland to show that endemic goiter in the eastern, southeastern and central parts of Finland may be caused by something other than iodine deficiency. He suggested a goitrogenic factor contained in cattle fodder and in cow's milk. Rats fed ad libitum a standard diet that provided each rat with 150 μg of iodine per day (about 50 times the daily requirement) in addition to milk obtained in a goitrous area had thyroid glands which were about twice as large as those in the animals fed the same standard diet but with milk from a nongoitrous area. The difference in weights of the thyroid glands was reportedly confirmed in another study utilizing a ration that provided each rat with 14 μg of iodine per day.[127] The rat-feeding studies of Peltola were repeated by Virtanen and co-workers.[129] Although they received milk from the same dairy in the goitrous area as Peltola, they found no enlargement of the thyroid glands of their rats.

Another group developed a sensitive analytic method for L-5-vinyl-2-thiooxazolidone.[120] By this procedure, they found 3 μg per ml of press juice from the green parts of marrowstem kale which, according to Clements and Wishart,[122] was the source of goitrogen in the Tasmanian and Australian milk. Winter rape and Swede turnips contained 33 and 32 μg per ml respectively. Further study showed that the goitrogen was unstable in fresh milk. Heating, which destroyed peroxidases, preserved the compound. The highest concentration of the goitrogen in milk when cows were fed marrowstem kale, winter rape or Swede turnips was 20 μg per liter. According to the Finnish investigators, this concentration is too low to produce any goitrogenic action.[129]

The work of Clements and Wishart, involving a determination of ^{131}I uptake by the thyroids of two subjects after ingesting milk from goitrous areas of Tasmania, was repeated by Finnish workers.[130] Twenty-two normal subjects drank, at one time, 1.5 to 2.2 liters of milk from cows fed large amounts of turnip or rape greens. This did not change the accumulation of ^{131}I by the thyroids of these normal subjects. Approximately 100 times the amount of L-5-vinyl-2-thiooxazolidone and thiocyanate present in the milk had to be given before any effect could be demonstrated on the ^{131}I uptake by the thyroids of these subjects.

From these studies, it would appear that the goitrogens present in natural products play a minor role, if any, in the development of human endemic goiter. Even the possibility that these compounds may influence the cattle feeding directly on the plants seems remote, since the Finnish investigators do not refer to the presence of enlarged thyroids among dairy cows in the goitrous areas.

Allergens

Allergic reactions to substances in food are spontaneous, peculiar to certain humans and rarely demonstrable in lower animals; hence, there are no good animal models for evaluating such reactions. The most common affliction caused by a food allergy is of the skin and respiratory tract; the GI tract is less frequently involved. Occasionally food allergy affects the central nervous system and produces a manifestation similar to migraine headaches or, in the most severe form, it may predispose to convulsive seizures. Aberrant behavior in patients has been described as being associated with allergic disorders. Infants and children may complain of abdominal distress, and occasionally the genital and urinary tracts as well as the cardiovascular system may be involved. The allergic response of individuals is evaluated by skin tests. This is accomplished by subcutaneous injection or patch testing of extracts of the suspected materials; if the individual is sensitive, a response is elicited after a specific period of time.

The Graminaceae family is comprised of a group of foods that commonly produce allergenic responses in people. These staple foods include barley, corn, oats, rice, rye and wheat; of this group, wheat is the most common offender. Vegetables comprise a large group of allergenic foods that vary considerably in importance. Legumes are the most important, and the soybean has also been described in some cases as an allergen when used as a milk substitute.[131] Fruits, particularly strawberries, are allergenic to some people; bananas and pineapples are allergenic but considerably less so than strawberries.[132] Additional miscellaneous food allergens are found in chocolate, coffee, tea, carbonated beverages, beer, alcoholic distillates, condiments and flavors, yeast and molds.

One of the better understood forms of food allergies is so-called celiac disease or gluten enteropathy, an adverse response by certain individuals to certain fractions of wheat gluten. This disease has many of the symptoms seen in patients with idiopathic and tropical sprue.[133] A number of early investigators reported that the elimination of wheat from the diet produced an improvement in the condition of celiac patients. Even the so-called banana diet, as originally proposed by Haas,[134] was one that completely eliminated wheat.[135] The dramatic response observed by the Dutch investigators with one of their pediatric patients when wheat gluten was added to or removed from the diet was enough to establish this protein as the dietary factor associated with the characteristic symptoms.[136,137] When wheat gluten

is removed from the diet improvement occurs in all aspects of the disease, but it may require as long as a year before the individual is completely restored to normal functioning.[133]

A description of the clinical aspects of gluten enteropathy and its dietary treatment are given in Chapter 31B. Much attention has been focused on the constituents of gluten and their relation to the intestinal changes,[138-143] but the exact composition of the deleterious gluten fraction is still uncertain.

Saponins

The saponins have been identified in at least four hundred different species belonging to more than eighty different plant families. These toxins, which occur as glycosides, have a bitter taste and characteristically hemolyze red blood cells. Although saponins have been studied from the point of view of hemolytic activity and, in some cases, for their therapeutic properties those occurring in foods and feeds have been studied very little. The nutritional significance of soybeans and alfalfas in which saponins occur makes this area one of potential significance to human populations.

Alfalfa saponins are comprised of at least three different types, and soybean saponins have been separated into five fractions which differ in their activity.[144,145] The two major classes of saponins, according to structural formulas, are the triterpenoids found in sugar beets and the steroid saponins represented by dioscin. Saponins are also present in spinach, asparagus and horse chestnut.[146] In addition, they are widely used in soft drinks, beers, confections and other food products because of their ability to stabilize aqueous solutions and suspensions of oil or powders. Saponins, particularly those in several species of Dioscorea, are major sources of starting material for the commercial synthesis of progesterone and other steroid products.[147]

Saponins inhibit cholinesterases, trypsin and proteinase. The hemolytic effect may be the only one of concern to public health. Much of the important data about saponins and public health is covered in the review by George.[146]

Oxalates

Increased interest in oxalates occurred in the 1930s when spinach was considered a valuable addition to the diet of children.[148] Analyses of foods showed that oxalic acid made up about 10 per cent of the dry weight of such foods as spinach, New Zealand spinach, Swiss chard, beet tops, lamb's-quarters, poke, purslane and rhubarb.[149] This was primarily in the form of insoluble calcium oxalate crystals, demonstrable in microscopic sections of the leaves.[150] Foodstuffs of animal origin contain only small amounts of oxalates.[151] Both animal studies[148,149] and clinical trials with children[152] indicate that calcium in spinach is not available, especially when the calcium content of the diet is close to the minimum requirement. The presence of soluble oxalates in foods may decrease the absorption of calcium from other foods.[152]

Animal studies have illuminated some aspects of the human problem with oxalates. When the diet was adequate in the nutrients required by the rat (e.g. 0.61 per cent calcium, 0.71 per cent phosphorus, 20 per cent casein, 8 per cent yeast), the addition of 0.9 per cent potassium oxalate did not influence growth rate of weanling rats nor their bone ash level during 10 weeks of study.[153] When the level of potassium oxalate was raised to 2.5 per cent, bone ash was reduced slightly without any change in growth rate. On the basis of Kohman's analyses,[149] the 2.5 per cent potassium oxalate would be equivalent to about 13 per cent dried spinach. Similar results were obtained when 10 children (5 to 8 years of age) were fed common foods to which 100 gm canned spinach was added.[154] Over a period of 60 to 85 days,

the retention of calcium, phosphorus and nitrogen was not influenced by the spinach added to the diet, when compared to the preceding control period.

A more direct toxic effect has been associated with the ingestion of rhubarb leaves. The leaves contain about 3 to 4 times as much oxalic acid as the stalks.[150] A number of cases of poisoning reportedly due to this food have appeared, most of them during World War I[148] but others more recently. One of the more recent involved four 3- to 6-year-old children who ate the raw leaves and stalks.[155] One of these children had convulsions. Individuals who develop mild symptoms of oxalic acid poisoning following the ingestion of rhubarb complain of gastroenteritis with abdominal pain, diarrhea and vomiting—occasionally hematuria, convulsions, collapse, noncoagulability of blood and coma are also seen.[150] The Dieffenbachi plant commonly displayed in homes and offices may pose a danger to small children.[156]

The problem of oxalate poisoning is even more acute and severe in certain western states where a range crop, the halogeton, may contain as much as 37 per cent oxalic acid on a dry weight basis.[157] Its use as fodder for sheep has resulted in large numbers of deaths. According to one report, the most effective means of preventing mortality is to provide another source of feed, such as alfalfa pellets containing 15 per cent calcium carbonate, when sheep are grazing in areas heavily infested with the halogeton plant.[158]

Although the most obvious effects of oxalates are on calcium metabolism, it is still not certain that this is the primary locus of action. As far as calcium absorption is concerned, there is evidence that animals become adapted to the presence of oxalates in the ration. This was shown by the change in the negative calcium balance during the first few days after the ration fed to cattle was supplemented with small amounts of soluble oxalate. Thereafter, the calcium balance gradually became positive.[159] Improvement in calcium balance was associated with the metabolism of the oxalate to carbonate. Some pharmacologists[160] claim that the toxicity of oxalates can be overcome completely by administering calcium salts. Other investigators[158] claim that sheep given large amounts of oxalates did not recover when infused with calcium gluconate; the calcium merely prolonged life for a few days.

An interesting endemic episode of calcium oxalate stones in children has been described in Thailand.[161] This disease arises from the high content of oxalates in native food products and highly effective preventive and therapeutic measures have been used to diminish the effects of oxalates in human populations of the affected areas, particularly the young.

Citral

While attempting to produce glaucoma in experimental animals, Leach and Lloyd[162] reported that a single subcutaneous dose of 10 μg of citral (an unsaturated aldehyde) raised the ocular tension of an adult rabbit. A similar effect was produced in monkeys by the oral administration of 2 to 5 μg a day for 2 weeks. At the same time, some monkeys were fed orange peel, which is a good source of citral. Both the citral and the orange peel diets were reported to produce changes in the eyes of the monkeys similar to those seen in vitamin A deficiency. Large doses of vitamin A or sulfhydryl-containing substances such as cysteine hydrochloride were reported to reverse the action of citral. On this basis, these authors suggested that citral is an antagonist to vitamin A.[163]

Subsequent work of two other groups has not clarified the relationship of citral to vitamin A. Moore[164] points out the similarity in the structures of the vitamin and citral. On that basis he suggests that citral might function as an antimetabolite. Evidence to support this suggestion came from work with tissue cultures of chick embryo trachea, esophagus, cornea and

skin. Aydelotte[165] demonstrated an antagonistic action between citral and vitamin A. However, no attempt was made to overcome completely the citral effect by adding large doses of vitamin A, and for this reason it is impossible to accept the investigator's conclusion "that citral may be a competitive inhibitor of vitamin A." It should be pointed out that the effect of citral on the intraocular pressure of rabbits could not be duplicated by another group of investigators[166] using doses as high as 26 mg of citral per rabbit.

Pyridoxine Antagonist

The presence of a growth-depressing factor in linseed meal was recognized more than 40 years ago. This inhibitory factor could be destroyed by autoclaving or incubating the meal after it was moistened with water or 50 per cent ethyl alcohol. That the growth inhibitor was a pyridoxine antagonist became evident when extra amounts of this vitamin added to the raw linseed meal ration produced normal growth in chicks.[7]

The isolation of this inhibitor has been achieved by Klosterman, Lamoureux and Parsons[167] who showed that the compound, 1-(n-γ-L-glutamyl) amino-D-proline, exists in flaxseed. The active part of the molecule appears to be 1-amino-D-proline, which forms a stable derivative with pyridoxal phosphate. Linatine was the name given to this compound. It is present in linseed meal at a concentration of about 100 ppm.

Thiaminase

The initial interest in this enzyme stemmed from the thiamin deficiency which appeared among foxes fed frozen carp as part of their ration.[7] With the recognition that this enzyme was distributed in a wide variety of fishes,[168-171] there was a possibility that some individuals consuming large amounts of seafood might develop a thiamin deficiency. The closest approach to such a condition is Haff, or

Yuksov, disease, reported from a number of areas in northern Europe among people consuming perch, bream and lake trout.[172] Although some investigators have suggested a relation between Haff disease and thiaminase present in the fish consumed by these individuals, such a relationship may be more apparent than real because: (1) the symptoms appear within 24 hours after eating the fish, (2) the urine has a brownish-black color and (3) recovery is usually complete 24 hours after eating the fish.[173] A deficiency of thiamin would not be associated with any of these characteristics.

A more direct association between the consumption of a food containing thiaminase and a consequent deficiency involves bracken fern. This plant (Pteridium aquilinum), which grows in upland pastures or in open woods, remains green even when most forage crops have succumbed to drought. If, at such times, monogastric animals consume considerable amounts over a period of a few weeks, they exhibit symptoms of thiamin deficiency about four weeks after first eating the fern.[174] Most of the reported cases have involved horses and, even with animals of that size, only four weeks were required for a deficiency to become manifest. Complete recovery occurs if supplemental thiamin is given before the condition becomes terminal.

Bracken fern is known to be carcinogenic for cattle, guinea pigs, rats[175] and mice. In a study to determine whether this activity was related to its thiaminase content, Pamukcu, Yalciner, Price and Bryan fed the fern to two groups of rats, one of which received, in addition to the common diet, once-weekly subcutaneous injections of 2 mg thiamin hydrochloride.[176] Interestingly, both male and female rats receiving the supplemental thiamin developed a statistically significant higher incidence of intestinal tumors, extremely high in both groups. The authors suggest that thiamin administration perhaps altered the absorption, distribution, metabolism or excretion of the bracken fern carcinogen by the host.

In regard to bracken, the young sprouts of some ferns (fiddlehead greens) are eaten as a delicacy by a number of populations. Studies in our laboratories demonstrated no effects when fed to rats for as long as two years at concentrations of 10 per cent of the diet.[175] This is in contrast to reports of others who claim, without evidence, that the young sprouts are a health hazard.[176]

Thiamin-destroying factors are being found in ever-greater numbers of plants normally used as food by human subjects, but the significance of these observations has still to be established. In one study, antithiamin activity was found in 31 vegetables and 18 fruits, with the highest activity in blackberries, black currants, red beets, Brussels sprouts and red cabbage.[177] A report from Japan[178] points out that some ferns, including bracken, have enjoyed a popularity as edible foods in various parts of the Orient. This report states that it is commonly recognized that dimness of vision results from eating large amounts of bracken fern in the early spring. How this disturbance might relate to a thiamin deficiency is not clear.

The potentially disturbing feature about the thiaminases found in many plant products is the fact that there appear to be at least two different types—one heat labile, the other heat stable.[178] The latter seems to be resistant to drying, is probably of small molecular weight, requires oxygen for its action and has an activity optimum at pH 8. Although our present knowledge indicates that these thiamin-destroying factors are primarily of theoretical interest, individuals who, because of unusual circumstances, consume large amounts of spinach, cabbage and blackberries may develop a thiamin deficiency.

Cycad

Cycads are palm-like trees consisting of nine species growing mainly in the tropics and subtropics. The use of cycads by the peoples on various southwest Pacific islands stems from the fact that these are some of the few plants capable of surviving adverse climatic conditions. Prior to and during World War II, they provided a source of calories during droughts and following severe typhoons and served as a supplement when food supplies became low because of military action.[179]

Widespread interest in cycad toxicity developed when amyotrophic lateral sclerosis was associated with consumption of flour prepared from cycad nuts. The incidence of amyotrophic lateral sclerosis is 100 times greater among the Chamoro Guamanians than among the inhabitants of the United States or Europe. Human patients suffering from amyotrophic lateral sclerosis become progressively paralyzed and die about five years after the onset of symptoms. There is presently no known cure for this disease. In an attempt to determine the etiology of amyotrophic lateral sclerosis, investigators at the National Institutes of Health were impressed by the reported similarity of this disease to the paralytic symptoms seen in cattle and sheep that had eaten cycads.[179] The people of Guam use the seeds of the cycad both as an emergency source of food and to a lesser extent as a regular part of their diet. The starchy center or the kernels of the seeds are used in thickening various dishes (soups, tortillas, fruit desserts), while the outer husk of the seed is used as a confection.

The Guamanians have recognized for many years that the kernels of Cycas circinalis are toxic. They attempt to eliminate the toxin by soaking the kernel in vats of water for 7 to 10 days. The water may be changed several times during a soaking period. After soaking, the kernels are dried in the sun and then ground to a powder similar to that of wheat flour.[180]

The question has arisen as to whether or not the soaking process completely removes the toxic agents from the cycad kernel. The results of a long-term study indicated that the processed kernel was relatively safe for rats.[181] In contrast to the processed kernel, the unprocessed kernel is toxic when fed to rats at high levels, and carcinogenic when fed at lower levels over a 5- to 7-month period. Benign and malignant tumors developed, mainly in the liver and kidneys of the latter animals. None of these rats or any of those fed the processed kernel developed neurologic symptoms.[182] Furthermore, none of the other animals, including cows, horses, swine and guinea pigs, developed neurologic disturbances when fed the unprocessed kernels. Microscopic examination of the brain and spinal cord of these animals revealed no lesions that could be traced to cycad kernels.[183]

The neurologic disturbances originally described by Australian investigators as occurring in cattle grazing on cycad leaves[184] have also been described among cattle grazing in the highlands of the Dominican Republic.[185] These cattle exhibited a "goose-stepping" gait with posterior weakness and ataxia. Destruction of myelin was demonstrated around single nerve fibers in the fasciculus gracilis, dorsal spinocerebellar, lateral corticospinal, ventral corticospinal and medial longitudinal fasciculus tracts. A compound isolated from the cycad kernel tentatively described as a new amino acid, α-amino-β-methylaminoproprionic acid,[186] produces neurologic disturbances when injected into chicks.

The neurologic symptoms in animals are associated more with consumption of the leaves of these plants than of the nuts. Another part of the cycad (Cycas circinalis), the husk, is chewed fresh by the Guamanians to relieve thirst, or dried and eaten as candy. The husk is not processed except for drying.[179] When the dried husk was fed to rats, acute toxicity symptoms appeared within a few days. The rats exhibited an increase in hemoglobin and hematocrit concentrations. When fed husks as 6 per cent or more of the diet, the animals died in about 10 days from massive hemorrhages into the gastrointestinal tracts and pancreatic necrosis. Other symptoms included ascites, an intense yellow color of the urine and edema under the skin near the sternum. Rats fed lower concentrations (0.5 to 1.0 per cent of husks) developed tumors in the liver, kidneys and other internal organs similar to those fed the unwashed cycad kernels.

The toxic substance in cycad stems and cycad seeds (Cycas revoluta) has been identified as methylazoxymethanol-β-glucoside. The aglycone of this glucoside, methylazoxymethanol, is common to the glycosides present in other species of cycad.[187,188] The latter glycosides have sugars other than glucose linked to the aglycone.

The beta glycoside linkage in cycad explains why the glycoside is nontoxic when injected into conventional animals[190] or fed to germ-free animals.[191] Liberation of the active aglycone requires a beta glucosidase present in bacterial but not in mammalian cells. When the bacterial action in the gastrointestinal tract is circumvented by parenteral injection or by feeding to germ-free animals, cycasin remains intact and, as such, is nontoxic. A possible exception to the absence of beta glucosidases in mammalian tissues comes from the observation that cycasin injected into day-old rat pups was toxic.[192] These animals developed kidney tumors about five months following a single injection. The nature of the induction of cancer in rats under these conditions requires clarification. When pregnant rats are fed either unprocessed kernel or cycasin, the fetuses show typical toxic effects.[183,193] The transplacental transfer of the toxic agent was sufficient to produce liver tumors at a later date in the progeny of the pregnant rats. The toxic factor can also be transferred from dam to young through the milk in several species including rats, cows and pigs.[183] Excretory products of the young rats, consumed and processed by their dams, may have been passed to the young in the mother's milk.

The public health implications of these findings are difficult to evaluate. Even if human beings are susceptible to the carcinogenic agents in the cycad, it is likely that most of these compounds have been removed during processing. There is a possibility, however, that the compounds (in the unprocessed husk) may be consumed by both pregnant and lactating women and the active principles transferred to the fetuses or nursing infants. Further exposure may derive from the transmission of these compounds through cow's milk consumed by infants and children where cycad plants are endemic.

Ultrastructural observations of the phloem of coconut palms with "hartrot" disease in Surinam revealed plant-infecting flagellate Phytomonas in mature sieve tubes. The occurrence of these flagellates in the phloem as the disease progresses suggests that the organisms may be pathogenic to the palms. The public health significance of this interesting observation is worthy of investigation.

Herbal Intoxication

There has been a remarkable increase in the use of herbal products in recent years. These include capsules, teas, cigarettes and other smoking mixtures advertised as "natural and legal drugs" or "herbal highs."[194] Such products are available in health food stores and markets as well as by direct mail order from importers or suppliers. Many of the preparations contain significant amounts of psychoactive substances, the use of which has resulted in intoxications requiring clinical attention.

There are at least 192 distinct herbs commercially available for smoking as cigarettes or as blended smoking mixtures. The most common of those which contain psychoactive materials are spearmint, thyme, rosemary, yerba santa, mullein and damiana. Many of these are advertised as nontobacco substitutes; some are advertised as mimicking the effects of marihuana. A variety of clinical symptoms have been associated with smoking these mixtures, including a pervasive "spaced-out" sensation, ataxia, slurred speech, blurred vision, dilated pupils, and dry mouth and throat. One such product, "mint bidis," imported from India, results in such responses; analysis of the cigarettes revealed that a single cigarette contained 16 μg of atropine and 65 μg of scopolamine. Another cigarette made from Datura stramonium contained 250 μg of atropine and 220 μg of scopolamine. Some patients have consumed cigarettes in quantities to provide as much as 0.7 mg total alkaloids per day.

Teas are popular with a significant segment of the population of the United States and currently there are 396 distinct herbs and spices commercially available for use singly or as blended mixtures. Psychoactive agents are present in at least 43 of these, but generally in lower concentrations than in cigarettes. A leading product, kavabava tea, associated with confusion, ataxia, impaired breathing, dimmed vision, dulled hearing and hallucinations, is made from crushed roots of the kava plant, Piper methysticum, indigenous to islands of the South Pacific. Nutmeg tea may result in symptoms of nausea, dryness of mouth and throat, drowsiness, rapid pulse, flushed skin, disturbed vision, incoherent speech, vertigo and hallucinations.[195]

Tea is also made from Datura stramonium or jimsonweed. It results in ataxia, restlessness, blurred vision and severe hallucinations, much as the cigarette made from the same plant. The tea made from Datura stramonium contains large amounts of atropine and scopolamine, and the symptoms are typical of stramonium poisoning.

Another interesting tea that is widely advertised and consumed is made from the root bark of the sassafras tree, Sassafras albidum. The major constituent in sassafras tea is safrole (4-albyl, 1, 2-methylene-dioxybenzene), an hepatocarcinogen for laboratory animals. Aqueous and alcoholic extracts of sassafras root bark elicit a variety of pharmacologic responses in mice, including central nervous system depression, hypothermia, hypersensitivity, ptosis and ataxia.[196]

In addition to the disturbing clinical symptoms and intoxications, herb teas may change the bioavailability of foods and theraupetic drugs consumed concomitantly. The use of herbal cigarettes, teas and capsules is to be discouraged.

Mushrooms

Under ordinary circumstances, the consumption of the inky cap mushroom Coprinus atramentarius produces no unpleasant reactions. However, if an alcoholic beverage is drunk during or shortly after a meal that includes this mushroom, the face of the drinker and perhaps other parts of his body soon become purplish-red.[197] Apparently, this mushroom contains a compound with an action similar to that of Antabuse (disulfiram). To date the compound has not been isolated, but indirect evidence suggests it is not disulfiram.[198]

Poisoning from the ingestion of other types of mushrooms has occurred for many centuries.[199,200] In the United States, less than 2 per cent of the cases reported to the National Clearinghouse for Poison Control Centers involved mushrooms.[201] A partial explanation for the few cases of mushroom toxicity stems from the fact that only a few species are toxic. For instance, although there are over 800 species of these plants in New England, only 53 are considered poisonous.[202]

In the 37-year period following 1924, there were 24 deaths in the United States attributable to mushroom poisoning.[202] Half of these were associated with the eating of mushrooms of the Amanita species and the others with Gyromitra esculenta or unidentified species. The fatalities resulted when the mushrooms were collected by the individual or someone other than a commercial producer. There was one nonfatal epidemic in which canned mushrooms imported from Taiwan produced headaches and varied neurologic disturbances in 55 of 80 women who ate a soup prepared from them.[203] In the latter cases, the symptoms appeared within minutes after eating the soup, and resembled those attributable to Amanita muscaria.

Apparently, there is considerable variability among individuals to mushroom toxicity. Part of this results from:

1. Difficulty in classifying the mushrooms. The Amanita, among which are some of the more poisonous mushrooms, pose the greatest taxonomic problems.[200] For many years, the white, yellow, green, gray, brown and black mushrooms that resembled the phalloides were believed to be variants of the same species. More recently, it has been recognized that these are different species and that they differ markedly in their content of toxins.[204]

2. Development of sensitivity to the mushroom or variation in its toxicity. For the same mushroom, Gyromitra esculenta, there are reports that it can be eaten once without any disturbances, but frequently on the second or third consumption toxic manifestations follow.[205] Another report states that this same mushroom has caused poisoning in persons who had eaten it for years without ill effect, and small, localized groups of cases have occurred more frequently in some years than others.[202] Presumably, this variability in toxicity was due to "climatic or other undetermined factors." Recent studies of the same species of mushrooms collected in the same park show a variability in toxin concentration from none to a high value.[204]

3. Individual predilection to mushroom toxicity. Some people are able to eat mushrooms with impunity, while others develop severe toxicity when eating the same kind.[203,206,207]

In the United States, two of the more toxic mushrooms are Amanita phalloides and A. muscaria.[174] The toxic principles in these two differ in that the former contains cyclopeptides and the latter alkaloid-like compounds. The ingestion of A. phalloides and its close relatives accounts for most of the fatal cases of mushroom poisoning.

Most of the toxic mushrooms contain more than one toxic compound. For instance, the A. phalloides mushrooms contain at least five toxins that are related biochemically since they are all cyclopeptides that have only a few amino acids, some of which do not occur in proteins.[208] Each of the toxins contains one sulfur atom which is not present as a sulfhydryl group. At least two of these toxins (α- and β-amanitine) are heat stable and, for them, there is no effective antidote.[201] Treatment of patients with severe poisoning after eating these mushrooms involves careful fluid and electrolyte therapy.[200] Although an antitoxin against Amanita phalloides was reportedly prepared at the Pasteur Institute in France as long ago as 1925, its use in other countries appears to have been extremely limited since the best that can be said for it is that there is no clear record of its effectiveness in man.[209]

The symptoms associated with the ingestion of the toxic A. phalloides mushroom do not appear for 10 to 20 hours. At that time, the individual suddenly experiences severe abdominal pain, vomiting and diarrhea. Excessive thirst develops with anuria. There is no hemoglobinuria. The patient rapidly loses strength and may die within 48 hours after eating large quantities of the mushrooms. In less severe cases, jaundice, cyanosis and marked coldness of the skin may appear after 2 to 3 days, with death occurring on the sixth to eighth day. Autopsy reveals fatty degeneration and necrosis of the liver and kidney, degeneration of areas in the central nervous system and hemorrhagic areas in various organs.[173,199] Animal studies have shown that one of the major disturbances following the ingestion of these mushrooms involves a reduction in liver glycogen level and the failure of this to be restored following glucose therapy.[208] Despite these biochemical studies, the mechanism whereby the toxins of A. phalloides produce their effects is obscure.

The other important mushroom toxicant is muscarine, which is found in Amanita muscaria, from which it was isolated in 1869,[209] Amanita pantherina and certain species of the Boletus, Russula and Clitocybe genera.[201] Muscarine is a heat-stable quaternary ammonium base which resembles choline esters in some of its actions. Most of its effects are attributable to stimulation of the parasympathetic postganglionic nerves.[209] Frequently, within minutes to at most a few hours after eating these mushrooms, the individual exhibits excessive salivation and lacrimation, contracted pupils that do not respond to light, nausea and frequent vomiting, and excruciating abdominal pains with severe diarrhea; dizziness and confusion may appear, with convulsions in the more advanced state.[199] In one group of women who presumably had consumed mushrooms containing muscarine the symptoms were limited to headaches, malaise and muscular tingling, especially of the facial muscles.[203] Atropine is the specific antidote, and must be given in sufficiently large doses (0.5 to 15.0 mg subcutaneously every 4 hours) to dilate the pupils and inhibit sweating.[209]

Domestically cultivated varieties of mushrooms (Agaricus bisporus) are free of any toxic substance. The more poisonous species are not amenable to cultivation. Safety dictates that mushrooms should be purchased in the marketplace rather than harvested from the forest.

TOXINS OF MARINE ORIGIN

Paralytic Shellfish Poisoning (PSP)

Mussels, clams, and occasionally scallops and oysters from both the Atlantic and Pacific coastal areas and from such other areas as South Africa, New Zealand, Belgium, Germany, France, England and Ireland have produced poisoning in man.[210] Poisoning is associated with the growth in the water of dinoflagellates. These unicellular organisms produce a poison that is retained in the dark gland or hepatopancreas of the mussel or other shellfish feeding on them. The shellfish show no disturbance as a result of the toxin; however, when the contaminated seafood is eaten by man, symptoms of toxicity usually develop in 1 to 3 hours.[211]

The symptoms associated with paralytic shellfish poisoning include a numbness of the lips and fingertips, an ascending paralysis and finally, in severe poisoning, death from respiratory paralysis is reported to be about 8.5 per cent.[210] Death may occur in 3 to 20 hours after eating the shellfish. Should the person survive the first 24 hours, the prognosis for his complete recovery is good. In most areas, the poisoning is confined to local residents who dig for their own shellfish. In the Alaskan coastal area, the problem becomes of more importance to general public health, since the shellfish from this area are canned or frozen and widely distributed. Hazardous levels of PSP accumulate when the dinoflagellate undergoes rapid growth (i.e. "blooms") in the area where shellfish are feeding. The increase in organisms and the changes associated with this are referred to as the "red tide." As a protective measure along United States and Canadian coastal waters, a quarantine is posted whenever the toxicity of the shellfish becomes dangerous. The toxicity is determined by injecting an aqueous extract of the shellfish into mice.[210,211] Even this measure is not completely adequate, since sampling of shellfish from various areas in the same region may suggest low levels of toxicity while other areas nearby may have highly toxic shellfish. This was evident when 32 persons in one region became ill before testing indicated that a quarantine should have been established.[210]

Ordinary cooking procedures reduce the toxicity, but not enough to make the seafood safe for eating. Since about 95 per cent of the poison is concentrated in the digestive organs or dark meat,[211] removal of those tissues would make the seafood safe; the white meat contains no poison. The toxicity disappears from mussels once the dinoflagellates leave the water. The

Alaskan butter clams, on the other hand, retain their toxicity for long periods of time. The source of the poison in the Alaskan clams is not known for certain, since the water where these clams grow contains large numbers of plankton, but none of these appears to be toxic.[211] That an organism comparable to the dinoflagellates is probably responsible is suggested by the isolation of the same toxic compound from butter clams and the dinoflagellates.[212]

The compound isolated from both the Alaskan butter clams and axenic cultures of the dinoflagellates has been given the name *saxitoxin*. This word comes from the scientific name for the butter clams, Saxidomus giganeus. The toxin appears to block nerve transmission in the motor axon and not at the end-plate, presumably by blocking the increase of sodium conductance normally associated with excitation. On the basis of experiments with cats, it was estimated that the lethal dose of this toxin for an adult would be 0.4 mg given intravenously.[213] Orally, the toxic dose has been suggested as 8 mg.[214]

Squid and Octopus

Fresh squid and octopus have produced a seasonally occurring toxicity among the inhabitants of certain areas in Japan. This toxicity involves primarily the gastrointestinal tract, and recovery usually occurs within 48 hours. The nature of the toxin appears to be unknown.[210]

Allergic Reactions

This problem is subject to a great deal of conflicting testimony, partly because of the psychoneurotic factor in many allergic reactions[215,216] and the confusion in classifying fish by the lay public. The commercial classification of fish frequently differs from that recognized by the ichthyologists. A related problem exists among the solutions used in testing for food sensitivity. Antigenically, the same preparation from a variety of sources exhibited a remarkable lack of uniformity in antigenic components.[217]

Fish and shellfish are known to serve as powerful allergens which, in some persons, may produce almost explosive reactions.[210] These reactions include urticaria, angioneurotic edema, gastrointestinal disturbances and migraine; asthma and coryza are seen less frequently. Attempts have been made to classify fish on the basis of those to which an allergic individual might be sensitive, e.g. those allergic to cod might also react to trout, carp, herring and sardines. Whether such a classification will survive is doubtful since there are reported cases of allergies to one specific type of seafood with no reactions to other closely related species.[210,216]

Fish and Iron Deficiency

A report from Norway[218] indicated that when mink were fed certain species of raw fish (coal fish, Gadus virens, or whiting, Gadus merlangus), they became severely anemic and died. Parenteral iron therapy cured this anemia. Another report[219] suggested that the substance making the dietary iron unavailable was located primarily in the viscera. This substance was inactivated by cooking. More than a simple sequestering of iron appears to be involved in this problem, however. When the offspring of mink that had developed anemia on the raw-fish ration were fed the same diet as their parents, they all developed anemia.[219] On the other hand, when young from "anemia-resistant" parents were fed the raw-fish ration, few, if any, developed anemia.

Not only may genetic factors be involved in this condition, but species differences may also exist.[220]

Mercury in Fish

The United States Food and Drug Administration adopted, in May of 1969, a safe-level guideline of 0.5 parts per million (ppm) mercury in fish[221] which applied to all fish in interstate commerce. The 0.5

ppm level was an interim guideline for internal use in deciding when to charge that a fish product was adulterated under the federal Food, Drug and Cosmetic Act, but it has remained in effect since its original application.

The action by the FDA was taken following reports of methylmercury poisoning in Japan and Sweden.[221-226] The level of 0.5 ppm for methylmercury in fish was based on a careful review of the limited information available to the FDA at that time. A major part of these data was observation of clinical symptoms and blood levels of mercury in victims of the Minamata Bay incident.[223] Further data were developed from the calculations made by the Swedish Expert Committee,[227] who accepted 30 μg Hg per day as the upper limit of acceptable daily intake.

To better understand the current state of concern about potential or real poisoning from mercury in fish, a brief reference to developments of the problem over the past 20 years is in order.

In 1953, in Japan, villages around Minamata Bay were confronted with a mass outbreak of a progressive toxicologic disease that resulted in blindness, deafness, incoordination and intellectual deterioration (characteristics of the Hunter-Russell syndrome, but not recognized as such at the time[228]). This disease was subsequently designated "Minamata disease." In these villages along the shore of the Minamata Bay, 121 persons developed the disease between 1953 and 1960. Of the total number affected, 23 were infants and 46 died.[229] A similar outbreak occurred in the villages along the Agano River in Niigata with 47 officially documented cases, 6 of whom died.[230] Investigations of the outbreaks around Minamata Bay and along the Agano River identified the cause as heavy consumption of fish contaminated with methylmercury. It was significant that the infants who contracted the disease had not eaten any of the fish themselves, but that their mothers had eaten varying quan-

tities of contaminated fish while pregnant. The mothers had exhibited no symptoms themselves, but the methylmercury circulating in their blood streams was easily transferred through the placenta to the developing fetuses.[231,232]

Pathologic examination of deceased patients revealed a reduction of brain cells in the cerebrum and cerebellum which helped to explain the ataxia, convulsions, numbness of limbs and mouth, constriction of the visual field and difficulty in speaking. A search of the literature revealed a report describing symptoms of poisoning by the methylmercury resembling those observed in the Japanese endemic.[228] An analysis for mercury in fish and in tissues from victims of the disease revealed that both contained remarkably high levels of mercury, as much as 24 ppm in small crabs taken from the Bay, and as much as 144 ppm in kidneys of people who had succumbed to the disease. Human patients suffered damage to bone marrow, lymph nodes, nerve fibers, liver and kidneys, but the most catastrophic effects of the poisoning occurred in the brain.[229] The Japanese investigators fed some of the local fish to experimental animals and observed toxicologic symptoms and pathologic lesions similar to those observed in people who had succumbed to the disease.[229]

The Japanese investigators traced the contaminating methylmercury from shellfish and finfish back through the waters of the Bay to the effluent pipes and the sludge expelled from the principal industry in the village which, a year before the first people became ill, had started producing acetaldehyde and vinyl chloride with the aid of mercury compounds as catalysts.[222,223] During the reactions, some of the mercury was converted to methylmercury and discharged with other wastes into Minamata Bay. Here, the fish and shellfish, feeding on contaminated marine life and pumping water through their gills, absorbed and concentrated the methylmercury into their tissues. Subsequent to this epidemic, it has been determined that even under natural conditions the ability of fish to concentrate mercury from their immediate environment can create public health problems. The larger, more aged fish such as swordfish and tuna constitute primary potential sources of poisoning. To refrain from eating these species unless certified as free of significant mercury contamination assures safety to the consumer. In the United States a case report of possible mercury poisoning from fish[233] has not been documented and recent deliberations cast doubt on the validity of this presumption.

Results of studies by Clarkson,[234] just beginning to emerge, indicate that populations with high exposure to methylmercury from fish over long periods of life may be in jeopardy. These studies on fishermen and their families in Peru and perhaps in Samoa may indicate clinical symptoms of methylmercury poisoning from eating large amounts of fish taken from normal marine environments with standard background levels of mercury. A few of the subjects have complained of symptoms when their body burdens of methylmercury were less than 10 mg. The investigators feel that they can detect a toxic response with certainty when the body burden has reached 25 mg of mercury. This figure compares well with the 30-mg body burden calculated by the Swedes from the Japanese data.

These longitudinal studies indicate that problems may arise in selected human populations from methylmercury poisoning when fish with normal background levels of methylmercury are consumed in large quantities over extended periods of time.

METALS, METALLOIDS AND OTHER CHEMICALS

The largest part of the total body burden of most metals in biologic species is traceable to diet from sources which include constituents of rocks and minerals that weathered to produce the soil, water erosion of soil particles, metals as added ingredients or impurities in fertilizers, pesticides containing metals (arsenic, lead, copper, mercury, manganese and zinc), metals in manure and sludge and those present in airborne dust (industrial and mining wastes, fossil fuel combustion products, wind-eroded soil particles, radioactive fallout, pollen, sea spray, meteoric and volcanic material). Plants may grow normally but contain levels of selenium, cadmium, molybdenum or lead that are toxic to animals. Plants exclude arsenic, beryllium, nickel, zinc and mercury by minimizing their absorption from soil.[235]

The most important toxic action of metals is enzyme poisoning. Mercury, lead, copper, beryllium, cadmium and silver have been found to inhibit alkaline phosphatase, catalase, xanthine oxidase and ribonuclease in fish. Some metals act as antimetabolites, e.g. arsenate substituting for phosphate. Metals may form precipitates or chelates with essential metabolites; they may catalyze the degradation of essential metabolites and metals such as gold, cadmium, copper, mercury, lead and uranium and may react with cell membranes to alter their permeability or even rupture them. Some metals may replace structurally or electrochemically important elements in cells—lithium substituting for sodium, calcium for potassium and strontium for cadmium.[235]

The two naturally occurring toxic metals in foods believed to be of most practical importance are mercury and selenium, although mercury, lead and cadmium are the most serious environmental pollutants. Mercury is toxic, volatile and widely distributed over the surface of the earth. It undergoes methylation which increases its toxicity and mobility in aquatic and animal circulatory systems.

Selenium

Selenium is essential for domestic animals but the margin of safety is relatively narrow. A low level of selenium is essential to prevent myopathies, liver injury and congenital abnormalities in domestic and laboratory animals and poultry. There is little reason to believe that humans differ appreciably in this regard; however, data are lacking. High dietary selenium is toxic to animals, and a defined set of signs and lesions has been established for acute and subacute exposure to toxic concentrations in several species. Chronic, long-term studies have been limited primarily to feeding studies in the rat, and these have involved relatively high concentrations of the element.[236,237]

Inorganic and organic forms of selenium are readily absorbed from the gastrointestinal tract of animals. Selenite is absorbed more rapidly by monogastric animals than by ruminant animals, perhaps because of bacterial reduction of selenite to elemental selenium or other insoluble forms in the ruminant gastrointestinal tract.

Selenite and selenate are distributed largely to the liver, kidneys, muscle mass, gastrointestinal tract and blood. Chronic administration of selenium results in increased concentration in the testes. The principal route of excretion is via the urine. Fecal excretion by rats is small under most situations. Small amounts of selenium are found in bile, pancreatic excretions and saliva. At higher levels, selenium is incorporated into molecules normally served by sulfur; it is methylated by mammalian tissues in an apparent detoxication process. Selenite and selenate are metabolized to trimethylselenonium ion, $(CH_3)_3Se^+$, which is the principal excretory product for selenium in urine.

The toxicity of selenium can be altered extensively by interactions with sulfate, methionine, cystine, mercury, lead, zinc, cadmium, copper, arsenic and vitamin E, but little is known about these interactions. Human toxicity has resulted primarily from acute industrial exposure.[238] There is little evidence that human populations living in affected areas are as affected by selenium deficiency or toxicity as animals are. The difference between man's and domestic animals' susceptibility to chronic selenium poisoning is unlikely to be associated with a higher tolerance in the human species, since species differences in tolerance to selenium appear to be small. Absence of obvious signs of chronic selenosis in man in seleniferous areas is probably attributable to the wide geographic source of many of the foods composing modern human dietaries and the fact that most of these foods, unlike animal feeds, are subject to modification by processing and cooking.

The minimum dietary level of selenium, which results in accumulation in the tissues of animals and ultimately produces signs of toxicity, is about 3 to 4 ppm of the dry diet. This is probably the minimum toxic or the maximum safe level for man, although the nature of the rest of the diet, particularly its protein and sulfate contents, can greatly influence toxicity. Thus 10 ppm Se in a 20 per cent protein diet has no adverse effects.[239] Increasing the concentration of sulfate up to 0.87 per cent of a sulfate-free diet progressively decreased the growth inhibition induced in young rats by 10 ppm Se, as selenite or selenate.[236] However, inorganic sulfate is much less effective in protecting against organic forms of selenium, such as occur largely in foods, than against inorganic forms.

Epidemiologic studies with children and experimental studies with animals have indicated that above-normal intakes of selenium during the development period of the teeth increase the incidence of cavities.[241] The results reported would be more convincing if the actual selenium intakes of the children in the different groups had been measured; more evidence is needed before the caries-enhancing effect of selenium is fully established and its mode of action understood.

Early studies in rats suggested that selenium was a carcinogen but there has been little support from later investigations.[237] Furthermore, limited epidemiologic evidence suggests that selenium may be a possible protective agent against human cancer.[242] The important questions of selenium and cancer and of selenium and dental caries clearly need further study, but the fact that the FDA now permits the addition of selenium salts to poultry and swine feeds indicates that scientific judgment has concluded that this element is not carcinogenic.

Arsenic

Arsenic is widely distributed in the waters of the United States, but generally in low concentrations (10 to 22 ppb). In a few instances, arsenic concentrations reach significant, even toxic levels. The two most widely studied geographic localities with arsenic levels sufficient to result in public health hazards are Antofagasta, Chile, and the southwest coast of Taiwan.[243] Both were associated with arsenic in drinking water supplies which, over many years of exposure, resulted in cutaneous lesions, skin cancer and cancer of the lung.[244,245] Other conditions attributed to arsenic in human populations include neuropathy, an increase in myocardial infarcts (heart attacks) and vascular injury leading to gangrene and "blackfoot." Industrial exposures with serious public health consequences have been reported from the United States, Sweden, Japan and Germany.

There is some pollution of streams and lakes with arsenic from fertilizers and detergents manufactured from phosphate rock rich in arsenic, but the extent of this source is unknown. Shellfish concentrate arsenic. It is found also on fruit sprayed with arsenical insecticides and in apple cider and wine.[246] Arsenicals as growth promotors in food animals are permitted and controlled by the FDA, but the potential for exposure from this source is an unknown quantity.

From all sources, the general public of the United States consumes a calculated daily intake of 0.137 to 0.330 mg of arsenic. Epidemiologic studies have clearly shown that chronic excessive consumption of arsenic results in cutaneous lesions, including skin cancer, and, in some cases, lung cancer.[244] However, the lack of uniformity of design and other defects in the studies indicate a need for international agreements on the best methods for collecting and disseminating data for more accurate evaluation from one location to another.

There is little information about arsenic in marine organisms or about methylation-demethylation processes in marine and terrestrial organisms. Likewise, the uptake of arsenic by plants is poorly understood, although it appears to be related to the amount of soluble arsenic in the soil, the nature of the soil and the species of plant.

There is speculation that interactions between arsenic and other metals and irritating substances, such as sulfur dioxide, may be important in overall effects on humans exposed to environmental contaminants.

Kinetics and metabolism studies of arsenic in man have been neglected, although it appears that urinary excretion of arsenic is mainly in the form of methylarsenic and dimethylarsenic acid; much of a single dose is excreted within 24 hours.

Arsenic compounds in animals are fetotoxic in high doses and teratogenic in lower concentrations. They are also associated with chromosomal aberrations in man.

Arsenic is the only known human carcinogen for which an animal model has not been found; this has greatly hampered investigations into arsenic metabolism and carcinogenicity.

Lead

Classic lead poisoning has been well known for centuries and has been described by many investigators and clinicians.[248] Concern has grown in recent years, however, as to whether the increased use and dissemination of lead through the environment is resulting in subclinical disease and in a long-term adverse effect on the health of human populations. Food has been a major source of human intake of lead through contamination from lead-containing vessels, lead pottery glazes and pesticides entering the food chain; however, these sources have decreased recently. Shellfish may concentrate lead from contaminated water.

Most human foods under standard environmental conditions contain less than 1 ppm Pb. Cow's milk may contain 0.02 to 0.08 ppm Pb, and muscle meats approximately 0.1 ppm.[247,248] Lead has a marked affinity for bone, which sometimes contains between 5 and 20 ppm on the fresh basis.[248] Little is known of the natural levels of lead in foods of plant origin; these must be quite low, however, because average intakes from food by adult man have been variously estimated to range from 0.22 to 0.4 mg Pb per day, approximately 0.3 to 0.5 ppm of the dry diet. In addition, smaller amounts of lead are ingested with drinking water, and inhaled from the atmosphere and from cigarette smoke. As a result of such activities, the current average daily adult intake of lead from all food sources in the United States has been estimated to be about 300 micrograms.[250]

Cadmium

Daily intakes of cadmium by human adults have been estimated as 0.2 to 0.5 gm, with considerable variation, according to sources and types of food. These estimates now appear to be much too high. A mean total cadmium content of 0.013 mg was recently reported for school lunches served to sixth-grade children in 300 U.S. schools.[250] The total dietary cadmium intakes of institutionalized children (ages 9 to 12 yrs) in 28 U.S. cities were found to average 0.092 mg per day, with a range of 0.032 to 0.158 mg per day.

Oysters are exceptionally rich in cadmium, with levels of 3 to 4 ppm compared with levels of one tenth or one hundredth as much in most other foods.[251] Appreciable amounts of cadmium may also be obtained from the air and the water supply. Soft water remaining overnight in galvanized or black polyethylene pipes can take up 0.15 to 1.1 μg Cd per liter, although total intakes from these sources are calculated to supply no more than 1 to 2 μg Cd per day. The cadmium level in the air of 28 U.S. cities was shown to range from undetectable to as high as 0.06 μg Cd per cu mm of air.[250]

Whether cadmium intakes from the food, air, and water supply present any long-term hazards to human health is speculative, at best. Outbreaks of acute cadmium poisoning, accompanied by nausea, vomiting, diarrhea and prostration, have been reported from the consumption of jellies and ices containing 15 to 530 ppm Cd derived from cadmium-plated trays and vessels and from consumption of lemonade containing 100 ppm Cd that had been in contact for some hours with cadmium-plated vessels. It appears that 15 ppm is necessary to produce mild symptoms of cadmium poisoning in man.[253]

A progressively increasing incidence of systolic hypertension develops in rats exposed to 5 ppm Cd in the drinking water from the time of weaning. However, the animals must be constantly exposed to the cadmium for 1 year or more and must have accumulated considerable quantities of cadmium in their kidneys if hypertension is to appear and to be sustained. The pathologic changes associated with cadmium hypertension in rats include renal, arterial, arteriolar and glomerular lesions; these are indistinguishable from those accompanying benign hypertension from other causes.

The relationship of cadmium to hypertension in man is unknown; however, some hypertensive patients exhibit a higher than normal urinary excretion of a range of metals, especially cadmium, and carry significantly higher renal cadmium concentrations and a higher Cd:Zn ratio in their tissues than do similar normotensive individuals.[254]

Other Trace Elements

Elements classified as trace elements have regained a position of prominence recently because of recognition that their excess or unbalanced concentration in food and water can produce adverse effects on human health. Zinc, copper, manganese and selenium all have relatively narrow margins of safety, and the presence of one of these elements often can make one or more of the others available[250] (Chap. 9B).

ORGANIC CONTAMINANTS

Pesticides, especially the chlorinated hydrocarbons along with polychlorinated biphenyls, chlorinated dibenzo-p-dioxins and chlorinated dibenzofurans, are widespread in our environment and result in pathologic changes in animals.[256,257]

One of the most characteristic responses to most organochlorides is a stimulation of the drug-metabolizing enzymes of the liver.[258] The induction of enzymes in this manner may have important implications for human health, but currently little is known about the nature of this response. Pesticides are used in large quantities in areas of the world where malnutrition and disease are widespread. As a result, selected pesticides must be considered a potential problem in those areas of the United States where malnutrition is prevalent. An excellent review of the impact of pesticides in protein-deficiency states has recently been published.[259] For example, it is known that poor-quality protein impairs

microsomal enzyme induction and thus potentiates metabolic response to DDT and lindane.

Dieldrin and DDT aggravate the deleterious effects of essential fatty acid deficiency in the rat. Dieldrin partially offsets the effects of thiamin deficiency, but does not prevent the effect to riboflavin and pyridoxine deficiency. Hypovitaminosis C impairs the induction of hepatic microsomal enzymes. Studies with guinea pigs have shown that this leads to a requirement of higher dietary levels of ascorbic acid in order to prevent scurvy.[260] Clearly, this area requires extensive support for a broad-based research effort on the potential hazards of such important chemicals to man.

TOXINS FROM ANIMAL FOODSTUFFS

Factors in animal foodstuffs which have a potential for inducing toxic responses in man and animals have generally been treated in a superficial manner in most comprehensive treatises devoted to the general topic of naturally occurring toxicants. This reflects a lack of interest and research in this area of food safety. Naturally occurring toxicants in animal tissues are limited mainly to avian and fish eggs and to some shellfish and amphibia. There are many examples, however, of toxicity caused by the introduction of man-made chemicals into meat and dairy products.

Milk and Dairy Products

Since some segments of the population of the United States are "vegetarian" and depend on dairy and vegetable sources for their food needs, there is a need for more data about how milk products affect selected, hypersensitive individuals or those with enzyme deficits. Milk and dairy products are of concern, then, because of the intolerance of some individuals to constituents in milk and milk products (i.e. milk proteins, lactose). In addition, milk can contain estrogens, plant substances, nitrates and nitrites, antibiotics, pesticides, radionuclides and mycotoxins as contaminants. Further, as noted below, cheese can contain a number of amines that are pharmacoactive and cause serious problems in people who are sensitive to them. Those amines of importance are norepinephrine, epinephrine and 5-hydroxytryptamine (serotonin).[261]

Cheese. The presence of various symptoms in patients receiving monoamine oxidase inhibitors is an illustration of a food toxicity seen in special groups of people. These individuals complain of hypertension, severe headache and palpitation. Initially, these disturbances were considered side effects of the monoamine oxidase inhibitors. It was almost 10 years after the introduction of these drugs that the "side effects" became associated with the consumption of cheese.[262]

The monoamine oxidase inhibitors are used to treat patients in depressive states. These drugs inhibit the enzyme that "destroys" serotonin, norepinephrine and related neurohormonal compounds. As a result of this and possibly other reactions, the drugs produce a euphoric state.

Tyramine in cheese is a potent vasopressor substance. Under normal circumstances, it is metabolized through the action of monoamine oxidases. When the activity of these enzymes is inhibited by drugs, the tyramine from the cheese acts to produce severe hypertension and its sequelae. A few fatalities have occurred in patients treated with one of the monoamine oxidase inhibitors after eating cheese.[263-267]

Tyramine is formed by the decarboxylation of tyrosine. This and other amino acids are liberated during the ripening of cheese by bacteria acting on the peptides formed from the action of renin on casein.[262] Other foods normally contain pressor amines without the intervention of bacterial action. One of these is broad beans (Vicia faba L.) which also precipitate

headaches, palpitation and hypertensive crises in patients treated with monoamine oxidase inhibitors.[268,269] In this case, the pressor amine responsible for the difficulties is 3,4-dihydroxyphenylalanine (dopa).

The concentration of tyramine in cheese is related to ripening or maturation time, bacterial flora and manufacturing process. Cheddar cheese is reported to contain sufficient tyramine to produce a hypertensive crisis in patients treated with monoamine oxidase inhibitor. Different samples of cheese vary considerably in their tyramine content.[262] Only limited information is available as to the dose of pressor amines that is dangerous for patients being treated with the monoamine oxidase inhibitors. Tyramine is one twentieth to one fiftieth as active as epinephrine in producing hypertension, and it has been proposed that 25 mg of tyramine constitutes a hazard for patients treated with monoamine oxidase inhibitors. On this basis, 4 of 22 samples of cheese approached that value in an average serving of 50 gm. The concentration of tyramine in these cheeses ranged from 0 to 1 mg per gm.[262] Another report suggested that only 6 mg of tyramine by mouth was sufficient to produce a blood pressure increase in patients treated with monoamine oxidase inhibitors. This amount of tyramine could be obtained by ingesting 20 gm of ordinary cheddar cheese or a glass of Chianti wine.[270]

In normal individuals, there is a dramatic rise in the urinary excretion of p-hydroxyphenylacetic acid after eating cheese. This acid is probably derived from tyramine by oxidation with monoamine oxidase and aldehyde oxidase.[136] Unfortunately, this work was not extended to include patients treated with monoamine oxidase inhibitors. It was reported that, in subjects who received one of these inhibitors for two weeks, the concentration of 5-hydroxytryptamine in the brain was twice that of those not receiving the inhibitor.[138]

Lactose and Lactase Deficiency. The intestinal mucosa of man contains a number of disaccharidases, many of which can be influenced by disease or dietary habits.[271,272] Lactase deficiency is the most common of all disaccharidase deficiencies, and, although it occurs in infants, it is also frequently manifested in childhood, adolescence or adulthood.[273] A number of studies have been published concerning lactase intolerance and lactase deficiencies in population groups.[274] In the United States, there is a high prevalence of lactose intolerance among blacks; the reported figure varies between 70 and 95 per cent.[275,276] This compares to an incidence of between 6 and 10 per cent in the white population. On the basis of published reports and documented data, it must be concluded that lactose intolerance and lactase deficiency may be far more widespread among apparently normal subjects than had previously been realized.

Lactase deficiency is not restricted to the United States; it has been reported in virtually every country in the world and is particularly prevalent in South African tribes and in Great Britain, Greece, Asia and India.[277] The clinical manifestations of lactose intolerance are reviewed in Chapter 32B.

Eggs

Eggs often cause allergic disorders in children and in adults; these generally consist of urticaria and asthma.[278] For these people, eggs must therefore be excluded from the diet if the disease syndrome is to be avoided. Egg albumin has many constituents which inhibit trypsin, and a basic protein, avidin, binds biotin, a member of the vitamin B group, and makes it unavailable.[279] In man, those who subsist on a diet low in biotin may conceivably develop a dermatitis if they consume large amounts of raw egg white.

Egg yolks sometimes contain estrogen activity of unknown origin. Eggs from chickens that have been given antibiotics should not be used for human consumption.[280] In addition, pesticides have been detected in eggs.[281] The well-known high concentration of cholesterol in egg yolks may contribute to cardiovascular disease in some human patients, and this is a source of public health concern.

SUMMARY

This chapter assembles data which clearly indicate that, while food is essential to life, it is the most complex chemical mixture to which man and animals are exposed and may contain substances that are harmful when ingested. Whether the substances are natural and native to a particular food or whether they are included as nonintentional additives does not alter their effects on biologic systems. Progress in nutrition, food science technology and toxicology now permits us to consider interactions of nutrients and chemicals as an area of high priority. To identify real or potential problems and to understand interactions may help unravel the enigma of some of our important chronic diseases.

BIBLIOGRAPHY

1. Crampton and Charlesworth: Br. Med. Bull., *31*, 209, 1975.
2. Report of the ARC/MRC Committee on Food and Nutrition Research. London, Her Majesty's Stationery Office, 1974, p. 170.
3. Liener (Ed.): *Toxic Constituents of Plant Foodstuffs.* New York, Academic Press, 1969.
4. Pusztai: Nutr. Abstr. Rev., *37*, 1, 1967.
5. Read and Haas: Cereal Chem., *15*, 59, 1938.
6. Ham and Sandstedt: J. Biol. Chem., *154*, 505, 1944.
7. Mickelsen and Yang: Fed. Proc., *25*, 104, 1966.
8. Osborne and Mendel: J. Biol. Chem., *32*, 369, 1917.
9. Mitchell and Smuts: J. Biol. Chem., *95*, 263, 1932.
10. Barnes and Kwong: J. Nutr., *86*, 245, 1965.
11. Kwong and Barnes: J. Nutr., *81*, 392, 1963.
12. O'Dell and Savage: Proc. Soc. Exp. Biol. Med., *103*, 304, 1960.
13. Oberleas, Muhrer and O'Dell: J. Anim. Sci., *21*, 57, 1962.
14. Forbes: J. Nutr., *82*, 225, 1964.
15. Lease, Barnett, Lease and Turk: J. Nutr., *72*, 66, 1960.
16. McCarrison: Indian J. Med. Res., *21*, 179, 1933.

17. Sharpless, Pearsons and Prato: J. Nutr., *17*, 545, 1939.
18. Halvorson, Zepplin and Hart: J. Nutr., *38*, 115, 1949.
19. Wilgus, Gassner, Patton and Gustavson: Nutrition, *22*, 43, 1941.
20. Van Wyk, Arnold, Wynn and Pepper: Pediatrics, *24*, 752, 1959.
21. Ripp: Am. J. Dis. Child., *102*, 106, 1961.
22. Sarett: Pediatrics, *24*, 855, 1959.
23. Anderson and Howard: Pediatrics, *24*, 854, 1959.
24. Kunitz: J. Gen. Physiol., *30*, 291, 1947.
25. Back and Mamen: Ann. N.Y. Acad. Med., *146*, 361, 1968.
26. Jones, Moore and Stein: Biochemistry, *2*, 66, 1963.
27. Honavar and Sohonie: J. Sci. Ind. Res. (India), *18C*, 202, 1959.
28. Tobishka, J.: *Die Phythamagglutinine*. Berlin, Akademie Verlag, 1964.
29. Stillmark: Arch. Pharmakol. Inst. Dorpat., *3*, 59, 1889.
30. Liener: Am. J. Clin. Nutr., *11*, 281, 1962.
31. Jaffe: *Hemagglutinins and Toxic Constituents of Plant Foodstuffs* (Liener, Ed.). New York, Academic Press, 1969, p. 69.
32. Nowell: Cancer Res., *20*, 462, 1960.
33. Liener and Pallansch: J. Biol. Chem., *197*, 29, 1952.
34. Shepherd: Pediatrics, *24*, 854, 1959.
35. Shepard, Pyne, Kirschvink and McLean: N. Engl. J. Med., *262*, 1099, 1960.
36. Hydovitz: N. Engl. J. Med., *262*, 351, 1960.
37. Strong: Nutr. Rev., *14*, 65, 1956.
38. Gardner and Sakiewicz: Exp. Med. Surg., *21*, 164, 1963.
39. Selye: Rev. Can. Biol., *16*, 1, 1957.
40. Dastur and Iyer: Nutr. Rev., *17*, 33, 1959.
41. Stockman: J. Pharmacol. Exp. Ther., *37*, 43, 1929.
42. Lewis, Fajans, Esterer, Shen and Oliphant: J. Nutr., *36*, 537, 1948.
43. Geiger, Steenbock and Parsons: J. Nutr., *6*, 427, 1933.
44. Ressler, Redstone and Erenberg: Science, *135*, 188, 1961.
45. Ressler: J. Biol. Chem., *237*, 733, 1962.
46. Roy, Nagdrajan and Gopalan: Curr. Sci. (India), *32*, 116, 1963.
47. Murti, Seshadri and Venkitasubramamian: Phytochemistry, *3*, 72, 1964.
48. Adie, Rao and Sarma: Curr. Sci. (India), *32*, 153, 1963.
49. McKay, Lalich, Schilling and Strong: Arch. Biochem. Biophys., *52*, 313, 1954.
50. Duprey and Lee: J. Am. Pharm. Assoc., *43*, 61, 1954.
51. Duprey and Lee: Nutr. Rev., *21*, 28, 1963.
52. Schilling and Strong: J. Am. Chem. Soc., *77*, 2843, 1955.
53. Weaver and Spittel: Proc. Staff Meet. Mayo Clin., *39*, 485, 1964.
54. Zinkham et al.: Bull. J. Hopkins Hosp., *102*, 169, 1958.
55. Beutler: In *The Metabolic Basis of Inherited Disease* (Stanbury, Wyngaarden and Fredrickson, Eds.). New York, McGraw-Hill, 1966.
56. Beutler: Br. Med. J., *2*, 1140, 1965.
57. Iranian Institute Nutrition: First Report of the Symposium on Research Relating to Favism in Iran, Teheran, August, 1965.
58. Lin and Ling: J. Formosan Med. Assoc., *61*, 484, 1962.
59. Lin and Ling: J. Formosan Med. Assoc., *61*, 490, 1962.
60. Lin and Ling: J. Formosan Med. Assoc., *61*, 579, 1962.
61. Bull, Culnenor and Dick: *The Pyrrolizidine Alkaloids*. New York, John Wiley and Sons, 1968.
62. Selzer and Parker: Am. J. Pathol., *27*, 885, 1951.
63. Liener (Ed.): *Toxic Constituents of Plant Foodstuffs*. New York, Academic Press, 1969, p. 408.
64. Newberne and Rogers: Plant Foods for Man, *1*, 23, 1973.
65. Svobody and Reddy: Cancer Res., *32*, 908, 1972.
66. Newberne: Cancer Res., *28*, 2327, 1968.
67. Allen, Chesney and Frazee: Toxicol. Appl. Pharmacol., *23*, 470, 1972.
68. Newberne, Wilson and Rogers: Toxicol. Appl. Pharmacol., *18*, 387, 1971.
69. Rogers and Newberne: Toxicol. Appl. Pharmacol., *18*, 356, 1971.
70. Schoental: Isr. J. Med. Sci., *4*, 1133, 1968.
71. Mattocks: Nature, *232*, 476, 1971.
72. White and Mattocks: Xenobiotica, *1*, 503, 1971.
73. IARC Monograph No. 10, Lyon, France, 1976, p. 333.
74. Shank: In *Trace Substances and Health: A Handbook* (Newberne, Ed.). New York, Marcel Dekker, 1976.
75. Krishnamachari, Nagarajan, Bhat and Tilak: Lancet, *1*, 1061, 1975.
76. Newberne: Environ. Health Perspect., *9*, 23, 1974.
77. WHO Environmental Health Criteria for Mycotoxins, Vol. 1—Aflatoxins, January, 1977, p. 116.
78. Patterson: Food Cosmet. Toxicol., *11*, 287, 1973.
79. Newberne and Rogers: J. Natl. Cancer Inst., *50*, 439, 1973.
80. Newberne, Harrington and Wogan: Lab. Invest., *15*, 962, 1966.
81. Rogers and Newberne: Cancer Res., *29*, 1965, 1969.
82. Rogers and Newberne: Nature, *229*, 62, 1971.
83. Sinnhuber, Wales, Engelirecht and Amend: J. Natl. Cancer Inst., *41*, 711, 1968.
84. Sinnhuber, Lee, Wales, Landers and Keyl: J. Natl. Cancer Inst., *53*, 1285, 1974.
85. Newberne: Cancer Detect. Prevent., *1*, 129, 1976.
86. Hamilton and Harris: Poultry Sci., *50*, 906, 1971.
87. Edds, Nair and Simpson: Am. J. Vet. Res., *34*, 819, 1973.
88. Pier, Heddleston, Cysewkki and Patterson: Avian Dis., *16*, 381, 1972.

89. Thurston, Deyoe, Baetz, Richard and Booth: Am. J. Vet. Res., *35*, 1097, 1974.
90. Purchase and Vorster: S. Afr. Med. J., *42*, 219, 1968.
91. Kiermeier and Mucke: Z. Lebensmit. Untersuch. Forsch., *150*, 137, 1972.
92. Jung and Hanssen: Food Cosmet. Toxicol., *12*, 131, 1974.
93. Alpert, Hutt, Wogan and Davidson: J. Natl. Cancer Inst., *50*, 549, 1973.
94. Campbell, Caedo, Bulatao-Jayne, Salamat and Engel: Nature, *227*, 403, 1970.
95. Peers and Linsell: Br. J. Cancer, *27*, 473, 1973.
96. Shank, Bhamarapravati, Gordon and Wogan: Food Cosmet. Toxicol., *10*, 171, 1972.
97. Van Rensburg, Van der Watt, Purchase, Pereira Coutinho and Markham: S. Afr. Med. J., *48*, 2508, 1974.
98. Shank, Bourgeois, Keschamras and Chandavimol: Food Cosmet. Toxicol., *9*, 501, 1971.
99. Joffe: In *Mycotoxins* (Purchase, Ed.). Amsterdam, Elsevier, 1974.
100. Birmingham, Key, Tubich and Perone: Arch. Dermatol., *83*, 74, 1961.
101. Scheel, Perone, Larkin and Kupel: Biochemistry, *2*, 1127, 1963.
102. Van der Merwe, Scott and Thatcher: J. Chem. Soc., 7083, 1965.
103. Van der Merwe, Steyn, Fourie, Scott and Theron: Nature, *205*, 1112, 1965.
104. Krogh: In *Mycotoxins* (Purchase, Ed.). Amsterdam, Elsevier, 1974.
105. Markovic: Urol. Int., *27*, 130, 1972.
106. Steyn and Holzapfel: J. S. Afr. Chem. Inst., *20*, 186, 1967.
107. Steyn: In *Microbial Toxins*, Vol. VI (Ciegler, Kadias and Ajl, Eds.). New York, Academic Press, 1971, p. 71.
108. Theron, Van der Merwe, Liebenberg, Joubert and Nel: J. Pathol. Bacteriol., *91*, 521, 1966.
109. Nel and Purchase: J. S. Afr. Chem. Inst., *21*, 87, 1968.
110. Pitout: Biochem. Pharmacol., *18*, 485, 1969.
111. Smalley and Strong: In *Mycotoxins* (Purchase, Ed.). Amsterdam, Elsevier, 1974.
112. Smalley: J. Am. Vet. Med. Assoc., *163*, 1278, 1973.
113. Mirocha, Pathre, Schauerhamer and Christensen: Appl. Environ. Microbiol., *32*, 553, 1976.
114. Mirocha and Christensen: Annu. Rev. Phytopathol., *12*, 303, 1974.
115. Stob, Baldwin, Tuite, Andrews and Gillette: Nature, *196*, 1318, 1962.
116. Urry, Wehrmeister, Hodge and Hidy: Tetrahedron Let., *27*, 3109, 1966.
117. Kurtz, Nairn, Nelson, Christensen and Mirocha: Am. J. Vet. Res., *30*, 551, 1969.
118. Bailey, Cox, Morgareide and Taylor: Toxicol. Appl. Pharmacol., *37*, 144, 1976.
119. Greer: Physiol. Rev., *30*, 513, 1950.
120. Van Etten: In *Toxicant Constituents of Plant Foodstuffs* (Liener, Ed.). New York, Academic Press, 1969.
121. Kjaer: In *Comparative Phytochemistry* (Swaine, Ed.). New York, Academic Press, 1966.
122. Clements and Wishart: Metabolism, *5*, 623, 1956.
123. Clements: Med. J. Aust., *2*, 894, 1954.
124. Greer: Borden Rev. Nutr. Res., *21*, 61, 1960.
125. Roche and Lissitsky: *Endemic Goitre*. Geneva, WHO, 1960, p. 351.
126. Peltola and Krusius: Acta Endocrinol., *33*, 603, 1960.
127. Peltola: Acta Endocrinol., *34*, 121, 1960.
128. Kreula and Kiesvaara: Acta Chem. Scand., *13*, 1375, 1959.
129. Virtanen, Kreula and Kiesvaara: Z. Ernährungswiss., Suppl. 3, 23, 1963.
130. Vilkki, Kreula and Piironen: Ann. Acad. Sci. Fenn., *2*, 110, 1962.
131. Perlman: *Toxic Constituents of Plant Foodstuffs*. New York, Academic Press, 1969, p. 319.
132. Fries and Glazer: Allergy, *21*, 169, 1950.
133. Frazer: Adv. Clin. Chem., *5*, 69, 1962.
134. Haas: Am. J. Dis. Child., *28*, 421, 1924.
135. Weijers and Van de Kamer: Am. J. Clin. Nutr., *17*, 51, 1965.
136. Dicke, Weijers and Van de Kamer: Acta Paediatr., *42*, 34, 1953.
137. Weijers, Van de Kamer and Dicke: Adv. Pediatr., *9*, 277, 1957.
138. Van de Kamer and Weijers: Acta Paediatr., *44*, 465, 1955.
139. Weijers and Van de Kamer: Acta Paediatr., *44*, 536, 1955.
140. Weijers and Van de Kamer: Acta Paediatr., *48*, 17, 1959.
141. Messer, Anderson and Hubbard: Gut, *15*, 259, 1964.
142. Frazer: Proc. R. Soc. Med., *49*, 1009, 1956.
143. Heiner, Lahey and Wilson: Am. J. Dig. Dis., *9*, 786, 1964.
144. Pederson, Aimmer, McAllister, Anderson, Wilding and Taylor: Crop Sci., *7*, 349, 1967.
145. Birk: In *Toxicant Constituents of Plant Foodstuffs* (Liener, Ed.). New York, Academic Press, 1969.
146. George: Food Cosmet. Toxicol., *3*, 81, 1965.
147. Preston, Haun, Garvin and Daum: Econ. Bot., *18*, 323, 1964.
148. Tisdall, Drake, Summerfeldt and Jackson: J. Pediatr., *11*, 374, 1937.
149. Kohman: J. Nutr., *18*, 233, 1939.
150. Jeghers and Murphy: N. Engl. J. Med., *233*, 208, 1945.
151. Zarembski and Hodgkinson: Br. J. Nutr., *17*, 627, 1962.
152. Editorial: J.A.M.A., *109*, 1907, 1937.
153. MacKenzie and McCollum: Am. J. Hyg., *25*, 1, 1937.
154. Bonner, Bates, Horton, Hunscher and Macy: J. Pediatr., *12*, 188, 1938.
155. Kalliala and Kauste: Nutr. Abstr. Rev., *35*, 485, 1965.
156. Drach and Maloney: J.A.M.A., *184*, 1047, 1963.
157. Cook and Gates: J. Range Manag., *13*, 97, 1961.
158. Cook and Stoddart: Utah Agric. Exp. Sta. Bull. 364, 1953.
159. Telepatra, Ray and Sen: J. Agric. Sci., *38*, 163, 1948.

160. Sollmann: *Manual of Pharmacology*. Philadelphia, W.B. Saunders, 1948.
161. Valyaseni and Dhanamitta: Am. J. Clin. Nutr., 27, 877, 1974.
162. Leach and Lloyd: Trans. Ophthalmol. Soc. U.K., 76, 453, 1956.
163. Leach and Lloyd: Proc. Nutr. Soc., 15, 15, 1956.
164. Moore: *Vitamin A*. Amsterdam, Elsevier, 1957.
165. Aydelotte: J. Embryol. Exp. Morphol., 11, 279 and 621, 1963.
166. Rodger, Saiduzzafar and Grover: Am. J. Ophthalmol., 50, 309, 1960.
167. Klosterman, Lamoureux and Parsons: Biochemistry, 6, 170, 1967.
168. Deutsch and Hasler: Proc. Soc. Exp. Biol. Med., 53, 63, 1943.
169. Melnick, Hochberg and Oser: J. Nutr., 30, 81, 1945.
170. Jacobsohn and Azevedo: Arch. Biochem., 14, 83, 1947.
171. Hilker and Peter: J. Nutr., 89, 419, 1966.
172. Shewan: In *Fish as Food*, Vol. 2 (Borgstrom, Ed.). New York, Academic Press, 1962.
173. Berlin: Acta Med. Scand., 129, 560, 1948.
174. Kingsbury: *Poisonous Plants of the United States and Canada*. Englewood Cliffs., Prentice-Hall, 1964.
175. Newberne: J. Natl. Cancer Inst., 56, 551, 1976.
176. Pamukcu, Yalciner, Price and Bryan: Cancer Res., 30, 2671, 1970.
177. Kundig and Somogyl: Int. Z. Vitaminforsch., 34, 135, 1964.
178. Fujiwara and Matui: J. Biochem., 40, 427, 1953.
179. Whiting: Econ. Bot., 17, 271, 1963.
180. Campbell, et al.: J. Nutr., 88, 115, 1966.
181. Yang, et al.: J. Nutr., 90, 153, 1966.
182. Laqueur, Mickelsen, Whiting and Kurland: J. Natl. Cancer Inst., 31, 919, 1963.
183. Mickelsen, et al.: Fed. Proc., 23, 1363, 1964.
184. Edwards: J. Bur. Agric. W. Aust., 1, 225, 1894.
185. Mason and Whiting: Fed. Proc., 25, 533, 1966 (abstract).
186. Bell and Vega: Fed. Proc., 26, 322, 1967 (abstract).
187. Nishida, Kobayashi and Nagahama: Bull. Agric. Chem. Soc. Japan, 19, 77, 1955.
188. Riggs: Chem. Ind., 35, 926, 1956.
189. Cooper: J. Proc. R. Soc. (New South Wales), 74, 450, 1941.
190. Nishida, Kobayashi, Nagahama, Kojima and Yamane: Seikagaku (Biochemistry), 28, 218, 1956 (in Japanese).
191. Laqueur: Fed. Proc., 23, 1386, 1964.
192. Magee: *Fourth Conference on the Toxicity of Cycads* (Whiting, Ed.). Bethesda, National Institutes of Health, 1965.
193. Spatz and Laqueur: Fed. Proc., 25, 662, 1966 (abstract).
194. Siegel: J.A.M.A., 236, 473, 1976.
195. Weil: *Ethnopharmacologic Search for Psychoactive Drugs* (Halmstedt and Kline, Eds.). USPHS, Publication 1647, 1967, p. 188.
196. Segelman, Segelman, Karliner and Sofia: J.A.M.A., 236, 477, 1976.
197. Kingsbury: *Poisonous Plants of the United States and Canada*. Englewood Cliffs, Prentice-Hall, 1964, p. 96.
198. Weir and Tyler: J. Am. Pharm. Assoc., 49, 426, 1960.
199. Van der Veer and Farley: Arch. Intern. Med., 55, 773, 1935.
200. Grossman and Malbin: Ann. Intern. Med., 40, 249, 1954.
201. Cann and Verhulst: Am. J. Dis. Child., 101, 127, 1961.
202. Buck: N. Engl. J. Med., 265, 681, 1961.
203. Rose and Rieder: Ann. Intern. Med., 64, 372, 1966.
204. Tyler, Benedict, Brady and Robbers: Pharm. Sci., 55, 590, 1966.
205. Smith: *Mushrooms in Their Natural Habitat*. Portland, Sawyer's Inc., 1949, p. 152.
206. Murrill: Mycologia, 2, 255, 1910.
207. Deerness: Mycologia, 2, 75, 1911.
208. Wieland and Wieland: Pharmacol. Rev., 11, 87, 1959.
209. Grollman: *Pharmacology and Therapeutics*. Philadelphia, Lea & Febiger, 1962.
210. Halstead: *Fish as Food*, Vol. 2 (Borgstrom, Ed.). New York, Academic Press, 1962.
211. Schantz: Ann. N.Y. Acad. Sci., 90, 834, 1960.
212. Schantz, et al.: Biochemistry, 5, 1191, 1966.
213. Kao and Nishiyama: J. Physiol., 180, 50, 1965.
214. Meyer: N. Engl. J. Med., 249, 843, 1953.
215. Burden: Ann. Intern. Med., 43, 1283, 1955.
216. Fenton: In *Practice of Allergy* (Vaughn and Black, Eds.). St. Louis, C.V. Mosby Co., 1948.
217. Cohen: J. Allergy, 30, 267, 1959.
218. Helgebostad and Martinsons: Nature, 181, 1660, 1958.
219. Stout, Oldfield and Adair: J. Nutr., 70, 421, 1960.
220. Gjönnes and Helgebostad: Acta Vet. Scand., 6, 239, 1965.
221. Kolbye: Testimony Subcommittee on Energy, National Resources and the Environment of the Senate Committee on Commerce, May 8, 1970.
222. Irukayama: Kumamoto Med. J., 15, 57, 1962.
223. Katsuna (Ed.): *Minamata Disease*. Study Group of Minamata Disease, Kumamoto University, 1968.
224. Kurland, Faro and Siedler: World Neurol., 1, 370, 1960.
225. Lofroth: Bull. No. 4, Ecological Research Committee, Swedish National Science Research Council, 1969.
226. Johnels and Westermark: In *Chemical Fallout* (Miller and Berg, Eds.). Springfield, Charles C Thomas, 1969, p. 221.
227. Berglund, Berlin and Mirke: *Nord. Hyg. Tidskr. Suppl. 4*. Stockholm, National Institute of Health, 1971.
228. Hunter, Bomford and Russell: Q. J. Med., 33, 193, 1940.
229. Takeuchi: Paper presented at International Conference of Environmental Mercury Contamination, Ann Arbor, 1970.
230. Wallace, Shults, Fulkerson and Lyon: Oak Ridge National Lab.–National Science Foundation Environmental Program, March 1971.

231. Suzuki, Miyama and Katsunuma: Bull. Environ. Contam. Toxicol., 5, 502, 1971.
232. Matsumoto, Koya and Takeuchi: J. Neuropathol. Exp. Neurol., 24, 563, 1965.
233. Korns: Nutr. Today, 7, 21, 1967.
234. Clarkson: Personal communication, 1976.
235. Lisk: New York J. Med., 71, 2541, 1971.
236. Halverson and Monty: J. Nutr. 70, 100, 1960.
237. Harr, Bone, Tinsley, Weswig and Yamamoto: Selenium in Biomedicine (Muth, Ed.). Westport (Conn.), AVI Press, 1967.
238. Underwood: Toxicants Occurring Naturally in Foods, 2nd ed. NAS/NRC, 1973, p. 58.
239. Smith: U.S. Public Health Report, 54, 1441, 1939.
240. Moxion: Science, 88, 81, 1938.
241. Hadjimarkos: Caries Res., 3, 14, 1969.
242. Shawberger and Frost: Can. Med. Assoc. J., 100, 682, 1969.
243. Frost: Fed. Proc., 26, 194, 1967.
244. Bennett and Heyman: Principles of Internal Medicine, 5th ed. (Harrison, et al., Eds.). New York, McGraw-Hill, 1966, p. 1405.
245. Pelfrine: J. Toxicol. Environ. Health, 1, 1003, 1976.
246. Schroeder and Balassa: J. Chronic Dis., 19, 85, 1966.
247. Cantarrow and Trumper: Lead Poisoning. Baltimore, Williams & Wilkins, 1944.
248. Murthy, Rhea and Peeler: J. Dairy Sci., 50, 651, 1967.
249. Kehoe, Cholak and Storey: J. Nutr., 19, 579, 1940.
250. NAS/NRC: Geochemistry of the Environment, Vol. I, 1974, p. 53.
251. Murthy, Rhea and Peeler: Environ. Sci. Technol., 5, 436, 1971.
252. Gleason, Grosselin, Hodge and Smith: Clinical Toxicology of Commercial Products: Acute Poisoning. Baltimore, Williams & Wilkins, 1969.
253. Fassett: Cadmium, Metallic Contaminants and Human Health (Lee, Ed.). New York, Academic Press, 1972.
254. Heyden: J. Chronic Dis., 29, 149, 1976.
255. NAS/NRC: Geochemistry of the Environment, Vol. II, 1977.
256. Nisbet and Sarofim: Environ. Health Perspect, 1, 21, 1972.
257. Kosza, et al.: J. Toxicol. Environ. Health, 1, 689, 1976.
258. Schulte-Hermann: CRC Crit. Rev. Toxicol., 3, 97, 1974.
259. Boyd: Protein Deficiency and Pesticide Toxicity. Springfield, Charles C Thomas, 1972.
260. Wagstaff and Street: Toxicol. Appl. Pharmacol., 19, 10, 1971.
261. Sapieka: Toxic Constituents of Animal Foodstuffs. (Liener, Ed.). New York, Academic Press, 1974, p. 1.
262. Blackwell and Mabbitt: Lancet, 1, 938, 1965.
263. Read and Arora: Lancet, 2, 587, 1963.
264. Mann: Lancet, 2, 639, 1963.
265. Foster: Lancet, 2, 587, 1963.
266. Womack: Lancet, 2, 463, 1963.
267. Blackwell: Lancet, 2, 414, 1963.
268. Blomley: Lancet, 2, 1181, 1964.
269. Hodge, Nye and Emerson: Lancet, 1, 1108, 1964.
270. Horwitz, Lovenberg, Engelman and Sjoerdsma: J.A.M.A., 188, 1108, 1964.
271. Holzel, Schwartz, and Suitcliffe: Lancet, 1, 1126, 1959.
272. Dahlquist: J.A.M.A., 195, 225, 1966.
273. Cook and Kajubi: Lancet, 2, 275, 1966.
274. Huang and Bayless: N. Engl. J. Med., 276, 1283, 1967.
275. Cuatrecasis, Lockwood and Caldwell: Lancet, 1, 14, 1965.
276. Bayless and Rosensweig: J.A.M.A., 197, 968, 1966.
277. Patworden and White: Toxicants Occurring Naturally in Foods, 2nd ed. NAS/NRC, 1973, p. 477.
278. Mansmann: Foods as Antigens and Allergens. NAS/NRC Publication No. 1354, 1966, p. 72.
279. Ambrose: Foods as Antigens and Allergens. NAS/NRC Publication No. 1354, 1966, p. 105.
280. World Health Organization: WHO Research Report Series. 260, 1963.
281. Dunache and Fletcher: Nature, 212, 1062, 1966.

Chapter *13*

EFFECT OF PROCESSING ON THE NUTRITIONAL VALUES OF FOODS

Benjamin Borenstein

The interest in nutrient stability during food processing has concentrated on vitamins on the assumption that many of the vitamins can be seriously depleted by leaching, heat degradation, light and oxidation. Although this assumption is valid, food processing per se in most cases does not significantly decrease the nutritional value of foods with respect to vitamins, minerals, proteins or fats. This does not mean, however, that food composition handbook values for fresh foods can be used to calculate the nutrient content of diets or that the food supply is liberal in all nutrients.

Storage of fresh vegetables can cause degradation of vitamin C and handbook values used to estimate nutrient contents of foods and diets do not usually take storage losses or home preparation losses into account. The effect of home preparation procedures on vitamin C was summarized by Harris:[1]

> Fifty-three per cent of ascorbic acid in cole slaw was lost in two hours when vinegar was used on cole slaw. Cucumbers lost 22 per cent ascorbic acid during slicing, 33–35 per cent during standing for one hour and 41 per cent to 49 per cent during standing for three hours. Cucumber salads lost 33 per cent in the same period, while tomato salads lost 8 per cent. Cantaloupe slices lost 35 per cent ascorbic acid during 24 hours of refrigeration. Orange juice held at 48°F lost 17 per cent thiamine in 24 hours.

The above losses are atypically high for most nutrients but indicate the difficulty in calculating the actual nutrient content of diets. With some reservations, a generalization can be made that minerals, carbohydrates, lipids, protein, vitamin K, and niacin are stable ($\geq$ 85 per cent retention) during processing and storage of foods. Vitamins A, D, E, B_6, B_{12}, riboflavin, pantothenic acid and folacin may be somewhat less stable and thiamin and ascorbic acid are most likely to be seriously depleted by processing, storage and home preparation of foods.

Losses in nutritive value of foods are greater, in many cases, during final preparation in institutions and homes than during commercial processing and storage. These losses are caused both by destruction of the more labile vitamins and by leaching of water-soluble compounds. Leaching of stable vitamins can be as significant as destruction, and this problem is exacerbated by lengthy cooking and holding times in institutional feeding.[2] The importance of institutional feeding to nutritional status is growing with the increase in fast food establishments, school feeding, nursing homes and day-care centers. An extreme example of undesirable food preparation resulted in one of the earliest cases of diagnosed folacin deficiency in man.[3] In this case, an individual subsisting on restaurant hamburgers, doughnuts and coffee had megaloblastic anemia definitely traced to folacin deficiency. The hamburgers were thin and kept on a hot plate for several hours prior to consumption and had little residual folate.

VITAMINS

The most significant vitamin losses in food processing occur during the milling of wheat to 70 to 75 per cent extraction white flour. These are mechanical separation losses rather than destruction and are approximately 70 to 80 per cent for thiamin, riboflavin, niacin, vitamin B_6 and other nutrients.

Ascorbic Acid

As mentioned earlier, handbook values for the vitamin content of foods must be viewed with a critical eye. Mashed potatoes are a potentially good source of vitamin C, but dehydrated potato flakes reconstituted and held on a steam table for an hour have no residual C activity. Canned and frozen concentrated orange juices are a good source of vitamin C, but pasteurized orange juice packaged in milk cartons is a variable and possibly poor source of C. Actual assays of the latter indicated 18 to 35 mg per 100 gm[4] as compared to the USDA Handbook #8 value of 50 mg per 100 gm.[5]

The lack of ranges in handbooks can be misleading. USDA Handbook #8 reports an average of 16 mg vitamin C per 100 gm of canned tomato juice,[5] but a study in 1971 of 130 samples from canneries around the country reported an actual range of 1 to 25 mg per 100 gm with a mean of 13.4 mg per 100 gm.[6] In a recent report the Kirk group studied the kinetics of ascorbic acid degradation in tomato juice as a function of temperature, pH and copper concentration and evolved a mathematical model to predict ascorbic stability in tomato juice.[7]

Ascorbic acid is a moderately strong reducing agent (redox potential +0.127 v at pH 5), hence, it is readily oxidized during food processing and storage. Copper and iron are effective oxidation catalysts at levels as low as 0.5 ppm. At food concen-

trations, stability is superior at pH 3 to 5 to that at pH 6 to 7. Ascorbic acid is more stable in concentrated solutions under anaerobic conditions and the pH optimum is closer to neutrality. It reacts readily with anthocyanin pigments which occur widely in fruits and vegetables. Prune juice which contains both high iron and anthocyanins exhibits poor vitamin C stability.

Thiamin

As stated earlier, ascorbic acid and thiamin are the most unstable vitamins during processing. Thiamin is more stable than thiamin pyrophosphate, the form which may account for over 50 per cent of the native vitamin in specific foods. Thiamin is readily degraded in neutral and alkaline solutions even at low temperatures, so stability in high pH foods is poor. Therefore, it is completely degraded in chocolate cake (pH 8.0) compared to 75 to 80 per cent retention in white bread (pH 5.8). Sulfite used in food processing can split thiamin into its pyrimidine and thiazole constituents. For this reason the USDA does not permit use of sulfite in meat products. The sensitivity of thiamin to sulfite is shown by the comparative losses when cabbage is blanched with and without sulfite—45 and 15 per cent respectively.[8]

Brine grading and blanching of green baby lima beans prior to freezing cause thiamin losses of 20 to 65 per cent, depending on variety, year and other factors. Canned vegetables and fruits stored for one year at 65°F show low losses of thiamin; at 80°F losses are 15 to 25 per cent.[9] Thiamin and other water solubles are distributed between the solids and liquid in canned vegetables. The liquid generally contains approximately 30 per cent of the available thiamin.

Retention of thiamin in cooked and processed meats ranges from 40 per cent for irradiation products to about 85 per cent for mild cured products. Cooking meat under home preparation conditions produces variable results; retention of 40 to 100 per cent has been reported. Roasting temperature of beef and pork is a significant variable. High oven temperature decreases retention—62 per cent retention at low temperature versus 51 per cent at high temperature. This subject is well reviewed by LaChance and Erdman.[10]

A 3-year freezer-storage study on thiamin, riboflavin and niacin in beef indicated that stability depends on prefreezing aging treatment, but the vitamins were essentially stable.

Cow's milk contains approximately 0.4 mg per liter total vitamin B_1 activity, 50 to 70 per cent as thiamin plus thiamin pyrophosphate (cocarboxylase) and protein-bound thiamin. Ten per cent of the thiamin is destroyed during pasteurization and 30 per cent or more in heat processing evaporated milk. High-temperature short-time pasteurization decreases thiamin content only 3 to 4 per cent. Spray-dried milk powder has minimal losses of 5 to 15 per cent.

Riboflavin

This vitamin is heat stable in acid solution and in the presence of mild oxidizing agents, but it is very sensitive to light, particularly at neutral and alkaline pH. In neutral solution it is moderately heat stable. Its retention (75 to 90 per cent) during brine grading and blanching of lima beans is superior to and less variable than that of thiamin.[11] Retention in blanched cabbage was 80 per cent and losses during cabbage dehydration were negligible. Riboflavin is stable in the processing and cooking of meat (approximately 90 per cent retention). Roasting beef and pork results in retention of 70 to 90 per cent if the drippings are discarded. The drippings contain 15 to 20 per cent of the original vitamin. Although the vitamin is light sensitive, it is important to note that it is stable in white bread wrapped in clear cellophane. It is stable in home cooking procedures.

Pasteurization and sterilization of milk cause less than 10 per cent degradation in milk products. Light exposure of fluid milk can cause losses of 20 to 80 per cent in two hours, depending on temperature, surface area exposed and light intensity. Fluorescent light is less harmful than sunlight.[12] The greatest destruction is caused by light in the range of 420 to 560 nm.

Niacin

This is the most stable vitamin. It has excellent heat and light stability in the entire pH range of foods. It should be remembered, however, that niacin leaches readily in blanching and washing operations and is thus reduced both in frozen and canned vegetables. It can be enzymatically degraded in aging meats.

Vitamin B_6

Pyridoxine is stable to heat in acidic and alkaline solutions, but is light sensitive at $pH \geq 6.0$. Pyridoxal, a major form in milk and other foods, is heat labile. Vitamin B_6 retention in cooking meat ranges from 45 to 80 per cent. There is 20 to 30 per cent destruction in cooking vegetables, and similar loss in canning. In milling wheat, 75 to 90 per cent of the vitamin B_6 is lost.[14] Bread baking losses range from 1 to 17 per cent. Vitamin B_6 is stable during milk pasteurization and during manufacture and storage of milk powder. Canned evaporated milk retains 50 to 65 per cent of its initial content during heat processing. Sweetened condensed milk, which has a milder heat treatment, retains about 80 per cent. Vitamin B_6 in milk is light sensitive, with 21 per cent loss after eight hours in sunlight.

Pantothenic Acid

This is stable at pH 5 to 7, but is more heat sensitive at pH 3 to 4. It occurs widely in foods primarily as coenzyme A, a conjugated nucleotide. Although the available data suggest it is one of the most unstable vitamins in food processing and storage, the data base is inadequate. Blanching of baby green lima beans preceded by brine grading causes losses of 27 to 35 per cent. Pantothenic acid is stable to home cooking procedures in the preparation of frozen lima beans, with 90 per cent retention with cooking in a minimum of water and 70 per cent retention in an excess of water. Roasting meat causes degradation of only 7 to 10 per cent pantothenic acid, but the meat drippings contain 20 to 25 per cent of the original content. Cooking rice causes some leaching or destruction.

Vitamin A

This vitamin and its precursors occur in animal source foods primarily as retinyl palmitate and as provitamin A carotenoids in plant products. Beta-carotene is the most important indigenous provitamin A carotenoid because of its relatively good conversion and widespread occurrence in foods. In plant products, the carotenoids are either complexed with proteins or are in solution or colloidal dispersion in lipoid chromoplasts. They are reasonably stable in almost all food products and processes, but a notable exception is dehydrated foods exposed to air. Freeze-dried carrots bleach completely to white on air exposure for 1 to 2 weeks. Extended cooking of green, yellow and red vegetables causes cis-trans isomerization of both beta- and alpha-carotene. The cis isomers have lower biologic values than the trans and, hence, processing can lower the provitamin A biologic value (green vegetables 15 to 20 per cent reduction, yellow and red vegetables 30 to 35 per cent).[15] Conversely, cooking of high-fiber foods, e.g. carrots, probably increases absorption of carotenes. The total net effect of processing on the provitamin A value of vegetable products— negative effect of cis-trans isomerization plus positive effect of increased absorption of carotenes—is not known.

Vitamin A_1 occurs in marine fish-liver oils, in the livers of most land vertebrates and in butter fat and eggs. Vitamin A_2 (containing two double bonds in the ionone ring) occurs only in fresh-water fish oils. Frying calf or chicken liver causes vitamin A losses of 10 to 20 per cent. Sunlight rapidly destroys the vitamin A in whole milk in clear glass containers.[16]

Folacin

The stability of folacin is affected by the conjugate form present in foods. The mono-glutamate (unconjugated) form is moderately heat stable in acid solution and at neutrality. The tri- and hepta-glutamate conjugates are heat unstable. Free folic acid is stable during milk pasteurization. Boiling milk for 5 seconds decreases free folic acid activity 40 to 90 per cent. Native total folacin levels are about the same in baked bread as in the initial dough mix.[17] This is because folacin increases during dough proofing by yeast synthesis and approximately the same amount is destroyed during baking. Added free folic losses average about 10 per cent during different bread-baking procedures.[17] Thin hamburgers held warm for several hours have little residual folate. Folacin is stabilized by ascorbate and destruction is catalyzed by copper.

Vitamin B_{12}

Vitamin B_{12} has moderate to good heat stability at pH 4 to 5. Retorting at high pH causes rapid destruction, as does exposure to light. Pasteurizing milk has no effect on B_{12} content. Evaporated milk has losses of 70 to 90 per cent, and spray-dried milk losses of 20 to 35 per cent. Ferrous salts catalyze destruction.

There is a current controversy on the possible effect of consuming 0.5- to 1.0-gm quantities of ascorbic acid with meals on the stability of the B_{12} contained in the meals. The Herbert group reported that megadoses of vitamin C may destroy substantial amounts of vitamin B_{12} in food.[18] Other researchers believe this is an analytic problem caused by inadequate B_{12} extraction during analysis of B_{12} rather than by degradation in the GI tract.[19] A more recent report by Herbert et al.[19a] indicates that destruction of serum B_{12} can occur during the heating step in analysis because of high serum ascorbate levels and that destruction is prevented by the addition of KCN.

Biotin

While there are little data on biotin stability in foods, all evidence indicates good stability. Evaporated and powdered milk incur losses of 10 to 15 per cent during processing. Biotin is stable during home cooking of frozen baby lima beans and does not leach in cooking water. In nature, biotin is usually bound. A protein complex, avidin, occurring in egg whites reacts with and inactivates biotin. Avidin is denatured by heat so that cooked egg white is not a biotin antivitamin.

Other Fat-soluble Vitamins

Vitamin D is sensitive to both oxygen and light. Analysis of D compounds is quite difficult at food occurrence levels and conclusions about D stability require replicate assays. *Vitamin K* compounds are light sensitive. Vitamin K_1, which occurs in green plants, is the predominant form in foodstuffs. *Alpha-tocopherol*, the most important tocopherol with respect to vitamin E activity, is an effective fat phase antioxidant and can oxidize readily. Oxidation is catalyzed by very low levels of copper. Bunnell et al.[20] reported the alpha-tocopherol and total tocopherol contents of a wide variety of foods and showed that the ordinary processes used in preparing foods for the table do not involve large losses. However, these authors found significant losses of tocopherol during the storage of foods which had been cooked in vegetable oil. High losses occurred in a relatively short time even during freezer storage at $-12°C$. The researchers also found almost complete loss of the tocopherols in various cooking oils heated to high temperature. Vegetable oils are the major dietary sources of vitamin E, and it is important that oil refiners monitor and minimize vitamin E losses during refining steps.

MINERALS

The literature on the effects of processing and home preparation on minerals in food is sparse. The two major theoretical results are changes in bioavailability and leaching of water solubles, but little specific information is available.

Intestinal tract absorption of minerals depends on the oxidation state of the cation, whether the cation is bound to organic compounds, the type of binding and the type of anions present in the food and in the GI tract during digestion. Insoluble compounds such as iron phytates and iron oxalates are poorly absorbed. Zinc in cow's milk is bound to high-molecular-weight protein fractions. In contrast, zinc in human milk is bound to low-molecular-weight fractions and has greater bioavailability than that in cow's milk as measured by treatment of infants with acrodermatitis enteropathica, a genetic disease causing zinc deficiency.[21]

One study revealed that the processing of raw peanuts into peanut butter resulted in the following mineral losses: calcium 3 per cent, magnesium 6 per cent, iron 19 per cent, copper 10 per cent, zinc 12 per cent.[22]

The cooking water of legumes contains measurable amounts of all studied minerals—calcium, copper, iron, magnesium, phosphorus, potassium, sodium and zinc—and surprisingly high amounts of magnesium, phosphorus and potassium, but the data indicating this are presented in a manner that the per cent of leaching cannot be determined.[23]

Iron

Oxidation of ferrous to ferric iron during bread baking would decrease iron bioavailability, but most of the work on this subject is on enriched bread and the effects on native iron have not been thoroughly determined. In one study, iron in unenriched dough was present in both the ferrous and ferric states and baking resulted in the oxidation of ferrous iron to ferric.[24] Only 2 per cent of the iron in spinach is absorbed by man because it is present primarily as insoluble oxalates. There are no data which demonstrate the effect of processing or cooking on iron absorption from spinach.

Hodson reported that in canned liquid-formula diet iron absorption was increased by product storage.[25] He found that ferric orthophosphate, which was the preferred iron source organoleptically, was dissolved and reduced to the ferrous state during 2 to 5 months of storage. He concluded the product had the high absorption characteristics attributed to the ferrous ion even though it was fortified with ferric orthophosphate, which is poorly absorbed.

PROTEIN AND AMINO ACIDS

The amino acid content of a protein need not quantitatively reflect its nutritive value since the limiting step in the utilization of certain proteins is their digestibility. Processing can both increase and decrease digestibility of protein. Heat-induced denaturation can increase the ease with which the protein is hydrolyzed by intestinal tract proteases, but heat can also degrade protein quality and block the epsilon amino group of lysine in intact protein, thus preventing hydrolysis by trypsin.

Another factor in the case of certain seed proteins—lima beans, soybeans and black-eyed peas—is the occurrence of trypsin inhibitors. These are generally inactivated by mild heat treatment, resulting in higher protein utilization.

A new area of research is the study of lysinoalanine, which forms in proteins subjected to alkali treatment. This compound, which is not hydrolyzed, is believed to cause severe growth retardation and may occur in processed protein products other than those treated with alkali. It had a nephrotoxic effect when fed to rats in one study but additional work is necessary.[26] Alkaline treatment of corn to prepare tortilla flour and hominy resulted in approximately 15 per cent losses of arginine and cystine and both laboratory-prepared and commercial tortillas contained lysinoalanine.[26a] The degradation of arginine and cystine presumably caused a loss in protein quality, although this was not measured.

The significance of this loss in protein quality to an individual consumer must be evaluated in context with the fact that alkaline treatment of corn increases the bioavailability of the bound niacin which would otherwise not be nutritionally available. To early Central American Indian tribes subsisting largely on lime-treated corn, the release of bound niacin may have been essential to survival.

In addition, food storage may decrease protein quality by the nonenzymatic browning reaction of reducing sugars with protein,[27] but it is difficult to evaluate the practical significance of this reaction in foods. Potato protein contains satisfactory ratios of the nutritionally limiting amino acids in most human diets—lysine, threonine, tryptophan and methionine. Theoretically, therefore, potato chips with a 5 per cent protein content may be a good protein source, but there are no data on the effects of frying and browning reactions on the quality of potato chip protein.

The protein quality of biscuits supplemented with milk powder before baking is considerably lower than that of biscuits plus unbaked milk powder, apparently because lysine incorporated in the milk powder protein becomes less biologically available upon baking. Analysis of protein hydrolysates of bread indicated that lysine, phenylalanine, tyrosine and serine were degraded 5 to 17 per cent during baking.[28]

One study indicated that lysine was 18 per cent more available in soy meal than in meal further processed into soy isolate.[29]

This substantiates the need for processors to monitor protein quality as they develop new soy analogs. Another study[30] concluded that heating commercially available soy isolates increased their protein efficiency ratio values and they were better substrates for enzymatic hydrolysis. Heating a mixture of protein isolate and glucose decreased the protein efficiency ratio to 0.87, compared with 0.95 for the unheated mixture. Supplementation of soy isolate with methionine after the heat treatment increased the level of liver glutamic-oxalacetic transaminase, indicating that methionine is a limiting amino acid in the heated isolate for the rat.

FAT

Vegetable oil refining, i.e. removal of free fatty acids, bleaching and deodorization, almost completely removes the carotenes and reduces the tocopherols in oils. The tocopherol losses are minimal under proper processing conditions. These losses do not affect the quality of the triglycerides per se. Hydrogenation of oils to produce a variety of products with improved oxidative stability and the desired firmness for shortenings and margarine decreases the essential fatty acid content of these products, both by reduction and positional and geometric isomerization of linoleic and linolenic acids. Hydrogenation also causes the reduction of linoleic acid to trans-oleic (elaidic) acid, which does not occur naturally in vegetable oils. Cow's milk fat contains about 8 per cent trans acids and ruminant animal fats contain about 5 to 10 per cent trans acids.

Although hydrogenation is controlled by processors to minimize isomerization and formation of elaidic acid, its consequences still need review. Formation of elaidic acid can be circumvented in some products by blending unhydrogenated oil with highly hydrogenated fat (containing little trans acids) and then interesterifying to produce the desired physical properties for shortening or margarine.[31] The resulting blend contains high levels of polyunsaturated fatty acids and low levels of trans fatty acids.

Trans fatty acids are metabolized completely by rats and there is no good experimental evidence of any harmful effects. In one major study 46 generations of rats were maintained with no adverse effects on a diet in which the sole source of fat was a hydrogenated margarine fat containing 7 per cent cis-9, cis-12-linoleic acid, 3 per cent isomers of linoleic acid and 35 per cent elaidic acid.[32] In more recent work the emphasis has been on rate of metabolism of trans versus cis acids and on comparative distribution in tissues. In rabbits dietary elaidic acid is incorporated into all serum lipid and lipoprotein fractions and into adipose tissue. In the serum the triglycerides contain the greatest amount of elaidic acid, followed by the phospholipids; cholesterol esters contain the least. The triglycerides of high-density lipoproteins contain less elaidic acid than the triglycerides of the other lipoproteins. Adipose tissue contains a high level of elaidic acid, possibly at the expense of oleic acid. More linoleic acid is incorporated in the serum phospholipids and the serum cholesterol esters of the trans-acid-fed rabbits.[33] Although these differences indicate that elaidic acid is not necessarily the metabolic equivalent of oleic acid, there is no indication of a biologic effect. Similarly, there is evidence that positional isomers of oleic acid (cis-Δ 9) are metabolized at a different rate from oleic acid as measured by comparative incorporation into egg lipids when the compounds are fed to laying hens.[34] No information is available on the significance of these rate differences.

It is generally agreed that three types of degradation changes can occur in fats and oils: (1) autoxidation (temperature up to 100°C), (2) thermal polymerization (200 to 300°) and (3) thermal oxidation (~200° with air). Many published nutrition studies on the effects of heated fats are based on findings with severely treated oils atypical of commercial and consumer practice. Such work is not of practical significance since such severely damaged oil is not consumed in the diet.[35] The main symptoms observed in animal feeding experiments after ingestion of such overheated fats are decreased absorption of the fats and unsaturated fatty acids, growth depression which may be related to decreased food intake, decreased food efficiency, decreased motility of the GI tract, disturbances in chylomicron formation, enlarged livers and kidneys and reduced fat stores of the body.[35]

Many decomposition products of severely heated fats have been isolated and identified. In one study cottonseed oil was kept at 182°C for six 8-hour periods. After conversion to methyl esters, the distillable non-urea adductable fraction (DNUA) was separated into 136 components. Esters of alicyclic fatty acids made up 34 per cent of the characterized material. These cyclic materials are probably responsible for the toxic effects seen when DNUA is isolated and fed to rats.[36]

Heating corn oil, cottonseed oil, safflower oil and shortening for 7.5 hours to fry potatoes caused linoleic acid losses of 4 to 11 per cent.[37] Oxidative rancidity results in a gradual loss of essential fatty acid activity in a fat and also an increase in the concentration of fatty acid peroxides which may be more or less toxic, accompanied by destruction of carotenoids, vitamin A, tocopherols and vitamin E. Such oxidation may occur at any stage of storage, processing or use of fats and oils. It also causes rancidity, so that the consumer is not likely to consume badly oxidized fat.

Thermal polymers, however, cannot be readily tasted, and any process in which thermal polymerization is suspected should be thoroughly checked. A significant drop in the iodine value of fats and oils occurs with thermal polymerization. It is therefore easy for a processor to monitor potential polymerization by measuring the iodine value. This is not currently feasible for individual fast food restaurants, and additional work is necessary in this area of food supply.

Highly unsaturated oils have a shorter shelf-life during home storage than do products such as olive oil and cottonseed oil. Tocopherols are vegetable oils' natural antioxidants. Animal fats contain very low tocopherol levels and may have a short oxidative shelf-life even though they have low unsaturated fatty acid levels.

BIBLIOGRAPHY

1. Harris: In *Nutritional Evaluation of Food Processing* (Harris and Von Loesecks, Eds.). New York, John Wiley & Sons, 1960.
2. Ang, et al.: J. Food Sci., *40*, 997, 1975.
3. Zalusky and Herbert: N. Engl. J. Med., *265*, 1033, 1961.
4. Borenstein: Unpublished material.
5. Watt and Merrill: *Composition of Foods*. Agriculture Handbook No. 8. Washington, USDA, 1963.
6. Farrow, et al.: *Nutritive Value of Canned Tomato Juice*. Berkeley, National Canners Assoc. Western Regional Lab., 1971.
7. Lee, et al.: J. Food Sci., *42*, 640, 1977.
8. Mallette, et al.: Ind. Eng. Chem., *38*, 437, 1946.
9. Sheft, et al.: Ind. Eng. Chem., *41*, 144, 1949.
10. LaChance and Erdman: In *Nutritional Evaluation of Food Processing* (Harris and Karmas, Eds.). Westport (Conn.), Avi Publishing Company, 1975.
11. Cook, Gunning and Uchimoto: J. Agric. Food Chem., *9*, 316, 1961.
12. Sattar and de Man: J. Can. Inst. Food Sci. Technol., *6*, 170, 1973.
13. Lushbough, et al.: J. Nutr., *67*, 45, 1959.
14. Polansky and Toepfer: Cereal Chem., *46*, 664, 1969.
15. Sweeney and Marsh: J. Am. Diet. Assoc., *59*, 238, 1971.
16. Thompson and Erdody: J. Inst. Can. Sci. Technol. Aliment., *7*, 157, 1974.
17. Keagy, Stokstad and Fellers: Cereal Chem., *52*, 348, 1975.
18. Herbert and Jacob: J.A.M.A., *230*, 241, 1974.
19. Newmark, et al.: Am. J. Clin. Nutr., *29*, 645, 1976.
19a. Herbert, et al.: Am. J. Clin. Nutr., *31*, 253, 1978.
20. Bunnell, et al.: Am. J. Clin. Nutr., *17*, 1, 1965.
21. Eckhert, et al.: Science, *195*, 789, 1977.
22. Galvao, Lopez and Williams: J. Food Sci., *41*, 1305, 1976.
23. Meiners, et al.: J. Agric. Food Chem., *24*, 1126, 1975.
24. Windle, Nimmo and Lew: Cereal Chem., *53*, 671, 1976.
25. Hodson: J. Agric. Food Chem., *18*, 946, 1970.

26. Woodward, et al.: Food Cosmet. Toxicol., *15*, 109, 1977.
26a. Sanderson, et al.: Cereal Chem., *55*, 204, 1978.
27. Schnickels, Warmbier and Labuza: J. Agric. Food Chem., *24*, 901, 1976.
28. McDermott and Pace: Br. J. Nutr., *11*, 446, 1957.
29. Sarwar, Shannon and Bowland: J. Inst. Can. Sci. Technol. Aliment., *8*, 137, 1975.
30. Shemer and Perkins: J. Nutr., *104*, 1389, 1974.
31. Melnick and Gooding: U.S. Patent 2, 921, 855, January 19, 1960.
32. Alfin-Slater, et al.: J. Nutr., *63*, 241, 1957.
33. Schrock and Conner: Am. J. Clin. Nutr., *28*, 1020, 1975.
34. Mounts: Lipids, *11*, 676, 1976.
35. Perkins: Rev. Fr. Corp., Gras, *23*, 313, 1976.
36. Artman and Smith: J. Am. Oil Chem. Soc., *49*, 318, 1972.
37. Kilgore and Bailey: J. Am. Diet. Assoc., *56*, 130, 1970.

Chapter 14

CHEMICAL ADDITIVES IN FOODS

Bernard L. Oser

Many factors have contributed to the radical changes in the food consumption pattern of the American public in this modern age of urbanization. The grocery store has given way to the self-service supermarket with its vast array of packaged and frozen foods, household servants and cooks have virtually disappeared and women are increasingly finding employment outside the home. More and more meals are eaten in restaurants and fast-food establishments, and food preparation has become centralized in industrial and institutional kitchens.

As a consequence, the responsibility for the processing and packaging of wholesome, nutritious and palatable foods of uniform and stable composition, of good keeping quality throughout the channels of distribution, and convenient to store and prepare, has fallen largely upon scientists and technologists associated with the food industries. To achieve these objectives and to maintain quality control and assurance require a high degree of technologic skill and, inevitably, the judicious use of chemicals.

Scientists are well aware of the fact that all natural foods are complex mixtures of chemicals, many of which can be demonstrated to be toxic in excessive dosage. The deliberate addition of chemicals to food, however, is often looked upon with concern by the laity. It is not surprising, therefore, that strict legislative controls be adopted to ensure protection of the public health. Even such traditional methods of chemical preservation as the use of s[...] smoke and spices have come under regu[...] tory scrutiny in the light of mode[...] methods for the toxicologic assessment[...] safety.

The avenues by which chemicals n[...] enter the food supply are best illustra[...] by the definition of food additives in [...] federal Food, Drug and Cosmetic Act:

> . . . any substance the intended use of wh[...] results or may reasonably be expected to res[...] directly or indirectly, in its becoming a com[...] nent or otherwise affecting the characteris[...] of any food (including any substance inten[...] for use in producing, manufacturing, pack[...] processing, preparing, treating, packag[...] transporting, or holding food; and includ[...] any source of radiation intended for any s[...] use . . . .[1]

Under the law, all such additives must[...] safe for use, including several classes[...] substances exempt from certain of [...] regulatory requirements for prior [...] proval as defined in the Act. In [...] broadest sense a food additive is intend[...] either to introduce some desired or ess[...] tial characteristic in or on the food itself[...] to facilitate its production, processing[...] distribution. The benefit or functio[...] values of the manifold uses of food [...] ditives may be classified as

1. Nutritional, including the enhancem[...] and/or stabilization of nutrients.
2. Technologic, including the use of chem[...] to affect pH adjustment, emulsificat[...] rheologic properties, etc.
3. Sensory, to impart or improve organole[...] qualities and increase acceptability[...] esthetic appeal.

4. Economic, to prevent or reduce waste and spoilage due to bacterial or fungal infestation, enzymatic fermentation and putrefaction.
5. Utilitarian, to facilitate convenience in converting the commercial, industrially produced item to the ready-to-serve food.

The statutory definition includes not only substances introduced intentionally into food to achieve desired purposes but those which become components of foods indirectly and unintentionally, such as through contact with equipment or containers. It is imperative to recognize that incidental or accidental chemical contaminants are not food additives. In rare cases, where some degree of contamination is unavoidable, tolerances or guidelines have been established limiting their presence in foods.

Examples are mercury in fish, lead in evaporated milk and aflatoxin in peanuts. Major sources of indirect additives are metallic, paper or plastic containers, or packaging materials, the surfaces of which come into direct contact with food but are not intended to have any effect in or on the food itself. Under federal law, additives to food are not permitted if their use is unsafe, deceptive or not in accord with good manufacturing practice. The legal definition makes no distinction between natural substances, such as spices and essential oils, and synthetic chemicals, even though the latter may be identical in composition with naturally occurring substances.

The basic purpose of the food additive amendment to the Food, Drug and Cosmetic Act is to require approval by the Food and Drug Administration of the evidence establishing the safety of use of a food chemical prior to introduction into the channels of interstate commerce. Several classes of substances, as indicated above, are not included in the category of food additives as defined in the statute, because their regulatory control is exercised under other sections of the Act. For example, to the extent that pesticide chemicals are used in production, storage and transportation of raw agricultural commodities, they are defined as "economic poisons" under the federal Insecticide, Fungicide and Rodenticide Act.[2] Pesticide residues present in processed foods as ready to eat, at levels not greater than those permitted in the raw agricultural commodities, are exempt from the legally defined category of food additives. However, when the concentration of a pesticide residue in a processed food exceeds the tolerance set for the raw agricultural commodity, the food is adulterated unless it conforms to a specific food additive regulation. A similar exemption applies in the case of a dye, pigment or other coloring substance, provided that, when added or applied to a food, it conforms to the color additive regulations prescribed for its safe use.

The legal definition of food additives excludes substances used in accordance with sanctions or approvals granted prior to enactment of the food additives amendment. This exemption covers substances permitted in foods under definitions and standards of identity established by the Food and Drug Administration and those permitted by the Department of Agriculture under the Poultry Products Inspection Act or the Meat Inspection Act. Also included under the "prior sanction" exemption are substances granted specific approval for use by the FDA through direct communication with individual firms before enactment of the food additives amendment.

The major category of substances not encompassed under the food additives definition is that of those deemed to be generally recognized as safe (GRAS) under the conditions of intended use, in the judgment of scientists qualified by training and experience to evaluate food safety. The law provides that these scientists base their assessments upon scientific procedures or, in the case of substances used prior to 1958, upon "experience based on common use in food." "'Scientific procedures' include those human, animal, analytical, and other scientific studies, whether published or unpublished, appropriate to establish the safety of a substance."[3] The necessary expertise has been described as encompassing sufficient training and experience in biology, medicine, pharmacology, physiology, toxicology, veterinary medicine or other appropriate science to recognize and evaluate the behavior and effects of chemical substances in the diet of man and of animals. General recognition of safety is not the prerogative of any special group of scientists, in government or out, so long as these qualifications are met. For example, the Flavor and Extract Manufacturers' Association has published long lists of substances used in food flavors which a panel of independent scientists has evaluated as GRAS.[4,5]

Publication of a "complete" GRAS list by the Food and Drug Administration is not mandatory. Shortly after enactment of the food additives amendment, the Food and Drug Administration promulgated a partial list of substances and their respective uses for review by appropriately qualified scientists. This was eventually published (and dubbed the "white list") as Section 121.101 (now recoded as Part 182) of the Code of Federal Regulations.[6] In accordance with the recommendation made at the White House Conference on Food, Nutrition and Health in 1969, this GRAS list, as well as other substances believed to have prior sanction, is being reviewed at the present writing from the standpoint of current usage and criteria for safety evaluation. When the review and assessment will have been completed, it is expected that a revised GRAS list will be published by the Food and Drug Administration and substances not included thereon either will be subject to specific food additive regulations or will be dropped from use.

In accordance with a pronouncement of the Food and Drug Administration, certain restrictions have been imposed on the eligibility of substances for classification as GRAS.[7] The following criteria have been adopted:

1. Any substance of natural biological origin that has been widely consumed for its nutrient properties in the United States prior to January 1, 1958, without known detrimental effect, for which no health hazard is known, and which has been modified by processes first introduced into commercial use after January 1, 1958, which may reasonably be expected significantly to alter the composition of the substance.

2. Any substance of natural biological origin that has been widely consumed for its nutrient properties in the United States prior to January 1, 1958, without known detrimental effect, for which no health hazard is known, that has had significant alteration of composition by breeding or selection after January 1, 1958, where the change may be reasonably expected to alter the nutritive value or the concentration of toxic constituents.

3. Distillates, isolates, extracts, and concentration (sic) of extracts of GRAS substances.

4. Reaction products of GRAS substances.

5. Substances not of a natural biological origin, including those for which evidence is offered that they are identical to a GRAS counterpart of natural biological origin.

6. Substances of natural biological origin intended for consumption for other than their nutrient properties.

In addition to the above, GRAS classification requires that the substance be of suitable purity, meet applicable food grade specifications, perform its intended function and be used at a level no higher than needed to achieve its purpose. Any substance not meeting these criteria will require a food additive regulation. It is noteworthy that under this broad classification foods themselves, if they become components of other foods, can actually be considered as additives unless otherwise exempt.

This new interpretation of the requirements for GRAS status raises a number of questions which will doubtless have to be resolved in the coming years.

PESTICIDES

Under the Food, Drug and Cosmetic Act, a pesticide chemical is an economic poison as defined under the Federal Environmental Pesticide Control[2] Act:

> . . . (1) any substance or mixture of substances intended for preventing, destroying, repelling, or mitigating any pest and (2) any substance or mixture of substances intended for use as a plant regulator, defoliant or desiccant.

Generally speaking pests include, but are not limited to, insects, rodents, nematodes, fungi and weeds.

The production of an adequate food supply and its protection against predators and spoilage would not be possible without the use of pesticides. It has been estimated that man has been deprived of a fifth to a half of the total world food production through infestation and spoilage. A great variety of pesticide chemicals are used, each with its own particular spectrum of activity against specific insects, mites, blights, weeds or other agricultural pests. Legal tolerances have been established which limit the concentration of residue that may remain in or on a raw agricultural commodity, after allowing appropriate intervals between the last application and harvesting and other "good agricultural practices" such as washing, waxing and stripping of outer leaves. The practical efficacy of pesticides from the standpoint of the protection of agricultural productivity and the safety of applicators and farm workers is subject to approval by the Environmental Protection Agency, which issues regulations governing their use. (Foods that are processed, fabricated or produced by milling, freezing, dehydration or cooking are excluded from the category of raw agricultural commodities and are subject to the provisions of the Food, Drug and Cosmetic Act.) In the event that pesticide residues may remain after harvesting, the determination of safety and the setting of tolerance limits are the prerogatives of the Department of Health, Education and Welfare, i.e. the Food and Drug Administration. Tolerances for pesticide residues on agricultural crops are set at levels far below the experimentally determined "no-adverse-effect" level in animals and are designed to assure the safety of foods as ready to eat.

A number of pesticides were originally approved for use on the ground that no residue remained on the fruits or vegetables, and hence it was not necessary to establish tolerances. Later, it was found by the use of more sensitive analytic procedures that demonstrable amounts of these substances, albeit only minute traces, were present. Consequently, the regulations of the Food and Drug Administration requiring prior proof of safety were invoked. Many of these substances were thought to be present in toxicologically inconsequential amounts. The problem of how to deal with "zero tolerance" or "no residue" regulations became highly controversial when it was later discovered by new, exquisitely sensitive analytic procedures that traces of certain potentially carcinogenic pesticides were present in previously undetectable amounts. After numerous unsuccessful efforts to cope with this problem, the Food Protection Committee, in 1969, proposed "Guidelines for Estimating Toxicologically Insignificant Levels of Chemicals in Food,"[8] variations of which are in current use. They take into account chemical structure in relation to known or assumed metabolic fate, toxicologic data on the substance and on structurally analogous compounds and estimated intake in the human diet.

COLOR ADDITIVES

For regulatory purposes, a color is distinguished from a food additive and is defined[9] as a material which "(A) is a dye, pigment, or other substance made by a process of synthesis or similar artifice, or extracted, isolated, or otherwise derived, with or without intermediate or final change of identity, from a vegetable, animal, mineral, or other (sic) source, and (B) when added or applied to a food, drug, or cosmetic, or to the human body or any part thereof, is capable (alone or through reaction with other substance) of imparting color thereto; . . . "color" includes black, white, and intermediate grays." This broad definition includes both natural and artificial substances.

Many natural materials have been used for ages as food colorants, e.g. annatto, carmine, paprika, saffron and turmeric. When used to impart color, certain nutrients (β-carotene and riboflavin) are regarded as color additives, as are also fruit and vegetable juices, carrot oil, grape skin extract and beet powder.

With the advent of synthetic organic colors the so-called coal-tar colors came into use. The Food and Drug Act of 1906 provided that they be "harmless and suitable" and certified for purity. When the 1938 Act was passed 17 such artificial colors were permitted for food use; 2 were added later. Because of demonstrated adverse reactions in man or experimental animals, or the presence of questionable impurities in certain of these substances, the list has been whittled away to the point where (as of April 1978) less than half remain, only a few have been added, all are provisionally listed and several more are likely to be banned. The color additives now permitted for food uses under "good manufacturing practice" and subject to certification are: FD&C Yellow No. 5, Red No. 3, Red No. 40 and Blue No. 1, and, for restricted use, Orange B (for coloring casings for frankfurters and sausages), and Citrus Red No. 2 (on skins of mature oranges not intended for processing). The aluminum or calcium lakes of these colors are also certifiable. FD&C Blue No. 2, Yellow No. 6 and Green No. 3 are included among the provisionally listed food colors.

Because of the paucity of synthetic colors, increasing interest is being directed toward the production of purified natural coloring agents of appropriate hue, inten-

sity, stability and safety for food use. Pigments or dyes used in the fabrication of containers or packaging materials which do not impart visually detectable color to foods contained therein are not considered to be color additives but, if analytically detectable, may be "food additives."

The usual evidence to demonstrate safety of food colors under the conditions of intended use is a prerequisite for listing. Because certain azo dyes and other synthetic colors are, or are derived from, chemicals with structures which suggest potential carcinogenicity, the toxicologic evaluation of food colors places great emphasis on chronic feeding studies in at least two species of laboratory animals.

Certification by the Food and Drug Administration requires that a sample of each production batch must be sent to Washington to be examined for identity and purity according to prescribed specifications, whereupon the batch is assigned a certification number, permitting shipment in interstate commerce.

FUNCTIONAL CATEGORIES OF FOOD ADDITIVES

Direct Additives

Additives that are purposefully and intentionally introduced into foods to achieve specific effects during production or processing or to impart or retain desired characteristics are classified as "direct" additives. Many of these have been exempt from food additive regulations on the ground that they are generally recognized as safe under the conditions of intended use. However, since these substances are currently under review and evaluation, no distinction will be made here between those that are GRAS and those subject to specific regulations. The introduction to a 1965 publication of the Food Protection Committee outlined briefly the technologic uses of food chemicals. It was followed by a well-indexed listing of substances in 12 functional categories and the approximate levels of use of each substance in the major food groups.[10] Subsequently, in connection with the new GRAS review, this Committee subdivided and extended both the food groups and the functional categories. For the purpose of setting limitations and tolerances where necessary, the Food and Drug Administration adopted these classifications as shown in Tables 14–1 and 14–2, respectively.[3]

In the context of this book, it may be appropriate to elaborate on those functional aspects of food additives which relate directly to nutrition. The "Nutrient Supplements" in Table 14–2 refer specifically to vitamins, minerals and amino acids used to enhance or restore the levels present in natural or processed foods (Table 14–3). When used for other purposes, these substances are subject to food additive regulations, unless GRAS or otherwise exempt for such uses. For example, ascorbic acid and tocopherol are included among GRAS chemical preservatives, and calcium citrate and sodium phosphate among sequestrants.

Vitamin potencies of natural foods are subject to regional and seasonal variations and to losses due to processing. In these cases, enrichment or fortification with nutrients is commonly employed. Government regulations applicable to a number of foods, especially those intended for special dietary uses, prescribe ranges and limits for nutrient content. Moreover, many nonstandardized foods for which claims are made must meet requirements for nutritional labeling in terms of "U.S. Recommended Daily Allowances."[13] To maintain uniformity in compliance with food standards and labeling, supplementation with synthetic nutrients is often necessary. Enrichment of flour and bread with B vitamins and iron and fortification of milk with vitamin D are classic examples of the use of nutritional additives. The FDA now intends to specify which foods are appropriate vehicles for fortification, and to what degree.

In this connection reference must be made to substances which have the effect of stabilizing nutrients subject to rancidity or oxidative degradation. Examples are antioxidants (e.g. BHA, BHT and tocopherols) and chelating agents (e.g. ethylenediaminetetraacetates and citric acid) which sequester pro-oxidative metal ions.

Food technologists have recently developed novel food products from soybeans and other sources, in semblance of animal

Table 14–1. Food Categories[11]

(1)   Baked goods and baking mixes, including all ready-to-eat and ready-to-bake products, flours, and mixes requiring preparation before serving.

(2)   Beverages, alcoholic, including malt beverages, wines, distilled liquors, and cocktail mix.

(3)   Beverages and beverage bases, nonalcoholic, including only special or spiced teas, soft drinks, coffee substitutes, and fruit and vegetable flavored gelatin drinks.

(4)   Breakfast cereals, including ready-to-eat and instant and regular hot cereals.

(5)   Cheeses, including curd and whey cheeses, cream, natural, grating, processed, spread, dip, and miscellaneous cheeses.

(6)   Chewing gum, including all forms.

(7)   Coffee and tea, including regular, decaffeinated, and instant types.

(8)   Condiments and relishes, including plain seasoning sauces and spreads, olives, pickles, and relishes, but not spices or herbs.

(9)   Confections and frostings, including candy and flavored frostings, marshmallows, baking chocolate, and brown, lump, rock, maple, powdered, and raw sugars.

(10)   Dairy product analogs, including non-dairy milk, frozen or liquid creamers, coffee whiteners, toppings, and other non-dairy products.

(11)   Egg products, including liquid, frozen, or dried eggs, and egg dishes made therefrom, i.e., egg roll, egg foo young, egg salad, and frozen multi-course egg meals, but not fresh eggs.

(12)   Fats and oils, including margarine, dressings for salads, butter, salad oils, shortenings, and cooking oils.

(13)   Fish products, including all prepared main dishes, salads, appetizers, frozen multi-course meals, and spreads containing fish, shellfish, and other aquatic animals, but not fresh fish.

(14)   Fresh eggs, including cooked eggs and egg dishes made only from fresh shell eggs.

(15)   Fresh fish, including only fresh and frozen fish, shellfish, and other aquatic animals.

(16)   Fresh fruits and fruit juices, including only raw fruits, citrus, melons, and berries, and home-prepared "ades" and punches made therefrom.

(17)   Fresh meats, including only fresh or home-frozen beef or veal, pork, lamb or mutton and home-prepared fresh meat-containing dishes, salads, appetizers, or sandwich spreads made therefrom.

(18)   Fresh poultry, including only fresh or home-frozen poultry and game birds and home-prepared fresh poultry-containing dishes, salads, appetizers, or sandwich spreads made therefrom.

(19)   Fresh vegetables, tomatoes, and potatoes, including only fresh and home-prepared vegetables.

(20)   Frozen dairy desserts and mixes, including ice cream, ice milks, sherbets, and other frozen dairy desserts and specialties.

(21)   Fruit and water ices, including all frozen fruit and water ices.

(22)   Gelatins, puddings, and fillings, including flavored gelatin desserts, puddings, custards, parfaits, pie fillings, and gelatin base salads.

(23)   Grain products and pastas, including macaroni and noodle products, rice dishes, and frozen multi-course meals, without meat or vegetables.

(24)   Gravies and sauces, including all meat sauces and gravies, and tomato, milk, buttery, and specialty sauces.

(25)   Hard candy and cough drops, including all hard type candies.

(26)   Herbs, seeds, spices, seasonings, blends, extracts, and flavorings, including all natural and artificial spices, blends, and flavors.

(27)   Jams and jellies, home-prepared, including only home-prepared jams, jellies, fruit butters, preserves, and sweet spreads.

(28)   Jams and jellies, commercial, including only commercially processed jams, jellies, fruit butters, preserves, and sweet spreads.

(29)   Meat products, including all meats and meat containing dishes, salads, appetizers, frozen multi-course meat meals, and sandwich ingredients prepared by commercial processing or using commercially processed meats with home preparation.

(30)   Milk, whole and skim, including only whole, lowfat, and skim fluid milks.

(31)   Milk products, including flavored milks and milk drinks, dry milks, toppings, snack dips, spreads, weight control milk beverages, and other milk origin products.

(32)   Nuts and nut products, including whole or shelled tree nuts, peanuts, coconut, and nut and peanut spreads.

(33)   Plant protein products, including the National Academy of Sciences/National Research Council "reconstituted vegetable protein" category, and meat, poultry, and fish substitutes, analogs, and extender products made from plant proteins.

(34)   Poultry products, including all poultry and poultry containing dishes, salads, appetizers, frozen multi-course poultry meals, and sandwich ingredients prepared by commercial processing or using commercially processed poultry with home preparation.

(35)   Processed fruits and fruit juices, including all commercially processed fruits, citrus, berries, and mixtures; salads, juices and juice punches, concentrates, dilutions, "-ades," and drink substitutes made therefrom.

(36)   Processed vegetables and vegetable juices, including all commercially processed vegetables, vegetable dishes, frozen multi-course vegetable meals, and vegetable juices and blends.

(37)   Snack foods, including chips, pretzels, and other novelty snacks.

(38)   Soft candy, including candy bars, chocolates, fudge, mints, and other chewy or nougat candies.

(39)   Soups, home-prepared, including meat, fish, poultry, vegetable, and combination home-prepared soups.

(40)   Soups and soup mixes, including commercially prepared meat, fish, poultry, vegetable, and combination soups and soup mixes.

(41)   Sugar, white, granulated, including only white granulated sugar.

(42)   Sugar substitutes, including granulated, liquid, and tablet sugar substitutes.

(43)   Sweet sauces, toppings, and syrups, including chocolate, berry, fruit, corn syrup, and maple sweet sauces and toppings.

Table 14–2. Functional Categories[11]

(1) "Anticaking agents and free-flow agents": Substances added to finely powdered or crystalline food products to prevent caking, lumping, or agglomeration.

(2) "Antimicrobial agents": Substances used to preserve food by preventing growth of microorganisms and subsequent spoilage, including fungistats, mold and rope inhibitors, and the effects listed by the National Academy of Sciences/National Research Council under "preservatives."

(3) "Antioxidants": Substances used to preserve food by retarding deterioration, rancidity, or discoloration due to oxidation.

(4) "Colors and coloring adjuncts": Substances used to impart, preserve, or enhance the color or shading of a food, including color stabilizers, color fixatives, color-retention agents, etc.

(5) "Curing and pickling agents": Substances imparting a unique flavor and/or color to a food, usually producing an increase in shelf life stability.

(6) "Dough strengtheners": Substances used to modify starch and gluten, thereby producing a more stable dough, including the applicable effects listed by the National Academy of Sciences/National Research Council under "dough conditioner."

(7) "Drying agents": Substances with moisture-absorbing ability, used to maintain an environment of low moisture.

(8) "Emulsifiers and emulsifier salts": Substances which modify surface tension in the component phase of an emulsion to establish a uniform dispersion or emulsion.

(9) "Enzymes": Enzymes used to improve food processing and the quality of the finished food.

(10) "Firming agents": Substances added to precipitate residual pectin, thus strengthening the supporting tissue and preventing its collapse during processing.

(11) "Flavor enhancers": Substances added to supplement, enhance, or modify the original taste and/or aroma of a food, without imparting a characteristic taste or aroma of its own.

(12) "Flavoring agents and adjuvants": Substances added to impart or help impart a taste or aroma in food.

(13) "Flour treating agents": Substances added to milled flour, at the mill, to improve its color and/or baking qualities, including bleaching and maturing agents.

(14) "Formulation aids": Substances used to promote or produce a desired physical state or texture in food, including carriers, binders, fillers, plasticizers, film-formers, and tableting aids, etc.

(15) "Fumigants": Volatile substances used for controlling insects or pests.

(16) "Humectants": Hygroscopic substances incorporated in food to promote retention of moisture, including moisture-retention agents and anti-dusting agents.

(17) "Leavening agents": Substances used to produce or stimulate production of carbon dioxide in baked goods to impart a light texture, including yeast, yeast foods, and calcium salts listed by the National Academy of Sciences/National Research Council, under "dough conditioners."

(18) "Lubricants and release agents": Substances added to food contact surfaces to prevent ingredients and finished products from sticking to them.

(19) "Non-nutritive sweeteners": Substances having less than 2 percent of the caloric value of sucrose per equivalent unit of sweetening capacity.

(20) "Nutrient supplements": Substances which are necessary for the body's nutritional and metabolic processes.

(21) "Nutritive sweeteners": Substances having greater than 2 percent of the caloric value of sucrose per equivalent unit of sweetening capacity.

(22) "Oxidizing and reducing agents": Substances which chemically oxidize ro reduce another food ingredient, thereby producing a more stable product, including the applicable effect listed by the National Academy of Sciences/National Research Council under "dough conditioners."

(23) "pH control agents": Substances added to change or maintain active acidity or basicity, including buffers, acids, alkalies, and neutralizing agents.

(24) "Processing aids": Substances used as manufacturing aids to enhance the appeal or utility of a food or food component, including clarifying agents, clouding agents, catalysts, flocculents, filters aids, and crystallization inhibitors, etc.

(25) "Propellants, aerating agents, and gases": Gases used to supply force to expel a product or used to reduce the amount of oxygen in contact with the food in packaging.

(26) "Sequestrants": Substances which combine with polyvalent metal ions to form a soluble metal complex, to improve the quality and stability of products.

(27) "Solvents and vehicles": Substances used to extract or dissolve another substance.

(28) "Stabilizers and thickeners": Substances used to produce viscous solutions or dispersions, to impart body, improve consistency, or stabilize emulsions, including suspending and bodying agents, setting agents, jelling agents, and bulking agents, etc.

(29) "Surface-active agents": Substances used to modify surface properties of liquid food components for a variety of effects, other than emulsifiers, but including solubilizing agents, dispersants, detergents, wetting agents, rehydration enhancers, whipping agents, foaming agents, and defoaming agents, etc.

(30) "Surface-finishing agents": Substances used to increase palatability, preserve gloss, and inhibit discoloration of foods, including glazes, polishes, waxes, and protective coatings.

(31) "Synergists": Substances used to act or react with another food ingredient to produce a total effect different or greater than the sum of the effects produced by the individual ingredients.

(32) "Texturizers": Substances which affect the appearance or feel of the food.

Table 14–3.   Nutrients and/or Dietary Supplements[12]

Alanine	Manganese citrate
Aminoacetic acid (glycine)	Manganese gluconate
Arginine	Manganese glycerophosphate
Ascorbic acid	Manganese hypophosphite
Asparagine	Manganese sulfate
Aspartic acid	Manganous oxide
Biotin	Mannitol
Calcium carbonate	Methionine
Calcium citrate	Niacin
Calcium glycerophosphate	Niacinamide
Calcium oxide	D-Pantothenyl alcohol
Calcium pantothenate	Phenylalanine
Calcium phosphate	Potassium chloride
Calcium pyrophosphate	Potassium glycerophosphate
Calcium sulfate	Potassium iodide
Carotene	Proline
Choline bitartrate	Pyridoxine hydrochloride
Choline chloride	Riboflavin
Copper gluconate	Riboflavin-5-phosphate
Cuprous iodide	Serine
Cystine	Sodium pantothenate
Ferric phosphate	Sodium phosphate
Ferric pyrophosphate	Thiamin hydrochloride
Ferric sodium pyrophosphate	Thiamin mononitrate
Ferrous gluconate	Threonine
Ferrous lactate	Tocopherols
Ferrous sulfate	α-Tocopherol acetate
Folic acid	Tryptophane
Glutamic acid	Tyrosine
Glutamine	Valine
Histidine	Vitamin A
Inositol	Vitamin A acetate
Iron reduced	Vitamin A palmitate
Isoleucine	Vitamin B_{12}
Leucine	Vitamin D_2
Linoleic acid	Vitamin D_3
Lysine	Zinc chloride
Magnesium oxide	Zinc gluconate
Magnesium phosphate	Zinc oxide
Magnesium sulfate	Zinc stearate
Manganese chloride	Zinc sulfate

protein foods. These "texturized plant proteins" or "analogs" are required to supply not only proteins of comparable biologic value but all the other principal vitamins and minerals characteristic of the genuine foods.

As the commonly quoted aphorism puts it, "To be nutritious, food must be eaten." The role of additives in imparting or enhancing hedonic value should not be underestimated. Acceptability by the consumer—using this term in its literal sense—requires that food be esthetically attractive and organoleptically appealing. Whether prepared commercially or in the home, satisfactory flavor, taste, texture and color are as important attributes of foods as their nutritional composition—and are more readily recognized and appreciated by the average consumer.

Flavoring agents comprise by far the largest single category of direct food additives. They are used not only to impart aromatic and taste properties to foods but also to mask objectionable organoleptic qualities and to adjust for variations in flavor intensity of natural foods. They include spices and herbs, essential oils, oleoresins, extracts, gums, balsams and a large number of chemical substances isolated from natural sources or produced synthetically; in either case, when known by its chemical name a substance is generally classed as "synthetic." Many of the latter are counterparts of naturally occurring components of fruits, berries and other plant parts used as or in foods. More than 1400 natural and "synthetic" flavoring substances have been determined to be safe under the conditions of use.[4,5,14] Among the most common are vanillin, citral, eugenol, diacetal, cinnamic aldehyde, menthol, methyl anthranilate and methyl salicylate.

Texturizing agents are used to retain the firmness or crispness of pickled or canned vegetables. Among them are alums (potassium or sodium aluminum sulfate) used in pickling cucumbers and several calcium salts in canned peas, tomatoes and potatoes.

Other substances are used for miscellaneous purposes, such as to impart clarity or foaming property to beverages, to inhibit foaming during processing or filling operations and as propellant gases in aerosol containers.

Indirect Additives

Modern methods of distribution of foods from growers and processors to retail outlets demand packaging in containers of great variety and size. The materials of which they are composed include wood, glass, paper, paperboard, metals, plastics, cotton and rubber. The largest single group of indirect additives includes the components of food packaging materials which "may reasonably be expected to result . . . in (their) becoming a component . . . of any food."[1] Resins and lacquers are applied as coatings to metallic containers; waxes and synthetic polymeric resins are used to coat paperboard and other types of fiber packaging materials. A multitude of chemical components are used to impart stability, flexibility, grease resistance, moisture repellency, clarity, color or other physical properties to containers. The components of cap liners and of adhesives employed in the fabrication of food containers also fall within the class of indirect additives.

The passage of the food additives amendment raised the question, for the first time in many instances, of whether or not any of the components of food packaging materials might "reasonably be expected" to become components of food. In certain cases, it was regarded as expedient by the industries concerned to include all substances then in use in the manufacture of food packages as potential food additives; hence a number of "omnibus" regulations were promulgated covering paper and paperboard containers, plastics and resins, rubber, cap lacquers and adhesives, to cite a few.

Processing aids, such as defoaming, wetting or washing agents, may, in some cases, remain in or leave residues on foods and most of these come under food additive regulations. Fumigants and residues of extraction solvents also belong in this category, as do filtration aids (e.g. fuller's earth) and synthetic polymers used as ion exchange resins.

Other types of indirect additives are those contained in foods derived from livestock and poultry which may have been given feed containing growth promoting agents, e.g. coccidiostats, antibiotics, organic arsenicals, etc. The use of veterinary drugs for the prevention or treatment of diseases such as mastitis in cows or blackleg and coccidiosis in poultry raises the possibility that residues may be transmitted to foods (meat, milk, eggs) derived from animal sources. Regulations for the use of drugs in food-producing animals take into consideration the safety of residues of the drugs or their metabolites in food for man. Where relevant, withdrawal intervals are required prior to the collection of milk or eggs, or the slaughter of cattle, hogs or poultry for food use.

LEGAL AND SAFETY ASPECTS

Unless the use of a substance satisfies one of the statutory exemptions from the definition of a food additive, it is subject to the issuance of a regulation by the Food and Drug Administration specifying the permitted conditions of use. Any person may petition for such a regulation but, once issued, anyone may use the substance as identified, in the manner described. It falls upon the petitioner however to supply the required information upon which an appraisal of the safety under conditions of use may be made. The petition must contain:[15,16]

1. The name and all pertinent information concerning such food additive, including, where available, its chemical identity and composition.
2. A statement of the conditions of the proposed use of such additive, including all directions, recommendations and suggestions proposed for the use of such additive, and including specimens of its proposed labeling.
3. All relevant data bearing on the physical or other technical effect such additive is intended to produce, and the quantity of such additive required to produce such effect.
4. A description of practicable methods for determining the quantity of such additive in or on food, and any substance formed in or on food, because of its use.
5. Full reports of investigations made with respect to the safety for use of such additive, including full information as to the methods and controls used in conducting such investigations.

Difficulties are frequently encountered in defining the chemical identity of a substance, particularly if it is of natural origin, sufficiently to ensure uniformity and reproducibility. The lack of suitably specific or sensitive analytic methods to detect and determine the presence of minute traces, e.g. of packaging "migrants" or other indirect additives, may present obstacles to the granting of petitions. However, the most critical information—that relating to toxicologic evaluation—is more often than any other factor responsible for rejection or delays in approval of petitions. The type of data generally required are:

1. Acute oral toxicity tests in a minimum of two species of animals one of which should be a nonrodent (excluding rabbits). In addition to mortality data (usually expressed as the LD_{50}) premortal signs of toxicity and gross postmortem examinations should be recorded.
2. Short-term oral toxicity studies (at least 90 days in rodents and 6 months in nonrodents) at multiple dosage levels, with observations of growth, physical appearance and behavior, efficiency of food utilization, hemocytologic and hemochemical changes, urine analyses, tests of hepatic and renal function and, postmortem, gross autopsies, including the weighing of all major organs, and histopathologic examinations. The short-term tests may be extended to provide reproductive or teratogenic data in rodents. The animals may be bred through two pregnancies, some of the females being delivered by cesarian section to permit ob-

servation of implantation and resorption sites, corpora lutea, prenatal mortality and teratologic abnormalities, as revealed upon examination of soft and skeletal tissues. In addition, observations are recorded for efficiency of fertilization, gestation and lactation, live and still births, postnatal growth and survival.

3. Long-term oral toxicity studies in at least two species, one a nonrodent. These are generally run for two years, a major part of the life cycle of the rodent (but not, of course, of the dog or primate). The observations are similar to those made in the short-term tests and are repeated entirely or in part at 3, 6, 9, 12, 18 and 24 months. Premortal signs and age at death or sacrifice of moribund animals are recorded. The study may be designed to yield additional data on reproduction and lactation efficiency by increasing the number of pregnancies in the parent or first generation, and continuing the study into several successive generations. More specific data on teratogenetic potential are obtained by administering test dosages to different groups prior to, during or after the most critical period of fetal organogenesis, viz. the second trimester of pregnancy.

The main purpose of long-term studies in rodents is to reveal the possibility of a carcinogenic effect, particularly in the highest dosage group. This is ideally set at the maximum level which will permit a sufficient number of the animals to survive beyond 1.5 years for statistically valid comparison of tumor incidence between the test and control groups. Examinations of microscopic sections for neoplastic changes are made by light microscopy, occasionally supplemented by electron microscopy.

Some investigators are recommending tests for mutagenic potential, particularly where carcinogenic or teratogenic effects are found or suspected. However, methodology currently available in this field is still under study, and interpretation in relation to human health hazard has not been sufficiently well established. The methods vary widely in principle and, in order to develop a body of data on the subject, it was proposed that at least three basic procedures be employed: (1) in vivo cytogenetic study involving karyotyping for the detection of chromosomal aberrations, (2) the host-mediated assay in which mutagenic changes are observed in neurospora or E. coli injected intraperitoneally into treated animals and (3) the dominant lethal test in which treated males are mated with untreated females.[17] Recent developments in toxicologic methodology have been introduced into the procedures for safety evaluation of food components. These are exemplified in a proposed System for Food Safety Assessment[18] which incorporates metabolic and pharmacokinetic tests as well as "short-term" predictive tests for mutagenicity and carcinogenicity. However, these have not as yet been evaluated to the point of adoption for regulatory purposes.

Proper evaluation of the safety of a food chemical under the conditions of intended use takes into account:

1. The food consumption pattern of the population concerned, with particular reference to the amount, frequency and duration of intake of the substance in question and of chemically and pharmacologically related substances.
2. The maximum no-adverse-effect level in test animals, with particular reference to a species where metabolic handling of the substance is similar to that in man.
3. The application of a suitable safety factor, i.e. a fraction of the maximum no-adverse-effect dose in the test animal expressed in terms of mg per kg body weight (or per square meter of body surface) per day.

Where legal tolerances are set, they are based not on the maximum safe levels estimated from animal studies but on the limits established by good manufacturing (or agricultural) practice, and, of course, at levels not exceeding safe limits in the total diet.

Under the federal Food, Drug and Cosmetic Act, no food additive is permitted if its use would be considered deceptive or, for whatever reason, unsafe. By statutory definition, a substance is unsafe "if it is found to induce cancer when ingested by man or animal, or if it is found, after tests which are appropriate for the evaluation of the safety of food additives, to induce cancer in man or animal. . . ." (the so-called Delaney clause). It is this provision that-led to the outlawing of oil of sassafras and safrole, the characteristic flavor ingredient of root beer, oil of calamus used in vermouth, several food colors, cyclamates, and, more recently, the proposed banning of saccharin, the last remaining non-nutritive sweetener.

This legal mandate recognizes no specific experimental conditions for determining the carcinogenic potential of a substance; any dose, no matter how large, administered to any species of animal, no matter how frequent or prolonged, might condemn a substance as a carcinogen. Literal interpretation of this provision of the law makes no allowance for minute or unavoidable traces of added potential carcinogens. Problems have arisen in cases where permitted uses of such substances, e.g., as pesticides or constituents of packaging materials, were predicated on non-detectability only to have more sensitive analytic methodology later reveal the presence of traces as low as parts per trillion, i.e. below toxicologically significant levels. Unavoidable traces of the mycotoxin aflatoxin or the polycyclic hydrocarbon benzo-α-pyrene, both known carcinogens, are present in peanut butter and smoked meats, respectively. Various foods naturally contain traces of cancer-inducing substances, but escape legal prohibition because these substances are not "added." These are examples of how the legal concept of "zero tolerance" or "no residue" has been found to be scientifically untenable. The Food and Drug Administration has administratively taken the pragmatic position, in certain cases, of setting "actionable" limits on the presence of such carcinogens, taking cognizance of the sensitivity of currently available analytic methodology.

In the view of many responsible scientists, the Delaney clause should be amended, or regulations adopted, to permit greater latitude and discretion on the part of those qualified by scientific training and experience. On the other hand, some contend that the principle of "zero tolerance" implicit in this statute should be extended to prohibit potential teratogens and mutagens and other agents believed to be etiologically related to chronic or irreversible pathologic states. This is one of numerous controversies among scientists and regulatory agencies both here and abroad surrounding the use of food additives.

Whatever the outcome, the review of GRAS substances by the FDA should have a major impact on the regulatory control of food additives. The identity, purity, chemical composition and technologic uses of hundreds of GRAS and "prior-sanctioned" substances, as well as updated information on potential intake levels based on literature reviews, food industry practices and current U.S. food consumption patterns, are being studied by expert committees under the auspices of the Life Sciences Branch of the Federation of American Societies for Experimental Biology and, in the case of flavors, by the Flavor and Extract Manufacturers' Association.

BIBLIOGRAPHY

1. Federal Food, Drug and Cosmetic Act, as amended October 1976, Sec. 201(s).
2. Federal Insecticide, Fungicide, and Rodenticide Act (Federal Environmental Control Act of 1972).
3. Code of Federal Regulations, Title 21, Chapter 1, Subpart A, Sec. 170.3.
4. Recent progress in the consideration of flavoring ingredients under the food additives amendment. III GRAS substances. Food Technol., 19, 151, 1965; IV-X, ibid., 1968-77.
5. Oser and Hall: Criteria employed by the expert panel of FEMA for the GRAS evaluation of flavoring substances. Food Cosmet. Toxicol., in press.
6. Code of Federal Regulations, Title 21, Chapter 1, Part 182, Subparts A–H.
7. Code of Federal Regulations, Title 21, Chapter 1, Part 170, Subpart B, Sec. 120.30 (f) (1).

8. Evaluating the Safety of Food Chemicals. Washington, National Academy of Sciences–National Research Council, Food Protection Committee, Food and Nutrition Board, 1970.

9. Federal Food, Drug and Cosmetic Act. Sec. 201 (t)(l).

10. Chemicals Used in Food Processing. Washington, National Academy of Sciences–National Research Council, Publication No. 1274, 1965.

11. A Comprehensive Survey of Industry on the Use of Food Chemicals Generally Recognized as Safe. Washington, National Academy of Sciences/National Research Council, 1972.

12. Adapted from Code of Federal Regulations, Title 21, Chapter 1, Part 21, Sec. 172, Subpart D, and Sec. 182, Subpart F.

13. Code of Federal Regulations, Title 21, Chapter 1, Subchapter B, Sec. 105.3 (b).

14. Code of Federal Regulations, Title 21, Chapter 1, Sec. 172.510 and 172.515.

15. Federal Food, Drug and Cosmetic Act as amended October 1976, Sec. 409(b)(2).

16. Code of Federal Regulations, Title 21, Chapter 1, Part 171, Subpart A, Sec. 171.1.

17. Food and Drug Administration Advisory Committee on Protocols for Safety Evaluations: Panel on Reproduction Report on Reproduction Studies in the Safety Evaluation of Food Additives and Pesticide Residues. Toxicol. Appl. Pharmacol. 16, 264, 1970.

18. Proposed System for Food Safety Assessment. The Scientific Committee, Food Safety Council, Food Cosmet. Toxicol., 16, (Suppl. 2), 1978.

Chapter 15

RADIOACTIVITY IN FOODS

C. L. Comar
and
J. C. Thompson, Jr.

There is little doubt that atomic energy is assuming an important role in our civilization, and it is appropriate that possible hazards be evaluated. Although present environmental radiocontamination and exposure of the population are caused almost entirely by fallout from nuclear weapons, peacetime operations may become increasingly important as sources. In addition to fallout, small quantities of radioactive materials are released into the environment as a result of such operations as mining of uranium and thorium ore, nuclear fuel processing, reactor installations in power plants, submarines, ships and aircraft (normal operations and accidents), and applications of radioisotopes in medicine, industry and agriculture.

Radioactivity from environmental contamination reaches the human population primarily in food. However, at the present time it can be concluded that there is no reason for any change in our nutritional habits or food technology as a result of such contamination. Research must continue, nevertheless, so that remedial measures can be implemented to minimize the intake of radioactive contamination should this ever become necessary.

RADIOISOTOPES OF POTENTIAL HAZARD

The relative hazard of radioactive materials is governed by the amount released into the environment, physical half-life, efficiency of transfer through the food chain to the human diet, degree of absorption by the body and length of time retained in the body. Because of these factors the list of potentially hazardous radioisotopes is reduced considerably, with those of greatest immediate concern being the radioisotopes of iodine, barium, strontium and cesium. Extensive data are available on the passage of these radioactive materials through food chains and their metabolism in the human body.[1-5] Table 15-1 summarizes their characteristics from the standpoint of environmental contamination. Other radioisotopes found in peaceful nuclear operations such as ^3H, ^{85}Kr, ^{51}Cr, ^{65}Zn, ^{55}Fe, ^{60}Co, ^{54}Mn, etc. may be important under certain conditions but will tend to follow similar contamination patterns. Unique pathways and characteristics might require special considerations under some conditions, but such radioisotopes are intensively studied before releases are permitted. This is especially true under the National Environmental Protection Act of 1969, which requires environmental impact statements for actions which may affect the environment. This Act has proven to be a most effective instrument in requiring the consideration and implementation of alternatives to provide minimal environmental insults or to justify actions where feasible alternatives

Table 15–1. Comparison of Radioisotopes in Environmental Contamination

	Iodine 131	Barium 140	Strontium 89	Strontium 90	Cesium 137
Physical half-life	8 days	13 days	51 days	28 years	30 years
Metabolic behavior	Collects in thyroid	Like calcium, collects in bone	Like calcium, collects in bone	Like calcium, collects in bone	Like potassium, collects in muscle
Removal rate from body	Fast	Slow	Slow	Slow	Relatively fast
Main pathways in food chain*	A → V → C → M → Man	A → V → C → M → Man	A → V, A → S ⇌ V → Man, C → M → Man	(see Strontium 89)	A → V → C → M → Man, C → MP
Samples for monitoring radioisotope levels	Vegetation, milk, and thyroid	Vegetation and milk	Soil, vegetation, milk, dairy products, bone and aquatic food	Soil vegetation, milk, dairy products, bone and aquatic food	Vegetation, milk, dairy products, meat and whole body

* A = atmosphere, V = vegetation, M = milk, S = soil, C = cattle, MP = meat products.

do not exist. In the administration of this Act there has been a definite attempt at balancing long-term social and economic benefits with overall environmental quality.

The radioisotopes of iodine collect in the thyroid gland and those of barium concentrate in bone. Since the major isotopes of both of these elements have short physical half-lives they can be dangerous only during certain periods, depending on the frequency and nature of production and contamination. Experience has indicated that ^{131}I may be most important shortly after tropospheric and local fallout and release from reactor accidents. However, under normal operating conditions the release of ^{131}I to the environment from nuclear reactors is seldom discernible, even in cattle thyroid sampling networks designed to provide first indications of exposures to the surrounding environment.

Long-lived [129]I is also being studied but is not regarded as a potential hazard because of the low release levels. Barium 140 is of much less concern because it is transmitted less efficiently through the food chain. Strontium 89, which is produced in higher activities than ^{90}Sr, may be the more hazardous shortly after production, whereas ^{90}Sr with a much longer half-life becomes more dominant with time. The radioisotopes of strontium are cumulative in bone. Cesium 137, which follows potassium in metabolism, is considered less of a hazard than ^{90}Sr because cesium is turned over relatively rapidly in the body, is not selectively concentrated in any one part of the body and does not pass appreciably from soil to plant in the food chain.

Insofar as other radionuclides are concerned, [14]C (half-life of about 5,700 years) is of greatest interest because carbon is such an important constituent of living matter. Little attention has been given to the movement of ^{14}C in the food chain because its specific activity in the population can be estimated directly from its specific activity in atmospheric carbon dioxide, which is essentially the sole precursor of carbon in food and body tissues. The extent of contamination is most conveniently expressed in terms of naturally occurring levels of ^{14}C, which have always existed as a result of the action of cosmic ray neutrons on carbon atoms. It is estimated that the peak excess atmospheric ^{14}C activity occurred during the period from 1963 to 1965 when levels were more than 100 per cent greater than normal atmospheric levels. Following this peak, which resulted from nuclear testing, the levels declined to about 70 per cent excess in 1970. This decline will continue so that by the year 2000 the excess levels will be about 3 per cent.[2,3,4,6] Such large reductions are brought about mainly by movement between reservoirs (i.e. exchange between atmosphere, biosphere and ocean-surface layer); further decreases will occur only by radioactive decay.[2] Estimated ^{14}C production by the nuclear power industry through the year 2000 will be approximately 10 per cent of the levels produced from weapons testing or 0.3 per cent of the natural level.[3] Carbon 14 is expected to produce about the same amount of total harm as ^{90}Sr but, because of its long half-life, its effects will be spread over thousands of years. However, ^{14}C may turn out to be the most important radionuclide released in the nuclear fuel cycle.

A few radionuclides are considered potentially more significant in relation to seafoods than to the terrestrial food chain: cerium 144, zinc 65, iron 55, iron 59 and cobalt 60. The exposure of the human population to these radionuclides and to others that have been detected in air, rain or tissues, such as sodium 22, manganese 54, tritium and plutonium, is considerably less than exposure to the radionuclides listed in Table 15–1.[2] This pattern is expected to continue with doses from peaceful uses seldom approaching the levels received from fallout testing.

Considerable concern has been expressed about the presence of plutonium in the environment as an integral part of the nuclear power cycle. Much emotion and public uncertainty have been aroused about the availability, toxicity and hazard of plutonium to human health. Plutonium 239 is the main isotope of concern because of its half-life (24,390 years) and its abundance resulting from reactor production. Plutonium emits alpha radiation which penetrates matter very poorly but which is highly carcinogenic when deposited in or on living tissue. Plutonium usually exists as plutonium dioxide, which is highly insoluble in water and body liquids. It tends to adsorb onto undigested food and is, therefore, poorly absorbed from the gastrointestinal tract. Also, it migrates very slowly in soil and is not readily taken up by plants from the soil (1/1000th to 1/100,000th of soil levels). Thus, the main pathway to humans is via inhalation. The major sources of plutonium continue to be the approximately five tons released during weapons testing and distributed as worldwide fallout. The peak levels resulting from those tests occurred in 1963-1964, when average inhaled levels were 12 picocuries (pc) per person and body burdens were 4 pc per person.[8] More recent observations for 1972 to 1974 indicate average annual dietary intakes of 1 to 2 pc per year as typical, with 30 per cent coming from grain products, 21 per cent from meat, fish and eggs, 17 per cent from vegetables, 17 per cent from fruit, 9 per cent from water and 6 per cent from dairy products.[9]

Pathways in the Food Chain

Radioactive contaminants are transferred to man by means of specific pathways through the terrestrial and aquatic food chains. Terrestrial food chains are the main sources of radiocontaminants and their generalized pathways are illustrated in Figure 15–1. Specific pathways for barium, iodine, strontium and cesium are described in Table 15–1. Aquatic food chains follow the same general principles, with many interrelationships among water, vegetation, animals and man. However, the aquatic food chains have not contributed significant amounts of radiocontaminants because of normal dilution factors and a limited intake of aquatic food products.

Fallout from the atmosphere can be retained by above-ground plant parts, such

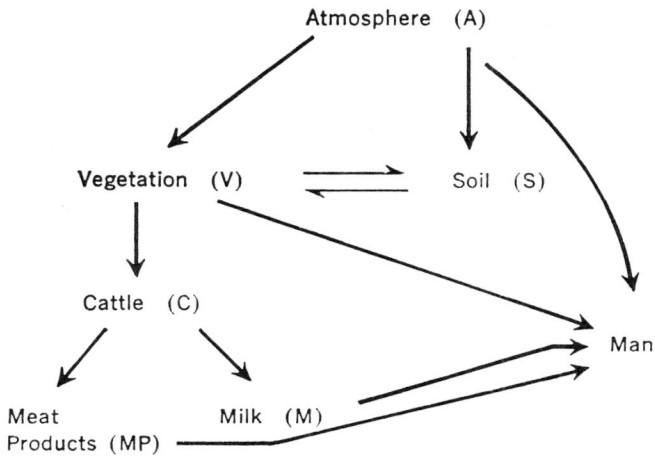

Fig. 15–1. Diagram of main terrestrial food chains by means of which environmental radioactive contaminants reach the human population.

as leaves, fruits or seeds, or it can be absorbed directly by basal parts and surface roots of plants. In addition, radioactive contaminants can enter the soil and pass through the roots into plants just like any soil nutrient. Man ingests the radioactive material both by direct consumption of plant materials and by consumption of products from animals that have eaten contaminated forage.

Radioiodine is deposited from the atmosphere on the surface of vegetation which is grazed by dairy animals, and the ingested radionuclide is secreted into milk. Exposure of man to ^{131}I also occurs by consumption of fruits and vegetables; however, such exposure is usually minor, because of the time delay. Also, the surface area of these products, as consumed by man, is very small compared to the surface area grazed by an animal, and most often the surface contamination of fresh fruits and vegetables is removed by washing or skinning before consumption. Man inhales ^{131}I present in air, but observations have shown that this route of contamination is relatively unimportant. Thus, one item of the diet, fresh milk, is by far the most important source of ^{131}I for the human population, although locally grown produce consumed within a short time could be a significant contributor.[7,10,11]

Radiostrontium is available to man primarily through the consumption of dairy products and foods of plant origin. Two major pathways form the routes for intake: (1) surface contamination of plants (fallout-rate dependent) and (2) soil uptake (cumulative dependent). The relative importance of these two routes varies, depending upon the magnitude of fallout rate, soil reservoir, crop characteristics and time pattern of contamination. In 1958, for example, surface contamination of cereals was quite evident, and in some areas as much as 80 per cent of the radiostrontium in food had originated as surface contamination. By 1960, the general contribution from surface contamination

had declined to approximately 20 per cent.[12] Increased fallout rates from nuclear testing in 1961 and 1962 again raised the contribution from surface contamination to more than 50 per cent.[2,12,13] However, with the cessation of above-ground nuclear testing the fallout rate has dropped and the soil reservoir has become the main source of radioactivity in foods.

The movement of strontium radionuclides from soil to man is interrelated with and, to some extent, governed by the simultaneous movement of calcium. For this reason, levels of ^{90}Sr are often expressed in terms of "strontium units," namely, picocuries of ^{90}Sr per gm of calcium.

It must be emphasized that the important factors are the amounts of ^{90}Sr and of calcium in the total diet. For example, if foodstuff A were to contain 10 pc of ^{90}Sr per gm of calcium and contributed 0.1 gm of calcium, whereas foodstuff B were to contain 1 pc of ^{90}Sr per gm of calcium and contribute 1 gm of calcium to the diet, it could be said that both foodstuffs were equally important contributors, even though foodstuff A was 10 times more contaminated than foodstuff B. Thus, no judgment can be made from analytic values on a single constituent of the diet; it is necessary to consider the total diet.

In regard to the deposition of ^{90}Sr in the human population, two practical generalizations can be made:

1. Calcium is preferentially utilized relative to ^{90}Sr in practically every step of the food chain from vegetation to human bone, thus providing a biologic barrier against [90]Sr.
2. Food processing that involves washing or discarding of outer layers of plant foods serves as a mechanical barrier.

Were it not for these processes the ^{90}Sr of the human population would be several times higher than it is now.

A word should be said about milk, because in the United States dairy products are the largest single source of dietary calcium. Attention has been focused on milk because it has been the most important single item used for analysis and evaluation of food contamination. This is because milk is produced regularly all year round, is convenient to handle, can be readily sampled so as to represent large or small areas and contains the most important radiocontaminants. It must be emphasized that the use of milk as an indicator food does not mean that milk is a major factor in determining total ^{90}Sr intake. As a matter of fact, because the dairy cow secretes, in proportion to the amounts ingested, 10 times as much calcium as strontium into the milk, the calcium originating from the milk will be the least contaminated of all food sources of calcium.

For ^{137}Cs, the direct contamination of plant materials is the most important route of contamination, since this element is fixed in the soil and generally rendered unavailable for root uptake. Aquatic pathways have been a minor contributor, because of the dilution factors normally existent in most bodies of water. However, with more widespread peaceful uses of nuclear energy in small confined bodies of water, coupled with a natural tendency for ^{137}Cs to be concentrated in certain tissues, there will be greater need for closer evaluation of ^{137}Cs levels in aquatic organisms. Similar care will have to be exercised for other radionuclides planned for release to the aquatic environment, where the ecosystems are not as well defined or characterized as they are for the terrestrial environment.

RADIOISOTOPE LEVELS

The pattern of the levels of radioisotopes in the biosphere (soil-plants-animal products-man) can be understood only in terms of the timing and size of the nuclear explosions that produced them. Table 15-2 presents such data.[14,16,18] Thus, radionuclide levels arising from tests subsequent to the 1958 moratorium would be expected to exceed

Table 15–2. Fission Yields of Nuclear Explosions[14,16,18]

Period	Total by Period	Cumulative Total
	(Megatons)	
1945–1956	52	52
1957–1958	40	92
1959–1960	Test moratorium	
1961	25	117
1962	76	193
1963–1976	Underground tests primarily, except those by France and China which have been less than 5-megaton fission yield.	

the highest levels observed in 1959 because of the cumulative soil contribution and an increased fallout rate which resulted from the intensity of testing during 1961–1962. An understanding of the pathways, weapons yield, production and distribution patterns is necessary to estimate accurately future levels of radioactivity.

Because of the transient nature of ^{131}I in milk, very few measurements were made of levels resulting from tests prior to 1957; limited data were reported during 1957 to 1959. After the disappearance of the ^{131}I from the 1958 tests, none was observed until the resumption of nuclear testing by Russia in 1961. Monitoring networks began to record ^{131}I in milk by mid-September and continued to detect appreciable levels until late December. Values as high as 730 pc ^{131}I per liter of milk were observed, with monthly averages of 80, 100, 65 and 14 for the September-to-December period; values were less than 10 pc per liter during the next 4 months.[16] Increased testing by both the United States and Russia in the spring of 1962 caused ^{131}I levels in milk to rise again, with monthly averages in the United States rising from 20 in May to 70 pc per liter in November.[16] Such averages do not indicate the variability in ^{131}I deposition, since milk from some individual collection stations exceeded 700 pc per liter during the summer of 1962. Daily averages or values from individual dairy herds were even higher in certain locations. However, by February 1963 the average ^{131}I levels in the United States were again below 10 pc per liter or undetectable except for localized contamination from ventings of underground tests and some limited contamination from the French and Chinese above-ground testing programs.[16]

Dietary levels of ^{90}Sr, which are expressed as pc of ^{90}Sr per gm of calcium, have been estimated at approximately 0.4, 2, 4, 5, 7, 12, 18, 11, 7, 11, 22, 26, 21, 15, 12, 12, 11, 8, 8, 7, 6, 6, 6, 6, for each year from 1953 to 1976, respectively.[14-18] Values are predicted to be less than 10 throughout the next several decades, assuming no large-scale atmospheric testing. An indication of the typical contributions of various foods is given in Table 15–3.[18] No significant differences in ^{90}Sr/Ca values have been found for typical infant, teenage or adult diets. The breast-feeding of infants, however, should give an appreciable reduction of ^{90}Sr intake during the first few months of life. From observations and knowledge of metabolism, it can be assumed that the value of ^{90}Sr per gm of calcium in the human population will be no greater than one-fourth of the value of the total diet.[2]

The most extensive data are those on levels of ^{90}Sr in milk. In general, the values for milk are expected to be about 30 to 60 per cent of the values for total diet, depending upon the relative importance of the rate-dependent versus cumulative-dependent pathways.[19] In regard to variability, it appears that in any one month the highest value observed in the country might be 10 times the lowest; however, there is less variation in the total diet and in the levels found in the human population, presumably because the individual consumes food that originates from many areas.

Because the amount of rainfall is an important factor governing the fallout rate, the Federal Radiation Council has considered the country to be divided into "wet" and "dry" areas.[14] The "wet" region includes all states bordering on and extending east of the Mississippi River as well as the far northwest. The "dry" region includes the Great Plains, intermountain and southwest states where average rainfall is generally less than 30 inches per year. As an example, the ^{90}Sr content of milk in the wet area is usually 1½ to 2 times higher than that in the dry area.

Typical values for ^{137}Cs in the human diet also reflect the importance of the rate-dependent pathway with average daily intakes (Chicago 1961–1976) of 67, 92, 150, 202, 132, 54, 33, 33, 28, 25, 24, 17, 11, 14, 14 and 9, respectively.[18] In terms of the relative contributions from various foodstuffs, Table 15–4 shows the range for

Table 15–3.   Typical Contributions of Various Foods to the Total Strontium 90 of Diet in New York City for 1960-1976[18]

	Picocuries of ^{90}Sr/Day		Percentage Contribution	
	Average 1976	Range 1960–1976	Average 1976	Range 1960–1976
Milk	2.9	2.9–16.6	34	31–56
Flour and cereals	1.0	1.0– 8.5	12	11–28
Vegetables	2.4	2.1– 5.4	28	13–34
Fruits	1.7	0.8– 2.9	20	7–22
Meats, fish and eggs	0.3	0.2– 1.2	3	2–5
Water	0.3	0.3– 1.8	3	3–6
Total daily ^{90}Sr intake	8.6	8.6–30.6	—	—

Table 15–4.   Typical Contributions of Various Foods to the Total ^{137}Cs of Diet in Chicago for 1960–1976[18]

	Picocuries of ^{137}Cs/Day		Percentage Contribution	
	Average 1976	Range 1961–1976	Average 1976	Range 1961–1976
Milk	1.8	1.8–66	20	20–42
Flour and cereals	1.4	1.4–32	15	14–31
Vegetables	1.9	0.8–13	20	03–20
Fruits	0.7	0.7–16	07	07–26
Meat, fish and eggs	3.5	2.9–53	38	17–38
Total	9.3	9.3–202		

the major diet categories from 1961 to 1976 in Chicago diets.[18] Products of animal origin (milk, meat, eggs) contributed from 50 to 70 per cent of the ^{137}Cs intake, with the remaining contributions divided among grains, fruits and vegetables. Values for ^{137}Cs in picocuries per liter of milk averaged 65, 10, 10, 44, 114, 94, 52, 29, 11, 12, 8, 9, 9, 6, 3 and 2 in the nationwide milk network for 1959 through 1974, respectively.[16]

Levels have declined with time as a result of the cessation of nuclear testing, with the rate of decline lagging considerably behind the decrease in the fallout rate. It has been suggested that, in permanent pastures, an interaction with organic matter prolongs the availability of ^{137}Cs to plant roots by reduction of binding by clays. Levels in the human population, expressed in terms of picocuries per gram of potassium have ranged from 2 to 140 over the time span 1953 to 1976, with the highest levels occurring during the 1963–1966 period.[22,23] In general, it appears that the levels in the body lag behind those in the diet by about 4 months and that the ^{137}Cs/K ratio in the body is about three times the ratio in the diet.

Considerable attention has been given to the situation in some arctic regions where the ^{137}Cs levels in food and man are 100 or more times greater than those in the northern temperate latitudes. This is primarily the result of accumulation of fallout on lichens and other native vegetation which grow slowly and are grazed by reindeer and caribou. The meat from these animals constitutes a large part of the diets of arctic populations.

Recent concerns for radioactive releases from nuclear reactors and nuclear fuel reprocessing facilities have intensified efforts to minimize such releases and expand monitoring programs. These efforts have been instituted because of the one major difference between radioactivity from fallout and peaceful releases: the problem of worldwide fallout distribution as compared to the local distribution problem inherent with reactor releases. The widespread contamination patterns of fallout permitted generalizations to be drawn for wide regions with much less sampling rigor required. Localized peace-time releases require more intensive efforts to detect changes that may occur over time and to determine unique critical organisms or pathways that were heretofore relatively unimportant. Operating experiences to date indicate that releases in most instances have been well within authorized levels, usually resulting in dose rates at the boundary zones which are 1 to 5 per cent of the normal background levels in the area. Special consideration is being given to the aquatic environment, because of the different pathways and interrelationships to other releases and contaminants in this medium. However, it must be pointed out that these releases are generally much lower than the levels already experienced from fallout releases.[20,21]

BIOLOGIC CONSEQUENCES OF ENVIRONMENTAL RADIOCONTAMINATION

From the knowledge of the amounts of radioactivity present in man's body, reasonable estimates can be made of the radiation dosage that is delivered. Whereas there is a considerable body of information on the effects of radiation on man and animals, it has been impossible to detect any biologic effects at levels of radiation and dose rates as low as those resulting thus far from nuclear testing or from commercial nuclear power releases, which are much lower than fallout levels.[24,25] Thus, the best basis for estimating the effect of man-made radiation exposure on man is a comparison with the levels of natural background radiation to which the human population has always been exposed. Such a comparison is presented in Tables 15-5[2] and 15-6.[25]

These dosages take into account exposure from radionuclides of strontium, cesium and carbon, which are the elements of primary concern as potential long-term hazards. Thyroid doses from ^{131}I (half-life, 8 days) are not included, because peak

Table 15-6. Comparative Environmental Radiation in the United States (Whole-body Dose) Estimated 1970-2000[25]

Source	1970	2000
	(millirem/person/year)	
Natural (subtotal)	130	130
Cosmic	45	45
External gamma	60	60
Internal	25	25
Fallout (subtotal)	4	4.99
External gamma	0.89	0.90
Inhalation	0.04	0.04
Ingestion	3.07	4.05
Other (subtotal)	0.060	0.451
Nuclear reactors	0.002	0.174
Fuel reprocessing	0.0008	0.202
Worldwide ^{3}H	.045	.026
Worldwide ^{85}Kr	0.0004	0.037
AEC installations	0.012	0.012
Total all sources	134.060	135.441

dose rates persist only for a short period of time and these are discussed later. The most authoritative estimates of the consequences of such radiation exposure are shown in Table 15-7, where comparisons are made between the natural incidence and the potential effects from 5 rem per generation (a level that assumes maximum permissible man-made radiation exposures for the population at large or 170 millirem per person per year over a 30-year reproductive period).[15]

Table 15-5. Estimates of Worldwide Average Dose Commitments from Man-made Environmental Radiation and Annual Doses from Natural Background[2]

	Gonads	Bone-living Cells	Bone Marrow
	(mrad)		
Dose Commitments			
Atmospheric tests (before 1971)	120	180	160
Cratering experiments (before 1972)	2×10^{-2}	2×10^{-2}	2×10^{-2}
Electrical power (dose commitments per year)			
1970	9×10^{-4}	9×10^{-4}	9×10^{-4}
2000	2×10^{-1}	2×10^{-1}	2×10^{-1}
	(mrad/year)		
Annual Doses			
Natural background	93	92	89

Table 15–7. Estimated Consequences of Radiation Exposure[15]

Disease Classification	Current Incidence	Effect per One Million Population from Five (5) rem per Generation* First Generation	Equilibrium
Dominant diseases	10,000	50–500	250–2500
Chromosomal and recessive diseases	10,000	Relatively slight	Very slow increase
Congenital anomalies	15,000 ⎫		
Anomalies expressed later	10,000 ⎬	5,500	50–5000
Constitutional and degenerative diseases	15,000 ⎭		
Totals	60,000	60–1000	300–7500

* The estimated fraction of this attributable to nuclear power is less than 0.006 based on 1 millirem per year over a 30-year reproductive generation.

Since ^{131}I is the fallout radionuclide most likely to produce the greatest radiation exposures within short times (up to several weeks) after nuclear detonations, it is of interest to consider estimated radiation dosages and possible biologic effects. The dose to the thyroid of infants 6 to 18 months was estimated to range from 0.03 to 0.65 roentgens in 1961 and 1962, as determined from high and low individual stations of the Public Health Service Pasteurized Milk Nework. It has been estimated that a small number of infants conceivably could have received doses from 10 to 30 times the average.[14] Because the dose is inversely related to the size of the thyroid gland, the exposure of adults would be about one-tenth the values cited for infants.

In May 1953, local areas in Utah were reported to have received unusual amounts of fallout from the Nevada test site, with reconstructed estimates of thyroid dose ranging from less than 10 rad to above 400 rad. Examinations in 1965 and subsequent follow-ups of school children from the areas in question have revealed no thyroid abnormalities that can be ascribed specifically to radiation. Experience is available on the relatively high exposures (up to 1,000 rad or more) of the thyroid gland of human beings by virtue of: (1) diagnostic and therapeutic x-ray treatment, (2) diagnostic and therapeutic use of ^{131}I, (3) exposure of a Marshallese population and (4) exposures at Hiroshima and Nagasaki. In general, it appears that radioactive iodine, delivering dosages of several hundred rad to the thyroids of infants or young children, will produce a high incidence of thyroid nodules, whereas the incidence of cancer has not been observable and must be extremely low.[7]

On the basis of this and estimates presented in Table 15–7, it is generally agreed that health risks from present and anticipated levels of environmental radiocontamination are probably not zero, but are too small to justify individual anxiety or attempts to modify dietary intakes.

GOVERNMENTAL RESPONSIBILITY AND REMEDIAL MEASURES

Although there need not be individual anxiety about fallout, there must be concern and interest on the part of officials and scientists who have authorized responsibility. There are two interrelated areas of consideration: (1) the establishment of radiation standards or levels as guidelines at which remedial actions should be recommended, and (2) the development of remedial or preventive measures to reduce the exposure of the population to radioactive contamination.

Radiation Standards

It is necessary that an official body stipulate some level or range of radiocontamination at which preventive or remedial action should be given serious considera- tion. To the Federal Radiation Council falls the crucial and difficult task of setting radiation standards. This body, which was created in 1959, is comprised of representatives from all the national agencies that have an interest in any aspect of radiation. Its major function is to advise the President with respect to radiation matters directly or indirectly affecting health, including guidance for all federal agencies in the formulation of radiation standards and in the establishment and execution of programs of cooperation with states.[14] The formation of the Environmental Protection Agency (EPA) has resulted in numerous organizational realignments within the federal government. Among them is the shifting of responsibilities of the Federal Radiation Council to the EPA. Although these changes have altered the functional aspects of the Council, the basic philosophy for radiation protection is still maintained in accord with, and mutually compatible with, guidance from the National Council on Radiation Protection and Measurements (NCRP) and the International Commission on Radiological Protection (ICRP).

In 1960, the Federal Radiation Council provided the general philosophy for radiation protection. The term *radiation protection guide* (RPG) was introduced and defined as "the radiation dose which should not be exceeded without careful consideration of the reasons for doing so: every effort should be made to encourage the maintenance of radiation doses as far below this guide as practicable." RPGs were developed for radiation workers, for individuals in the population and for suitable samples of exposed population groups. The RPG for whole-body exposure of individuals in the general population (exclusive of natural background and

deliberate exposure of patients by practitioners of the healing arts) was established as 0.5 rem per year. The value was set at one-third of this dose, or 0.17 rem per year, for suitable samples of exposed population groups. These guides were considered appropriate for normal peacetime operations and were not to apply to contamination produced by weapons testing.

In 1961, in order to provide guidance for agencies in developing appropriate programs for control of intake of radioactivity from the environment, the Federal Radiation Council described a graded approach for various radionuclides. Three ranges of transient rates of daily intake were determined, with various actions outlined for each range. The objective of this approach was to limit the intake of radioactive materials so that the specified RPGs would not be exceeded. Table 15–8 presents an outline of the ranges and recommended actions for ^{89}Sr, ^{90}Sr and ^{131}I. The upper limit of Range II is based on an

Table 15–8. Federal Radiation Council Recommended Daily Intake Ranges and Action Criteria to Remain Below Radiation Protection Guides[14]

	Daily Intake Levels (pc/day)		
	Range I	Range II	Range III
^{89}Sr	0–200	200–2000	2000–20,000
^{90}Sr	0– 20	20– 200	200– 2000
^{131}I (infant)*	0– 10	10– 100	100– 1000

Action Criteria	
Range I	Surveillance adequate to provide reasonable confirmation of calculations.
Range II	Active surveillance and controls so that exposures will not exceed upper limit of Range II.
Range III	Active surveillance and controls designed to return levels of radioactive intake to Range II or lower.

* Ranges designed for the most susceptible group. Adult levels would be increased by a factor of 10.

annual RPG considered as an acceptable risk for a lifetime.

Since ^{131}I is the only radionuclide which has attained levels near the established guidelines, the status in regard to radiation standards is discussed in terms of this radionuclide. In brief, the Federal Radiation Council guidance for ^{131}I is represented by an annual average intake of 100 pc per day or an annual intake of 36,500 pc as the upper level of so-called Range II, above which the application of control measures is to be considered. Although the guidelines were originally presented with appropriate qualifications, especially restricting their application to normal peacetime industrial operations, there seemed to be an understanding in the minds of most individuals that these standards should also apply to fallout. In the fall of 1962, concentrations in milk in some areas of the country approached the levels at which action appeared to be warranted by the Federal Radiation Council guidelines. As a matter of fact, at least one state undertook to reduce the ^{131}I levels in commercial fresh milk by arranging for farmers to utilize stored feed instead of pasture for dairy herds.[26]

In response to this situation, the Federal Radiation Council issued an official statement on September 17, 1962, which affords some clarification and from which the following excerpts are taken:[27]

> In some localities in the United States, average annual intake values of radioactive iodine have approached the upper level of Range II, and, in one locality, have slightly exceeded Range II. This had led to actions and proposed actions involving countermeasures or preventive health measures. The Federal Radiation Council does not recommend such actions under present circumstances.
>
> The Council believes, based on competent scientific advice, that any possible health risk which may be associated with exposures even many times above the guide levels would not result in a detectable increase in the incidence of disease.
>
> The Radiation Protection Guides are not a dividing line between safety and danger in

actual radiation situations nor are they alone intended to set a limit at which protective action should be taken. As applied to fallout, guides can be used as an indication of when there is need for detailed evaluation of possible exposure risks and when there is need to consider whether any protective action should be taken under all the relevant circumstances.

> Radiation exposures anywhere near the guides involve risks so slight that countermeasures may have a net adverse rather than favorable effect on the public well-being. The judgement as to when to take action and what kind of action to take to decrease exposure levels involves consideration of all factors.

In view of the misunderstanding regarding the application of radiation protection guides, the Federal Radiation Council considered the problems of fallout from nuclear tests and in 1964–1965 established *protective action guides* for ^{131}I, ^{89}Sr, ^{90}Sr and ^{137}Cs. These set forth the projected absorbed doses of individuals in the general population that warrant protective action

Table 15–9. Federal Radiation Council Protective Action Guides and Action Criteria—Acute Localized Event[14]

	Annual Projected Dose	
	Individual (rad)	Population (rad)
^{89}Sr, ^{90}Sr, ^{137}Cs		
Category I	10*	3
Category II	5	2
Category III	0.5	0.2
^{131}I		
Category I	30	10

Protective Actions

Category I
  (1) Remove cattle from pasture to stored feed.
  (2) Switch to uncontaminated milk by changes in processing or distributing with diversion or disposal of contaminated milk.
Category II
  (1) Modify animal feed utilization, food processing and marketing practices.
  (2) Diversion of crops to remove radionuclides from food chain areas.
  (3) Destruction of selective food or feed crops.
Category III
  (1) Action to be determined on a case-by-case basis.

* Total dose must not exceed 15 rad.

following a contaminating event. Categories were developed for acute contaminating events and are shown in Table 15–9 along with some of the protective actions considered appropriate for the given categories. The relationships between the levels of radionuclides in food products and the projected doses to the population are also discussed in the referenced publications but are too complex to be presented here. Similarly complex release criteria are in effect for peaceful uses of nuclear energy including special release restrictions for nuclear-powered reactors, fuel fabrication plants and nuclear fuel reprocessing plants. Basically, the restrictions limit effluent releases so that annual whole-body dose rates for individuals do not exceed 5 per cent of background levels.[28] In a 1977 action, the Environmental Protection Agency proposed limited releases of ^{85}Kr, ^{129}I and transuranics and proposed limited annual radiation doses of 25 millirem whole body and 75 millirem thyroid for individual members of the public.[29]

It is important to keep clearly in mind the difference between "local" fallout and "worldwide" or stratospheric fallout. The levels for Categories I and II of Table 15–9 are likely and the actions proposed are feasible only for local fallout. Effective protective action to cope with worldwide fallout conditions could be achieved only by long-term changes in: (1) agricultural practices, (2) food processing practices or (3) basic dietary habits. The Federal Radiation Council concluded that, while surveillance of worldwide contamination should be continued, the health risks therefrom over the next several years would be too small to justify protective action.

Remedial Measures

It is prudent that knowledge be obtained to cope with any foreseeable contingencies and research must be done on preventive measures.[30] The fact that such work is under way, however, should not be interpreted by the lay public to indicate that these measures are needed or desirable under existing conditions. In general, any remedial measure, to be useful, must fulfill certain requirements:

1. It must be effective in removing contamination.
2. It must be safe in that the health risk from its use must be less than that from the radiocontaminant.
3. It must be practical from the standpoint of application.
4. The responsibility for the application must be defined, since this cannot be left to the individual but has to be done on a national or state basis.
5. The impact on the public must be considered so that there is no panic that could lead to malnutrition, with a deleterious effect that might far outweigh the expected benefits from the removal of the radiocontaminant.

Specific comments on remedial measures are limited here to ^{131}I, since this radionuclide, if any, will probably be the first to require action. Remedial measures for ^{131}I are relatively simple because of its short half-life and because it reaches the public primarily in a single identifiable food, milk. Measures that have been proposed are as follows, starting with the most practical.[30]

Use of Stored Feed Instead of Pasture for Dairy Cows. The practicability of this procedure depends first of all upon the availability of stored feed (usually over 20 days old) in a given location at the needed time. Another problem is the time element. The peak of ^{131}I in milk is usually reached within a few days after deposition and, unless animals are transferred to stored feed within that time, the procedure may be of little avail. This means that plans must be made well ahead of time so that they can be put into effect immediately upon notification.

Use of Evaporated or Powdered Milk for Young Children and Pregnant and Lactating Women. This approach would be quite effective but there would undoubtedly be a public relations problem in that many individuals in the rest of the population would also want to stop using fresh milk. The feasibility would depend upon the available stores and production capacity for such products.

Use of Other Stored Milk Products. The feasibility of this measure would depend upon the maintenance and availability of large enough stores of such items as refrigerated, frozen or canned milk.

Pooling of Milk. Theoretically, the ^{131}I level in milk from regions of high contamination can be reduced by pooling with milk from regions of low contamination. Limiting factors would be the necessary assay of milk supplies and logistics.

Addition of Stable Iodine to Human Diet. Increased levels of stable iodine in the diet will reduce the deposition of ingested ^{131}I in the thyroid. However, the consensus of medical opinion is that there would be certain health risks in the use of stable iodine on a population-wide basis.

Other Measures. Strontium 90 decontamination is a much more difficult problem and as yet there are no preventive or remedial measures that fulfill the criteria of effectiveness, safety and feasibility, except possibly the removal of ^{90}Sr from milk by ion exchange. This process has been demonstrated on a commercial scale and could be initiated as a part of most milk plants at costs approaching 1 cent per quart. However, this measure would be regarded as an emergency capability which would have little application under current and expected contamination levels. Similar techniques have also been explored for ^{137}Cs and ^{131}I with comparable results. Other research is being continued on the possibilities of soil control, liming of soils and addition of stable calcium to dairy rations and human diets.

SUMMARY

In regard to environmental radiocontamination there seems to be general agreement about the following: (1) the behavior of radioactive materials in their movement from the site of production through the atmosphere and the food chain to reach the human population, (2) the levels of radiation exposure of the population from given amounts and patterns of nuclear testing and (3) the maximum biologic effects that can be expected from a given degree of environmental contamination.

There are areas of uncertainty that require continued research and attention. These include among others: (1) the significance of local regions of high fallout that might result from combinations of circumstances, such as high rainfall, low soil calcium and local distribution from underground bursts or accidental releases from nuclear facilities, (2) more detailed knowledge on the biologic and social consequences of radiation exposure of large populations and special-risk population components (e.g. the developing fetus, the sick, the young, the aged) and (3) the development of effective and feasible preventive and remedial measures for the reduction of exposure from environmental contamination.

It seems clear that any use of nuclear energy or radiation probably involves a biologic cost to the individual or society, even though the harm may not be observable. There is little question that the benefits from controlled peacetime applications of nuclear energy more than justify its use. This is especially true if the total environmental costs of alternatives are fully considered in terms of the effects on plants, animals and man. Many comparative studies have been made of alternative energy sources which show nuclear power to have decided advantages in terms of total environmental impact (i.e. air emissions, water emissions, solid wastes, land impacts and occupational health factors).[21,31-34]

The effects of environmental radiocontamination from nuclear explosions prior to 1970 are small enough so that individual anxiety is not warranted, and any individual action to reduce exposure is likely to be detrimental as well as futile. Nevertheless, in regard to weapons tests, there are too many intangibles to permit a logical evaluation of both sides of the fundamental equation—benefit versus cost.

BIBLIOGRAPHY

1. Comar, Goldblith, Kraybill, Reitemeier and Shank: Health Phys., 9, 569, 1963.
2. Reports of the United Nations Scientific Committee on the Effects of Atomic Radiation. General Assembly 17th Session, Suppl. No. 16 A/5216, 1962; 19th Session Suppl. No. 14A/5814, 1964; 21st Session, Suppl. No. 14A/6314, 1966; 24th Session, Suppl. No. 13A/7613, 1969; 27th Session, Suppl. No. 25A/8725, 1972.
3. Hayes: Health Phys., 32, 215, 1977.
4. Russell: Radioactivity and Human Diet. Oxford, Pergamon Press, 1966.
5. Comar: Annu. Rev. Nucl. Sci., 15, 175, 1965.
6. Health and Safety Laboratory: United States Atomic Energy Commission, New York Operation Office, HASL Report 243, 1971, p. I–3.
7. Report of the Subcommittee of the National Academy of Sciences-National Research Council Advisory Committee to the Federal Radiation Council on Pathological Effects of Thyroid Irradiation, 1967.
8. Comar: Plutonium: Facts and Inferences. Electric Power Research Institute Special Report, EPRI EA-43-SR, 1976.
9. Health and Safety Laboratory: Energy Research and Development Administration, HASL Report 306, 1976.
10. Wasserman, Lengemann, Thompson and Comar: In Radioactive Fallout, Soils, Plants, Foods, Man (Fowler, Ed.). Amsterdam, Elsevier, 1965, p. 236.
11. Thompson: Health Phys., 13, 883, 1967; 14, 483, 1968.
12. Agricultural Research Council Radiobiological Laboratory: Report for 1964–1965, ARCRL 14, 75, 1965.
13. Russell: Health Phys., 11, 1305, 1965.
14. Federal Radiation Council Reports No. 1, 1960 through No. 7 1965. Washington, U.S. Government Printing Office.
15. Report of the Advisory Committee on the Biological Effects of Ionizing Radiations (BEIR). National Academy of Sciences—National Research Council, 1972.
16. Public Health Service: Radiological Health Data, Monthly Reports, 1, No. 1, 1960 through 15, No. 12, 1974.
17. Kulp and Schulert: ^{90}Sr in Man and his Environment, Vol. III. New York, Publications Geochemical Laboratory, Columbia University, 1961.
18. Health and Safety Laboratory: United States Atomic Energy Commission and Energy Research and Development Administration, HASL Reports 111, 1961 through No. 318, 1977.
19. Michelson, Thompson, Hess and Comar: J. Nutr., 78, 371, 1962.
20. Technical Reports, Northeastern Radiological Health Laboratory BRH/NERHL 70–1, 70–2, 70–3; Division of Environmental Radiation BRH/DER 70-2.
21. Hart, Ritchie and Varnadore (Eds.): Symposium on Population Exposures. Health Physics Society Eighth Midyear Topical Symposium, 1974.
22. Gustafson and Miller: Health Phys., 16, 167, 1969.
23. Shukla, Dombrowski and Cohn: Health Phys., 24, 555, 1973.
24. Joint Committee on Atomic Energy Hearings: Environmental Effects of Producing Electric Power, 91st Congress of the United States, 1969.
25. Environmental Protection Agency: Comparative Radiation Doses in the U.S. 1970–2000 EPA Report ORP/CSD 72–1, 1972.
26. Utah State Department of Health: Utah's Experience with Radioactive Milk, 1962.
27. Public Health Service: Radiobiological Health Data, Monthly Reports, 3, No. 11, 1962.
28. Federal Register, 36, No. 111, 1962.
29. U.S. Environmental Protection Agency: 1976 Environmental Radiation Protection Requirements for Normal Operations of Activities in the Uranium Fuel Cycle 40CFR190: Final Environmental Statement, Vol. 1 EPA Report 520/4-76-016, Washington.
30. National Advisory Committee on Radiation: Radioactive Contamination of the Environment: Public Health Action, 1962. Washington, Public Health Service.
31. Council on Environmental Quality: Energy and the Environment, 1973.
32. Sagan: Human and Ecologic Effects of Nuclear Power Plants. Springfield, Charles C Thomas, 1974.
33. Beckmann: The Health Hazards of Not Going Nuclear. Boulder, Golem, 1976.
34. Comar and Sagan: Health effects of energy production and conservation. Annu. Rev. Energy, 1, 581, 1976.

Part III

Interrelations of Nutrients and Metabolism

Chapter 16

HORMONAL CONTROL OF NUTRIENT METABOLISM

Albert B. Eisenstein
and
Sant P. Singh

The ability of animals to utilize carbohydrate, protein and fat as fuel provides the energy necessary to maintain life. Each of these essential nutrients has a specific and important role as a source of energy which complements that of the others. Carbohydrate (glucose) is used by all tissues as fuel and some, e.g. the brain and the erythrocyte, are almost totally dependent on a constant supply of glucose. Unfortunately, the capacity for storage of carbohydrate is small, so that after 24 hours of starvation the depots are exhausted. Protein catabolism begins after only a few hours of food deprivation and yields amino acids, which are directed into the pathway of carbohydrate synthesis in liver and kidney. Thus the supply of glucose is replenished. During starvation, fat tissue is broken down with release of fatty acids, glycerol and ketone bodies. Muscle can use fatty acids and ketone bodies almost exclusively to provide energy. In the chronically starved animal metabolic adjustments occur which are designed to protect protein stores, since loss of approximately half the body protein is incompatible with life. The brain develops the capacity to use ketone bodies as fuel; hence the need for protein catabolism, with conversion of amino acids to glucose, is lessened. When the food supply is plentiful protein synthesis occurs as new tissues are formed and old tissues replaced. If caloric intake is greater than energy expenditure, fatty acids are synthesized and stored as triglycerides in fat depots.

The synthesis and catabolism of carbohydrate, protein and fat are influenced by many hormones. These agents control nutrient metabolism in a variety of ways. Certain hormones increase the supply of substrate for synthetic processes, while others act on specific enzymatic reactions which regulate the flow of intermediates along biochemical pathways. Transport of substrate across the cell membrane is an important action of several hormones. Some complex metabolic processes are stimulated by one hormone and inhibited by another: thus fine adjustments in the rate or direction of the reactions are possible. In this chapter, we have not attempted to consider every hormone known to influence these processes but have tried to deal with those that appear to have the most significant roles.

PROTEIN METABOLISM

Hormonal Effects on Body Protein Distribution

Corticosteroids. A major action of the adrenal glucocorticoids is to induce protein catabolism in peripheral tissues. Cortisone administration results in increased nitrogen excretion because of loss of protein from the carcass, whereas the protein content of liver and other viscera increases.[1] Amino acids liberated as a result of protein breakdown in the periphery are transported to the liver, where they may be utilized in the synthesis of new protein. Not only is there protein synthesis but the total nucleic acid content of the liver also increases, primarily because of a rise in RNA content.[2] The responses to cortisone and to protein feeding are similar, in that both lead to increased liver protein and RNA.[3]

Insulin. Early evidence that insulin has an important role in protein synthesis was provided by the observation that the ingestion of sugar by animals or human subjects produced a prompt, but temporary, lowering of the plasma amino acid concentration. The concentrations of all amino acids were not altered to the same extent, but they were removed from plasma in the relative proportions needed for protein formation in muscle.[4] In studies utilizing labeled amino acids, carbohydrate-fed animals demonstrated increased incorporation of amino acids into muscle protein, but liver protein formation was not affected. The lowering of the plasma amino acid concentration which follows glucose administration results in reduced hepatic urea production and a diminished supply of amino acids for protein synthesis in tissues other than muscle.[3] It was soon realized that the influence of carbohydrate feeding on protein synthesis was the result of the action of insulin, since the effect of sugar ingestion on plasma amino acid concentration is abolished in diabetic animals. Furthermore, insulin causes a rapid fall in the blood amino acid level and stimulates in vitro uptake of amino acids by muscle, liver and other tissues. Insulin enhances the uptake of amino acids in vivo within a few minutes after injection, whereas the in vitro action of the hormone in liver has a delayed onset and takes several hours to reach its maximum. The rapid uptake of amino acids induced by insulin in vivo appears to be caused by hormonal action on muscle.

Anabolic Hormones (Androgens and Growth Hormone). The nitrogen-retaining effect of insulin is shared by androgens and growth hormone (GH). Animals receiving a normal diet respond to testosterone with an increase in protein content of muscle, liver and other viscera. If the androgenic steroid is given to fasting animals or those on a protein-free diet, there is acceleration of protein loss from liver but protein degradation in muscle is slowed.[5,6] Growth hormone also exerts a preferential effect on protein synthesis in muscle, as shown by the finding that the relative size of certain muscles is increased more following administration of the hormone than is that of the liver, other muscles and viscera. Furthermore, treatment of animals with GH increased the incorporation of labeled amino acids into muscle protein and reduced conversion to liver protein.

Catabolic Hormones (Thyroid Hormones, Estrogens). Short-term thyroxine (T_4) administration to animals leads to an increase of liver protein and RNA while there is a concomitant loss of protein from muscle. If treatment with T_4 is continued both liver and carcass are reduced in size, but the liver is less affected than are peripheral tissues.[3] Thyroid hormones act on liver to produce increased uptake of amino acids and enhance incorporation of amino acids into protein by liver microsomes.[7]

Large doses of estrogens cause nitrogen loss from the animal body, but their effect seems to be indirect since it is abolished by adrenalectomy.

Hormonal Effects on Protein Metabolism

Insulin. Although the profound influence of insulin on glucose utilization was recognized before effects of the hormone on protein metabolism were detected, it is now apparent that the action of insulin on the latter process is as important as is its role in carbohydrate metabolism. Insulin affects protein and amino acid metabolism in several ways: (1) It promotes cellular uptake of amino acids by stimulating transport, thus reducing blood amino acid levels; (2) it enhances the incorporation of amino acids into tissue protein; (3) it acts to induce synthesis of certain hepatic enzymes and to suppress synthesis of others;[8] (4) it inhibits protein degradation.

Insulin lowers blood amino acids in normal as well as in diabetic humans and animals. The time required to lower the blood level is similar to that for glucose. Lotspeich[9] reported that insulin lowered the blood level of the 10 essential amino acids in normal, fasted dogs, and noted that the pattern of decrease of individual amino acids corresponded to their relative concentrations in muscle protein. Valine, leucine, isoleucine, methionine, tyrosine and phenylalanine showed the largest changes. Other investigators found plasma amino acid levels to be higher in diabetic rats than in controls, with leucine, isoleucine and valine showing the most striking changes.

Muscle incubated in vitro liberates amino acids, the rate of release of which is depressed by the addition of insulin to the incubation mixture. A similar effect on amino acid release from the isolated liver has been observed. Studies of the human forearm in which physiologic amounts of insulin were infused through the brachial artery demonstrated inhibition of net output from muscle of leucine, isoleucine, methionine, tyrosine, phenylalanine and threonine.[10] In addition to reducing amino acid release, insulin also stimulates the accumulation of these compounds, as shown by an increased uptake of various amino acids, including α-aminoisobutyric acid, which is a nonutilizable compound. While insulin inhibits efflux of amino acids from muscle, Adibi has reported that glucose lowers amino acid levels in plasma, liver and muscle, through a mechanism independent of its effect on insulin secretion.[10a] It was suggested that glucose, by direct or indirect action on peripheral tissues, contributes to the production of hypoaminoacidemia.

Insulin added to isolated muscle preparations promotes incorporation of labeled amino acids into tissue protein.[10b] This stimulatory effect is not restricted to muscle but also occurs in adipose tissue, mammary gland slices, costal cartilage, bone marrow cells and leukocytes, as well as other tissues.[8] Insulin stimulates the incorporation of naturally occurring amino acids into protein by tissues of normal animals except for the liver, in which action of the hormone is evident only in diabetic preparations. Wool and Krahl[11] showed that, if amino acids were accumulated by the diaphragm in vivo, subsequent exposure to insulin in vitro increased their incorporation into protein. Furthermore, there is increased conversion of amino acids synthesized in muscle into tissue protein. Thus it is clear that insulin stimulates protein synthesis as well as amino acid uptake.

In searching for the primary action of insulin, various investigators have examined the effect of the hormone on RNA synthesis. Wool and others[12,13a–d] have shown that insulin stimulates incorporation of labeled precursors into nucleic acid, although Manchester could not completely confirm these observations.[8] Despite the fact that insulin increases RNA synthesis in muscle, the increase is not a requisite for hormone-mediated stimulation of protein synthesis. This was shown by the observation that actinomycin, an inhibitor of RNA synthesis, did not impair the ability of insulin to increase protein formation.[13e]

Although the effects of insulin in muscle are quite apparent, it has been more difficult to clarify the role of the hormone in hepatic protein metabolism. Liver slices from diabetic rats show decreased capacity to incorporate amino acids into protein, a defect which can be corrected by insulin treatment. However, addition of insulin to livers of diabetic animals in vitro does not restore the depressed rate of protein synthesis unless the diabetes is mild and glucose is also present. In microsomes prepared from diabetic liver, amino acid incorporation into protein is impaired and can be restored to normal by prior administration of insulin.[14a,b] Kletzien recently studied the effects of insulin on amino acid transport in cultured rat liver cells by assessing the uptake of α-aminoisobutyric acid.[14c] Following the addition of insulin to cultured liver cells, there was an increased influx of α-aminoisobutyric acid (AIB) reflected in a higher initial rate of amino acid transport as well as in an increased accumulation of AIB at later time points. Uptake of the amino acid by cultured hepatocytes was blocked by cycloheximide; thus transport is dependent on protein synthesis.

Activities of a number of hepatic enzymes are altered in experimental diabetes. Glucokinase, glycogen synthetase, phosphofructokinase, pyruvate kinase and pentose shunt enzymes are depressed in diabetic liver, whereas glucose-6-phosphatase, fructose-1, 6-diphosphatase, phosphoenolypyruvate carboxykinase and pyruvate carboxylase are increased. These abnormalities are corrected by insulin administration. The increase in activity of the first group of enzymes after insulin treatment facilitates disposition of glucose through oxidation and storage, while the reduced activity of the second group lowers the elevated gluconeogenesis found in diabetes. Insulin causes glycogen deposition in liver by increasing glycogen synthetase activity and decreasing phosphorylase activity. Insulin rapidly elevates activity of a phosphatase that dephosphorylates glycogen synthetase, thereby converting the enzyme to its active form.[14d]

The long-term effects of insulin on glycolysis and gluconeogenesis are caused, at least in part, by its influence on synthesis of important regulatory enzymes, such as pyruvate kinase, pyruvate carboxylase, phosphofructokinase and fructose diphosphatase.[14d] Insulin also has acute effects on the activities of glycolytic and gluconeogenic enzymes in liver. Since rate-limiting reactions in glycolysis are at the phosphofructokinase, glucokinase and pyruvate kinase steps, and insulin causes rapid changes in the activities of these enzymes, the effects of the hormone on glycolysis may be explained.

Glycolytic enzymes of fat and muscle and gluconeogenic enzymes of the renal cortex are affected by insulin and glucagon in a manner similar to liver enzymes. Insulin increases the activities of phosphofructokinase and pyruvate kinase and decreases the activity of fructose diphosphatase.[14d]

Although there is evidence that insulin acts directly to induce synthesis of certain enzymes (e.g. glucokinase) and to suppress formation of others, it has not been established that the hormone regulates liver carbohydrate metabolism by primary control of enzyme synthesis and degradation. Of added significance are reports which describe insulin stimulation of RNA polymerase activity, of liver cell hyperplasia and of DNA synthesis.[15] The relationship of these alterations to the changes in enzyme levels in diabetes and after insulin treatment remains to be elucidated.

Growth Hormone (GH). Many early clinical and experimental observations pointed to an important role for GH in protein metabolism. Hypophysectomy is followed by abrupt cessation of growth in young animals and by weight loss in adults. The decline in weight following pituitary removal is accompanied by negative nitrogen balance which persists for several weeks before nitrogen equilibrium is regained. Forced feeding prevents weight loss in hypophysectomized rats; however, carcass analysis has revealed that nitrogen storage is slight and that there is an abnormal accumulation of fat.[16] Administration of GH to intact or hypophysectomized rats results in increased body weight accompanied by a rise in water and protein content and loss of fat. It has been shown that the increases in tissue protein content brought about by GH treatment result from enhanced protein biosynthesis and not from reduced protein breakdown.

Subsequently, GH was found to stimulate incorporation of labeled amino acids into liver protein, while hypophysectomy has the opposite effect. Amino acid conversion to protein in a cell-free system containing liver microsomes and cell sap is less than normal if the tissue is taken from hypophysectomized rats. Treatment of the animals with GH before removal of the liver restores the incorporating activity of this system. Separation of the system into microsomes and cell sap shows that hypophysectomy and GH treatment of rats affect the ability of the microsomal fraction, not that of the cell sap, to incorporate amino acids into protein.[17]

Injection of amino acids into the rat and study of liver cell fractions confirm the in vitro observation that GH increases the amino acid-incorporation capacity of microsomes. GH also enhances amino acid incorporation into protein by the isolated diaphragm of hypophysectomized rats when the hormone is added to the incubation medium.[17a] Hjalmarson and Ahren investigated the effects of GH on uptake of AIB by diaphragms of normal and hypophysectomized rats.[17b] Their results demonstrated that muscle of hypophysectomized rats is far more responsive to GH than is normal diaphragm. The insensitivity of normal muscle is related to the fact that this tissue has been exposed to GH secreted in vivo.

In order to assess the metabolic effects of GH in rats, Nutting determined the ability of ovine GH to stimulate amino acid uptake and protein synthesis in diaphragm muscle.[17c] GH stimulated α-aminoisobutyric acid (AIB) uptake in diaphragms from fed, intact rats 7 to 24 days old but did not influence AIB transport in diaphragm from younger or older rats. When rats were fasted for 24 hours, muscle responsiveness to GH was considerably increased. GH stimulated AIB uptake of 4- to 23-day-old fasted rats, with the greatest effect occurring on day 15. Leucine incorporation into protein by rat diaphragm exposed to GH was also elevated on the fifteenth day. These results suggest that rat

diaphragm muscle first becomes sensitive to GH at about 4 to 7 days (AIB transport) but that further development may be necessary for protein synthesis to be stimulated.

Efforts to uncover the mechanisms by which GH stimulates protein synthesis have focused on the effects of the hormone on RNA metabolism. Not only is there a fall in protein content and in the capacity for protein synthesis in the hypophysectomized animal but there is also a decline in RNA content and in its rate of synthesis. Treatment with GH returns RNA synthesis to normal. Ribosomes prepared from liver of hypophysectomized rats have an impaired capacity to incorporate amino acids into protein, even though they have an RNA content similar to that found in ribosomes from normal rats.[18] Although it was thought that GH might stimulate synthesis of messenger RNA, no such specific effect has been discovered. Instead, GH administration stimulates synthesis of all types of RNA and enhances RNA polymerase activity.[15] The manner by which GH stimulates RNA synthesis in liver and other tissues is not known. There is a lag period of 3 to 5 hours before hormone-induced RNA synthesis is clearly evident in rat liver; thus it is likely that other events may precede this action of the hormone.[18a] It is of interest that liver RNA synthesis is also stimulated by feeding large amounts of amino acids. The observation that GH promotes amino acid incorporation into protein in the presence of actinomycin D indicates that RNA synthesis may not be required in order for the hormone to exert its characteristic effects.

Adrenal Cortical Steroids. Removal of the adrenals from fasting rats results in prompt reduction of nitrogen excretion and a decline of blood glucose and liver glycogen. Replacement therapy with corticosteroids restores urinary nitrogen to the previous level and corrects abnormalities of carbohydrate metabolism.[19a] These observations demonstrate the important influence of corticosteroid hormones on protein metabolism. Also, many investigations have shown that cortical steroids promote protein catabolism and interfere with protein synthesis.

Muscle Protein. Engel studied the effects of corticosteroids on protein metabolism by determining the rate of urea formation in nephrectomized rats. Urea production was not altered for 2 to 3 hours after hormone administration; then it rose and remained elevated for 3 to 6 hours.[19b] Engel believed the increased urea formation to be caused either by accelerated protein catabolism or the inhibition of protein anabolism. Similar conclusions were reached by Friedberg and Greenberg, who observed decreased plasma amino acids after adrenalectomy and increased plasma, muscle and liver amino acids following administration of a lipid extract of adrenal cortical tissue.[20] More recent data reveal that cortisol or cortisone administration results in increased levels of free amino acids in muscle and reduced capacity of muscle to concentrate amino acids. The accumulation of free amino acids in muscle of corticosteroid-treated animals appears to be the result of inhibition of protein synthesis.[21] Other investigators found that the increase of individual amino acids in plasma during ACTH treatment of dogs parallels the proportions of the same amino acids in muscle, indicating muscle to be their source.

Bondy determined the effects of adrenal cortical extract (ACE) and adrenalectomy on the accumulation of amino acids in the plasma of eviscerated rats.[22] ACE produced a greater increase of plasma amino nitrogen (N) in 3 hours than occurred in saline-treated controls, while adrenalectomy resulted in a much diminished rise of plasma amino N. Of added importance was the finding that glucose administration abolished the accumulation of amino acids induced by ACE. Since glucose does not alter amino acid metabolism, its effect appears to be that of inhibition of ACE-induced protein breakdown. It is now generally recognized that muscle is the chief site of protein breakdown and liberation of amino acids following corticosteroid administration.

Muscle protein formation, as measured by the incorporation of radioactive amino acids, is raised soon after adrenalectomy and is reduced when animals are treated with glucocorticoids.[23] Weinshelbaum and Wool studied ^{14}C phenylalanine incorporation into heart muscle of adrenalectomized rats. Adrenalectomy increased amino acid incorporation into muscle protein, with the greatest effect occurring in the microsomal fraction.[23a] Hydrocortisone administration decreases phenylalanine incorporation equally in all subcellular fractions of heart muscle. Kostyo used diaphragms from normal and adrenalectomized rats to evaluate the effects of adrenal steroids on muscle protein metabolism.[23b,c] After 2 to 3 hours of preincubation with $10^{-5}M$ corticosterone, uptake of α-aminoisobutyric acid by diaphragm was reduced. Simultaneously, the glucocorticoid-treated muscle became less able to incorporate ^{14}C methionine into tissue protein. Adrenal cortical hormones also depress amino acid incorporation into protein by spleen, lymphocytes, reticulocytes, bone cells and thymus tissue.

Although these findings demonstrate that corticosteroids interfere with protein synthesis in certain tissues, the mechanism by which these agents act is not understood. It is possible that steroids suppress RNA formation, since they reduce RNA polymerase activity in thymus nuclei and, as a result, there is decreased incorporation of labeled precursors into RNA.

Liver Protein. In contrast to their effects in muscle, adrenal cortical hormones enhance amino acid trapping by the liver. Noall et al.[24] demonstrated that cortisol administration to rats led to a marked increase in hepatic uptake of α-aminoisobutyric acid (AIB) within a few hours after the hormone was given. Weber found that injection of corticosteroids into fed rats produced a rapid increase of the free amino nitrogen level in liver.[25] Others observed elevation of only selected amino acids in liver after cortisol injection into fasting rats, indicating that the nutritional state of the animal influences hormone response. Addition of glucocorticoid to isolated, perfused rat livers stimulates transport of AIB from medium into liver, although there is a lag period of about 1 hour before the effect is apparent.[26]

Although glucocorticoid administration causes increased N excretion due to protein loss from the animal carcass, protein content of the liver and other viscera increases.[27] Deposition of protein in liver following adrenal steroid treatment is affected by the amount of energy provided by diet, with greater protein synthesis occurring when caloric content of the diet is high. This finding suggests that the capacity of liver to utilize amino acids derived from peripheral tissue catabolism depends upon a constant and adequate caloric intake. The increase in liver protein synthesis resulting from steroid administration is accompanied by an increase in tissue RNA content.

Synthesis of Liver Enzymes. Tryptophan pyrollase (TP) was the first liver enzyme found to be induced by glucocorticoids. Activity of the enzyme is stimulated by corticoids as well as by its substrate, tryptophan. The mechanisms by which cortisone and tryptophan elevate TP are different, since the effects of these agents are additive. Using immunochemical methods, Feigelson and Greengard demonstrated that both hormone and substrate increase TP concentration in proportion to the rise of enzyme activity.[28] Cortisol has been shown to increase synthesis of the enzyme, whereas tryptophan has little effect on amino acid incorporation into enzyme protein. Tryptophan stabilizes the enzyme by causing a great decline in the rate of degradation.[29]

Tyrosine transaminase (TT) concentra-
tion in liver is elevated quickly and markedly in response to glucocorticoids. In contrast to TP, which is stabilized by tryptophan, TT is not affected in this manner by tyrosine nor does substrate induction of the enzyme occur. Kenney has shown that the rate of TT synthesis is accelerated four- to fivefold by corticosteroids.[29] Increased synthesis is apparent within 1 hour after injection and the elevated rate is maintained for an additional 4 to 5 hours. Induction of TT is due to a direct action of glucocorticoids on the liver, since the steroids stimulate enzyme activity in isolated perfused rat liver. Levitan and Webb made the intriguing observation that, as TT activity of rat liver rises during the first 4 hours after corticosteroid treatment, enzyme degradation is turned off.[29a] This suggests an interaction between enzyme degradation and synthesis.

Corticosteroids also cause elevation of glutamic-alanine transaminase (GAT) levels; however, the rise of enzyme activity is much slower than that of TP or TT. Enzyme activity increases about fivefold after several days of steroid treatment.[30] Glucocorticoids increase activity of pyruvate carboxylase (PC), phosphoenolpyruvate carboxykinase (PEPCK), glucose-6-phosphatase (G6Pase) and fructose-1,6-diphosphatase (FDPase), enzymes which are considered to regulate the rate of gluconeogenesis. As Kenney has made clear, even though activity levels rise there is no direct evidence to demonstrate that enzyme synthesis is responsible for the increases.[29] Furthermore, the enhanced PEPCK activity produced by cortisol can be reproduced by the administration of glucagon. The cortisol-induced rise of PEPCK is blocked by the administration of glucose or insulin, both of which suppress glucagon secretion, thus raising the possibility that glucocorticoids do not affect PEPCK directly but act by causing release of glucagon.[29]

Since corticosteroids stimulate synthesis of certain enzymes, intensive investigation to uncover the mechanism by which this effect is mediated has been conducted. It has been learned that glucocorticoids influence hepatic RNA metabolism in several ways.[29] Synthesis of nuclear RNA occurs prior to the first elevation of induced enzymes. All types of RNA—ribosomal, transfer and "DNA-like"—are elevated by cortisol, suggesting that the hormone actually affects precursor pools and not true synthesis of RNA. This question has not been conclusively answered. The activity of RNA is elevated by the hormone. The significance of the increase in RNA synthesis that occurs following cortisol administration is unclear.[29]

Corticosteroids and Protein Metabolism in Man. The catabolic and antianabolic actions of glucocorticoids on protein metabolism are responsible for many of the characteristic clinical features of Cushing's syndrome. Loss of protein leads to wasting of bone matrix and osteoporosis. Atrophy of skin and supporting tissue and increased capillary fragility are evidenced by ecchymoses and cutaneous striae, which are commonly present. There is often poor wound healing in hyperadrenocorticism. Muscle wasting and weakness may be so pronounced that the patient has difficulty in rising from a squatting position. A chronic excess of corticoid hormones, whether of endogenous or exogenous origin, inhibits growth in children.

Despite clinical evidence of protein wasting, patients with Cushing's syndrome remain in nitrogen balance if the diet contains 1 gm of protein per kg of body weight. Ingestion of a high-protein diet, whether it contains adequate calories or not, results in positive nitrogen balance, while a low-protein diet is associated with negative nitrogen balance, regardless of caloric content.[31] The administration of testosterone to patients with Cushing's syndrome induces positive nitrogen balance and improves skin thickness and strength.

Thyroid Hormones. Short-term administration of thyroxine (T_4) leads to an increase in liver protein and RNA and a loss of protein from the carcass. If hormone treatment is prolonged, protein depletion is general, although loss from the liver is less than that from peripheral tissues. Foley[32] found an increased amino acid concentration in venous blood draining the forearm of human subjects treated with thyroid hormone. The catabolic effect of T_4 on peripheral protein stores is similar to that of corticosteroids; however, the adrenal steroids reduce amino acid transport into muscle and decrease muscle protein synthesis, whereas T_4 does not have these effects. In the livers of rats receiving T_4 the level of all amino acids was increased but, in the carcass, only histidine, lysine and tryptophan concentrations were elevated.[33] These changes are different from those observed after corticosteroid administration, since the latter hormone increases free amino acids in the carcass rather than in the viscera.

An effect of thyroid hormones on protein synthesis was demonstrated by the observation that triiodothyronine (T_3) increased incorporation of amino acids into protein by isolated liver microsomes and mitochondria. This enhancement of protein synthesis could not be demonstrated in the presence of actinomycin, suggesting that the hormonal effect was mediated by stimulating RNA formation.[15] Recently, specific nuclear binding sites for iodothyronines have been recognized in liver and there is substantial evidence that thyroid hormones initiate their effects by augmenting the transcription of genetic information. In thyroidectomized rats injected with T_3, the first biochemical change in liver is increased incorporation of orotic acid into rapidly labeled nuclear RNA. This is soon followed by stimulation of RNA polymerase and, later, by increased rates of protein synthesis and oxygen consumption. It has been proposed that the effects of thyroid hormone are largely caused by new protein synthesis brought about by enhanced transcription of DNA.[34,34a]

Thyroid hormone administration leads to increased formation of specific hepatic proteins, e.g. glycerophosphate dehydrogenase and carbamyl phosphate synthetase.

Androgenic Hormones. A stimulatory effect of androgenic hormones on growth and protein metabolism has been long recognized. The androgens do not have a uniform effect on all organs and tissues, but are particularly active on genital structures. In seminal vesicles, testosterone increases the RNA-DNA ratio, the activity of amino acid-activating enzymes and the incorporation of amino acids into protein.[16] Androgens appear to act at the transcriptional level rather than at the translational level.

Muscle is also a major site of androgen action, although not all muscles respond to the hormones in a similar manner. In the guinea pig, masticatory muscles are more sensitive to androgens than are other skeletal muscles. The response of hepatic protein metabolism to androgenic steroids is less clear than is that of muscle. Testosterone administration to rats eating a normal diet causes protein retention in liver, as well as in other viscera, and muscle; however, in fasted, castrated guinea pigs testosterone stimulates liver protein breakdown, while it acts to conserve muscle protein. Some investigators have been unable to detect an effect of androgens on liver protein metabolism.

Many observations demonstrate that androgens stimulate muscle growth. Female animals and castrated males have smaller muscles, with reduced contents of protein and DNA, than do normal males. When androgens are administered to castrated animals, protein is deposited in muscle. In studies of the mechanism by which androgens exert their anabolic action, it has been found that testosterone administration does not elevate muscle DNA content nor are there changes in the number of muscle

cells. The increased muscle weight induced by androgenic hormones results from growth of individual muscle fibers and not from formation of new fibers. Furthermore, following castration, muscle fiber size is decreased but there is no change in the number of fibers.[35] Androgens do not affect all muscles in the same manner, as indicated by the increased sensitivity of temporal and masseter muscles in guinea pigs and of perineal muscles in rats.

Androgen administration enhances incorporation of ^{14}C-labeled amino acids into muscle protein in normal or castrated rats and also stimulates amino acid uptake by isolated muscle strips. Breuer and Florini[36] found muscle ribosomes from castrated animals to be less active in protein synthesis than ribosomes from normal animals or castrated animals treated with androgens. These investigators also observed that actinomycin D prevented androgen stimulation of ribosome activity. While RNA content and ribosome activity are reduced by castration, replacement therapy with androgens results in increased RNA polymerase activity. Liao et al. suggested that RNA synthesized as a result of androgen treatment may be primarily ribosomal.[37a-c] These investigators showed that actinomycin inhibits the hormonal effect on RNA synthesis but does not alter the basal level of nuclear RNA formation.

Glucagon. *Amino Acid Metabolism.* Glucagon influences amino acid metabolism by liver in at least three ways: (1) Membrane transport is stimulated, (2) protein synthesis is inhibited and protein catabolism accelerated and (3) glucose synthesis from amino acids is enhanced.[38] Glucagon increases gluconeogenesis by perfused liver from mixtures of amino acids with a concomitant rise of urea formation. Glucagon induces a threefold increase in conversion of alanine to glucose, an action which can be reproduced by the perfusion of liver with 1 mM cyclic AMP (adenosine-3',5'-monophosphate). Mallette[39] studied the influence of glucagon on hepatic amino acid metabolism by perfusing livers with medium containing amino acids in normal plasma concentrations. He demonstrated that glucagon induced: (1) increased intracellular utilization of glycine, alanine, glutamate and phenylalanine for gluconeogenesis, (2) intracellular production of leucine, isoleucine and valine, a result of protein degradation and (3) enhanced cellular uptake of several amino acids, a result of action of the hormone on membrane transport. The increases of gluconeogenesis and ureogenesis are accompanied by rises in activities of several hepatic enzymes involved in glucose and urea synthesis. Glucagon also stimulates activities of aromatic amino acid transaminases, as well as those of enzymes specific for catabolism of amino acids.[38] The action of glucagon on hepatic enzymes is reduced by glucose administration, suggesting an inhibitory influence of insulin.

The actions of glucagon on amino acid metabolism have been extensively studied in fasted human subjects. Plasma glucagon rises during the first 3 or 4 days of starvation, while glucose and insulin levels are reduced. The early rise of glucagon relative to insulin is associated with accelerated gluconeogenesis, increased urea excretion and enhanced splanchnic amino acid extraction.[38] Felig showed that splanchnic extraction of alanine increases from 43 per cent in the postabsorptive state to 71 per cent on day 3, and after 6 weeks returns to 53 per cent.[40] During the first few days of food deprivation, glucagon secretion is elevated, resulting in a marked increase in the conversion of amino acids to glucose by the liver. It is through this mechanism that fuel is provided to the central nervous system and other tissues. However, as starvation becomes more prolonged, the brain adapts by developing the capacity to use ketone bodies as an energy source; hence there is a lesser need for a high rate of gluconeogenesis. Such adaptation is important, since the need for amino acids is

diminished and muscle protein degradation is reduced.

Protein Metabolism. Glucagon stimulates liver protein catabolism in the intact animal and in isolated tissue preparations. This overall effect is manifested by augmented urea formation, reduced liver protein content and increased release of amino acids from liver. The elevated protein catabolism can be suppressed by the administration of insulin or a mixture of amino acids. Mortimore's group has shown that glucagon inhibits liver protein synthesis despite the fact that the hormone induces synthesis of some liver enzymes.[41] These apparently paradoxical observations are thought to represent two distinct effects of the hormone. The mechanism by which glucagon suppresses protein synthesis has not been established, although there is some evidence that factors concerned with elongation or termination of peptide chains may be involved.

CARBOHYDRATE METABOLISM

Insulin. The discovery that insulin lowers the blood sugar in man and animals focused attention on the effects of this hormone on carbohydrate metabolism. Although the decline of blood glucose which follows insulin administration has attracted major attention, the hormone also stimulates glycogen synthesis, promotes glucose oxidation and has important influences on the metabolism of proteins and lipids.

Many attempts to explain the blood sugar-lowering effects of insulin have been made. Levine and associates[42,43] demonstrated that insulin accelerates the membrane transport of sugars by determining the effects of the hormone on the disposition of nonmetabolizable analogs of glucose. The most detailed studies of the role of insulin in the membrane transport of sugars were conducted with the perfused rat heart preparation. Insulin increases sugar transport fourfold in normal hearts and up to six- or sevenfold in hearts from diabetic animals.[44] The onset of hormone action is rapid, with accelerated transport evident within 1 to 2 minutes after the hormone is introduced into the perfusion fluid and reaching a maximum 15 to 20 minutes later. Insulin not only promotes the transport of nonutilizable sugars into the muscle cell but has a similar effect on the movement of glucose across the cell membrane.[44] Transport of glucose into skeletal and heart muscle, fat cells and fibroblasts is stimulated by insulin; however, entry of glucose into hepatic cells does not depend on this hormone. Glucose utilization by brain tissue was previously thought to proceed without being mediated by insulin; however, recent data demonstrate a requirement for insulin in glucose utilization by the hypothalamus.[45] The mechanism by which insulin stimulates glucose transport has not been elucidated but it is believed that it acts on a carrier substance present in the membrane.[46]

Cuatrecasas has demonstrated that insulin combines with specific receptors on fat cells and hepatocytes and that action of the hormone on glucose uptake by these cells depends upon this reaction.[47,48] The insulin receptor has been isolated, highly purified and demonstrated to be a glycoprotein. Reduced numbers of insulin receptors are present in insulin-resistant tissues of diabetic humans and rodents. Several investigators have observed a strong inverse correlation between the concentration of insulin in blood and the number of insulin receptors in liver, fat, muscle and blood cells.[48]

Insulin causes glycogen deposition in the liver, an effect which depends on activation of glycogen synthetase and inactivation of phosphorylase. Glycogen synthetase exists in two forms: One (D) depending on glucose-6-phosphate for its activity and the other (I) active in the absence of glucose-6-phosphate. Glycogen phosphorylase also exists in active and inactive forms. Insulin administration promotes rapid changes in both the hepatic glycogen synthetase and phosphorylase systems in the dog, monkey, rat and other animals.[49,50] Insulin causes rapid decreases in phosphorylase activity and more gradual increases in synthetase I activity in vivo; however, the hormone effect is of brief duration.[50]

Insulin not only promotes disposition of intracellular glucose by stimulating glycogen synthesis but it also acts to accelerate glycolysis. Glucokinase, which is involved in the initial enzymatic reaction of glycolysis in liver (phosphorylation), depends on insulin for maintenance of activity. In the absence of insulin or in subjects who are fasting or ingesting a carbohydrate-free diet, glucokinase activity drops to low values within 48 hours.[51] When insulin levels are reduced, activity of phosphofructokinase is diminished in both liver and muscle, so that glucose utilization is diminished. Insulin administration restores glucokinase and phosphofructokinase levels to normal and suppresses the activities of gluconeogenic enzymes, so that cellular uptake of glucose is increased and glucose synthesis is reduced.

Glucagon. The role of glucagon is as significant as that of insulin. Glucagon provides glucose for the organism when there is need for this substance as an energy source. How does the hormone of the pancreatic alpha cell act to make glucose available so that it may be utilized? It has long been known that glucagon is a powerful glycogenolytic agent in liver, and a good deal has been learned about its mechanism of action. Glucagon stimulates production of cyclic AMP (cAMP) by activating the enzyme adenyl cyclase. cAMP promotes the conversion of inactive phosphorylase to active phosphorylase, an enzyme which participates in the breakdown of glycogen to glucose.[50] Sokal[52] demonstrated that glucagon is a more potent glycogenolytic agent than epinephrine and believes that it is the only humoral factor which could serve as a physiologic regulator of hepatic glycogenolysis. The hormone is effective in the liver at a concentration of 3×10^{-11}M; its onset of action is rapid and its duration is short. In addition to a stimulatory effect on glycogen degradation, glucagon reverses the activation of glycogen synthetase induced in dog liver by administration of glucose and insulin.[53] This action prevents glucose from being stored in liver and it remains available for use as fuel.

Glucagon also provides glucose for the organism through a powerful stimulation of hepatic gluconeogenesis. Glucagon enhances glucose formation from amino acids, especially alanine, and from lactate and pyruvate.[54] The hormone produces its effects when present in physiologic concentration. Early studies of the stimulation of gluconeogenesis by glucagon in perfused rat liver indicated that regulatory events occur at early reactions in the biosynthetic pathway, i.e. between pyruvate and phosphoenolpyruvate. Glucagon also inhibits hepatic glycolysis. It has been suggested that hormonal regulation of hepatic carbohydrate metabolism involves complex regulation of several gluconeogenic and glycolytic enzymes.[55] The action of glucagon on gluconeogenesis can be totally reproduced by cAMP and the evidence indicates that glucagon acts to promote gluconeogenesis by activating adenylate cyclase in the plasma membrane. Insulin causes a reduction of cAMP levels and, thus, gluconeogenesis is inhibited.

Glucagon not only alters activities of enzymes involved in glycogen deposition (glycogen synthetase) and breakdown (phosphorylase) but also affects enzymes concerned with glycolysis and gluconeogenesis. Taunton reported that glucagon rapidly increases activity of hepatic fructose diphosphatase in the rat and decreases activities of phosphofructokinase and pyruvate kinase.[56] They also found these actions to be reversed by insulin. Blair and co-workers observed reproducible regulation of hepatic pyruvate kinase by glucagon, cyclic AMP and insulin in perfused rat liver.[55]

Glucagon and insulin are counterregulatory hormones in control of carbohydrate metabolism. Insulin enables glucose to penetrate into the cell where it may be used to provide immediate energy or stored for subsequent use. It is also the signal which directs the liver to turn off the glucose-producing machinery (gluconeogenesis). Glucagon is secreted when glucose is in short supply, i.e. during starvation, with hypoglycemia and after exercise.

Protein feeding also stimulates the pancreatic alpha cell to secrete glucagon in both normal and diabetic humans and animals.[57,58] The response of the alpha cell to protein feeding is of great importance inasmuch as such a meal, unless accompanied by carbohydrate ingestion, constitutes a state of glucose need. Glucagon causes prompt release of glucose through hepatic glycogenolysis and stimulates gluconeogenesis.

Although it may at first appear paradoxical, glucagon secretion is increased in diabetes mellitus, despite elevated blood sugar values.[59] The rise in glucagon secretion probably occurs because glucose utilization is diminished.

Catecholamines. Epinephrine influences carbohydrate metabolism in several ways. The catecholamine stimulates glycogenolysis in muscle, although the physiologic importance of glycogen as a reserve fuel varies with different types of muscle. The metabolic need for endogenous carbohydrate is greater in skeletal than in cardiac muscle, which preferentially uses fatty acids and ketone bodies as fuel. Human skeletal muscle has a high capacity for oxidation of fatty acids and ketone bodies, although glucose is an energy source during brief periods of vigorous activity. In addition to activating glycogenolysis, catecholamines also inhibit glycogen synthesis in skeletal muscle. The catecholamines stimulate glycogenolysis in muscle by stimulating adenylate cyclase activity, which leads to increased cyclic AMP formation. The end-result of this action is that phosphorylase b (the inactive form of the enzyme) is converted to phosphorylase a, which catalyzes breakdown of muscle glycogen to glucose.

The classic action of epinephrine and other catecholamines on liver carbohydrate metabolism is stimulation of glycogenolysis. The catecholamines activate membrane-bound adenylate cyclase, resulting in intracellular accumulation of cyclic AMP. Sutherland demonstrated that cyclic AMP causes activation of phosphorylase, the enzyme which catalyzes conversion of liver glycogen to glucose. Fain has described another mechanism by which catecholamines increase glycogenolysis (and gluconeogenesis) and does not involve cyclic AMP.[60] The evidence cited is that propranolol blocked epinephrine-stimulated elevation of cyclic AMP in perfused rat liver, but did not block the increase of hepatic phosphorylase in vivo or in perfused liver. In addition, phenylephrine, a predominantly alpha agonist, increased glycogen phosphorylase activity in perfused liver but did not cause a rise in cyclic AMP. Fain interpreted these data as evidence that epinephrine-induced hepatic glycogenolysis is not a classic beta response and probably occurs independently of cyclic AMP.[60]

Epinephrine and other catecholamines are potent stimulators of hepatic gluconeogenesis as well as glycogenolysis. The catecholamines promote gluconeogenesis by enhancing cyclic AMP formation, and an epinephrine-responsive adenylate cyclase system, separate from the glucagon responsive enzyme, has been demonstrated.[61] Both glucagon and epinephrine stimulate cAMP formation, but the effect of glucagon is far greater than that of epinephrine.[62] Although glucagon and epinephrine appear to act at the same regulatory site in glycose biosynthesis,[63] recent evidence suggests that epinephrine accelerates gluconeogenesis by a mechanism independent of cyclic AMP that does not involve cyclic GMP, Ca flux or K flux.[60]

Catecholamines impair peripheral utilization of glucose by inhibiting pancreatic insulin secretion and by causing a rise of the glucose-6-phosphate level. Hexokinase activity is inhibited when glucose-6-phosphate accumulates; hence glycolysis is diminished.

Corticosteroid Hormones. Adrenalectomy of previously pancreatectomized animals causes decreased nitrogen and glucose excretion which is restored to normal by use of corticosteroid preparations. Recently, evidence has been obtained that adrenal steroids act in conjunction with glucagon to augment the rate of glucose synthesis in perfused liver of adrenalectomized rats and that neither hormone alone will stimulate glucose formation.[54] Glucose release is restored to normal by adding glucagon to the perfused liver of adrenalectomized rats, if the animal is pretreated with dexamethasone or if dexamethasone is included in the perfusion medium.[54,64] The view that adrenal steroids exert a permissive action on gluconeogenesis has been expressed.

Adrenal glucocorticoids are also concerned with glycogen synthesis. Administration of cortisol, or other active glucocorticoid, causes glycogen deposition in the livers of normal or adrenalectomized animals. Glycogen synthetase activity is depressed in fasted, adrenalectomized rats and is restored to normal by corticosteroid administration. Adrenal steroid stimulation of glycogen synthetase requires about 4 hours to reach its maximal level; however, in the presence of glucose, activation occurs within several minutes. There is also evidence that glucocorticoid hormones inhibit glucose utilization. Fain[65] observed that the addition of dexamethasone to incubated rat adipose tissue resulted in diminished uptake of ^{14}C-glucose, decreased oxidation of glucose to CO_2 and diminished conversion of glucose to glycerol and fatty acids. Although several investigators have found decreased uptake of glucose by certain tissues (skin, fat and thymocytes) soon after glucocorticoid administration, muscle uptake remains normal and there is no significant overall decrease in glucose uptake by peripheral tissues.[66]

Thyroid Hormones. Thyroid hormones affect glucose synthesis and glycogen degradation as well as glucose oxidation and absorption. Glycogen content of the liver is markedly decreased in thyrotoxicosis and by pharmacologic doses of thyroid hormones administered to animals. Thyroid hormones modify actions of other hormones on carbohydrate metabolism, especially the catecholamines. For example, when the level of T_4 is raised, the glycogenolytic and lipolytic effects of epinephrine and norepinephrine are potentiated. The synergistic action of T_4 and the catecholamines is thought to result from their common action of stimulating adenyl cyclase to produce cAMP. As mentioned previously, cAMP activates phosphorylase, one of the enzymes involved in glycogen degradation.

Thyroid hormones increase the supply of glucose for oxidation by their catabolic action on liver glycogen and by enhancing glucose synthesis in liver.[67] The mechanism of action of thyroid hormones on gluconeogenesis is not fully understood, but it is known that substrate supply to the liver is increased because of accelerated peripheral protein breakdown, with release of amino acids. Augmented glucose production may also be promoted by an increased availability of glycerol as a result of the accelerated lipolysis of the hyperthyroid state. This suggestion is supported by the observation that perfused livers of thyroxine-treated rats exhibit increased glucose formation from glycerol.[68] There are reports that T_4 administration results in increased activity of hepatic enzymes concerned with gluconeogenesis; however, this is probably a response to the acceleration of gluconeogenesis, rather than an initial action of the hormone.

Most patients with hyperthyroidism show a marked loss of glucose tolerance. The peak glucose concentration in blood,

which occurs 30 to 60 minutes after glucose injection, is far higher in hyperthyroid subjects than in controls. The plasma glucose level declines rapidly, so that by 3 hours after sugar administration the concentration is the same as in normal volunteers.[69] Plasma insulin values are also markedly elevated in thyrotoxic patients after glucose administration. Like glucose, the peak insulin level is attained within 60 minutes and returns to normal by 180 minutes.[69] Although the incidence of diabetes is increased in hyperthyroidism, the abnormality of glucose tolerance has been attributed to the more rapid intestinal absorption of sugar. In hypothyroidism, absorption of a glucose load from the intestine is delayed. Glucose oxidation is enhanced when the T_4 level is elevated. Disposal of glucose via the Embden-Meyerhof pathway and the hexose monophosphate shunt is augmented.

Growth Hormone (GH). A single intravenous injection of growth hormone into hypophysectomized animals or humans produces prompt hypoglycemia from direct stimulation of glucose uptake and utilization in peripheral tissues. This insulin-like action is an acute effect which is not sustained when repeated injections of somatotropin (growth hormone) are given. The insulin-like effect of growth hormone can be readily demonstrated in isolated tissues of hypophysectomized animals.[70] Growth hormone does not produce hypoglycemia in normal subjects.

Chronic administration of growth hormone to normal animals or man results in elevation of the fasting blood glucose level. The rise of blood sugar occurs because of augmented hepatic glucose output resulting from accelerated glycogenolysis. Long-term treatment with growth hormone also causes a rise in concentration of blood insulin; however, the mechanism by which this hormone effect is produced is not apparent. Animals treated chronically with growth hormone demonstrate a marked decrease in the sensitivity of peripheral tissues to the stimulatory effects of insulin on glucose uptake and utilization. This action of GH is probably the result of reduced phosphorylation of glucose, which has been observed in heart and diaphragm muscle.[70] Growth hormone may exert its inhibitory effect on phosphorylation by stimulating the release of fatty acids from adipose depots. Fatty acids and ketone bodies impair glucose utilization by skeletal and heart muscle.[71]

Acute administration of growth hormone to normal human subjects is followed by a short-lived fall of plasma free fatty acids and a more prolonged decrease of glucose. The decline of blood sugar is secondary to stimulation of the pancreatic beta cells by the pituitary hormone. Prolonged growth hormone administration produces hyperglycemia in animals and man, despite enhanced insulin secretion, and frank diabetes mellitus may be produced. If treatment with GH is continued, permanent diabetes and degenerative changes in the B-cells result. It is evident that GH induces resistance to the blood sugar-lowering action of insulin. This is at least partially because of the increased concentration of plasma fatty acids. In patients with acromegaly the incidence of diabetes mellitus may exceed 20 per cent.[72] In many other acromegalics whose blood sugars are within normal limits, plasma insulin values are markedly elevated, especially after glucose ingestion. Thus, insulin resistance not only occurs after experimental administration of growth hormone but also is a natural phenomenon. The marked elevation of pancreatic insulin secretion that occurs in the acromegalic indicates that growth hormone has a trophic effect on the pancreatic islets.

FAT METABOLISM

Fat metabolism is in constant flux as fatty acids are synthesized and esterified into triglycerides, while existing triglycerides are hydrolyzed into fatty acids and glycerol which serve as body fuel. Lipid synthesis (lipogenesis) and lipid breakdown (lipolysis) are influenced by the balance between calorie intake and calorie expenditure. When food is freely available, lipogenesis is greater than lipolysis; during food deprivation lipogenesis is inhibited and lipolysis is increased. Several hormones play key roles in the regulation of lipid synthesis, breakdown and utilization.

Two kinds of action need to be considered in regard to hormonal influences on lipid metabolism. Acute effects are manifest within a short period after hormone administration and are of brief duration. Long-term actions are manifest over a period of days and are reflected by alterations in metabolic activity and/or the capacity of tissues to respond to acute influences. Among the hormones that induce acute changes in fat metabolism are insulin, glucagon and catecholamines. Glucagon and catecholamines bind to fat cell membrane receptors,[73,74] leading to increased adenylate cyclase activity and elevated intracellular cyclic AMP. The increased level of cAMP activates the enzyme triglyceride lipase, which enhances triglyceride hydrolysis.

Long-term effects of hormones on lipid metabolism may involve other mechanisms. For example, adrenalectomy reduces the effectiveness of signal transmission from cell membrane receptors to adenylate cyclase, thereby reducing responsiveness to other hormones.[75] In contrast, thyroid hormones and growth hormone enhance adenylate cyclase in the fat cell and render the adipocyte more sensitive to acute effects of catecholamines and other hormones.[76] In addition, the number of receptor sites on the fat cell membrane varies with diet and alterations of the physiologic state,[77] influencing the effects of hormones on the adipocyte.

Insulin exerts acute as well as chronic effects on adipose tissue. Under acute conditions insulin decreases cyclic AMP,[78] an alteration which correlates with antilipolytic and lipogenic actions of the hormone. Over a longer period, insulin increases activities of lipogenic enzymes and decreases the adipose tissue response to lipolytic hormones.

Insulin. Insulin promotes lipogenesis and inhibits lipolysis. The importance of these actions is evident in fed and fasted states. During feeding, elevated levels of blood insulin stimulate lipid synthesis and deposition, while, in the fasted state, low levels of blood insulin enhance lipid mobilization. The fall in insulin, coupled with a normal or elevated level of glucagon, is perhaps the major mechanism that results in lipid mobilization to provide energy during fasting.[80]

Adipose tissue is a major organ for insulin action and functions to synthesize and store lipids as well as to mobilize this stored fuel for the provision of energy. Synthesis of fatty acids and their esterification require glucose utilization; therefore, lipogenesis is influenced by the rate of glucose metabolism. Insulin stimulates carrier-mediated transport of glucose and its utilization in the fat cell.[81] Increased glucose utilization promotes lipid synthesis in the following manner: (1) by supplying acetyl coenzyme A, a precursor of fatty acids, (2) by providing α-glycerophosphate for esterification of fatty acids to form triglyceride and (3) by generating triphosphopyridine nucleotide (NADPH) which is necessary for crotonyl-CoA-butyryl-CoA hydrogenation, an important step in fatty acid synthesis. In addition, insulin stimulates lipogenesis by two other mechanisms: (1) It activates pyruvate dehydrogenase, an enzyme required for conversion of glucose to acetate and hence to fatty acids[82] and (2) by inhibiting lipolysis, it reduces the concentration of palmityl CoA, an inhibitor of lipogenesis.[83]

Fatty acids stored as triglycerides in adipose tissue arise from two sources: preformed fatty acids which are taken up from blood and those synthesized from glucose carbon. The preformed fatty acids are transported from the gastrointestinal tract and liver to adipose tissue, either as chylomicrons or very-low-density lipoproteins (VLDL). Hydrolysis of chylomicrons and VLDL is mediated by the enzyme lipoprotein lipase, which is located on the cell surface of capillary endothelium. Insulin is important in maintaining and stimulating the activity of lipoprotein lipase.[84] In response to its effect on lipoprotein lipase, hydrolysis of circulating triglycerides is accelerated and, consequently, transport of fatty acids into adipose tissue is increased. In addition, insulin has a direct stimulatory effect on free fatty acid (FFA) uptake by adipose tissue. During insulin lack, lipoprotein lipase activity is low and uptake of circulating FFA by adipose tissue is diminished.[85]

Insulin inhibits lipolysis, which occurs in adipose tissue constantly and concurrently with lipogenesis. The dynamic summation of these two reactions determines the functional state of adipose tissue. Hydrolysis of stored triglycerides into FFA and glycerol is catalyzed by a hormone-sensitive enzyme, triglyceride lipase, also known as depot fat lipase. Glycerol diffuses out of the adipocyte, as it cannot be utilized within the fat cell because of lack of glycerolkinase. FFA may be released into the circulation or reesterified into triglycerides. The antilipolytic action of insulin is partly due to its stimulatory effect on reesterification of FFA. Insulin also retards lipolysis by direct inhibition of triglyceride lipase, which apparently results from reduced adipocyte cyclic AMP. Butcher et al. showed that insulin decreased catecholamine-stimulated cyclic AMP in the adipose cell;[86] however, it is not clear whether insulin can lower the basal level of cyclic AMP. Furthermore, the mechanism by which insulin lowers cyclic AMP is not understood; it could decrease the activity of adenylate cyclase and/or increase the activity of phosphodiesterase.[87] During insulin lack, glucose utilization is decreased and, as a result, the amount of α-glycerophosphate becomes insufficient for triglyceride formation. The FFA diffuse out of fat cells into the circulation; thus lipids are mobilized from adipose tissue. It should be noted that, under certain select conditions, lipid mobilization is increased and not decreased by unphysiologically high concentrations of insulin.[88]

In humans, liver as well as adipose tissue is a major site of lipid synthesis. In addition to de novo synthesis, liver removes a large proportion of the circulating FFA delivered to it from adipose tissue. At low plasma FFA levels the rate of hepatic uptake is low, while at high plasma levels of FFA it is elevated. In liver, FFA are oxidized to CO_2 or ketone bodies, or incorporated into triglyceride, phospholipids and cholesterol esters. Insulin stimulates fatty acid synthesis in a manner similar to that observed in adipose tissue. During insulin deficiency hexose monophosphate shunt activity is impaired and, as a result, NADPH is not provided for fatty acid synthesis.[89] Lipid synthesis is also retarded by the lack of citrate and isocitrate, which occurs secondary to decreased glucose utilization. Lastly, the activity of fatty acid synthetase is impaired during insulin deprivation.[90] Unlike adipose tissue, however, liver contains glycerol kinase, which phosphorylates glycerol to yield glycerolphosphate, permitting lipogenesis to occur without insulin when the flow of FFA and glycerol to liver is adequate. During insulin deficiency, lipolysis in adipose tissue is stimulated and large amounts of FFA and glycerol reach the liver where FFA are converted into ketone bodies and released into the circulation. Accumulation of ketones, elevated levels of total blood lipid, rise in plasma FFA and occurrence of fatty liver in individuals with insulin deficiency are all reflections of deranged metabolism.

Glucagon. Pancreatic glucagon was discovered in 1923,[91] but its importance in metabolic regulation did not come under intense study until recent years. The role of glucagon in the metabolic derange-ments of diabetes mellitus is currently a subject of controversy.[92,93] Glucagon is a potent stimulus of lipolysis in adipose tissue and thus there is release of FFA and glycerol for utilization by liver and other tissues. The mechanism of hormone action involves cyclic AMP formation via activation of the adenylate cyclase system. Intravenous administration of glucagon in man produces a transient decline in FFA level, followed by a prolonged rise.[94] The early depression of plasma FFA is due to glucagon-induced insulin secretion. In previous studies, pharmacologic amounts of glucagon were used to demonstrate its lipolytic effect. More recent work shows that physiologic concentrations of glucagon also enhance lipid mobilization in man,[95] although this effect has not been substantiated by all investigators.[96] One reason for the difficulty in delineating the physiologic role of glucagon is the simultaneous presence of the counterregulatory hormone insulin. Nonetheless, it is clear that glucagon can modulate lipid mobilization, although the action is ordinarily not apparent in the presence of insulin.

In liver, glucagon stimulates fatty acid oxidation and ketogenesis and inhibits triglyceride release.[97] These effects are influenced by the plasma concentration of FFA as hepatic uptake of FFA is proportional to the circulating FFA. Glucagon has little if any effect on hepatic uptake of FFA. Oxidation of FFA and ketogenesis are regulated by the enzymatic activity of carnitine acyltransferase, an enzyme activated by glucagon.[98] Insulin counteracts the ketogenic action of glucagon by a direct hepatic effect and by limiting substrate available for ketogenesis. A recent study showed a close correlation between blood levels of glucagon and ketone bodies and postulated that glucagon excess, in addition to insulin lack, might play a role in hyperketonemia.[99]

Unger has suggested that the ratio of insulin to glucagon in blood is important for metabolic homeostasis.[100] Insulin, mole for mole, has more antilipolytic activity than glucagon has lipolytic action. In contrast, the stimulatory effect of glucagon on hepatic glucose release is greater than the inhibitory action of insulin.[101] An increase in glucagon relative to insulin favors catabolic processes. This is important in fasting, when fuel mobilization is essential. Glucagon stimulates glycogenolysis and gluconeogenesis.[102] The preponderance of glucagon relative to insulin is also associated with an increase in hepatic fatty acid oxidation and ketone body concentration in blood.[103] Conversely, after a carbohydrate meal, there is an increase in insulin relative to glucagon in blood, resulting in increased glucose utilization and decreased gluconeogenesis and fatty acid oxidation in the liver. The antilipolytic and lipid synthetic actions of insulin serve to convert energy ingested as carbohydrate to a storage form as lipid.

Catecholamines. Epinephrine and norepinephrine are potent lipolytic agents which induce a prompt rise in plasma FFA.[104] Effects of catecholamine-induced lipolysis become evident in tissues which normally take up considerable amounts of FFA. Liver, kidney, lung, heart and skeletal muscle utilize FFA as a major source of energy. As circulating FFA levels rise, fatty acid uptake and oxidation by tissues are increased, since these events, in part, depend upon the blood levels. The increase in fatty acid oxidation may account for the calorigenic action of epinephrine and norepinephrine and also for the accompanying hypermetabolism. Catecholamines also stimulate the conversion of glucose into lipids.[105] However, stimulation of lipogenesis is of lesser magnitude than that of lipid mobilization.

The lipolytic action of catecholamines is the result of an increase in formation of cyclic AMP from ATP.[106] Adenylate cyclase enzyme systems catalyze the formation of cyclic AMP from ATP; catecholamines and other lipolytic hormones, including ACTH, TSH and glucagon, stimulate adenylate cyclase and, thus, promote cyclic AMP formation. Cyclic AMP activates a lipase that induces hydrolysis of triglyceride to fatty acids. The hormone-sensitive lipase activated by cAMP is present not only in adipose tissue but also in liver, heart and skeletal muscle. In vitro studies show that the catecholamine effect on lipolysis is biphasic, apparently because of biphasic production of cyclic AMP.[107] The two phases are termed lipolysis I and lipolysis II. Propranolol inhibits lipolysis I but not lipolysis II. Age abolishes the lipolysis I response; in old rats only high concentrations of epinephrine cause lipid mobilization. Insulin inhibits catecholamine-induced lipolysis I but augments lipolysis II.[108] Butcher et al.[109] reported that insulin at low concentration decreases intracellular cyclic AMP, but at high concentrations increases the nucleotide level. This is because of an inhibition of adenylate cyclase which disappears at high concentrations of insulin. It has been speculated that the lipolytic effect of high insulin concentrations might be a causal factor of lipoatrophy at the site of insulin injections and of elevated plasma FFA in obesity.[110]

Exercise, cold exposure and emotional stress evoke a strong sympathetic nervous system response associated with an elevation of plasma FFA. Lipid mobilization appears to occur in response to the catecholamine release. Adipose tissue is rich in autonomic nervous system fibers and contains significant stores of norepinephrine. Both exercise and cold exposure require energy which is provided through catecholamine-induced lipid mobilization.

Adrenal Cortical Steroids. Glucocorticoids produce increased carbohydrate stores at the expense of body proteins and fats. The catabolic influence of glucocorticoids on tissue proteins provides precursors to meet the needs of gluconeogenesis. In regard to fat metabolism, glucocorticoids exert a permissive action on lipolysis, leading to increased levels of FFA and glycerol.[111] In adrenalectomized rats, catecholamine-induced lipolysis is diminished, an aberration which is corrected with cortisol. Adrenal glucocorticoids are similarly required for the maximal lipolytic action of growth hormone. The lipid-mobilizing effect of cortisol is blocked by inhibitors of protein and RNA synthesis.[112]

Glucocorticoids also inhibit lipid synthesis. Lipogenesis is depressed in alloxan diabetic rats; however, after adrenalectomy lipid formation returns to a nearly normal level.[113] Administration of cortisol to adrenalectomized, diabetic rats causes a reduction of hepatic lipid synthesis. The inhibitory influence of glucocorticoids on hepatic fat synthesis becomes evident within 2 to 6 hours and occurs concomitantly with enhanced glucose synthesis from pyruvate. Not all investigators agree that glucocorticoids depress hepatic lipid formation. For example, Hays and Hill[114] showed that chronic cortisone treatment enhanced triglyceride-synthesizing activity as well as acyl CoA synthetase activity in hepatic microsomes. Hepatic oxidation of FFA is also inhibited by glucocorticoids and conversely increased by adrenalectomy. Finally, under certain conditions, glucocorticoids stimulate triglyceride release from liver. Experiments with isolated, perfused rat liver have shown the cortisol concentration necessary to stimulate triglyceride release from liver of normal or adrenalectomized animals to be quite specific. When the critical level of cortisol was exceeded, hepatic triglyceride release was diminished.[115] Chronic treatment with glucocorticoid leads to hyperlipemia and fatty liver. These changes result from enhanced fat mobilization, increased circulating FFA and enhanced uptake by liver.

In humans, intravenous injection of cortisol is followed by a 30 per cent decline in blood free fatty acids lasting about 90 minutes. Subsequently, FFA rise progressively until, 3 hours after hormone injection, the level is about 35 per cent greater than the control value.[116] Prolonged steroid treatment results in elevated plasma lipids. When circulating corticosteroid levels are increased in human subjects with Cushing's syndrome or those treated with steroids, an increase in total body fat mass and changes in fat distribution occur.[117] Chronic corticoid excess leads to obesity and fat accumulation in the face, supraclavicular areas, over the lower cervical vertebrae and in the trunk. The explanation of this curious predilection for fat deposits is not known. Alterations in fat distribution cannot be explained by the lipogenic effect of the associated hyperinsulinemia, since insulin-mediated obesity is generalized. An increase in body weight caused by elevated fat stores is partially counterbalanced by the protein catabolism that occurs in Cushing's syndrome.

Adrenocorticotropin (ACTH). One of the prominent extra-adrenal actions of ACTH is its fat-mobilizing activity. Administration of ACTH to intact or adrenalectomized animals increases lipolysis, an action which does not depend on stimulation of the adrenal cortex.[118] In consequence, plasma FFA increase after ACTH administration and there is an elevation of liver lipid content and increased ketone formation. The fat mobilization induced by ACTH is mediated through cyclic AMP, which activates triglyceride lipase in adipose tissue.

Growth Hormone. Growth hormone promotes lipid mobilization from adipose tissue, an action associated with increased FFA uptake and oxidation in muscle and ketogenesis in liver.[119] The rise of plasma FFA and ketones reduces glucose uptake by muscle and explains, in part, the well-recognized peripheral antagonism between growth hormone and insulin. Lipolysis induced by GH differs from that of other lipolytic hormones (e.g. catecholamines, ACTH, glucagon) in requiring at least one hour before the effect can be observed. Furthermore, GH appears to require glucocorticoids for maximal effect on FFA mobilization. The lipolytic actions of GH and glucocorticoids are unique in that they are blocked by inhibitors of RNA and protein synthesis—actinomycin, puromycin, cyclohexamide, ultraviolet light and x rays.[120] Growth hormone increases protein synthesis via DNA-dependent RNA synthesis, which leads to enhanced lipolysis through an as yet unclear mechanism. In most previous studies, pharmacologic amounts of GH have been used to demonstrate the action of GH on lipid metabolism. Recently, Gerich et al.[95] showed that physiologic levels of GH are lipolytic and can lead to ketosis under appropriate conditions, especially during insulin deficiency. Nonetheless, the physiologic significance of growth hormone influence on lipid mobilization under normal conditions has not been defined.

Acute administration of growth hormone results in a transient fall of plasma FFA in humans. Furthermore, growth hormone exerts an immediate antagonism to epinephrine-induced lipolysis in epididymal fat pad excised from hypophysectomized rats.[121] This antilipolytic action is in accord with other early responses to growth hormone, all of which are insulin-like in nature. They include a fall in blood glucose and amino acid levels, enhanced uptake of amino acids by muscle and accelerated glucose uptake and utilization by adipose cells and muscle. These early effects disappear within a few hours, but can be prolonged by inhibitors of RNA and protein synthesis. A recent study suggests that the transient, immediate, antilipolytic effect of growth hormone is the result of inhibition of protein kinase activity.[122]

Growth hormone not only stimulates lipolysis but also inhibits lipogenesis. Hypophysectomized or normal rats injected with GH exhibit reduced incorporation of carbon from glucose and amino acids into fatty acids. The underlying mechanism appears to be intimately connected to the associated declines of glucose

uptake and oxidation.[119] In short, growth hormone exerts catabolic effects on fat metabolism and this is evident in patients with acromegaly, who exhibit decreased total body fat. The rise of body weight in these patients results from increased lean body mass.

Thyroid Hormones. A major effect of thyroid hormones on lipid metabolism is to enhance mobilization of FFA from adipose tissue and to increase FFA oxidation. Rich et al.[123] first observed elevated plasma FFA levels in hyperthyroid subjects and also showed that administration of triiodothyronine (T_3) to normal individuals produced a rise of plasma FFA levels. Adipose tissue from thyrotoxic rats incubated in vitro releases FFA into the medium at an accelerated rate and exhibits an exaggerated response to epinephrine-induced lipolysis. Conversely, lipolysis and the effectiveness of catecholamines in mobilizing FFA are impaired in thyroid-deficient animals. Other studies have shown that fat mobilization by glucagon, TSH, ACTH, GH and dibutyryl cyclic AMP is also facilitated by thyroid hormones.[124] A definite underlying mechanism for the activated lipolysis has not been established, although involvement of cyclic AMP has been suggested. Krishna et al.[125] suggested that the response involved increased activity of plasma membrane adenyl cyclase. Fat cells isolated from hypothyroid rats show an increase in membrane-bound phosphodiesterase which can restrict cyclic AMP-induced lipolysis. It has been suggested that thyroid hormones exert a primary effect on mitochondrial energy metabolism and that the lipolytic action is secondary to this.[126]

In hyperthyroidism, delivery of FFA to peripheral tissue and the liver is increased. As a result, uptake and oxidation of FFA by various organs are proportionately increased. In hyperthyroid patients and animals, the respiratory quotient is lower than in normal subjects, indicating preferential oxidation of fat. Biosynthesis of fatty acids is increased by thyroid hormones. In vivo conversion of ^{14}C-acetate into fatty acids is greater in liver of thyrotoxic rats than in that of normal animals. Conversely, fatty acid synthesis is reduced in thiouracil-fed rats. Lipid synthesis is decreased in hypothyroid individuals but is restored to normal by administration of thyroid hormones. Some investigators claim that fat synthesis is decreased by thyroid hormones; however, there is little support for this finding.

Thyroid-hormone enhancement of fat catabolism outweighs its influence on fat synthesis. In thyrotoxicosis, weight is lost and the fat content of the body is below normal. Serum cholesterol is decreased because of an accelerated cholesterol breakdown which is greater than the enhancement of cholesterol biosynthesis. In hypothyroidism lipolysis is diminished in response to fasting or administration of epinephrine or growth hormone; the serum lipid changes include increases in cholesterol, total lipids, phospholipids, betalipoproteins and, in severe cases, even prebetalipoproteins.

BIBLIOGRAPHY

1. Clark: J. Biol. Chem., 200, 69, 1953.
2. Goodlad and Munro: J. Biochem., 73, 343, 1959.
3. Munro: In Mammalian Protein Metabolism, Vol. 1 (Munro, Ed.). New York, Academic Press, 1964.
4. Munro and Thomson: Metabolism, 2, 354, 1953.
5. Kochakian, Tillotson and Austin: Endocrinology, 60, 144, 1957.
6. Blanpin and Aschkenasy: C. R. Soc. Biol., 142, 997, 1959.
7. Roche, Dumazert, Emond and Roger: C. R. Soc. Biol., 136, 326, 1942.
8. Manchester: In Diabetes Mellitus (Ellenberg and Rifkin, Eds.). New York, McGraw-Hill, 1970.
9. Lotspeich: J. Biol. Chem., 179, 175, 1949.
10. Pozefsky, Felig, Tobin, Soeldner and Cahill: J. Clin. Invest., 48, 2273, 1969.
10a.Adibi, Morse and Amin: J. Lab. Clin. Med., 86, 395, 1975.
10b.Jefferson and Robertson: Diabetes, 21 (Suppl. I), 341, 1972.
11. Wool and Krahl: Nature, 183, 1399, 1959.
12. Wool: Am. J. Physiol., 199, 719, 1960.
13a.Herrera and Renold: Biochim. Biophys. Acta, 44, 165, 1960.
13b.Mayne and Barry: J. Biochem., 99, 688, 1966.
13c.Davidson and Goodner: Diabetes, 15, 835, 1966.
13d.Mayne and Barry: Biochim. Biophys. Acta, 138, 195, 1967.
13e.Wool, Stirewalt, Kurihara, Low, Bailey and Oyer: Recent Prog. Horm. Res., 24, 139, 1968.
14a.Korner: J. Endocrinol., 20, 256, 1960.
14b.Robinson: Proc. Soc. Exp. Biol. Med., 106, 115, 1961.
14c.Klotzien, Pariza, Becker, Potter and Butcher: J. Biol. Chem., 251, 3014, 1976.
14d.Taunton, Stifel, Greene and Herman: J. Biol. Chem., 249, 7228, 1974.
15. Manchester: In Mammalian Protein Metabolism, Vol. 4 (Munro, Ed.). New York, Academic Press, 1970.
16. Leathem: In Mammalian Protein Metabolism, Vol. 1 (Munro, Ed.). New York, Academic Press, 1964.
17. Korner: Nature, 181, 422, 1958.
17a.Korner: Prog. Biophys., 17, 61, 1967.
17b.Kjalmarson and Ahren: Acta Endocrinol., 54, 645, 1967.
17c.Nutting: Endocrinology, 98, 1273, 1976
18. Korner: J. Biochem., 81, 292, 1961.
18a.Talwar, et al.: Recent Prog. Horm. Res., 31, 141, 1975.
19a.Long, Katzin and Fry: Endocrinology, 26, 309, 1940.
19b.Engel: Recent Prog. Horm. Res., 6, 277, 1951.
20. Friedberg and Greenberg: J. Biol. Chem., 168, 405, 1948.
21. Munro: In Mammalian Protein Metabolism, Vol. 4 (Munro, Ed.). New York, Academic Press, 1970.
22. Bondy, Ingle and Meeks: Endocrinology, 55, 355, 1954.
23. Noall, Riggs, Walker and Christensen: Science, 126, 1002, 1957.
23a.Weinshelbaum and Wool: Nature, 191, 1401, 1961.
23b.Kostyo: Endocrinology, 76, 604, 1965.
23c.Kostyo and Rodmond: Endocrinology, 79, 531, 1966.
24. Noall, Riggs, Walker and Christensen: Science, 126: 1002, 1957.
25. Weber, Srivastava and Singhal: J. Biol. Chem., 240, 750, 1965.
26. Bass, Chambers and Richtarik: Life Sci., 4, 266, 1963.
27. Clark: J. Biol. Chem., 200, 69, 1953.
28. Feigelson and Greengard: J. Biol. Chem., 237, 3714, 1963.
29. Kenney: In Mammalian Protein Metabolism, Vol. 4 (Munro, Ed.). New York, Academic Press, 1970.
29a.Levitan and Webb: J. Mol. Biol., 48, 339, 1970.
30. Segal and Kim: Proc. Natl. Acad. Sci., 50, 912, 1963.
31. Kreisberg, Owen and Siegal: Med. Clin. North Am., 54, 1473, 1970.
32. Foley, London and Prenton: J. Clin. Endocrinol. Metab., 26, 781, 1966.
33. Wellers and Leblane: C. R. Soc. Biol., 160, 1785, 1966.
34. Tata: Prog. Nucleic Acid Res., 5, 191, 1966.
34a.Oppenheimer: N. Engl. J. Med., 292, 1063, 1975.

35. Young: In *Mammalian Protein Metabolism,* Vol. 4 (Munro, Ed.). New York, Academic Press, 1970.
36. Breuer and Florini: Biochemistry, *4*, 1544, 1965.
37a. Liao, Lin and Barton: J. Biol. Chem., *241*, 3869, 1966.
37b. Liao, Barton and Lin: Proc. Natl. Acad. Sci., *55*, 1593, 1966.
37c. Liao and Lin: Proc. Natl. Acad. Sci., *57*, 379, 1967.
38. Marliss, Aoki and Cahill: In *Glucagon, Molecular Physiology, Clinical and Therapeutic Implications* (Lefebore and Unger, Eds.). New York, Pergamon Press, 1972.
39. Mallette, Exton and Park: J. Biol. Chem., *244*, 5713 and 5724, 1969.
40. Felig, Owen, Wahren and Cahill: J. Clin. Invest., *48*, 584, 1969.
41. Woodside, Ward and Mortimore: J. Biol. Chem., *249*, 5458, 1974.
42. Levine, Goldstein, Klein and Huddlestun: J. Biol. Chem., *179*, 985, 1949.
43. Levine and Goldstein: Recent Prog. Horm. Res., *11*, 343, 1955.
44. Park, et al.: Recent Prog. Horm. Res., *17*, 493, 1961.
45. Debons: Am. J. Physiol., *217*, 1114, 1969.
46. Levine: In *Diabetes Mellitus* (Ellenberg and Rifkin, Eds.) New York, McGraw-Hill, 1970.
47. Cuatrecasas: Proc. Natl. Acad. Sci., *63*, 450, 1969.
48. Maugh: Science, *193*, 220, 1976.
49. Villar-Palasi and Larner: Annu. Rev. Biochem., *39*, 639, 1970.
50. Curnow, Rayfield, George, Zenser and De Rubertis: Am. J. Physiol., *228*, 80, 1975.
51. Sharma, Menjeshwar and Weinhouse: J. Biol. Chem., *238*, 1342, 1963.
52. Sokal and Ezdinli: J. Clin. Invest., *46*, 778, 1967.
53. Bishop and Larner: J. Biol. Chem., *242*, 1354, 1967.
54. Eisenstein and Strack: Endocrinology, *83*, 1337, 1968.
55. Blair, Cimbala, Foster and Morgan: J. Biol. Chem., *251*, 3756, 1976.
56. Taunton, Stifel, Greene and Herman: Biochem. Biophys. Res. Commun., *48*, 1663, 1972.
57. Unger and Orci: Physiol. Rev., *56*, 778, 1976.
58. Eisenstein and Strack: Diabetes, *25*, 51, 1976.
59. Unger, Agiular-Parada, Muller and Eisentraut: J. Clin. Invest., *49*, 837, 1970.
60. Fain, Tolbert, Pointer, Butcher and Arnold: Metabolism, *24*, 395, 1975.
61. Bitensky, Russell and Robertson: Biochem. Biophys. Res. Commun., *31*, 706, 1968.
62. Exton and Park: Adv. Enzyme Regul. *6*, 391, 1968.
63. Exton and Park: Pharmacol. Rev., *18*, 181, 1966.
64. Friedman, Exton and Park: Biochem. Biophys. Res. Commun., *29*, 113, 1967.
65. Fain: J. Biol. Chem., *239*, 958, 1964.
66. Steele: In *Handbook of Physiology*, Section 7, Endocrinology (Greep and Astwood, Eds.). Washington, American Physiological Society, 1975.
67. Murad and Freedland: Proc. Soc. Exp. Biol. Med., *124*, 1176, 1967.
68. Freedland and Krebs: Biochem. J., *104*, 45P, 1967.
69. Eisenstein: Unpublished observations.
70. Kostyo and Reagan: Pharmacol. Ther. B, *2*, 591, 1976.
71. Randle, Garland, Hales and Newsholme: Lancet, *1*, 785, 1963.
72. Boshell and Chaudalia: In *Diabetes Mellitus* (Ellenberg and Rifkin, Eds.). New York, McGraw-Hill, 1970.
73. Birnbaumer: Biochim. Biophys. Acta, *300*, 129, 1973.
74. Birnbaumer and Rodbell: J. Biol. Chem., *244*, 3477, 1969.
75. Exton, Freidman, Wong, Brineaux, Corbin and Park: J. Biol. Chem., *247*, 3279, 1972.
76. Robinson, Butcher and Sutherland: In *Cyclic AMP* (Robinson, Ed.). New York, Academic Press, 1971, p. 285.
77. Livingston, Cuatrecasas and Lockwood: J. Lipid Res., *15*, 26, 1974.
78. Zinman and Hollenberg: J. Biol. Chem., *249*, 2182, 1974.
79. Yen and Steinmetz: Horm. Metab. Res., *4*, 331, 1972.
80. Felig: N. Engl. J. Med., *283*, 149, 1970.
81. Avruch, Carter and Martin: In *Endocrine Pancreas*, Vol. 1 (Steiner and Freinkel, Eds.). Washington, American Physiological Society, 1972.
82. Taylor, Mukherjee and Jungas: J. Biol. Chem., *248*, 73, 1973.
83. Weber, Lea and Stamm: Lipids, *4*, 388, 1969.
84. Bagdade, Porte and Bierman: N. Engl. J. Med., *276*, 427, 1967.
85. Kessler: J. Clin. Invest., *42*, 362, 1963.
86. Butcher, Maird and Sutherland: J. Biol. Chem., *243*, 1705, 1968.
87. Keirn, Freeman and Bitensky: Am. J. Med. Sci., *268*, 62, 1964.
88. Kono and Barham: J. Biol. Chem., *28*, 7417, 1973.
89. Siperstein and Fagan: J. Clin. Invest., *37*, 1185, 1958.
90. Lakashmanan, Nepokroeff and Porter: Proc. Natl. Acad. Sci., *69*, 3516, 1969.
91. Murlin and Kimball: J. Biol. Chem., *58*, 321, 1923.
92. Unger and Orci: Lancet, *1*, 14, 1975.
93. Sherwin, Fisher, Hendler and Felig: N. Engl. J. Med., *294*, 455, 1976.
94. Lipsett, Engel and Bergenstal: J. Lab. Clin. Med., *56*, 342, 1960.
95. Gerich, et al.: J. Clin. Invest., *57*, 875, 1976.
96. Pozefsky, et al.: Diabetes, *25*, 128, 1976.
97. Heimberg, Weinstein and Kohout: J. Biol. Chem., *244*, 5131, 1969.
98. McGarry, Wright and Foster: J. Clin. Invest., *55*, 1202, 1975.
99. Alberti, Christensten, Iversen and Orskov: Lancet, *1*, 1307, 1975.
100. Unger: Diabetes, *20*, 834, 1971.
101. Linjenquist, et al.: J. Clin. Invest., *53*, 190, 1974.

102. Marliss, Aoki, Unger, Soeldner and Cahill: J. Clin. Invest., *49*, 2256, 1970.
103. McGarry, Robles-Valdes and Foster: Metabolism, *25*, 1387, 1976.
104. Steinberg: Pharmacol. Rev., *18*, 217, 1966.
105. Winegrad: Vitam. Horm., *20*, 141, 1964.
106. Butcher: N. Engl. J. Med., *279*, 1378, 1968.
107. Allen, Hillman and Ashmore: Biochem. Pharmacol., *18*, 2233, 1969.
108. Miller and Allen: J. Lipid Res., *14*, 331, 1973.
109. Butcher, Baird and Sutherland: J. Biol. Chem., *243*, 1705, 1968.
110. Desai, Li and Angel: J. Lipid Res., *14*, 657, 1973.
111. Goodman: Endocrinology, *86*, 1064, 1970.
112. Fain: Science, *157*, 1062, 1967.
113. Gurin and Brady: Recent Prog. Horm. Res., *8*, 571, 1953.
114. Hays and Hill: Biochim. Biophys. Acta, *98*, 646, 1965.
115. Klausner and Heimberg: Am. J. Physiol., *212*, 1236, 1967.
116. Dreiling, et al.: Metabolism, *11*, 572, 1962.
117. Lamberts and Birkenhager: J. Clin. Endocrinol. Metab., *42*, 864, 1976.
118. Engel: Vitam. Horm., *19*, 189, 1961.
119. Goodman and Schwartz: In *The Pituitary Gland and Its Neuroendocrine Control*, Part 2, Vol. 4. Washington, American Physiological Society, 1974.
120. Fain, Dodd and Novak: Metabolism, *20*, 109, 1971.
121. Goodman: Metabolism, *19*, 849, 1970.
122. Birnbaum and Goodman: Endocrinology, *99*, 1336, 1976.
123. Rich, Bierman and Schwartz: J. Clin. Invest., *38*, 275, 1959.
124. Caldwell and Fain: Endocrinology, *89*, 1195, 1971.
125. Krishna, Hynie and Brodie: Proc. Natl. Acad. Sci., *59*, 884, 1968.
126. Fain: Pharmacol. Rev., *25*, 67, 1973.

Chapter *17*

PHYSIOLOGY OF HUNGER AND SATIETY

Jean Mayer

REGULATION OF CALORIC INTAKE AND WEIGHT: MORPHOLOGIC ASPECTS AND POSSIBLE MECHANISMS

Anatomic Basis

Gastrointestinal Tract. Haller was the first to suggest (in his *Elementa Physiologica*, in 1777) that hunger was a gastric sensation. In his chapter *"Famis causa proxima"*—the immediate cause of hunger —he stated that hunger sensations were results of the excitation of stomach nerves. For over a century and a half this theory was generally accepted. It was only in 1911 that it was tested experimentally by Cannon and Washburn,[3] who showed that hunger sensations appeared simultaneously with contractions of the stomach. The hunger contractions were further investigated by Carlson,[4] who found that during starvation the tonus of the empty stomach and the frequency and intensity of its contractions became progressively more pronounced, at least until the fourth day. The desire for food decreased. These gastric hunger contractions are relatively powerful; they occur in series of from 20 to 70 and last usually between half an hour and an hour and a half; they alternate with periods of quiescence. The contractions are seen in newborn babies before any food has been consumed. Their presence is general in land vertebrates, whether homeotherms or poikilotherms.

Hunger contractions are present even when there is some food in the stomach. The only time when the fundus does not exhibit them is immediately after a large meal. They occur after isolation from the brain and spinal cord, though at longer intervals and with less vigor. They are inhibited by a variety of stimuli: by the tasting or chewing of a palatable food, or even of an inert substance such as paraffin wax (unless the contractions have become tetanic in nature), by stimulation of the gastric mucosa by ice-cold water, acid, alcohol, cigarettes, tightening of the belt, vigorous muscular exercise, sudden application of cold, emotions such as fear or rage, epinephrine, glucagon or intravenous glucose, given under conditions such that normal utilization takes place. Inhibition of gastric contractions can be brought about also by irrigation of the duodenum by glucose. That this inhibition persists when the stomach is denervated or in autotransplanted denervated gastric pouches has led to the postulation of secretion of a chalone by the duodenum or the liver. Interesting modifications of gastric tone take place in disease: duodenal ulcer and diabetes cause an increase, pulmonary tuberculosis and vitamin B_1 deficiency, a decrease.

Carlson considered that the vagi were the main, if not the only, afferent pathways for the gastric hunger impulses and that the "primary hunger center" must therefore be the "sensory nuclei of the vagi" in the medulla (fasciculus solitarius). The existence of pressure- or tension-sensitive receptors in the stomach wall has been demonstrated.

The possible relation of intestinal phenomena to hunger has attracted some attention. The forward movement of food in the small intestine has been studied by a number of authors, in particular by Quigley.[5] The character of the peristaltic movement has been shown to be dependent on the composition of the chyme. The small intestine, like the stomach, obtains its supply of extrinsic nerve fibers from two sources: a bulbar autonomic (parasympathetic) supply by way of the vagi and a thoracic autonomic (sympathetic) supply by way of the splanchnic nerves and the superior mesenteric ganglia. Stimulation of the vagi causes contraction or increased tonus in the musculature of the intestine; stimulation of the splanchnic nerves generally inhibits tonus. Psychologic states and stimulation of portions of the cerebral cortex may produce contraction or relaxation of the walls of the small and large intestines. Epinephrine, as does splanchnic stimulation, inhibits intestinal movements; oxygen, organic acids and bile increase

them. The sensory fibers from the intestine are carried by the vagus and the splanchnic nerves.

Central Nervous System. Autopsies of patients with hypothalamic obesity suggested a role for the hypothalamus in the control of food intake. Experimental work by investigators on both sides of the Atlantic eliminated the pituitary from consideration as the prime suspect in the development of adiposity. The work of Hetherington and Ransom[6] and Brobeck and co-workers[7] demonstrated that bilateral involvement of the ventromedial nuclei causes hyperphagia in the rat. It has since been shown that, in that species, unilateral destruction of the ventromedial nucleus may cause slow development of obesity.[1,2]

Hypothalamic obesity has been produced in the mouse by Mayer and his associates;[8] in that species, bilateral involvement of the ventromedial area is necessary for even the slightest degree of hyperphagia to appear. Obesity follows superficial lesions of the base of the anterior hypothalamus in the monkey, and lesions caudal to the paraventricular nuclei in the dog. Conversely, Anand and Brobeck[9] found that, in rats, bilateral destruction of more lateral parts of the

REGULATION OF ENERGY EXCHANGE

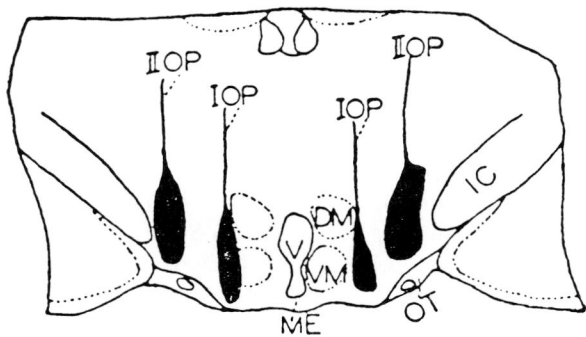

Fig. 17–1. Transverse section through tuberal region of hypothalamus. Medial lesions (I OP) induced hyperphagia and obesity, while lateral lesions (II OP) abolished feeding. ME, median eminence; OT, optic tract; IC, internal capsule; DM, dorsomedial nucleus; VM, ventromedial nucleus; V, third ventricle. (From Anand and Brobeck, Yale J. Biol. Med., 24, 123, 1951.)

hypothalamus is followed by complete cessation of eating (Fig. 17–1). Teitelbaum and Stellar[10] have confirmed this finding, though noting that this inhibition may be temporary with resumption of eating dependent on the nature and consistency of the food presented.

Morrison and Mayer,[11] noting that lesions in the lateral hypothalamus or subthalamus at the same rostrocaudal level as the ventromedial nucleus cause both aphagia and adipsia, tried to see whether these two responses were separate consequences of the lesions. They found that the patterns of food or water exchange cannot be reproduced by deprivation of sham-operated rats of either food or water. Daily water intubation facilitated the "escape" from inhibition of eating and drinking. Localization of "aphagic" and "adipsic" lesions did not completely coincide and their histologic location suggested that the median forebrain bundle was as important as the lateral area proper in the control of water and food intake.[12] Morgane[13,14] in a careful anatomic analysis of this phenomenon has concluded that lesions causing aphagia may interfere with at least two systems of fibers, of which the more important is lateral to the median forebrain bundle; only destruction of this system (and of the median area of the pallidum) causes an irreversible aphagia.

Other areas have also been shown to interfere with the regulation of food intake; bilateral damage to the ventromedial portion of the thalamus, of the rostral mesencephalic nuclei, of the temporal area of the amygdala or the hippocampus causes hyperphagia. Destruction of the frontal area of the amygdala or the hippocampus decreases food intake. Separation of the frontal lobes from their thalamic connections in rats, frontal lobotomy in man and selective decortication in various types of animals also lead to hyperphagia.

Stimulation of various areas of the central nervous system has also proved re-

warding. Larsson,[15] for example, studied the results of electrical stimulation of the hypothalamus and the medulla and of intrahypothalamic injections in sheep and goats. He found that stimulation of the hypothalamus, just caudal to the optic chiasma backward throughout the hypothalamus, lateral to the sagittal level, through the columna fornicis descendens and the mammillothalamic tract resulted in hyperphagia. The most pronounced effect was obtained by stimulation of the region of the lateral hypothalamic nucleus, anterior to the columna fornicis descendens or at the same transverse level as this tract. Rumination was seen on electrical stimulation of the same structures as gave hyperphagia. Mastication, licking and swallowing could be elicited as single effects without the simultaneous occurrence of hyperphagia. These results were taken by Larsson to suggest that it is an oversimplification to speak of a mammillothalamic or an anterolateral hypothalamic "feeding center." Although electrical stimulation of both of these areas, particularly the latter, causes hyperphagia, the fact that extramasticatory and licking movements as well as hyperphagia are obtained diffusely in other areas supports the conclusion that centers directing feeding behavior and centers having to do with motivation to eat rest on centers which are in part different.

Finally, before leaving the anatomic description of central nervous areas involved in the regulation of food intake, it might be noted that some experiments performed by Sudsaneh and me,[16] described below, suggest that the ventromedial area of the hypothalamus exercises some measure of control over gastric contractions.

The use of the behavioral techniques developed by B. F. Skinner and his associates has facilitated the definition of the role of central neural structures in the regulation of food intake. It is also opening a trail which may some day give a precise metabolic and neurologic basis to the concepts of hunger, satiety, appetite and specific appetites. An early experiment was that by Anliker and me, which compared the feeding behavior of normal animals with that of animals with various types of hyperphagia.[17] This clearly demonstrated that, as previously suggested by Brobeck[7] and by Miller, Bailey and Stevenson,[18] the ventromedial area appears to act as a "satiety" brake inhibiting constantly activated lateral "feeding" areas. (Similar techniques have permitted Rozin and Mayer[19] to study the characteristics of the regulation of food intake in the fish.)

Again on the basis of results obtained by behavioral techniques, Teitelbaum[20,21] has suggested that qualitative effects on taste were necessary concomitants of the destruction of the ventromedial area or of lateral hypothalamic lesions. Animals with ventromedial hypothalamic lesions cease to be hyperphagic if presented with diets the consistency or taste of which they do not like. Under such conditions, they may eat less than normal animals. The significance of this interesting observation is difficult to evaluate. Lesions performed with stereotaxic instruments are notoriously complex, and it may well be that Teitelbaum was studying the effect of the destruction of a number of anatomically contiguous centers; the fact that animals can maintain their weight when feeding themselves through a gastric fistula suggests that taste (if not exaggeratedly aversive) is not an essential component in the regulation of food intake, although it obviously is one of the factors influencing food intake at a given time.

Another important behavioral technique which has contributed to our knowledge of central nervous areas involved in the regulation of food intake is that of Olds, who combined lever pressing for food with autoexcitation of a number of central areas, in the rat.[22] The autoexcitation of certain areas (corresponding roughly to parasympathetic nuclei) acts as an additional reward and leads the animal to a tremendous increase in the rate of lever pressing. The autoexcitation of other areas (corresponding roughly to the areas in which Hess has obtained stimulation of the sympathetic system) acts as a negative reinforcement and decreases rates of lever pressing. The combination of Olds' autoexcitation technique with the use of an electric grid permitting the examination of the circumstances under which the drive to eat is particularly intense has allowed Morgane[23] to explore the role of the ventromedial area, the pallidum, the median forebrain bundle and the lateral areas. His results seem to indicate that the lateral area should be subdivided into at least two subareas, an extreme lateral one— excitation of which leads to extreme rates of lever pressing for food, to considerable hyperphagia and to the crossing of the electrified grid to obtain food, even when the animal is fed—and the properly lateral area, excitation of which leads to some hyperphagia, even in fed animals, but not to the crossing of the grid. These experiments, together with those on the effect of lateral lesions, suggest the presence in the lateral hypothalamus of two systems of fibers, one having to do with purely quantitative aspects of the regulation of food intake (and presumably subject to ventromedial "satiety" inhibition) and one with more qualitative aspects of appetite, the relation of which to the ventromedial area is still obscure.

Physiologic Mechanisms of Regulation

Gastric Contractions as a Basis or a Component of Hunger and of Short-term Regulation of Food Intake. The views of Carlson[4] on the relations among gastric pangs, hunger and the regulation of food intake are summarized in his well-known book *The Control of Hunger in Health and Disease.* They constitute the oldest attempt to account experimentally for these phenomena. For Carlson, the consciousness of gastric sensations carried by the vagi is the kernel to the problem. Hunger is defined by him as "a more or less uncomfortable feeling of tension and pain referred to the region of the stomach." While he considers that an explanation of hunger pangs is an explanation of hunger, he does recognize that "many apparently normal persons experience in hunger, besides the gnawing pressure-pain sensation in the stomach, a feeling of weakness, 'emptiness,' headache and sometimes nausea," but calls these states or symptoms "accessory hunger phenomena" because "they are not always present in hunger and their relative preponderance depends on the length of starvation and on some individual peculiarity in the person. It must be admitted, however, that in some individuals these accessory phenomena appear to overshadow, if not entirely to suppress, the pressure-pain sensations from the stomach." In turn, Carlson, struck by the fact that insulin hypoglycemia leads to gastric contractions and hunger feelings, postulated that blood glucose levels were involved in the occurrence of hunger.

The theory received wide, if temporary, acceptance. Although the existence of hunger pangs has been abundantly confirmed, accumulating facts led observers to doubt whether gastric movements provided a sufficient basis for Carlson's generalizations. For example, Adolph[24] showed, by diluting the ration of animals with inert material, that the bulk of the diet—in spite of its effect on the stomach—had only a transient influence on food intake. Complete bilateral vagotomy, which abolishes the motor response to insulin hypoglycemia, does not prevent or even impair the augmentation of food intake produced by insulin administration.

The existence of patients in whom bilateral vagotomy has been performed for the treatment of gastric ulcers enabled Grossman and Stein[25] to extend these findings to human subjects; they found that the sensations of hunger (including feelings of emptiness and weakness) continued to occur after complete vagotomy. In those persons in whom epigastric pangs of distress

associated with individual gastric sensations were a part of the sensation-complex of hunger, vagotomy—by abolishing the contractions—eliminated that particular sensory component. Though the removal of this fraction of the sensory complex was recognized by the subject, it did not delay hunger or change the response to it. Vagotomy actually simply shifted the emphasis to the extragastric components, in particular the feelings of weakness and emptiness associated with the desire for food.

Incidentally, the observation of Grossman and Stein appeared to disprove not only the essential nature of gastric contractions as a basis of hunger and regulation of food intake (the two concepts are not separated by Carlson) but Carlson's suggested mode of perception of these contractions as well. In two patients who had undergone sympathectomy, persisting gastric contractions were no longer associated with a feeling of distress. Grossman and Stein concluded that the splanchnic nerves are the afferent pathways for the distress associated with gastric hunger contractions and that no such pathway exists in the vagus nerves.

With the decrease of the significance of hunger pangs, interest in their causation died and stayed dormant for several decades. Scott[26] and his associates could find no correlation between blood sugar levels and the onset and prevalence of hunger contractions. Experimental work on the testing of the glucostatic hypothesis (see below) has revived interest in both the contractions and their control by showing the negative correlation between gastric hunger contractions and glucose utilization, by demonstrating the striking effect of glucagon in inhibiting gastric contractions and, finally, by indicating that gastric hunger contractions may be in part under the control of the ventromedial hypothalamic area.

It is legitimate to conclude from these studies, and from more recent ones conducted in my own laboratory on the nature and timing of hunger sensations in men, women and children, that hunger pangs are an important component of the sensory complex identified subjectively as hunger. At the same time, in spite of the metabolic and neural concomitants of hunger contractions, available evidence makes it impossible to base a mechanism of regulation of food intake exclusively or even principally on their perception. It remains true, however, that any theory purporting to interpret the regulation of food intake which cannot account for the occurrence of hunger pangs is doomed at the outset.

Thermostatic Component in the Regulation or the Limitation of Food Intake. Brobeck,[27] struck by the fact that the hypothalamus appears able to deal with a number of different stimuli which affect feeding behavior and to make suitable adjustments of food intake, hypothesized that a number of such stimuli may operate through their effect on the heat balance of the body. He accordingly advanced a thermostatic hypothesis which postulated that "animals eat to keep warm and stop eating to prevent hyperthermia." The actual experimental evidence for his view rested first on the observation that short-term exposure to high environmental temperature is followed by reduction of food intake. Kennedy,[28] however, has indicated that, under experimental conditions not dissimilar to those in which Brobeck's animals were placed, dehydration and pyrexial tissue breakdown may have played a major part in weight loss following acute exposure to heat. Acute exposure to cold also caused depression of food intake at first. Working with hypothalamic, hyperphagic rats, Kennedy demonstrated that in the long run—and as long as his animals stayed within the range of adaptation—they showed similar rates of weight gain at high and at low temperatures.

Another piece of evidence used in sup-port of a thermostatic scheme is the fact that a change from a high-carbohydrate to a high-fat diet usually increases food intake and a change to a high-protein diet usually decreases it. The specific dynamic action of protein is higher than that of carbohydrate, which in turn is greater than that of fat. This was taken by Brobeck to indicate that modifications of intake follow perceptions of differences in specific dynamic action. It must be noted, however, that the specific dynamic action of a dietary mixture cannot be calculated by adding the specific dynamic actions of its constituents if these were fed singly, but is usually lower and far less sensitive to changes in composition (within the usual range) than would be the case if the specific dynamic action were additive for the various nutrients. It has been repeatedly shown that, in most strains, the effect on total caloric intake of changing from a high-carbohydrate to a high-fat diet is transient (though there are strains of animals which continue to eat more on a high-fat diet, as do certain types of obese animals).

Finally, there is no doubt that diets very high in protein do reduce the food intake of normal animals. The problem of the mechanism of this effect has been recently reexamined in my laboratory.[29] The fact that the effect is as marked, at a protein level of over 60 per cent, in animals in which the ventromedial hypothalamus has been damaged shows that the effect is not mediated through the hypothalamic "satiety" centers. Above the 60 per cent level, and as the proportion of protein in the diet is further increased, food intake decreases in such a way that the protein intake remains constant, giving an appearance of regulation based on protein intake. Inasmuch, however, as protein levels appear to have little or no effect in the 8 to 60 per cent range (which encompasses the range of protein levels normally encountered by rats living on natural foods rather than on semisynthetic laboratory diets), it seems doubtful that this interpretation is the cor-

rect one. It appears more likely that we are
dealing here with a safety-valve effect,
which indeed could be based on an abnormally high specific dynamic action (or
excessive blood amino acids, or other
mechanisms), which limits food intake
when more than a given amount of protein
is ingested but which does not come into
play at lower levels. This safety mechanism
would have to be situated elsewhere than
at the ventromedial (satiety) centers. (Incidentally, it is possible that below a certain
minimum intake of protein some other
mechanism comes into play to decrease
hunger. In man, Dole and his co-workers[30]
have obtained spontaneous reduction on
diets excessively low in protein.)

Perhaps the most cogent experimental
argument in favor of the existence of a
thermostatic influence on feeding is the
observation of Andersson and Larsson[31]
that refrigeration of the preoptic area
causes feeding in a fed goat. Cessation of
feeding is observed in this animal, even
when fasted for a prolonged period, when
the preoptic area is warmed. The effect of
cooling and warming on drinking behavior
is the opposite of that on eating. While the
effects demonstrated by Andersson and
Larsson are clear-cut, the fact that the
differences of temperature used in the
experiment are enormous (of the order of
10°C in the vicinity of the thermode, of 1 to
1.5°C at a distance of 6 mm) casts some
doubt on the applicability of the results
under physiologic conditions. Results obtained in several laboratories, mine in particular, indicate, incidentally, that the temperature of the ventromedial area remains
remarkably constant in a variety of nutritional situations.

I feel that a thermostatic factor is an
important component in the hunger-
satiety mechanism. I am inclined to believe
that, while progressive exposure to cold
may have a facilitatory effect on feeding
(over and beyond its effect on energy requirements) and exposure to heat, particularly if sudden, a clearly inhibitory effect

on feeding, variation in heat balance is
probably not the agency through which
metabolic requirements influence food intake to ensure caloric homeostasis. On the
other hand, it appears that an elevation of
body temperature may exert a safety-valve
effect (similar to that demonstrated for
very-high-protein diets) which overrides
any other factor which might promote
feeding, to prevent any further heat load
on an already overloaded organism.

**Souleirac's Theory of Regulation of
Carbohydrate Appetite by Intestinal Absorption.** Souleirac limited himself to the
study of appetite for carbohydrate in rodents. However, his numerous publications, later collected in book form, deserve
a somewhat detailed analysis. His work[32]
has the original merit of being directed
toward the quantitative account of a qualitative appetite, and thus provides facts
which may eventually be used to integrate
taste and calorie intake. Souleirac was
struck by the observation that phlorhizin,
which, according to Carlson, increases gastric contractions, inhibited appetite for
carbohydrate. Thyroidectomized and adrenalectomized animals, both of which
present hypoglycemic tendencies, also
show diminished appetite for carbohydrate. The observation led to a search for
possible correlations between carbohydrate appetite and physiologic characteristics. Using a self-selection method,
Souleirac systematically examined the
quantitative and qualitative variations of
uptake of different types of sugar after
removal of the anterior pituitary, thyroid,
and adrenal glands, alloxanization of the
pancreas, and administration of the corresponding hormones: anterior and posterior pituitary extracts, thyroxin, "cortine"
and desoxycorticosterone and insulin. He
concurrently studied the modifications of
taste threshold for carbohydrates and the
effect of the endocrine disturbances just
listed on the intestinal absorption of carbohydrates. Similar studies were made
after administration of epinephrine, er-

gotamine, pilocarpine, acetylcholine and atropine, after spinal section in the cerebral region and hypothalamic lesions, or after administration of glucose, riboflavin and phosphate. The effects of cold and physical exercise also were examined. Estimations of blood glucose and of serum amylase were made after these procedures.

Souleirac found that there was no correlation between either absolute blood sugar level or the level of serum amylase and carbohydrate consumption. On the other hand, he found that all hormones with an effect on carbohydrate metabolism modified the taste threshold for glucose, though the interpretation of the modifications was difficult. By contrast, the correlation between the taste for carbohydrates and the intestinal absorption of carbohydrates was clear-cut. Any condition which increased intestinal absorption increased consumption and, conversely, if carbohydrate absorption was decreased carbohydrate intake was decreased. For instance, injections of glucose depressed absorption of glucose and glucose intake, phlorhizin and thyroidectomy decreased glucose absorption and intake, and insulin and alloxan diabetes increased glucose absorption and intake. The only exception was provided by atropine, which slightly decreased the proportional absorption of glucose from the intestine but considerably increased the total. Souleirac explains the effect of atropine by the intense thirst it produces.

Although the facts invoked by Souleirac are clear enough as far as they go, it seems regrettable that no data are ever given on the caloric intake of the experimental animals, but only on the amount of carbohydrate solution ingested. The omission is all the more regrettable because the solid food available, cereals and greens, constituted a high-carbohydrate diet. It would help to know also the fluid (water) consumption in the different experimental situations.

Examination of the available informa-tion raises the question, not discussed by Souleirac, of how the organism detects the fact that carbohydrate is being absorbed. Souleriac observed that spinal section at the level of the sixth to seventh cervical vertebra did not eliminate the response of the carbohydrate intake to endocrine stimulation, but then it would not interrupt splanchnic sensory connections. The increased intake after atropine treatment could conceivably lend itself to an interpretation based on the effect of the drug on the vagus. The fact that vagotomy and sympathectomy, which would seem to eliminate afferent impulses from the intestine to the central nervous system, while eliminating hunger pangs do not eliminate feelings of emptiness, weakness and desire for food[25] makes it unlikely that the regulation of food intake is based exclusively, or even primarily, on awareness of intestinal absorption. A humoral or hormonal intermediary could, of course, operate independently of intermediary nervous pathways, but there is no indication of the existence of such a link with the higher centers.

Souleirac suggests that the effect of the hypothalamus on the regulation of food intake is mediated through intestinal absorption. Excitation of the hypothalamus would bring about a diminution of carbohydrate absorption and consumption; the action of the hypothalamus would be antagonistic to that of the pituitary and the balance between these organs would determine carbohydrate intake. While, in Souleriac's experiments, consumption of sugar solution increased after hypothalamic lesions, it is difficult to appreciate the significance of his finding, as it cannot be compared with the increases in total food and water consumption which follow the operation. The incidental finding that unilateral lesions lead to increased carbohydrate consumption is of interest in the light of the fact that slow development of obesity follows the production of unilateral hypothalamic lesions in the rat.[2]

Thus, the facts presented by Souleirac, although offering an undeniable challenge, do not appear to support the mechanism he wants to base them on. His observation that any modification of carbohydrate metabolism can affect appetite, and even taste, is in agreement with the postulation of the glucostatic theory. It appears doubtful, however, whether, strong though the appetite for carbohydrate (or protein or salt) may be, hunger and the regulation of food intake are simply summations of selective hungers and partial regulations. Such selective appetites do exist and can be extremely compelling; the "salt wars" are bloody illustrations of their strength. However, compelling though such appetites are, they do not appear to overrule general regulation. Men and animals will, it is true, eat after satiety has apparently been obtained if the supplement offered is particularly appetizing or contains a nutrient of which they have been deprived, yet no mammal will increase its food consumption from, say, a low-protein diet simply to satisfy a need for protein or a specific amino acid.

Glucostatic Component of the Regulation of Food Intake. The glucostatic mechanism in the regulation of food intake, proposed by Mayer and his co-workers in the early fifties,[2] postulated that, in the ventromedial (satiety) hypothalamic centers (and possibly in other central and peripheral areas as well), glucoreceptors existed sensitive to blood glucose in the measure that they utilize it. This concept was based on the facts that the central nervous system is dependent for its function on the availability of glucose, that carbohydrates are preferentially oxidized and are not stored to any appreciable amount, so that their depletion is rapid, and that, in the interval between meals, there is an incomparably greater proportionate drop of carbohydrate reserves than of reserves of proteins and fat. Only intake of food will replenish fully these depleted stores. Furthermore, carbohydrate

metabolism is not only regulated by a complex edifice of endocrine interrelationships it is, in turn, a regulator of fat oxidation and fat synthesis, of protein mobilization and breakdown and of protein synthesis; thus, a mechanism of regulation of food intake based on glucose utilization could be—as it should be—successfully integrated with energy metabolism and its components. Such a theory also permitted successful interpretation of the known effects of cold, exercise, diabetes mellitus, hyper- and hypothyroidism and other metabolic changes, provided the additional postulate was made that carbohydrate metabolism in the ventromedial area differed from that in the brain in general. In particular, it was postulated that the ventromedial area was highly glucoreceptive and, unlike the rest of the brain, would show varying rates of utilization. Such a theory could also account for such facts as the self-perpetuating effect of hyperphagia, which of itself causes a rapid utilization of glucose.

Early experimental work designed to test the theory has often been misinterpreted and, apparently not infrequently, continues to be misinterpreted. Because of the (then) insuperable difficulty in measuring glucose utilization in the ventromedial area and the postulate that, in general, ventromedial utilization must parallel peripheral utilization, an attempt was made by Mayer and Van Itallie to correlate hunger feelings (and later, by Stunkard, gastric contractions) with diminished peripheral glucose utilization in an easily accessible area, i.e., the forearm. Utilization was measured by capillary-venous (or arteriovenous) differences (or "Δ-glucose"); in patients at rest, variations of blood flow were not taken into effect. It was found that, in general, there was a satisfactory degree of correlation between small Δ-glucose and the appearance of subjective feelings of hunger and of gastric contractions. (That the correlation is far from perfect, even when carotid-jugular vein determinations are made, is emphasized in recent work.) It was also shown, in particular by Stunkard and Wolff,[33] that, whenever glucose utilization is proceeding satisfactorily, a slow intravenous glucose infusion in hungry individuals eliminates both the feeling of hunger and gastric contractions. In diabetics, and in hunger diabetes, glucose infusion does not affect hunger to a similar degree.

While other authors at times have not observed the correlation between cessation of hunger and rises in glucose utilization,[34] they may have been operating under some of the conditions described by Van Itallie[35] when peripheral glucose arteriovenous differences are not reliable indices of overall glucose utilization by the body, much less by the satiety mechanisms: such conditions include changes in circulation dynamics because of increase in blood flow, rapid rises in blood glucose, certain effects of insulin and the presence of overriding dominant conditioning. Again, the peripheral arteriovenous differences, although still associated in the thinking of many workers with the foundation of the glucostatic theory, have never really held any direct significance in it and were used in this early work "merely to obtain more reliable information about the changes which take place in carbohydrate supply than is available from arterial or venous glucose alone."[35]

It is interesting to note that Van Itallie and Hashim[36] have shown the reciprocal relation of blood nonesterified fatty acid levels and arteriovenous glucose differences. While these authors point out that it is unlikely that nonesterified fatty acid levels per se act directly as a signal to the food regulatory centers, their work provides yet another indirect way to evaluate patterns of metabolic utilization and their possible correlation with the hunger-satiety balance.

Major recent developments have entirely altered the status of our knowledge in this field by developing means of assessing, much more directly, hypothalamic events in the regulation of food intake, rather than having to rely on mere statistical correlations: the effect of glucagon on hunger feelings and gastric contractions and the role of the ventromedial area in the regulation of gastric contractions, the elucidation of the mode of action of gold thioglucose, the demonstration of the special characteristics of the metabolism of the ventromedial hypothalamic area and the determination of the electrical activity of the ventromedial hypothalamic area under the influence of variations of blood metabolites, glucose in particular.

Action of Glucagon. Hypothalamic Glucostatic Control of Gastric Hunger Contractions. Stunkard, Van Itallie and Reiss[37] made the interesting observation that the injection of 2 mg of glucagon reproducibly eliminates gastric contractions (and hunger sensations) in human subjects. Their results demonstrated that the elimination of gastric contractions lasts as long as glucose utilization proceeds actively and ceases when it is reduced, even though the absolute level of blood glucose is still well above the fasting level.

Stunkard also had the opportunity to observe a patient who had lost practically all of his brain cortex in an accident and was incapable of feeding himself.[38] After one week of fasting, he exhibited almost continuous gastric contractions. A variety of treatments, including the infusion of amino acids and induction of pyrexia (by rolling the patient in an electric blanket), did not inhibit gastric contractions. The only treatment (with the exception of food) which proved effective in inhibiting gastric contractions was the administration of glucagon.

Mayer and his co-workers found that in rats, too, intravenous injections of glucagon inhibit gastric hunger contractions. The dose found to be 100 per cent effective in a large series of animals was 75 μg. The inhibition starts between 45 and 60

seconds after the administration of glucagon. By the time inhibition takes place, the
glucose in the blood has already risen
considerably from the control fasting
values and inorganic phosphorus has decreased, indicating active utilization. Blood
glucose continues to increase as inorganic
phosphorus returns to the fasted level and
gastric hunger contractions appear.[16]

Mayer and Sudsaneh[16] found that rats in
which the ventromedial hypothalamic area
has been destroyed show no significant
difference in their pattern of fasting contractions from that seen in normal animals.
The inhibitory response to epinephrine
and to norepinephrine is normal. On the
other hand, the intravenous administration of 75 μg of glucagon almost invariably
fails to produce complete inhibition of
hunger contractions in animals with lesions
of the ventromedial nuclei, whether the
animals are allowed to become and remain
obese or whether they are reduced to their
preoperative weight after demonstrating
this hyperphagia. Response of the animals
to prolonged exposure to cold is delayed,
on the average, by 100 per cent. The
failure of the animals to respond to glucagon and the delay in response to prolonged exposure to cold are obviously not
caused by refractoriness of gastric contractions as such. The finding may be interpreted as indicating that the ventromedial
area does exercise a definite measure of
control over gastric hunger contractions
and does so in response to an increase in its
glucose utilization. An anatomic basis for
such a mechanism may be provided by the
existence of the bundles of Schultze which
seem to originate in the general area of the
ventromedial hypothalamus and go down
to the roots of the vagus.

Mode of Action of Gold Thioglucose. In
1949, Brecher and Waxler[39] observed a
syndrome of hyperphagia and obesity in
mice after a single intraperitoneal or subcutaneous injection of gold thioglucose.
The observation was confirmed by Marshall, Barrnett and Mayer,[40] who showed

that gold thioglucose caused extensive
damage to the ventromedial area and, in
varying degree, to the supraoptic nucleus,
the ventral part of the lateral hypothalamic
area, the arcuate nucleus and the median
eminence. Marshall and Mayer[41] showed
that there was minimal impairment of
functions other than the regulation of food
intake, unlike that which is observed with
stereotaxic lesions. Gold thioglucose-obese
animals, unlike animals made obese by
stereotaxic lesions, will frequently mate
and rear their young. As do stereotaxic
hypothalamic animals, such animals show
impairment of satiety mechanisms as well
as impaired reaction of the regulation of
food intake to cold, exercise, and caloric
dilution. Mayer and Marshall[42] later showed
that gold thiogalactose, gold thiosorbitol,
gold thiomalate, gold thioglycerol, gold
thiocaproate, gold thioglycoanilide and
gold thiosulfate did not produce the brain
damage which follows gold thioglucose
administration. Hyperphagia and obesity
were not seen following such treatments,
even though toxicity of such compounds is
similar to that of gold thioglucose. It was
also shown that, in the rat, gold thioglucose
caused lesions which were similar to those
seen in the mouse. The fact that simultaneous administration of sodium thioglucose protects animals against hypothalamic
damage is probably traceable to competitive inhibition. On the basis of these observations, Mayer suggested that the toxic
gold moiety of accumulated gold thioglucose destroyed the ventromedial neurons
specifically because of the affinity of these
cells for the glucose component of the
molecule, in accordance with the general
proposal that glucose is a cardinal activator
of the satiety center.

Debons and co-workers,[43] using
radioautographics and neutron-activating
analytic techniques, confirmed and considerably extended these conclusions. The
Brookhaven co-workers first determined
the gold content of the rostral, middle, and
caudal portions of brains for controls.

They found that some gold accumulated in the brains of all gold-treated animals with, however, notable differences in the localization of the gold. Animals treated with gold thiomalate failed to show any hypothalamic localization of the gold. Animals which received gold thioglucose but failed to become obese had a lesser total gold content of the brain, and the amounts of gold localized in the medial sections were less than those in animals which developed the hyperphagic syndrome.

In gold thioglucose-treated animals, radioautographic localization of gold activity was found consistently in four regions. The greatest concentration was in the hypothalamus, chiefly at the lateral angles and the floor of the third ventricle. (Histologically, this region consisted of collapsed glial scar tissue and, in some instances, showed cystic changes.) There was also a second and discrete concentration of radioactivity in the midline dorsal and cephalad to the optic chiasma and immediately dorsal to the anterior commissure, a third in the caudal portion of the septum and ventral hippocampal commissure and a fourth labeled area in the hindbrain in the midline at about the level of the vestibular nuclei in the floor of the fourth ventricle. The fact that gold thioglucose, but not gold thiomalate, administration leads to such localization, even though gold diffused throughout the brain in either case, was taken by the authors as a probability that the gold moiety is responsible for the focal accumulation of sufficient gold in the hypothalamus to produce a destructive lesion, which can result in hyperphagia and obesity.

Luse, Harris and Stohr,[44] in electron microscopy studies of the early lesion, noted that gold thioglucose brought about initial changes in the hypothalamic oligodendroglia cells followed by focal neuronal degeneration. Luse and Harris suggest that the oligodendroglia cells, within certain areas of the central nervous system, share a high degree of specificity to glucose.[45]

Debons and his colleagues[43] point out that, while it is true that the foci of gold accumulation in the hindbrain, in the hippocampal commissure, and above the optic chiasma are at sites where lesions have been reported by Perry and Liebelt,[46] this by no means proves the suggestion of these authors that such extrahypothalamic lesions indicate that gold thioglucose passes through deficient areas in the blood-brain barriers and is not selectively accumulated at "glucoreceptor" sites. Indeed, they add, in view of the extreme chemical specificity demonstrated for the gold thioglucose molecule, consideration must be given to the possibility that the sites of extrahypothalamic gold accumulation may themselves be glucoreceptive areas.

Arees and Mayer[47] have subjected Perry and Liebelt's hypothesis, that a nonspecific weakness in the blood-brain barrier in the ventromedial areas is responsible for the gold thioglucose effect, to critical experimental test. They purposely increased the permeability of the blood-brain barrier in the cortex by inducing a local (electrolytic) lesion. It has often been demonstrated that many substances, such as dyes, electrolytes, or more complex molecules, which do not enter an intact brain will readily enter at the site of any focal lesion. Their test demonstrated that such lesions do not increase brain permeability to gold thioglucose.

More important, they were able to demonstrate that a reasoning based on the existence of glucoreceptors permitted the discovery of important new facts. They showed that destruction of cells with special affinity for glucose and a special role in the regulation of food intake made it possible to locate and stain nerve fibers the functions of which had hitherto only been postulated.

It is well known that destruction of neurons causes their axons to degenerate.

This process, which is believed to occur over the course of several days, is referred to as secondary or Wallerian degeneration. Degenerating axons, whether or not myelinated, are more argyrophilic than normal fibers. A number of silver techniques have been devised to take advantage of this characteristic and to stain fiber pathways. Arees and Mayer[47] used a modification of one technique, that used by Heimer[48] in 1967, which stains both the degenerating fibers and their points of termination (*boutons terminaux*). They reasoned that tracing axons of neurons which were selectively destroyed by gold thioglucose (either because the neurons are glucoreceptors or because they are in close topologic and functional relationship to the glucoreceptors) would enable them to define fibers involved in the regulation of food intake. Indeed, they found that they could demonstrate the hitherto unseen (though universally postulated) fibers connecting the ventromedial area and the lateral area. The axons extended from the ventromedial area in a dorsolateral and slightly rostral direction and terminated in the medial half of the lateral area. Most fibers passed ventral to the fornix bundle, whereas those coming from the most dorsal boundary of the lesion passed just dorsal to the bundle. Some isolated fibers appeared to traverse the fornix bundle directly. Termination degeneration was lightest in the rostral and caudal regions of the lateral hypothalamus and heaviest in its middle region. No terminal degeneration was observed in the lateral half of the lateral hypothalamus.[49] The last finding is perhaps related to behavioral evidence, particularly that already cited obtained by Morgane,[13] which suggests that this area has to do with qualitative aspects and is not subject to ventromedial inhibition.[23]

As mentioned previously, Sudsaneh and Mayer[16] have shown that destruction of the ventromedial area eliminates the inhibition of gastric hunger contractions brought about by administration of glucagon and the consequent hyperglycemia and increase in glucose utilization. The fact that gastric hunger contractions continued to be responsive to epinephrine and norepinephrine suggested that they are not refractory to local agents. These authors proposed[16] that the glucoreceptor system in the ventromedial area involves the dorsal longitudinal fasciculus (bundle of Schultze). The demonstration by Ridley and Brooks[50] that destruction of the ventromedial area also eliminates the gastric acid secretion which normally follows hyperglycemia was seen as perhaps involving the same structure.

Arees and Mayer[47] found that the lesions brought about in the ventromedial area by gold thioglucose do cause the degeneration of the bundle of Schultze. This descending pathway was shown to terminate in the central gray region of the mesencephalon at the level of the superior colliculus, indicating that the axons linking the ventromedial area to the nucleus of the vagus, as are those linking it to the lateral area, are part of the glucoreceptor system.

Finally, it is interesting to note that the fact that mercury thioglucose can replace gold thioglucose in the production of ventromedial lesions[51] confirms the general character of the findings obtained with gold thioglucose.

Special Metabolic Characteristics of the Ventromedial Area. A number of recent experiments have emphasized the metabolic heterogeneity of the hypothalamus and the special metabolic characteristics of the ventromedial area. Larsson,[52] seeking to test the glucostatic hypothesis, reasoned that the hunger state must be accompanied by changes in the concentration of compounds through which brain tissue, which cannot burn or store fat, can nonetheless achieve some energy storage in the form of phosphagens (creatine phosphate) and adenosine triphosphate. We would expect rates of incorporation of glucose and phosphorus to be particularly affected in the ventromedial area, if it was designed to be sensitive to the rate of utilization of glucose. These workers studied the incorporation of glucose labeled with ^{32}P and ^{14}C in three areas, one including the "feeding" and satiety areas and two situated directly above the optic chiasma, the upper one cutting across the columna fornicis. In hungry rats the sample including the feeding area showed a preferential uptake of ^{32}P, indicating an increase of physiologic activity over that in the fed state. In the fed state, by contrast, activity of the two control regions was enhanced, whereas that of the feeding area was proportionally decreased. Experiments with ^{14}C-labeled glucose showed the same type of response. In hungry rats the region that included the feeding area had a greater uptake of glucose than the control areas. Although these studies demonstrated that various parts of the hypothalamus differ in their metabolic reactions, interpretation was difficult because the experimental samples studied and compared with "control" areas included both the ventromedial and lateral areas, as well as other structures presumably not directly concerned with the regulation of food intake.

Chain, Larsson and Pocchiari,[53] in a subsequent study, confirmed differences in the fate of radioactive glucose, particularly in the labeling of amino acids, in different parts of the rabbit brain. Andersson, Larsson and Pocchiari[54] extended the findings and mapped the incorporation of ^{14}C-labeled alanine, aspartic acid, glutamic acid, gamma-aminobutyric acid, glutamine, and arginine in the hypothalamus of the goat, again demonstrating differences in uptake in various parts of the brain. Interpretation of the results, beyond the demonstration of heterogeneity of the hypothalamus, is again difficult. The fact that alloxan diabetes eliminates the sensitivity of the ventromedial area to gold thioglucose, indicating the insulin dependence of the area,[55] has already been mentioned.

Anand,[56] studying glucose and oxygen uptake of various parts of the hypothalamus in the monkey, arrived at more clear-cut results because of the better anatomic definition of his sample. He found that, in the fed animals, there is a relative increase in oxygen and glucose uptake per unit of nucleic acid by the satiety (ventromedial) region as compared with that of the feeding center. In the starved animal, the brain's uptake of oxygen and glucose is less than that of the feeding region. In this experiment, the arteriovenous glucose difference was low in the starved animals and high in those that had been fed. Anand concluded that the results demonstrated an increase in activity of the satiety centers in the fed state, accompanied by an increase in the uptake of glucose, and presumably determined by the changes in availability of glucose. He stated:

> . . . the medial regions are activated as a result of changes in the levels of the blood sugar produced by food intake, which subsequently produces satiety and abolition of further eating by inhibiting the lateral mechanisms. The electroencephalographic recordings from feeding and satiety centers under conditions of hyperglycemia lend further support to this hypothesis, as changes in the activity of satiety centers are more pronounced than changes in the activity of feeding centers.[56]

Perhaps the most direct and striking demonstration of the existence of hypothalamic glucoreceptors regulating food intake, and of their special metabolic character, was the finding by Glick and Mayer[57] that infusion of minute amounts of phlorhizin into the cerebral ventricles of rats (in the vicinity of the hypothalamus) causes dramatic hyperphagia. Phlorhizin is a drug that interferes with cellular transport of glucose in a variety of tissues (kidney, intestine, red cells and, under certain conditions, skeletal muscle).[58] The amounts given were less than those necessary for system effect. The duration of the hyperphagia is a function of the dose. While these findings do not specifically indicate where the glucoreceptive cells are, they point out again the idiosyncrasies of hypothalamic glucoreceptors, inasmuch as other cells in the central nervous system tissue have not been shown to be affected by phlorhizin.

Electroencephalographic Determinations. Anand and his co-workers[59] have evaluated, in rats and monkeys, the role of changes in the blood levels of glucose in various hypothalamic areas. Electrodes were implanted in the lateral, ventromedial, and various control areas of the hypothalamus. Still other electrodes were implanted in the cortex. Connections were brought through the skin at the back of the neck. Four or five days after the operation, hyperglycemia was produced by the intravenous injection of concentrated glucose solution. The consequent rise in blood glucose caused an increase in the frequency of encephalographic waves from the ventromedial (satiety) area (from 6 or 7 per second to 9 or 10 per second). The glucose injection was followed by a drastic decrease in activity in the lateral (feeding) area, with reductions in potential of two-thirds or more being noted. Electric activity of control areas in other parts of the hypothalamus was not affected. Conversely, hypoglycemia (produced by intravenous injection of insulin) caused a reduction in frequency of ventromedial waves (from 6 or 7 per second to 2 or 3). Activity in the feeding area was increased.

Changes in blood amino acid and blood lipid concentrations did not affect the electric activity of the satiety and feeding centers. An increase in glucose utilization after the consumption of a meal was similarly found to be associated with a doubling of the frequency of ventromedial pulsation and a decrease in the activity of the feeding centers.

Effect of Glucose on Activity of Single Neurons in the Hypothalamus. In an impressive series of experiments utilizing 109 mongrel dogs and 47 cats, the effect of glucose and insulin on the electric activity of single hypothalamic neurons was examined by Anand and his collaborators,[60] with striking results. The experiments were well controlled—for example, in osmolarity of solutions infused. Microelectrodes were placed in the required sites under vision by a micromanipulator. The femoral vessels were cannulated for blood sampling and infusions.

The response of single neurons in the feeding centers to glucose infusion showed a decrease in spike frequency. In the satiety centers the spike frequency was markedly increased. This increase in the spike frequency of the neurons of the satiety center and the decrease in the feeding centers occurred within 5 to 15 minutes after glucose infusion. The change in spike frequency was sustained for a period lasting half an hour to an hour, with the maximum occurring about half an hour after infusion. A second infusion two hours after the first caused a lesser change in the spike frequency. Other hypothalamic areas did not respond to glucose infusion, nor did the satiety areas respond to saline infusions. The response of single satiety-center neurons to insulin infusion is a transitory increase followed by a prolonged decrease in spike frequency. The changes in spike frequency when glucose and insulin were perfused were much more closely correlated with arteriovenous differences than with glucose levels, suggesting to the Indian workers that the activity of the satiety centers is much more closely correlated to glucose utilization than to absolute blood glucose levels, and that their reaction to insulin makes their metabolism representative of that of extracerebral tissues.

The glucostatic mechanism appears to be one of the essential processes through which metabolic requirements influence the feeding mechanism and through which energetic homeostasis is maintained. There are, of course, many other factors that influence food intake at a given time.

A thermostatic component, sensitive to elevations of body temperature, may act on a safety valve situated in another hypothalamic area to shut off feeding behavior.[61] Other safety valves may be similarly sensitive to protein imbalance,[62] to excessively high intakes of protein,[62] to gastric distention and to dehydration. Metering of food intake by the mouth or the pharynx, taste, emotions and habits may at a given moment also influence intake. Long-term factors, such as the state of the adipose tissue, also appear to regulate food intake. (It may well be, however, that, because of the relation of free fatty acid release to the size and metabolic state of fat cells, and because of the mutual interrelation of glucose and fatty acid availability, the particular factor is mediated through the glucostatic mechanism.)

LONG-TERM REGULATION OF FOOD INTAKE AND BODY WEIGHT

While the likelihood of the existence of a long-term mechanism of regulation of intake and body weight, correcting the errors of the short-term mechanism, comes out very strongly from the experiments of Gasnier and A. Mayer, the mechanism of such a regulation (the existence of which has since been postulated by a number of authors, in particular G. C. Kennedy[63]) is still unclear. Experiments conducted in my laboratory indicate that the efficiency of food utilization by an animal which has once been obese and then reduced is greater than before obesity had taken place. This would suggest that, as postulated by Kennedy, adipose tissue does play a considerable role in long-term homeostasis and that perhaps the level of enzymatic activity within this tissue tends to be more self-perpetuating than that of the fat content. It is of course possible that the long-term mechanism works through short-term components: more rapid uptake of nutrients, in particular glucose, could take place whenever the steric hindrance caused by accumulated fat in the

adipose tissue is relieved by fat loss. Quaade has pointed out some of the effects on heat load of the body caused by the insulation caused by increased adipose tissue.[64]

HUNGER AND SATIETY SENSATIONS IN MAN

Until a 1965 study conducted by Mayer, Monello and Seltzer,[65] there had been a complete dearth of systematic information on the sensory aspects of hunger and satiety in man. While much remains to be found, this study provided 400 elements of information each on 800 persons, adults and adolescents, obese and nonobese. The study revealed the existence of a multiplicity of sensations recognized by various individuals as hunger signals, with significant differences being found between age groups, the sexes and individuals. There is also an element of variability in the timing and the sequence of hunger sensations. Changes in moods associated with changes in the state of nutrition and degrees of urge are also more complex and more variable than hitherto recognized.

A major finding of the study was that, while hunger is associated with sensations which increase in number and intensity as deprivation progresses, satiety—the cessation of the urge to eat—is not necessarily associated with any specific sensation, nor does it coincide simply with the disappearance of hunger sensations. It is often associated, particularly in adults, with changes in mood. In growing youngsters and some adults, while sensations of gastric fullness frequently accompany satiety, this is by no means general, even in individuals in whom it is a frequent concomitant of satiety. The sensory picture is thus not inconsistent with the phenomenon of satiety being dependent on events occurring largely at the subconscious or unconscious level, such as the hypothalamic level. It is obvious, however, that the timing of satiety is too rapid to make it dependent on "metabolic" monitoring of the food ingested. A more likely physiologic explanation is the possible presence of subsidiary chemoreceptors in the gastrointestinal tract and, perhaps, a reflex secretion of glucagon with, as a result, an indirect effect on the ventromedial hypothalamus. (Incidentally, comparison between the hunger and satiety pictures in obese and nonobese individuals suggests that abnormalities of satiety may be more prevalent than abnormalities of hunger.)

Work by Schachter[66] suggests that obese individuals are responsive to "outside" cues, while normal-weight subjects respond to "inside" cues. In a society which is highly punitive toward the obese,[67] it seems possible that individuals whose physiologic regulatory systems are inadequate are driven to meter the intake which they will allow themselves through "outside" cues. These may form a more or less logical system "built in" as a result of information (or misinformation) concerning the caloric value of food. The observations of Schachter can, therefore, be interpreted as demonstrating that many obese subjects have a physiologically deranged regulatory mechanism, compensated for by psychologic methods, rather than proving a psychogenic etiology of their obesity.

CONCLUSION

The existence of a regulation of food intake—perhaps mediated by a long-term and a short-term mechanism—which ensures homeostasis is clear. In addition to metabolic influences, probably mediated through a glucostatic component acting on the ventromedial hypothalamic area, with a thermostatic component acting perhaps on another area (preoptic?) as a safety valve, also acting on various areas are a number of factors—gastric contractions (probably in part regulated through the hypothalamus), gastric distention, metering by mouth and pharynx, water balance, extremes of environmental temperature (acting above and beyond their effect on energy balance), a host of psychologic factors (taste, habits and emotions) and social and cultural habits and pressures which at a given moment will influence the subject to increase or decrease intake. These various factors interact. For example, taste may be in part dependent on the physiologic state.[68] It seems to me, having studied a large number of forms of experimental and human hyperphagias and anorexias, that the wonder is not that there should be a great diversity of disturbances in the regulation of food intake, producing many different types of obesities and excessive thinness, but rather that in most animals and men, with feeding behavior subject to so many influences, the mechanism of regulation of food intake works as extraordinarily well as it does.

BIBLIOGRAPHY

1. Gasnier and Mayer: Ann. Physiol. Physiochem. Biol., *15*, 145, 157, 186, 195, 210, 1939.
2. Mayer: Nutr. Abstr. Rev., *25*, 597, 871, 1955.
3. Cannon and Washburn: Am. J. Physiol., *29*, 441, 1911–12.
4. Carlson: *The Control of Hunger in Health and Disease*. Chicago, University of Chicago Press, 1914.
5. Quigley: Ann. N. Y., Acad. Sci., *63*, 6, 1955.
6. Hetherington and Ranson: Am. J. Physiol., *136*, 609, 1942.
7. Brobeck: Physiol. Rev., *26*, 541, 1946.
8. Mayer, French, Zighera and Barrnett: Am. J. Physiol., *182*, 75, 1955.
9. Anand and Brobeck: Yale J. Biol. Med., *24*, 123, 1951.
10. Teitelbaum and Stellar: Science, *120*, 894, 1954.
11. Morrison and Mayer: Am. J. Physiol., *191*, 248, 1957.
12. Morrison, Barrnett and Mayer: Am. J. Physiol., *193*, 230, 1958.
13. Morgane: Am. J. Physiol., *201*, 420, 1961.
14. Morgane: J. Comp. Neurol., *117*, 1, 1961.
15. Larsson: Acta Physiol. Scand., *32*, (Suppl. 115), 1, 1954.
16. Mayer and Sudsaneh: Am. J. Physiol., *197*, 274, 1959.
17. Anliker and Mayer: Am. J. Clin. Nutr., *5*, 148, 1957.
18. Miller, Bailey and Stevenson: Science, *112*, 256, 1950.
19. Rozin and Mayer: Am. J. Physiol., *201*, 968, 1961.
20. Teitelbaum and Epstein: Psychol. Rev., *69*, 74, 1962.
21. Teitelbaum and Epstein: *First International Symposium on Olfaction and Taste*. Oxford, Pergamon Press, 1963.

22. Olds: Science, *127*, 315, 1958.
23. Morgane: Science, *133*, 887, 1961.
24. Adolph: Am. J. Physiol., *151*, 110, 1947.
25. Grossman and Stein: J. Appl. Physiol., *1*, 263, 1948.
26. Scott, Scott and Zuckhardt: Am. J. Physiol., *123*, 423, 1938.
27. Brobeck: Yale J. Biol. Med., *20*, 545, 1948.
28. Kennedy: Proc. R. Soc. B, *137*, 535, 1950.
29. Krauss and Mayer: Nature, *200*, 123, 1963.
30. Dole, Schwartz, Thayson, Thorn and Silver: Am. J. Clin. Nutr., *2*, 381, 1954.
31. Andersson and Larsson: Acta Physiol. Scand., *52*, 75, 1961.
32. Souleirac: Bull. Biol. Fr. Belg., *81*, 274, 432, 1947.
33. Stunkard and Wolff: J. Clin. Invest., *35*, 954, 1956.
34. Bernstein and Grossman: J. Clin. Invest., *35*, 627, 1956.
35. Van Itallie: Ann. N. Y. Acad. Sci., *63*, 89, 1955.
36. Van Itallie and Hashim: Am. J. Clin. Nutr., *8*, 587, 1960.
37. Stunkard, Van Itallie and Reiss: Proc. Soc. Exp. Biol. Med., *89*, 258, 1955.
38. Stunkard: Am. J. Clin. Nutr., *5*, 203, 1957.
39. Brecher and Waxler: Proc. Soc. Exp. Biol. Med., *70*, 498, 1949.
40. Marshall, Barrnett and Mayer: Proc. Soc. Exp. Biol. Med., *90*, 240, 1955.
41. Marshall and Mayer: Am. J. Physiol., *178*, 271, 1954.
42. Mayer and Marshall: Nature, *178*, 1399, 1956.
43. Debons, Silver, Cronkite, Johnson, Brecher, Tenzer and Schwartz: Am. J. Physiol., *202*, 743, 1962.
44. Luse, Harris and Stohr: Anat. Rec., *139*, 250, 1961.
45. Luse and Harris: Arch. Neurol., *4*, 139, 1961.
46. Perry and Liebelt: Proc. Soc. Exp. Biol. Med., *106*, 55, 1961.
47. Mayer and Arees: Fed. Proc., *27*, 1345, 1968.
48. Heimer: Brain Res., *5*, 86, 1967.
49. Arees and Mayer: Science, *157*, 1574, 1967.
50. Ridley and Brooks: Am. J. Physiol., *209*, 319, 1965.
51. Sandrew and Mayer: Fed. Proc., *31*, 397, 1972.
52. Larsson: Acta Physiol. Scand. *32* (Suppl. 115), 7, 1954.
53. Chain, Larsson and Pocchiari: Proc. R. Soc. Lond. (Biol.), *152*, 283, 1960.
54. Andersson, Larsson and Pocchiari: Acta Physiol. Scand., *51*, 314, 1961.
55. Debons, Krimsky and Likuski: Am. J. Physiol., *214*, 652, 1968.
56. Anand: Am. J. Clin. Nutr., *8*, 529, 1960.
57. Glick and Mayer: Nature, *219*, 1374, 1968.
58. Lotspeich: Harvey Lect., *56*, 63, 1960–61.
59. Anand, Dua and Singh: Electroencephalogr. Clin. Neurophysiol., *13*, 54, 1961.
60. Anand, Chhina, Sharma, Dua and Singh: Am. J. Physiol., *207*, 1146, 1964.
61. Brobeck: Yale J. Biol. Med., *20*, 545, 1948.
62. Krauss and Mayer: Am. J. Physiol., *209*, 479, 1965.
63. Kennedy: Proc. R. Soc. B, *14*, 578, 1952–53.
64. Quaade: Lancet, *2*, 429, 1963.
65. Mayer, Monello and Seltzer: Postgrad. Med., *37*(6), A97, 1965.
66. Schachter: Science, *161*, 751. 1968.
67. Monello and Mayer: Am. J. Clin. Nutr., *13*, 35, 1963.
68. Titlebaum and Mayer: Experentia, *19*, 539, 1963.

Chapter *18*

NUTRITION IN RELATION TO IMMUNITY

A. E. Axelrod

Much attention has been directed toward the possibility of a relationship between nutritive state and resistance-susceptibility to infection. With this in mind, many experimentalists have sought for dietary factors that could influence the resistance or susceptibility of a host to infectious disease. Many of these studies have certainly been motivated by the hope that suitable manipulation of the diet might influence the incidence and course of an infection for the benefit of the host. However, these interrelationships have proven to be exceedingly complex.

The determinants of resistance to infectious disease are multiple in nature and include the classic antigen-antibody interaction (acquired immunity). In many instances, this reaction may represent a most significant part of the intricate mechanism involved in resistance to infection. In this chapter, we shall discuss only the interdependence between nutrition and actively acquired immunity, i.e. specific immunity attributable to the presence of antibody formed by the animal in response to antigenic stimulus.

STATUS PRIOR TO 1955

This subject has been discussed fully in a review paper appearing in 1955[1] and there is little need to recapitulate the material in detail. A brief summation of the field as it existed in 1955 is, however, in order. From a morass of data accumulated by numerous investigators, the significant fact emerged that certain nutrients could play an important role in the process of antibody formation. Apparently a severe protein deficiency, as well as deficiencies of pyridoxine, pantothenic acid and pteroylglutamic acid, produced the most consistent deleterious effects upon antibody formation. However, the need for certain other dietary components, particularly members of the vitamin B complex, also could be demonstrated clearly on occasion.

A state of inanition usually accompanies the deficiencies under consideration. It became extremely important, therefore, to determine whether the effects observed in a particular deficiency were actually caused by specific absence of the nutritional factor or by the nonspecific effects of caloric restriction (inanition). The accumulated evidence argued strongly against any significant role of inanition per se and supported the viewpoint that the phenomena observed were attributable specifically to deficiency of the nutrient in question. This conclusion has been further strengthened by numerous observations showing little correlation between growth and antibody responses of experimental animals in various deficiency states.

This latter observation has served as the basis for the suggestion that antibody response might be utilized as a more sensitive criterion of nutritional adequacy than the frequently employed growth response. It was recognized that the serum antibody level, utilized as a measure of antibody response, probably reflects an equilibrium between the rate of antibody synthesis and release from the sites of synthesis on the one hand and the rate of destruction of circulating antibody on the other. A change in any one of these factors could obviously affect the content of circulating antibodies. Thus, it became important to evaluate the effects of a nutritional deficiency upon antibody *release* and *degradation* before any positive statements could be made regarding any direct relationship between nutritional factors and antibody synthesis. Such experiments were conducted and suggested that the decreased level of circulating antibody in the vitamin deficiencies could not be attributed to a faulty release mechanism or to excessive destruction of antibody. It seemed more likely, though not definitely proven, that there was a disturbance in the process of antibody synthesis.

CURRENT STATUS

Immune Responses—Experimental Animals

Studies conducted in the main between 1955 and 1971 and summarized in the previous edition of this series[2] have corroborated the earlier observations of the inhibitory effects of nutritional deficiencies upon *antibody production* in experimental animals. In these studies, experimenters have utilized a wide range of antigenic stimuli—various vaccines, bacterial and nematode antigens, heterologous erythrocytes, swine influenza virus, ovalbumin, horse serum, synthetic peptides and a variety of experimental animals: rats, mice, guinea pigs, swine, rabbits, chicks, dogs and monkeys. In a number of cases, vitamin and amino acid metabolic antagonists were employed to advantage in the production and exacerbation of these deficiency states.

A deficiency of thiamin was generally without effect, whereas the most reproducible and extensive changes were observed in deficiencies of pyridoxine, pantothenic acid and folic acid. Occasional deleterious effects were noted in deficiencies of vitamins A and D and riboflavin. Reports on the role of vitamin C have been conflicting. In our laboratory,[3] we failed to demonstrate any effect of severe scurvy in guinea pigs upon primary or secondary circulating antibody formation to diphtheria toxoid. Many studies emphasized the harmful effects of specific amino acid deficiencies in experimental animals. As might be expected, the dietary balance of amino acids was shown to play a significant role in the determination of immune response. In some instances, decreased serum antibody formation was associated with a decreased production of antibody-forming cells of the spleen. A series of observations on the effects of large dosages of various vitamins administered to animals maintained on normal diets during the periods of active immunization produced conflicting results.

Early work with diphtheria toxoid had demonstrated a requirement for a number of vitamins, particularly those of the B complex, in antibody synthesis in the rat. In a continuation of these studies, we found that deficiencies of the amino acids tryptophan and methionine markedly inhibit antibody response. Deficiencies of vitamin E and choline were without effect. The absence of any deleterious action of a choline deficiency is of some interest, since this deficiency state produced a marked weight loss as well as an extreme hemorrhagic condition of the kidney. A similar lack of correlation between antibody response and severity of the symptomatology of deficient animals has been noted frequently.

Marked decreases in the avidity of serum antibody were observed in rats with pyridoxine and pantothenic acid deficiencies. Thus, in these deficiency states, there was a qualitative difference in the type of antibody formed as well as a diminution in the total quantity of antibodies produced. This qualitative change is manifested by a lowered ability of the antibody to combine with the antigen, and probably results from the synthesis of altered antibody molecules. The effect of a pyridoxine deficiency upon circulating antibody formation has been studied in the guinea pig.[4] Pyridoxine deficiency was produced in very young guinea pigs by feeding a highly purified diet lacking pyridoxine. The deficiency state was produced in more mature animals by administering the pyridoxine antagonist, deoxypyridoxine, to guinea pigs receiving the pyridoxine-deficient diet. Pyridoxine deficiency produced by either of these procedures depressed both circulating antibody formation and the degree of the early, Arthus-type skin hypersensitivity reaction to diphtheria toxoid. The latter reaction, edema and necrosis at the site of the injection, is associated with circulating antibodies.

Further studies were designed to investigate the role of nutritional factors in the various phases of the anamnestic response (reappearance in the blood of preexisting antibodies in response to a nonspecific antigen) to diphtheria toxoid in the rat.[5] Deficiencies of pantothenic acid, biotin, pyridoxine and tryptophan produced marked inhibition of the secondary (booster) as well as of the primary response to this antigen, the inhibition of the booster response being most pronounced. Intensive nutritional therapy, given only during the secondary phase, failed to elicit antibody formation. In no case was an anamnestic effect seen in the animals given supplement, despite their immediate and marked growth response to the nutritional therapy. Repeated injections of diphtheria toxoid were unable to overcome the inhibitory effect of a pyridoxine deficiency induced by dietary means or by the administration of the pyridoxine antagonist. Thus, it seems clear that adequate nutrition during the primary phase is essential for the attainment of a satisfactory booster response. Subsequent experiments demonstrated that a pyridoxine deficiency induced by the administration of deoxypyridoxine during the secondary phase could significantly inhibit the secondary response. This inhibition was apparent 3 days after the booster injection. It should be stressed that these animals received adequate diets during the primary phase and were, therefore, permitted to initiate the events which, under normal circumstances, would be triggered by the secondary stimulus to accelerate the processes of antibody synthesis. A pyridoxine deficiency in the secondary phase inhibited this normal sequence. It was felt that these results could be ascribed to the deleterious effects of an acute pyridoxine deficiency upon the lymphoid apparatus. Thus, the successful attainment of a satisfactory anamnestic response to diphtheria toxoid in the albino rat required a state of adequate nutrition during both the primary and secondary phases of this process. Control experiments demonstrated again that inanition was not a factor in these studies. It was further noted that the high content of circulating antibody produced by anamnesis in normal animals was not affected by a subsequent acute deficiency of pyridoxine.

The studies described thus far utilized only particulate antigens. To obtain further information regarding the specificity of these deficiency effects, we repeated these experiments with a nonparticulate antigen. Influenza virus was chosen, since it represents a nonparticulate antigen of clinical interest the corresponding serum antibody of which can be readily determined by a specific neutralization procedure. Antibody formation to this virus was markedly diminished in both pantothenic acid- and pyridoxine-deficient rats.[6] Of considerable interest was the observation that antibody synthesis was not impaired in rats with severe thiamin deficiency. Inanition was without effect. These results paralleled our previous observations with other antigens and further emphasized the general nature of this phenomenon as well as the specificity of action of the vitamins as regards antibody production.

It is conceivable that the impairment of antibody production in the vitamin-deficient animals may be traced to a disturbance in some phase of antigen metabolism. It, therefore, seemed appropriate to investigate antigen metabolism in these deficiency states (Pruzansky and Axelrod, unpublished observations). A heterologous serum protein, bovine gamma globulin, was utilized as a model to investigate the metabolic fate of an antigen. ^{131}I-labeled bovine gamma globulin was injected intravenously into riboflavin-, pyridoxine- and pantothenic acid-deficient rats and into control rats pair-fed with the riboflavin-deficient group. Since the rates of removal of bovine gamma globulin from the blood were essentially the same in the various groups, it was felt that the mechanism involved in the removal of a foreign protein (and presumably also of an antigen) from the blood is not impaired in these vitamin deficiencies.

We have shown (Axelrod and Seaborn, unpublished observations) that splenic cells from pyridoxine-deficient rats treated with diphtheria toxoid, in contrast to those removed from normal immunized rats, were unable to produce antibody when passively transferred to normal nonimmunized rats. Utilizing the procedure of Jerne et al.[7] for the estimation of individual antibody-synthesizing cells, we have shown that the number of antibody-producing splenic cells following antigenic stimulus is markedly diminished in pyridoxine deficiency.[8] This decreased cellular immune response was independent of the inanition associated with the deficiency and was restored to normal by the administration of pyridoxine shortly before immunization. Accumulation of antigen by rat spleen did not appear to be deranged in pyridoxine deficiency.

Mechanism of Action of Pyridoxine. The precise role of pyridoxine in the sequence of events leading to its various effects upon immune phenomena has not been elucidated. Since antibodies are proteins, we considered the possibility that the inhibitory effect of the deficiency upon antibody synthesis could be a reflection of the requirement for this vitamin in the general process of protein biosynthesis. Our experiments to this end have shown that pyridoxine deficiency in the rat produces a consistent decrease in incorporation of L-valine-1-^{14}C into proteins of liver, spleen and serum.[9] Incorporation into proteins of subcellular fractions, i.e. nuclear, mitochondrial, microsomal and soluble fractions, is affected in a similar manner. Incorporation by deficient animals ranged from 50 to 75 per cent of that of controls. Simple inanition was without effect and the diminished rate of incorporation was restored by administering pyridoxine 24 hours before injection of labeled valine. Utilizing a cell-free system capable of incorporating amino acids, we have since demonstrated that ribosomes isolated from liver or spleen of pyridoxine-deficient rats exhibit a decreased capacity for incorporating DL-leucine-1-^{14}C from that of ribosomes isolated from corresponding tissues of normal rats.[10]

The relation of pyridoxine to protein biosynthesis and the known profound effects of pyridoxine deficiency upon cellular growth suggest a role for this vitamin in metabolism of nucleic acids. At the enzymatic level it has been established that pyridoxal phosphate is involved in the production of "active formaldehyde," via conversion of serine to glycine, and that this C_1 unit participates in biosynthesis of purine bases and of thymidylic acid from deoxyuridine-5'-phosphate. Our results indicate that pyridoxine-deficient rats possess fewer cells and less DNA per milligram of splenic tissue than do normal rats. Studies on incorporation of labeled precursors of nucleic acids provide evidence for a decreased biosynthesis of DNA and RNA in pyridoxine deficiency.[11]

Our next series of experiments dealt with effects of pyridoxine deficiency upon polysomes and messenger RNA, components which play a fundamental role in protein biosynthesis.[10] These experiments clearly indicate that a pyridoxine-deficient rat possesses fewer polysomes per unit of liver or spleen tissue than a corresponding control. Accordingly, the decreased incorporation of amino acids into protein by ribosomes isolated from liver and spleen of pyridoxine-deficient rats may be attributed to the decreased level of polysomes in these animals. These results suggest a decreased biosynthesis of RNA, particularly messenger RNA, in pyridoxine deficiency. This suggestion was investigated by determining incorporation of orotic-6-^{14}C acid into RNA associated with ribosomes. A decrease in RNA, particularly messenger RNA, synthesis in pyridoxine deficiency was shown.

Apparently pyridoxine deficiency impairs nucleic acid synthesis, with subsequent deleterious effects upon cell multiplication and protein biosynthesis. The adverse effects of pyridoxine deficiency upon immune responses can be explained on this basis. It is known that administration of an antigen stimulates an intensive multiplication of host cells in certain organs concerned with immune responses, e.g. spleen, lymph nodes. Although the mechanism of antigenic activity in this proliferation process is not clear at present, there is no doubt that requirements for DNA are increased at this step of the immune response. Since pyridoxine is required for DNA synthesis, its relative absence would represent a decisive deterrent to antibody synthesis. Furthermore, an accelerated production of specific mRNA would be expected to accompany synthesis of antibody by immunologically competent cells. Accordingly, a lack of pyridoxine would be manifested by a decreased rate of mRNA synthesis and, ultimately, by inhibition of the immune response. Thus, the deleterious effects of pyridoxine deficiency upon development of an immune response could be visualized at the sites of cellular proliferation as well as indicated by the synthetic capacities of the cell.

Mechanism of Action of Pantothenic Acid.
Previous investigations have demonstrated an impairment of antibody response to a variety of antigenic stimuli in pantothenic acid-deficient rats. The molecular basis of this impaired response is not clearly defined. Since antibodies represent a class of proteins, efforts have been directed toward elucidation of the role of pantothenic acid in protein synthesis.[12] We have demonstrated a decreased incorporation of intravenously injected labeled amino acids into serum albumin in this deficiency state, thus implicating pantothenic acid as a significant factor in the metabolism of protein other than circulating antibodies. However, we could find no evidence for the malfunctioning of the enzymatic processes involved in protein synthesis. Thus, hepatic polysomal profiles and in vitro incorporation of labeled amino acids by a polyribosomal system were not affected in the pantothenic acid-deficient rats. Similarly, the synthesis of nascent polypeptides remained normal in deficient rats receiving an intravenous pulse of radioactive amino acids. Since our data indicate that the decreased rate of incorporation of amino acids in vivo in pantothenic acid-deficient rats is not the result of decreased synthesis of protein in liver, we have considered the possibility that the defect may be the inability to secrete newly synthesized proteins into the extracellular compartment.

Cell-mediated Immunity. Investigations of the relationship between nutritional state and cell-mediated immunity have assumed considerable prominence.

Pyridoxine-deficient guinea pigs inoculated with Mycobacterium tuberculosis, BCG, exhibit depressed delayed-hypersensitivity skin reactions to the allergen, purified protein derivative (PPD).[13] Deoxypyridoxine treatment of previously sensitized animals also depresses skin reactivity. However, in vitro tests and passive transfer experiments have demonstrated that cells of the pyridoxine-deficient animals are sensitive to PPD. Thus, the sensitization mechanism is not inhibited by the deficiency at the cellular level, even though ability to respond to the allergen is affected. One can speculate that pyridoxine or its coenzyme is an essential component in the sequence of reactions between sensitized cell and antigen. Later studies[14] have shown that a pyridoxine deficiency affects, in parallel manner, both systemic and skin reactivity to PPD, rendering unlikely the possibility that the decreased skin reactivity to PPD of pyridoxine-deficient guinea pigs results from skin abnormalities produced by the lack of pyridoxine. Since similar results were obtained with killed BCG as an immunizing agent, it would appear that impairment of growth of BCG in pyridoxine-deficient animals is not a dominant factor in the production of depressed reactivity. Animals immunized with BCG during a state of pyridoxine deficiency rapidly acquired reactivity when supplied with pyridoxine. Neither skin nor systemic reactivity is affected in inanition controls or in ascorbic acid-deficient animals. Anaphylactic sensitivity to bovine serum albumin is not depressed in pyridoxine-deficient guinea pigs. The differential effect of pyridoxine deficiency upon endotoxin and PPD reactivity in the guinea pig permits the conclusion that differences in basic mechanisms must be involved.[15]

Host nutrition is a factor of crucial significance in the development of hypersensitivity phenomena. The inhibitory effect of a pyridoxine deficiency has already been cited. Mueller et al.[16] have demonstrated that ascorbic acid deprivation in the guinea pig can abolish tuberculin sensitivity, as measured by the PPD skin reaction. Supplementation with ascorbic acid restores sensitivity. Evidence has also been presented[17] that ascorbic acid deficiency interferes with actual induction of delayed hypersensitivity rather than with skin reactivity. Results of passive transfer experiments and studies of the in vitro mitotic response of lymphocytes suggest, however, that delayed tubercular hypersensitivity is

not qualitatively lost at the cellular level in scorbutic guinea pigs.[18,19] Perhaps the scorbutic state affects the tuberculin skin response at a more "peripheral" level, possibly in the inflammatory response. The tuberculin reaction can also be inhibited by administration of the folic acid antagonist, amethopterin.[20] Passive transfer experiments with lymph node cells suggest that amethopterin does not inhibit tuberculin sensitization of cells, but probably suppresses multiplication of cells altered by contact with tuberculin.[21] This antagonist is also capable of suppressing the development of delayed skin hypersensitivity and the specific febrile response to ovalbumin and diphtheria toxoid.[22]

Studies on the effects of 6-mercaptopurine and methotrexate on passive delayed hypersensitivity reactions indicate that, in the guinea pig, the suppression of delayed cutaneous hypersensitivity reactions by these compounds is caused primarily by an immunosuppressive and not by an anti-inflammatory reaction.[23]

Experimental allergic encephalomyelitis (EAE) is a specific manifestation of hypersensitivity which may have an autoimmune basis. It is, therefore, of considerable interest to note that the course of development of this disease is amenable to nutritional manipulation. In 1957, Schneider et al.[24] reported that susceptibility of homozygous BSVS mice to acute disseminated encephalomyelitis is nutritionally dependent, folic acid and vitamin B_{12} being the most effective factors studied. Supplementation of a highly purified diet with these vitamins restored in great measure the susceptibility of mice to this disease. Biotin was less effective. This study was followed by the observations that EAE is suppressed in scorbutic guinea pigs[16] and in guinea pigs treated with amethopterin.[25] The protective effect of amethopterin is reversed by folinic acid.

Studies on skin homotransplantation afford another illustration of the possible usefulness of an induced vitamin deficiency state in preventing or diminishing the extent of a hypersensitivity reaction. It is generally agreed that the failure of an homologous transplant arises from an acquired immune response, perhaps of the delayed hypersensitivity type, in the recipient to the antigens of the donor tissue. The subsequent antigen-antibody interaction is assumed to effect the rejection of the donor tissue. On this basis, a successful transplant would be established if the immune response of the host could be blocked. The soundness of this hypothesis has been verified.[26,27] A high proportion of successful skin homotransplants can be achieved in pyridoxine-deficient rats of certain strains. We have achieved partial tolerance to skin grafts in normal rats by utilizing a state of immunologic inertness induced by pyridoxine deficiency.[28] In these experiments, microsomal ribonucleic acid extracts derived from splenic cells of a normal rat, which later served as the skin donor, were administered to a pyridoxine-deficient rat of another strain. Skin homografting was performed after the ribonucleic acid-treated recipient had received intensive pyridoxine therapy. Later experiments[29] showed that the biologic effects of these extracts could be ascribed to their ribonucleic acid content. The ribonucleic acid effect was manifested only when administered during a state of pyridoxine deficiency.

Tolerance of CBA J mice to skin grafts from C3H/HeJ mice has been achieved by injection of C3H/HeJ splenic cells into pyridoxine-deficient CBA J recipients.[30] Skin grafting was performed subsequent to pyridoxine therapy. Similar experiments conducted in our laboratory with mice of C57 B1/6J strain have indicated that the dose of splenic cells required for induction of tolerance in C57 B1/6J females to C57 B1/6J male skin isografts can be reduced if the cells are administered to recipient females in a state of pyridoxine deficiency.[31] In this sex-linked histocompatibility system, a male skin isograft transplanted to a female behaves as a

homograft and is rejected. The ability of a pyridoxine deficiency to prolong viability of grafts has since been demonstrated in mice with skin[32,33] and ovarian[34] grafts and in dogs with skin grafts.[35]

Administration of semicarbazide to rats receiving a pyridoxine-deficient diet improved survival of skin homografts.[36,37] Pyridoxine deficiency alone[36,37] or deoxypyridoxine plus a pyridoxine-deficient diet[37] had little effect. Smellie and Moore[38] have presented results which suggest that semicarbazide plus a pyridoxine-deficient diet may cause significant prolongation of canine renal homotransplants. Treatment with amethopterin has been reported to enhance survival of skin,[39] lung,[40] marrow[41,42] and tumor[43] grafts. The inactivity of this antagonist has been noted in skin[44] and renal[45] homografts.

Humoral Immunity: Effects of Various Nutrient Deficiencies. *Protein Deficiency.* Continued attention has been given to the effects of protein deprivation upon formation of circulating antibodies in experimental animals. Protein or specific amino acid deprivation generally had an inhibitory effect.[46-53] In some instances, the inhibitory effect of protein deficiency was associated with changes in the cells involved in the immune process.[46-48,50,53-55] A chronic protein deficiency had a differential effect on the humoral antibody response depending on the nature of the antigen.[48] Michalek et al.[56] observed that protein malnourishment of rat dams led to decreases in the level of colostrum and milk IgG2A and in the serum levels of IgG2A of the developing offspring. The progeny of female rats fed diets deficient in lipotropes,[55] protein[55] or pyridoxine[57] exhibited impaired humoral immune responses. Price and Bell[58] have demonstrated that the immunologic response of protein-deficient mice is conditioned by the antigen dose, the presence of adjuvant and the age of the animal, as well as by the duration and time of initiation of deprivation. Chronic moderate protein restriction in

NZB mice contributed to the maintenance of antibody responses to sheep red blood cell antigens and interfered with changes of immunoglobulin levels with age.[59] Neither serum immunoglobulins nor antibody responses to tetanus toxoid, sheep red blood cells or bacteriophage ΦX174 were affected in the marasmic pig.[60] However, a decreased humoral immunity was evidenced by the delayed appearance of IgG antibody after immunization with bacteriophage ΦX174 and sheep red blood cells and decreased antibody titers against erythrocyte A antigen. Impaired circulatory antibody response and impaired production of antibody-forming cells were observed in calorically restricted female rats and in their first- and second-generation offspring.[61]

Tocopherol Deficiency. Tengerdy and co-workers have reported that supplementation with vitamin E of diets fed hens and mice can stimulate the humoral immune response and the production of antibody-forming cells.[62,63] Campbell et al.,[64] utilizing an in vitro cellular system, demonstrated that vitamin E can stimulate production of antibody-forming cells by nonadherent cells. The adjuvant activities of ubiquinone-7,[65] coenzyme Q_{10}[66] and certain metabolites of ubiquinone, α-tocopherol and phylloquinone,[65,67] have been demonstrated. The stimulatory activity of large amounts of vitamin A has created considerable interest among immunologists; this subject has been reviewed by Stark.[68] Recent studies have demonstrated an enhancing action of high doses of vitamin A upon humoral response[69,70] and production of antibody-forming cells.[71] The rejection time of skin grafts was also reduced.[69]

Mineral Deficiencies. The function of minerals in antibody synthesis has been a neglected area of research. However, recent reports have demonstrated the deleterious effects of a magnesium deficiency upon serum immunoglobulins[72,73] and circulating antibody following immunization

with sheep red blood cells.[74] Decreased formation of antibody-forming cells has been observed in magnesium[73] and zinc deficiencies,[75] while circulating antibody formation decreased with decreasing amounts of dietary iron.[76] In mice, dietary supplementation with sodium selenite enhanced the amount of circulating antibodies and antibody-forming cells following immunization with sheep red blood cells.[77,78]

Other Vitamin Deficiencies. Further studies have been conducted in our laboratory on the mechanism of action of pantothenic acid at the cellular level.[79] These studies demonstrated a marked inability of pantothenic acid-deficient rats to produce splenic antibody-forming cells to the stimulus of sheep erythrocytes. This defect was corrected by therapy with pantothenic acid. These studies provided no evidence for a disturbed metabolism of the antigen in this deficiency. Thus, as is the case in pyridoxine deficiency, the decreased production of circulating antibody in pantothenic acid deficiency appears to be the result of decreased production of antibody-forming cells. In similar experiments with rats deficient in thiamin, riboflavin, biotin or folic acid, we found that the number of antibody-forming cells was reduced in all deficiency states, with thiamin deficiency having the least effect.[79a] Of particular note was the observation that thiamin deficiency also had the least effect upon production of circulating antibodies. Studies on the effects of deficiency states upon the formation of background plaque-forming cells in nonimmunized rats revealed, surprisingly enough, an increased number of such cells in pantothenic acid, pyridoxine and riboflavin deficiencies.[80] The significance of this observation is not understood at this time. Decreased levels of B cells have been observed in blood, lymph node and spleen of pyridoxine and pantothenic acid-deficient rats (South and Axelrod, unpublished observations).

Cell-mediated Immunity. In this area the effects of protein-calorie malnutrition have received the greatest attention. Reduction in number or functional activity of T-lymphocytes involved in cell-mediated immunity has been indicated in this deficiency.[46,50,51,55,81] Various parameters of cell-mediated immunity—cutaneous hypersensitivity, homograft rejection and reactivity in the mixed leukocyte reaction—were shown to be decreased in marasmic piglets[60] and atrophy of lymphoid tissue, leading to impaired ability of the host to recover from viral disease, has been noted in marasmic mice.[82] Conversely, normal or increased activity has been observed in various processes related to the development of cell-mediated immunity as a consequence of protein-calorie malnutrition, i.e. graft versus host reactions,[48,59,83] proliferative response after in vitro stimulation of lymphocytes with antigen, phytohemagglutinin or concanavalin A,[48,59,84] skin homograft rejection[48,85] and cellular immunity to allogenic mouse tumor cells.[49,51,59]

Studies of other deficiency states revealed that the number and function of T cells were decreased in scorbutic monkeys,[86] although the deficient animals were capable of developing delayed hypersensitivity to BCG. Impairment in several parameters related to cellular immunity was observed in thoracic-duct lymphocytes obtained from vitamin B_6-deficient rats.[87] Similar findings were noted in thoracic-duct lymphocytes from progeny of vitamin B_6-deficient mothers.[88] Rats with a congenital vitamin B_6 deficiency showed impaired ability to be sensitized to BCG.[89]

Immunocompetence in Humans: Nutritional Effects

In the previous edition of this series[2] we reviewed the relationship of malnutrition in the human to the acquired immune response and concluded that such a relationship remained indeterminate and that the inconsistent pattern of the reported results might reflect: (1) the type and strength of the antigenic stimuli employed, (2) the difficulties inherent in the control and evaluation of nutritional status in man and (3) frequent concomitant infections. We have since seen an upsurge in activity in this area and these recent developments will be discussed in this section.

The effects of protein-calorie malnutrition (PCM) upon the serum levels of various classes of the immunoglobulins have been investigated. In some studies, the serum levels of different immunoglobulin fractions were either unaffected or increased in the deficiency,[90–100,133,136–139] while in others decreases in certain classes were observed.[91,94,101,102,137] High immunoglobulin levels have been found in the intestinal contents of malnourished children.[103] It appears that the IgA of the intestinal contents is produced locally. Then again, decreased amounts of secretory IgA have been noted in nasal washings of children with PCM[104] and in nasopharyngeal secretions of malnourished children after immunization with a single dose of live attenuated measles or poliovirus vaccine.[105] Circulating antibody responses to a variety of specific antigens have been unaffected[98,102,105,106,138] or decreased by protein-calorie deficiency.[90,96,97,99,102,106,107]

Cell-mediated immunity, as reflected by delayed skin hypersensitivity reactions to a number of antigens, evaluation of circulating T cells determined by rosette formation and lymphocyte response to mitogens—generally phytohemagglutinin—determined by blast cell formation or synthesis of DNA, has been investigated in protein-calorie malnutrition. With few exceptions,[107,109] cell-mediated immunity as measured by one or more of these three parameters was impaired in the deficiency.[90,94,96,98,102,106–118,133–135,138]

The relationship of fetal malnutrition to resistance to infection in low-birth-weight infants has stimulated interest in the immunocompetence of these infants. Chandra[119,120] has observed that the antibody response to tetanus toxoid and S. typhosa was comparable to that of healthy neonates, but that antibody response to poliovirus vaccine was impaired. Cell-mediated immunity determined by number of peripheral T cells, sensitization to dinitrochlorobenzene and lymphocyte response to phytohemagglutinin was diminished. Ferguson[108] has also noted a depressed number of T cells in low-birth-weight infants.

Decreases in various parameters of cell-mediated immunity have been observed in vitamin A[121] and folic acid deficiencies,[122,135] while no effect of a vitamin B complex deficiency was seen.[121] Studies of a patient with hereditary deficiency of transcobalamin II have implicated vitamin B_{12} in the processes of humoral and cellular immunity.[123] Clinical scurvy has no effect upon the antibody response to typhoid antigens.[124] Linoleic and arachidonic acid deficiencies inhibit the human lymphocyte response to various antigens.[125,126] Interest in a possible relationship between iron deficiency and the immune response derives from the reported susceptibility of iron-deficient children to intercurrent infection. Humoral immunity as determined by levels of serum immunoglobulins[127,128] and antibody responses to specific antigens[128] was unaffected in iron deficiency. In contrast, the parameters of cell-mediated immunity—delayed cutaneous hypersensitivity, T cell enumeration and lymphocyte response to phytohemagglutinin or specific antigens—were generally decreased in iron deficiency.[121,127,131] However, comparable decreases in skin sensitization to dinitrochlorobenzene[122] and lymphocyte response to phytohemagglutinin[122,130,135] were not observed in other studies.

SUMMARY

The detrimental effects of specific dietary deficiencies upon the development of acquired immunity—both humoral and cell mediated—in experimental animals have been amply documented. In particular, the requirements for amino acids and certain members of the vitamin B complex are well recognized. However, under some circumstances, a decreased protein intake can lead to an increased immune response. These requirements are certainly influenced by various factors, such as the type and strength of the antigenic stimulus, the host species, the nutritional balance of dietary amino acids and the extent of dietary deprivation. It is also evident that the degree of dietary restriction, particularly of protein, may have a differential effect upon the humoral and cell-mediated immune responses. In some deficiency states, the type as well as the total amount of antibody protein can be affected. The anamnestic (booster) response seems to be particularly sensitive to the absence of required nutrients. In a number of instances, the decreased immune response resulting from a nutritional deficiency is associated with a decrease in number and function of the responsible cellular types that can be corrected by appropriate nutritional therapy.

In experimental animals, the relationship of ascorbic acid and the fat-soluble vitamins A, D and E to the immune response requires further clarification with more extensive and more rigidly controlled experimentation. Reports on the stimulatory effects of large doses of vitamins A and E, as well as vitamin B_{12} and coenzyme Q, upon the immune response are of interest in their possible application to the human. The role of minerals—magnesium, zinc, iron and selenium—in the immune response is beginning to achieve recognition.

In man, there has been a preponderance of experiments in recent years purporting to establish a relationship between protein-calorie malnutrition and the immune response. These clinical investigations have been fraught with the difficulties attendant upon the frequent concurrent infections and the existence of multiple rather than single, well-defined deficiency states in the subjects. Large variations in the degree of malnutrition were inevitably present and, in many instances, precise measurements of nutritional status were not feasible. In view of these inherent difficulties in the control and evaluation of nutritional status, the indeterminate nature of endemic infections and variations in response to different antigenic stimuli, it is not surprising that reports in this area have been conflicting. There are observations of decreases in serum immunoglobulin levels, while frequently the immunoglobulins were unaffected or even increased. This latter circumstance may be related to intercurrent infection. The reports of decreased levels of secretory IgA in children with protein-calorie malnutrition assume a particular relevance as an explanation of the increased incidence of infection in these individuals.

Reports on the effects of protein-calorie malnutrition on the antibody response to various antigens have also been erratic. In some instances the deficiency had no effect upon antibody response while in others a depression was observed. The implication of these findings to mass immunization programs must be considered. With but few exceptions, cell-mediated immunity was impaired in deficient subjects. This expressed itself as: (1) failure to develop cutaneous hypersensitivity to various allergens and to tuberculin, (2) decreased T-cell formation and (3) inhibition of the lymphocyte transformation induced by phytohemagglutinin. These parameters of T-cell function reflect a severe depression of the thymolymphatic system.

A decreased activity of cell-mediated immunity has been found in vitamin A, folic acid and vitamin B_{12} deficiencies in human subjects, while clinical scurvy has no effect on the antibody response to typhoid antigen. Considerable interest has been evinced in the relation of iron deficiency to the immune response. Whereas humoral immunity in these subjects appears to be unaffected, various manifestations of cell-mediated immunity, with some exceptions, generally are decreased.

It is evident that the decreased immune responses associated with nutritional deficiencies may have a deleterious effect upon resistance to infection. However, the role of these nutrients in immunologic processes may have broader significance to the phenomena of aging and tumorogenesis. A considerable body of evidence indicates that the aging process can be influenced by a variety of dietary modifications. A deterioration of various immunologic systems also occurs with aging. The possibility that modifications in the metabolic activity of certain nutrients occurring with advancing age produce immunologic changes associated with or influencing the phenomenon of aging is an interesting speculation. This possibility is amenable to experimental verification which requires as a basis more detailed information on the precise mechanism of action of these nutrients in the immune process.

The growth and survival of a tumor may be influenced by the type and magnitude of the host's response to specific tumor antigens. This constitutes the basis of the "surveillance" reaction, which prevents tumor initiation and proliferation via a cell-mediated immune response. On the other hand, the surveillance reaction may be inhibited by "blocking" (humoral) antibodies resulting from the stimulus of tumor antigens. The complexity of the interrelationship between nutrition and tumorogenesis is manifested by the possibility that specific nutrients may influence either or both of these immune processes. Thus, an observed decrease in tumor incidence in malnutrition could result from a decreased formation of blocking antibody or from an increased activity of T-cell function, with a resultant increased tumor surveillance. Experimental evidence exists to support both of these possibilities.

It is important to recognize the possibility that a nutritional deficiency may produce abnormalities in the maturation of cells responsible for the immune response which may continue to affect the immunocompetence of these cells long after apparent recovery from the deficiency. Such nutritional insults could occur in the fetus, as a consequence of poor maternal nutrition, or in early postnatal existence. It is a matter of concern whether prolonged or permanent impairment of immunocompetence occurs, with possible long-term effects on immunity to infection, incidence of neoplasia, hypersensitivity reactions, autoimmunity and even the aging process itself. There is experimental evidence to buttress the reality of these possibilities and to suggest that these effects may persist into subsequent generations.

The relevance of the relation of nutrition to immunity and its ramifications in experimental animals and human subjects have been stressed in this chapter. However, we should also recognize the potential application of the nutritionally deficient animal model in studies of the mechanisms of the immune response. Advantages of these animal models reside in the ability to maintain rigid control over both nutritional and infectious state. Deficient experimental laboratory models, exhibiting varying modifications of the immune response, should be useful in exploring the interactions of the diverse cell populations and humoral factors involved in the development of immunocompetence. It also remains to be determined whether the effects of deficiency states may be mediated via the adrenal or the thymus. Both of these organs are affected by nutritional deficiencies and the secretions of both have been implicated in the mechanisms of the immune response.

BIBLIOGRAPHY

1. Axelrod and Pruzansky: Vitam. Horm., *13*, 1, 1955.
2. Axelrod: In *Modern Nutrition in Health and Disease*, 5th ed. (Goodhart and Shils, Eds.). Philadelphia, Lea & Febiger, 1973, pp. 493–505.
3. Kumar and Axelrod: J. Nutr., *98*, 41, 1969.
4. Axelrod, Hopper and Long: J. Nutr., *74*, 58, 1961.
5. Axelrod: Am. J. Clin. Nutr., *6*, 119, 1958.
6. Axelrod and Hopper: J. Nutr., *72*, 325, 1960.
7. Jerne, Nordin and Henry: In *Cell Bound Antibodies* (Amos and Koprowski, Eds.). Philadelphia, Wistar Institute Press, 1963, p. 109.
8. Kumar and Axelrod: J. Nutr., *96*, 53, 1968.
9. Traketellis and Axelrod: J. Nutr., *82*, 483, 1964.
10. Montjar, Axelrod and Trakatellis: J. Nutr., *85*, 45, 1965.
11. Traketellis and Axelrod: Biochem. J., *95*, 344, 1965.
12. Roy and Axelrod: Proc. Soc. Exp. Biol. Med., *138*, 804, 1971.
13. Axelrod, Trakatellis, Bloch and Stinebring: J. Nutr., *79*, 161, 1963.
14. Trakatellis, Stinebring and Axelrod: J. Immunol., *91*, 39, 1963.
15. Stinebring, Trakatellis and Axelrod: J. Immunol., *91*, 46, 1963.
16. Mueller, Kies, Alvord and Shaw: J. Exp. Med., *115*, 329, 1962.
17. Mueller and Kies: Nature, *195*, 813, 1962.
18. Zweiman, Schoenwetter and Hildreth: J. Immunol., *96*, 296, 1966.
19. Zweiman, Besdine and Hildreth: J. Immunol., *96*, 672, 1966.
20. Friedman, Buckler and Baron: Fed. Proc., *20*, 258, 1961.
21. Friedman and Buckler: Fed. Proc., *22*, 501, 1963.
22. Friedman, Buckler and Baron: J. Exp. Med., *114*, 173, 1961.
23. Borel, Fauconnet and Miescher: Int. Arch. Allergy, *33*, 583, 1968.
24. Schneider, Lee and Olitsky: J. Exp. Med., *105*, 319, 1957.
25. Brandriss: Science, *140*, 186, 1963.
26. Axelrod, Fisher, Fisher, Lee and Walsh: Science, *127*, 1833, 1958.
27. Fisher, Axelrod, Fisher, Lee and Calvanese: Surgery, *44*, 149, 1958.
28. Axelrod and Lowe: Proc. Soc. Exp. Biol. Med., *108*, 549, 1961.
29. Lowe and Axelrod: Transplantation, *3*, 82, 1964.
30. Axelrod and Trakatellis: Proc. Soc. Exp. Biol. Med., *116*, 206, 1964.
31. Trakatellis and Axelrod: Proc. Soc. Exp. Biol. Med., *132*, 46, 1969.
32. Hargis, Wyman and Malkiel: Int. Arch. Allergy, *16*, 276, 1960.
33. Herr and Coursin: J. Nutr., *88*, 273, 1966.
34. Parkes: Nature, *184*, 699, 1959.
35. Humphries, Harms and Moretz: J.A.M.A., *178*, 490, 1961.
36. Moore: Nature, *215*, 871, 1967.
37. Moore: J. Cardiovasc. Surg., *9*, 63, 1968.
38. Smellie and Moore: Surg. Gynecol. Obstet., *128*, 81, 1969.

39. Berenbaum: Nature, *198*, 606, 1963.
40. Blumenstock, Collins, Thomas and Ferrebee: Surgery, *51*, 541, 1962.
41. Thomas, Collins, Herman and Ferrebee: Blood, *19*, 217, 1962.
42. Uphoff: Proc. Soc. Exp. Biol. Med., *99*, 651, 1958.
43. Uphoff: Transplant. Bull., *28*, 110, 1961.
44. Brooke: Transplant. Bull., *26*, 453, 1960.
45. Zukoski, Lee and Hume: J. Surg. Res., *2*, 44, 1962.
46. Aschkenasy: Immunology, *24*, 617, 1973.
47. Nasseri, Mohagheghpour and Khakpour: Nutr. Metab., *17*, 347, 1974.
48. Cooper, Good and Mariani: Am. J. Clin. Nutr., *27*, 647, 1974.
49. Jose and Good: Nature, *231*, 323, 1971.
50. Jose, Stutman and Good: Nature, *241*, 57, 1973.
51. Jose and Good: J. Exp. Med., *137*, 1, 1973.
52. Malavé and Layrisse: Cell. Immunol., *21*, 337, 1976.
53. Law, Dudrick and Abdou: Ann. Surg., *179*, 168, 1974.
54. Mathur, Ramalingaswami and Deo: J. Nutr., *102*, 841, 1972.
55. Gebhardt and Newberne: Immunology, *26*, 489, 1974.
56. Michalek, Rahman and McGhee: Proc. Soc. Exp. Biol. Med., *148*, 1114, 1975.
57. Debes, Kirksey and Clark: Fed. Proc., *34*, 914, 1975.
58. Price and Bell: Immunology, *32*, 65, 1977.
59. Fernandez, Yunis and Good: J. Immunol., *116*, 782, 1976.
60. Lopez, Davis and Smith: Pediatr. Res., *6*, 779, 1972.
61. Chandra: Science, *190*, 289, 1975.
62. Tengerdy and Heinzerling: Ann. N.Y. Acad. Sci., *203*, 177, 1972.
63. Tengerdy, Heinzerling, Brown and Mathias: Int. Arch. Allergy, *44*, 221, 1973.
64. Campbell, Cooper, Heinzerling and Tengerdy: Proc. Soc. Exp. Biol. Med., *146*, 465, 1974.
65. Imada, Azuma, Kishimoto, Yamamura and Morimoto: Int. Arch. Allergy, *43*, 898, 1972.
66. Bliznakov, Casey and Premuzic: Experientia, *26*, 953, 1970.
67. Sugimura, Azuma, Yamamura, Imada and Morimoto: Int. J. Vitam. Nutr. Res., *46*, 192, 1976.
68. Stark: In *Frontiers of Biology* (Neuberger and Tatum, Eds.). New York, American Elsevier, 1972, pp. 394–408.
69. Jurin and Tannock: Immunology, *23*, 283, 1972.
70. Leutskaya and Fais: Biochim. Biophys. Acta, *475*, 207, 1977.
71. Cohen and Cohen: J. Immunol., *111*, 1376, 1973.
72. Alcock and Shils: Proc. Soc. Exp. Biol. Med., *145*, 855, 1974.
73. Elin: Proc. Soc. Exp. Biol. Med., *148*, 620, 1975.
74. McCoy and Kenney: J. Nutr., *105*, 791, 1975.
75. Fraker and Luecke: Fed. Proc., *36*, 1176, 1977.
76. Nalder, Mahoney, Ramakrishnan and Hendricks: J. Nutr., *102*, 535, 1972.
77. Spallholz, Martin, Gerlach and Heinzerling: Proc. Soc. Exp. Biol. Med., *143*, 685, 1973.
78. Spallholz, Martin, Gerlach and Heinzerling: Infect. Immun., *8*, 841, 1973.
79. Lederer, Kumar and Axelrod: J. Nutr., *105*, 17, 1975.
79a. Kumar and Axelrod: Proc. Soc. Exp. Biol. Med., *157*, 421, 1978.
80. Koros, Axelrod, Hamill and South: Proc. Soc. Exp. Biol. Med., *152*, 322, 1976.
81. Nejad and Mohagheghpour: Nutr. Metab., *19*, 158, 1975.
82. Woodruff and Woodruff: Proc. Natl. Acad. Sci., *68*, 2108, 1971.
83. Bell and Hazell: J. Exp. Med., *141*, 127, 1975.
84. Kramer, Good and Finstad: Fed. Proc., *36*, 1218, 1977.
85. Parkayastha, Kapoor and Deo: Indian J. Med. Res., *63*, 1150, 1975.
86. Hsu: Fed. Proc., *36*, 1177, 1977.
87. Robson and Schwarz: Cell. Immunol., *16*, 135, 1975.
88. Robson and Schwarz: Cell. Immunol., *16*, 145, 1975.
89. Davis: Clin. Res., *22*, 227A, 1974.
90. Law, Dudrick and Abdou: Ann. Intern. Med., *79*, 545, 1973.
90a. Schopfer and Douglas: Clin. Immunol. Immunopathol., *5*, 21, 1976.
91. Kamel, Ramly, Khattab, Shousha, Shaker and Raziky: In *Proceedings Western Hemisphere Nutrition Congress*, III. Mount Kisco, Futura Publishing, 1971, p. 350.
92. McFarlane, Reddy, Adcock, Adeshina, Cooke and Akene: Br. Med. J., *4*, 268, 1970.
93. Watson and Freesemann: Arch. Dis. Child., *45*, 282, 1970.
94. McMurray, Reyes and Watson: Fed. Proc., *36*, 1171, 1977.
95. Munson, Franco, Arbeter, Velez and Vitale: Am. J. Clin. Nutr., *27*, 625, 1974.
96. Coovadia, et al.: Am. J. Clin. Nutr., *27*, 665, 1974.
97. Mathews, Mackay, Tucker and Malcolm: Am. J. Clin. Nutr., *27*, 908, 1974.
98. Neumann, et al.: Am. J. Clin. Nutr., *28*, 89, 1975.
99. Suskind, et al.: Am. J. Clin. Nutr., *29*, 836, 1976.
100. Sirisinha: In *Protein-Calorie Malnutrition* (Olson, Ed.). New York, Academic Press, 1975, p. 369.
101. Aref, Badr El-Din, Hassan and El-Araby: J. Trop. Med. Hyg., *73*, 186, 1970.
102. Chandra: J. Pediatr., *81*, 1194, 1972.
103. Bell, Turner, Gracey, Suharjono and Sunoto: Am. J. Clin. Nutr., *29*, 392, 1976.
104. Sirisinha, Suskind, Edelman, Asvapaka and Olson: Pediatrics, *55*, 166, 1975.
105. Chandra: Br. Med. J., *2*, 583, 1975.
106. Reddy, Jagadeesan, Ragharamulu, Bhaskaram and Srikantia: Am. J. Clin. Nutr., *29*, 3, 1976.
107. Jose, Welch and Doherty: Aust. Paediatr. J., *6*, 192, 1970.
108. Ferguson, Lawlor, Neumann, Oh and Stiehm: J. Pediatr., *85*, 717, 1974.
109. Schlesinger and Stekel: Am. J. Clin. Nutr., *27*, 615, 1974.

110. Smythe, et al.: Lancet, 2, 939, 1971.
111. Sellmeyer, Bhettay, Truswell, Meyers and Hansen: Arch. Dis. Child., 47, 429, 1972.
112. Edelman, Suskind, Olson and Sirisinha: Lancet, 1, 506, 1973.
113. Geefhuysen, Rosen, Katz, Ipp and Metz: Br. Med. J., 4, 527, 1971.
114. Bang, Mahalanabis, Mukherjee and Bang: Proc. Soc. Exp. Biol. Med., 149, 199, 1975.
115. Bistrian, Blackburn, Scrimshaw and Flatt: Am. J. Clin. Nutr., 28, 1148, 1975.
116. Chandra: Br. Med. J., 3, 608, 1974.
117. Grace, Armstrong and Symthe: S. Afr. Med. J., 46, 402, 1972.
118. Vithayasai: In Protein-Calorie Malnutrition (Olson, Ed.). New York, Academic Press, 1975, p. 383.
119. Chandra: Lancet, 2:1393, 1974.
120. Chandra: Am. J. Dis. Child., 129, 450, 1975.
121. Bhaskaram and Reddy: Br. Med. J., 3, 522, 1975.
122. Gross, Reid, Newberne, Burgess, Marston and Hift: Am. J. Clin. Nutr., 28, 225, 1975.
123. Hitzig and Kenny: Clin. Exp. Immunol., 20, 105, 1975.
124. Hodges, Hood, Canham, Sauberlich and Baker: Am. J. Clin. Nutr., 24, 432, 1971.
125. Mertin: Br. Med. J., 4, 357, 1973.
126. Mertin, Shenton and Field: Br. Med. J., 2, 777, 1973.
127. Macdougall, Anderson, McNab and Katz: J. Pediatr., 86, 833, 1975.
128. Chandra and Saraya: J. Pediatr., 86, 899, 1975.
129. Srikantia, Prasad, Bhaskharam and Krishnamachari: Lancet, 1, 1307, 1976.
130. Joynson, Jacobs, Walker and Dolby: Lancet, 2, 1058, 1972.
131. Fletcher, Mather, Lewis and Whiting: J. Infect. Dis., 131, 44, 1975.
132. Kulapongs, Vithayasai, Suskind and Olson: Lancet, 2, 689, 1974.
133. Schopfer and Douglas: Clin. Immunol. Immunopathol., 5, 21, 1976.
134. Abbassy, et al.: J. Trop. Med. Hyg., 77, 13, 1974.
135. Burgess, Vos, Coovadia, Smythe, Parent and Loening: S. Afr. Med. J., 48, 1870, 1974.
136. Rosen and Geefhuysen: S. Afr. Med. J., 45, 980, 1971.
137. Samuel, Patel and Mankodi: Indian J. Med. Res., 60, 1278, 1972.
138. Feldman and Gianantonio: J. Pediatr., 78, 899, 1971.
139. Alvarado and Luthringer: Clin. Pediatr., 10, 174, 1971.

Chapter 19

NUTRITION AND CELL GROWTH

Myron Winick
and
Jo Anne Brasel

During the past years new techniques in biology have made it possible to study cellular growth of organs in a quantitative manner. In 1962 Enesco and LeBlond serially measured DNA content of a number of rat organs.[1] Since DNA content per diploid cell is a constant for any particular species,[2] these investigators were able to calculate the number of cells in the various organs of the rat at any particular time, simply by dividing the total DNA content analyzed by 6.2 picograms (pg) (the DNA content of all diploid rat cells). Once the number of cells is determined, the weight per cell, the total protein content per cell or the total lipid content per cell can be determined by either weighing the organ or ascertaining the total protein or lipid content of the organ and dividing by the number of cells. This can be expressed as a weight/DNA, protein/DNA or lipid/DNA ratio.

Thus by simple biochemical techniques it has become possible to follow growth by monitoring the contribution made by increase in cell number and the contribution attributable to increase in cell size. It should be recognized that total DNA content, while accurately reflecting cell number, in no way differentiates one cell type from another. In addition, although the ratios as outlined above give an overall average for these materials per cell, no single cell may actually contain this quantity of material. Individual cells, especially when differing in type, might vary widely in their composition of either proteins or lipids.

Within these limitations, however, this "chemical" approach to cellular growth has allowed certain generalizations which have given rise to an overall picture of growth on a cellular level.

NORMAL CELLULAR GROWTH

Careful examination of all non-regenerating organs by these methods reveals three distinct phases of growth. The first is characterized by a proportional increase in weight, protein and DNA content; the number of cells is increasing whereas the ratios and the size of the individual cells are not changing. Simple hyperplasia is occurring. This phase ends as the rate of net DNA synthesis begins to slow while weight and protein content continue to increase, giving rise to a transitional phase of hyperplasia and concomitant hypertrophy which lasts until net DNA synthesis stops. After this point, all growth is by hypertrophy. Finally when weight stabilizes and net protein synthesis stops, growth is finished.[3]

These data allow us to view the overall growth of any organ as a continuous accretion of protoplasm made up of water, proteins and in some cases lipids. The ultimate packaging of this protoplasm into individual cells depends on the rate of DNA synthesis. At present the mechanisms controlling the period during which DNA may be synthesized by an organ and the mechanisms governing the rate of synthesis during that period are largely unknown.

Brain

In whole rat brain DNA synthesis and hence cell division stops at about 20 days of age. Total protein continues to increase until about 99 days of age when the brain reaches its final size. However, more detailed examination reveals that different regions have their own patterns of cellular growth.[4] In the cerebrum, DNA synthesis continues until about 21 days postnatally. After this the cells continue to accumulate protein and lipid. Total cerebral lipid content is achieved somewhat later and total protein content around 99 days of age. In the cerebellum, DNA synthesis stops at 17 days postnatally. Net protein synthesis actually becomes negative for a short period after this and the size of the individual cerebellar cells decreases. This decrease in cell size probably reflects the maturation of larger, more primitive cells into smaller, more mature ones. In the brain stem, total cell number is increased to 14 days of age. Thereafter there is an enormous increase in the protein/DNA ratio. This increase probably reflects an increase not only in the size of the brain stem cells but also in growth, myelination and enlargement of neuronal processes from other brain regions into the brain stem. The hippocampus is an area which demonstrates a type of cellular growth unique to central nervous system. There is a discrete rise in DNA content between the 14th and 17th day of life. The increase corresponds to a migration of neurons from under the lateral ventricle into the hippocampus, which occurs on the 15th day after birth in the rat.[5]

The ultimate cellular makeup of the various regions depends, then, on the rate of cell division within the particular region, the time that cell division stops, the type of cells dividing and whether or not cells are migrating to or from the region.

In human brain the sequence of events is not as clearly defined as in rat brain. Studies initially indicated that DNA synthesis was linear prenatally, began to slow down shortly after birth and reached a maximum around 8 to 12 months of age.[6] More recent studies have tended to modify these results somewhat and would extend the time beyond the first year of life.[7] Moreover, Dobbing and Sands[8] have shown that two peaks of DNA synthesis may occur normally in human brain. The first peak is reached at about 26 weeks of gestation and the second around birth. They have interpreted these results as corresponding to the peak rate of neuronal division and the peak rate of glial division respectively.

There are still few data on the cellular growth of various regions of human brain. The data available would indicate that the rate of cell division postnatally is about the same in cerebrum and cerebellum and stops at about the same time in both areas, that is, between 12 and 15 months of age.[9] The number of cases studied, however, is too small to attempt too precise a statement.

In the brain stem, DNA synthesis continues at a slow but rather steady rate until at least 1 year of age. The exact cell types involved and the migratory patterns of the cells in the developing human brain are not as clearly worked out as in the rat brain. For obvious reasons, radioautography cannot be done. What is known, then, is the result of careful histologic and histochemical examination of brains of fetuses of various ages. In a series of elegant studies Duckett and Pearse[10] have shown that during fetal life the brain not only increases linearly in weight but also undergoes a series of biochemical changes. Glycolysis is present during the second month of fetal life, oxidative mechanisms appear during the third month and activity and localization of a number of enzymes reach a mature pattern during the seventh month of fetal life.

In addition there is evidence that the presence of acetylcholinesterase indicates tissue excitability.[11] The activity of this enzyme is localized in neurons of the anterior horn of the spinal cord as early as the 10th week of embryonic life, according to Duckett and Pearse.[12] This correlates well with the time that movement of the lower limb can be elicited by proper stimulation.[13]

Two specific cell types, the Cajal-Retzius cells[14] and the monamine oxidase cells,[15] are present only in fetal life, disappearing before birth. Their function is unknown. Serial analysis of lipids in human brains would indicate that the lipid/DNA ratio rises shortly after birth until at least 2 years of age. This is reflected in a rise in both the cholesterol/DNA and phospholipid/DNA ratios.[16] Thus postnatal lipid synthesis is occurring at a more rapid rate than DNA synthesis. This is undoubtedly related to the rapid myelination which is occurring during this period of life.

Although the descriptive work in human brain would suggest that cellular growth is governed by the same principles as those governing cellular growth in rat brain, more data are needed to complete the picture. Indirect measurements have been used to follow normal growth of human brain. The most common of these is cranial circumference. Some correlations have been made between increase in cranial circumference and cellular growth of the brain. Approximate formulas have been worked out relating head circumference to brain weight, protein and DNA content during the first year of life.[17]

In summary, normal cellular growth of mammalian brain is made up of an early proliferative phase in which cell division predominates and the quantity of protein and lipid per cell remains relatively constant. The rate of proliferation of cells appears to be separated into two peaks:

one probably neuronal and the other glial. At the same time, cells migrate from certain regions of the brain to other regions. In human brain, there is evidence that certain cell types appear and disappear during this early phase of growth.

Later growth is characterized by a slowing and finally a cessation of cell division in spite of a constant rate of net protein synthesis, except in the cerebellum, and an increasing rate of myelin synthesis. Finally myelination is completed and net protein synthesis stops. The mechanisms controlling the rate of cell division and the migratory patterns of cells are just beginning to be investigated.

Skeletal Muscle

Various aspects of skeletal muscle growth have been reviewed by Widdowson[18] and Mastaglia.[19] Quantitatively, skeletal muscle is the most important soft tissue of the body; at birth it accounts for 25 per cent of body weight and by adulthood approximately 40 per cent. The muscle fibers arise from the fusion of the long, narrow multinucleated myoblasts. Contrary to previous belief, the number of muscle fibers does increase after birth; the age at cessation of fiber formation is not known but is said to be between birth and 4 months by Montgomery.[20] However, Adams and De Rueck[21] have reported that fiber number increases up to the middle of the fifth decade.

Growth in muscle mass has been assessed by creatinine excretion. In normal children on a low-creatinine diet Graystone[22] has determined that each gram of urinary creatinine excreted per 24 hours is the equivalent of 20 kg of muscle mass.

The work of Cheek[23] demonstrates that from 5 to 18 years muscle mass in males increases more than fivefold and in females approximately fourfold. The amount of muscle per unit height is similar in the two sexes until 13 years of age, when the male adolescent growth spurt begins and proportionately more muscle tissue is deposited in the male per unit height gained. From 11 to 17 years the male doubles his muscle mass; the female doubles hers from 9 to 15 years. The difference in ultimate muscle mass achieved is importantly related to the continued growth in the male between 13 and 18 years, a time when only small increments in muscle mass are noted in the female.

Widdowson et al.[24] have directly measured the DNA content of gastrocnemius muscle from human fetuses; levels rise from 10 to 15 mg at 15 weeks gestation to 160 mg at 25 weeks and approximately 300 mg at birth. Determination of muscle nuclear number during postnatal growth has been made largely from extrapolation of information from biopsy samples. Earlier it had been held that muscle fiber nuclei did not undergo mitosis, yet both histologic and biochemical studies demonstrated an increase in muscle nuclear number. It is now felt that the additional subsarcolemmal nuclei arise from mitosis and incorporation of undifferentiated mononucleated satellite cells into the muscle fiber.[25] Since muscle tissue contains both fiber and nonfiber nuclei and since skeletal muscle may not be homogeneous in composition throughout the body, it is important to deal with these issues before citing the data derived from biopsy.

In one study of four different limb muscles in male rats at three different ages, Enesco and Puddy[26] determined that 35 per cent of the nuclei consistently lay outside the fiber. Therefore, under these circumstances an increase in DNA content, even if uncorrected for nonfiber nuclei, would proportionately reflect growth in muscle fiber nuclei. The constancy of DNA concentration in muscles throughout the body has also been studied. Cheek et al.[27] report that DNA concentrations among four muscles of the Sprague-Dawley rat and among five muscles of the young macaque monkey are in agreement. Yet Enesco and Puddy[26] found agreement in only certain muscles of the Sherman rat;

additionally, the extent of agreement varied with age and disease states. No systematic study of DNA concentration in various muscles at different ages has been carried out in the human. Thus, although the importance of the human data derived from biopsy material should not be underestimated, it must be recalled that the validity of the extrapolation methodology has not been unequivocably established in man.

The work of Cheek[23,28] and of Cheek and Hill[29] utilized biopsy extrapolation methodology in which the DNA concentration in gluteal or abdominal rectus muscle samples was multiplied by the amount of muscle mass derived from creatinine excretion. Forty normal male subjects from infancy through 16 years and 23 normal female subjects from 3 to 17 years were studied; there are essentially no data, however, for either sex between 18 months and 5 years. The data reveal a 14-fold increase in muscle nuclear number in males from 2 months to 16 years; this increase is not achieved by a steady accumulation of new nuclei with time. Three separate linear equations were derived for males 0.18 to 1.5 years, 5 to 10.5 years and 10.5 to 16 years. The slopes of these three separate lines are, in general, similar to those for postnatal growth in height and weight, that is, the slope or rate of accumulation of new nuclei is greater in infancy than in the middle childhood years, while at adolescence the slope again increases. From 5 to 10 years the increase is from 0.90×10^{12} to 1.22×10^{12} nuclei, from 10 to 16 years from 1.22 to 3.10×10^{12} nuclei. The data over this entire age span can also be expressed as a cubic equation.[29] The pattern of muscle nuclear growth in female subjects over the age of 5 years is linear through adolescence; in contrast to males no acceleration in nuclear accumulation occurs at adolescence. At 16 years of age the equation would predict a nuclear number of 1.96×10^{12} in females, a value of 63 per cent of the male figure. Since muscle mass of the female is approximately 80 per cent of the male value at this age,[23] the nuclear density must be less in the female. This is, in fact, confirmed by protein/DNA ratios, which are slightly greater in females during the childhood years.[28] With further growth of muscle mass in males beyond 16 years of age, it is likely that nuclear density and protein/DNA ratio will equal or exceed the values in females.

The protein/DNA ratio has been used to assess average cell size or cell mass in skeletal muscle even though the muscle fibers are multinucleated structures in which the individual nuclei are believed to be only diploid in nature. In this context the protein/DNA ratio can be considered an index of the average mass or protein content per "diploid cell unit," even though this unit has no physical membrane boundaries. Widdowson et al.[24] determined protein/DNA ratios in the fetal muscle samples. The increases before 30 weeks of gestation were modest compared to the sharp increases noted in the last 10 weeks. The values for the gastrocnemius at 40 weeks are in accord with values in abdominal rectus muscles obtained by Cheek[28] in older infants, which suggests that the rapid growth phase initiated in utero persists for some period after birth. In five adult gastrocnemii the protein/DNA ratio ranged from 121 to 280;[24] the value reported by Cheek[28] for adolescents is approximately 300 for both sexes and one might wonder if the adult values reflect some degree of involutional atrophy.

Liver

Mammalian liver grows by increasing the number and size of its cells, by forming multinucleate cells and by forming other cells with single nuclei containing tetraploid and octaploid amounts of DNA. Human liver growth is no exception, and several studies of the ploidy development in humans have been reported.[30-32] The data of Swartz[31] reveal that until 6 years of age the liver contains essentially only diploid (2N) nuclei; between 6 and 10 years mitotic figures are noted in liver tissue and a rare tetraploid (4N) cell may be encountered. During the pubertal years a definite tetraploid class of cells is established, and until 20 years both 2N and 4N cells are present. With cessation of body growth, beginning after 20 years, a definite octaploid (8N) nuclear class is noted. From then until death all three classes exist in the liver, with the number of 4N and 8N cells increasing slowly with advancing age. Even in adulthood, however, over 80 per cent of the nuclei are of the 2N class. The frequency of polyploid nuclei is independent of sex. There are differing reports as to whether the frequency of binucleate cells is proportionate to the extent of nuclear ploidy or not and whether the male displays more binucleate cells than the female.

Since polyploidy is an established, age-dependent feature of liver growth, the use of the protein/DNA ratio as an index of cell size must be reexamined. Epstein[33] determined cell volume in mammalian liver samples and found that the volume is directly proportional to cell ploidy regardless of whether the cell contains one or more diploid nuclei of variable ploidy. This is consistent with the operation of gene dosage in the control of rates of synthesis of cell constituents in polyploid liver cells. Therefore, even in mature liver, the protein/DNA ratio is a valid index of the average cell mass per "diploid cell unit."

Data on total liver DNA and protein content during normal human development are scanty. Widdowson et al.[24] have published data from a number of fetuses plus values from 5 adults. At 13 to 14 weeks gestation total liver DNA is approximately 13 mg, at 20 to 22 weeks 130 mg, at 30 weeks 320 mg and at birth approximately 600 mg. The adult values ranged from 2,770 to 4,600 mg, indicating that considerable DNA synthesis accompanies postnatal liver growth. A certain but unknown portion of the DNA in liver is due to hematopoietic tissue, especially before and shortly after birth. The protein/DNA ratios in fetal liver were stable at approximately 13 between 15 and 30 weeks gestation and then more than doubled to nearly 30 at birth; the mean adult value was 56 with a range from 52 to 64. Thus postnatal growth in liver is accomplished by proportionately greater increases in "diploid cell units" than in mean cell size.

Placenta

Since placenta is readily available for study, abnormalities in fetal growth that are paralleled in the placenta can be investigated using this tissue. With this in mind, placental growth has been examined in the normal rat and human and under certain abnormal conditions known to affect the growth of the fetus.

Using radioautography, Jollie has demonstrated that labeled mitotic figures do not appear in the trophoblastic layer of rat placenta after the 18th day of gestation.[34] Our own studies demonstrate that, although weight, protein and RNA rise linearly until the 20th day, DNA fails to increase after the 17th day owing to a cessation of DNA synthesis.[35] Thus three phases of cellular growth may be described in rat placenta just as in the other organs of the rat. From 10 days until about 16 days of gestation DNA synthesis and net protein synthesis are proportional and cell number increases, whereas cell size is unchanged. This is the period of pure hyperplasia. From 16 to 18 days, as a consequence of a slowing in the rate of DNA synthesis with protein synthesis continuing at the same rate, hyperplasia and hypertrophy are occurring together. Finally, around 18 days, cell division stops altogether. Weight and protein still continue their linear rise. The ratios rapidly increase. Hypertrophy is occurring alone.

Maturational changes occur throughout gestation. Therefore, growth by cell division is not necessary for certain of these maturational changes to occur. During the final period of hypertrophy certain electron microscopic changes take place in the rat placenta. There is a reduction of the "placental barrier" with the appearance of endothelial and trophoblastic fenestrations. Increased micropinocytotic activity, irregularities at the inner plasma membrane and the appearance of large vacuoles can all be seen in the so-called element III. Approximation of inner and outer membranes at points of constriction and formation of pedicle-like foot processes also occur.[34]

Concomitant with these morphologic changes, profound functional changes also take place. There is a change in the selectivity of transportable materials and an increase in the transport rate of certain materials. Also glycogen, which had previously been deposited in copious amounts, rapidly becomes depleted.[36]

Although the exact timing of events is not as clear as with the rat, available data indicate that the human placenta grows in a qualitatively similar manner. Placenta is the only human tissue in which cellular growth has been studied throughout its entire life span. Therefore, it is not known whether the sequence to be described is characteristic for other human tissues. However, studies cited in the previous section would indicate that human brain grows in a qualitatively similar manner.

At least until the fetus reaches 3,500 gm, fetal weight gain is accompanied by a linear increase in the weight of the placenta. In addition both total protein and RNA increase linearly to term. DNA, however, ceases to increase after the placenta reaches about 300 gm. This corresponds to a fetal weight of about 2,400 gm or a gestational age of 34 to 36 weeks.[37] Thus, as was previously demonstrated in the rat, cell division ceases before term. In the human this appears to be about the 35th week of gestation.

Although the cellular events are similar

during the growth of human and rat placenta, there is one quantitative difference: the RNA/DNA ratio is twice as high in the rat. The reason for this difference is unknown, but it may result from increased connective tissue within the human placenta. Fibroblasts contain relatively little RNA. Possibly the trophoblasts contain equal quantities of RNA in both species.

In summary, the normal cellular growth of tissues proceeds through an orderly sequence of changes as maturation progresses. Therefore, the time at which a stimulus is exerted may be as important as the nature of the stimulus itself. The same stimulus acting early might interfere with cell division, whereas later it cannot. Conversely, the nature of the cellular effects produced might give a clue to the time an unknown stimulus was most active. In any event, the DNA, RNA and protein content of the tissues can be examined under conditions known to affect growth. The similarity in the growth pattern between rat and human tissues also suggests the possibility of using the rat as an experimental model.

EFFECTS OF MALNUTRITION ON CELLULAR GROWTH

Brain

The most common method employed in altering the nutritional status of neonatal rats is to vary the number of pups nursing from a single mother. The normal rat liter consists of from 8 to 12 pups and therefore a nursing group of 10 animals has arbitrarily been considered as normal. Malnutrition is imposed by increasing the size of the nursing group to 18 animals and overnutrition by decreasing the size to 3 animals.

More recently, other methods of undernutrition have been employed. Protein restriction in the lactating mother reduces the quantity of milk produced without altering its composition. Allowing the

animals to nurse for only a single 8-hour period per day also reduces the quantity of milk consumed. All of these methods produce a total caloric restriction as well as a restriction in individual nutrients, the most notable of which is protein. Thus far, all three methods have produced comparable results on brain growth and we will, therefore, examine them together.

In order to produce qualitative changes in the milk without changing the quantity produced, the nursing animal must be artificially fed. Two procedures have been employed: repeated tube feeding and gastrostomy with continuous infusion of liquid. Both are time consuming, extremely tedious and technically quite difficult. At present no data on cellular growth of the brain are available from these feeding techniques, although Miller has extensively used the former to study protein synthesis in developing liver.[38]

Employing the "large and small litter" technique, McCance and Widdowson[39] demonstrated a number of years ago that growth rate of the nursing pups was inversely proportional to the number of animals in the group. Moreover, they demonstrated the weight of the brain was reduced in the undernourished animals and increased in the overnourished animals. Perhaps the most important finding in these experiments was that, no matter what the state of nutrition after weaning, the undernourished animals never attained normal size and their brains never recovered normal weight. Other experiments with neonatal pigs confirmed these results.[40] Profound growth retardation in the pigs was produced in the neonatal period and complete recovery in either body size or brain size could not be obtained even when maximum nutritional rehabilitation was attempted.

Previous studies had indicated that undernutrition later during the growing period of the rat would retard growth but that nutritional rehabilitation could restore normal body weight and brain weight.[41]

The determining factor in recoverability appeared to be the time at which malnutrition occurred. The earlier the undernutrition, the less likely was recovery after discontinuing the stimulus. Thus there is something different about early growth from later growth which allows the older animal to recover from malnutrition.

The studies of normal cellular growth outlined above suggest a possible explanation. Early organ growth is primarily caused by cell division and an increase in the number of cells. Later organ growth is caused by hypertrophy with individual cells already present becoming larger. When the original McCance and Widdowson experiments were repeated and compared with animals undernourished at two later times during the growing period, it became clear that, if malnutrition were imposed during the proliferative phase of growth, the rate of cell division was slowed and the ultimate number of cells reduced.[42] Moreover this change was permanent and could not be reversed once the normal time for cell division had passed. In contrast, undernutrition imposed during the period when cells are normally enlarging will curtail this enlargement, but on subsequent rehabilitation the cells will resume their normal size. These experiments demonstrated that total brain cell number could be permanently reduced by undernourishing the rat during the first 21 days of his life and that no matter what is attempted thereafter this reduction in cell number would persist.

If the reduction in brain size in the animals reared in litters of 18 was caused by reduced cell number, what about those reared in litters of 3? When these experiments were performed,[43] it became clear that these overnourished animals had an increased number of brain cells when compared to brains of animals nursed in normal-sized litters. Thus the number of cells attained by the developing rat brain depends, in part, on the nutrition of the animals during the period of time when brain cells actively are undergoing proliferation. Subsequent experiments have demonstrated that the rate of cell division can actually be manipulated in either direction by changing the state of nutrition during the proliferative phase.[44] Thus undernutrition for the first 9 days of life produced a deficit in brain cell number which can be entirely overcome by overnourishing the animal for the next 12 days. It should be noted here that, as pointed out earlier, we cannot differentiate one cell type from another with these methods. It is therefore possible that the deficit is made up by proliferation of a different cell type than was inhibited during the earlier restriction.

Malnutrition during the first 21 days of life also inhibits lipid synthesis in whole rat brain. The rate of cholesterol and phospholipid synthesis is reduced and the total brain quantity of these materials lowered.[45] This reduction is proportional to the reduction in DNA or cell number and, hence, the ratios of these lipids to DNA or the amount of these lipids per cell is unchanged. If the malnutrition continues beyond the proliferative phase of growth, the continued inhibition of lipid synthesis will result in a reduced lipid content per cell. Enzymes involved in lipid synthesis, such as galactocerebroside sulfokinase, are also reduced in activity by malnutrition during the first 10 days of life.[46]

Regional patterns of cellular growth are also modified by malnutrition during the nursing period.[47] The cerebellum, where the rate of cell division is most rapid, is affected earliest (by 8 days of life) and most markedly. The cerebrum, where cell division is occurring at a slower rate, is affected later (at 14 days of life) and less markedly. The effects produced include a reduced rate of cell division in both areas and a reduction in overall protein synthesis and in the synthesis of various lipids. In addition to these effects on areas of rapid cell division, the increase in DNA content which normally appears in the hippocampus between the 14th and 17th day is delayed and perhaps even partially prevented. It would appear from these data that those regions in which the rate of cell division is highest are affected earliest and most markedly and that cell migration is also curtailed. Whether this is actually an interference with migratory patterns or an inhibition of cell division at the source below the lateral ventricle is not fully known, but data to be discussed shortly strongly suggest that the latter accounts for at least some of the reduced cell number in the hippocampus. Regional patterns of lipid synthesis and the effects of malnutrition on these patterns have not been clearly established. What data are available,[48] however, suggest that areas where myelination is most rapid are most vulnerable to the effects of early malnutrition.

In all of the discussion to this point, individual cell types have not been considered. At present, three types of studies have been conducted on malnourished animal brains during rapid growth: (1) careful histologic examination, employing a variety of special stains, (2) histochemical examination in an attempt to differentiate effects on patterns of specific enzyme development, and (3) radioautographic studies to determine the effect of undernutrition on the division of particular cell types. Unfortunately the same species have not been employed in all of these studies, which makes cross-comparisons difficult.

Histologic changes have been observed in the central nervous systems of rats,[49] pigs and dogs[50] reared after weaning on protein-deficient diets. Both neurons and glia in spinal cord and medulla degenerate. These changes persist even after intensive rehabilitation with a protein-rich diet lasting for as long as 3 months. The changes could be made more severe either by beginning the restriction at an earlier age or by extending the duration of the deficient diet. In pigs it has also been demonstrated that severe undernutrition early in life produces histologic changes in

the cortex itself. Neurons in the gray matter are reduced in number and appear swollen. More recently histochemical changes have been described in the brains of rats submitted to early malnutrition.[51] The appearance of a variety of enzymes, demonstrable by special staining techniques, is delayed and the ultimate quantity obtained is reduced. Thus early malnutrition produces specific histologic and histochemical changes within the cells of the central nervous system. Again, the earlier the malnutrition, the more severe is the damage and the more likely it is to persist.

Radioautographic studies indicate that in neonatal rats malnourished for the first 10 days of life only glial cell division is inhibited in the cerebrum since neuronal cell division ceases prior to birth. In the cerebellum, the rates of cell division of external granular cells, internal granular cells and molecular cells are reduced. In addition, the rate of cell division in neurons under both the third and lateral ventricle is decreased.[15] The reduction in neurons under the lateral ventricle explains, at least in part, the reduced DNA content in hippocampus 5 days later, since these are the cells which are destined to migrate into the hippocampus.

The effect of malnutrition on the human brain has been studied only to a limited extent.[9,16] The data indicate that in marasmic infants who died of malnutrition during the first year of life, wet weight, dry weight, total RNA, total cholesterol, total phospholipid and total DNA content are proportionally reduced. Thus the rate of DNA synthesis is slowed and cell division curtailed, resulting in a reduced number of cells. Since the reduction in the other elements was proportional to the reduction in DNA content, the ratios are unchanged and, hence, the size of cells or the lipid content per cell is not altered. Again it is to be emphasized that these are "average" cells, and it is quite possible that certain cells, i.e. those with lipid being actively deposited, are being affected differently than those in which this is not occurring. If the malnutrition persists beyond about 8 months of age not only is the number of cells reduced but the size of individual cells is also reduced. In addition the lipid per cell is reduced.

Recent data suggest that the ganglioside content and concentration of human brain be reduced by early malnutrition. Since gangliosides are localized within dendritic arborizations, the data suggest that there may be a reduction in such arborizations in the brains of children who suffer severe early malnutrition.[52]

Thus in human brain there is a similar type of response to malnutrition. During proliferative growth cell division is curtailed; during hypertrophic growth the normal enlargement in cells is prevented.

It is obviously not possible to collect recovery data in infants, but indirect data suggest that the situation might be similar to the situation in animals. Since head circumference was correlated with these cellular parameters and was reduced in proportion to the reduction in the number of cells in these infants, their head circumferences were appropriate for their brain sizes and cell number and reduced for their ages. In similar children recovering from this type of severe marasmus, this reduced head circumference persisted even after maximum rehabilitation until they were at least 5 years old. Regional effects of malnutrition in the human have been studied and the data indicate reduction in cell number will occur in cerebrum, cerebellum and brain stem in children who die of marasmus during the first year of life.[9] Thus available data indicate that the effects of malnutrition on human brain are qualitatively similar to the effects on rat brain. However, the quantitative events have still not been worked out.

Skeletal Muscle

During hyperplastic growth in the rat, protein-calorie malnutrition results in a retardation in the rate of DNA synthesis in the gastrocnemius muscle.[53] There is little change in the protein/DNA ratio, and the number of nuclei remain reduced even after adequate refeeding. Malnutrition in the more mature postpubertal animal[53] results in a reduced protein/DNA ratio only, and this change is reversed with refeeding.

In muscle of young rats fed a diet low in both calories and protein, Hill et al.[54] have found a reduction in both DNA content and protein/DNA ratio. By contrast, when the animals were restricted in calories but were fed adequate protein, less reduction in either muscle growth or muscle nuclear number was noted. In these animals the protein/DNA ratios were either normal or slightly increased. These authors postulate that reducing caloric intake will affect DNA replication primarily, while reduction of both caloric and protein intake has more serious effects on intracellular protein synthesis as well.

In laboratory studies, a specific type of malnutrition can usually be produced. In clinical studies, however, patients rarely exhibit pure marasmus or pure kwashiorkor, but present a picture of mixed protein-calorie malnutrition. In the literature on muscle growth in human malnutrition, the age of onset, duration of malnutrition, severity of malnutrition and type of dietary deficiency are variable, and hence it is difficult to generalize regarding effects on cellular growth of muscle. It seems clear, however, that whether estimated from cadaver analysis,[55] biopsy specimen,[56] limb measurements,[57] or creatinine excretion,[57-59] muscle growth is more severely and disproportionately reduced than the reduction in total body weight alone would indicate. Loss of total body potassium[59] and muscle tissue protein[55,56] can often be severe. Concomitantly, there is an increase in total body water when compared to body weight which is primarily due to expansion of the extracellular fluid compartment.

Undernutrition in the immature human

subject[60,61] reduces muscle nuclear number, as well as total muscle mass, when values are compared to age-mates; nutritional rehabilitation will restore these deficits toward normal. Overnutrition in early childhood increases total muscle mass[62] and muscle nuclear number;[63] reduction in body weight associated with some loss of muscle mass would not be expected to alter muscle nuclear number but might well decrease the average protein/DNA ratio. One of the greatest difficulties in interpreting these data lies in the fact that it has been assumed, a priori in some instances, that the ratio of fiber to nonfiber nuclei, the constancy of DNA concentration among the various muscle groups and the ratio of 1 gm creatinine per 20 kg muscle mass pertain in disease as well as in health. This may not be so; indeed, there is some evidence to the contrary.[26,64,59] With these caveats in mind, the following generalization can be made. Since the increase in nuclear number occurs throughout prenatal and postnatal growth through adolescence, this process is likely to be vulnerable to nutritional insults occurring at any time during this period. The human data support this, but whether the absolute values reported for muscle DNA content or nuclear number are, in fact, accurate awaits further confirmation of the validity of the methodology in subjects with altered nutrition.

Placenta and Fetus

During intrauterine life all organs of the fetus are in the hyperplastic phase of growth. At no other time should the organism be more susceptible to nutritional stresses, and yet only recently has any information about fetal malnutrition been forthcoming. This is true probably for two reasons, one operational and the other philosophical: (1) the relative inaccessibility of the fetus for experimental manipulation, and (2) the generally accepted view of the fetus as the perfect parasite, extracting its needs from its mother. Recently, as researchers have ventured to study the uterus, this widely accepted viewpoint is being challenged. Fetal malnutrition may result from reduced maternal circulation, inadequate nutrients within the maternal circulation or faulty placental transport of specific nutrients. The first two situations are now being extensively investigated in experimental animals.

The supply of blood to a single fetus in an animal delivering a litter of fetuses may be reduced spontaneously. It is not uncommon to see a "runt" in a litter of dogs or cats, and it is common knowledge that these animals will survive only with special care and that they will never reach the same final size as their littermates even if this special care is given. Occasionally the same situation occurs in a litter of pigs. Widdowson has studied the cellular changes which take place in the organs of these spontaneously occurring runt pigs. Her findings indicate that cell division has been curtailed in heart, kidney, brain and skeletal muscle, the only organs thus far studied. Cell size was also reduced in all organs studied when compared to littermate controls.[65]

In the rat, blood supply can be artificially reduced by clamping the uterine artery supplying one uterine horn. Using this technique, Wigglesworth[66] has compared the growth of the fetuses in the ligated horn to that of the fetuses in the unligated horn. Growth rate was reduced in proportion to the distance of the particular fetus from the ligated artery. Those at the uterine end closest to the ligation generally died. Progressing farther from the ligated uterine artery and closer to the intact ovarian artery, growth rate increased. More recently the cellular growth of various fetal organs, including placenta, has been studied in surviving animals within the ligated horn. Ligation on the 13th day of gestation will affect the rate of cell division in placenta and all fetal organs except the brain. Ligation on the 17th day will curtail cell division in the fetal organs, again sparing brain, but in placenta cell size will be reduced with cell number remaining normal.[67]

Thus in currently available animal studies in which blood supply has been either artificially or spontaneously curtailed, the rate of cell division in fetal organs excluding brain has been retarded. Placenta, moreover, responds in a manner that might have been predicted from the earlier studies involving early postnatal malnutrition. Ligation during the period of hyperplasia results in reduced cell number, whereas ligation during hypertrophy results in reduced cell size. Therefore, by determining the final effect on placental growth at delivery, it may be possible to pinpoint the time at which a stimulus producing such a result must have been active. As we shall see, this possibility may have relevance in the human, where placenta is the only tissue readily available for study.

Another abnormality was defined in placentas from the ligated horns: elevation of total organ RNA content and hence an elevation of the RNA/DNA ratio or RNA per cell.[67] Such elevations in tissue RNA/DNA have been described in several tissues under a variety of circumstances. Clamping the aorta results in an increased RNA/DNA ratio in the left ventricle.[68] Repeated nerve stimulation results in an elevation of the RNA/DNA ratio in the innervated muscle,[69] injection of estrogen results in an increased RNA/DNA ratio in the uterus and removal of one kidney will result in an increased RNA/DNA ratio in the contralateral kidney.[70] The exact significance of this change is unknown, but it has been described under conditions requiring increased protein synthesis. This increase in placental RNA/DNA ratio may, therefore, represent an abortive attempt by placental cells to increase their rate of protein synthesis secondary to the stress of vascular insufficiency. Further evidence that this may be occurring comes from the

fact that the activity of alkaline RNase (an enzyme involved in RNA catabolism) is elevated in placentas within the ligated horn. This suggests that the overall turnover of RNA is increased under these conditions.[71]

Maternal protein restriction in rats will also retard both placental and fetal growth. In placenta, cell number (DNA content) was reduced by 13 days after conception, cell size (protein/DNA ratio) remained normal and the RNA/DNA ratio was markedly elevated. Retardation in fetal growth first became apparent at 15 days, followed by a progressive decrease in cell number in all the organs studied. By term there were only about 85 per cent of the number of brain cells in control animals.[67] These data agree with previous data of Zamenhof[72] which showed a similar reduction in total brain cell number in term fetuses with mothers exposed to a slightly different type of nutritional deprivation. Thus the cellular changes produced by severe prenatal food restriction are reflected in the placenta even earlier than in the fetus, but retardation of cell division in all fetal organs, including brain, can be clearly demonstrated.

By employing radioautography after injecting the mother with tritiated thymidine, cell division can be assessed in various discrete brain regions. Differential regional sensitivity can be demonstrated in this way by the 16th day of gestation in the brains of fetuses of protein-restricted mothers. The cerebral white and gray matter are mildly affected. The area adjacent to the third ventricle and the subiculum are moderately affected, whereas the cerebellum and the area directly adjacent to the lateral ventricle are markedly affected.[73,74] These data again demonstrate that the magnitude of the effect produced on cell division is directly related to the actual rate of cell division at the time the stimulus is applied. Moreover, they demonstrate that the maternal placental barrier in the rat is not effective in protecting the fetal brain from discrete cellular effects caused by maternal food restriction.

The subsequent course of animals born of protein-restricted mothers can be examined. Lee and Chow have reported that even if these animals are raised normally on foster mothers they demonstrate a permanent impairment in the ability to utilize nitrogen.[75] Data from our own laboratory demonstrate that if the animals are nursed on normal foster mothers in normal-sized litters they will remain with a deficit in total brain cell number at weaning. Thus we can again see early programming of the ultimate number of brain cells. This program, moreover, is written in utero in response to maternal nutrition.

These same newborn pups of protein-restricted mothers may be subjected to postnatal nutritional manipulation. If they are raised in litters of 3 on normal foster mothers until weaning, the deficit in total number of brain cells may be almost entirely reversed.[73] Although quantitatively the number of cells approaches normal, qualitatively the deficit at birth might well be made up by an increase in cell number in areas different from those most affected in utero. Thus although it may appear that optimally nourishing pups after exposing them to prenatal undernutrition will reverse the cellular effects, this may not actually be so in specific brain areas.

Perhaps the most analogous situation to the situation in humans is exposing these pups, malnourished in utero, to subsequent postnatal deprivation. These animals can be raised on foster mothers in groups of 18. Animals so reared show a marked reduction in brain cell number by weaning. This effect is much more pronounced than the effect of either prenatal or postnatal undernutrition alone.[76,77] Animals subjected to prenatal malnutrition alone, as previously described, show a 15 per cent reduction in total brain cell number at birth. Animals subjected only to postnatal malnutrition show a similar 15 to 20 per cent reduction in brain cell number at weaning. In contrast, the "doubly deprived" animals demonstrate a 60 per cent reduction in total brain cell number by weaning. These data demonstrate that malnutrition applied constantly throughout the entire period of brain cell proliferation will result in a profound reduction in brain cell number, greater than the sum of the effects produced during various parts of the proliferative phase. It would appear that the duration of malnutrition as well as the severity during this early critical period is extremely important in determining the ultimate cellular makeup of the brain.

Experiments by Widdowson[65] in the guinea pig demonstrate that caloric restriction during gestation markedly reduces birth weight of the offspring and curtails the rate of cell division in the brain. In the skeletal muscle not only is there a reduction in cell number but the actual number of muscle fibers is also reduced, and each muscle fiber has an increased number of nuclei. These animals when fed normally after birth fail to recover normal height or weight.[65]

The animal data, then, clearly demonstrate that undernutrition from either reduced blood supply or reduced availability of nutrients will curtail placental and fetal growth, retard the rate of cell division in various fetal organs and result in an animal the organs of which contain fewer cells. Evidence also indicates that animals born after developing in this type of intrauterine environment will carry these cellular deficits for the rest of their lives. However, the two types of "malnutrition" produce very different effects on brain. In the vascular insufficiency model brain is spared, whereas in the maternal malnutrition model brain is markedly affected.

Human placenta goes through the same three phases of growth as those described for the organs of the rat. Cell division ceases at about 34 to 36 weeks of gestation, whereas weight and protein increase until nearly term.[37] Placentas from infants with "intrauterine growth failure" show fewer cells and a larger RNA/DNA ratio than controls.[78] Fifty per cent of placentas from an indigent population in Chile showed similar findings.[76] Placentas from a malnourished population in Guatemala had fewer cells than normal.[79] In a single case of anorexia nervosa in which a severely emaciated mother carried to term and gave birth to a 2,500-gm infant, the placenta contained less than 50 per cent of the expected number of cells.[76] Thus both vascular insufficiency and maternal malnutrition will curtail cell division in human placenta. The cellular makeup of the placenta in both of these situations strongly suggests that both stimuli have been active for some time prior to the 34th to 36th week of gestation. In addition, more recent data demonstrate that placentas from malnourished women show an increased activity of alkaline RNase, similar to that described in the rat models.[80]

The effects of these stimuli on the cellular growth of the fetus are more difficult to assess. Indirect evidence suggests that cell division in the human fetus may be retarded by maternal undernutrition. Fetal growth is retarded and birth weight reduced.[81] If available data on infants who died after exposure to severe postnatal malnutrition are examined, three separate patterns emerge. Breast-fed infants malnourished during the second year have a reduced protein/DNA ratio but a normal brain DNA content. Full-term infants who subsequently died of severe food deprivation during the first year of life had a 15 to 20 per cent reduction in total brain cell number. Infants weighing 2,000 gm or less at birth who subsequently died of severe undernutrition during the first year of life showed a 60 per cent reduction in total brain cell number.[76] It is possible that these children were deprived in utero and represent a clinical counterpart of the "doubly deprived" animal. It is also possible that

these were true premature infants and that premature infants are much more susceptible to postnatal malnutrition than are full-term infants.

Other Tissues

The normal cellular growth patterns for most of the organs of the rat have been worked out. In general, weight and protein continue to increase until about 100 days of age. By contrast, DNA reaches a maximum before this in all organs. The time at which it does so varies with the particular organ. In brain and lung DNA reaches a maximum at about 21 days of life, in liver, spleen and kidney at about 40 days, in submaxillary gland at about 45 days and in heart at about 65 days. Malnutrition during the period of hyperplastic growth results in a reduced number of cells in all of these organs.

In the human, cellular growth patterns have been studied in 16 organs during normal fetal development. The data indicate that total cell number, as measured by total organ DNA content, increases in all organs from 13 weeks of gestation until term. Cell size, as measured either by weight/DNA or protein/DNA ratio, remains unchanged throughout gestation in heart, kidney, spleen, thyroid, thymus, esophagus, stomach, large and small intestines and tongue. In brain, lung, liver, adrenal gland and diaphragm, cell size increases slowly from the beginning of the seventh month of gestation until term.

More limited data during the first year of life demonstrate that cell number continues to increase rapidly in heart, liver, kidney and spleen. Heart cell size begins to increase after three months of age, whereas in kidney, liver and spleen cell size does not change during the first year.

Children who died of marasmus during the first two years of life showed marked reductions in cell number in all organs studied. As described in a previous section, brain cell size was also reduced when the malnutrition extended into the second year. In contrast, cell size in the other organs was not significantly reduced even if the malnutrition persisted beyond the first year.

BIBLIOGRAPHY

1. Enesco and LeBlond: J. Embryol. Exp. Morphol., 10, 530, 1962.
2. Boivin, Vendrely and Vendrely: C.R. Acad. Sci., 226, 1061, 1948.
3. Winick and Noble: Dev. Biol., 12, 451, 1965.
4. Fish and Winick: Pediatr. Res., 3, 407, 1969.
5. Altman and Das: J. Comp. Neurol., 126, 337, 1966.
6. Winick: Pediatr. Res., 2, 352, 1968.
7. Dobbing: Reported at Symposium of The American Pediatric Society, Atlantic City, May 1970.
8. Dobbing and Sands: Nature, 226, 639, 1970.
9. Winick, Rosso and Waterlow: Exp. Neurol., 26, 393, 1970.
10. Duckett and Pearse: Proceedings Fifth International Congress Neuropathology. ICN Series No. 100. Amsterdam, Excerpta Medica, 1966, p. 738.
11. Nachmansohn: In Modern Trends in Physiology and Biochemistry (Barron, Ed.). New York, Academic Press, 1952, p. 38.
12. Duckett and Pearse: Anat. Rec., 163, 59, 1969.
13. Auguslinsson: In The Enzymes, Vol. 1 (Sumner and Myrbäck, Eds.). New York, Academic Press, 1950, p. 443.
14. Duckett and Pearse: J. Anat., 102, 183, 1968.
15. Duckett and Pearse: Rev. Can. Biol., 26, 173, 1967.
16. Rosso, Hormazabal and Winick: Am. J. Clin. Nutr., 23, 1275, 1970.
17. Winick and Rosso: In Brain Function and Malnutrition: Neuropsychological Methods of Assessment (Prescott, Read and Coursin, Eds.). New York, John Wiley & Sons, 1975, p. 41.
18. Widdowson: In Scientific Foundation of Paediatrics (Davis and Dobbing, Eds.). Philadelphia, W. B. Saunders, 1974, p. 153.
19. Mastaglia: In Scientific Foundation of Paediatrics (Davis and Dobbing, Eds.). Philadelphia, W. B. Saunders, 1974, p. 348.
20. Montgomery: Nature, 195, 194, 1962.
21. Adams and DeRueck: In Basic Research in Myology. Proceedings of the II International Congress on Muscle Diseases, Part I, ICN Series No. 294. Amsterdam, Excerpta Medica, 1973.
22. Graystone: In Human Growth (Cheek, Ed.). Philadelphia, Lea & Febiger, 1968.
23. Cheek: In Control of Onset of Puberty (Grumbach, Grave and Mayer, Eds.). New York, John Wiley & Sons, 1974, p. 426.
24. Widdowson, Crabb and Milner: Arch. Dis. Child., 47, 652, 1972.
25. Moss and Leblond: J. Cell. Biol. 44, 459, 1970.
26. Enesco and Puddy: Am. J. Anat., 114, 235, 1964.
27. Cheek, Holt, Hill and Talbert: Pediatr. Res., 5, 312, 1971.
28. Cheek: In Human Growth (Cheek, Ed.). Philadelphia, Lea & Febiger, 1968.
29. Cheek and Hill: Fed. Proc., 29, 1503, 1970.
30. Leuchtenberger, Leuchtenberger and Davis: Am. J. Pathol., 30, 65, 1954.
31. Swartz: Chromosoma, 8, 53, 1956.
32. Ranek, Keiding and Jensen: Acta Pathol. Microbiol. Scand., 83, 467, 1975.
33. Epstein: Proc. Natl. Acad. Sci., 57, 327, 1967.
34. Jollie: Am. J. Anat., 114, 161, 1964.
35. Winick and Noble: Nature, 212, 34, 1966.
36. Correy: Am. J. Physiol., 112, 263, 1935.
37. Winick, Coscia and Noble: Pediatrics, 39, 248, 1967.
38. Miller: Fed. Proc., 29, 1497, 1970.
39. McCance and Widdowson: Proc. R. Soc. Lond., 156, 326, 1962.
40. Widdowson and McCance: Proc. R. Soc. Lond., 152, 88, 1960.
41. Jackson and Steward: J. Exp. Zool., 30, 97, 1920.
42. Winick and Noble: J. Nutr., 89, 300, 1966.
43. Winick and Noble: J. Nutr., 91, 179, 1967.
44. Winick, Fish and Rosso: J. Nutr., 95, 623, 1968.
45. Davison and Dobbing: Br. Med. Bull., 22, 40, 1966.
46. Chase, Dorsey and McKahnn: Pediatrics, 40, 551, 1967.
47. Fish and Winick: Pediatr. Res., 3, 407, 1969.
48. Culley and Lineberger: J. Nutr., 96, 375, 1968.
49. Platt: Proc. R. Soc. Lond., 156, 337, 1962.
50. Platt, Heard and Steward: In Mammalian Protein Metabolism, Vol. II (Munro and Alison, Eds.). New York, Academic Press, 1964.
51. Zeman and Stanbrough: J. Nutr., 99, 274, 1969.
52. Dickerson: Personal communication.
53. Winick: Pediatr. Clin. North Am., 17, 69, 1970.
54. Hill, Holt, Parra and Cheek: Johns Hopkins Med. J., 127, 146, 1970.
55. Waterlow: West Indian Med. J., 5, 167, 1956.
56. Hagerman and Villee: Physiol. Rev., 40, 313, 1960.
57. Standard, Wills and Waterlow: Am. J. Clin. Nutr., 7, 271, 1959.
58. Cheek, Hill, Cordano and Graham: Pediatr. Res., 4, 135, 1970.
59. Alleyne: Clin. Sci., 34, 199, 1968.
60. Graham, Cordano, Blizzard and Cheek: Pediatr. Res., 3, 579, 1969.
61. Cheek, Hill, Cordano and Graham: Pediatr. Res., 4, 135, 1970.
62. Forbes: Pediatrics, 34, 308, 1964.
63. Cheek, Schultz, Parra and Reba: Pediatr. Res., 4, 268, 1970.
64. Beach and Kostyo: Endocrinology, 82, 682, 1968.
65. Widdowson: Presented at Symposium on Fetal Malnutrition, New York, 1970.
66. Wigglesworth: J. Pathol. Bacteriol., 88, 1, 1964.
67. Winick: In Diagnosis and Treatment of Fetal Disorders (Adamson, Ed.). New York, Springer-Verlag, 1968, p. 83.
68. Gluck, et al.: Science, 144, 1244, 1964.
69. Logan, Mannell and Rossiter: J. Biochem., 51, 482, 1952.
70. Karp, Brasel and Winick: Am. J. Dis. Child., 121, 186, 1971.

71. Velasco, Brasel, Sigulem, Rosso and Winick: J. Nutr., *103*, 213, 1973.

72. Zamenhof, Van Marchens and Margolis: Science, *160*, 3823, 1968.

73. Winick: Am. J. Obstet. Gynecol., *109*, 166, 1971.

74. Winick and Velasco: In Proceedings Eighth International Congress Nutrition, Prague, 1969. ICN Series No. 213. Amsterdam, Excerpta Medica, 1970.

75. Lee and Chow: J. Nutr., *87*, 439, 1965.

76. Winick: Fed. Proc., *29*, 1510, 1970.

77. Winick, Fish and Rosso: J. Nutr., *95*, 623, 1968.

78. Winick: J. Pediatr., *71*, 390, 1967.

79. Dayton, Filer and Canos: Fed. Proc., *28*, 488, 1969.

80. Velasco, Rosso, Brasel and Winick: Am. J. Obstet. Gynecol., *123*, 637, 1975.

81. Smith: J. Pediatr., *30*, 229, 1947.

Part IV

Malnutrition

Chapter 20

VITAMIN ANALYSES IN MEDICINE

Herman Baker,
Oscar Frank
and
Seymour H. Hutner

When some diseases were first recognized as deficiencies of one or another vitamin, the vitamins were assayed mainly by their effect upon growth and health of one or another laboratory animal. Vitamin deficiencies underlie numerous diseases; numerous diseases induce vitamin deficiencies. Hypovitaminosis may reflect decreased dietary intake, absorption defects, decreased hepatic avidity, storage and conversion to active metabolic forms, excess utilization, destruction or excretion. Vitamin demands increase in liver disease, pregnancy, hyperthyroidism, growth, neoplasia, anemia and tissue repair.[1-4] Some drugs act as antimetabolites which interfere with normal vitamin metabolism.[5] Their structural similarity to cell components enables them to compete for vitamin-dependent sites in metabolism; in this manner they can cripple or distort metabolism. Some antimetabolites may substitute for the vitamin in a coenzyme, thereby producing a faulty enzyme which blocks or modifies a specific biosynthetic pathway.[6]

Vitamins are organic substances required in minute quantities the effects of which derive from their catalytic activity. Elucidation of their structure and then practical synthesis are exciting chapters in chemistry and microbiology. Their identification as prosthetic groups of enzymes fulfilled the revolution in biochemistry begun by Sir Frederick Gowland Hopkins.

Vitamins can be determined by the tools of analytic chemistry, but, while such methods are widely used in industrial production, the minute quantities in body fluids and tissues limit the purely chemical approach to a few vitamins. Microchemical methods, based on the most sensitive colorimetric and, in particular, fluorometric techniques, are in use for determination of thiamin, riboflavin, ascorbic acid and some of the fat-soluble vitamins. Vitamin D, on the other hand, is determined by animal assay or, indirectly, by use of alkaline phosphatase. Its metabolism in man is being studied with the use of ^{14}C or ^{3}H vitamin D.[7] Radioisotope assays are proving valuable for vitamin D and its hormonal forms, since no microbiologic assay is available for any of these compounds.

Since vitamins, especially the water-soluble ones, enter into the coenzymes for fundamental cellular mechanisms, they are required by invertebrates and by unicellular organisms such as bacteria, and most algae, which, like man, depend on outside sources of these factors. One way to analyze circulating vitamins is to measure enzyme function. Since many enzymes have vitamin-containing coenzymes, prolonged vitamin deficit diminishes coenzyme synthesis. Apoenzyme deficiency also diminishes enzyme activity, independent of vitamin concentration.[8] The analysis of circulating enzyme activity as a measure of vitamin status is not accurate in the presence of apoenzyme deficits; this was shown in liver disease.[8,9] For example, vitamin B_6 (as pyridoxal phosphate) is a coenzyme for a large number of reactions involving amino acids. This is because pyridoxal phosphate is a general "claw" which grasps the amino acid molecule. If one suffers from a B_6 deficiency, any enzyme requiring pyridoxal phosphate as a coenzyme is supposedly affected and, as B_6 deficiency increases, inhibition of the appropriate enzymes also increases. However, all B_6-dependent enzymes are not affected *equally* because there is an equilibrium between enzyme $\rightleftarrows$ apoenzyme + coenzyme and the affinities of the different apoenzymes for the coenzyme vary.

In moderate deficiency, where some coenzyme is present but the amount is limited, those enzymes in which apoenzyme and coenzyme have a high affinity will be least affected, while those with a low affinity may be almost completely inactivated; the available supply of coenzyme will be preferentially distributed and, as a deficiency increases, reactions are eliminated in turn, but not all together. In general, reactions most essential to life tend to be last eliminated.[9a] Therefore, the choice of enzymes as a measure of vitamin status does not permit a safety time factor in which to reverse the vitamin depletion before untoward clinical signs appear.

The measure of the circulating vitamins per se permits detection of vitamin deficiency before biochemical and clinical signs appear; decrease in circulating vitamin titer is the earliest warning signal of impending biochemical and clinical deficiency. For example, the plasma ascorbate level fell to zero after 41 days of ascorbate depletion, whereas clinical signs of scurvy did not appear for 134 days.[9b] In a study on folate, the first sign of impend-

ing biochemical and clinical folate deficiency was a depressed serum folate level. It took approximately 14 to 18 weeks for the biochemical lesion to appear and 20 weeks for the clinical symptoms to appear; depressed folate levels were apparent after 3 weeks. It therefore seems that there is still ample storage of vitamin-containing enzymes to maintain biochemical functions (enzymes), but the earliest sign of enzymatic malfunction remains the depressed circulating vitamin level.[220]

Before the introduction of microbiologic assays for B_{12} in human serum, deficiency could be diagnosed only by signs of hematologic stimulation upon administration of liver extracts or B_{12} preparations. A similar problem was presented by folic acid.[10] Because folic acid is metabolically related to vitamin B_{12}, microbiologic assays had to be devised for differential diagnosis. This has been solved not only for the B_{12}-folic acid duo but also for thiamin, biotin, pantothenic acid, riboflavin, nicotinic acid, folinic acid and vitamin B_6.[1] These additions to the diagnostic armory have proved their value for assaying vitamins in biologic fluids and tissues.

Use of protozoa to assay biologically active materials is not so well known, for historic reasons, as the use of bacteria or fungi. Protozoan assays have several advantages over other biologic, physical or chemical assays.[1] These include unusually high sensitivity and specificity, especially for vitamins and organic nutrients, fewer restrictions on size or physical state of the molecule to be assayed and marked sensitivity to many pharmacologically interesting compounds. Because of their ability to obtain exogenous metabolites by phagocytosis and pinocytosis, as well as by diffusion, osmosis and active transport, particle-ingesting protozoa may be used to assay soluble vitamins and vitamins in particulate form, including small molecules such as nicotinic acid and bulky ones such as B_{12}. Protozoan assays are easy to do and require minimal space and inexpensive materials, and environmental conditions can be easily controlled.

Except for the Lactobacillus casei method for detecting folate activity, bacteriologic assays for vitamins have not been successful for assay in biologic fluids and tissues;[1,11] they proved to be either insensitive or nonspecific. Introduction of protozoa-based techniques met the practical needs,[1] since the protozoa have a sensitivity and specificity for vitamins much like man's.[1,12] By conjoint use of adequate chemical methods for β-carotene, vitamins A, C and E, vitamin imbalances can be gauged in many metabolic and nutritional diseases.[2]

The development of protozoan techniques for such purposes introduces a new chapter in vitaminology. As nutritional biochemistry deepens into insights of intracellular happenings, the need arises to detect essential metabolites as components of enzymes or of complex cofactors for enzymes with tools mimicking metazoan metabolic patterns. As noted, vitamins function as parts of enzymes. If the enzyme mediates electron transfer, one finds nicotinic acid or riboflavin; carboxylation or decarboxylation, thiamin or biotin; 1-carbon transfer, folic acid and B_{12}; 2-carbon transfer, pantothenic acid; 3-carbon transfer or synthesis of a single carbon group, B_{12}; and nitrogen transfer, vitamin B_6. On a microscale, protozoa respond to a great variety of vitamins in most of their molecular forms with a comprehensiveness matching chick or rat assays.[12] The criticisms that protozoa generally grow more slowly than bacteria and that radioactive tracers such as $^{60}CoB_{12}$ are faster analytic tools are of minor importance; more valid comparisons are with the growth rate of the chick or rat. The economy of the protozoan assay and freedom from radioactivity hazards are important factors.

The increasing use of broad-spectrum antibiotics has deterred some workers from use of microbiologic assays because of a fear that tissues and tissue fluids may contain concentrates of the antibiotic that may inhibit the assay organism. This fear is groundless. It stems from ignoring both the thermolability of nearly all antibiotics and the prescribed procedures for preparation of samples. The preliminary autoclaving used to liberate protein-bound vitamins will destroy all commonly used antibiotics except gentamicin. Where the antimicrobial agent is thermostable, as are the sulfonamides, inclusion of the appropriate metabolic target—in this case, p-aminobenzoic acid—in the basal medium obviates the difficulty. Use of "aseptic addition" methods[12a] may save an hour or two, but introduces variability in liberation of vitamins as well as susceptibility to interference by antimicrobial agents. This belief is supported by the finding[12b] that in the L. casei assay for folates simple heating of serum and whole blood eliminated all interference from chloramphenicol. Also, the aseptic addition is an unnecessary step which adds nothing to accuracy or sensitivity and introduces a possibility of serious mechanical error. It is rare for that matter, thanks to the sensitivity of the assays, especially those based on protozoa, that interfering substances are not diluted out in diluting the sample to bring it within the assay range.

It should be remembered that, in dealing with a microanimal such as Tetrahymena which requires all the B vitamins except B_{12}, a simple, uniform methodology suffices for the several assays based on these deficiencies; even the same basal medium, aside from adjustments in the vitamin block, can be used. Radioimmune assays require different reagents, notably binding factors, for each different assay.

For a while, many investigators needed convincing about the applicability of protozoa not only for assaying vitamins but also for detecting drug toxicity. The excellent reproducibility, sensitivity and metabolic similarity to man and metazoa have made certain protozoa favorable reagents for such use.[1] For example, Ochromonas malhamensis has a B_{12} requirement seemingly identical to man's;[1] this is now the official method in Britain for measuring vitamin B_{12} and has replaced Lactobacillus leichmannii, chicks and rats for practical purposes. It is in routine use for monitoring the industrial production of B_{12}. We have given elsewhere many of the biochemical applications of microbiologic assays,[1,13] so we shall keep theory brief while showing how microbial vitamin assays serve as an increasingly valuable clinical tool for investigating nutritional status, notably vitamin interrelationships.

We shall also discuss briefly the value of accurately charting vitamin involvement in metabolic processes for evaluating malnutrition, keeping in mind that body vitamins are commonly determined by assessment of biologic fluids and tissues. Laboratory tests assume a correlation between the amount of nutrient in tissues, blood or urine and bodily function. Their usefulness, therefore, depends in large measure on establishing such a relationship and finding the range in which changes in concentration can be interpreted. In all instances, however, the usefulness of various tests designed for nutritional investigation rests with an appreciation of the distinction between those techniques which reflect only the supply of nutrients to the body and those which indicate abnormal metabolism brought about by the nutritional deficiency.[1] In selecting an appropriate method for studying a nutritional problem, it is necessary to have clearly in mind the objectives of the investigation. These objectives fall into three categories: clinical diagnosis, fundamental research and nutritional survey work.[1,14]

In this section, we shall describe application of methods for the analysis of vitamins in biologic fluids and tissue; methods for vitamin analyses in pharmaceutic preparations and foodstuffs have been treated extensively by others.[15]

Many laboratories use variations of the assays referred to here and elsewhere.[1] More significance should be attached to the usefulness of *differentials* permitted by a specific assay than to the absolute values; absolute values may deviate with varied methods. It is important to establish a normal range of a method, so that laboratory-to-laboratory variations in obtaining absolute values do not alter the conclusions, e.g. ability to identify vitamin imbalance.

The development of protozoan assay techniques[1] for nutritional surveys brings a new realism to analytic survey procedures. Inadequacies in methodology hampered previous studies of this sort; some methods were not sensitive nor specific enough, making indirect methods necessary. In many instances, the fluid analyzed—urine—did not yield data correlating well with vitamin status, owing to large variations in these 24-hour samples.

Many investigators report results as the ratio of a particular metabolite in the urine to urinary creatinine.[15a] However, large diurnal and day-to-day variations in urinary creatinine excretion have been charted, suggesting that creatinine values should be used with caution.[15b] Data thus gathered permitted only rough estimates of nutritional status. However, with specific and sensitive protozoan techniques, blood and plasma values could now serve as an index of vitamin status. Earlier we had seen no gross circulating diurnal variations in vitamin titers, as frequently seen in urine specimens, except when dietary intakes were designed to cause gross vitamin overload. Once blood, serum, plasma or tissue is collected, the specimens can be stored frozen and shipped for assay; the vitamin titers do not significantly vary in specimens so handled.[1,52]

The easier quantitative determinations of vitamins in body fluids and tissues permitted by protozoan techniques should elucidate the significance of vitamins not merely in classic nutritional deficiencies but in the wider field of metabolic disturbances generally. Overt vitamin deficiencies are produced by malabsorption, by inhibitors of vitamin function and sometimes strikingly by drugs and other toxic substances. Vitamin deficiencies may appear whenever an individual's metabolism is so deranged as to require enhanced quantities of a vitamin to cure or to counteract certain symptoms; a B_6-dependent infant is a good example.

As with other constituents of blood or serum, deviation of vitamin titers from the normal range can mean different things: reduced intake or absorption, increased utilization, increased demand, increased excretion. All decrease titers; their opposites increase. In our studies we were able

Table 20–1.   Some Clinical Conditions Warranting Vitamin Assessment

Vitamin	Conditions Warranting Assessment
Vitamin B_{12} Folic acid	Macrocytic anemia (differential diagnosis) Suspected malnutrition (food faddism) Neurologic involvement Alcoholism Liver disease (viral) Gastrointestinal disease and surgery Drug abuse Pregnancy
Vitamin B_6	Microcytosis with normal iron Neurologic signs (convulsive seizures, peripheral neuropathy) Malnutrition Alcoholism Liver disease Pregnancy
Thiamin	Cardiomyopathy Neurologic involvement (peripheral neuropathy) Alcoholism Malnutrition Liver disease Drug abuse
Niacin Biotin Riboflavin Pantothenic acid	Malnutrition Dermatologic and oral lesions Glossitis and cheilosis Neurologic involvement ("burning feet" syndrome) Alcoholism Liver disease
Vitamin A and β-carotene	Xerosis and dermatitis Liver disease Malnutrition GI surgery and suspected malabsorption
Vitamin C (ascorbic acid)	Frank scurvy (bleeding gums, loosened teeth, corkscrew hairs) Petechiae and ecchymosis Malnutrition, especially heavy reliance on canned food
Vitamin E	Liver disease Hemolytic anemias GI disease and surgery Malnutrition, food faddism and especially reliance on preserved and cooked foods

to recognize subtle nutritional deficiency states lacking overt signs, i.e. subclinical nutritional deficiencies.[52,225] Subclinical malnutrition, as the very phrase implies, is not obvious—but it exists; it warns of approaching biochemical and clinical lesions. It remains to be determined how malnutrition due to subclinical deficiencies contributes to ill health or aging.

A vitamin is often the etiologic focus of a disease, e.g. vitamin B_{12} and folic acid in macrocytic anemias. Because of the obvious importance for diagnosis and therapy, determination of the "nucleogenic" vitamins B_{12} and folic acid is a necessity in the routine of clinical hematology. Where connections between vitamins and a disease are less clear, a wide field remains for discovery of correlations between physiologic or pathologic events and vitamin and enzyme content of body fluids and tissues.

A glance at vitamins in clinical practice reveals a wide panorama with attractive opportunities in hepatic conditions, renal dialysis technique, oxalosis and calculus disease, obscure but widely spread neurologic diseases and many dermatologic disorders. Astute clinical observations combined with knowledge of vitamin metabolism could make vitamin analysis a powerful tool.

The potential importance of an apparently wide variation in individual human nutritional needs has become evident not only in our studies but in those of others. Because the concept of extreme human variability tends to destroy the orderliness of science, this subject has been overlooked. Many diseases have their roots in faulty nutrition, but once the extreme variability of human need is recognized medical scientists may have a better understanding of a host of diseases of unknown etiology. In any event, once the analytic facility for vitaminology is set up, it can be turned into a valuable tool for diagnosing a variety of metabolic imbalances.[1,2]

A vitamin profile is in order for patients with signs of malnutrition, alcoholism, liver disease, pre- and posthyperalimenta-

Table 20–3. Interpretation of Vitamins in Total 24-hour Urine*

Vitamin	Normal Range	Mean
ng		
Vitamin B_{12}	5–25	12
μg		
Biotin	6–50	29
Total folates	2–10	8
Thiamin	90–500	180
Niacin	300–1500	600
Riboflavin	200–1500	675
Vitamin B_6	20–120	36
mg		
Pantothenate	1–15	4
Vitamin C	10–100	39

* Values reflect metabolically active forms of the vitamin, not catabolic forms. This information is based on observations in over 300 subjects with no clinical disease or overt malnutrition. Protozoal and chemical methods were used for vitamin estimation; Lactobacillus casei for folate estimations. From Baker and Frank.[1]

Table 20–2. Interpretation of Circulating Vitamin Values*

Vitamin	Deficient	Low	Normal
pg/ml			
Vitamin B_{12}	80	80–100	100–800
Biotin	160	160–200	200–500
ng/ml			
Folate	3	3–5	5–24
Thiamin	20	20–25	25–72
Riboflavin	80	80–100	100–500
Pantothenate	160	160–200	200–800
Vitamin B_6	25	25–30	30–80
μg/ml			
Niacin	2.8	2.8–3.5	3.5–7.0
μg/100 ml			
Vitamin A	20	20–25	25–75
Carotenes	32	32–40	40–150
mg/100 ml			
Vitamin C	0.2	0.2–0.4	0.4–1.5
Vitamin E	0.4	0.4–0.6	0.6–1.2

* Based on information from over 300 subjects with no clinical diseases or overt malnutrition. Protozoal and chemical methods were used for vitamin determinations; Lactobacillus casei was used for folate estimation. From Baker and Frank.[1]

tion, gastrointestinal disorders, some hematologic diseases and suspected nutritional neuropathies and hematologic complications of pregnancy; specifics are listed in Table 20–1. A suggested guide to the interpretation of circulating vitamin and urine data, based on our experiences[1,2] (see other references to Baker et al, Frank et al, Leevy et al.) is given in Table 20–2 and Table 20–3.

VITAMIN A AND CAROTENE

The chemistry, metabolism and new researches in vitamin A have recently been treated in great detail.[16,17] A ready reference for many of the analytic procedures adopted for vitamin A has also been published.[18]

Many macro- and microphysiochemical methods[1,15] can be used for determining vtiamin A and carotenes in a wide variety of materials; the choice depends on the materials to be assayed. Bioassays and thin-layer chromatography[15,20] have been widely used for assaying vitamin A and carotenes, but these methods have little value in estimating the vitamin in small samples of biologic fluids and tissues. The most widely used system for such purposes depends on a series of color reactions to demonstrate the presence of vitamin A or carotenes. The best-known method is based on the Carr-Price reaction[19]—a reaction between the carotenes or vitamin A and $SbCl_3$ in chloroform. This reaction yields a blue color in the presence of extracts of carotene and vitamin A-containing substances. Maximum blue color is reached after 5 seconds and, as the blueness then drops quite rapidly, the measurement must be carried out during this short interval; the reaction is, therefore, carried out directly in the spectrophotometer. Measurement of maximum light absorption can be carried out with any spectrophotometer or similar optical apparatus. With this method, the constants for carotene and vitamin A are usually uniform from one instrument to another.

In serum, the fractionation or concentration of vitamin A and carotenoids is unnecessary.[21] A combined determination is made by means of the blue color with $SbCl_3$ at various wavelengths. Human serum contains vitamin A, carotenoids and small amounts of free carotene. Since carotenoids also react with $SbCl_3$ with a blue color, corrections become necessary when determining vitamin A.[1]

Most procedures customarily employ serum or plasma. Care must be taken not to use hemolyzed samples, since it has been shown[22,23] that hemolysis of blood gives very high values for vitamin A but not for carotene.[24] This method[1] is useful for determining vitamin A in lyophilized tissues.[1,16] A new colorimetric procedure for macro- and microanalysis of serum vitamin A has been introduced.[25] This method is based on the blue color produced by trifluoroacetic acid with vitamin A.

An additional means for estimating vitamin A is the ratio in plasma of retinol to retinol-binding protein. Vitamin A is transported in plasma by a specific binding protein (RBP); approximately 90 per cent of the total vitamin A measured in serum circulates as RBP. RBP is complexed with a second protein, prealbumin A (PA), to form RBP-PA.[25a] Over a wide range of plasma values there is correlation between RBP and plasma vitamin A.[25b] Serum RBP levels are decreased in both chronic and acute liver disease and markedly elevated in renal failure.[25c] Plasma RBP is measured by radioimmune assay[25b] as yet too complex for routine use.

Samples for assay may be stored frozen without loss of vitamin activity. Use of conical glass-stoppered centrifuge tubes minimizes evaporation and also ensures good packing of the centrifuged, precipitated protein.

The determination of vitamin A is restricted largely to serum or plasma studies, since this vitamin is not normally present in sufficient amounts to be measured in the urine of most animals. Injury to the kidneys or the action of certain drugs may cause its excretion in the urine.[18] In the blood both vitamin A and β-carotene are found. Tests of vitamin A absorption in terms of "tolerance curves" have been employed in examining the nutritional state of individuals, especially in cases of celiac disease. As a measure of the storage of this vitamin, the assay of the vitamin A content of liver biopsy material has been used in certain select cases. Normal values for carotene range between 40 to 150 μg per 100 ml of serum and for vitamin A 25 to 75 μg per 100 ml of serum. In a study of vitamin A levels in infants and children,[26] the average fasting level under 6 months of age was found to be 24 μg; it was 32 μg in the group 6 months to 1 year and 38 μg in children over 1 year. The serum carotene level is rather high toward term in pregnancy.[27] In cord blood it is about 25 per cent of that in the maternal blood.[28] The serum vitamin A level is about 25 per cent lower toward term in pregnancy.[27,28] In cord blood it is about 50 per cent of that in maternal blood.[28,28a]

Infants and young children[1] have only a limited capacity for converting carotene into vitamin A. Conversion of carotene is also limited in diseases of the intestine, liver and kidney and in diabetes. In hypothyroidism conversion is almost completely blocked.[1] How vitamin A is derived from carotene is still receiving intensive research; opinions vary as to mechanisms.

A significant seasonal variation has been reported for carotene but not for vitamin A.[29] It was noted in a study of nutrient intake and serum levels that the serum level of carotene reflected the nutrient intake of carotene, but that the serum level of vitamin A did not reflect the nutrient intake of vitamin A.[30] There appears to be no significant difference between fasting and random sampling of blood on the vitamin A level, provided that no form of vitamin A concentrate has been ingested.

Following a single oral dose of vitamin A in oil or in aqueous dispersion, the level of vitamin A in the blood rises to a maximum in about 3 hours for the latter and 5 hours for the former menstruum, and in both cases returns to normal in approximately 24 hours.[26] The magnitude of the response to the test dose is greater with vitamin A dispersed in aqueous media; however, in normal subjects, total absorption is essentially the same.

The relationship between serum levels and liver stores has been examined using the fluorescence microscopy method.[31] Good correlation between liver stores and serum levels of this vitamin was found; low serum vitamin A reflects low intake and also depleted liver stores.[31a] Serum levels of vitamin A and carotene have been called an expression of liver function.

It is believed that the vitamin A alcohol level of the blood is a better index of hepatic storage and vitamin A nutrition than is the total vitamin A level.[32] The latter is influenced by a postprandial rise, whereas the alcohol level is not. In the fasting state, 80 per cent of the vitamin A circulates in the blood as the alcohol form. The elevation of blood vitamin A in the postprandial state is caused largely by an increase in the ester form. The ester variety disappears in about 24 hours after the ingestion of the vitamin. The separation of the ester and alcohol form is carried out best by the chromatographic absorption method.[18]

VITAMIN D

Vitamin D deficiency can be defined biochemically as a disease in which the calcification process cannot keep pace with the synthesis of the organic matrix of bone.[33] The current methodology and metabolism-involving studies of vitamin D have been reviewed in excellent treatises.[34,35] In determining the state of nutrition with vitamin D, reliance must be placed on such indirect methods as blood levels of calcium, inorganic phosphate and alkaline phosphatase. No satisfactory chemical methods are available to measure either the concentration of this vitamin, its provitamin or a metabolic product.

In rickets there is generally a decreased blood level of inorganic phosphorus and an associated rise in alkaline phosphatase activity. Alteration of serum calcium is not so consistent, but there is generally a low level. These changes are, however, not specific for vitamin D deficiency. In uncomplicated cases of hyperactivity of the parathyroid, an elevated serum calcium is generally associated with a decreased level of serum phosphate. The alkaline phosphatase is increased above normal in various conditions other than rickets— hyperparathyroidism, Paget's disease, osteomalacia and metastatic carcinoma.

One of the difficulties with chemical methods is in separating interfering substances such as cholesterol and retinol which have chemical and physical properties similar to vitamin D;[35] a further complication is the small amounts of vitamin D which occur in biologic fluids and tissues. Thus, any reagent to be used for vitamin D detection must be extremely sensitive and specific for vitamin D. Since there is no such reagent, work has centered around the separation of vitamin D from cholesterol and retinol by a variety of chromatographic and photometric procedures[36–38] as well as by thin-layer chromatography;[39] they all suffer from a variety of limitations.

The use of alkaline phosphatase as a means of evaluating the state of vitamin D nutrition[40] has become popular, especially in survey studies. This method requires only 5 to 20 μl of serum. The reagent, sodium p-nitrophenyl phosphate, is a colorless compound but, with the splitting off of the phosphate group, the chromogenic salt of p-nitrophenol is liberated. This product of the phosphatase reaction on the reagent serves directly as a measure of enzymatic activity. One p-nitrophenyl phosphate unit is equivalent to 1.8 Bodansky units; one King-Armstrong unit is equivalent to 7.3 units of p-nitrophenyl phosphate. The normal level of serum alkaline phosphatase is given as 1.5 to 4.0 Bodansky units for the adult and 5 to 14 units for the child.

Most of the procedures for the determination of inorganic phosphorus in blood or serum use protein-free serum or blood extracts.[41] The extract is treated with molybdate in acid solution, forming phosphomolybdate. This is reduced by excess molybdate to give a blue color. Normal serum inorganic phosphorus levels range between 3 to 4.5 mg per 100 ml for adults and 4 to 6 mg for children. Serum calcium has also been used. An empiric rule for determining if a child is rachitic is to calculate the product of the serum phosphorus and serum calcium. If it is below 30, rickets is present or will develop; if it is above 40, it will not.

A bioassay for vitamin D in sera of animals and humans has also been used.[42] Thomas et al.[43] assayed the sera of 18 normal subjects and found them to contain between 0.7 and 3.1 I.U. of antirachitic activity per ml. The predominant antirachitic activity was associated with the alpha globulins of serum.

In adults, the body's needs for vitamin D are usually met by its own synthesis. Liver oils are rich in vitamin D: tuna, 7,000 to 50,000 I.U. per gm; cod, 60 to 300 I.U. per gm. The mammalian liver contains little vitamin D.[43a] Recent reports[43b] indicate that the active circulating form of vitamin D_3 is 25-hydroxycholecalciferol; this form is activated by the liver. Another, more potent form is believed to be 1,25-dihydroxycholecalciferol. This form is synthesized by the kidney from 25-hydroxycholecalciferol and returned to the circulation to activate bone formation.

A masterly review of this subject has appeared.[43c] Competitive binding assays for serum 25-hydroxycholecalciferol[43d,e] and 1,25-hydroxycholecalciferol[43f] have appeared; all use tritiated compounds and are not yet routine methods.

VITAMIN E (TOTAL TOCOPHEROLS)

There are many methods for determining vitamin E;[1,15,44-47] all are either biologic or chemical. The former measure biopotency of tocopherols without quantitating the tocopherols and take longer to complete.

The standard biologic method is the rat antisterility assay, in which female rats are depleted of vitamin E and mated with normal males. The material to be tested is administered in divided doses for some days after conception; the standard is given the same way. The rats are autopsied after 20 days of pregnancy and the numbers of living fetuses, dead fetuses and resorption sites are recorded.[46] The chemical methods are not all suitable for determining vitamin E in all types of samples, e.g. in biologic fluids and tissues. Determination of tocopherol in animal tissues can be carried out by means of column[47] or thin-layer chromatography,[48] but these are not suitable for large-scale nutrition studies involving biologic fluids. Another method involves the oxidation of tocopherol to tocopherol quinone, but this is not practical because of the interference of carotene and the rigid controls necessary for precise results.

An oxidimetric color reaction employs the Emmerie-Engel reaction.[49] This is based on the reduction of ferric ions to ferrous ions, which form a red color with a,a'-dipyridyl. Reading the reaction at 520 nm in a suitable instrument yields the results. This method has advantages over other techniques: It is rapid, reproducible and well suited to determine tocopherols in microquantities.[44] All the tocopherols give maximum color in the short time before measurements are made. The procedure measures total tocopherols in serum, plasma or tissues.[44] Tocopherols and carotenoids are extracted into xylene and the optical density of the extract is read at 460 nm to measure carotenoids. This reading is subtracted from that at 520 nm.[1] The maximum peak of absorption for tocopherols is at 520 nm and is developed 1.5 minutes after adding reagents.[1] Some workers use direct measurement for vitamin E in blood at 295 nm, but this is not recommended;[1] the low extinction value of tocopherol and interfering substances make it impractical. Serum or plasma may be stored frozen for 1 month without loss of tocopherol activity. When measuring vitamin E in tissue, it is important to know how results are affected by interfering substances, e.g. steroids in liver tissue.[1] Extraction by column chromatography and determination of vitamin E by gas-liquid chromatography aid in standardizing the technique when tissue vitamin E analysis is undertaken.

A procedure to determine 1 to 20 μg of α-tocopherol, extracted from 0.5 to 1.5 gm of animal tissue, by means of chromatographic techniques and the Emmerie-Engel reaction has been described.[1] This is an accurate and reproducible method for the determination of tocopherol in macro- and microquantities of plasma.[1,50] Many workers have found it useful in population and experimental studies of plasma tocopherol.[1,51,52]

In rats with experimentally induced vitamin E deficiency the erythrocytes are abnormally susceptible to hemolysis by H_2O_2.[53] In man[54] it has been shown that, in a variety of clinical conditions, the degree of hemolysis by this test is inversely related to the serum tocopherol concentration. Normal adults usually have serum tocopherol levels greater than 0.5 mg per 100 ml and it has been shown that, at and above this level, relatively little hemolysis (<20 per cent) occurs.[55,56]

VITAMIN K

There are several methods for vitamin K determination in pharmaceutic preparations and extracts from biologic materials. The Irreverre-Sullivan reaction is particularly useful for testing the fractions from column chromatography.[57,58] The K vitamin may be differentiated from other quinones by spectrography or by a color test;[58] biologic methods use chicks which are better suited for animal assays than are laboratory mammals.

Vitamin K is required to maintain normal plasma levels of the protein prothrombin (factor II) and of the other clotting factors, VII, IX and X,[59] apparently by mediating synthesis of a unique component γ-carboxyglutamate.[60a] Thus the prominent sign of vitamin K deficiency is prolonged time for clotting. The clinical manifestation is hemorrhage.

In general, prothrombin is measured by its ability to form thrombin which reacts with fibrinogen to form a clot. Actually, in most cases, prothrombin activity, not its concentration, is measured. An excellent discussion of the various methods used has been detailed.[59,60] For clinical purposes, the plasma prothrombin time of Quick, with various modifications, has been used widely.[60] This test is carried out by placing fresh blood in a tube containing a measured amount of thromboplastin. A clot normally should form in 25 to 40 seconds. In general, if the prothrombin clotting time is not greater than 20 to 25 per cent above normal, bleeding does not occur on the basis of prothrombin deficiency.

In view of the number of variable factors other than prothrombin content that influence the prothrombin time,[60a] plus the variety of methods used in determining it,[60] it is not surprising that it is difficult to define a prothrombin concentration below which hemorrhage will occur. Many believe that a concentration between 5 to 10 per cent of normal is a safe range.

THIAMIN

The many methods proposed for the analysis of thiamin can be classified into animal, microbiologic, chemical or physical; each has certain advantages and disadvantages.[1]

Chemical, microbiologic and erythrocyte transketolase methods are the most fre-

quently used for measuring thiamin in biologic fluids and tissues.

The chemical assay for thiamin depends upon the alkaline oxidation of thiamin by ferricyanide into thiochrome, which exhibits an intense blue fluorescence in ultraviolet light and can, therefore, be measured fluorometrically; the details of this reaction have been reviewed.[61] As with all fluorometric determinations, selection of appropriate purification procedures and blanks is most important. A purification method using synthetic zeolite Decalso has been modified for nutrition surveys.[62]

The assay of blood for thiamin by the thiochrome method presents problems,[63,64] since hematin catalyzes the destruction of thiochrome in alkaline solutions.[65] This seems to have been circumvented by removal of the hematin by precipitation with trichloroacetic acid. The retention of thiamin in proteins precipitated with trichloroacetic acid and incomplete hemolysis of red cells may limit the usefulness of this procedure;[66,67] also, the supernatants from trichloroacetic acid precipitates show a marked increase in fluorescence upon storage, which necessitates their analysis for thiamin immediately after preparation.[68] A macro-[69] and microprocedure[70] for thiamin in blood, employing the thiochrome method, has been reported and reviewed in detail.[65] Urine contains free thiamin so that it can be diluted and assayed directly by the thiochrome method, without prior treatment. A method for tissue thiamin has been described which permits the differentiation between thiamin and thiamin disulfide content by the thiochrome procedure.[71]

The main drawback of the thiochrome procedure is interference by fluorescing of nonthiamin substances; this is seen especially with urine. Its adequacy in detecting thiamin deficiency has been questioned by nutritional survey teams.[72] The measurement of red-blood-cell transketolase activity has been proposed for thiamin assay;[73,74] several modifications have been used.[74a,b] Transketolase is a thiamin-dependent enzyme. It catalyzes transfer of a 2-carbon fragment from a ketose to the aldehydic carbon of the aldose. The method involves incubation of hemolyzed washed red blood cells in a buffered medium with an excess of ribose-5-phosphate, both in the presence and absence of excess thiamin pyrophosphate. Disappearance of ribose-5-phosphate[73] by condensation with a 2-carbon intermediate to yield sedoheptulose-7-phosphate[74] is the indicator of thiamin activity.

Microorganisms which require thiamin fall into five categories. They may require (1) intact thiamin, (2) the pyrimidine moiety, (3) the thiazole moiety, (4) either the pyrimidine or the thiazole moiety and (5) both moieties. Man and other animals utilize only intact thiamin. Hence, the assay organism must respond only to the intact vitamin for use in assessing thiamin status. Compared with chemical methods, microbiologic assay methods for thiamin are more sensitive, more specific and require less equipment and material for assay—important considerations when many biologic samples are to be analyzed.

Microbiologic methods based on lactobacilli and yeast[65,75,76] suffer from poor reproducibility, partly because nonchemically defined media are used; also, lactobacilli are often stimulated nonspecifically by substances in biologic materials,[77,78] since these stimulants are inadequately supplied in published basal media. The phytoflagellate Ochromonas danica requires intact thiamin.[1] It does not respond to the thiazole or pyrimidine moieties as do the yeasts,[79,80] nor can it combine the thiazole and pyrimidine moieties.[80] It is a photosynthetic microanimal with a mammalian-like requirement for not only thiamin but also biotin.[1] It can assay 100 pg per ml of thiamin in biologic fluids and tissues. It also uses aseptically added thiamin pyrophosphate (cocarboxylase). Its metazoan-like permeability, as inferred from its sensitivity to a wide variety of antimetabolites, coupled with counteraction of these growth inhibitors by appropriate metabolites, makes it also a versatile instrument for mode-of-toxicity drug studies.[81,82] The medium supports heavy, rapid growth and is not appreciably stimulated by natural fluids such as blood. The method based on O. danica has been successful for assaying biologic fluids and tissues; others have confirmed it.[83]

Lactate and pyruvate blood levels are of little value, especially in mild thiamin deficiency and severe liver disease.[84,85] Transketolase values are of little diagnostic usefulness during severe liver disease; levels are low and never recover, even after thiamin treatment.[85,86] This prompted reports that a transketolase apoenzyme deficiency exists in severe liver disease.[85,86] Transketolase level is useful only in frank, long-standing thiamin deficiency,[84] when transketolase levels are invariably low but increase after thiamin treatment.

We have seen thiamin-normal individuals who show no increase in transketolase activity when thiamin pyrophosphate (TPP) is added to the red cell hemolysate.[86,87] In contrast, in thiamin deficiency the introduction of TPP into the hemolysate increased the transketolase activity, indicating the thiamin deficiency. We have also seen some thiamin-deficient individuals who, when treated with thiamin, do not show any increases in their deficient transketolase levels. Only upon the introduction of exogenous TPP into the hemolysate does transketolase activity increase, indicating a phosphorylating defect of administered thiamin in vivo. We have observed another group which, when treated with thiamin, still have deficient transketolase activity, despite TPP added in vitro. Most of the members of the latter group had liver disease. In some instances the transketolase level returned to normal when positive nitrogen balance was restored. This group thus seemed to have an apotransketolase deficiency, i.e. an inability to form or couple the protein moiety of the enzyme to the coenzyme.[87]

A better approach for determining

thiamin status is an assay for the intact vitamin, an assay which is sensitive and specific and which permits the earliest evaluation of total thiamin status and not of one of the many thiamin-dependent enzymes which depend on apoenzyme as well as coenzyme. Also, these enzymes may or may not be important in assaying thiamin nutrition (see beginning of chapter for discussion of enzyme assays). Blood thiamin, as measured with O. danica, seems to be a more sensitive indicator of thiamin deficiency. This is especially true in severe liver disease.[1,2,88]

A method for measuring tissue saturation with thiamin involves the determination of half-disappearance of intravenously administered thiamin. The faster the thiamin disappearance, the more depleted are the tissue stores.[88]

Thiamin excretion tests have been carried out either in the fasting state or for varying periods of time following oral or parenteral administration of this vitamin; microbial methods,[1-3,65,88] automated thiochrome methods[89] and ^{35}S thiamin HCl[90] have been used. With the thiochrome method an interfering fluorescent substance called F_2 is present in the urine.[91] This material has been identified as N'-methylnicotinamide.[92] There is now reason to believe that there are other extraneous substances in urine that also contribute to this fluorescence.[86] One of the most troublesome problems in the determination of urinary thiamin has been how to obtain a satisfactory blank.

A colorimetric method[93] uses p-aminoacetophenone, which couples with thiamin to produce an insoluble purple-red compound. Such substances as uric acid and ascorbic acid interfere with the development of the color and the removal of these interfering substances is difficult. The method also is not sensitive for material with a low content of thiamin.

The load test method has also been used, but there is considerable disagreement as to the level of excretion which indicates a deficiency state. A variety of forms of

thiamin are present in urine: thiamin, thiochrome, cocarboxylase and various degradation products, such as thiazole and pyrimidine moieties.[94] A method for determining the metabolites of thiamin in urine has been designed.[95] This method is based on the fact that bakers' yeast can synthesize thiamin from equal molar concentrations of pyrimidine and thiazole.

In our experience[1,96] and those of others,[97] it was found that an oral dose of thiamin made little change in the amount of thiamin in blood, whereas there was the expected increase in urinary excretion. When comparing oral absorption of thiamin[1,3] we have consistently found that thiamin propyldisulfide is better absorbed than thiamin hydrochloride. Circulatory and urinary thiamin levels are increased approximately tenfold with thiamin propyldisulfide. In contrast, thiamin hydrochloride will produce only slight increases in circulating levels and approximately threefold increase in urinary levels.

The amount of cocarboxylase in whole blood varies directly with the amount of total thiamin, as determined by biologic methods, and also with the degree of tissue saturation.[98] The decarboxylation of pyruvic acid requires the coenzyme cocarboxylase (thiamin pyrophosphate), and a deficiency of thiamin results in an elevation of blood pyruvic acid. The elevation of blood pyruvic levels, however, is not a specific indicator of thiamin lack, since other pathologic conditions are associated with an increase in the amount of this substance in blood. Except in severe thiamin deficiencies, the determination of fasting pyruvic levels in blood is not a reliable indicator of thiamin deficiency.[99]

Since both lactic and pyruvic acid are normally formed during carbohydrate metabolism, it was thought that the determination of the level and ratio of pyruvic and lactic acid in blood might be a reliable aid in evaluating thiamin nutrition. A test based on the fact that the rate of breakdown of pyruvic acid is directly related to the metabolic load of glucose and lactic acid was proposed.[100] Accordingly, the simultaneous determination of these three constituents under proper conditions was used to provide information regarding thiamin nutrition. The validity of such a test depends on pyruvate and lactate levels; these are not reliable in the case of thiamin evaluations.[84,99]

In conclusion, our experience shows that the protozoan method utilizing Ochromonas danica is best suited for determining metabolically active thiamin in man and animals; it is simple and unequivocal.[1]

Urinary load tests are of little value in grading the severity of a deficiency, not only of thiamin but of most vitamins. Considerable variation has been reported in the results from individuals supposedly under similar conditions.[99] These divergencies may be explained in part by: (1) differences in absorption from the gastrointestinal tract, (2) various renal threshold levels, (3) differences in the rate and volume of urine excreted, (4) inadequate emptying of the bladder, (5) varying amounts of the test dose administered and (6) different degrees of tissue breakdown as the result of the deficiency state. All these factors must be considered when urinary excretion studies are used to evaluate the nutrient state. Since we know so little about the renal threshold and metabolism of these nutrients, estimations upon urine, with or without test doses, are not valuable for assessing nutrition.[101]

BIOTIN

There are no chemical methods for biotin assay[102] but many biotin-requiring microorganisms are available: Saccharomyces cerevisiae,[103] Lactobacillus casei,[104] Lactobacillus arabinosus (now L. plantarum ATCC #8014),[105] Micrococcus sodonensis,[106] Neurospora crassa[107] and Rhizobium trifolii.[108] None has been applied satisfactorily for assaying biotin in biologic fluids. Lactobacillus casei is not specific because it requires certain uniden-

tified factors which affect the validity of biotin assays, particularly if the sample is low in biotin and relatively potent in unknown factors. S. cerevisiae, since biotin is strongly but variably spared by aspartic acid, oleic acid and pimelic acid, is thus not specific in its biotin requirement[109] despite its development as an ultramicroassay for biotin.[110] Because the flagellate Ochromonas danica has a specific and sensitive biotin requirement,[111] as do man and animals, it has been utilized as a reagent for biotin in blood, serum, urine, brain and liver tissue;[1] it has also been used in nutrition surveys for biotin.[1,2,52,84] The other method widely used utilizes Lactobacillus plantarum;[105] unlike O. danica it has its drawback as to specificity.

Pimelic acid, aspartic acid, Tween 80, alone or in combination, do not stimulate growth of O. danica;[111] these compounds spare biotin as an essential medium for some yeasts and lactobacilli.[112] Desthiobiotin, the sulfur-free analog of biotin, competitively inhibits the growth of O. danica.[111] Because O. danica is phagotrophic, it presumably ingests and digests low-molecular forms of biotin, e.g. biocytin; other organisms cannot use biocytin.[113]

RIBOFLAVIN

As with most vitamins, the first assays developed for riboflavin depended on the biologic response of animals.[114]

Until recently none of the laboratory procedures available has been entirely satisfactory for measuring riboflavin in biologic fluids and tissues.[115] Microbial and chemical methods have been used for riboflavin assay,[65,116] but, because of interfering substances and technical difficulties, these techniques have not been used widely for biologic fluids and tissues. Such difficulties have restricted riboflavin estimation to urinary excretion, in terms of μg per gm of creatinine, with inconsistent results. A detailed description of the more common methods for riboflavin analysis has been published.[116a]

The fluorometric method has been widely applied.[117] It has been used to measure free riboflavin, riboflavin 5-phosphate (FMN) and flavin adenine dinucleotide (FAD) in natural products as well as biologic fluids.[65,118] The most widely used assays are microbial and the most specific of these uses Tetrahymena thermophila WH$_{14}$ (ATCC #30008), a ciliate. This method gives excellent correlation with the more cumbersome fluorometric assays.[1,119] T. thermophila responds equally on a molar basis to riboflavin, FMN and FAD. The growth curve for riboflavin is superimposable on those for FMN and FAD when molarities are taken into account. Therefore T. thermophila permits estimation of total riboflavin.

The riboflavin requirement for T. thermophila is specific, sensitive, rapid and reproducible enough for assay of large numbers of biologic fluids and tissues.[1,52,84] Traces of fatty acids result in too-high riboflavin values when other assay organisms[116,120,121] are used—an obvious drawback when dealing with fatty acid and lipid-rich fluids and tissues. In assay of fluids and tissues for riboflavin by the Lactobacillus casei method,[120] growth stimulation and drift in blood and tissues were noted.[119] Tween 80 (polyoxyethylene sorbitan mono-oleate) lessened but did not eliminate drift. Presumably, traces of other fatty acids and other compounds in the fluids and tissues were stimulating L. casei, thus yielding falsely high riboflavin values. Obviously, removal of traces of fats from 1-ml aliquots of biologic fluids would entail great losses of sample material and time, especially if many samples were to be assayed. The Lactobacillus medium gave high blanks.[119]

Since T. thermophila in riboflavin-limited media is not stimulated by fats in blood and tissues or by ingredients in the medium, use of T. thermophila obviates the drawbacks listed for lactobacilli.[1,78] The T. thermophila method[119] has proved readily adaptable to routine or large-scale assays,[1,2,52,106] not only because it is sensitive and specific for riboflavin but also because it is simple, inexpensive and requires few precautions.

The fluorometric procedure is too slow and poorly suited for large-scale studies because of the involved preliminary procedures before determinations can be made.[118] Special precautions must be taken: Tissues have to be finely ground at 0 to 4°C, centrifugation must be at 4°C and, until neutralized, the samples must be kept as cold as possible to prevent hydrolysis of flavin adenine dinucleotide. Other sample aliquots must then be kept at room temperature in the dark for 2 days to complete hydrolysis of FAD to FMN; then, after incubation and neutralization, care must be taken to protect the samples from light, since both riboflavin and FMN are more sensitive to destruction by light in the concentrated salt solution needed for the final fluorometric determination. Caution must be taken to dilute the samples properly to prevent interference from other substances present. The calculations are laborious. Considering the lengthy preliminary procedures and the extra precautions necessary for fluorometric analysis, with only a slight gain in sensitivity, e.g. 0.1 ng per ml with the fluorometric analysis versus 0.5 ng per ml with the T. thermophila assay (values practically meaningless in analysis of biologic fluids and tissues), the T. thermophila method has fewer pitfalls and permits more assays per unit effort.

In a preliminary survey of riboflavin disappearance in 32 randomly selected subjects, after intravenous administration of 5 mg of flavin mononucleotide, the half-time clearance for riboflavin in 27 subjects with riboflavin levels above 100 ng per ml was slower than in 5 subjects with levels below 80 ng per ml.[119] Clearance of intravenously administered riboflavin may be useful as a rapid measure of tissue avidity for riboflavin: the more depleted the riboflavin tissue pool, the quicker is the clearance of administered riboflavin from the circulation.

Methods have been developed for the determination of riboflavin in urine based on the use of either microbiologic[1,120] or fluorometric procedures.[118] The latter methods involve measuring the fluorescence produced by the flavin in urine when subjected to light of prescribed wavelengths. The quantity of riboflavin in urine can also be assayed by measuring the rate of acid produced by Lactobacillus casei. The high levels of urea cause lowering of the titrimetric microbiologic results with L. casei.[99]

Extensive investigations have been carried out in the hopes of correlating urinary riboflavin excretion with nutritional status. Some of the various methods employed have determined the amount of urinary riboflavin excreted in, for example, 1 hour while fasting, during 24 hours and after the administration of load tests.[99] There is no consistent agreement among workers in the interpretation of their results.[122] It has been demonstrated that not only is the excretion of riboflavin affected by the dietary intake but it is proportional to the volume of urine excreted and inversely related to the level of protein intake.[123]

The value of load tests in appraising riboflavin nutrition has not been settled. It is unlikely that urinary excretion is an accurate estimation of riboflavin nutrition, since changes in tissue saturation are expected with different levels of intake.[124]

There is a wide variation for serum riboflavin values. The total riboflavin content of red blood cells[125] or whole blood[119] is considered to be a reasonable, sensitive and practical index of riboflavin nutritional status.

An enzymatic approach utilizing $NADPH_2$-dependent glutathione reductase from red cells has been proposed for measurement of riboflavin status in man.[74b,125a,b,c] The enzyme has FAD as a cofactor and reflects riboflavin status (see earlier critique on enzyme assays). However, the specificity of the erythrocyte glutathione reductase activity may be altered by other diseases, for example, hematologic disease, and by riboflavin antagonists and other pharmacologic agents. The effects of other vitamin deficiencies, for example, B_6,[116a] on the enzyme activity remains uncertain. Care is needed in interpreting glutathione reductase activity in diabetics. Alterations appear related to lesions in carbohydrate metabolism; thus, diabetics may have *increased* erythrocyte glutathione reductase activity, which is, supposedly, unrelated to riboflavin metabolism.[116a] There seems to be no abnormal metabolite in the urine of riboflavin-deficient subjects which could serve as a marker for a riboflavin-deficient state.

NIACIN (NICOTINIC ACID)

Recognition that many bacteria require niacin for growth has resulted in the development of microbial assay methods for niacin and closely related niacin-active compounds. Many methods are not specific,[117] causing drifts in organism growth because of an incomplete medium or stimulatory substances in the unknown sample. The use of Tetrahymena thermophila has obviated these objections. The protozoan is sensitive and specific for niacin and niacinamide.[1,126] Microbial assay methods are particularly well adapted to the simultaneous assay of many samples. The microbial method used by many investigators employs Lactobacillus plantarum ATCC #8014.[126,127] L. plantarum responds to niacin, niacinamide and nicotinuric acid;[117] nicotinuric acid is not biologically active. Hence T. thermophila has a higher specificity.

There are several chemical methods for niacin determination.[128,129] Most are based on the use of organic reagents which yield colored niacin derivatives that can be quantitated photometrically; most are plagued by extraction difficulties as well as by a lack of specificity for niacin. The two principal metabolites of niacin and niacinamide excreted in urine of man are N'-methylnicotinamide (MN) and the 6-pyridone of MN. MN reacts with ketones in alkaline solutions to produce a green fluorescent compound. An excess of acid converts this compound to another more stable substance with a blue fluorescence that may be measured with a fluorophotometer. The pyridone does not interfere with MN determinations. The original method[130] and modifications[127] have been used. This method measures non-metabolic catabolites of niacin. Most niacin in blood and tissues is found as NAD, $NADH_2$, NADP and $NADPH_2$. Chemical methods used for niacin determinations in blood[131] and tissues[132] depend on the highly fluorescent products formed with both pyridine nucleotides after proper extraction.

An enzymatic-fluorometric method for the determination of pyridine nucleotides in tissue has been developed which is based on the observation that a neutralized alkaline extract of tissues contains $NADH_2$ and $NADPH_2$ plus smaller amounts of NAD and NADP which arise from auto-oxidation. The auto-oxidation was compensated for by adding simultaneously alcohol dehydrogenase and acetaldehyde, to completely oxidize the $NADH_2$ to NAD and glucose-6-phosphate, and glucose-6-phosphate dehydrogenase to reduce all of the NADP to $NADPH_2$. The NAD and $NADPH_2$ are measured fluorometrically.[133,134] This method has been extremely useful for studying alcoholism.[135] The NAD/NADH ratio permits an indirect measure of alcohol dehydrogenase activity as well as a measure of alcohol oxidation in vivo.[135]

The number of products of niacin metabolism that appear in the urine are many and they vary from species to species. The end-products of niacin metabolism in man are MN and its pyridone. In addition to these and other derivatives, a number of intermediates on the tryptophan-niacin pathway are excreted; therefore, MN excretion is particularly susceptible to the influences of non-nutritional factors. Since both MN and the pryidone depend on methylation for their formation, a lower excretion might be expected no matter what the niacin intake is, if insufficient methyl groups are available.[136]

Workers disagree on what percentage of niacin is excreted as MN.[99] They also have diverging views regarding the significance of 24-hour urinary excretion studies. One group contends that the determination of MN for a 24-hour period is of little help in evaluating niacin nutrition. Another group feels that there is reasonably good correlation between the excretion of this compound and dietary and clinical findings.[99] The different findings in different studies undoubtedly are the result in part of the variety of methods used, as well as of inter- and intraindividual variations. Differences among persons in methylating ability may also partly account for variance. At present, the excretion levels of MN in the urine during fasting and after administration of load test doses of niacin are the only chemical procedures available for appraising niacin nutrition.

There is an acute need for more accurate methods for estimating body niacin. Assay with T. thermophila can fill this void. Use of T. thermophila permits a wider assay range and more comprehensive responses than does the use of Lactobacillus plantarum. In our hands the range of L. plantarum was 3 to 30 ng per ml, as compared with 1 to 300 ng per ml for T. thermophila. Some naturally occurring niacin derivatives were tested with T. thermophila;[126] only niacin and niacinamide permitted full growth. 1-Methylnicotinamide and 1-ethylnicotinamide showed some activity, but compounds having other modifications of the carboxyl groups did not elicit growth. Trigonelline (the betaine of nicotinic acid), which has no animal activity, proved inert for T.

thermophila. The organism's requirement seems to parallel that of higher animals. MN and its 6-keto derivatives, some of the principal excretion products in man, are not active for T. thermophila.

The cellular components of whole blood contribute the greatest niacin activity. Such results are to be expected since red blood cells contain much NAD and NADP activity.[137-139] The chief excretory products of nicotinic acid in human urine include nicotinuric acid (nicotinoylglycine) and N'-methylnicotinamide (MN). Tetrahymena thermophila does not respond to either compound, whereas L. plantarum does,[140] another point of specificity favoring T. thermophila, if it is assumed that clinical status is reflected by niacin activity rather than by niacin plus its catabolic derivatives. Highly pigmented urines do not interfere with this assay as they do with the MN determination.[130]

The biosynthesis and metabolism of nicotinic acid in disease have received little attention; metabolic studies deal mainly with normal animals and man.[1,226,227] After a tryptophan load dose, the main catabolites in the urine are nicotinuric acid, MN, nicotinamide, quinolinic acid, kynurenine, 6-pyridone, anthranilic acid and 3-hydroxyanthranilic acid.

VITAMIN B$_6$

Vitamin B$_6$ can be determined microbiologically, enzymatically or chemically.[14,74b,141,142] Some chemical analyses are done by measuring the fluorescence of the cyanohydrin of pyridoxal.[143] Chromatographic methods have also been used.[15,144] Microbiologic determinations can be carried out with Escherichia coli mutants, Saccharomyces carlsbergensis 4228, Streptococcus faecalis, and Lactobacillus casei.[142,145] The above organisms lack sensitivity and specificity when detecting vitamin B$_6$ in biologic fluids, nor have the results been correlated with the clinical signs of B$_6$ deficiency. Indirect methods for determining B$_6$ status in biologic fluids include the

transaminase method, the xanthurenic acid-kynurenine method and a method utilizing circulating leukocytes. The transaminase system is based on the dependence on pyridoxal-5-phosphate of the alanine (SGPT) and aspartic (SGOT) transaminases in the serum. B$_6$ deficiency results in decreased plasma alanine and aspartic transaminases;[74b] the alanine enzyme appears to be more sensitive.[146] Three other enzymatic methods have been developed for the estimation of pyridoxal phosphate in biologic materials. One is based on tyrosine decarboxylase and the liberation of CO_2.[147] Another method measures pyridoxal phosphate enzymatically by estimating activity of a tyrosine decarboxylase preparation that has pyridoxal phosphate as a cofactor.[147a] The third depends on the tryptophanase-catalyzed breakdown of tryptophan to indole, pyruvic acid and ammonia.[148]

It seems probable that, using the enzyme methods, only free pyridoxal phosphate or that loosely bound to protein is measured. Thus, any pyridoxal phosphate bound with holoenzymes would not be measured.[99] A disturbance of B$_6$ metabolism, through derangement of tryptophan metabolism, gives rise to excretion of excess xanthurenic acid in the urine, and some workers have used xanthurenic acid excretion as an index of B$_6$ status in man. There is disagreement about the validity and specificity of the xanthurenic acid titer as an index of B$_6$ deficiency,[149] e.g. high xanthurenic acid levels in human urine have been found, unrelated to pathologic or clinical changes due to B$_6$ deficiency.[150] Riboflavin deficiency also produces high urine levels of tryptophan catabolites.[9a] Nongravid women[151] and women in the last trimester of pregnancy[152] have been reported to excrete tryptophan catabolites equivalent to 2 to 3 times the tryptophan intake even though the absorption of vitamin B$_6$ was normal. Marked increases in xanthurenic acid excretion occur in toxemias of pregnancy[153] although xanthurenic acid itself is not toxic.[149] Elderly subjects were found to excrete about twice as much xanthurenic acid as young subjects in a 24-hour period after tryptophan loading, a defect abolished by vitamin B_6 therapy.[154] The tryptophan load test is not a real test of absolute B_6 deficiency. An intake of 10 gm DL-tryptophan upsets the amino acid balance and causes a severe stress that does not exist under normal conditions.[155] A methionine-loading test for determining B_6 adequacy has been proposed.[155a] During B_6 depletion, methionine loading (3 gm L-methionine orally) induced a marked excretion of cystathionine which was prevented by B_6 supplementation.[155a,b] Pregnant women excreted much cystathionine after methionine loading; the ratio of cystathionine/cysteine sulfinic acid was elevated.[155a]

The leukocyte method estimates pyridoxal phosphate in isolated leukocytes; it is based on a coenzyme-catalyzed tyrosine decarboxylase system from S. faecalis.[156] A comparison of pyridoxal phosphate content of circulating leukocytes in nonpregnant women, women at term and umbilical cord blood showed higher values in nonpregnant controls; cord blood showed the highest values.[157] Enough data are not yet at hand to evaluate this method.

4-Pyridoxic acid has frequently been used as an indicator of B_6 status.[142,160] It is the principal excretion product from B_6 ingestion in man.[149,158] However, it has been reported that, in subjects on a normal diet, pyridoxic acid excretion accounted for only about half the intake of vitamin B_6.[159] This method is, therefore, not a totally reliable indicator of B_6 status.

The increased urinary excretion of oxalate in B_6-deficient rats and man[161] suggests the possible use of urinary oxalate as a criterion of B_6 adequacy.

Tetrahymena thermophila has been used to assay for vitamin B_6.[1,162] Its vitamin requirements cannot be bypassed, e.g. its vitamin B_6 requirement cannot be satisfied or even spared by amino acids, including D-alanine, effective for such bacteria as Streptococcus faecalis and Lactobacillus casei.[142,163] Response to D-alanine also makes Saccharomyces carlsbergensis unreliable for assaying B_6 in blood.[163] Because T. thermophila has a lesser response to pyridoxol (pyridoxine), it has been criticized as being less valuable for assaying B_6 in plants where pyridoxol predominates. This does not detract from its use for assaying B_6 in biologic fluids and tissues were pyridoxal and pyridoxamine predominate.

Measurement of vitamin B_6 activity using enzyme systems involves knowledge of two variables: (1) concentration of coenzyme pyridoxal phosphate and (2) concentration of apoenzyme. Normal enzyme activity would indicate adequate concentration of both components, but decreased activity could mean a decrease in either or both. Since T. thermophila has a mammalian-like requirement for vitamin B_6, it permits a direct measure of all metabolically active vitamin B_6 in man, rather than merely a determination of the function of individual enzymes which may not give a true reflection of the vitamin B_6 status.

With Tetrahymena thermophila the B_6 distribution in blood was studied.[162] In 15 normal subjects, the ratio of plasma to red cells ranged between 1.5 and 4.6. The mean B_6 for whole blood is 37 ± 6, for red cells 20 ± 3 and for plasma 59 ± 13 ng per ml. Tetrahymena thermophila, like man and animals, does not utilize B_6 in the presence of B_6 antagonists.[162] It is inhibited by D-, L-, and DL-penicillamine and isonicotinic acid hydrazide; penicillamine is the more potent B_6 antagonist.

PANTOTHENIC ACID

Chemical and animal methods for pantothenate assay are unsuited for biologic materials.[164,165] Saccharomyces carlsbergensis, Lactobacillus plantarum,[1,166] Lactobacillus casei, Acetobacter suboxydans[15] and Tetrahymena thermophila[1,166] have been used. S. carlsbergensis lacks specificity; this yeast produces its own pantothenate.[165] L. casei was replaced by L. plantarum because L. casei needs a complex medium for growth and is stimulated by fatty material in biologic materials when assaying for pantothenate.[166] Pantothenyl alcohol is inactive for A. suboxydans but pantoic acid is very active,[15] so that the alcohol must be hydrolyzed to pantoic acid before using this assay. T. thermophila is used[166] when nonspecific contamination from natural products becomes a drawback.[13] Pantothenol and pantoyl lactose (with or without the addition of D-alanine) and coenzyme A are inactive for Tetrahymena[167] and L. plantarum; neither of which is stimulated by fats.[1]

There is no free pantothenate in blood; it is all bound. The vitamin can be released by an alkaline phosphatase and an enzyme from avian liver.[165] This liberates pantothenate from coenzyme A in a variety of foods and tissues. Treatment with diastase gives more reliable results than autolysis, acid hydrolysis, treatment with mylase P or combinations of diastase and papain or liver enzyme and alkaline phosphatase.[166] Diastase is free from pantothenate contamination. The other enzymes contain enough pantothenate to make results unreliable. In urine, the vitamin is unbound; results show no increase with enzyme hydrolysis. Pantothenic acid shows the same concentration in blood and cerebrospinal fluid.[1]

L. plantarum and T. thermophila are reliable reagents for pantothenate in tissues and biologic fluids.[165,166,168] Results with both organisms are similar.[1,166]

VITAMIN C (ASCORBIC ACID)

Vitamin C is the only water-soluble vitamin for which there is no microbial assay. Biologic assays generally have been replaced by chemical methods. Biologic tests are used now only to ensure that ascorbic acid is being measured.

Methods for determining ascorbic acid are many.[169,170] The methods of choice for determination of ascorbic acid status in humans involve plasma or serum ascorbic acid concentration[1] and white blood cell-blood platelet ascorbate concentration, which is more closely related to tissue stores.[1] Two types of procedures are used: One is based upon the oxidation of ascorbic acid by 2,6-dichlorophenolindophenol and the other upon the color formed by treating with 85 per cent H_2SO_4, the derivative produced by coupling oxidized ascorbic acid with 2,4-dinitrophenylhydrazine.[170] Titration and colorimetric techniques using 2,6-dichlorophenolindophenol suffer from interference from pigments and extraneous reducing substances in biologic fluids.[99] A modified method, using a combination of the two procedures,[171,172] has been devised and has served well in large-scale nutrition surveys and clinical situations.[2,52]

Samples for total ascorbate assay are best stored frozen, after precipitation of protein and separation of the acid extract containing the ascorbate. Ascorbate remains stable for two months when treated in this way. Samples not so treated should be processed within two weeks of freezer storage. Some solutions used in the procedure are labile and are best made fresh if the test is done infrequently.

Polarography and spectrophotometry have been used to measure ascorbate. Polarography offers no advantages over the chemical methods. Spectrophotometric methods are not adequate because of the weak absorption of ascorbate and prevalence of interfering substances.[169] Enzymatic and chromatographic assays have been used;[169] however, they have limited use in biologic materials. The most satisfactory chemical assays are based on reduction of 2,6-dichlorophenolindophenol or the formation of a colored dinitrophenylhydrazine derivative.[170] Dichlorophenolindophenol is blue in neutral and pink in acid solutions. In acid extracts ascorbic acid reduces dichlorophenolindophenol, at pH

1 to 4, to the colorless leuco form. Thiosulfate, ferrous, cuprous, stannous salts and heated sugar solutions (reductones) interfere with this method because they also reduce indophenol.

The dinitrophenylhydrazine methods are sensitive and specific for ascorbate.[170] The reaction depends upon the coupling of 2,4-dinitrophenylhydrazine to the keto groups of carbon 2 and 3 of diketogulonic acid to form a bis-2,4-dinitrophenylhydrazone—an osazone. In strong acid the osazone rearranges to a stable reddish-brown product which can be measured photometrically. Ascorbic acid must first be oxidized to dehydroascorbate for this reaction to occur. In the modified method,[1] 2,6-dichlorophenolindophenol is used as the *oxidizer*. We found dichlorophenolindophenol to be superior to activated charcoal or copper:[1] copper ions caused precipitate to form in the extracts. The use of dichlorophenolindophenol simplifies the method, especially for large-scale studies. The strong acid medium permits the dehydroascorbate to be hydrolyzed to diketogulonic acid so that hydrazone formation can take place.[173] Other reductones react slowly with dinitrophenylhydrazine and their osazones are unstable in high acid concentrations. Addition of thiourea as a reducer increases specificity by avoiding interference from nonascorbate chromogens.[1]

A 3-hour incubation of the acidic extracts at 37°C works well. Five per cent metaphosphoric acid has been used to extract ascorbic acid, precipitate protein, inactivate the enzymes which oxidize ascorbate acid and produce the required acidic milieu for the analysis.[170] We have found 5 per cent trichloroacetic acid (TCA) equally effective.[1] Once ascorbate is extracted with TCA, it can be stored frozen before assay. We have obtained excellent recoveries of ascorbate (96 to 102 per cent) and no gross errors as a result of the formation of chromogenic materials with sugars or glucuronic acid.

In adults, plasma ascorbate levels of 0.4 to 1.4 mg per 100 ml reflect a daily ascorbate intake of 70 mg or more; less than 0.2 mg per 100 ml indicates less than a 25-mg daily intake of ascorbate. In children, a plasma concentration of approximately 1.0 mg per 100 ml indicates an ascorbate intake of about 1.5 mg per kg body weight, whereas ascorbate intake of 0.2 mg per kg will give serum ascorbate levels of 0 to 0.1 mg per 100 ml.

When tissues are saturated with vitamin C, the plasma ascorbate levels lie between 0.8 to 1.5 mg per 100 ml; the whole blood levels are between 1.0 to 1.5 mg per 100 ml and the buffy coat ascorbate levels are between 25 to 35 mg per 100 ml.

A wide variety of load test methods for the analysis of ascorbic acid nutrition has been proposed. In general, individuals with low intakes of ascorbic acid excrete less of a given dose than do those on an adequate or saturating intake. The load test provides a fairly good index of tissue depletion and parallels moderately well the fasting plasma levels. However, the load test does not distinguish between varying degrees of deficiency states. The sensitivity of load tests may be increased if larger doses are administered.[99]

The known products of ascorbic acid catabolism do not offer great possibilities for assessment of ascorbic acid status, partly because ascorbic acid is basically a carbohydrate and many of its known metabolic products can arise from other sources. The products of ingested ascorbate excreted in urine are primarily oxalate, 2,3-diketogulonic acid, ascorbic acid and dehydroascorbic acid.[174] On an individual basis, all patients with scurvy will have serum ascorbate levels of zero, but not all persons with zero ascorbic acid levels will have scurvy.[1] Increased amounts of ascorbate are excreted in urine with increasing intake.[228]

Complete elimination of vitamin C from the diet, as seen by us in 5 patients on a complete restriction of food and vitamins, resulted in a serum ascorbate of zero within 35 to 40 days; the whole blood levels reached zero in about 80 to 90 days, and the white cell levels reached zero in 100 to 120 days. When the white cell level reached zero, clinical scurvy became manifest. White cell ascorbate seems best to reflect tissue stores, while plasma levels reflect intake within the preceding weeks.[1] Nevertheless, vitamin C levels in plasma, whole blood and white blood cells all correlate.[228a]

VITAMIN B$_{12}$

Most studies agree that protozoan methods are the most sensitive and specific way to measure metabolically and clinically active forms of B$_{12}$ in biologic fluids and tissues or in B$_{12}$-containing products.[1,2,12] These methods employ the protozoans Euglena gracilis or Ochromonas malhamensis.[1] Such methods can be used to follow B$_{12}$ metabolism in vitro or in vivo.[1,2,175]

Assay of vitamin B$_{12}$ by physiochemical means is difficult because B$_{12}$ occurs in exceptionally low concentrations in nature. Such assays are usually carried out on relatively concentrated solutions of the vitamin, e.g. pharmaceutical preparations and B$_{12}$ feed concentrates, and then only when the B$_{12}$ is freed from interfering impurities.[15]

The availability of ^{57}Co, ^{58}Co, ^{60}Co-vitamin B$_{12}$ has permitted the wide application of tracer techniques for detecting B$_{12}$.[176] They are more expensive and less adaptable to routine use than the microbiologic ones with discrepancies between results.[177-179] Since the Schilling test is biologic, the factors influencing reproducibility are multiple and not all apparent.[180] Radioactivity techniques require close cooperation between patient and analyst throughout. The Schilling test, for example, requires that the patient fast for 12 hours and drink no water for 4 hours before the test. After the radioactive oral dose, the patient must wait 90 to 120 minutes for the intramuscular dose of non-labeled vitamin B$_{12}$ and the urine must be

carefully collected for 24 hours after the load doses.[1] In the B$_{12}$ absorption feces test, the feces must be diligently collected by the patient for 1 to 7 days after a radioactive load dose.[1] In the hepatic-uptake test,[181] the radioactivity after an oral dose is measured with a surface scintillation counter over the liver after the radioactivity has disappeared from the intestine, either spontaneously or after purgation. Indeed, in these tracer tests, the patience of patient and tester is critical.

The measurement of serum vitamin B$_{12}$ level by radioisotope dilution with albumin-coated charcoal has been introduced[182] and has been adapted to intrinsic-factor assay.[183] This method is based on the adsorption of free B$_{12}$ by albumin-coated charcoal. Residual B$_{12}$ is then determined directly by radioactivity counts with the use of labeled B$_{12}$. Charcoal absorption of B$_{12}$ has been used for the isotopic determination of B$_{12}$ binding capacity and concentration in biologic fluids.[184] Another method uses zinc sulfate instead of charcoal.[185] Validity of the charcoal assay of bound B$_{12}$ or B$_{12}$ binding capacity of body fluids is questionable, especially when dealing with gastric materials.[181] Isotope methods give higher values than microbial assays and therefore obscure the "true B$_{12}$" value as well as diagnosis.[181a] Evidence has recently been presented to explain why routinely used radiodilution methods yield inappropriately high values for cobalamins.[181c] It was shown that R proteins (cobalamin-binding protein in human gastric juice that is devoid of intrinsic factor activity, designated as protein R because of its rapid mobility on electrophoresis) provided in several assay kits bind a wide variety of biologically inactive cobalamin analogs besides vitamin B$_{12}$ present in serum. These inactive analogs are present in sufficient concentration to interfere substantially with the radiodilution assay for vitamin B$_{12}$ when pure R protein is used as the binder in that assay. As a result, biologically inactive cobalamin analogs present in human plasma can mask vitamin B_{12} deficiency because current radioisotope dilution assays are not specific for true vitamin B_{12}.[181c] Much data show almost invariable correlation between clinical vitamin B_{12} deficiency and low serum vitamin B_{12} activity as measured with protozoan reagents, e.g. *Euglena gracilis* and *Ochromonas malhamensis*.[1,181d] This reliability appears not true of the radiodilution assays tested.[181d] Tracer methods also require expensive radioisotopes, counters and larger samples[181b] and risk raising the radiation background on prolonged use.

Biochemical tests for B_{12} have been introduced. Some workers have found an increased urinary excretion of amino-imidazole-carboxamide (AIC) in patients with untreated pernicious anemia;[186] however, this test is not specific for B_{12} deficiency, since high AIC is also excreted during folate deficiency[187] and other unrelated stress situations.[188] Proper propionic metabolism depends on the B_{12} coenzyme for conversion of malonyl CoA to succinyl CoA. In severe deficiency propionic acid excretion rises and falls after B_{12} treatment. Folate deficiency does not affect this pattern.[188] Such results indicate that methylmalonyl CoA isomerase is lowered in B_{12} deficiency; hence, methylmalonic acid (MMA) excretion should increase. This reasoning has been substantiated: MMA excretion is indeed high during a B_{12} deficiency.[189] There seems to be no correlation between urinary titer of MMA and degree of hematologic or neurologic abnormalities. In some patients, MMA excretion continued even after the hematologic abnormalities and serum vitamin B_{12} returned to normal.[190] Other workers have used preloading with saline or valine as a means of increasing MMA excretion during B_{12} deficiency;[191] preloading with propionic acid does not seem suitable.[190] Unfortunately the MMA excretion method is complex and not accurate.[192]

Lactobacillus lactis was the first microorganism used to identify the then unknown vitamin B_{12} in the refined liver extracts used for treating pernicious anemia.[1] L. lactis Dorner (ATCC 8000), L. leichmannii, and *Escherichia coli* mutants have also been used to assay for vitamin B_{12}.[193,194] When the lactic acid bacteria are used, deoxyribosides replace B_{12} in the assay and can invalidate results.[12] Methionine will do the same when the E. coli mutant or thermophiles are used for B_{12} assay.[12] Bacterial assays thus lack specificity.[1,12]

Although B_{12} can be assayed biologically with mice, rats, chicks and radio cobalt, the protozoan method of assay is preferred because of its economy, sensitivity— detects 1 pg B_{12} per ml—and relative freedom from stimulation in biologic fluids and tissues. As inferred in the beginning of the chapter, ordinary antibiotics do not interfere with protozoan assay methods if the original directions are followed.[1] Neither deoxyribosides nor methionine can replace the B_{12} requirement.[1,12] Euglena gracilis is not as specific for B_{12} as O. malhamensis.[1,12] Serum and blood from normal subjects have a growth-promoting effect on Euglena above that seen with Ochromonas.[193] The reason for such stimulation is obscure, since no known pseudoforms of B_{12} have yet been found in biologic fluids. That the O. malhamensis method is superior for assay of B_{12} in natural materials was made clear by the agreement of Ochromonas and chick assays.[1,12] When Ochromonas, Euglena, L. leichmannii and E coli assays for B_{12} in blood, serum and urine were compared, Ochromonas was the most dependable.[195] Serum or whole blood can be assayed, which simplifies the procedure.[1]

The specific vitamin B_{12} requirement of O. malhamensis still remains undisputed: It is exactly like man's and is unlike Euglena's.[1,12] B_{12} was the only vitamin to overcome the antagonistic action of various thyroactive compounds on the growth of O. malhamensis.[196] These findings suggested that O. malhamensis, like animals, could be used as an indicator of thyroactive substances and thyroid antagonists in man.[1] Because of its simplicity, specificity and freedom from pitfalls, we routinely use O. malhamensis for assaying B_{12}.[1]

FOLATES

Chick assays were probably the first determinations of what is now called folic acid (pteroylglutamic acid, PGA). Like all animal assays they were costly and time consuming. Chemical methods are not useful for unfractionated biologic materials.[1] They are applicable mainly to pharmaceutic preparations, particularly those having folic acid as sole active constituent. Chromatographic methods are valuable for differentiating folates in biologic fluids when coupled with appropriate microbial assay systems.[197]

Indirect methods for determining folate status have been proposed.[197–199] One depends on estimating the formiminoglutamic acid (FIGLU) arising from histidine catabolism. FIGLU is normally converted into glutamic acid by donating its formimino group to tetrahydrofolate (THF). In severe folate deficiency no acceptor THF is available; hence, large amounts of FIGLU are excreted. Urocanic acid, the precursor of FIGLU, is also excreted in folate deficiency. Many methods are available for estimating FIGLU[192,199] and urocanic acid.[192,197,199] Both tests are nonspecific for folate deficiency;[192,199] abnormal urinary excretion of histidine catabolites is found in patients with vitamin B_{12} deficiency as well as in folic-deficient patients.[192,199] Indeed, many pregnant women with folate megaloblastic anemias, as proven by treatment, excreted *normal* amounts of FIGLU.[200] Folic acid abolishes the excretion of abnormal histidine catabolites, but so does vitamin B_{12}, methionine or glycine.[192,199,201] Increased excretion of histidine catabolites is, therefore, not a specific index of folate deficiency. Alanine interferes with the FIGLU deter-

mination[202] and makes determinations unreliable.

Another indirect test proposed to detect folate deficiency is one which measures excretion of 4(5)-amino-5(4)-imidazole-carboxamide (AIC). AIC, as the ribotide, is formylated in vivo to yield formamido-imidazole carboxamide ribotide, an intermediate in purine synthesis. The formyl group is donated by N^{10}-formyl-THF. In folate deficiency, this conversion should be crippled because N^{10}-formyl-THF is lacking; the substrate AIC accumulates.[192] However, AIC is increased in B_{12} as well as folate deficiency.[203,204] This test,[205] like that for FIGLU, does not distinguish between folate and B_{12} deficiency.[192,199]

Recently tritiated folic acid became available, making possible a nonmicrobiologic method for studying folic metabolism. This technique has been used to monitor uptake, metabolism and excretory products of folic acid.[192,199,206] The ^{3}H-labeled compounds excreted after intravenous ^{3}H-folate were N^{10}-formyl folate, p-amino-benzoylglutamate, and PGA. The N^5-methyl-THF that was also excreted was not labeled but was displaced from the liver and did not arise from the administered labeled folic acid.[199,207]

Nearly all microbiologic assays for folate activity have used Streptococcus faecalis, Lactobacillus casei, and Pediococcus cerevisiae.[1,199] Earlier it appeared that these organisms did not lend themselves to detecting folic acid deficiency in man, e.g. in one study using S. faecalis there was no detectable activity in the fasting serum of humans.[208] Our own studies confirm this.[209] Administration of a loading dose of folic acid with subsequent assay by S. faecalis has been used as a workable means of detecting folic acid deficiency, but this technique has drawbacks.[210] Because of the multiplicity of folic acid factors reported in whole blood, the microbiologic assay for folic acid in *whole blood*, not serum, is regarded as valueless.[1] Our results show that almost no administered folic acid is taken up by the red cell, despite high plasma folate which serves to saturate the tissue (liver) stores.[138,139] Low red cell folates persist despite saturation of tissue and *plasma* with administered folate; only a new generation of red cells would show increased folate. Plasma folates accurately mirror tissue stores.[88] We therefore chose serum, not whole blood, for assaying the folate status of man.[1,11] Red blood cells contain a multiplicity of materials which stimulate growth of folate requirers. They also contain many forms of folypolygluta- mates which are not detectable unless properly deglutamylated to free folate.[211] Anticoagulants also affect folic acid activity.[212] Serum apparently is low in these folic bypassing substances, but may be rich in some PGA polyglutamates or N^5-methyltetrahydrofolic acid, available to L. casei only.[213,214] Streptococcus faecalis is inferior to L. casei in its utilization of N^5-methyl-THF[1,193,199] and the PGA poly- glutamates.[1,11,199] In short, ability to utilize PGA polyglutamates may underlie the superiority of L. casei over S. faecalis.[1,11,199,215,216]

In 1945 an L. casei method for detecting folic acid was described[217] but was virtually unused for biologic fluids until 1959. Our experience with L. casei then showed that serum L. casei activity correlated with the clinical picture, even though we did not know then to which folate in serum the bacterium was actually responding.[11,212,218] The clinical worth and specificity of this L. casei method[11] have been confirmed.[199,218,219,220]

Since this L. casei method was intro- duced, minor modifications have been advocated.[12a,199,219,221–223] They do not materially affect the end result.

The L. casei serum folate method has been extremely useful as a tool in studying folate metabolism. Combined with S. faecalis and P. cerevisiae, these assays yield a picture of total folates, one comprising oxidized and reduced mono- and polyglu- tamates.[1]

An oral folic acid tolerance test based on L. casei has been developed and applied to investigation of intestinal absorption of fo- lates in normal subjects, patients with fo- late deficiency anemia and patients with folate malabsorption associated with sprue.[224,224a,224b] The sensitivity of this test eliminates the need for priming doses of folic acid and urinary collections, needed for other tests,[199] and permits a direct assessment of folate absorption in various clinical conditions.

Detection of folic acid activity in biologic fluids and tissues is of the utmost impor- tance; it pinpoints the cause of the megaloblastic anemias, e.g. it distinguishes between vitamin B_{12} and folate deficien- cies. Because morphology of the abnormal red cell does not help diagnose the specific vitamin deficiency, assay methods must be relied on for the differential diagnosis. The L. casei method,[1] unlike the FIGLU method, defines specifically the folate status[1,2] in man, and has been useful in studying many aspects of folate metabo- lism. This method for detecting folate activity in biologic fluids and tissues has proven the most reliable.[1,2,52,106,199] It pro- vides an easy, fast (overnight) detection of specific folate deficiency,[1,199] including, importantly, subclinical folate de- ficiency.[220] As noted earlier, if the proce- dure is followed as detailed[1] antibiotics in the specimen are destroyed by the auto- claving steps; other heat-stable drugs that might inhibit growth of L. casei are ren- dered harmless by dilution. Tracer methods for serum folate requiring folate binders have been described.[229,230] Consid- ering cost, efficiency, accuracy and speed they offer little advantage over the L. casei method.[1] These tracer methods are not yet perfected and many pitfalls still exist.[231–233] For example, folate binders used in serum radioassay can cause artifactually low serum folate values when compared to the L. casei assay.[234] Also, some unsaturated binding proteins may have little affinity to bind methyltetrahydrofolate, which, as mentioned, is the major constituent of serum folate.[235]

Considering all of the above, it appears that the advantages of using a radioisotope to assay serum folate are exaggerated. When the tracer method works, the time involved and the accuracy are comparable to the L. casei assay but the cost is considerably higher.[236]

BIBLIOGRAPHY

1. Baker and Frank: In *Clinical Vitaminology: Methods and Interpretation*. New York, Interscience Publishers, 1968.
2. Baker and Frank: World Rev. Nutr., *9*, 124, 1968.
3. Leevy and Baker: Med. Clin. North Am., *54*, 467, 1970.
4. Kaminetsky and Baker: Clin. Obstet. Gynecol., *20*, 363, 1977.
5. Pratt: In *Chemotherapy of Infection*. New York, Oxford University Press, 1977.
6. Karnofsky and Young: Fed. Proc., *26*, 1139, 1967.
7. Avioli: In *The Fat Soluble Vitamins* (DeLuca and Suttie, Eds.). Madison, University of Wisconsin Press, 1970, p. 159.
8. Fennelly, Frank, Baker and Leevy: Am. J. Clin. Nutr., *20*, 946, 1967.
9. Banyl: Am. J. Clin. Nutr., *23*, 52, 1970.
9a.Dalgleish: In *The Scientific Basis of Medicine Annual Reviews*. London, Athlone Press, 1961, p. 127.
9b.Crandon, Lund and Dill: N. Engl. J. Med., *223*, 353, 1940.
10. Kahn: Med. Clin. North Am., *54*, 631, 1970.
11. Baker, Herbert, Frank, Pasher, Hutner, Wasserman and Sobotka: Clin. Chem., *5*, 275, 1959.
12. Ford and Hutner: Vitam. Horm., *13*, 101, 1955.
12a.Herbert: J. Clin. Pathol., *19*, 12, 1966.
12b.Cooper and Jonas: J. Clin. Pathol., *26*, 963, 1973.
13. Hutner, Cury and Baker: Anal. Chem., *30*, 849, 1958.
14. Pearson: In *The Vitamins*, Vol. 7 (György and Pearson, Eds.). New York, Academic Press, 1967, p. 1.
15. Strobecker and Henning: In *Vitamin Assay Tested Methods*. Weinheim, Verlag Chemie, 1965, p. 33.
15a.Wilson, et al.: Am. J. Clin. Nutr., *15*, 29, 1964.
15.bClarke, Cosgrove and Morse: Am. J. Clin. Nutr., *19*, 335, 1966.
16. Schwieter and Isler: In *The Vitamins*, Vol. I, 2nd ed. (Sebrell, Jr., and Harris, Eds.). New York, Academic Press, 1967, p. 5.
17. Roberts and DeLuca: In *The Fat Soluble Vitamins* (DeLuca and Suttie, Eds.). Madison, University of Wisconsin Press, 1969, p. 227.
18. Roels and Makadevan: In *The Vitamins*, Vol. III, 2nd ed. (György and Pearson, Eds.). New York, Academic Press, 1967, p. 139.
19. Carr and Price: Biochem. J., *20*, 497, 1926.
20. Bolliger: In *Thin-Layer Chromatography* (Stahl, Ed.). New York, Academic Press, 1965, p. 220.
21. Inhoffer and Pommer: In *The Vitamins*, Vol. I (Sebrell, Jr., and Harris; Eds.). New York, Academic Press, 1954, p. 87.
22. Sobel and Snow: J. Biol. Chem., *171*, 617, 1947.
23. Bieri and Schultze: Arch. Biochem. Biophys., *34*, 273, 1954.
24. Utley, Brodovsky and Pearson: J. Nutr., *66*, 205, 1958.
25. Neeld and Pearson: J. Nutr., *79*, 454, 1963.
25a.Smith and Lindenbaum: Am. J. Clin. Nutr., *27*, 700, 1974.
25b.Smith, Raz and Goodman: J. Clin. Invest., *49*, 1754, 1970.
25c.Smith and Goodman: J. Clin. Invest., *50*, 2426, 1971.
26. Kagen: Nutr. Symp. Ser., *7*, 31, 1953.
27. Hummel: J. Biol. Chem., *180*, 1225, 1949.
28. Nordmann, Arnaud and Nordmann: Clin. Chim. Acta, *12*, 304, 1965.
28a.Baker, Frank, Thomson, Langer, Munves, DeAngelis and Kaminetzky: Am. J. Clin. Nutr., *28*, 59, 1975.
29. Raiha: Pediatrics, *32*, 1025, 1963.
30. Merrow, Krause, Browe, Newhall and Pierce: J. Nutr., *46*, 445, 1952.
31. Popper: Physiol. Rev., *24*, 205, 1944.
31a.Underwood, Siegal, Weisell and Doblinski: Am. J. Clin. Nutr., *23*, 1037, 1970.
32. Popper, Steigmann, Dublin, Dymewicz and Hesser: Proc. Soc. Exp. Biol. Med., *68*, 676, 1948.
33. DeLuca, Weller, Blunt and Neville: Arch. Biochem. Biophys., *124*, 122, 1968.
34. DeLuca, and Suttie (Eds.): In *The Fat-Soluble Vitamins*. New York, Academic Press, 1969, p. 1.
35. Kodicek, and Lawson: In *The Vitamins* (György and Pearson, Eds.). New York, Academic Press, 1967, p. 211.
36. Theivagt and Campbell: Anal. Chem., *31*, 1375, 1959.
37. Strobecker and Pies: Arch. Pharm., *294*, 800, 1961.
38. Osadca and DeRitter: Feedstuffs, *35*, 26, 1963.
39. Heaysman and Sawyer: Analyst, *89*, 529, 1964.
40. Bessey, Lowry and Brock: J. Biol. Chem., *164*, 321, 1946.
41. György (Ed.): In *Inorganic Phosphate in Whole Blood and Serum*. New York, Academic Press, 1951.
42. Warkany, Guest and Grabill: J. Lab. Clin. Med., *27*, 557, 1942.
43. Thomas, Morgan, Connor, Haddock, Bills and Howard: J. Clin. Invest., *38*, 1078, 1959.
43a.Dam and Sondergaard: In *Nutrition*, Vol. 2 (Beaton and McHenry, Eds.). New York, Academic Press, 1964, p. 2.
43b.Norman: Am. J. Clin. Nutr., *24*, 1346, 1971.
43c.DeLuca and Schnoes: Annu. Rev. Biochem., *45*, 631, 1976.
43d.Haddad and Chyn: J. Clin. Endocrinol., *33*, 992, 1971.
43e.Belsey, DeLuca and Potts: J. Clin. Endocrinol. Metab., *38*, 1046, 1974.

43f. Eisman, Hamstra, Kream and DeLuca: Science, *193*, 1021, 1976.
44. Quaife, Scrimshaw and Lowry: J. Biol. Chem., *180*, 1229, 1949.
45. Freed: In *Methods of Vitamin Assay*. New York, Interscience Publishers, 1966, p. 363.
46. Bunnell: In *The Vitamins*, Vol. 6. New York, Academic Press, 1967, p. 261.
47. Bieri, Pollard, Prange and Dam: Acta Chem. Scand., *15*, 783, 1961.
48. Bollinger: In *Dunnschicht-Chromatographie* (Stahl, Ed.). Berlin, Springer, 1962, p. 217.
49. Emmerie and Engel: Recueil Trav. Chim. Pays-Bas, *60*, 104, 1941.
50. Haskin and Schuttringer: Am. J. Clin. Nutr., *19*, 137, 1966.
51. Bieri, Teets, Belavady and Andrews: Proc. Soc. Exp. Biol. Med., *117*, 131, 1964.
52. Baker, Frank, Feingold, Christakis and Ziffer: Am. J. Clin. Nutr., *20*, 850, 1967.
53. György and Rose: Ann. N. Y. Acad. Sci., *52*, 231, 1949.
54. Gordon and Nitowsky: Am. J. Clin. Nutr., *4*, 391, 1956.
55. MacKenzie: Pediatrics, *13*, 346, 1954.
56. Binder and Spiro: Am. J. Clin. Nutr., *20*, 594, 1967.
57. Irreverre and Sullivan: Science, *94*, 497, 1941.
58. Dam and Sondergaard: In *The Vitamins*, Vol. 6 (György and Pearson, Eds.). New York, Academic Press, 1967, p. 245.
59. Suttie: In *The Fat Soluble Vitamins* (DeLuca and Suttie, Eds.). Madison, University of Wisconsin Press, 1969, p. 447.
60. Page and Culver (Eds.); In *Syllabus of Laboratory Examinations in Clinical Diagnosis*. Cambridge, Harvard University Press, 1962, p. 186.
60a. O'Reilly: Annu. Rev. Med., *27*, 245, 1976.
61. Maier and Metzler: J. Am. Chem. Soc., *79*, 4386, 1957.
62. Manual for Nutrition Surveys, International Committee on Nutrition for National Defense. Washington, U.S. Government Printing Office, 1963, p. 136.
63. Burch, Bessey, Love and Lowry: J. Biol. Chem., *198*, 477, 1952.
64. Pence, Miller, Dutcher and Thorp: J. Biol. Chem., *158*, 647, 1945.
65. Pearson: In *The Vitamins*, Vol. 7. (György and Pearson, Eds.). New York, Academic Press, 1967, p. 53.
66. Baker, Pasher, Frank, Hutner, Aaronson and Sobotka: Clin. Chem., *5*, 13, 1959.
67. Mickelson and Yamamoto: In *Methods of Biochemical Analysis*, Vol. 6 (Glick, Ed.). New York, Academic Press, 1958, p. 191.
68. Dube, Johnson, Yu and Storvich: J. Nutr., *48*, 307, 1952.
69. Rindi and Perri: Int. Z. Vitaminforsch, *32*, 398, 1962.
70. Burch: In *Methods in Enzymology*, Vol. 3 (Colowick and Kaplan, Eds.). New York, Academic Press, 1957, p. 946.
71. Bonvicino and Hennessy: Int. Z. Vitaminforsch., *30*, 89, 1959.
72. Interdepartmental Committee on Nutrition for National Defense: Nutrition Survey. The Kingdom of Thailand. Washington, Department of Defense, 1962.
73. Brin: Ann. N. Y. Acad. Sci., *98*, 528, 1962.
74. Dreyfus: N. Engl. J. Med., *267*, 596, 1962.
74a. Warnock: Clin. Chem., *21*, 432, 1975.
74b. Bayoumi and Rosalki: Clin. Chem., *22*, 327, 1976.
75. Edwards, Kaufman and Storvich: Am. J. Clin. Nutr., *5*, 51, 1957.
76. Banhidi: Acta Physiol. Scand., *50*, 1, 1960.
77. Drebil, Evans and Neven, Jr.: J. Bacteriol., *74*, 818, 1957.
78. Hutner, Cury and Baker: Anal. Chem., *30*, 849, 1958.
79. Krampitz and Woolley: J. Biol. Chem., *152*, 9, 1944.
80. Baker, Frank, Fennelly and Leevy: Am. J. Clin. Nutr., *14*, 197, 1964.
81. Frank, Baker, Ziffer, Aaronson, Hutner and Leevy: Science, *139*, 110, 1963.
82. Hutner, Provasoli and Baker: Microchem. J., *1*, 95, 1961.
83. Myint and Houser: Clin. Chem., *11*, 617, 1965.
84. Fennelly, Frank, Baker and Leevy: Br. Med. J., *2*, 1290, 1964.
85. Fennelly, Frank, Baker and Leevy: Proc. Soc. Exp. Biol. Med., *116*, 875, 1964.
86. Cole, Turner, Frank, Baker and Leevy: Am. J. Clin. Nutr., *22*, 44, 1969.
87. Baker: Am. J. Clin. Nutr., *20*, 543, 1967.
88. Leevy, Baker, ten Hove, Frank and Cherrick: Am. J. Clin. Nutr., *16*, 339, 1965.
89. Pelletier and Medere: Fed. Proc., *30*, 522, 1971.
90. Thomson, Baker and Leevy: J. Lab. Clin. Med., *76*, 34, 1970.
91. Najjar and Wood: Proc. Soc. Exp. Biol. Med., *44*, 386, 1940.
92. Mickelson, Condiff and Keys: J. Biol. Chem., *160*, 361, 1945.
93. Alexander and Levi: J. Biol. Chem., *146*, 399, 1942.
94. Pearson: Am. J. Clin. Nutr., *20*, 514, 1967.
95. Ziporin, Nunes, Powell, Waring and Sauberlich: J. Nutr., *85*, 287, 1965.
96. Sorrell, Frank, Aquino, Thomson, Howard and Baker: Am. J. Clin. Nutr., *25*, 125, 1972.
97. Burch, Bessey, Love and Lowry: J. Biol. Chem., *198*, 477, 1952.
98. Goodhart and Sinclair: J. Biol. Chem., *132*, 11, 1940.
99. Krause: In *Modern Nutrition in Health and Disease*, 4th ed. (Wohl and Goodhart, Eds.). Philadelphia, Lea & Febiger, 1968, p. 531.
100. Horwitt and Kreisler: J. Nutr., *37*, 411, 1949.
101. Sinclair: N. Engl. J. Med., *245*, 39, 1951.
102. György and Langer, Jr.: In *The Vitamins*, Vol. 2 (Sebrell and Harris, Eds.). New York, Academic Press, 1968, p. 280.
103. Hertz: Proc. Soc. Exp. Biol. Med., *52*, 15, 1943.
104. Schull and Peterson: J. Biol. Chem., *151*, 201, 1943.
105. Wright and Skeggs: Proc. Soc. Exp. Biol. Med., *56*, 95, 1944.

106. Aaronson: J. Bacteriol., *69*, 67, 1955.
107. Hodson: J. Biol. Chem., *157*, 383, 1945.
108. West and Woglom: Cancer Res., *2*, 324, 1942.
109. The Association of Vitamin Chemists, Inc.: In *Methods of Vitamin Assay* (Freed, Ed.). New York, Interscience Publishers, 1966, p. 245.
110. Glick and Ferguson: Proc. Soc. Exp. Biol. Med., *109*, 811, 1962.
111. Baker, Frank, Matovitch, Pasher, Aaronson, Hutner and Sobotka: Anal. Biochem., *3*, 31, 1962.
112. Terroine: Vitam. Horm., *18*, 1, 1960.
113. Wright, Cresson, Skeggs, Peck, Wolf, Wood, Valiant and Folkers: Science, *114*, 635, 1951.
114. Bliss and György: In *The Vitamins*, Vol. 7 (György and Pearson, Eds.). New York, Academic Press, 1967, p. 134.
115. Goldsmith: In *Nutrition*, Vol. 2 (Beaton and McHenry, Eds.). New York, Academic Press, 1964, p. 109.
116. Barton-Wright: In *Microbiological Assay of the Vitamin B-Complex and Amino Acids*. London, Pitman, 1952, p. 35.
116a. Baker and Frank: In *Riboflavin* (Rivlin, Ed.). New York, Plenum Press, 1975, p. 49.
117. Freed: In *Methods of Vitamin Assay*, 3rd ed. New York, Interscience Publishers, 1966, p. 150.
118. Burch: In *Methods in Enzymology*, Vol. 3 (Colowick and Kaplan, Eds.). New York, Academic Press, 1957, p. 960.
119. Baker, Frank, Feingold, Gellene, Leevy and Hutner: Am. J. Clin. Nutr., *19*, 17, 1966.
120. Snell: In *The Vitamins*, Vol. 3 (Sebrell and Harris, Eds.). New York, Academic Press, 1954, p. 372.
121. Horwitt: In *Modern Nutrition in Health and Disease* (Wohl and Goodhart, Eds.). Philadelphia, Lea & Febiger, 1960, p. 335.
122. Rivlin: N. Engl. J. Med., *283*, 463, 1970.
123. Sarett, Klein and Perlzweig: J. Nutr., *24*, 295, 1942.
124. Mickelson: In *Present Knowledge of Nutrition*. New York, The Nutrition Foundation, Inc., 1967, p. 61.
125. Bessey, Horwitt and Love: J. Nutr., *58*, 367, 1956.
125a. Glatzle, Korner, Christeller and Wiss: Int. J. Vitam. Res., *40*, 166, 1970.
125b. Tillotson and Baker: Am. J. Clin. Nutr., *25*, 425, 1972.
125c. Sharada and Bamji: Int. J. Vitam. Res., *42*, 43, 1972.
126. Baker, Frank, Pasher, Hutner and Sobotka: Clin. Chem., *6*, 572, 1960.
127. Goldsmith and Miller: In *The Vitamins*, Vol. 7 (György and Pearson, Eds.). New York, Academic Press, 1967, p. 139.
128. Friedemann and Frazier: Arch. Biochem., *26*, 361, 1950.
129. Official Methods of Analysis, Association of Official Agricultural Chemists. Washington, 1960, p. 660.
130. Huff and Perlzweig: J. Biol. Chem., *167*, 157, 1947.
131. Levitas, Robinson, Rosen, Huff and Perlzweig: J. Biol. Chem., *167*, 169, 1947.
132. Fergelson, Williams and Elvehjem: J. Biol. Chem., *185*, 741, 1950.
133. Lowry, Roberts and Kapphahn: J. Biol. Chem., *224*, 1047, 1957.
134. Lindall and Lazarow: Metabolism, *13*, 259, 1964.
135. Lieber: In *The Biological Basis of Medicine*, Vol. 5 (Bittar and Bittar, Eds.). New York, Academic Press, 1969, p. 318.
136. Ellinjer and Coulson: Biochem. J., *38*, 265, 1944.
137. Hoagland, Ward and Shank: J. Biol. Chem., *241*, 2367, 1966.
138. Baker, Frank, Thomson and Feingold: Am. J. Clin. Nutr., *22*, 1469, 1969.
139. Sorrell, Frank, Aquino, Thomson and Baker: Am. J. Clin. Nutr., *24*, 924, 1971.
140. Leder and Handler: J. Biol. Chem., *189*, 889, 1951.
141. Storvich, Benson, Edwards and Woodring: In *Methods of Biochemical Analysis*, Vol. 12 (Glick, Ed.). New York, Interscience Publishers, 1964, p. 183.
142. Sauberlich: In *The Vitamins*, Vol. 7 (György and Pearson, Eds.). New York, Academic Press, 1967, p. 169.
143. Toepfer, Polansky and Hewston: Anal. Biochem., *2*, 463, 1961.
144. Korytnyk, Fricke and Paul: Anal. Biochem., *17*, 66, 1966.
145. Anderson, Peart and Fulford-Jones: J. Clin. Pathol., *23*, 232, 1970.
146. Cinnamon and Beaton: Am. J. Clin. Nutr., *23*, 696, 1970.
147. Umbreit, Bellamy and Gunsalus: Arch. Biochem., *7*, 185, 1945.
147a. Hamfelt: Clin. Chim. Acta, *10*, 48, 1964.
148. Wada, Morisue, Sakamoto and Ichibara: J. Vitaminol., *3*, 183, 1957.
149. Leitch and Hepburn: Nutr. Abstr. Rev., *31*, 389, 1961.
150. Gassman, Knapp and Gartner: Klin. Wochenschr., *37*, 189, 1959.
151. Marquez and Reynolds: J. Am. Diet. Assoc., *31*, 1116, 1955.
152. Turner and Reynolds: J. Am. Diet. Assoc., *31*, 1119, 1955.
153. Wachstein and Gudartis: J. Lab. Clin. Med., *42*, 98, 1953.
154. Ranke, Tauber, Hornick, Ranke, Goodhart and Chow: J. Gerontol., *15*, 41, 1960.
155. György: Vitam. Horm., *22*, 885, 1964.
155a. Krishnaswamy: Int. J. Vitam. Nutr. Res., *42*, 468, 1972.
155b. Park and Linkswiler: J. Nutr., *100*, 110, 1970.
156. Boxer, Pruss and Goodhart: J. Nutr., *63*, 623, 1957.
157. Wachstein, Moore and Graffeo: Proc. Soc. Exp. Biol. Med., *96*, 326, 1957.
158. Holtz and Palm: Pharmacol. Rev., *16*, 113, 1964.
159. Reddy, Reynolds and Price: J. Biol. Chem., *233*, 691, 1958.
160. Huff and Perlzweig: J. Biol. Chem., *155*, 345, 1944.
161. Gershoff: Vitam. Horm., *22*, 581, 1964.

162. Baker, Frank, Ning, Gellene, Hutner and Leevy: Am. J. Clin. Nutr., *18*, 123, 1966.

163. Haskell and Wallnofer: Anal. Biochem., *19*, 659, 1967.

164. Hubbard, Hintz, Libby and Sutor: J. Assoc. Off. Agric. Chem., *48*, 1217, 1965.

165. Bird and Thompson: In *The Vitamins*, Vol. 7 (György and Pearson, Eds.). New York, Academic Press, 1967, p. 209.

166. Baker, Frank, Pasher, Dinnerstein and Sobotka: Clin. Chem., *6*, 36, 1960.

167. Dewey and Kidder: Proc. Soc. Exp. Biol. Med., *87*, 198, 1954.

168. Malgras, Meyer and Pax: Ann. Inst. Pasteur, *93*, 792, 1957.

169. Knox and Groswami: Adv. Clin. Chem., *4*, 121, 1961.

170. Roe: In *The Vitamins*, Vol. 7 (György and Pearson, Eds.). New York, Academic Press, 1967, p. 27.

171. Roe: In *Methods of Biochemical Analysis*, Vol. 1 (Glick, Ed.). New York, Interscience Publishers, 1954, p. 134.

172. Schwartz and Williams: Proc. Soc. Exp. Biol. Med., *88*, 136, 1955.

173. Penny and Zilva: Biochem. J., *37*, 403, 1943.

174. Baker, Hodges, Hood, Sauberlich and March: Am. J. Clin. Nutr., *22*, 549, 1969.

175. Baker and Frank: In *The Vitamins*, Vol. 7 (György and Pearson, Eds.). New York, Academic Press, 1967, p. 293.

176. Rosenthal: In *The Vitamins*, Vol. 2 (Sebrell and Harris, Eds.). New York, Academic Press, 1968, p. 151.

177. Reizenstein: Blood, *27*, 744, 1966.

178. Woodliff and Armstrong: Med. J. Aust., *1*, 1023, 1966.

179. Mahmud, Ripley and Doscherholmen: J.A.M.A., *216*, 1167, 1971.

180. Lawar, McCracken, Miller and Goldsmith: Am. J. Clin. Nutr., *16*, 402, 1965.

181. Glass: Physiol. Rev., *43*, 529, 1963.

181a. Raven, Robson, Morgan and Hoffbrand: Br. J. Haematol., *22*, 21, 1972.

181b. Britt, Bolton, Cull and Spray: Br. J. Haematol., *16*, 457, 1969.

181c. Kolhouse, Kondo, Allen, Podell and Allen: N. Engl. J. Med., *299*, 785, 1978.

181d. Cooper and Whitehead: N. Engl. J. Med., *299*, 816, 1978.

182. Lau, Gottlieb, Wasserman and Herbert: Blood, *26*, 202, 1965.

183. Gottlieb, Lau, Wasserman and Herbert: Blood, *25*, 6, 1965.

184. Grossowicz, Sulitzeam and Merzbach: Proc. Soc. Exp. Biol. Med., *109*, 604, 1962.

185. Hift: S. Afr. J. Med. Sci., *29*, 84, 1964.

186. Luhby and Cooperman: Lancet, *2*, 138, 1962.

187. Herbert, Streiff, Sullivan and McGeer: Lancet, *2*, 45, 1964.

188. Coward and Smith: Clin. Chem. Acta, *12*, 206, 1965.

189. Barness, Young, Mellman, Kahn and Williams: N. Engl. J. Med., *268*, 144, 1963.

190. Kahn, Williams, Barness, Young, Shafer, Vivacqua and Beaupre: J. Lab. Clin. Med., *66*, 75, 1965.

191. Gompertz, Jones and Knowles: Lancet, *1*, 424, 1967.

192. Johns and Bertino: Clin. Pharmacol. Ther., *6*, 372, 1965.

193. Baker and Sobotka: Adv. Clin. Chem., *5*, 215, 1962.

194. Skeggs: In *The Vitamins*, Vol. 7 (György and Pearson, Eds.). New York, Academic Press, 1967, p. 278.

195. Baker, Frank, Pasher and Sobotka: Clin. Chem., *6*, 578, 1960.

196. Baker, Frank, Pasher, Ziffer, Hutner and Sobotka: Proc. Soc. Exp. Biol. Med., *107*, 965, 1961.

197. Blakley: In *The Biochemistry of Folic Acid and Related Pteridines*. New York, Wiley Interscience Division, 1969, p. 32.

198. Ellegaard and Esmann: Lancet, *1*, 308, 1970.

199. Chanarin: In *The Megaloblastic Anaemias*. Philadelphia, F. A. Davis Co., 1969.

200. Chanarin: Proc. R. Soc. Med., *57*, 384, 1964.

201. Eichhorn and Rutenberg: Lancet, *2*, 906, 1965.

202. Cooperman, Luhby and Singer: Proc. Soc. Exp. Biol. Med., *131*, 434, 1969.

203. McGeer, Sen and Grant: Can. J. Biochem., *43*, 1367, 1965.

204. Herbert, Streiff, Sullivan and McGeer: Lancet, *2*, 45, 1964.

205. Luhby and Cooperman: Lancet, *2*, 1381, 1962.

206. Cherrick, Baker, Frank and Leevy: J. Lab. Clin. Med., *66*, 446, 1965.

207. McClean and Chanarin: Blood, *27*, 386, 1966.

208. Chanarin, Anderson and Mollin: Br. J. Haematol., *4*, 156, 1958.

209. Baker, Frank, Gellene and Leevy: Proc. Soc. Exp. Biol. Med., *117*, 492, 1964.

210. Girdwood: Br. Med. Bull., *15*, 14, 1959.

211. Bird, McGlohon and Vaitkus: Can. J. Microbiol., *15*, 465, 1969.

212. Hutner, Nathan and Baker: Vitam. Horm., *17*, 1, 1959.

213. Larrabee, Rosenthal, Cathou and Buchanan: J. Am. Chem. Soc., *83*, 4094, 1961.

214. Herbert, Larrabee and Buchanan: J. Clin. Invest., *41*, 1134, 1962.

215. Baker, Frank, Feingold, Ziffer, Gellene, Leevy and Sobotka: Am. J. Clin. Nutr., *17*, 88, 1965.

216. Jeejeebhoy, Pathare and Noronba: Blood, *26*, 354, 1965.

217. Teply and Elvehjem: J. Biol. Chem., *157*, 303, 1945.

218. Herbert, Baker, Frank, Pasher, Sobotka and Wasserman: Blood, *15*, 228, 1960.

219. Herbert: J. Clin. Invest., *40*, 81, 1961.

220. Herbert: Trans. Assoc. Am. Physicians, *75*, 307, 1962.

221. Waters and Mollin: J. Clin. Pathol., *14*, 335, 1961.

222. Hansen: In *On the Diagnosis of Folic Acid Deficiency*. Goteborg, Orstadius Baktryckeri AB, 1964.

223. Chanarin, Kyle and Stacy: J. Clin. Pathol., *25*, 1050, 1972.

224. Baker, Frank, Sobotka, Ho, Cohen, Janowitz, Ziffer and Leevy: J.A.M.A., *187*, 159, 1964.
224a. Baker, Frank, Zetterman, Rajan, ten Hove and Leevy: Am. J. Clin. Nutr., *28*, 1377, 1975.
224b. Baker, Jaslow and Frank: J. Am. Geriatr. Soc., *26*, 218, 1978.
225. Baker, Frank and Hutner: Science, *169*, 313, 1969.
226. Okuda: J. Biochem., *48*, 13, 1960.
227. Reddi and Kodicek: Biochem. J., *53*, 286, 1953.
228. King: J.A.M.A., *142*, 563, 1950.
228a. Andrews and Brook: Lancet, *1*, 1350, 1966.
229. Rothenberg, DaCosta and Rosenberg: N. Engl. J. Med., *286*, 1335, 1972.
230. Waxman and Schreiber: Blood, *42*, 281, 1973.
231. Mortensen: Clin. Chem., *22*, 1408, 1976.
232. Kamen and Casten: Clin. Chem., *22*, 1408, 1976.
233. Zettner: Clin. Chem., *22*, 1410, 1976.
234. Paine, Hargrove, Jr. and Eichner: Arch. Intern. Med., *136*, 756, 1976.
235. Eichner, McDonald and Dickson: Am. J. Clin. Nutr., *31*, 1988, 1978.
236. O'Donnell, Tennant and Jones: J. Clin. Pathol., *30*, 1175, 1977.

Chapter 21

RADIOLOGIC FINDINGS IN NUTRITIONAL DISTURBANCES

Robin C. Watson,
Herman Grossman
and
Morton A. Meyers

The roentgenographic findings in nutritional disorders are somewhat varied: They may be distinctive, as in scurvy or rickets, but they are often nonspecific, as in osteoporosis and osteomalacia, and the diagnosis may depend upon secondary manifestations.[1-3] Also, it must be pointed out that any radiographic abnormality occurs only in the face of prolonged deficiency or excessive intake. In all probability the most striking changes are seen in this day and age as the result of malabsorption rather than deficient intake. However, particularly in underdeveloped areas, the latter is still a dominant factor. Generally, the earliest and most specific findings are seen in the child and adolescent, rather than in the adult, although with gastrointestinal abnormalities this probably is reversed.

OSTEOPOROSIS

Over the years there has been a considerable blurring of the meaning of "osteoporosis," which has become a vague, all-embracing word.[4,5]

In the normal subject there is a balance between osteoporosis and osteolysis and an adequate degree of bone mineralization. Osteoporosis represents a breakdown in this mechanism; there is a defect in osteogenesis while osteolysis proceeds at the normal rate and the process of bone mineralization is unimpaired. The result is that there is an overall loss of bone mass with respect to the volume of bone present, and the bone elements, therefore, become sparse and brittle.

Radiographically the cortical bone thins, with an overall loss of bone density, and the distance between the normally mineralized longitudinal, but thin, trabeculae increases (hence the term porotic), while there is a concomitant loss of transverse trabeculae.[6] These changes are usually first apparent in the spine; however, in advanced cases, the process may be seen to involve all bones. Fractures resulting from the brittle quality of the bone are common and deformities may result. Most often seen are crush fractures of the spine with collapse of the vertebral end-plates and anterior wedging of the bodies, resulting in increased lordotic curves. Pseudo-fractures are not seen in this condition.

Osteoporosis may be seen in relation to:

1. Senile and postmenopausal patients
2. Malnutrition
3. Hypovitaminosis C
4. Endocrine disorders, such as Cushing's disease, acromegaly, hypothyroidism and hyperthyroidism.
5. The congenital defect of osteoporosis imperfecta.
6. Idiopathic conditions

Difficulty in interpretation results from the fact that there must be extensive loss of the mass of bone before this becomes radiographically apparent. Furthermore, the findings are nonspecific and there is no way of differentiating, say, postmenopausal osteoporosis from that found in multiple myeloma.

Osteoporosis is, perhaps, most often seen in elderly patients, often in reduced circumstances, in whom there is an associated dietary insufficiency, including that of vitamin C. Although there are perhaps fewer of these individuals than in the past, they exist in both rural and urban areas.

SCURVY

Abnormalities in the skeleton in infantile scurvy have been studied by Park.[7] There is a disturbance of endochondral bone growth, with subperiosteal hemorrhagic manifestations occurring without associated trauma. The bone changes occur quite symmetrically throughout the skeleton and are more widely distributed than are gross subperiosteal or intramedullary hemorrhages. As are the changes in rickets, those of scurvy are most marked where growth in length is normally most rapid: at the sternal end of the middle ribs, the lower end of the femur, the upper end of the humerus, both ends of the tibia and fibula, the lower end of the radius and ulna, in approximately the order given.

The columns of cartilage cells in the proliferative cartilage in infantile scurvy tend to be irregular rather than linear. Whether this change represents a purely scorbutic process or whether it depends in part on an associated or antecedent rickets is not entirely certain. Scurvy interferes with the mechanism for removal of calcified cartilage matrix; it suppresses the formation of new trabeculae and, wherever there is bone already formed, resorption proceeds. These changes, morphologically important in themselves, affect the structure of bone also from a functional point of view by diminishing its capacity to withstand mechanical stress.

Roentgenographic changes are often diagnostic or suggestive. The costochondral junctions of the ribs are wide (Fig. 21–1*A* and *B*). The abrupt bony swelling culminates in a ridge where bone and cartilage meet. The sternochondral plate

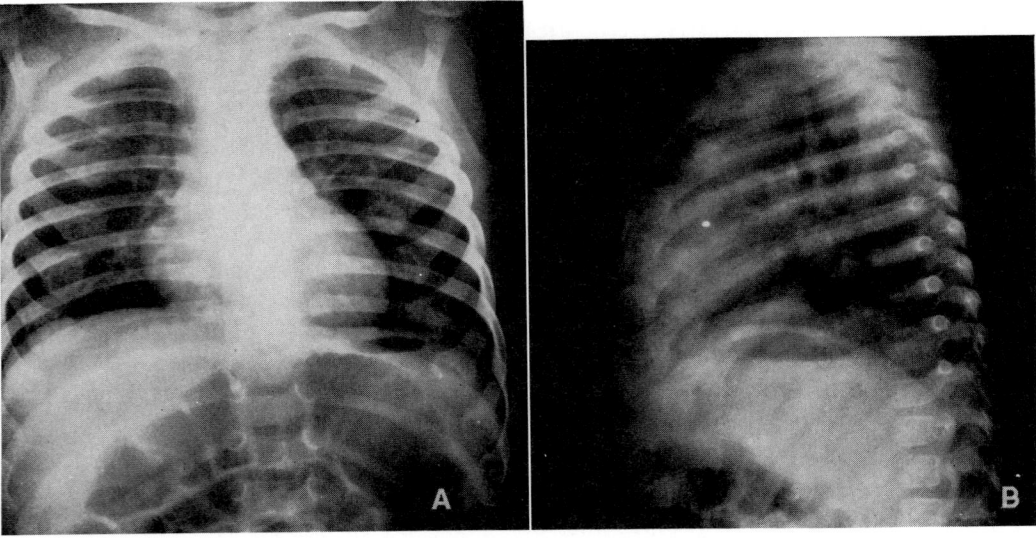

Fig. 21–1. Twenty-seven-month-old male with scurvy. Frontal and lateral chest roentgenograms demonstrate bony swelling at the costochondral junctions of the ribs.

may be displaced posteriorly by atmospheric pressure where the cartilage has been pushed backward at the line of its separation from the bony shaft.

In the early stages, the changes in the bone are nonspecific, presenting poorly discernible trabeculae and thin cortices. As the disease progresses a thick white line at the metaphysis (Figs. 21–2, 21–3) develops. Spurs develop at the cartilage shaft junction and subepiphyseal atrophy casts a transverse line or band of diminished density[8] (Fig. 21–2). This zone of rarefaction is a linear break in the bone proximal and parallel to the white line. Peripheral metaphyseal clefts, the so-called corner sign, are characteristic of scurvy[7] (Fig. 21–3). Ossification centers have central

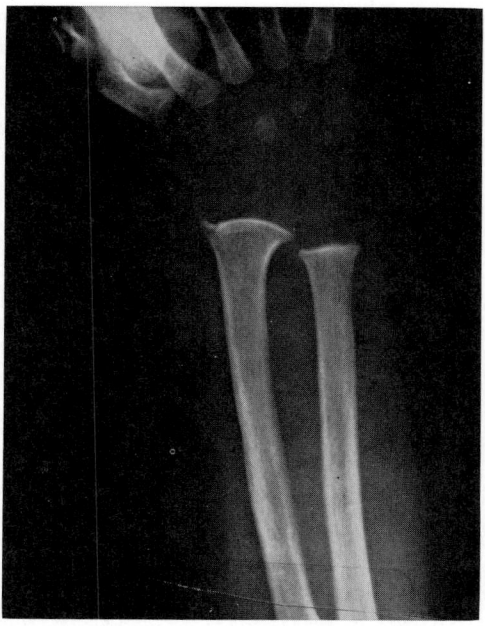

Fig. 21–3. Eight-month-old female with scurvy showing dense white lines and rarefaction at the distal ends of the radius and ulna. The "corner sign" of scurvy, noted at the distal lateral aspect of the radius, is the result of a defect at the angle between the provisional zone of calcification and the cortex.

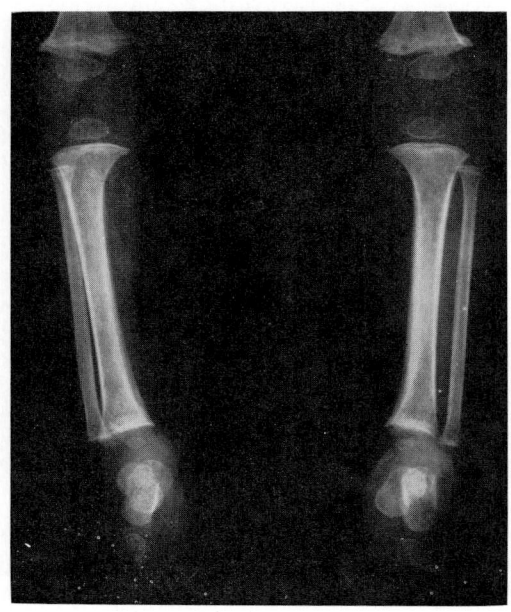

Fig. 21–2. Ten-month-old male with scurvy demonstrating a thick white line at the metaphyses of the long bones of the knees. Linear breaks are present in the bones proximal and parallel to the white lines of the distal femurs. Spurs are present and best seen at the ends of the femurs and medial aspect of the right tibia. The ossification centers have central rarefaction with heavy ring shadows on the margins. Periosteal new bone is along the medial aspects of the tibias.

rarefaction with heavy ring shadows (Fig. 21–2) on the margins. Epiphyseal separation may occur along the line of destruction, with linear displacement or compression of the epiphysis against the shaft.

Subperiosteal hemorrhages often appear on the larger long bones[8,9] (Fig. 21–4A and B). During healing the elevated periosteum becomes calcified (Fig. 21–4B), creating a heavy shell of subperiosteal bone. This shell of bone gradually shrinks and forms a new cortex. Subperichondrial hemorrhages over the epiphysis are said not to occur in scurvy.

OSTEOMALACIA

In most countries osteomalacia is now considered to be the adult form of rickets. It represents an abnormality of the mineralizing process while both os-

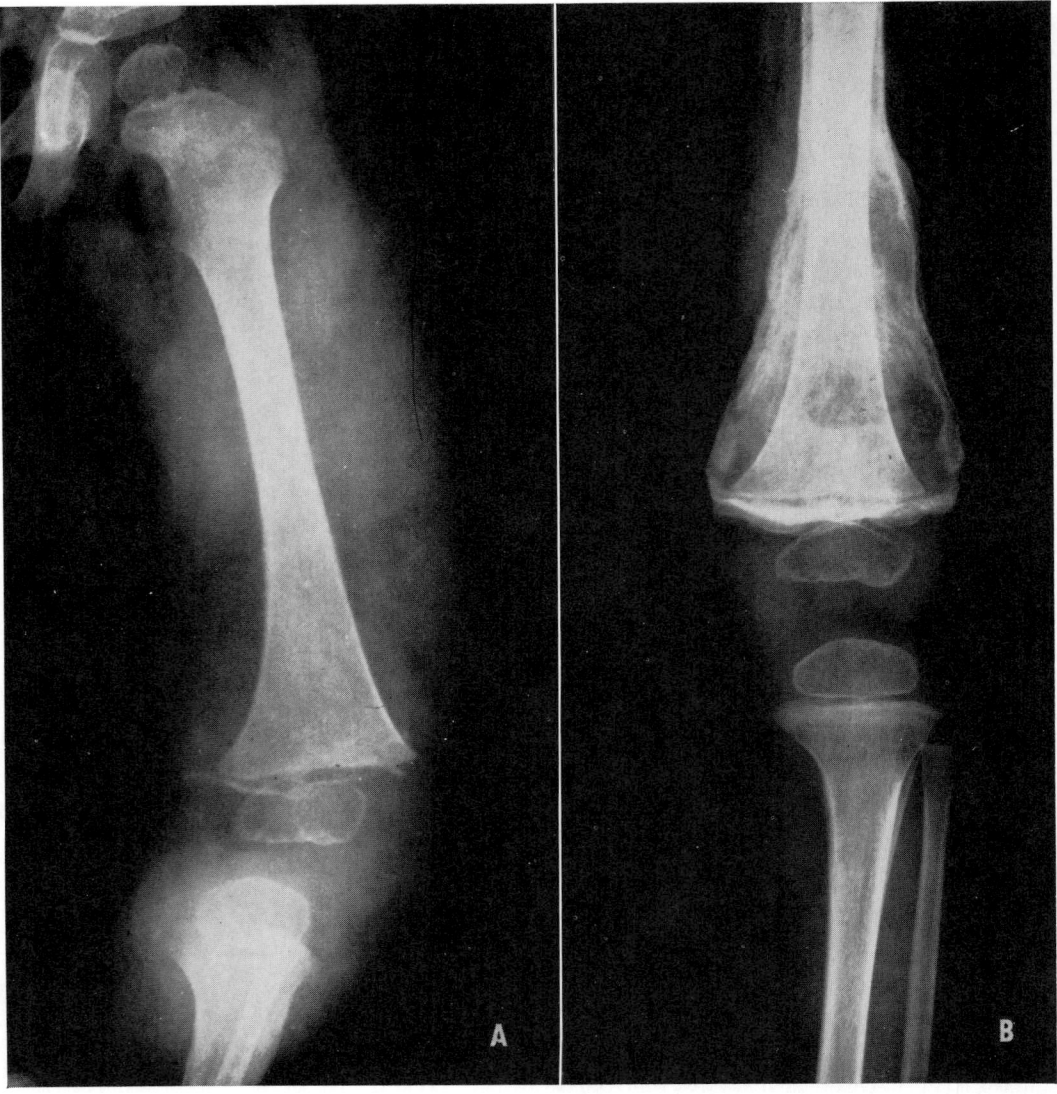

Fig. 21–4. Twelve-month-old male with healing scurvy. *A*: Fracture of the provisional zone of calcification of the distal femur with early calcification. Displacement of the soft tissues is due to hematoma which has not begun to calcify. *B*: Extensive calcification of elevated periosteum after 2 weeks of vitamin C therapy.

teogenesis and osteolysis proceed at a normal rate.[10] The result of the mineral deficiency is that the bone becomes soft and pliable. Whereas in osteoporosis the thin and brittle bones fracture easily, in osteomalacia there is more likely to be bending of the bony structures. The bone mass is still of normal volume, but there is a loss of bone density.[11]

Most often osteomalacia is related to malabsorption as a result of a variety of conditions: sprue, steatorrhea, pancreatic insufficiency, Crohn's disease, gastric or small bowel resections, fistulas or chronic ulcerative colitis. Radiographically the bone density is decreased; however, this may be hard to recognize. The trabeculae are poorly defined and coarse, with widening of the intertrabecular spaces. The most striking feature is that, in areas of stress, pseudofractures appear as thin radiolucent lines extending across the cortex at right angles to the long axis of the bone.[12] These fractures are most often symmetrical and bilateral. With treatment, the margins become sclerotic, but angulation often occurs at the site. One theory is that the fractures are related to pulsating periosteal blood vessels; however, this seems unlikely. In partially treated or untreated cases, these zones of lucency remain for considerable periods of time. The bones most commonly affected are the first or lower ribs, the public rami, the transverse processes of the lumbar vertebra, the lateral scapular borders, the tibiae and fibulae and the shafts of the femoral necks. In chronic and untreated cases, gross skeletal deformities may result.

RICKETS

Rickets, a disease of infancy and childhood, is a metabolic disorder of bone characterized by formation of normal collagen, matrix and osteoid with a disturbance in calcium and phosphorus metabolism which prevents the normal deposition of calcium salts in the growing parts of the skeleton. The skeleton becomes weak, is unable to withstand the stress and strain to which it is ordinarily subjected and yields and deforms. For the development of ordinary rickets, a deficiency must exist both in the short ultraviolet radiations of the sun and in the vitamin D present in certain foods. Osteomalacia is merely deficiency rickets occurring after endochondral growth has come to an end.

The roentgenograms give the most accurate information regarding rickets. The costochondral junctions, the most actively growing bones, are not accessible for clear radiographic study early in the course of rickets. The lower end of the femur is too thick and the junction of the epiphysis with the diaphysis is too uneven for slight changes to show distinctly. The lower ends of the radius and ulna are most useful for the study of rickets by x-ray pictures because of their small size and convenient location. Significant changes are often visible in the ulna when the radius appears to be normal.

The changes at the cartilage shaft junction are characterized by total or partial lack of calcification of the terminal segment of the shaft. This "invisible" provisional zone of calcification is seen only in rickets (Fig. 21–5*A*). Cupping, spreading, cortical spurs and fraying at the ends of bones are also seen in rickets, but not one of these changes itself is characteristic of rickets, since it may be seen in other conditions such as congenital syphilis or scurvy.

Cupping may not be evident until treatment is begun, because of the lack of lime salts in the organic tissue which forms the cup (Fig. 21–5*B* and *C*). Cupping may be seen in scurvy, to a slight degree, in the ulnae of young, especially premature, infants whose bones are growing rapidly.

Cortical spurs are linear shadows which extend as prolongations of the shadows of the cortex along the sides of the proliferative cartilage[13] (Fig. 21–5*B*). They are not always in the direct line of the cortex but are external to it, since they lie in the perichondrial-periosteal layer which envelops the cortex. Such shadows may be found on one or both sides; they may be straight and in line of the cortex or they may arch outward. The shape and direction of the spurs are determined by the configuration of the proliferative cartilage. X-ray films often show the spurs lying external to the cortex, overlapping and seeming to splint the cartilage shaft junction. This represents a new cortical layer forming outside the old. Spur formation also occurs in congenital syphilis.

Fraying consists of thread-like calcified shadows extending from the end of the

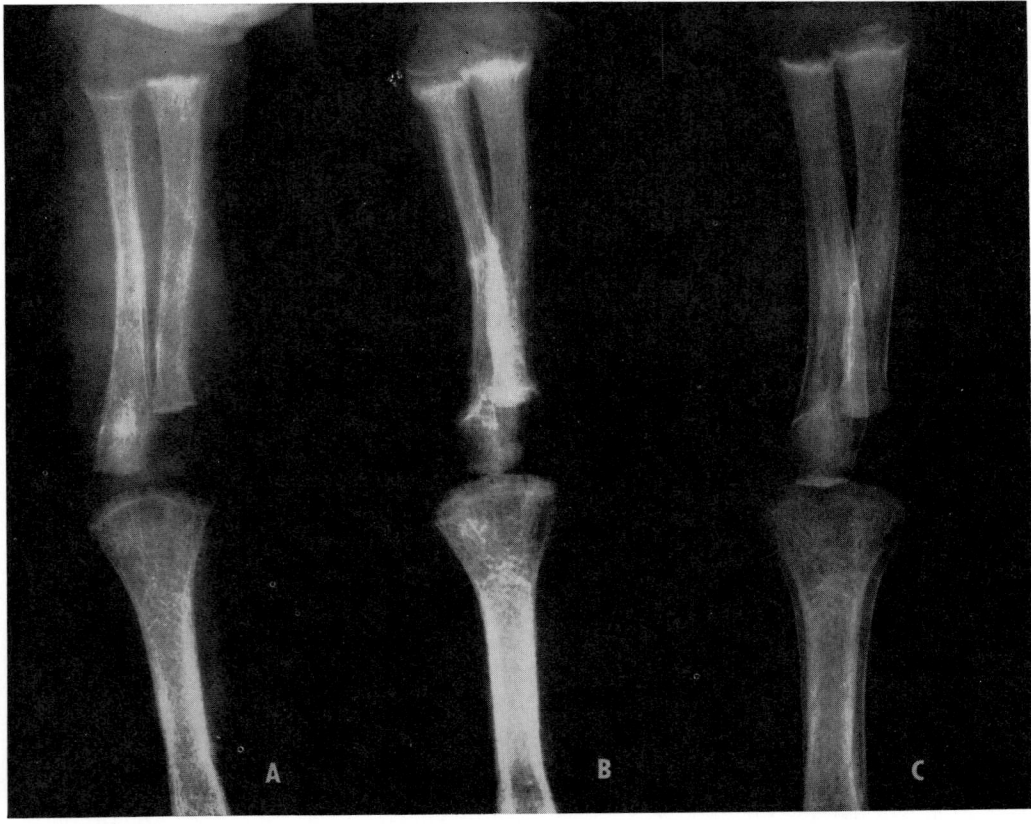

Fig. 21-5. A 10-month-old male during various stages of rickets. *A:* Noncalcified provisional zone. Fraying of the distal humerus. Strands of calcified osteoid projecting from the sides of the bone. *B:* Cupping, spread metaphysis, fraying and cortical spurs. Transverse linear recalcified density develops in rachitic metaphysis. A fracture in the midshaft of the radius. Greenstick fractures are common in the long bones. *C:* Metaphyseal spongiosum recalcifies and fuses with that of the provisional zone of calcification. Diffuse layer of recalcified cortex.

shaft into the transparent cartilage[14] (Fig. 21-5B). These frayed densities are neither straight nor parallel but extend in various directions, exactly as would be expected from the disorder in the underlying pathologic condition.

In severe rickets the shaft of the bone shows a diffuse rarefaction caused by the loss of lime. The cortex may be thin and, in places, invisible. Strands of osteoid may extend from the poorly defined cortex to the almost invisible periosteum, which contains enough lime salts to cast hair-like shadows sticking out from the sides of the bones (Fig. 21-5A). Other changes in the shaft which may be visible are complete or partial fracture, callus formation, curvature of the shaft, with great thickening on the concave side, or displacement of the epiphysis on the diaphysis.

Healing rickets is first observed in the provisional zone of calcification. A transverse linear recalcified density develops in the rachitic metaphysis beyond the visible end of the shaft and at a level the epiphyseal plate would have reached in the absence of rickets (Fig. 21-5B). As healing continues, the new provisional zone of calcification thickens. The metaphyseal spongiosum also recalcifies and fuses with that of the provisional zone of calcification. The cortex heals more slowly and is less conspicuous roentgenographically. However, when layers of osteoid have been deposited under the periosteum, recalcification of this osteoid discloses a diffuse layer or cortex, which may be of uniform density or lamellated (Fig. 21–5C).

Complete healing can be achieved in deficiency rickets. Distortion and sclerosis in the bone remain visible in the same level of the shaft for years and cortical thickening on the concave surfaces of curvature deformities may also remain. Most bowing and angulation deformities result from displacement of the epiphyseal cartilage. Angulation deformities may also be secondary to pathologic fractures.

Rickets may be distinguished from scurvy by the tenderness and pain present with scurvy, which exceeds anything found in rickets. The various hemorrhagic phenomena seen with scurvy do not occur in rickets. Difficulty may be encountered in distinguishing the enlargement of the costochondral junctions found in scurvy from that found in rickets and differentiation may be impossible.

Vitamin D and C deficiencies occur commonly together, since both vitamins must be given as accessories to the diet. If one is not given, it often happens that the other is omitted also. The association is thus due to chance, not to any interrelationship between the two vitamins in a chemical sense. However, a deficiency in one vitamin may prevent deficiency in the other from expressing itself by characteristic symptoms and signs. If vitamin D deficiency is sufficiently severe and prolonged, the lattice of calcified matrix framework, which is a characteristic feature of scurvy, cannot form at all or forms imperfectly. In scurvy the collapse of the brittle lattice framework is responsible for the fractures and the development of subperiosteal hemorrhage—and probably the pain and tenderness. Thus, as a result of suppressing the development of the lattice, vitamin D deficiency may prevent or mod-

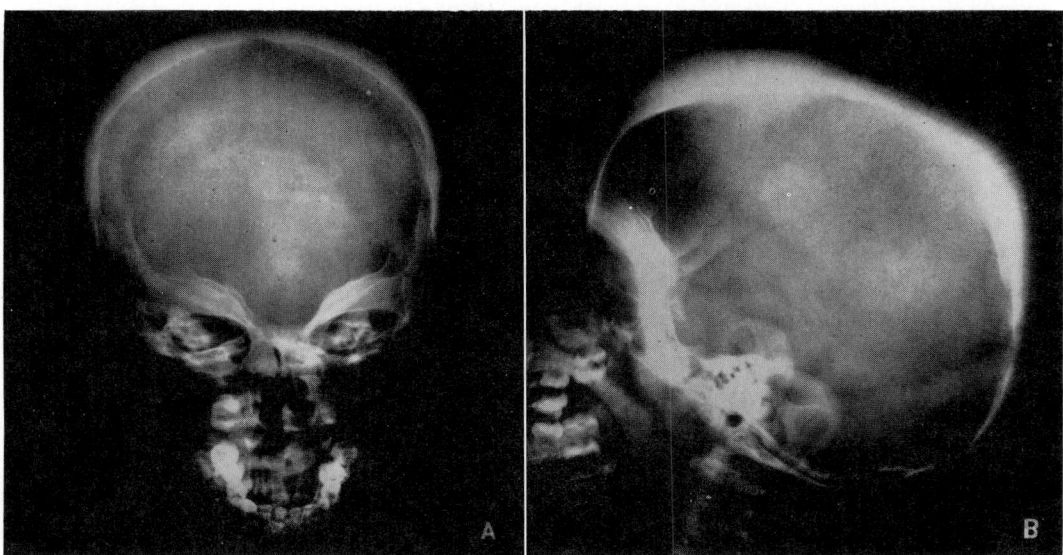

Fig. 21–6A and B. Frontal and lateral views of the skull in a young child with iron deficiency anemia demonstrating nonuniform widening of the diploic space with a "hair-on-end" appearance. (Courtesy of Dr. Philip Lanzkowsky.)

ify important symptoms of scurvy, typical roentgenographic signs and characteristic histology.

IRON DEFICIENCY ANEMIA

Roentgenographic changes in the skeleton in association with congenital hemolytic anemia result from increased proliferation of hematopoietic tissue in the bone marrow.

In 1936 Sheldon[15] first described a child with changes in the skull in association with iron deficiency anemia. In the 1960s many other reports[16-20] described such changes. Lanzkowsky[21] reported several children with iron deficiency anemia who had changes in the metacarpals as well as in the skull.

The degree of change in the roentgenograms of the skull and metacarpals is variable. Children with marked changes are similar to those seen with severe congenital hemolytic anemias. The diploic space of the skull is widened in a nonuniform man-

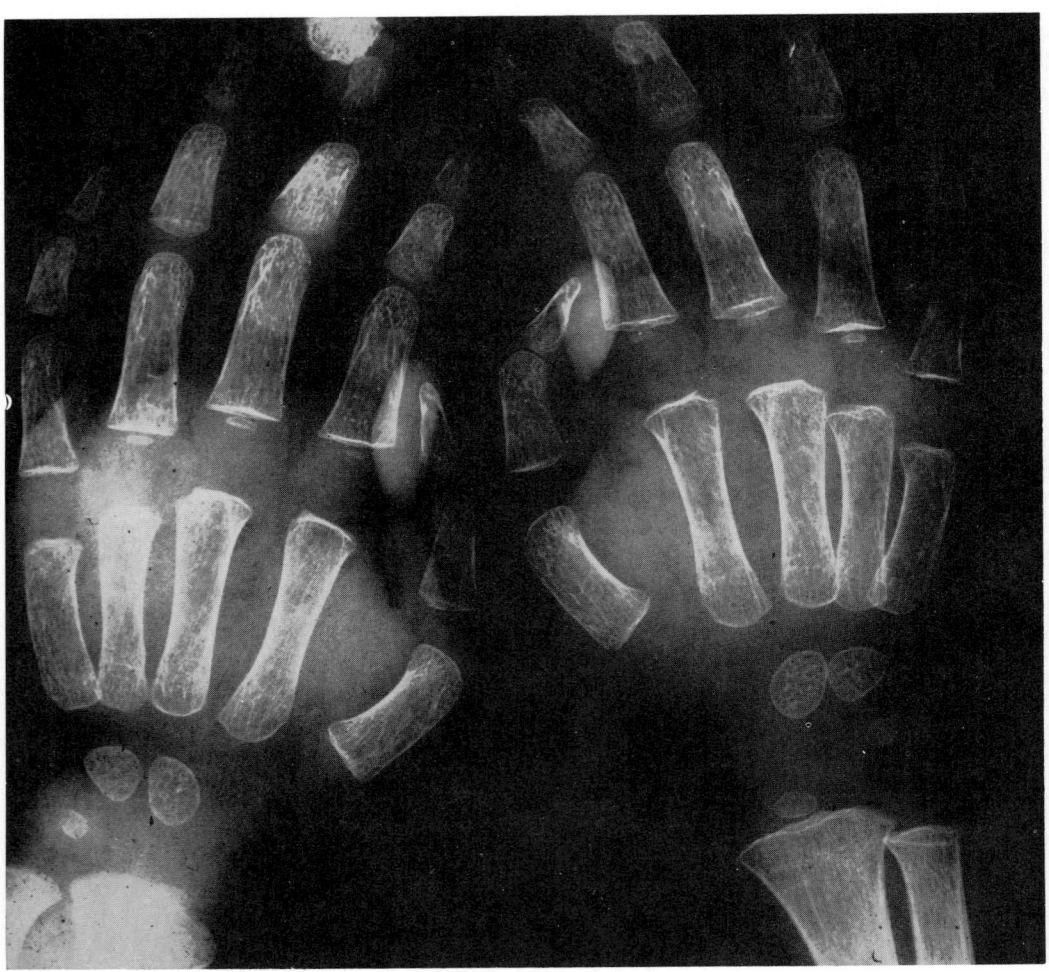

Fig. 21–7. The hands of a child with iron deficiency anemia, demonstrating widening of the metacarpals, prominent trabeculae of the bones of the hands and thin cortices. (Courtesy of Dr. Philip Lanzkowsky.)

ner. The squama occipitalis is usually not wide, a result of normally deficient marrow in this portion of the skull. The trabeculae may be perpendicular to the inner table, presenting a radial pattern which may have a "hair-on-end" appearance (Fig. 21–6A and B).

Involvement of the long bones has been described in only a few patients.[21,22] The metacarpals show widening from expansion of the medullary space, prominent trabeculae and thinning of the cortices (Fig. 21–7).

HYPERVITAMINOSIS A

Early roentgenographic findings of chronic vitamin A poisoning may be limited to widened sutures in the skull and a bulging anterior fontanelle (Fig. 21–8A and B). The long bones (Fig. 21–9A and 21–10) may be normal at this stage of the disease. The 2-year-old patient represented in Figures 21–8 to 21–10 was seen for anorexia and vomiting. Because her

fontanelle was full, a skull x-ray film was taken and demonstrated sutural diastasis. The dense line at the metaphyses of all long bones suggested lead poisoning. The history of a "poor eater" raised the possibility of pica, but careful questioning revealed that "extra" cod liver oil had been given, 100,000 units of vitamin A and 15,000 units of vitamin D, 1 to 3 times a day, intermittently during the previous 6 months. Serum vitamin A level was elevated. The dense line was considered to be caused by excess vitamin D. Two weeks after the diagnosis and the cessation of vitamin A, cortical hyperostosis was present on the ulnae (Fig. 21–9B) and the fibulae. The bone changes are usually symmetric. Three weeks after admission to the hospital the serum vitamin A became normal but the hyperostosis continued.

When soft tissue swellings are noted in association with clinical symptoms of vitamin A toxicity (e.g. anorexia, pruritus, alopecia, desquamation of the skin) cortical

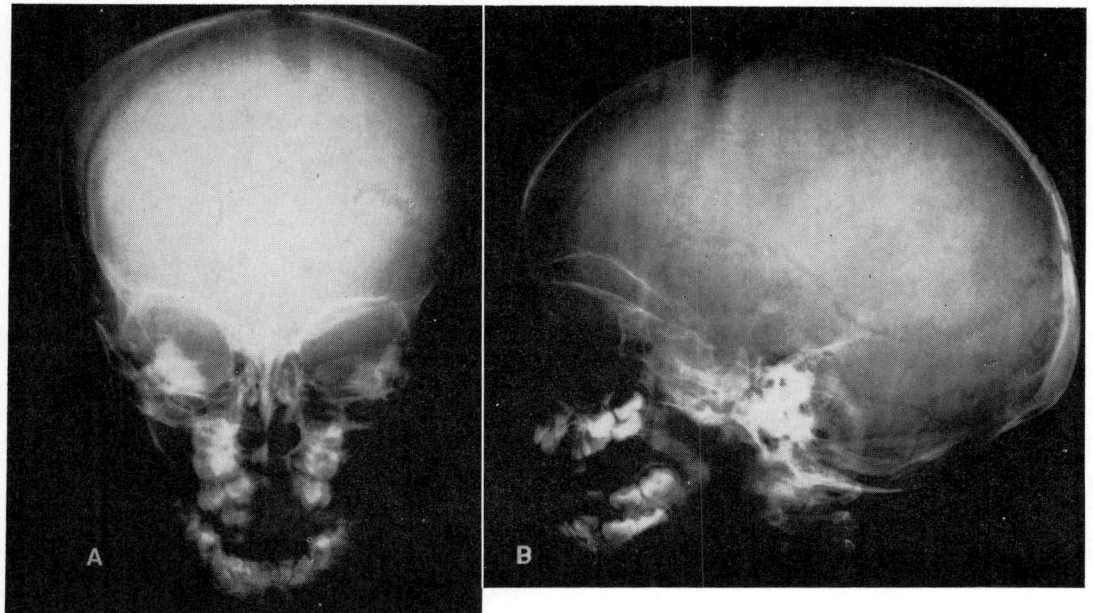

Fig. 21–8A and B. Skull of a 2-year-old female, in frontal and lateral projections, with hypervitaminosis A showing wide sagittal and coronal sutures.

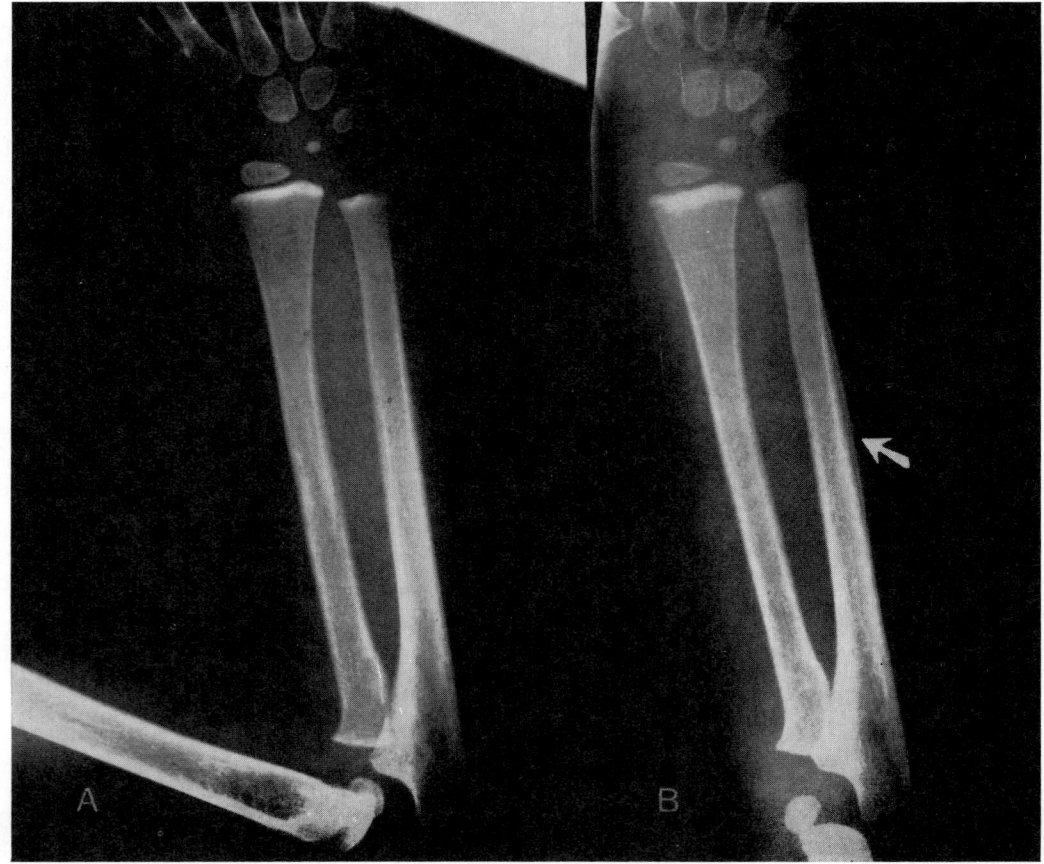

Fig. 21-9. Same patient as in Figure 21-8. *A*: Dense line at the distal end of radius and ulna. No subperiosteal new bone. *B*: Three weeks later periosteal new bone seen on the lateral aspect of the ulna.

thickening of long bones is present (Fig. 21-11*A*). Although vitamin A then is eliminated from the diet, the changes in the bones continue. The subperiosteal new bone continues to thicken (Fig. 21-11*B*). These cortical thickenings usually stop short of the ends of the shafts. In some patients metaphyseal cupping, splaying of the affected end of the shaft, hypertrophy of the contiguous epiphyseal ossification center and premature fusion of this center with the shaft are found (Fig. 21-11*B* and *C*). Premature fusion of the center with its shafts is most often seen at the distal ends of the femurs and results in arrested

growth, with permanent shortening of the affected bones. Although these changes at the metaphyses and epiphyses were demonstrated in experimental animals,[23,24] it was not until Pease[25] reported 7 patients in 1962 that this complication of vitamin poisoning was universally accepted. Cortical hyperostosis of ribs (Fig. 21-12) also occurs with vitamin A poisoning.

Caffey[26] reviewed the many diseases which cause cupping of the metaphyses. He believes that the basic defect is a reduced growth in the arterial segment of the epiphyseal plate. The "walls" of the cup are dependent on the periosteal and

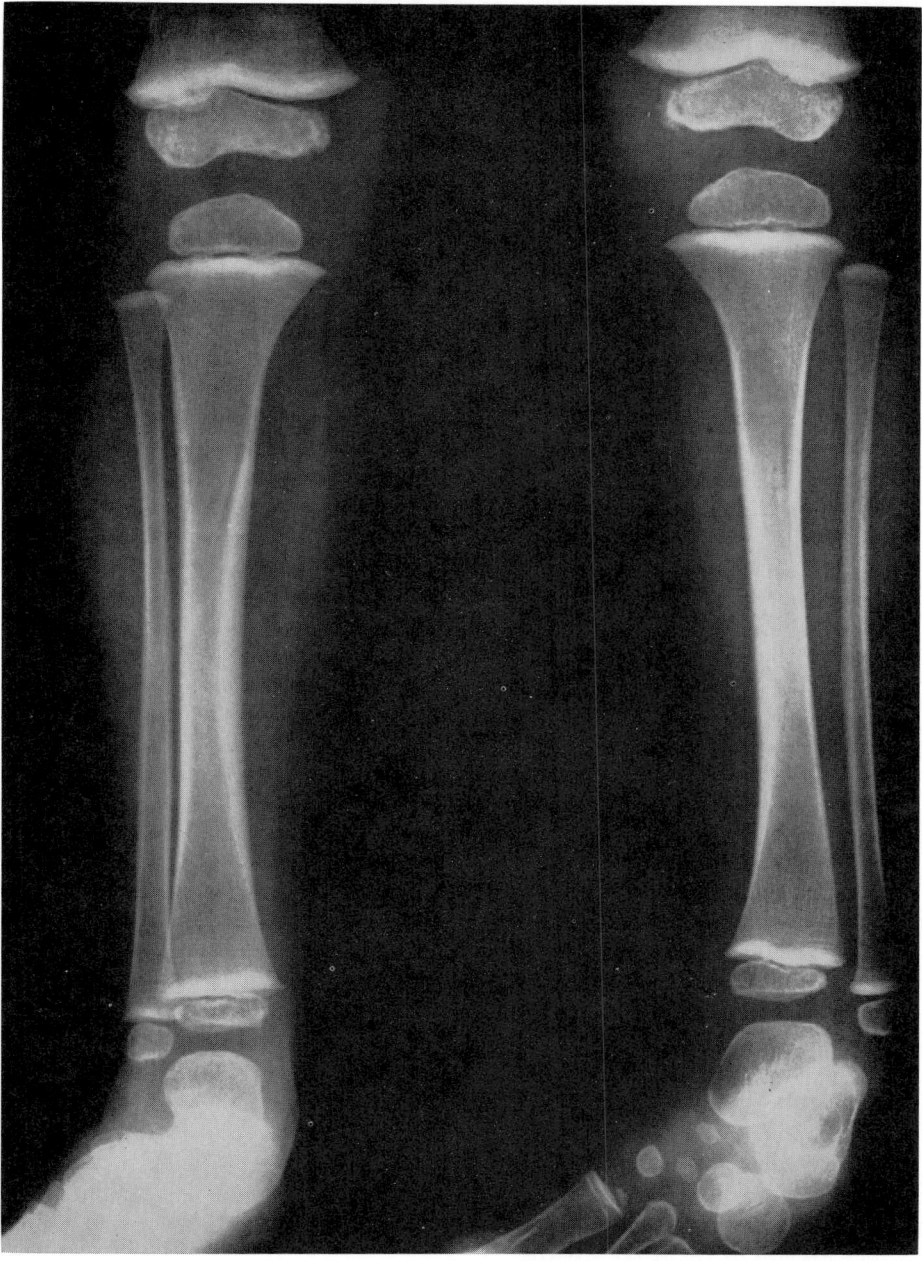

Fig. 21–10. Same patient as in Figure 21–8. Initial roentgenograms of the metaphyses at the knees and ankles demonstrate dense lines. No periosteal new bone is present.

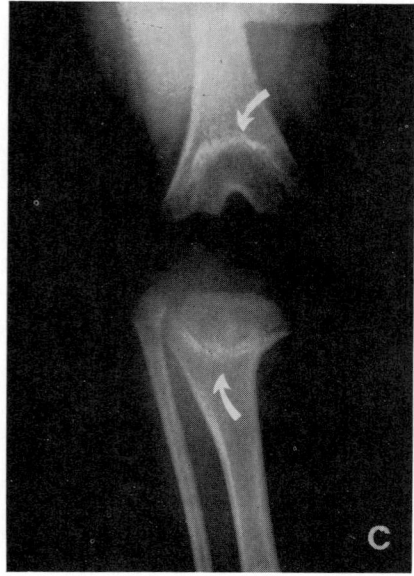

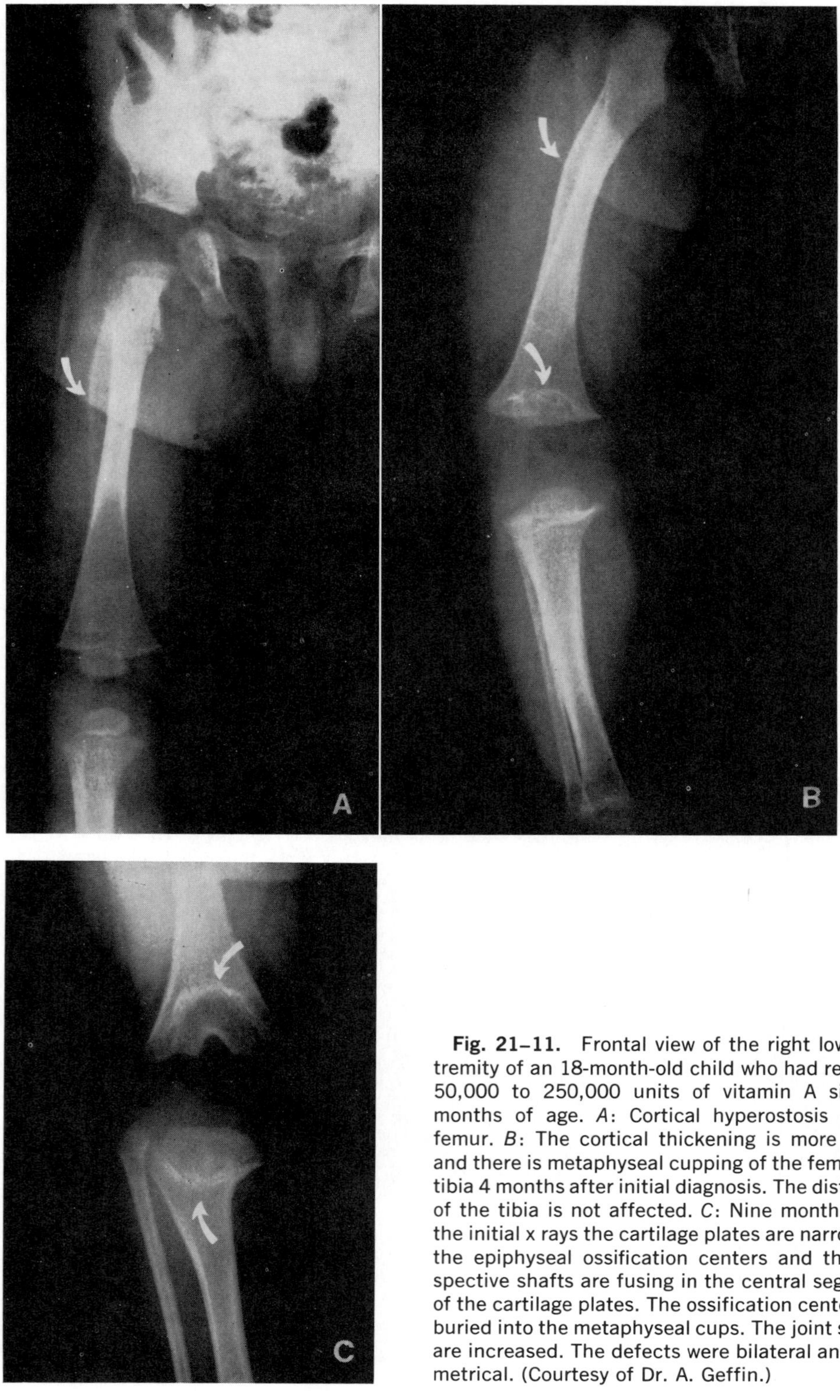

Fig. 21–11. Frontal view of the right lower extremity of an 18-month-old child who had received 50,000 to 250,000 units of vitamin A since 3 months of age. *A*: Cortical hyperostosis of the femur. *B*: The cortical thickening is more dense and there is metaphyseal cupping of the femur and tibia 4 months after initial diagnosis. The distal end of the tibia is not affected. *C*: Nine months after the initial x rays the cartilage plates are narrow and the epiphyseal ossification centers and their respective shafts are fusing in the central segments of the cartilage plates. The ossification centers are buried into the metaphyseal cups. The joint spaces are increased. The defects were bilateral and symmetrical. (Courtesy of Dr. A. Geffin.)

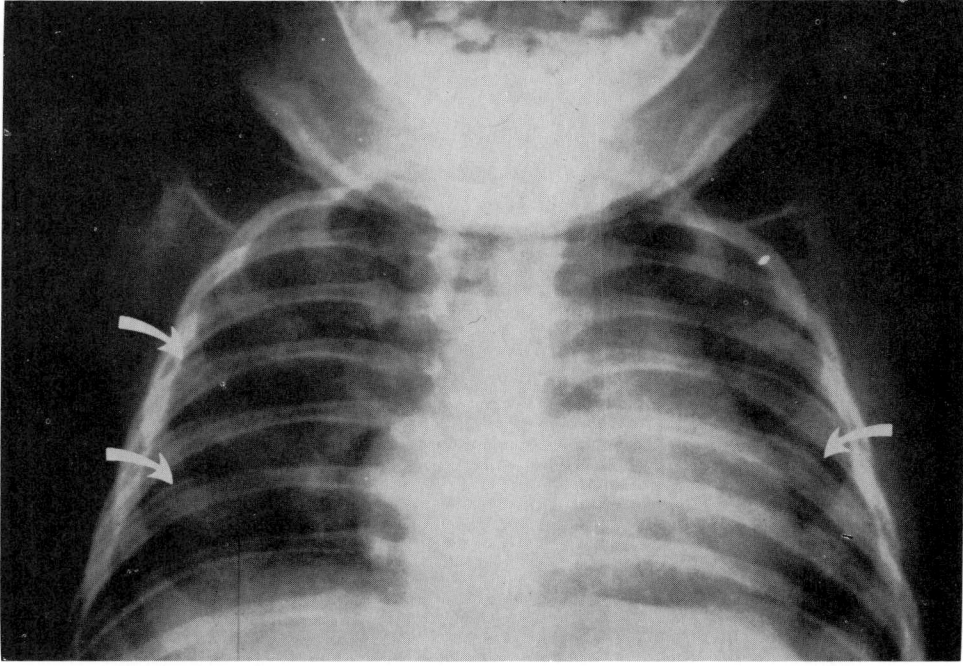

Fig. 21–12. Same patient as in Figure 21–11. Chest roentgenogram shows cortical hyperostosis of many ribs caused by vitamin A poisoning.

metaphyseal arteries, not on the epiphyseal arteries, and, therefore, the peripheral zones of the bones continue to grow. Caffey suggests that in vitamin A poisoning spontaneous immobilization is caused by exquisite pain and hyperesthesia. Immobilization causes slowing and stagnation of the blood, which lead to thrombosis of the arteries of the epiphyseal plate.

HYPERVITAMINOSIS D

In the presence of an excess of vitamin D an increased mobilization of mineral occurs with secondary hypercalcemia and phosphatemia.[27] Calcific deposits occur in the renal tubules with secondary renal failure, and sometimes death results. In the growing child the zone of provisional calcification becomes relatively dense in comparison to the adjacent metaphyseal region. In addition, extensive periarticular and vessel calcification may be present with, in some cases, premature vascular calcification.[28,29] When the calcium intake is correspondingly high, thickening of the bony cortex may result so that, instead of decreased density, the bones may in fact be more dense. Distinguishing between this entity, hypercalcemia and hypovitaminosis D can be difficult radiographically.

SUTURAL DIASTASIS FOLLOWING RAPID WEIGHT GAIN

Sutural diastasis has been considered a sign of acute raised intracranial pressure in children, especially under the age of 10 years. Capitanio and Kirkpatrick[30] described 3 children with nutritional deprivation who developed increased head circumference and cranial sutures following the correction of malnutrition. In 1970, two other reports[31,32] added 9 more children with these changes related to nutrition. The increased head circumference

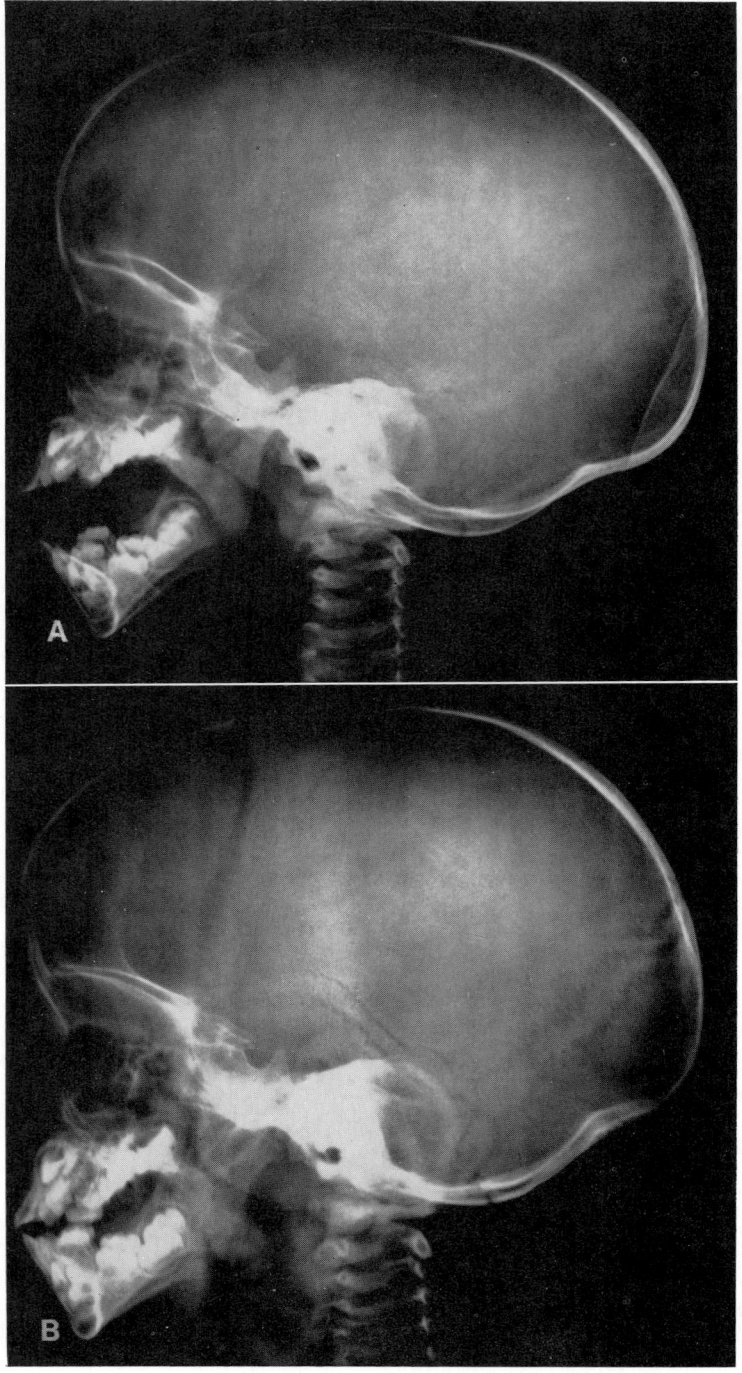

Fig. 21–13. Thirty-month-old male hospitalized for failure to thrive. *A*: Lateral skull roentgenogram at time of admission is normal. *B*: Two months later, when the child had gained weight and was well, the lateral skull roentgenogram demonstrates wide coronal and lamboid sutures.

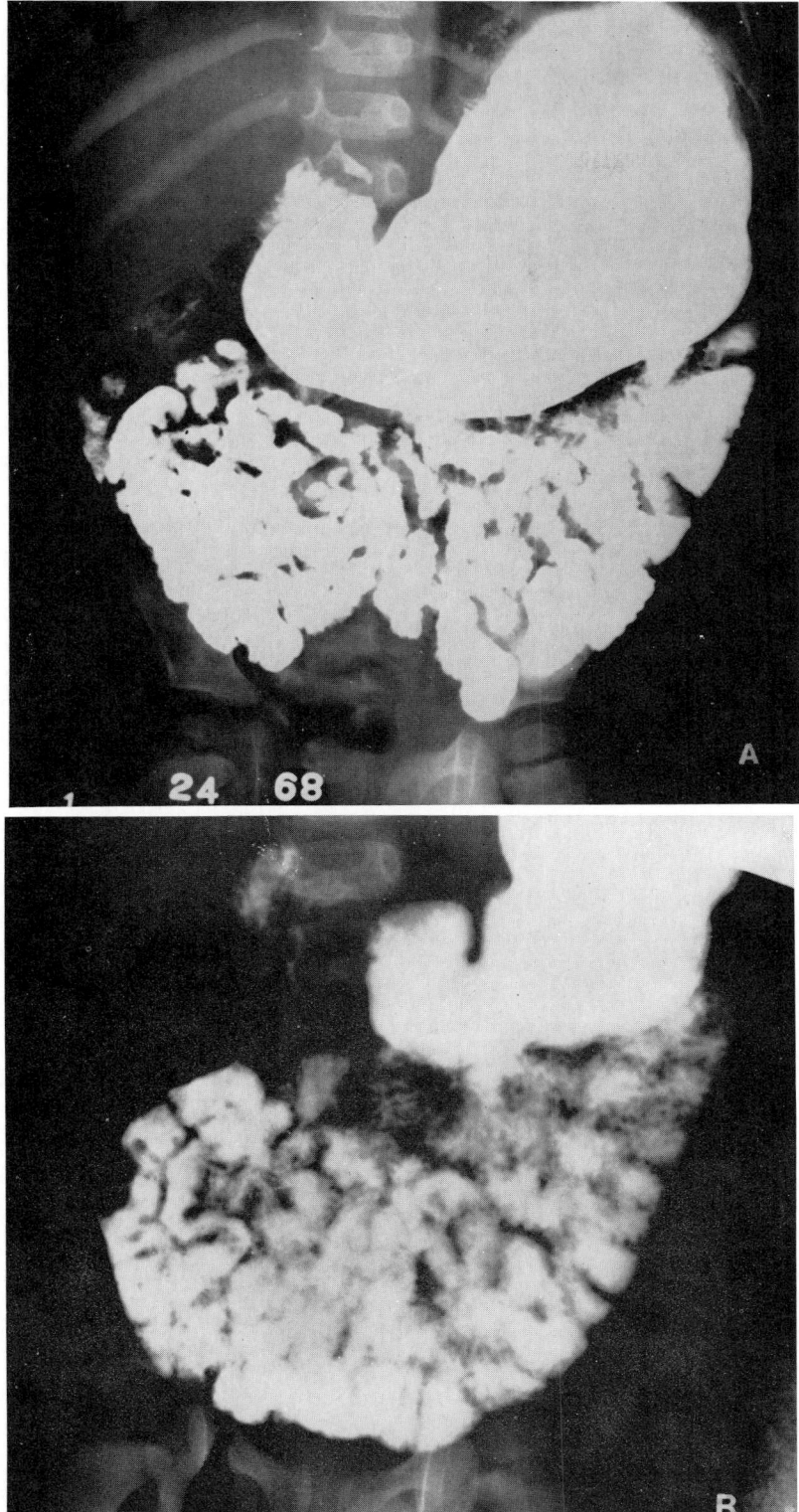

Fig. 21–14. *A*: Gastrointestinal series 2 weeks after admission demonstrates a large stomach and separated loops of small intestine with thickened valvulae connivents. *B*: Four weeks after the original study, when the patient was well, repeated intestinal studies show the small intestine to be normal.

and separation of the cranial sutures (Fig. 21–13*A* and *B*) are caused by cellular growth of the brain when nutrition is improved in previously malnourished young children.[33] Although the sutural diastasis simulates increased intracranial pressure, there are no abnormal neurologic signs or symptoms. No increased intracranial pressure has been noted, and, in the one patient who had a pneumoencephalogram, the lateral ventricles were normal.

Distention of the stomach may be apparent on abdominal roentgenogram in nutritional deprivation. One patient had a small bowel study done as part of the workup for "failure to thrive." Thickened valvulae conniventes and separation of loops, noted (Fig. 21–14*A*) on an early examination, were normal (Fig. 21–14*B*) on an examination 1 month later. The pathogenesis of the gastrointestinal changes is not known, but it was thought that these findings were the result of edema although the serum albumin was normal.

MILK-ALKALI SYNDROME

With excessive ingestion of milk and alkali, usually related to peptic ulcer disease, insoluble calcium and phosphate precipitates may occur,[34] resulting in a renal tubular deposition of calcium with visible demonstration of nephrocalcinosis. To a certain extent the condition can be relieved by limiting the intake of calcium. Soft tissue calcification, usually periarticular in nature, is also a feature of this syndrome; however, the most common finding is that of calculi within the upper urinary tracts.[35]

FLUOROSIS

When fluorine is used to excess, probably above levels of 4 million ppm in water, or in the treatment of osteoporosis, multiple myeloma or Paget's disease, certain side effects may be demonstrated.[36] Arguments persist as to the exact mechanism by which fluorine exerts its effects, but in all probability it acts by decreasing the solubility of bone salts, thus impairing the process of osteolysis. Radiographically thickening and coarsening of the trabeculae and similar changes in the cortex are seen. The overall result is one of increased density of the bony structure, although the underlying abnormality is sometimes difficult to visualize. Similar changes, of course, are seen in cases of myelosclerosis and myelofibrosis.

LEAD AND BISMUTH

Both these heavy metals have an affinity for bone and act by replacing calcium. In these days the effects of bismuth are rarely seen, as it is seldom used for the treatment of syphilis in the growing child except when the mother has been treated during pregnancy. However, cases of lead poisoning still present themselves where eating of lead paint has been the causative factor. In the growing child deposition of heavy metals is principally seen in the region of the metaphyses of long bones, particularly where there is accelerated growth, i.e. the knee, ankle and wrist. Intoxication makes itself evident by zones of increased density in this region. Confirmation may be obtained by the visualization of heavy metal content in the GI tract, together with widening of the skull sutures, indicating increased intracranial pressure.

GASTROINTESTINAL DISTURBANCES

While the clinical presentation of gastrointestinal abnormalities that may lead to nutritional disturbances is often nonspecific, gastrointestinal contrast studies may be crucial in making the correct initial diagnosis, in outlining the site and extent of disease or in indicating the likely underlying entities requiring further investigation. In many of these conditions x-ray interpretation relies upon subtle but characteristic findings. It must be emphasized that x-ray abnormalities may reflect pathologic anatomic changes or physiologic disturbances.

Malabsorption Syndrome

Sprue. This group of diseases includes celiac diseases of children, nontropical sprue (gluten-induced enteropathy, idiopathic steatorrhea) and tropical sprue. Characteristic radiologic changes in the small intestine are present in almost all patients during the active phase of the disease.[37,38] The sine qua non of this deficiency state includes: (1) dilatation of small bowel loops, either diffusely or more marked in the middle and distal jejunum, and (2) hypersecretion, shown by dilution of the barium suspension often with striking flocculation and segmentation (Fig. 21–15A and B).

Frazier et al.[39] have shown that the classic "deficiency pattern" of segmentation within the small bowel is not necessarily associated with disordered motor function of the intestinal wall but is dependent upon the quality of the contents of the intestinal lumen. The loops are flaccid and contract poorly, so that the transit time through the small bowel may be delayed. Little intrinsic change occurs in the mucosal folds. Their appearance is dependent upon the amount of secretions and peristaltic disorder. Short nonobstructive intussusceptions may transiently occur.[40]

The peculiar relationship of sprue and lymphosarcoma of the bowel[41] must be kept in mind. Not only may lymphoma demonstrate sprue-like malabsorption[42] but the incidence of lymphoma complicating well-documented chronic cases of adult celiac disease is about 7 per cent.[43] Roentgenographic study may be helpful in the distinction.[38]

Malabsorption and a sprue-like

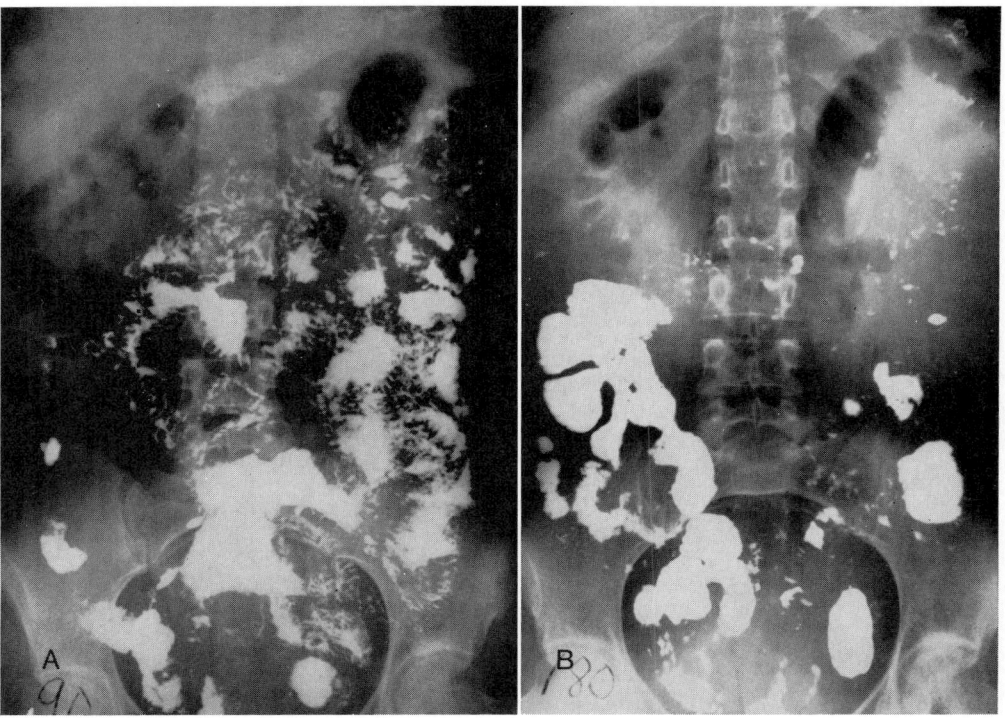

Fig. 21–15. Nontropical sprue. *A*: At 90 minutes, conspicuous fragmentation and flocculation of the barium suspension are seen. Disordered motor activity is apparent. *B*: At 180 minutes, segmentation of the contrast within ileal loops occurs, further reflecting hypersecretion.

radiologic pattern may result from vascular insufficiency of the small bowel.[44,45] This must be suspected clinically if malabsorption appears in middle or later life, particularly if accompanied by abdominal angina or manifestations of atherosclerotic occlusive disease elsewhere. Abdominal aortography and selective arteriography may be crucial in establishing the diagnosis. Revascularization procedures have been shown to reverse the steatorrhea.[45]

Whipple's Disease (intestinal lipodystrophy). While the multisystem involvement of this disease is shown by the major clinical manifestations of diarrhea, steatorrhea, arthralgias, increased skin pigmentation, lymphadenopathy and serous effusions, the intestinal symptoms are usually predominant by the time the diagnosis is established.

Small intestinal series demonstrate definite thickening of the mucosal folds in the jejunum and duodenum and only oc-

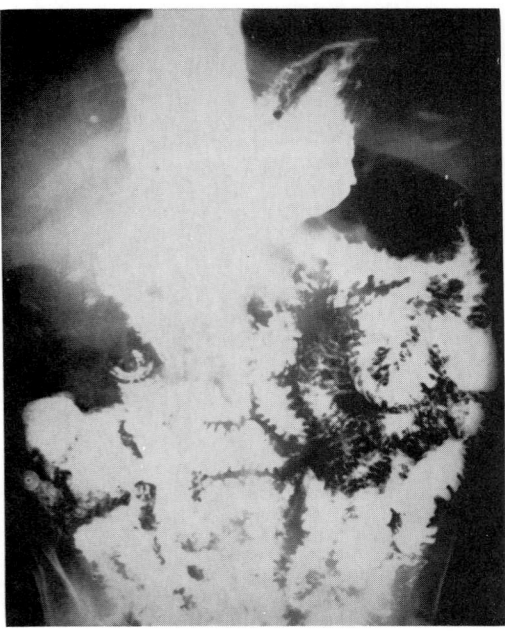

Fig. 21-16. Whipple's disease. Markedly prominent valvulae conniventes without hypersecretion or dilatation.

casionally in the ileum (Fig. 21-16). The coarsened folds are frequently wild and redundant in outline and may present slightly nodular contours. No significant hypersecretion or dilatation is shown; any flocculation or segmentation is minimal. There is normal peristaltic activity and transit time from stomach to cecum is within normal limits.[46,47]

The diagnosis can be established by intestinal mucosal or lymph node biopsy. The small bowel villi are swollen and the lamina propria is infiltrated with macrophages containing PAS-positive bodies. These have been shown to be bacteria.[48] Improvement in the radiologic picture may parallel the clinical remission on long-term antibiotic therapy.[47]

Scleroderma (diffuse systemic sclerosis). The hallmarks of sclerodermatous involvement of the alimentary tract are dilatation and a marked diminution in peristaltic activity. These reflect the underlying pathologic changes of collagen replacement of the muscular layers. Bacterial overgrowth in the intestinal lumen is now recognized as a major cause for steatorrhea in patients with scleroderma.

The esophagus is most commonly involved and presents hypomotility and some dilatation. Poor drainage results, and characteristic roentgenographic findings include failure of the esophagus to empty on prone films and stasis even in the erect position, with air-fluid levels (Fig. 21-17A).

In the intestines, large flaccid loops are seen without hypersecretion. The dilatation may appear most striking in the descending duodenum (Fig. 21-17B). Transit time is often markedly prolonged. Colonic dilatation and hypotonicity may also be present, with characteristic secondary pseudosacculations projecting from the antimesenteric border of the transverse colon (Fig. 21-17C).

Amyloidosis. The presence of malabsorption in some patients with amyloidosis has been well established.[49] In a report

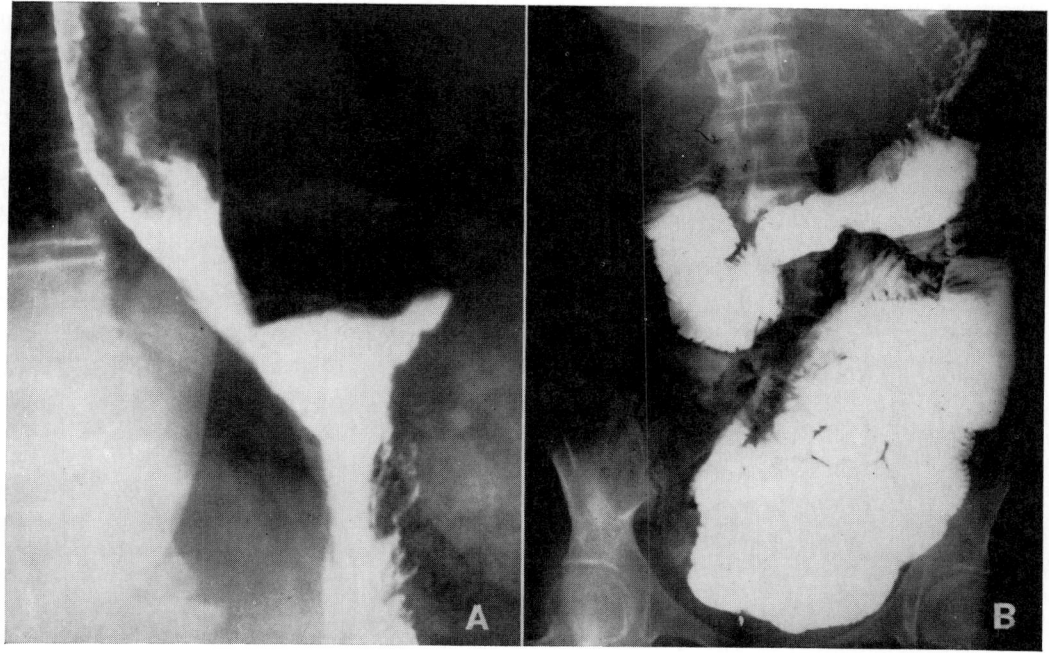

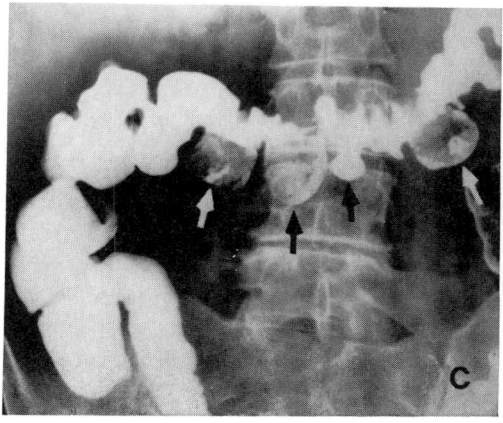

Fig. 21–17. Scleroderma. A: Despite a nonobstructed lumen, differential fluid levels persist in the esophagus and stomach in the upright position. B: Diffuse involvement of the small bowel results in gross dilatation, most evident in the descending duodenum and jejunum. C: Asymmetric involvement of the colon is shown by large wide-mounted pseudosacculation (arrows).

from the Mayo Clinic, Herskovic et al.[50] reviewed 103 patients with amyloidosis and were able to find 6 with documented steatorrhea. With known gastrointestinal involvement, the incidence of malabsorption may approach 50 per cent.[51] Radiologically, markedly diminished motility, conspicuous valvulae conniventes and, rarely, tumor-like deposits scattered throughout the intestinal tract may be present.[51]

Disaccharidase Deficiency. This is probably the most common abnormality of the small bowel in man, the only known mammal in whom lactase activity in the small intestine is maintained after weaning. Diarrhea, cramps and flatulence after milk ingestion clinically indicate the disorder, which can be easily confirmed roentgenologically.[52,53] When 50 gm of lactose are added to the usual barium mix-

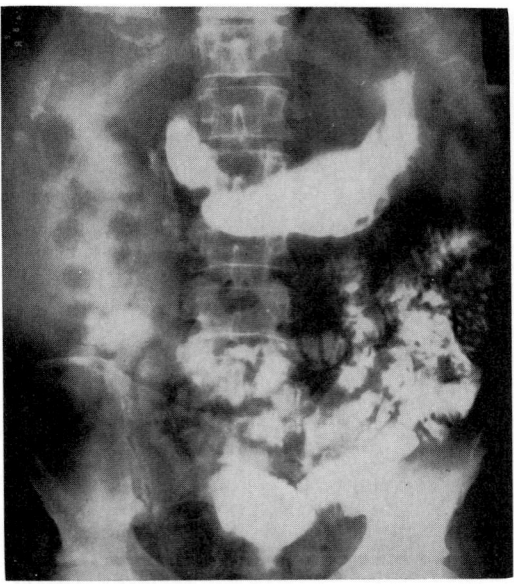

Fig. 21-18. Lactase deficiency. A barium-lactose mixture results in progressive dilution and hypermotility.

ture, characteristic changes occur in the small bowel series. These include dilution of the barium, particularly noticeable in the ileum and colon, and dilatation of the small bowel (Fig. 21-18). These effects are secondary to the ingress of water into the bowel lumen in response to the osmotic forces of the disaccharide. Rapid intestinal motility accompanies the dilatation.

Intestinal lactase deficiency occurs on a genetic basis and is also common in a variety of intestinal disorders. This radiologic technique is the most valuable screening aid for it. The addition of lactose to the barium sulfate mixture does not interfere with the examination of the small bowel in patients without disaccharidase deficiency. When a lactase deficiency is discovered, a conventional small bowel examination with barium alone is indicated to identify any morphologic abnormality.[53]

Small Bowel Resection. The severity of malabsorption after small bowel resection generally depends on the extent and site of resection, presence of the ileocecal valve and the condition of the remaining small bowel and other digestive organs.[54] These parameters of the "short-gut syndrome" can be evaluated by roentgenographic study (Fig. 21-19). On occasion, the exact extent of resection performed in the past is not known when malabsorption becomes a serious problem of management. Since the normal length of small intestine is variable, more important than knowledge of the length of bowel *removed* is an accurate appraisal of the length in the *remaining* functioning loops.

This is best accomplished by measurements derived from x-ray study after the passage of an opaque tube. This obviates the inaccuracy inherent in measuring the continuity of superimposed barium-filled loops.

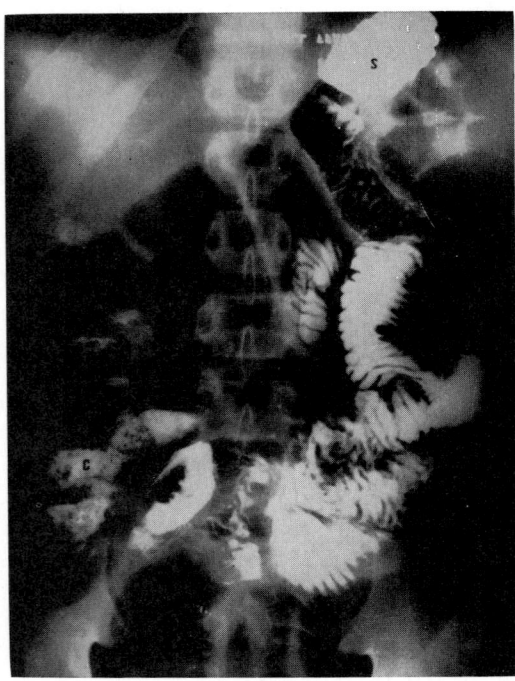

Fig. 21-19. Massive small bowel resection for volvulus following gastrojejunostomy. Few small bowel loops, primarily jejunal as shown by their mucosal pattern, remain between the stomach pouch (S) and the cecum (C).

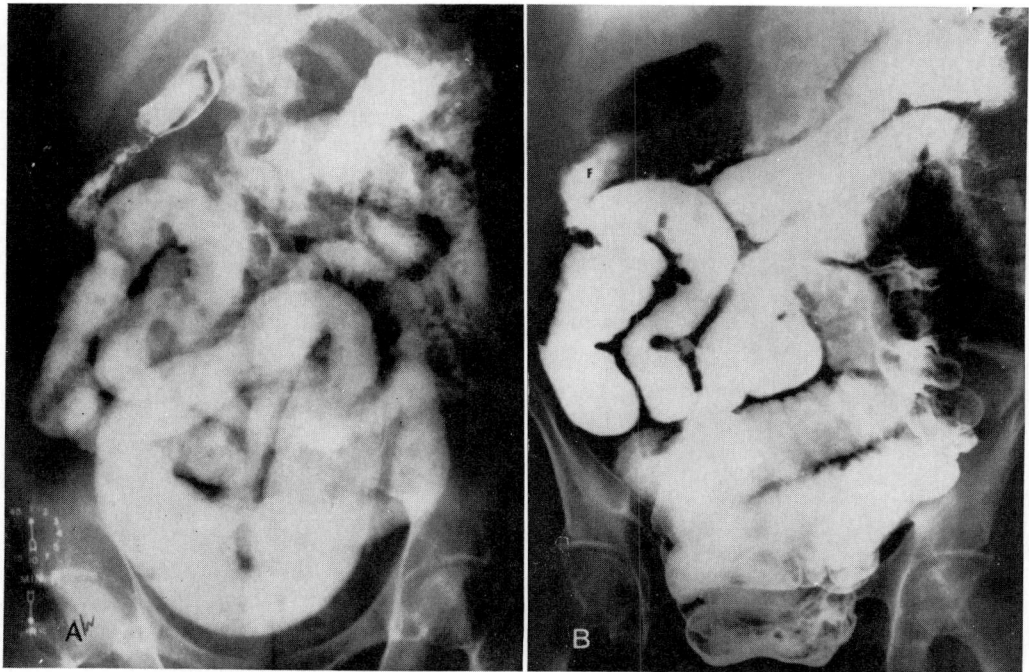

Fig. 21–20. Enteric fistula producing malabsorption following ileotransversostomy. *A*: Dilatation and hypersecretion of small bowel loops. While there is no flocculation or segmentation, these changes constitute a sprue-like pattern. *B*: During another examination, the fistula (F) between the distal ileum and descending duodenum is demonstrated.

Enteric fistulas (Fig. 21–20*A* and *B*) and inadvertent gastroileostomy[55] result in a similar condition by bypassing the absorptive mechanisms of the small bowel.

Diverticula, Blind Loops and Strictures. Common to all these conditions, which may result in malabsorption, is stasis of intestinal contents and bacterial overgrowth. Normally, the small bowel flora consists of predominantly gram-positive and anaerobic organisms. The ileocecal valve serves to separate two distinct groups of organisms: above, mainly streptococci, lactobacilli and fungi; below, coliforms, bacteroides and anaerobic lactobacilli.[56] In a variety of disease states, an overgrowth of bacteria—especially the anaerobic bacteroides, lactobacilli and clostridia—may occur and cause steatorrhea by deconjugating and/or dehydroxylating primary bile salts in the intestinal lumen.[57]

Diverticulosis of the small bowel is readily recognized as multiple outpouchings without gross intrinsic contractility from the mesenteric borders of the loops. Blind loops may be a result of (side-to-side) intestinal anastomoses, an obstructed postoperative loop, as in the afferent-loop syndrome following a Billroth II gastrojejunostomy (Fig. 21–21), multiple strictures of the intestine, as in the stenotic phase of regional enteritis,[38] or post-radiation changes (Fig. 21–22). In radiation enteritis, lymphatic dilatation, bowel thickening and avascularity may also contribute to the malabsorption.[58]

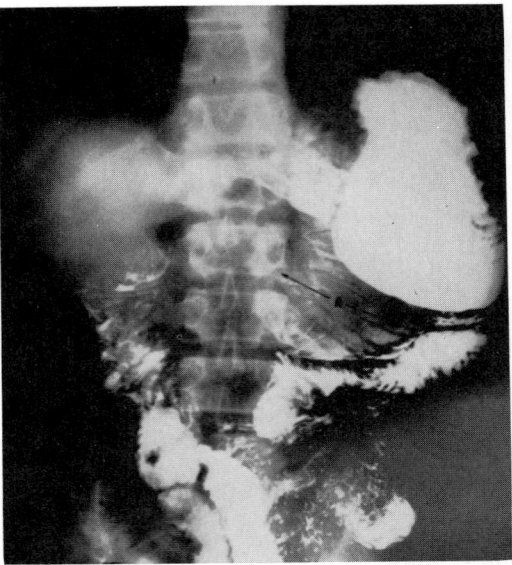

Fig. 21–21. Afferent loop syndrome. The massively distended, obstructed afferent loop following a Billroth II gastrojejunostomy constitutes a blind loop leading to malabsorption.

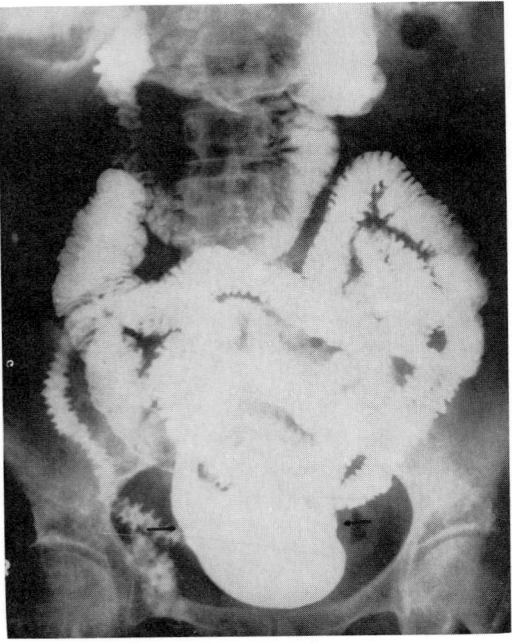

Fig. 21–22. Blind loop secondary to radiation effects. Stasis within a fixed, distended loop as a consequence of multiple strictures.

Parasitic Diseases. The enteritis caused by infestation with Giardia lamblia[59] or Strongyloides stercoralis[60] is reflected by roentgenographic alterations, which may first draw the attention of the clinician to the diagnosis.

Dysgammaglobulinemia. Hypogammaglobulinemia may underlie a clinical pattern of repeated infections and chronic or intermittent diarrhea and mild steatorrhea. In 1966, Hermans and his co-workers[61] noted the association of nodular lymphoid hyperplasia of the small intestine, with or without giardiasis, in cases of dysgammaglobulinemia with a disproportionate deficiency of the IgA and IgM components. These nodular hyperplastic lymphoid follicles in the lamina propria can be recognized as tiny, 1- to 3-mm filling defects, primarily in the duodenum and jejunum[62] (Fig. 21–23A and B). Their recognition may be an important clue in directing the clinician to evaluation of the gamma globulins and to intestinal biopsy for information necessary in management.

Uncommon Constitutional Disorders. In recent years, a number of uncommon systemic diseases in which malabsorption may be a significant complication have been recognized. Radiologic abnormalities in the gastrointestinal tract have been noted or are a conspicuous feature in the Canada-Cronkhite syndrome,[63] mastocytosis,[64] Degos' disease,[65] abetalipoproteinemia (Bassen-Kornzweig syndrome),[66] and Waldenstrom's macroglobulinemia.[67]

PROTEIN-LOSING ENTEROPATHY

There is now widespread recognition that excessive gastrointestinal protein loss is a major cause of hypoproteinemia seen in association with a wide variety of disorders. Loss of protein secondary to exudation through an inflamed or ulcerated mucosa (as in regional enteritis or ulcerative colitis) or secondary to obstructed outflow of the gastrointestinal lymphatics (as in lymphoma or Whipple's disease) is well

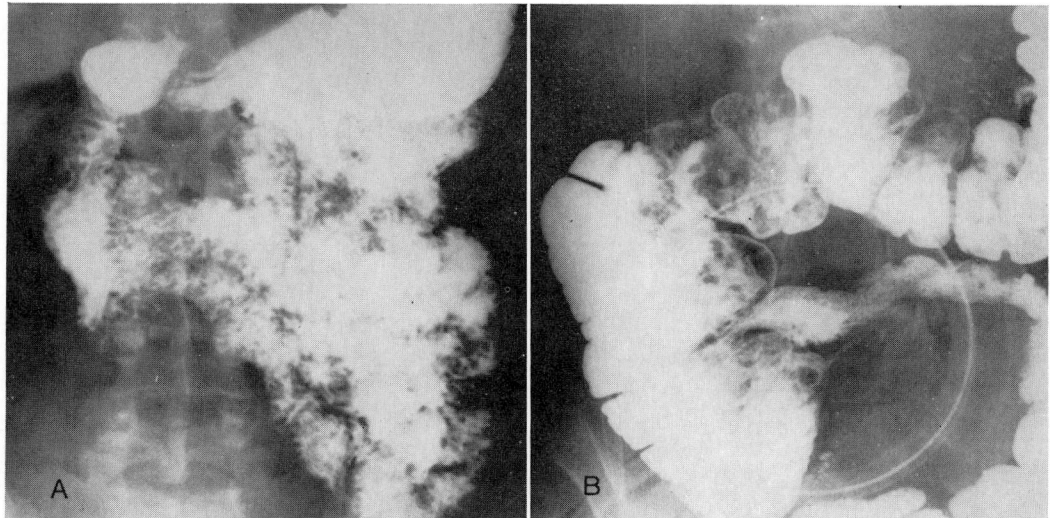

Fig. 21–23. Nodular lymphoid hyperplasia of the small intestine associated with hypogamma-globulinemia. Two different cases illustrate multiple punctate to nodular submucosal filling defects in the jejunum *(A)* and terminal ileum *(B)*.

known. In an excellent review, Waldmann[68] has compiled over 40 such gastrointestinal disorders and emphasizes that, in many of these patients with clearly defined gastrointestinal tract diseases, hypoproteinemia and edema may be the only clinical manifestations.

Giant Hypertrophy of the Gastric Mucosa (Menetrier's disease). Massively enlarged gastric rugae may be the site of loss of plasma proteins, particularly albumin, into the lumen.[69] They characteristically are more prominent along the greater curvature and usually do not extend to involve the gastric antrum. The hypertrophied folds maintain pliability and are not nodular or ulcerated (Fig. 21–24).

Intestinal Lymphangiectasia. This syndrome reflects a generalized disorder of the development of lymphatic channels. First defined by Waldmann in 1961, it is characterized by excessive loss of serum protein into the intestine with massive edema (often asymmetric), chylous effusions, hypoalbuminemia and hypogammaglobulinemia. The dilated lymphatic

vessels invariably present in the intestinal wall may leak protein through an intact epithelium or may rupture and discharge their contents into the lumen of the gut. Isotopic studies are helpful in document-

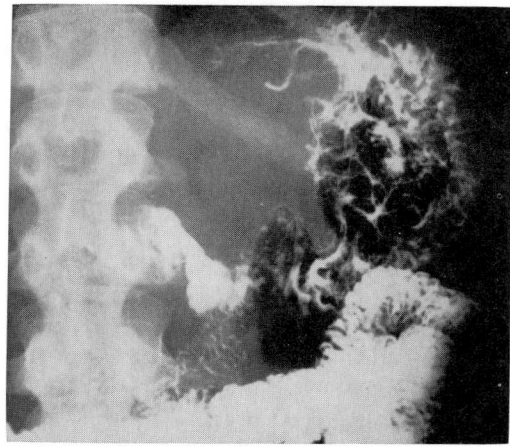

Fig. 21–24. Menetrier's disease. Markedly enlarged gastric folds, particularly prominent in the upper two-thirds of the stomach.

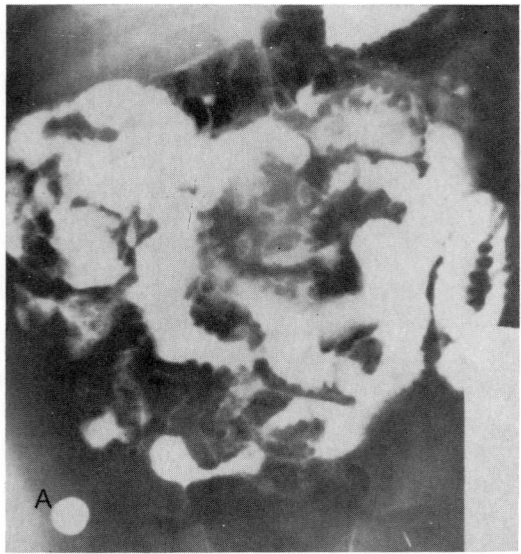

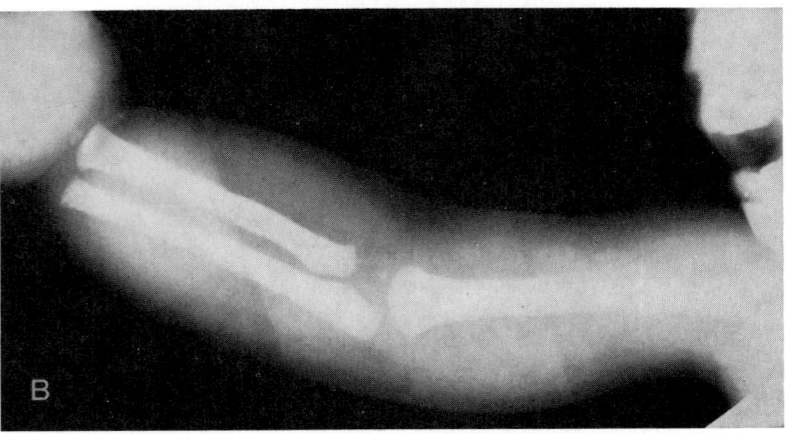

Fig. 21–25. Intestinal lymphangiectasia. Three-year-old child with severe protein-losing enteropathy. *A:* Prominent mucosal folds within mildly dilated small bowel loops containing increased secretions. *B:* Edematous involvement of right upper extremity.

ing the serum protein loss into the intestine.

The condition is being recognized with increased frequency, and x-ray study plays an important role in its diagnosis. The characteristic appearance in the small bowel series consists of enlargement of the valvulae conniventes of both jejunum and ileum, increased secretions and minimal or absent dilatation of the bowel (Fig. 21–25*A*

and *B*). The fold enlargement may assume a "cobblestone" pattern. Punctate filling defects occasionally seen may represent the enormously enlarged villi secondary to dilated submucosal lymphatics.[70]

Hypoalbuminemia itself, below a level of 2.5 gm per 100 ml resulting from other causes (e.g. nephrosis or hepatic cirrhosis), may result in edema of the bowel with diffusely thickened intestinal folds[71] but

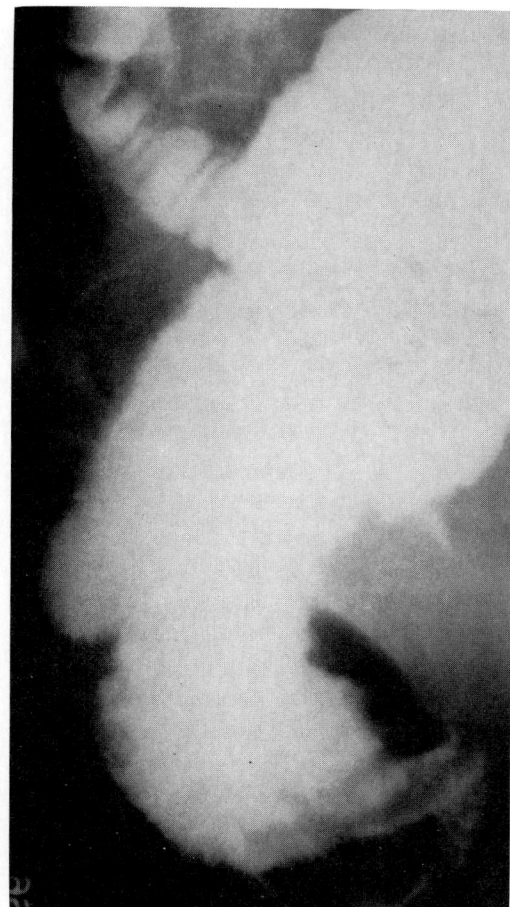

Fig. 21–26. Villous adenoma of rectum. Large circumferential mucosal mass with diffusely irregular contours.

usually does not exhibit increased intraluminal secretions.

Lymphangiographic findings support the concept that this disease is a systemic lymphatic dysplasia.[70,72] In the lower extremities, either hypoplasia of lymph vessels or dilated varicose lymphatics are present. In the abdomen, hypoplasia of lymph nodes or moderate contrast reflux into mesenteric lymphatics, associated with possible obstruction of the cisterna chyli and enlarged lymph nodes, has been demonstrated.

Villous Adenoma of the Colon. Among the neoplasms of the gastrointestinal tract which may produce excess secretion of mucus to result in severe protein loss, villous adenoma of the colon is one of the most prominent. It is most common in the rectum, where, because of its usual soft consistency, it may be easily missed on digital palpation. On barium enema examination, it is revealed by its characteristically irregular polypoid or flame-shaped contours as the contrast agent fills in the interstices between its frond-like projections (Fig. 21–26).

BIBLIOGRAPHY

1. Gould: Am. J. Med. Sci., *223,* 569, 1952.
2. Barnett and Nordin: Br. J. Radiol., *34,* 683, 1961.
3. Shapiro: Clin. Radiol., *13,* 238, 1962.
4. Harrison, Fraser and Mullan: Lancet, *1,* 1015, 1961.
5. Park: Pediatrics, *33* (Suppl.), 815, 1964.
6. Steinbach: Radiol. Clin. North Am., *2,* 191, 1964.
7. Park, Guild, Jackson and Bond: Arch. Dis. Child., *10,* 265, 1935.
8. McLean and McIntosh: Am. J. Dis. Child., *36,* 875, 1928.
9. Kato: Radiology, *18,* 1096, 1932.
10. Albright, Burnett, Parson, Reifenstein and Roos: Medicine, *25,* 399, 1946.
11. Lasser: *Dynamic Factors in Roentgen Diagnosis.* Baltimore, Williams & Wilkins, 1967.
12. Milkman: Am. J. Roentgenol., *32,* 622, 1934.
13. Park: Harvey Lect., *34,* 157, 1938–39.
14. Park and Jackson: J. Pediatr., *13,* 748, 1938.
15. Sheldon: Proc. R. Soc. Med., *29,* 743, 1936.
16. Shahidi and Diamond: N. Engl. J. Med., *262,* 137, 1960.
17. Britton, Canby and Kohler: Pediatrics, *25,* 621, 1960.
18. Moseley: J. Mt. Sinai Hosp., *29,* 109, 1962.
19. Burko, Mellins and Watson: Am. J. Roentgenol., *86,* 447, 1961.
20. Ryan: Med. J. Aust., *1,* 844, 1962.
21. Lanzkowsky: Am. J. Dis. Child., *116,* 16, 1968.
22. Holt and Hodges: *Year Book of Radiology,* 1958–1959 Series. Chicago, Year Book Medical Publishers, 1958, p. 51.
23. Wolbach: J. Bone Joint Surg., *45,* 171, 1947.
24. Maddock, Wolbach and Maddock: J. Nutr., *39,* 117, 1949.
25. Pease: J.A.M.A., *182,* 980, 1962.
26. Caffey: Am. J. Roentgenol., *108,* 451, 1970.
27. Christiansen, Liebman and Sosman: Am. J. Roentgenol., *65,* 27, 1951.
28. Bauer and Freyberg: J.A.M.A., *130,* 1208, 1946.
29. Danowski, Winkler and Peters: Ann. Intern. Med., *23,* 22, 1945.
30. Capitanio and Kirkpatrick: Radiology, *92,* 53, 1969.

31. Sondheimer, Grossman and Winchester: Arch. Neurol., 23, 314, 1970.
32. DeLevie and Nogrady: J. Pediatr., 76, 523, 1970.
33. Wincik and Rosso: J. Pediatr., 14, 774, 1969.
34. Wenger, Kersner and Palmer. Am. J. Med., 24, 161, 1958.
35. Burnett, Commons, Albright and Howard: N. Engl. J. Med., 240, 787, 1949.
36. Leone, Stevenson, Hilbish and Sosman: Am. J. Roentgenol., 74, 874, 1955.
37. Laws, Booth, Shawdon and Steward: Br. Med. J., 1, 1311, 1963.
38. Marshak and Lindner: Semin. Roentgenol., 1, 138, 1966.
39. Frazier, French and Thompson: Br. J. Radiol., 22, 123, 1949.
40. Ruoff, Linder and Marshak: Am. J. Roentgenol., 104, 525, 1968.
41. Sherlock, Winawer, Goldstein and Bragg: Progress in Gastroenterology, Vol. II. New York, Grune & Stratton, 1970, pp. 367–391.
42. Sleisenger, Almy and Barr: Am. J. Med., 15, 66, 1953.
43. Harris, Cooke, Thompson and Waterhouse: Am. J. Med., 42, 899, 1967.
44. Shaw and Mayard: N. Engl. J. Med., 258, 874, 1958.
45. Watt, Watson and Haase: Br. Med. J., 3, 199, 1967.
46. Clemett and Marshak: Radiol. Clin. North Am., 7, 105, 1969.
47. Rice, Roufail and Reeves: Radiology, 88, 295, 1967.
48. Trier, Phelps, Edelman and Rubin: Gastroenterology, 48, 684, 1965.
49. Gilat and Spiro: Am. J. Dig. Dis., 13, 619, 1968.
50. Herskovic, Bartholomew and Green: Arch. Intern. Med., 114, 629, 1964.
51. Legge, Carlson and Wollaeger: Am. J. Roentgenol., 110, 406, 1970.
52. Laws and Neale: Lancet, 2, 139, 1966.
53. Preger and Amberg: Am. J. Roentgenol., 101, 287, 1967.
54. Winawer, Broitman, Wolochowo, Osborne and Zamcheck: N. Engl. J. Med., 274, 72, 1966.
55. Katz and Karp: Am. J. Roentgenol., 99, 162, 1967.
56. Gorbach, Plaut, Nahas, Weinstein, Spanknebel and Levitan: Gastroenterology, 53, 856, 1967.
57. Rosenberg, Hardison and Bull: N. Engl. J. Med., 276, 1391, 1967.
58. Tankel, Clark and Lee: Gut, 6, 560, 1965.
59. Marshak, Ruoff and Lindner: Am. J. Roentgenol., 104, 557, 1968.
60. Louisy and Barton: Radiology, 98, 535, 1971.
61. Hermans, Huizenga, Hoffman, Brown and Markowitz: Am. J. Med., 40, 78, 1966.
62. Hodgson, Hoffman and Huizenga: Radiology, 88, 883, 1967.
63. Orimo, Fujita, Yoshikawa, Takamoto, Matsuo and Nakao: Am. J. Med., 47, 445, 1969.
64. Clemett, Fishbone, Levine, James and Janower: Am. J. Roentgenol., 103, 405, 1968.
65. Strole, Clark and Isselbacher: N. Engl. J. Med., 276, 195, 1967.
66. Stacy and Loop: Am. J. Roentgenol., 92, 1072, 1964.
67. Khilnani, Keller and Cuttner: Radiol. Clin. North Am., 7, 43, 1969.
68. Waldmann: Gastroenterology, 50, 422, 1966.
69. Reese, Hodgson and Dockerty: Am. J. Roentgenol., 88, 619, 1962.
70. Shimkin, Waldmann and Krugman: Am. J. Roentgenol., 110, 827, 1970.
71. Marshak, Khilnani, Eliasoph and Wolf: Am. J. Roentgenol., 101, 379, 1967.
72. Bookstein, French and Pollard: Am. J. Dig. Dis., 10, 573, 1965.

Chapter 22

MALNUTRITION IN HOSPITAL PATIENTS: ASSESSMENT AND TREATMENT

C. E. Butterworth, Jr.
and
Roland L. Weinsier

Precise information on the frequency and severity of nutritional imbalance in hospitalized subjects is scarce because of human variables, wide differences in the duration of illness and metabolic problems associated with the disease itself, or with its treatment. However, we are learning that malnutrition is widespread among patients hospitalized longer than two weeks, that much of it is avoidable and that in some cases the disease or its treatment is associated with specific patterns of nutritional imbalance. Recent improvements in enteral and parenteral nutrition therapy have demonstrated dramatically the benefits to be derived from providing an adequate supply of nutrients during medical and surgical illnesses.

In 1965 Leevy and co-workers[1] first called attention to the rather common occurrence of hypovitaminemia among a random sample of patients in a large municipal hospital. These studies were extended by Bollet and Owens in 1973,[2] who compared a number of nutritional parameters in 51 hospital employees (controls) with 351 patients on the medical service. Patients were selected and evaluated according to seven separate diagnostic categories. It was observed that hemoglobin was below normal in 45 per cent of patients, serum albumin in 35 per cent, vitamin C in 26 per cent and vitamin A in 20 per cent. Body weight was below desirable standards in 24 per cent.

Bistrian et al.,[3,4] employing a series of anthropometric and laboratory measures of nutritional status, concluded that protein-calorie malnutrition affects 44 per cent of general medical patients and as many as 50 per cent of surgical patient populations.

In a recent prospective study[5] baseline observations were made on each of 134 consecutive patients admitted to a general medical service. Of 44 patients remaining two weeks or longer, deterioration was observed in a number of important parameters: 79 per cent showed a decline in arm muscle circumference (average 1.2 cm), 74 per cent lost weight (average 4.5 kg), the hematocrit fell in 64 per cent (average 8 per cent) and the serum albumin declined in 47 per cent of the subjects (average 0.4 gm per dl). It is remarkable that in this group many nutritional parameters were abnormal at the time of discharge or transfer and in many cases were worse than at the time of admission. It is worthy of emphasis that the population at risk is large and the percentage figures are high.

Although the word *iatrogenic* means physician-induced (Gr. *iatros*, physician, + Gr. *genesis*, production), its use in connection with malnutrition does not imply malicious intent or callous disregard for a patient's welfare. Nevertheless, malnutrition does occur because of what the physician does or does not do. To a considerable extent, physician-induced malnutrition is the result of inappropriate emphasis on a complex modern treatment program while fundamental principles of nutrition remain in the background. Examples include: undue reliance on antibiotics without regard for host factors in resisting infection, prolonged use of mechanical life-support systems and the performance of surgical procedures without careful consideration of the patient's ability to heal wounds and resist complications. It is paradoxical that many cases of nutritional failure encountered among hospital patients are due to spectacular successes in other fields. Patients tend to live longer and exhaust their nutritional reserves. Whatever the cause, the end-result is the same: Many patients fail to receive the full benefit of existing nutrition knowledge.

While it is understandable that science does not advance uniformly on all fronts, the present situation underscores the basic importance of nutrition in a wide variety of medical disciplines. It further suggests that neglect of nutrition education in medical schools over the past few decades has been costly. In addition, a number of organizational or administrative deficiencies contribute to suboptimal delivery of nutrition care in the hospital setting (Table 22–1).

IDENTIFYING THE "HIGH-RISK" AND MALNOURISHED PATIENT

For many years malnutrition has been considered synonymous with vitamin deficiency syndromes. Although these "classical" far-advanced syndromes are occasionally encountered and should not be missed, overt vitamin deficiencies are best regarded as rare medical curiosities. By contrast, protein-calorie malnutrition (PCM), formerly thought to be a problem only of poorer populations, is being recog-

Table 22–1.   Undesirable Practices Affecting the Nutritional Health of Hospital Patients*

Failure to record height and weight.

Rotation of staff at frequent intervals.

Diffusion of responsibility for patient care.

Prolonged use of glucose and saline intravenous feedings.

Failure to observe patients' food intake.

Withholding meals because of diagnostic tests.

Use of tube feedings in inadequate amounts, of uncertain composition and under unsanitary conditions.

Ignorance of the composition of vitamin mixtures and other nutritional products.

Failure to recognize increased nutritional needs due to injury or illness.

Performance of surgical procedures without first making certain that the patient is optimally nourished, and failure to give the body nutritional support after surgery.

Failure to appreciate the role of nutrition in the prevention of and recovery from infection; unwarranted reliance on antibiotics.

Lack of communication and interaction between physician and dietitian. As staff professionals, dietitians should be concerned with the nutritional health of *every* hospital patient.

Delay of nutrition support until the patient is in an advanced state of depletion which is sometimes irreversible.

Limited availability of laboratory tests to assess nutritional status; failure to use those that are available.

* From *Nutrition Today*, March-April, 1974. Reprinted with permission of the publisher.

Table 22-2. The High-risk Patient

Gross underweight: weight-for-height below 80 per cent of standard

Gross overweight: weight-for-height above 120 per cent of standard (The risk is due to the tendency to overlook protein and calorie requirements in the acutely ill obese patient.)

Recent loss of 10 per cent or more of usual body weight

Alcoholism

No oral intake (n.p.o.) for over 10 days on simple intravenous solutions

Protracted nutrient losses
    Malabsorption syndromes
    Short-gut syndromes/fistulas
    Renal dialysis
    Draining abscesses, wounds

Increased metabolic needs
    Extensive burns, infection, trauma
    Protracted fever

Intake of drugs with antinutrient or catabolic properties: steroids, immunosuppressants, antitumor agents

---

nized in our hospitals in one-fourth to one-half of medical and surgical patients whose illnesses have required hospitalization for two weeks or longer.[3,4] High priority should, therefore, be given to the identification, treatment and, ultimately, the prevention of protein and calorie deficiencies.

Patients with malnutrition, particularly protein-calorie malnutrition, do not tolerate illness well. They tend to have delayed wound healing and greater susceptibility to infection and other complications. Thus, early identification of the patient at risk, and the assurance of adequate protein and calorie supplies, may serve to prevent a prolonged and complicated, or even catastrophic, hospital course. The "high-risk" patient, nutritionally, tends to exhibit one or more of the eight characteristics listed in Table 22-2. The presence of any one of these is a warning that a patient is at increased risk of PCM. Their absence, however, does not mean PCM does not exist or cannot occur.

Protein-calorie Malnutrition

Protein-calorie malnutrition is a diagnostic category that encompasses two,

often distinctly different, disease processes: marasmus and kwashiorkor.

1. Marasmus or simple starvation

    Marasmus is basically a clinical diagnosis based on the physical findings of severe fat and muscle wastage in the chronic setting of inadequate intake of calories. Diminished skinfold thicknesses reflect the loss of calorie reserves, and reduced arm circumference with temporal and interosseus muscle wastage reflects the resorption of protein from the parietal and visceral muscles, including the heart. The laboratory picture is relatively unremarkable other than occasionally revealing a serum albumin reduced to about 2.8 gm per 100 ml. In most cases of marasmus immunocompetence, wound healing and the ability to handle short-term stress are reasonably well preserved despite the morose appearance.

2. Kwashiorkor or acute visceral attrition

    In contrast to marasmus, kwashiorkor is largely a laboratory diagnosis based on the sharp decline of serum albumin and lymphocyte count in the acute setting of protein-poor intake and stress. In children, the situation is often one of being fed a starchy, low-protein diet under the stress of growth and parasitic or viral infection. In adults, kwashiorkor typically occurs in the hospitalized patient who is unable to eat and is under the stress of an acute illness or major surgery. The time course of development may be as short as two weeks.

The clinical findings are often few. Fat reserves and muscle mass tend to be normal, giving the deceptive appearance of adequate nutrition. Useful signs that support the diagnosis of kwashiorkor include easily pluckable hair, edema and delayed wound healing. Characteristic laboratory changes include severely depressed levels of serum proteins, such as albumin (<2.8 gm per 100 ml) and transferrin (<150 mg per 100 ml). Associated with this visceral protein depletion is a depression of cellular immune function as reflected by lymphopenia (<1200 cells per cu mm in adults, higher at younger ages) and skin anergy.

Once the diagnosis of kwashiorkor is made, the prognosis for recovery is poor without aggressive nutrition support. Dehiscence of surgical wounds is likely, host defenses are compromised and death from gram-negative septicemia or overwhelming fungal infection may occur despite antibiotic therapy.

The combined form of PCM (marasmic kwashiorkor) develops when acute stress of illness or surgery supervenes on the chronically starved patient. As expected, this is an extremely serious, life-threatening situation because of the high risk of infections and other complications. As with kwashiorkor, the necessity for vigorous nutritional therapy is urgent. It is of utmost importance to separate the forms of protein-calorie malnutrition in order to develop the appropriate nutritional support plan.

The characteristic features of marasmus and kwashiorkor are summarized in Table 22-3.

Bodily Defenses

The bodily defenses are divided into three main categories—mechanical, cellular and humoral.

1. Mechanical: The body is protected from microbial invasion by intact epithelial surfaces, mucous barriers, digestive enzymes and secretory antibodies. These cells, like all others, require an adequate supply of nutrients for their growth, turnover and function.
2. Cellular: Cellular defense mechanisms are mediated by lymphocytes and plasma cells, the exact functions and modes of action of which are not well understood, and by polymorphonuclear leukocytes, which have the ability to ingest and destroy bacteria or foreign bodies.

Table 22-3. Protein-calorie Malnutrition

	Marasmus	*Kwashiorkor*
Clinical setting	↓ Calories	↓ Protein + stress
Time course to develop	Months—years	Weeks—months

Clinical features	Starved appearance
	  weight/height
	    < 80% std
	  triceps skinfold
	    < 3 mm
	  midarm muscle circumference
	    < 15 cm
		Well nourished appearance
		  hair easily pluckable
		  edema

Laboratory findings	Serum albumin > 2.8 gm per 100 ml	Serum albumin <2.8 gm per 100 ml Serum transferrin < 150 mg per 100 ml Lymphocytes <1200 cells per cu mm Nonreactive skin tests
Clinical course	Reasonably preserved responsive-ness to short-term stress	↓ Wound healing ↓ Immunocompetence ↑ Infectious/other complications
Mortality rate	Low (unless related to underlying disease process)	High

3. Humoral: Humoral defense mechanisms are mediated by gamma globulins and other plasma proteins which aid in the destruction of microorganisms. Some antibodies appear in secretions, such as tears, colostrum and intestinal mucus.

There is ample evidence that in protein-calorie malnutrition all three defense systems are impaired. Thus, in addition to other serious disorders, the body is open to infection at a time when it is least able to cope with it. Presently, the most useful findings suggesting altered defense mechanisms are lymphopenia (<1500 cells per cu mm) and unreactivity to tuberculin, Candida and dinitrochlorobenzene skin tests. These results should be regarded as possible manifestations of impaired cell-mediated immunity from PCM.

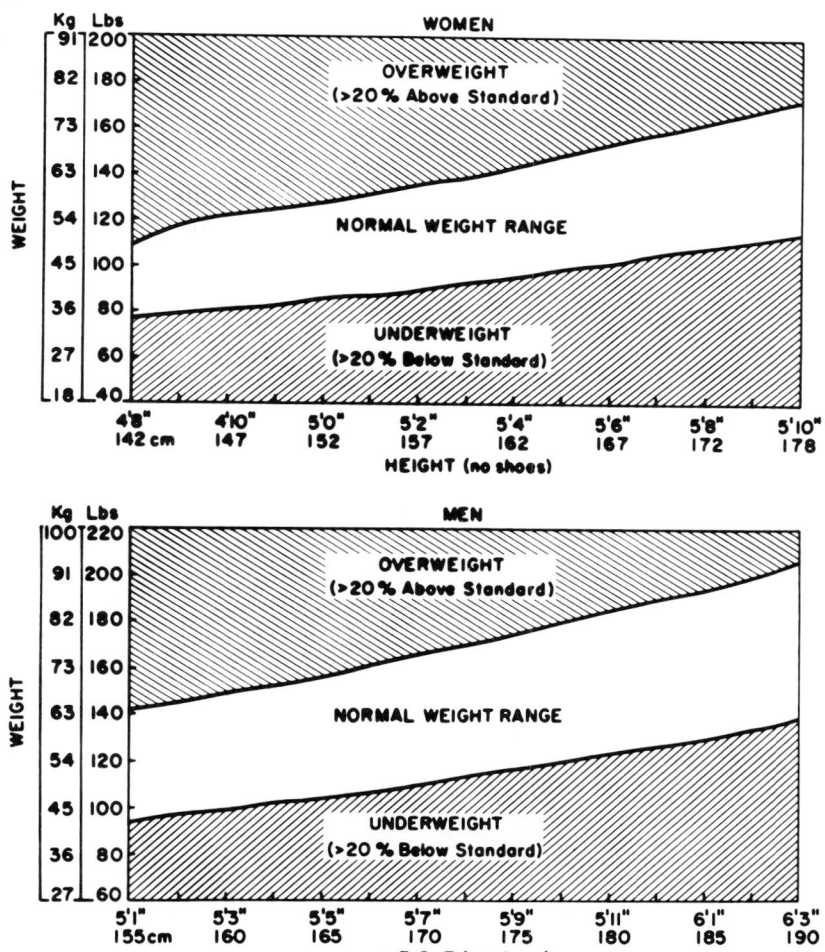

Fig. 22–1. Weight/height reference graphs. Patients 20 per cent or more above standard are likely to be grossly overweight, regardless of body frame. Patients 20 per cent or more below standard are likely to be grossly underweight and at high risk of nutritional deficiency. (Data adapted from Metropolitan Life Insurance Company, Build and Blood Pressure Study, 1959, and reprinted from Weinsier, Butterworth and Sahm: *Handbook of Clinical Nutrition.* Birmingham, University of Alabama Department of Nutrition Sciences, 1977.)

Evaluation of Nutrition Status

To assess the nutritional status of every hospitalized patient should be as fundamental a part of the workup as listening to the heart or obtaining a urinalysis. There are three key components; anthropometric measurements, the clinical examination and laboratory data.

Anthropometrics. On admission, or as soon thereafter as feasible, *weight and height* are taken and plotted on the weight/height reference graph (Fig. 22–1). This is routinely done on pediatric wards to document growth rate, but it is equally important among adults to document nutritional risk on admission and change in status with hospitalization. Body weight is one of the most convenient and useful indicators of nutritional status. Weight loss that is not secondary to fluid loss is an ominous sign in the hospitalized patient. It often reflects

use of body protein (i.e. muscle and organ tissue) as a metabolic fuel, which occurs quickly when calorie intake is severely restricted. This is the case in patients maintained on intravenous solutions of 5 to 10 per cent glucose. The obese patient can suffer extreme protein-calorie malnutrition under such circumstances while maintaining an appearance of being well fed. In general, the acutely ill obese patient should not be treated with calorie restriction. On the other hand, weight maintenance may falsely suggest adequate nutritional status if edema, a common feature of PCM, replaces fat and muscle tissue.

Skinfold thickness is a good indicator of body fat (calorie) reserves since approximately 50 per cent of the adipose tissue is located in the subcutaneous area. Not only are skinfolds easy to measure but they are likely to obviate the confusion arising from

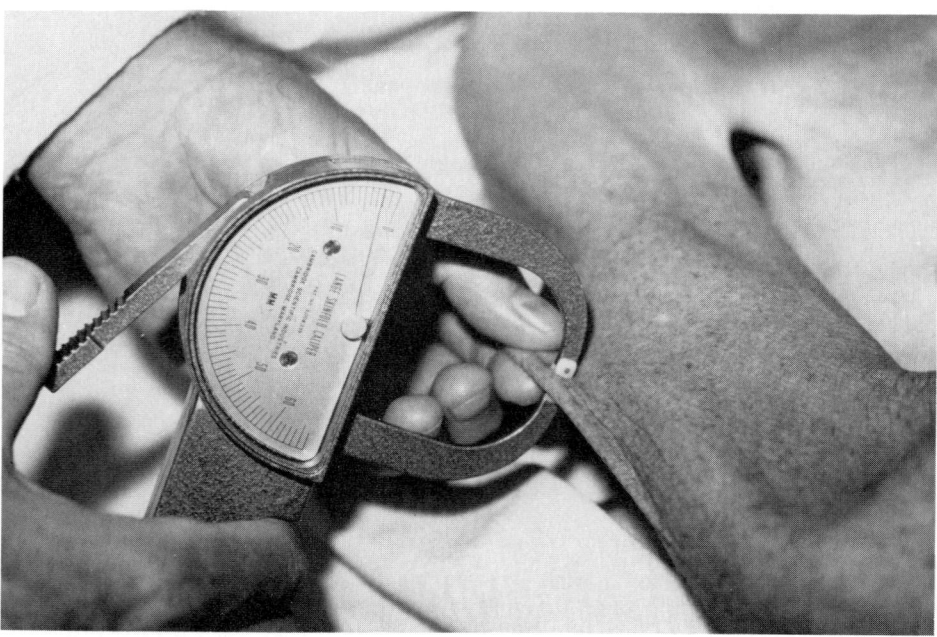

Fig. 22–2. Lange skinfold calipers in use for measurement of triceps skinfold thickness. In this patient the reading of 2 mm is in the "minimal fat reserves" range and indicates far advanced depletion of subcutaneous fat stores, as seen in protein-calorie malnutrition. (From Weinsier, Butterworth and Sahm: *Handbook of Clinical Nutrition.* Birmingham, University of Alabama Department of Nutrition Sciences, 1977.)

dramatic weight changes with fluid shifts. The triceps skinfold is a convenient site and is considered to be representative of the fatness of the entire body.[6] The proper technique is to grasp a fold of skin on the posterior aspect of the arm midway between shoulder and elbow, gently pulling it away from the underlying muscle (Fig. 22–2). The caliper is applied and the reading taken after about 3 seconds. The average of 3 readings is then recorded on the reference graph (Fig. 22–3). Either Lange or Harpenden calipers are suitable for this purpose since both are designed to exert uniform pressure over a wide range of thicknesses. Cheaper calipers are now be-

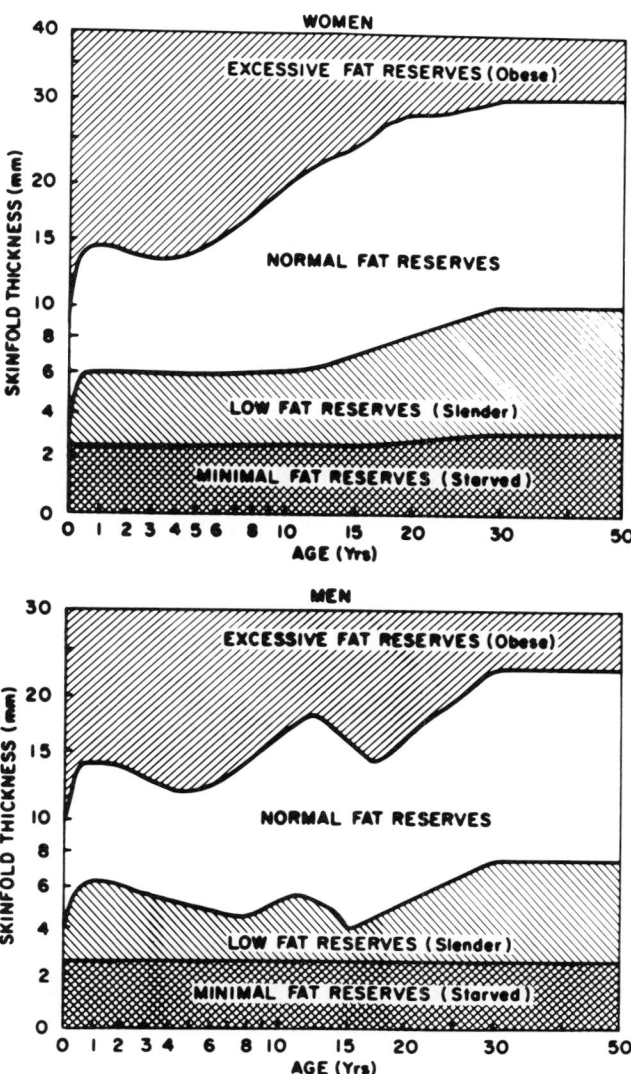

Fig. 22–3. Triceps skinfold reference graphs (all ages). (Adapted from data of Seltzer and Mayer,[9] Tanner and Whitehouse[10] and Frisancho,[11] and reprinted from Weinsier, Butterworth and Sahm: *Handbook of Clinical Nutrition*. Birmingham, University of Alabama Department of Nutrition Sciences, 1977.)

coming available, but their accuracy must be tested before and with use. In the absence of calipers, skinfold thickness can be estimated with the fingers, knowing that 1 mm is about the thickness of a dime. Other sites (e.g. subscapular, abdominal, hip, thigh) can also be used to assess fat loss or gain during the course of hospitalization. Legs and dependent areas are more likely to show accumulation of edema and are less desirable test areas.

The *midarm muscle circumference* (MAMC) reflects both caloric adequacy and muscle mass. A soft tape measure is used to mea-

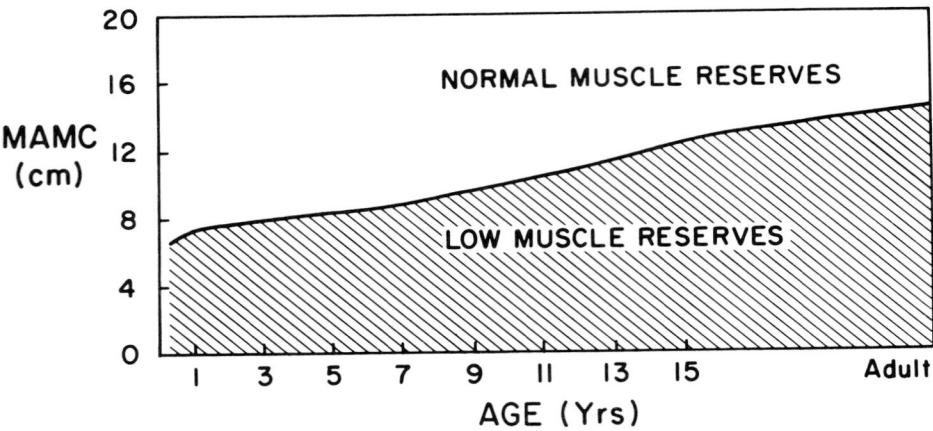

Fig. 22–4. Midarm muscle circumference (MAMC) reference graph, both sexes, all ages (MAMC = arm circum. − 3 × skinfold [cm]). Patients with values in the "low muscle reserves" area are likely to be severely malnourished. It is possible, however, to fall in the "normal" range and be depleted. (Data adapted from Frisancho[11] and reprinted from Weinsier, Butterworth and Sahm: *Handbook of Clinical Nutrition.* Birmingham, University of Alabama Department of Nutrition Sciences, 1977.)

Table 22–4.   The Clinical Nutrition Examination

Clinical Finding	Consider Deficiency	Comment
Hair, nails		
Hair easily pluckable, sparse, straight, depigmented, dull	Protein	
Spoon-shaped nails	Chronic iron	
Brittle, ridged lined nails	Nonspecific	
Skin		
Petechiae, purpura, corkscrew hairs	Ascorbic acid	
Pigmentation, desquamation	Niacin (pellagra)	Sun-exposed areas; symmetric
Follicular keratosis	Vitamin A	Keratin plugs in follicles
Dry, scaling	Nonspecific	
Subcutaneous fat loss	Calories	Minimal fat reserves if triceps skinfold ¼" between fingers
Eyes		
Dull, dry conjunctiva	Vitamin A	
Blepharitis	B-complex	
Ophthalmoplegia	Thiamin	Wernicke's syndrome; prompt treatment necessary

Table 22-4.   Continued

Clinical Finding	Consider Deficiency	Comment
Perioral		
Angular fissures, scars	B-complex, iron, protein	Also seen with ill-fitting dentures
Cheilosis	B-6, niacin, riboflavin, protein	
Oral		
Ageusia, dysgeusia	Zinc	Also associated with altered sense of smell
Glossitis, depapillation	Niacin, riboflavin, B_{12}, folate, iron	
Swollen, bleeding gums	Ascorbic acid	
Glands		
Parotid enlargement	Protein	
"Sicca" syndrome	Ascorbic acid	
Thyroid enlargement	Iodine	
Heart		
Small heart, decreased output	Protein	
Enlargement, tachycardia, high-output failure	Thiamin	"Wet beriberi"
Sudden failure, death	Ascorbic acid	
Abdomen		
Hepatomegaly (fatty)	Protein	
Muscles, extremities		
Muscle wasting evident in temporal area, dorsum of hand between thumb and index finger		
Calf muscles	Protein-calorie	
Pain in calves, weak thighs	Thiamin	
Edema	Protein, thiamin	
Bones, joints		
Epiphyseal thickening, deformities	Vitamin D (rickets)	
Bone pain (adult)	Osteomalacia	Repeated pregnancies with poor Ca^{++} intake, no sun, steatorrhea
Bone pain (child)	Ascorbic acid	Subperiosteal hemorrhage
Arthralgias	Ascorbic acid	
Neurologic		
Ophthalmoplegia, footdrop	Thiamin	Wernicke's encephalopathy
Confabulation, disorientation	Thiamin	Korsakoff's psychosis
Decreased position, vibratory sense, ataxia	B_{12}	Subacute combined cord degeneration
Weakness, paresthesias of legs	Thiamin, pyridoxine, pantothenic acid, B_{12}	Nutritional polyneuropathy, esp. with alcoholism
Other		
Delayed healing and tissue repair (e.g. wound, infarct, abscess)	Vitamin C, zinc, protein, calories	

sure the circumference of the upper midarm. The contribution of the underlying fat tissue is then removed by the following formula:

$$\text{MAMC} = \text{arm circumference} - 3.14 \times \text{skinfold (in cm)}$$

The MAMC can be plotted on the reference graph (Fig. 22–4). Protein and calorie deficiency can also be judged by visual observation of muscle wastage in the temporal, scapular, pelvic and calf areas. Disuse atrophy, of course, can produce similar changes but is less likely to affect the temporal muscles.

Clinical Examination. Clinical findings suggestive of vitamin, mineral and protein-calorie deficiencies are outlined in Table 22–4.

Laboratory Data. A number of routine laboratory procedures available in most hospitals can yield remarkably accurate information about nutritional status (Table 22–5). The key is merely the adoption of a slightly different approach to the interpretation of laboratory results. As an example,

abnormally low levels of serum albumin, lymphocytes and transferrin and a negative PPD skin test may each have a separate explanation. Collectively, however, they may well represent PCM of the kwashiorkor type. Put in the clinical setting of an acutely ill patient, edematous, with easily pluckable hair and without protein intake for several weeks, the diagnosis of protein-calorie malnutrition is clear-cut.

APPROACH TO THE MALNOURISHED PATIENT

The Feeding Triangle

There are three major routes for supplying nutrients: oral, gastric and intravenous. Every patient can be nourished by at least one of the three routes, and in many cases two approaches can be used complementarily. In a patient who cannot or will not eat, the nasopharyngeal route can be used, while oral intake is encouraged. If

Table 22–5. Routine Laboratory Tests in Nutrition Assessment

Albumin, low serum	Protein-calorie	Protein-losing enteropathy, hepatic dysfunction and nephrotic syndrome may be absent
Albuminuria, mild	Protein-calorie	No renal abnormalities
Anemia		
normocytic	Protein	
microcytic	Iron, copper, pyridoxine	
macrocytic	Folate (in months), B_{12} (in years), ascorbic acid	
Calcium, low serum	Vitamin D, calcium	Also seen with fat malabsorption; hypomagnesemia
Carotene, low serum		Suggestive of fat malabsorption
Creatinine, low serum	Muscle wastage	
Lymphopenia (<1500 per cu mm)	Protein-calorie	Impaired cell-mediated immunity
Phosphate, low serum	Vitamin D, phosphate	Also seen with phosphate-binding antacids
Prothrombin deficiency	Vitamin K	In malabsorption, biliary obstruction, sterile bowel
Skin tests (unreactivity to PPD, Candida, DNCB)	Protein-calorie	Impaired cell-mediated immunity
Transferrin or TIBC, low	Protein-calorie	Also seen in liver disease and infection
Transferrin or TIBC, high	Iron	
Urea, low serum	Low protein intake	

necessary, the same individual may be given supplemental calories, protein, vitamins and electrolytes through a peripheral intravenous line. The chronically depleted, starved patient who is beginning to eat may temporarily need additional nutrient input, which can be supplied peripherally. When the decision is made to use a "central line" for total parenteral nutrition (TPN), it is generally because of unavailability of both the oral and gastric routes. Recall, however, that the *only* difference between peripheral and central intravenous feeding with regard to nutrient input is the final glucose concentration, not the protein, vitamin or mineral content.

There are few set rules dictating the route or routes to be used for a particular case. In general, the most physiologic route (i.e. oral) is preferred. Too often, however, weight is lost and protein-calorie deficiency occurs while the physician waits for the appetite to improve; the postoperative patient is a typical example. The second choice is nasopharyngeal tube feeding, effective in many patients who have inadequate intake because of depressed appetite or inability to eat. If this approach is effective but must be continued for longer than 2 or 3 weeks, then a feeding esophagostomy or gastrostomy should be considered. In patients with PCM of the marasmic type (simple starvation), oral and/or tube feeding may well be adequate therapy. In the case of kwashiorkor, however, a more aggressive approach is often needed. Here, immunologic competence is failing, wound healing is defective and resistance to stress and infection are so altered that the patient is likely to die without immediate and intensive nutrition support, which may best be achieved by TPN. The indications and procedures for TPN are reviewed in Chapter 37.

Tube feeding by nasopharyngeal tube or gastrostomy is the method of choice in individuals with a normal GI tract. The approach to tube feeding is outlined below.

Tube Feeding

The Nasopharyngeal Tube. A #8 French infant tube or a soft mercury-weighted 2.4 mm tube is recommended for use with most formulas. Such thin polyethylene, Silastic or nylon tubing can be left in place for weeks at a time without patient discomfort or damage to the mucous membranes of the nose and throat. Small-gauge tubing of the type designed for catheterizing blood vessels has been used successfully for the administration of nonviscous solutions.

Continuous Feeding. When malnutrition is severe, appetite is poor and bowel function compromised, the continuous drip method is preferred, using the closed, sterile systems whenever possible. Ready-to-use formulas in sterile containers may be infused by gravity or pump in a fashion similar to IV infusions. The advantages of continuous feeding over bolus feeding include: (1) facility in administering larger daily volumes and with greater reliability, (2) less chance of acute abdominal distention and resultant aspiration or osmotic overload and (3) less chance of bacterial overgrowth in closed continuous flow system. Reflux and stagnation may occur frequently with clamped tubes despite water flushes after each feeding.

Guidelines

1. Use an infusion pump whenever available to ensure a constant flow rate.
2. In general, avoid diluting formulas. (Diluting often entails bacterial contamination of the hanging "culture media" which may be a cause of diarrhea.)
3. Do not hang even sterile formulas longer than 12 hours to minimize bacterial overgrowth, unless a container is used which has a separate compartment filled with ice.
4. Begin infusion at approximately 20 ml per hr and check for gastric retention (>100 ml) after 8 hours. If absent, progress stepwise to 40 ml per hr × 8 hours, 60 ml per hr and then 80 ml per hr. (In the alert patient, it is not usually necessary to check for retention thereafter unless there is abdominal distention or subjective discomfort.)

Flow rate should not exceed approximately 200 ml per hr. (For higher calorie inputs, a more concentrated formula can be used.)

5. In a patient with an altered state of consciousness or depressed gag reflex, keep the head elevated during high-rate infusions.

6. Change infusion set daily.

7. Wean to solid foods by first stopping the infusion for 1 hour before and after each meal, and then by infusing only between 8 p.m. and 8 a.m.

Bolus Feeding. Intermittent or bolus feeding has the primary advantage of permitting the patient mobility. This is particularly the case in gastrostomy patients requiring long-term liquid feedings.

Guidelines

1. Start at approximately 50 ml every 2 hours, using undiluted formula, over 8 hours. (Hold feedings if retention >100 ml). Progress at 8-hr intervals to boluses of 100 ml, 150 ml, etc. Night feedings may be spaced or eliminated to permit patient rest and avoid aspiration.

2. Feed patient in the sitting position whenever possible.

3. Flush line with water after each infusion and clamp tightly.

4. Rinse syringe after each infusion and discard daily.

5. Do not allow opened formula to sit at room temperature over 4 hours.

6. Wean to solid foods by holding feeding preceding each meal.

Troubleshooting Problems of Tube Feeding. *Diarrhea* should not be considered a usual accompaniment of formula feeding. Possible causes include bacterial overgrowth of the formula (a good culture medium at room temperature), too rapid feeding and osmotic overload (especially with formulas high in mono- and disaccharides), and lactose or milk intolerance. If diarrhea occurs, follow the guidelines with regard to avoiding contamination, continue the same formula but step back to a much lower rate and volume, using the continuous drip method, and question the patient for milk intolerance. If diarrhea persists, then switch formulas empirically and look for other causes.

Retention is loosely defined as more than about 100 ml gastric contents 2 hours after the last feeding. Rule out hypokalemia, effect of drugs, obstruction and ileus. Keep the patient sitting or semisitting during and after feeding and mobilize if possible. Problems of retention tend to be fewer with continuous feeding.

Hyperglycemia and hyperosmolar, nonketotic coma may occur with hyperosmolar or concentrated formulas principally as a result of solute overload and inadequate hydration. Blood and urine glucose levels should be monitored frequently in the initial days of feeding to detect diabetes and appropriate adjustments in formula, water volume and insulin made as indicated. Daily weights are mandatory.

Protein-calorie Requirements

Caloric requirements of the average adult patient who is at normal weight can be only grossly approximated on the basis of the rule of 30 kcal per kg body weight. For the underweight patient or one who is moderately hypermetabolic 2,500 to 3,000 calories will meet daily needs; occasionally requirements of 4,000 or more and rarely to 8,000 calories per day are found in severely traumatized or hypermetabolic patients. Because of wide variations in caloric need, the only guide to caloric requirements should be frequent measurements of body weight or anthropometrics.

Optimal protein intake, as for calories, can be only approximated and is usually based on the Recommended Dietary Allowance guidelines of 0.8 gm per kg body weight per day for an average adult. Larger amounts of 1 to 2 gm per kg or above may be required under conditions of protein wastage (e.g. burns, enteropathy, drainage of wounds or secretions), whereas daily amounts of 0.3 to 0.5 gm per kg or less may be recommended for cases of renal or hepatic insufficiency. Two points should be remembered: (1) The serum urea/creatinine ratio may rise with excess protein and fall with inadequate

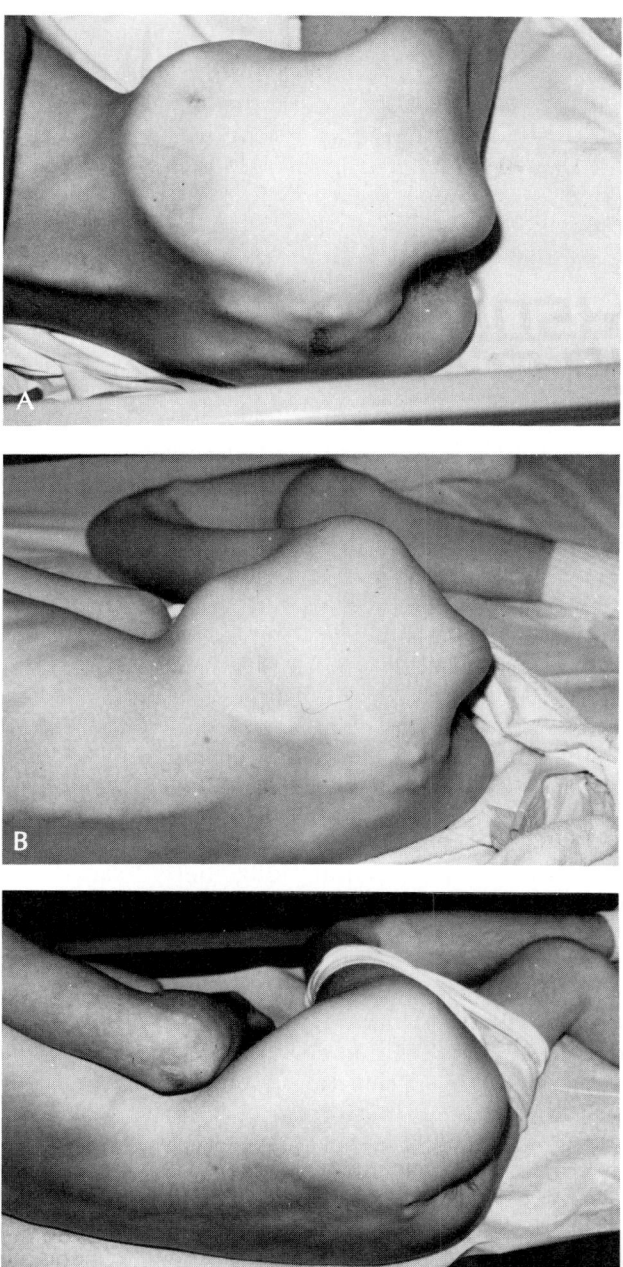

Fig. 22–5. Progressive repletion of fat and muscle reserves in a 19-year-old male hospitalized for depressed skull fracture and other injuries sustained in a motorcycle accident. Preadmission weight was 130 lb by history; height was 5'7" and serum albumin was normal. Because of the altered state of consciousness, no food was taken by mouth, and body weight fell 45 lb in 26 days (1¾ lb/day) while receiving IV solutions of 5 per cent dextrose. With total parenteral nutrition and subsequent gastrostomy feeding, a steady rise in triceps skinfolds (TSF), midarm circumference (MAC) and serum albumin (Alb) was achieved (Table 22–6). The decubitus ulcer healed spontaneously. Higher neurologic functions improved concurrently, allowing transfer to a rehabilitation facility after 7 weeks of nutritional therapy. The patient became able to feed himself regular meals and was discharged 15 weeks after the initial injury with continuing improvement in neurologic status.

protein. Urea reflects rate of protein catabolism as well as renal function, whereas creatinine reflects only renal function. (2) Nitrogen balance = nitrogen intake (i.e. protein/6.25) − nitrogen losses (via urine, stools and bodily drainage, if present). A 3-day average should be zero or positive.

Adequate intake of protein does not necessarily mean that it will be deposited as muscle tissue in proportion to its intake, because inactive muscle cannot make full use of the bathing nutrient solution. Therefore, it is important that muscular activity be emphasized to patients. Active exercises under the guidance of a physical therapist can be a valuable adjunct in the rehabilitation of patients receiving special nutrition therapy. It should be remembered that excessive feedings of protein cannot force the regeneration of denervated muscle.

Figure 22–5 is an example of reversing protein-calorie malnutrition that developed in a hospitalized patient. Being able to recognize and treat the malnourished patient entails relatively little sophistication but a reassessment of priorities and hospital procedures. With this will come the more important aspect of nutrition support—the prevention of iatrogenic malnutrition.

PREVENTION OF HOSPITAL MALNUTRITION

The physician clearly occupies a central role in the prevention of hospital malnutrition, but perhaps equally important is the organization of the entire health-care team, including nurses, dietitians, pharmacists, laboratory scientists and administrators. Another key element is *awareness* by all concerned of the continuing nutritional needs of the patient under the prevailing conditions of the illness. The central role of energy sources and of essential and nonessential nutrients to the metabolic function of various tissues cannot be overemphasized. While some of these requirements can be met from endogenous reserves, there are limits to the reserves and the capacity to mobilize them. The basic doctrine of "Do for the patient what he cannot do for himself" is perfectly applicable here. Related to this is the concept of *nutritional equilibrium* and the importance of providing nutrients appropriate to the situation. It is a challenge to the ingenuity of the various members of the health-care team to anticipate requirements and attempt to provide for them, or to detect incipient deficiencies and devise means to restore equilibrium to the system.

It is beyond the scope of this chapter to outline specific details of therapy, and much of this is given in other chapters. However, it is appropriate to suggest that steps be taken to avoid the undesirable practices listed in Table 22–1. Particular attention must be given to requirements for energy (for example, there is an increase of approximately 10 per cent in daily calorie consumption for each degree of temperature elevation above 37°C). Attention must also be given to fluid, electrolyte and protein losses from wounds, fistulas and suction tubes. Relatively large

Table 22–6. Sequential Changes in Body Weight, Total Serum Protein, Albumin, Triceps Skinfold Thickness (TSF) and Midarm Circumference (MAC) Prior to and during Nutritional Rehabilitation of Patient Shown in Figure 22–5.

(Standard)	Weight (130)	TSF (12.5)	MAC (29.3)	TSP/ALB (6/3.5)
5–03–76				7.5/4.3
5–29–76	85	2.5	19.5	7.8/2.7
6–04–76	82			7.0/2.3
6–11–76		2.5	19.5	7.4/2.5
6–23–76	80			
7–01–76	84	2.0	18.5	
7–09–76		3.0	18.5	
7–12–76	85			
7–19–76	89			7.0/3.0
8–03–76	94			7.3/3.5
8–09–76	101	5.0	22.5	
9–23–76	114	9.0	24.0	

amounts of protein of high biologic value are lost in tubes of blood sent to the laboratory for analysis; this loss should be kept to a minimum.

An important contribution to the prevention of hospital malnutrition can be made by a well-organized nutrition committee. Such a committee, supported by the chief of staff or administrator, can do much to coordinate the needs, activities and talents of various staff units, including representatives from pharmacy, nursing and dietetics as well as from major subspecialties of medicine and surgery, to increase the efficiency of delivering nutrition support to the patient population. It can, for example, centralize certain services, design uniform systems for order writing and record keeping, standardize practices for enteral and parenteral feeding and assist in the procurement, distribution and maintenance of constant-infusion pumps.

Many large hospitals have found it desirable to identify an interdisciplinary team to supervise nutrition services, particularly parenteral nutrition, throughout the hospital, and to serve as consultants to various units. It would also seem desirable to identify certain nursing units or wards as having special expertise in caring for the growing number of patients for whom nutritional support is a major problem.

Administrative policies and staff procedures should be reviewed frequently to eliminate obstacles. The feeding of patients should take precedence over feeding hospital employees. When patients are unable to feed themselves, volunteer workers or family members can be mobilized to carry out this important task. Diet prescriptions, tube feedings and intravenous infusion orders should be reviewed frequently (e.g. every 3 days) to determine if they are suited to the patient's needs. Specially trained nurses and dietitians should be available to help physicians monitor patient status, keep records and maintain communication lines between the patient and all others involved in the delivery of nutrition services. Considerably greater effort needs to be expended in the area of patient education. A period of hospitalization can be a valuable learning experience. It is an opportunity to demonstrate meal patterns, portion sizes and other aspects of applied nutrition. Hasty, last-minute diet instructions given at the time of discharge must be condemned and avoided; they can lead only to serious misunderstanding, frustration, treatment failure and early readmission. It must be remembered that newly diagnosed medical illness or a recent surgical procedure may impose drastic revisions in life style.

Cost Effectiveness of Improved Nutrition

For the last several decades, nutritional factors have not figured prominently in health statistics. There has been a tendency to record only specific terminal events on death certificates, without adequate exploration of underlying factors among which the patient's nutritional status might have been crucial. For example, the death rate from measles and its complications during 1962 was 268 times as great in Guatemala as in the United States. When a protein-rich food supplement was provided in children less than 5 years old, the measles mortality rate was reduced to one-third of the rate observed in unsupplemented children.[7] It therefore becomes necessary to look beyond ordinary and conventional

Table 22–7. Mechanisms of Drug-nutrient Interaction

Decreased intestinal absorption

Increased renal excretion

Direct competition

Displacement from carrier protein

Interference with synthesis of enzyme, coenzyme or carrier

Hormonal effects on genetic systems (e.g. vitamin and mineral binders)

Effects due to vehicle or to components in drug formulation

Table 22–8. Effects of Drugs on Nutritional Status*

Drug	Nutrient(s) Affected	Presumed Mechanism of Action	Possible Clinical Consequences
Antacids	Phosphate	Decreased absorption	Hypophosphatemia
Colchicine	Vitamin B_{12}	Intestinal malabsorption; mucosal damage	Macrocytic anemia; neurologic dysfunction
PAS	Vitamin B_{12}	Intestinal malabsorption; mucosal damage	Macrocytic anemia; neurologic dysfunction
5-Fluorouracil	Protein	Intestinal malabsorption; mucosal dipeptidase activity	Altered mucosal structure and function; amino acid imbalance
Metformin Phenformin	Glucose Vitamin B_{12} Disaccharides	Intestinal malabsorption	↓ Blood glucose Vitamin B_{12} deficiency ?
Cholestyramine	Triglyceride (also calcium soaps, fat-soluble vitamins)	Intestinal malabsorption (due to bile acid sequestration)	Steatorrhea; tetany; deficiency of fat-soluble vitamins
Neomycin	Triglyceride, (fat-soluble vitamins)	Bile acid sequestration; mucosal damage	Steatorrhea; tetany; deficiency of fat-soluble vitamins
Thiazide	Sodium, potassium	Increased urinary excretion (also impaired GI transport)	Hypokalemia, muscle weakness, etc.
Ethanol	Zinc Magnesium	Increased zinc loss in urine (?) Increased Mg loss in urine (?)	Zinc deficiency Magnesium deficiency
Aspirin Barbiturates Paraldehyde Hydantoins Aminopyrine Ether	Vitamin C	Increased urinary excretion (probably due to displacement from binding sites)	Clinical or subclinical vitamin C deficiency (scurvy)
Penicillamine	Vitamin B_6	Increased urinary excretion due to chelation of vitamin	Mood changes; peripheral neuritis; convulsions
Methotrexate Pyrimethamine Triaminopteridine Trimethoprim	Folate " " "	Direct antagonism; competition for active site on enzyme due to similarities in chemical structure	Reduced serum folate level; macrocytic anemia; megaloblastic bone marrow
Isoniazid	Vitamin B_6 Tryptophan Niacin	Direct antagonism; competition for active site on enzyme due to similarities in chemical structure	Peripheral neuritis; convulsions; pellagra-like syndrome
Chloramphenicol	Phenylalanine	Compete for attachment to tRNA	Abnormal protein synthesis
α-Methyldopa	Vitamin B_6	Metabolic antagonism	B_6 may nullify beneficial effect of drug in Parkinson's disease

Table 22–8. Effects of Drugs on Nutritional Status*

Drug	Nutrient(s) Affected	Presumed Mechanism of Action	Possible Clinical Consequences
Coumadin	Vitamin K	Suppresses synthesis of vitamin K-dependent coagulation factors	Hypoprothrombinemia; hemorrhage if excessive
Oxyphenbutazone	Vitamin K	Enhances coumadin effect by displacing it from albumin-binding site	Less coumadin required
Barbiturates	Vitamin K	Lowers coumadin effect by induction of hepatic enzymes to inactivate	More coumadin required
Ethanol	Vitamin B_6	Impaired conversion of pyridoxine to pyridoxal phosphate	Impaired iron utilization for heme synthesis; ringed sideroblasts in bone marrow
Ethanol	Folate	Uncertain	Increased requirement; megaloblastic anemia; F.A.-responsive impairment in iron utilization
Ethanol	Magnesium	Excessive Mg loss in urine	Hypomagnesemic tetany
Oral contraceptive agents (OCA)	Vitamin A	Impaired hepatic storage; increased plasma binding	Uncertain
OCA	Copper	Increased plasma ceruloplasmin	?
OCA	Iron	Increased transferrin	?
OCA	Folate	Increased folate binding protein	?
OCA	Vitamin B_6	Altered B_6 and tryptophan metabolism	Mood changes; abnormal protein metabolism
OCA	Vitamin B_{12}	Reduced serum concentration	Uncertain
OCA	Folate	Reduced red cell concentration	Megaloblastic anemia; other effects?
OCA	Zinc	Reduced serum concentration	Uncertain
Diphenyl hydantoin Primidone	Folate	Uncertain	Macrocytic anemia
Tetracyclines	Calcium	Drug binds to Ca in bones	Growth retardation in premature infants; pigmentation of teeth
Tricyclic antidepressants Imipramine	Various	Stimulate appetite	Weight gain

*For further discussion on this topic, see Butterworth,[9] Hathcock and Stanasyet,[10] Theuer,[11] Roe[12] and Hathcock and Coon.[13]

diagnoses to demonstrate a relationship between nutritional status and the outcome of an illness. One can proceed only on the basis of logic until better statistics are available to document a correlation between malnutrition and length of hospital stay or eventual outcome. Nevertheless, there are clear indications that undernutrition is associated with poor wound healing and with increased susceptibility to infection. The cost and frequency of these two complications alone should make it worthwhile to attempt to prevent them through nutrition support, thereby shortening the overall period of hospitalization.

> In 1975, for the ninth consecutive year, total hospital expenditures increased at an annual rate of more than 10 per cent. Total expenditures were $48.7 billion—17.6 per cent higher than in 1974. This represented the largest one-year increase of the decade from 1965 to 1975.[8]

Total hospital expenditures in this country in 1975 were $48,700,000,000. There were 170 admissions to the hospital per 100,000 population, for an average stay of 7.7 days. It does not seem unreasonable to suggest that improved nutrition services in the hospital (and clinics) could reduce both the admission rate and duration of hospital stay by 10 per cent. This could represent a saving to the nation of some 5 to 10 billion dollars annually. Total hospital expenditures in 1976 were $55,700,000,000. It is worthy of emphasis that complications arising from malnutrition tend to be long and costly, e.g. infections, decubitus ulcers, wound dehiscence and massive gastrointestinal hemorrhage. Such catastrophes are better prevented than treated.

Drug-nutrient Interaction

Iatrogenic malnutrition may occur as a result of drugs prescribed for the treatment of an illness. In some cases interaction between drugs and nutrients is an intentional part of drug design; in others it is an undesirable and sometimes unexpected side effect. In any event the physician should be alert to the possibility of nutrient imbalance caused by medications so that undesirable effects can be prevented or minimized. Table 22–7 summarizes some of the mechanisms by which drugs may interact with nutrients. Table 22–8 summarizes some of the known interactions between drugs and nutrients and presents the presumed mechanism of action and possible clinical consequences, where information is available.

BIBLIOGRAPHY

1. Leevy, et al.: Am. J. Clin. Nutr., *17*, 259, 1965.
2. Bollet and Owens: Am. J. Clin. Nutr., *26*, 931, 1973.
3. Bistrian, et al.: J.A.M.A., *230*, 858, 1976.
4. Bistrian, et al.: J.A.M.A., *235*, 1567, 1976.
5. Weinsier, Hunker, Krumdieck and Butterworth: Am. J. Clin. Nutr., *32*, 418, 1979.
6. Mayer (Ed.): *Overweight: Causes, Cost, and Control.* Englewood Cliffs, Prentice-Hall, 1968, p. 31.
7. Scrimshaw, Salomon, Bruch and Gordon: Am. J. Trop. Med. Hyg., *15*, 625, 1966.
8. American Hospital Association: *Hospital Statistics.* Chicago, 1976.
9. Butterworth: J. Am. Diet. Assoc., *62*, 510, 1973.
10. Hathcock and Stanasyet: Hosp. Pharm., *9*, 373, 1974.
11. Theuer: J. Reprod. Med., *8*, 13, 1972.
12. Roe: *Drug-induced Nutritional Deficiencies.* Westport, Avi Publishing Co., 1976.
13. Hathcock and Coon: *Nutrition and Drug Interrelations.* New York, Academic Press, 1978.

Chapter *23*

CLINICAL MANIFESTATIONS OF CERTAIN CLASSICAL DEFICIENCY DISEASES

Harold H. Sandstead

The classical deficiency diseases of beriberi, pellagra, scurvy and rickets occur infrequently in the North America of today. Such has not always been the case. Prior to the discovery of the vitamins and the subsequent elucidation of their roles in human nutrition, these diseases were more prevalent. In fact, their near disappearance from the scene of American medicine is largely the result of the striking advances in communication, education, food technology and public health which began with World War II and have accelerated in pace ever since. The modern student is thus often unaware of the impact these diseases have had and, in fact, still have on large segments of the world's population. It is the intent of this chapter to briefly review the history of these diseases and their clinical features. Details of their biochemistry are considered elsewhere in conjunction with discussions of the metabolism and requirements for specific vitamins.

Today in North America and northern Europe, these diseases, when they occur, usually are associated with social or medical pathologic conditions of some variety. In contrast to other regions of the world, they seldom occur primarily. In addition, they almost never are caused by a single deficiency, except under experimental conditions. Thus, they are, in fact, mixed deficiency syndromes with "major" manifestations reflecting derangements induced by lack of the most limiting nutrient and "minor" manifestations induced by the associated deficiencies.

Examples of social pathology often associated with these diseases include alcoholism, social isolation, food faddism, ignorance and neglect of individuals unable to care for themselves, such as small children or the elderly. Medical causes that may contribute to their occurrence include intestinal malabsorption syndromes, senility, psychosis and iatrogenic factors. In the technologically less advanced parts of the world, social factors such as customs, taboos, poverty, lack of education, primitive agricultural practices and poor systems of food delivery and storage play a much greater role in their genesis.

It is evident, therefore, that, when they occur, these syndromes are the consequence of a variety of factors which ultimately result in the patient not having access to, not eating or not utilizing a diet adequate in all nutrients. The complexity of their pathogenesis, therefore, must be kept in mind when one is confronted with a patient with clinical manifestations consistent with one of them. Only by determining the root cause can recurrence be prevented. In addition, an understanding of underlying causes will make it possible for the physician and public health worker to prevent their occurrence in the first place.

BERIBERI

Beriberi is an ancient disease that has been endemic in the Orient for over 4,000 years. Although it generally occurs in populations whose staple is polished rice, it has been observed in individuals subsisting on unenriched white flour.

Clarification of the cause of beriberi began toward the end of the last century with the studies of Takaki, Director General of the Japanese Naval Medical Service. He conducted a clinical trial in which he added meat, milk and barley to the polished rice diet of sailors to see if he could prevent the occurrence of beriberi during a long voyage. His success led to improvement of the diet of the navy and near disappearance of the disease among Japanese sailors. Antedating the concept of vitamins by roughly 25 years, he attributed the prevention to the increased dietary protein.[1]

Unaware of Takaki's observations, a Dutch physician, Eijkman, working in Java during the 1890s, discovered that feeding polished rice to fowl produced a fatal polyneuritis. Influenced by the discoveries of Pasteur and Koch, he at first thought the disease infectious. Later he attributed it to a toxic effect of the starch in the polished rice, which could be overcome by a substance in the husk.

Eijkman's successor, Grijns, extended the studies on the "factor" and enunciated the concept that beriberi was caused by a deficiency of a heat-labile substance present in the husks of grain.[1] Clinical studies were inconclusive until 1910, when Frazer and Stanton clearly affirmed that "beriberi is a disorder of metabolism" resulting from a lack of a substance extractable from rice that is essential for nerve tissue. Soon after this, Vedder, a U.S. Army physician, enlisted the help of Williams, a chemist, to help in the search for the unknown factor.

Many years later, Williams and his associates isolated and subsequently synthesized thiamin. The German chemist Casimir Funk also searched for the factor. His studies led him intuitively to propose in 1912 that the missing factor was a "vital amine" and to coin the word *vitamine*. The vitamin concept was thus born.[1]

Clinically, beriberi, like many other diseases, presents a spectrum of manifestations. Their presence seems in part to be determined by the chronicity of the deficiency, its severity and stress factors which may acutely increase the rate of metabolism and thus the thiamin requirement of the patient.[2] Thus, individuals subsisting on a diet of 0.2 to 0.3 mg of thiamin per 1000 calories, which is slightly less than the thiamin requirement, may gradually become depleted and develop peripheral neuropathy. The extremities of maximal use are most affected. Paresthesia, hyperesthesia, anesthesia, formication and weakness are experienced. Initially, the deep tendon reflexes are increased; later they may be absent. The muscles are often tender and may atrophy. Foot and wrist drop occur. Fatigue, decreased attention span and impaired capacity to work are striking. This type of beriberi is so-called dry or atrophic beriberi.

If the patient has been subsisting on something less than 0.2 mg of thiamin per 1,000 calories, deficiency will be more severe and he will develop so-called subacute or wet beriberi. In addition to neurologic manifestations, cardiovascular signs and symptoms will be more apparent. Dependent edema may be seen. The heart is often enlarged, with the right side particularly prominent and the pulmonary second sound accentuated. With the slightest effort, tachycardia occurs. The patient complains of palpitation and dull precordial and epigastric pain. The venous pressure is often increased while the circulation time may be shortened or normal, through arteriovenous shunting. Digestive disturbances with anorexia and constipation commonly occur. The anorexia may be quite striking. As the disease advances, the neurologic manifestations become increasingly evident.

Fulminant cardiac failure may be precipitated in the above types of patients by physiologic stress which increases the rate of metabolism, even if the individual has shown little previous evidence of thiamin deficiency. This type of cardiac failure has been given the colorful name of "Shoshin beriberi" after the region in China where it was studied. Patients so afflicted rapidly succumb with cardiac failure which seems to be primarily right-sided. Systolic hypotension, venous distention and peripheral cyanosis are prominent. Pulmonary congestion is reported to occur late in the illness and the patients are said to expire in extreme agony and fully conscious.[2]

In the western world, where thiamin-deficiency heart disease is most often associated with alcoholism, the cardiac features of the illness are similar to those observed in Oriental beriberi.[3] Such patients typically have been drinking heavily and eating little for some weeks, thus depleting their body stores of thiamin. (Such depletion can be produced experimentally in man in roughly 12 to 14 days.) Often they are also deficient in calories, protein, other B vitamins, minerals such as magnesium, potassium and zinc, and ascorbic acid. In addition to cardiac failure, they may display a variety of neurologic abnormalities attributable to thiamin deficiency: peripheral neuropathy, myelopathy, cerebellar signs and Wernicke's encephalopathy or its residual effects.[4]

It is generally held that the cardiac failure of thiamin deficiency is of the high-output variety. However, it should not surprise the clinician to find an occasional patient with low-output failure which is responsive to thiamin. Biochemically and physiologically, such a phenomenon is quite understandable as the cardiac metabolism of pyruvate is grossly compromised by thiamin lack.[5] Further evidences of myocardial injury in thiamin deficiency are nonspecific electrocardiographic abnormalities. In thiamin-deficient experimental animals similar physiologic derangements have been produced, both with and without microscopic pathology.[6,7] The essential factors influencing the incidence of morphologic injury are the severity and the acuteness of the deficiency.

The superimposition of the toxic effects of alcohol or other toxic substances such as cobalt on the myocardium may cause some clinical confusion; therefore, it is essential that the patient's response to therapy with thiamin be the principal diagnostic criterion. Patients with heart failure due to thiamin deficiency do not respond to digitalis or diuretics. In contrast, therapy with thiamin (5 to 10 mg 3 times daily) is followed by a rapid disappearance of tachycardia, ventricular gallop and other evidences of congestive failure. Unfortunately the response of the neurologic lesions may be slow, in contrast to the myocardiopathy. This poor response reflects the limited regenerative capacity of nervous tissue.

The most acute type of thiamin deficiency, Wernicke's encephalopathy,[4] is rare in the Orient. It occurs primarily in alcoholics and in patients with pernicious vomiting, such as that which may occur in pregnancy or following surgery on the gastrointestinal tract. Acute administration of glucose to such severely deprived patients may precipitate the encephalopathy. Manifestations range from mild confusion to coma. Ophthalmoplegia with sixth nerve weakness and lateral and/or vertical nystagmus are seen. Cerebellar ataxia is often evident. If untreated, death is common. If the patient survives, damage to the cerebral cortex may result in a psychosis (Korsakoff's). Retentive memory and cognitive function are severely impaired. Confabulation is a common characteristic.

Because of the high mortality, morbidity

and sequelae of Wernicke's encephalopathy, it is imperative that thiamin be included in the therapeutic regimen of all patients admitted to hospitals for the various illnesses associated with alcoholism. In addition, thiamin, as well as the other vitamins, should be given to those who are unable to eat for any extended period and those who are severely hypermetabolic. Thus iatrogenic disease due to thiamin deprivation or other vitamin deficiencies can be avoided.

Though infantile beriberi is rarely if ever seen in the Occident, it still occurs in the Orient in regions where enrichment of rice with thiamin has not been instituted. In these places, beriberi is still an important cause of infant death. Nursing babies whose mothers subsist largely on polished rice and who show evidence of thiamin deficiency are particularly at risk. Typically, the infants become ill between the first and fourth month of life.[8]

The clinical onset of infantile beriberi may be sudden. It may appear as acute cardiac failure in a previously healthy-appearing child. In other babies, the signs may be primarily neurologic, with aphonia (silent crying) or features suggestive of meningitis. In some infants, the signs may be intermittant. In others, death is prompt. Recovery is often rapid and dramatic following administration of thiamin.[9]

The diagnosis of thiamin deficiency can be made more rapidly and objectively today than in the past. Advantage is taken of the role of thiamin pyrophosphate in the transketolase reaction of the pentose shunt (see Chapters 6E and 20). The activity of the enzyme in erythrocytes is determined with and without added thiamin pyrophosphate. If the baseline activity is low and addition of thiamin pyrophosphate causes a striking increase, this is interpreted as metabolic evidence consistent with thiamin deficiency.[10,11,11a] The diagnosis can be established unequivocally by a subsequent therapeutic trial and documentation of the clinical and biochemical responses.

Thiamin status may also be assessed by measurement of the urinary excretion of the vitamin. This has been a useful technique for assessing the thiamin status of populations. For technical reasons, it generally has not been utilized for evaluation of individuals. Further discussion of the biochemical assessment of thiamin status is presented in Chapters 6E and 20.

PELLAGRA

Pellagra is a mixed deficiency disease, the major manifestations of which are primarily results of a deficiency of niacin or its precursor tryptophan. Classically it occurs seasonally, is often chronic and tends to recur. Historically it appears to be a relatively new disease in that it was not recognized by European physicians or in the Middle East until after the introduction of corn (maize). It seems probable, however, that populations subsisting on Sorghum vulgare have suffered from the disease from antiquity. This supposition is based on Sandwith's description of pellagra in noncorn-eating Egyptians from upper Egypt, and on his report that physicians who had been working in India recognized the disease when shown photographs of his Egyptian experience.[12] The fact that pellagra continues to occur today among Indians who live on Sorghum vulgare (Joware)[13] is also supportive. Whether pellagra occurred in the preColumbian new world is unknown.

The association of pellagra with maize was reported in the middle of the 18th century by Casal and Frapollie.[14] Casal noted its seasonal occurrence, the relation of the dermatitis to sunlight and described the good therapeutic effect of milk.[15]

The first clear enunciation of the relationship between a poorly balanced diet and pellagra was by Cerri in 1795.[15] His observations were generally disregarded for 120 years until Goldberger reported his classical studies in the early 1900s. The dilemma and confusion of scientists prior to Goldberger are well presented in Roberts' text Pellagra, which appeared in

1913.[12] At that time, pellagra had reached epidemic proportions in the southeastern United States and affected an estimated 10,000 persons nationally.

The careful epidemiologic and experimental studies of Goldberger disproved the infection and toxin hypotheses and established that the disease was caused by a lack of some nutrient or nutrients in the corn on which the populace subsisted. He favored a deficiency of cystine and/or tryptophan.[15,16] Despite Goldberger's observations and the subsequent efforts of others, pellagra continued to be a serious public health problem throughout the south until after 1938 when Elvehjem et al.[17] isolated niacinamide from liver and demonstrated that it would cure black tongue in dogs. Of interest is the fact that Funk[18] had isolated niacin in 1912 and had suggested that it might be lacking from the diet of pellagrins. Other major factors in the eradication of pellagra were enrichment of foods such as bread with niacin and the social and economic changes which occurred throughout the country during and subsequent to World War II.[16] Since that time, in the United States and northern Europe, it has become a disease of the alcoholic, the elderly recluse and others with bizarre eating habits. It may also rarely occur in patients with malabsorption syndromes, thyrotoxicosis, diabetes mellitus, neoplasia and serotonin-producing tumors (carcinoid).

The multiple-deficiency aspects of pellagra emerged when it became possible to treat pellagrins specifically with niacin. Examples of other nutrients which the pellagrin may lack include protein, riboflavin, pyridoxine, thiamin, folic acid, vitamin A, magnesium, potassium, iron and zinc. The presence of these associated deficiencies contributes to some of the clinical findings noted below.

The clinical features of classical endemic pellagra were graphically described and related to the gross and microscopic pathology by Roberts in 1913.[12] More recently, Follis[19] reviewed the pathologic condition. While the disease adversely affects all systems of the body, the most striking symptoms and signs involve the integument, nervous system and gastrointestinal tract. Generally the patients are apathetic and anorexic, have neurasthenia and complain of intermittent pain in their extremities and body. They appear pale and may have severe weight loss. If the disease has been chronic, the skin over exposed surfaces and pressure points may be thickened, hyperkeratotic and hyperpigmented without evidence of inflammation, while moist areas, such as the vulva and scrotum, may be macerated and erythematous. When deficiency is severe, the rash may resemble a severe burn and may be secondarily infected. Areas classically involved are the backs of the hands, the elbows, the neck (Casal's necklace) and the anterior chest.

Neurologic manifestations may be a prominent feature. Peripheral neuropathy, myelopathy and encephalopathy may all occur. In less severe disease, peripheral nerve abnormalities may predominate. Both sensory and motor modalities may be affected. With increased chronicity and, presumably, more severe deficiency, myelopathy, which may progress to full-blown combined cord degeneration, may occur.[12,19] Involvement of the brain may result in mania and, shortly before death, in seizures and coma. Prior to the availability of specific therapy, the psychiatric aspects of pellagra accounted for a high percentage of admissions to mental institutions in endemic areas.

The gastrointestinal tract is affected from mouth to anus. The mouth shows a number of nonspecific lesions which emphasize the multiple-deficiency aspects of the disease: cheilosis, angular fissures, atrophy of the epithelium of the tongue with associated pain and inflammation. Hypertrophy of the fungiform papillae may also occur, as may gastric achlorhydria. In some patients, the small intestinal mucosa is atrophic and may be inflamed; in others, the small intestine appears histologically normal. Nonspecific colitis with bleeding may occur, while the rectum and anus are inflamed and painful. Malabsorption of fat and other nutrients can occur in association with diarrhea, though in other patients the diarrhea is watery and not laden with fat.

Clinically less striking aspects include anemia, which may be macrocytic and responsive to folic acid, or hypochromic, microcytic and responsive to iron.[15] In some patients the anemia is mixed. The reproductive system may also be involved, resulting in amenorrhea and an apparent increased incidence of abortion.[12]

The biochemical pathogenesis of pellagra has been a fertile area of research. After the relationship between tryptophan and niacin became known (60 mg tryptophan is equivalent to 1 mg of niacin),[15] it was evident that Goldberger had been partially correct in his supposition that the quality of the dietary protein consumed is an important factor in the genesis of the disease.[16] In addition, it has been shown that, while the niacin in corn and other cereals such as wheat, rice and barley is present in amounts sufficient to prevent pellagra, it is firmly bound to indigestible constituents in the grain and is, therefore, poorly available to man and other monogastric animals. The alkaline treatment of corn, which is common in Latin America, improves this availability. Such treatment coupled with the consumption of coffee, which may contain significant amounts of niacin depending on the roast, presumably explains the rarity of pellagra among the corn-eating peasants of the region.[15] A third factor in pathogenesis may be the amino acid pattern of certain grains. Studies by Gopalan et al.[20,20a] suggest that the high leucine content of Sorghum vulgare induces an amino acid imbalance which apparently may produce pellagra in man and black tongue in dogs. It is thus evident that the biochemical etiology of pellagra is complex and that several characteristics of the food consumed interact to produce the disease.

The diagnosis of pellagra is usually straightforward in patients with the rash. If, however, the skin has not been exposed to sunlight or to minor trauma, the rash may be minimal or absent. Then, with only neurologic and/or gastrointestinal manifestations, the diagnosis may be obscure. A careful dietary history will usually resolve the issue. In general, an intake of less than 9.0 mg of niacin daily, or less than 4.4 mg per 1,000 calories, including that formed from tryptophan, is inadequate. If facilities allow, the measurement of the 24-hour urinary excretion of N^1-methyl nicotinamide and pyridine in patients fed a diet containing 10 mg of niacin and 1,000 mg of tryptophan is also informative. Patients with pellagra excrete less than 3.0 mg on this regimen, while well-nourished individuals excrete more than 7.0 mg.[15] Unfortunately, a more rapid laboratory method for niacin assessment, analogous to the erythrocyte transketolase assay for thiamin status, is not available. (For further discussion of the biochemistry of niacin and diagnosis of deficiency, see Chapters 6G and 20.)

Treatment of patients with pellagra should, in addition to nutrients, include attention to the various distressing manifestations noted above. Nutrient therapy includes 300 to 500 mg of niacinamide daily in divided doses plus administration of the other nutrients often deficient in such patients. The diet, at least initially, should be soft so as to be easily eaten while the patient is acutely ill.

SCURVY

Scurvy is perhaps the oldest well-described deficiency disease, in that it is referred to in the Ebers Papyrus and by Hippocrates.[21] Its occurrence among soldiers and explorers doubtless influenced the course of history, because those so afflicted were unable to carry out their intentions. Thus, it contributed to the failure of certain crusades,[22] frustrated long sea voyages and land explorations and, through its occurrence in the French navy, may have contributed to Nelson's triumph over Napoleon.[23]

The first clear-cut formulation of the cause of scurvy is attributed to Bachstrom, who, in 1734, noted that those who abstained from fresh vegetables and fruits developed the disease. He is said to have been the first physician to discard the "humor concept" in favor of the hypothesis that lack of a specific type of food could result in disease.[21] It should be noted, however, that Lancaster, a British sea captain, had demonstrated the preventive value of lemon juice 134 years earlier[21] and that the French explorer Cartier had learned 200 years previously of the curative value of a decoction of pine needles and bark.[22] Contemporary with Bachstrom, James Lind, a British naval physician, conducted a controlled therapeutic experiment on scorbutic sailors which conclusively demonstrated the preventive and curative value of citrus fruit. He published his findings and recommendations in 1753. Forty-two years later, the Admiralty followed his advice,[22] a decision which, as noted above, may have changed the course of history.

Scurvy among infants became a severe clinical problem in the late 19th century, when pasteurization and the boiling of infant formulas became the vogue. It continued to be not uncommon in this age group until the evolution of modern pediatric feeding practices. This was in spite of the fact that Waugh and King[24] had isolated and crystallized vitamin C from lemons in 1932, and had shown it to be identical with the "hexuronic acid" of Szent-Györgyi.[25] The following year Reichstein et al.[26] accomplished its synthesis.

Today scurvy is rare where modern medicine is practiced and nutrition education has had an impact. When it occurs, it is usually the result of self-neglect by individuals who, because of psychiatric difficulty, age, alcoholism or ignorance, are unable or unwilling to care for themselves. In infants, it is found, except in a rare instance, only among the artificially fed; its occurrence reflects a lack of understanding on the part of mothers of the nutritional needs of children. An unusual cause of scurvy today is the sudden discontinuance of megadoses of ascorbic acid and its continued increased degradation by enzymes previously induced by the high intake.

The clinical manifestations of scurvy appear to reflect the role of the vitamin in the metabolism of mesenchymal cells, which form connective tissue, osteoid and dentin.[27] Osteoblastic activity is retarded, new wounds do not heal and old wounds open up. In addition, it appears from animal studies that scurvy may impair the production of vasohumoral agents by the kidney.[28] Such a phenomenon might allow an abnormal distribution of blood flow in capillary beds, resulting in engorgement and subsequent extravasation. In addition, because of impaired collagen formation, the supporting matrix for the capillary bed may be inadequate.

Under usual circumstances, the onset of clinical scurvy in adults is delayed for 4 to 5 months from the time dietary vitamin C is restricted. The severity of the restriction and the previous body stores of the individual dictate the time of onset. Plasma concentrations of ascorbic acid, on the other hand, reflect the recent intake of the vitamin and fall to low levels in 3 to 4 weeks. A decline in white blood cell–platelet vitamin C occurs more slowly, reaching low levels after 20 to 24 weeks. This decrease is believed to reflect tissue saturation, as signs of clinical scurvy appear roughly two weeks after the white blood cell–platelet concentration of the vitamin has become negligible.[29]

In infants, scurvy occurs most commonly between the 5th and 24th month of age; the peak incidence is between 8 and 11 months. The time of onset reflects the body stores at birth, the duration of nursing, which provides adequate ascorbic acid, the rate of growth and its duration and the vitamin C content of the infant's food.

Early symptoms in adults include anorexia, weakness, neurasthenia and aching in the joints and muscles. One of the first specific clinical signs is an increased prominence of the hair follicles on the thighs and buttocks, caused by keratin plugging of the lumens. Hairs within the follicles become coiled and fragmented and have a characteristic corkscrew appearance after they erupt. Perifollicular hemorrhages ultimately result in the deposition of brown pigmentation. With time, the purpuric lesions coalesce and form ecchymoses which spread from the lower extremities to the rest of the body, particularly those areas exposed to trauma. Hemorrhage may also occur in muscles, in and around joints, in gastrointestinal mucosa, in the kidneys and into the pericardium. The gingiva at the base of teeth becomes hemorrhagic and finally necrotic. This abnormality first appears at the base of the molars. The interdental papillae become swollen and bluish red in color and may become secondarily infected. With time, the teeth fall out. A curious finding is the hemorrhage which may occur in old scars, premonitory of their subsequent dehiscence. Death may occur suddenly once the clinical signs have become extensive and severe.

In infants, the clinical features are somewhat different from those of adults. The onset is usually insidious. Failure to thrive may be an early clue. Commonly, the infant is irritable, with tender extremities and pseudoparalysis. Purpuric lesions, which may be overlooked, are also present. If teeth are erupting, hemorrhage of the adjacent gum may be seen. A striking finding is the apprehension of the infant when it is handled. Other hemorrhagic manifestations include epistaxis, retrobulbar hemorrhage, hematuria and bloody diarrhea.

X-ray examination of the extremities often reveals a ground-glass appearance of the bones with a thinning of the cortex. A radiolucent area may surround the epiphy-seal plate. The center of ossification may be displaced. Following initiation of treatment, calcification of the periosteum will outline the subperiosteal hemorrhage. The radiolucency noted above initially affects the shaft, giving rise to the "corner sign" of Park; this is seen at the lateral margin of the junction between the metaphysis and epiphysis. The absence of calcification in this region is starkly apparent and constitutes an early roentgenographic sign of the disease.[29] Radiographic examination of the chest shows findings analogous to the extremities. The external appearance and palpation of the costochondral junctions are characteristic. Posterior subluxation of the sternum results in the sharp end of the ribs being palpable, while the displaced cartilages are related to the ends of the ribs in a manner analogous to a bayonet attached to a rifle (see also Chapter 21).

Anemia occurs in both adult and infantile scurvy. While in experimental subhuman primates it is clear that ascorbic acid has a sparing effect on the folic acid requirement, and will prevent the occurrence of megaloblastic anemia,[30,31] this relationship is more obscure in man.[32,33] This is probably related to the fact that single nutrient deficiencies are rare in man. Thus, the anemia associated with human scurvy may have components of iron, folic acid and ascorbic acid deficiencies simultaneously, in addition to reflecting the effects of infections which may be present.

The prevention and treatment of scurvy are straightforward; therefore, the disease should occur only on rare occasions in modern society. Ten mg of ascorbic acid daily will prevent the disease in infants and adults. Several times this amount is provided by a diet containing a mixture of fresh fruits and vegetables. Animal sources which contain significant amounts of ascorbic acid are liver and raw milk. Because the vitamin is readily destroyed by heat, oxygen and storage, the content of ascorbic acid in processed foods is significantly decreased. To correct for this loss, ascorbic acid is often added to processed foods normally considered important sources of the vitamin. (For further discussion of the laboratory diagnosis of scurvy and the biochemistry of ascorbic acid, see Chapters 6K and 20.)

RICKETS AND OSTEOMALACIA

Rickets and osteomalacia are diseases of the skeleton characterized by decreased deposition of calcium in osteoid. The failure of calcification causes a decreased structural rigidity of bone. Skeletal deformities, which are clinical hallmarks, are the consequence of the soft bones.

One of the earliest "modern" descriptions of rickets is the medical thesis prepared by Whistler in 1645.[34] He described the softness of the bones, their contorted shapes, the rachitic rosary and other chest deformities. He also alluded to the poor muscular development, delayed tooth eruption and poor nutritional status of the children. A more comprehensive description, *De Rachitide*, was published by Glisson in 1650. From these texts it may be inferred that rickets was a serious and common affliction of children in the northern Europe of that day.

The relationship of the deformities to decreased bone mineral was documented in 1842 by Marchand.[35] Sixteen years later a clear description of the morphologic pathology was provided by Müller.[35] By the turn of the century, the failure of rachitic children to absorb calcium and phosphorus was appreciated. Experimental animal studies reported in 1921 documented the predictive value of the product of the serum calcium and phosphorus concentrations in the diagnosis of the disease.[36] The same year Park and Howland described the curative effects of vitamin D.[37]

Since these early days, it has become evident that rickets and osteomalacia may be caused by a variety of etiologies other than lack of exposure to ultraviolet light or dietary inadequacy of vitamin D. Certain of these causes are inborn errors of metabolism; others are related to disorders of gastrointestinal function, to substances toxic to the kidney or gastrointestinal tract or to drugs which alter the metabolism of vitamin D, such as corticosteroids or diphenylhydantoin. Today, these "metabolic" causes are more commonly implicated than is dietary deficiency. The near elimination of dietary rickets in advanced countries may be credited to a general appreciation of the causes of the disease, its prevention and cure and the implementation of vitamin D enrichment. Dietary rickets is still found in countries where children are customarily shielded from the sun, vitamin D enrichment of food is not practiced and fish oils or vitamin preparations containing vitamin D are not given. The same is true of osteomalacia in women who, because of custom, continue to wear heavy veils.

Classically, dietary rickets was a disease of temperate countries. Long winters, with little ultraviolet light because of the angle of the sun, cloud cover and smog over industrial centers, resulted in a high incidence of the disease. From 1901 to 1908, in Dresden, 94 per cent of 287 autopsied children under 2 years of age were rachitic.[38] A similar study on material obtained in Baltimore from 1926 to 1942 showed that more than 50 per cent of the children had been affected. When grouped by age according to month, severe rickets was found in 12 to 43 per cent.[35] Today the disease is rare in Baltimore.

Rapid growth increases the susceptibility of premature infants and babies to rickets.[39] One of the earliest signs is craniotabes. The normal remodeling of bone results in removal of hydroxyapatite. Failure to calcify new osteoid results in a softening of the skull and delayed closure of the fontanelles. The habitual position of the child molds the skull with resultant flattening of the chronically dependent surface, usually the occiput. Thickening (bossing) of the skull over the frontal and parietal eminences also occurs. This may be particularly impressive in infants with anemia, giving the skull the appearance of a hot cross bun.

The shafts of the extremities are also soft. In response to the influence of gravity and position, they may become severely misshapened. Epiphyseal growth and the failure of calcification result in knobby deformities at the ends of the long bones. Displacement of the epiphysis may occur. Thus, posterior tilting of the lower tibial epiphysis by the weight of the foot results in initiation of the classical saber-shin deformity, and displacement of the distal radial and ulnar epiphysis by the weight of the infant on his pronated hand results in a conspicuous bulging at the wrist.[39]

Dentition typically is delayed; teeth may erupt out of order. While the enamel of deciduous teeth is unaffected, permanent teeth formed during the rachitic interval may be severely injured. The enamel is thin, pitted and sometimes absent.

Enlargement of the costochondral junctions, the so-called rachitic rosary, is an early sign of rickets. Occasionally, posterior displacement of the sternum occurs in response to force exerted by the diaphragm and intercostal muscles, thus forming a trough. In other instances, the sternum may move anteriorly, forming a pigeon breast. With softening, the inferior ribs may bend inward, forming a Harrison's groove. If the ribs become very soft, the bellow function of the chest may be severely compromised. Later in life, rachitic deformities of the chest may limit pulmonary function.

Just as the chest and extremities are twisted, so is the spine. Early in life a dorsolumbar kyphosis occurs. Later, after the child begins to walk, the kyphosis may disappear and severe lordosis develop. The deformity of the back and twisting of the tibia and femur grossly alter the gait, so that the patient may waddle in a manner similar to that seen with congenital dislocation of the hips.

The musculature of the rachitic child is often hypotonic. Potbelly is common. Motor development may be retarded. Other nutrient deficiencies may be present, but are inconsistent. The presence of scurvy, because of its effect on the metabolism of osteoblasts, retards the development of rickets.[35]

X-ray abnormalities occur in both the epiphysis and shaft. The junction of the epiphysis and metaphysis typically shows a concave cupping of the metaphysis, with spreading of the junction. The inner margin of the cup is often fringed and stippled. Stippling reflects the incomplete deposition of calcium and phosphorus that occurs in early rickets.

The x-ray abnormalities in the shaft reflect the normal remodeling of bone and subsequent failure of calcification. Osteoid is not radiopaque; therefore, the trabeculae appear coarse and the cortex is thin. In extreme instances, the bone is nearly translucent.

When vitamin D is given, calcium is deposited in the provisional zone of cartilaginous calcification. Thus an opaque line (Müller's line), separate from the rest of the metaphysis, appears on the x-ray film.

Osteomalacia is metabolically identical to rickets except that it occurs in adults. Because longitudinal growth has stopped, only the shafts of the long bones and flat bones, such as the pelvis, are affected. The remodeling process results in softening, and distortion of the shape of the bone. When fractures occur they probably result from an associated osteoporosis. Some of the most distressing signs of the disease are the pelvic deformities which occur in women as a consequence of multiple pregnancies and lactation, low dietary calcium and nonexposure to ultraviolet irradiation. Even today, osteomalacia of this etiology is said to be endemic in northern India, Japan and northern China.[40]

X-ray findings in osteomalacia reflect resorption of bone and failure to calcify osteoid. Gross asymmetric deformity of the pelvis with narrowing of the outlet is typical. Minute ribbon-like pseudofractures of long bones also occur (for additional discussion of x-ray findings in rickets and osteomalacia, see Chapter 21).

The pathogenesis of dietary rickets and osteomalacia seems to be roughly as follows.[39] Deficiency of vitamin D, either of dietary origin or due to lack of ultraviolet irradiation, results in decreased absorption of dietary calcium and phosphorus. As a result, hydroxyapatite formation is decreased and plasma levels of calcium tend to decline. In response to the lowering of plasma calcium, the parathyroid glands release parathormone. Bone resorption and phosphate excretion are accelerated through the influence of the hormone. Thus the plasma concentration of ionized calcium is maintained. In bone, calcification of cartilage and new osteoid is inhibited and bones become soft. Flat bones and the shafts of long bones become distorted in both children and adults. In children, the cartilaginous growth sites on the ends of bones overgrow, resulting in knobby deformities.

From this simple scheme, the expected serum concentrations of calcium, phosphorus and alkaline phosphatase which occur in rickets and osteomalacia can be predicted.

In infants and children, serum calcium may be normal or low; phosphorus is low and alkaline phosphatase is quite elevated. In adults, serum calcium is usually normal to low-normal. Serum phosphorus is low and alkaline phosphatase is increased. Because the methods of analysis and expression of results differ in various laboratories, numerical values have not been given.

Rickets or osteomalacia due to other causes such as renal tubular defects, familial hypophosphatemia, inborn errors of vitamin D metabolism, intestinal malabsorption of fat, chronic renal failure, or cadmium poisoning (itai-itai disease) is morphologically and clinically similar to the dietary disease. When related to intestinal malabsorption, not only is vitamin D absorption decreased but calcium malabsorption may be so severe as to be little affected by endogenous vitamin D derived from ultraviolet irradiation.

As a consequence of abnormalities in renal tubular phosphate reabsorption, severe depletion in the anion may occur. Serum levels may be low enough to impair the formation of hydroxyapatite. Renal tubular acidosis promotes calciuria, thus decreasing the amount of calcium available for bone. This form of rickets is vitamin D resistant. In chronic renal failure and itai-itai disease, impaired synthesis of 1-25 dihydroxycholecalciferol is responsible for impaired intestinal absorption of calcium. Low dietary calcium also seems to be a contributing factor.

The prevention and treatment of dietary rickets are straightforward. Enrichment of milk with 400 I.U. of vitamin D per quart has been shown to be an effective preventive measure. This level of intake has been suggested as the recommended daily allowance for children. Treatment requires the administration of both vitamin D and calcium. Three thousand to 5000 I.U. of vitamin D and 1 to 2 pints of milk daily are usually sufficient. In instances of vitamin D resistance, considerably larger amounts are required (up to 500,000 I.U. daily). In patients with intestinal malabsorption syndrome and osteomalacia, severe restriction of dietary fat to less than 30 gm daily may be required to correct the malabsorption of calcium. Replacement of much of the dietary fat with medium-chain triglycerides is an alternative way of improving intestinal fat absorption and decreasing fecal calcium loss. Prevention of excessive losses of calcium in the feces will often allow restoration of bone, if several grams of calcium are given daily. Modest amounts of vitamin D (±5000 I.U.) will also facilitate the process. If it is not possible to decrease the dietary fat, large doses of vitamin D (50,000 to 100,000 I.U.) may have a salutary effect. (For discussion of the management of the osteomalacia which may be associated with chronic renal failure, see Chapter 33.)

Details of the biochemistry of vitamin D and its active metabolites are presented in Chapter 6B, as is additional information concerning dietary sources and human requirements.

BIBLIOGRAPHY

1. Williams. *Toward the Conquest of Beri Beri*. Cambridge, Harvard University Press, 1961.
2. Platt: Fed. Proc., *17*, 8, 1958.
3. Blankenhorn: Circulation, *11*, 288, 1955.
4. Victor and Adams: Am. J. Clin. Nutr., *91*, 379, 1961.
5. Olson: Fed. Proc., *17*, 24, 1958.
6. Hundley: Fed. Proc., *17*, 27, 1958.
7. Follis: Fed. Proc., *17*, 23, 1958.
8. Burgen: Fed. Proc., *17*, 39, 1958.
9. Ramalingaswami: Fed. Proc., *17*, 44, 1958.
10. Brin, Dibble, Peel, McMullen, Brouquin and Chen: Am. J. Clin. Nutr., *17*, 240, 1965.
11. Warnock: J. Nutr., *100*, 1057, 1970.
11a. Vo-Khactu, Clayburgh and Sandstead: J. Lab. Clin. Med., *83*, 983, 1974.
12. Roberts: *Pellagra*. St. Louis, C. V. Mosby, 1913.
13. Gopalan and Srikantia: Lancet, *1*, 954, 1960.
14. Majors: *Classic Description of Disease*, 3rd ed. Springfield, Charles C Thomas, 1945, p. 607.
15. Goldsmith: In *Nutrition, a Comprehensive Treatise II*. (Beaton and McHenry, Eds.). New York, Academic Press, 1964, p. 109.
16. Sydenstricker: Am. J. Clin. Nutr., *6*, 409, 1958.
17. Elvehjem, Madden, Strong and Wooley: J. Biol. Chem., *123*, 137, 1938.
18. Funk: *The Vitamins*. Baltimore, Williams & Wilkins, 1922.
19. Follis: *Deficiency Disease*. Springfield, Charles C Thomas, 1958, p. 316.
20. Gopalan, Belvady and Krishmanurthi: Lancet, *2*, 956, 1969.
20a. Gopalan, Kamala and Rao: Vitam. Horm., *33*, 505, 1975.
21. Friedman and Jolliffe: In *Clinical Nutrition*, 2nd ed. (Jolliffe, Ed.). New York, Hoeber Medical Division, Harper & Row, 1962, p. 656.
22. Majors: *Classic Description of Disease*, 3rd ed. Springfield, Charles C Thomas, 1945, p. 585.
23. Davidson: In *Textbook of Medicine*, 11th ed. (Beeson and McDermott, Eds.). Philadelphia, W. B. Saunders, 1963, p. 1218.
24. Waugh and King: J. Biol. Chem., *97*, 325, 1932.
25. Szent-Györgyi: Biochem. J., *22*, 1387, 1928.
26. Reichstein, Grussner and Oppenhauer: Helv. Chem. Acta, *16*, 1019, 1933.
27. Follis: *Deficiency Disease*. Springfield, Charles C Thomas, 1958, p. 175.
28. Akers and Lee: Proc. Soc. Exp. Biol. Med., *82*, 195, 1953.
29. Woodruff: In *Nutrition, a Comprehensive Treatise II* (Beaton and McHenry, Eds.). New York, Academic Press, 1964, p. 265.
30. May, Nelson, Lowe and Salmon: Am. J. Dis. Child., *80*, 191, 1950.
31. Woodruff, Dutra, Misra and Darby: Fed. Proc., *17*, 498, 1958.
32. Zuelzer, Hutoff and Apt.: Am. J. Dis. Child., *77*, 128, 1949.
33. Vilter, Woolford and Spies: J. Lab. Clin. Med., *31*, 609, 1946.
34. Majors: *Classic Description of Disease*, 3rd ed. Springfield, Charles C Thomas, 1945, p. 594.
35. Follis: *Deficiency Disease*. Springfield, Charles C Thomas, 1958, p. 361.
36. Howland and Kramer: Am. J. Dis. Child., *22*, 105, 1921.
37. Park and Howland: Bull. Johns Hopkins Hosp., *32*, 341, 1921.
38. Schmorl: Cited by Follis: *Deficiency Disease*. Springfield, Charles C Thomas, 1958, p. 380.
39. Park: In *Clinical Nutrition*, 2nd ed. (Jolliffe, Ed.). New York, Hoeber Medical Division, Harper & Row, 1962, p. 506.
40. Snapper: In *Clinical Nutrition*, 2nd ed. (Jolliffe, Ed.). New York, Hoeber Medical Division, Harper & Row, 1962, p. 261.

Chapter 24

PROTEIN-CALORIE MALNUTRITION*

Fernando E. Viteri
and
Benjamin Torún

Large segments of the world's population live under conditions where the availability and intake of food are inadequate for their needs.[1] This is the case in many developing areas where food consumption is deficient both in quantity and quality. Insufficient food intake leads to chronic caloric deficiency, and ingestion of foods with insufficient protein concentration induces protein deficiency in vulnerable groups. This is particularly true when the protein is of poor quality, as is the case with most vegetable proteins. The problem with the latter is that the bulk of the food often imposes a limit to its intake. Also, amino acid deficiencies further limit the utilization of such protein sources, so that small children cannot satisfy their naturally elevated nitrogen and specific amino acid requirements.

These dietary factors, associated with many other health problems to be described later, lead to primary chronic protein-calorie malnutrition (PCM). In conditions conducive to primary PCM, the intakes of other essential nutrients, such as vitamins and minerals, are also generally low; however, serious manifestations of their specific clinical deficiencies are less common than might be expected because, when the calorie and protein intake is the limiting factor, the requirements for other nutrients diminish. Nevertheless, in PCM, vitamin or mineral deficiencies may become overt.

Primary PCM should be differentiated from secondary PCM, which is the consequence of a primary disease that leads either to inadequate food intake or utilization or to increased nutritional requirements. Examples of secondary PCM are psychologic disorders, obstructive gastrointestinal lesions, primary malabsorptive problems, diseases inducing cachexia of metabolic, infectious or neoplastic origin and endocrine disorders.

This chapter deals only with primary PCM, that is, the situation where energy and protein intake are apparently the most limiting factors in malnutrition.

EPIDEMIOLOGIC AND ETIOLOGIC CONSIDERATIONS

All developing areas of the world have several common characteristics, among which are low weight of newborn babies, high disease prevalence, small physical size of inhabitants, elevated mortality rates,

---

*Scientific articles published on this subject are much more numerous than those cited in the present chapter. However, because of limited space, the reader is often referred to some comprehensive reviews on the subject. Publications cited at the beginning or at the end of paragraphs or sections are general references for the topic dealt with. Through these, as well as through the more recent specific articles cited, many other important references may be easily located by those interested in a deeper approach to the subject.

Table 24–1.   Mortality Rates of Children 0-4 Years of Age*

Age	Guatemala (1965)	%	U.S.A. (1967)	%	Ratio Guatemala/U.S.A.
	A. Infant mortality (deaths/1000 live births)				
0–28 days	35.9	39.1	16.6	73.8	2.2
1–11 months	55.9	60.9	5.9	26.2	9.5
1 year	91.8	100.0	22.5	100.0	4.1
	B. Mortality in children between 1 and 4 years of age (deaths/1000 children of the corresponding age)				
1 year	50.0		1.4		35.7
2 years	35.2		0.9		39.1
3 years	24.9		0.7		35.6
4 years	15.6		0.6		26.0
1–4 years	30.3		0.9		33.7

* Compounded from data published by the Pan American Health Organization: *Las Condiciones de Salud en las Américas 1965–1968*. Washington, Organización Panamericana de la Salud, Septiembre 1970 (Publicación Científica No. 207), and INCAP.[3]

particularly during infancy and early childhood (Table 24–1) and, as a consequence, short life expectancy. The main reasons for these characteristics are undernutrition and poor environmental health. These situations lead to decreased productivity and increased waste of human and economic capital, including food. This perpetuates and often aggravates underdevelopment, thus worsening nutrition and health and, therefore, establishing a vicious cycle. This general picture, associated with a large concentration of still unproductive young people, provides the background for underdevelopment.

The magnitude of the problem varies from area to area. As an example, we cite the figures obtained from a survey of the Central American region where, by projecting to the total population of the area the prevalence obtained from a statistically representative sample of all of the 2.5 million children below 5 years of age, 1.6 million could be categorized, on the basis of body weight, as suffering from or as having had undernutrition. Nearly one-third of them had been or were moderately or severely malnourished (second- and third-degree undernutrition) at the time of the survey.[3] These findings are presented in Table 24–2.

Mild and moderate forms of adult undernutrition are more difficult to recognize but are also prevalent in developing areas. The manifestations of chronic PCM in this age group are more evident in terms of performance than in symptoms or clinical signs.

In adult males engaged in agricultural practices requiring intensive physical effort, caloric intake is often insufficient and leads to chronically limited energy expenditure in order to maintain a delicate energy balance. This results in suboptimal work performance, inadequate interactions with other family members or poor participation in community programs after working hours. In adult women, chronic undernutrition results in inadequate reproductive performance, which includes little weight gain during pregnancy, delivery of small-for-date babies and inadequate milk production in terms of both quantity and quality.[5,6]

A high proportion of newborns with low weight at birth is associated with a higher incidence of infant mortality.[7] Inadequate quantity and quality of woman's milk in groups of low socioeconomic condition are important factors in infant malnutrition.

Protein-calorie malnutrition should then be considered a social disease affecting

Table 24–2. Children Below 5 Years of Age in Central America, 1965–67, Presenting Growth Retardation which, by the Gómez* Classification, Could be Cataloged as Malnourished†

Country	Total Population below 5 Years of Age	1st, 2nd, and 3rd Degree Malnourished		Malnourished					
				1st Degree		2nd Degree		3rd Degree	
		No. of Cases	%	No. of Cases	%	No. of Cases	%	No. of Cases	%
Costa Rica	294,300	153,200	52.0	117,900	40.0	31,300	10.6	4,000	1.4
El Salvador	554,400	380,000	68.5	244,600	44.1	116,900	21.1	18,500	3.3
Guatemala	833,400	611,660	73.4	380,100	45.6	197,700	23.7	33,860	4.1
Honduras	346,900	221,300	63.7	143,000	41.2	71,200	20.5	7,100	2.0
Nicaragua	287,500	148,800	51.8	112,300	39.1	32,400	11.3	4,100	1.4
Panama	207,900	104,947	50.4	84,625	40.7	18,990	9.1	1,332	0.6
Total	2,524,400	1,619,907	64.2	1,082,525	42.9	468,490	18.6	68,892	2.7

* Gómez, et al.[2]

† Numbers are extrapolations from a statistically representative sample.

families, communities and geographic areas because of the negative effects that mild-to-moderate PCM of adults has on the well-being of the children and the development of the community.

In these settings, the few subjects who develop severe PCM with clinical manifestations must be interpreted as index cases which point at a widespread underlying nutritional problem. Thus, the fact that over 8 per cent of all adults admitted to public hospitals in countries such as Guatemala have moderate-to-severe primary PCM strengthens the concept that the poor functional performance of underprivileged populations is closely related to underlying mild-to-moderate PCM.

From the epidemiologic point of view, PCM can be conceived as the consequence of the interaction of the environment on the host through an agent which, in this case, is the deficient availability of calories and protein at the cell level. The environment, host and agent factors are interwoven.

Environment

This can be considered at two levels: (1) macroenvironment, at a regional or na-

tional level and (2) microenvironment, at the family and individual level.

In the developing areas, the macroenvironment is that of poverty, not only in the strict economic sense but also in the more important concept of human resources. Both are the cause and the consequence of lack of education, unsatisfactory health of the population, poor communications, low productivity, unfavorable economic balance and inadequate utilization of natural resources; all of these factors lead to inadequate food production, conservation, distribution and consumption.

The microenvironment constituted by the family, which is the biologic unit in terms of nutrition, receives the impact of the macroenvironment and further limits the availability of nutrients to the host. The factors operating at this level are meager purchasing power, faulty concepts of food utilization that lead to poor food consumption practices and inadequate distribution of available nutrients among the members of the family. The latter is particularly evident in the case of small children and when disease strikes a member of the family whose food intake is very often thereby drastically restricted.

Host and Agent

Maternal malnutrition and infectious episodes during pregnancy are frequently the cause of prematurity and small born-at-term infants, as well as of poor nursing performance. Children already at a nutritional disadvantage are the victims of poor feeding practices, especially in those regions where breast-feeding is being replaced early in life by artificial formulas in the face of prevailing inadequate education, hygiene and economic resources. All of these factors must be adequate to allow successful artificial feeding.

Inadequate feeding takes place at a time when nutritional requirements are high per unit of body weight. The consequence is an increasing number of infants who suffer from early protein-calorie malnutrition, particularly in urban areas. The most common type of severe malnutrition at this age is that of nonedematous PCM, due to a predominant caloric deficiency.[9]

Even when properly breast-fed, complementary feeding practices for the child are poor, and induce some degree of PCM after the first 3 or 4 months of life. When weaning occurs, most children are fed diets that provide insufficient amounts of calories and proteins. Others receive only starchy gruels or high-carbohydrate low-protein diluted cereal drinks, which accentuate protein deficiency. Table 24–3 presents the median nutrient intake of rural Central American children, expressed as per cent of the recommended allowances for each age group.

It is important to realize that, in the developing areas, children are smaller in size than those of the same age in the developed areas; consequently, their actual requirements are somewhat reduced. Nonetheless, a decreased food intake for age, even when it could be fairly satisfactory for size, perpetuates undernutrition. If, at this time, the child is forced-fed diets high in calories but low in protein, he becomes acutely protein-deficient in spite of being fat. This severe protein deficiency

Table 24–3. Median Nutrient Intake as Per Cent of Recommended Allowances of Nutrients Consumed by Preschool Children in the Rural Area of Guatemala*†

Nutrients	Age Groups (years)			
	1 (38)‡	2 (43)	3 (34)	4–5 (14)
Calories	63	66	80	48
Proteins	79	74	108	67
Calcium	72	69	101	72
Iron	56	71	103	66
Vitamin A¶	24	30	25	20
Thiamin	100	92	128	68
Riboflavin	50	46	50	31
Niacin	42	50	68	39
Vitamin C	40	60	56	20

* Over 90 per cent of preschool children consumed less calories and over 60 per cent consumed less protein than the recommended allowances. The calories and protein consumption was lower than recommended in 80 per cent and 40 per cent of the families, respectively.
† Modified from Flores, Menchú, Lara, and Guzmán: Arch. Latinoam. Nutr., 20, 41, 1970.
‡ Figures in parentheses represent the number of children.
¶ Vitamin A intake has improved, especially in the older preschoolers, since sugar fortification with this vitamin was begun in 1976.

gives rise to edematous PCM of the "sugar-baby" type.[10] More often, infants become the victims of mild-to-moderate repeated infections[11] and, by the time they are weaned, develop a common diarrhea syndrome known as "weanling diarrhea."[12]

After weaning, children eat little or no milk and other animal products and they are fed the usual family foods, frequently in insufficient amounts, because of poor availability of food and incorrect cultural practices in child feeding. Also, after weaning, children living in these environments frequently suffer from acute infections. As a consequence, their nutritional condition rapidly deteriorates. Those children who prior to weaning were growing at a slower rate and very often were somewhat underweight for their height become frankly undernourished. Those who follow this path develop the edematous type of PCM, but at the same time are somewhat emaciated. They suffer from a predominant protein deficiency, superimposed on various degrees of caloric deficit.

The majority of children, however, do not develop a severe degree of PCM and, through a series of adaptive mechanisms, remain in a state of mild-to-moderate protein-calorie malnutrition. This condition is characterized only by growth retardation and by periods wherein they have a mild weight-for-height deficit, with or without traces of edema. Children who survive the critical weaning and preschool periods continue to grow at a slower rate and their calorie and protein requirements per unit of body mass rapidly decrease. Their daily diets continue to be low in both calories and protein, but they usually can procure more food and often have already had most of the common childhood infectious diseases. Thus, these children can progress into adulthood without further serious risks of becoming severely undernourished. However, if a severe infection or diarrhea supervenes, they can still develop severe PCM, regardless of age. Among the common childhood infections, measles and whooping cough are well known to precipitate severe protein-calorie malnutrition. In children and adults, repeated acute diarrheal episodes, chronic malaria, schistosomiasis and massive infestations by hookworm, Trichiuris trichiura or Strongyloides, plus other stresses such as acute food shortage and severe physical or psychologic stresses, can induce severe PCM.

PHYSIOPATHOLOGY AND ADAPTIVE RESPONSES IN CALORIE AND IN PROTEIN DEFICIENCY

Through a series of physiologic mechanisms, the body tends to maintain a dynamic equilibrium. A typical example is the tendency toward caloric equilibrium: After the ingestion of a meal energy is stored, mostly in the form of high-energy phosphates, fat and glycogen, which are drawn upon to obtain energy during the daily regular and relatively short periods of fasting and during periods of increased energy expenditure.

With longer periods of calorie and/or protein restriction, the body progressively adapts itself in order to maintain as adequate a functional status as the limited supply of nutrients allows. Consequently, in the process leading to PCM, the body is dynamically adapting to it and continues to do so throughout, until the individual is "maximally adapted." This adaptation results in a decreased nutrient demand and in the attainment of nutritional equilibrium compatible with a lower level of cellular nutrient availability. If, at this point, the supply of nutrients becomes persistently lower than that to which the body can adapt, death supervenes. However, although in most instances the nutrient supply is low, it is not so inadequate as to cause death and the individual is thus able to live in a state adapted to the diminished intake. In this process, most functions are altered and have the following characteristics: (1) They are more susceptible to being overwhelmed by an overloading mechanism, which brings about decompensation or failure of adaptation and consequently poses a threat to the life of the host. In other words, the adapted PCM individual is a labile, functionally fragile subject. (2) Because of their dynamic nature, the degree of functional alteration generally correlates with the degree of protein depletion. This correlation is also influenced by the rate at which depletion occurs, or at which repletion takes place during nutritional rehabilitation.[13]

The adaptive metabolic processes in both calorie and protein malnutrition occur by hormonal interaction, by servomechanisms at the cellular level and by as yet poorly understood generalized body reactions. Briefly, calorie deficit induces the hormonal adaptations described in

Table 24–4. Schematic Hormonal Adaptive Mechanisms in Malnutrition

			Hormonal Activities in	
Hormone	Stimulus	Result	Calorie Deprivation	Protein-calorie Deprivation
Insulin	↑ Glucose ↑ amino acids	↑ Protein synthesis (muscle) ↑ Growth ↑ Lipogenesis	Decreased	Decreased
Growth hormone	↓ Glucose ↑ amino acids	↑ Protein synthesis (body) ↑ Growth ↑ Lipolysis ↓ Urea synthesis	Variable, generally normal	Increased

Glucocorticoids	↓ Glucose
	↓ amino acids
		↑ Protein catab-
		   olism (muscle)
		↑ Protein turnover
		   (viscera)
		↑ Neoglucogenesis
		↑ Lipolysis
			Increased	Variable, generally normal

Thyroid hormones	↑ Energy
	  metabolism
		Energy homeo-
		   stasis
		↑ Protein turnover
			Decreased	Decreased

Table 24–4, which lead to increased fat mobilization from adipose tissue.

During the initial phases of deficiency, the individual shows decreased physical activity and a lower basal energy expenditure per unit of lean body mass. The body composition is progressively altered by decreasing adiposity at a fast rate and lean body mass at a slower rate. Muscle catabolism produces an increased efflux of amino acids, primarily as alanine. As the caloric deficit becomes severe, basal energy expenditure may be normal or even increased per unit of lean body mass, which then decreases at a faster rate.[13–15]

Protein deficit usually occurs together with caloric inadequacy and the hormonal changes are generally similar to those observed in caloric deprivation; often, fasting circulating growth hormone levels are higher in protein deprivation than in caloric deficit[16,17] and glucocorticoids are not increased in the former, although free cortisol is higher than normal, resulting in functional hypercorticism[18] (Table 24–4). Somatomedin levels are low in PCM, espe-

cially in cases with severe protein deficiency.[19] In protein deficit there are also cellular adaptation mechanisms not directly hormonally mediated but induced by the poor availability of amino acids, causing decreased protein synthesis at the ribosomal level. The result of both mechanisms of adaptation are an internal shift in protein metabolism to an increase in muscle protein catabolism and, therefore, a relative increase in amino acid availability at the visceral level. The composition of the free amino acid pool is altered. There is a decrease in both the synthesis and the catabolism of total body proteins, the latter predominating over the former.

The most significant change in protein metabolism is a marked recycling of amino acids. The end-result is a longer half-life of some proteins, such as albumin, and a generally decreased protein and amino acid turnover. In addition, the internal body distribution of protein changes. This is the case with albumin, which diminishes more in the extravascular than in the intravascular space. Urea synthesis decreases and simple nitrogen-containing compounds, such as urea, apparently are more efficiently utilized as sources of nitrogen. In terms of body composition, a progressive reduction in lean body mass occurs, resulting primarily from muscle, and probably also from skin, protein loss. Visceral protein is initially reduced ("labile protein") but then becomes stable or may even regain some of its total mass. As the body protein turnover and total body protein mass decrease, basal oxygen consumption also decreases.[13,20,21]

These adaptations, which lead to the sparing of body protein, are easily upset by forced calorie intake, primarily in the form of carbohydrates such as starch gruels. Hormonal adaptation mechanisms are "fooled" and, as a consequence, internal amino acid and protein shifts are impaired, thus inducing visceral amino acid depletion and a breakdown of adaptation. Infections leading to disease and other stresses also upset adaptation by causing anorexia and markedly reduced food intake in the face of increased energy and protein needs. Fever increases energy waste and is accompanied by large nitrogen losses and shifts toward amino acid utilization for energy purposes. Amino acid utilization is also diverted for increased synthesis of special proteins, such as gamma globulins (antibodies).[22,23] This probably also reflects a breakdown of the amino acid-sparing adaptive mechanisms described.

An important finding in most investigations of the hormonal status in PCM is that hypophyseal functional capacity is unimpaired. Another important concept must be kept in mind in explaining metabolic adaptations: Hormonal effects may not be wholly explained by circulating levels of hormones and metabolites. Cellular responses to hormonal stimulation, as well as hormonal metabolism, may be markedly altered in PCM.

When the adaptive mechanisms are maintained, the impact of PCM is diminished and the length of time that an individual takes to go from mild to severe protein-calorie malnutrition is prolonged. Of course, the individual has to sacrifice certain functions and some nutrient reserves and, for this reason, becomes more susceptible to injuries which a well-nourished individual can withstand with little repercussion. Total body K content is reduced.[24-26] Total circulating hemoglobin is reduced pari passu with decreased body oxygen demands. Red cell production is diminished and hemodilution takes place.[13,14,27] Cardiac work decreases, as does functional reserve,[28] and central circulation takes precedence over peripheral circulation. Cardiovascular reflexes are altered, leading to postural hypotension and diminished venous return. Hemodynamic compensation in severe PCM occurs primarily from tachycardia rather than from increased stroke volume. The renal plasma flow, glomerular filtration rate and tubular function decrease. As a consequence, in severe cases, the renal concentrating ability and acidification mechanisms are impaired.[29] Before this occurs, chronic sodium retention and increased serum and urine antidiuretic activities lead to relatively increased total and extracellular body water.[30] Intracellular water is reduced in absolute terms because of losses in lean body mass, but intracellular overhydration may be present.[24,26,31] Physical strength is diminished, further inducing a reduction in the physical working capacity.[32,33]

Other alterations not directly correlated with the degree of protein deficit, but always present in advanced protein deficiency, include impaired intestinal absorption, moderately decreased capacity to transport protein-bound substances in blood, reduced gonadal function and lowered resistance to infection. The immune systems affected in severe PCM include those mediated by cells: antibodies, phagocytes, complement and other nonspecific factors including lysozyme.[34] Moderate

PCM and fetal malnutrition, as well as other specific nutrient deficiencies, appear to have profound effects on cell-mediated immunity.

Impaired intestinal absorption of lipids and disaccharides and a decreased rate of glucose absorption occur in severe protein deficiency; the greater the protein deficit, the greater the functional impairment. A decrease in gastric, pancreatic and bile production is also observed, with normal to low enzyme and conjugated bile acid concentrations. These alterations further impair the absorptive functions. Protein-deficient individuals are diarrhea-prone because of these alterations and possibly also because of irregular intestinal motility and gastrointestinal bacterial overgrowth. Diarrhea per se aggravates the malabsorption.[35-40]

Finally, a generalized decrease in nervous system function is clearly apparent in severe PCM.[41,42] The etiology of these alterations has not been elucidated. Several explanations have been proposed, among others decreased brain potassium content and catecholamine production, reduced number of cells in the central nervous system when malnutrition occurs before 6 to 8 months of age and small cell size when it occurs at a later age.[43-45]

Decompensation from severe calorie deficiency occurs from inability to maintain internal energy supply and results in hypoglycemia, hypothermia, impaired circulatory and renal functions, acidosis, coma and death. In the case of decompensation from protein deficiency, visceral functional failure also results from unavailability of amino acids. At the same time, an accelerated tissue breakdown takes place. The resulting alterations are failure of the liver to synthesize certain proteins such as albumin, several clotting factors and transport proteins, leading to fatty liver, increased free circulating cortisol, hemorrhagic diathesis, and jaundice in extreme cases; various degrees of renal failure with acidosis, as well as water and sodium retention, frankly decreased cardiac work and tissue anoxia with pulmonary congestion occur. All of these factors lead to the development of clinical edema and, in extreme cases, skin lesions with hemorrhagic phenomena. In addition, fluid leakage into the gastrointestinal tract,

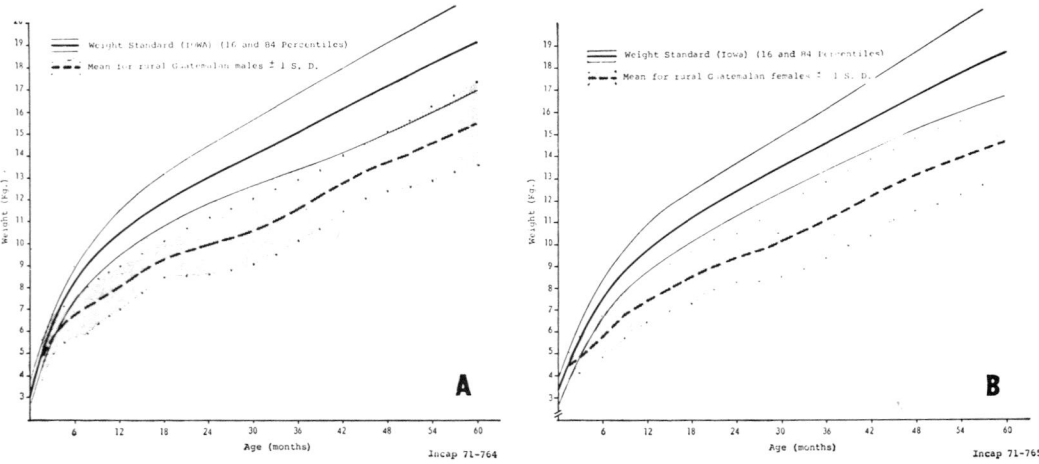

Fig. 24–1. Weight of rural Guatemalan male and female children below 5 years of age, in relation to that of U.S.A. children. Number of Guatemalan children in the sample: 431 males and 436 females. (From INCAP.[3])

increased susceptibility to pulmonary infections, water and electrolyte disturbances with hypokalemia and hypomagnesemia, frank central nervous system depression and death can result.[46–48]

DIAGNOSTIC CHARACTERISTICS OF PROTEIN-CALORIE MALNUTRITION

The clinical and biochemical picture of PCM varies according to its severity and to the characteristics of the host, the environment and the agent.

Chronic Mild-to-moderate PCM[49]

Clinical. It is obvious that the severe syndromes of edematous and nonedematous PCM, recognized as kwashiorkor and marasmus, respectively, represent the critical end of a spectrum of varying degrees of deficiency.

However, before these severe stages are reached, children survive with insufficient calories, protein or both, a situation which does not allow them to grow and develop at the rate to be expected from their genetic potential. A long-standing restriction would be clearly manifested by a retardation in height and weight gain (Figs. 24–1 and 24–2). This reduced size may be a life-saving device to allow the children to survive on the restricted food available to them.

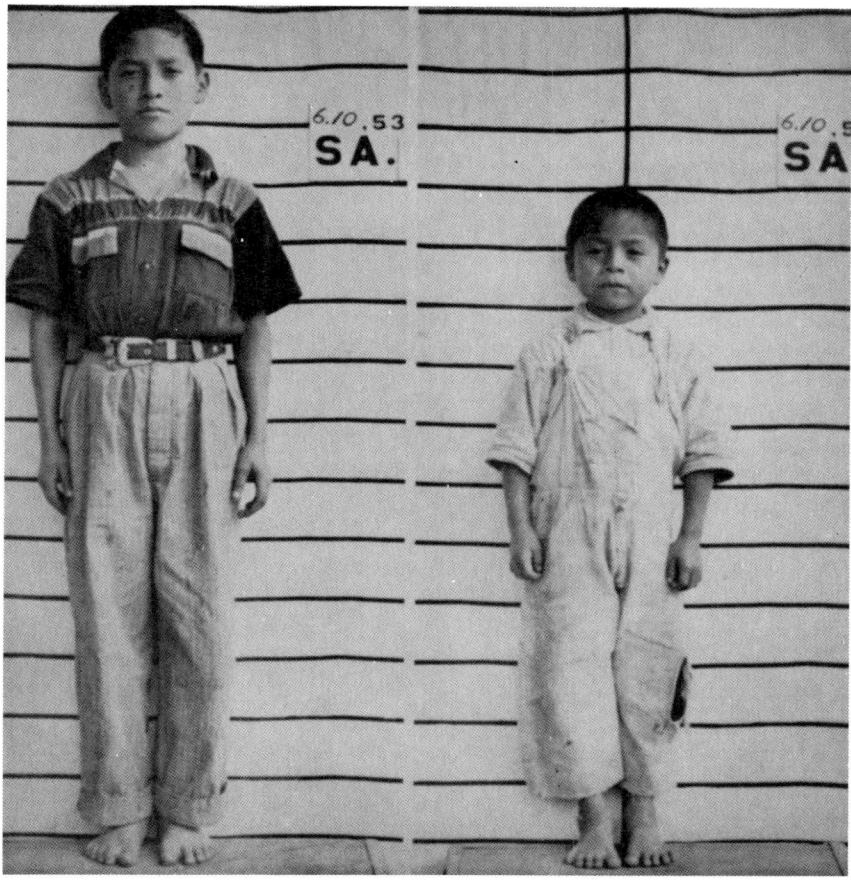

Fig. 24–2. Appearance of two 10-year-old children in the rural Central American region. The one at the left has always been well nourished. The one at the right has been mild-to-moderately malnourished.

Under these chronic conditions, it is generally observed that body mass, although markedly retarded for the chronologic age of the child, is adequate for its height. However, these children may be chronically affected by temporary periods of weight-for-height deficits. As judged by body composition studies, bone maturation and biochemical measurements, the malnourished child is not a small version of his well-nourished counterpart of equivalent chronologic age. He shows an immaturity in biologic development compatible with his retarded physical size. This includes deficits in lean body mass and adiposity, with relative overhydration affecting primarily the extracellular space. Without knowing the actual age of the subject, it is often difficult or even impossible to determine the presence or extent of malnutrition.

Other characteristics of such cases, which are more difficult to attribute exclusively to nutrition, are reduced physical activity, mental apathy, frequent episodes of ill-defined sickness, anorexia and diarrhea and a higher fatality rate from common infectious diseases.

It has been shown that an association exists between retarded physical growth and development and some tests of psychomotor and mental development.[50-52] The isolated effect of malnutrition as a cause of this phenomenon is strongly suggested by data derived from animal experimental work. Direct proof does not exist in humans, although studies are now under way from which an answer to this question is expected. Nevertheless, it is beyond doubt that the responsible factor is the complex of social deprivation, of which nutrition is one of the most important components.[53]

Chronic PCM in adults generally results in marked leanness (Fig. 24–3), which, in severe cases, can reach a state resembling cachexia. Because their protein requirements per unit of body mass are much smaller than those of children, the main

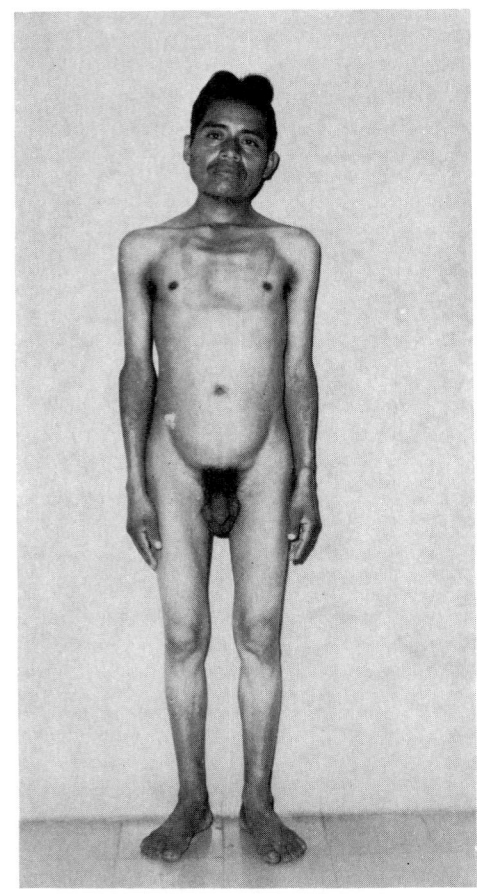

Fig. 24–3. Mild-to-moderate malnourished 36-year-old man.

manifestations are of primary calorie deficiency. Thus, physical activity and capacity for prolonged physical work are reduced, perhaps as a mechanism to maintain caloric equilibrium on low food intake. Changes in body composition similar to those described for children can also be observed.[32,33]

Biochemical. Because of the characteristically low protein intake, subjects have a low excretion of urea N per unit of creatinine[54] and a somewhat abnormal plasma free amino acid pattern with a decrease of the branched essential amino acids.[55,56] It has been reported also that they excrete a lower amount of hydroxy-proline in the urine, in good agreement with the slow growth rate.[57] Slight decreases in transferrin and albumin serum levels have been reported.[58,59] If lean body mass is reduced for height, this is manifested by a decreased creatinine/height index.[60]

Severe Protein-calorie Malnutrition

Clinical. *Nonedematous PCM.* Severe calorie deficiency is clinically recognized in children by the syndrome identified as marasmus in most parts of the world, or nonedematous severe PCM (Fig. 24–4). The child is frankly small for his age, looks emaciated and, in extreme conditions, reduced to "skin and bones" because of an essentially total absence of adipose tissue. His skin is usually dry and "baggy," wrinkles easily and has lost its turgor. The hair is sparse, thin and dry, and can be pulled

out easily; it loses its normal sheen and acquires a dull brown or reddish yellow color, giving it a lifeless appearance. The face resembles that of a monkey, with sunken cheeks in extreme cases, because of the disappearance of the Bichat fat-pad. The child is weak and looks hypotonic, and his pulse, blood pressure and temperature may be low. He is sensitive to cold temperature, cries easily and is often found retracted from his environment, sucking one or more fingers. His viscera are small and lymph nodes are easily felt. Soon after therapy is initiated the child becomes alert and interested in his environment. In adults, extreme emaciation is characteristic of calorie deficit (Fig. 24–5).

Common complicating features are eye lesions, due to hypovitaminosis A, and skin infections. The classical cases suffer from constipation and are ravenously hungry, but diarrhea, anorexia and vomiting, with

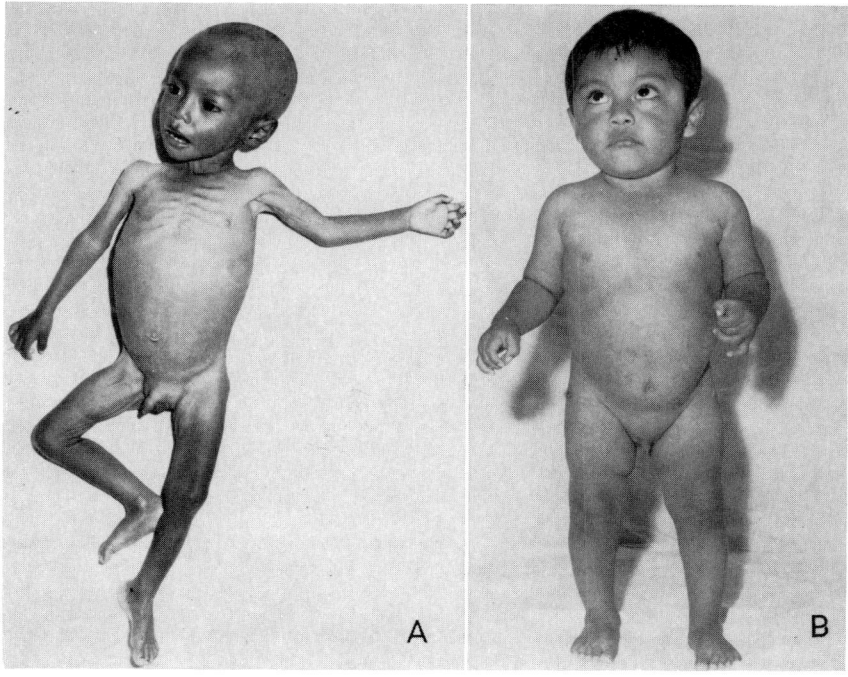

Fig. 24–4. Twenty-one-month-old child with severe nonedematous PCM (marasmus) on admission to the hospital and 4 months later, when fully recovered.

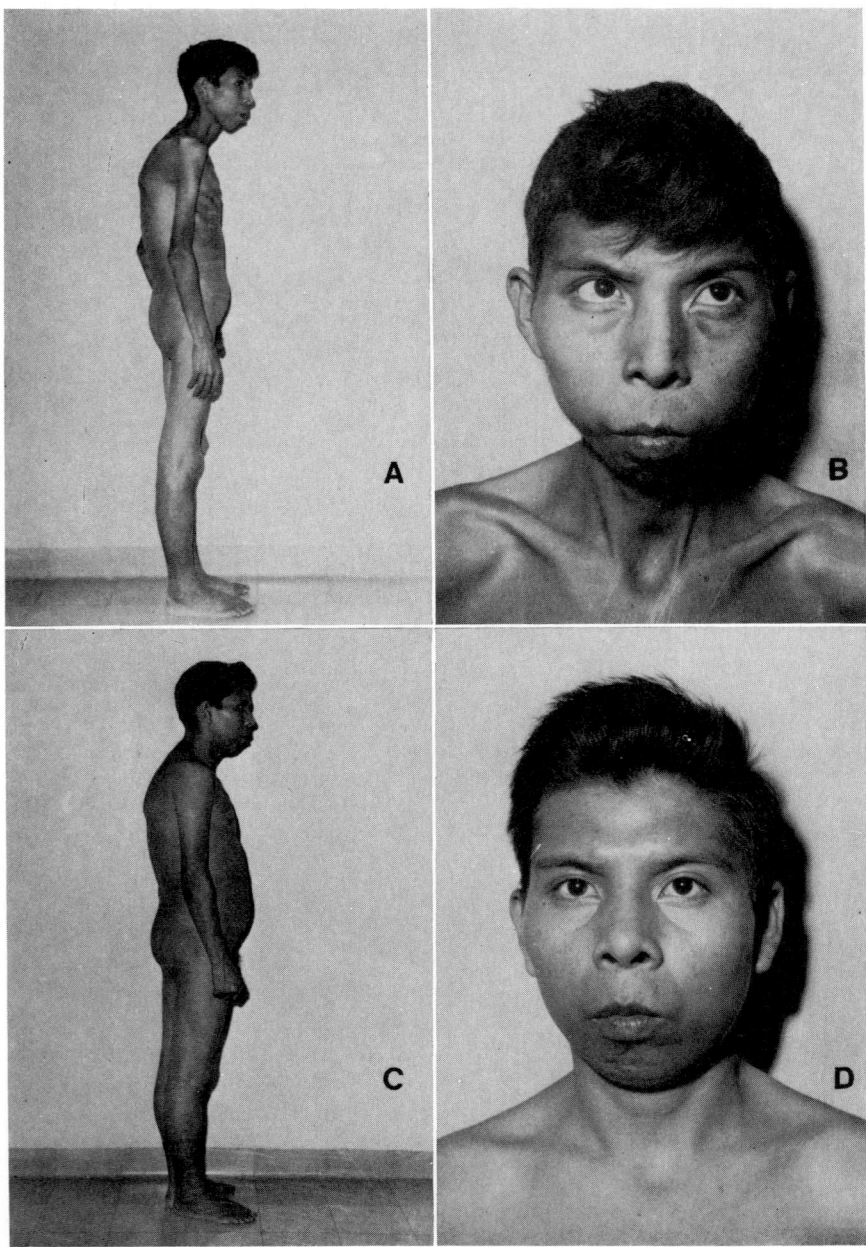

Fig. 24–5. Twenty-nine-year-old man with severe nonedematous PCM on admission to the hospital and 3 months later, when fully recovered.

dehydration, are not rare; dehydration, acidosis and electrolyte imbalances may, in fact, cause death. Postmortem examination shows only generalized atrophy, without fatty liver. Clinically and post mortem, the child has no edema, although his total body water is increased for his size.[15,24]

Edematous PCM. The child with acute severe protein deficiency of the sugar-baby type (Fig. 24–6) is usually almost normal in height for age; his body fat is normal or increased, but flabby, and he is clinically edematous. The edema may be located only in the lower segments of the body, through the action of gravity, but generally his face is swollen, his cheeks look heavy and his eyelids are swollen shut. He is pale and the skin shines in the edematous areas. In other parts of his body the skin may be dry and atrophic or have large asymmetric confluent areas of hyperpigmentation and

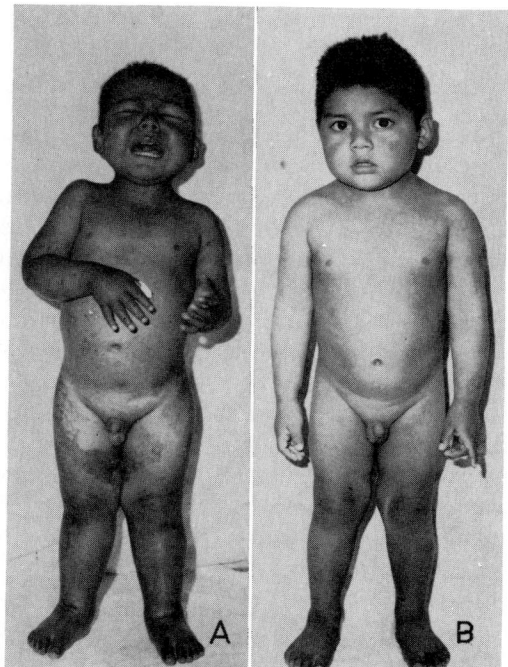

Fig. 24–6. Thirty-six-month-old child with severe edematous PCM and preservations of adiposity (kwashiorkor) on admission to the hospital and 4 months later, when fully recovered.

hyperkeratosis. A peeling type of desquamation occurs in these areas, leaving underneath a fine, atrophic pinkish skin. Hair is atrophic, dry, depigmented and has a reddish tint, falls off easily and breaks upon rolling between the fingers. Often, zones of alopecia are noted. The nails are brittle and have horizontal grooves. The general appearance is that of a hypotonic, miserable-looking child. He is apathetic and irritable at the same time. In the severest cases his apathy is profound. Anorexia is almost universal. Hepatomegaly is frequent, as are a swollen stomach and intestinal loops. Diarrhea is almost always present. Frequent complications are eye lesions due to vitamin A deficiency, cheilitis and cheilosis, as well as other manifestations of deficiencies of the vitamin B complex. Upper respiratory infections and dehydration, even in the presence of edema, are common and often lead to death. Intestinal motility is irregular, and these children often become dehydrated before they pass a huge liquid stool. As the child begins to recover he loses his edema and remains fat and flabby. This appearance often misleads the clinician who may consider him recovered because his weight may be normal. In fact, he is still severely protein deficient in terms of lean body mass.

Pulmonary edema with bronchopneumonia, septicemia, gastroenteritis and water and electrolyte imbalances are the most common causes of death. At autopsy, generalized edema, visceral and muscle atrophy and severe fatty liver are found. Red bone marrow is centripetally retracted.

Most cases of severe malnutrition, both in children and adults, fall between these two extremes of pure caloric and pure protein deficiency. In these cases, a moderate-to-severe protein deficit may be superimposed on a severe degree of calorie deficiency, and vice versa (Fig. 24–7). These subjects, suffering from severe PCM with edema, together with pure

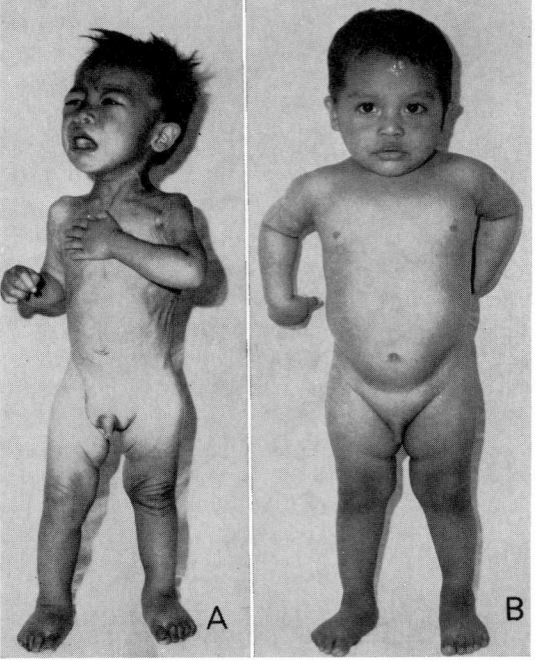

Fig. 24-7. Twenty-five-month-old child with severe edematous PCM superimposed on chronic caloric deficit. In addition to being edematous, he appears wasted (marasmus-kwashiorkor). Pictures were taken on admission to the hospital and 4 months later, when fully recovered.

protein deficiency, have been identified with kwashiorkor. Clinical edema constitutes the main characteristic for diagnosis. The mixed PCM cases have also been identified with a variety of terms, among which are pluricarential syndrome in Central America, undernutrition in other Latin American regions, and protein malnutrition in certain African and Asian countries.[1,48,49] In adults, a predominant protein deficiency can also lead to edematous PCM (Fig. 24-8).

Biochemical. In severe protein-calorie malnutrition several biochemical alterations can be observed. Many of these distinguish between the *edematous* and the *nonedematous* types.

Proteins and Nitrogenous Compounds.
The child who has reached the severe stage

of edematous PCM has been submitted to a severe negative protein balance.[61,62] Consequently, his total body nitrogen is markedly reduced. Different organs share this protein loss to different extents.[63-65] The liver rapidly loses a fraction of proteins, while the loss of muscle protein is progressive and, because of the large muscle mass, accounts for the major protein loss. Kidney, brain and endocrine organs seem to retain their protein more efficiently. However, the importance of these different losses in terms of organ function cannot be derived from their relative magnitudes. A low ratio of protein to DNA is found in muscle, liver and brain, indicative of intracellular protein loss.[44,66] In nonedematous PCM these changes are moderate, becoming severe only in the most advanced stages.

The concentration of several protein fractions in the body fluids is low. (Although present in both types of PCM, edematous and nonedematous, the changes to be described are more pronounced in the first type. In the second, they may be totally absent.) The concentration of total proteins is reduced, mainly due to a decreased albumin concentration. The concentration of beta-globulins is also decreased. The gamma-globulin fraction concentration is either normal or increased; therefore, the per cent contribution to the total plasma proteins is always high.[48] Some plasma proteins with very specific functions may also be decreased. Among them, those associated with the transport of other nutrients and hormones are particularly important: transferrin,[58,67] ceruloplasmin,[67] retinol-binding protein (RBP),[68] alpha- and beta-lipoproteins,[69] thyroxin,[70,71] and cortisol-[72,73] and aldosterone-binding proteins.[74] Impaired blood transport may attain significance in the development of secondary metabolic abnormalities, as has been shown in the case of lipids and vitamin A.[75] The blood concentration of urea nitrogen is low, as is its excretion in the urine. This reflects the

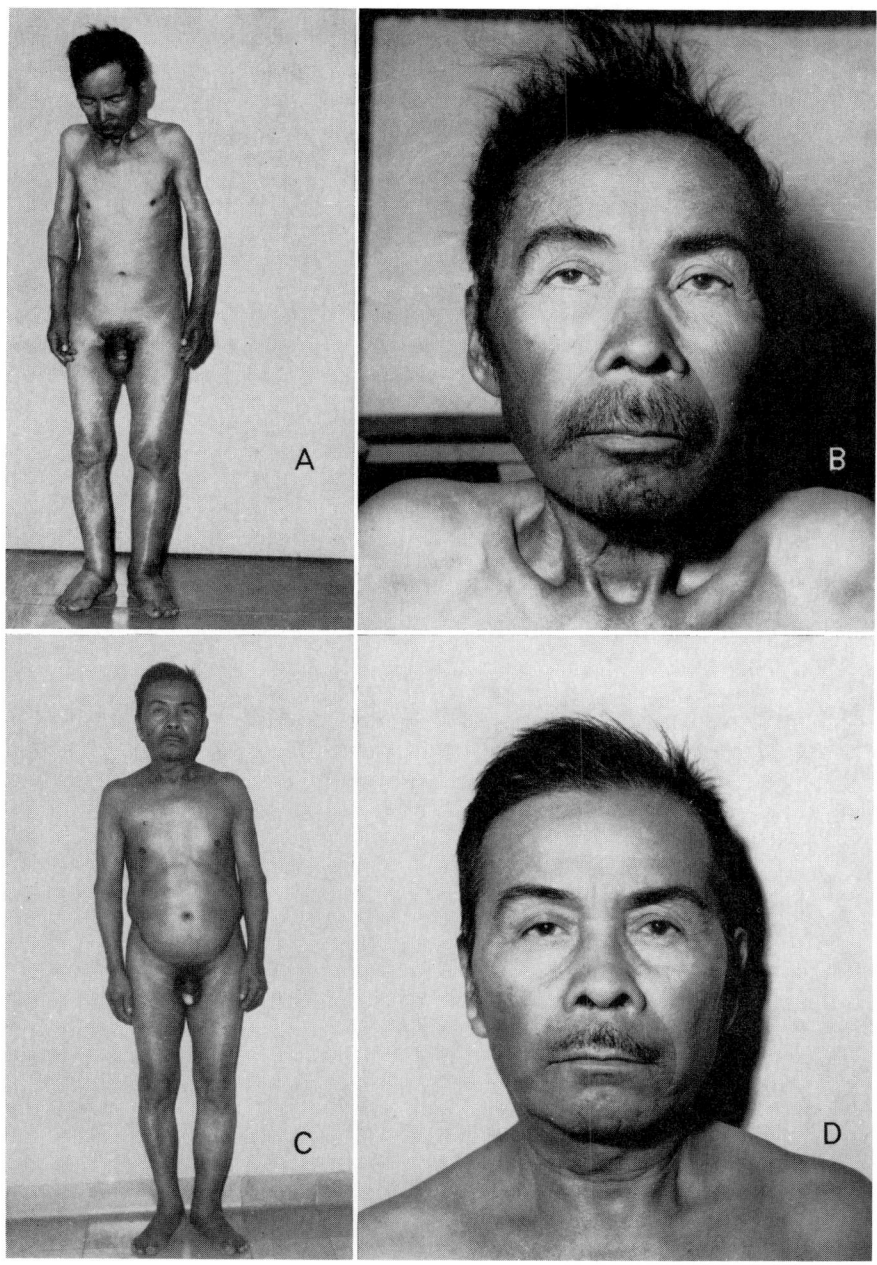

Fig. 24–8. Forty-six-year-old man with severe edematous PCM on admission to the hospital and 3 months later, when fully recovered.

low catabolic rate of body proteins and decreased urea synthesis, which are characteristic of primary protein deficiency.[20,76,77] When calories are the most limiting factor, urea production is increased because body protein catabolism is elevated.[78]

The excretion of urinary creatinine is decreased,[79,80] a consequence of the decrease in muscle tissue and lean body mass.[81,82]

The plasma free-amino acid pattern is abnormal in edematous PCM. A lowered concentration of valine, leucine, and isoleucine is characteristic, as is also a very low tyrosine concentration.[83,84] The ratio of the branched essential to nonessential amino acids is low. Another finding, which is very characteristic, is a low tyrosine/phenylalanine ratio, as a result of a deficiency in phenylalanine hydroxylase.[85] In nonedematous PCM, plasma amino acid alterations may be absent.[55]

Hemoglobin concentration is variable, but often it is around 8 to 10 gm per 100 ml because of hemodilution. Generally, the cells are normochromic and normocytic. Hypochromia can be present if a severe iron deficiency exists from other causes. Mild to overt megaloblastosis can occur because of folate deficiency.[86] The great majority of subjects are not anemic but physiologically adapted to the decreased oxygen demands.[14,27] Leukocytosis can occur if infection is present. Leukopenia and thrombocytopenia generally indicate the presence of gram-negative septicemia.

Although it has been observed that urinary amino acid excretion is abnormal, no consistent pattern seems to be evident. The abnormal metabolites ethanolamine and beta-aminoisobutyric acid have been detected, suggesting a defect in transmethylation.[87] Excretion of urocanic acid has been shown to be abnormal after a histidine load.[88]

Carbohydrates. Usually blood glucose is normal. However, there is an increased tendency to hypoglycemia upon fasting. This is compatible with the finding that liver and muscle glycogen stores are normal or low.[89] Some alterations revealed by clinical laboratory studies suggest abnormal metabolic handling of glucose. Glucose tolerance tests give a diabetic type of curve, and insulin secretion is low.[90,91] Impaired glucose utilization, glycogenolysis and glycolysis have also been demonstrated. In addition, there are isolated pieces of evidence of impaired enzymatic steps along the glucose oxidation, the Krebs cycle and the galactose-to-glucose conversion paths.[89,92,93]

Lipids. Steatorrhea is a characteristic of edematous PCM, even when the diet is practically devoid of fat.[94] Lipid absorption is reduced.[95] Low levels of many serum lipid fractions, neutral fat, cholesterol, particularly its esters, vitamins A and E and phospholipids have been demonstrated. These findings suggest that the changes in specific plasma proteins and physical chemical structure of the lipid-protein complexes account for impaired blood transport.[75,96,97] In fact, there is direct evidence for decreased lipoproteins as well as for decreased RBP, the specific vitamin A-binding protein.[68] A great part of the fatty liver may well be the consequence of inability to mobilize fat.[97]

Vitamins.[98] Signs of water-soluble vitamin deficiencies vary with the local dietary patterns, but, even when intakes are low, serum concentrations of thiamin, riboflavin, vitamin C, niacin metabolites and folates may well be within the normal range, and overt clinical signs of deficiency of these factors are rarely seen. Vitamin B_{12} serum levels are often found to be high. All of the above findings suggest that, although the supply of these vitamins may be low, tissue demands are also decreased.

In the edematous type of PCM (kwashiorkor), serum levels of vitamins A and E are consistently lower than normal. In the case of vitamin A, poor vitamin intake and defective absorption and transport explain these alterations. This explanation may well apply also to vitamin E. All levels rise rapidly with therapy.

Water and Electrolytes.[47,99-101] Hypo-osmolarity is a common finding. Serum sodium levels are from normal to low. Potassium and magnesium serum levels are not decreased, except when excessive losses of the cations occur through diarrhea and vomiting. In such cases, hypokalemia is accompanied by a loss of potassium from specific tissues such as muscle and brain.[26,102] This results in a decreased cellular potassium/nitrogen ratio. Mild acidosis is also common, on account of a decrease in the renal acidification mechanisms. Total serum calcium is somewhat low, primarily because of the protein-bound fraction.

Enzymes. The activity of several serum enzymes such as amylase, pseudocholinesterase and alkaline phosphatase is reduced. Their drop is consistent with and quite parallel to that of albumin, so that they may be normal in nonedematous PCM.[48,103] Serum transaminases are elevated and reflect increased tissue transaminase activity and leakage from the cells.[104] Around 15 hepatic enzymes have been studied,[105,106] including dehydrogenases, oxidases and esterases. Of these, 4 are clearly decreased in the edematous type of PCM—xanthine oxidase, glycolic acid oxidase, d-amino acid oxidase and cholinesterase. It has been pointed out that these enzymes are not involved in fundamental physiologic functions and seem to be of relatively little importance. On the other hand, cytochrome c reductase, a key enzyme in electron transport, is well preserved.

More complex systems, which depend on the integrity of the mitochondria, have been studied. Oxidative phosphorylation is somewhat reduced, and phosphate uptake into phosphatides is about half the value seen in recovered children.[61]

Enzymatic changes in liver and PMN leukocytes have been studied comparatively.[107] It has been found that not only

are changes in both tissues similar but that they are characteristically different in the edematous and nonedematous types. In summary, these changes are: increased activity of fumarase and aconitase, decreased activity of isocitric dehydrogenase, glutamic dehydrogenase and aldolase in the edematous malnourished child with the reverse being true of the nonedematous patients. Muscle creatine phosphokinase activity has been found to be consistently low in children with the edematous type, while in those suffering from the marasmic type low or normal values can be observed.[108]

It is impossible to separate the effects of protein deficiency per se on enzymes from changes in activity, which may reflect changes in functional pattern in response to adaptation. In general, the latter interpretation seems more plausible. Measurements done in vitro with reconstructed systems tell nothing about subcellular structure changes, which may alter linking of enzymes with their substrates and cofactors. These could well involve alterations in membrane structure at the cellular and subcellular level.

TREATMENT

Chronic Mild-to-moderate Protein-calorie Malnutrition in Children

Because the children are not only physically retarded but also proportionally immature, their protein and calorie intake should be calculated on the basis of their height, that is, as if the child were well-fed but younger, of an age for which his height would correspond to the 50th percentile. This means a higher calorie and protein intake per kg of body weight than that of children of the same chronologic age. These intakes, therefore, will promote a retention of energy and protein to permit catch-up in growth and development. Of course, they should contain the appropriate concentrations of all the other essential nutrients. When marked deficiencies of other nutrients are also prevalent, administration of specific supplements is called for.

Severe Protein-calorie Malnutrition

The severe, uncompensated forms of PCM require medical guidance during the initial phases of treatment.[109,110] Whenever possible, children with noncomplicated PCM should be treated on an outpatient basis,[111,112] Hospitalization in pediatric wards increases the risk of cross-infections. The presence of the mother or another close relative in the hospital is highly desirable.

Mortality in severe, uncompensated PCM is high even with hospitalization, ranging from 11 to 50 per cent depending on the center where treated and on certain characteristics of the patients, such as those listed on Table 24–5. In most cases the cause of death is a complication rather than PCM per se, but such complications do not have such high mortality in well-nourished patients.

Table 24–5. Characteristics of Severely Protein-calorie Malnourished Children which Carry a Poor Prognosis

Stupor or coma.
Age less than 6 months.
Weight-for-height deficit greater than 40 per cent.
Severe, protracted diarrhea.
Infection, primarily bronchopneumonia or measles.
Hemorrhagic tendency. Purpura is usually associated
   with septicemia.
Severe eye lesions.
Extensive exudative or exfoliative dermal lesions.
Extensive and deep decubitus ulcers.
Dehydration and electrolyte disturbances, particularly
   hyponatremia, hypokalemia and probably hypo-
   magnesemia.
Clinical jaundice or increased serum bilirubin and/or
   frankly elevated serum glutamic-oxaloacetic and
   glutamic-pyruvic transaminases.
Hypoglycemia and/or hypothermia.
Total serum proteins below 3 gm per 100 ml.
Severe anemia with clinical signs of hypoxia.
Severe tachycardia, signs of heart failure and/or re-
   spiratory distress.

The treatment of severe PCM may be divided into two phases:

1. That oriented toward saving the patient's life by bringing him back to his adapted stage.
2. The rehabilitation or "consolidation of cure" phase. At this stage, body protein and energy repletion for the patient's height should be achieved.

The main objectives of the initial treatment are: therapy of infection and correction of water and electrolyte imbalances as well as of other factors which lead to decompensation.

Maintenance of adequate urinary output is of primary importance. Preferably this is accomplished by oral therapy, keeping in mind the fact that the severely PCM individual is hypo-osmolar.[99] In addition to hypo-osmolarity, other peculiarities of the severely malnourished patient that must be taken into account to correct and/or maintain his electrolyte balance are: (1) total body potassium depletion, frequently without hypokalemia, because of intracellular potassium depletion, (2) mild-to-moderate metabolic acidosis, which tends to disappear when electrolyte balance is reestablished and the patient receives dietary or parenteral energy and (3) increased tolerance to hypocalcemia, partly because of the acidosis, which produces a relative increment in ionized Ca^{++}, and partly because of hypoproteinemia (when present), which makes less protein available to bind Ca^{++}.

As plasma proteins increase, hypocalcemia and even tetany may appear if calcium intake is inadequate.

If there is adequate diuresis, the diet should also provide from 6 to 8 mEq per kg body weight per day of K. If needed, the potassium concentration can be increased to supply 10 mEq per kg per day body weight to replace actual K losses from diarrhea or vomiting, which are usually 40 mEq per liter. Sodium intake should be sufficient to replace losses (about 35 mEq/L from diarrhea and 12 mEq/L from emesis), but otherwise it should be relatively low (3 to 5 mEq per kg per day) because PCM patients have an excess of body sodium. Diets very low in sodium, however, hamper both renal function and normalization of intracellular electrolyte composition.[113] An excess of sodium and osmolar overloads can easily induce cardiac failure. Magnesium should also be administered, particularly when diarrhea and vomiting occur. Usually 1 ml of Mg $SO_4 \cdot 7H_2O$, 50 per cent solution IM every 12 to 24 hours, is adequate. This therapy is important if tetany, oculogyric crises, tremor and bizarre neurologic signs occur in the initial phases of realimentation. In patients with tetany, calcium gluconate should also be administered intravenously, 0.5 to 1 gm slowly in 1 hour. Unless severe, acidosis should not be treated. Usually, renal function will handle acid-base balance efficiently.

If needed, intravenous therapy can and should be used, following the general outline described for oral rehydration, except that K therapy should not exceed 6 mEq per kg per day. Osmolarity should be kept at around 280 mOs per liter, and sodium must be kept low. Administration of plasma or other "protein-rich" fluids is contraindicated, except when severe intravascular dehydration (hypovolemia) with shock is present. Shock due to severe dehydration or gram-negative septicemia should be treated as if the individual were not malnourished. In some of these cases blood transfusions are indicated, but hemoglobin concentrations should be brought only to 10 gm per 100 ml or less, which are commonly the hemoglobin levels these children achieve from adaptation. Transfusions of packed red cells are indicated only when severe anemia is present and cardiorespiratory failure is imminent. Again, hemoglobin concentrations should be brought only to about 10 gm per 100 ml.

Infection should be treated vigorously and, if possible, with the help of a laboratory, so that the infective organisms can be isolated and their sensitivity to antibacterial agents determined. When there is a choice, the use of antibiotics that inhibit protein synthesis should be avoided.

A free airway with adequate lung ventilation is essential. When pneumonia is present, oxygen therapy and even tracheostomy may have to be undertaken, because it often happens that these patients are weak and cannot clear their airways satisfactorily.

When severe hepatic failure occurs it should be treated accordingly, as is done when cardiac failure supervenes. Diarrhea is treated mainly by diet. No anticholinergic drugs are used. Another general rule is to protect the PCM patient from exposure to cold and hypothermia, and from hypoglycemia. Hypoglycemia is prevented by avoiding prolonged periods of fasting. If a patient cannot be fed by mouth, intravenous infusions should provide 20 to 30 kcal per kg per day body weight as glucose.

During this initial phase of therapy a diet based on high-quality protein, such as milk-casein mixtures (to reduce lactose loads), casein alone, egg or fish protein, is recommended. During this phase a cautious handling of the nutrition aspect is essential. This demands patience, and personnel must be conscious of the fact that the most common causes of death are the complications and not malnutrition per se. Drastic therapeutic nutritional measures, such as high protein or calorie load from the start, may precipitate death by posing an "iatrogenic" overload on enzymatic and various physiologic functions which had reached maximal adaptation in several weeks or even months in the process of progressive malnutrition. This cautious dietary approach should provide initially, in children, around 1 gm protein and 80 to 100 kcal per kg per day: 20 per cent of the calories should be derived from fat. After 2 to 4 days, the protein and energy contents of the diet should increase gradually, as shown in Table 24–6, until they provide

Table 24–6.   Example of a Dietary Therapeutic Regimen for Children Based on Dry Skim Milk, Sugar and Vegetable Oil*

Days from Beginning of Treatment	Protein (gm)	Energy (kcal)	Milk (gm)	Sugar (gm)	Oil (ml)	Water (ml)
1	0.8–1	80–100	3	17	2	100
3	1.5–2.5	110–120	6	20	2	130
5	2.5–3.5	140–150	9	20	4	150
7	3.5–4.5	150–160	12	20	4	160
12 (marasmus‡)		175‡			6‡	
17		195			8	
22		215			11	
	3.5–4.5	‡	12	20	‡	160

* All amounts per kg body weight per day. The liquid formula must be supplemented with adequate levels of vitamins, minerals and electrolytes.

‡ Marasmic patients may require more than 150 to 160 kcal per kg per day. Vegetable oil 2 to 3 ml per kg per day at 5-day intervals should be added until the rate of weight gain becomes adequate.

3 to 4 gm protein and 120 to 160 kcal per kg per day. Twenty to 40 per cent of the energy then should come from fat, preferably of vegetable origin with a high content of polyunsaturated fatty acids (e.g. corn or cottonseed oils). Marasmic patients may need a higher energy intake to recover. In these cases, 20 to 25 kcal per kg per day should be added to the diet as vegetable oil at 5-day intervals, until weight gain becomes adequate. In a few instances this may require 200 or more kcal per kg per day and, even though a mild steatorrhea may develop, this regimen should be maintained. The example shown in Table 24–6 is based on a liquid diet. Children who can eat solids should receive a varied diet, aiming at the same levels of protein and energy intakes.

In the adult, the therapeutic scheme is the same but the diet should initially provide around 0.6 gm protein and 50 kcal per kg per day and eventually reach 3 to 4 gm protein and 80 to 100 kcal.

Vitamins, including folate, should be administered from the beginning, to meet recommended allowances. On admission, the routine administration of a single high dose (20,000 μg) of water-dispersible vitamin A is recommended to avoid acute eye lesions resulting from vitamin A deficiency when high calorie and protein diets are initiated and there is greater physiologic demand for the vitamin. This is followed by a daily oral dose of 1500 μg.

The diet should also provide from 4 to 5 mEq per kg body weight per day of K, 3 to 5 mEq per kg per day of Na and adequate amounts of magnesium, calcium and phosphorus. Iron, in amounts from 16 to 32 mg, as $FeSO_4$, is routinely administered by mouth as soon as increased protein-calorie intakes are begun, in order to supply the excess requirements for this mineral produced by the rapid increase in total circulating hemoglobin.

With this regimen, the severely malnourished subjects begin a smooth recovery: They start to lose edema and to gain body mass; their general state shows the first signs of improvement and anorexia is replaced by an increased appetite; then the patient may begin to eat a more varied diet. Serum and urine values also start a trend toward normal and the hematologic status initiates recovery. All of these changes are accompanied by a rise in nitrogen and energy retention. Except for sodium, mineral retention also increases. Rapid changes in weight should be avoided, particularly a rapid loss of edema. Usually within 2 to 3 weeks of therapy serum composition returns to normal limits, and consolidation of cure begins.

The second phase of therapy is accomplished only by dietary means. The patients should by then be receiving a complete mixed diet, providing the protein and calorie levels reached in the later phase of the initiation of therapy. A systematic program of psychosocial stimulation and progressive physical activity should be undertaken.[114,115] In children this can be accomplished through games that require frequent walking, preferably uphill, running, jumping and climbing. In adults it can be accomplished through exercise that imposes a gradual increment in cardiorespiratory work load. Complete calorie and protein repletion generally is accomplished in a 6- to 12-week period, depending on the deficits at the start of treatment. Calorie repletion is judged by weight for height, and is considered achieved when this index is 0.90 or more,

based on the 50th percentile of normal well-nourished populations. It is a mistake to use weight for age as an indicator of nutritional recovery. A child who is stunted in height would have to become obese in order to reach a normal weight for age. Generally, in nonedematous PCM, normalization of weight for height is reached later than normalization of the creatinine/height index an indicator of protein repletion.[60] In edematous PCM the opposite occurs. These changes are illustrated in Figures 24–9 and 24–10. Some children, however, stabilize at a creatinine/height index lower than 0.9, though fully recovered from PCM according to other indicators.

PREVENTION

Prevention can be approached by (1) measures to decrease the risk of individuals reaching severe PCM and (2) improvement of the general nutritional status of

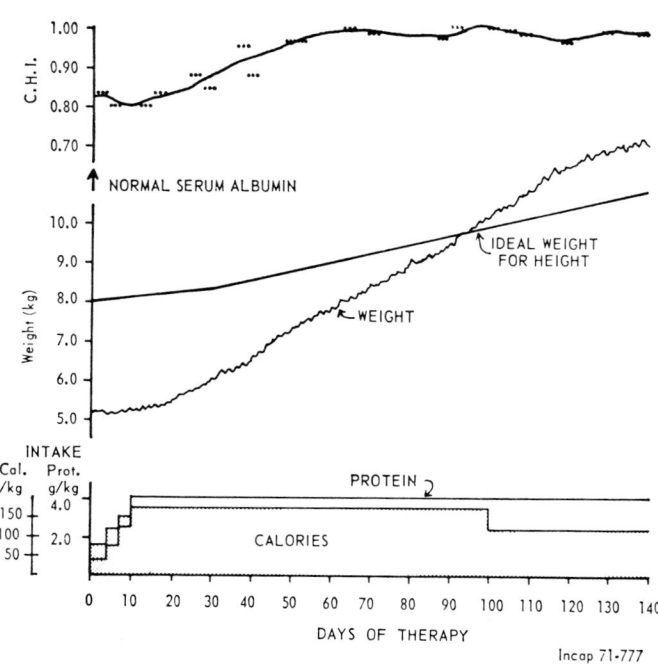

Incap 71-777

Fig. 24–9. Clinical record of a 16-month-old child during recovery from nonedematous PCM. His lean body mass (CHI) reached normal levels before his weight for height was normal.

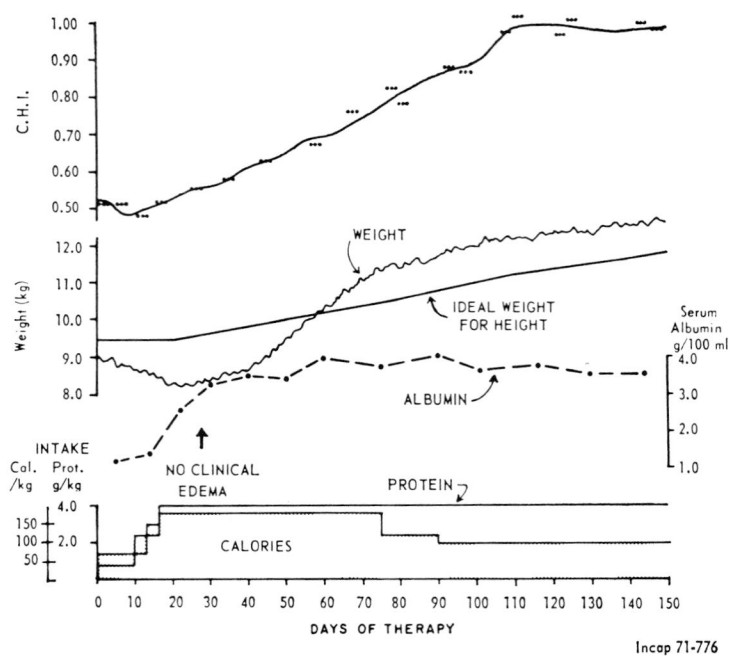

Fig. 24–10. Clinical record of a 20-month-old child during recovery from edematous PCM. His lean body mass (CHI) reached normal levels after his weight for height was normal.

the population, so that even chronic mild-to-moderate PCM cases become rare.

The first is amenable to some direct actions: (1) fostering of maternal lactation and adequate supplementation practices during infancy, (2) food supplementation programs of vulnerable groups, such as pregnant and lactating women, children up to school age and above, if possible, and physically hard-working men, (3) improvement of sanitary conditions and (4) specific nutrition education. For this last objective, nutrition education and recuperation centers have been instituted in several countries.[116] Their main objective is to educate the parents of chronic mild-to-moderate PCM children by having them participate actively in the nutrition rehabilitation of their own children. These centers must (1) be located in the community and be adapted to the local environment, (2) be supported by each community, (3) see that children are rehabilitated

by the proper feeding of locally available foods and (4) see that mothers are rotated in the care of the children, so as to have direct experience of the benefits that adequate nutrition brings to their children. Experience is accumulating on the effects of these specific preventive measures, indicating that they appear to fulfill their goals.[117]

Improvement of the general nutritional status of the population, so that malnutrition is eradicated, requires a complex approach.[118] This is inseparable from the acceleration of socioeconomic development; the actions to bring it about are beyond the scope of this chapter.

BIBLIOGRAPHY

1. Scrimshaw and Béhar: Fed. Proc., *18* (Suppl. 3), 82, 1959.
2. Gómez, Ramos Galván, Frenk, Cravioto-Muñoz, Chávez and Vásquez: J. Trop. Pediatr., *2*, 77, 1956.

3. Evaluación Nutricional de la Población de Centro América y Panamá. Guatemala. Instituto de Nutrición de Centro América y Panamá (INCAP): Oficina de Investigaciones Internacionales de los Institutos Nacionales de Salud (EEUU); Ministerio de Salud Pública y Asistencia Social. Guatemala, Instituto de Nutrición de Centro América y Panamá, 1969.

4. Viteri and Torún: Bol. Of. Sanit. Panam., 78, 58, 1975.

5. Lechtig, Delgado, Martorell, Yarbrough and Klein: In *Perinatal Medicine* (Rooth and Bratterby, Eds.). Stockholm, Almqvist and Wiksell, 1976, p. 208.

6. Lindblad and Rahimtoola: Acta Paediatr. Scand., 63, 125, 1974.

7. Mata, Urrutia, Kronmal and Joplin: Am. J. Dis. Child., 129, 561, 1975.

8. Viteri, Béhar and Alvarado: Rev. Col. Med. (Guatemala), 21, 137, 1970.

9. Soriano: Rev. Chil. Pediatr., 39, 475, 1968.

10. Waterlow: *Fatty Liver Disease in Infants in the British West Indies* (Medical Research Council Special Report Series No. 263). London, Her Majesty's Stationery Office, 1948.

11. Mata, Urrutia and Gordon: Trop. Geogr. Med., 19, 247, 1967.

12. Gordon, Chitkara and Wyon: Am. J. Med. Sci., 245, 345, 1963.

13. Viteri and Alvarado: Rev. Col. Med. (Guatemala), 21, 175, 1970.

14. Viteri and Pineda: In *Famine. A Symposium Dealing with Nutrition and Relief Operations in Times of Disaster* (Blix, Hofvander and Vahlquist, Eds.). Uppsala, Almqvist and Wiksells, 1971.

15. Kerpel-Fronius, Varga and Kun: Ann. Pediatr. (Switzerland), 183, 1, 1954.

16. Parra, Garza, Garza, Saravia, Hazlewood and Nichols: J. Pediatr., 82, 133, 1973.

17. Parra, Klish, Cuellar, Serrano, García, Argote, Canseco and Nichols: J. Pediatr., 87, 307, 1975.

18. Alleyne and Young: Clin. Sci., 33, 189, 1967.

19. Grant, Hambley, Becker and Pimstone: Arch. Dis. Child., 48, 596, 1973.

20. Waterlow, Alleyne, Chan, Garrow, Hay, James, Picou and Stephen: Arch. Latinoam. Nutr., 16, 175, 1966.

21. Waterlow and Alleyne: Adv. Protein Chem., 25, 117, 1971.

22. Beisel: Annu. Rev. Med., 26, 9, 1975.

23. Cohen and Hansen: Clin. Sci., 23, 351, 1962.

24. Frenk, Metcoff, Gómez, Ramos-Galván, Cravioto and Antonowicz: Pediatrics, 20, 105, 1957.

25. Alleyne: Clin. Sci., 34, 199, 1968.

26. Nichols, Alvarado, Hazlewood and Viteri: J. Pediatr., 80, 319, 1972.

27. Viteri, Alvarado, Luthringer and Wood: Vitam. Horm., 26, 573, 1968.

28. Viart: Am. J. Clin. Nutr., 30, 334, 1977.

29. Gordillo, Soto, Metcoff, López and García Antillón: Pediatrics, 20, 303, 1957.

30. Srikantia: In *Calorie Deficiencies and Protein Deficiencies* (McCance and Widdowson, Eds.). London, J. & A. Churchill, 1968, p. 2033.

31. Brinkman, Bowie, Friss-Hansen and Hansen: Pediatrics, 36, 94, 1965.

32. Keys, Brozek, Hanschel, Mickelsen and Taylor: *The Biology of Human Starvation*, Vol. II. Minneapolis, University of Minnesota Press, 1950, p. 1002.

33. Viteri: In *Amino Acid Fortification of Protein Foods*. Report of an International Conference Held at the Massachusetts Institute of Technology, September 16 to 18, 1969 (Scrimshaw and Altschul, Eds.). Cambridge, MIT Press, 1971, p. 350.

34. Suskind (Ed.): *Malnutrition and the Inmune Response*. New York, Raven Press, 1977.

35. Viteri, Flores, Alvarado and Behar: Am. J. Dig. Dis., 18, 201, 1973.

36. Bowie, Barbezat and Hansen: Am. J. Clin. Nutr., 20, 89, 1967.

37. Barbezat and Hansen: Pediatrics, 42, 77, 1968.

38. Schneider and Viteri: Am. J. Clin. Nutr., 27, 777, 1974.

39. Schneider and Viteri: Am. J. Clin. Nutr., 27, 788, 1974.

40. Viteri and Schneider: Med. Clin. North Am., 58, 1487, 1974.

41. Geber and Dean: Courrier (Paris), 6, 3, 1956.

42. Scrimshaw and Gordon (Eds.): *Malnutrition, Learning and Behavior*. Cambridge, MIT Press, 1968.

43. Hoeldtke and Wurtman: Fed. Proc., 30, 459, 1971.

44. Winick and Rosso: In *Protein-Calorie Malnutrition* (Olson, Ed.). New York, Academic Press, 1975, p. 93.

45. Dobbing: Pediatrics, 53, 2, 1974.

46. Wayburne: In *Calorie Deficiencies and Protein Deficiencies* (McCance and Widdowson, Eds.). London, J. & A. Churchill, 1968, p. 7.

47. Garrow, Smith and Ward: *Electrolyte Metabolism in Severe Infantile Malnutrition*. London, Pergamon Press, 1968.

48. Trowell, Davies and Dean: *Kwashiorkor*. London, Edward Arnold Ltd., 1954.

49. Viteri, Béhar, Arroyave and Scrimshaw: In *Mammalian Protein Metabolism*, Vol. II (Munro and Allison, Eds.). New York, Academic Press, 1964, p. 523.

50. Cravioto, DeLicardie and Birch: Pediatrics, 38 (Suppl., II), 319, 1966.

51. Klein, et al.: Bol. Of. San. Panam., 10, 301, 1976.

52. Tizard: Br. Med. Bull., 30, 169, 1974.

53. Canosa: In *Malnutrition, Learning, and Behaviour*. Proceedings of an International Conference Cosponsored by the Nutrition Foundation Inc. and the Massachusetts Institute of Technology, Held at Cambridge, Massachusetts, March 1–3, 1967 (Scrimshaw and Gordon, Eds.). Cambridge, MIT Press, 1968, p. 389.

54. Arroyave: In *Mild-Moderate Forms of Protein-Calorie Malnutrition*. Symposia of the Swedish Nutrition Foundation I. Bastad, August 29–31, 1962 (Blix, Ed.). Uppsala, Almqvist and Wiksells, 1963, p. 32.

55. Whitehead: In *Calorie Deficiencies and Protein Deficiencies* (McCance and Widdowson, Eds.). London, J. & A. Churchill, 1968, p. 109.

56. Arroyave: In *Protein Calorie Malnutrition* (von Muralt, Ed.). Berlin, Springer-Verlag, 1969, p. 48.

57. Whitehead: Lancet, 2, 567, 1965.
58. McFarlane, Ogbeide, Reddy, Adcok, Adeshina, Gurney, Cooke Taylor and Mordie: Lancet, 1, 392, 1969.
59. Hansen: In Calorie Deficiencies and Protein Deficiencies (McCance and Widdowson, Eds.). London, J. & A. Churchill, 1968, p. 33.
60. Viteri and Alvarado: Pediatrics, 46, 696, 1970.
61. Waterlow, Cravioto and Stephen: Adv. Protein Chem., 15, 131, 1960.
62. Waterlow: In Protein-Calorie Malnutrition (Olson, Ed.). New York, Academic Press, 1975, p. 23.
63. Garrow, Fletcher and Halliday: J. Clin. Invest., 44, 417, 1965.
64. Halliday: Clin. Sci., 33, 365, 1967.
65. Milward: Clin. Sci., 39, 591, 1970.
66. Mendes and Waterlow: Br. J. Nutr., 12, 74, 1958.
67. Lahey, Béhar, Viteri and Scrimshaw: Pediatrics, 22, 1958.
68. Smith, Goodman, Arroyave and Viteri: Am. J. Clin. Nutr., 26, 982, 1973.
69. Cravioto: Bol. Med. Hosp. Infant. Mex., 15, 805, 1958.
70. Graham and Blizzard: In Endocrine Aspects of Malnutrition (Gardner and Amacher, Eds.). Sta. Ynez (California), Kroc Foundation, 1973, p. 205.
71. Graham, Baertl, Claeyssen, Suskind, Greenberg, Thompson and Blizzard: J. Pediatr., 83, 321, 1973.
72. Alleyne and Young: Clin. Sci., 33, 189, 1967.
73. Leonard and MacWilliam: J. Endocrinol., 29, 273, 1964.
74. Leonard and MacWilliam: Am. J. Clin. Nutr., 16, 360, 1965.
75. Arroyave, Wilson, Méndez, Béhar and Scrimshaw: Am. J. Clin. Nutr., 9, 180, 1961.
76. Picou and Taylor-Roberts: Clin. Sci., 36, 283, 1969.
77. Picou and Phillips: Am. J. Clin. Nutr., 25, 1261, 1972.
78. Reddy, Belavady and Srikantia: Indian J. Med. Res., 51, 952, 1963.
79. Standard, Wills and Waterlow: Am. J. Clin. Nutr., 7, 271, 1959.
80. Arroyave, Wilson, Béhar and Scrimshaw: Am. J. Clin. Nutr., 9, 176, 1961.
81. Alleyne, Viteri and Alvarado: Am. J. Clin. Nutr., 23, 875, 1970.
82. Picou, Reeds and Jackson: Pediatr. Res., 10, 184, 1976.
83. Holtz, Snyderman, Norton, Roitman and Finch: Lancet, 2, 1343, 1963.
84. Arroyave, Wilson, Funes and Béhar: Am. J. Clin. Nutr., 11, 517, 1962.
85. Cravioto: Am. J. Clin. Nutr., 11, 484, 1962.
86. Adams and Scragg: J. Pediatr., 60, 580, 1962.
87. Edozien and Phillips: Nature, 191, 47, 1961.
88. Whitehead and Arnstein: Nature, 190, 1105, 1961.
89. Alleyne and Scullard: Clin. Sci., 37, 631, 1969.
90. James and Coore: Am. J. Clin. Nutr., 23, 386, 1970.
91. Becker, Pimstone, Hansen, Buchanan-Lee and MacHutchon: S. Afr. Med. J., 43, 1154, 1969.
92. Gillman, Gillman, Scragg, Savage, Gilbert, Trout and Levy: S. Afr. J. Med. Sci., 26, 31, 1961.
93. Metcoff, Frenk, Yoshida, Torres-Pinedo, Kaiser and Hansen: Medicine, 45, 365, 1966.
94. Van der Sar: Dos. Neerl. Indones. Morb. Trop., 3, 25, 1951.
95. Jayasekera, De Mel and Collumbine: Ceylon J. Med. Sci., 8, 1, 1951.
96. Schwartz and Dean: J. Trop. Pediatr., 3, 23, 1957.
97. Flores, Sierralta and Mönckeberg: J. Nutr., 100, 375, 1970.
98. Olson (Ed.): Protein-Calorie Malnutrition. New York, Academic Press, 1975.
99. Metcoff, Frenk, Gordillo, Gómez, Ramos Galván, Cravioto, Jeneway and Gamble: Pediatrics, 20, 317, 1957.
100. Caddell and Goddard: N. Engl. J. Med., 276, 533, 1967.
101. Nichols, Alvarado, Rodríguez, Hazlewood and Viteri: J. Pediatr., 84, 759, 1974.
102. Garrow: Lancet, 2, 643, 1967.
103. Arroyave, Feldman and Scrimshaw: Am. J. Clin. Nutr., 6, 164, 1958.
104. McLean: Clin. Sci., 30, 129, 1966.
105. Waterlow: Fed. Proc., 18, 1143, 1959.
106. Bruch, Arroyave, Schwartz, Padilla, Béhar, Viteri and Scrimshaw: J. Clin. Invest., 36, 1579, 1957.
107. Pineda: In Calorie Deficiencies and Protein Deficiencies (McCance and Widdowson, Eds.). London, J. & A. Churchill, 1968, p. 75.
108. Contreras, Pineda, Viteri and Arroyave: Fed. Proc., 30, 231, 1971.
109. Garrow, Picou and Waterlow: West Indian Med. J., 11, 217, 1962.
110. Torún and Viteri: Rev. Col. Med. (Guatemala), 27, 43, 1976.
111. Jelliffe and Jelliffe: J. Pediatr., 77, 895, 1970.
112. Cook: J. Trop. Pediatr., 17, 15, 1971.
113. Nichols, Alvarado, Kimsey, Hazlewood and Viteri. In Endocrine Aspects of Malnutrition (Gardner and Amacher, Eds.). Sta. Ynez (California), Kroc Foundation, 1973, p. 363.
114. Viteri: Am. J. Clin. Nutr., in press.
115. Torún and Viteri: Am. J. Clin. Nutr., in press.
116. Bengoa: J. Trop. Pediatr., 10, 63, 1964.
117. Beghin and Viteri: J. Trop. Pediatr., 19, 404, 1973.
118. Bengoa. In Protein Calorie Malnutrition (Olson, Ed.). New York, Academic Press, 1975, p. 435.

Chapter 25

OBESITY

Jean Mayer

Obesity is a pathologic condition characterized by an accumulation of fat much in excess of that necessary for optimal body function. As such, it is distinct from "overweight," which is defined as body weight much in excess of average. Both these definitions contain an element of imprecision, from the physiologic and the anatomic viewpoints. For example, populations which expect to be subjected at regular intervals to scarcity of food may consider a certain measure of obesity as desirable, indeed as necessary for survival. Such considerations, however, no longer apply to the United States, where longevity is greatest when obesity is least. The definition of overweight given above makes no mention of body type. A professional football player may be muscular and lean at a weight for his height which is clearly excessive when seen on a physically inactive executive. At the risk of being trite, let us emphasize at the outset of this chapter the importance of careful physical examination of the patient: If a man, woman or child looks fat when undressed, he or she probably is too fat. Visual judgment by an experienced observer is a more reliable method than the automatic application of height-weight tables, at least when the degree of overweight is not extreme. Obviously, however, we need quantitative data on both obesity and overweight if we are to carefully follow individual patients and relate weight and fat content to disease in population groups.[1]

DIAGNOSIS AND ESTIMATION OF OBESITY

A number of methods have been developed for the estimation of body fat (Chapter 1). The execution of some of these methods is too complex for the practicing physician or nutritionist. We shall, therefore, concentrate, in this chapter, on the two basic methods, determination of weight and its relation to height, age and body type and skinfold determinations.

Height-weight Tables

The appearance of the naked patient is the usual basis for the diagnosis of obesity by the experienced clinician and, as a qualitative guide, is usually reliable. When a quantitative estimate is desired, the patient's weight is usually compared with the "standard" weight for his height as given by one of several tables. For children and adolescents, the standard is usually an average weight for height, age and sex. The numerous tables available include the Baldwin-Wood, Bayer and Bayley, Stuart, Hathaway, Falkner, etc. Some of these show percentiles as well as medians. (See Chapter 1 for discussion of height-weight tables and Appendix for table of desirable weights for adults.) The Wetzel grid defines channels expressing percentiles of weight for height, independent of age.

Limitations of Tables. It is obvious that, if overweight (weight in excess of average) is marked, obesity (excessive fatness) is present. For moderate degrees of overweight, however, obesity may be by no means clear. College football linemen are generally overweight; they are generally not obese. Conversely, some extremely sedentary persons can be obese without being markedly overweight. Without a more direct measurement of adiposity, the diagnosis of obesity cannot be certain.

Epidemiologic data have shown that properly defined variations in body structure are important not only in terms of defining obesity but also possibly in terms of longevity. Analysis of the data of the Build and Blood Pressure Study, 1959,[2] tends to suggest this. In general, for each broad height category, mortality increased as weight increased. These data have been interpreted to mean that increased overweight is responsible for increased mortality. However, since persons who have the lowest weight for height (referred to by the life insurance companies' actuaries as underweights) and who must be for the most part dominant ectomorphs (rather than emaciated mesomorphs and endomorphs) have the highest longevity, it appears that this body type is associated with a longer-than-average life expectancy. The significant association of obesity with bones and muscles larger than average which Seltzer and Mayer[3,4] have demonstrated in females suggests that, at least among females, there may be an association between increased mortality and body type, irrespective of adiposity. Gertler and White[5] and Spain, Bradess and Greenblatt[6] also have suggested the association of certain body types with specific diseases. The ultimate answer to the question of the relation of obesity to mortality may lie in treating each type of body build separately and in correlating the extent of adiposity of each category of body build with mortality and disease manifestations.

While one cannot quarrel with the general concept that excessive weight gain after growth has ceased is bad for the patient, it appears questionable to base the diagnosis of obesity and the prescription of an ideal weight for a given patient on height-weight tables, even those as seemingly sophisticated as the ones derived from the Build and Blood Pressure Study, 1959. A knowledge of the patient's actual fatness is preferable not only from the viewpoint of diagnosing obesity but also because it emphasizes that component of body weight which can, in fact, be modified.

Measurement of Skinfold Thickness

Measurements of skinfold thickness appear to be the simplest and most practical available method of determining the extent of obesity. These measurements, obtained by using a suitable caliper on selected sites, have been shown by comparison with results of other methods to give a good indication not only of subcutaneous fat (about 50 per cent of the total fat) but also of total body fat. The technique is simple and the caliper relatively inexpensive. With proper directions and a minimum of demonstration by an experienced person, the physician can obtain reproducible measurements with the skinfold caliper.

Standardization of skinfold calipers has become a necessary requirement for universal comparability of fatfold measurements and conversion to total body fat. The accepted national recommendation is a caliper designed to exert a pressure on the caliper face of 10 gm per sq mm and with a contact surface of 20 to 40 mm.[7]

The skinfold measurement to be obtained is the (doubled) thickness of the pinched "folded" skin plus the attached subcutaneous adipose tissue. The person making the measurement pinches up a full fold of skin and subcutaneous tissue with the thumb and forefinger of his left hand at a distance about 1 cm from the site at which the calipers are to be placed, pulling the fold away from the underlying muscle. The fold is pinched up firmly and held while the measurement is being taken. The calipers are applied to the fold about 1 cm below the fingers, so that the pressure on the fold at the point measured is exerted by the faces of the caliper and not by the fingers. The handle is released to permit the full force of the caliper arm pressure, and the dial is read to the nearest 0.5 mm. Caliper application should be made at least twice for stable readings. If the folds are extremely thick, dial readings should be made 3 seconds after applying the caliper pressure.

Sites Measured for Skinfold Thickness. Various workers have used a number of sites, including the triceps, subscapular, abdominal, hip, pectoral and calf areas. For the general population, the Committee on Nutritional Anthropometry of the National Research Council has recommended the triceps and the subscapular skinfolds as good indexes of an individual's overall fatness.[8]

The triceps skinfold is located at the back of the right upper arm midway between the acromion and olecranon processes. The midpoint can be marked with the aid of a steel tape. The arm should hang freely during the skinfold measurement. Because of the gradation of subcutaneous fat thickness from shoulder to elbow, location of the midpoint is somewhat critical.

The subscapular skinfold is located just below the angle of the right scapula (shoulder and arm relaxed). The fold is picked up in a line slightly inclined in the natural cleavage of the skin. Because the subcutaneous fat is fairly uniform in this region, precision of location is less critical.

The work of Seltzer, Goldman and Mayer,[9] among others, indicates that for obese individuals the triceps skinfold, which is the easiest to measure, is also the most representative of body fatness. No special advantage is gained in utilizing any skinfold in addition to the triceps skinfold.

Criterion for Obesity. Extensive data on the distribution of triceps skinfold values, such as those obtained by Young and Blondin[10] and Novak,[11] allow determina-

tion of the normal variation of such skinfolds in our population (at least for Caucasian subjects). The next step, setting up a cutoff point for obesity, is obviously arbitrary. Because of its association with certain body types, the distribution of fatness within the general population may not be strictly monomodal; it does, however, represent a continuum, and any cutoff point would be a practical rather than a theoretically based selection. Furthermore, while this selection may represent a common fat content, it may not represent a common risk, because the significance of a given

Table 25–1. Obesity Standards for Caucasian Americans[1] (minimum triceps skinfold thickness in millimeters indicating obesity)[2]

Age (years)	Skinfold Measurements	
	Males	*Females*
5	12	14
6	12	15
7	13	16
8	14	17
9	15	18
10	16	20
11	17	21
12	18	22
13	18	23
14	17	23
15	16	24
16	15	25
17	14	26
18	15	27
19	15	27
20	16	28
21	17	28
22	18	28
23	18	28
24	19	28
25	20	29
26	20	29
27	21	29
28	22	29
29	23	29
30–50	23	30

[1]Adapted from Seltzer and Mayer.[7]
[2]Figures represent logarithmic means of the frequency distributions plus 1 S. D.

body fat content may differ with body type. Finally, it must be noted that the relation of skinfold thickness to body fat content is virtually independent of height.[12] This permits giving a single value for each sex and age as a cutoff point.

Based on these considerations, Seltzer and Mayer have recommended that, in the American population, the diagnosis of obesity in individuals less than 30 years old be reserved for those persons in whom the triceps skinfold is greater than 1 S.D. from the mean.[7]* Furthermore, the standard established for subjects 30 years old should be applied to men and women in the 30- to 50-year age group. Table 25–1 shows the details of this definition in numerical terms.

The very definition of standard deviation signifies that 16 per cent of the present American population less than 30 years of age is obese. Experienced workers in the field, whatever the basis for their criteria, recognize at least a similar proportion as obese.†

PREVALENCE OF OBESITY

Children and Adolescents

We have no satisfactory national statistics for the prevalence and incidence of obesity in the general population. However, a number of reports point to a steady increase in prevalence both in children and adults. For example, a 1952–53 study showed more than 10 per cent of the boys and girls examined in the public schools of Newton-Brookline, Massachusetts, to be obese by the definition chosen—that is,

they were in Channel A-4 or above on the Wetzel Grid.[13] Actually, a more specific definition of obesity, which should be based on body fat, would have shown that a number of boys and girls in Channel 3 had as great a proportion of body fat as those in Channel 4 and were, therefore, obese. In general, more children tended to be stocky than slender and more girls than boys ranged from stocky to obese. The obese children in high school with records from the first grade fell mainly into three groups. One-half of the obese girls and nearly one-half of the obese boys showed persistent obesity throughout their school years. About one-third of the boys and girls became obese in the sixth to eighth grades. There also were those who showed year-to-year variation, especially in the junior high groups.

A survey of the school in the late 1960s showed an increase in prevalence of obesity by over 20 per cent. Similar studies show increases of the same order for urban children. Children living in the country, particularly in areas where the climate is conducive to outdoor activity throughout the entire year, tend to be leaner.

Adults

Selective Service data show that the weight of draftees for any given height and age has increased during the past 50 years. A comparison of army inductees from World War I, World War II and 1957–58 reveals that in each period they were taller and heavier than their predecessors. Height increased a total of 1.2 inches, and weight increased 18 pounds.[14]

The 1959 Build and Blood Pressure Study of the Society of Actuaries produced new tables of average weight based on 5 million insured persons.[2] These new figures are more nearly representative of the general population than the previously used 1912 life insurance tables, because the new data include overweight persons rated as substandard risks because of weight only. Nevertheless, the figures do

---

*The triceps skinfold frequency distribution is typically skewed to the right. To normalize the distribution, the logarithmic mean rather than the arithmetic mean is determined before establishing the cutoff point. This prevents very obese members of the population from unduly influencing the determination of the mean.

†This does not mean that a physician may not consider some patients whose skinfolds are slightly below our cutoff points to be too fat for their body builds. Our criteria define frank obesity.

not represent a general population based on a nationwide probability sample.

These tables of average weight indicate that men tend to weigh 1 to 5 pounds more than shown in the earlier tables, and women 2 to 6 pounds less. The increase in average weight is greatest for short men at most ages, with the greater differences occurring after age 45 for tall men and men of medium height. The decrease in average weight reflected on the new tables is greatest for younger women, with the differences from the previous years becoming less with advancing age. Average weight increases with age, increasing rapidly in men who are in their 20s and early 30s and most rapidly in women in their mid-30s and 40s.

The prevalence of weight deviation from desirable or best weight for ages 20 to 69 is shown in the following Metropolitan Life Insurance Co. data[15,16] (Table 25–2).

The table shows a considerable increase of overweight with advancing years. The greatest increase occurs from the 20s to the 30s. However, the percentage of overweight men remains fairly constant after the 30s, while it continues to rise among women. The proportion of persons 20 per cent above best weight is the same for men and women in the 20s and 30s: Both are respectively 12 and 25 per cent over-

weight. Although the proportion continues to rise with advancing age, only about one-third of the older men are overweight compared with nearly one-half of the older women. One is tempted to conclude that, contrary to some published articles, men may be doing a better job at keeping weight down with advancing years than women.

Data on height, weight and selected body dimensions have been published by the National Center for Health Statistics, Public Health Service.[14] The height and weight data are presented as averages for age and sex and also selected percentiles by age and sex. The data are descriptive of the adult, civilian, noninstitutional population of the United States. They are not evaluated in terms of underweight, overweight or desirable weight. Neither are they analyzed for association with morbidity or mortality. However, it is interesting to note that these 1960–62 averages show the population to weigh more than does the 1959 Build and Blood Pressure Study. A maximum average weight for men occurs between ages 35 to 54 and a maximum average for women between ages 55 to 64. Women, according to these data, thus appear to achieve maximum weights about two decades later than do men, and have a greater relative gain with age. Within each age group, the average weight for both men and women tends to increase with increasing height.

Data from the Manhattan Mental Health Study suggest that there is less overweight among the high socioeconomic class, particularly among the women in that class,[17] than in the lower classes. There is less correlation between overweight and class among the men, but even there the prevalence of overweight increases as socioeconomic status decreases except, perhaps, for the lower group, constituted of laborers.

ETIOLOGY

As recently as 15 years ago, obesity was dealt with clinically as an almost exclusively

Table 25–2. Percentage of Persons Deviating from Best Weight[1]

Age (years)	Men		Women	
	10–19% Above Best Weight	20% or More Above Best Weight	10–19% Above Best Weight	20% or More Above Best Weight
20–29	19	12	11	12
30–39	28	25	16	25
40–49	28	32	19	40
50–59	29	34	21	46
60–69	28	29	23	45

[1]Adapted from Metropolitan Life Insurance Co.[16]

psychologic problem. The rationale was simple: Obesity is caused by overeating. Overeating is due either to lack of self-control—that is, gluttony—or to more serious abnormalities of personality.

Fortunately, the intervening years have seen knowledge progress on a wide front. Oversimplifications are no longer tenable by those who are concerned with the problem and its prevention and management. Advances in scientific knowledge have not resulted in any "magic bullet" based on diagnosis of specific neurophysiologic or biochemical disturbances. However, the progress witnessed does open avenues for exploration and affords a more comprehensive understanding of the complexities involved.

Obesity, the result of a positive caloric balance, can be the outcome of a number of disturbances (Table 25–3). The variations in causes and subsequent manifestations indicate that not all obesity can be considered the same. For this reason, some investigators have come to use the plural term "obesities" rather than "obesity."

Obesity can be classified according to etiology, or underlying causes, or it can be classified according to pathogenesis—changes in the mechanisms involved in the development of obesity, such as the impairment of a physiologic or biochemical process. Both classifications are intimately involved in the regulation of food intake.[1]

Genetic Factors in Obesity

In laboratory animals the role of genetic factors is clear-cut. The hereditary obese hyperglycemia syndrome of mice is an example of metabolic obesity. Other examples of hereditary obesity are: the yellow obesity, a dominant syndrome seen in mice heterozygous for this gene;[18] the New Zealand obesity, a recessive syndrome of obesity and diabetes that differs in many ways from the obese hyperglycemia syndrome (to cite one difference, the affected animals will mate),[19] and a genetically controlled spontaneous degeneration of the ventromedial area of the hypothalamus.[20] Other examples of genetic obesity in various types of laboratory and farm animals have been discussed in previous papers.[21,22]

Familial Occurrence in Man. The demonstration of the hereditary nature of familial obesity in man is much more difficult. That obesity does "run in families" is well established. In a series of over 1000 obese patients in Vienna,

Table 25–3. Types of Human Obesity

Genetic: A multiplicity of genes have been studied by Newman, von Verschuer. Bauer, Gurney, Rony, Angel, and others; in congenital adipose macrosomia; in monstrous infantile obesity; associated with Laurence-Moon-Biedl syndrome; associated with hyperostosis frontalis interna; associated with von Gierke's disease; in familial hypoglycemosis (congenital lack of alpha cells)

Of hypothalamic origin: In dystrophia adiposogenitalis, with discrete or diffuse hypothalamic injury; occasionally with panhypopituitarism and narcolepsy; Kleine-Levin syndrome

Of other central nervous system origin: After frontal lobotomy; in association with cortical lesions, in particular bilateral frontal lesions

Of endocrine origin: With insulin-producing adenoma of islands of Langerhans, with diffuse hyperplasia of islets and in association with diabetes; with chromophobe adenoma of pituitary gland without hypothalamic injury; in Cushing's syndrome (hyperglycocorticoidism); from treatment with cortisone or ACTH; in Bongiovanni-Eisenmenger syndrome; in disorders of reproductive system; gynandrism and gynism; aspermatogenic gynecomastia without aleydigism; male hypogonadism (sometimes with bulimia); postpubertal castration; menopause; ovarian disorder; paradoxical (Gilbert-Dreyfus) disorder

Otherwise induced: By immobilization in adults and children; by psychic disturbances; by social and cultural pressure

Bauer[23] found that one or both parents were obese in 73 per cent of cases. This figure is close to that of 69 per cent found by Rony[24] for a series of 250 patients in Chicago. In his studies in Philadelphia, Angel[25] reported that half the offspring of obese-average parents were obese, as were two-thirds of the offspring of obese-obese matings. Eighty per cent of the obese children had at least one fat parent; the parents of 25 per cent of the obese children were both obese. Gurney,[26] in a previous survey of a similar population, had found that only 9 per cent of the children of average-weight parents were overweight. Fellows,[27] studying the overweight fraction of a life insurance sample, observed that 58 per cent of the mothers and 43 per cent of the fathers were or had been overweight. Dunlop and Lyon,[28] studying a group of obese subjects in Edinburgh, reported that 69 per cent had at least one overweight parent (in 39 per cent, mothers only; in 12 per cent, fathers only; in 18 per cent, both parents overweight).

Ellis and Tallerman[29] stated that 30 of 50 very obese children studied (60 per cent) had a parent or sibling similarly affected; 13 (26 per cent) had grossly overweight mothers, 6 (12 per cent) grossly overweight fathers, and in 3 cases (6 per cent) both parents were grossly overweight. Iversen,[30] following 40 obese children, found that in 78 per cent (31 cases) one or both parents were obese. In only 10 per cent (4 cases) was there no obesity in parents or siblings. Our own studies in Boston[3] also show a high degree of correlation between overweight in parents and in children.

Ethnic Differences. Interpretation of these data is difficult since cultural background interacts with genetics to determine the incidence of overweight. Angel[25] reported that the sizable obese group he studied showed a relative excess of first- and second-generation Americans: 42.7 per cent had American-born parents (more than half "old Americans"), 8.7 per cent were American-born with one foreign

parent and one American-born parent, an unusual 35 per cent were American-born of foreign-born parents and 13.6 per cent were foreign-born. On the other hand, although it has been claimed on the basis of small samples that children of southern European[25] and Jewish[29] stock have an unusually high incidence of obesity, studies in Boston did not confirm this. Fry[31] did not find any significant association between ethnic (white) origin and severity of obesity. Johnson et al.[3] did not observe any significant difference between the incidence of obesity in two well-to-do suburbs of Boston: Brookline (mostly Jewish) and Newton (mixed background). The fact that in the southern United States overweight is more prevalent in black females than in black males[32] may be the result of a socioeconomic situation in which black men are still frequently employed in jobs entailing physical labor while black women no longer are, but are not yet subjected to social pressure for weight control. On the other hand, this difference between the white and the black population may be determined, at least in part, by genetic factors.

Several factors emphasize the importance of two tools—the study of twins and the study of sex ratios—that are applicable to problems of genetic factors in human obesity: the possible interaction of environmental and genetic factors, the mixed genetic background of most human groups, particularly in Europe and North America, the fact that human genetics deals with generations with life expectancies similar to those of the geneticists, and the fact that some of the most useful tools of genetics (for example, parent-offspring and brother-sister mating) are not applicable to human studies.

Evidence from Studies of Twins. Siemens' Zwillings-Pathologie, the study of diseases in twins,[33] provides much more cogent evidence of the importance of genetic factors in the etiology of at least some forms of obesity than do simple demonstrations of familial association. The method is, briefly, as follows: Assuming that it is possible to diagnose with accuracy identical (monozygous) and fraternal (heterozygous) twins, it is then reasonable to say that pathologic and other characteristics are hereditary which, if they occur at all, are always or nearly always present in both members of identical twin pairs, but rarely or never appear in both members of fraternal twin pairs. (This statement does not imply the reverse—that is, that characteristics found in members of both types of pairs are not hereditary.) The twin method has been applied by Newman, Freeman and Holzinger[34] to measurable characteristics such as height, weight and intelligence quotient. In this case, comparison of the variability of the quantity measured in identical twins and in fraternal twins permits a preliminary assessment of the role of heredity and environmental factors. (A comparison of variability among siblings and persons of the same age and sex obviously leads to a far less clear-cut distinction between environmental and hereditary causation.)

The study of Newman et al. bore on a large number of subjects, identical and fraternal twins and siblings of like sex. Variability of weight was included among the many physical and mental characteristics compared.[34] The correlation between identical twins for weight was found to be extremely high (0.973), exceeded only (and barely) by that for standing height (0.981), higher than right-finger and left-finger ridges (0.919 and 0.931) and intelligence characteristics (Binet, 0.910, Woodward-Mathews, 0.562). The ratio of standard errors of weight estimate for fraternal twins to identical twins is 2.2 (22.96 pounds for fraternal-twin weights as compared to 10.33 pounds for identical-twin weights), of the same order as height or head length and superior to all such ratios for mental traits. When twins and siblings are paired (the siblings being taken at comparable age), the mean pair difference in weight of siblings is 10.4

pounds (with 32.5 per cent differing by more than 12 pounds), that of fraternal twins is 10.0 pounds (with 34.5 per cent differing by more than 12 pounds) and that of identical twins 4.1 pounds, with only 2 per cent differing by more than 12 pounds.

Verschuer,[35] studying 57 pairs of identical twins from 3 to 51 years of age, found weight somewhat more variable than other physical characteristics, but still similar from twin to twin. The average variation amounted to only 2.58 per cent. A separate calculation for identical twins reared and living in identical environments and for those reared and living in dissimilar environments showed the average percentage variation in body weight to be 1.39 per cent for the first group and 3.6 per cent for the second. These results tend to demonstrate that, whereas environmental factors have a role in the control of body weight, genetic factors are of paramount importance.

Suggestive of the importance of genetic factors in the etiology of human obesity is the finding[25,26] that segregation can be shown to take place in the transmission of obesity. If the various types of mating—stout-stout, stout-nonstout, and nonstout-nonstout—are considered, the variability of weight of the offspring is relatively small for the first type (most of the offspring—73 per cent in this study—stout), least for the third type (almost none of the offspring—9 per cent in this study—stout) and largest for the matings of stout-nonstout (offspring divided between obese—41 per cent—and nonobese—59 per cent). This is interpreted by Gurney as showing that stout persons carry gametes for slenderness, whereas slender ones rarely carry gametes for stoutness.

Evidence from Sex Ratios of Children. Perhaps the most striking indication of genetic determination in human obesity is the demonstration by Angel[3] that the sex ratios of children in the various types of matings (as characterized by weight) are statistically different from those for the population as a whole.

Evidence from the Study of Adopted Children. Finally, a study by Withers[36] attempts to differentiate genotype from phenotype in yet another way. He studied the possible correlation of overweight in adopted children and in their adoptive parents, and compared it to the correlation observed between weights of natural children and their biologic parents in a South London suburb. The weight picture in natural children was found to be correlated to the weights of the biologic parents; that in the adopted children showed no correlation. The evidence that genetic factors dictate predisposition to overweight— and to a significant extent its occurrence— in a society where food is abundant and hard physical labor unnecessary is, I believe, convincing, although the data that would permit the elucidation of the mechanism of hereditary transmission are still missing.

Somatotype, Obesity and Genetics. Seltzer and Mayer,[4] studying the somatotypes of obese adolescent girls, showed that they differed from the nonobese population in features other than amount of fatty tissue. Obesity did not occur in all varieties of physical types; it occurred more often in some physical types than in others. The obese adolescent girls appeared to be more endomorphic, somewhat more mesomorphic and considerably less ectomorphic than the nonobese girls of comparable age drawn from the general population. The obese series was somatotypically more homogeneous and invariable than the general population, as manifested by the absence of subjects low in endomorphy and high or even moderate in ectomorphy. In nonanthropologic language, the obese group was remarkable for large skeleton and muscle mass, which seemed to be present in spite of the extreme inactivity of these obese adolescent girls,[37] and by the absence of narrow, elongated extremities (very few girls with long, tapered fingers are obese).

In adults the problem is more complex, since in that population group one must deal with physical types that are prone to a relatively sudden blossoming into middle-age obesity. The results[38] show that, in the adult age group as well, the obese are not, as far as body build is concerned, identical to the nonobese in body components other than fat, but are once again more endomorphic, more mesomorphic and considerably less ectomorphic.

If there is a close correlation between obesity and body types in adolescents, this obviously argues further for the genetic determination of obesity, in that the hereditary nature of body build has been repeatedly demonstrated. For example, Withers[36] has attempted to determine, in the working-class population of a South London suburb and in samples from a boys' and a girls' school in a London borough, the extent and manner in which endomorphy, mesomorphy and ectomorphy were transmitted from parents to children. Several findings stood out when the results obtained in both studies were collated: The father definitely contributed mesomorphy to his sons, and the mother contributed endomorphy to her sons. The father may also have transmitted his mesomorphy or ectomorphy to his daughters, and the mother her endomorphy or ectomorphy to her daughters, though the size of the population studied was too small to establish these correlations definitely.

Traumatic Factors

Experimental obesity has been produced in animals by both physiologic and psychic trauma. For example, obesity may be produced by creating hormonal imbalances in animals. Likewise, animals can be punished until they overeat: soon they learn to overeat and, with removal of punishment, continue to overeat for a while.

Again, identification of an exact human counterpart type of obesity is elusive. However, studies of obese persons make it clearly evident that overeating is frequently associated with emotional trauma. The onset of obesity in a number of subjects can be identified with some particular stress period.[1] In some instances, this is self-limiting, disappearing with disappearance of the stress, but in others the overeating and the obese condition remain.

Human obesity resulting from physiologic trauma is less clearly evident.

Environmental Factors

Such factors as culture, activity and diet all exert at least a permissive effect on the development of obesity.[1,21,22] The nature of the diet, which in the present-day United States of America tends to be a concentrated source of calories, and the lack of opportunity to exercise in our cities are important elements in the etiology of obesity. This is particularly true if heredity or certain responses to stress predispose an individual to obesity.

The possible role of a particular type of diet in the etiology of obesity is frequently expressed as an important factor. A study of body fat, diet and physical activity reveals little correlation between caloric intake and degree of body fatness. It reveals no correlation between degree of body fatness and the frequency of eating, nor between the degree of body fatness and the consumption of one-half of the total daily calories at one meal.[39]

The one general difference in this country between the food habits of people who are or are not obese is that the obese tend to "overeat" in the evening.[39]

PATHOGENESIS

An alternate classification of obesities relates to the actual mechanism involved within the individual.[22] Two categories of classification have been suggested, regulatory obesity and metabolic obesity.

Regulatory Obesity

In regulatory obesity the primary impairment is in the central mechanism regulating food intake.[1,22] Metabolism of the extracerebral tissue is normal except to the extent that it is modified by hyperphagia

or by extreme adiposity. Experimental examples are the hypothalamic obesities induced in animals by surgical intervention or by gold thioglucose, or the obesities from thalamic or frontal lesions or from forcing or conditioning an animal to overeat. In human subjects, this regulatory type of obesity might be likened to that resulting from immobilization or from extreme sedentariness.

A decreased tendency to move about is a common finding in studies of obese adults and obese children. A number of recent studies have demonstrated the extreme inactivity of most obese children.

A study of incidence and prevalence of obesity in two suburban school systems showed that excessive weight gain among obese children generally occurred in the winter. This suggested that inactivity might be a major factor in the development of obesity.[13] A more detailed study comparing the food intake and activity schedules of 28 obese girls and 28 nonobese girls showed that the obese girls ate less but exercised strikingly less than the nonobese.[40] Similar studies with similar results have been conducted on other groups.[41] A new technique developed for time/motion studies in industry and involving the analysis of sample 3-second motion pictures (30,000 were taken and analyzed) has demonstrated unequivocally that obese girls both devote less time to exercise than nonobese girls and expend far less energy during scheduled exercise periods.[37] Conversely, a number of experiments have demonstrated that increased exercise in obese children does not generally increase their food intake and is, therefore, an effective weight control measure.[42]

There is convincing evidence that, to a large degree, inactivity antedates the development of obesity in an individual. Physiologic causes may be involved. In most obese youngsters, psychologic traumas consequent to the obesity seem to operate to make the inactivity self-perpetuating. Obese children, and obese girls in particular, show many of the characteristics of minority groups—obsessive concern with their condition, passivity, withdrawal and expectation of rejection. These result in unhappiness, social isolation—and growing inactivity.

Metabolic Obesity

In contrast to regulatory obesity, where the excessive food intake is caused by an error in the central mechanism, metabolic obesity is that type where the overeating results from an abnormality in the metabolism of fats and carbohydrates.[1,22] A number of experimental examples of metabolic obesity have been studied in great detail in this writer's laboratory.

In animals with metabolic obesity, one may observe an increase in lipogenesis over that seen in normal animals. This type of obese animal will make more fat even though it may not "overeat"—in fact, even in the presence of fasting.

Examples of decreased fat mobilization or oxidation have also been described in the metabolic type of obesity. While it is likely that similar examples exist in man, these have not yet been documented.

RISKS OF OBESITY

The increase in mortality in the obese is well known and is summarized in Table 25–4. The effects of obesity on established disease are also important and are discussed in the next section under "indications for weight reduction."

TREATMENT OF OBESITY IN ADULTS

Medical History and Basic Data

It is essential that, in the medical history, particular attention be given to the age of onset of obesity and its past course; the psychologic aspects and prognosis are quite different in persons who become obese in their adult years than in those who were obese as children and as adolescents. Persons who were obese as youngsters are much more likely to be obsessively concerned with self-image and to view their obesity as a badge of shame rather than as a medical problem which can be attacked by rather simple means, they are more likely to have failed repeatedly to control their weight in the past and are more likely to be victims of as yet little understood physiologic or psychologic abnormalities.[43] While the classic "endocrine" abnormalities are rare, the possibility of hypothyroidism, hyperadrenocorticism and, in the male, hypogonadism should be ruled out. The possible occurrence of abnormal fluid retention also should be ruled out. Dietary habits should be investigated thoroughly, together with the familial psychologic and economic background. Patterns of hunger and satiety should be understood and their modification, when the patient is on a reducing diet, followed,[44] as they form the basis of decisions on the division of the calories allotted in the reducing diets among the proper number of meals and snacks. The actual time spent in activities not involving sitting or lying down, and some idea of the vigor with which these activities are pursued, should be known. These elements, together with the sex of the patient and his or her size and age, form the basis of the estimate of the daily caloric requirements for energy balance.

As regards psychologic data, it is important, before searching for possible psychogenic factors, to evaluate as carefully as possible the psychologic effects of obesity on the patient. The psychologic impact on the patient of newly discovered pathologic conditions (e.g., diabetes, hypertension) ought also to be appraised in terms of their possible effect on motivation.

Indications for Weight Reduction

Outside of some (rare) situations involving either somatic or psychiatric problems, weight reduction is desirable in all obese individuals. The attitude that, in the absence of any clear reason for reducing the

Table 25-4. Principal Causes of Death Among Men and Women Rated for Overweight. Attained Ages 25-74 Years

Ratio of Actual to Expected Deaths According to Estimates of Contemporaneous
Mortality Experience on Standard Risks

Metropolitan Life Insurance Company, Ordinary Department Issues of 1925 to 1934,
Traced to Policy Anniversary, 1950

	Men		Women	
Causes of Death	Deaths	Per Cent Actual of Expected Deaths	Deaths	Per Cent Actual of Expected Deaths
Principal cardiovascular-renal diseases	1,867	149	1,103	177
Organic heart disease, diseases of the coronary arteries and angina pectoris	1,377	142	697	175
Organic heart disease	748	*	515	*
Coronary disease and angina pectoris	629	*	182	*
Cerebral hemorrhage	247	159	226	162
Chronic nephritis	243	191	180	212
Cancer, all forms	385	97	476	100
Stomach	62	85	34	86
Liver and gallbladder	33	168	46	211
Peritoneum, intestines and rectum	103	115	93	104
Pancreas	19	93	21	149
Respiratory organs	39	78†	—	—
Breast	—	—	81	69
Genital organs	—	—	132	107
Uterus	—	—	103	121
Leukemia and Hodgkin's disease	26	100	23	110
Diabetes	205	383	235	372
Tuberculosis, all forms	24	21	20	35
Pneumonia, all forms	98	102	78	129
Cirrhosis of the liver	96	249	32	147
Appendicitis	76	223	41	195
Hernia and intestinal obstruction	39	154†	31	141†
Biliary calculi and other gall-bladder diseases	32	152†	30	188†
Biliary calculi	19	206	50	284
Ulcer of stomach and duodenum	30	67	—	—
Puerperal conditions	—	—	43	162
Suicide	63	78	23	73
Accidents, total	177	111	74	135
Auto	76	131	27	120
Falls	32	131	—	—

* Satisfactory basis for comparison not available.

† Based on mortality rates on Standard risks for 1935-39.

Note: Percentages which have been underlined indicate statistically significant deviations from experience on standard risks.

patient, he or she should be left alone is a counsel of laziness. Should one wait for hypertension or diabetes or immobilization consequent to the superimposition of excess weight on arthritis to do something about the problem? Furthermore, the patient's general fitness is visibly improved, his employability is increased in both government and industry and, in a society which, for better or for worse, puts a great deal of emphasis on appearance, his social acceptability—and, in some cases, his happiness—is improved.

In some serious conditions indications for weight reduction are particularly pressing.

Respiratory Difficulties. The work of breathing is increased if considerable additional weight is carried on the chest wall. Excessive adipose tissue also increases the complexity of the problem of keeping the whole body oxygenated. Obese people consequently have diminished exercise tolerance and may show great difficulty in normal breathing, particularly in the presence of any—even mild—respiratory infection. At the extreme, very marked obesity may lead to the Pickwickian syndrome where, through decreased ventilation, accumulation of carbon dioxide in blood leads to lethargy and somnolence. Lowered oxygenation of arterial blood may also lead to reactive polycythemia, which may compound the possibility of thrombosis and abnormal blood clotting. Cardiac enlargement and congestive heart failure may also result from pulmonary difficulties caused by extreme obesity. The removal of obesity is essential to the treatment of the Pickwickian syndrome.[45] It can aid greatly the treatment of congestive heart failure.

Hypertension. While it is true that in some early reports the correlation between obesity and hypertension was exaggerated by the use of pressure cuffs of ordinary size, which excessively compressed the tissues in the upper arm, even when a cuff of proper size is used a significant association

between obesity and hypertension is seen. In general, it can be said that hypertension is more prevalent among obese than among nonobese persons and that obese hypertensives show greater morbidity and mortality rate and, in particular, greater risk of coronary heart disease than nonobese hypertensives (or than obese nonhypertensives).[46,47]

The effects of weight reduction on hypertension are by no means universally evident but, when there is a change, it tends to be favorable, with the drop in blood pressure a function of the drop in body weight. Recent experience shows that, in large groups of hypertensives, at least half—and in some instances as many as 75 per cent—of the patients experience significant decreases in blood pressure (20 mm Hg systolic or 15 mm Hg diastolic) if they lose at least 15 pounds. While certain authors have claimed that the most important effect of weight reduction regimens is the curtailment in sodium chloride which accompanies the caloric restriction, it appears that this is only one of the variables involved. There is no doubt that, whatever the mechanisms involved, hypertension in an obese patient is a compelling indication for weight reduction. The favorable effect of weight reduction on the survival of postcoronary patients is well documented.[47,48]

Endocrine and Metabolic Disturbances. Hirsutism and menstrual irregularities, much more frequent among obese women than among nonobese, can often be mitigated by sufficient weight loss. There are somewhat conflicting reports on the association of obesity with high cholesterol levels, triglycerides and fatty acids.[1] It is possible that such conflicts arise from a lack of differentiation of the phase of obesity (active weight gain, static obesity) and from our inability at present to differentiate among various forms of obesity. It can be stated in general that, while abnormal plasma lipid levels frequently fail to respond to weight reduction, any response which takes place, particularly in blood cholesterol level, tends to be favorable, i.e., the abnormally high lipid level is decreased temporarily or permanently.

There is a high prevalence among obese subjects of impaired glucose tolerance and of hyperglycemia. This type of maturity-onset "diabetes," which often responds dramatically to weight reduction, may be less likely to lead to vascular degeneration than juvenile, "nonobese" types of diabetes.[49] Nevertheless, avoiding the need for insulin, preventing skin and other infections related to hyperglycemia and avoiding the risk of acidosis provide strong indications for immediate institution of weight reduction in such patients.

Other Pathologic Conditions. Serious difficulties in reproduction associated with obesity can often be diminished or eliminated by weight reduction. The risk of toxemia and delivery problems can be decreased if the woman's weight is controlled, preferably by reduction before the beginning of pregnancy (See Chapter 26 for discussion of obesity and pregnancy.) Infertility in obese men may be the result of excessively high temperature of the scrotum, if it is surrounded by folds of adipose tissue.

While there is a significant association between obesity and gallbladder disease, there is as yet no documented evidence that, once the disease is present, it is ameliorated by weight reduction.

Certain skin problems may similarly be mitigated or eliminated by weight reduction. Obesity, because it restricts normal heat loss by the body, tends to promote excessive perspiration. Contact or friction between moist skin areas in adjacent folds often leads to rashes, inflammation and furuncles. While obesity per se probably does not cause varicose veins, weight reduction considerably lessens the risk of ulcers and other skin complications in women who have varicose veins.

A number of bone and joint diseases are greatly benefited by weight reduction, which decreases the pressure on the damaged structure and facilitates mobility. Rupture of intravertebral disks and osteoarthritis are examples in point.

In spite of steady advances in anesthesiologic and surgical techniques, obese patients still have an increased risk at operation and, if possible, should be reduced before elective procedures.

Finally, especially in adolescents but also in many obese adults, particularly in women, the adverse psychologic effects of obesity—"losing one's looks," anxiety about its effects on marital relationships, etc.—may, by themselves, constitute a pressing medical indication for weight reduction.

Contraindicatons to Weight Reduction

Certain diseases, in particular tuberculosis, gout and diverticulitis, are often quoted as examples of conditions in which weight reduction is contraindicated. Actually, weight reduction, if needed, can be accomplished safely in these diseases if done very gradually with a sensible dietary regimen. Weight reduction is contraindicated in Addison's disease, regional ileitis and ulcerative colitis; obesity is, however, rarely associated with these diseases.

Cases in which rapid weight loss was associated with profound depression or acute psychosis have received wide attention and have frequently been cited as illustrating the dangers attendant on weight reduction. While such cases are indeed documented, the following points must be made: (1) The occurrence of depression or psychosis during weight reduction is very rare, (2) the patients had manifestly unstable personalities before the reduction therapy, (3) treatment was usually aimed at a rapid rate of weight loss and was based on a drastic curtailment of food intake, rather than aimed at a slow rate of weight loss with the combination of increased exercise and a moderate diet to create the caloric deficit necessary for weight loss. In the enormous majority of cases, the physician need not fear such drastic psychologic complications of treatment, although regular checks of the patient's outlook and a careful examination of the degree of hunger and fatigue experienced, with proper remedial measures if both appear excessive, are essential parts of the sound therapy of obesity.

Methods of Weight Reduction

It cannot be emphasized enough that the various methods which we are about to examine are not alternative methods. Diet and exercise are complementary measures in establishing the caloric deficit. The manipulation of the dietary schedule and the use of formula diets are directed at making the limitation in caloric intake more acceptable. Salt restriction may help to provide a more even rate of weight reduction, by avoiding excessive fluid retention. Psychologic support is always an essential element of any long-term therapy.

Dietary Regimen. A proper diet must provide all necessary nutrients, other than calories, in sufficient amounts, be palatable, easily available from the viewpoints of economics and convenience and limited in calories, so as to permit the desired caloric deficit. Ideally, the diet must help in the reeducation of the patient, so that, by increasing somewhat the size of the portions, it will provide a proper maintenance diet when the desired weight has been obtained.

The determination of the desired deficit is based on the fact that a pound of fatty tissue is the caloric equivalent of approximately 3500 calories. This means that a daily deficit of 500 calories will lead, over a long enough period, to an average rate loss of 1 pound a week, a deficit of 1000 calories to a loss of 2 pounds. This rate of 2 pounds a week is, incidentally, as much as should be lost by a patient not under close, frequent medical supervision. If patients are extremely obese and are followed carefully, both metabolically and psychologically, greater rates of weight loss can be obtained safely, at least at the beginning of the reduction regimen, but indications for such a rapid rate must be pressing (e.g., impending surgery).

It is generally true that, in ambulatory, busy patients, a caloric intake of less than 1500 calories for men and 1000 for women is poorly tolerated over long periods. An increased rate of energy expenditure through stepped-up physical activity makes it possible to obtain a caloric deficit of 500 or 1000 calories per day without having to cut food intake below those (low) limits.

Once the rate of weight loss has been decided (e.g. 2 pounds per week, tantamount to a deficit of 1000 calories per day), a guess is made as to the requirements to maintain the patient, given his or her size and pattern of activity. Let us assume that the best guess is 2200 calories. Adding an hour of walking to the usual activity pattern will bring it to 2500 calories. The diet should be geared then to provide 1500 calories, with the intake adjusted as the results of the trial become available over, say, a 2-week period.

Determining the caloric content of the diet is but one aspect of dietary prescription. Knowledge of the patient's familial and economic status, his usual eating pattern, his tastes and the capabilities of the person who does the marketing and cooking are necessary before the choice of foods to be included in the diet can be made (always remembering that the more varied a diet, the greater are the chances that it will be nutritionally adequate, thus eliminating the need for nutritional supplement such as vitamin pills).

Education of the patient on the caloric content of the various foods in various-sized portions is essential not only to the success of the weight reduction program but also to the success of the subsequent maintenance program. Models are necessary in demonstrating the size of portions. Such expressions as an "average" potato or an "average" serving of lean meat are understood to mean widely different sizes by various individuals.

The distribution of the food in a number of meals and snacks is a matter for individual prescription and experimentation; a "good" reducing diet is one on which the patient does not become too hungry. Knowing the normal pattern of hunger and satiety of the patient, a guess can be made as to the number of meals and snacks which will prevent excessive hunger. If hunger does develop once caloric restriction is instituted, further fragmentation of the daily food allowance may help to mitigate the problem.

There is at present no evidence available to support the idea that some of the extreme diets recently popularized have any advantage over a calorically restricted, balanced, "normal" diet. A low-protein, low-fat, "rice" type of diet was popular a few years ago, followed by a very-low-protein diet, dubbed the "Rockefeller" diet by its promoters. The very-high-protein, moderate-carbohydrate diet has been recommended by a number of groups in part on the basis of a misconception of the order of magnitude of the specific dynamic action of proteins in a mixed diet. The high-fat, low-carbohydrate (or carbohydrate-free) diet reappears every now and then under a variety of names—the DuPont or Pennington or Mayo diet. With alcohol added, it has become the "drinking man's diet." Again, advocates of these diets, who are sincere, are apparently misguided on a number of counts. While it is true that a high-fat diet depresses fat synthesis, it by no means prevents fat deposition when fat is copiously available in the diet. Fat does have "satiety" value, but so do other foods. A carbohydrate-free, high-fat diet does cause an immediate weight loss (over and above the steady decrease from caloric deficit), but this is because of partial dehydration and is of no lasting significance in a program designed to reduce adiposity, not simply to decrease weight, per se, over the short term. A diet high in fat, where calories and alcohol can be consumed ad libitum, not only tends to make patients fat (and inebriated) but also may be highly atherogenic.

A balanced diet, containing no less than 12 to 14 per cent of protein, no more than 30 per cent of fat (with saturated fats cut down) and the rest carbohydrates (with sucrose cut down to a very low level), provided by foods of sufficient variety is infinitely preferable to the fad diets mentioned (and their congeners, the grapefruit diet, the banana diet, the hard-boiled-egg diet, etc.).

Formula diets have become popular in the past 15 or so years. Whether purchased in liquid form or as powders to be suspended in water, their main advantage is that they provide strictly established amounts of food (3 times 300 calories or 4 times 225 calories per day, in general) and thus provide a simple, rigid regimen which does not need to be based on any knowledge of foods and food values. While this is often an advantage at the beginning of the reducing period (2 to 4 weeks), it should not delay the dietary education which, sooner or later, is absolutely necessary to carry the patient over a prolonged weight reduction period and through the maintenance, lifelong phase. The enormous majority of patients do not, in fact, stay exclusively on such formula diets, and as the formula diet is supplemented by other foods its intrinsic value is lost. Formula diets may, nevertheless, be found useful during maintenance, as the exclusive replacement of one meal a day.

According to Van Itallie and Yang,[53] although some consider a low-calorie diet consisting entirely of protein to be uniquely advantageous in preserving body nitrogen, it has yet to be shown that protein alone is more effective in this regard than an isocaloric mixture of protein and carbohydrate. A number of deaths have been associated with liquid-protein modified-fast diets,[54] although a cause-and-effect relationship has not been proven.

Generally these products are hydroly-sates, made largely from cowhides, collagen and gelatin, to which saccharin and artificial flavor have been added. The protein is of low biologic value.

Bulk-producing agents (such as methyl-cellulose) have not been shown to have any special merit. Apples, celery, raw carrots or salads are more palatable, more likely to become parts of a lifelong dietary pattern and, thus, are superior on all counts to artificial bulk-producing agents. Work done in our laboratory suggests that bulky foods may be particularly valuable as satiety adjuncts, not so much because of their stomach-filling role but because they slow down the course of the meal and provide time for satiety phenomena to supervene.

Artificial sweeteners are questionable adjuncts to reducing diets. There is little to say for the extensive consumption of sucrose, an "empty" source of calories which, in large amounts, may excessively stimulate insulin production. The use of sugar in the numerous cups of tea and coffee often consumed by reducing patients and the use of sugar-containing soft drinks should be strictly eliminated. If reducing patients have to drink a number of cups of coffee a day (a questionable practice for some patients on other grounds) it would be preferable to drink it black. The use of artificial sweeteners should not be recommended.

Strict restriction of salt is a therapeutic procedure which should be prescribed only if the clinical picture warrants it. On the other hand, cutting down on salt intake decreases the tendency to excessive fluid retention seen in many reducing obese subjects, particularly middle-aged and older women and sedentary individuals. It may also have some effectiveness in the prevention of hypertension. However, weight reduction without salt restriction will lower the blood pressure in overweight hypertensives.[55] Salt restriction is a much sounder and safer way to prevent excessive water retention during weight reduction

than the use of diuretics which, if prolonged, may cause renal damage. It is unfortunate that certain "reducing" pills containing diuretics (ammonium chloride) are still available for over-the-counter sale. Patients ought to be warned against such preparations.

Exercise. The value of exercise in the prevention of obesity and the treatment of moderately obese persons in otherwise good health is well established.[1,50] Its value in the prevention of heart disease is also well established.[1,51,52] Let it be recalled simply that exercise is the great variable in energy expenditure. The caloric expenditure in exercise is proportional to the duration of the exercise; it is also proportional to the weight of the subject, so that an obese person will use up proportionately more calories to perform the same task than will a thin one. The caloric expenditure increases rapidly with the intensity with which the exercise is performed. Exercise does not increase voluntary food intake until it has reached a certain critical duration and intensity, depending on the individual.

While obviously a very obese subject, even one in good cardiovascular state, should not be put suddenly to exercise, it is a good idea to start him walking every day and to increase the duration and eventually the intensity of the exercise as his weight reduction progresses. An understanding of the schedule and of the mode of life of the patient is necessary if exercise is going to be built into his daily life. Advantage of every opportunity for walking, stair climbing, etc., can be taken, to restore mobility in patients used to the constant use of automobiles and elevators.

The physician must remind the patient that the insulation provided by the excessive adiposity will restrict his rate of heat loss on hot days, so that particular caution must be exercised in the summer to interrupt the exercise with sufficient rest periods and to keep hydrated (preferably with water!).

Thyroid Preparation. There is still too much thyroid hormone prescribed for obese patients (usually in the form of desiccated thyroid) without any clear indication that patients are in a hypothyroid state. Such medication is based on the misconception that most obese patients are hypometabolic, an old idea originating from relating basal oxygen consumption to body weight. At present, sophisticated methods (I uptake, PBI determinations, etc.) should be used before a diagnosis of hypothyroidism is arrived at and acted on. The administration of thyroid hormone is in part self-defeating anyway, as it depresses endogenous thyroid secretion, and such depression is very slow to reverse. If large doses are given, tachycardia, palpitation, nervousness and insomnia appear, creating an unpleasant and potentially dangerous situation.

Other Methods. A number of "heroic" measures, such as total fasting, have been advocated. Published reports, including reports of accidents during total fasting, do not impel us to look at this method favorably, although there may be situations, such as impending surgery, where the risk of total fasting for a hospitalized patient, under close laboratory and psychologic supervision, may be less than that of continued extreme obesity. If surgery is contemplated, it is important that the patient have a week of moderate feeding at the end of the fasting period and immediately before the operation. Patients ought to be strongly warned against self-administered total fasting, because of dangers to themselves (as well as to others, if they drive a car!). Also, the prognosis for the long-term maintenance of the reduced weight achieved by fasting for periods of two months or more is not good. Johnson and Drenick[56] followed 121 patients for 7.3 years and found that, although fast-induced weight losses were maintained by "the great majority" for 1 to 1½ years, 50 per cent of the group had reverted to the original admission weight within 2 to 3 years and, by the end of the follow-up period, less than 10 per cent weighed less than they had originally.

Surgical procedures which permit temporary bypass of part of the small intestine have been used in "intractable" obesity. In patients on whom adequate follow-ups are available, the experience has been miserable. Not only did the patients exhibit serious difficulties while the shunt lasted (including some cases of uncontrollable hypocalcemia) but the weight was generally recovered rapidly after the shunt was discontinued.

Psychologic Support. The physician should be concerned with certain psychologic aspects of the therapy of obesity. In order of increasing diagnostic and therapeutic difficulty, these are:

Psychology of Weight Reduction. The physician should ease the discomforts attending the continued sensations associated with a prolonged period of caloric deficit, such as mitigating hunger and fatigue by appropriate measures and counseling, and fixing realistic short-term and long-term targets, arriving at the latter by his clinical judgment based on the actual body structure of the patient and his mode of life and capabilities.

Psychology of Being Obese. Particularly in patients who were obese in adolescence, when the body image appears to be developed, a galaxy of psychologic traits appears to result from the obesity-obsessive concern with self-image, such as passivity, expectation of rejection and progressive withdrawal, which must be coped with if the patient is to be a happy, well-adjusted person. Many of these psychologic effects of obesity may tend to make the obesity self-perpetuating.

Psychologic Factors Leading to Obesity. These are the least known and thus are particularly difficult to deal with adequately. Anxieties and stresses which burden an obese patient may be instrumental, if the patient is otherwise predisposed to obesity by genetics and by constitution, in causing overeating and immobilization and, hence, weight accumulation. The development of new interests can be useful, particularly in middle-aged women with little to do outside of the home, much time on their hands and a tendency to view their interpersonal relationships in terms of sitting down together at meals.

TREATMENT OF OBESITY IN CHILDREN AND ADOLESCENTS

We have seen earlier that the concept of childhood obesity as "puppy fat" which, left to itself, will disappear does not correspond to the facts as we know them. Treatment of obesity in children and adolescents is desirable but must be conducted with the thought in mind that any drastic caloric reduction may be accompanied by cessation of growth and, therefore, be essentially self-defeating. The following additional considerations should be kept in mind.

An obese child is not necessarily an otherwise well-fed child. There is evidence, for example, that a low serum iron, indicative of a tendency toward anemia, is of much more common occurrence among fat adolescents than among normal-weight young people of the same age.[57] Similar observations have been made concerning fat babies.

Moderately obese children and adolescents are generally characterized by intakes not in excess of the average for their age, sex and height but by drastically reduced energy expenditure. In fact, many such moderately obese youngsters may be eating somewhat less than average, but are incredibly inactive. Under these conditions, to further reduce intake in an effort to cause weight loss (or at least fat loss) may compromise growth in length. Considerable measures of success have been achieved in weight reduction programs conducted in summer camps[58] and in a school[42] where a program of vigorous *daily* physical activity was instituted, with food

habits improved by careful painstaking instruction but without prescribed caloric restriction.

In the case of extremely obese children, a degree of caloric restriction can usually be imposed without resultant impairment of growth. As with adults, instruction on diets must be conducted with food models or with real food portions, so that the concept of portion size is firmly understood. In general, small children are best indoctrinated with their mothers present. Older children and adolescents should be seen separately from their parents. If, as is often the case, the parents also have a weight problem, it is often effective to make both dieting and exercise a family affair. The obese child, often a lonely, unhappy person isolated from his or her contemporaries by the early and massive discrimination against the obese characteristic of our society, should receive as much encouragement and companionship from his family as possible.

It may be useful to restate that an estimation of fat, rather than weight, is particularly important during growth. Whereas, in adults, a weight gain usually means accumulation of fat, in growing youngsters it may mean true (protein) growth, growth and fat accumulation, fat accumulation alone and even, in some cases (particularly during the puberty "growth spurt" of boys), growth with loss of fat. It is, therefore, essential to supplement the readings of the scale with careful examination of the patient and, preferably, with skinfold measurements.

BIBLIOGRAPHY

1. Mayer: *Overweight: Causes, Cost and Control.* New York, Prentice-Hall, 1968.
2. Build and Blood Pressure Study, 1959. Chicago, Society of Actuaries, 1959.
3. Seltzer and Mayer: J.A.M.A., *201*, 221, 1967.
4. Seltzer and Mayer: J.A.M.A., *189*, 677, 1964.
5. Gertler and White: *Coronary Disease in Young Adults.* Cambridge, Harvard University Press, 1954.
6. Spain, Bradess and Greenblatt: Am. J. Med. Sci., *229*, 294, 1955.

7. Seltzer and Mayer: Postgrad. Med., *38*, A101, 1965.
8. Committee on Nutritional Anthropometry, Food and Nutrition Board, National Research Council (Keys, chairman). Recommendations concerning body measurements for the characterization of nutritional status. In *Body Measurements for Human Nutrition* (Brozek, Ed.). Detroit, Wayne University Press, 1956.
9. Seltzer, Goldman and Mayer: Pediatrics, *36*, 212, 1965.
10. Young, Tensuan, Sault and Holmes: J. Am. Diet. Assoc., *42*, 409, 1963.
11. Novak: Ann. N.Y. Acad. Sci., *110*, 545, 1963.
12. Garn and Haskell: Dis. Child., *99*, 746, 1960.
13. Johnson, Burke and Mayer: Am. J. Clin. Nutr., *4*, 231, 1956.
14. National Center for Health Statistics: Weight by height and age of adults, U.S. 1960–62. Vital and Health Statistics. Public Health Service Publication No. 1000–Series 11, No. 14. Washington, U.S. Government Printing Office, 1966.
15. Friis-Hansen: Pediatrics, *28*, 169, 1961.
16. Metropolitan Life Insurance Co., N.Y.: Frequency of overweight and underweight. Stat. Bull., *41*, 4, 1960.
17. Moore, Stunkard and Stole: J.A.M.A., *81*, 962, 1962.
18. Carpenter and Mayer: Am. J. Physiol., *193*, 499, 1958.
19. Bielschowsky and Bielschowsky: Aust. J. Exp. Biol. Med. Sci., *34*, 181, 1956.
20. Vidal and di Roberti: Medicina, *3*, 185, 1943.
21. Mayer: Physiol. Rev., *33*, 472, 1953.
22. Mayer: Nutr. Abstr. Rev., *25*, 597, 1955.
23. Bauer: *Constitution and Disease: Applied Constitutional Pathology*, 2nd ed. New York, Grune & Stratton, 1945.
24. Rony: *Obesity and Leanness*. Philadelphia, Lea & Febiger, 1940.
25. Angel: Am. J. Phys. Anthropol., 7, 433, 1949.
26. Gurney: Arch. Intern. Med., *57*, 557, 1936.
27. Fellows: Am. J. Med. Sci., *181*, 301, 1931.
28. Dunlop and Murray Lyon: Edinburgh Med. J., *38*, 561, 1931.
29. Ellis and Tallerman: Lancet, *2*, 615, 1934.
30. Iversen: Acta Paediatr. Scand., *42*, 8, 1953.
31. Fry: Am. J. Clin. Nutr., *1*, 453, 1953.
32. Hundley: *Weight Control*. Ames, Iowa State College Press, 1956.

33. Siemens: *Einfuhrung in die allgemeine und spezielle Vererbungspathologie des Menschen: Ein Lehrbuch fur Studierende und Arzte*. Berlin, Springer, 1923.
34. Newman, Freeman and Holzinger: *Twins: A Study of Heredity and Environment*. Chicago, University of Chicago Press, 1937.
35. von Verschuer: Dei vererbungsbiologische Zwillingsforschung: Ihre biologischen Grundlagen: Studien an 102 eineiigen und 45 gleichgeschlechtlichen zweieiigen Zwillingsund an 2 Drillingspaaren. Ergeb. Inn. Med. Kinderheilkd., *31*, 35, 1927.
36. Withers: Eugenics Rev., *56*, 81, 1964.
37. Bullen, Monello, Cohen and Mayer: Am. J. Clin. Nutr., *12*, 1, 1963.
38. Seltzer and Mayer: J. Am. Diet. Assoc., *55*, 457, 1969.
39. Beaudoin and Mayer: Fed. Proc., *11*, 436, 1952.
40. Johnson, Burke and Mayer: Am. J. Clin. Nutr., *4*, 37, 1956.
41. Stefanik, Bullen, Heald and Mayer: Res. Q., *32*, 229, 1961.
42. Seltzer and Mayer: Am. J. Public Health, *60*, 679, 1970.
43. Monello and Mayer: Am. J. Clin. Nutr., *13*, 35, 1963.
44. Monello and Mayer: Am. J. Clin. Nutr., *20*, 253, 1967.
45. Walker: Arch. Intern. Med., *93*, 951, 1954.
46. Bjerkedal: Acta Med. Scand., *159*, 13, 1957.
47. Mayer: Postgrad. Med., *46*, 195, 1969.
48. Marks: Diabetes, *11*, 544, 1962.
49. Hundley: J. Am. Diet. Assoc., *32*, 417, 1956.
50. Mayer: Ann. N.Y. Acad. Sci., *131*, 502, 1965.
51. Mayer: J. Am. Diet. Assoc., *52*, 13, 1968.
52. Mayer: Med. Today, *2*, 25, 1968.
53. Van Itallie and Yang: N. Engl. J. Med., *297*, 1158, 1977.
54. Anon: J.A.M.A., *238*, 2680, 1977.
55. Reisin, Abel, Modan, Silverberg, Eliahou and Modan: N. Engl. J. Med., *298*, 1, 1978.
56. Johnson and Drenick: Arch. Intern. Med., *137*, 1381, 1977.
57. Seltzer, Wenzel and Mayer: Am. J. Clin. Nutr., *13*, 343, 1963.
58. Bullen, Monello, Cohen and Mayer: Am. J. Clin. Nutr., *12*, 1, 1963.

Part V

Nutrition during "Physiologic" Stress

Chapter 26

NUTRITION IN PREGNANCY

C. E. Gibbs
and
Joseph Seitchik

Pregnancy consists of two fundamental and interdependent anabolic processes: (1) maternal physiologic and metabolic adaptations and (2) growth and maturation of the fetus and placenta. The conceptus is entirely dependent upon the mother for nutrients, and the maternal adaptations, which involve most organs, are induced by the conceptus. Because pregnancy consists of the accretion of mass in the form of increased maternal red blood cells, plasma and interstitial fluid volumes, increased weight of the uterus, breasts, fetus, placenta and amniotic fluid, it is presumed that a constant supply of nutrients and calories is required to support growth. Human fetal or neonatal death or damage resulting from severe calorie and protein deficits is demonstrable from clinical experience.[1,2] The impact of lesser degrees of nutritional deficit on fetal health is more difficult to identify[3,4] because of the ability of the mother to provide nutrients from catabolism of her own tissues[5,6] and the ability of the placenta to adapt functionally to an adverse environment.[7,8]

Successful outcome of the pregnancy may also be determined by the prepregnant nutritional condition of the mother. Within stable cultures with little in-migration, the highest fetal and neonatal losses occurred in women of shortest stature[2] whose fathers had the lowest paying jobs,[9] suggesting that restricted nutrition sufficient to reduce growth in height of the mother during childhood can limit adult reproductive capacity. Women who were lean prior to pregnancy had smaller newborns at term than those who were obese.[10,11] Although unproved in humans, protein-calorie restriction in animals, particularly rodents,[12] will result in neonates with fewer cells in many organs, particularly brain, and these animals will manifest learning disabilities if they survive (see Chapter 19). Contrariwise, Cahill[13] notes that the black bear "gestates, delivers, and nurtures her cub during a prolonged period of total starvation." Applying the results of animal experiments, particularly those obtained in species where pregnancies are characterized by brief duration and large litters, to those of human pregnancy may be illogical,[14a,14b,14c] but the possibility exists that limited nutrition of the fetus resulting from maternal malnutrition may produce permanent neonatal disability. This suggestion alone provides sufficient incentive to provide each pregnant woman with an optimal diet during her pregnancy.

The ideal pregnancy diet is undefined because ethical considerations preclude the necessary experiments. Study of changes in body composition and metabolism, the estimation of nutritional requirements from these data and clinical observations represent the only methods available. The techniques include the measure of changes in total body weight, body water, body density, oxygen consumption and protein, fat and minerals such as calcium, sodium and potassium during pregnancy,[15] as well as the assessment of newborn size, body composition and balances.[4] These studies have been conducted upon white women in the United States and Britain almost exclusively and should not be applied rigidly to all ethnic groups. The egalitarian concept of an "average woman" is appropriate for a particular ethnic group because such values are obtained by measurement. The elitist concoction of the "ideal woman," which represents an extrapolation of data derived from Scottish women, seems inapplicable to the Watusi or pygmy. The ill-considered application of this conceit can result in obstetric pathology.[16]

STATUS DURING PREGNANCY

The average woman in the United States gains about 11 kg during pregnancy.[17] Although considerable variation may be observed, maternal weight is usually added by increments of 1 to 1.5 kg in the first trimester, 4 to 5 kg from 14 to 27 weeks and 5 kg during the last 13 weeks. The approximate mean weights of known components are: fetus 3,400 gm, placenta 650 gm, amniotic fluid 800 gm, uterus 1,000 gm, breasts 400 gm, maternal blood 1,250 gm, maternal interstitial fluid 1,500 gm, for a total of 9 kg. Calculations for the extra calories required for the assembly and maintenance of the conception and the maternal anatomic and physiologic adaptations to pregnancy amount to 27,000[18,19] to 31,000[15] kcal for the whole pregnancy. These caloric needs are lowest during the first 20 weeks—approximately 60 to 70 kcal per day—and rise to 220 to 230 kcal per day at term.

As emphasized by Emerson and co-workers, the caloric requirements of pregnancy are small in comparison to those for resting metabolism, 1,200[20] to 1,470[5] per day, or for activities, 600[5] to 1,000[4] kcal per day. The total is estimated to be between 2,070 and 2,260 kcal per day. If the difference between the 9-kg weight of the identified changes in pregnancy and the 11 kg actually gained is stored fat accumulated during the first 30 weeks of pregnancy, then an additional 19,000 kcal will be required, or about 100 extra kcal per day.

Two important modifiers of the total calories recommended for pregnant women need to be considered in giving dietary advice to an individual patient: the antepartum obesity or leanness of the patient and her physical activity demands, particularly in the latter half of pregnancy. When compared to women of average weight and average weight gain, lean mothers (<110 pounds) who gain little during pregnancy (<10 pounds) produce excessive numbers of low-birth-weight (<2,500 gm) infants.[10,11] The cause of inadequate weight gain during pregnancy is difficult to identify in most cases. In some, the lack of increase in fat-free solids or body cell mass, despite adequate nutrition, suggests that the fault is with the conceptus—failure to provide adequate stimulation for complete maternal adaptations and/or failure to grow adequately. There is no evidence that providing such patients with an overabundance of calories will correct the deficiency. Contrariwise, the patient who has suffered prepregnant chronic protein and/or caloric malnutrition should benefit from correction of her dietary deficiencies during pregnancy.[21]

The data of Niswander indicate that low prepregnancy weight combined with low weight gain during pregnancy is more common and produces a greater incidence of adverse effects in black than in white women. The black group has lower economic status, perhaps implying that poor nutrition prior to pregnancy may be of more importance than low prepregnant or small intragestational weight gain per se.

Physical activity studies of pregnant women have established that *non*weight-bearing activities utilize only slightly more calories[22,23] than do the same activities in the nonpregnant state. Weight-bearing activities during pregnancy require many more calories than they do in the prepregnant state, because the pregnant woman usually weighs more and thus does more work for the same activity.[24,25] Our study[26] (Fig. 26–1) of nonpregnant, midpregnant, late-pregnant and puerperal women walking on a treadmill at the rate of 1½ miles per hour on a 6 per cent grade for 20 minutes demonstrates that the cost of working in excess of the patient's sitting basal caloric need is determined by the patient's weight and not by pregnancy. In a study of a few nulligravidas, Taggart[15] suggested that women in late pregnancy spare calories by reducing their physical activities, particularly "outside walking and strenuous activity," and by increasing time spent in bed. Women who continue to work at jobs requiring considerable weight-bearing should receive diets with increased calories and should be encouraged to spend more of their leisure time in bed or in quiet sitting. The recommendations of the Food and Nutrition Board[20] for energy and various nutrients are listed in Table A–1 in the Appendix.

Often ignored in demographic studies of pregnancy weight gain is the fact that obese nondiabetic patients produce excessive numbers of overweight newborns for their gestational ages.[27] Infants large for their gestational ages at term suffer several

The Energy Cost of Walking

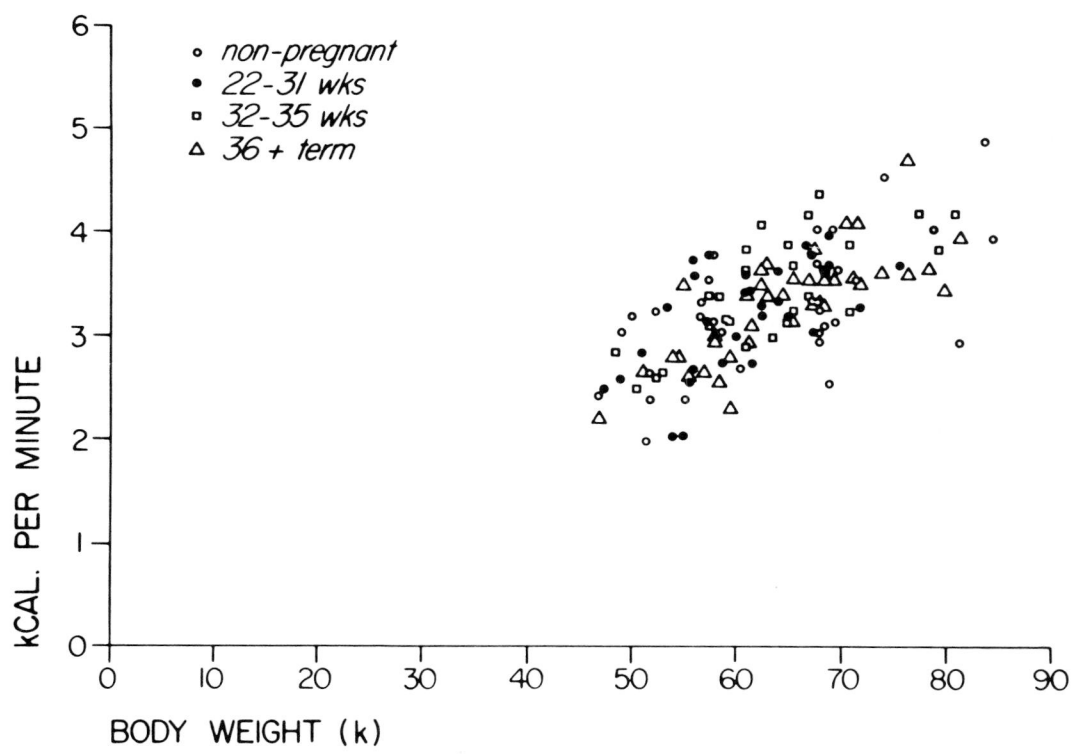

Fig. 26–1. Kilocalories expended per minute by nonpregnant and pregnant women at different stages of pregnancy walking at 1½ mph on a 6 per cent grade (see text). (From Seitchik.[26])

times the neonatal mortality rate of their average-size-for-gestation peers.[28] It has not been demonstrated that weight reduction by controlled diets reduces the incidence of overweight newborns for obese women. Studies which actually have measured body fat during pregnancy demonstrated that weight loss or small weight gain can be accomplished in a few obese women without detriment to the conceptuses.[5,6] Further, in otherwise healthy obese white women (weight 150 to 190 pounds), the mean birth weights were well within the usual range, and birth weight was insignificantly influenced by the mother's weight gain or even loss during the pregnancy. Obesity is a handicap in maintaining health and achieving longevity, and there is no evidence to suggest that obese women cannot restrict calories during pregnancy provided that the other necessary nutrients are provided.[5,29]

Protein needs are poorly defined because of differences between the results of nitrogen balance studies and body composition analyses. Early balance experiments suggested that, when pregnant women are provided with calories and protein, they accumulate quantities of nitrogen far in excess of the needs of their conceptuses and maternal adaptations.[30] Later research suggested that excess protein nitrogen is accumulated modestly[31,32] and, possibly, not at all.[33,34] Estimates of the protein mass from the components known to be accumulated during pregnancy are: fetus 440 gm, placenta 100 gm, amniotic fluid 3 gm, uterus 166 gm, breasts 81 gm, maternal blood 135 gm, for a total of 925 gm. The peak accretion rate is reached in the last trimester and approximates 6.1 gm per day. Assuming a biologic value of 70 to the protein ingested, the actual dietary need for extra protein required by pregnancy would be 8.7 gm per day. This is considerably less than the 30 gm recommended by the Food and Nutrition Board's RDA.[20]

Two physiologic phenomena suggest that recommended increases in dietary protein of the order of 8 to 9 gm per day may be insufficient for pregnant women. Urinary excretion of some essential amino acids is increased during pregnancy as a result of reduced renal tubular reabsorption.[35] The mechanism inducing this altered renal function with loss of amino acids is unknown, but it may result from the increased availability of plasma corticoids.[36] Amino acids transported by the placenta to the fetal circulation are used both for tissue anabolism and as an energy source. Approximately 50 per cent of the O_2 consumption of the ovine fetus is accounted for by the uptake of glucose,[37,38] and 25 per cent by the oxidation of lactate provided by the placenta.[39] The remaining 25 per cent is utilized in the catabolism of amino acids.[40] Thus, the RDA recommendation of 30 gm extra protein per day may be excessive and costly, but seems far safer than the marginal and possibly inadequate suggested increase of 8.5 gm.

Pritchard and McDonald[41] have emphasized the high incidence of gastrointestinal disorders, and Page[42] the muscle cramps induced by large quantities of milk in the diets of pregnant women. The former results from lactose intolerance, rather common in minority groups, and the latter from high phosphate intakes. Education of pregnant women to sources of high-quality proteins other than milk should be emphasized in prenatal care. Adequate quantities of calories added to the diets (40 gm protein and 1,500 cal) of malnourished pregnant women markedly reduced the frequency of low-birth-weight infants regardless of the protein content of the supplement.[43]

Anemias in Pregnancy

Pregnancy demands an increased supply of iron for hemoglobin synthesis because of a 30 per cent increase in the total number of maternal red blood cells, requiring 500 mg of iron, and the needs of the fetus and placenta, requiring an additional 300 mg.[44] There are two primary sources from which to meet these needs: body stores and dietary ingestion. Iron stores may be depleted prior to pregnancy and, consequently, this resource may be limited. Absorption of iron from the intestine appears to be enhanced in the latter two-thirds of the pregnancy.[45,46]

Folic acid is a cofactor in DNA synthesis and requirements are, therefore, increased whenever there is rapid cell production, as in pregnancy. Usual dietary sources are leafy vegetables, kidney, liver and peanuts. Cooking may reduce the folic acid content of foods.[47]

Iron deficiency anemia was the most common nutritional deficiency encountered in a 10-state nutritional survey.[48] As many as 25 per cent of low-income pregnant women may have hemoglobin levels below 10 gm per 100 ml during pregnancy. The causes of this deficiency are often depleted stores, an increased demand and a modest dietary intake of iron. Black individuals appear to have slightly lower hemoglobin and hematocrit values than white persons, even when income differences are eliminated. Garn et al.[49] have shown the difference may be close to 0.9 gm of hemoglobin or 2.6 per cent for the hematocrit and suggest that there may be race-specific norms for these two determinations.

Folic acid deficiency may be obscured by an associated iron deficiency. The anemia of folic acid deficiency and iron deficiency will not be corrected by adequate iron supplementation alone.

Routine iron and folic acid supplementation will be discussed in a subsequent paragraph. Specific deficiency states should be determined by appropriate clinical tests which do not usually include evaluation of iron stores by bone marrow examination.[44,47] Correction of iron deficiency anemia is possible by oral ingestion of 180 to 200 mg of elemental iron daily.[44] Rarely, the parenteral route is necessary. Folic acid deficiency is easily corrected by 1 mg or less of folic acid daily.[50]

Adolescent Pregnancy

The health problems of pregnant adolescents and their newborns have received considerable attention in recent years. The possible roles which maternal nutrition may play in the causes and effects of these problems are being investigated.[51] King et al.[52] assessed the nutritional status of a small group of poor and pregnant teenagers; using intake measurements, they found considerable deficiencies in calcium, iron, vitamin A and calories. Morse et al.[53] compared biochemical findings in three age groups of pregnant women, one of which was composed of adolescents. No specifically low levels were found in any of the three groups, but the youngest had a tendency toward lower levels than the other two groups.

Many difficulties are associated with the nutritional evaluation of adolescent patients.[54] For example, concern is expressed that the early adolescent growth spurt might be competitive with pregnancy for the available nutritional resources.[51] It is probable, however, that even the youngest pregnant women (under 16) achieve most, if not all, of their growth prior to the conception.[55]

Effort invested in nutritional assessment and counseling of these very young pregnant women may pay big dividends over the years, being profitable not only for the immediate pregnancy but for the child as it develops and for the mother in subsequent gestations. In a recent study[56] it was found that young pregnant patients of one ethnic group had very little accurate information concerning foods and nutrition.

Vitamin Deficiencies

Clinical vitamin deficiencies (aside from folate) are not commonly perceived in pregnant women in the developed countries. However, low serum levels may be common. Biochemical determinations of 13 vitamins were done in 174 pregnant women and in 68 of their newborns by Baker et al.[57] They noted levels believed to be below normal in one or more women not on supplements for 8 of the 13 vitamins. Supplementation reduced this number. Similar findings were present in some of the infants at birth. Another investigation found significant red blood cell folate deficiency in 30 per cent of 110 poor New York women.[58] The ascorbic acid levels were found to be low in many pregnant women studied in the 10-state nutritional survey.[48]

Toxic Agents and Malformation

Following the thalidomide catastrophe there has been much interest in the production of fetal anomalies by agents ingested during pregnancy. Most of this interest is centered around various drugs, but some foods have also been investigated. The great geographic differences in the frequency of neural tube defects (anencephaly), for example, have led to considerable work regarding the possible effects of potatoes[59,60] and of tea.[61] No significant relationship has been established with these or any other foods.

Pica

Pica, the craving for unnatural foods, is seen occasionally in pregnant women and is often associated with iron deficiency anemia.

Whether or not the ingestion of clay and/or starch in large amounts is a result of or causes this anemia is unclear, but most authors[62,63] have noted correction of the anemia results in a reduction of the phenomenon. Luke,[64] in a nice review of the subject, stresses the nutritional aspects of this interesting disorder. The 2:00 a.m. cravings for pizza or pickles encountered in healthy pregnant patients pose no nutri-

tional threats and, when convenient, may be satisfied.

DIET MANAGEMENT

Normal Pregnancy and Nutritional Assessment

The aim of a pregnancy diet is to supply, in the foods most available and acceptable to the patient, the recommended daily allowances of the needed calories and nutrients.[20] Those giving prenatal educational services should be aware of the cultural traditions of their patients regarding foods and weight gain, as well as the accuracy of the information they possess. For instance, many patients still are hesitant to eat well during pregnancy and need to be encouraged to do so.

Weight gain should be seen as a result of achievement of good nutritional goals. When excess calories are supplied, fat storage is usually experienced; this should be interpreted in the light of the individual's prepregnant weight. A person beginning her pregnancy underweight may have a useful gain in excess of the physiologic 11 kg mentioned previously. On the other hand, obese patients may be allowed a calorie reduction to 1,800 cal per day if it is accompanied by adequate supplies of proteins and other nutrients. This may have the effect of weight stabilization throughout pregnancy with an overall loss after delivery of 7 to 8 kg.

When *nausea and vomiting* of pregnancy occur, food should be supplied in 5 to 6 small feedings daily; in late pregnancy this schedule may again be useful.

A pregnant women should have an assessment of her nutritional status early in the antepartum course. Aubrey, Roberts and Cuenca[65] have reported their experience with a rather detailed scheme. Most physicians will make the assessment using weight at the onset of pregnancy, the absence or presence of food fads and gastrointestinal disorders, and the blood hemoglobin and hematocrit. Monitoring of weight changes is critical throughout pregnancy: a normal weight gain is a favorable index of the patient's nutritional status. The hemoglobin and hematocrit are usually repeated one or two times also.

Nutritional Supplements. The increased demand for iron described above probably is best met by supplementation with a ferrous salt. The recommended daily allowance in normal pregnancy is 18+ mg of elemental iron.[20] This cannot be met by normal diet and, therefore, supplementation with 60 to 100 mg of additional elemental iron is recommended.[41] There is some disagreement about the need for additional calcium. Hytten[66] believes that natural foods in a normal diet contain sufficient calcium for pregnancy. Pitkin[67] states that there is an increased calcium absorption in pregnancy and indicates that the 1200 mg of the RDA are easily met by a diet containing milk and/or cheese. When these two foods are minimal or absent, however, or specifically avoided as in the markedly lactose-intolerant individual, he recommends supplementation with 2 gm of a nonphosphate calcium salt daily. Duggin et al.,[68] as a result of careful balance studies in 7 women, recommend supplementation at the 2-gm level for all pregnant women. Folic acid supplement, at the rate of 800 μg a day, has been recommended for normal pregnant women.[41] This amount of the nutrient may be added without a prescription to vitamin-mineral preparations designed for pregnant or lactating women.[69] Folic acid can be added to foods with resulting improvement in a folate-poor population.[70,71]

Fluoride Supplementation. The effect of prenatally administered fluoride, either by water fluoridation or by fluoride in the form of vitamin-mineral supplements, is chiefly on the deciduous teeth of the newborn. The degree of caries prevention is probably not significantly enhanced over fluoride administration begun soon after birth. Because efficacy has not been proven, the Food and Drug Administration ban on prenatal tablets containing fluoride is still in effect.[69] There is no evidence, however, that prenatal fluoride supplementation is harmful.

Hypertensive Disorders

Elevated blood pressure is commonly encountered in obstetric patients. When it is an acute illness related only to pregnancy, it is termed pregnancy-induced hypertension (PIH), but when it is associated with convulsions it is termed eclampsia. PIH may occur spontaneously in an otherwise normal pregnant woman or it may be superimposed on chronic hypertensive or renal disorders which may be obscure. Of whatever cause, the hypertensive complications of pregnancy (toxemia of pregnancy) are a major cause of perinatal and maternal morbidity and mortality.[41]

For more than a generation the role of nutrition in the cause and treatment of PIH has engaged the minds of many persons. Evidence in support of a nutritional etiology for this disorder includes the high occurrence rate among poor women, geographic patterns coinciding with areas of known deficiency disease and/or low per capita income and nutritional disorders, such as anemia, occurring in the same population group. A specific nutritional deficiency, such as of a protein or vitamin, has not been identified. Obesity is not considered a cause, although chronic hypertensive vascular disease does occur in obese patients. Limiting weight gain during pregnancy does not prevent PIH and, in fact, may do harm to mother or baby.

PIH often is associated with marked changes in renal function, which may lead to excessive extravascular fluid retention (edema) in the presence of significant hemoconcentration. Fluid and/or sodium restriction, with or without diuretics, may not only fail to relieve the edema but may potentiate the hemoconcentration and thus the pathophysiology. The modest increase in extravascular fluid experienced in normal pregnancy does not lead to PIH and is not indicative of disease.

Until such time as the issues are clarified concerning the relationship between nutrition and PIH, it would appear that the best policy is to: (1) assure optimum caloric, protein and vitamin intake for all patients, (2) except under very unusal circumstances, allow normal sodium ingestion along with increased amounts of fluid intake, (3) avoid all diuretics.

Diabetes

The proper management of the pregnant diabetic includes an appropriate dietary prescription and schedule. As many of these patients are obese, there will be considerable temptation to reduce their caloric intake. It should be kept in mind that these pregnant women have the same nutrient needs as nondiabetics, and good nutrition should be assured.[72] It will often be necessary to adjust the diet to changing time schedules and to variable portions, because insulin requirements frequently change throughout pregnancy and control often becomes increasingly difficult. Frequent consultation among physician, dietitian and patient is necessary.

Gastrointestinal Shunts for Obesity

Bypass or shunting operations have been performed in the treatment of severe obesity. A few patients have become pregnant after such surgery. Olow et al.[73] reported their experience with 4 such patients who ate normal pregnancy diets with supplementation. Three of the 4 lost weight and the other's weight remained unchanged throughout the pregnancy. The 4 infants appeared normal and weighed between 2,700 and 3,600 gm. Taylor and O'Leary,[74a] however, in a review of a total of 13 infants born to parents with the bypass, indicated that 7 were of low birth weight. They believe that this might be related to the interval between operation and pregnancy, and suggest postponing pregnancy until after the second postsurgical year. Savel et al. reviewed 56 fullterm pregnancies in 44 patients and agree with this conclusion.[74b] Although experience is limited, it would appear that proper management of these patients would include careful monitoring of dietary intake of protein, supplementation with all the necessary vitamins and minerals and monthly hemoglobin and hematocrit determinations as a simple biochemical assessment of nutrition. Although the theory is untested, it is likely that lactation and breast feeding would not be harmful if a well-nourished infant is delivered.

Lactation

Milk letdown induced by oxytocin occurs following the initiation of lactation and is stimulated by suckling. Although the mechanism is obscure, continued milk production thereafter depends primarily on suckling and removal of the milk from the gland-duct system.

For most nutrients breast milk is not influenced significantly by the maternal diet. Protein content usually remains constant as long as maternal lean body tissues are maintained, even in the face of marked reduction of dietary protein.[75] Likewise, considerable variation in fluid intake will not change the volume of milk produced nor is the calcium content modified by dietary calcium. The type of fat in the milk may vary with the type of fat in the diet, but generally the caloric value of the milk remains constant as long as sufficient maternal resources are present.[75] Watersoluble vitamins appear in breast milk and, when the maternal diet and stores of these vitamins are depleted, the milk will become deficient. The child who is entirely dependent upon mother's milk for these nutrients might exhibit a vitamin deficiency. The fat-soluble vitamins are not excreted in the milk, nor are iron and fluoride.[76]

About 900 kcal are required to produce a liter of human milk. About one-third of these calories can be obtained from the maternal stores laid down during pregnancy. The remainder should come from dietary additions. About 100 calories should be supplied by protein. In addition, slight increases in water-soluble vitamins, folate, calcium, phosphorus and iodine are advisable[20] (Table A–1, Appendix). Most of the additional requirements for lactation can be met by a quart of milk a day.

Considerable research has been conducted on the metabolic effects of the sex steroids in oral contraceptives and the possible impact of these effects on the nutrition of the nursing infant.[77] In a recent statement of the National Research Council[78] these research efforts were discussed and analyzed. Although some reports indicate that the drugs may have some effect on the metabolism of vitamins B_6, B_{12}, A and C and on iron and copper, no particular nutritional hazards were identified nor does the report suggest any specific nutritional therapy or dietary management.

BIBLIOGRAPHY

1. Smith: J. Pediatr., 30, 229, 1947.
2. Lechtig et al.: Am. J. Obstet. Gynecol., 125, 25, 1976.
3. Osofsky: Am. J. Obstet. Gynecol., 105, 1150, 1969.
4. Habicht et al.: Size at Birth. Ciba Foundation Symposium 27. Amsterdam, Associated Scientific Publishers, 1974.
5. Emerson, Poindexter and Kothari: Obstet. Gynecol., 45, 505, 1975.
6. Seitchik: Obstet. Gynecol., 29, 155, 1967.
7. Tominaga and Page: Am. J. Obstet. Gynecol., 94, 679, 1966.
8. Beischer et al.: J. Obstet. Gynaecol., Br. Commonw., 77, 398, 1970.
9. Thompson and Billewicz: Proc. Nutr. Soc., 22, 55, 1963.
10. Peckham and Christianson: Am. J. Obstet. Gynecol., 111, 1, 1971.
11. Niswander et al.: Obstet. Gynecol., 33, 482, 1969.
12. Winick: In Nutrition and Fetal Development. New York, John Wiley and Sons, 1974.
13. Cahill: Pediatrics, 50, 357, 1972.
14a. Maternal Nutrition and the Course of Pregnancy. National Research Council, Committee on Maternal Nutrition, Food and Nutrition Board. Washington, National Academy of Sciences, 1970.
14b. Riopelle, Hale and Watts: Hum. Biol., 48, 203, 1976.
14c. Cheek, Holt, London, Ellenberg, Hill and Sever: Am. J. Clin. Nutr., 29, 1149, 1976.
15. Hytten and Leitch: In The Physiology of Human Pregnancy, 2nd ed. Oxford, Blackwell Scientific Publications, 1971.
16. Sambhi: Int. J. Gynecol. Obstet., 2, 51, 1973.
17. Chesley: Am. J. Obstet. Gynecol., 48, 565, 1944.
18. Emerson, Saxena and Poindexter: Obstet. Gynecol., 40, 786, 1972.
19. Emerson et al.: Obstet. Gynecol., 43, 354, 1974.
20. Recommended Dietary Allowances, 8th rev. ed. Washington, National Academy of Science, 1974.
21. Naeye, Blane and Paul: Pediatrics, 52, 494, 1973.
22. Bader et al.: J. Clin. Invest., 34, 1524, 1955.
23. Seitchik: Am. J. Obstet. Gynecol., 97, 701, 1967.
24. Teruoka: Arb. Physiol., 1, 259, 1933.
25. Widlund: Acta Obstet. Gynecol. Scand., 25, Suppl. 1, 1945.
26. Seitchik: Unpublished data.
27. Kerr: J. Obstet. Gynaecol., Br. Commonw., 69, 988, 1962.
28. Lubchenko, Searls and Brazie: J. Pediatr., 81, 814, 1972.
29. Jacobson et al.: Am. J. Obstet. Gynecol., 83, 1609, 1962.
30. Hunscher et al.: J. Biol. Chem., 99, 507, 1933.
31. Calloway: In Nutrition and Fetal Development (Winick, Ed.). New York, John Wiley and Sons, 1974.
32. King, Calloway and Margen: J. Nutr., 130, 772, 1973.
33. Zuspan and Goodrich: Am. J. Obstet. Gynecol., 100, 7, 1968.
34. Buckingham and Barnes: Surg. Forum, 6, 471, 1955.
35. Page et al.: Am. J. Obstet. Gynecol., 68, 110, 1954.
36. Zimmerman, Seal and Doe: J. Clin. Endocrinol. Metab., 27, 397, 1967.
37. Boyd et al.: Am. J. Physiol., 225, 897, 1973.
38. Tsoulos et al.: Am. J. Physiol., 221, 234, 1971.
39. Bard et al.: Nature, 254, 710, 1975.
40. Gresham et al.: Pediatrics, 50, 372, 1972.
41. Pritchard and Macdonald: In Williams Obstetrics, 15th ed. New York, Appleton-Century-Crofts, 1976.
42. Page and Page: Obstet. Gynecol., 1, 94, 1953.
43. Lechtig et al.: Am. J. Dis. Child., 129, 553, 1975.
44. Scott and Pritchard: Clin. Perinatol., 1, 491, 1974.
45. Svanberg: Acta Obstet. Gynecol. Scand., 48 Suppl., 1, 1975.
46. Van Campen: Fed. Proc., 33, 100, 1974.
47. Kitay and Harbort: Clin. Perinatol., 2, 255, 1975.
48. Ten State Nutrition Survey. Washington, HEW Pub. No. (H.S.M.) 72–8129, 1972.
49. Garn et al.: Am. J. Clin. Nutr., 30, 461, 1977.
50. Pritchard, Scott and Whalley: J.A.M.A., 208, 1163, 1969.
51. Weigley: J. Am. Diet. Assoc., 66, 588, 1975.

52. King et al.: Am. J. Clin. Nutr., *25*, 916, 1972.
53. Morse et al.: Am. J. Clin. Nutr., *28*, 1000, 1975.
54. McGanity: In *Nutrient Requirements in Adolescence,* WS 115 N974, 1973 (McKigney and Munro, Eds.). Cambridge, MIT Press, 1976.
55. Thomson: In *Nutrient Requirements in Adolescence,* WS 115, N974, 1973 (McKigney and Munro, Eds.). Cambridge, MIT Press, 1976.
56. Cardenas, Gibbs and Young: J. Am. Diet. Assoc., *69*, 262, 1976.
57. Baker et al.: Am. J. Clin. Nutr., *28*, 59, 1975.
58. Herbert et al.: Am. J. Obstet. Gynecol., *123*, 175, 1975.
59. Sever: Teratology, *8*, 319, 1973.
60. Nevin and Merrett: Br. J. Prev. Soc. Med., *29*, 111, 1975.
61. Fedrick: Proc. R. Soc. Med., *67*, 356, 1974.
62. Bronstein and Dollar: J. Med. Assoc. Ga., *63*, 332, 1974.
63. Whitlam: The problem of pica. Med. J. Aust., *2*, 541, 1975.
64. Luke: Am. J. Mater. Child Nurs., *2*, 97, 1977.
65. Aubry, Roberts and Cuenca: Clin. Perinatol., *2*, 207, 1975.
66. Hytten: Practitioner, *212*, 495, 1974.
67. Pitkin: Am. J. Obstet. Gynecol., *121*, 724, 1975.
68. Duggin et al.: Lancet, *2*, 926, 1974.
69. Federal Register, October 20, 1966.
70. Colman et al.: Am. J. Clin. Nutr., *28*, 465, 1975.
71. Colman et al.: Am. J. Clin. Nutr., *27*, 339, 1974.
72. Davidson: Postgrad. Med. J., *59*, 114, 1976.
73. Olow et al.: Acta Chir. Scand., *142*, 82, 1976.
74a. Taylor and O'Leary: Obstet. Gynecol., *48*, 425, 1976.
74b. Savel, Simon and Maxon: Obstet. Gynecol., *52*, 585, 1978.
75. Filer: Clin. Perinatol., *2*, 253, 1975.
76. Oseid: Clin. Obstet. Gynecol., *18*, 149, 1975.
77. Barsivala and Virkar: Contraception, *7*, 307, 1973.
78. *Oral Contraceptives and Nutrition.* National Research Council, Committee on Nutrition of the Mother and Preschool Child. Washington, National Academy of Sciences, 1975.

Chapter 27

NUTRITION IN INFANCY AND ADOLESCENCE

Selma E. Snyderman

The physician who is responsible for the diet of infants and children faces different problems in different countries and population groups. In underdeveloped countries and among the underprivileged ignorance of nutrition is profound and malnutrition is widespread; the problem is to provide adequate intakes of calories and specific nutrients. In well-developed countries, and particularly in the United States, the reverse is the case. The public has been made overconscious of nutrition—concerned about nutrients which are of no practical importance: the problems by and large are those of overnutrition and the task of the physician is to reeducate people as to what is important and what is not. Our basic knowledge—and it is far from complete—will be considered in the light of: (1) the nutritional requirements of the normal child, (2) the extent to which a margin of safety beyond these levels is desirable to promote health and (3) nutrition in pathologic conditions in which increments or decrements of particular nutrients are indicated.

PECULIARITIES OF NUTRITION IN EARLY LIFE

The phenomenon of growth involves more than an increase in size; it involves changes in function and in body composition which are reflected in nutritional requirements. These differences in requirements are seen particularly during the period of infancy, for it is then that growth is most rapid and that most of the chemical maturation is accomplished. In terms of body weight the infant needs more of all nutrients. Not only does he require the nutrients for growth but, in addition, because of his higher metabolic rate and more rapid turnover of nutrients, his requirements for maintenance are higher than those of the adult. His relatively large surface area involves relatively greater losses of heat and water through the skin. The development of the skeleton imposes special nutritive requirements. The absence of teeth requires that his food be finely subdivided. In contrast to these handicaps there are certain nutrients in regard to which he is in a favored position, having received during fetal life a surplus which is stored in the liver and which will tide him over the early months. Iron, copper and vitamin A are in this category.

Energy Requirements

The caloric requirements of the newborn infant are 2 to 3 times as great as those of the adult in terms of body weight. Average figures for boys are given in Figure 27–1, which also indicates the distribution of calories needed during the period of growth. The basal heat production of the infant is high, partly because of his relatively greater body surface, which favors loss of heat by conduction and convection, and partly because of his larger proportion of active metabolic tissue. It should be pointed out that what is commonly

CALORIC REQUIREMENTS DURING CHILDHOOD

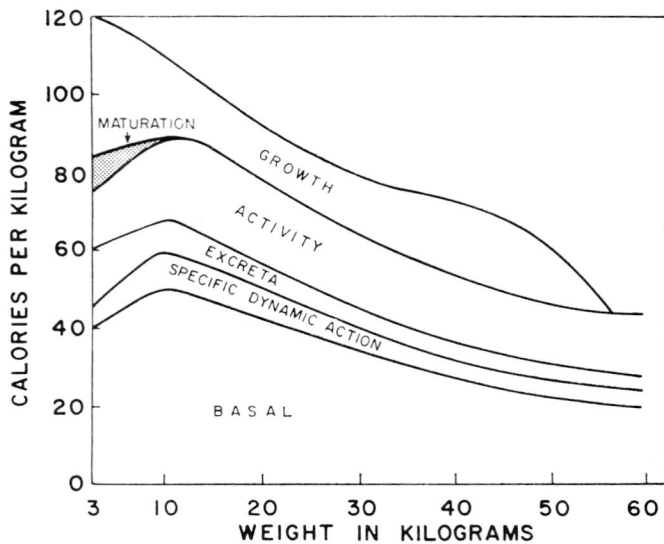

Fig. 27–1. Caloric requirements per kilogram throughout childhood. The ordinate under the upper curve shows the average requirement in calories per kilogram. The space between the curves indicates the allowance for the various factors which make up the total. (Modified from Barnett: *Pediatrics*, 15th ed. New York, Appleton-Century-Crofts, 1972.)

referred to as basal metabolism—namely, metabolism under conditions of rest—is actually not basal in the growing child, for it represents the requirement for growth as well as for maintenance. Energy required for growth is greatest in the newborn period, decreasing rapidly during the first year and more gradually up to the time of puberty, when a spurt in growth occurs. A special requirement for chemical maturation quite apart from that demanded by increase in body size exists in infancy. The requirement for activity is surprisingly great, particularly in small infants; crying alone has been shown to double the metabolic rate.[1] The energy lost in the excreta is somewhat greater in early infancy than later; this, however, represents only a small fraction of the total energy requirement. There is considerable variation in the caloric requirements of individual infants, chiefly because of differences in activity. A placid infant may thrive on as little as 70 kcal per kg, whereas one who cries a great deal may require 130 kcal or even more.

Protein Requirements

Protein is required for maintenance (wear and tear) of tissues, for growth of new tissues and for maturation of tissues. At birth, roughly 2 per cent of the body consists of nitrogen, as contrasted with a trifle over 3 per cent for the adult. Most of this change occurs during the first year. The zone of requirements for high-quality protein at different ages is shown in Figure 27–2. It would appear that breast milk, which commonly furnishes an intake ranging between 2.0 and 2.5 gm per kg, provides only a small margin of safety; however, its quality, constancy of composition and regularity of administration render this small margin adequate. Cow's milk was

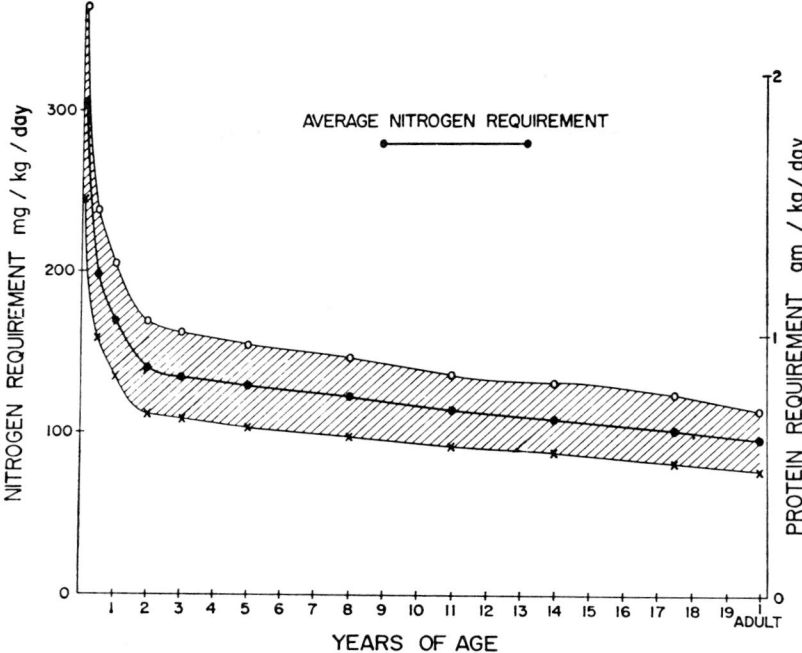

Fig. 27–2. The average nitrogen requirement during childhood. The shaded zone is designed to cover individual variations. The upper border of the zone represents a level of intake upon which virtually all individuals (95 per cent of the population) can be expected to thrive. The lower figure represents a figure below which a normal individual cannot be expected to thrive. (From Holt and Synderman: Nutr. Abstr. Rev., *35*, 1, 1965.)

formerly regarded as considerably inferior to breast milk in biologic value and for this reason higher protein intakes have been commonly given. Recent work, however, has shown that when cow's milk is processed to avoid curd indigestion the protein is utilized virtually as efficiently as that of breast milk, and that intakes greater than 2.5 gm per kg are not necessary even in the early months of life.

As infancy advances the curve of protein requirement falls off sharply, more sharply than the curve for caloric requirement. The reason for this is that activity is now the major function for which calories are required, and activity, unlike growth and maintenance, does not involve additional expenditure of nitrogen.[2] The widely used formula that 15 per cent of the total calories should consist of protein, a

proportion which obtains in most American diets at all ages, appears to provide well in excess of minimal requirements in infancy and even more as the child grows older. It should be borne in mind, however, that in the case of older children taking a mixed diet an allowance must be made for irregularities of intake and deficiencies of mastication. An increase of 25 per cent to cover this is not excessive.

Beyond this, an allowance must finally be made for protein quality on diets in which a major portion of the protein is of vegetable origin. On mixed American and European diets increasing the intake by the factor 1.2 should suffice, but as the quality of the protein declines, as may be the case in underdeveloped areas where the chief reliance is upon a single vegetable protein, the quantity may need to be doubled. This may not be practicable because of the large quantity of food required; in such situations manifestations of protein deficiency are commonly encountered.

Amino Acid Requirements

It has been generally accepted since the time of Mendel[3] that the limiting factors in protein diets are the essential amino acids, from which it follows that adequacy of a diet could be obtained by providing a diet which met the minimum requirements of each essential amino acid. Much effort has been expended in determining individual requirements of the essential amino acids at different ages so that these figures could be applied in practical dietetics. It now appears that the figures are of limited usefulness, since they were determined under special conditions and are not applicable to many other conditions. The amino acid requirements of adults[4-26] and older children[27-31] were determined under conditions of maximum sparing of the essential amino acids, generous caloric intakes and generous provision of "unessential" nitrogen (unessential amino acids and ammonium salts) to minimize the utilization of essential amino acids for energy or for the synthesis of unessential amino acids. The figures obtained no doubt represent close approximations to absolute minima but, when applied to natural diets of high protein quality, it appears that these minimum figures may have to be doubled or more than doubled before the protein needs of the organism are met.[32] The limiting factor in most human diets appears to be not an essential amino acid but nitrogen—essential or unessential.[33,34] As the quality of the protein diet deteriorates, the discrepancy between the adequacy of the diet and the minimal essential amino acid requirement values diminishes and, of course, when it comes to the seriously deficient proteins upon which Mendel's concept was based, the essential amino acids are indeed limiting.

The studies of essential amino acid requirements of infants[35-44] were not determined under conditions of maximum sparing, the experimental diets employed being based on the pattern of human milk. The values obtained, though of greater practical value, may not represent absolute minimal requirements.

Amino Acid Patterns and Biologic Values

There is no doubt that the nutritional quality of a protein food or a protein diet is determined by its amino acid *pattern* and primarily by its pattern of essential amino acids. Supplementation of a diet with a single amino acid will often result in improved growth performance. In the past, this phenomenon has been attributed to an effect of the supplement upon the *content* of that particular amino acid in the diet; a deficiency was being met. However, with our growing knowledge of interrelations among amino acids, particularly the competition of certain related amino acids for transport systems, it seems that the benefits of supplementation can be attributed to correction of an amino acid imbalance rather than to meeting a deficiency in an absolute requirement—to an approach to a more ideal amino acid pattern.

A number of efforts to delineate an ideal amino acid pattern as a standard of reference have been made. In a consideration of the subject by a joint committee of FAO and WHO[32] the conclusions were reached that no artificial pattern was superior to that of whole egg or human milk and that it was not possible to say that the pattern of one of these foods was superior to that of the other.

Several scoring procedures have been devised to evaluate the nutritional quality of a diet from its amino acid pattern. Although of some value, these procedures, as we have pointed out elsewhere, are subject to considerable errors. As a guide to the quality of the protein of a diet it is necessary to evaluate that diet by criteria discussed elsewhere in this volume, notably those based on nitrogen balance (biologic value and net protein utilization). It is preferable that such data be determined for the species under consideration and the time of life for which their application is desired. Although there is marked parallelism between protein quality as evaluated in the rat and man, there are notable exceptions. The rat, for example, makes a rather poor showing on human milk.

Fat Requirement

There is a dietary requirement for essential fatty acids. Undesirable consequences have followed the long-continued use of fat-free diets. Chwalibogowski[45] fed two infants on a fat-free diet for over a year. Their clinical courses and development did not appear abnormal, but there was some evidence of rickets. Hansen and Wiese[46] maintained a child with chylothorax on a fat-free diet for 2 years and observed increased frequency of skin infections and the development of eczema. Later they studied a large group of infants[47] maintained on a fat-free diet in whom scaly dermatitis developed; a number of infants also had loose stools and unsatisfactory weight gain. These manifestations were cured by the addition of small amounts of polyunsaturated fatty acids to the diet. The essentiality of linoleic acid has been emphasized by the appearance of symptoms of deficiency during the use of fat-free intravenous nutrition in young infants.[48,49] Although the exact requirement for linoleic acid is not known, there is evidence that when it comprises 1 per cent of the caloric intake fatty acid deficiency is prevented.[50]

The older pediatric literature contains many references to the deleterious action of volatile (short-chain) fatty acids, and their higher concentration in cow's milk was long blamed for some of the shortcomings of artificial feeding. It now appears, however, that the short-chain fats are digested as well as, if not better than, their long-chain analogs. Short-chain fats and fats containing unsaturated linkages are somewhat more readily absorbed.[51,52] In feeding normal infants it appears desirable to include a certain amount of fat in the diet, but a strong case for feeding particular fats cannot be made, for the differences are small. In conditions of steatorrhea, however, the superior absorption of certain fats such as medium-chain triglycerides appears to have some practical advantage.

There has been a good deal of interest, recently, in the possible prevention of arteriosclerosis later in life by altering the fat intake in infancy. The cholesterol content of human milk is considerably higher than that of cow's milk, and this is reflected in the plasma cholesterol level of infants; that of artificially fed infants is significantly lower.[53] Although it has been suggested that a higher cholesterol intake may be beneficial, in that it may stimulate the development of homeostatic mechanisms for the control of cholesterol levels,[54,55] there is no evidence that adults who were breast fed have lower cholesterol levels than those who were not.[56] The intake of considerable amounts of cholesterol in infancy has also been advocated as necessary for myelin formation; this could be questioned, since the infant brain can synthesize cholesterol from glucose.[57] On the other hand, there is no information about the late beneficial results of limitation of fat intake in infancy and, in addition, this may be difficult to accomplish because the low satiety value of skim milk may result in a high protein intake and an excessive renal solute load.

Carbohydrate Requirement

Although infants have been fed on carbohydrate-free diets for many months,[45] this is not a practical procedure. The development of ketosis is difficult to avoid. As a rule, roughly half of an infant's caloric requirement is supplied as carbo-hydrate.

Mineral Requirements

These are, for the most part, not accu-rately defined. With the exception of iron, the breast-fed infant appears to be adequately provided with minerals, and it may be assumed that the quantities in-gested are well above his minimal re-quirements. A 12-pound infant ingesting 800 ml breast milk per day would receive the quantities of minerals indicated in Table 27-1. Deficits of these minerals do not ordinarily arise from inadequate in-take; they may, however, result from pathologic processes in which there are abnormal losses of electrolytes from the gastrointestinal tract, kidney and, at times, skin. A dietary requirement for oxidized sulfur does not appear to exist. If the protein intake is adequate, oxidation of the sulfur derived from the sulfur-amino acids will meet all the body's needs for sulfur.

The only important mineral deficiency likely to be encountered in the normal infant is that of iron. This may be the most common nutritional deficiency of infancy; the exact prevalence depends on the criteria used for diagnosis.[58] The iron con-tent of both cow's and breast milk is simi-lar, 0.5 to 1 mg per 100 calories. The much lower incidence of iron deficiency in breast-fed infants is presumably related to the better absorption of the iron. It is current practice to give supplemental iron either in the formula or as a reinforced cereal. An iron intake of 1 mg per kg per day, to a total of 15 mg, has been recom-mended.[59] This fulfills the requirement and allows for variations in absorption and in iron stores. This supplementation should be initiated before 4 months of age.

Under exceptional circumstances, when a milk-free diet must be used, fortification of the diet with calcium may be advisable. An intake of 200 to 300 mg per day appears to be adequate.

A factor complicating the exact deter-mination of mineral requirements is the phenomenon of "supermineralization." When more mineral is given more is re-tained, and the body may become, for a time at least, somewhat richer in mineral. This phenomenon is particularly striking with calcium and phosphorus, and it ap-pears that hyperalimentation of these ele-ments may temporarily increase their stor-age in the bones. Whether this is beneficial or not is not established. Although claims have been made that a generous calcium intake prevents osteoporosis in later life, some observations made in animals[60,61] suggest that calcium more rapidly acquired during the growth period is more loosely held in adult life and may predispose to senile osteoporosis. Evidence that this holds for man is not available.

The requirements of children for the trace elements—copper, manganese, cobalt, selenium, silicon, vanadium and zinc—are not known with accuracy. The possibility that zinc deficiency may occur with some degree of frequency in arti-

Table 27-1.   Infant Mineral Intake from Breast Milk

	mg/day	mg/kg/day	mM/day	mM/kg/day	Per Cent of Intake Retained*
Na	120	21.6	5.2	0.95	40–55
K	420	75.7	10.8	1.96	20–30
Ca	250	45.0	6.2	1.13	15–20
Mg	30	5.4	1.2	0.22	20–30
Cl	330	59.2	8.4	1.53	20–30
P	200	36.0	6.4	1.16	15–20

* According to Swanson: Am. J. Dis. Child., 43, 10, 1932.

ficially fed infants has been suggested by the findings of reduced plasma zinc levels and a slower rate of growth; the condition was corrected with the use of a zinc supplement.[62] Although the zinc content of human and cow's milk is similar, zinc deficiency has not been described in breast-fed infants; zinc may be more readily available since it is bound to a low-molecular-weight fraction.[63] Iodine is discussed elsewhere (Chapter 9, Section B).

The intake of fluoride has recently assumed considerable importance. An excess of this element leads to discoloration and mottling with increased brittleness of the dental enamel (fluorosis), whereas a deficiency predisposes to dental caries. The margin of safety between the two is relatively small. It has been estimated that, if drinking water contains less than 1 ppm of fluoride, cariogenic effects may be expected. A concentration between 1.0 and 1.5 ppm is thought to be ideal.[64] Concentrations up to 2 ppm may lead to white mottling; beyond this level, brown mottling and fragility of teeth may be encountered. Milk itself may contain as much as 2 ppm of fluoride, but this does not lead to fluorosis since the fluoride exists in an insoluble form. The control of the fluoride content of drinking water has become a public health problem (see Chapter 30); it is of particular importance during the period of dental development.

Vitamin Requirements

The requirements of infants for the vitamins which are established as dietary essentials are as follows:

Vitamin A	Not accurately known 1,500 I.U. per day is definitely protective
Vitamin C	25–35 mg per day[65,66]
Vitamin D	200 I.U. per day[66]
Thiamin	0.20 mg per day[67]
Riboflavin	0.50 mg per day[68]
Pyridoxine	0.50 mg per day[69]

The requirement for nicotinic acid is a conditional one. If the intake of tryptophan is sufficient, it appears that the nicotinic acid required can be synthesized from this source. However, when the protein intake is marginal, nicotinic acid must be supplied as such. The requirement is commonly expressed in terms of niacin equivalents, 60 mg of tryptophan being equivalent to 1 mg niacin. The requirement for choline is also conditional. With a sufficient intake of methionine the needs of the body for additional choline appear to be insignificant, but when the intake of methionine is limited choline becomes a dietary factor of importance. The quantitative relationships between these conditionally required factors and their antecedents remain to be accurately defined.

It would appear that extremely small amounts of folic acid and B_{12} are needed by the human organism. B_{12} requires no consideration in the infant's diet, nor does folic acid, provided the diet contains an adequate amount of vitamin C and antibiotics are not being given.

In infant feeding ascorbic acid and vitamin D are the chief vitamins which merit concern. Milk provides limited amounts of these vitamins, and in sterilization much of the ascorbic acid is destroyed; hence, it is regarded as good practice to provide the daily requirement by means of a vitamin supplement or by orange or tomato juice. A number of proprietary feedings are now fortified with adequate amounts of C.

Vitamin D should be supplied, since neither human or cow's milk can be relied on completely to furnish adequate amounts of this vitamin. An explanation for the lower incidence of rickets in breast-fed infants has been found recently: Vitamin D is present as a water-soluble conjugate with sulfate.[70]

Vitamin A deficiency is seen in infants only under exceptional circumstances, as when skim milk has been employed for feeding for a prolonged period.

On the basis of the peroxide reaction,[71] it has been claimed that vitamin E deficiency exists in many premature infants and in certain forms of steatorrhea, notably cystic fibrosis of the pancreas.[72] As yet it has not been possible to establish beyond question clinical benefit from supplementation with vitamin E in these conditions. Instances of a macrocytic anemia with multinucleated erythroblasts in the bone marrow have been reported in patients with kwashiorkor[73] who have responded to the administration of vitamin E and some of its congeners. A symptom complex consisting of edema, anemia, reticulocytosis and thrombocytosis, which is responsive to vitamin E therapy, has been described. It occurred in small premature infants fed a proprietary formula supplemented with iron and with a high content of polyunsaturated fatty acids. Presumably, the increased vitamin E requirement associated with this type of fat was further increased by oxidation by the iron in the gastrointestinal tract.[74]

Vitamin K deficiency occurs in various clinical conditions associated with malabsorption from the intestine, liver disease or prolonged oral antibiotic therapy. It is commonly recommended that a single dose, not to exceed 2 mg, be given after birth as prophylaxis for hemorrhagic disease of the newborn.

At one time pyridoxine deficiency was observed in infants given a proprietary feeding which had been subjected to unusual thermal treatment.[69] This defect was soon corrected and, with the recognition of this possible deficiency, it appears unlikely that it will recur.

Water Requirement

The infant is peculiarly susceptible to lack of water. His obligatory water loss through the kidney and the skin is considerably greater than that of the adult, and in addition he is far more subject to pathologic processes causing water loss, notably vomiting and diarrhea. Symptoms of dehydration appear rapidly and have serious consequences. For the healthy infant in a temperate climate, the minimum water requirement is probably in the neighborhood of 75 ml per kg. A daily intake of 150 ml per kg (2¼ ounces per pound) may be regarded as providing an adequate margin of safety,[75] but under subtropical or tropical conditions it may have to be increased to 175 ml per kg or even more.

INFANT AND CHILD FEEDING

Overnutrition in Childhood

The emphasis on nutrition in well-developed countries has all been directed to the prevention of dietary deficiencies, the objective being to meet nutritional requirements and to provide, in addition, a generous margin of safety. This margin of safety has a twofold purpose: to compensate for the defects in our knowledge of requirements and to build up stores of specific nutrients that can be drawn upon to combat future situations of stress. The possibilities of overnutrition with specific nutrients have received relatively little attention. An approach to an optimal diet—or rather an optimal range of nutrient intakes—requires a critical consideration of the risks as well as the advantages of generous margins for safety.

Needs for specific nutrients must be established by surveys in which both physical status and dietary intake are measured. Laboratory criteria of deficiency, when applied, must be based not on deviations from an average of a healthy population but on correlations with clinical deviations from health. Generosity in a margin of safety should bear some relation to the risk of deficiency. Finally, the extent to which effective reserves can be stored by a generous diet must be critically examined. In the case of calories, reserves of flesh can be accumulated that are effective against future situations of caloric deficit. When it comes to specific nutrients, this does not necessarily follow. Much has been written about protein "reserves" but, if reserves are to be defined as "a moiety retained by intakes above the minimal adequate that is effective against some form of stress," evidence of the reality of protein reserves is difficult to find. Halac[76,77] and Holt et al.[78] were unable to demonstrate such reserves in rats. Carbohydrate reserves in the form of glycogen are real but transitory. Fat reserves in the form of adipose tissue are synonymous with caloric reserves.

The situation as to reserves of minerals and vitamins is far from clear, and needs much further study. That fat-soluble vitamins can be stored in body fat for long periods is clear enough, but in the case of the water-soluble vitamins the quantities stored effectively and their duration in the body are still largely unknown; the same is true for the minerals. Even when it can be shown that the body contains more of a particular nutrient after a high intake, it does not follow that this constitutes a useful reserve. With deprivation it may be excreted faster and the end-result may be no different.

The effects of overnutrition in the pediatric age group have received some attention. Obesity in the infant is said to predispose to obesity in the older child and adult, often causing psychologic problems and, in many instances, being caused by them. A vicious cycle may thus develop, the remote results of which, as far as health is concerned, become apparent only in adult life. Obesity occurring before puberty seems to be associated with a marked degree of fat cell hyperplasia, while that developing later is accompanied by cell hypertrophy.[79] The relationship of this hyperplasia to predisposition to obesity later in life needs further clarification.

Overnutrition with protein, apart from specific hypersensitivities to foods, may, under certain circumstances, cause difficulty. "Protein fever,"[80] described in infants on high-protein diets, was actually dehydration fever, the result of an increased demand for water to excrete urea. A sudden shift from a low- to a high-protein intake may cause difficulty, because increased activity of the enzymes of the urea cycle, a needed response to a high-protein intake, has not had time to take place. Temporary loss of appetite and failure to gain weight may occur.

The pediatric literature contains many references to fat intolerance attributed to an excess of fat in the diet, the presenting symptom being steatorrhea. At the present time, it is more generally believed that the loss of intestinal tolerance for fat is not induced by fat feeding but is merely demonstrated by it. Steatorrhea per se is not an indication for reducing the fat intake. The fat lost in the stool does no harm in transit; it does not appear to wash out other nutrients.[81] The real indications for reducing the fat intake are ketosis, lipemia and fatty liver.

An excessive proportion of carbohydrate in the diet of infants and young children led to a syndrome described by German pediatricians as Mehlnährschaden, a picture which we now describe as kwashiorkor or prekwashiorkor and which we attribute to a deficiency of protein rather than to an excess of carbohydrate.

Acute toxic episodes occur occasionally as a result of ingesting a large quantity of some mineral. Occasionally, the use of an iron tonic in excess gives rise to hemosiderosis.

Hypervitaminosis is seen particularly with the fat-soluble vitamins, which cannot be readily excreted in the urine. Hypervitaminosis A, though relatively uncommon, is seen from time to time as the result of the administration of a vitamin concentrate in spoonful rather than drop quantities. Hypervitaminosis D, common for a time in England and on the continent of Europe, is today less common, now that attention has been called to it. Hemolytic disease of the newborn, from excessive vitamin K administration, is now rarely seen. The tolerance of the body for water-soluble vitamins is such that large excesses can be taken with apparent impunity.

Little is known about possible remote effects of overnutrition of specific nutrients in humans. It may be suspected that untoward results such as those observed in animals[82] may occur, but the evidence is not at hand.

Breast Feeding

Many good and some poor arguments are adduced in support of breast feeding, and the subject is surrounded with a certain amount of emotionalism. For most mothers, successful nursing is a satisfying emotional experience and, for that reason, it is to be encouraged unless there are reasons to the contrary. From the point of view of the welfare of the child, the writer is not impressed with the views of certain psychiatrists that failure to nurse at the mother's breast will cause emotional deprivation and subsequent psychologic maladjustment. The advantage to the child is in the somatic field. The strongest argument for maternal nursing is that it is a relatively foolproof method. When artificial feeding is carried out under ideal conditions—by an intelligent and careful mother or nurse, under experienced medical guidance and with a milk supply that is beyond question—the risk is negligible, but under less ideal conditions the infant may suffer and the morbidity and mortality of the artificially fed infant may run far ahead of the breast fed. It is obvious that in some countries, in some areas and with some groups of people the encouragement of nursing is a matter of the greatest importance. A rare contraindication to the use of breast milk is the onset of hyperbilirubinemia, from the presence of pregnane-3 (alpha), 20 (beta)-diol. This steroid inhibits hepatic glucuronyl transferase activity in the newborn.[83]

Breast Feeding versus Breast Milk. The question of the extent to which the overall superior results with breast feeding is due to the safety of the method or to the superior nutritional qualities of breast milk is much debated. Adequate data on infants artificially fed on human milk obtained from a breast-milk dairy would settle the matter, but such data are not available. In their absence, conclusions must be drawn from data where artificial feeding is carried out under ideal circumstances and from biochemical and nutritional studies of the two milks. As stated above, the results of ideal artificial feeding appear to be comparable to those of breast feeding. It can be stated with assurance that the important nutritional differences have been overcome. It is possible, however, that factors of minor importance remain to be discovered in which breast milk may possess some small advantage. One or two claims for such substances[84,85] have recently been made, but await confirmation. The possibility that local immunity of the gastrointestinal tract may be enhanced by cellular and secretory immune factors contained in breast milk[86–88] has recently received a good deal of attention and is presently under study.

Practical Considerations in Breast Feeding. If the mother is healthy and the child is receiving an adequate quantity of milk—something that can be determined by periodic weighing before and after nursing—it can be assumed that he will be adequately nourished. After the second month, a supplement of iron should be provided, usually in the form of solid food, since human milk is deficient in iron and the hepatic stores present at birth have been exhausted. Vitamin supplements providing C and D are commonly given to breast-fed infants, not so much because of the risk of deficiency during this period as because of the risk that, at weaning, these supplements may be overlooked unless they have become habitual.

Details of the technique of breast feeding may be found in standard pediatric texts.

Artificial Feeding

Successful artificial feeding with cow's milk involves three problems: (1) meeting the nutritional requirements of the child, (2) avoiding certain mechanical difficulties of digestion caused by the curd of the milk and (3) avoiding pathogenic microorganisms. The bacteriologic problem is solved by heat treatment of the milk—pasteurization, boiling or autoclaving—and by scrupulous care of the utensils, nipples and bottles, all of which are heat sterilized. Cleanliness on the part of the mother or nurse in preparing and giving the feeding is also essential.

The curd problem, too, is conveniently solved by heating the milk. This causes the lactalbumin to coagulate in fine particles; the subsequent coagulation of the casein in the infant's stomach occurs about these micelles and the resulting curd is friable and easily digestible rather than tough and resistant. The beneficial effect varies with the amount of heat applied. Pasteurization improves the digestibility of the curd, but does not overcome the difficulty as completely as does boiling or autoclaving.

Table 27–2. Average Percentage Composition of Mature Breast Milk and Cow's Milk*

Constituents	Breast Milk (per cent)		Cow's Milk (per cent)	
Water	87.6		87.2	
Total solids	12.4		12.3	
Protein	1.1		3.3	
Casein		0.4		2.7
Lactalbumin		0.4		0.4
Lactoglobulin		0.2		0.2
Fat	3.8		3.8	
Lactose	7.0		4.8	
Ash	0.21		0.71	
Sodium		.015		.058
Potassium		.055		.138
Calcium		.034		.126
Magnesium		.004		.013
Iron		.00021		.00015
Chlorine		.043		.100
Phosphorus		.016		.099
Sulfur		.014		.030
Vitamin content per 100 ml				
Vitamin A	53.00 μg		34.00 μg	
Carotenoids	27.00 μg		38.00 μg	
Thiamin	16.00 μg		42.00 μg	
Riboflavin	43.00 μg		157.00 μg	
Nicotinic acid	172.00 μg		85.00 μg	
Pyridoxine	11.00 μg		48.00 μg	
Pantothenic acid	196.00 μg		350.00 μg	
Folic acid	0.18 μg		0.23 μg	
Choline	9.00 mg		13.00 mg	
Inositol	39.00 mg		13.00 mg	
Biotin	0.40 μg		3.50 μg	
B_{12}	0.18 μg		0.56 μg	
Vitamin C	4.30 mg		1.80 mg	
Vitamin D	0.4–10.0 I.U.†		0.3–4.0 I.U.†	
Vitamin K	26 D.G. units‡		100 D.G. units‡	
Calories per ounce	22		21	
Calories per 100 ml	71		69	

* Taken largely from National Research Council Bulletin No. 254, 1953.
† International units
‡ Dam-Glavind units

However, terminal sterilization by raising the milk to the boiling temperature in the feeding bottles is routine practice, so that, even when fresh pasteurized milk is used, the subsequent heat treatment takes care of the curd problem. The all-important consideration is the nutritive property of the feeding, a consideration of which demands some knowledge of the differences between cow's milk and breast milk.

Differences between Breast Milk and Cow's Milk. As is shown in Table 27–2, cow's milk is richer in protein by reason of its higher content of casein; it is comparable in fat content, although the content of polyunsaturated fatty acids is sometimes lower. It contains considerably less sugar (lactose). Its mineral content is higher, individual minerals being from 3 to 5 times as abundant as in breast milk. Most vitamins, too, are present in higher concentrations in cow's milk, exceptions being vitamins C and D and nicotinic acid.

Provided the bacteriologic problem and the mechanical problem of the curd are taken care of by the heat treatment, undiluted and unmodified cow's milk can be and often is used for infant feeding and with success. Such difficulties as are attributed to it are of a minor nature. It may require a few days for the infant to adapt to the higher protein intake if a change to whole cow's milk is suddenly made. It has also been pointed out[89,90] that, because of the higher protein and mineral content of cow's milk, infants so fed have a greater obligatory water requirement for renal excretion; hence, with the same fluid intake they have a slightly smaller margin of safety against dehydration. For these reasons, and also because of tradition based on experience before the curd problem was solved, the general practice has continued of diluting cow's milk to reduce its protein content, the caloric deficit being made up with a carbohydrate supplement.

Modified Milks. In the United States, formulas employing diluted evaporated milk supplemented with sugar were the most common form of artificial feeding until about ten years ago. Most recently a number of ready-to-feed products have been introduced and widely accepted. Their great convenience and almost universal use in hospitals have stimulated the use of these feedings. They are available both in disposable bottles that supply a single feeding and more recently in 32-ounce containers. Although the latter form has reduced the cost somewhat, it is still considerably more expensive than formulas prepared at home using evaporated milk.

Commonly used and convenient modifications are the following:

```
Evaporated milk  . . . . . . . . . . . . . . 3 oz
Water  . . . . . . . . . . . . . . . . . . . . . 7 oz
Cane sugar  . . . . . . . . . . . . . . . . . . ½ oz
                                              10 oz


Whole milk  . . . . . . . . . . . . . . . . . 7 oz
   (or reconstituted whole milk
   prepared from milk powder)
Water  . . . . . . . . . . . . . . . . . . . . . 3 oz
Cane sugar (1 tbsp)  . . . . . . . . . ½ oz
                                              10 oz
```

These formulas, approximately isocaloric with breast milk, furnish 20 calories to the ounce. The percentage distribution of calories in breast milk, cow's milk and in a widely employed modification is as follows:

	P	F	C
Breast milk	8%	50%	42%
Cow's milk	20%	51%	29%
Common milk modification	15%	35%	50%

The range in percentage distribution of calories which can be used successfully in infant feeding is a wide one, there being no need to simulate closely the composition of breast milk, as was once thought necessary. By tradition, more protein is commonly given to artificially fed infants, but, as pointed out above, the difference in biologic value between the proteins of breast milk and cow's milk is a negligible one. Experience with feedings providing only 10 per cent of the calories as protein has been altogether satisfactory.

Carbohydrates commonly used as supplements in artificial feeding are cane sugar, lactose and maltose-dextrin mixtures. There would seem to be little choice among them. Starch and cereals may also be used, although their absorption is slightly less complete.

The heat treatment used in destroying bacteria in milk and in rendering the curd more digestible also exerts some untoward effects on the nutritive properties of the milk, which may have to be repaired. Most important is the loss of vitamin C; much of this is lost during pasteurization and more during terminal sterilization; hence, all artificially fed infants should be given a supplement of 25 mg ascorbic acid in some form. Boiling the milk destroys some thiamin, and autoclaving even more; this vitamin is, however, amply supplied in cow's milk and, unless autoclaving has been unduly prolonged (a half hour or more), the loss is not serious. Autoclaving milk also causes some destruction of pyridoxal, the chief form of vitamin B_6 present in milk. As ordinarily carried out in the processing of evaporated milk, the loss is not serious. At high temperatures several of the amino acids, notably lysine, may react with the lactose of the milk, forming compounds which render the amino acid unutilizable by the body although still present by analysis. This so-called Maillard or "browning" reaction assumes significant proportions only when liquid milk has been subjected to autoclaving for a half hour or more. The possibility of thermal inactivation of a fraction of the protein is, however, a reason for using a protein intake slightly higher than that of breast milk. In the preparation of evaporated milk it has been estimated that about 11 per cent of the lysine has been inactivated.[91] Lysine is, however, present in cow's milk protein in a somewhat higher concentration than in breast milk protein and does not appear to be a limiting amino acid.[92]

A number of ready-to-use formulas are now available. They are usually modifications of nonfat cow's milk with vegetable oil and added lactose or corn syrup solids. The "humanized" products imitate the composition of breast milk by adding demineralized whey and modifying the mineral content. Several products supplemented with iron are also available. Sufficient vitamins are added to all so that such supplementation is unnecessary when the infant is taking enough of the formula. All of these products are nutritionally adequate, and the superiority of the humanized products is questionable. Any advantage to whey protein for the full-term infant has not been demonstrated; however, the reduced mineral content may be a consideration in the feeding of infants with special problems, such as renal or cardiac disease.

Practical Infant Feeding. Feedings for an entire day are usually prepared at one time and put into the feeding bottles, which are then terminally sterilized by standing in boiling water for 10 minutes and refrigerated until used. The necessity of carrying out this procedure has been recently questioned. Under standard conditions prevailing in American cities (a pure municipal water supply and excellent milk hygiene), there would beem to be a minimal risk of contaminating a feeding with a pathogenic organism. Fischer[93] observed no untoward effects from omitting terminal sterilization in data obtained in Philadelphia under conditions of good pediatric care and Vaughan[94] showed that no differences could be obtained even in an underprivileged group in Georgia. Other pediatricians,[95] however, have viewed this innovation with alarm. Before feeding the infant the bottle is commonly warmed to body temperature, although it has been shown that such warming also is unnecessary.[96]

The technique of feeding is important. The rubber nipple (which must be sterilized before use) must have an opening wide enough to permit the milk to drop out of the bottle without shaking. Smaller nipples cause the baby to suck in much air and may lead to vomiting. It is also important to hold the bottle at such an angle that the nipple is always full of milk and to hold the baby vertical for a few moments after feeding to enable him to "burp" and bring up swallowed air. Regularity of feeding, though it need not be made a fetish, on the whole is to be desired, as it is with breast feeding. Some latitude may, however, be given the child as to the quantity he takes at each feeding. As a rule his appetite is an excellent guide to follow.

In planning artificial feeding for a baby one should: (1) estimate the caloric requirements from the weight (roughly 100 calories per kg), (2) estimate the daily quantity of formula needed from a knowledge of the calories furnished by the formula, (3) divide this by the number of feedings desired.

Most babies will require 6 feedings a day, which may be given at 4-hour intervals around the clock. At the age of 2 months a night feeding can usually be omitted and only 5 feedings given. It is wise to check the calculation of the formula to make sure that an adequate protein allowance (2.5 gm per kg) and water allowance (150 per kg) are provided.

An initial artificial feeding is always in the nature of an experiment. An individual baby may need more or less than the calculated requirement. A steady weight gain and the appearance of health are the best indications of success. *Provided air swallowing and consequent distention of the stomach are avoided,* the baby's appetite can usually be relied upon as to the quantity of food needed. If he steadily refuses some of his bottle, he probably needs less and, if he drinks it ravenously and cries before mealtime, he probably needs more.

The artificially fed infant should be given a supplement containing 25 mg ascorbic acid and vitamin D in some form to ensure an intake of 400 I.U. a day. A need for other vitamin supplements on an ordinary milk formula has not been established. Cereals and homogenized baby foods can be fed by spoon at any age, replacing a portion of the formula feeding, but there is no particular advantage in giving them to small infants. Their purpose is twofold: to provide iron and to educate the child to accept solid foods. Since the iron stored at birth takes care of the needs of the early weeks, a good case cannot be made for giving iron before the age of 2 months. Training to eat solid foods is likewise readily accomplished at the age of 3 or 4 months; it should not be delayed beyond the first half year.

On the other hand, there is no advantage to the very early introduction of solid foods; this practice has been increasing since many parents seem to consider it an important milestone in the infants' developmental progress. The possibility that such foods provide a surfeit of calories and lead to obesity has been suggested by a number of individuals.[97,98] A great variety of canned meats, vegetables, fruits and soups is now available for infants. As these are introduced, calculation of calories becomes highly inaccurate and feeding by appetite becomes the rule.

By the age of 7 or 8 months it should be possible to reduce meals to 4 a day, the last one being milk alone, and by the age of a year 3 meals a day should suffice. As teeth come in, the need for homogenized foods disappears.

Digestive Disturbances

A discussion of the causes, pathologic physiology and therapy of acute and chronic digestive disturbances is beyond the scope of this chapter. These disturbances provide some of the most difficult problems with which the physician has to deal. In the presence of vomiting, oral alimentation is out of the question and, in the case of diarrhea, its value is limited by the hyperperistalsis. Parenteral nutrition must be relied on to replete stores of water and electrolyte, to correct abnormalities of acid-base equilibrium and to supply needed calories.

In conditions of acute dehydration and shock, restoration of the circulation is the matter of first concern. An electrolyte solution, preferably with an excess of fixed base, should be given without delay and followed by a transfusion of whole blood or plasma to maintain plasma volume. The repair of extracellular fluid deficits requires the further administration of an electrolyte solution, to which potassium may be added, when it is clear that the kidneys are functioning; Darrow's solution[99] is satisfactory for that purpose. The severity of the dehydration can only be guessed at from clinical appearances and intensive treatment must be continued until the signs of dehydration—particularly lack of skin turgor—have disappeared.

There are, however, limits to the rate at which intravenous fluid can be safely administered. A 5-kg infant should rarely receive more than 1,500 ml by vein a day, given by continuous drip or by intermittent push infusions. This corresponds to a rate of about 1 ml per minute for a continuous drip. A more rapid rate, not exceeding 15 to 20 ml per minute, may be employed with push infusions in which a fraction—not exceeding 250 ml—may be given at one time.

Parenteral Nutrition. This becomes important whenever the requirements of the body cannot be met by the oral route. To the extent that the organism cannot be nourished parenterally, it must live on its own tissues. It is the general experience, particularly with infants, that most of the fatalities which occur in severe digestive disorders are the result of nutritional failure. The chief minerals of intracellular fluid, potassium, magnesium and phosphorus, must be given cautiously, for only a limited rise in their concentrations in the plasma can be tolerated. Considerable experience has been obtained in recent years

in the parenteral administration of potassium, largely as a result of the pioneer work of Darrow. Much can be done to restore the diminished cell concentrations of this element, which occur in conditions of dehydration and in other pathologic states, by giving infusions with several times the concentration of potassium found in extracellular fluid. Provided the kidneys are functioning, as much as 35 mEq per liter may safely be given. Potassium so given may at times serve to replete the deficit of sodium from the cells.

Unfortunately, the restoration of the K/Na balance in the cells is not a simple matter. Active metabolic processes are concerned in maintaining the differences in concentration inside and outside the cell; when these are deranged the cell may not be able to accept potassium[100] presented to it in the extracellular environment. Nevertheless, the provision of this element, as in Darrow's solution,[99] permits the cell to accept it when it can. Signs, symptoms and biochemical changes of magnesium depletion and its therapy are discussed in Chapter 7, Section B.

The recent introduction of total parenteral nutrition (hyperalimentation) routines has made it possible to maintain even the smallest infant on intravenous feeding for prolonged periods. The insertion of a catheter into the superior vena cava and the use of a peristaltic pump to control the speed of delivery have allowed the use of hypertonic dextrose solutions which ensure adequate caloric intake. In addition to protein hydrolysate solutions or amino acid mixtures, fat, electrolytes and vitamins, various trace elements and intravenous fat should be given on a regular basis as the situation demands. Normal growth and development, as well as adequate nitrogen retention, have been attained in these infants.[101-103] Nutritional and procedural aspects of this method of feeding are considered in Chapter 37.

It should be pointed out that the administration of plasma or whole blood, valuable though it may be in maintaining plasma volume, is of negligible importance from the point of view of providing nitrogen for nutritional purposes. The proteins so administered have slow turnover rates, and it is only as they are degraded that the constituent amino acids become available. Amino acids given as such can, however, be rapidly used.

Oral Feeding in Digestive Disturbances. Vomiting presents an obvious barrier to oral alimentation, but the situation in the case of intestinal disturbances—acute and chronic diarrheas—is not so obvious and has provoked differences of opinion in regard to management. Restriction of the oral intake has been the policy generally favored. In its support were the observation that it resulted in decreased stooling and stool losses and the general philosophy that rest favored recovery of a disordered function.

The philosophy of rest, however, has not gone unchallenged. Coleman[104] and Dubois[105] some years ago questioned the value of resting the intestine in typhoid fever, and their results have revolutionized the dietary treatment of that disease. Likewise in the pediatrics field, Schick and Wagner[106] in studying chronic intestinal indigestion (celiac disease) concluded that the therapy of use was preferable to that of rest of the disordered function. Their work was supported by the subsequent observations of McCrae and Morris[107] in celiacs and by Black et al.[108] on sprue in adults, all of which pointed to the conclusion that, regardless of stooling, the administration of fat in steatorrhea improved fat absorption.

There has, however, been little direct evidence with which to answer the two leading questions involved: (1) What is the effect of feeding on absorption of the food itself and of other substances and (2) how does oral feeding affect the duration of the digestive disorder? If feeding increases the net loss of caloric food or of water and electrolyte, or if it delays recovery, it is contraindicated, and if it does none of these things and favors absorption it would seem to be indicated. The studies of Chung[81] on infantile diarrhea, carried out at different levels of food intake, failed to reveal any "washing out" of minerals or other foodstuffs caused by food administration; the amount of each foodstuff absorbed—whether calorigenic foodstuff, mineral or water—was found to be roughly proportional to the intake. The administration of food increased stool volume and stooling, but in every instance, and for every food ingredient studied, either net absorption was increased or loss was decreased.

A study designed to evaluate the effect of feeding on the duration of infantile diarrhea was made by Chung and Viscorova,[109] who treated alternate cases: (1) by a conventional plan of initial starvation with a gradual resumption of food and (2) by offering full caloric feeding from the start. The duration of the disorder was found to be identical in the two groups, indicating that the duration of the disturbance is not influenced by the feeding. Similar observations have been made by others.

A series of studies of various forms of steatorrhea—celiac disease,[110] cystic fibrosis of the pancreas, biliary atresia[111] and steatorrhea of prematurity[112]—was carried out by a group at New York University with a view to determining the effect of varying fat intakes. Similar observations on the steatorrhea of kwashiorkor were made by Gomez et al. in Mexico.[113] Although the stool fat output increased with increasing fat intake, fat absorption was correspondingly increased and only clinical benefit was observed. The conclusion drawn from these studies was that intestinal intolerance in these states was not induced or indeed affected in any way by the administration of the poorly tolerated foodstuff. The increased stooling was interpreted as a *demonstration of existing intolerance* rather than as a relapse.

These recent observations serve to support the views expressed in former years by Dubois,[105] Schick,[106] Park[114] and others, and would seem to point to a more liberal oral feeding policy than has generally prevailed. It is of course quite possible, particularly in the chronic disorders, to feed these patients satisfactorily without using the poorly tolerated foodstuff to any great extent. It is, however, not necessary to do so, nor should the conclusion be hastily drawn that relapses when they occur are caused by breaches of a prescribed diet. In celiac disease in particular such untoward events occur quite independently of the diet employed. The idea of "food intoxication" once widely held is now largely abandoned. It is believed that the manifestations of food intoxication accompanying a digestive upset are not caused by food but by dehydration associated with electrolyte losses and derangements of electrolyte metabolism. However, it would seem wise to initiate oral feeding after severe diarrhea with a lactose-free formula. The appearance of temporary lactase insufficiency after an acute gastrointestinal infection has been documented on numerous occasions.[115]

The Allergic Infant

Food allergy presents a special problem in infant feeding. It may be observed even in the breast-fed infant. Hypersensitivity to the natural proteins of the mother's own milk has not been observed, but in rare instances[116] proteins ingested by the mother find their way unsplit into the milk in biologic traces and, when the sensitivity of the infant is extreme, they produce symptoms. The mother herself may not be sensitive to the offending protein. Elimination of the particular food from the maternal diet is followed by the disappearance of the symptoms.

Hypersensitivity to one of the proteins of cow's milk—usually lactalbumin—is somewhat more frequently encountered and may be found in all degrees of severity. Idiosyncrasy of an extreme degree is rare, but dramatic in its manifestations. A single drop of cow's milk may lead within a few minutes to urticaria, asthma, acute gastrointestinal symptoms and shock of alarming proportions. Fatalities have been reported. In these circumstances the elimination of cow's milk from the diet must be scrupulously done. Goat's milk is often well tolerated by these infants, but at times there is sensitivity to this also and a milk-free diet must be given. Such extreme sensitivity is not permanent. By means of desensitization procedures, in which small graded nonreactive doses are given, it appears that a complete tolerance can be established though this may require a year or more.

Lesser grades of food intolerance—sometimes to milk, eggs, wheat or other protein foods—are also recognized; the symptoms are usually gastrointestinal or cutaneous (usually urticaria) and they develop less promptly than in the extreme cases. Rubin[117] and others[118] have reported acute diarrheas resulting from milk allergy in the newborn period; usually the symptoms are less acute. Subjecting milk to autoclaving temperatures often denatures the lactalbumin to such an extent that it can be tolerated and a milk-free diet is not required. In older subjects the celiac syndrome has been related by several investigators to intestinal allergy to wheat gluten.[119]

Aside from the clearly demonstrable cases, there is a wide zone in which respiratory, digestive and cutaneous manifestations are not so strikingly related to allergy. It is our opinion that the diagnosis of food allergy is often uncritically made and food unnecessarily restricted. It should be appreciated that a positive skin test is not synonymous with clinical allergy; such tests are frequently encountered in normal subjects. Elimination tests—elimination diets—are needed to establish the diagnosis. Only when the symptoms can repeatedly be made to disappear on removal of the dietary antigen and to recur when it is restored to the diet, *other factors remaining constant*, is a causal relationship justified. In our experience, it is only in the exceptional case of digestive disturbance in early life that the diagnosis of allergy can be sustained by an environmental test. It is also a mistaken notion that a child's distaste for a particular food, such as spinach, indicates that he is allergic to it. An article of food to which a patient is hypersensitive is as a rule eaten with enthusiasm, even when—as in older subjects—its relation to forthcoming symptoms is known.

The construction of a complete elimination diet free from all antigenic protein has been solved by a preparation in which all nitrogen is supplied in the form of amino acids and nonantigenic polypeptides. The suspected food or foods can be added to this one at a time for diagnostic purposes. When cow's milk allergy is demonstrated there are now many milk-free feedings that are available; complete feedings based on meat or soybean protein may be employed, as well as the protein hydrolysate.

Some allergic patients appear to be benefited by a reduction in the carbohydrate of the diet, for which fat is substituted. The underlying mechanism is not clearly understood, but appears to be related to a loss of fluid, chiefly extracellular, which occurs under these circumstances and which limits inflammatory reactions.

The Premature Infant

The premature infant presents peculiar nutritional problems. His caloric requirements are high and he absorbs certain foodstuffs—notably fats and fat-soluble vitamins—poorly. He is known to have a greater need for vitamin C than the mature infant, and it seems likely that other special nutritive requirements exist. He often regurgitates and aspirates his food with serious consequences. It is in the smallest premature infants that these difficulties are most often encountered.

The small premature infant is born with negligible reserves of body fat and is poorly equipped to withstand caloric deprivation, yet it is often impossible to feed him maintenance diets for some days; one must proceed cautiously. If medical complications prevent early feeding, intravenous therapy should be used. The tendency of the premature infant to develop symptomatic hypoglycemia can be prevented by the use of intravenous glucose.

The basal energy requirement of the premature is as high and perhaps higher than that of the full-term infant and his growth rate is more rapid; the caloric loss in the excreta—largely unabsorbed fat—is also greater. These problems are, however, partly compensated for by the low activity of these infants, so that the total caloric requirement is only moderately elevated. Most of these infants will gain well on 125 calories per kg, some on less than this.

The composition of the premature infant's feeding has been a controversial matter. In years past, breast milk has been regarded as the ideal food and the results with it appeared to be satisfactory. The avidity with which these infants retain protein,[120] however, suggested that the low protein content of breast milk might be suboptimal. The question is still unsettled. Higher protein intakes than that of breast milk will lead to increased nitrogen retention, but whether or not this is advantageous from the point of view of health is not established.

More recently, breast milk has again been advocated for the premature infant because of several purported advantages. Its possible role in preventing gastrointestinal infections has already been noted and it has been suggested, but not proved, that it may be instrumental in preventing necrotizing enterocolitis in this vulnerable group. Certain advantages for the quality of the protein have also been claimed. The premature infant does have poor development of a number of enzyme systems, including that involved in the synthesis of cystine from methionine, thus making cystine at least partially essential.[121] This, however, is not a definitive argument in favor of breast milk, which has a higher cystine content than cow's milk, since there is some degree of enzyme activity present and this, in addition to the cystine content of cow's milk, is sufficient to meet the requirement of the premature infant. The higher content of taurine which results in higher plasma taurine levels[122] has also concerned those who advocate the use of human milk for premature infants. The adverse effect of such a "deficiency" has not been demonstrated for the human infant; moreover the higher plasma levels in breast-fed infants may simply represent an impaired ability to degrade this amino acid.

By and large premature infants absorb fat poorly, although this steatorrhea is not apparent clinically. Tidwell and Holt[123] showed that it could be substantially reduced by substituting more unsaturated fats for butter in the feeding. Because of the limited absorption of fat, low-fat feedings have frequently been advised.[124] However, it now appears that unabsorbed fat in the intestine is completely innocuous. Morales et al.[112] have shown the interesting fact that the percentage of fat absorbed by premature babies remains relatively constant regardless of the intake. They were able to increase the total fat absorbed by increasing the fat intake without untoward effects, thereby achieving a total fat absorption comparable to that of full-term infants. This also is true for the fat-soluble vitamins which, like fat, are poorly absorbed; the absorption defect is met by increasing the intake.

Premature infants have a peculiar need for vitamin C, particularly when relatively high-protein feedings are given. Levine and Gordon[125] demonstrated that, unless this vitamin was generously supplied, a characteristic defect of aromatic amino acid metabolism appeared, with the excretion of so-called tyrosyl compounds (hy-droxyphenyllactic acid and hydroxphenylpyruvic acid) in the urine. It has been subsequently demonstrated that ascorbic acid activates p-hydroxyphenyl-pyruvic acid hydroxylase, the enzyme necessary for further degradation of these metabolites of tyrosine. A special requirement of the premature infant for vitamin E has been suggested. Both the anemia of prematurity[126] and a syndrome[127] consisting of edema, skin changes, elevated platelet count and morphologic changes in the red blood cells have been attributed to deficiency of this vitamin.

In summary, the feeding of the premature infant should provide, as soon as this can be tolerated, a caloric intake of 125 calories per kg. This can be accomplished satisfactorily by cow's milk mixtures as well as by breast milk. The defect of fat absorption can be overcome in several ways: by giving more protein and carbohydrate, by giving more fat or a more readily absorbable fat. An increased requirement for fat-soluble vitamins is best established for vitamin D, of which the intake should be no less than 1,000 I.U. per day. Single-dose therapy of 300,000 units has also proved safe and effective, lasting several months. A daily supplement of 100 mg of ascorbic acid given for the early weeks is adequate to control tyrosyluria, even on a relatively high-protein intake.

Peculiarities of the mineral requirements of the premature infant are not known to exist. Although the so-called anemia of prematurity[128] is a common event, this appears to differ in no sense from the physiologic anemia of the newborn and early infancy. Until recently it has been maintained that exogenous iron, though absorbed, was not readily utilized until the end of the second month of life. However, Gorten, Hepner and Workman[129] showed with labeled iron that even young premature babies will utilize such iron for hemoglobin synthesis without difficulty.

The feeding of premature infants is

rendered difficult by their imperfectly developed reflexes. Sucking and swallowing are often imperfectly performed by the small premature, who must in consequence be tube fed. A small rubber catheter introduced at mealtime was formerly in general use, but in recent years this has largely been replaced by a small polyethylene catheter[130] which can be left in place continuously. Regurgitation of food presents a greater danger of aspiration in the premature than in the mature infant, because the coughing reflex is often imperfectly developed. The use of a continuous oral drip or of small frequent feedings helps to reduce the volume of food in the stomach at any one time and thereby minimizes the risk of aspiration. Feeding by gastrostomy to avoid the risk of aspiration has been introduced recently.[131] Its recommendation as a routine procedure will have to await more extensive data. Total parenteral nutrition offers an alternative route of feeding when necessary.

The Older Child

The presumption that nutritional deficiencies are not common among children in the United States has been borne out by three large nutritional surveys[132-134] that included a total of over 10,000 children. Several interesting features did, however, become apparent. Iron deficiency and iron deficiency anemia were the most common nutritional deficiencies; the use of improved biochemical techniques such as the ferritin assay has demonstrated how prevalent iron deficiency is.

There were few clinical findings indicative of malnutrition. The most striking was the smaller size of children below the poverty level, compared to those above that level; the difference in weight was much less than the difference in height. This difference in stature was not related to protein intake which, throughout all surveys, was 1.5 to 2 times that of the Recommended Dietary Allowance; in addition,

virtually no evidence of depressed serum albumin levels was found. The smaller size of these children is not adequately explained. Although it might be related to a deficient energy intake, other nonnutritional factors such as genetic background, the rate of infections or other socioeconomic conditions may play an important role.

The other deficiency that was found in these surveys was that of vitamin A, which was especially prevalent in certain segments of the population such as the Mexican-American children of the southwest.

Anorexia is an exceedingly common condition said to occur in nearly 50 per cent of American homes. The difficulty usually arises from rigid ideas on the part of the parents, or perhaps the grandparents, as to what the child should eat and, more particularly, the quantity he should eat—these being at variance with the child's appetite. Coaxing and forcing of food effectively destroy the appetite and a vicious cycle is started. In some instances, this situation leads to psychogenic vomiting. Often the child learns to capitalize on the concern of the parents regarding his nutrition. He enjoys being the center of attention and may hold out for special privileges in return for eating. The therapy is simple, but sometimes difficult to carry out in a home where there are opinionated adults. It is to set before the child a well-balanced diet, sweets being withheld until protein foods are eaten. Comments on the desirability of eating are withheld and after a limited time—no longer than 20 minutes—the meal, if uneaten, is quietly removed; no food is offered until the next meal, when a similar procedure is followed. A few strong-willed children will resist until the third day, but most of them will become hungry and capitulate before this, often eating ravenously foods which previously they were unwilling to touch.

Pica, which involves the eating of dirt or of any inedible material, though uncommon, presents a serious problem. Its cause is not understood. The theory that the habit starts from an effort to compensate for some dietary deficiency is not established in man, although this has been observed in experimental animals. The habit, seen particularly in urban ghetto areas, has been related to emotional deprivation.[135] The danger from the ingestion of toxic substances is a serious one, the most frequent difficulty arising from the ingestion of lead from paint or plaster. The habit may be difficult to break and requires careful supervision.

Except in a few notable instances—pica, certain acute illnesses, certain mental deficiencies, and a few situations of bad conditioning—the *appetite of the infant* remains an excellent guide to his dietary needs, a far better one than is generally supposed. The observations of Clara Davis,[136] in which a group of normal children were allowed to select their own diets from 8 months of age onward for several years, bear eloquent testimony to this fact. Marked irregularities in the intake of particular foods were observed, a single food often being ingested in large quantities for a time; such dietary enthusiasms corrected themselves, however, and over a long period the intake proved to be a balanced one. The health record of these children was impressive. It is unfortunate that sweets were not included in this classical study for there is evidence that a "sweet tooth," if uninhibited, also tends to correct itself in time.

Several *dietary trends* may have some impact on the nutrition of children. Food faddism, which is extended to include children of all ages, may vary from the liberal diet of the lacto-ovovegetarian to the very restricted Zen macrobiotic diet. The use of the lacto-ovovegetarian diet has not been associated with nutritional problems, while the Zen diet has resulted in severe nutritional failure in young children.[137] The strict vegan diet, which excludes all foods of animal origin, may be adequate if it is carefully chosen; special attention must be paid to the iron and vitamin B_{12} content.

Changing *patterns of food consumption* also play a role in the nutrition of the child. The typical meal of fast-food establishments, although monotonous, is nutritionally adequate, with the exception of a low vitamin C intake and a surfeit of calories. The effect of the increasing use of convenience foods on the nutrition of the child has not as yet been evaluated, although it might be expected also to provide excessive calories.

Unsolved Problems of Infant Nutrition

In spite of the notable advances in infant feeding made during the past half century, many nutritional problems contributing heavily to infant mortality and morbidity remain unsolved. Frank nutritional failure is still responsible for most of the deaths in infantile diarrhea. Uncertainty still prevails as to the cause of many of these diarrheas. Undiscovered microbial agents—producing enteral or parenteral infection for which no specific therapy is available—are doubtless responsible for many of these; their discovery is important. A knowledge of the mechanism whereby an infection, enteral or parenteral, damages the assimilatory mechanisms of the intestine would be invaluable. A temporary deficiency of disaccharide-splitting enzymes appears to explain certain cases of poor carbohydrate assimilation. A knowledge of the steps involved in assimilatory mechanisms, of the enzymes and coenzymes concerned, might make it possible to restore function even if the damaging agent could not be eliminated. A perfect parenteral feeding would eliminate the immediate need of the digestive tract; our present materials have well-recognized imperfections. Good criteria for the adequacy of specific nutrients, especially protein, are needed. The long-range effects of overnutrition in infancy merit further study.

The largest infant mortality problem, that of the smallest premature infants, may well be due to nutritional failure. Obvious causes of death are not found at autopsy and the diagnosis of physiologic immaturity is used to cloak our ignorance. A more precise definition of immaturity in terms of defective tissue enzymes and coenzymes might lead the way to replacement of some of the latter at any rate. It is quite possible that the small premature infant needs a variety of accessory substances which the mature infant can manufacture for himself. Their discovery might permit these subjects to survive without difficulty.

Finally it is possible that many diverse diseases of known and unknown origin may exert baneful effects upon intermediate metabolism that are as yet unsuspected. Accessory cofactors—unessential for the normal individual but essential for the disease state—remain to be discovered.

NUTRITION IN ADOLESCENCE

The nutritional requirements of the adolescent are conditioned primarily by the *pubertal growth* spurt. During this period, which in an individual child may be much more striking than average figures indicate, there is an increase in the apparent basal metabolic requirement which, as pointed out, includes the growth requirement. There is also an increased demand for calories and for nitrogen. The increased caloric need is ordinarily reflected in the appetite. Unless additional food is provided at mealtime, the individual of necessity eats between meals. These between-meals snacks have been considered by many to be detrimental, resulting in the ingestion of "empty calories." However, an analysis of the composition of such snacks, based on data obtained in the 10-state nutritional survey, demonstrated that this was not the case.[138] Such foods were far from empty and provided considerable amounts of protein, vitamin A, riboflavin, ascorbic acid and calcium. Although the total consumption of iron and calcium was considered to be low, it was calculated that there would still be the same degree of deficiency of these two minerals if all caloric intake had occurred at mealtime. Exceptionally, the increase in appetite is inadequate and one observes a spindly individual who compensates for his or her increased caloric need by taking little exercise. Gephart[139] found the caloric consumption of boys at boarding school to be surprisingly large—much of it outside the dining room.

The need for additional nitrogen at the pubertal growth spurt has been stressed particularly by Johnston.[140] The additional caloric need and nitrogen need are thought to be proportional. Both are correlated with physiologic events, menarche in girls and the adolescent growth spurt in boys.[141] Failure to meet the additional requirement for protein at this time is believed to be an important cause of loss of resistance to infections, particularly tuberculosis. The loss of resistance at this time of life is seen particularly in the female, whose growth spurt is more rapid, though less prolonged (Fig. 27–3). Factors other than nutrition may, however, have some influence on loss of resistance, such as the hormonal changes occurring at this time. The practical consideration would seem to be the maintenance of an adequate protein intake with the first evidences of puberty. The maintenance of an adequate diet is often difficult in girls, who often attempt to achieve artificial standards of slimness by ill-advised dietary restrictions.

Although the need for sufficient protein and calories has been recognized, there have not been exact definitions of the nutritional requirements of the prepubertal growth spurt and of the change in body composition that occur at this time. That certain deficiencies of intake, notably those of vitamin A, riboflavin, calcium and iron, do occur was documented in the 10-state nutritional survey. These deficiencies were related to a depression of the growth spurt in a more detailed analysis of the Texas

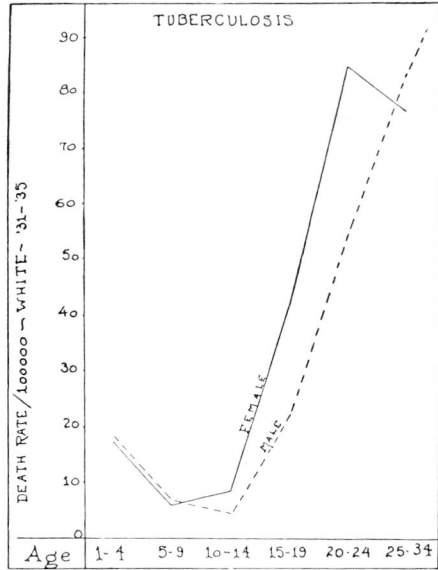

Fig. 27–3. Mortality rates in tuberculosis. Note the sharp rise in adolescence, the increase occurring first in the female, corresponding with the sex differences in pubertal phenomena. (From Johnston: *Nutritional Studies in Adolescent Girls and Their Relation to Tuberculosis.* Springfield, Charles C Thomas.)

portion of the survey.[142] The effect of nutritional intake on the growth spurt had previously been demonstrated in Japanese children; a delayed and smaller growth spurt was observed during World War II when food intake was inadequate.

An extreme form of malnutrition, *anorexia nervosa*, is seen particularly in adolescence, although not confined to this time of life. The term implies a neurosis, and there is no question that this is the explanation for most of the patients, in whom a psychologic disturbance is often apparent. We are not, however, inclined to accept the view that all nonfatal cases exhibiting extreme anorexia and malnutrition should be regarded as neuroses in contrast to Simmonds' disease, where the syndrome is brought about by total destruction of the pituitary. There is some evidence for the existence of transitory or

incomplete pituitary lesions which may induce this picture. Such cases have been observed post partum (Sheehan's syndrome) and it may be that the endocrine changes at puberty induce similar changes. Such extreme forms of anorexia and malnutrition require expert psychotherapy, but forced feeding is at times necessary.

Obesity, although prevalent at all ages, may be a special problem in the adolescent. Recent analyses have documented the fact that children from higher socioeconomic classes tend to be larger and heavier than those from lower-income classes. However, there is a striking reversal at adolescence; the poorer girl becomes fatter and remains so, while the higher-income girl becomes leaner and maintains this throughout adult life. Another factor in obesity is particularly apparent at this age. Children of obese parents tend to be fatter at all ages, but this trend is most marked during the second decade of life. By the age of 17, children of two obese parents are three times as fat as those of two lean parents.[143] The dietary management of obesity is discussed elsewhere (Chapter 25), but the psychologic factors at this period of life merit special attention. This is particularly true when an attitude of defeatism develops. This may result in withdrawal from social and athletic activities, overindulgence in foods and the development of a vicious cycle.

The problem of *simple goiter* or adolescent goiter is related to diet at this time of life. The classical work of Marine and his co-workers[144] served to relate this condition to a suboptimal intake of iodine. The demand for thyroid hormone is increased at the time of puberty and, in the presence of an iodine shortage, the gland responds by simple hypertrophy. The evidence cited by Marine et al. consisted of the demonstration of low iodine in the soil areas where adolescent goiter was more prevalent and a reduction of goiter when the iodine intake was increased. Exception to this concept has been taken by

Greenwald,[145] who points to a number of discrepancies in the iodine content of the soil and the incidence of goiter, and particularly to variations in the incidence of goiter in the same locality from time to time. Goitrogenic substances in foods and drugs may perhaps play a role in the incidence of this disorder. The beneficial effect of iodine is, however, a fact beyond question, both prophylactically and therapeutically (Chapter 9, Section A). Endemic goiter is seen particularly in isolated communities, usually in mountainous regions some distance from the sea. The development of transportation invariably results in a sharp decrease in its incidence. Food with a higher iodine content begins to come in from other places and there is a greater tendency for the inhabitants themselves to travel.

NUTRITION IN PATHOLOGIC STATES

A number of pathologic conditions are seen in early life which present nutritional problems because of derangements of metabolism. Some of these represent inborn errors and others are acquired.

Anomalies of Amino Acid Metabolism

A number of these respond to restriction of a specific amino acid or of protein intake. Some respond to pharmacologic doses of vitamins. These and other inborn errors of metabolism are discussed in Chapter 39.

High-protein diets may be useful in any condition associated with abnormal loss of protein from the body. One chronic situation where such loss from the bowel may not be readily appreciated is cystic fibrosis of the pancreas. In certain hypoglycemic states, such as the Von Gierke type of glycogen storage disease, the blood sugar can be maintained by giving additional protein meals, a procedure which may help restore the normal growth of the child.

Anomalies of Carbohydrate Metabolism Correctable by Diet

Of particular importance in this group is galactosemia, a congenital condition involving a deficit in the enzyme system which converts galactose to glucose.

Analogous to the above condition is hereditary fructose intolerance, a rare familial condition presenting similar symptoms and caused by an enzymatic block in the conversion of fructose to glucose.[146]

An inherited deficiency of one of the sugar- or starch-splitting enzymes in the gastrointestinal tract may result in a diarrhea severe enough to interfere with growth. The specific defect can be demonstrated by following the blood sugar curve after loading with the appropriate carbohydrate. A complete remission can be obtained by omitting the proper carbohydrate from the diet. Specific inabilities to utilize lactose, maltose, sucrose and starch[147] have been reported.

Anomalies of Fat Metabolism

Several disorders of fat metabolism occur in children which may be influenced by dietary therapy. The separation of idiopathic familial hyperlipemia into two forms is based on the response to diet: one responds to fat[148] and the other to carbohydrate restriction.[149] Low-fat intake reduces the plasma lipid level and the number of attacks of acute abdominal pain to which individuals of the first group are subject. Carbohydrate-induced hyperlipemia occurs in children rarely. Familial hypercholesteremia occurs in the pediatric age group;[150] the response of atheromatous lesions to dietary therapy has not been significant.

The demonstration of a metabolic error in the catabolism of phytanic acid in Refsum's disease[151] makes dietary treatment of this rare neurologic disorder possible.[152] Since phytanic acid is of exogenous origin, restriction of foods containing this 20-

carbon branched-chain fatty acid is indicated.

Anomalies of Vitamin Metabolism

Familial vitamin D-resistant rickets[153] is an inherited metabolic disease associated with marked hypophosphatemia in the presence of relatively normal serum calcium and only slight to moderate elevation of the alkaline phosphatase. The clinical manifestations of rickets are variable. The fundamental defect is an impairment of the renal tubular reabsorption of phosphate as a result of an insensitivity to the action of vitamin D or one of its metabolites. Extremely large doses of vitamin D (50,000 to 500,000 units daily) are required. Since these amounts are close to the toxic range, and often beyond it, treatment should be carefully monitored by frequent serum calcium determinations and by roentgenograms of the long bones. Recently, impaired conversion of 25-hydroxycholecalciferol to 1,25-dehydroxycholecaliciferol has been found to be the difficulty in certain of these patients.[154] The treatment in these individuals is the administration of the active form of the vitamin.

The clinical features of vitamin B_6 dependency are limited to the central nervous system and include hyperirritability, convulsions with electroencephalographic changes and a significant elevation of the spinal fluid protein.[155] The disease appears to be an inborn error of metabolism of a brain enzyme dependent on vitamin B_6, the exact nature of which has not yet been elucidated. Symptoms may appear within a few hours or days after birth and are controlled specifically by the administration of large amounts of pyridoxine. Therapy must be continuous; symptoms have recurred promptly on withdrawal of the vitamin even after several years of continuous therapy.

Supplementation of the diet with vitamins A, D and E is required in the malabsorption syndromes with poor fat absorption. Steatorrhea is the only indication for vitamin E supplementation known at present.

States Requiring Adjustment of the Mineral Intake

Since there are a number of such states, space will be taken only to mention them. Situations in which additional sodium is required include Addison's disease, the salt-losing form of the adrenogenital syndrome, congenital tubular renal acidosis (Lightwood's syndrome)[156] and hypotonic dehydration. Potassium supplementation is needed in the acute diarrheas, congenital alkalosis with diarrhea, congenital renal alkalosis, aldosteronism, periodic familial paralysis (hypokalemic type) and diabetic coma. Sodium restriction is used in nephrotic and cardiac edema and potassium restriction is indicated in anuria. Calcium supplementation is necessary in the various forms of tetany. Restriction of calcium intake is indicated in idiopathic hypercalcemia (Lightwood[157] and Fanconi[158]) and in prolonged immobilization, where bone decalcification may result in elevation of the serum calcium levels.

Two unusual clinical conditions have recently been related to defects in mineral metabolism. Acrodermatitis enteropathica, characterized by a typical dermatitis and chronic diarrhea, is the result of zinc deficiency[159] probably resulting from defective uptake of this mineral by gastrointestinal mucosa. The low plasma and urinary zinc levels as well as the clinical abnormalities all respond promptly to relatively small quantities of oral zinc. Menkes syndrome (progressive cerebral degeneration, bone changes, pili torti and arterial disease) is the manifestation of copper deficiency resulting from defective intestinal absorption;[160] presumably there is derangement in activity of a number of copper-dependent enzymes. Therapeutic results with parenteral copper administration have not been good;[161] this may be a reflection of the age at which therapy was instituted. The effect of treatment from the first days of life has not yet been evaluated.

BIBLIOGRAPHY

1. Murlin, Conklin and Marsh: Am. J. Dis. Child., 29, 1, 1925.
2. Protein Requirements. Nutritional Studies #16. Rome, Food and Agriculture Organization of United Nations, 1957.
3. Mendel: Harvey Lect., 10, 101, 1914.
4. Rose, Johnson and Haines: J. Biol. Chem., 182, 541, 1950.
5. Rose, Haines, Warner and Johnson: J. Biol. Chem., 188, 49, 1951.
6. Rose, Haines and Warner: J. Biol. Chem., 193, 605, 1951.
7. Rose, Warner and Haines: J. Biol. Chem., 193, 613, 1951.
8. Rose, Haines and Warner: J. Biol. Chem., 206, 421, 1954.
9. Rose, Lambert and Coon: J. Biol. Chem., 211, 815, 1954.
10. Rose, Leach, Coon and Lambert: J. Biol. Chem., 213, 913, 1955.
11. Rose, Borman, Coon and Lambert: J. Biol. Chem., 214, 579, 1955.
12. Rose, Coon, Lockhart and Lambert: J. Biol. Chem., 215, 101, 1955.
13. Rose, Eades and Coon: J. Biol. Chem., 216, 225, 1955.
14. Leverton, Gram, Chaloupka, Brodousky and Mitchell: J. Nutr., 58, 59, 1956.
15. Leverton, Gram, Brodousky, Chaloupka, Mitchell and Johnson: J. Nutr., 58, 83, 1956.
16. Leverton, Johnson, Pazur and Ellison: J. Nutr., 58, 219, 1956.
17. Leverton, Johnson, Ellison, Geschwender and Schmidt: J. Nutr., 58, 341, 1956.
18. Leverton, Ellison, Johnson, Pazur, Schmidt and Geschwender: J. Nutr., 58, 355, 1956.
19. Mertz, Baxter, Jackson, Roderick and Weis: J. Nutr., 46, 313, 1952.
20. Swendseid, Williams and Dunn: J. Nutr., 58, 495, 1956.
21. Swendseid and Dunn: J. Nutr., 58, 507, 1956.
22. Jones, Baumann and Reynolds: J. Nutr., 60, 549, 1956.
23. Clark, Yess, Vermillion, Goodwin and Mertz: J. Nutr., 79, 131, 1963.
24. Clark, Yang, Walton and Mertz: J. Nutr., 71, 229, 1960.
25. Clark, Reitz, Vacharotayan and Mertz: J. Nutr., 78, 173, 1962.
26. Clark, Mertz, Kwong, Howe and DeLone: J. Nutr., 63, 71, 1957.
27. Nakagawa, Takahashi and Suzuki: J. Nutr., 71, 176, 1960.
28. Nakagawa, Takahashi and Suzuki: J. Nutr., 73, 186, 1961.
29. Nakagawa, Takahashi and Suzuki: J. Nutr., 74, 401, 1961.
30. Nakagawa, Takahashi, Suzuki and Kobayashi: J. Nutr., 77, 61, 1962.
31. Nakagawa, Takahashi, Suzuki and Kobayashi: J. Nutr., 80, 305, 1963.
32. Joint FAO/WHO Expert Group on Protein Requirements. Geneva, 1963.
33. Snyderman, Holt, Dancis, Roitman and Balis: J. Nutr., 78, 75, 1962.
34. Hundley, Sandstead, Sampson and Whedon: Am. J. Clin. Nutr., 5, 316, 1957.
35. Pratt, Snyderman, Cheung, Norton and Holt: J. Nutr., 56, 231, 1955.
36. Snyderman, Pratt, Cheung, Norton and Holt: J. Nutr., 56, 253, 1955.
37. Snyderman, Norton, Fowler and Holt: Am. J. Dis. Child., 97, 175, 1959.
38. Snyderman, Holt, Smellie, Boyer and Westall: Am. J. Dis. Child., 97, 186, 1959.
39. Snyderman, Boyer and Holt: Am. J. Dis. Child., 97, 192, 1959.
40. Snyderman, Roitman, Boyer and Holt: Am. J. Dis. Child., 102, 157, 1961.
41. Snyderman, Boyer, Phansalkar and Holt: Am. J. Dis. Child., 102, 163, 1961.
42. Snyderman, Boyer, Roitman, Holt and Prose: Pediatrics, 31, 786, 1963.
43. Snyderman, Boyer, Norton, Roitman and Holt: Am. J. Clin. Nutr., 15, 313, 1964.
44. Snyderman, Boyer, Norton, Roitman and Holt: Am. J. Clin. Nutr., 15, 322, 1964.
45. Chwalibogowski: Acta Paediatr., 22, 110, 1937.
46. Hansen and Wiese: Fed. Proc., 5, 233, 1946.
47. Hansen et al.: Pediatrics, 31, 171, 1963.
48. Paulsrud: Am. J. Clin. Nutr., 25, 897, 1972.
49. Caldwell: J. Pediatr., 81, 894, 1972.
50. Ballabriga and Martinez: Symposium on Nutrition in Early Life. Lund, 1975.
51. Holt, et al.: J. Pediatr., 6, 427, 1935.
52. Snyderman, Morales and Holt: Arch. Dis. Child., 30, 83, 1955.
53. Darmady, Fosbrooke and Lloyd: Br. Med. J., 2, 685, 1972.
54. Reiser and Sidelman: J. Nutr., 102, 1009, 1972.
55. Hahn and Kirby: J. Nutr., 103, 690, 1973.
56. Friedman and Goldberg: Am. J. Clin. Nutr., 28, 42, 1975.
57. Plotz, Kabara, David, Le Roy and Gould: Am. J. Obstet. Gynecol., 101, 534, 1968.
58. Owen, Lubin and Garry: J. Nutr., 76, 563, 1971.
59. Committee on Nutrition: Pediatrics, 58, 765, 1976.
60. Henry and Kon: Br. J. Nutr., 7, 147, 1953.
61. Gershoff, Legg and Hegsted: J. Nutr., 64, 303, 1958.
62. Walravens and Hambridge: Am. J. Clin. Nutr., 29, 1114, 1976.
63. Eckhert, Sloan, Duncan and Hurley: Science, 195, 7891, 1977.
64. New York Academy of Medicine Committee on Public Health Relations: Bull. N. Y. Acad. Med., 28, 275, 1952.
65. Hamil, Reynolds, Poole and Macy: Am. J. Dis. Child., 56, 561, 1938.
66. Recommended Dietary Allowances. Washington, National Research Council Food and Nutrition Board, 1974.

67. Holt, et al.: J. Nutr., *37*, 53, 1949.
68. Snyderman, et al.: J. Nutr., *39*, 219, 1949.
69. Report of the Tenth M. & R. Pediatric Research Conference: *Vitamin B₆ in Human Nutrition.* Columbus, M. & R. Laboratories, 1953.
70. Lakdawala and Widdowson: Lancet, *1*, 167, 1977.
71. Gyorgy, Cogan and Rose: Proc. Soc. Exp. Biol. Med., *81*, 536, 1952.
72. Nitowsky, Gordon and Tildon: Bull. Johns Hopkins Hosp., *98*, 361, 1956.
73. Majaj, Dinning, Azzam and Darby: Am. J. Clin. Nutr., *12*, 374, 1963.
74. Ritchie, Fish, McMasters and Grossman: N. Engl. J. Med., *279*, 1185, 1968.
75. Pratt, et al.: Pediatrics, *1*, 181, 1948.
76. Halac: Am. J. Clin. Nutr., *9*, 557, 1961.
77. Halac: Am. J. Clin. Nutr., *11*, 574, 1962.
78. Holt, Halac and Kajdi: J.A.M.A., *181*, 699, 1962.
79. Knittle, Ginsberg-Fellner and Brown: Am. J. Clin. Nutr., *30*, 762, 1977.
80. Hoag, Rivkin, Levine and Wilson: Am. J. Dis. Child., *34*, 150, 1927.
81. Chung: J. Nutr., *33*, 1, 1953.
82. Ross: Fed. Proc., *19*, 1190, 1959.
83. Arias, Gartner, Seifter and Furman: J. Clin. Invest., *43*, 2037, 1964.
84. Gyorgy: Pediatrics, *11*, 98, 1953.
85. Mellander: Ups. Läkeref. Forhandl., *52*, 107, 1947.
86. Goldman and Smith: J. Pediatr.,*82*, 1082, 1973.
87. Willis, Bullen and Williams: Br. Med. J., *111*, 691, 1973.
88. Warren, Lepaw and Baitch: Pediatrics, *34*, 4, 1964.
89. Pratt and Snyderman: Pediatrics, *11*, 65, 1953.
90. Calcagno and Rubin: Pediatrics, *13*, 193, 1954.
91. Mauron: Arch. Biochem., *59*, 433, 1955.
92. Harper: J. Nutr., *67*, 109, 1959.
93. Fischer and Whitman: J. Pediatr.,*55*, 116, 1959.
94. Vaughan, et al.: J. Pediatr., *61*, 547, 1962.
95. Report of Committee on Fetus and Newborn: Pediatrics, *28*, 675, 1961.
96. Holt, Davies and Hasselmeyer: J. Pediatr., *61*, 566, 1962.
97. Shukla, Forsyth and Andersen: Br. Med. J., *4*, 504, 1972.
98. Taitz: Br. Med. J., *1*, 315, 1971.
99. Darrow: J. Pediatr., *28*, 515, 1946.
100. Kauhtio and Hallman: Acta Paediatr., *39*, 328, 1950.
101. Wilmore and Dudrick: J.A.M.A., *203*, 140, 1968.
102. Filler, Erakles, Rebin and Das: N. Engl. J. Med., *281*, 589, 1969.
103. Dudrick, et al.: Ann. Surg., *169*, 974, 1969.
104. Coleman: J.A.M.A., *69*, 320, 1917.
105. Dubois: Arch. Intern. Med., 10, 177, 1912.
106. Schick and Wagner: Zeitschr. Kinderheilkd.,*35*, 263, 1923.
107. Macrae and Morris: Arch. Dis. Child., *6*, 75, 1931.
108. Black, Fourman and Trinder: Lancet, *1*, 574, 1946.
109. Chung and Viscorova: J. Pediatr., *33*, 14, 1948.
110. Chung, Morales, Snyderman, Lewis and Holt: Pediatrics, 7, 491, 1951.
111. Krahulik, Shoob, Morales, Snyderman and Holt: J. Pediatr., *41*, 774, 1952.
112. Morales, et al.: Pediatrics, *6*, 86, 1950.
113. Gomez, et al.: Lancet, *2*, 121, 1956.
114. Park: N. Y. J. Med., *24*, 921, 1924.
115. Sunshine and Kretchmer: Pediatrics, *34*, 38, 1964.
116. Lyon: Am. J. Dis. Child., *36*, 1012, 1928.
117. Rubin: Am. J. Med. Sci., *200*, 385, 1940.
118. Rothman: Am. J. Dis. Child., *86*, 201, 1953.
119. Dicke, Weyers and Van de Kamer: Acta Paediatr., *42*, 34, 1953.
120. Rubner and Langstein: Arch. Ges. Physiol., *39*, 39, 1918.
121. Snyderman: *Metabolic Processes in the Foetus and Newborn Infant.* Leiden, Stenfert Kroese, 1971.
122. Rassin, Sturman, and Gaull: Pediatr. Res., *11*, 449, 1977.
123. Tidwell, Holt, Farrow and Neale: J. Pediatr., *7*, 481, 1935.
124. Gordon and McNamara: Am. J. Dis. Child., *62*, 328, 1941.
125. Levine, Marples and Gordon: J. Clin. Invest., *20*, 209, 1941.
126. Oski and Barness: Am. J. Dis. Child., *67*, 1045, 1965.
127. Hassan, et al.: Am. J. Clin. Nutr., *9*, 147, 1966.
128. Mackay: Arch. Dis. Child., *10*, 195, 1935.
129. Gorten, Hepner and Workman: J. Pediatr., *63*, 1063, 1963.
130. Kunz: Pediatrics, *41*, 84, 1952.
131. Steigman: Am. J. Dis. Child., *100*, 794, 1961.
132. Owens, Kram, Garry, Lowe and Lubin: Pediatrics, *53*, 597, 1974.
133. Garn and Clark: Pediatrics, *56*, 306, 1975.
134. Preliminary Findings of First Health and Nutrition Examination Survey. Washington, Department of Health, Education and Welfare, Publ. No. 74, 1970.
135. Millican and Laurie: In *The Child in His Family.* New York, John Wiley and Sons, 1970.
136. Davis: Am. J. Dis. Child., *36*, 651, 1928.
137. Robson: Pediatr. Clin. North Am., *24*, 189, 1977.
138. Thomas and Coll: Nutr. Rev., *31*, 137, 1973.
139. Gephart: Boston Med. Surg. J., *176*, 17, 1917.
140. Johnston: Ann. N. Y. Acad. Sci., *69*, 881, 1958.
141. Heald: *Adolescent Nutrition and Growth.* New York, Appleton-Century-Crofts, 1969.
142. McKigney and Munro: *Nutritional Requirements in Adolescence.* Cambridge, M.I.T. Press, 1975.
143. Garn and Clark: Pediatrics, *57*, 443, 1976.
144. Marine: Medicine, *3*, 453, 1924.
145. Greenwald: Trans. Am. Goiter Assoc., 369, 1950.
146. Levin, Oberholzer, Snodgrass, Stimler and Wilmers: Arch. Dis. Child., *38*, 220, 1963.
147. Weijers and Van De Kamer: Acta Paediatr., *52*, 329, 1963.
148. Holt, Aylward and Timbres: Bull. Johns Hopkins Hosp., *64*, 279, 1939.
149. Knittle and Ahrens: J. Clin. Invest., *43*, 485, 1967.

150. Rausen and Adlersberg: Pediatrics, *28*, 276, 1961.
151. Steinberg, et al.: J. Clin. Invest., *46*, 313, 1967.
152. Eljjarn, et al.: Lancet, *1*, 691, 1966.
153. Winters, Graham, Williams, McFalls and Burnett: Medicine, *37*, 97, 1958.
154. Fraser, Kooh, Kind, Holick, Tanaka and De Lucca: N. Engl. J. Med., *289*, 817, 1973.
155. Scriver: Pediatrics, *26*, 62, 1960.
156. Lightwood, Payne and Black: Pediatrics, *12*, 628, 1953.
157. Lightwood: Arch. Dis. Child., *27*, 302, 1952.
158. Fanconi and Girardet: Helv. Paediatr. Acta, 7, 314, 1952.
159. Moynahan: Lancet, *2*, 399, 1974.
160. Danks, Campbell and Stevens: Pediatrics, *50*, 188, 1972.
161. Bucknall, Haslam and Holtzman: Pediatrics, *52*, 653, 1973.

Chapter 28

NUTRITION FOR THE AGING AND THE AGED

Donald M. Watkin

Aging is a process beginning with conception and continuing until death. The aged are those persons in whom at least 65 per cent of the total changes associated with biologic aging have already occurred, assuming the life span (defined as the oldest age to which any member of a given species has survived) of man to be approximately 114 years.[1]

In man, aging is so modified by disease that its truly uncomplicated course is unknown. When an elderly man dies he dies from disease or accident, although his demise may euphemistically be attributed to "old age." Prior to death the aged display interindividual variations far greater than those observed in younger populations because of both hereditary differences in aging patterns and differences in the lifetime accumulation of insults from environmental hazards, disease and trauma. These variations are reflected in the variety of values reported as minimum requirements for specific nutrients among the aged. Such reports emphasize the fact that nutritional recommendations directed at the aged as a class must be couched in terms so general as to be meaningless. Older individuals may or may not have special nutritional needs. If they do, these special needs spring from medical, psychologic, social and economic factors as varied as the fingerprints of the aged themselves. Good nutrition for today's aged requires attention to the specific needs of each individual.

Although there is little evidence in man that nutrition can influence aging per se, certain animal studies (v.i.) suggest that caloric undernutrition increases the life span and may influence the aging of collagen, while others point to perinatal nutrition as a determinant of some aspects of aging after maturity.[1q] Good nutrition plays its most significant role during youth and middle age in the prevention of those diseases which ultimately manifest themselves as serious disabilities among the aged.

Basically, ideal nutrition for an elderly person in good health differs insignificantly from that of younger individuals, assuming in both cases that caloric intake is proportional to energy expenditure.[1b] Organ systems and metabolic processes normally have sufficient reserve so that decrements in efficiency associated with physiologic aging require no compensatory adjustments in nutrient intake. Rarely, however, are elderly men and women unafflicted by disabilities.[1u] Often these are complicated further by socio-economic problems.

Consider for a moment the plight of an elderly man who is edentulous and whose dentures are of an improper, painful fit.[1v] If barred by economic reasons from consulting a dentist, he may resort to the simple expedient of eating only those foods which can be consumed without teeth. His economic position and living arrangements may make it impossible for him to purchase and prepare well-balanced diets and dietary supplements, of which many suitable for his dentition are now on the market. Instead he may revert to such standbys as bread, mashed potatoes and other easily swallowed, high-carbohydrate, low-protein foods.

Consider the case of an elderly woman crippled by arthritis and living alone. Merely going to a store to buy food may be an insurmountable task. Even opening food containers, let alone preparing meats and vegetables, may be painful and disagreeable. As being alone and eating alone compound her misery, she soon may revert to easily prepared foods which furnish calories but do little to supply the protein, minerals and vitamins needed for proper nutrition.

Consider the elderly patient with myocardial insufficiency whose diet should be low in salt, the elderly patient with hypercholesterolemia who has been advised to restrict his intake of saturated fats, the elderly diabetic who needs a carefully planned daily menu of 6 feedings, the elderly cancer patient whom surgery has left with a colostomy or the elderly cirrhotic who has been told to eat a sodium-restricted regimen quantitatively low in protein but containing protein of the highest biologic value.

Consider the 19-year-old whose cervical fracture sustained in an auto accident produced instant aging, telescoping 80 years into a few milliseconds.[1c] Plagued by paralysis, cachexia, neurogenic dysfunction of the bladder and bowel, bone dissolution leading to osteopenia, pathologic fractures and renal lithiasis, pulmonary insufficiency, cardiovascular instability, anemia, carbohydrate intolerance, upper gastrointestinal hemorrhage, pressure ulcers of the skin, severely restricted vocational opportunities and negligible pension rights, he is almost totally dependent upon others.

Obviously, solutions exist on paper for all these individuals and for many more with conditions amenable to nutritional therapy. However, their transformation into practice requires their being tailored to the individual, his environment, the social conditions under which he lives and his financial resources, all of which demand an interdisciplinary approach by physicians, nutritionists, hospital and visiting nurses, social workers and, when necessary, personnel of appropriate governmental and nongovernmental agencies providing health and other supportive services.

The food industry, through the introduction of protective foods processed to provide long shelf-life in any climate, packed in single-meal units in easy-to-open containers labeled in large letters and marketed on a sufficiently large scale to ensure a truly low retail price, could help solve the practical problem of providing balanced diets for the great majority of the aged. Incidentally, marketing experience indicates that food products labeled "for the aged" are not accepted by older people. This unwillingness to identify themselves with products obviously prepared for them does not prevent the aged from consuming large quantities of baby and junior foods, the purchase of which can always be explained as being for grandchildren. These purchases indicate a need, either real or conceived out of fear or ignorance, for inexpensive single-service, easily opened foods of high nutritional quality and requiring minimal effort in preparation and eating.

Nutrition in the perinatal stage of the aging process has attracted attention for its influence on the physical and behavioral growth and development of children.[1d-i] Less well recognized and investigated is the influence of perinatal nutrition on senescent changes occurring in adult life. Animal studies[1j-r] in short-lived species have shown altered age-related patterns correlated with the quality of perinatal nutrition. Similar prospective studies in man would require many decades, while retrospective studies face methodologic obstacles of such magnitude that their credibility is seriously in doubt. Nonetheless, animal investigations and epidemiologic studies[1s-t] provide evidence supporting a high index of suspicion that perinatal nutrition may condition the aging process in adult life. Prospective studies of the outcomes of pregnancies in women addicted to alcohol lend support to this theory.[1w]

Preventive nutrition for aging should begin, of course, before birth and continue through childhood and adolescence. Preschool and elementary school nutrition education programs are commonplace. Less common, however, are secondary school and college programs. In universities, in business and among the professions, preventive nutrition is neglected entirely or acknowledged but sidetracked in deference to matters of presumed higher priority. Even in the armed forces, where the means of indoctrinating troops with preventive nutrition is at hand, more attention is paid to food industry lobbyists, worried mothers, congressional complaints and the unthinking cravings of youth than to disease prevention by nutritional means. The lack of knowledge regarding preventive nutrition is no more evident than among many United States Peace Corps volunteers whose first realization of the interrelation between nutrition and health has come when they have encountered malnutrition in developing countries. Lack of appropriate concern for preventive nutrition by government agencies has manifested itself not only in the defense establishment (v.s.) but even in the National Aeronautics and Space Agency, where hardware considerations and astronaut whims have received higher priority. Other agencies are no less remiss.[2,2b]

These examples highlight the need to seize every opportunity to teach young men and women, to indoctrinate them with and to habituate them to the virtues and the substance of preventive nutrition. Nowhere is this more evident than in consideration of nutrition for the elderly.[2c]

NEW POTENTIAL FOR NUTRITIONAL GERONTOLOGY

The low positions assigned nutrition and gerontology in rank order of priorities have severely limited resources apportioned to amelioration of human needs in both fields.[2c] These restricted resources have made impossible simultaneously meeting the exigencies of those already old while protecting the future interests of young generations, including the unborn and those yet to be conceived.

Recent developments are the harvest of seed planted years ago in hostile environments by those whose vision included faith in an eventual change in majority attitudes toward the poor, the hungry and the old. In the United States of America, the 1969 White House Conference on Food, Nutrition and Health (WHCFNH) (in itself an underscoring by the federal government of the decisive role nutrition plays in national ecology[2a]) stressed gerontology by incorporating into its own structure a Panel on Aging. Community and statewide preliminary conferences and special task force meetings, all incorporating considerations of nutrition and aging in their agendas, culminated in the Washington WHCFNH in late November and early December 1969.

The final report of the Panel on Aging comprised 11 recommendations, each in turn comprising varying numbers of specific components. These have been published.[2a] Developments in the year following the 1969 WHCFNH have been reported.[2d] Subsequent developments leading to the national Nutrition Program for Older Americans (NPOA), authorized by Title VII of the Older Americans Act of 1965, as Amended, have also been reported.[2c] The growth of and concepts underlying the NPOA have been described.[2e]

In addition to the success of the NPOA, the almost ninefold increase in funding for food stamps since the WHCFNH in 1969 has drastically changed the potential for adequate nutrition for the aged American.[2f]

Concern for nutrition among the aged and the aging has not been confined to the United States. In the USSR, interest in the notorious longevity of certain Transcaucasian peoples has focused on their lifelong activity and dietary practices.[2g] In other industrialized nations, well-subsidized projects provide adequate nutrition as part of national health and social security programs.[2h] While the aged in technically underdeveloped societies represent comparatively low percentages of total populations, their presence has not gone unnoticed by the public or by specialists in development planning.[2i]

In such developing societies, great concern for nutrition during the pregnancy of mothers and the early lives of children has been manifest for years. As these concerns are translated into effective programs, their impact on aging throughout life may become more evident, and more nongenetically elite[2j] may survive into advanced old age. The challenge for these societies is to plan well enough to leapfrog over the errors committed by presently developed societies into a more promising 21st century.

THE AGING PROCESS

The lack of evidence in adult man that nutrition can influence the aging process per se has been mentioned. This statement can be better understood if the nature of aging can be more clearly defined. Whether to regard aging as an indication of pathology or to look upon it as a normal process is to indulge in semantics. That aging occurs in man whether or not it is accompanied by disease is a prima facie assumption.

Cell Loss

Aging has been attributed in large measure either to losses of cells by organ systems or to reduction in the cellular metabolism of tissues with age.[2k] Much convincing evidence exists to support the concept of cell loss with increasing age. Histologists can distinguish old from young tissues, especially those of heart, skeletal muscle, brain, cartilage and kidney, which have no capacity for regeneration, by the reduction with age in the number of functioning parenchymal cells.[21] Reduction in the volume of specific muscles in old rats has been interpreted as cell loss.[3] The number of nonglial cells per unit of cerebral cortex decreases with advancing age, the greatest slope being between 45 and 55.[3a] However, several brain stem structures show no reduction in cell number with age.[3b]

In man, reductions in organ or organ system functions are commonly found in aging. These have been directly associated with demonstrable cell loss. For example, linear reductions in discrete renal functions[4,5] between age 30 and 90 indicate loss of functioning nephrons, a loss corroborated by quantitative counts in histologic sections.[6] Age-related decrements in body water, unaccompanied by decrements in oxygen consumption per unit of body water,[7] similarly suggest cell loss. Body composition studies[8–11] have revealed decreased fat-free and total-body weight in advanced age. Studies of total-body potassium, measured either by ^{42}K dilution techniques[12,12a] or by estimation of ^{40}K radiation in a whole-body counter,[13,13a,b] have revealed age-related decrements suggesting cell loss.

Virtually all these data represent observations on age differences among groups of subjects representing different age categories. The data have, therefore, a built-in bias resulting from selective mortality, a bias which would be eliminated were it possible to assemble serial measurements on the same subject as that subject grows older.[13c]

Longitudinal studies in man designed to overcome this bias began following World War II.[13d,e,f] Among the valuable data collected are those indicating intraindividual decrements in height beginning at age 25, and in weight beginning at age 55.[13g] In spite of the institution of these longitudinal studies, meaningful data continue to be scarce, even for those parameters now subject to measurement in man. Hence, most data presently available are still based on cross-sectional studies. Interpretations derived from such information should be accepted with reservations.

Reduced Cellular Metabolism

While the bulk of evidence from cross-sectional studies supports the concept of cell loss with aging, the possibility remains that reduced organ or organ system performance may result in part from reduced cellular metabolism with age. When enzyme activity in the heart, kidney and liver of young and old rats was measured and related to the deoxyribonucleic acid (DNA) content of tissues,[14-18] no decrements in alkaline and acid phosphatase, succinoxidase, pyrophosphatase, pseudocholinesterase or D-amino acid oxidase were found. One enzyme, cathepsin, however, showed increased activity with aging. Other enzyme studies during protein deprivation and refeeding showed little evidence of decrements in protein synthesis in senescence.[19] In fact, these and other studies showing increased tryptophan peroxidase activity with age in rat liver,[20] and increased ribonucleic acid (RNA) in the cells of aged mice[21] have even suggested increased protein turnover with age.

Reductions of succinoxidase activity in whole tissue homogenates led to speculation that mitochondria (which contain essentially all succinoxidase activity) might lose enzyme activity with age. However, studies of isolated liver and kidney mitochondria[17,22] failed to reveal decrements with age, leading to the suggestion that impaired cellular enzyme activity may result from a loss of mitochondria from cells rather than from changes in the enzyme activity of mitochondria themselves.

Studies in 193 men aged 21 to 95, mentioned briefly above,[7] showed no decrement in oxygen consumption with age per unit of body water, although body water per square meter of body surface decreased with age. These observations suggest that functioning cells are lost as man ages but that the oxygen uptake of functioning cells in old men is no different from that in young. This clinical evidence, combined with the fact that even the maximum observed decrements in enzyme activity in animal tissues cannot account for the well-documented organ and organ system decrements in function, which may reach 60 per cent,[23] leads to the conclusion that cell death continues to be the major phenomenon responsible for the functional impairment accompanying the aging process.

Biochemical Mechanisms Underlying Cell Death

Knowledge of possible biochemical mechanisms underlying cell death has increased with recent advances in understanding of the role of deoxyribonucleic acid (DNA) and ribonucleic acid (RNA) in protein synthesis. One hypothesis in explanation of cell death has been proposed by Wulff et al.[21-23]

These authors attribute aging to the accumulation of somatic mutations in DNA. This in turn yields defective RNA which is incapable of producing enzymes which can synthesize proteins from available amino acids. A cell will survive until functional enzymes fall below a critical level, at which point cell death ensues.

The factors which may be responsible for errors in the synthesis of nucleic acids and proteins have been reviewed by Medvedev.[24] He includes random error in RNA replication from DNA, radiation, micro-emission of heat and radiant energy, blocking of active groups, microdenaturation, incorporation of analogs and products of side reactions, and changes in ratio of substrates during the synthesis of RNA and proteins. These factors act on DNA and RNA in different ways.

The synthesis of DNA is relatively unaffected. In addition, natural selection rapidly eliminates any negative characteristics arising from errors in synthesis and spares positive characteristics for future reproduction. Unlike DNA synthesis, RNA and protein synthesis are relatively unsheltered, a situation leading to damaged molecules which are retained and accumulated in cells.[24a,b] Since proteins are extremely specific for each function performed and since they cannot replicate themselves, changes in proteins form the molecular basis for cell death and eventually for death of the individual.

Medvedev suggests that aging is associated with a gradual weakening of the hereditary control of protein synthesis, i.e. cellular RNA replication of DNA becomes less exact with the passage of time.[24,24a,24b] The process of aging could be altered, therefore, by eliminating the responsible factors mentioned above or creating conditions unfavorable to the production and accumulation of damaged molecules. This might be done by eliminating or segregating the altered RNA templates so that only the correct RNA could function in protein synthesis. The rate of autoreproduction of correct RNA templates might be increased. Medvedev's suggestion[24] that tests be run on the immunization of young animals by proteins derived from the aged with a view toward the elimination of altered proteins by autoimmune reactions in the young can be challenged by more recent considerations of immunologic phenomena.[24c]

Immune responses or the lack thereof have been implicated as potentially causative factors in aging.[24d,e] Immune responses decline with aging, while autoim-munity, i.e. the production of antibodies by the host against antigens produced by the same host, increases. Manipulation of two elements of the environment, body temperature and nutrition, have been shown to influence the relation of immune responses to age.

In fish, Liu and Walford[24f,g] have shown prolongation of life, collagen changes suggesting a slowing of the aging process and favorable changes in immune and autoimmune antibody responses when the ambient temperature of the poikilothermic Cynolebias alloffi is reduced from 20° to 15°C. The greatest influence on longevity was obtained when the fish lived at 20°C for the first 8 months of life and at 15°C for the remainder, suggesting that the lower temperature may influence favorably production of autoantibodies which could be expected to increase during the latter phase of life.

Caloric undernutrition, first demonstrated to increase longevity in fish[24h] and rats[24i] by McKay and colleagues, has been a mystery in regard to its mechanism of action for decades.[24j] However, Walford[24k] has suggested that the causes of this prolongation of life may be immunologic. Data supporting this hypothesis have been obtained in mice in studies by Jose et al.[24l] and by Walford et al.,[24m] who have shown that both dietary protein deficiency and calorie deficiency result in diminished humoral and cellular immune responses in young animals. The latter study also showed greater immune responses in 1-year-old mice fed low-protein, low-calorie diets than in animals fed diets containing higher protein and calorie levels, indicating a delay associated with the low-protein and -calorie diet in the usual decrements in immune functions and increments in autoimmunity with advancing age.

As noted by Walford,[24n] these observations will have meaning only if the same diets prolong the lives of mice. Nonetheless, they do show a profound effect of dietary restriction on immune function in mice. Fernandez et al.[24o,p] have demonstrated that high, as opposed to low, fat diets promote autoimmunity, decrease cell-mediated immunity and shorten the lives of mice prone to autoimmune disease.

By whatever method it is brought about, extension of the time period during which DNA effectively governs protein synthesis provides a major avenue of research into deceleration of the aging process.

In 1963 and 1964, Medvedev[24q,r] postulated a process he calls "active aging." This implies a marked group of "aging" genes activated at a predetermined stage of life. These genes would increase the rate of molecular reproduction, incorporate "noise" into the system and cause aging as a special case of random morphogenesis. This programmed aging would act in determining life span independently of previously mentioned mutagenic factors. Medvedev sees in "active aging" a mechanism for preventing the accumulation of mutations which, if allowed to continue indefinitely, could be lethal for a given species. In addition, Medvedev[24s] proposes that not only error-producing but also error-correcting systems exist. Repairs to DNA, in which endonucleases recognize injuries and excise them and DNA polymerases fill the gaps, using information on the complementary strands (double-stranded breaks cannot be repaired) and ligases to rejoin the ends, have been studied in detail, as have repairs occurring at the time of DNA replication when segments of a strand complementary to the damaged areas are read and new segments are inserted. Repair mechanisms have been summarized by Sinex.[24t]

The observation of a positive correlation between DNA repair activity and the longevity of various animal species, including man, has been made by Hart and Setlow.[24u,v] Using the ability of dermal fibroblasts to perform unscheduled DNA synthesis after ultraviolet irradiation as a measure of excision repair, they observed the greatest activity in cells from man, elephants and cows, the least in cells from shrews, mice and rats, and an intermediate state in cells from hamsters. Hart has suggested[24w] that repair activity might be increased and/or prolonged by the type of undernutrition first described by McCay.[24h,i]

Another model theory of aging as a process has been presented by von Hahn.[24x,y] According to him, the aging of DNA appears to consist in large measure of the stabilization of the Watson-Crick double helix by firm binding of histone, as opposed to the temporary binding of histone to DNA which characterizes normal repression of RNA synthesis. Since local unwinding of the double helix is necessary for the transcription of genetic information, the firmer binding of histones could interfere with the transcribing mechanism, prevent the formation of RNA and enzymes and result in cell death.

Maturation of Collagen as an Index of Biologic Age

The above discussion of nucleic acid metabolism applies particularly to the labile proteins. Certain proteins—collagen and elastin, for example—have half-lives long enough to preclude their being turned over at all.[25-27] Verzár[28] has studied the maturation of collagen as an objective index of biologic age as distinguished from calendar age of men and animals. He observed that tendons from the tails of 30-month-old, senile rats showed greater contractility on heating to 65°C than did tendons from the tails of 5-month-old rats. Verzár[28,28a] and Chvapil,[29] using heat, sodium perchlorate, and 7M urea-induced contraction of tendon, have also observed a prolonged relaxation time in old collagen, as opposed to young. Chvapil[29] used this technique to quantify the impact of nutrition on molecular aging. In animals with lives prolonged by feeding restricted diets, as first described by McCay,[30] he found tendons with biologic age younger than the animals' calendar age. Holeckova, Chytil and Chvapil[31] also observed that fibers from the tail tendons of wild Norway rats showed a lower biologic age than fibers from the tail tendons of domesticated animals of the same calendar age. Chvapil and Holeckova[32] later showed that intermittent feeding and fasting of Wistar rats led to an inhibition of the normally occurring age-related increase in stability of collagen in domesticated rats.

Molecular Aging of Collagen

The increased tension of biologically older collagen fiber has been attributed by Verzár,[28,28a] Bjorksten[33] and Piez[33a] to the increased number of hydrogen and ester bonds forming cross-links between molecules within the fiber. The increased number of cross-links in aging collagen are attributed by Verzár to the random contact between collagen molecules bathed in body fluids as they are shuttled about by Brownian movements. In a lifetime, during which collagen is neither renewed nor replaced, cross-links between molecules would accumulate in increasing numbers.

Confirmation of this hypothesis exists in the lower solubility of old collagen during thermally induced contraction at 65°C,[34] suggesting an increase in the number of cross-links in older fibers. With aging, more ester (as opposed to hydrogen) bonds requiring hexose molecules for formation have been postulated.[33,35] While these changes were once regarded as evidence of deterioration with advancing age, Verzár[28a] and Piez[33a] now suggest they represent a continuing and perhaps genetically programmed maturation process. Hamlin and Kohn[35a,b] have shown, in studies with human diaphragm tendon, that collagen becomes progressively more resistant to digestion by bacterial collagenase, so predictably, in fact, that the resistance of tendon collagen to collagenase can be used in determining human chronologic age.

Milch et al.[36,36a,b] have identified as al-dehydes intermediary metabolites which stabilize the lattice structure of collagen against the adverse effects of pH or collagenase activity. Of the several carbohydrate metabolites studied, only those with aldehyde structure promote stability; others disrupt the collagen lattice structure. Among the aldehydes, glyceraldehyde, the major intermediary metabolite found in all known carbohydrate metabolic pathways, is the most potent stabilizer of collagen under conditions approximating those of extracellular body fluid. This research may lead to the means of preventing cross-link formation and thereby of slowing down the molecular aging of collagen.[28] While agreement exists that stable cross-linkages increase with advancing age, their exact nature remains undefined.[36c]

The apparent reduction in cross-linkages in the tendons of rats the lives of which have been prolonged by underfeeding or whose biologic ages have been reduced by intermittent feeding and fasting suggests the role of nutrition in influencing the molecular aging process.

Since collagen constitutes 40 per cent of all protein in the body,[28] and since collagen is an important component of connective tissue on which all cells depend for contact with the external environment, molecular aging of collagen would seem to deserve a high priority in considerations of overall aging in man. However, ionizing radiation which shortens life and produces changes resembling aging[37] has been reported by Verzár[28] to have no effect on the biologic age of rat tail tendon fibers. Although this lack of effect has not been found by Baily,[38] the lack of agreement may be related to methodologic differences (irradiation in the wet in vivo or the dry state) or to the fact that Verzár measured a net effect of both scission and formation of cross-linkages within the collagen molecules.[39] In any event, the lack of a conclusive effect of radiation on collagen aging, along with the impossibility of explaining cell death (except by invoking oxygen and nutrient transport failure) on the basis of collagen aging, suggests that deterioration of RNA and labile protein synthesis with age remain the more significant problems at this time.

AGING AND SPECIFIC NUTRIENTS

Protein

Various investigators, using conventional nitrogen balance techniques, have found increased,[40–43,43a,b] decreased[44–46] and similar[47,48,48a] minimum protein requirements for the aged when compared to the young. Adherents to the "allowance"[49] principle have seized upon this large intergroup variability to insist on a standard of protein intake for the elderly high enough to include even those who obviously deserve to be treated as special cases.

Among the evidence supporting a higher dietary protein allowance for the aged is the observation that serum albumin falls with aging, while serum globulins show a compensatory rise.[50–54] Most authors have blamed reduced protein synthesis by the liver for the lowered albumin content. However, Acheson and Jessop[54] found lower serum albumins among those with histories of low-protein intake and noted an age-related increase in γ-globulin which was reversed only in extreme old age. The success in increasing low albumin concentrations, encountered in a variety of conditions in all age groups, with diets containing ample quantities of high-quality protein has led to the inference that high-protein diets are desirable for the aged.

The varied results of nitrogen balance studies and the nonspecificity of serum albumin as an index of protein needs have led to additional methods of investigation of alterations in protein metabolism with advancing age.

Anabolic Hormones. The changes in nitrogen balance accompanying administration of anabolic hormones have been described by several investigators[55–59] whose work has suggested a superiority of male over female hormones in inducing nitrogen retention. Watkin et al.[60] studied nitrogen balances in eight elderly men on high- and low-protein diets before, during and after androgen administration. The androgen induced somewhat greater retention on the high- than on the low-protein diet, and the increment achieved by androgen administration on the low-protein regimen was less than the increment achieved by a high-protein diet alone. A variance analysis[61] performed on data from the four men fed high- and the four fed low-calorie diets during these studies showed no effect of the calorie difference, but revealed a marked effect of the protein level. A modified t-test analysis was performed to assess the role of dietary protein level on the response to androgen administration. This analysis revealed a significant effect of hormone therapy on nitrogen balance at both levels of protein intake.

Of far greater significance, however, was the influence of the dietary protein level itself. The analysis revealed no significant hormone-protein interaction. From those studies, it was concluded that a high-protein diet is a far greater stimulus to nitrogen retention than either added calories or androgenic hormone. These studies confirmed the ability of aged men to retain nitrogen when fed diets containing adequate protein. The problems of side effects,[62] cost and inconvenience of taking anabolic hormone preparations suggest the desirability of using increased dietary protein when greater protein anabolism is desired.

Changes in Protein Intake. Another approach has compared the metabolic responses of older and younger subjects to abrupt changes in protein intake. During investigations in four elderly and three middle-aged men, Watkin, Silverstone and Shock[63] studied whether old subjects retained their ability to adapt to sudden changes in dietary protein level. Diets were changed from medium- (7.0 gm nitrogen per day) to low- (4.3 gm nitrogen per day) to high- (13.3 gm nitrogen per day) protein content. After shifting from the medium- to the low-protein diet, the elderly men reached a minimal level of nitrogen loss in 10 days and the middle-aged men in 14. When the dietary protein was raised from the low to the high level, the elderly retained more nitrogen than the middle-aged men, both during the first 5 days and for 30 days after the change. No statistically significant differences in cumulative nitrogen balances, however, were found after any shift in dietary protein level.

Similar observations were made by Couch et al.[64,187] in a 70-year-old man subjected to complete nitrogen withdrawal while he consumed a 2,800-calorie diet containing all essential nutrients except amino acids. Well within the 12-day period of nitrogen deprivation, the subject reduced his urinary nitrogen to 2.5 mg per day, a level comparable to that observed in younger subjects.[65] When L-amino acids in the casein pattern were subsequently added to the basic regimen, he responded with strongly positive nitrogen balances.

In studies of elderly men and women on protein-free diets, Scrimshaw et al.[65a] and Uauy et al.[43b] have described prompt reductions in urinary nitrogen losses to levels averaging 1.5 gm per day from women averaging 76 years of age and 2.4 gm per day from men averaging 70 years of age. Such values differ insignificantly from those found in young persons studied under similar conditions.

These studies provide convincing evidence that the aged can adapt successfully to protein withdrawal. The positive nitrogen balances following the addition either of more dietary protein or of L-amino acids indicate as well that protein synthesis in the aged increases rapidly when additional amino acid substrate is supplied in the diet.

Amino Acid Metabolism. The increased availability of pure amino acids and the development of chromatographic methods for the measurement of amino acids in biologic materials have made possible quantitative studies of amino acid metabolism in men of all ages. Those performed in the aged have added immeasurably to the information previously available,[66,67] which had revealed deficiencies of methionine and lysine in diets self-selected by older individuals.

In the first of a series of investigations, Tuttle et al.[68] studied five men aged 52 to 68 whose protein nitrogen intake was kept at 7.0 gm per day and whose calorie intake (30 to 40 calories per kg) was sufficient to maintain constant weight. After a 12-day control period, the subjects were given an L-amino acid mixture based on the composition of 18.75 gm of egg protein containing, in addition to the eight essentials, the L-forms of histidine, cystine and tyrosine. The test mixture was supplemented with glycine to bring the nitrogen intake up to that of natural food (7.0 gm per day). Although the mixture contained amounts of amino acids in excess of the quantities required for nitrogen equilibrium in young adults, all five older men went into negative nitrogen balance while receiving it. In addition, three subjects also went into negative nitrogen balance when fed egg protein in an amount duplicating the essential L-amino acid content of the amino acid mixture. These findings suggested that the minimum requirement for one or more of the essential amino acids is higher in older men or that the nonessential nitrogen source (glycine) may not be so well utilized by the aged as by the young for the synthesis of nonessential amino acids.

Minimum Requirement for Essential Amino Acids. Results of these investigations must be viewed in the light of others of slightly different design in which no increase in requirement for aged men was observed. Watts et al.,[69] using the nitrogen balance technique, measured the minimal amount of essential amino acids needed for nitrogen equilibrium in six men ranging from 65 to 84 years of age. The authors also compared nitrogen balances in this aged group with those observed[70] in a group of 25-year-old men when both groups received the FAO reference and the milk patterns of essential amino acids. Positive balances at the 200-, 280- and 360-mg tryptophan levels of the FAO pattern were in marked contrast to findings by Tuttle et al.[68] and, in the author's opinion, cannot be simply explained by differences in experimental design. The minimum requirements of only two of the aged men while being fed the FAO patterns were slightly in excess of Rose's *minimum* for young men.[71]

When these same aged men were fed essential amino acids in the milk pattern, Watts et al. observed methionine requirements ranging from 0.29 to 0.60 gm methionine, as opposed to the 2.4 to 3.0 gm requirement reported by Tuttle et al.[72] All of the aged men were in nitrogen equilibrium on amino acid mixtures containing approximately half the methionine required for nitrogen equilibrium in 25-year-old men. The authors concluded that their studies indicate no higher requirement for men over 65 years of age than for men of 25.

Amount of Amino Acids in Relation to Total Nitrogen Content of Diet. Tuttle et al.[73] also studied the relation of the essential amino acid requirements of older men to the total nitrogen content of their diet. Previous studies[74] had indicated that men over 60 could maintain nitrogen equilibrium on 1.5 gm of essential nitrogen with amino acids proportioned in the egg pattern if the total nitrogen intake was 3.5 gm per day. The same men went into negative nitrogen balance when total nitrogen was raised to 7.5 gm per day. When the essential nitrogen component was raised to 3.0 gm, their nitrogen balance again became positive. When the total nitrogen content was increased to 15 gm daily by the addition of glycine and diammonium citrate,

their nitrogen balance again became negative.[73]

The authors suggest that this dependence of essential amino acid requirement on total nitrogen intake may be characteristic of older men, since similar dependence has not been observed in younger men and women.[75] They also point out that these observations, combined with those of food intake studies[66,67] showing self-selection of proteins low in biologic value by the aged, could justify an upward revision for dietary protein allowances for the elderly.

Source and Quantity of Nonessential Nitrogen. Other studies[76,77] in normal male and female subjects aged 20 to 24 fed limiting amounts of essential amino acids had revealed that the source as well as the quantity of nonessential nitrogen influenced nitrogen retention. Hence, Tuttle et al.[78] investigated the effect of the kind of dietary nonessential nitrogen fed on the dietary essential amino acid requirement in a group of six older men ranging in age from 50 to 70 years, with an average age of 63. Nitrogen balance was measured while the subjects received three different levels (1.2, 1.8 and 2.4 gm amino acid nitrogen per day) of purified essential L-amino acids in whole egg pattern proportions supplemented by either glycine alone or by a mixture of nonessential L-amino acids in whole egg protein proportions in amounts needed to maintain total nitrogen intake at 7 gm daily. When the nonessential amino acid mixture replaced glycine as a source of supplemental nitrogen, greater nitrogen retention was observed in five out of the six subjects. Despite this increased retention, the requirement for nitrogen equilibrium still was greater than 1.2 gm of essential amino acid nitrogen daily in all but one subject. One additional subject achieved nitrogen equilibrium when the essential amino acid nitrogen intake was 1.8 gm daily. However, 2.4 gm daily were required to achieve nitrogen equilibrium in all subjects.

These studies demonstrate clearly the great variability in amino acid requirement among the aged. They suggest that the nonessential as well as the essential amino acid composition of the diet may influence nitrogen retention. They also point toward the possibility of a failure of certain nonessential synthetic pathways with advancing age. Although they suggest an increased requirement for essential amino acids for the aged, the differences in experimental design between this study and that in younger men[79] leave room for some doubt and suggest the desirability of additional investigation.

Requirement for Specific Amino Acids. In studies of requirements for specific amino acids, Tuttle et al.,[72] Swendseid and Tuttle[80] and Tuttle et al.[81] have investigated the dietary requirement for methionine in six men aged 58 to 73 (average age 64) and for lysine in four men aged 53 to 64 (average age 59). The diets contained essential L-amino acids (except for cystine and methionine in the study of methionine requirement and for lysine in the study of lysine requirement) in the proportions of whole egg protein in amounts equivalent to 2.4 gm of essential amino acid nitrogen daily. They also contained 17 gm of nonessential L-amino acids proportioned in the whole egg protein pattern and enough additional glycine to bring the total dietary nitrogen up to 7 gm per day.

Four men tested were in negative nitrogen balance on 2.1 gm or less of methionine daily. One of two subjects tested was in positive nitrogen balance on 2.4 gm methionine daily, one of three on 2.7 gm daily, and all of three on 3.0 gm daily. These estimates are well in excess of requirements ranging from 0.8 to 1.1 gm daily proposed by various investigators[82,83] for young men and women, and also in excess of the 0.29 to 0.60 gm daily noted by Watts et al. (v.s.). However, since the diets contained less than 50 mg cystine daily (all in the low-protein food present in the basal diet), the possibility exists that the increased requirement comes not from the need for sulfur-containing amino acids per se but rather from a decreased efficiency of conversion of methionine to cystine.

Two of four subjects tested retained nitrogen on 1.4 gm lysine daily. The two subjects in negative balance on this amount (the two men in the group over 60) retained nitrogen when 2.8 gm lysine were fed daily. Even 1.4 gm lysine daily is well in excess of the 0.8 to 0.9 gm daily proposed as the requirement for the young by other investigators.[77,82]

The authors conclude that, under the experimental conditions imposed, elderly men require more than twice the amount of methionine and lysine needed for nitrogen equilibrium or retention in young adults.

Tontisirin et al.[83a,b] have estimated requirements of healthy elderly subjects for tryptophan and threonine, using the intake beyond which plasma concentrations no longer fell with gradual reductions in intake of the amino acid under study as indicative of the minimum daily requirement of that amino acid. They interpreted their data to indicate a mean minimum tryptophan requirement of 2 mg per kg body weight per day in the elderly, as opposed to previously determined minima of 3 mg per kg per day in young men[83c] and of 4 mg per kg per day in children with Down's syndrome.[83d] In regard to threonine, they interpreted their data to indicate a minimum requirement of 7.6 ± 2.2 mg per kg per day for one male and 12 female elderly persons, and 6.8 ± 1.7 mg per kg per day for young men, a difference without statistical significance.

Young et al.[48a] have argued that such data suggest that the minimum amino acid requirement per unit of total body protein increases with age, since lean body mass is reduced and the proportion of body fat increased among the aged. They maintain that preliminary data on a valine response curve in the elderly also suggest that the minimum valine requirement per unit of cell mass may be higher among the elderly, although no differences from young adults on the basis of 1 mg per kg body weight were observed.

Plasma Amino Acids. Data[74] which make direct comparisons between young and old subjects on the same diet are confined to one tabulation in which four college students were found to have total essential amino acid concentrations of 92 μ moles per 100 ml and an essential/nonessential (E/N) ratio of 48, whereas five men over 60 were found to have total essential amino acid concentrations of 87 μ moles per 100 ml and an E/N ratio of 45. Both groups were consuming a 7-gm nitrogen diet.

Swendseid[74] tentatively regards the low E/N ratio as an indicator of inadequate protein nutritional status, provided disease states and dietary intake are given adequate consideration or are controlled.[84] Since most of the increase in nonessential amino acids is confined to asparagine-glutamine and alanine, all actively involved in transamination,[84a] Swendseid also raises the question of whether the plasma concentrations of these amino acids would increase if metabolic processes were unable to supply adequate amounts of the keto acids necessary to synthesize these amino acids,[74,84b] as might occur if a calorie deficit were combined with a low-protein diet. Some preliminary evidence[84c,d] supporting this concept has been obtained in elderly, obese but otherwise healthy subjects undergoing starvation for 28 days. In contrast to the elderly men fed calorically adequate diets containing 3.5 gm of nitrogen, these men showed an approximately 30 per cent increase in branched-chain amino acids (valine, leucine, isoleucine) for 3 weeks, followed by a fall to normal or low values at the end of 4 weeks. The initial rise in the branched-chain acids was accompanied by a decrease in nonessential amino acids. The fate of the nonessentials during the fourth week in these preliminary studies was not reported.

Young[43a] has reported plasma concentrations of branched-chain amino acids in 19 healthy young men and 11 healthy elderly women consuming an "adequate free-choice diet." Blood samples were drawn after a 10-hour overnight fast. No significant differences in mean concentrations of leucine, isoleucine, valine or the leucine/valine ratio were found.

Ackerman and Kheim[84e] have reported levels of the essential amino acids valine, methionine, leucine, isoleucine, phenylalanine and lysine to be lower in the elderly than in young adults. Theimer[84f] also has reported reduced concentrations among the elderly for most plasma amino acids.

In contrast, Wehr and Lewis[84g] have reported 12 of 18 free amino acids in plasma from fasting elderly subjects to be elevated, with the concentration of ornithine significantly higher in the old than in young control subjects. Armstrong and Stave[84h] have found increased concentrations of alanine, citrulline, cystine and tyrosine but decreased serine concentrations in older persons.

These varying reports deserve relatively little attention unless derived from studies with persons of matched sexes and constant dietary intakes during comparative studies. In addition, the elderly should not be lumped together as a homogeneous group but rather studied by cohorts varying in age by at least five years. Excessively obese or emaciated persons should not be included in such studies.

Protein Synthesis in Aging. Sharp et al.[85] fed ^{15}N-tagged yeast to four elderly women (average age 66) and to one young man and one young woman (both aged 24). During 5 days following the feeding of the tagged yeast, they observed retentions of absorbed ^{15}N of 49.1 per cent in the elderly and 57.6 per cent in the young subjects. Based on the amount of ^{15}N absorbed, the amount of nitrogen (both fed and recycled) used for protein synthesis was 0.204 gm per kg per day in the elderly and 0.284 gm per kg per day in the young subjects. The mean ^{15}N half-life was 61 days in the elderly and 86 days in the young. The turnover of ^{15}N (protein/

nitrogen) in the young was about one and one-half times that in the elderly. The authors concluded that the rate of protein synthesis is slowed by physiologic aging.

Another study of the rates of amino acid incorporation into protein was performed by Tschudy et al.[86] in a 54-year-old woman with lymphosarcoma during an inactive phase of her disease. The study was designed to measure the effect of variations in the protein calorie/total calorie ratio in the diet, and the differences between inactive and active phases of the disease. The incorporation rate was increased significantly only when both total calories and protein calories were simultaneously raised. This increased rate was associated with a more rapid metabolic pool turnover with the higher calorie intake but was unaccompanied by more nitrogen retention than when the patient was on an equally high-protein but lower-calorie diet.

One year later, the patient was again studied,[87] this time with active neoplastic disease. She was unable to consume more than the low-calorie, low-protein regimen of the previous investigations. The rate of nitrogen incorporation into protein and the metabolic pool turnover rate were both increased to values equivalent to those observed on the high-calorie, high-protein diet of the earlier study. This investigation clearly indicates both that dietary intake must be carefully standardized among subjects and that disease must be excluded from all subjects if changes in rates of protein synthesis are to be correlated with aging per se and not with some extraneous factor.

Using their application[88] of the continuous infusion of ^{15}N-glycine developed by Picou and Taylor-Roberts,[89] Winterer et al.[90] have estimated the protein synthesis and breakdown in healthy elderly people aged 65 to 91 years and compared the results with data derived from studies in young adults receiving adequate amounts of dietary protein. Their estimates suggest lower values among the elderly, the differ-

ences being of relatively low statistical significance (p=<0.05) when the data are expressed in terms of gm per kg body weight per day. The rates, regardless of age, were lower in women than in men, but the differences among age groups were identical for men and women. The number of subjects in each group was small and variances in the data, especially for the elderly men, were large.

The authors also related the synthesis and breakdown of protein (1) to muscle mass, using urinary excretion of creatinine as an index, (2) to fat-free body cell mass estimated by whole-body [40]K measurements and (3) to calories of basal energy expenditure. Their data, some reported in preliminary form,[48a,43a,b] showed that whole-body protein synthesis and breakdown were 40 to 68 per cent greater in old than in young adults when related to creatinine excretion, 10 to 14 per cent greater when related to whole-body [40]K measurements, and 2 to 24 per cent greater when related to basal caloric expenditure.

The authors[48a,43a,b,88] interpret these findings as reflections of a lower contribution of muscle to whole-body protein synthesis and breakdown in elderly than in young adults. Since protein turnover is more rapid in visceral organs than in muscle, and since the quantity of muscle diminishes with age, they believe their findings suggest a relatively greater contribution in the elderly by visceral tissues to whole-body protein metabolism.

Using urinary excretion of [1]N-methylhistidine as a quantitatively accurate indicator of the breakdown of muscle protein, the same authors have observed that the daily rate is lower in old than young adults. Assuming (1) a known [1]N-methylhistidine concentration in the mixed protein of adult human muscle (in a recent publication,[43] although not in some preceding it,[48a,43a] stated to be 4.2 μM per gm of muscle protein), (2) an equal daily breakdown of myofibrillar and sarcoplasmic proteins and (3) the equality of synthesis and breakdown rates over short time periods, they maintain that muscle breakdown and synthesis account for 27 per cent of whole-body protein breakdown and synthesis in young adults (both sexes), but for only 20 and 16 per cent in older men and women, respectively. These latest figures suggest decrements in muscle contribution of 26 per cent for males and 41 per cent for females, when young and old adults are compared.

The authors maintain that such computations support the thesis that protein metabolism in muscles accounts for a lower proportion of the total-body protein turnover in the elderly than it does in the young. They speculate that the greater contribution of visceral organs to total-body protein metabolism might indeed reduce needs for exogenous sources of nitrogen and amino acids.[48a]

In summary, the dietary protein needs of adult man have yet to be related satisfactorily to the aging process. The existence of great variation in protein requirements for nitrogen equilibrium among the aged is the only conclusive fact arising from many balance investigations. Age-related studies of serum proteins and of adaptations to protein withdrawal and to refeeding have led to no conclusions which could be related to aging per se. Studies using pure L-amino acids which have indicated greater requirements among the aged are counterbalanced by others of slightly different design in which indications of marked differences in amino acid requirement were not demonstrated. All these investigations show marked interindividual variation among the aged. Differences based on age alone in the E/N ratios in plasma are so small as to lack significance. Turnover studies provide some evidence of slower protein synthesis, but even this must be tempered by considerations of the sex and body composition of the elderly subjects studied and by the nature of the tagged protein fed. Obviously a clear answer to the question of protein requirement must await more carefully controlled investigations in larger numbers of elderly and young subjects unimpaired by disease. Even more desirable would be longitudinal studies in the same subjects conducted at stated intervals over a span of many years.[13c]

Fat

Relating the aging process per se to quantitative or qualitative intake of dietary fat is complicated in man by the ubiquitous nature of the disease atherosclerosis. Since diagnosis of the presence, let alone quantification of the extent, of atherosclerosis is virtually impossible in man short of autopsy or clinical indications of important vascular occlusions, experimental work in human subjects who are guaranteed free of atherosclerosis cannot be performed. The best compromise has been work in population groups known by experience to have low mortality rates attributable to and little autopsy evidence of atherosclerosis. Often these groups habitually consume diets low in total fat and/or diets containing fat a high percentage of which is in the form of unsaturated oils.[91,92,93,93a,b,94,94a] However, since these same population groups often live under environmental circumstances which preclude optimum personal hygiene, public sanitation and preventive and curative medicine, they form a poor group in which to conduct studies relating dietary fat to aging per se.

Many carefully controlled clinical investigations[94b–d,95,95a–c,96,96a–c,97–100,100a–h] have left little doubt that substitution of unsaturated for saturated fats will depress serum cholesterol concentrations as well as those of other serum lipids which have been correlated in surveys of population groups with clinical evidences of atherosclerosis.[94,101,102] Consequently, it has been customary to recommend that the aged who statistically have a great prevalence of atherosclerosis adhere to diets moderate in total fat, a high percentage of which should be in the form of unsaturated oil. However, recent commentators on the lipid hypothesis and on dietary intervention in the prevention of coronary heart disease[102a-e] have raised issues of validity, especially as to recommendations for those who are 55 or older. Available data suggest that little can be accomplished for those in late maturity and old age who have waited until those ages to pay heed to nutritional factors influencing cardiovascular diseases.

Of greater importance are efforts directed at the prevention of atherosclerosis through the use of similar measures throughout youth and middle age. Despite strong circumstantial evidence in favor of restricting total fat and of substituting unsaturated for saturated fats, the Committee on Dietary Fat Levels of the Council on Foods and Nutrition of the American Medical Association[103] has cautioned that no direct causal relationship between dietary or serum lipids concentrations and atherosclerosis has been proved. The committee recommends that any manipulations with dietary fat be regarded as experimental procedures as far as the prevention and treatment of atherosclerosis are concerned.

In commenting on the *Dietary Goals for the United States* promulgated by the Select Committee on Nutrition and Human Needs of the United States Senate,[103a] the American Medical Association has reasserted its view that the above statement of its position remains valid.[103b]

The final report (1968) of the U.S. National Diet-Heart Study (1963–1965)[100a,103c] on the feasibility of studying the effects of low-fat, low-cholesterol, high-polyunsaturated-fatty acid diets on serum cholesterol concentrations in both free-living and closed populations includes the recommendation that a 5-year, major definitive study of the effects of diet on the primary prevention of myocardial infarction be planned and put into operation as soon as possible. Such a study, had it been

successfully completed, would have provided data on which to base further recommendations on the use of diet control as a public health measure in the prevention of myocardial infarction and other manifestations of atherosclerosis. As observed in the final report,[100a] such data would have had profound implications for major food processors in the United States and abroad. Properly designed, it would have provided data relative to the impact of nutrition, if any, on the aging process per se. However, the high cost and doubts about the impact of the proposed diet led to the study being cancelled;[103d,103e] hence, the role of diet in the prevention of atherosclerosis remains in question. Its role in the prevention of the disease among the elderly, with one possible exception (v.i.), seems insignificant.

At this point, it should be reemphasized that prevention or treatment of atherosclerosis is not prevention of aging. Atherosclerosis is a disease; aging is for the time being an inexorable biochemical process. It may, at some future date, be demonstrated that the biochemical changes associated with aging may be related to those leading to the disease atherosclerosis. The influence of quantitative and qualitative changes in dietary fat on plasma amino acid concentrations[103f] suggests other relationships between dietary lipids and aging. For the present, however, it is well to remember that progress in understanding the aging process, progress which may well cause the aging process to submit to modification by man, is more likely to come from studies in basic chemistry, physics and mathematics[21,24,28,29,31,32,104,104a] than from investigations primarily aimed at modifying a widespread chronic disease.

During the past decade, interest in the Fredrickson classification of serum lipid and lipoprotein patterns in persons with familial hyperlipoproteinemia has spread beyond academic centers to become a diagnostic reality in the evaluation of all age groups.[104b,c] The dietary management of each of the six types affords a means of protecting those affected from premature disability and death. The interrelationships of each of the types to aging as a biologic process remain to be explored.

As mentioned above, one possible exception to the general rule that plasma lipid concentrations are not predictors of risk from coronary artery disease has resurfaced after lying dormant for over a quarter century.[104d] High-density lipoproteins, also designated α-lipoproteins and α-cholesterol, have been found to be more predictive of coronary artery disease than other lipid parameters[104e-h] and to retain this predictive quality beyond age 55. The correlations are inverse, i.e. the higher the concentration of high-density lipoproteins the lower is the incidence of coronary heart disease. Glueck et al.[104i] have noted that high-density lipoprotein concentrations characterize long-lived families.

How these observations relate to nutrition has yet to be explored in detail, although, in one study among men of Japanese ancestry living in Hawaii,[104j] the investigators have reported that moderate alcohol consumption, up to 60 ml per day mainly from beer, was positively correlated (r = 0.28) with high-density lipoprotein levels and hence with lower incidence rates for coronary heart disease.

Although the mechanisms underlying the inverse correlation of high-density lipoprotein concentrations to coronary heart disease (and obesity[104e]) are not fully understood, various investigators have suggested that the lipoproteins serve as scavengers, removing cholesterol from deposits[104k] and interfering with the uptake of excess cholesterol by cells.[104l,m]

Carbohydrate

Carbohydrate once was called the "Cinderella of human nutrition,"[105] in large measure because it was a nutrient the physiologic role of which in human nutrition had been overlooked or given scant attention. As far as aging and its associated diseases are concerned, carbohydrate has received far less attention than either protein or fat. Studies applying various tolerance tests suggested[106,107,107a,b] that man's ability to metabolize carbohydrate is reduced with advancing age. Andres and Tobin[107b] and Andres[107c] have presented an oral glucose tolerance test nomogram by which performance on tolerance tests may be judged in the light of the subject's age. They recommend that this standard be used instead of an arbitrary number applying to all ages, and warn against classifying middle-aged and elderly subjects as diabetics on the basis of poor performances on tolerance tests alone. A substantial literature exists[46,107d-k] suggesting that diets high in carbohydrate improve the clinical and biochemical states of diabetics, many of whom are elderly.

Concern has been expressed by many authors about the "empty calories" found in the high-carbohydrate diets of certain categories of the aged.[108-110] Gustafsson et al.[111] presented strong evidence that consumption of large amounts of carbohydrate-containing foods, especially those which adhere for long periods on tooth surfaces, leads to a high caries rate in susceptible persons.

When carbohydrate is present as a high percentage of total calories in man's diet, lactescence appears in serum, associated with a rise in the concentrations of S_f 20–400 β-lipoproteins.[112] This has been attributed to the accumulation of triglycerides synthesized endogenously from carbohydrate.[104b,112] Increasing the frequency of carbohydrate ingestion daily from 3 to 6 or more times clearly results in reduced insulin requirements in diabetics.[113-115] Also, in studies with isocaloric, isonitrogenous diets, frequent carbohydrate ingestion has resulted in lower serum cholesterol concentrations and greater nitrogen retention than similar quantities ingested 3 times daily.[115]

The fact that carbohydrate is receiving increased attention is indicated by the plethora of studies dealing with its metabolism which have appeared in recent years. While the effects of carbohydrates on lipid metabolism in animals were observed previously,[115a] attention more recently has been stimulated by the papers of Yudkin[115b,c,d] and others[115e-k] indicting refined carbohydrates for hypertriglyceridemia and hypercholesterolemia and for an increased incidence of ischemic heart disease in man.[115d,l,m] The majority of studies have suggested that highly refined carbohydrates, particularly sucrose, when substituted isocalorically for complex carbohydrates such as starch, lead to an increase in the concentrations of serum cholesterol and serum triglycerides.[115i-o]

Findings such as these, coupled with the sharp rise in consumption of refined sugar[115p] in the American diet, have led to the recommendation in *Dietary Goals for the United States*[103a] that refined sugar consumption be reduced by about 40 per cent so that it would account for only about 15 per cent of total energy intake (goal 5). However, the first goal suggested increasing consumption of complex carbohydrates—fruits, vegetables and whole grains—to account for approximately 55 to 60 per cent of total energy intake. This would be achieved by application of goal 2, the reduction of fat calories from over 40 to approximately 30 per cent of energy intake.

Minerals

Calcium. As is atherosclerosis, osteoporosis is often regarded as a manifestation of the aging process.[116,116a,b] In its primary type, it is, however, a disease which much experimental and epidemiologic evidence relates to negative calcium balances, small in quantity but continued over long periods of time.[117-120a] This evidence is contradictory to the long-standing hypothesis of Reifenstein and Albright[55] that osteoporosis is associated with lack of adequate protein matrix. Therapy also has changed in that greater calcium intake, the

ingestion of strontium[120b] and the use of sodium fluoride[120c-h] have tended to supplant estrogen and androgen therapy. However, no single therapeutic regimen is clearly ascendant, leading many cautious investigators to acknowledge the pluralistic etiology of this disease.[116a,120i,j] Exton-Smith,[120k] in agreement with Garn et al.,[120l,m] has concluded that bone loss in old age cannot conclusively be related to calcium intake in adult life, but that considerable evidence exists relating the amount of bone present in old age directly to the skeletal mass at maturity.

Developments in the intermediary metabolism of vitamin D[120n-p] have led to clinical investigations suggesting an association between age and plasma concentrations of 1,25 $(OH)_2$ vitamin D[120q] and an association between plasma concentrations of 1,25 $(OH)_2$ vitamin D and the presence of osteoporosis.[120r] New, simpler techniques to replace the presently complex assay for 1,25 $(OH)_2$ D are being developed and should lead to collection of much more detailed information than is available at this time.[120s]

Since kidney is the site of action of 25-hydroxy vitamin D_3-1α-hydroxylase, the enzyme catalyzing the formation of 1,25 $(OH)_2$ vitamin D_3 from its precursor 25 (OH) vitamin D_3, it is tempting to speculate that the normal bone loss associated with women over 40 and men over 50[120t] may be associated with the decrements with age in numbers of nephrons as indicated by the linear fall in discrete renal functions with biologic aging in man.[4,5] Data to support such speculation may be found in observations on patients with renal disease. Bone disease appears when glomerular filtration rates fall below 30 ml per minute,[120u] but intestinal calcium absorption declines linearly with renal impairment.[120v] Assays for 1,25 $(OH)_2$ vitamin D in nephrectomized patients reveal undetectable concentrations.[120w,x] Kidneys in patients with end-stage renal failure are incapable of synthesizing 1,25 $(OH)_2$ vitamin D. Dramatic improvement in calcium absorption and suppression of parathyroid hormone activity have been observed on treatment with 1,25 (OH)$_2$ vitamin D$_3$ or with 1α-(OH) vitamin D$_3$ (a synthetic precursor of the natural compound which is converted into 1,25 (OH)$_2$ vitamin D$_3$ via a route circumventing renal 1α-hydroxylation).[120y,z]

These investigations have raised anew the question of the optimum calcium intake for man, and particularly for the elderly. Hegsted et al.[121] observed metabolic equilibrium for calcium among prisoners in Peru accustomed to calcium intakes as low as 0.2 to 0.3 gm daily. Walker[122] also has observed adaptation to low-calcium diets. Malm,[123] working with elderly men, observed successful adaptation to diets containing from 0.9 down to 0.45 gm daily. Smith et al.[120i] found higher serum calcium and phosphorus concentrations and greater antirachitic activity in the sera of Puerto Rican than in those of Michigan women, suggesting that sunlight exposure may be related to lower prevalence rates for osteoporosis in tropical climates. Calkins,[124] studying an aging male while in a metabolic research unit and later when the man worked on his own farm, found increased retentions of calcium, phosphorus and nitrogen during the second phase of the investigation. Hence, environment[120i] and activity[116a,b] are additional variables which must be standardized in comparing metabolic phenomena in individuals or groups.

Higher calcium requirements for the aged than for the young have been reported.[125–127] On the other hand, no differences in requirements for old and young have been reported by others.[47,123] Calcium was not stored in one investigation[47] despite retention of large amounts of phosphorus and nitrogen. Similar findings were observed[60] in old men retaining large amounts of nitrogen and phosphorus at two dietary protein levels, both with and without a potent

synthetic androgen. By a reevaluation of data collected from seven sources, Harrison[128] has inferred that there is little difference in the efficiency of calcium absorption among old men, young adults and older children, although his evaluation revealed a very high calcium absorption efficiency among infants.

Lutwak et al. have presented impressive evidence that bone resorption in human periodontal disease and in experimental models in animals can be prevented or reversed by adequate calcium intakes. They suggest that bone loss can be prevented at any age and in a variety of physiologic states (e.g. post-traumatic immobilization) by the provision of calcium in at least the recommended daily allowance, if not higher, in the dietary regimen.[128-a,b,c,d]

Albanese et al.[120t,128e] have developed radiographic methods for quantitative evaluation of bone loss in both the middle phalanx of the fifth digit and in the alveolar ridges of the mandible and maxilla. They found peak densities in women aged 35 to 45 and in men a decade older, with progressive declines thereafter. In controlled dietary studies they demonstrated a 12 to 30 per cent increase in coefficients of bone density after 24 to 48 months of administering supplements containing 750 mg of calcium and 375 I.U. of vitamin D. The diets prior to supplementation averaged 450 mg of calcium. These data have led the authors to press for a higher recommended dietary allowance[49] for calcium for both the aging and the aged.

On the whole, present evidence suggests that the calcium requirements of the aged in good health are at least equivalent to those of younger adults. Data on bone mineralization in old age,[129,130,131] data on osteoporosis (v.s.) and long-term negative calcium balances, occasioned either by deficient intake in earlier adulthood or by some as-yet-undefined metabolic defect associated with aging, indicate a need in many aged persons for greater dietary intakes of calcium. This in turn implies a need for greater consumption of milk, a product which is often unpopular among or too expensive for the aged. The problem of unpopularity may be resolved by education campaigns and the issue of cost by the use of powdered skim milk. The availability of milk in the nutrition program authorized by Title VII of the Older Americans Act (NPOA) has led to dramatic increases in milk consumption by eligible participants aged 60 and over. A Limited Use Supplemental Food (LUSF), based on powdered skim milk to which carbohydrates, vitamins and trace elements are added has been introduced and overwhelmingly accepted by NPOA participants.[131a]

When milk or milk products are absolutely contraindicated, calcium gluconate or lactate may be needed to rectify a continued negative calcium balance. Attention to dietary calcium intake should be matched by encouragement of physical activity, the anabolic consequences of which have already been mentioned (v.s.).

Phosphorus. Dietary phosphorus has gained new significance as a result of some studies in rodents and primates[132] suggesting that an increase may lead to greater protection against caries in childhood and adolescence. Animal studies suggest a similar role for phosphorus in improving bone structure. However, increasing the phosphorus content in the diets of the aged has yet to be undertaken experimentally and should be approached with considerable caution in view of the linear decrements in renal function associated with the aging process after age 30. Hyperphosphatemia is a common companion of azotemia in renal disease. Lives have been saved in acute situations, or prolonged in chronic renal disease, by the prescription of high-carbohydrate, low-protein, low-phosphorus diets such as the rice diets.[46] When only conventional diets are available, phosphorus absorption may be prevented by the administration of two hourly, 30-ml doses of aluminum hydroxide gel, a procedure that will reduce urinary phosphorus concentration practically to zero and keep serum phosphorus concentrations in the normal range.[133,133a] The high-phosphorus diets associated with the ingestion of large amounts of meat and soft drinks by some segments of the population lower the dietary calcium/phosphorus ratio and may predispose those affected to osteopenia unless sufficient calcium is included in the diet to maintain a ratio of one or higher.[133b]

Fluorine. When consumed by children under five in drinking water with a concentration of one part per million (ppm), fluorine will protect teeth from dental caries during childhood and adolescence and preserve them for use throughout adulthood and into old age.[134,135] Scientific data to support the contention of certain groups that fluoridation of drinking water in the recommended concentration is harmful have not been presented.

As mentioned in the discussion of calcium (v.s.), sodium fluoride in doses ranging from 50 to 150 mg per day[135a] has been under investigation as a treatment for osteoporosis. Both epidemiologic evidence[120h] and clinical investigation by balance study and bone density techniques[120e] have indicated a potential role for fluoride in prevention and treatment. Not all investigators have been enthusiasts,[120j,135b] the favorable effects being transitory or negligible in their hands. Toxic manifestations of sodium fluoride therapy (anorexia, epigastric pain, ectopic calcification, optic neuritis and retinal damage)[135a,b] serve as reminders that it is still an experimental procedure. The potential hazards of the fluoride content of bones incorporated into whole fish flour has been investigated and found to be of no great physiologic significance.[135c,d]

At the Mayo Clinic, combination therapy comprising 50 mg of sodium fluoride and 1 gm of calcium as calcium carbonate daily and 50,000 I.U. of vitamin D twice weekly has been under investigation.[135e] Calcium intake is regarded as the key ingredient in the prevention of osteoporosis, with the combination regimen reserved for therapy of symptomatic disease.

Iron. Aged males and postmenopausal females without blood loss from disease may develop iron deficiency on the basis of inadequate intake alone if the deficient diet is consumed over many years. However, physicians must assume that older persons who are iron deficient are bleeding and seek causes for bleeding before assuming a priori that dietary lack of iron is at the root of the problem.[135f] Parenteral iron is usually contraindicated by its inconvenience and expense, not to mention its potential carcinogenicity.[136]

Iodine. This element is essential to the proper function of the thyroid gland throughout life. If iodinized salt is contraindicated as a source of iodine because of diets restricted in sodium, other iodine-containing medications should be administered to provide the appropriate amount. However, caution in prescribing iodinized salt or other iodine-containing preparations must be exercised, since iodine used in animal feed and animal medications and in food and dairy-product processing is entering the food chain in such amounts that dietary iodine intake in North America is generally in excess of the RDA of 100 to 300 μg per day.[136a]

Sodium. Although sodium is an essential component of any diet, its restriction in therapeutic diets has caused it to become a household term to patients with congestive heart failure, hypertension, cirrhosis of the liver with ascites and other conditions associated with the retention of extracellular fluid. Among mature and elderly adults whose physicians prescribe low-sodium diets, two problems arise: (1) It is difficult for a patient to secure meals low in sodium if he eats in restaurants or with others who practice no sodium restriction and (2) by lowering the palatability of diets, sodium restriction may lead to lowered food con-

sumption and therefore to deficiencies in the intake of other essential nutrients.

The first problem is related to the general one of obtaining proper nutrition counseling and appropriate, low-cost foods as discussed in detail above. The second requires reeducation of the patient and, if necessary, the substitution of other sodium-free flavoring agents and condiments. Of paramount importance, however, is motivating the patient to adhere to his diet, and this is a task requiring great ingenuity on the part of the physician and all others in the patient's immediate environment.

Management of many conditions in which rigorous sodium restriction was once indicated has been made far simpler through the introduction and widespread use of diuretic drugs.[136b] By substituting moderate for rigorous sodium restriction, compliance with dietary regulation improves. However, compliance with drug dosage instructions may continue to be a problem not only among the elderly but with patients of all ages.

Hypernatremia is a serious and usually preventable problem seen not infrequently in patients whose medical conditions require feedings administered by tube.[137] If the tube feedings are high in protein and salt, the resulting load of urea and salt which must be excreted increases the obligatory renal water loss sufficiently to produce a negative water balance and hypernatremia. Hence, great care must be given to the water requirements of tube-fed patients, especially to those who are obtunded or comatose and unable to respond to the sensation of thirst. If hypernatremia occurs, the appropriate treatment is the administration of water, enough to add 4 per cent of the body weight in kg for each 10 mEq/liter increase in serum sodium above normal.[138]

Potassium. Potassium is so widely distributed among natural foods that primary potassium deficiency is virtually unknown. Potassium is so effectively excreted that excessive intake rarely causes difficulty in healthy man.[138a] In disease states, however, both hypo- and hyperkalemia may occur, the former in association with gastrointestinal losses and the latter with renal insufficiency. Hypokalemia can be corrected by parenterally administered solutions containing potassium salts and/or by the oral administration of potassium-containing foods. Hyperkalemia can be treated by administration of pure carbohydrate and fat, either orally or parenterally, supplemented by appropriate vitamins. Such regimens reduce potassium intake and also minimize tissue breakdown, an endogenous source of potassium.[139] Hyperkalemia may be attacked more directly by infusions of insulin and glucose or by the administration of sodium polystyrene sulfonate, a cation exchange resin prepared in the sodium phase with exchange capacity in vivo of approximately 1 mEq potassium per gm. This resin when given to normal men over a period of a week may result in a loss of total body potassium of greater than 10 per cent, with associated deterioration of myocardial performance, delay in cellular glucose uptake and retention of water.[139a] In either the hypo- or the hyperkalemic state, monitoring serum potassium concentrations by flame photometry or electrocardiography is required for guidance in prescribing control measures.

Vitamins

Socioeconomic conditions and reduced physical activity among the aged may lead to sharp curtailment in intake of vitamin-containing foods. The high costs of protective foods and of dietary supplements may eliminate these as sources of vitamins for the poor. Also, various diseases capable of inducing secondary deficiencies are more common among the aged. It is not surprising, therefore, that many authors have postulated and some have sought evidence for vitamin deficiency among the elderly.

Water-soluble Vitamins. According to one group of investigators, B-complex vitamins and ascorbic acid supplements have resulted in improved "general vitality and vigor" among the aged studied.[140] According to others, administration of B-complex vitamins and ascorbic acid has resulted in improvement in symptoms previously attributed to nonspecific senility and cerebral atherosclerosis.[141,142] One psychiatrist, influenced by these reports, has blamed further dietary restrictions superimposed on an already borderline vitamin reserve for acute psychotic episodes in elderly adults.[143] Rafsky and Newman have reported greater ascorbic acid needs,[144] greater quantities of thiamin for "saturation"[145] and lower blood thiamin concentrations and urinary thiamin excretions[146] in the elderly fed diets qualitatively adequate for young adults. However, Horwitt et al.,[147] in a classical series of carefully controlled metabolic studies in institutionalized subjects, have failed to reveal differences in thiamin and riboflavin excretion between young and old. No correlation between age and urinary excretion has been found in studies during which test doses of various B-complex vitamins were administered.[148–150]

Vitamin B_{12} was found by Watkin et al.[151] to be retained in greater amounts by old than by young men when test doses were administered parenterally at four different dose levels. Old and young subjects alike had received good diets adequate in vitamin B_{12} for many months.

Ascorbic acid has achieved notoriety by virtue of Pauling's assertions that it affects morbidity from diseases ranging from the common cold[152] to neoplasias.[153] In one portion of a large nutrition survey in Wales, Burr et al.[154] confirmed previous reports[155–160] of lower plasma and leukocyte ascorbic acid concentrations in older persons than among the general population. Their data displayed a progressive decline with advancing age in both sexes, with men having consistently lower concentrations than women even when the analyses were controlled for fresh fruit and vegetable consumption and for smoking. No correlations were observed between ascorbic acid concentrations and the presence of chronic illnesses, anemias, body weights or skinfold thicknesses.

Persons habituated to high ascorbic acid intakes have higher rates of the vitamin's metabolism and excretion, a high incidence of scurvy when intake is reduced to the recommended dietary allowance[49] and plasma concentrations insignificantly higher than those of persons not receiving nondietary ascorbic acid.[161]

Another risk lies in the false-negative stool occult blood tests caused by ingestion of nondietary ascorbic acid.[162] In aging populations, where testing stools for occult blood is a desirable screening and management tool for alimentary tract pathology, false-negative tests could lead to serious consequences for patients consuming large doses of nondietary ascorbic acid.

A third potential risk is suggested by Herbert and Jacob,[163] who observed in vitro "destruction" of 50 to 95 per cent of the vitamin B_{12} content of a meal by 0.5 gm of ascorbic acid. Jacob et al.[163a] reported low serum B_{12} concentrations in veterans with spinal cord injuries and neurogenic dysfunction of the bladder who were taking 0.5 gm ascorbic acid daily to acidify their urine in a gesture at control of urinary tract infections. Vitamin B_{12} deficiency in patients ingesting 1.0 gm daily of ascorbic acid for three or more years has been reported by Hines.[163b] The findings of Herbert and Jacob[163] have been challenged by Newmark et al.,[163c] who attributed the reported "destruction" of B_{12} to methodologic problems.

A fourth difficulty is the potential increase in risk of urinary tract uric acid stones occasioned by the marked increase in uric acid clearance observed with either single large (4.0 gm) or chronically administered (8.0 gm daily) doses of ascorbic acid.[163d] In addition, the associated reductions in serum uric acid concentrations may invalidate measurements used in the diagnosis of gout. Ascorbic acid acts on the renal tubule to produce uricosuria.

Yet another problem is the increased risk of erythrocyte hemolysis in patients receiving pharmacologic doses of ascorbic acid,[163e] especially in those with glucose-6-phosphate dehydrogenase deficiency.[163f]

Fat-soluble Vitamins. Deficiencies in fat-soluble vitamins among adults in the United States are usually secondary to consumption of low-fat diets, to the interference with absorption caused by habitual ingestion of mineral oil as a laxative[164] or to diseases characterized by steatorrhea.[165,166] The aged who are clinically free from disease and who consume an adequate diet show few evidences of fat-soluble vitamin deficiencies.

There are no age-related decrements in plasma vitamin A and carotene concentrations.[167] Absorption of vitamin A by the intestine is unchanged by aging.[168] A significant decline in visual sensitivity, revealed by light threshold, has been observed.[169] However, no correlation between light threshold and serum vitamin A concentrations and no improvement in light threshold after administration of 100,000 I.U. vitamin A daily for as long as 76 days has been demonstrated.[170]

Diseases preventing absorption of vitamin D, calcium and phosphorus may lead to senile osteomalacia. Immediate therapy consists of administration of vitamin D, calcium and phosphorus, while the ultimate objective is correction of the illness responsible for the secondary deficiency. An inverse relation of exposure to sunshine and the prevalence of involutional osteoporosis has been proposed by Smith et al. (v.s.).[120i] Treatment of rheumatoid arthritis with massive doses (150,000 to 500,000 I.U. daily) of vitamin D has led to vitamin D intoxication.[171-173] Signs and symptoms have included metastatic calcification, hypercalcemia, azotemia, renal insufficiency, weakness, lassitude, anorexia, visual disturbances, anemia, dermatitis and inflammation and fatty deposits in the sclerae.

Except for individuals with bizarre eating habits,[174] primary vitamin K deficiency is not observed in adults. Man obtains the vitamin not only in his food but also from synthesis by the intestinal microflora. Hence, various diseases and types of therapy which interfere with fat absorption also interfere with absorption of vitamin K. In addition, sulfa drugs and antibiotics, if taken in amounts large enough to substantially reduce the number of intestinal microflora, will reduce the amount of vitamin K available for absorption.

No convincing evidence of any significant effect of supplemental, nondietary vitamin E on aging in man or animals has been presented.[175] Tappel,[176] observing mice fed a basic mouse diet with 0.3 per cent vitamin E added (equivalent to a human taking 2,000 I.U. daily or 150 times the 1974 RDA for a year) found no differences from control mice in walking capacity, coordination, renal and muscle membrane functions and mortality. The mice receiving supplemental vitamin E did demonstrate about one-half as much accumulation of fluorescent ("aging") pigment products as did the control mice. Williams et al.[176a] and Haeger[176b] have reported that 400-mg doses of vitamin E daily for at least three months diminish the severity of symptoms of intermittent claudication. However, apart from these reports of a partial success, evidence of the ineffectiveness of vitamin E in treating or preventing heart disease or other vascular ailments is overwhelming.[175,176]

Water

Although potable water is available in most parts of the United States, it is an inexpensive nutrient which the aged, through custom or distaste, consume in less than optimum quantities. Water can be a useful aid in washing down partially masticated food which might otherwise prove too difficult to eat. When consumed in copious amounts, it reduces the osmotic work of the kidney. In patients subject to renal and vesical lithiasis, such as those confined to bed or paralyzed by accident or disease, water intakes as high as 4 liters daily are needed to prevent stone formation. Water has been suggested as a means of improving elimination.[177]

Water need not be taken in pure form. The aged often find it more acceptable in soups, juices, milk products, soft drinks, alcoholic beverages, tea and coffee. In prescribing such easily ingested and pleasant liquids, care must be taken to avoid overconsumption of pure appetite-satisfying calories and the consequent exclusion of protective foods from the diet.

The dangers of hypernatremia during tube feeding of obtunded and comatose patients with formulas prepared with insufficient water have already been mentioned (v.s.).

Rarely, hyponatremia may result from overhydration[177a,b] but it usually suggests abnormal renal capacity to dilute urine.

When total body sodium is low, the associated arterial hypovolemia stimulates the release of antidiuretic hormone (ADH) and decreases renal plasma flow (RPF) and glomerular filtration rate (GFR) so that more filtrate is reabsorbed proximal to the sites of urinary dilution. This form of hyponatremia responds to isotonic saline, since the isotonic solution removes the stimulus to ADH release, corrects the renal hemodynamics and hence remedies the causes of abnormal water retention.

When total body sodium is high, as in patients with generalized edema, hyponatremia results from a decrease in the "effective" arterial blood volume which stimulates excess ADH secretion and decreases RPF and GFR, with enhanced sodium and water resorption proximal to the distal tubule where dilution occurs. In this case, both sodium and water should be restricted, the latter to no more than insensible losses. The underlying cardiac, renal or hepatic disease should be vigorously treated. Hypertonic saline is definitely proscribed.

Unfortunately, the most common cause of hypotonic hyponatremia in persons with normal body sodium is the syndrome of inappropriate secretion of ADH (SIADH), the causes of which are nonosmolar stimuli to ADH release: emotional stress, pain, hypovolemia, CNS disease, pulmonic infections, and many anesthetics and drugs, including narcotics, barbiturates, antidepressants, an hypolipidemic agent (clofibrate), oral hypoglycemic agents, antitumor agents and even diuretics.[177c,d] It is also seen in patients with neoplasms which themselves produce ectopic hormones with ADH activity[177e] and in patients receiving exogenous ADH. Since these conditions, diseases and drugs are all present or potential companions of old age, SIADH is a frequent problem among the elderly. If edema of the brain cells is a serious symptomatic complication, appropriate treatment consists of osmotically dehydrating the edematous cells by giving hypertonic saline with the dosage calculated on the basis of total body water. In the absence of cerebral symptoms, SIADH may be managed by water restriction alone and, if possible, removal of the causal stimuli.

Some patients appear to reset their osmoreceptors so that they maintain homeostatically lower than normal serum sodiums. These persons usually have conditions causing great debility. Treatment should be directed at the underlying process, since the hyponatremia itself requires no therapy. Prognostic implications in this condition are usually grave.

The water content of diets has received increasing attention with respect to its effect on the utilization of other nutrients by and on the body composition of growing animals.[178,179] Such effects have not been investigated in controlled studies in older animals or in aged man. Most research protocols have permitted ad libitum water intakes, thereby precluding any preliminary evaluation from work already completed. In view of the great variance associated with most parameters by which nutritional status is assessed in the aged, control of the water intake variable is recommended in future studies.

Calories

Calories have already received attention either in general discussion of nutrition and aging or under the respective headings of their components, protein, fat and carbohydrate. Mention has been made of the influence of under- or intermittent feeding on the aging of collagen. Note has been taken of the differences observed when isocaloric diets are fed as three meals or are taken as numerous small feedings throughout the day. Mention must be made also of the impressive role of caloric restriction in the prevention of chronic illness, well documented in man by the morbidity and mortality statistics among the overweight.[180]

In animals, calorie restriction has long been associated with greater longevity than has ad libitum feeding.[181,181a–c,182a–h] Ross[182c] demonstrated that the age of the rat at which dietary restriction begins is an important determinant of longevity. Restricting food intake from 21 to 70 days only, even though ad libitum feeding ensued throughout life, increased life duration. The adverse effects of ad libitum feeding early in life were partially overcome by restriction imposed at 70 days of age. Ross found the level of restriction most favorable for longevity to change with age. Rats severely restricted from age 21 days until death lived longest. When the same severe restriction was imposed later in life (300 days), life expectancy decreased; in somewhat older rats (365 days), life duration was drastically shortened. However, in these same older rats the length of life could be extended when less severe degrees of restriction were imposed.

In seeking a practical means of ascertaining the optimum nutrition for rats of various ages, Ross et al.[182e–g] turned to the self-selection method of feeding. Weaned rats were permitted to choose from three different complete purified isocaloric diets containing adequate amounts of minerals, vitamins and trace elements. The percentages of protein were 10, 22 and 51, and of carbohydrate 70.5, 58.5 and 29.5, respectively. Ross[182h] has summarized the many details of his studies. From them, he has derived a mathematical model best explaining variances in length of life. It incorporates seven variables describing dietary behavior and associated growth responses:[182g,h] (1) absolute and (2) relative preferences for protein between the 43rd and 49th day of life, (3) the efficiency with which food consumed is converted to body mass between the 49th and 98th day of life, (4) body weight at 119 and (5) 133 days, providing a measure of absolute change in weight between the two ages, (6) the time required to double a body weight of 250 gm and (7) the age at attaining a weight of 500 gm.

From their model, Ross et al. have concluded that feed efficiency and rates of growth early in life are inversely related to longevity. Low-protein, high-carbohydrate intakes early in life and high-protein, low-carbohydrate intakes later in life seem to be associated with shorter lives. After 400 days of age, the dietary protein or carbohydrate contribution to longevity is negligible. The variable contributing most to the variance in longevity is the number of days required to double the specified body weight. Maximum body weight during maturity is unrelated to length of life, supporting the concept that dietary habits and growth responses early in life are those which relate most to longevity.

Of special interest is the observation by Ross and Bras[182e] that rats nourished by self-selection had from 2 to 5 times the rates of tumors and of kidney, heart and prostate disease as did rats fed each of the same diets singly.

Although not altering the morbidity from radiculoneuritis,[183] calorie restriction has afforded protection against almost every disease afflicting the rat.[184]

Since calorie balance is dependent on thermodynamic equilibrium between food intake and energy expenditure, it is obvious that there should be a progressive decline in calorie ingestion to correspond with the progressive decline in physical activity beginning in the third decade and continuing throughout life if weight gain or, more important, an increase in the ratio of fat/nonfat tissue in the body is to be avoided. Also, even though restriction of calorie intake seems to be the most effective way to avoid calorie accretion, equilibrium still is the result of balanced forces, indicating that reasonable activity can be used effectively in achieving optimum calorie nutrition in the aging and the aged and in taking advantage of its anabolic properties[124] and its ability to clear lipids from the blood.[185]

The influence of physical exercise on coronary artery collateralization has been examined by Ferguson et al.[186] and Conner et al.[186a] In studying patients with proven coronary artery disease, both groups failed to demonstrate any increase in coronary collateralization attributable to exercise training programs per se. Nonetheless, subjectively, patients experienced an increased sense of well-being, greater self-esteem and more confidence in their ability to cope with and enjoy life. The failure to demonstrate increased collateralization may have been of methodologic origin. Using more modern methods,[186b,c,d] more specific data regarding collateralization might have been obtained.

DRUG-NUTRIENT INTERACTIONS

Drugs are part of the modern world scene not only among youth but also among the aging and the aged. While many drugs are prescribed properly, many are self-procured or prescribed for psychologic rather than pharmacologic impact. Regardless of how obtained, drugs influence the nutrition of the aging and the aged. This vast subject has been reviewed in depth by Roe.[186e]

CONCLUDING COMMENTS

This chapter has been designed to acquaint its readers with various aspects of gerontology that involve considerations of nutrition. Gerontology, the study of aging, is quite distinct from geriatrics, the treatment of diseases in the aged. Today, few clues exist as to methods of altering the process of aging by nutritional means.[24j,187] Most existing evidence reviewed here points to intrauterine and postnatal periods of life as those during which nutrition has most impact on aging as a biologic process. For the moment, prevention of chronic illness by nutritional planning from youth through late maturity promises the greatest rewards in terms of a healthy, active old age. For the aged, recent moves by government and private agencies promise to relieve the burdens of hunger and poverty, leaving the elderly and their champions more opportunity to lend their support to the funding of investigations benefiting future aged—but obviously not those who are old today.

The large interindividual variations in aging patterns and the infinite variety of physical and emotional insults during long lives make general recommendations for the aged as a class meaningless and mere grist for the mills of food faddists. Physicians and other health professionals informed in the role of nutrition in the management of health and disease, who can offer the aged individualized medical care and a sympathetic understanding of the biologic and socioeconomic aspects of being old, have no replacements.

BIBLIOGRAPHY

1. McWhirter and McWhirter: *The Guinness Book of World Records.* 14th ed. New York, Bantam, 1976, pp. 25–29.
1a.Watkin: Am. J. Public Health, *55*, 548, 1965.
1b.Schettlein-Gsell: Europa Med., *1*, 177, 1964.
1c.Watkin: In *Proceedings of the Joint Meeting of the U.S. Veterans Administration Spinal Cord Injury Centers and the International Medical Society of Paraplegia,* Boston, October 1971 (Talbot, Ed.). Washington, U.S. Veterans Administration, 1972.
1d.Vega and Robles: Salud Publica Mex., *4*, 385, 1962.
1e.Cravioto: Am. J. Public Health, *53*, 1803, 1963.
1f.Ramos-Galván, Vega and Cravioto: Bol. Med. Hosp. Infant. Mex., *21*, 157, 1964.
1g.Cravioto and Robles: Am. J. Orthopsychiatry, *35*, 449, 1965.
1h.Cravioto, Delicardio and Birch: Pediatrics, *38*, 319, 1966.
1i. The Nutrition Foundation: *Proceedings of an International Conference on Malnutrition, Learning and Behavior,* Cambridge, March, 1–3, 1967 (Scrimshaw and Gordon, Eds.). Cambridge, MIT Press, 1968.
1j. Barnes, Cunnold, Zimmerman, Simmons, MacLeod and Krook: J. Nutr., *89*, 399, 1966.
1k.Winick and Noble: J. Nutr., *91*, 179, 1967.
1l. Hseuh, Augustin and Chow: J. Nutr., *91*, 195, 1967.
1m.Guthrie and Brown: J. Nutr., *94*, 419, 1968.
1n.Howard and Granoff: J. Nutr., *95*, 111, 1968.
1o.Knittle: J. Nutr., *102*, 427, 1972.
1p.Roeder and Chow: Am. J. Clin. Nutr., *25*, 812, 1972.
1q.Kahn: Am. J. Clin. Nutr., *25*, 822, 1972.
1r.Barrows: Am. J. Clin. Nutr., *25*, 829, 1972.
1s.Watkin, et al.: Encuesta de Nutrición, República del Paraguay, Mayo-Agosto de 1965. Programa de Nutrición, Centro Nacional para el Control de Enfermedades Crónicas. Bethesda. Servicio de Salud Pública, Departamento de Salud, Educación y Bienestar de las EE. UU., 1967, pp. 1–482.
1t. Chow, Blackwell, Blackwell, Hou, Anilane and Sherwin: Am. J. Public Health., *58*, 668, 1968.
1u.Watkin: Ann. N. Y. Acad. Sci., *300*, 290, 1977.
1v.Toga, Nandy and Chauncey (Eds.): *Geriatric Dentistry: Clinical Application of Selected Biomedical and Psychosocial Topics.* Lexington (Massachusetts), D. C. Heath and Company, 1979.
1w.Ouellette, Rosett, Roseman and Weiner: N. Engl. J. Med., *297*, 528, 1977.
2. Mayer: Med. News, *1*, 11, 1966.
2a.White House Conference on Food, Nutrition and Health. Final Report and Addendum. Washington, Superintendent of Documents, U.S. Government Printing Office, 1969.
2b.Richmond (Chairman): *The Role of the Federal Government in Nutrition Education.* Subcommittee on Domestic Marketing, Consumer Relations, and Nutrition of the Committee on Agriculture, U. S. House of Representatives, Committee Print 86–248 0. Washington, U. S. Government Printing Office, 1977.
2c. Watkin: World Rev. Nutr. Diet., *26*, 26, 1977.
2d.Watkin: Med. Clin. North Am. *54*, 1589, 1970.
2e. Watkin: J. Am. Geriatr. Soc., *26*, 193, 1978.
2f. Feldman: Food Nutr., *6*, 2, 1976.
2g.Leaf: Nutr. Today, *8*, 4, 1973.

2h. Division of Community Health Services, U. S. Public Health Service, in cooperation with the Medical Care Section, American Public Health Association: *Medical Care in Transition*, 1949–1962. Washington, U. S. Government Printing Office, 1964.

2i. Watkin: World Rev. Nutr. Diet., *16*, 46, 1973.

2j. Watkin: In *Vitamins for the Elderly: Report of the Proceedings of a Symposium held at the Royal College of Physicians, London, on 2nd May, 1968* (Exton-Smith and Scott, Eds.). Bristol, John Wright & Sons, Baltimore, Williams & Wilkins, 1968.

2k. Shock: In *Age with a Future*. Copenhagen, Munskgaard, 1964.

2l. Oliver: In *Geriatric Medicine*, 2nd ed. (Steiglitz, Ed.). Philadelphia, W. B. Saunders, 1949.

3. Yiengst, Barrows and Shock: J. Gerontol., *14*, 400, 1959.

3a. Brody: In *Proceedings of the 7th International Congress of Gerontology*, Vol. 8. Wien, Medical Akad. Wien, 1966.

3b. Brody: *Proc. 9th International Congress of Gerontology*, Vol. 1. Kiev, 1972, p. 228.

4. Davies and Shock: J. Clin. Invest., *29*, 496, 1950.

5. Watkin and Shock: J. Clin. Invest., *34*, 969, 1955 (abstract).

6. Andrew, Shock, Barrows and Yiengst: J. Gerontol., *14*, 405, 1959.

7. Shock, Watkin, Yiengst, Norris, Gaffney, Gregerman and Falzone: J. Gerontol, *18*, 1, 1963.

8. Pett and Ogilvie: Hum. Biol., *28*, 177, 1956.

9. Norris, Shock and Landowne: J. Gerontol., *13*, 437, 1958.

10. Alvarez: Geriatrics, *15*, 671, 1960.

11. Norris, Lundy and Shock: Ann. N. Y. Acad. Sci., *110*, 623, 1963.

12. Sagild: Scand. J. Clin. Lab. Invest., *8*, 44, 1956.

12a. Moore, Olesen, McMurrey, Parker, Ball and Boyden: *The Body Cell Mass and its Supporting Environment*. Philadelphia, W. B. Saunders, 1963.

13. Allen, Anderson and Langham: J. Gerontol., *15*, 348, 1960.

13a. Meneely, Heyssel, Ball, Weiland, Lorimer, Constantinides and Meneely: Ann. N. Y. Acad. Sci., *110*, 271, 1963.

13b. Forbes and Reina: Metabolism, *19*, 653, 1970.

13c. Shock: In *Aging of the Lung* (Cander and Mayer, Eds.). New York, Grune and Stratton, 1964, p. 1.

13d. Stone and Norris: J. Gerontol., *21*, 575, 1966.

13e. Rose: Hum. Dev., *8*, 158, 1965.

13f. Rose and Bell: *Predicting Longevity: Methodology and Critique*. Lexington (Massachusetts), Heath Lexington Books, 1971.

13g. Shock: In *Nutrition and Old Age* (Carlson, Ed.). Uppsala, Almquist & Wiksell, 1972, pp. 12–23.

14. Barrows: Fed. Proc., *15*, 954, 1956.

15. Barrows, Yiengst and Shock: J. Gerontol., *13*, 351, 1958.

16. Falzone, Barrows and Shock: J. Gerontol., *14*, 2, 1959.

17. Barrows: In *The Biology of Aging*. Symposium No. 6 (Strehler, Ed.). Washington, American Institute of Biological Science, 1960, p. 116.

18. Barrows, Roeder and Falzone: J. Gerontol., *17*, 144, 1962.

19. Barrows and Roeder: J. Gerontol., *16*, 321, 1961.

20. Rivlin and Knox: Am. J. Physiol., *197*, 65, 1959.

21. Wulff, Quastler and Sherman: Proc. Natl. Acad. Sci., *48*, 1373, 1962.

22. Wulff, Quastler and Sherman: J. Gerontol., *19*, 294, 1964.

23. Wulff, Samis and Falzone: Adv. Gerontol. Res., *2*, 37, 1967.

24. Medvedev: Usp. Sorrem. Biol., *51*, 299, 1961.

24a. Medvedev: In *Biological Aspects of Aging* (Shock, Ed.). New York, Columbia University Press, 1962, p. 255.

24b. Medvedev: In *Biosynthesis of Proteins and Problems of Ontogenesis*. Moscow, Gosudarstvennoe Izdatelstvo Meditsinskoy Literaturi, 1963, p. 377.

24c. Ram: J. Gerontol., *22*, 92, 1967.

24d. Yunis (Chairman): Symposium on the Immunopathology of Aging, 57th Annual Meeting of the Federation of American Societies for Experimental Biology, Atlantic City, April 16, 1973. Fed. Proc., *33*, 2017, 1974.

24e. Makinodan: In *Handbook of the Biology of Aging* (Finch and Hayflick, Eds.). New York, Van Nostrand Rheinhold Company, 1977, pp. 379–408.

24f. Liu and Walford: Nature, *212*, 1277, 1966.

24g. Liu and Walford: Gerontologia, *18*, 363, 1972.

24h. McKay, Dilley and Crowell: J. Nutr., *1*, 233, 1929.

24i. McKay, Crowell and Maynard: J. Nutr., *10*, 63, 1935.

24j. Watkin: In *Nutrition, Longevity, and Aging* (Rockstein and Sussman, Eds.). New York, Academic Press, 1976, pp. 47–66.

24k. Walford: *The Immunologic Theory of Aging*. Copenhagen, Munksgaard, 1969.

24l. Jose and Good: J. Exp. Med., *137*, 1, 1973.

24m. Walford, Liu, Mathies, Gerbase-Delima and Smith: Mech. Aging Dev., *2*, 447, 1973/4.

24n. Walford: Fed. Proc., *33*, 2020, 1974.

24o. Fernandez, Yunis, Smith and Good: Proc. Soc. Exp. Biol. Med., *139*, 1189, 1972.

24p. Fernandez, Yunis, Jose and Good: Int. Arch. Allergy, *44*, 770, 1973.

24q. Medvedev: Zh. Vsesouz. Himich. Obshch. Mendel., *8*, 384, 1963.

24r. Medvedev: In *Advances in Gerontological Research* Vol. 1 (Strehler, Ed.). New York, Academic Press, 1964, p.181.

24s. Medvedev: Ninth Ciba Foundation Lecture on Research on Aging. In *Aspects of the Biology of Aging*. 21st Symposium Society Experimental Biology (Woolhouse, Ed.). New York, Academic Press, 1967.

24t. Sinex: In *Handbook of the Biology of Aging* (Finch and Hayflick, Eds.). New York, Van Nostrand Rheinhold Company, 1977, pp. 37–62.

24u. Hart and Setlow: Proc. Natl. Acad. Sci. *71*, 2169, 1974.

24v. Hart and Setlow: Basic Life Sci., *5B* 801, 1975.

24w. Hart: Personal communication.

24x. von Hahn: J. Gerontol., *21*, 291, 1966.

24y. von Hahn: *Proceedings of the 7th International Congress of Gerontology.* Vol. 8, Wein, Medical Akademy Wein, 1966, p. 243.
25. Neuberger, Perrone and Slack: Biochem J., *49*, 199, 1951.
26. Slack: Nature, *174*, 512, 1954.
27. Thompson and Ballou: J. Biol. Chem., *223*, 795, 1956.
28. Verzár: Sci. Am., *208*, 104, 1963.
28a. Verzár: Exp. Gerontol., *3*, 69, 1968.
29. Chvapil and Hruza: Gerontologia, *3*, 241, 1959.
30. McKay: In *Cowdry's Problems of Aging* (Lansing, Ed.). Baltimore, Williams and Wilkins, 1952, p. 139.
31. Holeckova, Chytil and Chvapil: Cas Lék Cesk., *100*, 612, 1961.
32. Chvapil and Holeckova: Physiol. Bohemoslov., *11*, 505, 1962.
33. Bjorksten, quoted by Verzár: Sci. Am., *208*, 104, 1963.
33a. Piez: Annu. Rev. Biochem., *37*, 547, 1968.
34. Meyer and Verzár: Gerontologia, *3*, 184, 1959.
35. Gallop, Seifter and Meilman: Nature, *183*, 1659, 1959.
35a. Hamlin and Kohn: Biochim. Biophys. Acta, *236*, 458, 1971.
35b. Hamlin and Kohn: Exp. Gerontol., 7, 377, 1972.
36. Milch: Gerontologia, 7, 129, 1963.
36a. Milch and Murray: Proc. Soc. Exp. Biol. Med., *111*, 551, 1962.
36b. Milch, Murray and Kenmore: Proc. Soc. Exp. Biol. Med., *111*, 554, 1962.
36c. Balazs: In *Handbook of the Biology of Aging* (Finch and Hayflick, Eds.). New York, Van Nostrand Rheinhold Company, 1977, pp. 222–240.
37. Dougherty: Fed. Proc., *20* (Suppl. 8), 3, 1961.
38. Baily: *Abstracts of Papers Presented at the International Collagen Symposium.* The Hague (Scheveningen), The Netherlands, August 23–25, 1963. New York, Stratton Intercontinental Book Corp., 1963.
39. Braams: Int. J. Radiat. Biol., 7, 29, 1963.
40. Kountz, Hofstatter and Ackermann: Geriatrics, *2*, 173, 1947.
41. Kountz, Hofstatter and Ackermann: Geriatrics, *3*, 171, 1948.
42. Kountz, Hofstatter and Ackermann: J. Gerontol., *6*, 20, 1951.
43. Kountz, Ackermann, Kheim and Toro: Geriatrics, *8*, 63, 1953.
43a. Young: In *Nutrition, Longevity, and Aging* (Rockstein and Sussman, Eds.). New York, Academic Press, 1976, pp. 67–102.
43b. Uauy, Scrimshaw and Young: Publication No. 3309, Department of Nutrition and Food Science, M.I.T., Cambridge, 1977.
44. Schulze: Altersforschung, *8*, 64, 1954.
45. Schulze: In *Old Age in the Modern World.* Third Congress of International Association of Gerontology, 1954. London, E. and S. Livingstone, 1955, p. 127.
46. Watkin, Froeb, Hatch and Gutman: Am. J. Med., *9*, 441, 1950.
47. Bogdonoff, Shock and Nichols: J. Gerontol., *8*, 272, 1953.
48. Horwitt: J. Am. Dietet. Assoc., *29*, 443, 1953.
48a. Young, Perera, Winterer and Scrimshaw: In *Nutrition and Aging* (Winick, Ed.). New York, John Wiley & Sons, 1976, pp. 77–118.
49. Food and Nutrition Board, National Academy of Sciences–National Research Council: *Recommended Dietary Allowances,* 8th ed. Washington, National Academy of Sciences, 1974.
50. Morgan, Murai and Gillum: J. Nutr., *55*, 671, 1955.
51. Herbeuval, Cuny, Manciaux and Hansen: In *Old Age in the Modern World.* Third Congress of International Association of Gerontology, 1954. Edinburgh, E. & S. Livingstone, 1955, p. 574.
52. Karel, Wilder and Beber: Am. Geriatr. Soc., *4*, 667, 1956.
53. Eastman: J. Am. Geriatr. Soc., *10*, 633, 638, 1962.
54. Acheson and Jessop: Gerontologia, *6*, 193, 1962.
55. Reifenstein and Albright: Clin. Invest., *26*, 24, 1947.
56. Kountz: Ann. Intern. Med., *35*, 1055, 1951.
57. Ackermann, Toro, Kountz and Kheim: J. Gerontol., *9*, 450, 1954.
58. Bogdonoff, Shock and Parsons: J. Gerontol., *9*, 262, 1954.
59. Kountz, Kheim, Toro, Ackermann and Toro: J. Am. Geriatr. Soc., *7*, 757, 1959.
60. Watkin, Parsons, Yiengst and Shock: J. Gerontol., *10*, 268, 1955.
61. Watkin: Ann. N.Y. Acad. Sci., *69*, 902, 1958.
62. Watkin: In *The Physician and the Total Care of the Cancer Patient.* New York, American Cancer Society, 1962, p. 135.
63. Watkin, Silverstone and Shock: Fed. Proc., *24*, 629, 1965 (abstract).
64. Couch, Watkin, Rosenberg, Smith, Winitz, Otey, Birnbaum and Greenstein: Fed. Proc., *19*, 13, 1960 (abstract).
65. Scrimshaw, Hussein, Murray, Rand and Young: J. Nutr., *102*, 1595, 1972.
65a. Scrimshaw, Perera and Young: J. Nutr., *106*, 665, 1976.
66. Mertz, Baxter, Jackson, Roderick and Weis: J. Nutr., *46*, 313, 1952.
67. Albanese, Higgons, Orto and Zavattaro: Geriatrics, *12*, 465, 1957.
68. Tuttle, Swendseid, Mulcare, Griffith and Bassett: Metabolism, *6*, 564, 1957.
69. Watts, Mann, Bradley and Thompson: J. Gerontol., *19*, 370, 1964.
70. Watts, Tolbert and Ruff: Can. J. Biochem., *42*, 1437, 1964.
71. Rose: Fed. Proc., *8*, 546, 1949.
72. Tuttle, Swendseid and Bassett: Fed. Proc., *19*, 11, 1960 (abstract).
73. Tuttle, Swendseid, Mulcare, Griffith and Bassett: Metabolism, *8*, 61, 1959.
74. Swendseid: In *Symposium on Protein Nutrition and Metabolism.* Special Publication No. 4 (Kastelic, Draper and Broquist, Eds.). Urbana, University of Illinois College of Agriculture, Agricultural Experiment Station, 1963, p. 37.
75. Swendseid, Feelery, Harris and Tuttle: J. Nutr., *68*, 203, 1959.

76. Swendseid, Harris and Tuttle: J. Nutr., *71*, 105, 1960.
77. Clark, Yess, Vermillion, Goodwin and Mertz: J. Nutr., *79*, 131, 1963.
78. Tuttle, Bassett, Griffith, Mulcare and Swendseid: Am. J. Clin. Nutr., *16*, 225, 1965.
79. Swendseid, Watts, Harris and Tuttle: J. Nutr., *75*, 295, 1961.
80. Swendseid and Tuttle: In *Progress in Meeting Protein Needs of Infants and Preschool Children*, Publication No. 843. Washington, Natl. Acad. Sci.–Natl. Res. Council, 1961, p. 323.
81. Tuttle, Bassett, Griffith, Mulcare and Swendseid: Am. J. Clin. Nutr., *16*, 229, 1965.
82. Rose: Nutr. Abstr. Rev., *27*, 631, 1957.
83. Reynolds, Steel, Jones and Baumann: J. Nutr., *64*, 99, 1958.
83a.Tontisirin, Young, Miller and Scrimshaw: J. Nutr., *103*, 1220, 1973.
83b.Tontisirin, Young, Rand and Scrimshaw: J. Nutr., *104*, 495, 1974.
83c.Young, Hussein, Murray and Scrimshaw: J. Nutr., *101*, 45, 1971.
83d.Tontisirin, Young and Scrimshaw: Am. J. Clin. Nutr., *25*, 976, 1972.
84. Swendseid, Tuttle, Figueroa, Mulcare, Clark and Massey: J. Nutr., *88*, 239, 1966.
84a.Karlson: *Introduction to Modern Biochemistry*. New York, Academic Press, 1963, p. 153.
84b.Swendseid, Villalobos and Drenick: Fed. Proc., *23*, 448, 1964 (abstract).
84c.Swendseid, Friedrich and Tuttle: Fed. Proc., *20*, 8, 1961 (abstract).
84d.Tuttle, Swendseid, Friedrich and Griffith: Fed. Proc., *21*, 395, 1962 (abstract).
84e.Ackerman and Kheim: Clin. Chem., *10*, 32, 1964.
84f.Theimer: Naturwissenschaften, *51*, 465, 1964.
84g.Wehr and Lewis: Proc. Soc. Exp. Biol. Med., *121*, 349, 1966.
84h.Armstrong and Stave: Metabolism, *22*, 571, 1973.
85. Sharp, Lassen, Shankman, Hazlet and Lendis: J. Nutr., *63*, 155, 1957.
86. Tschudy, Bacchus, Weissman, Watkin, Eubanks and White: J. Clin. Invest., *38*, 892, 1959.
87. Watkin: Am. J. Clin. Nutr., *9*, 446, 1961.
88. Steffee, Goldsmith, Pencharz, Scrimshaw and Young: Metabolism, *25*, 281, 1976.
89. Picou and Taylor-Roberts: Clin. Sci., *36*, 283, 1969.
90. Winterer, Steffee, Perera, Uauy, Scrimshaw and Young: Exp. Gerontol., *11*, 79, 1976.
91. Bronte-Stewart, Keys and Brock: Lancet, *2*, 1103, 1955.
92. Zarkovic, Levi, Radovanovic and Plecas: Acta Med. Jugosl., *9*, 129, 1955.
93. Keys, Anderson, Fidanza, Keys and Swahn: Clin. Chem., *1*, 34, 1955.
93a.Keys, et al.: J. Clin. Invest., *25*, 1173, 1956.
93b.Keys: J. Chronic Dis., *4*, 364, 1956.
94. Keys: J.A.M.A., *164*, 1912, 1957.
94a.Sacks, Costelli, Donner and Kass: N. Engl. J. Med., *292*, 1148, 1975.
94b.Kinsell, Partridge, Boling, Margen and Michaels: J. Clin. Endocrinol., *12*, 909, 1952.
94c.Kinsell, Michaels, Partridge, Boling, Balch and Cochrane: J. Clin. Nutr., *1*, 224, 1953.
94d.Ahrens, Blankenhorn and Tsaltas: Proc. Soc. Exp. Biol. Med., *86*, 872, 1954.
95. Ahrens, Tsaltas, Hirsch and Insull: J. Clin. Invest., *34*, 918, 1955.
95a.Beveridge, Connell and Mayer: Can. J. Biochem. Physiol., *34*, 441, 1956.
95b.Bronte-Stewart, Antonis, Eales and Brock: Lancet, *1*, 521, 1956.
95c.Keys, Anderson and Grande: Lancet, *1*, 66, 1957.
96. Ahrens, Insull, Blomstrand, Hirsch, Tsaltas and Peterson: Lancet, *1*, 943, 1957.
96a.Malmros and Wigand: Lancet, *2*, 1, 1957.
96b.Brown and Page: J.A.M.A., *168*, 1989, 1958.
96c.Ahrens, Insull, Hirsch, Stoffel, Peterson, Farquhar, Miller and Thomasson: Lancet, *1*, 115, 1959.
97. Jolliffe and Rinzler: Postgrad. Med., *29*, 569, 1961.
98. Jolliffe, Maslansky, Rudensey, Simon and Faulkner: Circulation, *24*, 1415, 1961.
99. Christakis, Rinzler, Archer, Winslow, Jampel, Stephenson, Friedman, Fein, Kraus and James: Am. J. Public Health, *56*, 299, 1966.
100. Leren: Acta Med. Scand., Suppl. 466, 1966.
100a.American Heart Association: *The National Diet Heart Study: Final Report*. New York, American Heart Association, 1968.
100b.Turpeinen, Miettinen, Karvonen, Roine, Pekkarinen, Lehtosuo and Alivirta: Am. J. Clin. Nutr., *21*, 255, 1968.
100c. Medical Research Council: Lancet, *2*, 693, 1968.
100d.Dayton, Pierce, Hashimoto, Dixon and Tomiyasu: Circulation, *40* (Suppl. II), 1, 1969.
100e.Grundy and Ahrens: J. Clin. Invest., *49*, 1135, 1970.
100f. Miettinen, Turpeinen, Karvonen, Elorsus and Paavilainen: Lancet, *2*, 835, 1972.
100g.Bierenbaum, Fleischman, Raichelson, Hayton and Watson: Lancet, *1*, 1404, 1973.
100h.Frantz, Dawson, Kuba, Brewer, Gatewood and Bartsch: Circulation, *51, 52* (Suppl. II), 4, 1975.
101. Groen: Medicine, *38*, 1, 1959.
102. Albrink: Am. J. Med., *31*, 4, 1961.
102a.Kannel, Castelli, Gordon and McNamara: Ann. Intern. Med., *74*, 1, 1971.
102b.Ahrens: Ann. Intern. Med., *85*, 87, 1976.
102c.Hazzard: In *Nutrition, Longevity, and Aging* (Rockstein and Sussman, Eds.). New York, Academic Press, 1976, pp. 143–195.
102d.Bilheimer: N. Engl. J. Med., *296*, 508, 1977.
102e.Mann: N. Engl. J. Med., *297*, 644, 1977.
103. Council on Foods and Nutrition, American Medical Association, Committee on Dietary Fat Levels (Hand, Chairman). J.A.M.A., *181*, 411, 1962.
103a.McGovern (Chairman), Select Committee on Nutrition and Human Needs of the United States Senate: *Dietary Goals for the United States*. Washington, U. S. Government Printing Office, Stock No. 052-070-03913-2, 1977.
103b.American Medical Association: Statement of the American Medical Association Submitted to the Select Committee on Nutrition and Human

Needs of the United States Senate re *Dietary Goals for the United States*, April 18, 1977.

103c. Page and Brown: Circulation, *37*, 313, 1968.

103d. Ahrens: Report of the Diet-Heart Review Panel of the National Heart Institute. New York, American Heart Association, 1969.

103e. Task Force on Arteriosclerosis, National Heart and Lung Institute: Report Vol. 1, June. Bethesda, National Heart and Lung Institute, 1971.

103f. Mellinkoff, Frankland, Schwabe, Kellner, Greipel and McNoll: Am. J. Clin. Nutr., *16*, 232, 1956.

104. Szilard: Proc. Natl. Acad. Sci., *45*, 30, 1959.

104a. National Institute on Aging: *Special Report on Aging: 1977.* Washington, U. S. Government Printing Office, DHEW Publication No. (NIH) 77–1121, 1977.

104b. Fredrickson and Levy: In *The Metabolic Basis of Inherited Disease*, 3rd ed. (Stanbury, Wyngaarden and Fredrickson, Eds.). New York, McGraw-Hill, 1972, pp. 545–614.

104c. Levy, Fredrickson, Shulman, Bilheimer, Breslow, Stone, Lux, Sloan, Krause and Herbert: Ann. Intern. Med., *77*, 267, 1972.

104d. Barr, Russ and Eder: Am. J. Med., *11*, 480, 1951.

104e. Rhoads, Gulbrandsen and Kagan: N. Engl. J. Med., *294*, 293, 1976.

104f. Miller, Forde and Thelle: Lancet, *1*, 965, 1977.

104g. Gordon, Castelli, Hjortland, Kannel and Dawber: Am. J. Med., *62*, 707, 1977.

104h. Kannel and Gordon: In *Proceedings of a Conference on the Epidemiology of Aging*. Bethesda, National Institute on Aging, 1977.

104i. Glueck, Fallat, Spadafora and Gantside: Circulation, *52* (Suppl. II), 272, 1975.

104j. Yano, Rhoads and Kagan: N. Engl. J. Med., *297*, 405, 1977.

104k. Bondjers and Bjorkerud: Proc. Eur. Soc. Clin. Invest., *9*, 51, 1975.

104l. Miller and Miller: Lancet, *1*, 16, 1975.

104m. Carew, Kaschinsky, Hayes and Stainberg: Lancet, *1*, 1315, 1976.

105. Passmore: In *Diet and Bodily Constitution* (Wolstenholme and O'Connor, Eds.). London, J. and A. Churchill Ltd., 1964, p. 59.

106. Smith and Shock: J. Gerontol., *4*, 27, 1949.

107. Silverstone, Brandfonbrener, Shock and Yiengst: J. Clin. Invest., *36*, 504, 1957.

107a. Swerdloff, Pozefsky, Tobin and Andres: Diabetes, *16*, 161, 1967.

107b. Andres and Tobin: *Proceedings 9th International Congress of Gerontology, Vol. 1.* Kiev, 1972, pp. 276–280.

107c. Andres: Med. Clin. North Am., *55*, 835, 1971.

107d. Sansum, Blatherwick and Bowden: J.A.M.A., *86*, 178, 1926.

107e. Himsworth: Clin. Sci., *2*, 67, 1935.

107f. Himsworth: Lancet, *2*, 171, 1939.

107g. Kempner, Peschel and Schlayer: Postgrad. Med., *24*, 359, 1958.

107h. Brunzell, Lerner, Hazzard, Porte and Bierman: N. Engl. J. Med., *284*, 521, 1971.

107i. Anderson, Herman and Zakim: Am. J. Clin. Nutr., *26*, 600, 1973.

107j. Weisner, Seeman, Herrera, Assal, Soeldner and Gleason: Ann. Intern. Med., *80*, 332, 1974.

107k. Kiehm, Anderson and Ward: Am. J. Clin. Nutr., *29*, 895, 1976.

108. Pyke and Harrison: Lancet, *2*, 461, 1947.

109. Ohlson, et al.: Am. J. Public Health, *40*, 1101, 1950.

110. Vinther-Paulsen: J. Gerontol., *5*, 331, 1950.

111. Gustafsson, Quensel, Lanke, Lundquist, Grahenen, Bonow and Krasse: Acta Odontol. Scand., *11*, 232, 1954.

112. Ahrens, Hirsch, Oette, Farquhar and Stein: Trans. Assoc. Am. Physicians, *74*, 134, 1961.

113. Ellis: Q. J. Med., *3*, 137, 1934.

114. Cohn and Joseph: Metabolism, *9*, 492, 1960.

115. Cohn, Joseph and Allweiss: Am. J. Clin. Nutr., *11*, 356, 1962.

115a. Portman, Lawry and Bruno: Proc. Soc. Exp. Biol. Med., *91*, 321, 1956.

115b. Yudkin: Lancet, *2*, 155, 1957.

115c. Yudkin: Lancet, *1*, 1335, 1963.

115d. Yudkin and Roddy: Lancet, *2*, 6, 1964.

115e. Keys, Anderson and Grande: J. Nutr., *70*, 257, 1960.

115f. Grande, Anderson and Keys: J. Nutr., *86*, 313, 1965.

115g. Cohen: Am. Heart J., *65*, 291, 1963.

115h. Antar, Ohlson and Hodges: Am. J. Clin. Nutr., *14*, 169, 1964.

115i. Hodges and Krehl: Am. J. Clin. Nutr., *17*, 334, 1965.

115j. MacDonald and Braithwaite: Clin. Sci., *27*, 23, 1964.

115k. Kuo and Bassett: Ann. Intern. Med., *62*, 1199, 1965.

115l. Yudkin: Am. J. Clin. Nutr., *20*, 108, 1967.

115m. Yudkin and Morland: Am. J. Clin. Nutr., *20*, 503, 1967.

115n. Kaufman, Poznanski, Blondheim and Stein: Am. J. Clin. Nutr., *18*, 261, 1966.

115o. Lopez, Hodges and Krehl: Am. J. Clin. Nutr., *18*, 149, 1966.

115p. Page and Friend: In *Sugars in Nutrition*. New York, Nutrition Foundation, 1974, pp. 93–107.

116. Dallas and Nordin: Am. J. Clin. Nutr., *11*, 263, 1962.

116a. Smith and Frame: N. Engl. J. Med., *273*, 73, 1965.

116b. Smith and Whyte: Clin. Orthop., *65*, 81, 1969.

117. Nordin: Lancet, *1*, 1011, 1961.

118. Nordin: Am. J. Clin. Nutr., *10*, 384, 1962.

119. Whedon: Fed. Proc., *18*, 1112, 1959.

120. Lutwak and Whedon: Borden Rev. Nutr. Res., *23*, 45, 1962.

120a. Lutwak and Whedon: DM, April 1, 1963.

120b. Shorr and Carter: Bull. Hosp. Joint Dis., *13*, 59, 1952.

120c. Rich and Ensinck: Nature, *191*, 184, 1961.

120d. Rich, Ensinck and Ivanovich: J. Clin. Invest., *43*, 545, 1964.

120e. Rich and Ivanovich: Ann. Intern. Med., *63*, 1068, 1965.

120f. Cohen and Gardner: N. Engl. J. Med., *271*, 1129, 1964.

120g. Cohen and Gardner: J.A.M.A., *195*, 962, 1966.

120h.Bernstein, Sadowsky, Hegsted, Guri and Stare: J.A.M.A., *198*, 85, 1966.

120i. Smith, Rizek and Frame: Am. J. Clin. Nutr., *14*, 98, 1964.

120j. Rose: Proc. R. Soc. Med., *58*, 436, 1965.

120k.Exton-Smith: Am. J. Clin. Nutr., *25*, 853, 1972.

120l. Garn, Rohmann and Wagner: Fed. Proc., *26*, 1729, 1967.

120m.Garn, Rohmann and Nolan: In *Relation of Development and Aging* (Birren, Ed.). Springfield, Charles C Thomas, 1964.

120n.DeLuca and Schnoes: Annu. Rev. Biochem., *45*, 631, 1976.

120o.DeLuca: Clin. Endocrinol., 5, 97s, 1976.

120p.Haussler and McCain: N. Engl. J. Med., *297*, 974, 1041, 1977.

120q.DeLuca: Personal communication, 1977.

120r.Gallagher, et al.: Clin. Res., *24*, 580A, 1976.

120s.Brumbaugh, et al.: Biochemistry, *13*, 4091, 1974.

120t. Albanese: *Bone Loss: Causes, Detection and Therapy*. New York, Liss, 1977.

120u.Pitt and Haussler: Skelet. Radiol., *1*, 191, 1977.

120v.Werner, et al.: Calcif. Tissue Res., *21*, Suppl. 210, 1976.

120w.Haussler, et al.: Clin. Endocrinol., 5, 151s, 1976.

120x.Haussler, et al.: In *Vitamin D: Biochemical, Chemical, and Clinical Aspects Related to Calcium Metabolism* (Norman, et al., Eds.). Berlin, Walter deGouyter, 1977, pp. 473–482.

120y.Brideman, et al.: J. Clin. Invest., *57*, 1540, 1976.

120z.Davie, Chalmers, Hunder, Pelc and Kodiak: Ann. Intern. Med., *84*, 281, 1976.

121. Hegsted, Moscosco and Collazos: J. Nutr., *46*, 181, 1952.

122. Walker: Metabolism, *3*, 114, 1955.

123. Malm: *Calcium Requirement and Adaptation in Adult Men*. Oslo, Oslo University Press, 1958.

124. Calkins: Personal communication.

125. Ohlson, Roberts, Joseph and Nelson: J. Am. Diet. Assoc., *24*, 286, 1948.

126. Roberts, Kerr and Ohlson: J. Am. Diet. Assoc., *24*, 292, 1948.

127. Ackermann and Toro: J. Gerontol., *8*, 289, 1953.

128. Harrison: Fed. Proc., *18*, 1085, 1959.

128a.Lutwak: J. Am. Geriatr. Soc., *17*, 115, 1969.

128b.Henrikson, et al.: Sven. Tandlak. Tidskr., *63*, 323, 1969.

128c.Krook, et al.: J. Nutr., *101*, 233, 1971.

128d.Lutwak, et al.: Isr. J. Med. Sci., 7, 504, 1971.

128e.Albanese, Edelson, Lorenze, Woodhull and Wein: N. Y. State J. Med., *25*, 326, 1975.

129. Weidmann: Biochem. J., *69*, 338, 1958.

130. Gitlin, Kamholtz and Levine: J. Gerontol., *13*, 43, 1958.

131. Vose, Stover and Mock: J. Gerontol., *16*, 120, 1961.

131a.Watkin: *Resumos Temas Livres, XI Congresso Internacional de Nutrição*, Rio de Janeiro, 1978. Rio de Janeiro, Comissão Executiva do XI Congresso Internacional de Nutrição, 1978, p. 737.

132. Harris: Fed. Proc., *18*, 1100, 1959.

133. Watkin and Steinfeld: J. Natl. Cancer Inst., *33*, 169, 1964.

133a.Fletcher, Jones and Morgan: Q. J. Med., *32*, 321, 1963.

133b.Lutwak, Singer and Urist: Ann. Intern. Med., *80*, 630, 1974.

134. Arnold, Dean, Jay and Knutson: Public Health Rep., *71*, 652, 1956.

135. U.S. Public Health Service: Public Health Rep., *71*, 963, 1956.

135a.Rich: J.A.M.A., *196*, 1165, 1966.

135b.Higgins, Nassim, Alexander and Hilb: Br. Med. J., *1*, 1159, 1965.

135c.Spencer, Osis, Wiatrowski and Samachson: J. Nutr., *100*, 1415, 1970.

135d.Spencer, Samachson, Fowler and Kulka: Am. J. Clin. Nutr., *24*, 311, 1971.

135e.Jowsey: In *Nutrition and Aging* (Winick, Ed.). New York, John Wiley and Sons, 1976.

135f.Crosby: N. Engl. J. Med., *297*, 543, 1977.

136. Fielding: Br. Med. J., *5295*, 1800, 1962.

136a.Life Sciences Research Office, Federation of American Societies for Experimental Biology: *A Review of the Significance of Untoward Reactions to Iodine in Foods*. FDA Contract No. FDA 71–294. Washington, Division of Nutrition, Bureau of Foods, Food and Drug Administration, 1974.

136b.Freis: Arch. Intern. Med., *133*, 982, 1974.

137. Leaf: N. Engl. J. Med., *267*, 24, 1962.

138. Bondy: *Year Book of Medicine, 1963–1964 Series*. Chicago, Year Book Medical Publishers, 1963, p. 680.

138a.Schultze: Arch. Intern. Med., *131*, 885, 1973.

139. Schneckloth, Dustan and Corcoran: Metabolism, *6*, 723, 1957.

139a.Das: Ph.D. thesis. Cambridge, Massachusetts Institute of Technology, 1967.

140. Stephenson, Penton and Korenchevsky: Br. Med. J., *2*, 839, 1941.

141. Wexberg: Am. J. Psychiatry, *97*, 1406, 1941.

142. Jolliffe: J.A.M.A., *117*, 1496, 1941.

143. Overholser: In *Geriatric Medicine*, 2nd ed. (Stieglitz, Ed.). Philadelphia, W. B. Saunders, 1949.

144. Rafsky and Newman: Am. J. Med. Sci., *201*, 749, 1941.

145. Rafsky and Newman: Gastroenterology, *1*, 737, 1943.

146. Rafsky and Newman: Geriatrics, *2*, 101, 1947.

147. Horwitt, Liebert, Kreisler and Wittman: Bull. Natl. Res. Coun. (U.S.), *116*, 1948.

148. Lossy, Goldsmith and Sarett: J. Nutr., *45*, 213, 1951.

149. Schmidt: J. Gerontol., *6*, 132, 1951.

150. Schmidt: J. Gerontol., *6*, 369, 1951.

151. Watkin, Lang, Chow and Shock: J. Nutr., *50*, 341, 1953.

152. Pauling: *Vitamin C and the Common Cold*. San Francisco, W. H. Freeman, 1970.

153. Cameron and Pauling: Proc. Natl. Acad. Sci., *73*, 3685, 1976.

154. Burr, Elwood, Hole, Hurley and Hughes: Am. J. Clin. Nutr., *27*, 144, 1974.

155. Kataria, Rao and Curtis: Gerontol. Clin., *7*, 189, 1965.

156. Bowers and Kubic: Br. J. Clin. Pract., *19*, 141, 1965.

157. Griffiths, Brocklehurst, Scott, Marks and Blackley: Gerontol. Clin., *9*, 1, 1967.

158. Woodhill: Int. J. Vitam. Res., *40*, 520, 1970.
159. Milne, Lonergan, Williamson, Moore, McMaster and Percy: Br. Med. J., *4*, 383, 1971.
160. Loh and Wilson: Int. J. Vitam. Res., *41*, 259, 1971.
161. Rhead and Schrauzer: Nutr. Rev., *29*, 262, 1971.
162. Jaffe, Kasten, Young and MacLowry: Ann. Intern. Med., *83*, 824, 1975.
163. Herbert and Jacob: J.A.M.A., *230*, 241, 1974.
163a.Jacob, Scott, Brenner and Herbert: In *Proceedings of the 16th Annual Meeting, American Society of Hematology*, Chicago, December 1–4, 1973. Thorofare, Charles B. Slack, Inc., p. 125.
163b.Hines; J.A.M.A., *234*, 24, 1975.
163c.Newmark, Scheiner, Marcus and Prabhudesai: Am. J. Clin. Nutr., *29*, 645, 1976.
163d.Stein, Hassan and Fox: Ann. Intern. Med., *84*, 385, 1976.
163e.Mengel and Greene: Ann. Intern. Med., *84*, 490, 1976.
163f.Campbell, Steinberg and Bower: Ann. Intern. Med., *82*, 810, 1975.
164. Alexander, Lorenzen, Hoffman and Garfinkel: Proc. Soc. Exp. Biol. Med., *65*, 275, 1947.
165. Sleisenger: N. Engl. J. Med., *265*, 49, 1961.
166. di Sant' Agnese and Jones: J.A.M.A., *180*, 122, 1962.
167. Kirk and Chieffi: J. Nutr., *36*, 315, 1948.
168. Yiengst and Shock: J. Gerontol., *4*, 205, 1949.
169. Birren, Bick and Fox: J. Gerontol., *3*, 267, 1948.
170. Birren, Bick and Yiengst: J. Exp. Psychol., *40*, 260, 1950.
171. Freeman, Rhoads and Yeager: J. Lab. Clin. Med., *31*, 480, 1946.
172. Bauer and Freyberg: J.A.M.A., *130*, 1208, 1946.
173. Donegan, Messer and Orgain: Ann. Intern. Med., *30*, 429, 1949.
174. McCollum and McCollum: In *Food: The Yearbook of Agriculture, 1959* (Stefferud, Ed.). Washington, U.S. Government Printing Office, 1959, p. 138.
175. Expert Panel on Food Safety and Nutrition and the Committee on Public Information, Institute of Food Technologists: A scientific status summary. Nutr. Rev., *35*, 57, 1977.
176. Tappel: Nutr. Today, *8*, 4, 1973.
176a.Williams, Fenna and Macbeth: Surg. Gynecol. Obstet., *132*, 662, 1971.
176b.Haeger: Am. J. Clin. Nutr., *27*, 1179, 1974.
177. White: Geriatrics, *13*, 819, 1958.
177a.Swanson and Iseri: N. Engl. J. Med., *258*, 831, 1958.
177b.Langgard and Smith: N. Engl. J. Med., *266*, 378, 1962.
177c.Moses and Miller: N. Engl. J. Med., *291*, 1234, 1974.
177d.Schrier and Berl: N. Engl. J. Med., *292*, 81, 141, 1975.
177e.Odell: In *Textbook of Endocrinology*, 5th ed. (Williams, Ed.). Philadelphia, W.B. Saunders, 1974, pp. 1105–1116.
178. Cizek. Am. J. Physiol., *197*, 342, 1959.
179. Keane, Smutko, Krieger and Denton: J. Nutrition, *77*, 18, 1962.
180. Dublin and Marks: Hum. Biol., *2*, 159, 1930.
181. McCay, Dilley and Crowell: J. Nutr., *1*, 233, 1929.
181a.McCay, Crowell and Maynard: J. Nutr., *10*, 63, 1935.
181b.McCay, Sperling and Barnes: Arch. Biochem., *2*, 469, 1943.
181c.McCay: Am. J. Public Health, *37*, 521, 1947.
182. Ross: Fed. Proc., *18*, 1190, 1959.
182a.Ross: J. Nutr., *25*, 197, 1961.
182b.Ross: J. Nutr., *97* (Suppl. 1), 565, 1969.
182c.Ross: In *Diet and Bodily Constitution* (Wolstenholme and O'Conner, Eds.). London, J. & A. Churchill, Ltd., 1946, p. 90.
182d.Ross: In *Symposium on Nutrition and Aging* (Watkin, Ed.). Am. J. Clin. Nutr., *25*, 834, 1972.
182e.Ross and Bras: Nature, *250*, 263, 1974.
182f.Ross and Bras: Science, *190*, 165, 1975.
182g.Ross, Lustbader and Bras: Nature, *262*, 548, 1976.
182h.Ross: Nutr. Rev., *35*, 257, 1977.
183. Berg, Wolf and Simms: J. Nutr., *77*, 439, 1962.
184. Berg and Simms: J. Nutr., *71*, 255, 1960.
185. Nikkilä and Konttinen: Lancet, *1*, 1151, 1962.
186. Ferguson, Petitclerc and Choquette: Am. J. Cardiol., *34*, 764, 1974.
186a.Conner, LaCamera, Swanick, Oldham, Holzaepfel and Lyczkowskyj: Med. Sci. Sports, *8*, 145, 1976.
186b.Borer, Bacharach, Green, Kent, Epstein and Johnston: N. Engl. J. Med., *296*, 839, 1977.
186c.Holman: N. Engl. J. Med., *296*, 876, 1977.
186d.Borer: In *Proceedings of a Symposium on Exercise in the Elderly–Its Role in Prevention of Physical Decline and in Rehabilitation*. Bethesda, National Institute on Aging, 1977.
186e.Roe: *Drug-Induced Nutritional Deficiencies*. Westport (Connecticut), AVI Publishing Company, 1976.
187. Watkin: World Rev. Nutr. Diet., *6*, 124, 1966.

Chapter *29*

FOOD AND NUTRITION RELATING TO WORK, EXERCISE AND ENVIRONMENTAL STRESS

Maurice E. Shils

Nutritional requirements can be affected by the degree of physical activities imposed by work and sport and by certain environmental stresses. This chapter considers this subject and reviews the types of changes, if any, that may be indicated by various activities in different environmental situations. It also reviews the corollary questions of effects of variations in dietary composition and of nutritional deficiencies on physical performance.

NUTRITIONAL REQUIREMENTS FOR WORK

Energy Expenditure

Metabolic Basis. Beginning with Lavoisier's published investigations (1783–85) on the nature of respiration and energy exchange, a series of studies in man on work and energy expenditure[1,2] culminated in the fundamental studies of Voit and Pettenkoffer, Rubner and his students, Magnus-Levy and DuBois and Lusk on energy exchanges and the energy value of foods.

Regnault and Reiset in 1849 were the first to devise a closed system for respiration studies with which they determined with considerable accuracy the relation between oxygen absorbed and carbon dioxide exhaled, i.e. the respiration quotient (R.Q.). They demonstrated that the R.Q. varied from 0.62 to 1.04 when different foods were fed to experimental animals.[1] Such studies were extended to man by Pettenkofer and Voit in their respiration chamber under various dietary conditions and at rest and exercising. Samples of air entering and leaving the room were continually analyzed for carbon dioxide and water; the gain in CO_2 and water by the whole volume of outgoing air gave the amount of these materials eliminated by the subject. The oxygen consumption was then estimated by the difference.[2] Atwater later designed a method for the direct determination of oxygen consumption by an individual in the respiration chamber.

Rubner, in turn, determined the calorific values of constituents of urine and feces. This afforded the basis for demonstrating that the caloric value of protein when metabolized in the body was 4.1 kcal per gm in contrast to 5.36 kcal per gm obtained in the bomb calorimeter. The difference resulted from the incomplete oxidation in the body of the nitrogen in amino acids. Rubner further demonstrated that 100 gm of fat yielded the same number of calories as 211 gm of protein, 232 gm of starch, 234 gm of cane sugar and 256 gm of glucose. Calculations were then possible for calorie intake and expenditure. Rubner made the important observation that the heat value of metabolism in a resting animal is proportional to the area of the body surface.

His studies indicated that carbohydrate and fat were interchangeable in metabolism on the basis of energy-equivalents, i.e. 100 kcal derived from fat have the nutritive equivalent of 100 kcal as carbohydrate; this is the isodynamic law of Rubner. When 100 kcal in the form of meat were ingested by a dog the heat production (energy metabolism) was increased by 30 kcal over the values obtained with the same animal at rest and fasting. When 100 kcal were given as sucrose or as fat, the increase in metabolism was only 5.8 kcal and 4.0 kcal, respectively. Any increase in protein intake led to proportionate increases in the magnitude of metabolism. Rubner termed this effect "specific dynamic action."[2a]

Rubner assigned the caloric values of 1 gm of carbohydrate at 4.1 kcal, 1 gm of fat at 9.3 kcal and 1 gm of protein at 4.1 kcal. Atwater assigned the figures of 4, 9 and 4 kcal per gm for carbohydrate, fat and protein, respectively, on the basis of absorption efficiency coefficients.

It has been customary to express the energy content of foods and the energy requirements of man and animals in terms of the thermochemical kilocalorie (kcal or large calorie). Energy values by international agreement are now expressed in joules.[2b] During an interim period both systems are in use. The factor for converting kcal to kilojoules (kJ) is 4.184, e.g. 1 kcal = 4.2 kJ and 1 kJ = 0.239 kcal. The energy content of diets and energy requirements of humans usually exceed 1000 kJ and are generally expressed as megajoules (MJ) where 1 MJ = 1000 kJ = 239 kcal.

Zuntz was the first to introduce a relatively portable apparatus which could determine the respiratory exchange in men under a great variety of circumstances and in relatively short periods of time. Magnus-Levy carried this apparatus to the bedside and made the pioneer respiratory metabolism investigations in a great number of diseases. In 1906 he defined basal metabolism (Grundumsatz) as the "energy exchange by which the normal functions of the organs may be maintained when under conditions of greatest possible relaxation." In practice this was measured 12 hours after the last meal when the subject was resting, relaxed and avoiding all muscular movement.

In 1891 Rubner demonstrated that the heat production of a dog as directly measured in a chamber calorimeter was essentially identical with the heat production measured by gaseous exchange with the Voit apparatus (indirect calorimetry) utilizing calculations of urine and fecal contents. The validity of his method was proven for man by Atwater and later by others.

These studies laid the basis for the study of energy expenditure and requirements in various activities and various metabolic states. Knowing the metabolic substrate or type of food consumed, the calories produced, the oxygen consumed and the carbon dioxide produced, it is relatively simple to calculate the heat production from either the oxygen consumption or the CO_2 production of the individual. With knowledge of the oxygen consumption and CO_2 production (the R.Q.), it is possible to estimate, within certain limits, not only the heat produced by an individual but also the nature of the food mixture from which this heat was derived. The details of such computations of energy expenditures in metabolic processes are given elsewhere.[3,4]

Instrumentation. The original methods for measuring respiratory exchange as the basis for energy expenditure calculations required restrictive laboratory or bedside apparatus. The development of the Douglas bag (1911) and later the apparatus of Benedict and Parmenter (1928) permitted studies with more mobile subjects, although they were still bulky and unwieldy. The Douglas bag used the open-circuit method where all expired air was collected in the bag carried by the subject; this air was then taken to the laboratory for analysis. The Benedict-Parmenter respiration calorimeter employed the closed-circuit method: the subject rebreathed the same air, with CO_2 being absorbed into chemicals, and the volume of oxygen consumed from the bags was measured during performance of the task.[5]

The development of a lightweight (8-lb) portable respirometer, designated the Max Planck Institute respirometer or the Kofranyi-Michaelis respirometer, has facilitated the obtaining of data on energy expenditure by workers.[4,5] This unit measures the volume of expired air directly and simultaneously diverts a small fraction into a rubber bladder for subsequent analysis. However, it has a limited sample storage capacity and offers considerable respiratory resistance at ventilation rates much above 25 to 30 liters per minute;[6] others consider it useful with ventilations up to 60 to 80 liters per minute.[7] A number of studies of various activities of industrial workers have been carried out using these techniques. Wolff[5,8] has designed an instrument (the Integrating Motor Pneumotachograph) which measures instantaneous flow (rather than direct volume) which is integrated with respect to time; sampling is achieved by diverting a small fraction of air passing through the flowmeter and storing it for subsequent analysis. Its usefulness in physiologic studies in polar expeditions has been described.[9]

A pneumotachograph based on flow measurements but with instantaneous volume indication suitable for on-line laboratory experiments was introduced by Fleish.[10]

Originally, measurements of oxygen or carbon dioxide were chemical. Although there were refinements and the development of micromethods[4] reduced the volumes required for gas samplings,[4] the procedures were relatively time consuming. With the development of various physical methods of gas analysis (e.g. an oxygen meter based on the magnetic susceptibility of O_2 molecules and analysis for CO_2 based on its infrared absorption), improved recording systems and small rugged telemet-

ering units, rapid continuous and distant measurements became possible.[5] A combination of sophisticated analytic equipment for gas analysis with other instrumentation for continuous measurements of temperature, heart rate and respiratory rate connected to computers allows detailed and rapid analysis of the different phases in each breath and of the effects of work, dietary and metabolic changes and disease.[11] Energy expenditure may be calculated from continuous heart rate recordings[12,13] and this technique has been applied clinically.[14]

Using one or another of the methods for estimating energy expenditure at rest and with various activities, data have been accumulating on such expenditures as sleep, personal care, walking, climbing, running, recreational activities, domestic and office work and a large variety of laboring activities, ranging from light to heavy and including agriculture, lumbering and fishing as well as industrial work and military activities. The reader is referred to published tables for data on energy expenditure in specific activities.[4,15,16]

Numerous efforts have been made to estimate activities over the day as the basis for setting standards for caloric needs of individuals and population groups. The most reliable method is based on continuous direct measurements over the entire 24 hours, but this is obviously a technique applicable to very few subjects. The more usual summation of expenditures is obtained by direct measurement of the energy cost of each of the individual activities over the day together with either time-motion studies or the diary method which indicates the period of time spent in each type of activity. The sum of the individual energy costs plus the 24-hour basal metabolic rate and specific dynamic action value (approximately 9 to 10 per cent of the caloric intake) give the total daily expenditure. Such a procedure has been outlined in some detail.[4]

The Committee on Calorie Requirements of the Food and Agriculture Organization of the United Nations[17,18] developed formulas for calculating the caloric requirements of populations and population groups by establishing "reference standards" for men and women and adjusting the requirements of individuals differing from the references with respect to their age (25 years), body size (65 kg and 55 kg for male and female, respectively), environmental temperature and activity. The mean caloric requirements of the reference men and women involved in a degree of activity corresponding to an occupation in light industry were 3,200 and 2,300 per day, respectively, in the 1950s[17,18] and were reduced to 2,700 and 2,000 kcal, respectively, in the 1974 report[19] (Appendix Table 7). The Food and Nutrition Board of the National Research Council, beginning with its 1953 revision of the Recommended Dietary Allowances, adopted references as a basis for caloric requirements. In successive revisions it has progressively changed the caloric requirements so that they stand presently at 2,700 and 2,100 kcal, respectively, for men and women (not pregnant or lactating) weighing 70 and 58 kg, respectively, in the age range of 23 to 50 years[20] (Appendix Table 1). Older men and women have somewhat reduced caloric allowances. Data on energy expenditure for various activities and the distribution of activity over the 24 hours are given in Appendix Tables 6 to 8.

Energy Expenditure and Body Size. In the standards referred to above, body size is taken to affect energy expenditure. Weight is used as the "basis of adapting allowances for differences in size, provided the individuals are not appreciably over or under their ideal weights."[20] Durnin has reviewed the relations of body weight, body fat and the activity factor in energy balance.[21] Body weight bears a close relationship to the total fat content of the body, but the fat-free mass is surprisingly constant. Oxygen consumption per kg body weight per minute for men and women walking with and without various additional loads is variable for individuals but there is no difference between the sexes. While gross body weight is a reasonable parameter in assessing the cost of moving the body, Durnin points out that the correlations are not high even when the activity groups are rather restricted. Consequently, if the assessment of an individual's energy requirement is based on body weight, a considerable error is likely to be introduced. Variations in body weight may not be of equal significance; data are now available showing an inverse relation between degree of obesity and amount of physical activity.

Energy Expenditure over 24 Hours. Based on daily energy expenditures of a fairly large number of men and women, Durnin found that on the average 34 per cent of the day (almost exactly 8 hours) was spent in bed and this accounted for 17 to 22 per cent of the total daily energy output. For men the correlation coefficient between the physical activity required by their work and the total energy intake or expenditure was quite high (=0.7), whereas this relationship was only 0.07 between physical activity in the nonwork period and total energy intake or expenditure. The physical activity involved in the occupation was responsible for determining about 50 per cent of the total energy requirements.

Although occupation is of major significance in relation to the energy requirement, it often accounts for only a minor proportion of that energy. For many occupation groups, the energy expended in nonworking, nonsleeping time is greater than that expended in work.[21] There was a negative correlation (−0.11) between activity at work and during nonworking time.[21]

Sitting occurs much of the day and accounts for from 15 to 37 per cent of total energy; it also takes up a considerable part of the working time in groups involved in "moderately heavy" or "heavy" occupations.[21] Standing has relatively little importance for most people.

Energy Expenditure and Food Intake. When groups of subjects are surveyed there is good agreement between estimates of food intake and energy expenditure. When results for individuals are examined, there are frequently considerable differences between intake and expenditure. In the studies of Edholm on soldiers, no relationship was evident when individual daily intake was compared with daily energy expenditure.[22] Over a period of one week, there was a significant correlation between the two but there was also considerable scatter, some individuals having marked surplus and others a deficit. When calorie balances were compared with weight changes a significant correlation was again found, but there was also a very large scatter. Food intake was not significantly correlated with body weight.[22,23] The discrepancies noted in some individuals even over a week between diet intake and energy expenditure should result in corresponding weight gains or losses. However, the daily weight changes were frequently too large to be explicable in terms of deficits or excesses of calories and must have occurred through changes in total body water. Edholm suggested that, for a significant number of individuals, any regulatory mechanism must operate over a relatively long time period.[22]

Gradation of Work and Endurance Limit

Christensen[24] suggested the following definitions of different grades of work:

> Unduly heavy—
>   energy expenditure over 12.5 kcal per min
> Very heavy—
>   energy expenditure over 10.0 kcal per min
> Heavy—
>   energy expenditure over 7.5 kcal per min
> Moderate—
>   energy expenditure over 5.0 kcal per min
> Light—
>   energy expenditure over 2.5 kcal per min

The energy expenditures of most of Christensen's grades apply only to rates of work which are carried on continuously for periods of a few minutes and must be interspersed with rest pauses. Hence, these definitions need to be considered in relation to work capacity in order to give information on average daily rates of work. Lehmann[25] and Müller[26] have considered this problem in the light of their studies on German workers. They set a figure of 4 kcal per min net or 5 kcal per min gross (i.e. including energy of basal metabolism) as the upper limit of energy available from foodstuff oxidation, and they term this value the *endurance limit*.

The upper level of work at which glucose is utilized completely and at which no oxygen debt accumulates in the body is termed the *aerobic capacity*. At this rate of energy expenditure the circulation can provide the working muscles with all the oxygen they need at the moment. The higher the degree of physical fitness, the higher is the aerobic capacity. A healthy man, without training, should be able to walk at 4 mph within aerobic capacity, i.e. at 5 kcal per min and with an O_2 consumption of slightly over 1L per min. When the individual is working at higher rates and up to maximum capacity, the O_2 supply to tissues becomes insufficient to allow complete glucose oxidation and energy is provided, in part, by the anaerobic conversion of glucose into lactate with accumulation of the latter and, in part, by hydrolysis of high-energy phosphate bonds. During the recovery period the lactate is removed by oxidation and organic phosphates are resynthesized. The extra O_2 uptake after exercise is termed the *oxygen debt*. Work physiologists often express the severity of a specific type of work or exercise as a percentage of the maximum oxygen consumption ($\dot{V}_{O_2}$ max) of the individual performing the work.

Work at 5 kcal per min gross for an 8-hour shift equals 2,400 kcal and probably represents the upper rate of daily energy expenditure that can be maintained at a steady rate in heavy industry. Müller[26] estimated that only about 4 per cent of the 25 million workers in West Germany work to this degree and Passmore and Durnin[27] state that it is slightly higher than the rates recorded for British coal miners at the time of their study. At this rate of 5 kcal per min for 8 hours, if 500 kcal are allowed for 8 hours in bed and 1,400 kcal for the additional 8 hours off work, the total 24-hour energy expenditure is 4,300 kcal.

For work requiring expenditure above the endurance limit, increased rest pauses or increased absences from work occur. For such work Müller[26] makes the point that many small rest pauses relieve fatigue much more than a few long pauses.

Figures given in various tables of requirements, standards or allowances are merely approximations of value as guides in estimating needs of groups. The requirements of the individual worker may vary greatly from the average for his occupation. This is exemplified in a study of coal miners where the average caloric expenditure for an 8-hour shift was 2,002 kcal but the range was from 1,587 to 2,394.[28] To the factors of size, age, sex and environment are added the variations in specific job situations and differences in activities among individuals on and off the job—all of which greatly influence the overall calorie requirements.[15,16,21,29]

Energy Deficiency

Caloric deficiency resulting from inadequate food supply is one problem that the employed American has never had to face even in time of war. The so-called food shortages which have developed from time to time and which caused some difficulties in certain industries in World War II did not involve calorie insufficiency, but rather an inability on the part of workers to get certain types of foods to which they felt they were entitled or which they believed they needed. For the majority of workers shortages of *calories* in the form of the more expensive animal products such as meat, milk and eggs could be met easily by increasing consumption of cereals, legumes and other plant materials. Such a shift in dietary pattern, particularly if it were a pronounced one, would raise the problems of ensuring an adequate intake of other nutrients and, equally important, of maintaining morale. Even mild, involuntary changes in the food pattern of a country are not taken lightly.

The effects of true deficiency in man have been studied under conditions of actual food shortages and in experimental situations, and a large literature exists.[30-36] In both acute starvation and semistarvation of some duration in adults, physiologic, psychologic and some psychomotor changes sooner or later become marked while tests of intellective function show much less deterioration.[37-39] The effects of deprivation in children are discussed in Chapters 19 and 24. The degree of change in the various functions depends upon the severity of the calorie deficit, its duration and the individual concerned. Young men performing hard work while deprived of food but receiving adequate water develop, within 24 hours, dehydration, hypoglycemia and ketosis; these changes are accompanied by nausea, fatigue, poor work tolerance and impairment of speed and coordination.[30,37,38] It would appear that, when sufficient calories (e.g. 420 to 580 per day), NaCl and water are provided to prevent ketosis, serious dehydration and hypoglycemia under conditions of moderate energy output (3,200 to 3,600 kcal per day) and good motivation, performance capacity is well maintained for approximately 10 days, up to a weight loss of 10 per cent of the original body weight.[38,38a-38c] At some point between 10 and 16 per cent weight loss, rapid deterioration of maximum effort sets in.[30,38] Cardiovascular insufficiency, anemia and decreased strength and speed of muscular action in chronic semistarvation are additional limiting factors.[30]

With restriction of calorie intake in industrial situations, work output is curtailed accordingly. A demand for heavy work output during a period of serious calorie deficiency would not be tolerated by workers for more than a few days and then only under emergency conditions. An interesting example of the relation of productivity to food consumption was noted among German miners during World War II.[40] Young "cutters" in the coal mines had a daily output of 7.0 tons of coal per man on a total daily intake of 2,800 kcal, about 1,200 kcal above the estimated basal metabolic rate, or about 170 kcal expended per ton of coal mined. When 400 additional kcal were allowed, output increased to 9.6 tons per man or 155 kcal per ton. At this rate the men lost, on the average, 1.2 kg of body weight in 6 weeks. The extra kilocalories were raised to 800, whereupon the output increased to 10 tons per man and the body weight slowly returned to normal. Additional data on caloric intake and productivity during the war and in postwar Germany tend to confirm a close relationship when food is limited.[41]

The body adapts to certain degrees of chronic calorie restriction. In addition to a restriction of voluntary activity, there is decreased energy expenditure resulting from decreased basal metabolism and a decrease in the energy required to perform work. The reduction of basal metabolism is attributed to two factors, namely, shrinkage of the metabolizing body mass and decrease of the cellular metabolic rate.[30,42] Caloric deficiency is associated with altered thyroid hormone metabolism, resulting in increased formation of "reverse" triiodothyronine (rT_3).[43] There is evidence that, in subacute caloric deficiency (of approximately 3 weeks' duration), the decrease in basal metabolism results, for the most part, from the operation of the second factor,[42] whereas in chronic semistarvation the first factor is predominant.[30,42] The ability to preferen-

tially metabolize body fat, to utilize ketone bodies, to spare certain tissues and to decrease the work of the heart further aids in withstanding lack of calories. The calorie equivalent of weight change with calorie deficit is considered in Chapter 1.

Calorie-protein Relationships. The corollary question arises as to whether the composition of the low-calorie diet has any influence on the organism's resistance to the deficit. It has been demonstrated in short-term studies with rats[44] and dogs[45] that, when the caloric intake fell below 50 per cent of normal, dietary protein was used primarily for energy purposes; in rats subsisting on low-calorie diets a moderately high-fat content (15 per cent) spared dietary protein to a much greater degree than low-fat diets.[44] With respect to healthy, active men, when the daily caloric intake was somewhat below 900 kcal dietary protein was utilized as an energy source, producing a concomitant rise in urinary nitrogen.[46] At approximately 900 kcal, small amounts of dietary nitrogen (3 gm) partially decreased the negative balance; increasing the nitrogen did not improve the situation. Further increases in caloric intake resulted in improved nitrogen retention.

These studies point up an area of major importance with respect to maintenance of body tissues during caloric deficiency. Whereas body fat in previously well-nourished individuals is, in great part, a true energy reserve, body protein is not. The proteins and polypeptides in tissues have structural, enzymatic and hormonal roles; their depletion to supply energy would not appear in the interest of the individual. As described in Chapter 36, depletion of muscle and visceral protein in patients is associated with increased morbidity and mortality. Recent work has reemphasized the intimate relationship between energy intake and expenditure and protein intake and nitrogen balance.[36,47-50] In healthy (as well as in hypermetabolic, septic or traumatized patients) increased caloric intake spares body nitrogen when energy intake is inadequate; similarly, increasing the protein intake will overcome the negative nitrogen balance resulting from inadequate nonprotein calories. The use of amino acids or protein for purposes of "protein sparing" in patients in marked caloric deficiency is discussed in Chapter 36.

Water. Water exerts important effects in permitting maximal activity and the maintenance of body composition. It has been observed that there is an increase in nitrogen excretion during dehydration.[51] Active young men on a caloric-deficient protein-free diet had marked increases in urinary nitrogen on 900 ml of water daily; even on 1,800 ml the losses were greater than those on ad lib water intake. The increased urinary nitrogen, in turn, increased obligatory urine losses, accentuating the dehydration. The metabolic response was considered to be secondary to the stress of dehydration partly related to increased adrenal cortex activity. The importance of adequate water intake in improving performance in exhausting physical work has been shown with dogs[52] and man.[52a] Loss of water amounting to 4 to 5 per cent of body weight decreases the capacity for hard muscular work by 20 to 30 per cent. Even 2 to 3 per cent loss through exercise dehydration causes marked impairment in performance.[52b] In hot environments water becomes a major factor and this is considered below.

The Effects of the Frequency and Composition of Meals on Work Performance

Our custom of eating three meals a day probably is based more upon considerations of convenience than upon those of physiologic need. Experience in industry has shown the value to worker productivity of additional rest periods, particularly when associated with between-meal feedings. The view is widely held that between-meal snacks in themselves in-

crease work performance and lessen fatigue. This may be true, but there is no proof that frequent feedings increase physiologic capacity to perform the usual type of factory work. Undoubtedly, psychologic factors are important and account for some, if not all, of the beneficial results observed.

Haggard and Greenberg[53] performed experiments with employees in a shoe factory in which productivity was measured during periods when 3 or 5 meals per day were eaten, and concluded that 5 meals a day resulted in superior work performance (about 40 per cent increase in productivity). The study was not sufficiently well controlled to entirely rule out psychologic effects, as Ivy[54] pointed out. These criticisms, of course, do not dispose of the finding that there was increased production with an increase in the number of meals. There have been similar reports[52-57] of improved efficiency or well-being with increased meals but the "morale" factors have never been ruled out.

The productivity of seamstresses as influenced by different amounts and kinds of food consumed during the midmorning and midafternoon rest periods has been assessed.[58] No differences were noted in work output when the caloric intake was varied from 80 to 650 kcal and the type of food from a soft drink to a small meal. Less definite evidence indicated that omitting all food during the rest period did not decrease production; this particular aspect of the problem could not be thoroughly assessed because the women objected to being denied the opportunity to partake of food during the rest period. In the Hawthorn experiment,[59] when women engaged in assembling telephones were given extra snacks, their output increased; however, when they were given a rest period without food, their output also increased. Many other changes in working conditions increased output and it became apparent that an important general factor influencing productivity was the recognition by the worker that management was concerned about her welfare and views. Hutchinson advocated a regimen of 6 meals daily.[60] However, no convincing nutritional or physiologic evidence is given to support this proposal for the usual industrial situation.

Since an appreciable number of workers are believed to report for work without having eaten any breakfast or only a cup of coffee and toast or sweet bun, it is of some interest to note reports on attempts to assess the results of different types of breakfast and of no breakfast on test subjects. Tuttle and co-workers[61-63] found that maximum work output attainable on the bicycle ergometer within 1 minute or less was adversely affected by omission of breakfast or by the consumption of only black unsweetened coffee, as compared with performance with adequate breakfasts.

The addition of midmorning food intake when an adequate breakfast was eaten resulted in no advantage, but the midmorning intake improved performance in one-half of the patients who omitted breakfasts.[64] Whatever the nature of the physiologic and/or psychologic basis of the results, the results would appear to warrant consideration of the practical applications. A study of the short-term (2-day) effect of a "breakfast" consisting only of unsweetened black coffee showed the expected absence of a rise in blood sugar above the fasting level and a slight decline throughout the subsequent 3-hour period.[64] Unfavorable subjective symptoms were often reported in the morning, including hunger, weakness, headache and lassitude. When this type of breakfast was followed by a lunch consisting of a low-protein low-calorie sandwich and coffee, a transitory high blood sugar developed which dropped by the third hour to a level below that found during fasting. This fall in blood sugar was accompanied by subjective symptoms of hypoglycemia. An intake of 360 kcal at breakfast decreased the blood sugar drop after the low-protein luncheon, and increasing amounts of protein and fat were associated with improved sense of well-being and flatter blood sugar curves.

A study of the effect of omission of lunch and of three types of lunch (standard, high-fat and high-carbohydrate) on the ability of men to perform strenuous work revealed that the intake of meals affects performance and fatigue of visual functions.[65] No single type of meal (including no food at all) was superior or inferior for all of the functions measured in the fairly large battery of tests applied. However, it was concluded that, in general, the standard meal (carbohydrate 50 per cent, protein 12 per cent and fat 38 per cent of the 1,300 kcal) and the high-fat meal (fat supplying 83 per cent of the 1,400 kcal) were preferable for this type of work.

Pyke, who had considerable experience with industrial feeding in Great Britain, summarized his experience and views on the subject of feeding individuals doing moderate work by concluding:[66]

> (a) Provided the daily diet supplies the full needs for nutrients, the number of meals into which it is divided does not appear to be crucial.
> (b) The nutritionist must always remember that industrial efficiency is influenced by very many factors other than diet.

Until more definitive experimental work demonstrates the contrary, we concur with this view.

Effects of Specific Nutrients on Work Performance

Protein. Liebig's theory that protein was the fuel of muscular work was disproved in 1866; nevertheless the suggestion is occasionally made that persons engaged in hard work require increased protein. To evaluate such claims it is essential to establish: (1) whether energy intake is appropriate for the energy expenditure, (2) that the protein source(s) and intake are adequate to meet total nitrogen requirements and (3) the extent of muscle development associated with the work program. As noted above, dietary protein is utilized efficiently for protein synthesis only when caloric intake is adequate. Chittenden, in 1904, noted that men receiving adequate calories performed hard work in good health on a daily protein intake of only 50 to 60 gm.[67] In 1926 and 1927 it was again demonstrated that, in hard work, there is only a small increase in nitrogen excretion, indicating little change in protein catabolism,[68,69] and even that change may have been an indirect one.[69] Young men doing hard manual work over a period of two months accomplished as much and remained in as good physical condition with approximately 50 gm of protein daily as with approximately 160 gm.[70] There was no difference in physiologic work performance between groups of healthy men during intensive physical training subsisting on either 1.4 or 2.8 gm of protein per kg body weight. During the exercise periods of 40 days, caloric intake was increased by approximately 400 to 450 kcal per day to meet increased energy requirements. On the higher protein intake, nitrogen retention was greater but both groups were in positive nitrogen balance.[71] Others (cf[71]) have recommended that daily protein intakes be increased to 2.0 to 2.5 gm per kg based on changes (some transient) in hemoglobin and serum proteins during heavy physical activity.

Studies of total-body potassium (TBK) and nitrogen balance in a small number of men on 75 minutes of exercise at 2.9 kcal per min while on 0.5 gm per kg of high-quality protein and a mean caloric intake of 50 kcal per kg indicated a variable response: TBK decreased in all, whereas nitrogen balance varied from positive to negative with most subjects being in very slight negative balance.[72] Increasing the protein to 1 gm per kg increased TBK and positive nitrogen balance. An approximate increase of 10 per cent in calories in several

subjects on 0.5 gm per kg protein increased TBK and nitrogen retention. This study emphasizes that either increased calories or protein intake by exercising individuals on borderline low intakes of both may be beneficial.

There is a report indicating an *inverse* relationship between caloric intake and exercise-induced protein catabolism. On a normal caloric intake with 2 gm protein per kg there was no increase in protein catabolism with exercise; however, with increased intake of nonprotein calories (500 and 1,000 kcal) there were exercise-associated increased nitrogen and sulfur excretions.[72a] The metabolic basis for this effect is not known.

When semistarved men were given a protein supplement 50 per cent above their basic intake of 50 gm per day, there was no increase in work performance.[73] Metabolic studies were performed on two chronically underweight but physically fit young adult males with anorexia nervosa. Both lost weight during the study and were in negative nitrogen balance, but no change was noted in the urinary excretion of nitrogen during or after heavy exercise. The substrates used were, presumably, ketone bodies and muscle glycogen.[74]

Chronic severe malnutrition (i.e. serum albumin less than 2.2 gm per 100 ml and weight/height ratio below 30 kg per m) was associated with markedly reduced endurance. Total-body hemoglobin was highly correlated (r = 0.83) with $\dot{V}o_2$ max.[74a]

Protein-restricted rats had longer endurance swimming times than unrestricted controls; energy-restricted underweight rats had endurance times similar to those of controls.[75] Oxygen consumption by all undernourished groups was higher than that of controls during the exercise, and this finding suggests altered metabolism.

The amount of nitrogen excretion in sweat during heavy exercise bears a direct relation to protein intake. Increasing protein from 1.4 gm per kg to 2.8 gm per kg in one study quickly increased sweat nitrogen from an average of 1.74 gm per day to 2.67 gm (+53 per cent).[71] On diets containing 0.5, 12.0 and 96.0 gm of nitrogen per day, daily sweat nitrogen excretions averaged 112, 149 and 514 mg in balance studies.[76]

Carbohydrate and Fat. While glucose has received wide publicity as the "quick-energy" sugar, the fact is that, normally, hydrolysis of disaccharides, such as sucrose, and also the more complex carbohydrates takes place so rapidly in the digestive tract that differences between the rates of absorption and utilization of different sugars and starches are of no practical importance to the healthy individual. On the other hand, the view is held that a high-carbohydrate low-protein meal is conducive to the development, within a short time, of hypoglycemia with its attendant symptoms of hunger, weakness and fatigue, and that high-protein meals maintain blood sugar level and a feeling of well-being.[77] The calorie intake and ratio of carbohydrate to protein in the breakfast meal influence the postprandial blood glucose curve, with the higher protein intakes being associated with lower peaks and slower return to fasting levels.[61-64] Various investigators have challenged the acceptance of the idea of a hypoglycemic reaction as a normal response, since no hypoglycemic responses were observed in a large number of healthy individuals following high-carbohydrate meals.[78,79]

The roles of carbohydrate and fat metabolism and the effects of varying diet composition on efficiency of muscular work have received much experimental attention.

Fats and carbohydrates serve as energy fuels for the working muscles, and the relative contribution of each depends on both the work-load level and dietary intake. In 1901, Zuntz demonstrated that metabolism and the respiratory quotients of working muscles could be altered through changes in diet. He observed that fat was essentially the only source of energy for moderate exercise performed after consumption of a diet extremely high in fat. Carlson and Froberg found that fat contributed the major source of energy for physical work in their study of 12 men who walked 50 km daily during a 10-day fast. The energy contributed from glycogen stores under these circumstances would be negligible, especially after the first 1 to 2 days.[80]

Haldi and Wynn[78] observed that a high-carbohydrate meal taken 3 hours prior to a swimming contest was not any better than an isocaloric meal low in carbohydrate. They concluded that in brief periods of strenuous exercise muscular efficiency was dependent on the energy reserves and the training of the subject. During light work, Marsh and Murlin[81] found small differences in the average efficiencies of individuals consuming a normal, a high-carbohydrate and a high-fat diet (22.1, 22.7 and 21.5 per cent, respectively), but after 4 days on a high-fat diet a decrease in net efficiency was observed. These investigators concluded that the improved efficiency in exercise occurred when the percentage of fat calories in the diet was not too high.

Christensen and Hansen[82] have calculated, from R.Q. values, the energy derived from subjects consuming high-carbohydrate low-fat diets during exercise at a standard work level. The respiratory quotients after 1 week of this diet indicated that fat contributed 25 to 30 per cent of the metabolic fuel. When the diet was changed to a high-fat low-carbohydrate content, over 70 per cent of the metabolic fuel was contributed by fat. Work times were decreased on a high-fat diet and increased (two- to threefold) for men consuming a high-carbohydrate diet. R.Q. measurements indicated that athletes utilized both fat and carbohydrate during rest and light work but utilized an increased percentage of carbohydrate during heavy work. These studies amply demonstrate that the muscle can use different proportions of fat and carbohydrate for combustion during physical exercise.

Krogh and Linhard[83] studied oxygen consumptions and respiratory quotients during work and observed an increase of 11 and 8 per cent in the muscular efficiency when the subjects were consuming high-carbohydrate diets. Gemmill[84] criticized these results because the conclusions were based on extrapolated values. He calculated that the difference in efficiency was only 4.5 per cent. However, as has been pointed out elsewhere,[85] a 4.5 per cent increase in efficiency with the consumption of high-carbohydrate diets could result in a highly significant increase in performance.

On a normal intake, with work loads up to 60 per cent of maximal oxygen consumption, the R.Q. indicates that 50 to 60 per cent of the energy is derived from carbohydrate, but, as the work load is increased to above 90 per cent of maximal oxygen consumption, the contribution of carbohydrate increases to 100 per cent.

Muscle Glycogen. On a normal diet the glycogen stores in the viscera (primarily the liver) amount to approximately 1,800 kcal. Recent work indicates that greater quantities of glycogen may be stored in muscle on diets containing a high percentage of carbohydrate. There appears to be a great variation in the glycogen content of muscle with values ranging up to 5 gm per 100 gm tissue. This results in a fairly large potential of glycogen stores inasmuch as the adult body may contain approximately 30 kg of muscle. Muscle glycogen averaged 144, 87 and 43 mM glucose units per kg wet weight of vastus lateralis muscle at rest in men after a 3-day intake of high-carbohydrate, mixed and high-fat and protein diets, respectively. Froberg[86] determined the glyceride and glycogen levels in muscle biopsy tissues taken before and after exercise from the same subjects. His results indicate that tissue glyceride levels decrease by approximately 10 to 15 per cent during exercise, whereas glycogen

levels decrease approximately 70 per cent during this same time period. The R.Q. during exercise was close to 0.90 during the study, which indicates a large percentage of carbohydrate metabolism. It appears that tissue levels of free fatty acids and triglycerides or fat stores do not decrease to the critical level or become depleted as the glycogen stores do when the individual becomes exhausted.

When young men were exercised and the ingested diet and muscle glycogen levels were related to performance and endurance, it was found that performance time to exhaustion averaged 59, 126 and 189 min after 3 days on a high-fat high-protein diet, a mixed diet and a high-carbohydrate diet, respectively;[87,88] others have found the same general relation.[93] The ability to continue work at 75 to 80 per cent maximal capacity level was related to the muscle glycogen stores.[88,89,91] Hermansen et al.[88] showed that the depletion rate of glycogen in the working muscles was dependent on the relative work load. Eight physically conditioned young men were exercised for three 1-hour periods weekly, with varying work loads. Muscle glycogen content was reduced by 0.31, 0.83 and 1.83 gm per 100 gm of muscle per hr, at work levels of 25, 54 and 78 per cent of the maximal oxygen uptakes, respectively. It was observed that these stores were reduced during strenuous exercise, and, when the muscle glycogen fell to a critical level, work usually stopped or the physical activity rate was decreased. In this instance the R.Q. decreased, indicating an increased energy yield from free fatty acids. These studies show that the working muscles have a requirement for carbohydrate as an energy source and that carbohydrate was obtained directly from the muscle stores of glycogen.

Ahlborg et al.[89] and Hultman and Bergstrom[90] have observed that, after the muscle glycogen stores had been depleted by previous exercise, a high-carbohydrate diet for 1 to 3 days greatly enhanced the synthesis of muscle glycogen. When carbohydrate was given without any previous exercise, only a moderate increase in muscle glycogen stores occurred.[90]

An instructive study has been performed in which the subjects each acted as his own control during exhausting work before and after induced deficiencies of caloric sources.[92] Four healthy male subjects performed bicycle exercise for 1 to 1.5 hours with one leg until exhaustion. After 1 hour of rest identical work was performed with the other leg. The glycogen content of the quadriceps femoris muscle, determined from needle biopsy samples, decreased in connection with the exercise from 11.7 to 0.3 gm per kg muscle. The subjects were then given a no-carbohydrate diet and the experimental procedure was repeated the following day. The capacity for prolonged work was now markedly reduced with regard to work load as well as work time. Between the two 1-leg exercises on the second day nicotinic acid was given in amounts sufficient to block the release of free fatty acids (FFA) from the adipose tissue. This procedure resulted in a further decrease in working capacity. Muscle glycogen decreased during the exercises on the second day from a mean of 2.9 to 0.3 gm per kg. The calculated total energy outputs during exercise on the first day were 850 and 820 kcal during the first and second leg exercise, respectively. Corresponding values on the second day were 430 kcal (first leg, low glycogen and normal FFA release) and 220 kcal (second leg, low glycogen and reduced FFA supply). R.Q. decreased from 0.96 (day 1) to 0.77 at the first exercise on the second day. After administration of nicotinic acid, R.Q. increased to 0.84. The femoral arteriovenous glucose difference was higher during exercise performed after reduction of FFA supply. It was apparent that, when the glycogen stores are reduced, prolonged work can still be performed on submaximal levels (less than 60 to 70 per cent of the maximal oxygen uptake) provided the supply of FFA is adequate. Elimination of both muscle glycogen and exogenous FFA seriously impairs the ability for prolonged exercise.

Others have also noted that reduced carbohydrate combustion and increased fat utilization occurred only when muscle glycogen was markedly reduced by prior exercise and prior consumption of a low-carbohydrate high-fat and protein diet.[85a]

Histochemical studies were made of vastus lateralis muscle biopsy specimens for myosin ATPase and glycogen before, during and after exercise by men at 74 per cent of maximal oxygen capacity on three different diets.[85a] Two fiber types were identified on the basis of myosin ATPase activity and designated as FT (fast twitch) and ST (slow twitch) (termed red and white or Types I and II respectively, by others). Although a spectrum of oxidative capacities exists, the FT fibers generally have lower oxidative and higher glycolytic capacities than ST fibers. Glycogen depletion during exercise was less in FT than ST fibers after a 3-day intake of a mixed or high-carbohydrate diet but higher after a high-fat and protein diet. Only with the latter diet was there almost complete degradation of glycogen during exercise.

Rested and trained men subsisting on a mixed diet (40 to 60 per cent carbohydrate, 30 to 40 per cent fat and 10 to 15 per cent protein) had their muscle (vastus lateralis) glycogen measured in biopsy samples before and after a 10-mile run in 60 to 80 minutes (80 per cent $\dot{V}_{O_2}$ max) on three successive days.[92a] Muscle glycogen utilization was greatest during the first run; it was markedly less during the second and third runs and was associated with a marked reduction in muscle-glycogen concentration, decreased lactate accumulation and increased FFA levels.

The question of the rate of glycogen resynthesis after various degrees of exercise has been examined. When an individual had endurance exercise for 1 hour followed by intermittent maximal exercise for the second hour, muscle glycogen did not regain preexercise level until after approximately 46 hours.[92b] In another study, 3 subjects consumed a mixed diet of 3,100 kcal with 50 per cent in the form of carbohydrate; another 3 consumed the same diet and an additional 2,500 kcal as carbohydrate. They were then exercised on bicycle ergometers for 1 minute at 140 per cent $\dot{V}o_2$ max, followed by a 3-minute rest. This program was continued until the pace could not be continued for 30 seconds. Biopsy and analysis for glycogen at 0, 2, 5, 12 and 24 hours postexercise revealed glycogen at 28, 39, 53, 67 and 102 per cent of the preexercise level. There was no significant difference between the two dietary groups.[92c]

Glucose and Hormonal Changes. Present views on glucose metabolism hold that glucose which is transported into the muscle cell from the blood is phosphorylated very rapidly; since dephosphorylating enzymes are not present in these cells, the phosphorylated glucose must be catabolized or synthesized into glycogen since it cannot leave the cell as free glucose. In the liver cell, however, glucose can be transported in either direction. Hence, in the fasting individual, blood glucose concentration must be the result of the rate of glucose release from the liver and the rate of its uptake by the working muscle and other cells, since net glucose synthesis in other tissue is assumed to be small.

In most subjects in the postabsorptive state working at 50 and 70 per cent of maximal oxygen uptake in multiple exercise periods for 6 hours (by which time they were at or near exhaustion), blood glucose concentrations fell to an average of 62 per cent of preexercise values. This fall was accompanied by symptoms typical of hypoglycemia (dizziness, nausea, confusion, partial blackout) and disappeared within 15 minutes after stopping the exercise, at which time blood glucose rose. In these subjects plasma insulin levels were very significantly reduced in all subjects

whether or not the glucose levels fell (in some cases to 30 per cent of the preexercise level). The insulin decline was greater than that of the glucose during the first hour of work.[93]

It may be concluded that in work of prolonged duration without food intake the fall in blood glucose cannot be accounted for by insulin levels but rather by other factors, which may include catecholamines and glucagon. Consistent with the fall in insulin level is a marked rise in free fatty acids. The fall in insulin may be regarded as a protective mechanism restricting the rate of entry of glucose into working muscle and preserving blood glucose at a level assuring adequate supply to the central nervous system.

At more severe levels of work (77 per cent of maximal O_2 utilization) where exhaustion occurred in about 90 minutes, the fall in glucose was less.[94] When work was so extreme that it could be endured for only a few minutes, there was no significant fall in glucose.[91] At work rates tolerable for less than 1 minute, there was a marked rise in blood sugar.[95]

Although glycogen of muscle is the more readily available energy source in the working muscle, nevertheless some uptake of glucose by the muscle cell is obviously occurring despite decreased insulin levels. Hultman found that at the point of exhaustion splanchnic glucose output represented one-half of the total carbohydrate utilization.[94] In the studies of Wahren et al.[95a] with fasting men working moderately hard for 40 minutes on a bicycle ergometer, splanchnic glucose production rose two- to threefold during exercise, with a rapid return to baseline after exercise. This was associated with a gradual rise in arterial glucose to 11 per cent above the resting level after exercise stopped. Arterial insulin fell slightly during exercise but rose rapidly during recovery to levels two to three times basal levels. Arterial alanine rose markedly (with smaller increments occurring with methionine, phenylalanine and tyrosine) with exercise correlating directly with pyruvate. The augmented peripheral release during exercise supports the existence of a glucose-alanine cycle of importance in gluconeogenesis.

When trained men were studied during graded exercise at 47, 77 and 100 per cent $\dot{V}o_2$ max, glucagon concentration increased 35 per cent above rest to the heaviest work while norepinephrine increased fivefold and epinephrine sixfold.[95b] When the subjects performed prolonged work to exhaustion, glucagon increased threefold and epinephrine 20-fold above basal levels.

During exercise at approximately 30 $\dot{V}o_2$ max for 4 hours and the ingestion of 200 gm of glucose at 90 minutes, there was a 35 per cent rise in arterial glucose, a two- to threefold rise in arterial insulin and a 60 to 70 per cent fall in arterial FFA and glycerol.[95c] Glucagon, which rose fourfold in the control subjects not given glucose, failed to rise in the glucose-supplemented group.

Plasma Electrolytes and Protein. In sustained heavy work plasma K increased early and then fell, probably secondary to an aldosterone effect and associated with a large urinary excretion of K+ (115 mEq per 6 hr). Plasma inorganic phosphate either rose (on mixed or high-carbohydrate diets) or remained essentially unchanged on the high-fat diet.[93]

In untrained rats after short-term or exhausting exercise there were shifts of water from extracellular to intracellular compartments, with a significant decrease in plasma corticosterone. In trained rats corticosteroid level rose with exercise, with shifts to one extracellular compartment.[95d] Plasma Na fell in exhausting exercise in untrained rats, whereas it rose in trained rats. Plasma K increased with short-term exercise in both trained and untrained animals but not with exercise to exhaustion.

In men bicycling with increasing intensity on an ergometer, up to $\dot{V}o_2$ max in 9.5 to 10 minutes, there was a net decrease in total content of plasma protein, Na and Cl in the first 2 minutes of the postexercise period, primarily as the result of significant loss (13 to 15 per cent) of plasma fluid.[95e] Plasma K was increased at the end of exercise but fell below preexercise levels within 2 minutes. The volume Cl and K were still reduced at 25 minutes postexercise.

Alimentary Tract Functions. Numerous studies have indicated that the volume, osmolality and chemical composition of a test meal influence gastric emptying.[96a] Exercise was found to have no effect on gastric emptying until working intensity exceeded 70 per cent $\dot{V}o_2$ max. The rate of gastric emptying increased in proportion to volume of fluid ingested up to a maximum rate at a volume of 600 ml. Cold solutions emptied more rapidly than warm ones. The addition of even small amounts of glucose (i.e. > 139 mM) induced a marked reduction in the rate of gastric emptying.[96b] The rate of absorption of glucose, xylose, saline or water by the small intestine is not affected by fairly hard exercise over 1 hour;[96c] similarly, glucose taken during exercise was well absorbed and utilized.[95a,96d] Administration of glucose near the point of exhaustion during heavy work of several hours' duration enables the individual to continue work for another hour or more.[91]

Exercise in dogs decreased the gastric secretory responses to a meat meal or to pentagastrin in association with decreased gastric mucosal blood flow.[96d] The exercise also decreased fluid and bicarbonate secretion stimulated by a meat meal, secretin or intraduodenal installation of acid; biliary secretion was not affected.

The hemodynamic effects of light exercise were measured in subjects who were fasting or in the postprandial state following ingestion of carbohydrate-rich or protein-rich meals of approximately 1,200 kcal. There were significant increases in cardiac output and oxygen consumption with these meals during exercise which were of the same magnitude as at rest.[97]

While data are needed on the effects of higher work loads, the ingestion of meals prior to exercise may impose an increased load on the cardiovascular system.

The needs for water, carbohydrate or other foods during work vary with the conditions of work. Light to moderate exercise in a hot environment imposes a greater need for water and salt replacement than for carbohydrate. In a cool environment with appreciably less sweating, prolonged work of moderate to high degree requires water in relatively small amounts but may be benefited by intake of carbohydrate. The intake of a large volume of fluid in a short period may lead to a feeling of fullness and be associated with some discomfort.

Vitamins. The experimental evidence leaves little room for doubt that the earliest symptoms of human deficiencies of those water-soluble vitamins about which we know most are those of easy fatigability, anorexia, irritability and apathy. The ability to perform work efficiently is impaired in frank deficiency states; adequate therapy will restore work capacity toward normal levels, when permanent incapacity is not involved.

Simonson and co-workers[99] found no effect on 5 different types of muscular work from the addition of large amounts of the vitamin B complex to the usual diet of 12 healthy subjects. There was no beneficial effect of supplementation with 5 B-complex vitamins and ascorbic acid on muscular ability, resistance to fatigue, or recovery from exertion of healthy young men subsisting on diets considered to be adequate.[100] In experiments lasting 10 to 12 weeks and utilizing normal young men, it was found that intakes of thiamin at 4 different levels (from 0.23 mg per 1,000 kcal daily up to 0.63 mg per 1,000 kcal) exerted no beneficial effect on diets otherwise considered adequate. Muscular, neuromuscular, cardiovascular, psychomotor and metabolic functions tested "were in no way limited—(and) clinical signs, subjective sensations and state of mind, and behavior were likewise unaffected."[101] A level of 0.96 mg of thiamin per 1,000 kcal was allowed to the control subjects in these experiments. Supplementation with B-complex vitamins of a diet considered adequate did not increase the endurance of several subjects operating a bicycle ergometer.[102]

An experiment with 86 volunteer military personnel exposed to a cold environment revealed no significant difference in physical and psychologic performance in a 10-week test between supplemented and unsupplemented groups.[103] The supplementation consisted of large amounts of 7 B-complex vitamins and ascorbic acid. The basal diets were presumed to be adequate except for a 3-week period of moderate caloric deficit.

The addition of varying amounts of ascorbic acid to diets already adequately provided with this vitamin has been found to exert no detectable effects in terms of general well-being, physical vigor and efficiency for hard work.[104-106]

From 1941 to 1943 a combined study of dietary habits, clinical status and the effect of nutrient supplementation was conducted by Borsook and his associates on large numbers of aircraft workers in Southern California.[107] No significant specific therapeutic effects of a multiple vitamin-mineral supplement (vitamins A, D, C, B_1, riboflavin, niacinamide and calcium) were observed. However, the supplemented group was reported to show decreases in unauthorized absences and turnover rate as compared with the group receiving a placebo.

This evidence supports the general opinion that, once the vitamin requirements of the organism are met, there is no value in additional supply, i.e. "supernutrition" does not exist.

Effects of Low Nutrient Intake on Efficiency

This topic is a highly complex subject characterized by conflicting evidence and opinion. Johnson et al.[108] found that young men subjected to hard daily physical work and subsisting on a diet deficient in members of the B complex, notably thiamin, exhibited symptoms of easy fatigability, apathy, muscle and joint pains, anorexia, constipation and a marked deterioration in work performance within 1 week. Another group on the same diet supplemented with thiamin exhibited only a few mild subjective symptoms, but their performance during hard work also deteriorated. Administration of yeast restored both groups to normal within 4 days.

Foltz, Barborka and Ivy[109] studied the work performance on the bicycle ergometer of 4 medical students. When the thiamin intake was reduced from 0.43 to 0.59 mg per 1,000 kcal of food to 0.33 to 0.38 mg per 1,000 kcal, a decrease in appetite was noted within three weeks. After 1 month at this reduced thiamin intake a further decrease in thiamin intake was effected (0.17 to 0.21 mg per 1,000 kcal) but no additional changes were noted until 4 weeks later, at which time a decided decrease in appetite and work output occurred together with increased fatigue and muscle tenderness and a deterioration in mental attitude. The objective and subjective symptoms disappeared promptly after the addition of a yeast concentrate. Archdeacon and Murlin[110] noted a decrease in muscular endurance on the bicycle ergometer in two subjects on a diet low in the B complex vitamins (the thiamin intake being 0.27 mg per day or 0.09 mg per 1,000 kcal), the effect being observed within 10 to 14 days on the diet. Addition of the B complex in the form of whole wheat bread or thiamin in pure form resulted in a marked improvement in endurance. Pyridoxine added in one experiment had a similar effect but riboflavin had none.

These results are in marked contrast to those of Keys and co-workers. In one experiment[101] already mentioned, no decrease in work performance was noted on diets containing 0.23 mg thiamin per 1,000 kcal. In a later paper[111] the Minnesota investigators published the results of a study in which eight young men were studied before, during and after a 2-week period during which five were on a basal diet providing on the average 0.16 mg of thiamin, 0.15 mg of riboflavin and 1.8 mg of niacin per 1,000 kcal. These men also received placebos while three control subjects were given the same basal diet plus capsules containing a yeast concentrate and synthetic B vitamins. With an energy expenditure of 4,800 kcal during the experimental period, no differences were noted in endurance and in a variety of clinical, psychologic and biochemical tests. The length of time on a low B complex intake (0.185 mg thiamin, 0.287 mg riboflavin and 3.71 mg niacin daily per 1,000 kcal) was extended to 161 days and again no impairment of work performance was noted at a calorie intake and expenditure of 3,300 kcal.[112] A small increase in blood pyruvate indicated a borderline thiamin deficiency. Immediately thereafter the daily intake of two of the subjects (known as the restricted-deficient group) was restricted more severely to 0.008 mg thiamin, 0.013 mg riboflavin and 0.1 mg niacin per 1,000 kcal with a daily energy intake and expenditure of 4,000 kcal. Anorexia developed after the first week and by the end of the third week the subjects exhibited almost complete inability to take any food. Supplementation was begun with thiamin alone on the 24th day. Two additional men who had been on an adequate diet prior to ingesting the very deficient diet (the control-deficient group) exhibited anorexia to a lesser extent. Despite marked changes in general behavior and obvious signs of subjective distress, there were no significant changes in simple strength as measured by grip and back lift. Psychomotor tests of speed and coordination showed slight to marked deterioration. The restricted-deficient subjects showed a rapid and progressive deterioration and incapacity to perform brief severe work. Nausea developed on extreme exertion. Similarly this group was often unable to complete the prescribed daily exercise of moderately hard work, while the control-deficient group was able to perform both types of work. The administration of thiamin alone reversed the deterioration.

It is worth noting at this point that even severe thiamin deficiency does not cause any significant diminution in ability to perform intellectual tasks, although marked deterioration takes place in certain psychomotor and personality tests and endurance.[39,113,114]

We can only conjecture about the reasons for the discrepancy in results obtained in different laboratories with intakes of thiamin in the same range. There were obvious differences in the subjects, diets and experimental conditions. It cannot be overemphasized that, in the study of the effects of nutritional deficiencies upon functions of the human subject, careful consideration must be given to both psychologic and physiologic factors which may influence the results. Since subjective reactions and individual variability are serious complicating factors in such experiments, the greatest caution must be exerted in accepting the conclusions of experiments not rigidly controlled.

In the only report published on the effects of uncomplicated low-riboflavin intake on muscular performance, the Minnesota group[115] found no deleterious effects in three men after 84 days and, on another three men, after 152 days on a diet containing 0.99 mg riboflavin per day. This level of riboflavin will not cause the development of obvious clinical signs even over a period of 2 years in less active individuals.[116]

In a study[117] of experimental human ascorbic acid deficiency induced by a diet low in the vitamin, the first symptom was fatigue which appeared after 2 months. An impaired capacity for walking and running progressed during the 6-month deficiency period. A similar effect of vitamin C deficiency was noted by Farmer[118] in experiments with a group of young men existing for several months on a diet low in vitamin C.

In view of the ability of the body to store sufficient vitamin A so that deficiency signs may not occur for a year or more on a diet deficient in vitamin A,[119] it is not surprising that no decrease in ability to perform hard muscular exercise was noted in men kept on diets low in vitamin A for about 6 months.[120]

Do vitamin requirements increase as energy expenditure rises? From indirect data on human dietaries associated with the presence or absence of beriberi, and on the basis of animal experiments where the amounts of activity or the environmental temperature was varied or where experimental hyperthyroidism was induced, it has been concluded generally that the requirement for certain B-complex vitamins, particularly thiamin, is related to total metabolism.

Although work ability is markedly diminished in severe vitamin C-deficiency states,[117,118] it is doubtful that hard work brings on scurvy more rapidly. Experiments in which both sedentary and working men were kept on scorbutic diets for 8 weeks failed to show any difference between the groups.[105]

NUTRITION AS AFFECTED BY ENVIRONMENTAL STRESS

Influence of Cold Environment on Nutrient Requirements

This subject requires consideration of a number of factors. Caloric requirements and the general health of the individual will vary greatly depending on the degree of protection against cold. The efficiency of arctic protective clothing and the availability of heated base camps and mechanical transportation have done much to provide a less stressful microclimate in cold regions. Hence, the usual responses to cold (cutaneous vasoconstriction and metabolic responses including shivering and non-shivering thermogenesis) are greatly minimized—but not entirely overcome, since face and extremities are subjected to cooling. The physiologic effects of cold exposure and adaptation to cold have been discussed in some detail.[121] Where possible much of the time is spent in shelter, and caloric requirements will depend on the nature of the outdoor work and of the terrain.

The weight and "hobbling" effect of arctic clothing adds to caloric needs.[122] Gray et al. measured the energy expenditure by men doing hard physical work in three different environments while wearing standard arctic, temperate and desert clothing.[123] For a given amount of external work performed at a constant temperature, energy expenditure increased approximately 5 per cent when the clothing was changed from desert to temperate type and approximately another 5 per cent when it was changed from temperate to arctic. There were further small energy increments related to temperature decrease while working in the same clothing (i.e. 2 per cent going from 15.7° C to −26.2° C). Increase in energy expenditure as bulk of clothing was increased has also been observed, and this appeared to be more related to the "hobbling" effect than to the increased weight per se.[124,124a]

A review of energy intake and expenditure in various polar expeditions indicates an average daily expenditure during 8- to 10-hour sledging operations of 5,000 to 6,500 kcal for men of 70 to 80 kg—usually associated with mild weight loss—whereas in base camp daily expenditure is usually 1,500 kcal less.[126] On many polar expeditions mechanical transport is now replacing dog sledging. It would be expected that energy expenditure would therefore be less than in the days of running and pushing heavy sleds. However, in a study in which field parties drove in enclosed heated tractors, there were weight losses up to 6 kg associated with changes in skinfold thickness.[127] In another study in which men traveled in small open motorized toboggans over 900 km in Antarctica between October and December, they lost 4.4 to 9.2 kg in weight with evidence of loss of body fat.[128] The subjects were cold and shivering much of the time. The mean energy expenditure was estimated at 3,500 kcal.

In an analysis of voluntary caloric intake by soldiers stationed in various climates, an inverse linear function was noted between caloric intake and temperature.[122] Average daily intake varied from 4,400 kcal per man in the cold to 3,200 kcal in the tropics. The proximate composition of the diets consumed was much the same regardless of environment.[122,126]

Other data were obtained with military units in Alaska[129] and northern Canada[130] and in a comparative study of troops performing similar tasks in areas with mean temperatures of −22.5, −7.3, 72 and 90° F.[131] These reports agree that caloric consumption in cold and temperate climates was similar, especially when calculated on an equal weight basis. A similar conclusion is reached by others in a review of these and other studies.[125,132]

Under arctic and subarctic living conditions there is a tendency for the majority of men to gain weight;[126,131] isolation, boredom and other abnormal living conditions predispose to excessive food intake.[131]

Considerable attention has been directed to the question of whether diet composition affects the ability of the organism to withstand exposure to cold when environmental protection is inadequate and protective physiologic mechanisms become prominent. In human studies the cooling of the internal tissues of the body was found to be most rapid on a high-protein diet (41 per cent of calories as protein) and least on a high-fat diet (73 per cent of calories), with a high-carbohydrate diet (66 per cent of calories) not quite so effective as a high-fat diet.[133] The least favorable method of feeding tested was the high-protein diet with one meal (20 per cent of the day's calories) served during an 8-hour exposure, and the most favorable method was the high-fat diet with three meals (20 per cent) served during 8 hours of exposure. By a change from the first to the second diet plan, the decrement in rectal temperature was reduced by two-thirds (1.63° to 0.57° C) and the decrement in general psychomotor functioning by one-half.[134]

In an acute experiment at 7.5° C, seminude subjects were given test meals of 214 kcal as glucose, steak or glycine and sucrose, in an effort to determine whether specific dynamic action affected tolerance to cold. It was concluded that this was not effective.[135] An interesting and unexplained observation was a reduction of shivering in those subjects ingesting the glycine-sucrose test meal prior to cold exposure.

Beneficial effects of increased fat have been affirmed[136,137] and denied[138] in rat experiments. Wtih diets having 10 per cent fat, a level of protein of 40 per cent was appreciably more protective than one of 20 or 5 per cent.[139,140] Under severe cold stress, a purified diet also fed to rats conferred greater protection than did a commercial chow diet.[141] It may be concluded that modification of dietary protein, fat or carbohydrate has little or no influence on improving cold adaptation in man.

Criteria for the development of survival rations in various environmental situations have been discussed by Johnson,[142] who stresses the fact that ketosis secondary to inadequate calories or lack of carbohydrate is exacerbated with cold exposure, presumably as the result of increased caloric requirements. Factors affecting the severity of ketosis have been considered[143] and reemphasized in arctic survival studies.[144]

In relation to the caloric expenditure occurring in cold climates, it is probable that vitamin requirements are not markedly altered from those in temperate climates. Troops in an arctic environment subsisting on a diet meeting the recommended allowances of the National Research Council did not appear to be noticeably benefited by vitamin supplements.[145] A short-term (3-month) study of performance of young men under cold stress during "borderline" and high intakes of thiamin and ascorbic acid did not reveal any significant differences attributable to these vitamins.[147] In conformity with the animal experiments of Dugal et al.,[148] a decreased ascorbic acid excretion was noted in the urines of these men during cold stress. Dugal[149] has claimed an increased need for ascorbic acid in rats, guinea pigs and monkeys exposed to cold.

Similar studies on the nutritional requirements for resistance by the rat to cold stress have indicated that there is significant impairment in deficiencies of thiamin,[150] riboflavin,[151] pyridoxine,[152] vitamin A[153] and pantothenic acid.[154] A contributing, but not the sole factor in the decreased survival to cold is the impaired caloric intake by the deficient rats.[155]

These and other problems of cold acclimation have been reviewed.[155-157]

Requirements in Hot Environments

As the environmental temperature rises in relation to the body temperature, the flow of heat from the body to the environment is impeded. In an attempt to maintain its usual temperature, the body secretes sweat, the evaporation of which removes heat. The altered nutritional requirements during exposure to heat are quantitative rather than qualitative and acutely involve mainly water and sodium chloride.

Water and Salt. The capabilities of the body for sweat loss are great; for example, in one experiment in which young men were subjected to severe stress of temperature and work,[116] the maximum sweating rate was 4.2 liters per hour and some men completed 4 hours of work while sweating at rates of 3 liters per hour, a total amount equal to approximately 4 times the blood water. This high rate is not met in industry or in athletic performance except in exceptional short-term situations. The loss of 1 liter of water per hour for an 8-hour day occurs at times in certain heavy industries and, with this volume of water, a total of perhaps 10 to 20 gm of salt. In competitive distance running losses may exceed 2 liters per hr.[158]

A number of investigators have demonstrated that, in a matter of a few hours, the physical status and performance of subjects in a hot environment and doing hard work deteriorate (proceeding under severe conditions to actual collapse) when water is withheld.[159–163] Administration of water under these circumstances enables the body to maintain lower rectal and skin temperatures, more normal pulse rates, and mental efficiency. Symptoms of acute water lack during hard work in a hot environment appear to be the most rapidly induced of any deficiency syndrome. Recovery from the effects of dehydration following water ingestion is even more rapid.

Thirst is a reliable guide to water needs under most circumstances. However, men sweating even at moderate rates do not tend to drink water as fast as they evaporate it, although they usually make up the deficiency after the day's work.[164,165] When the heat load is high and continued, thirst may fail to ensure an adequate intake.[163,166] It has been recommended that men working in the heat replace the water lost in sweat by hour-to-hour ingestion of amounts more than sufficient to keep thirst quenched at all times.

Water balance is affected by dietary factors other than water intake, since renal function operates within certain physiologic limitations. Thus, as indicated below, salt depletion leads to body water loss, despite a good fluid intake. At the other extreme, diets imposing a high osmotic load on the kidney will increase the obligatory water loss. Starvation during water deprivation with its attendant metabolic changes leads to increased urine volume.[167] A number of nutritional and metabolic factors influence renal function and the ability to utilize water efficiently.

The effect of salt deficiency among industrial workers was first pointed out by Moss[168] in connection with "miners' cramps." Since then it has been noted in a variety of occupations among workers exposed to elevated temperatures. The basis of this deficiency is failure to replace adequately the sodium chloride lost in sweat, while the water loss is made good. Symptoms may include nausea, vomiting, vertigo, mental apathy, exhaustion, painful cramps and circulatory failure.

Workers in hot environments should have ready access to water at all times and they should be instructed as to the importance of frequent water and adequate salt intake. Since the average American's daily diet contains 10 to 15 gm of salt and since salt lost in sweat need not be replaced hourly, the salt consumed at mealtimes is adequate for most needs.

The same would appear to hold for salt replacement in most types of physical exercise where sweating is not excessive and prolonged. Claims have been made that the ingestion of a glucose-electrolyte solution by athletes exercising in a hot climate resulted in less rise in body temperature, rate of sweat loss and rise in serum Na than did the ingestion of water or hypotonic saline.[169] Others have concluded that the addition of electrolytes to drinking water is of minimal value for individuals exercising at 37 to 38°C and R.H. of 55 to 60 per cent at 50 to 60 per cent $\dot{V}o_2$ max with a daily weight loss of 3 per cent. The subjects taking only water maintained positive Na, K and Cl balances via dietary ingestion and renal conservation.[170]

With prolonged heavy sweating which could lead to loss of 8 per cent of body weight without adequate water replacement, Na losses could exceed 200 mEq per 24 hours. Although salt is provided by regular meals, continued losses will probably lead to negative salt balances. In such situations it is often desirable to ensure an increased intake of 1 gm of salt for each liter of water consumed above 4 or 5 liters per day; salt can also be supplied in the drinking water as an 0.1 per cent solution.

In dry desert air, sweat may evaporate as fast as it is produced. At 40° C $\pm$ 5° C, sweat rates have been recorded of 6 to 8 ml per min per square meter of body surface, equal to 0.7 to 1.0 liter per hour for men 70 to 80 kg.[171] At temperatures of 47° C (117° F) (e.g. Death Valley) sweat rates reached 13 to 14 ml per min per m²; despite this sweating rate with rapid evaporation, body temperature could not be maintained at a tolerable temperature.

The use of salt tablets is not desirable since they frequently cause gastric distress, nausea and vomiting in some individuals, especially during hard work and, more importantly, there is no assurance that those needing salt most will take the tablets.

Acclimatization to work in the heat is associated with a decrease in the sodium content of sweat. In order for this adaptive change to occur, there must be a salt deficit with its attendant changes. During acclimatization of young men in the heat while subsisting on a salt intake leading to deficits of 140 to 320 mEq, renal and sweat sodium outputs were greatly reduced, plasma sodium fell and urinary tetrahydroaldosterone increased three- to sixfold.[172] With this salt depletion and attendant water deficit, the subjects had lower sweat rates and skin temperatures, higher rectal temperatures and less efficient tissue heat conductance than during acclimatization with replacement of salt and water. When salt and water were replaced under the same conditions of heat and exercise, sodium was retained and plasma volume was believed to increase. There was no increase in urinary tetrahydroaldosterone or sodium and three of the five subjects had no reduction in sweat sodium. Thus, while severe prolonged salt depletion, especially in the heat, is dangerous, some degree of salt depletion accelerates acclimatization.

During a 7-day period of acclimatization on low Na intake (30 mEq per day), the Na content of sweat decreased steadily from the range of 30 to 65 mEq per liter to 10 to 25 mEq for the subjects. During this period the K concentration rose from 5 to 6.5 mEq per liter to 6.5 to 10.[172]

Physiologic features of responses to heat and of acclimatization are discussed in detail elsewhere,[172-175] as are the endocrine responses to heat stress[172,175] and the various types of heat illness.[175]

Energy Requirements. There have been conflicting opinions over the last 40 years concerning energy needs in a hot environment as compared to those in a temperate climate. The issue has been reviewed by Consolazio and Schnakenberg[176] and concerns the question of energy cost of performance of a specific task in the two environments. Comparative investigations conducted by the Army Institute of Medical Research have demonstrated that body temperature and heat rates were elevated in the hot environment, that metabolic rate was increased and that oxygen uptake was higher with work. The increased energy expenditures were not attributable to lack of training or heat acclimatization but, rather, to the increased heat load imposed by the ambient temperature and solar radiation on metabolic rate and by increased cardiac, ventilatory and sweating rates. Increasing the relative humidity at 37.8° C from 30 per cent to 70 per cent and 96 per cent did not further increase the heart or ventilation rates or oxygen uptake, although the body temperature increased slightly with increasing humidity.[176] These findings resulted in a revision of caloric allowances of the National Research Council/National Academy of Science with an increase of 0.5 per cent for each degree of temperature above 30° C. While there are some who challenge this concept,[177] other data support the need for increased energy expenditure at elevated temperature. At the same time it should be noted that actual work of individuals may be decreased as the result of decreased motivation and avoidance of work during the heat of the day or in hot industrial areas.

Heat Acclimatization and Work Efficiency. Acclimatization has been demonstrated to improve stability of the cardiovascular system and ability to dissipate heat from the body.[178,179] These events do not necessarily occur in parallel but, as acclimatization occurs, both processes are supportive of performance. Prior training at cool temperature (18 to 22° C) resulted in little or no improvement in heat (33.8° C db, 32.4° wb) before acclimatization; after acclimatization work was accomplished with an energy expenditure 5 to 8 per cent less.[180] Similarly, improvement in heat dissipation during acclimatization cannot be ascribed solely to work efficiency and sweating. Accompanying an improved surface transfer of heat is the changing state of the vascular contents. Whereas exercise training was shown to protect the vascular volume during heat exposure, a similar work load after heat acclimatization is accompanied by a marked expansion of plasma volume.[180]

Protein Intake. Varying the daily protein intake in successive 2-month periods from about 100 to 150 to 75 gm and back to 100 gm had no deleterious effect upon ability to march on a treadmill for relatively short periods in humid heat or to perform very hard work of short duration in a temperate environment.[181] Such data challenge the recommendation of Lusk[182] that a high-protein diet is contraindicated in hard work, especially in hot weather. Certainly, the fact is well established that acclimatized men in tropical areas who have access to meat eat it, often in large amounts, without obvious untoward reactions. Considerable quantities of nitrogen are lost under conditions that produce profuse sweating, with values averaging 149, 189 and 241 mg per hour during exposures to environmental temperatures of 70, 85 and 100° F for men performing moderate daily physical activities.[183] With acclimation at 100° F, nitrogen excretion in sweat decreased from 300 to 200 mg per hour. These sweat losses were not compensated for after acclimation by decreased nitrogen losses from the kidneys and alimentary tract. As a result, it was recommended that protein requirements be increased appropriately to compensate for nitrogen losses in sweat.

Heat-acclimatized men on borderline low intake of protein of excellent quality (0.7 gm of nitrogen per kg) with moderate activity exposed to temperatures of 34 to 37° C had reciprocal losses of nitrogen through the skin and in the urine; as skin losses increased, urine nitrogen decreased but total nitrogen losses did not increase.[184] Skin losses during the latter part of heat exposure fell from 12.3 mg per kg (15 per cent of the total urine and dermal N losses) to 4.1 mg per kg (4 per cent of the total N losses). The total dermal N losses were 650 to 750 mg per day with moderate sweat losses; these were similar to skin losses for acclimatized Tanzanian men under hot conditions.[185]

Other Dermal Losses. It has been stated above that water and salt are the substances of main concern where sweating is profuse and prolonged. However, this is not to be construed as meaning that other nutrients may not be lost in significant quantities. Dermal losses have been reviewed by Mitchell and Edman,[186] and further quantitative data on the content of sweat have been published.[187-190]

Free amino acids are lost in sweat. It has been estimated that, with a sweat volume of 3 liters per day, the loss of essential amino acids is not likely to exceed 1.5 gm.[191] The data of Consolazio et al.[187] support this figure and indicate that approximately one-third of the weight of amino acids lost is made up of essential amino acids. Acclimatization decreases the losses of amino acids to a moderate degree but they still approximate 13 per cent of the total nitrogen lost in sweat.

During profuse sweating at 100° F calcium losses via this route averaged 234 mg per day with evidence of decrease with acclimatization.[188] In 7.5 hours at 100° F, sweat excretions averaged 0.601 gm per hour for sodium, 0.125 gm per hour for potassium, 2.3 mg per hour for magnesium, 0.13 mg per hour for iron and 0.45 to 0.81 mg per hour for phosphorus.[183] Iron losses in sweat in acclimatized Tanzanian men were approximately 0.3 mg per day; such losses may be a significant factor in iron depletion with low dietary intake or absorption.[165] Magnesium losses in sweat in unacclimatized men during work in a hot environment averaged 0.28 mEq per liter with a range of 0.13 to 0.45.[192] Thus various mineral losses may be significant and this route of excretion must be appreciated in mineral balance studies, especially where profuse sweating occurs. It should be noted that, in many studies,[183,186–188] the composition of arm sweat was taken as representative of whole-body sweat.

Whole-body sweat during 1 hour of profuse sweating at 40 to 45° C at high humidity at 1.29 L per hr was found to contain an average of 41.2 μg per 100 ml of iron, of which 29.8 was in the cell-free fraction;[189] iron loss per hour was 0.53 ± 0.45 mg, considerably higher than that noted above. Calcium and magnesium losses were 0.33 and 0.13 mEq per liter respectively and 0.42 and 0.16 mEq per hour, respectively.[190]

Fat and Carbohydrate. Although there are no well-established figures for optimal intakes of fat or carbohydrates and we cannot speak of actual requirements for these nutrients, it appears that the usual pattern of dietary intake need not be altered in hot climates in order to perform work.[176]

Vitamins. At least two possibilities exist for changes in vitamin requirements of men at elevated temperature: losses in sweat and altered metabolic requirements. Losses of vitamins in sweat were studied in a number of laboratories during World War II.[146] The evidence supports the conclusion that, in absolute amounts and in comparison with the urinary excretion of the water-soluble vitamins, losses in sweat are not a significant factor in depleting the body's stores. There is no evidence that metabolic requirements are increased. On the contrary, the observed increased urinary excretion of pantothenic acid and ascorbic acid may mean a lower requirement at elevated temperatures. Some popularization of the belief that the need for ascorbic acid is increased has resulted from reports[193,194] of benefits from large amounts of vitamin C given to workers and from reports[195] that, in hyperpyrexia of infective or artificially induced origin, plasma ascorbic acid levels are reduced. However, Osborne and Farmer[196] were unable to find any reduction in plasma ascorbic acid in patients exposed to a temperature of 102° F in fever cabinets, and Abt and co-workers[197] concluded from studies on infectious diseases that hyperpyrexia alone did not affect the vitamin C reserves or utilization. No beneficial effect of large amounts of vitamin C was noted on the ability of young men to work in hot environments for short periods (3 hours to 4 days) nor were there any apparent effects on temperature, vasomotor stability, psychomotor or strength responses or resistance to heat exhaustion.[198]

Effects of Altitude

On acute exposure to high altitude the process of acclimatization begins and many of its physiologic responses give rise to unusual bodily sensations and symptoms, e.g. essential hyperventilation leads to a feeling of breathlessness and tachycardia may give rise to palpitation. These sensations are to be distinguished from the symptom complex that develops in susceptible subjects after a lag time of 6 to 96 hours—"acute mountain sickness"—which does not appear to be a direct result of hypoxia per se.[199] The most common symptoms of acute mountain sickness include anorexia, nausea and vomiting, disinclination to work, edema and muscular weakness.[199] Food intakes may be decreased by 25 to 50 per cent during acute altitude exposure[200] and loss of body weight occurs among newcomers and climbers at high altitude.[199] Negative nitrogen and water balances have been observed,[201] as have decreased blood electrolytes and electrolyte balances.[202] Consolazio et al. have attributed these altered metabolic and biochemical changes of acute mountain sickness to anorexia and subsequent caloric restriction rather than to hypoxia.[200] When highly motivated trained young men were abruptly transferred to high altitude and their calorie consumption was maintained, positive nitrogen and mineral balances were achieved, weight losses were greatly reduced, and normal blood electrolyte and fasting glucose levels were maintained. However, hypohydration occurred whether food intakes were adequate or not; this was attributed to an adaptive response to hypoxia.

Significant increases in oxygen uptakes, pulmonary ventilation and heart rates were increased at altitudes of 4,300 meters[203] (but not at 3,500 meters[204]) as compared to sea level in young men doing standardized submaximal and maximal work. These increases at 4,300 meters suggest an increased caloric need during acute. high-altitude exposure which may be secondary to the increased cost of cardiac and respiratory work and/or to decreased efficiency of work performance.

The suggestion made in 1908[205] that a high-carbohydrate diet would prove beneficial in alleviating symptoms of oxygen lack has been confirmed in rats[206] and man.[207–213] Significant gains in altitude tol-

erance for periods up to 6 hours could be accomplished in human subjects maintained at the equivalent of 15,000 to 17,000 feet by the ingestion of preflight and in-flight foods of high-carbohydrate content, in contrast with performance after the omission of a meal, after a single meal high in protein or after large amounts of fat.[207–209]

A comparative study was performed with young men exercising at sea level and after abrupt transfer to 14,000 feet while subsisting on one of two liquid diets of the same caloric value. Each diet had 12 per cent calories as protein but differed in carbohydrate and fat. On the higher-carbohydrate lower-fat intake (68 and 20 per cent of calories, respectively), the men had considerably better performance in heaviest work and less clinical symptoms at altitude as compared to those on the diet with 48 per cent of calories from carbohydrate and 40 per cent from fat.[210]

High-carbohydrate meals enhanced glucose metabolism at high altitude[212] and increased pulmonary diffusing capacity and work performance.[213]

With pressurized cabins in commercial and military planes, this aspect of diet would appear to have little practical significance in aviation. However with mountain climbers and newcomers at high altitude and with population groups subsisting at high altitudes, benefit may be derived from high-carbohydrate intake.

Pressurized cabins have reduced the earlier problems of abdominal pain occurring as the result of expansion of intestinal gases following rapid ascent at low pressures. To minimize this problem advice has been given to avoid carbonated beverages and melons,[214] fried meat, beans, cabbage, green leafy vegetables and raw fruit[215] in the hours just preceding ascent. The problem of intestinal gases has assumed new importance with the advent of prolonged flight in a closed system; this is considered in the next section.

There is no evidence that mild vitamin

deficiency states have any effect on human altitude tolerance.[216,217]

Food and Nutrition in Space Travel

This is an important area of consideration in the complex of biologic and engineering problems the solution of which has been essential to ensuring health and safety during travel in space.

Practical considerations stem from storage space and weight constraints on food, supplies and water and from problems of weightlessness, low pressure and food acceptability over periods of time in confined quarters. Developments in technology, packaging and preparative techniques of foods have been innovative.

Food Systems. On each successive flight in the U.S. manned space program, improvements have been introduced. Tubed semisolid foods were utilized in the earliest manned Mercury flights. Experience proved that weightlessness posed no problems in chewing, swallowing and digestion. The last Mercury flights utilized bite-sized precooked dehydrated foods which were rehydrated by saliva as chewed. To these were added compressed bite-sized foods. The evolution of space feeding concepts during the Mercury and Gemini space programs has been reviewed.[218]

The increased duration and complexity of the Apollo flights led to more advanced food systems and availability. The weight and volume of food and packages per man per day for the Apollo 7 mission were 872 gm and 2,558 cc respectively, whereas in the Apollo 14 mission they were 1,126 gm and 3,083 cc, respectively. A detailed description of the Apollo 14 food system is available.[219] Optimum utilization of weight and volume favors major emphasis on rehydratable food (resulting in weight reduction by approximately 80 per cent) as long as water is available from fuel cells and other sources and where weight and volume savings will translate into payload. To tubed semisolid and bite-sized precooked foods were added thermostabilized items

such as fruit, meat and fowl in flexible or rigid packages (consumed by using a conventional spoon) and rehydratable solid foods. The latter are packaged in flexible spoon-bowl packages and are rehydrated by injecting hot or cold water, as appropriate, into the package by means of a water gun inserted into a one-way spring-loaded water valve. After the food is rehydrated with water, the package is opened and the contents are eaten with a conventional spoon.[219] In-flight sandwich preparation was accomplished using bread baked from irradiated flour and thermostable sandwich spreads. The types and varieties of foods varied during the flight phases. Foods have been selected for flight use after careful consideration of the food preferences of each crew member. Despite this, preflight preferences have afforded a poor basis for predicting in-flight food consumption in Apollo lunar landing missions.[219] This finding necessitates an oversupply of foods to allow for in-flight shifts of food acceptance and consumption.

Food and nutrition systems had to be developed in the Apollo program for astronauts wearing pressure suits to be used during emergency decompression situations (fortunately never required) and during lunar surface explorations. The astronauts estimated that work periods up to 10 hours were within their physical capability in the pressure suits. However, periods longer than 4 hours required fluids and solid nutrients to ensure proper physiologic performance.[220] Fluids and food in dispenser systems were incorporated into the helmet neck ring of the space suit and the liquid was obtained by opening a check valve and sucking. Food was given in the form of bars of fruit, gelatin, sugar and water supplying 188 kcal in approximately 2 ounces.

Skylab flights of increasing duration (28, 59 and 84 days) in earth orbit led to further improvements in food systems.[221] A larger variety of foods was available. With the exception of beverages, foods were served for the first time entirely from open vessels, eaten with conventional utensils and in usual meal-like fashion, with several items available for simultaneous consumption. Foods were heated in a special food warmer tray to $65 \pm 3.3°$ C within 2 hours; this temperature is below the boiling point of $72.2°$ C in the total pressure of approximately 250 mm Hg prevailing in the space vehicle. Foods must be heated slowly in the absence of convection. There were repetitive 6-day food menu cycles, with the daily ration designed to provide at least 100 per cent of the Recommended Dietary Allowances.

Nutrition and Metabolism. In short space travels lasting a few days to a week, mild caloric imbalances and depletion would not be critical to performance. However, as the duration away from earth increases, it becomes essential to have sound imformation on nutritional requirements and metabolic changes of man in space.

The intake of Gemini astronauts ranged widely from day to day and mission to mission and was less than the 2,500 kcal provided.[222,223] An effort was made to perform nitrogen and mineral balance studies before, during and after the 14-day Gemini VII flight of December 1965.[224] Decreased in-flight food intake and other problems adversely affected the accuracy of the results and considerable individual differences were noted. There were small changes in calcium balance and losses of phosphate, potassium and nitrogen, presumably reflecting loss of muscle mass.[224] In the Gemini missions as a group, weight losses were approximately 3 to 8 per cent of the preflight weight with time of recovery after return related to flight duration.[225]

Measurements of in-flight food consumption on American Apollo and on Soviet Vostok, Voskhod and Soyuz missions[226] indicated that on these flights, as with Gemini missions, there were diminished energy intake and weight losses.

The estimated mean daily intake of the Apollo 7–11 crews was 1,680 kcal of the 2,300 kcal available. The Apollo 16 crew ingested a daily average of 2,005 kcal of the 2,633 kcal provided.[227] On Apollo 17 approximately 1,950 kcal were consumed per day of the 2,600 provided.[228] Caloric intake and body weight changes in Apollo 7–17 missions have been published.[226] Some of the decrease was secondary to the occurrence of anorexia and nausea in a fairly high proprotion of crewmen; however, those maintaining a good appetite also lost weight.

In the 28-, 59- and 84-day Skylab missions, all nine crew members were able to eat approximately the same quantities of food in flight as on the ground but with considerable day-to-day variation;[221] the daily preflight intake over 3 weeks averaged $3,128 \pm 441$ kcal, while inflight the average was $3,130 \pm 488$ kcal. Nevertheless, weight losses occurred in 8 of the 9 men ranging from 0.7 to 4.5 kg; the amounts were not related to the duration of flight. There were also body water losses in 8 of 9 men ranging from 0.5 to 2.0 liters.[230] The water loss was rapid in the first few days of flight. This was attributed to diuresis as a reflex reaction to a shift in body fluid toward the thorax.[230]

Total body volumes decreased but, since they were approximately proportional to weight losses, densities were unchanged.[230,231] The volume loss was most noticeable in buttocks and abdomen (presumably as the result of fat loss) and in the calves.

In the Gemini and Apollo missions decreases in total body potassium were noted. In the last two Apollo flights the diets were supplemented with potassium; nevertheless, the losses in total-body potassium continued.[230] In the Skylab flights, potassium losses were noted also. There was an average decrease in total-body exchangeable potassium of approximately 6.3 per cent. Potassium losses would be expected in light of the negative nitrogen balances. Modest negative shifts in sodium during flight were followed by marked sodium retention during the first few postflight days.

It might be assumed that activity in a weightless environment would require less energy expenditure than at 1 g because work associated with counteracting gravitational force would be eliminated. On the other hand, while locomotion in situations of reduced gravity demands less energy than at 1 g, tasks that ordinarily depend on friction for their reactive force require muscular work to supply that force. Very little basal energy expenditure on earth is referable to direct gravity effects. Circulatory work against hydrostatic pressure and the maintenance of upright posture impose minimal demands.[230]

Direct measurements of precise energy requirements in space missions have not been practical; however, food consumption, balance studies and anthropometric measurements as noted above have provided some relevant information. Pulse rate data and some information on oxygen consumption and carbon dioxide production have been obtained and several estimates of heat production have been made. There were no significant differences in energy requirements of astronauts undertaking controlled activities on the lunar surface from those doing similar ground-based tasks.[231] It has been concluded, however, that the precision associated with many of these measurements is poor, with a variation greater than the differences expected to exist between the cost of metabolic activity in space and on the ground.[226] In a specific work activity, i.e. pedalling a bicycle ergometer, in the Skylab there was no significant difference in metabolic efficiency from performing the same task on the ground.[231]

Current data suggest that energy requirements in space travel as performed to date are certainly not less and may be greater than on the ground.[224,231] There were data from Skylab suggesting that the energy needs may have decreased as flight time increased. It is clear from changes in weight and body composition that within a period of 84 days in space the crew members of Skylab had not reached equilibrium with their weightless environment.[230,231]

Because of potential bone demineralization associated with weightlessness, much attention has been devoted to this problem in all of the flight missions. A detailed review and evaluation of the literature on the effects of immobilization and efforts to reduce the consequent bone demineralization were made early in the space program.[232] The authors questioned the prevailing view on the primacy of physical stress on the skeleton through weight bearing as the controlling influence on skeletal mineralization. Newer evidence at that time suggested that physical and circulatory factors related to continuing muscle activity could be playing the dominant role in maintenance of skeletal mineralization.

In the Gemini VII flight, fecal calcium was increased in one man and urinary calcium increased during the latter part of the mission in the other.[224] In the Apollo 17 12.6-day lunar mission an attempt was made to perform a mineral balance study.[233] Constraints in time and equipment and loss of body weight of the crew made the study less than ideal. However, there were marked increases in urinary and small increases in fecal phosphorus losses for the 3-man crew over the premission control period and all were in negative phosphorus balance on intakes of 1,390 to 1,675 mg per day. In contrast, urine calcium did not increase but fecal calcium did; dermal losses were not measured. On the basis of published data of urine and stool calcium losses, there was a positive calcium balance on intakes of 640 to 730 mg per day. There was an average daily negative shift for calcium of 137 mg per day and for phosphorus of 250 mg per day. The ratio of phosphorus lost compared to calcium changes indicated a reduction in both bone and soft tissue, as would be expected in view of body weight deficits and negative nitrogen balances. Significant elevations in serum calcium have not been found.

The dietary and metabolic procedures used in studies on crew members in the Skylab flights were conducted with a reasonable degree of success despite the technical problems of assuring dietary control and collection of specimens.[234] In the first Skylab flight, the various influences of space flight induced significant losses of body calcium, phosphorus, nitrogen, potassium and magnesium as previously noted. There were appreciable increases in urinary calcium; the peak reached during the latter part of this 28-day flight was 80 per cent greater than the 28-day preflight control period in one crew member and more than double the control values for the two other men.

In the second Skylab flight urinary calcium increased significantly with considerable individual variation.[234] It remained elevated during flight and did not decline until the recovery phase began. Calcium balance became negative in all three crewmen as the result of increases in both urinary and fecal excretion. The mean shift in calcium balance from mean preflight values to the last 30 days in flight was −248 mg per day. These losses were similar to those which have been noted in immobilized subjects at bed rest. Preliminary data in the 84-day third Skylab flight indicate continuing calcium losses with no tendency for urinary calcium to decrease with continued flight. Urinary hydroxyproline, indicative of skeletal turnover, also increased with considerable individual differences. The mean increase in the first two flights was 33 per cent. Increases in urinary phosphorus were modest; the mean shift in phosphorus balance from the preflight mean for Skylab 2 was -222 mg per day.

In the second flight there was an appreciable decrease in food intake during the first 6-day period as a result of anorexia; however, as food intake improved and stabilized, nitrogen balances reached equilibrium or became slightly positive.[234] The mean shift in nitrogen balance from the preflight control periods to flight was −4.0 gm per day. Ready restoration of in-flight losses occurred postflight. The nitrogen intake in the three flights averaged 18.3 ± 3.8 gm per day, which was not significantly different from preflight intake;[221] nevertheless nitrogen retention was less in flight and increased with prolongation of flights. On the 84-day mission the three crew members had nitrogen losses of 193, 277 and 395 gm, respectively.[230]

Muscle and nitrogen losses occurred despite an exercise regimen on all flights which was extremely rigorous on the second and third flights. It appeared that some fat was deposited in adipose tissue as muscle atrophied.[231]

Absorptiometric measurements of bone mineral revealed changes in one crewman on the 59-day mission and in two on the 84-day mission equivalent to bone mineral mass losses of 4.5 to 7.4 per cent.[235]

Young rats orbited for 19.5 days aboard the Soviet Cosmos 782 biologic satellite formed significantly less periosteal bone than did control rats on the ground; there was evidence that a complete cessation of bone growth occurred. The defect in bone growth was corrected during a 26-day postflight period.[236] No significant changes in bone resorption were observed. The mechanisms of the observed changes are unknown, but increased glucocorticoid secretion has been suggested as a possible factor.

American and Russian astronauts have returned from space flight with a decrease in red cell mass from the preflight values.[237] This decrease has been variously ascribed to weightlessness, relative immobility, lack of atmospheric nitrogen and/or a high oxygen partial pressure. However, a decrease in red cell mass without signs of erythrocyte destruction and apparently resulting from erythroid suppression was also observed in Skylab crews, although they exercised and lived in an environment with partial oxygen pressure comparable to that at sea level and with significant amounts of nitrogen.[238] More recent considerations suggest that the decrease in plasma volume which occurs after insertion into orbit results in erythrocytosis and that this contributes to the decrease in red cell mass.[238,239]

Mice deprived of water for 24 hours developed an increase in hematocrit and loss of body weight comparable to that seen in men in space flight. The increase in hematocrit was secondary to a decrease in plasma volume and was associated with suppression of erythropoiesis; however, there was no significant change in the titer of a humoral regulator.[239] Hence, the reasons for depressed erythropoiesis remain unknown at this time.

Despite the various changes which have been noted, it is clear that with the relatively prolonged Skylab mission there was no marked deterioration. With improved food technology, emphasis on ensuring adequate nutrient intakes and increased exercise there was reasonably good adaptation to weightlessness and adequate readaptation to 1 g environment. However, further efforts are necessary to ensure homeostasis of all systems for much more prolonged flights, particularly with regard to calcium and nitrogen retention.

Intestinal "Gas." Intestinal bacteria form the inflammable gases hydrogen and methane as well as a number of malodorous and toxic compounds which cannot be allowed to accumulate in a closed space. Their removal is necessary as flights become longer and crews become more numerous. Intestinal gas formation is affected by the type and abundance of microflora, the substrates and psychic and somatic conditions affecting the gastrointestinal tracts. Studies of the volumes of hydrogen and methane passed rectally and by pulmonary ventilation indicate that there are very large differences among individuals on the same diet. There is

much less production with a bland formula of purified nutrients than with a diet of dehydrated or compressed foods. Appreciably larger volumes of these gases are *exhaled* through the breath than are passed in flatus.[240]

The forthcoming manned orbital space stations with space shuttle will provide opportunity for longer-term nutritional, metabolic and acceptability studies. Expendable food supplies will be available by periodic resupply vehicles and more sophisticated systems of rations and preparation will be tested.

The need for the most efficient planning of diets will become increasingly important with prolonged flights without periodic resupply. For example, an overestimate of 300 kcal per man day will waste 71 pounds of oxygen per man year while underestimates may shorten flight time.[222]

Regenerative Cycling Systems. A sealed ecology will be necessary for flights lasting years. Physicochemical regeneration systems appear suitable for the production of carbohydrates from carbon dioxide and waste materials.[241-242] Bioregenerative systems, utilizing algae, higher plants, bacteria, fungi and animals, will obtain their nutrients from human excreta and supplements as indicated. Prototypes of future dwellings in space are being tested. Two men have remained for 1½ months in an airtight chamber in the presence of green plants, including the unicellular alga chorella, which purified the atmosphere and provided a partial source of food.[243] An atmospheric balance was achieved between the oxygen needs of the men and the carbon dioxide level by a careful selection of plants in the chamber. Undoubtedly, in more sophisticated systems, bacterial fermentors will be utilized to convert human waste matter into mineral salts needed by the green plants which, in turn, will produce food and oxygen and take up CO_2.

Planning proceeds for solutions of multiple problems in space medicine and exobiology and for space colonization.[244,245] It is intriguing to speculate on what man's ingenuity will produce in meeting these nutritional and metabolic problems of life maintenance imposed by independent space travel.

NUTRITION AND SPORTS

Interest in the potentially beneficial role of diet and nutrition in the performance of athletic endeavors is being demonstrated by all variants of sports enthusiasts. These include the "joggers" of all ages and the amateur and professional athletes in competitive sports. The wish to perform at maximum efficiency, combined with the great desire for winning manifested by many in competitive sports, has led to a fairly widespread belief that one or more aspects of diet and nutrition may give the extra "edge" between winning and losing. Not infrequently programs related to diet have been developed by coaches and athletes which are based on little experimental evidence but nevertheless are dogmatically accepted as the proper procedure. Use of large amounts of high-protein foods, protein pills, anabolic steroids and vitamin dosages of varying potency have been and continue to be used, and now trace element supplements are emerging into the field of interest.

In recent years the experimental techniques used by work physiologists to study energy expenditure and the substrates used in physical activity of varying intensity, fluid and electrolyte requirements and the effect of food composition on work performance have been utilized increasingly in objectively developed studies of various sports activities, particularly those requiring either prolonged or intense exertion. Many of the basic observations in this field have been mentioned above in the section on the effects of specific nutrients on work performance and exercise; they should be reviewed by those interested in the relation of diet and nutrition to athletic performance, since they have direct relevance to this field.

For the individual who exercises for limited periods and does not expend energy anywhere near his maximal oxygen consumption in such exercise, the usual dietary procedures will permit adequate performance within the capability of that individual at a given stage of training. Various investigators have demonstrated that the total energy expenditure in running on a level surface is constant and independent of velocity for the given individual, i.e. pace has very little effect on the caloric cost of running. Hence, individuals in low-fitness categories expend almost as much energy as well-conditioned persons of similar weight running the same distance. Of more importance is the energy cost based on the weight of the runner. For example, a 54-kg (119-lb) man who runs 2.4 km (1.5 miles) in 10 minutes will expend approximately 120 kcal, while another man weighing 100 kg (222 lb) running the same distance at the same pace will utilize 219 kcal.[246] Running up a hill with an incline of 6 per cent (i.e. 6 feet of vertical lift for every 100 feet of horizontal distance) requires 35 per cent more energy than running on level ground.[247] Running down a similar grade, however, will reduce the effort only by 24 per cent. For the ordinary jogger the caloric expenditure is not great in running several miles and can be made up or exceeded with even one energy-rich snack.

Running a given distance requires more energy than walking that distance. Margaria et al.[248] found that the energy cost of running 1 km at any speed is approximately twice that of walking 1 km at the most economical speed,[249] whereas the cost of running per unit distance is independent of speed (assuming that one is running on level ground). Data have been published on the caloric cost of running.[4,15,16,246,247,250–253] Data are also available on the cost of walking,[4,15,16,248,250–253] swimming and other sports activities.[4,15,16]

As indicated in the section on diet and

exercise, the composition of the diet appears to have little influence on the performance in intense short-lived "sprint" running or swimming. In such situations the degree of training, the aerobic capacity and the efficiency in performance of work are critical. In prolonged exercise ready access to fuel substrates may become the dominant factor in performance. This area has been reviewed earlier in this chapter. It has been pointed out that muscle protein and dietary protein are not utilized significantly in performance of muscular work. At low intensities of work energy is mainly derived from lipids. However, with increasing work load and duration, the fraction of carbohydrate used as the primary energy source increases; as work intensity approaches 85 to 90 per cent of the maximum inspiratory oxygen volume capacity practically all of the energy is derived from carbohydrate. Training is of course important, since well-trained athletes perform at a given intensity of work with a lower respiratory quotient and lower lactate production than do untrained individuals doing the same work.

The primary source of carbohydrates for energy expenditure in hard work for prolonged periods is muscle glycogen but carbohydrate ingested during the exercise can be utilized. It has also been demonstrated that the previous diet and exercise schedule will influence to a marked degree the amount of muscle glycogen available for prolonged hard work. A number of investigators have indicated that, when a diet is taken by an individual who has not exercised, the type of diet has only a minor effect on the muscle glycogen concentration. However, when glycogen in the muscle has been depleted by exercise, the effect of diet composition may be quite marked. When the diet is high in fat and protein or there is little diet intake, there is only a slow rate of synthesis of glycogen and normal values may not be achieved for several days. On the other hand, ingestion of a carbohydrate-rich diet following glycogen depletion by exercise results in a rapid synthesis of glycogen to values which exceed the normal range. It has therefore been recommended by various investigators previously cited that before a period of hard exercise the glycogen stores in muscle and liver be filled by the methods outlined above.

While ingestion of carbohydrate in the form of glucose or sucrose will contribute to carbohydrates for energy expenditure during prolonged hard exercise, it is also clear that the ability to take in significant amounts of food or carbohydrate containing fluids during such exercise is relatively limited. It has been shown, for example, that in the first 10 km of a marathon race the runner may already have incurred a 1- to 1.5-kg fluid deficit since international marathon rules prohibit fluid intake before the first 10 km.[247] Observations made during marathon competition demonstrated that despite water deficits of 4 to 6 kg few runners were able to drink more than 300 ml of water and were physically incapable of consuming sufficient amounts of fluid to keep pace with sweat losses.[247] Marathon runners on a 2-hour treadmill study ingested 100 ml of fluid every 5 minutes for the first 100 minutes of exercise. Despite the 2 liters of fluid ingested, the men still had a 2-kg weight deficit.[247] Furthermore, at the end of 100 minutes of this program it became apparent that further attempts to ingest fluid would have been intolerable. Immediately following a run approximately 340 ml of the ingested volume were still in the stomach. As had been demonstrated earlier, even partial fluid replacement will contribute calories and will reduce the risk of overheating. Efforts to replace at least some of the fluid losses are important since dehydration undoubtedly decreases the capability for sustained hard work.

In the marathon runner during the early stages of competition, muscle glycogen furnishes up to 90 to 95 per cent of energy while fat provides only 10 per cent or less. However, as the run continues, an increasingly larger fraction of the energy is obtained from fats and proportionately less from carbohydrates, so that near the end of the 42 km (26+ miles) as much as 95 per cent of the runner's energy is derived from free fatty acids. Even with this dependency on free fatty acids, some muscle glycogen seems to be essential for sustained muscle effort. If a runner starts with low muscle or liver glycogen, or both, or if there is some interference with his capability of forming and utilizing free fatty acids, then he will be exhausted prematurely. Similarly, since the rate of glycogen utilization is greatest during the early stages of the prolonged exercise, the individual who selects too fast a pace during this period may drastically reduce his glycogen storage and limit his performance. In marathon runners and others with prolonged exertion (e.g. cross-country skiing), in good physical condition and well trained, the rate of oxygen utilization is not limited by oxygen transport since blood lactate measurements made at the finish of the race have demonstrated little if any lactic acid accumulation.

Bergström and Hultman[254] have pointed out that on the average 2.7 gm of cellular water are released when 1 gm of glycogen is broken down, and the aerobic metabolism of each gram of glycogen results in the formation of 0.6 gm of water. Thus, the breakdown of 1 gm of glycogen releases more than 3 gm of water. If an athlete metabolizes 500 gm of glycogen in the course of a prolonged competition, this will correspond to 1.5 liters of water which will be lost from cells and which will partly compensate for the evaporative water losses.

Since the sweat is hypotonic, that is, there is more water lost than sodium in relation to the concentration of plasma, there is a tendency toward hyperosmolality of the body fluids with sweating. Previous discussion has reviewed the changes in plasma potassium which occur with vigorous exercise. When 1 gm of glycogen is released 0.45 mEq of potassium are also released.[254]

As the result of the local increase in glycogen in muscle which is stored together with water, there may be a feeling of heaviness and stiffness in muscles. The effect may be restrictive to movement in athletes such as sprinters who need only limited amounts of glycogen during intense, short-lived maximum exertion.[254]

With respect to fluid or water ingestion, Bergström and Hultman suggest that the subject be well hydrated before the competition but not drink much fluid immediately before.[254] If possible, an isotonic solution of glucose or glucose with sodium chloride at approximately 15 to 30 mEq per liter should be ingested in small portions at intervals of 10 to 15 or 30 minutes so that the amount of fluid will not exceed 1 liter per hour. Since there is a tendency toward overheating with prolonged vigorous exercise there is advantage in having the fluid chilled to 8 to 12°C, since this can contribute to keeping the core temperature low. As has been mentioned earlier, cold fluids can be better absorbed than warm fluids. There is generally no need for replacement of intracellular electrolytes such as potassium or magnesium during a competition. Where the competition is carried out at an elevated temperature, heat acclimatization as well as physical training is beneficial.

There is no evidence that consumption of increased amounts of protein, vitamins or other minerals beyond those needed in ordinary nutrition are beneficial.

References additional to those given earlier in this chapter which review various aspects of exercise in addition to nutritional facets are given in recent publications.[255]

ENERGY EXPENDITURE IN THE ORTHOPEDICALLY HANDICAPPED

Decreased mobility and deformity of various joints of the trunk and lower extremities will interfere with normal movements and result in extra energy cost of such movements. A knee immobilized in a cast at 180°, 165°, or 150° will increase energy expenditure by 5 to 10 per cent and a knee immobilized at 135° increases expenditure by 25 to 35 per cent.[256] An individual with a unilateral below-knee amputation has the same increase in energy cost of walking as does an individual with ankle immobilization, that is, about 10 per cent.[256] There is also an increased cost of walking with above-knee prostheses; this increases with the age of the amputee and the weight of the prosthesis and is affected by the efficiency of design and stability of the prosthesis. Findings by Ganguli et al.[257] show that below-knee amputees with a patellar tendon-bearing prosthesis had an increase of approximately 0.2 to 0.3 kcal per kg per hour over controls walking normally at rates of 3 to 5 km per hour.

The alternatives to prosthetic ambulation are crutch walking and wheelchair use. Crutch walking requires nearly as much energy as prosthetic use. Wheelchair ambulation by amputees requires no more energy than normal walking at the same speeds. Clarke found that male paraplegic college students engaged in a variety of activities had an average daily caloric expenditure which was relatively uniform at 2,200 to 2,300 kcal, somewhat less than that expended by their normally walking classmates; this indicates the need for ensuring regular physical activity and conservative caloric intake in paraplegics to avoid overweight.[258] The energy cost of paraplegic ambulation using crutches is 2 to 4 times greater than that of a normal person walking at the same speed, and increases rapidly with small increases in speed.[259,260] The higher the neurologic level, the greater is the energy cost of ambulation for paraplegics at a given rate of speed. Training minimizes energy expenditure. Corcoran points out that energy cost of hemiplegic ambulation in one series averaged 64 per cent greater than normal for a given speed; the use of a short leg brace reduced this to 51 per cent above normal.[256] Because of this energy cost, hemiplegics decrease the walking speed to a point at which the energy demands are tolerable, usually from 1 to 2 miles per hour. At this rate the hemiplegics expend almost the same amount of energy as normal subjects walking at 3 miles per hour.

BIBLIOGRAPHY

1. McCollum: *A History of Nutrition*. Boston, Houghton Mifflin, 1957, Chap. 10.
2. Lusk: *Nutrition*. New York, P.B. Hoeber, 1933.
2a. For a modern biochemical interpretation of this term, see Hegsted: In *Present Knowledge in Nutrition*. New York, Nutrition Foundation, 1976, Chap. 1, and Barnes: Ibid, Chap. 2.
2b. Kleiber: J. Nutr., *102*, 309, 1972.
3. Peters and Van Slyke: *Quantitative Clinical Chemistry. Interpretations*, Vol. 1, 2nd ed. Baltimore, Williams and Wilkins, 1946, pp. 3–36.
4. Consolazio, Johnson and Pecora: *Physiological Measurements of Metabolic Functions in Man*. New York, McGraw Hill, 1963.
5. Kamon: Trans. N.Y. Acad. Sci. Ser. 2., *36*, 625, 1974.
6. Montoye, van Huss, Reineke and Cockrell: Int. Z. Angew. Physiol. Arb. Physiol., *17*, 28, 1958.
7. Consolazio and Johnson: Fed. Proc., *39*, 1444, 1971.
8. Wolff: Q. J. Exp. Physiol., *43*, 270, 1958.
9. Lewis and Masterton: Lancet, *1*, 1009, 1963.
10. Fleisch: Arch. Ges. Physiol., *209*, 713, 1925.
11. Kinney, Morgan, Domingues and Gildner: Metabolism, *13*, 205, 1964.
12. Goldsmith, et al.: J. Physiol. Lond., *189*, 35P, 1967.
13. Bradfield, Huntzicker and Freuhan: Am. J. Clin. Nutr., *22*, 696, 1969.
14. Warnold, Lundhold and Schersten: Cancer Res., *38*, 1801, 1978.
15a. Durnin and Passmore: *Human Energy Expenditure*. London, Heinemann, 1966.
15b. Passmore and Durnin: *Energy, Work and Leisure*. London, Heinemann, 1967.
16. Kottke: In *Metabolism* (Altman and Dittmer, Eds.), Bethesda, Federation American Societies Experimental Biology, 1968, pp. 355–361.
17. Report of Committee on Calorie Requirements: Food and Agriculture Organization of the United Nations. Washington, FAO Nutritional Studies No. 5, 1950.
18. Report of Committee on Calorie Requirements: Rome, FAO Nutritional Studies No. 15, 1957.
19. Passmore, Nichol and Rao: Handbook of Human Nutritional Requirements. Rome, FAO Nutritional Studies No. 28, 1964. Geneva, WHO Monogr. Ser. No 61, 1964, pp. 66.

20. National Research Council, Food and Nutrition Board: Recommended Dietary Allowances, 8th ed. Washington, National Academy of Sciences, 1974.

21. Durin: In *Regulation de L'Equilibre Energetique Chez L'Homme* (in English) (Apfelbaum, Ed.). Paris, Masson, 1973, pp. 141–148.

22. Edholm: In *Regulation de L'Equilibre Energetique Chez L'Homme* (in English) (Apfelbaum, Ed.). Paris, Masson, 1973, pp. 57–58.

23. Thomson, Billewicz and Passmore: Lancet, *1*, 1027, 1961.

24. Christensen: In *Ergonomics Society Symposium on Fatigue* (Floyd and Welford, Eds.). London, Lewis, 1953, pp. 93–108.

25. Lehmann: *Prakistiche Abreitsphysiologie*. Stuttgart, Thieme, 1953.

26. Müller: Q. J. Exp. Physiol., *38*, 205, 1953.

27. Passmore and Durnin: Physiol. Rev., *35*, 801, 1955.

28. Humphreys, Lind and Sweetland: Br. J. Indust. Med., *19*, 264, 1962.

29. Burk, Bonjer and van der Sluys: In *Physical Activity in Health and Disease* (Evang and Andersen, Eds.). Baltimore, Williams and Wilkins, 1966, p. 207.

30. Keys, et al.: *The Biology of Human Starvation*. Minneapolis, University of Minnesota Press, 1950.

31. Waterlow: Lancet, *2*, 1091, 1968.

32. Cahill: N. Engl. J. Med., *282*, 668, 1970.

33. Gardner and Amacher (Eds.): *Endocrine Aspects of Malnutrition*. Santa Ynez, Kroc Federation, 1973.

34. Felig, Marliss and Cahill: In *Regulation de L'Equilibre Energetique Chez L'Homme* (in English) (Apfelbaum, Ed.). Paris, Masson, 1973, pp. 83–92.

35. Suskind (Ed.): *Malnutrition and the Immune Response*. New York, Raven Press, 1977.

36. Wilmore: In *Clinical Nutrition Update: Amino Acids* (Greene, Holliday and Munro, Eds.). Chicago, American Medical Association, 1977, pp. 47–57.

37. Henschel, Taylor and Keys: J. Appl. Physiol., *6*, 624, 1954.

38. Taylor, Buskirk, Brozek, Anderson and Grande: J. Appl. Physiol., *10*, 421, 1957.

38a. Consolazio, et al.: Am. J. Clin. Nutr., *21*, 793, 803, 1968.

38b. Johnson, et al.: Am. J. Clin. Nutr., *24*, 913, 1971.

38c. Daws, et al.: J. Appl. Physiol., *33*, 211, 1972.

39. Brozek: Am. J. Clin. Nutr., *5*, 332, 1957.

40. Kraut and Müller: Science, *104*, 495, 1946.

41. Keller and Kraut: Work and Nutrition. In *World Review Nutrition and Dietetics*. Vol. 3. (Bourne, Ed.). New York, Hafner, 1962, pp. 67–81.

42. Grande, Anderson, and Keys: J. Appl. Physiol., *12*, 230, 1958.

43. Eisenstein, et al.: J. Clin. Endocr. Metab., *47*, 889, 1978.

44. Swanson: Fed. Proc., *10*, 660, 1951.

45. Rosenthal and Allison: J. Nutr., *44*, 423, 1951.

46. Calloway and Spector: Am. J. Clin. Nutr., *2*, 405, 1954.

47. Calloway: J. Nutr., *105*, 914, 1975.

48. Rao, Naidu and Rao: Am. J. Clin. Nutr., *28*, 1116, 1975.

49. Torun, Scrimshaw and Young: Am. J. Clin. Nutr., *30*, 1983, 1977.

50. Garza, Scrimshaw and Young: J. Nutr., *108*, 90, 1978.

51. Grande, Anderson and Taylor: J. Appl. Physiol., *10*, 430, 1957.

52. Young, Schafer and Price: J. Appl. Physiol., *15*, 1022, 1960.

53. Haggard and Greenberg: *Deit and Physical Efficiency*. New Haven, Yale University Press, 1935.

54. Ivy: J.A.M.A., *118*, 569, 1942.

55. Clarke, DeJongh and Jokl: Manpower, *1*, 30, 1943.

56. Haggard and Greenberg: J. Am. Diet. Assoc., *15*, 435, 1939.

57. Holmes, Pigot, Sawyer and Comstock: J. Ind. Hyg. Toxicol., *14*, 207, 1932.

58. Haldi and Wynn: J. Appl. Physiol., *2*, 269, 1949.

59. Roethlisberger and Dickson: *Management and the Worker*. Cambridge, Harvard University Press, 1946.

60. Hutchinson: Nutr. Abstr. Rev., *22*, 283, 1952.

61. Tuttle, Wilson and Daum: J. Appl. Physiol., *1*, 545, 1949.

62. Tuttle, Daum, Meyers and Martin: J. Am. Diet. Assoc., *26*, 332, 1950.

63. Tuttle and Herbert: J. Am. Diet. Assoc., *37*, 137, 1960.

64. Orent-Keiles, and Hallman: Circ. No. 827. Washington, U.S. Department of Agriculture, 1949.

65. Simonson, Brozek and Keys: J. Appl. Physiol., *1*, 270, 1948.

66. Pyke: *Industrial Nutrition*. London, Macdonald & Evans, 1950.

67. Chittenden: *Physiological Economy in Nutrition*. New York, Stokes, 1904.

68. Cathcart and Burnett: Proc. R. Soc. Lond., *B99*, 405, 1926.

69. Garry: J. Physiol., *62*, 364, 1927.

70. Darling, et al.: J. Nutr., *28*, 273, 1944.

71. Consolazio, et al.: Am. J. Clin. Nutr., *28*, 29, 1975.

72. Torun, Scrimshaw and Young: Am. J. Clin. Nutr., *30*, 1983, 1977.

72a. Molé and Johnson: J. Appl. Physiol., *31*, 185, 1971.

73. Garry, Passmore, Warnock and Durnin: Medical Research Council, Spec. Rep. Ser. No. 289. London, Her Majesty's Stationery Office, 1955.

74. Nelson, Hayles and Wahner: Mayo Clin. Proc., *48*, 549, 1973.

74a. Barac-Nieto, et al.: J. Appl. Physiol., *44*, 209, 1978.

75. Hansen-Smith, Maksud and vanHorn: Growth, *41*, 115, 1977.

76. Calloway, O'Dell and Margen: J. Nutr., *101*, 775, 1971.

77. Thorn, Quinby and Clinton: Ann. Intern. Med., *18*, 913, 1943.

78. Haldi and Wynn: Am. J. Physiol., *145*, 402, 1945–46.

79. Lundbaeck: Acta Physiol. Scand., 7, 29, 1944.
80. Carlson and Froberg: Metabolism, 16, 624, 1967.
81. Marsh and Murlin: J. Nutr., 1, 105, 1928.
82. Christensen and Hansen: Scand. Arch. Physiol., 81, 160, 1939.
83. Krogh and Linhard: Biochem. J., 14, 290, 1920.
84. Gemmill: In Physiology in Modern Medicine (Bard, Ed.). St. Louis, C.V. Mosby, 1956, Chap. 47.
85. Consolazio and Johnson: Am. J. Clin. Nutr., 25, 85, 1972.
85a.Gollnick, et al.: J. Appl. Physiol., 33, 421, 1972.
86. Froberg: In Biochemistry of Exercise, Vol. 3 (Poortmans, Ed.). Basel, Karger, 1969, pp. 100–113.
87. Bergström, Hermansen, Hultman and Saltin: Acta Physiol. Scand., 71, 140, 1967.
88. Hermansen, Hultman and Saltin: Acta Physiol. Scand., 71, 129, 1967.
89. Ahlborg, Bergström, Ekelund and Hultman: Acta Physiol. Scand., 70, 129, 1967.
90. Hultman and Bergström: Acta Med. Scand., 182, 109, 1967.
91. Rodahl, Miller and Issekutz: J. Appl. Physiol., 19, 489, 1964.
92. Pernow and Saltin: J. Appl. Physiol., 31, 416, 1971.
92a.Costill, Bowers, Branam and Sparks: J. Appl. Physiol., 31, 834, 1971.
92b.Piehl: Acta Physiol. Scand., 90, 297, 1974.
92c.MacDougall, Ward, Sale and Saltin: J. Appl. Physiol., 36, 538, 1974.
93. Pruett: J. Appl. Physiol., 28, 199, 1970.
94. Hultman: Scand. J. Clin. Lab Invest., 19 (Suppl. 94), 31, 1967.
95. Hermansen, Pruett, Osnes and Giere: Acta Physiol. Scand., Suppl. 330, 79, 1969.
95a.Wahren, Felig, Hendler and Ahlborg: J. Appl. Physiol., 34, 838, 1973.
95b.Gallo, Holst and Christensen: J. Appl. Physiol., 38, 70, 1975.
95c.Ahlborg and Felig: J. Appl. Physiol., 41, 683, 1976.
95d.Körge and Viru: J. Appl. Physiol., 31, 1, 1971.
95e.vanBeaumont, et al.: J. Appl. Physiol., 34, 102, 1973.
96a.Davenport: Physiology of the Digestive Tract, 3rd ed. Chicago, Year Book Medical Publishers, 1971, pp. 165–168.
96b.Castill and Saltin: J. Appl. Physiol., 37, 679, 1974.
96c.Fordtran and Saltin: J. Appl. Physiol., 23, 331, 1967.
96d.Costill, Bennett, Branam and Eddy: J. Appl. Physiol., 34, 764, 1973.
97. Dagenais, Oriol and McGregor: J. Appl. Physiol., 21, 1157, 1966.
98. Konturek, Tasler and Obtulowicz: J. Appl. Physiol., 34, 324, 1973.
99. Simonson, Enzer, Baer and Brown: J. Ind. Hyg. Toxicol., 24, 83, 1942.
100. Keys and Henschel: J. Nutr., 23, 259, 1942.
101. Keys, Henschel, Mickelsen, and Brozek: J. Nutr., 26, 399, 1943.
102. Foltz, Ivy and Barborka: J. Lab. Clin. Med., 27, 1396, 1942.

103. Ryer: Am. J. Clin. Nutr., 2, 97 and 179, 1954.
104. Johnson, Darling, Sargent and Robinson: J. Nutr., 29, 155, 1945.
105. Jokl and Suzmann: Proc. Transvaal Mine Med. Off. Assoc., 19, 19, 1939.
106. Gey, Cooper and Bottenberg: J.A.M.A., 211, 105, 1970.
107. Borsook, et al.: Milbank Mem. Fund Q., 21, 115, 1943; 23, 113, 1945; 24, 99, 1946; 24, 251, 1946.
108. Johnson, et al.: J. Nutr., 24, 585, 1942.
109. Foltz, Barborka and Ivy: Gastroenterology, 2, 323, 1944.
110. Archdeacon and Murlin: J. Nutr., 28, 241, 1944.
111. Keys, Henschel, Taylor, Mickelsen and Brozek: J. Nutr., 27, 485, 1944.
112. Keys, Henschel, Taylor, Mickelsen and Brozek: Am. J. Physiol., 144, 5, 1945.
113. Brozek, Geutzkow, Mickelsen and Keys: J. Appl. Physiol., 30, 359, 1946.
114. Brozek, J.: In Symposium on Nutrition and Behavior. Am. J. Clin. Nutr., 5, 109, 1957.
115. Keys, et al.: J. Nutr., 27, 165, 1944.
116. Horwitt, et al.: J. Nutr., 39, 357, 1949.
117. Crandon, Lund and Dill: N. Engl. J. Med., 223, 353, 1940.
118. Farmer: Fed. Proc., 3, 179, 1945.
119. Vitamin A Subcommittee, British Accessory Food Factors Commission: Nature, 156, 11, 1945.
120. Wald, Brouha and Johnson: Am. J. Physiol., 137, 551, 1942.
121. Webster: In Environmental Physiology (Robertshaw, Ed.). Baltimore, University Park Press, 1974, Chaps. 2 and 3.
122. Johnson and Kark: Science, 106, 378, 1947.
123. Gray, Consolazio and Kark: J. Appl. Physiol., 4, 270, 1951.
124. Belding, et al.: Quoted in Consolazio and Schnakenberg.[125]
124a.Teitelbaum and Goldman: J. Appl. Physiol., 32, 743, 1972.
125. Consolazio and Schnakenberg: Fed. Proc., 36, 1673, 1977.
126. Edholm and Goldsmith: Proc. Nutr. Soc., 25, 113, 1966.
127. Hicks: Med. J. Austr., 1, 86, 1966.
128. Boyd: Br. J. Nutr., 34, 191, 1975.
129. Rodahl: J. Nutr., 53, 575, 1954.
130. Le Blanc: J. Appl. Physiol., 10, 281, 1957.
131. Welch, Buskirk and Iampietro: Metabolism, 7, 141, 1958.
132. Consolazio: In World Review of Nutrition and Dietetics, Vol. 4 (Bourne, Ed.). New York, Hafner, 1963, pp. 55–77.
133. Keeton, et al.: Am. J. Physiol., 146, 66, 1946.
134. Mitchell, et al.: Am. J. Physiol., 146, 84, 1946.
135. Rochelle and Horvath: J. Appl. Physiol., 27, 710, 1969.
136. Johnson: Fed. Proc., 22, 1439, 1963.
137. Johnson, Passmore and Sargent: Arch. Intern. Med., 107, 43, 1961.
138. Rogers, Setliffe and Buck: Aerosp. Med., 39, 585, 1968.

139. Dugal, Leblond and Therien: Can. J. Res., *23*, 244, 1945.
140. LeBlanc: Can. J. Biochem. Physiol., *35*, 25, 1957.
141. Seller, You and Moffat: Am. J. Physiol., *177*, 367, 1954.
142. Beaton, J.R.: Can. J. Biochem. Physiol., *41*, 139, 1963.
143. Beaton, Feleki and Stevenson: Can. J. Physiol. Pharmacol., *42*, 533, 1964.
144. Heroux: Fed. Proc., *28*, 955, 1969.
145. Blair, Urbush and Reed: Quoted by Mitchell and Edman.[146]
146. Mitchell and Edman: *Nutrition and Climatic Stress.* Springfield, Charles C Thomas, 1951.
147. Glickman, Keeton, Mitchell and Fahnestock: Am. J. Physiol., *146*, 538, 1946.
148. Dugal and Therien: Can. J. Res., *25*, 111, 1947.
149. Dugal: In *Cold Injury, 2nd Conference.* New York, Macy, 1952, p. 85.
150. Ershoff: Arch. Biochem., *28,* 299, 1950.
151. Ershoff: Proc. Soc. Exp. Biol. Med., *79*, 559, 1952.
152. Ershoff: Proc. Soc. Exp. Biol. Med., *78*, 385, 1951.
153. Ershoff: Proc. Soc. Exp. Biol. Med., *79*, 580, 1952.
154. Ershoff: J. Nutr., *49*, 373, 1953.
155. International Symposium on Cold Acclimation: Fed. Proc., *5*, Suppl. Dec., 1960.
156. Moroso: Physiol. Rev., *46*, 67, 1966.
157. International Symposium on Altitude and Cold: Fed. Proc., *28*, Suppl. May-June, 1969.
158. Bergström and Hultman: J.A.M.A., *221*, 999, 1972.
159. Eichna, Ashe, Bean and Shelley: J. Ind. Hyg. Toxicol., *27*, 59, 1945.
160. Bean and Eichna: Fed. Proc., *2*, 144, 1943.
161. Brown: In *Physiology of Man in the Desert* (Adolph, et al., Eds.). New York, Interscience Press, 1947, Chap. 13.
162. Dill: *Life, Heat and Altitude.* Cambridge, Harvard University Press, 1939.
163. Pitts, Johnson and Consolazio: Am. J. Physiol., *142*, 253, 1944.
164. Adolph and Dill: Am. J. Physiol., *123*, 369, 1938.
165. Wheeler, El-Neil, Willson and Weiner: Br. J. Nutr., *30*, 127, 1973.
166. Rothstein, Adolph and Wills: In *Physiology of Man in the Desert* (Adolph, et al., Eds.). New York, Interscience Press, 1947, Chap. 16.
167. Gamble: Harvey Lect., *42*, 247, 1946–47.
168. Moss: Proc. R. Soc. Lond. B., *95*, 181, 1923–24.
169. Cade, et al.: J. Sports Med. Phys. Fitness, *12*, 150, 1972.
170. Costill, et al.: Aviat. Space Environ. Med., *46*, 795, 1975.
171. Dill, Hall and Van Beaumont: J. Appl. Physiol., *21*, 99, 1966.
172. Smiles and Robinson: Am. J. Physiol., *31*, 63, 1971.
173. Hales: In *Environmental Physiology* (Robertshaw, Ed.). Baltimore, University Park Press, 1974, Chap. 4.
174. Taylor: In *Environmental Physiology* (Robertshaw, Ed.). Baltimore, University Park Press, 1974, Chap. 5.
175. Knochel: Arch. Intern. Med., *133*, 841, 1974.
176. Consolazio and Schnakenberg: Fred. Proc., *36*, 1673, 1977.
177. Strydom, et al.: Fed. Proc., *25*, 1366, 1966.
178. Wyndham, Rogers, Senay and Mitchell: J. Appl. Physiol., *40*, 779, 1976.
179. Mitchell, et al.: J. Appl. Physiol., *40,* 768, 1976.
180. Senay and Kok: J. Appl. Physiol., *43*, 591, 1977.
181. Pitts, Consolazio, and Johnson: J. Nutr., *27*, 497, 1944.
182. Lusk: *The Science of Nutrition,* 4th ed. Philadelphia, W.B. Saunders, 1931.
183. Consolazio, et al.: J. Nutr., *79*, 407, 1963.
184. Huang, Lo and Ho: Am. J. Clin. Nutr., *28*, 494, 1975.
185. Weiner, Willson, El-Neil and Wheeler: Br. J. Nutr., *27*, 543, 1972.
186. Mitchell and Edman: Am. J. Clin. Nutr., *10*, 163, 1962.
187. Consolazio, et al.: J. Nutr., *79*, 399, 1963.
188. Consolzaio, et al.: J. Nutr., *78*, 78, 1962.
189. Vellar: Scand. J. Clin. Lab. Invest., *21*, 157, 1968.
190. Vellar and Askevold: Scand. J. Clin. Lab. Invest., *22*, 65, 1968.
191. Heir, Cornbleet and Bergeim: J. Biol. Chem., *166*, 327, 1946.
192. Beller, et al.: Aviat. Space Environ. Med., *46*, 709, 1975.
193. Anonymous: Science, *95*, (Suppl.), 12, 1942.
194. Holmes: Science, *96*, 384, 1942.
195. Ershoff: Physiol. Rev., *28*, 107, 1948.
196. Osborne and Farmer: Proc. Soc. Exp. Biol. Med., *49*, 575, 1942.
197. Abt, Hardy, Farmer and Maaske: Am. J. Dis. Child., *64*, 426, 1942.
198. Henschel, et al.: Am. J. Trop. Med., *24*, 259, 1944.
199. Heath and Williams: *Man at High Altitude. The Pathophysiology of Acclimatization and Adaptation.* New York, Churchill Livingstone, 1977.
200. Consolazio, Johnson, Krzywicki and Daws: Am. J. Clin. Nutr., *25*, 23, 1972.
201. Johnson, Consolazio, Matoush and Krzywicki: Fed. Proc., *28*, 1195, 1969.
202. Surks, Chinn and Matoush: J. Appl. Physiol., *21*, 1741, 1966.
203. Johnson, Consolazio, Daws and Krzywicki: Nutr. Rep. Int., *4*, 77, 1971.
204. Consolazio, Nelson, Matoush and Hansen: J. Appl. Physiol., *21,* 1732, 1966.
205. Boycott and Haldane: Am. J. Physiol., *37*, 355, 1908.
206. Campbell: Q. J. Exp. Physiol., *29*, 259, 1939.
207. King, et al.: Science, *102*, 36, 1945.
208. Eckman, et al.: J. Aviat. Med., *16*, 311, 1945.
209. Green, Butts and Mulholland: J. Aviat. Med., *16*, 311, 1945.
210. Consolazio, et al.: Fed. Proc., *28*, 937, 1969.
211. Hansen, Hartley and Hogan: J. Appl. Physiol., *33*, 441, 1973.

212. Johnson, Consolazio, Burk and Daws: Aerosp. Med., *45*, 849, 1974.
213. Dramise, et al.: Aviat. Space Environ. Med., *46*, 365, 1975.
214. Blair, Dern and Smith: J. Aviat. Med., *18*, 352, 1947.
215. Tillisch: Quoted by McFarland: *Human Factors in Air Transportation*, New York, McGraw-Hill, 1953.
216. Friedemann and Ivy: Q. Bull. Northwestern Univ. Med. Sch., *21*, 31, 1947.
217. Harris, Ivy and Friedemann: Q . Bull Northwestern Univ. Med. Sch., *21*, 135, 1947.
218. Nanz, Michel and LaChance: Food Technol., *21*, 52, 1967.
219. Smith, Huber and Heidelbaugh: Aerosp. Med., *42*, 1185, 1971.
220. Huber, Heidelbaugh, Rapp and Smith: Aerosp. Med., *44*, 905, 1973.
221. Smith, Rambaut and Stadler: COSPAR Life Sci. Space Res., *15*, 193, 1977.
222. Calloway: J. Am. Dietet. Assoc. *44*, 347, 1964.
223. Berry and Curtis: In *Progress in Atomic Medicine*, Vol. 2 (Lawrence, Ed.). New York, Grune and Stratton, 1968, pp. 217–264.
224. Lutwak, et al.: J. Clin. Endocrinol. Metab., *29*, 1140, 1969.
225. White, Berry and Hessberg: COSPAR Life Sci. Space Res., *10*, 47, 1972.
226. Rambaut, Heidelbaugh, Reid and Smith: Aerosp. Med., *44*, 1264, 1973.
227. Johnson, Rambaut and Leach: Nutr. Metab., *16*, 119, 1974.
228. Johnson, Leach and Rambaut: Aerosp. Med., *44*, 1227, 1973.
229. Berry and Homick: Aerosp. Med., *44*, 163, 1973.
230. Rambaut, et al.: Fed. Proc., *36*, 1678, 1977.
231. Rambaut, Leach and Whedon: In COSPAR Life Sci. Space Res., *15*, 187, 1977.
232. Birge and Whedon: In *Hypodynamics and Hypogravics* (McCally, Ed.). New York, Academic Press, 1968, pp. 213–235.
233. Rambaut, Leach and Johnson: Nutr. Metab., *18*, 62, 1975.
234. Whedon, et al.: Aviat. Space Environ. Med., *47*, 391, 1976.
235. Vogel and Whittle: In *Proceedings Skylab Life Sciences Symposium* (Johnston and Dietlein, Eds.). NASA, Houston, 1974, p. 387.

236. Morey and Baylink: Science, *201*, 1138, 1978.
237. Kimzey: J. Am. Med. Wom. Assoc., *30*, 218, 1975.
238. Johnson, Driscoll and LeBlanc: In *Proceedings Skylab Life Sciences Symposium*, Vol. 2. NASA, Houston, 1974, pp. 495–505.
239. Dunn: Aviat. Space Environ. Med., *49*, 990, 1978.
240. Calloway and Murphy: COSPAR Life Sci. Space Res., *7*, 102, 1969.
241. Shapira, Mandel, Quattrone and Bell: COSPAR Life Sci. Space Res., *7*, 123, 1969.
242. Calloway: COSPAR Life Sci. Space Res., *8*, 295, 1970.
243. Mishina: Aviat. Space Environ. Med., *48*, 776, 1977.
244. Douglas: Aviat. Space Environ. Med., *49*, 902, 1978.
245. Winkler: Aviat. Space Environ. Med., *49*, 898, 1978.
246. Harger, Miller and Thomas: J.A.M.A., *228*, 482, 1974.
247. Costill: J.A.M.A., *221*, 1024, 1972.
248. Margaria, Cerretelli, Aghemo and Sassi: J. Appl. Physiol., *18*, 367, 1963.
249. Dill: J. Appl. Physiol., *20*, 19, 1965.
250. Fellingham, Roundy, Fisher and Bryce: Med. Sci. Sports, *10*, 132, 1978.
251. Walt and Wyndham: J. Appl. Physiol., *34*, 559, 1973.
252. Cavagna, Heglund and Taylor: Am. J. Physiol., *233*, R243, 1977.
253. Pandolf, Givoni and Goldman: J. Appl. Physiol., *43*, 577, 1977.
254. Bergström and Hultman: J.A.M.A., *221*, 999, 1972.
255. Astrand: In *World Review of Nutrition and Dietetics* (Bourne, Ed.). New York, Karger, 1973.
256. Corcoran: In *Physiologic Basis of Rehabilitation Medicine* (Downey and Darling, Eds.). Philadelphia, W.B. Saunders, 1971, p. 195.
257. Ganguli, Datta, Chatterjee and Roy: J. Appl. Physiol., *36*, 440, 1974.
258. Clarke: Arch. Phys. Med. Rehabil., *47*, 427, 1966.
259. Clinkingbeard, Gersten and Hoehn: Am. J. Phys. Med., *43*, 157, 1964.
260. Gordon and Vanderwalde: Am. J. Phys. Med., *37*, 276, 1956.

Part VI

Nutrition in the Prevention and Treatment of Disease

Chapter *30*

NUTRITION IN RELATION TO DENTAL MEDICINE

James H. Shaw
and
Edward A. Sweeney

Dental medicine is that specialty of medicine concerned with the welfare of the teeth and the soft tissues of the oral cavity and with the diagnosis of systemic diseases that have oral manifestations. During the past three or four decades, it has become increasingly evident that nutrition plays just as important a role in the development and maintenance of the oral tissues as in the development and maintenance of tissues elsewhere in the body. Indeed, the tissue components of the mouth are little different from comparable tissues elsewhere in the body as far as their metabolic processes during development, growth and maintenance are concerned.

By reason of the specific location and function of the oral cavity, its tissues are subjected to a wider variety and probably a more stringent series of stresses than are tissues in other moist internal cavities of the body. Consider for example: the wide variety in physical texture of the food that has to be chewed into a form suitable for swallowing, the wide range of temperatures of common food components as ingested, the wide variety of chemical stimuli to which the tissues of the oral cavity are exposed periodically and the ideal circumstances for the growth and multiplication of the wide spectrum of microorganisms that reside therein. The subdivision of food by the teeth and the buffering and diluting capacity of the saliva greatly re-

duce the intensity of some of these stresses before the food materials are passed on to the lower areas of the gastrointestinal tract. The soft tissues are unusually susceptible to current metabolic abnormalities of nutritional origin. During the early years in which characteristic signs of individual nutrient deficiencies were being recognized, the soft tissues of the oral cavity were particularly important for study by reason of their susceptibility to nutritional disturbances and their ready accessibility for examination. The classical signs of nutritional deficiencies in oral tissues will not be discussed in this chapter since they are presented in detail in the chapters of this book concerned with the B complex deficiencies and with scurvy.

In contrast, the hard tissues of the oral cavity, the enamel, dentin and cementum, are much less influenced by postdevelopmental systemic disorders than by the systemic disorders which operate during the developmental period. To a certain degree, the dental hard structures are kymographs in which are recorded both physical and chemical evidence of the metabolic circumstances which were prevalent at the time the specific areas of these structures were elaborated and calcified. In addition, however, the integrity of the teeth is influenced to a large extent by the oral environment which surrounds their external surfaces on a current basis. In any discussion of the relationship of a specific diet to the integrity of the hard structures, both the dietary influences upon oral environment and upon the nutritional status as mediated through one or more systemic pathways must be considered and integrated.

Over the past three or four decades, an appreciable change has occurred in the type of nutritional disease manifestations observed by clinicians. At the beginning of this period frank nutritional deficiencies, pellagra, beriberi and rickets, were commonly seen in dental practices in large urban areas and in rural communities alike. During this period, because of the widespread increase in the attention focused on nutritional problems, particularly in the oral cavity, a striking decrease in oral manifestations of nutritional deficiency diseases has been observed in the average practice. Our attention is being directed in an increasing degree to those nutritional abnormalities which occur during development or over prolonged periods of adult life, but which are not detected until long after the actual conditions of nutrient imbalance may have begun. Such studies need to be made in a variety of the chronic diseases that plague the human race.

Some diseases of the oral cavity are particularly good examples of diseases which have delayed components. The incidence of tooth decay, in particular, has been shown to be related to specific nutritional abnormalities that occur during tooth development. The diseases of the periodontal tissues may likewise have nutritional components which are presently unknown or ill defined, but the prevalence of these diseases should spur investigators to pursue more diligently the possible ways in which these influences are mediated.

Before a discussion of the oral diseases that result from nutritional abnormalities, let us consider some of the present knowledge about the structure of the teeth and surrounding tissues, the uniqueness of these calcified tissues and some of the established facts concerned with the etiology of oral disease.

THE STRUCTURE OF TEETH

The teeth are composed of three highly calcified tissues: enamel, dentin and cementum (Fig. 30–1). Enclosed within these calcified tissues is a highly vascular connective tissue, the dental pulp, which is frequently called the "nerve" of the tooth because of its great sensitivity to heat, cold and other stimuli. Around the periphery of the pulp, in contact with the inner surface of the dentin, is a layer of cells, the odontoblasts, responsible for the formation of the dentin and the laying down of secondary dentin at a relatively slow rate throughout the life of the tooth. When these cells are stimulated by the proximity of a carious lesion, secondary dentin is formed more rapidly as a barrier between the lesion and the pulp. The odontoblasts are mesodermal in origin, as are the cementoblasts which are responsible for the deposition of cementum around the outer surfaces of the roots of the tooth. In contrast, the enamel is of ectomesenchymal origin, being formed by ameloblasts that persist as a portion of the enamel organ until the teeth begin to erupt into the oral cavity.

The teeth are retained in their bony sockets or alveolae by means of the highly fibrous tissue structure termed the periodontal membrane. The diseases which affect the integrity of this structure or of the bone surrounding the socket result in one or another type of periodontal disease and may progress sufficiently to cause loosening and loss of the teeth.

Early anatomic studies of the enamel with the light microscope led investigators to postulate that the smallest structural units of enamel were inorganic prisms surrounded and cemented together by a sheath of interprismatic cementing substance. Only 2 or 3 per cent of organic matter is present in the enamel. Almost all the rest is inorganic. The tiny amount of

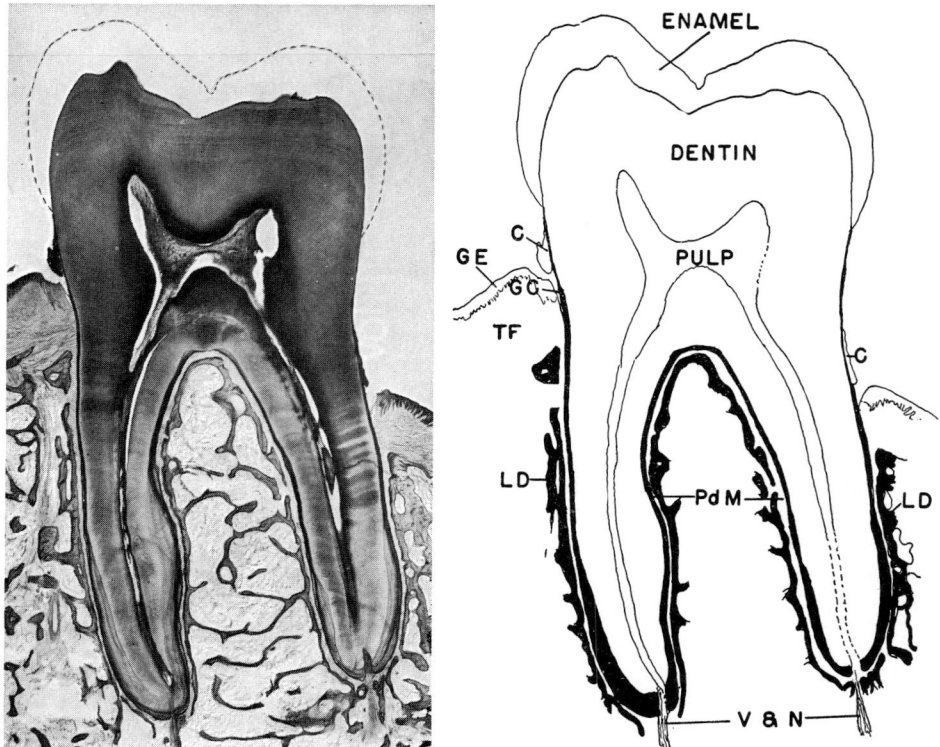

Fig. 30–1. Mesiodistal section of a lower molar tooth. (The enamel is disrupted by the evolution of gas bubbles during decalcification of the specimen.) Normally the gingival epithelium (GE) is in close apposition to the cervix of the tooth and acts as a barrier to decrease bacterial invasion of the underlying dermis. Transverse fibers (TF) form another barrier against bacterial penetration. In this case, a small amount of salivary calculus (C) was deposited and caused the formation of an abnormally deep gingival crevice (GC). This is the beginning of periodontoclasia which, at a later stage, causes destruction of the lamina dura (LD), a compact bony plate lining the alveolus as well as the periodontal membrane (Pd M) which attaches the entire tooth root to the surrounding bone. V and N = vessels and nerves supplying the dental pulp.

organic matter was originally believed to be contained in the interprismatic sheaths. However, recent observations made possible by the higher resolving power of the electron microscope indicated that this concept was unduly restricted. Instead, minute fibrils of organic matter have been observed to permeate each of the enamel prisms in extremely delicate and intimate fashion.[1] In addition, the interprismatic substance has been shown to have deposited within it an appreciable number of inorganic crystals.

The dentin is traversed by tubules which radiate from the pulp to the dentoenamel junction. Organic processes from the odontoblasts and nerve fibers actually penetrate the entire width of the dentin. It has been postulated that extracellular fluid may be transported from the pulp across the dentin by reason of these processes. The exact status of this hypothesis is indefinite at the present time. The organic content of dentin is much higher than that of enamel and approximates the concentration of the long bones.

The time intervals involved in the development of teeth are important considerations in any discussion of the relationship of nutrition to tooth development and to the later caries susceptibility of the teeth. The life history of a tooth may be divided into three main eras: (1) the period during which the crown of the tooth is forming and calcifying in the jaw, (2) the period of maturation when the tooth is erupting into the oral cavity and its root or roots are forming and (3) the maintenance period while it is in full function in the oral cavity. The length of time during which a human tooth is developing and maturing prior to its functional responsibilities is often forgotten. As an example let us consider the first permanent molar, the 6-year molar, which is one of our more important teeth by reason of its large masticating surface. Its histologic primordia begin to be elaborated about the 32nd week in utero. From then until 2½ to 3 years of age, the organic frameworks of the enamel and dentin in the crown are being deposited and calcified. By the end of the third year, the crown has attained its adult size but is not yet fully calcified. Eruption into the oral cavity begins between 6 and 7 years of age and its roots are completed around 9 to about 11 years of age. Thus 10 years elapse between the initiation of this tooth and the attainment of its final form. Comparable data for the primary and permanent teeth are presented in Table 30–1.

Dental Structure versus Other Body Tissues

In a discussion of nutritional influences upon teeth, we must recognize that at least three striking differences exist between the calcified tissues of the teeth and other tissues of the body. First, enamel contains no microscopically detectable capillary or lymphatic vessels to act as transport systems for nutrients. However, the intimate relationships between the organic and the inorganic components of enamel suggest that pathways for diffusion from saliva, and possibly blood, to the enamel may readily exist, even without any vascular or neural elements within enamel. The dentin likewise contains no formed vascular elements. However, its structure is such that it may lend itself more readily to a passage of extracellular fluids from the blood, by reason of dentinal tubules that traverse the dentin from the odontoblastic layer of the pulp to the dentoenamel junction.

Second, calcified dental tissues do not have a microscopically or chemically detectable ability to repair areas which are formed improperly or calcified inadequately during development, nor does the tooth have the ability to repair itself after a portion has been destroyed by tooth decay or by a mechanical injury. An exception to the latter statement may be the remineralization of those slightly decalcified superficial areas of the enamel where the organic matrix is intact, commonly referred to as "white spots." Lack of ability to repair dental tissues is in direct contrast to the long bones, where the haversian systems are continually being remodeled and replaced and where diseased or fractured areas heal. Yet, despite the above contrast, studies with radiotracer materials indicate that enamel and dentin are permeable to various inorganic ions. The inorganic elements of each area of mature teeth are capable of participating in an exchange process with comparable elements carried to the area by body fluids.[2] The observation in mature teeth that the interchange between normal and radioisotopic elements in the enamel takes place by reason of the contact of enamel with saliva is particularly interesting and thought provoking. In contrast, the interchange in the dentin occurs by reason of the ions brought to the dentin by the blood supply in the pulp or the periodontal membrane. Thus, saliva acts as the pathway by which systemic nutritional influences are communicated to the enamel.

In the third place, unlike other tissues,

Table 30–1. Chronology of Development of the Human Dentition*

	Primary Dentition								
	Calcification Begins		*Crown Completed*		*Eruption*		*Exfoliation*		
Tooth	*Maxilla*	*Mandible*	*Mandible (mo)*	*Maxilla (mo)*	*Maxilla (mo)*	*Mandible (mo)*	*Maxilla (yr)*	*Mandible (yr)*
Central incisors	14 wk in utero	14½ wk in utero	1½	2½	9⅓	7½	6–7	6–7
Lateral incisors	16 wk in utero	16½ wk in utero	2½	3	11	13¼	7–8	7–8
Cuspid	17 wk in utero	17 wk in utero	9	9	19½	19⅔	10–12	9–12
1st molar	5 wk in utero	15½ wk in utero	6	5½	15⅔	16	9–11	9–11
2nd molar	19 wk in utero	18 wk in utero	11	10	28	26½	10–12	10–12

	Permanent Dentition							
	Calcification Begins		*Crown Completed*		*Eruption*		*Root Completed*	
	Maxilla	*Mandible*	*Maxilla (yr)*	*Mandible (yr)*	*Maxilla (yr)*	*Mandible (yr)*	*Maxilla (yr)*	*Mandible (yr)*
Central incisors	3–4 mo	3–4 mo	4½	3½	7–7½	6–6½	10–11	8½–10
Lateral incisors	10–12 mo	3–4 mo	5½	4–4½	8–8½	7¼–7¾	10–12	9½–10½
Cuspid	4–5 mo	4–5 mo	5½–6½	5½–6	11–11⅔	9¾–10¼	12½–15	12–13½
1st premolar	1½–1¾ yr	1¾–2 yr	6½–7½	6½–7	10–10⅓	10–10¾	12½–14½	12½–14
2nd premolar	2–2¼ yr	2¼–2½ yr	7–8½	7–8	10¾–11¼	10¾–11½	14–15½	14½–15
1st molar[17]	32 wk in utero	32 wk in utero	4–4½	3½–4	6–6⅓	6–6¼	9½–11½	10–11½
2nd molar	2½–3 yr	2½–3 yr	7½–8	7–8	12¼–12¾	11¾–12	15–16½	15½–16½
3rd molar	7–9 yr	8–10 yr	12–16	12–16	20½	20–20½	18–25	18–25

* From Moyers, Hartsook, and Kapel: In *Growth and Development of Children,* 6th ed. (Lowrey, Ed.). Chicago, Year Book Medical Publishers, 1973.

the calcified tissues of teeth have a partial change of environment midway in their life history. During the developmental period, while the tooth is growing and calcifying, it has complete systemic contact through normal vascular and neural pathways. When the tooth begins to emerge into the oral cavity, the blood vascular supply to the enamel organ is severed, and the enamel surface comes in contact with that complex mixture of saliva, microorganisms, food debris, epithelial remnants, etc., which is typical of the oral cavity. Thus, instead of a systemic environment only, the erupted tooth has, in addition, an oral or external environment. The effects of this environment have to be studied and evaluated whenever a change in incidence of tooth decay results from a post-developmental dietary manipulation.

MODERN CONCEPTS OF DENTAL CARIES

During recent years a number of facts have been clearly established about the etiology of dental caries. Some of these pertain to concepts which have been postulated for generations from human studies but which have been demonstrated now beyond reasonable doubt by definitive experimental trials with laboratory animals.

Microorganisms are required to cause the destruction of tooth substance in the characteristic fashion termed "tooth decay." This point was established in studies with caries-susceptible rats that were maintained throughout life under germ-free circumstances.[3] In this experimental environment, these animals did not develop tooth decay when fed a caries-producing ration. The germ-free technique provides the opportunity to evaluate the microorganisms or groups of microorganisms which are responsible for the destruction of enamel and dentin in the characteristic manner defined as dental caries.

In one study Orland and co-workers[4] inoculated germ-free caries-susceptible rats with a mixed culture of enterococci and found that characteristic carious lesions developed in the sulci of the molars. Monoinoculation by several different microorganisms caused carious lesions in more recent studies. Keyes[5] has demonstrated that under certain experimental conditions dental caries in rats and hamsters can be considered to be an infectious and transmissible disease. Fitzgerald and Keyes[6] have induced experimental dental caries in a strain of caries-inactive hamsters maintained under conventional caging conditions by oral inoculation of single or pooled cultures of streptococci isolated from hamster carious lesions. Carious lesions have also been produced in rats that were maintained under germ-free conditions except for inoculation with a single strain of an oral streptococcus isolated from a rat[7] or with each of two strains of streptococci isolated from human carious lesions.[8] These cariogenic microorganisms stored intracellular iodophilic polysaccharide[9] and produced large quantities of extracellular nondialyzable capsules that may be important in enabling the microorganisms to adhere to tooth surfaces.[8] Some strains isolated from human carious lesions were immunologically similar to those isolated from oral cavities of rats and hamsters capable of causing carious lesions in these animals.[10]

Streptococcus mutans has received special attention in recent years, first by reason of the recognition that this microorganism was important in the causation of dental caries in hamsters. Later it was found to colonize tooth surfaces in infants soon after the tooth erupted[10a] and to be present in many carious lesions in children.[10b] S. mutans has the interesting ability to synthesize from dietary sucrose a polyglucose (dextran) which enables this organism to colonize surfaces of the teeth and form plaque thereon.[10c] Under this conglomerate the interaction between the metabolites of the microorganisms and tooth substance can occur to cause dental caries.

Clinical observations have indicated that the salivary glands are of considerable importance in the maintenance of teeth. Where salivary glands are congenitally missing or are destroyed by disease or radiation of the head and neck region, there is invariably an increased susceptibility to dental caries. Similarly, in experimental animals, the surgical removal of the major salivary glands results in spectacular increases in tooth decay.[11] Of the several salivary glands, the parotid and submaxillary have been shown to be most important in the rat, with the sublingual gland contributing relatively little to the maintenance of the teeth.[12] In human studies the quantity or consistency of the saliva has not yet been shown conclusively to have a definite relation to caries incidence except where xerostomia has been induced by surgical removal or radiologic destruction. The total amounts of certain salivary constituents secreted may be more important than the total volume in which they are secreted.[13]

The truism that "A clean tooth never decays," and the difficulty in obtaining such a condition have been demonstrated by experiments in rats where the diet was introduced directly into the stomach by a tube-feeding procedure.[14] The normal microbial oral flora were observed in those animals but no carious lesions developed. When the same caries-producing diet was eaten in the usual fashion by littermates, a high incidence of tooth decay was observed. Even when the supreme penalty of sialoadenectomy was imposed upon the tube-fed animals, no carious lesions developed. Of all the components of the diet, carbohydrate is essential in the oral cavity for the production of tooth decay. When a carbohydrate-free diet is fed for prolonged periods either to intact rats or to ones from which the principal salivary glands have been removed, no carious lesions develop.[15] If all the diet except the carbohydrate is introduced into the stomach by tube and only the carbohydrate

ingested orally, carious lesions developed at approximately the expected rate for rats that consume the entire diet by the normal route.[16] Likewise, when caries-susceptible rats consume a liquid diet, they have appreciably less tooth decay than when their littermate control rats consume the same ration in solid form.[17]

The frequency of eating and the length of time that a cariogenic diet is made available to rats each day are directly related to the amount of dental caries which develops during the experimental period.[17a] This laboratory observation has close parallels to epidemiologic studies in children, where correlations have been observed between frequency of eating cariogenic snacks and caries activity.

Extensive studies have been conducted in human populations in a mental institution in Sweden, where sucrose was fed in several forms at high levels to inmates for relatively prolonged periods of time.[18] When high amounts of sucrose were fed in solution at meals, the increase in dental caries incidence was barely perceptible. However, when sucrose was fed in the form of sticky candy such as caramels or toffees between meals, there were tremendous increases in the incidence of tooth decay. Comparable amounts of sugar in chocolates between meals or in bread at meals caused intermediate increases in dental caries incidence. As soon as the supplements were stopped, the frequency of appearance of new carious lesions decreased to the preexperimental level. These studies uniformly point toward the rate of oral clearance of carbohydrates and the frequency of their consumption as strong determining factors on the extent of tooth decay.

Mono- and disaccharides as the sole sources of carbohydrate in simple forms of purified diets usually cause a higher rate of dental caries in experimental animals than the same quantities of starches or dextrins.[19] However, where natural diets are used, other carbohydrates have been shown to be equally or more cariogenic than sucrose. In some experiments finely ground rice[20] and in other studies various forms of cooked cereals have been shown to be more cariogenic than sucrose.[21] Under some experimental conditions dietary sucrose permitted a more rapid progression of carious lesions than glucose and greater recoveries of cariogenic streptococci.[22] The latter microbiota produced large quantities of insoluble dextrans exclusively from sucrose, which enabled the microorganisms to adhere to and metabolize on tooth surfaces.[23,24] Under some conditions, the inclusion of a dextranase (glucosyl transferase) preparation in the drinking water and diet of hamsters caused a major reduction in plaque formation and caries activity.[25]

These studies led to the hypothesis that sucrose was uniquely cariogenic and that its replacement by other disaccharides or by monosaccharides in the human diet would be beneficial. Unfortunately some laboratory data do not support that position. For example, in the rat, other carbohydrates such as glucose and maltose were as cariogenic as sucrose and the mixed flora in these rats was able to form insoluble dextrans from glucose and maltose.[26] In addition, dextranase was not effective in white rats.[27] The likelihood is high in experimental animals that sucrose is of greater cariogenicity than other mono- and disaccharides only when S. mutans is the predominant cariogenic organism, as in the hamster and in rats inoculated heavily with the microorganism.

Whether sucrose in man is uniquely cariogenic in any sense other than that sucrose is the predominant simple sugar in human diets remains to be evaluated in clinical trials. Replacement of sucrose by glucose, fructose or maltose in the human diet does not seem likely to result in less caries. Various antibiotic materials such as penicillin, vancomycin, tetracyclines, dibasic ammonium compounds, chlorhexidine and urea have been shown to cause a reduced incidence in tooth decay among experimental animals and in some human subjects.[28-30]

Strong genetic traits toward caries resistance or caries susceptibility have been reported in animal strains in laboratories.[31,32] The mechanism by which these hereditary tendencies are mediated is unknown. However, it is important to notice that both oral environmental and nutritional variations may modify the degree of manifestation of the genetic tendency. For example, if a strain of rats is highly susceptible to tooth decay, the incidence of dental caries may be greatly reduced by any one of a number of the above variations induced in the oral environment. In addition, various nutritional influences imposed during tooth development may reduce the incidence of tooth decay below that which would be expected in this caries-susceptible strain if these nutritional influences had not been brought to bear during tooth development. Likewise a caries-resistant strain of rats will have an increased incidence of tooth decay if the salivary glands are removed or if a particularly cariogenic ration is fed.

An excellent description of the relationship between the genetic and environmental factors in experimental dental caries has been given by Larson.[33] The genetic determinism of the level of caries susceptibility in inbred strains of rats appeared to be strong.[34] Offspring of caries-susceptible parents were able to establish a caries-producing microflora with ease after various attempts to prevent the parents from passing on their flora to the next generation. Likewise, massive oral inoculations of flora from caries-active rats into offspring of caries-resistant parents had little influence on their rate of caries activity. Probably the most striking evidence of a genetic factor was provided by a double-mating of female rats from a white caries-susceptible strain with males of the same strain and males of a black, less caries-susceptible strain.[35] Despite the identical intrauterine environmental conditions, the heterozygotic offspring had a lesser dental caries incidence than the homozygotic littermates.

NUTRITIONAL INFLUENCES DURING TOOTH DEVELOPMENT

With this related background of information about the structure of teeth, the development of teeth and the etiology of dental caries, let us examine some of the specific known relationships between nutrition and dental caries as they are encountered in the three eras in the life history of an individual tooth. Unquestionably the most striking of these influences occur by reason of imposition of nutritional deficiencies during tooth development. Three classical examples exist in which specific nutritional deficiencies adversely influence the development of various areas of the teeth in ways that are histologically discernible: (1) avitaminosis-A, (2) scurvy and (3) rickets attributable to deficiencies of vitamin D, calcium or phosphorus or to a gross imbalance of the calcium/phosphorus ratio. In addition, inadequate levels of fluoride and disturbed calcium/phosphorus ratios during tooth development result in abnormalities of the chemical composition, at a submicroscopic level, which are related to caries susceptibility.

Vitamin A

Just as vitamin A deficiency influences the integrity of epithelial tissues throughout the entire body, this deficiency also influences the ameloblasts which are of epithelial origin. Early studies by Wolbach and Howe demonstrated that the deficiency of vitamin A in rodents resulted in degeneration and atrophy of the ameloblasts.[36,37] In the vitamin A-deficient animals, the first histologically visible change in the teeth was observed in the odontoblasts. Since the ameloblasts are responsible for the organization of the odontogenic epithelium, it is believed that the first evidence of abnormality in the ameloblasts during the early stages of the development of vitamin A deficiency is the loss of the physiologic ability to stimulate the development and arrangement of the odontoblasts from the connective tissue in the vicinity. Thus, the odontoblasts are not stimulated to differentiate and do not arrange themselves in normal fashion. Later, profound anatomic changes in the ameloblasts are observed. In late stages of this deficiency, the cells exhibit such a degree of squamous metaplasia that virtually no recognizable ameloblasts can be found. Consequently a great reduction occurs in the rate at which the organic matrix of enamel is formed. Various degrees of abnormality occur in the formation of the matrix. Enamel hypoplasia is a prominent manifestation of severe and prolonged vitamin A deficiency in experimental animals. Since the proliferative activity of the odontogenic epithelium does not cease in vitamin A deficiency, cords of these undifferentiated epithelial cells invade the pulpal tissue where they form isolated cell masses. Some of these cells retain the ability to stimulate the neighboring mesenchyma to abortive attempts at dentin formation; in this fashion numerous calcified concretions occur in the pulp of the teeth.

Repair patterns in the teeth of rodents recovering from vitamin A deficiency are both straightforward and rapid. The odontogenic epithelium regains its function and morphologic appearance; the formation of normal odontoblasts and the deposition and calcification of normal dentin follow. Where there has been an infolding of the odontogenic epithelium, recovery often results in tooth duplications and tumor-like formations.

Boyle has reported that similar changes occur in the developing dental tissues of a prematurely born vitamin A-deficient infant.[38] In additional cases of vitamin A deficiency in infants, Dinnerman has reported consistent abnormalities of structure and appearance in the enamel and the enamel-forming organs to those lesions observed in experimental animals.[39] In addition, the dentin was poorly calcified and contained scattered globules of unusual size; the predentin was extraordinarily wide. The other changes observed were entirely consistent with the descriptions in the literature for experimental animals.

No conclusive body of information indicates that enamel hypoplasia in human beings is directly attributable to vitamin A deficiency during tooth development. However, a linear enamel hypoplasia of deciduous incisor teeth has been reported in as many as 50 per cent of children from some developing countries which commonly have endemic vitamin A and protein-calorie deficiencies.[40,41] The etiology of this perinatally timed enamel hypoplasia may have its basis in the malnutrition-infection interrelationships. With a cariogenic diet these affected teeth demonstrate a high susceptibility to a type of decay which has been called odontoclasia.

Repeated demonstrations have been made of influences of vitamin A deficiency on epiphyseal bone formation. These changes were primary results of the general deficiency syndrome, since they occurred sufficiently early in the deficiency to precede the cessation of overall growth. The studies of Wolbach and Bessey have demonstrated that these are specific effects of vitamin A deficiency and that the nerve damage in these deficiency states is secondary to and caused by the bone changes.[42] Vitamin A is essential for the activity of the epiphyseal cartilage cells without which they are incapable of undergoing the normal sequence of growth, maturation and degeneration which is essential in the mechanism of endochondral or replacement bone growth. Since vitamin A deficiency suppresses the cartilage cell sequences, endochondral bone growth is retarded and finally ceases entirely if the deficiency persists. Remodeling sequences, involving concurrent resorption of bone

with bone deposition and replacement of cancellous bone by compact bone, cease to operate. A greatly reduced rate of resorption of trabecular bone with retardation and failure of haversian system formation results in an arrestment of compact bone formation. Eventually all skeletal growth dependent upon replacement of endochondral bone formation ceases. Appositional growth of bone of periosteal origin continues until inanition intervenes at a rate in conformity to the normal growth pattern at each particular site. Presumably the fact that growth of bone of periosteal origin continues is evidence that there is no fundamental error of calcification in the vitamin A-deficient rodent.

These effects upon bone growth in vitamin A deficiency are of potential interest for children's dentistry and orthodontics. No thorough investigation has been conducted to determine whether orthodontic problems may be related to nutritional deficiencies during development. Since vitamin A deficiency causes such a profound influence on bone development, some of the inadequate growth patterns which result in orthodontic problems may have had their origin in prolonged periods of subclinical deficiency—or deficiency of other nutritional elements such as protein-calorie malnutrition which cause reduced growth—during the developmental period of the child.

Vitamin C

Scurvy, the clinical entity which is attributable to vitamin C deficiency, has been described in detail in the chapter concerned with ascorbic acid. In frank vitamin C deficiency, the lesions of the gingiva are particularly striking[43] (Fig. 30–2).

It is noteworthy that these occur only when teeth are present and that the condition is remarkably consistent. The gingival lesions begin on the interdental papilla, first as hyperemia with dilated thin-walled vessels which have a tendency to hemorrhage. Disintegration of the epithelium

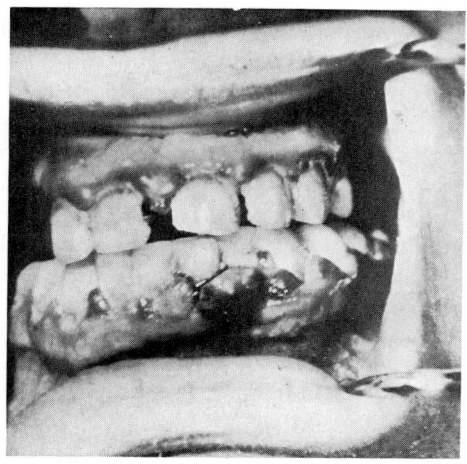

Fig. 30–2. Hemorrhagic gingivitis associated with avitaminosis C (scurvy). Note the swelling of the interdental papillae and the large hematoma between the lower left central and lateral incisors. (From Cahn: *Pathology of the Oral Cavity*. Baltimore, Williams & Wilkins, 1941.)

follows, and infection with ulceration, granulations and gangrene may result. The gums become inflamed and spongy and bleed easily. In cases of severe deficiency, these lesions become sufficiently extensive to obstruct mastication and are frequently accompanied by loosening of the teeth and tooth loss.

The deficiency of vitamin C primarily affects the ability of cells of connective tissue origin to elaborate their typical collagenous intercellular substances. The odontoblasts which form the dentin in developing teeth are of mesodermal origin and are readily affected by the deficiency of vitamin C. Wolbach and Howe have studied the pathogenesis of these changes extensively.[44] When guinea pigs are placed on a scorbutic diet, alterations soon appear in the odontoblasts which become atrophic and resemble the nearby pulp cells. There is a decrease in their orderly polar arrangement, a decrease in height and eventually a complete disorganization. The decreased height of the odontoblasts in mod-

erate deficiencies is believed to be sufficiently closely related to the vitamin C intake to permit this measurement to be used as a bioassay criterion.[45]

At the same time, the rate of dentin formation is sufficiently closely related to the amount of vitamin C consumed that it also can be used as a criterion for the bioassay of the vitamin C content of the diet.[46] The dentin which is formed is laid down irregularly with the dentinal tubules lacking their normal parallel arrangement. In severe deficiencies, dentin deposition stops entirely and the predentin becomes hypercalcified. At late stages in the deficiency the ameloblasts atrophy and hemorrhages occur. These changes have been interpreted to be caused by traumatic injury of the enamel organ as the result of inadequate support of the underlying dentin. Though the changes occur readily in the developing teeth of experimental animals, evidence has not been presented yet to indicate a similar occurrence in human teeth.

As would be expected, there is a rarefaction of the alveolar bone comparable to that seen in the ribs and bones of experimental animals and humans. The pathologic sequence in the destruction of the alveolar bone has been reported to closely resemble the changes observed in diffuse alveolar atrophy.[47] Weakness of the supporting bones, as well as the weakness of the collagen fibers in the supporting structures, allows for a greater mobility of the teeth and a decreased ability to withstand the mechanical stresses encountered in chewing.

The pathologic condition in the pulp and in the odontoblastic layer in human beings is nearly identical with the pathologic changes in the scorbutic guinea pig, according to Westin.[48] In the teeth of scorbutic adults the dentin is resorbed and porotic. The small amount of replacement dentin formed is of the osteodentin type. The pulp is atrophic and hyperemic. Degeneration of the odontoblasts, formation of cysts and foci of diverticuli-like regions of calcification were described.

Although the relationship of vitamin C deficiency to gingival changes and to bone pathology has been repeatedly demonstrated, there has never been a clear-cut demonstration of a relationship between scurvy and dental caries. A large experiment was conducted at an orphanage by Hanke in which the usual orphanage diet was daily supplemented with a pint of orange juice and the juice of 1 lemon for one year.[49] The experimental group of children evidently had a reduced incidence of new carious lesions in contrast to the control group of children which had had no citrus fruit supplementation.

In a recent study with institutionalized children, one orange was eaten at each of three meals per day for 44 weeks; no influence was observed on the scores for the gingival status, amounts of plaque and calculus, DMF surfaces or early demineralized areas.[49a] Furthermore, surveys by Westin,[50] Hess and Abramson,[51] and experiments by McBeath[52] and Grandison, Stott and Cruickshank[53] failed to demonstrate any difference in dental caries incidence between groups which received normal diets and those supplemented with considerable amounts of vitamin C.

Vitamin D, Calcium and Phosphorus

The first experimental production of rickets to demonstrate an influence upon tooth development was reported by Lady May Mellanby in 1918.[54] She observed that a deficiency of a fat-soluble vitamin, later designated as vitamin D, in young puppies had a profound effect on the developing enamel and dentin of the secondary teeth, on the rate of eruption and also on the position of the teeth in the jaw. When vitamin D deficiency was imposed upon a female dog during pregnancy, the primary teeth of the puppies had defects in structure and eruption was delayed.[55] However, the puppies from comparable dogs supplemented with adequate amounts of the fat-soluble vitamin had normal primary teeth.

The changes that occur in teeth during the rachitic process are appreciably less complex than those in bones. The first and most prominent change observed in rickets in rats is a calciotraumatic line, a line of disturbed calcification of the dentin.[56] This is accompanied by retardation in the formation of predentin and a pronounced disturbance in the calcification of the dentin. The latter is no longer homogeneously basophilic but is stippled by an irregular deposition of inorganic salts. Calcification of the cementum is likewise retarded.

Enamel hypoplasia does not occur except in the more severe cases of rickets in the dog, whereas inadequate calcification of both the enamel and dentin can be demonstrated at relatively mild levels of the rachitic process. Enamel hypoplasia has not been described in the rat as a result of rickets, but it is likely that a sufficiently severe deficiency over a prolonged period would cause this abnormality even in this species. In human beings, there is likely to be more than one cause of enamel hypoplasia (Figs. 30–3, 30–4). In a thorough survey of the case histories of individuals with enamel hypoplasia, Sarnat and Schour reported that only a small number of cases had any evidence of a rachitic process during tooth development.[57]

The bony structures supporting the teeth develop changes characteristic of those in bone elsewhere in the body. Wide osteoid borders are found on the trabeculae of the alveolar bone, and the number and size of the trabeculae are greatly decreased.

Mellanby has conducted a wide variety of studies to determine the extent to which there may be a correlation between the structure of human teeth as studied microscopically and the susceptibility to tooth decay.[58] In order to set up standards whereby such a comparison could be made, various stages of increasing severity

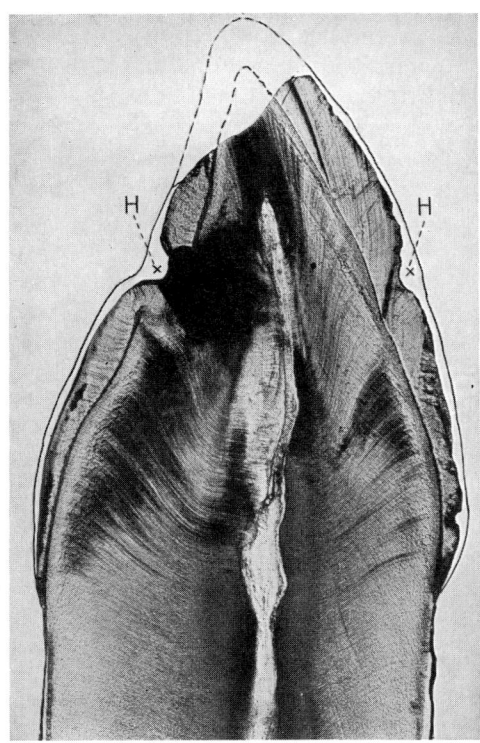

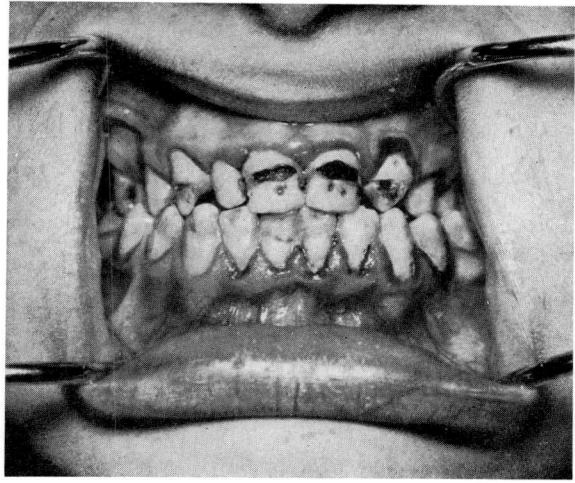

Fig. 30–4. Excessive enamel hypoplasia of the anterior teeth of a 16-year-old girl which may have been caused by severe malnutrition in early childhood. The marked gingivitis on lower anterior gingiva cleared up quickly as a result of vitamin C therapy. (From Cahn: *Pathology of the Oral Cavity.* Baltimore, Williams & Wilkins, 1941.)

Fig. 30–3. Section of an upper canine tooth. A severe systemic disturbance, which occurred when the patient was about 3 years old, caused the hypoplasia of the enamel (H). As shown by poor calcification and rills in the subsequently formed enamel (near the cervix of the tooth), the condition improved but did not become normal. Solid line = extent of normal enamel; dotted lines = loss of tooth structure from attrition.

of microscopic defects were described and correlated with the degrees of caries incidence in the same teeth. It should be clearly pointed out that the defects which Mellanby described—and which have come to be referred to as Mellanby hypoplasia—are visible only at a microscopic level and can be clinically discerned only by a careful exploration of the tooth surfaces with a sharp explorer. Thus this class of defects can be readily differentiated from those major areas of hypoplasia which are grossly visible upon clinical examination.

Mellanby reported that 78 per cent of primary teeth with well-calcified enamel and dentin were free from caries, while only 6 per cent of the teeth with appreciable degrees of microscopic abnormalities were free of tooth decay. Although these data have inherent assumptions, the overall trend of the material suggests a significant correlation between the structure of teeth as detected microscopically and the susceptibility to decay. However, this should not be interpreted to mean that grossly hypoplastic teeth will decay for that reason, nor is the corollary—that teeth that appear to be microscopically perfectly calcified will never decay—true. It is noteworthy to recall from histologic studies that perfectly formed teeth are rarely found in modern civilized populations. In contrast, the teeth of experimental animals rarely have developmental abnormalities unless a specific systemic disorder has been imposed during tooth development to alter the formation of organic matrix or its ability to calcify properly. The rhesus monkey is a particularly good example of this, for its teeth uniformly have a high degree of perfection in formation that is seldom equaled and never excelled in human teeth. The studies on the correlation between Mellanby hypoplasia and caries incidence have been extended to clinical surveys in the schools of London, England where oral examinations were made in 1929, 1943, 1945, 1947, 1949, 1951 and 1955.[59] A consistently high correlation between good tooth structure and freedom from caries was observed.

The effect of vitamin D supplementation upon the initiation and progress of carious lesions has been studied a great deal more intensively than the effect of any other essential nutrient. Studies were conducted by Mellanby and co-workers in England in a series of experiments which lasted from 1923 through 1936. The most extensive of these was conducted in three Birmingham children's institutions where the effect of supplements of cod liver oil and of irradiated ergosterol on dental caries incidence was evaluated.[60] The data obtained definitely pointed toward a lower incidence of new carious lesions and a lower rate of progress of existing lesions among the children in the group which received irradiated ergosterol and those in the group which received the cod liver oil supplement than in the children who received no vitamin D supplement. The reduction in dental caries incidence among the fully erupted teeth in the vitamin D-supplemented groups was statistically significant.

This experiment was not conducted for sufficiently long to give definitive results about the effect of the vitamin D supplements on the caries susceptibility of the developing teeth. In the small group of teeth that partially developed during the experiment, there was a trend toward a lower caries experience for the groups of children given the supplements. Data collected in clinical surveys have added sup-

porting evidence that inadequate vitamin D during tooth development results in a higher caries incidence.

For a variety of reasons these studies have been criticized. If they stood as the only evidence that an adequate amount of vitamin D during childhood was beneficial with respect to caries incidence, or if these investigators had claimed that vitamin D was the only nutrient involved, there would be reason to question the validity of the conclusions. However, a variety of studies have been conducted in the United States and Canada which corroborate the original observations made by Mellanby and co-workers.[61–63] In only a few experiments where the effect of vitamin D supplementation was studied were negative results found. It is interesting to note that some of these negative studies were conducted in older groups of children than in the remainder of the studies,[64] and that another one was conducted at such a high level of vitamin D supplementation as to raise a question as to whether the amount ingested was in the physiologic range of normalcy.[65] It is also noteworthy that none of the investigators who believed that vitamin D supplementation helped to reduce caries susceptibility claimed that this was the only reason for altered dental caries incidence, but rather that it was a partial means to cope with the problem.

Evidence from other types of studies also suggests that vitamin D is important for the maintenance of normal teeth in the child population. In a number of surveys efforts have been made to determine if there is any correlation between the incidence of dental caries and the number of hours of sunshine in a given community, the latitude of the locality and its winter temperature. For example, in a statistical evaluation which was based on a large compilation of dental caries data collected by the United States Public Health Service, Mills reported that there was a definite increase of dental caries among 12- to 14-year-old boys as the latitude increased.[66] This increase amounted to approximately 15 carious lesions per 100 children for each degree of latitude. Increases were reported from 289 decayed, missing or filled (DMF) teeth per 100 children in the cities between 25° and 36° latitude in the southern states to approximately 491 DMF teeth per 100 children in the cities between 43° and 46° latitude just south of the Canadian border.

On the basis of the same dental caries data, East has shown that there is a definite correlation between the mean annual hours of sunshine and the average incidence of tooth decay.[67] He observed the following relationship: the average DMF teeth per 100 boys was 290 in areas with 3,000 and more hours of sunshine per year and increased to a total of 486 in areas with less than 2,200 hours of sunshine annually. Other studies suggested a correlation between the dental caries incidence and the mean winter temperature, with a greater incidence of tooth decay when the winter temperature is lower. The most likely explanation of these effects would be an increased exposure of the children to sunlight, with a greater amount of vitamin D made available by reason of this exposure.

Other more subtle factors than the simple irradiation of the skin may contribute to this end-result. Although ethnic origin has been considered to some extent in these surveys, possible variations that might influence caries susceptibility on a regional basis have not been ruled out completely. In addition, variations in food patterns may influence the outcome and interpretation of the results. For example, throughout the southeastern states, where the caries incidence is generally lower than in the north, large amounts of a self-rising flour that contains appreciable supplements of inorganic phosphates are used. In the light of studies in experimental dental caries where the incidence of carious lesions was significantly reduced as a result of supplementation of the cariogenic diet with inorganic phosphates,

the increased phosphate consumption through the use of self-rising flour may affect caries incidence materially.[68,69]

Studies in rodents have shown that the calcium/phosphorus ratio of the diet during tooth development is an important factor in determining the composition of the inorganic fraction of the enamel and dentin. Sobel observed that a diet with a high calcium/phosphorus ratio resulted in the formation of teeth in the white rat and the cotton rat where inorganic components had a higher carbonate/phosphate ratio.[70,71] In contrast, the inorganic portion of the teeth of the animals which were fed a diet with a low calcium/phosphorus ratio during tooth development contained a much lower carbonate/phosphate ratio. In an experiment of this type conducted with cotton rats weaned at an early age, Sobel and co-workers reported that the animals with teeth which had the high carbonate/phosphate ratio were more susceptible to tooth decay than the teeth of the animals with the lower carbonate/phosphate ratio.[72]

The relation these studies may have to human beings is unknown. The calcium/phosphate ratios of the diets used by Sobel were appreciably more drastic than would ordinarily be encountered in human dietaries. The important contribution of these studies is the observation that the composition of the inorganic components of enamel and dentin varies depending upon the blood levels of the required elements, which in turn are dependent upon the amounts supplied by the diet. It may well be that human teeth are more sensitive during development and calcification to abnormalities in the calcium/phosphorus ratio of the diet than the rat, or it may be that other circumstances in the developing, calcifying tooth determine the extent to which calcium and phosphorus variations in the blood stream are reflected in an alteration in the composition of the inorganic components of the enamel and dentin.

Fluoride

Fluoride is the nutrient which has most clearly been demonstrated to reduce the caries susceptibility of teeth when consumed in optimal amounts during tooth development. No current chapter on the relation of nutrition to oral health would be complete without a discussion of the role of the fluorides in the etiology of dental caries. The fluorides are ubiquitous materials which occur in minute amounts in all foodstuffs and water supplies. Extensive surveys of the fluoride content of more than 130 foods are available. The majority of foods such as vegetables, meats, cereals and fruits contain between 0.2 and 1.5 ppm of fluorides. Outstanding exceptions to this lower range are the seafoods, the edible portions of which contain 5 to 15 ppm of fluoride, and tea leaves, which contain 75 to 100 ppm. A cup of tea will supply approximately 0.1 mg of fluoride. Reliable analyses of the fluoride contribution by foods in common human dietaries from areas as distant as Toronto, Minneapolis and Washington, D.C., indicate that an average diet supplies between 0.2 and 0.6 mg of fluoride daily, without the use of unusual amounts of either seafoods or tea.[73-75] Because of the widespread distribution of fluorides, production of a diet extremely low in fluoride is laborious. Schwarz used an ultraclean isolator system and a highly purified diet in which all ingredients including the amino acids had been purified to an extent not normally used in dietary studies.[76] Under these circumstances, young rats on the basal diet grew slowly and the orange pigment of the incisor enamel was not produced. The addition of 2.5 μg fluoride per gm of diet caused a significant increase in the rate of growth and the formation of normal amounts of the incisor pigment.[76]

In the data obtained from epidemiologic surveys in human populations and from rodent studies, there is a close correlation between the amount of fluoride ingested during tooth development and the amount of tooth decay occurring in the teeth after development is completed. The first convincing evidence of such a relationship was provided by Bunting and co-workers in 1929, who reported the results of a survey in Minonk, Illinois.[77] The amount of tooth decay among the children born and raised in this community was a great deal less than that of children who moved into Minonk after tooth development was complete. At the time of the survey, the investigators recognized that this striking difference must be related to the water supply, but the active agent was undefined. Later it was found that the drinking water contained 2.5 ppm of fluorides.

In 1939, more extensive information was provided by Dean and his collaborators as the result of a survey of 1,581 children in 4 communities in the Illinois area where the water contained varying amounts of fluorides.[78] Later a more comprehensive survey was reported for 4,425 children from 13 cities and 4 states by the same group of investigators.[79] The data from the latter study are presented in Table 30–2 in terms of the number of DMF permanent teeth observed in the 12- to 14-year-old children of these communities. Where the water contained 1 ppm of fluorides or more during tooth development, the children had a lower incidence of tooth decay than children in nearby communities where the water contained appreciably less than 1 ppm of fluoride. These findings have been corroborated by investigators in numerous areas of the United States, as well as in Canada, England, and numerous other countries.

Although these studies were concerned with the secondary teeth of the children, the primary teeth, likewise, have been shown to benefit from the ingestion of fluoride-bearing waters during tooth development.[80] In addition, it has been shown that the beneficial effect from the consumption of fluoride-bearing waters during tooth development remains into

Table 30–2.   A Comparison of the Fluoride Content of the Drinking Water and the Amount of Tooth Decay among 4,425 Children, 12 to 14 Years of Age in 13 Cities from 4 States.*

	Fluoride Content (ppm)	Number of Children Examined	Children With No Tooth Decay (per cent)	Average Number of Diseased Teeth per Child
Colorado Springs, Colo.	2.6	404	28.5	2.5
Galesburg, Ill.	1.9	273	27.8	2.4
East Moline, Ill.	1.2	152	20.4	3.0
Kewanee, Ill.	0.9	123	17.9	3.4
Pueblo, Colo.	0.6	614	10.6	4.1
Marion, Ohio	0.4	263	5.7	5.6
Lima, Ohio	0.3	454	2.2	6.5
Middletown, Ohio	0.2	370	1.9	7.0
Zanesville, Ohio	0.2	459	2.6	7.3
Quincy, Ill.	0.1	330	2.4	7.1
Portsmouth, Ohio	0.1	469	1.3	7.7
Elkhart, Ind.	0.1	278	1.4	8.2
Michigan City, Ind.	0.1	236	0.0	10.4

* Adapted from Dean, Arnold and Elvove.[79]

adult life.[81] Surveys in the United States, Argentina, England and Hungary have demonstrated that exposure to naturally borne fluorides during tooth development continues to manifest itself by a low incidence of tooth decay in adult life. On the basis of these and a great many other studies, there is no longer any doubt that water containing 1 ppm or more of fluorides has a definitely beneficial effect, when consumed during tooth development, upon the later caries susceptibility of the teeth. The ingestion of an optimal fluoride level during tooth development appears to be as effective in an area of relatively low caries incidence such as Hungary as in areas of high caries incidence such as England and the United States.

The fluoride content of teeth developed in areas where different amounts of fluorides were present in the water supply closely parallels the amount of fluorides in the water.[82] Where drinking water contained zero to 0.3 ppm of fluoride, as in Washington, D.C., the teeth of the native continuous residents had approximately 0.010 per cent of fluorides in the enamel and 0.024 per cent in the dentin. Where the water supply contained 1.0 to 1.2 ppm of naturally occurring fluorides, as in Aurora, Illinois, the teeth of comparable residents contained 0.014 per cent fluorides in the enamel and 0.036 per cent in the dentin. Comparable increases in bone fluoride occurred as the fluoride content of the water supply increased.

Presumably the caries resistance of the teeth is somehow related to their fluoride content. The exact nature of this relationship is not known. In an x-ray diffraction study of bone samples with various levels of fluoride, Zipkin, Posner and Eanes[83] observed that increasing fluoride concentrations were associated with increased "crystallinity" of the hydroxyapatite as evidenced by larger crystal size and more nearly perfect crystals. These changes in "crystallinity" would reduce the effective surface area of the crystals in a given weight of bone, reduce the reactivity of the crystals and provide less area for deposition and surface orientation of carbon dioxide and citrate, in particular. The inverse relationship between fluoride concentration and the carbonate and citrate concentrations in bone has been demonstrated.[84] Zipkin and Posner[85] postulated that, if this inverse relationship existed in enamel as well as in bone, a new concept could be introduced to explain the relationship between fluoride concentration in enamel and susceptibility to dental caries.

Further light is thrown upon this subject in studies by Jenkins and Speirs, who determined the level of fluoride content in various levels of the enamel.[86] They noted that the outer surface uniformly had a much higher fluoride level than the deeper layer. They also observed that this difference in distribution was detectable in unerupted as well as in erupted teeth. The latter observation indicates that this was a developmental arrangement of the concentration of fluoride, and not a distribution that took place after the teeth had erupted into the oral cavity by reason of contact with saliva. These observations have been corroborated by Brudevold and co-workers,[87,88] who also demonstrated a posteruptive acquisition of fluoride by the surface layers of enamel which increased in proportion to the amount of fluoride in the drinking water. Cooper and Ludwig[88a] observed decreases in the mesiodistal and buccolingual diameters and in cuspal height of molars in children who grew up in an area with fluoridated water in comparison with molars in children in a nearby town with low-fluoride water. This observation is consistent with earlier studies in rats and with the smaller crystal lattice in bones with elevated levels of fluoride. Optimal fluoride during tooth development has also been reported to result in more perfectly formed fissures between molar cusps.[88b]

In view of the beneficial influence of inorganic fluorides as introduced into water supplies by nature, the next step was to determine whether the introduction of comparable inorganic fluorides into low-fluoride waters would be equally efficacious. The first survey was begun at Grand Rapids, Michigan, in January 1945, where the fluoride content of the water supply was increased to 1.2 ppm under the joint sponsorship of the United States Public Health Service, the University of Michigan and the Michigan State Department of Health. Muskegon, Michigan, served as the control low-fluoride city. Soon after this, surveys were begun in a number of other cities. Some of the impressive data which are now available from the older surveys are presented in Table 30–3.[89]

The overall analysis of the data from these surveys indicates that the dental caries incidence in teeth formed during the survey period was on the average about 60 per cent lower than the caries incidence in otherwise comparable teeth formed prior to the increase in fluoride content of the water supply, or in those teeth formed in children in neighboring cities where the water supply did not have its fluoride content adjusted. As would be expected, the greatest benefits were in the youngest age groups and in the teeth of older children that were formed after fluoride adjustment occurred in the communal water supply. These facts are clearly shown in Figure 30–5 for the children of Newburgh and Kingston 10 years after fluoridation began in Newburgh.[90]

The high similarity of the data to those in communities where the fluoride is naturally borne is most striking. It is also noteworthy that no comparable decreases in dental caries incidence were noted in the children of nearby communities where the fluoride content of the communal waters had not been increased. The latter was true despite the use even on a limited scale of various toothpastes and other prophylactic measures which have been widely suggested as being highly beneficial for the reduction of dental caries incidence.

In rural areas or urban communities where the drinking water contains less than the optimal level of fluoride, supplemental drops or tablets may be provided daily throughout the period of tooth

Table 30–3. Reduction in Tooth Decay Observed in Various Fluoridation Study Projects*

Community	Fluoridation Date Started	Report Period (yr)	Age Group (yr)	Reduction in Decay† (per cent)
Grand Rapids, Mich.	Jan. 1945	8	6	70.8
			7	52.5
			8	49.2
			9	48.1
			13	39.7
Brantford, Ont.	June 1945	7	6	59.4
			7	69.5
			8	51.5
			9	46.2
			13	32.9
Newburgh, N. Y.	May 1945	7	6	69.4
			7	67.8
			8	40.4
			9	51.4
Evanston, Ill.	Feb. 1947	4	6	73.6
			7	56.4
			8	35.4
Sheboygan, Wis.	Feb. 1946	6	9–10 (4th grade)	35.3
			12–14 (8th grade)	29.7

* Adapted from Ast, Smith, Wachs and Cantwell.[90]
† Decayed, missing and filled teeth.

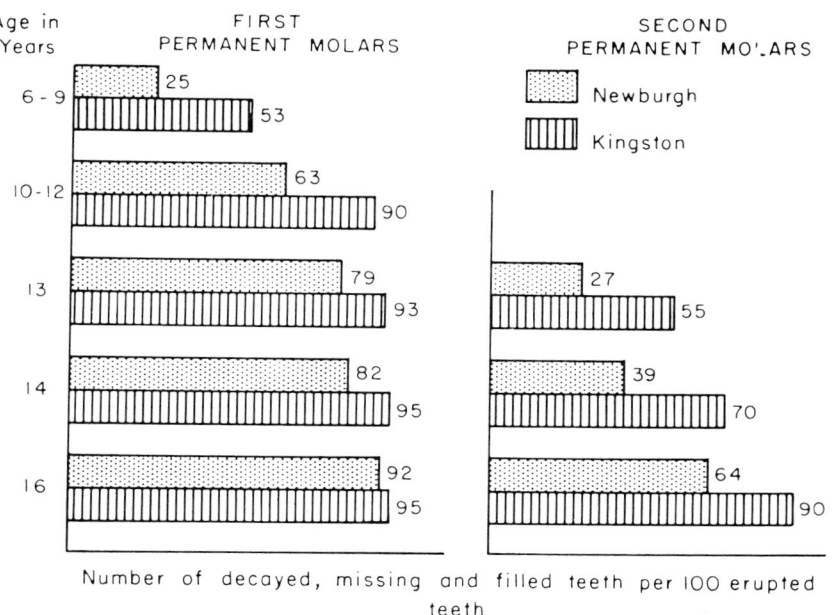

Fig. 30–5. The relation of added fluoride in the water supply for 10 years to the incidence of dental caries in first and second permanent molar teeth of children from 6 to 16 years of age. (From Ast, Smith, Wachs and Cantwell.[90] Courtesy of J. Am. Dent. Assoc.)

development. This procedure is as effective as water fluoridation provided it is followed faithfully from birth through the middle teens when the crowns of the teeth are fully formed. The recommended levels for daily supplementation are shown in Table 30–4.

On the basis of present knowledge, the most sensitive tissue in the body to excessive ingestion of fluorides is the ameloblastic layer which forms the organic framework of the enamel. When the drinking water of a community contains 2.5 ppm or more of fluorides, a manifestation known as mottled enamel (chronic endemic dental fluorosis) results.[91] This problem occurs only when the high fluoride ingestion takes place during the developmental period of the teeth, and cannot occur after tooth development has been completed. The degree of mottled enamel may vary from slight nonaesthetically significant amounts to an extensive chalkiness of the surface with large opaque areas which may erode rapidly and which in severe cases become heavily stained. Even severely mottled teeth are highly resistant to dental caries. In Figure 30–6, the freedom from fluorosis at optimal levels of fluoride in the water is clearly demonstrated.

As the fluoride content of the water increases, the severity and the extent of mottled enamel increase until at levels of 8 or 10 ppm in the communal water supply almost all of the individuals who grow up in the area have mottled enamel of such severity that it is aesthetically disfiguring. At fluoride levels from 2.0 ppm or more, the water supply is in need of treatment, either by the development of a new source, by adequate dilution with low-fluoride waters or by removal of the fluorides from the drinking water. However, on the basis of these epidemiologic surveys, fluorides contributing in the neighborhood of 1.2 ppm of fluoride to a water supply have definitely been shown to be of no detrimental public health significance with respect to the causation of mottled enamel in northern regions. In hotter climates, where the water consumption is appreciably higher, the optimal level of fluoride ingestion is in the neighborhood of 0.6 to 0.7 ppm.[92] Controlled fluoridation at the recommended levels has not resulted in any aesthetically disfiguring mottling among the children of any community.

Abnormalities other than those caused in the developing teeth by excessively high fluoride ingestion have been sought in various surveys in the United States and elsewhere throughout the world. Probably the most important and extensive surveys in which general systemic influence of fluoride ingestion was sought were made in 1943 and 1953 in Bartlett and Cameron, Texas.[93] The former community had a water supply that contained approximately 8 ppm of fluoride, whereas the latter community, situated some 30 miles distant, had a water supply with about 0.4 ppm

Table 30–4.   Appropriate Amounts for Supplemental Fluoride*

Patient's Age	Fluoride Content of Water, mg/liter (ppm)†			
	0.0–0.25	0.25–0.50	0.50–0.75	0.75+
0–12 mo	0.25 mg	0	0	0
12 mo–4 yr	0.50 mg	0.25 mg	0	0
4–8 yr	0.75 mg	0.50 mg	0.25 mg	0
8–12 yr	1.00 mg	0.75 mg	0.50 mg	0

* From Nikiforuk and Fraser: J. Can. Dent. Assoc., *30*, 67, 1964.

† The amount of fluoride prescribed varies according to the patient's age and the level of fluoride in the water supply. For example, a dosage of 0.25 mg per day is recommended for a 1-year-old child who lives in an area which has 0 to 0.25 ppm fluoride in its water supply.

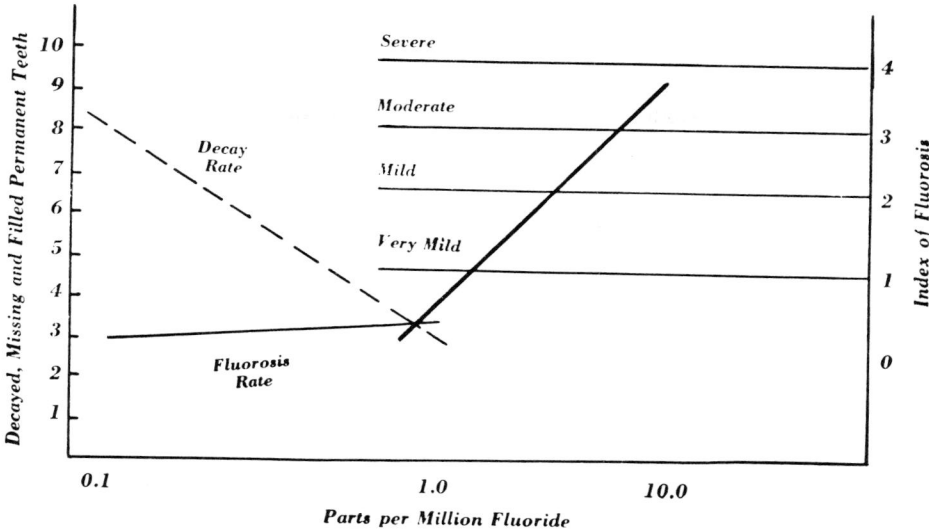

Fig. 30–6. Relation between DMF teeth (dotted line), severity of dental fluorosis (solid line) and fluoride concentration of the water expressed on a logarithmic scale. (Adapted from Hodge and Smith: In *Fluoridation as a Public Health Measure* (Shaw, Ed.). Washington, American Association for the Advancement of Science, 1954.)

fluoride. In 1943 a series of inhabitants who had resided at least 15 years in each community was selected at random and carefully examined by skilled physicians; 116 were examined in Bartlett and 121 in Cameron. These individuals ranged from 15 to 68 years of age in 1943; 57.8 per cent of the Bartlett participants and 47.2 per cent of those from Cameron were over 55 years of age. X-ray films of various portions of the skeletal system and full case histories were taken.

The data in these surveys indicated that there was no significant difference in any phase of health between individuals of one community and the other, with two exceptions. Many of the individuals who had resided in Bartlett during childhood had severely mottled teeth. In addition, a slightly higher incidence of cardiovascular disease was observed in Cameron. In all other regards, there were no detectable abnormalities that could be attributed to the different fluoride content of these two water supplies.

Though this survey is undoubtedly the most intensive of all that have been conducted, many other surveys on different phases of the fluoride problem as related to systemic disease have been conducted. In all cases, levels of 1.0 ppm or more, up to 8.0 ppm, in the United States have been shown to be negative with respect to any correlation of a systemic abnormality to the fluoride content of the water.

The case for both the dental benefits and the systemic safety of controlled fluoridation of public water supplies at recommended levels has been unequivocally established. Now new evidence is beginning to suggest that the ingestion of inadequate levels of fluoride over prolonged periods may be as disadvantageous for bone as for the development of caries-resistant teeth. Leone[94] reported the recognition of 279 cases of osteoporosis among 546 persons in a radiographic study in Framingham, Massachusetts, where the water supply contains 0.1 ppm fluoride. In addition, a higher frequency of other bone abnormalities was noted than had been observed in either Bartlett or Cameron, Texas.

Leone concluded that the data support "the hypothesis that disadvantageous effects on the bone structure of the adult population may be associated with the prolonged use of drinking water that contains an insufficient concentration of fluoride."

Bernstein et al.[95] conducted a survey in two towns in North Dakota where the water supplies contained 4.0 to 5.8 ppm fluoride and in three towns where they contained 0.15 to 0.30 ppm fluoride. The prevalence of reduced bone density was much higher in the low-fluoride than in the high-fluoride communities. In addition, the males in the low-fluoride towns had a much higher frequency of calcification of the abdominal aorta. In addition, Rich and Ensinck[96,97] have reported improvements in calcium balance in 6 patients with osteoporosis and one with Paget's disease when small amounts of fluoride were given orally in several divided doses daily. The average improvement in calcium balance was 802 mg per week for these patients during the 10th to 14th weeks of therapy. Jowsey and her co-workers[98] and Hanson and Roos[99] have also shown significant increases in bone mineral mass in patients with osteoporosis, using as much as 100 mg of sodium fluoride per day in combination with vitamin D and calcium supplementation. The use of calcium supplementation probably avoids the problem of osteomalacia associated with secondary hyperparathyroidism. Kyle et al.[99a] have also shown similar beneficial results in a number of patients with multiple myeloma using the same therapeutic regimen. Much more study needs to be given to this area of fluoride metabolism but these preliminary findings may indicate the existence of more widespread benefits of fluoride ingestion than had been previously expected.

It is noteworthy that over 3 million individuals in the United States have consumed natural fluoride-bearing waters in excess of 1.0 ppm for decades, and an additional 5 million individuals have consumed amounts between 0.5 and 1.0 ppm.[100] Already the fluoridation of community water supplies has been widely instituted throughout the United States and elsewhere in the world. As of December 31, 1975, fluorides were being added to the water supplies in cities and towns in the United States with a total population of 94,627,000.[101] In February, 1978, the water supply for the Metropolitan Water District of Greater Boston was fluoridated for 1,700,000 individuals. Many other communities are in some phase of equipment purchase and installation. Of the 12 largest cities in the United States, only Houston and Los Angeles do not currently fluoridate their water supplies.[101] There has yet to be any evidence presented to indicate that any individual in any age group has been harmed by ingestion of these water supplies.

Uncharacterized Relations

Another example of a developmental influence upon the teeth may be obtained from the extensive dental caries statistics that were collected on children from European countries during World Wars I and II (Fig. 30–7). Studies representing a total of about 750,000 children from 11 countries have been summarized and evaluated in detail by Sognnaes.[102] It is noteworthy that the reduction in dental caries experience in all these studies did not occur concurrently with the reduction in refined foods and sugar.

Possibly the most detailed data are available from the children in Norway where almost complete reduction in carbohydrate intake from sugar and highly refined flours occurred in 1939, yet the greatest increase in caries-free permanent teeth among 7-year-old children did not occur until 1945. Indeed, the reductions in 1940, 1941 and 1942 were relatively small. The attention of the reader should be drawn to the fact that all the teeth in this particular tabulation had been in the oral cavity for only 1 or 1½ years. The teeth that erupted

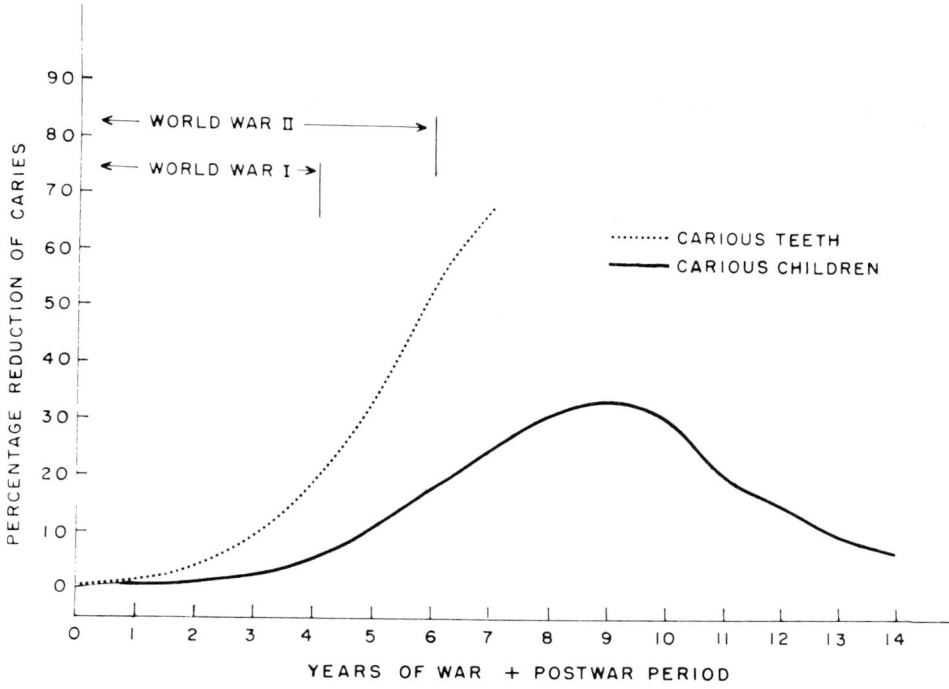

Fig. 30–7. The percentage reductions in decayed, missing, and filled teeth and of the number of children with carious lesions are plotted for the periods during World Wars I and II. The data on carious teeth represent averaged observations from Norway, Denmark, Finland, Sweden, and Britain. The curve for reductions in children with caries presents the averaged findings from Norway, Denmark, Britain, France, and Germany (From Sognnaes.[102])

6 to 8 years after hostilities enforced drastic changes in food habits were much more resistant to dental caries than the teeth that erupted during prewar and the earlier war years.

In World War I the maximum reduction in caries incidence was not observed until 1922 and 1923, that is, after the cessation of hostilities and the partial return of fine foods and sugar to the European diet. In the World War II period, the highest reduction in dental caries incidence was not reported until 1945. Thus, in both periods there was a 6- to 8-year lag in the attainment of maximum caries resistance. In other words, the teeth that were benefited most were those that were just beginning to form when the wartime dietary change was imposed.

This time lag obviously cannot be explained purely on the basis of alterations in the oral environment of teeth that have been in the oral cavity for short periods of time. Instead, the data point to strong effects of the diet during the war years on the development of teeth that are much more caries resistant than those developed by children consuming the typical prewar dietary foods.

The fact that these reductions in dental caries incidence were comparable for the two wars and in the several countries from which data are available suggests that the data have a high degree of validity. The active factor or factors in this effect on dental caries incidence are unknown. Along with the greatly reduced incidence of dental caries, Toverud[103] has reported that the permanent teeth erupted much later and that the primary teeth were retained in the mouth longer during the war years than in the prewar period.

Suggestions from other clinical surveys lend support to such developmental influences. In a survey conducted by Cohen[104] on a group of preschool children in New England where the proneness to develop carious lesions is high, it was noted that the 4- and 5-year-old children from families in the high socioeconomic group had a significantly lower incidence than children from less favored groups (Table 30–5). This difference between groups reflects good prenatal and pediatric care, including diet counselling, for the more favored groups. It is noteworthy that the dental caries experience among the preschool children in the high socioeconomic group compared favorably with the caries index in children of the same age in endemic fluoride areas and in areas where the communal water supplies have been fluoridated.

Similar results were observed in a clinic designed to give early pediatric care to children in two Norwegian communities. Toverud[105] reported that those children who received good care in their early years had a significantly lower incidence of tooth decay than similar children in the community who did not receive the services of this clinic or who did not seek help until later in their development.

This type of clinical information has been greatly strengthened by investigations with rodents and monkeys.[106,107] The ingestion of diets composed of natural foodstuffs during tooth development resulted in teeth that were much more resistant than the teeth of comparable experimental animals that developed during maintenance on diets composed of highly purified ingredients. Although the natural diet contained significantly more fluorides than the purified diet, other studies with rats have indicated that the difference in fluoride content of the two diets was insufficient to cause the different incidence of tooth decay.[108] Further experiments to determine the active agent in this study have shown that the influence is a result of the different mineral components of the two diets. When the mineral components of the natural diet were fed as the sole source of minerals in the purified diet, an appreciably lower incidence of tooth decay resulted.[109]

NUTRITIONAL INFLUENCES DURING TOOTH MATURATION AND MAINTENANCE

The maturation period of a tooth is the era about which we know the least. There are several demonstrations in the literature

Table 30–5. Average Number of Decayed, Extracted and Filled Teeth in Preschool Children of Different Socioeconomic Groups*

Socioeconomic Level	Age	Number of Children	Per Cent With One or More Defective Teeth	Average Number of Defective Teeth per Child
Low	4	135	84	3.90
	5	36	89	5.44
Medium	4	135	61	2.39
	5	36	69	3.06
High	4	77	53	2.03
	5	16	75	3.19
Total	4	347	68	2.89
	5	88	78	4.06

* From Cohen.[104]

that the caries susceptibility of the molar teeth of rodents decreases as the tooth age increases.[110-112] There are also clinical suggestions that, if a tooth is protected from decay during its early months in the oral cavity, it attains a greater degree of caries resistance and is less liable to be attacked by the carious process at later stages. These findings suggest a change in tooth structure or in permeability of the tooth after emergence into the oral cavity.

Studies with radioisotopes show that the recently erupted tooth has a high ability to incorporate inorganic ions into its structure. The rate at which this occurs is 10 to 20 times faster than the rate of exchange in teeth that have been in the oral cavity for appreciably longer periods of time.[113] In addition, the rate of exchange in recently erupted teeth is only about one-half the rate in developing crowns of teeth within the jaw. This small difference between unerupted and recently erupted teeth is in striking contrast to the concept that the enamel of erupted teeth is an inert region. Further radioisotope studies have shown that the inorganic components incorporated into enamel during maturation and during the maintenance period have their origin in the salivary secretions.

Another influence upon the maturation of teeth has been demonstrated in histologic studies. The teeth of rats exposed to a cariogenic diet during the early posteruptive period had enamel much more permeable to histologic stains than comparable teeth in animals fed their entire ration by stomach tube.[14]

The changes that take place during tooth maturation are influenced by the salivary secretions. In an experiment to study this relationship, rats were sialoadenectomized at various intervals after weaning.[114] The subjects in the several groups were maintained on a noncariogenic diet until the rats in the last group were sialoadenectomized. Then all subjects were transferred on the same day to a cariogenic diet on which they were maintained for the same length of time.

Under these circumstances, the rats which were sialoadenectomized at weaning had the highest incidence of carious lesions; their littermates which were sialoadenectomized after tooth maturation was complete had significantly less tooth decay. The mechanism by which this influence takes place is not known. Briner et al.[115] made an interesting observation concerning the presence of hypomineralized (and presumably developmentally immature) areas of the enamel in rat molars at the time of eruption. When a nutritionally adequate noncariogenic diet was fed, these hypomineralized areas slowly mineralized to sound enamel. However, where a soft, cariogenic diet was fed, these hypomineralized areas increased dramatically and in time progressed to form gross carious lesions. Furthermore, we do not know whether variations in the composition of the saliva, or in the quantity of the saliva, may alter the rate or extent of maturation. This relationship among saliva, maturation of teeth and caries susceptibility indicates a type of metabolic situation that could be altered by an adverse nutritional influence on the quantity or the quality of the saliva.

Strälfors[68] noted that the supplementation of cariogenic diets with phosphates caused major reductions in caries in the hamster. In addition, McClure[69] has demonstrated that supplementation of diets that cause smooth surface lesions with 1.6 per cent of dibasic sodium phosphate caused striking reductions in dental caries. Many additional studies on dietary phosphates and experimental dental caries have been conducted and are reviewed by Nizel and Harris.[116] Sodium trimetaphosphate has been the most effective of the many phosphates tested. While the influence of phosphates in reducing dental caries in laboratory animals has been consistent, human trials have been inconsistent; one indicated a good reduction[117] while two had negative results.[118,119] A recent study of a population normally consuming tortillas made from lime-soaked corn which contained large amounts of calcium and phosphate has shown a reduction in carious lesions in areas of the mouth which are not self-cleansing and where the susceptible enamel pits become plugged with calcified material.[120] A similar population primarily consuming bread served as a control group.

At present, there is no satisfactory explanation for the influences observed in these types of experimental studies. However, somewhere in them valuable clues are contained which are needed to explain how and why such postdevelopmental differences influence the initiation and progression of carious lesions. Possibly this information may clarify some of the seeming paradoxes seen in human populations.

In clinical investigations it is important, as well as difficult, during maturation and maintenance periods to attempt to evaluate the influence of a diet upon the dental caries incidence in terms of its two potential components: the oral environment and the systemic interrelationships. This evaluation is especially difficult in experiments or surveys with human subjects. Numerous surveys have been conducted to determine the incidence of dental caries among primitive populations and to determine the extent to which their dental caries experience has been modified as they came in contact with civilization.

Among the most definitive of these surveys were those in which the incidence of tooth decay in about 3,000 primitive and civilized groups of Eskimos in Greenland was studied.[121,122] The percentage of Eskimos with tooth decay in East Greenland varied from 4.3 for the males and 4.6 for the females at the isolated native settlements to 43.2 and 51.5, respectively, for the Eskimos residing in the neighborhood of trading stations. On the west side of Greenland, the incidence was much higher and varied from 31.8 per cent for the males and 44.4 per cent for the females in native settlements up to 83.3 and 90.5 per cent, respectively, for those residing in the immediate neighborhood of the trading

posts. It has been estimated that an average of 63 per cent of the total dietary intake of the western Greenlanders in 1930 was made up of imported foods, especially sugar and cereals, instead of the 17 per cent in 1901. In East Greenland, the natives in isolated settlements received relatively no imported food, and those at the trading stations a great deal less than their contemporaries on the western side of the island.

The data from this survey and numerous others point to the fact that the increasing use of foods associated with civilization has resulted in increased dental caries incidences among the populations using these diets. This increase has been widely interpreted to be mediated through changes in the oral environment. This may be true in the case of those who have adopted civilized foods after tooth development is complete. However, in the children of these areas, the consumption of the more refined foods during periods of tooth development probably has resulted in the formation of teeth that have a much higher caries susceptibility than the teeth of their ancestors. In addition, the teeth of the youngsters erupt into oral environments that are more cariogenic because of the greater availability of readily fermentable, adherent carbohydrates.

Numerous experiments have been conducted on the effect of the type and composition of children's diets on their dental caries experience in attempts to explore in specific terms the remarkably large differences between the caries index of different population groups as described in the Greenland survey above. One of the longest series of studies was that conducted by Boyd and co-workers at the State University of Iowa, who became interested in this problem in the course of their studies on the dietary control of diabetic children.[123,124] These workers reported that where careful control was maintained by the use of diets which were high in fat and protein and low in carbohydrates, with ample supplies of all basic nutrients, there was much less tooth decay than in children of the same area who were not under such dietary regimentation. Many of their cases were studied for prolonged periods of time. These workers noted that nonadherence to the dietary recommendations resulted within a few months in an increased incidence of tooth decay. They believed that the low incidence of decay which they observed in the diabetic children under dietary supervision was the result of the general nutritional adequacy of the diet and not of the control of the diabetic process itself.

Similar studies were conducted by Drain and Boyd[125] and by McBeath[126,127] in children in other institutions for normal youngsters. When the customary diets were supplemented with milk, butter and eggs in the first case, and milk, eggs, wheat, meat, vegetables, oranges, butter and cod liver oil in the second, they observed substantial reductions in the incidence of new cavities. In studies with outpatients, Howe and co-workers[128,129] and Livermore[130] reported a lower number of new carious lesions in the patients who were cooperative in accepting and following the recommendations made to them, but observed no reductions in uncooperative patients.

The general conclusions of these investigators implicated the nutritional improvement of the diets as the important factor in the causation of the reduced dental caries increments. They believed that the change in the oral environment occasioned by the relatively low carbohydrate content of the diet was less important than the improvement in nutritional adequacy.

Other workers approached this subject from a different point of attack by the addition of various amounts of carbohydrate to the diets of institutionalized children without any attempt to maintain diets of comparable nutritional acceptance.[131,132] In one survey conducted in an orphanage, the incidence of tooth decay at the beginning of the experiment was low, even though the amount of several nutrients in the diet was far below levels considered to be adequate. In 51 orphanage children who received approximately 3 pounds of candy per week, definitely increased annual increments of tooth decay were observed during this period of high-carbohydrate ingestion. Unquestionably, the nutritional adequacy of the diet decreased by reason of the large amount of candy provided for each child. At the same time, the oral environment must have contained a higher amount of readily fermentable carbohydrates during the period of carbohydrate administration than was the case prior to the experiment.

In experiments of either of the above types, there is no practical way in which the degree of influence of the oral and systemic factors can be eliminated, one from another, on the basis of the most detailed published data. This is largely true because strict precautions were not taken to hold constant factors other than those under investigation. This comment obviously does not question the reliability of the results nor the efficacy of the procedures described for the control of dental caries. The probable conclusion that should be drawn from the two series of experiments is that both systemic conditions and the oral environment were influenced by the dietary changes. Hence, the altered initiation and development of carious lesions were the end-products of changes in the two interrelated facets of the problem. However, from the results of the animal studies reviewed above, as well as from controlled clinical studies such as those at Vipeholm, Sweden,[18] there can be no question that the excessive consumption of carbohydrate-containing foods, especially those that are retained on the tooth surfaces, is responsible to a large degree for a high dental caries incidence in caries-susceptible populations.

Numerous surveys have indicated that the frequency of between-meal snacks is directly related to caries incidence. Hankin et al.[133] in a study on 910 Caucasian, Japanese and Hawaiian eighth-grade children, correlated the frequency of use of chocolate, caramels, toffees, hard candy, soft jelly candy, marshmallows and gum with the DMF teeth in all three ethnic groups. Likewise, Keene et al.[134] at the Great Lakes Naval Station reported that 825 caries-free recruits tended to consume more milk, meat and vegetables and less candy, desserts and snacks than 818 recruits with rampant caries.

Some studies in recent years have been interpreted to cast doubt on the relationship of sugar consumption to dental caries incidence. For example, Glass and Fleisch reported that the use of ready-to-eat cereals, regular or presweetened, did not cause an increase in caries.[135] The amount of cereal consumed was estimated on the basis of interviews of the parents by dietitians and on the amount of cereals delivered to the home divided by the number of family members over one year of age. According to their data, the highest amount of regular cereal consumed averaged 2.6 ounces per day and the highest amount of presweetened cereal averaged 2.2 ounces per day. Many of the children consumed far less cereal than this. If all of the presweetened cereal for the high consumer had been the type containing 45 per cent sugar, the amount of sugar contributed to the diet from that source would have been 1 ounce per day. In our culture, where average sugar consumption is about 2 lb per week, the ounce daily from a presweetened breakfast cereal was only one-fourth or one-fifth of the total. With many children consuming far less cereal, the likelihood that an effect on dental caries would be observed in this type of survey seems remote.

However, presweetened cereals and other foods and candies which contain high amounts of sugar cannot be absolved on the basis of this type of survey. Since approximately three-quarters of all sugars entering commerce are introduced into products during processing, the homemaker is greatly restricted in the ability to control the amount of sugar available for consumption by the family members. It is axiomatic that carious lesions cannot occur without fermentable carbohydrates and the appropriate microbial flora. As the availability and frequency of carbohydrate consumption increase, the potentiality for the development and progression of caries increases.

LESIONS OF THE ORAL MUCOUS MEMBRANES AND OF THE SUPPORTING STRUCTURES OF THE TEETH

In the diagnosis and treatment of the various diseases of the oral mucous membranes, and of the supporting tissues of the teeth, it is desirable for the examiner to thoroughly evaluate all local conditions which might subject the oral tissues to excessive physical or chemical trauma, and to ascertain the presence of any systemic abnormality, whether nutritional, infectious, endocrine, constitutional or psychologic, which might alter the resistance of the oral tissues. Certainly a thorough visual examination of the oral tissues, as well as of the eyes, hair and skin, should be made to ascertain if any classical signs of nutritional deficiency are present. The various criteria of these deficiencies have been described in detail in the particular chapters of this book pertaining to the specific deficiencies. When none of these signs is found to exist as an indication of frank deficiency, evidence of subclinical dietary deficiency should be sought through discussions with the patient about his diet and also by laboratory tests and whatever clinical methods of evaluation are applicable in each individual case. Frequently such subclinical deficiencies may predispose to a sufficiently low tissue tone and resistance to traumatic or infectious processes that ordinarily tolerable oral conditions become overwhelming in their impact.

There is an increasing concern among oral clinicians that many low-grade abnormalities of the oral tissues, such as mild gingivitis, are being dismissed as "normal" because of the frequency of their occurrence. The optimal goal to strive for is healthy tissue rather than any less satisfactory condition, even though the latter is much more commonly observed in the population seen by an oral clinician.

The maintenance of the integrity, physiology and anatomy of the oral tissues is a goal that is too rarely seen or achieved by treatment in clinical practice.

Gingivitis

Gingivitis is an inflammation of the gingivae, including the interdental papillae. There are three main types: (1) hemorrhagic gingivitis, (2) ulcerative gingivitis and (3) hypertrophic gingivitis.

Hemorrhagic Gingivitis. Hemorrhagic gingivitis, which can be local or general, is characterized by free bleeding, red gingiva and edematous interdental papillae. The epithelial lining of the gingival trough is thin and edematous and is usually infiltrated with polymorphonuclear leukocytes. Bordering the "rough" epithelium, numerous bacteria and fungi are found. The direct cause of hemorrhagic gingivitis is basically poor oral hygiene, but indirectly is dietary since the retention of food in the crevicular and interstitial areas favors an accumulation of those products of bacterial fermentation which can act as an irritant on the underlying tissues to produce typical inflammation and edema. Infrequent or poor dental care can contribute to the inflammatory process by failure to remove mineralized deposits which form from salivary calcium and phosphate on the teeth in the gingival area, and which serve as additional irritants for the initiation or progression of the gingivitis. Broken-down teeth, malformed and malplaced teeth and traumatic occlusion act as physically debilitating circumstances or as food traps. Finally, iatrogenic factors

must be included in this partial list of causes of gingivitis. Among these are improperly placed fillings, overhanging fillings, ill-fitting dentures and poorly constructed crowns and bridges. A predisposing systemic cause of hemorrhagic gingivitis occasionally appears to be avitaminosis C, although there unquestionably must be additional factors that are not presently recognized.

Acute Necrotizing Ulcerative Gingivitis (Trench Mouth, Vincent's Gingivitis). This acute and painful condition is characterized by the loss of the interdental papillae by reason of acute necrosis, pseudomembrane formation, bad breath, regional lymph node involvement, mild lymphocytosis (although not always), sometimes a rise in temperature and anorexia. It is particularly characteristic that the first site of attack is the interdental papillae and that all are not attacked simultaneously. Instead, various stages are noted, with some papillae being very slightly involved and others, often close at hand, being completely destroyed. When the process is allowed to go on without interruption, extensive loss of the interdental papillae is noted, with the formation of cup-like ulcers between the teeth. The lesion is characteristically sensitive to any pressure or instrumentation. Usually the rest of the gingiva is uniformly inflamed and appears clinically as a reddened zone rather sharply demarcated from the subjacent alveolar mucosa. However, Vincent's disease is occasionally localized to a specific area or tooth with no involvement of the remaining oral tissues.

While the direct cause of acute necrotizing ulcerative gingivitis is believed to be the fusospirochetal group of microorganisms, postulates have been made about various underlying causes that predispose toward this rapidly fulminating disease entity. No underlying causes have been characterized in sufficient detail to justify a sound working hypothesis, but an association appears to exist with psychologic and emotional stresses, such as those experienced by college students at examination times and during courtship difficulties. A complicating factor during such periods is the frequency of grossly abnormal dietary habits. In addition, abnormalities in the endocrine status during intensive stress are commonly involved.

The most satisfactory treatment appears to be a thorough combination of local treatment with adequate diet, antibiotics and the alleviation of any psychologic stress or constitutional disorder that may be superimposed upon the condition.

Hypertrophic Gingivitis. This condition may exist either in the acute or in the chronic form. Acute hypertrophy of the gingiva is caused by a rapid influx into the gingiva of inflammatory cells, hemorrhage or abnormal white blood cells. When confronted with the acute form of the disease, it is necessary to think of, and to rule out wherever possible, an acute inflammation such as periodontal abscess, scurvy, purpura or leukemia. It is noteworthy that acute hypertrophic gingivitis is relatively rare. Chronic hypertrophy of the gingiva is fairly common. At least one factor involved in the causation of hypertrophic gingivitis is the lack of masticatory function.

Conditioned gingival enlargement occurs when the systemic state of the individual is such as to exaggerate the usual response to local irritation. Such a response is seen in patients experiencing hormonal change, as for example in pregnancy and in both sexes at puberty. Exaggerated responses to local factors are also described in leukemia and vitamin C-deficiency states. Another example of the exaggerated response occurs in upward of 50 per cent of patients receiving diphenylhydantoin (Dilantin), usually for control of seizures. With scrupulous oral hygiene the changes are either rarely seen or are minimal in nature. The condition is characterized by excessive accumulation of collagen in the gingiva.

Neoplastic gingival enlargements, although accounting for a comparatively small percentage of oral tumors[136] (8 per cent), nonetheless comprise a rather sizable proportion of growths of the gingiva[137] (23 per cent). The remaining 77 per cent were shown to be inflammatory in nature. Early detection and proper disposition in this field of oral diagnosis may indeed be lifesaving.

Periodontitis

The most common type of periodontitis is that familiarly known as pyorrhea alveolaris. This is in reality a rarefying osteitis of the supporting bone of the teeth and is accompanied by pocket formations that sometimes become infected with a considerable amount of pus. This disease is probably a consequence of the failure to eliminate the gingivitis described in the preceding section. Local infection commonly plays an important role in the clinical course of the disease. There are two postulates as to how infection occurs. According to one school of thought, in order for there to be an infection in these areas bacteria may have to pass two barriers of defense in order to form pockets in the alveolar bone: the normal epithelial lining of the gingival crevice and the strong transverse fibers over the crest of the alveolus. The latter appear to resist invasion, even after the gingivae have been destroyed. A more prevalent view today is the one supported by the findings of Weinmann,[138] which indicate that chronic infection of the gingiva progresses, following the course of the blood vessels, into the bone marrow spaces and on the periosteal side of the alveolar bone. According to this view the infection penetrates directly into the periodontal membrane only in exceptional cases. Resorption of the alveolar crest from the gingival side leads to destruction, first, of the supporting alveolar bone, and then of the lamina dura with its insertions of the periodontal membrane.

Although relatively little is known about

the nature of systemic predisposing factors, it is likely that one or more systemic factors of nutritional and constitutional nature predispose toward the destruction of the tissues in this area. The main reason for believing in systemic influence of a presently unidentifiable nature is the observation that even after local conditions have been cleared up, periodontitis may continue to progress or may not regress. Various postulates concerning low-calcium intake, poor calcium utilization, avitaminoses C and D, deficiencies of the B complex and endocrine malfunction have been made. However, there is little evidence to support any of these hypotheses.

In experimental animals the only deficiency disease which has been reported to be comparable to periodontitis is scurvy in the guinea pig, in which Boyle and co-workers reported that prolonged vitamin C deficiency resulted in an absorption of the alveolar bone in a way that was characteristic of periodontitis in man.[47] However, in clinical trials human patients with various degrees of periodontitis have not uniformly responded to vitamin C therapy, even though the tissues were saturated by administering doses of 200 to 500 mg of ascorbic acid daily.

The only studies concerning vitamin D deficiency in relation to osteomalacia and to periodontitis have been those reported from Indian surveys by Taylor and Day.[139] They examined 22 Indian women who were suffering from clinical osteomalacia by reason of diets deficient in calcium and in vitamin D, and found that 11 of them had severe cases of periodontitis. In view of the high incidence of periodontal diseases of all types in India, it is questionable whether the high incidence of periodontitis among these women was attributable to the osteomalacia or was simply a manifestation that would have been expected in any group of Indian women of comparable age. However, more thorough clinical studies in this area are badly needed to provide definite information.

In the dog and in the monkey, various experiments in which B complex deficiencies were produced with resultant effects upon gingival inflammation and infection have been reported. Becks and Morgan described deficiencies in the filtrate fraction of the vitamin B complex, probably pantothenic acid deficiency and niacin deficiency, in which severe abnormalities were reported in the supporting structures of the teeth of dogs.[140] Likewise, in monkeys fed diets deficient in the B complex, Chapman and Harris have produced severe gangrenous lesions of the gingival tissue and osteitis of the alveolar bone with exfoliation of the teeth.[141] These observations suggest that there are predisposing nutritional factors, when the deficiencies are particularly severe, to produce clinical entities comparable in some degrees to periodontal destruction. However, comparable observations are not available in human surveys.

For the best treatment of periodontitis, local irritating factors must be removed by proper procedures, an attempt must be made to restore the gingiva to normal physiologic form and function and a program of home care to maintain the results of treatment must be conscientiously applied. Without proper oral hygiene, all other measures are futile. The most satisfactory benefit from local treatment will be achieved when there is an accompanying improvement in systemic conditions. Though there are no specific dietary entities which have been clearly shown to be related to clinical periodontitis, improvement of the diet in all regards is strongly indicated. The best prescription which can be given in these cases is the adherence to a fully adequate diet. Where there is reason to believe that one or more specific deficiencies exist in the patient, suitable therapeutic preparations should be given. Where there is no indication of specific deficiencies, general improvement of the diet will be found adequate, without supplementation by proprietary materials.

Noma (Cancrum Oris)

This particularly catastrophic gangrenous lesion has its initial origin in the gingival area of the oral cavity, even though it may ultimately involve the mucosa, cheeks, muscles and bone. Although the lesion is now rarely seen in Europe and North America, it is still prevalent in underdeveloped areas of the world where malnutrition and infection are major problems.[142]

The etiology of the lesion is somewhat obscure but usually involves a chronically malnourished child from 2 to 5 years of age who contracts an acute infection, often exanthematous such as measles or smallpox, which debilitates him further. Some days or a week after the precipitating systemic infection a gingival ulceration appears in the vicinity of the premolar-molar areas which within a few days spreads, becomes gangrenous and can eventually slough leaving large defects in the cheeks, lips and nose, often with large bony

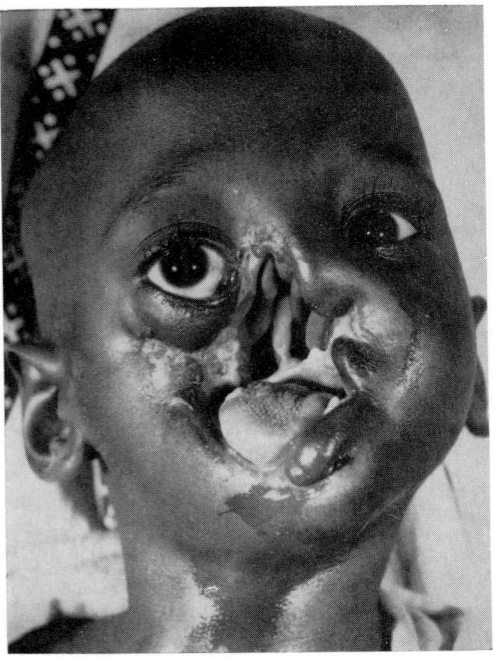

Fig. 30–8. Disfigurement in a case of noma. (Courtesy of Dr. Michael Tempest.)

sequestra. Almost certainly the lesion is an extreme expression of Vincent's disease since the same fusospirochetal organisms are found in the tissues from the noma lesion. This is further borne out by the finding of the same organisms in extraoral lesions which also occasionally occur. It seems that an acute fusospirochetal infection of the oral cavity which ordinarily is kept within bounds by the host's natural defense may assume a rampant, explosive character in the malnourished debilitated child. Noma formerly had a mortality of 70 to 90 per cent, but with antibiotic therapy this has been reduced to under 15 per cent. However, the severe disfiguring sequelae present formidable surgical and psychosocial problems (Fig. 30–8).

Relationship of Chewing Ability and Nutritional Status

Examples of an interrelationship between proper dentures and malnutrition have been reported. Mann and co-workers made a clinical study of 160 edentulous patients with a long-standing clinical record of multiple deficiency disease who had been under their observation for at least 3 years.[143] All had previous histories or present evidence of chronic pellagra, beriberi, scurvy or riboflavin deficiency. The identity of these deficiencies was established by the presence of characteristic mucosal membrane lesions of pellagra, of the nutritional peripheral neuritis of beriberi, of the gingival lesions of scurvy and of angular cheilosis and the ocular lesions of riboflavin deficiency.

The vertical dimension of the face had decreased in 140 out of the 160 cases. Fifty-seven of the 74 patients who had only 1 denture, or none, had monilial cheilitis. Fifty-two of the 66 patients who were wearing dentures with decreased vertical dimension gave evidence of monilial cheilitis. In contrast, only 7 of the 20 cases with a normal vertical dimension showed any evidence of angular cheilosis. Ninety-eight of the patients with a reduced vertical dimension complained of symptoms arising from the alimentary tract, "burning of the mouth and tongue, epigastric burning and pain, nausea and vomiting, intermittent diarrhea, cramping and anorexia." Only 8 of the 20 patients with a normal vertical dimension mentioned these subjective symptoms. In most of these cases, artificial dentures had been constructed poorly or of inferior materials. This resulted in much irritation that was ultimately augmented by the unsanitary condition of these appliances. Under these circumstances, in many of these patients, the consumption of adequate amounts of an adequate variety of foodstuffs was either difficult or impossible. When patients with a reduced vertical dimension were given riboflavin there was a reduction in the cheilotic lesions, but at no time did these lesions disappear if a reduced vertical dimension was still present. Niacin and pyridoxine did not have any effect on angular cheilosis, although they aided in the reduction of other symptoms characteristic of these particular deficiencies.

These data indicate the necessity to restore adequate dental function by well-fitted dentures that restore the normal vertical dimension. Even dentures that are perfect when originally fitted must be examined periodically to determine whether or not the alveolar ridges have been resorbed sufficiently to alter the original normal relationships. If such a reduction in dental function is allowed to persist, monilial cheilitis may result from the decreased vertical dimension of the face and a complex nutritional deficiency disease may arise from the inability to masticate an adequate amount or an adequate variety of food.

In a continuation of these studies, Greene and co-workers made a survey of the incidence of impaired mastication ability in 446 consecutive patients at the Nutrition Clinic of the Hillman Hospital in Birmingham, Alabama.[144] *Masticatory insufficiency* was the term used to describe a variable clinical condition that resulted from one reason or another in the inadequate ability to chew food. A patient was considered to be in the state of masticatory insufficiency if any one of the following conditions prevailed: (1) no natural teeth and artificial dentures that were inadequate or painfully fitting, (2) no natural teeth and no artificial dentures or only one denture or (3) less than 3 opposing serviceable natural masticating teeth and 3 opposing serviceable natural anterior teeth and no functional replacements in the form of dentures or bridges. Of these patients, 268 had no natural teeth. Only 49 of these edentulous individuals had well-balanced functional artificial dentures. Of the 178 individuals who still had some natural teeth, only 96 had well-balanced dentitions. Thus, 301 of the 446 patients had various degrees of masticatory insufficiency, and only 145 had natural or artificial well-functioning dentitions according to the definitions laid down by the investigators. The incidence of masticatory insufficiency was observed to increase appreciably with age.

A further problem with patients who have been edentulous for prolonged periods is the difficulty in designing and making dentures that are comfortable and masticatorily efficient. After prolonged periods of edentulousness, the mucous membranes of the mouth and lips are sufficiently atrophied and altered that the wearing of dentures is very difficult. In these cases in particular, there is a special necessity to correct the underlying nutritional disorders that have arisen over the edentulous period. Otherwise successful construction and fitting of the dentures in tissues with reduced viability and altered structure will increase the likelihood of unsatisfactory results.

Xerostomia (Dry Mouth)

While xerostomia is rare in young people, older individuals have gradually decreased salivary flows as a function of aging and the replacement of acinar tissue with oncocyte cell types. In the elderly, this gradual decrease in flow does not seem to provoke any serious consequences. However, in one form, Sjögren's syndrome, in addition to the usually profound xerostomia a decrease in lacrimation usually occurs which may lead to keratoconjunctivitis sicca. Frequently associated with this syndrome is evidence of autoimmune disease, usually rheumatoid arthritis. Sjögren's syndrome is generally believed to represent an autoimmune disorder.

Xerostomia has also been reported to occur in the following conditions: aplasia of one or more of the salivary glands, systemic diseases with an accompanying high fever or inducing a state of dehydration, menopause, psychic stimulation (fear, anxiety), certain drugs (atropine, antihistamines, rauwolfia alkaloids, sympathomimetic drugs) and post-radiation fibrosis of salivary glands.

Pain

Oral pain may vary from the annoyance of a "burning" sensation in the tongue to the excruciating manifestations of tic douloureux. The burning tongue is one of the most difficult problems with which the dentist and physician must cope. Each case is a diagnostic problem in itself. The condition is usually localized in the lateral margins and the tip of the tongue and is described as a peppery or burning sensation. This is commonly an early sign of pernicious anemia, and also occurs early in pellagra, sometimes in diabetes, early pregnancy and alcoholism. In all these situations a deficiency of one or more members of the vitamin B complex may be involved.

If the diagnosis of the underlying factor can be made, the burning tongue is easily corrected. If there is suspicion of faulty absorption of nutrients, the parenteral route is advisable. In all cases, treatment is likely to be prolonged. Various claims have been made for specific effects of thiamin chloride and of pyridoxine hydrochloride. However, there are no data to corroborate these statements with any degree of accuracy, although isolated cases may have responded to therapy in this line. From available data, it cannot be deduced that these are specific for the treatment of such sensations as are described under the terms burning tongue or tic douloureux. In these conditions, it is important to remember to treat local conditions that may contribute to the breakdown of the adjacent tissues but, in addition, systemic conditions of a rather general nature must be considered and evaluated. It is relatively rare that individual nutrients will be found to be responsible for any of these manifestations.

Summary of Dietary Treatment

By far the better means of treating dietary abnormalities that may accompany or predispose toward these local lesions of the oral mucous membranes or of the supporting structures of the teeth is the prescription of a well-balanced diet composed of the four basic food groups with a general distribution of the foods generously among the several groups. In cases where there is clear-cut evidence of prolonged deficiency of one or more nutrients, they should obviously be supplied in purified form in high enough amounts to replete the body supplies. However, by and large, this is neither necessary nor desirable. In addition, where there are cases of faulty absorption or excessive requirements by reason of peculiar constitutional circumstances or accompanying disease requirements, then supplementation also is in order. It is noteworthy too, in connection with postoperative healing, especially when there are extensive needs in the oral cavity, that a diet adequate with respect to all the nutrients should be prescribed.

SUMMARY

Our knowledge about the relationships of nutrition to the diseases of the oral cavity has been rapidly expanding during the past decades. This is best exemplified by the increased factual information about the relationship of nutrition to the development, the maturation and the maintenance of the teeth and to their caries susceptibility. Insofar as the influence of nutrition upon the lesions of the oral mucous membranes and of the supporting structures of the teeth is concerned, we still have a much smaller collection of established facts than is needed. It is not unreasonable to assume by reason of the rapidly expanding horizons in nutritional research that the next decade or two may well provide as many substantial answers to the latter category of oral problems as has been added to our pool of knowledge about tooth decay in the past decade or two. It is noteworthy, although not surprising in view of the chronic nature of most oral problems, that many of the nutritional problems of the mouth involve metabolic abnormalities which create predispositions to disease entities manifested years or decades later.

The best advice for any age group about the dietary regimen that will provide the best opportunity for normal oral tissues is simple and straightforward. Each of the basic four food groups should be represented liberally in each day's diet, and as many as possible in each of the day's three meals. The best selection of foods for dental health is one where as many foods as possible are purchased in their natural state without excessive refining and where the cooking procedures conserve the maximum of the original nutritive value. Attention should also be paid to the inclusion in the diet of a frequent and varied series of foods that require vigorous mastication as a means to stimulate and exercise the various tissues and organs involved in the comminution of food. In addition a liberal source of vitamin D should be provided daily throughout the entire period of an individual's growth and development. A minimum of sticky, adherent high-carbohydrate foods with a low rate of clearance from the oral cavity should be consumed. After eating foods with a slow oral clearance, the teeth should be cleaned thoroughly by the procedure recommended by the dentist. As between-meal snacks, fresh fruits, vegetables, fruit juices, milk and other dairy products are much to be preferred to sticky high-carbohydrate foods. In the overall nutritional planning for improved dental health, one of the most important facets to be considered is the fluoridation of public water supplies.

BIBLIOGRAPHY

1. Scott, Ussing, Sognnaes and Wyckoff: J. Dent. Res., *31*, 74, 1952.
2. Sognnaes and Shaw: J. Am. Dent. Assoc., *44*, 489, 1952.
3. Orland, Blayney, Harrison, Reyniers, Trexler, Wagner, Gordon and Luckey: J. Dent. Res., *33*, 147, 1954.
4. Orland, Blayney, Harrison, Reyniers, Trexler, Ervin, Gordon and Wagner: J. Am. Dent. Assoc., *50*, 259, 1955.
5. Keyes: Arch. Oral Biol., *1*, 304, 1960.
6. Fitzgerald and Keyes: J. Am. Dent. Assoc., *61*, 9, 1960.
7. Fitzgerald, Jordan and Stanley: J. Dent. Res., *39*, 923, 1960.
8. Gibbons, Berman, Knoettner and Kapsimalis: Arch. Oral Biol., *11*, 549, 1966.
9. Berman and Gibbons: Arch. Oral Biol., *11*, 533, 1966.
10. Zinner, Jablon, Aran and Saslow: Proc. Soc. Exp. Biol. Med., *118*, 766, 1965.
10a. Berkowitz, Jordan and White: Arch. Oral Biol., *20*, 171, 1975.
10b. Gibbons, dePaola, Spinell and Skobe: Infect. Inmun., *9*, 481, 1974.
10c. Gibbons and vanHoute: J. Periodontol., *44*, 347, 1973.
11. Weisberger, Nelson and Boyle: Am. J. Orthod. Oral Surg., *26*, 88, 1940.
12. Schwartz and Shaw: J. Dent. Res., *34*, 239, 1955.
13. Afonsky: *Saliva and its Relation to Oral Health.* Birmingham, University of Alabama Press, 1961, pp. 21–30.
14. Kite, Shaw and Sognnaes: J. Nutr., *42*, 89, 1950.
15. Shaw: J. Nutr., *53*, 151, 1954.
16. Haldi, Wynn, Shaw and Sognnaes: J. Nutr., *49*, 295, 1953.
17. Anderson, Smith, Elvehjem and Phillips: J. Nutr., *35*, 371, 1948.
17a. König, Schmid and Schmid: Arch. Oral Biol., *13*, 13, 1968.
17b. Shaw: Arch. Oral Biol., *13*, 1003, 1968.
18. Gustafsson, Quensel, Lanke, Lundqvist, Grahnen, Bonow and Krasse: Acta Odontol. Scand., *11*, 232, 1954.

19. Schweigert, Shaw, Phillips and Elvehjem: J. Nutr., 29, 405, 1945.
20. Stewart, Hoppert and Hunt: J. Dent. Res., 32, 210, 1953.
21. Constant, Phillips and Elvehjem: J. Nutr., 46, 271, 1952.
22. Krasse: Arch. Oral Biol., 10, 215, 223, 1965.
23. Wood and Critchley: Arch. Oral Biol., 11, 1039, 1966.
24. Gibbons and Banghart: Arch. Oral Biol., 12, 11, 1967.
25. Fitzgerald, Keyes, Stoudt and Spinell: J. Am. Dent. Assoc., 76, 301, 1968.
26. Shaw, Krumins and Gibbons: Arch. Oral Biol., 12, 755, 1967.
27. Guggenheim, König, Mühlemann and Regolati: Arch. Oral Biol., 14, 555, 1969.
28. Stephan, Fitzgerald, McClure, Harris and Jordan: J. Dent. Res., 31, 421, 1952.
29. Phillips: J. Am. Diet. Assoc., 26, 85, 1950.
30. Stephan and Miller: Proc. Soc. Exp. Biol. Med., 55, 101, 1944.
31. Hunt, Hoppert and Erwin: J. Dent. Res., 23, 205, 1944.
32. Hodge, Johansen, Hein and Maynard: J. Dent. Res., 32, 654, 1953.
33. Larson: In Environmental Variables in Oral Disease. Washington, AAAS Publication No. 181, 1966.
34. Shaw, Griffiths and Terborgh: Arch. Oral Biol., 7, 693, 1962.
35. Larson and Simms: Science, 149, 982, 1965.
36. Wolbach and Howe: J. Exp. Med., 42, 753, 1925.
37. Wolbach and Howe: Am. J. Pathol., 9, 275, 1933.
38. Boyle: J. Dent. Res., 13, 39, 1933.
39. Dinnerman: Oral Surg., 4, 1024, 1951.
40. Sweeney, Cabrerra, Urrutia and Mata: J. Dent. Res., 48, 1275, 1969.
41. Sweeney, Saffir and deLeon: Am. J. Clin. Nutr., 24, 29, 1971.
42. Wolbach and Bessey: Arch. Pathol., 32, 689, 1941.
43. Dalldorf: In The Vitamins. Chicago, American Medical Association, 1939, p. 339.
44. Wolbach and Howe: Proc. Soc. Exp. Biol. Med., 22, 400, 1925.
45. Crampton: J. Nutr., 33, 491, 1947.
46. Boyle, Bessey and Howe: Arch. Pathol., 30, 90, 1940.
47. Boyle, Bessey and Wolbach: J. Am. Dent. Assoc., 24, 1768, 1937.
48. Westin: Dent. Cosmos, 67, 868, 1925.
49. Hanke: Diet and Dental Health. Chicago, University of Chicago Press, 1933.
49a.Dilley, Koerber and Roche: J. Dent. Child., 44, 35, 1977.
50. Westin: Uber Zahnveränderungen in Fällen von Skorbut bei Homo. Vol. 2. Stockholm, A. B. Fahlcrantz, 1931.
51. Hess and Abramson: Dent. Cosmos, 73, 849, 1931.
52. McBeath: J. Dent. Res., 12, 723, 1932.
53. Grandison, Stott and Cruickshank: Br. Dent. J., 72, 237, 1942.
54. Mellanby: Lancet, 2, 767, 1918.
55. Mellanby: Br. Dent. J., 44, 1031, 1923.
56. Weinman and Schour: Am. J. Pathol., 21, 821, 1945.
57. Sarnat and Schour: J. Am. Dent. Assoc., 28, 1989, 1941; 29, 67, 1942.
58. Mellanby: Special Report Series, Medical Research Council, Report No. 191. London, His Majesty's Stationery Office, 1934.
59. Mellanby, Coumoulos, Kelley and Neal: Br. Med. J., 2, 318, 1957.
60. Committee for the Investigation of Dental Disease: Special Report Series, Medical Research Council, Report No. 211. London, His Majesty's Stationery Office, 1936.
61. Agnew, Agnew and Tisdall: J. Am. Dent. Assoc., 20, 193, 1933; J. Pediat., 2, 190, 1933.
62. McBeath: Am. J. Public Health, 24, 1028, 1933.
63. McBeath and Verlin: J. Am. Dent. Assoc., 29, 1393, 1942.
64. Anderson, Williams, Halderson, Summerfeldt and Agnew: J. Am. Dent. Assoc., 21, 1349, 1934.
65. Day and Sedwick: J. Dent. Res., 14, 213, 1934; J. Nutr., 8, 309, 1934.
66. Mills: J. Dent. Res., 16, 417, 1937.
67. East: Am. J. Public Health, 29, 777, 1939.
68. Strälfors: Sven. Tandläk. Tidskr., 49, 108, 1956.
69. McClure: J. Nutr., 65, 619, 1958.
70. Sobel and Hanok: J. Biol. Chem., 176, 1103, 1948.
71. Sobel and Hanok: J. Dent. Res., 37, 631, 1958.
72. Sobel, Hanok and Shaw: Abstracts, 124th Meeting American Chemical Society. Abstract No. 173, p. 72, 1953.
73. Armstrong and Knowlton: J. Dent. Res., 21, 316, 1942.
74. Ham and Smith: Can. J. Res., 28, 227, 1950.
75. McClure: Public Health Rep., 64, 1061, 1949.
76. Schwarz: Fed. Proc., 33, 1748, 1974.
77. Bunting, Crowley, Hard and Keller: Dent. Cosmos, 70, 1002, 1928.
78. Dean, Jay, Arnold, McClure and Elvove: Public Health Rep., 54, 862, 1939.
79. Dean, Arnold and Elvove: Public Health Rep., 57, 1155, 1942.
80. Dean: Public Health Rep., 53, 1443, 1938.
81. Russell and Elvove: Public Health Rep., 66, 1389, 1951.
82. McClure and Likins: J. Dent. Res., 30, 172, 1951.
83. Zipkin, Posner and Eanes: Biochim. Biophys. Acta, 59, 255, 1962.
84. Zipkin, McClure and Lee: Arch. Oral Biol., 2, 190, 1960.
85. Zipkin and Posner: International Association for Dental Research, 40th General Meeting. Preprinted abstracts, 28, 103, 1962.
86. Jenkins and Speirs: J. Physiol., 121, 21, 1953.
87. Brudevold, Gardner and Smith: J. Dent. Res., 35, 420, 1956.
88. Isaac, Brudevold, Smith and Gardner: J. Dent. Res., 37, 318, 1958.
88a.Cooper and Ludwig: N.Z. Dent. J., 61, 33, 1965.
88b.Simpson and Quiglia: Odontol. Rev., 20, 1, 1969.

89. Sognnaes, Arnold, Hodge and Kline: Washington, National Research Council, Publication No. 294, 1953.

90. Ast, Smith, Wachs and Cantwell: J. Am. Dent. Assoc., *52*, 314, 1956.

91. Moulton (Ed.): *Fluorine and Dental Health.* Washington, American Association for the Advancement of Science, 1942.

92. Galagan and Vermillion: Public Health Rep., *72*, 491, 1957.

93. Shaw (Ed.): *Fluoridation as a Public Health Measure.* Washington, American Association for the Advancement of Science, 1954.

94. Leone: Arch. Ind. Health, *21*, 324 and 326, 1960.

95. Bernstein, Sadowsky, Hegsted, Guri and Stare: J.A.M.A., *198*, 499, 1966.

96. Rich and Ensinck: Nature, *191*, 184, 1961.

97. Rich and Ensinck: Clin. Res., *10*, 118, 1962.

98. Jowsey, Riggs, Kelly and Hoffman: Am. J. Med., *53*, 43, 1972.

99. Hanson and Roos: Am. J. Roentgenol., *126*, 1294, 1976.

99a. Kyle, Jowsey, Kelly and Taves: N. Engl. J. Med., *293*, 133, 1975.

100. Hill, Jelinek and Blayney: J. Dent. Res., *28*, 398, 1949.

101. Fluoridation Census, 1975 Annual Edition. Dental Disease Preventive Activity, Bureau of State Services, Center for Disease Control, Public Health Service, Atlanta.

102. Sognnaes: Am. J. Dis. Child., *75*, 792, 1948.

103. Toverud: Milbank Mem. Fund Q., *34*, 354, 1956; *35*, 127 and 373, 1957.

104. Cohen: Personal communication, 1954.

105. Toverud: Br. Dent. J., *86*, 191, 1949.

106. Sognnaes: J. Am. Dent. Assoc., *37*, 676, 1948.

107. Shaw and Sognnaes: Unpublished data.

108. Shaw and Sognnaes: J. Nutr., *53*, 207, 1954.

109. Sognnaes and Shaw: J. Nutr., *53*, 193, 1954.

110. Hodge: J. Dent. Res., *22*, 275, 1943.

111. Braunschneider, Hunt and Hoppert: J. Dent. Res., *27*, 154, 1948.

112. Constant, Sievert, Phillips and Elvehjem: J. Nutr., *53*, 29, 1954.

113. Sognnaes, Shaw and Bogoroch: Am. J. Physiol., *180*, 408, 1955.

114. Fanning, Shaw and Sognnaes: J. Am. Dent. Assoc., *49*, 668, 1954.

115. Briner, Francis and Rosen: International Association for Dental Research, 43rd General Meeting. Abstract 210, 1965.

116. Nizel and Harris: J. Dent. Res., *43*, 1123, 1964.

117. Strälfors: J. Dent. Res., *43*, 1137, 1964.

118. Ship and Mickelsen: J. Dent. Res., *43*, 1144, 1964.

119. Averill and Bibby: J. Dent. Res., *43*, 1150, 1964.

120. Sutfin, Sweeney and Ascoli: J. Dent. Res., *49*, 772, 1970.

121. Pederson: Dent. Rec., *58*, 191, 1938.

122. Pederson: Dtsch. Zahn. Mund. Küferheilkd., *6*, 728, 1939.

123. Boyd, Drain and Nelson: Am. J. Dis. Child., *38*, 721, 1929.

124. Boyd: Am. J. Dis. Child., *66*, 349, 1943.

125. Drain and Boyd: J. Am. Dent. Assoc., *22*, 155, 1935.

126. McBeath: J. Dent. Res., *12*, 723, 1932.

127. McBeath: J. Dent. Res., *13*, 243, 1933.

128. Howe, White and Rabine: Am. J. Dis. Child., *46*, 1045, 1933.

129. Howe, White and Elliott: J. Am. Dent. Assoc., *29*, 38, 1942.

130. Livermore: Dent. Surg., *18*, 1169, 1942.

131. Koehne and Bunting: J. Nutr., *7*, 657, 1934.

132. Koehne, Bunting and Morrell: Am. J. Dis. Child., *48*, 6, 1934.

133. Hankin, Chung and Kaw: J. Dent. Res., *52*, 1079, 1973.

134. Keene, Shklair and Hoerman: In *Comparative Immunology of the Oral Cavity* (Mergenhager and Scherp, Eds.). Bethesda, Public Health Service Publication NIH73–438, 1973.

135. Glass and Fleisch: J. Am. Dent. Assoc., *88*, 807, 1974.

136. McCarthy: J. Am. Dent. Assoc., *116*, 16, 1941.

137. Bernick: Oral Surg., *1*, 1098, 1948.

138. Weinmann: J. Periodontol., *12*, 71, 1941.

139. Taylor and Day: Br. Med. J., *2*, 221, 1940.

140. Becks and Morgan: J. Periodontol., *13*, 18, 1942.

141. Chapman and Harris: J. Infect. Dis., *69*, 7, 1941.

142. Tempest: Br. J. Surg., *53*, 949, 1966.

143. Mann, Mann and Spies: J. Am. Dent. Assoc., *32*, 1357, 1945.

144. Greene, Dreizen and Spies: J. Am. Dent. Assoc., *39*, 561, 1949.

Chapter *31*

NUTRITION IN DISEASES OF THE GASTROINTESTINAL TRACT

A. *Nutrition in Diseases of the Stomach, Including Related Areas in the Esophagus and Duodenum*

Harry D. Fein

Of primary concern to the clinician are the appraisal and analysis of the complaints of his patients. Thus he must have fundamental knowledge of the mechanisms operative in the production of the symptoms related to the various organ systems. First there must be appraisal of the site of the stimulus responsible for the symptom and the pathway of impulses to the area of manifestation, second, appreciation and understanding of the pain threshold of the patient and, third, reaction to the registered impulses both emotional and physiologic. This will help to determine functional and/or structural changes and choice of appropriate treatment of the patient. The frequent association of functional disorders and symptoms related thereto with structural disease must be recognized. The mechanism of the physiologic derangement may be purely local, secondary to the disease per se, but more often it is mediated through autonomic-hypothalamic-cerebral pathways as a result of the emotional trauma incidental to the presence of organic disease of a more or less serious nature.

The stomach is the seat of dyspepsia, the symptom complex of disordered motility and the common denominator of most upper abdominal complaints. It may not be the lesion itself which produces the symptoms but the gastric or gastrointestinal neuromuscular dysfunction which the lesion initiates. Distant diseases can produce the same disturbances of the stomach's neuromuscular activity and therefore the same symptoms. The trigger mechanism may lie elsewhere in the abdomen, in the emotions or generalized throughout the body. Thus the patient with gastric cancer or pancreatic or biliary tract disease may have the same type of abnormal stomach sensations as the patient with peptic ulcer, neurosis or some generalized systemic infection or disease. As far as stomach complaints are concerned, the patient relates as much about the way his stomach is reacting to the disturbing disease as about the disease itself. Various affections of the stomach may cause anorexia and consequent nutritional impairment from restricted food intake. The stomach, in relation to its configuration and motility, is so complex that the proper interpretation of the result of its study is often difficult. This difficulty is reflected in the observation that opinion regarding diagnosis and treatment of stomach disease may vary from locality to locality and from gastroenterologist to gastroenterologist.

THE ROLE OF THE STOMACH IN NUTRITION

Cannon[1] has noted that Galen stated that the main functions of the stomach were to receive and retain food during the processes of chemical digestion and then to pass the changed material onward. Beaumont's experiments in 1825 made clear that this was indeed the case.[2] The stomach receives all types of food, acting as the great reservoir in the first or salivary stage of digestion. It maintains the second or gastric stage, where the ingested material is altered in such a way that the resultant chyme is discharged slowly and intermittently into the duodenum and small intestine without irritating those structures. This is accomplished by two types of motor activity, namely, tonus and peristalsis. The mechanism that regulates gastric emptying and determines the rate at which food leaves the stomach is complex, subject to many influences and as yet not fully understood.

The gastric juice represents a mixture of gastric secretion, saliva and intestinal contents refluxed from the duodenum. Clinically, the gastric secretion is a complex and variable mixture of water, inorganic ions, including hydrogen and bicarbonate (when acid is absent), and a number of organic constituents. Among the latter are several active enzymes and their precursors, three or more different mucins and their degradation products, the intrinsic factor of Castle and a variety of other substances derived in minute amounts from interstitial fluid and cellular degradation.[3]

Immunoelectrophoretic studies seem to have confirmed the existence of four pepsinogens and four pepsins.[4] The relative proportions of these may vary from person to person. In patients with normal gastric mucosa, the pepsin activity in gastric juice usually parallels the HCl output. The func-

tion of pepsin in the stomach is to hydrolyze proteins to proteoses and peptones, in preparation for further and more complete degradation in the intestine.

Mucous products are produced by various cells in the stomach. These are mucoproteins composed of mucopolysaccharide and protein moieties. They exist in visible and dissolved forms. The visible mucus covers the entire lining of the mucosa and forms the first line of defense for the gastric mucosa against mechanical, thermal and chemical trauma.

Of special interest to the clinician are the hormones and drugs which exert a stimulating or inhibitory action on gastric secretion. The hormone gastrin (peptides I and II), produced by the antrum of the stomach in response to vagal stimulation, distention by food and probably by exposure of the mucosa to the products of protein digestion, is the most potent stimulus to gastric secretion known. Histamine and its analog, betazole, are the best-known commercially available chemical stimulants of gastric secretion. Pentagastrin, a derivative of the active portion of the peptide hormone gastrin, is now also available. The stomach, which receives most prescribed medications, is subject to erosion, ulceration, hypersecretion and intolerance to drugs. The anti-inflammatory agents—the salicylates,[5] phenylbutazone, indomethacin, glucocorticoids and ACTH[6,7]—may be particularly injurious. Colchicine, para-aminosalicylic acid, tolbutamide and caffeine seem to facilitate ulcer formation by reducing mucosal resistance. Caffeine may also increase acid-peptic secretion, as do alcohol, aminophyllin, isonicotinic acid hydrazide and reserpine. Caffeine sustains and potentiates other stimuli of hydrochloric acid secretion and reduces mucosal regeneration.

Different foods, or their pleasurable or indifferent anticipation, may influence gastric secretion differently. Fatty foodstuffs exert an inhibitory effect on secretion by way of the gastrone mechanism. Carbohydrates, in the average diet, as a rule neither stimulate nor inhibit gastric secretion. Protein foods, such as meat, fish, chicken, cheese and milk, are stimulants of gastric acidity. The protein renders the gastric contents neutral or nearly so and thus antral hormone is liberated.

The motor functions of the stomach are among the most important in the alimentary tract. They are complex and not fully understood. The tonic and peristaltic activity of the empty stomach stops abruptly during the ingestion of food, thus permitting an increase in the intragastric volume under a relatively constant intragastric pressure (3 to 6 cm H_2O). Peristaltic activity resumes shortly thereafter with contractions limited to the pyloric region, followed in 5 to 10 minutes by waves originating higher in the fundus of the stomach. The mechanism that regulates gastric emptying and determines the rate at which food leaves the stomach is subject to many influences. There is a definite pattern of gastric emptying and, under physiologic circumstances, any variation in the rate of emptying results primarily from changes in stroke volume. At first the volume of the gastric meal decreases rapidly, and then with time more slowly, with the result that a comparatively constant percentage of the remaining meal is evacuated per minute.

In the normal stomach several factors are known to influence gastric emptying. The hypertonic stomach tends to be hypermotile and to empty more rapidly than the hypotonic one. Liquids leave the stomach more rapidly than do semisolids or solids, whether ingested separately or not, and the rate of emptying is much greater with large-sized meals. This is all relevant to the occurrence of a dumping-like syndrome, even in certain normal persons, after large meals, and the beneficial effect of small meals on some persons and on the number of stools in patients with diarrhea. Carbohydrates leave the stomach more quickly than proteins, and proteins leave more quickly than fats. Fats and fatty acids entering the intestine release enterogastrone, which acts to delay the evacuation of the stomach and to suppress its secretion. Hypertonic and hypotonic solutions remain in the stomach longer than isotonic solutions, probably to facilitate osmotic adjustment in the duodenum. A meal eaten at the time of marked hunger is generally evacuated more rapidly, probably because of increased tonus. Severe or protracted pain, especially of visceral origin, tends to decrease motor activity and evacuation. The emotional state may also markedly influence stomach activity. Generally, aggressive experiences are associated with increased motor activity, while depressive states result in decreased contractions and delayed evacuation of the stomach.

Disturbances of the vital functions of the stomach by disease or by partial or almost total removal of the stomach invariably result in local or generalized symptoms of varying degree. Stomach emptying and function may thus be altered by a variety of physiologic states. In addition systemic disorders such as hypokalemia, diabetic acidosis and neuropathy and uremia, as well as gastric ulcer itself, may result in gastric retention and decreased gastric secretion. Obstruction in the region of the pylorus from whatever cause partially or completely impairs gastric emptying.

The relation between nutrition and diseases of the stomach is a complex one. Diseases of the upper gastrointestinal tract may interfere with the actual intake of food by disturbing appetite, inducing nausea and vomiting, evoking pain or producing mechanical obstruction. Traditionally, the medical therapy of disorders of the upper gastrointestinal tract has been in a large measure dietetic, though now there is some question as to the importance of rigid prolonged dietary restriction in diseases such as peptic ulcer. Surgical therapy of the stomach may of itself lead to malfunction and nutritional disturbances requiring correction.

DYSPEPSIA

Dyspepsia may be defined as difficult or deranged digestion, a disordered state of the stomach in which its functions are disturbed. Ordinarily there is no awareness of digestive activity, except a sense of satisfaction. In the dyspeptic from whatever cause, a characteristic variety of complaints referable to the upper gastrointestinal tract are present: aerophagy, bitter taste, bad breath, anorexia, nausea, heartburn, acrid or fetid eructions, a sense of fullness or bloating especially after meals, epigastric distress or pain, substernal discomfort or pain, regurgitation and vomiting, rumination, so-called cardiospasm and dysphagia. Dyspepsia can thus be thought of under two main headings: (1) *organic dyspepsia*, which arises directly from organic disease of the upper gastrointestinal tract, reflexly from other parts of the intestinal tract or from organic disease elsewhere in the body, and (2) *functional dyspepsia*, which constitutes the majority of cases seen by the gastroenterologist, well over 50 per cent of any group.

Dyspepsia of reflex origin is quite frequent. Disease of the biliary tract, liver disease, diseases of the pancreas and enterocolonic disease, for example, may all reflexly affect gastric function and digestion, thus giving rise to any or many of the symptoms previously mentioned. A careful search must be made for disease or dysfunction in organs or organ systems other than the stomach. Dyspepsia may be secondary to one of many systemic diseases other than those found primarily in the gastrointestinal tract: atherosclerosis (generalized, coronary or cerebral), hypertensive vascular disease, chronic renal disease, diabetes and other metabolic or endocrine disturbances, blood dyscrasias, collagen disease, lymphomas and other malignant diseases.

Most primary functional derangements of the gastrointestinal tract can be attributed to emotional tension. Visceral responses to emotional trauma have been observed in a variety of subjects by endoscopic examinations, balloon techniques and radiologic study. Disturbances of motility, tonus, secretion and vascularity have been noted. Personality patterns and their expressions are determined by experiences in early life, so that emotional behavior occurring in association with disease or physiologic derangement is the result of a complex series of interactions.

Many conditioning factors will modify the character of the complaint. The disorders encountered as the result of emotional change may be classified into (1) hyperfunction, (2) hypofunction and (3) mixed types. As the result of one or a combination of these physiologic disorders, the patient may complain of a variety of symptoms—pain, pyrosis, dysphagia, abdominal fullness, anorexia, nausea, vomiting and the other symptoms previously listed under dyspepsia. In this group there will be a variety of diagnostic types: the psychoneurotic, the infantile, the dependent, the aggressive and the frustrated.

Treatment

The treatment of this functional group of dyspeptics requires great skill on the part of the physician. He must be versed in the functional physiologic disorders so that he is able to dissect out and recognize the nature of the problem, and recognize the presence of emotional aberrations and physiologic effects. Treatment must be directed to the patient as a whole, with warm sympathetic understanding. Treatment directed toward the involved organ per se is only palliative. A careful explanation of the mechanism for the production of the symptoms is of utmost importance. If no amelioration of emotional stress is achieved by specific therapy, or refractoriness is noted, psychiatric help should be sought.

A prudent bland diet (see Appendix Table 21) covers the average nutritional needs. It avoids the excessive amounts of saturated fats characteristic of the average American diet and highly spiced and seasoned foods and condiments. It provides for regularity of eating patterns. A general suggestion is the avoidance of stress at meals, haste in eating and bolting of food.

Tobacco, particularly cigarettes, is to be prohibited in such patients. It often causes pseudo-ulcer syndromes as well as interfering with appetite and normal digestion. Alcohol, as a general rule, is forbidden dyspeptic patients. There are some who can tolerate an occasional well-diluted alcoholic beverage and benefit from its relaxing effect. This may be permitted provided it is taken with food. The excessive use of coffee and other caffein-containing beverages is likewise discouraged.

The management of the dyspeptic patient presents many problems and the approach is not primarily a dietary one. If organic disease is present, resulting in reflex dyspepsia, treatment for the underlying condition is of paramount importance. The patient with functional dyspepsia requires special and individual attention.

DISEASE OF THE ESOPHAGUS

No attempt will be made to cover all the known diseases of the esophagus. Only those which interfere with nutrition, or those which disturb nutrition, will be considered. These are the ones that stem from derangements of motility or from reflux of acid into the esophagus, or those which cause obstruction to the free passage of food.

An understanding of the anatomy and physiology of the esophagus is important. This should include knowledge of the normal radiographic and endoscopic appearances and their relationship to the other mediastinal structures, because of possible involvement in diseases originating elsewhere. The only important function of the esophagus is to transmit food from the mouth to the stomach. Its secretory function appears to be minimal and it possesses no significant absorptive func-

tions. The normal motor activity and its upper and lower sphincters are dependent upon a series of stimulatory and inhibitory reflex neural actions. The tone of the lower esophageal sphincter is known to be influenced by the gastrointestinal hormones gastrin and secretin, insulin hypoglycemia and even cigarette smoking.[8,10] Presently it is felt that the intrinsic myogenic activity of the sphincter muscle is the basis for basal sphincter tone.

The function of the upper esophageal sphincter is to separate the cavity of the hypopharynx from the lumen of the esophagus except during swallowing, by remaining tonically closed. The sphincter is about 3 cm in length with an intrasphincteric resting pressure of 15 to 30 cm of water above atmosphere. Resting intraluminal pressure in the upper esophagus is a few cm of water below atmospheric pressure. Within 0.1 to 0.3 seconds after the onset of swallowing the upper esophageal sphincter begins to relax, permitting the bolus to pass into the upper esophagus.

The primary function of the lower esophageal sphincter is considered to be prevention of gastroesophageal reflux. As does the upper sphincter, the lower one remains in a state of chronic contraction except during the act of swallowing. The upper sphincter is composed of striated muscle, whereas the lower one is made up of smooth muscle. Functionally the two sphincters have a great deal in common. In normal individuals the high pressure zone of the lower sphincter is usually about 4 cm in length, with basal resting pressures of 15 to 20 cm of water. The basal resting pressure in the lower esophagus is 4 to 6 cm of water below atmospheric pressure and, in the fundus of the stomach, 6 to 8 cm of water above atmospheric pressure.

Achalasia

This is a generalized disorder of esophageal motility caused by a lack of integrated parasympathetic stimulation and associated with lack of tone, non-propulsive motility of the body of the esophagus and only brief partial receptive relaxation of the lower esophageal sphincter. The disorganized motility is the result of deranged postganglionic cholinergic innervation, with ganglion cell degeneration. The functional obstruction at or near the level of the hiatus esophagus eventually results in dilatation of the thoracic esophagus. Achalasia is widely distributed geographically; it rarely occurs in two or more members of the same family but it has been reported in children, siblings and twins.[11] It occurs with equal frequency in both sexes. Most commonly the onset of symptoms is during the fourth to sixth decade. Dysphagia occurs in nearly all patients, regurgitation in 70 per cent and substernal discomfort in about 30 per cent. Frequently the onset is abrupt and often follows a shock, emotional upset or food indiscretion. At the beginning the symptoms are intermittent; eating slowly and swallowing some water will relieve them. Later the dysphagia is more frequent and severe, followed by regurgitation. The rate of progression is unpredictable and depends on the extent of ganglion cell degeneration. Aspiration, particularly at night, may lead to serious pulmonary infections.

Reduction of food intake because of sitophobia (fear of eating) or loss of food by regurgitation of esophageal content results in marked weight loss. Anemia and other evidence of nutritional deficiency— glossitis, cheilosis and peripheral neuropathy—may be seen when the esophagus is markedly dilated. The diagnosis is not difficult to make, utilizing special radiographic and motility techniques. Carcinoma must be looked for, since its incidence is increased in long-standing achalasia. It must be differentiated from Chagas' disease, scleroderma, neuromuscular disorders, hypertensive gastroesophageal sphincter, presbyesophagus and diffuse esophageal spasm.

The most common complication is esophagitis. The diagnosis can be made only by endoscopy, when the characteristic changes of redness, inflammation, swelling, erosions and small ulcerations, up to the height of the area of retained food, can be seen. Hemorrhage, perforation and periesophagitis may complicate static esophagitis. The objective of treatment is to weaken the lower esophageal sphincter sufficiently to allow food to gravitate into the stomach without destroying the sphincter action of the vestibule. This is accomplished by forceful dilatation or by esophagomyotomy.

Once the diagnosis is established, the patient must be reassured with an explanation of the disorder. He must avoid emotional turmoil, especially at meals, and anxiety must be relieved by sedation. Faulty dietary and eating habits must be corrected. The patient should be instructed to eat slowly, chew food thoroughly, use liquids to wash down a mouthful of food and not eat before retiring. Nutritional supplements in liquid form may be freely used.

Before dilatation or surgery is attempted, the nutrition should be improved as much as possible. The diet should be semiliquid or liquid; in some instances, as in peptic ulcer disease, hourly feeding may be employed. Tube feedings may be necessary. In the markedly malnourished individual, total parenteral nutrition may have to be employed. Supplemental vitamins, iron by injection, transfusions and salt-poor albumin may also be necessary.

After satisfactory drainage of the esophagus has been achieved, the patient should be maintained on a bland diet for several weeks, avoiding alcohol, caffeinated drinks, spices, condiments, iced drinks and any mucosal irritants.

Reflux Esophagitis and Esophageal Ulcer

In 1935, Winkelstein[12] described peptic esophagitis as a new clinical entity. He emphasized the association of esophagitis with duodenal ulcer disease. Recently it has been recognized that reflux esophagitis may occur in the absence of duodenal ulcer or sliding hiatus hernia. The emphasis is upon reflux through an incompetent gastroesophageal sphincter. Mechanical factors such as hiatus hernia, patulous hiatus or nasogastric intubation may contribute to sphincter incompetence. The primary barrier to reflux is the intrinsic lower esophageal sphincter.

The symptoms are caused by reflux or the complications of esophagitis. Pain is noted in the low retrosternal area but may spread to the epigastrium and to the interscapular region, neck or even down both arms. It is a burning sensation, called heartburn, coming on shortly after eating and on bending over or lying down. The patient may be awakened by the discomfort. Regurgitation is common, and reflux symptoms are frequently precipitated by changes in position which compress the abdomen or increase intragastric pressure. Aerophagia and coexisting duodenal ulcer disease may confuse the picture. Reflux may also give rise to dysphagia because of esophageal spasm. Odynophagia, or painful swallowing, may occur during exacerbations of reflux esophagitis.

The complications, which may be troublesome and severe, include peptic ulcer of the esophagus, stenosis or stricture, bleeding, aspiration with its pulmonary complications, occasional perforation, Barrett's syndrome and Zenker's diverticulum. Medical therapy should include measures to prevent reflux. Tobacco, caffeine-containing drinks, fatty food and overdistention of the stomach should be avoided. These relax the lower esophageal sphincter. When the symptoms are severe the dietary management should be that of active symptomatic ulcer disease, starting with small frequent feedings on an hourly basis and then progressing to a graduated diet. The patient should avoid condiments, spices and extremes of hot and cold foods and drinks; he should abstain from alcohol and any ulcerogenic or irritating drugs.

The frequent and adequate ingestion of liquid antacids is recommended to neutralize esophageal contents (15 to 30 cc). Anticholinergic agents should not be given. Topical anesthetics before meals may help decrease the pain. Cholestyramine has helped in the control of bile acid reflux. Bethanechol, by increasing lower esophageal sphincter pressure and promoting gastric emptying, has been shown to be a helpful adjunct to the therapy of the patient with chronic gastroesophageal reflux (25 mg q.i.d.) who has failed to respond to the usual modalities of therapy. The H_2 receptor blocking agents, such as cimetidine, have also been shown to be effective in patients with chronic reflux. Sleeping with the chest elevated, blocks under the head of the bed or a device between the mattress and spring keeps the gastroesophageal junction higher than the level of the gastric contents and will help prevent reflux.

HIATUS HERNIA

This is defined as a protrusion of a portion of the stomach above the diaphragm into the chest, having passed through the normal esophageal hiatus. (It does not include congenital hernia or hernia through any other abnormal opening in the diaphragm.) Hiatus hernia is the most common structural abnormality affecting the upper gastrointestinal tract. It must be understood that hiatus hernia, like many other mechanical defects, causes illness or symptoms in only a small proportion of the people it affects. The frequency of recognizable hernias rises with age from 9 per cent in patients under the age of 40 to 69 per cent in those over 70.[13] The diagnosis is usually of clinical importance only when reflux of acid, which may lead to reflux esophagitis and even stricture, is present.

Several forms of hiatus hernia have been described. *Paraesophageal hernia* occurs when a portion of peritoneum enters the chest, followed by some of the greater curvature of the stomach. This is a relatively rare condition; it is not accompanied by reflux because the lower end of the esophagus remains beneath the diaphragm and the closing mechanism of the cardia is unimpaired. It is of importance when incarceration occurs and it becomes a surgical emergency. *Sliding hiatus hernia* is the common type of hiatus hernia. It is important because its presence interferes with the normal protective mechanisms around the cardia which prevent reflux into the esophagus. If the hernia is permanently fixed above the diaphragm, congestion of the gastric mucosa may result in gastritis and even ulcerations in the herniated sac. On occasion a true gastric ulcer may result.

Pyrosis or heartburn is probably the most common subjective complaint of the individual with hiatus hernia. It occurs most frequently with a direct sliding hernia, and reflux is considered to be the most common cause. It is not necessarily the amount of gastric acid that determines the occurrence of heartburn of reflux origin; this is more likely to be associated with the presence of duodenal ulcer. Pyrosis may occur with reflux in association with anacidity and in the achlorhydria associated with gastric resection. Gillison et al.[14] have suggested that regurgitation of bile and pancreatic secretions as a result of pyloric incompetency, if associated with hiatus hernia and reflux, may be a cause of heartburn and esophagitis. Heartburn may also occur in hiatus hernia in the absence of reflux. Changes in intraluminal pressure in relation to dilatation or spasm, localized or diffuse, may give rise to the sensation.

Pain

Some patients also complain of actual pain, with or without pyrosis. The pain is described as a lump, ball, pressure, tightness or fullness. It is often initiated by or aggravated by eating particularly large meals, emotional upsets or physical exer-

tion after eating. Discomfort may also be felt in the region of the pharynx and be misinterpreted as being caused by intrinsic disease in that region.

Dysphagia, or a sense of food sticking in the esophagus, is less common. It is more common in paraesophageal hernias or when some degree of stricture is present with a direct sliding hernia.

Bleeding

This may be secondary to esophagitis or erosions in the gastric pouch in the chest. A slow ooze is most common and may amount to 15 ml per day. Among the most common causes of asymptomatic gastrointestinal blood loss anemia in a person over 40 is hiatus hernia. The bleeding may also be massive, usually short lived, not repeated and often associated with the ingestion of salicylates.

Chronic Lung Disease

A common complication of hiatus hernia and peptic esophagitis, as well as of obstructive disease of the esophagus, is chronic lung disease because of nocturnal regurgitation and aspiration.[15] This complication requires surgical correction.

Treatment

Therapy of symptomatic hiatus hernia is primarily medical and conservative, as for peptic esophagitis. Dietary management is important. Weight reduction is essential for the obese patient. Fats may lower the lower esophageal sphincter pressure just as proteins tend to maintain it. Weight should be lost gradually. In the presence of active symptoms, the diet should be bland. Small frequent feedings are desirable; certainly the evening meal should be small. Eating during the evening and before retiring is not desirable and should be prohibited in the patient with night distress. Avoidance of physical exercise or effort or reclining after meals should be practiced.

Antacids are of the greatest value. They neutralize the hydrochloric acid in the stomach and raise the lower esophageal sphincter pressure by increasing the amount of circulating gastrin.[16] They may be given hourly if necessary. On occasion an aluminum gel combined with magnesium hydroxide before meals may be helpful. An aluminum gel with sodium bicarbonate and magnesium trisilicate combined in tablets and chewed and swallowed with water after meals may also be beneficial, especially in the patient with associated esophagitis. Anticholinergics are contraindicated, but mild sedation in liquid form is of value.

Elevating the head of the bed or placing devices between the spring and mattress, as in the treatment of peptic esophagitis, is advised.

Operation is not advised initially in the absence of an urgent surgical complication. Medical therapy should be pursued. Only when severe symptoms persist in spite of good conservative management or in the presence of complications, such as stenosis or persistent ulceration in the esophagus or gastric pouch, should surgery be advised. Chronic bleeding giving rise to chronic anemia which cannot be overcome by iron administration and massive bleeding may be considered as possible surgical indications. The risk of surgery in the elderly is so great that palliative treatment should be pursued, even though it does not bring about complete relief. Stricture, when present, has in many instances been successfully treated with bougie dilatation, without surgery, and this should be tried.

GASTRITIS

Gastritis is at least as common as gastric and duodenal ulcer combined. The thinking regarding diffuse gastric mucosal disease has in the past been confused, but it is much less so now because of direct observation made feasible by the advances in endoscopy, gastric photography and gastric biopsy. There is little dispute about acute gastritis. The more clinically impor-

tant chronic gastritis, however, has been more actively studied and debated.

Acute gastritis may be divided into four types: (1) simple exogenous, (2) corrosive, (3) infectious (hematogenous) and (4) phlegmonous. The acute simple variety is frequent at any age and is characterized by malaise, anorexia, nausea and vomiting. It may be due to infection with a specific microorganism or a virus. The disease may last from one to several days and, if food cannot be taken orally, the patient may be sustained by intravenous fluids. The immediate therapy of acute corrosive gastritis must combat collapse and consists of intravenous feedings until oral intake becomes feasible.

Acute infectious or hematogenous gastritis is a form of acute gastritis arising from toxins or bacteria entering the stomach from the blood stream. Avoidance of food may be helpful to the patient, but starvation must not be allowed. If oral intake can be instituted a bland diet should be given; otherwise intravenous feedings should be used. Acute phlegmonous gastritis is a rather rare purulent diffuse or localized inflammation of the gastric wall. General supportive measures and specific therapy for the underlying disease are indicated. At times surgery may be necessary.

Chronic nonspecific gastritis is clinically more important than the acute variety. Based on gastroscopic observations it may be divided into three types: (1) Superficial gastritis is a form in which the mucosa is reddened, edematous and covered with adherent mucus; mucosal hemorrhages and small erosions are frequent. (2) Atrophic gastritis is characterized by a thinned, gray or greenish-gray hemorrhagic mucosa; the atrophy usually is distributed irregularly, but the entire stomach may be affected. (3) Hypertrophic gastritis presents a dull spongy or nodular appearing mucosa, the rugae are irregular, thickened or nodular and hemorrhages and superficial erosions are frequent. Gastritis occurring after gastroenterostomy or partial gastric resection combines the manifestations of all three types. Menetrier's disease (giant gastric rugae) is noted most commonly in the midportion of the stomach along the greater curvature, although there may be diffuse involvement.

The etiology and pathogenesis of chronic gastritis are not known. Dietary indiscretions, alcohol, tobacco, coffee, infections and nutritional deficiencies have been implicated, but the evidence is inconclusive. All types of chronic gastritis are observed in association with peptic ulcer, but atrophy is more frequent in gastric than in duodenal ulcer, whereas hyperplastic mucosa is more common in duodenal than in gastric ulcer. Atrophy of the gastric mucosa is invariably present with pernicious anemia and gastric polyposis and is not infrequently found with sprue, pellagra and iron deficiency anemia. A possible immune mechanism in the development of gastric atrophy has been suggested.[17]

The consequences of chronic nonspecific gastritis are not known. The course seems to be persistent or recurrent with unpredictable variations in type, severity and distribution in the same person. Minor surface alterations, such as erosions, hemorrhages and hyperemia, usually heal completely. Severe and complete atrophy of the stomach generally tends to continue unchanged. In elderly patients, especially women, deficiency of vitamin B_{12} may develop, but it does not progress to pernicious anemia. The associated clinical manifestations include weakness, loss of memory, mental depression, paresthesias and abdominal discomfort with flatulence. These symptoms frequently respond to treatment with vitamin B_{12}. Deficiencies of iron and other vitamins also may be associated with atrophy of the gastric mucosa. The most frequent complaints are loss of appetite, fullness, belching, vague epigastric pain, nausea and vomiting. These are also the symptoms of functional distress;

they may be relieved by the use of a bland diet, antispasmodic drugs and hydrochloric acid.

PEPTIC ULCER

An important cause of sickness and death, peptic ulcer has been the subject of millions of dollars of research and the cause of many more millions lost in illness and nonproductiveness. It affects about 10 per cent of the world's population. It is most often found in patients with rheumatoid arthritis, chronic obstructive pulmonary disease and, probably, cirrhosis, especially after a portacaval shunt. Chronic peptic ulcer develops when acid-pepsin gastric juice destroys the mucosa, the submucosa and sometimes the muscular layer of the digestive tract. The areas of the digestive tract affected can include the lower portion of the esophagus, the stomach, the first portion of the duodenum, the jejunum after gastroenterostomy, Meckel's diverticulum containing functioning gastric glands and the lower duodenum and jejunum in the patient with the Zollinger-Ellison syndrome.

The ulcers usually occur along the lesser curvature of the stomach or in the duodenal bulb. Peptic ulcer is of itself a benign disease. It can occur at any time from infancy to later in life. The highest incidence occurs between ages 45 and 55. Gastric ulcer, duodenal ulcer and perforation occur more often in men than in women, although the relative frequency varies with the type of ulcer, the geographic location and the patient's age.

The exact etiology of peptic ulcer is not understood. It is clear, however, that ulcers occur when an imbalance exists between acid-pepsin secretion and mucosal resistance. Patients with a family history of peptic ulcer and patients with blood group O are at high risk. Close relatives of patients with ulcer have approximately three times as many ulcers as members of the general population. Relatives of patients with duodenal ulcers will tend to have duodenal ulcers; relatives of patients with gastric ulcers will tend to have gastric ulcers. Patients with blood group O develop duodenal ulcer more often than do patients with blood groups A, B, and AB.

Gastric ulcer and duodenal ulcer, the two principal types of peptic ulcer, differ in location, pathogenesis, malignant potential and association with drug ingestion. Both gastric and duodenal ulcers are characterized by high recurrence rates. Periods of symptomatic ulcer pain lasting up to several weeks are typically interspersed with longer asymptomatic intervals.

Most gastric ulcers arise at the border between acid-secreting (oxyntic gland) mucosa and antral (pyloric gland) mucosa on the lesser curvature of the stomach. Almost invariably they are found in an area of gastritis on the antral side of this border. However, gastric ulcers may occur in the distal antrum or pyloric channel and ulcerogenic drugs may produce ulcer in gastric mucosa free of gastritis. The gastritis of gastric ulcer patients usually involves the entire antrum. Some patients have gastritis that invades the acid-secreting portion. Extensive invasion causes the antrum to enlarge by metaplasia. It also causes the ulcer to develop at the new higher antral border. The chronic gastritis found in most gastric ulcer patients is probably the result of excessive reflux of duodenal contents into the stomach. It is caused by a defect in motor activity, such as incompetence of the pyloric sphincter. Bile and pancreatic juice repeatedly attack the gastric mucosa, leading to chronic gastritis. Mucosa affected by chronic gastritis shows a lowered resistance to acid pepsin, and the ulcer formation process is facilitated.

Much research is being conducted on the hypersecretion of acid, but little is understood about the function of normal mucosa and the factors that control tissue resistance to acid. At least four factors influence gastroduodenal mucosal resistance: (1) the integrity of mucosal cells, (2)

the equality of epithelial regeneration, (3) the mucosal barrier and (4) the blood supply. When one of these factors is impaired or when such irritants as aspirin, alcohol, antihypertensive drugs, caffeine, adrenal steroids and other anti-inflammatory drugs or bile acids come in contact with the mucosa, the normal barrier to diffusion of hydrochloric acid into the mucosa is damaged. Among the factors that contribute to impaired mucosal resistance in patients with gastric ulcer are: (1) poor nutrition, (2) low mucosal blood flow and (3) a defect in the antral inhibition of gastric secretion.

Duodenal ulcer, a common disease as previously stated, is less common now than it was 20 years ago, though the reason for this decreased incidence is not clear. Men are affected 2 to 3 times more frequently than are women, and the average age of the ulcer patient has increased. Psychologic factors may play some role in the pathogenesis of duodenal ulcer, but no distinct personality type is free of the disease. Also, it is difficult to relate specific stressful situations to the appearance or recurrence of symptomatic ulcers. The best-defined functional abnormalities in duodenal ulcer patients are an increased capacity to secrete acid and pepsin and a loss of normal autoregulation of acid secretion by a low pH of the gastric contents. Consequently, patients with duodenal ulcer disease deliver larger acid loads to the duodenum, on the average, than do normal subjects.

The duodenal mucosa has not been studied extensively in patients with duodenal ulcer. Some patients who secrete large quantities of acid do not develop duodenal ulcers, while some who secrete normal amounts of acid do develop them. Thus there must be factors that alter resistance or susceptibility to ulceration in specific patients, but these factors are not yet understood. No systematic biopsy studies have been carried out to determine whether ulcer patients have underlying mucosal changes of "duodenitis" similar to the gastritis found in gastric ulcer patients. Serum and antral concentrations of gastrin are relatively normal. This peptide hormone is known to be a potent stimulant of acid secretion by the parietal cells of the stomach.

Medical Management

The controversy regarding physiologic gastric rest by dietary control in ulcer patients started during the 19th century. Some advocated an empty stomach, whereas others advocated hourly feedings of milk or milk combinations in an attempt to achieve neutralization of the free hydrochloric acid. The Sippy regimen of hourly milk combinations was interspersed with antacid powders.[18] The value of strict dietary control in the management of peptic ulcer is not entirely settled. Many dietary concepts have been examined, some endorsed and some condemned on the basis of individual experiences, controlled studies or statistical analysis. A basic dietary formulation acceptable to all physicians and to all patients, and applicable to all phases of ulcer disease, has not yet evolved.[19-21]

Most physicians agree that a dietary regimen of the Sippy type is unnecessary, except in the acute phase of the active ulcer, when there is some justification for the traditional dietary modifications.

The overall aim of dietary control is to provide "physiologic rest" for the stomach, reduce mechanical trauma, minimize the effects of the ingesta on the chemical phase of gastric secretion and, most importantly, provide nourishment with maximum neutralizing capacity. Known stimulants of gastric secretion, such as alcohol and caffeine-containing beverages, should be avoided. Direct mucosal irritants, such as black pepper, chili, vinegar, mustard, pickles and irritating spices, should be eliminated entirely.

Small frequent feedings provide the most consistent buffering effects. In addition, total bulk is adjusted to avoid the distention stimulus to the antral gastric mechanism. Studies by Code et al. leave little doubt that all foods stimulate the production of gastric juice.[22] The secretory pattern for each food is rather characteristic, similar patterns being obtained with the bread and cereal group, fruit and vegetables, milk and dairy products and the meat, fish and egg group. Protein is the most important acid stimulator of the foods tested. The highest acid secretory equivalent values are found in meat, fish and dairy products. The least stimulating foods, the carbohydrates and fats, are also the least neutralizing. The more effective neutralizers, amphoteric proteins, are the strongest secretogogues.

The following dietary principles should be acceptable in all instances relating to ulcers. The diet should be adequate to meet in full the nutritional needs of the patient with a margin of safety to compensate for various stresses, undernutrition, growth, development and normal physical activity. Caloric inadequacy for periods of 7 to 10 days during the management of the acute phase of ulcer disease presents no real nutritional deficiency or dietary problem. Obesity should be corrected because of its well-known harmful physical effects. Psychologic factors should be recognized. The creation of the proper atmosphere at mealtimes certainly has favorable motor and secretory influences. Any concomitant diseases requiring dietary regulation—protein restriction in liver and renal disease, limitation of sodium, control in diabetes, restriction of gluten in patients with gluten enteropathy—must obviously be taken into consideration.

The literature has emphasized the hazards of diets high in saturated fats and cholesterol in the high-risk coronary-ulcer group. Excessive cholesterol and triglycerides in the blood may predispose to atherosclerosis and, therefore, increase the incidence of coronary artery disease and possibly cerebrovascular episodes. In studies of patients and of postmortem data, the incidence of myocardial infarction was found to be twice as high in patients with peptic ulcer who had been treated with a Sippy diet or milk products as it was in those who did not follow such a diet, or in control subjects without ulcer. The incidence of myocardial infarcts, in general, is higher in patients with chronic peptic ulcer disease than in subjects without ulcer. Studies have shown that diets in which 40 per cent of the calories are derived from fat, mainly saturated, produce high levels of serum cholesterol, whereas equicaloric polyunsaturated vegetable oil reduces serum cholesterol. The desirability of restricting saturated fat in the ulcer program is obvious.[23-29]

The following dietary regimens are suggested, depending upon the phase of the ulcer disease.

Diet in Clinically Active Uncomplicated Ulcer. During the first 2 or 3 days the diet should be extremely bland, consisting of frequent feedings (hourly or 2-hourly) of milk interspersed with a nonabsorbable antacid preparation (Diet I, Appendix Table 22). The patient may take additional feedings and antacids during the night if awake and exhibiting distress.

Skim milk should be used when fat restriction and/or caloric restriction is desired. To relieve the monotony of plain milk, a mixture of milk with one of the many flavored prepared dried protein powders may be made up or one of the prepared liquid nutritional supplements may be used. This will increase the nutritional and caloric value of the drink. Supplemental vitamins should be given at this time, if not included in adequate amounts in the commercial formula.

The average ulcer patient without complications will be quickly relieved of his pain in a matter of a few days. Particularly if nocturnal pain has disappeared, the diet may be advanced to include cereal, toast, soft-boiled eggs, creamed soups, cottage cheese, pureed or well-cooked vegetables,

cooked or stewed fruits, Jell-O, custard, plain puddings or plain crackers and cookies as tolerated (Diet II, Appendix Table 23). If the patient remains symptom-free, he is advanced to a full bland or convalescent ulcer diet (see Appendix Table 21 for bland diet with between-meal feedings).

It is of the utmost importance that the ulcer patient does not allow long periods to elapse without having something to eat or drink; he must learn to take something between meals. The type and amount of nourishment can be regulated so as to gain weight if indicated, maintain weight or even lose weight if necessary.

Any strict diet for long periods of time may deprive the patient of nutrients, and many ulcer diets eliminating fresh vegetables, juices and fruits have induced borderline ascorbic acid deficiencies. This is less evident now with the administration of supplemental vitamins. Strict diets are self-defeating in many patients. When we prescribe a regimen, we want the patient to follow it, have the ulcer heal as thoroughly as possible and not recur. In terms of these objectives, what are the effects of eliminating most tasty foods and insisting on minced and pureed foods?

Most ulcer regimens are full of regulations; it is difficult for the patient to observe them for more than a few weeks or months. It is probably unsound, as well as unrealistic, to add to his difficulties by requiring observance of rigid dietary rules which are not supported by sound rationale. Following a rigid dietary requirement for all time certainly has not been shown to prevent recurrences of the ulcer disease or its complications.

In the case of the acutely symptomatic active peptic ulcer a planned regimen may be desirable. It results in rapid improvement in over 80 per cent of the patients in a short time. Many ulcer patients improve within 24 to 48 hours with a change in environment. Regular administration of antacids after meals, cimetidine before meals and at bedtime and the discreet use of sedatives should supplement the dietary regimen. Anticholinergics are now less commonly used.

The mainstay of traditional therapy for peptic ulcer is neutralization of the gastric contents with antacids. The safest and most effective antacids are magnesium hydroxide and aluminum hydroxide. Calcium-containing antacids stimulate rebound acid secretion and should be avoided. Milk, the traditional "antacid," has been found not a good antacid because liquids are emptied rapidly from the stomach, milk has a relatively low buffering capacity and it is a relatively potent stimulant of gastric acid secretion.

The major problem in antacid therapy is rapid emptying of antacids from the stomach. The duration of neutralization is prolonged considerably when solid food is present in the stomach at the time antacids are given. The intragastric pH is maintained at higher levels when antacids are given 1 and 3 hours after meals than when the same doses are given hourly on an empty stomach. Today, peptic ulcer patients are allowed to eat regular meals of whatever foods they select, except the known gastric irritants and foods which they have learned result in obvious symptoms.

The most promising new agents for control of gastric acid secretion are those antihistamines known to be H_2-receptor antagonists, specifically cimetidine.[30,31] The conventional antihistamines, which are H_1-receptor antagonists, do not block histamine-stimulated gastric acid secretion, but the H_2-receptor antagonists are potent inhibitors of all forms of gastric acid secretion. They antagonize stimulation of gastric acid secretion produced by gastrin, food or insulin hypoglycemia. Cimetidine is now widely used in the treatment of the symptomatic peptic ulcer patient.

The effects of anticholinergic agents appear to be additive to those of the H_2-receptor antagonists. A combination of these agents and oral antacids may permit marked neutralization of gastric contents over most of each 24-hour period. This type of regimen offers the best theoretical hope for increasing ulcer healing, particularly in the chronic recurrent or refractory ulcer patients.

Management of the Obese Patient with Ulcer Disease. The ulcer patient who is obese is subject to the same complications of degenerative disease that pertain to other overweight patients. In addition, he represents an additional serious risk if surgical intervention is contemplated for his ulcer or its complications. If too-rapid weight reduction is attempted by sharp caloric restriction, there may be an exacerbation or recurrence of ulcer symptoms. During the course of weight reduction adjunctive measures, such as the conventional antacid therapy (nonabsorbable alkalies), cimetidine and the anticholinergic drugs, may be employed, even though the ulcer may not be active or symptomatic.

Dietary Management of Upper Gastrointestinal Hemorrhage. Whatever may be the source of bleeding, the patient should be started on a diet close to normal as soon as nausea and hematemesis have stopped. Experience from many quarters has shown that bleeding patients progress more satisfactorily when fed than when starved. There is nothing to suggest that hunger contractions or the dyskinesias produced by blood in the stomach are any more beneficial to a bleeding patient than physiologic peristalsis. The empty stomach is far from a resting stomach. Early feeding should start with milk, custards, Jell-O, and other bland foods as tolerated, along with frequent antacid administration and cimetidine q.i.d. This should progress rapidly to a full bland diet as soon as possible.

The initial recommendation of early feeding in cases of hemorrhage was made by Lenhartz in 1904. He recommended the use of small hourly feedings during the first day, in an effort to neutralize the acid and facilitate healing of the ulcer. Meulengracht perpetuated and reinforced this regimen and, in 1934, recommended the use of more sizable meals composed of high-calorie pureed foods with between-meal feedings of milk.[32] He presented good evidence that hemorrhage may be controlled while feeding an abundant diet. Thus, nutrition is maintained, loss of weight is prevented, convalescence is shortened and blood regeneration is favored. The patient does not complain of constant hunger and is more satisfied and, above all, the mortality rate is lower than under the older starvation method.

If the bleeding has been severe and patient tolerance is diminished, it may be desirable to limit the feedings during hemorrhage. A diet such as that suggested for active peptic ulcer disease may be employed and rapidly added to as tolerated. Pain is not a feature in hemorrhage; in fact pain, if it had been present, usually disappears or markedly diminishes with the onset of bleeding.

Anticholinergics do not appear to have any place in the treatment of the bleeding patient. Since they increase the heart rate, their use may make the evaluation of the patient more difficult. Cimetidine, orally or intravenously, is the drug of choice.

Obstruction at the Pylorus and the Duodenal Bulb. This type of obstruction is both a medical and surgical problem. The cause may not be evident or certain initially and every effort must be made to relieve the obstruction, if possible, in order to make a positive diagnosis. Peptic ulcer disease is the most common cause of pyloric obstruction and resulting gastric stasis, and accounts for approximately 80 per cent of the cases. The obstructing lesion is most often in the duodenum, but it may be in the pyloric channel or in the prepyloric antrum of the stomach. Next in order of frequency is gastric cancer, rarely pyloric muscle hypertrophy in the adult and, on occasion, prolapse of a gastric polyp into the duodenal bulb and malignant or inflammatory diseases of contiguous structures such as the biliary tract and pancreas.

Gastric juice contains high concentrations of chloride approaching 150 mEq per liter. It contains about 15 mEq of K+ per liter and the other cations are hydrogen and sodium which vary reciprocally. The chief hazard for the patient with pyloric obstruction and consequent vomiting, or suction via a nasogastric tube, is the loss of fluid and electrolytes in the gastric secretions and the accompanying systemic imbalance. Advanced pyloric obstruction exhibits the classic findings of hypochloremic-hypokalemic alkalosis with azotemia. The management of pyloric obstruction resulting from disease must be undertaken in the following manner: (1) restoration of fluid and electrolyte balance, (2) decompression of the dilated atonic stomach and (3) amelioration of the active ulcer disease. Since the secretions lost in pyloric obstruction result in essentially an isotonic contraction of body fluids, the administration of hypotonic solutions is dangerous and results in water intoxication. The need is for parenteral solutions of approximately isotonic concentration. The chief depletion is in Cl− and K+, but the latter should be given with caution and only after satisfactory urinary output is assured. It is best not to be too vigorous in attempts to restore fluid and acid-base balance and not to follow too rigid a schedule for correcting the calculated theoretical deficits.

The pyloric obstruction can be treated by intubation and constant suction. This should be maintained for no longer than 48 to 72 hours, since prolonged gastric suction further depletes a patient who is already in electrolyte imbalance, has lost weight and requires nourishment. Wilkinson advocated alternate nasogastric feedings and drainage.[33] Brown also uses alternate feeding and drainage, except that he suggests longer periods of feeding during the day and drainage during the night.[34] If the degree of obstruction is not too severe, the stomach may be aspirated night and morning, before bedtime and on arising, and the amount of aspirate measured and recorded. This is preferable, if possible, to intermittent or constant suction. The serial aspirations serve a twofold purpose, therapeutic and diagnostic. When the amount of accumulated fluid during the day is 250 ml or less, the night aspiration can be discontinued. Oral feedings can be started, with 30 to 60 ml of clear liquids given at hourly intervals along with antacids. If the underlying lesion is known or suspected to be peptic ulcer disease, cimetidine intravenously (300 mg q.6h.) and then orally should be started immediately. If this is well tolerated, the amounts can then be increased by small increments to 150 ml in each feeding. The saline test load can also be used every morning to determine if the obstruction is lessening: 450 ml of saline are instilled into the stomach via the nasogastric tube, the tube is clamped and, after 45 minutes, the remaining saline is withdrawn. Normally less than 50 ml should be recovered. If the patient is recovering from obstruction the residual volume should continue to lessen each day. When less than 50 ml is recovered the tube can be removed.

As soon as feasible, frequently within 48 hours, the next step in the program is started, namely, the treatment of the active peptic ulcer. The feedings are then changed to skim milk and, if tolerated, to whole milk, alternating with nonabsorbable antacids given at hourly intervals as outlined under treatment for any case of active ulcer. Anticholinergic and antispasmodic drugs have no place in the face of obstruction and should not be employed. If the patient continues to improve on this prescribed regimen, the diet can progress to one that is bland and high in proteins and carbohydrates. Fats should be avoided since they are poorly tolerated in the face of obstruction.

After 7 to 10 days of such treatment the radiographic study should be repeated. If the obstructing lesion was caused by mainly acute inflammation, spasm and edema, there will be considerable radiographic improvement; indeed, all signs of obstruction may be gone. However, if the obstruction was produced largely by the thick cicatricial tissue the persistent distortion will remain. Throughout this period, correction of electrolyte imbalance, anemia, if present, and maintenance of fluid intake must be accomplished by intravenous feedings. If the patient is badly nourished, has lost much weight and would represent an especially poor surgical risk, total parenteral nutrition should be employed.[35,36] The technique for the latter is covered in Chapter 37.

Surgical Management

The patient who does not respond to a medical regimen will require surgery. Rarely is pyloric stenosis an emergency. Correction of fluid and electrolyte imbalance, improvement in the patient's nutritional state plus decompression of the dilated stomach must always precede surgical intervention.

The peptic ulcer patient is not often presented for surgical intervention at the late date when he is so malnourished and in such a poor metabolic state that prolonged measures for improvement of his nutrition must be undertaken. If this is necessary, total parenteral nutrition is preferable to jejunostomy feedings. The latter are at best poorly tolerated. Presently TPN (total parenteral nutrition) has been developed so that the metabolic complications and risks of infection have been minimized.[24,25]

The principal effect of pyloric obstruction upon the prognosis at the present time is only the mortality that might be expected from an elective procedure if the patient is in good surgical hands, that is, if the patient is properly prepared preoperatively by the correction of malnutrition, anemia, azotemia, alkalosis and hypochloremia.

Evaluation of the various surgical procedures for peptic ulcer disease is an ongoing study. Limited gastric resection of 40 to 50 per cent, with removal of the antrum, combined with some form of vagotomy, or pyloroplasty with vagotomy, are presently the procedures of choice in the treatment of duodenal ulcer. The unpleasant side effects and complications are minimal. Perhaps, in gastric ulcer, when surgery is indicated, subtotal resection is the operation of choice. Vagotomy and pyloroplasty in the treatment of duodenal ulcer appear to be indicated in poor-risk patients, in underweight individuals, in young patients with complications of ulcer disease and in patients who have anatomic pathologic conditions which make resective surgery too hazardous.

In the next few years it is possible that application of potent inhibitors of gastric secretion, such as histamine H_2-receptor antagonists or certain prostaglandins, to the treatment of ulcer disease will decrease the incidence of complications of ulcer and markedly diminish the number of patients requiring surgery.

Diet and Surgical Treatment. Following surgery, how long should the patient remain on a restricted diet? There is no rationale for an indefinite period of rigid dietary restriction. A relatively bland diet is followed for several weeks postoperatively and then new foods are added as tolerated until a full regular diet is taken. Each patient must be evaluated individually.

It is generally recognized that the *dumping or postgastrectomy syndrome* is the outstanding complication associated with substantial or partial removal of the stomach. The syndrome has its onset 10 to 15 minutes after the ingestion of a meal and is characterized by abdominal fullness and distention followed by tachycardia, pallor, tachypnea, weakness, sweating and, in some instances, syncope. The intact stomach normally empties small quantities of food into the jejunum, permitting digestion of only small aliquots of food, and

guards against a massive and acute change in osmotic load. Following gastric resection, the capacity of the stomach as a reservoir has been reduced and ingested material enters the intestine in larger quantities and more rapidly. There is evidence that the dumping syndrome is associated with a shift of plasma water to the intestinal lumen to equalize increased intraluminal osmotic pressure. This results in a marked and precipitous drop in plasma volume. The acute increase in osmotic pressure in the intestinal lumen results from the rapid entrance of small molecular components from the stomach.[37,38] It has also been postulated that dumping is the result of intestinal distention and increased intraluminal pressure. This has not been confirmed by balloon studies. The blood sugar has also been implicated in dumping; it may rapidly develop a rise to hyperglycemic levels and then abruptly fall to hypoglycemic levels, but these changes do not appear to coincide with the clinical symptoms of dumping. Occasionally a patient may have symptoms of hypoglycemia a few hours after a meal; symptoms referable to this should not be confused with the dumping syndrome. The fall in potassium and the sometimes-seen nonspecific electrocardiographic changes are not fully clarified, since they are not necessarily temporally related to the dumping syndrome. Some believe that the symptoms are brought on by excessive serotonin output.

Since most dumping symptoms are more easily produced by carbohydrates than by protein or fat and are related to the quantity of food ingested, dietary management is of great importance in treating the postgastrectomy syndrome. Since carbohydrates are more rapidly hydrolyzed into smaller molecular particles than either proteins or fat, this is the basis for the concept that carbohydrates are the least desirable food for the patient with the dumping syndrome.

The dietary regimen recommended is designed to consider: (1) type of food ingested, (2) total quantity of food taken at any one time, (3) daily caloric requirement and (4) physical form of the food ingested. Carbohydrate food should be limited. The diet should be high in proteins and fats, with a caloric intake of 2,000 to 3,500 kcal per day. Feedings are recommended at frequent intervals, e.g. every 2 to 3 hours, to avoid overloading the stomach. The diet should be relatively dry, with restricted fluids at meals. Fluids may be taken more freely between meals. Sugar, sweets, candy, syrups and chocolate should be avoided. The patient with late postprandial dumping, in whom hypoglycemia is found, must shorten the intervals between meals and increase the protein and fat content. The ingestion of a readily assimilable source of sugar may be helpful. Some patients cannot achieve correction of the dumping syndrome by dietary means alone. If the symptoms are severe, further surgical correction may be necessary.

Nutritional Impairment Following Gastric Surgery. A nutritional defect following gastrectomy is the most common undesirable sequela; the more extensive the gastric resection the greater is the nutritional problem. This is generally seen as a failure to maintain or regain normal body weight or, more specifically, a lack of one or more essential nutritional factors. These problems are now encountered in a relatively small number of patients and rarely in the partially gastrectomized patient, who enjoys a healthy appetite, appears to have almost normal gastric capacities, consumes an essentially unrestricted diet and has normal bowel function.

The causes of deficient nutrition will vary from patient to patient. The chief cause is simple reduction in caloric intake, because of either early satiety, reflecting a diminished gastric reservoir, or actual fear of eating, because of the distressing postprandial symptoms. Others, as Goldstein,[39] implicate steatorrhea as a cause of weight loss, diarrhea and malnutrition in a far higher percentage of patients than is generally recognized. These observers do not negate the importance of decreased caloric intake as a factor in postgastrectomy malnutrition, but emphasize the added detrimental effects of malabsorption. Decreased pancreatic secretion as a cause of malabsorption has been suggested, but this has not been shown to be a significant factor; neither has rapid intestinal transit. There is some evidence to suggest that faulty mixing of food with pancreatic juice and bile may be a factor in postgastrectomy steatorrhea. This, too, has not been proven. In some cases afferent loop stasis and bacterial overgrowth have been implicated as causes of steatorrhea. These conditions, if present, would apply in only a small percentage of cases.

Anemia has been recognized as a complication of partial gastrectomy for many years, with numerous reports concerning its frequency, course and possible etiology. Some months or even years after surgery a varying percentage of individuals, up to 57 per cent, develop a mild iron deficiency anemia which usually responds to oral iron therapy. Women in their reproductive years develop this anemia oftener and sooner than postmenopausal women or men of comparable age. Some patients may develop a progressive fall in serum vitamin B_{12} levels as a result of impaired B_{12} absorption, but only a small number develop megaloblastic anemia. Occasionally megaloblastic anemia occurs as a result of folic acid deficiency. The incidence of postgastrectomy anemia due to both iron and vitamin deficiency seems to increase in the first postoperative decade. Inadequate food intake, chronic intermittent blood loss from the associated gastritis or gastrojejunitis and malabsorption of iron have each been blamed for the development of iron deficiency, while atrophy of the gastric mucosa is currently considered responsible for the development of most cases of vitamin B_{12} deficiency. Chronic malabsorption of calcium may lead to bone demineralization.

The management of the poorly nourished postgastrectomy patient is implied in the previous discussion. The designing of an acceptable, nutritious diet, along with a great deal of sympathetic understanding and encouragement, is essential (though many patients improve spontaneously with time). If a problem such as dumping exists, every effort should be made to ameliorate this condition. If steatorrhea, other than the very mildest form, is present, it should be treated. Symptomatic measures, including anticholinergics, psychotropic drugs, dietary manipulation and pancreatic enzyme administration, should be tried. In those cases where there appears to be a true intolerance for fat, a mixture of medium-chain triglycerides may be used. The patient should be assured adequate calcium and vitamin D intake. In those cases with obvious deficiency of iron, B_{12} or folic acid, these substances should be administered. Anabolic agents and supplemental vitamins should also be considered. In the suspected afferent loop stasis with bacterial overgrowth, antibiotics should be given, either in prolonged administration at reduced dosage or in repeated short courses. At best these cases are difficult to treat and every available means of nutritional and psychologic support should be tried.

MISCELLANEOUS DISEASES OF THE STOMACH AND DUODENUM
Crohn's Disease
(Nonspecific Granulomatous Inflammation)

In 1950, Comfort et al., in a report of 5 cases, established that nonspecific granulomatous inflammation of the stomach and the duodenum was the same condition as regional enteritis affecting other parts of the small intestine.[40] By 1967 approximately 62 cases had been recorded. Fielding et al. studied 12 patients

with gastroduodenal involvement followed between the years 1944 and 1969.[41] In Comfort's original paper, patients with this condition exhibited the following symptoms: continuous or intermittent upper abdominal pain made worse by food, systemic upset with fever, loss of weight and diarrhea, and finally a progressive stenosing lesion in the duodenum. Fielding and others found patients in whom the symptoms were relatively mild and, when related to food, were relieved by antacid therapy. Obstructive symptoms at some time during the course of the disorder were common and present in two-thirds of the patients followed. Hemorrhage may also occur. There is no special dietary regimen other than that used for the basic disease, i.e. a diet which is nutritionally balanced and easily tolerated without producing further gastrointestinal irritation and pain. Some patients with this disease do well on a regular selected diet, whereas others must follow a bland low-residue diet.

Menetrier's Disease

Menetrier's disease or giant rugal hypertrophy is characterized by large, prominent gastric folds found diffusely throughout the stomach or localized to the body. Inflammation need not be present, so the term giant hypertrophic gastritis is a misnomer. The markedly elongated gastric glands secrete a thick viscous mucus. This secretion is high in albumin content and may lead to hypoalbuminemia, peripheral edema and occasionally ascites. Menetrier's disease is considered to be a protein-losing gastropathy. There may be other symptoms, such as vague dyspepsia, and postprandial epigastric pain, which may or may not be relieved by food and antacids. In some instances, food may actually aggravate the pain. Anorexia, nausea and sometimes vomiting may be present with marked weight loss as a prominent feature.

The diagnosis is made by a combination

of radiography, gastroscopy, peroral biopsy of the stomach and cytology studies. Treatment is symptomatic with the administration of antacids and a high-protein diet, especially when hypoalbuminemia is present. Surgery may be necessary when intractable symptoms are present or if uncontrollable bleeding occurs.

Isolated Granulomatous Gastritis

An entity separate and distinct from Crohn's disease and sarcoidosis appears clinically as pyloric obstruction with radiologic features of antral narrowing simulating neoplasm. The treatment in these cases is that for pyloric obstruction or surgical intervention to establish a definite diagnosis, if this is impossible with the other diagnostic means available.

Eosinophilic Gastritis

This is a rare disorder, usually a part of a more diffuse process characterized by diffuse or circumscribed eosinophilic infiltration of the gastrointestinal tract. In both forms, the stomach is the organ most commonly involved. In the diffuse form, symptoms are predominantly those of long-standing partial and intermittent pyloric obstruction. The circumscribed form appears as an eosinophilic granuloma anywhere in the gastrointestinal tract. When it is present in the stomach the symptoms are not as marked or as acute as in the diffuse variety.

Biopsy is necessary for diagnosis and surgical resection of the isolated granuloma is curative. Steroids have been used with beneficial effect in the diffuse variety. No special dietary regimen is recommended, other than avoiding foods to which the patient may be allergic. A selected balanced diet that the patient can tolerate without further gastrointestinal irritation is recommended. If dietary restrictions must be imposed, then supplemental vitamins are recommended.

BIBLIOGRAPHY

1. Cannon: Am. J. Physiol., 1, 359, 1898.
2. Beaumont: Experiments and Observations on the Gastric Juice and the Physiology of Digestion. Plattsburg, F. P. Allen, 1833.
3. Hollander: Proceedings World Congress of Gastroenterology, Washington, 1958.
4. Rapp, Aronson, Burton and Grabar: J. Immunol., 92, 579, 1964.
5. Benson: Am. J. Dig. Dis., 16, 357, 1971.
6. Kirsner: In Textbook of Medicine (Beeson and McDermott, Eds.). Philadelphia, W. B. Saunders, 1967.
7. Wirts: In The Stomach. New York, Grune & Stratton, 1967.
8. Cohen and Lipshutz: J. Clin. Invest., 50, 449, 1971.
9. Castell: Gastroenterology, 61, 10, 1971.
10. Dennish and Castell: N. Engl. J. Med., 284, 1136, 1971.
11. Naeler, Schwartz, Stahl and Spiro: Ann. Intern. Med., 59, 906, 1963.
12. Winkelstein: J.A.M.A., 104, 906, 1935.
13. Pridie: Gut, 7, 188, 1966.
14. Gillison, de Castro and Nyhus: Surg. Gynecol. Obstet., 134, 419, 1972.
15. Pearson and Wilson: Thorax, 26, 300, 1971.
16. Castell and Levine: Ann. Intern. Med., 74, 223, 1971.
17. Doniach and Roitt: Semin. Hematol., 1, 313, 1964.
18. Sippy: In A Handbook of Practical Treatment, Vol. 3 (Musser and Kelly, Eds). Philadelphia, W. B. Saunders, 1912.
19. Ingelfinger: In Controversy in Internal Medicine. Philadelphia, W. B. Saunders, 1966.
20. Roth: In Controversy in Internal Medicine. Philadelphia, W. B. Saunders, 1966.
21. Dietary misconceptions: Nutr. Rev., 26, 1, 1968.
22. Code et al.: Gastroenterology, 39, 1, 1960.
23. Sandweiss, et al.: Harper Hosp. Bull., 17, 2, 1959.
24. Briggs, et al.: Circulation, 21, 538, 1960.
25. Sterner, et al.: J.A.M.A., 181, 186, 1962.
26. Katz, et al.: Nutrition and Atherosclerosis. Philadelphia, Lea & Febiger, 1958.
27. Jolliffe: Circulation, 20, 109, 1959.
28. Jolliffe, Rinzler and Archer: Am. J. Clin. Nutr., 7, 451, 1959.
29. Christakis, et al.: J.A.M.A., 198, 597, 1966.
30. Black, et al.: Nature, 236, 385, 1972.
31. Henn et al.: N. Engl. J. Med., 293, 371, 1975.
32. Meulengracht: Acta Med. Scand., 59, 375, 1934.
33. Wilkinson: Am. J. Dig. Dis., 9, 321, 1942.
34. Brown: Am. J. Dig. Dis., 4, 940, 1959.
35. Dudrick et al.: Med. Clin. North Am., 154, 577, 1970.
36. Shils: J.A.M.A., 220, 1721, 1972.
37. Roberts, et al.: Ann. Surg., 140, 631, 1954.
38. Clarke and Wimmer: Gastroenterology, 40, 803, 1961.
39. Goldstein: In The Stomach. New York, Grune & Stratton, 1967.
40. Comfort, Weber, Baggenstoss and Kiely: Am. J. Med. Sci., 220, 616, 1950.
41. Fielding, Toye and Cooke: Gut, 11, 1001, 1970.

B.   Nutrition in Diseases of the Intestines

Selwyn A. Broitman
and
Norman Zamcheck

Because the intestinal tract, particularly the small intestine, is the site of digestion and absorption of nutrients, diseases of the intestinal tract are promptly accompanied by alterations in general nutrition. The dynamic interrelationship existing between the gut mucosal pathobiology and host nutrition has been elucidated largely in animals.[1]* In recent years, Dubos,[2] Donaldson,[3] Sprinz[4] and others have emphasized the participation of the nutrition and metabolism of the gut flora in this complex dynamic interaction. Full understanding, therefore, of nutritional alterations in disease of the intestinal tract requires broad understanding of the biology of the gut itself, the nature of the previous diet of the patient and the gut flora, and knowledge of the normal and pathologic anatomy of the small intestine.

The influence of previous dietary experience on enzyme activity, i.e. enzyme adaptation, has been widely appreciated by chemists,[5] and has been studied in the gut. Deren and associates[6] showed that feeding carbohydrate influenced the disaccharidase activity of the small bowel in rats. The significance of this aspect of "diet" with respect to clinical disaccharide disorders, including malabsorption, is only beginning to be appreciated.

The most frequent clinical manifestations of disease of the intestine are diarrhea and steatorrhea and the consequent weight loss and nutritional deficien-

cies. Some patients with steatorrhea, however, may have little diarrhea. The clinical evidence may be manifest elsewhere, e.g. dermatitis and dementia (niacin deficiency), cheilosis and glossitis (riboflavin deficiency), bone marrow, e.g. macrocytic anemia (folic acid and vitamin B_{12} deficiency) and tetany (calcium and/or magnesium deficiencies), to mention only a few.

A few disorders have been characterized in part biochemically. The elucidation of vitamin B_{12} malabsorption in pernicious anemia is described in Chapter 6J. Gluten sensitivity, disaccharidase deficiencies, defect in trytophan metabolism in Hartnup disease, agammaglobulinemic states, abetalipoproteinemia are other examples. However interesting, this group provides a relatively small proportion of the patients seen clinically.

Most clinical disorders have in common an impairment in absorption. From the point of view of the nutritional consequences and nutrient needs, the specific pathologic process responsible for the impairment is less relevant. For successful treatment of the patient, however, nutritional management must be combined with a clear understanding of the site, etiology and extent of the gut disorder. Thus, bacterial diarrhea requires appropriate antibiotic therapy; gut enzymatic deficiencies require the elimination of the nonutilizable substrate; regional enteritis and ulcerative colitis often respond to corticosteroid therapy; parasites may be eliminated by specific drugs.

*Bibliographic numbers and references are grouped under the headings of specific subsections at the end of the chapter.

The attempt is made in this chapter to allude only to those aspects of clinical nutrition which seem most pertinent to the disorders discussed. Limitations of space permit only a survey of the subject.

The management of fulminant loss of the intestinal content presents one of the most challenging therapeutic problems in medicine. This is seen in cholera and other acute bacterial diarrheas, and in massive intestinal resection. The general principles of management, i.e. fluid, nutrition, electrolyte, mineral and vitamin replacement, apply similarly in all of these disorders. The more acute the diarrhea, the greater is the loss of water and electrolytes such as sodium, potassium, chloride and bicarbonate. The fluid loss in acute inflammatory states tends to resemble plasma and, accordingly, the losses of protein as well as of electrolytes become prominent. Quantitative aspects of replacement vary, depending upon the severity, the location of the lesion and the reduction of or interference with the absorbing apparatus. In the more chronic states, such as gluten enteropathy, steatorrhea tends to predominate, because intestinal transit time is sufficiently slow to permit absorption of most of the other nutrients. Fat generally being the most slowly absorbed, fat malabsorption and its consequences may be seen in those conditions in which malabsorption is less severe (also see Chapter 5). In each section below specific deficits and their replacement will be discussed individually.

MASSIVE RESECTION OF THE SMALL BOWEL

The clinical state, par excellence, which represents a severe quantitative reduction in the absorptive apparatus is *massive resection of the small intestine.* Many of the nutritional and physiologic disturbances encountered in this condition also occur in many other malabsorptive disorders of the small intestine. For this reason a large proportion of this section is devoted to it.

Within the past 10 years the nutritional needs of these patients have been elucidated. In several painstaking metabolic studies[1-3] resection of 50 per cent of the small bowel or less usually posed minimal difficulties. There are reports of patients surviving for long periods of time with as little as 8 to 18 inches of bowel remaining,[2,4] and Kinney et al. reported survival in one patient with only the duodenum and half the colon remaining.[2] The most common conditions requiring resection are mesenteric vascular occlusion, strangulated hernia or acute volvulus.

The resultant absorptive defects depend upon the degree of resection, the area resected, the presence or absence of the ileocecal valve, and the state of the remaining bowel. Gastric hypersecretion, diminished bile salt reabsorption and pancreatic insufficiency contribute to the malabsorption.

Proximal Resections

Resection of up to 8 feet of proximal jejunum may result in minimal malabsorption of fat or protein, since these can be handled by the large reserve capacity of the distal gut.[1] If the duodenum remains intact, there is no defect in absorption of folic acid,[5] glucose,[6] calcium[7,8] and probably no defect in absorption of the fat-soluble vitamins.[1] The ileum can assume some of the functions of the upper small bowel. However, when proximal resections exceed 8 feet, fat and protein absorption is impaired, as is absorption of calcium, magnesium and fat-soluble vitamins (A, D and K).

Distal Resections

A patient with a resected ileum who has an intact jejunum may require no specific diet therapy other than parenteral replacement of vitamin B_{12} and restriction of fat intake to 30 to 50 gm daily.[9] In the absence of the ileum, Booth[1] and Scheiner[9] have demonstrated the critical minimal amount of jejunum necessary for satisfactory absorption of water-soluble nutrients to be 1 to 4 feet. Since the ileum is the site of reabsorption of bile salts, its absence will cause fat malabsorption.[10,11] Rapid transit through the remaining jejunum contributes to losses of all nutrients, but particularly to losses of lipids. The longer the ileum remaining, the less rapid is the transit. The presence of the ileocecal valve is of utmost importance in slowing the transfer of materials from the small to the large bowel. In the absence of the ileocecal valve, segments of small bowel have been reversed and interposed between the distal small bowel and the cecum.[12] The size of this antiperistaltic segment seems to be of prime import, although the findings to date have not shown this to be a complete substitute for an ileocecal valve.

Carbohydrate

Digestion of carbohydrate is simpler than that of fat and protein and, hence, it is absorbed best in these patients. The simple sugars are easily absorbed throughout the small bowel and are carried away by the portal circulation. Carbohydrate absorption may not be accurately reflected by the oral glucose tolerance test or by absence of sugars in the stool, since gut bacteria and yeast metabolize them. The 3-0-methylglucose absorption test has been of value in assessing the absorptive capacities of the small bowel following resection.[3] This methylated sugar is absorbed in the same manner as glucose; it is not metabolized and consequently all that is absorbed appears in the urine within 24 to 48 hours. It was previously shown to have little value as a diagnostic test of carbohydrate malabsorption,[13] since it is virtually completely absorbed by even the diseased small bowel. However, in patients with resection, the percentage excreted yields an approximate index of that amount of bowel remaining with carbohydrate absorptive capacity.

The question of compensatory increase in carbohydrate absorption by the remaining small bowel has been raised repeatedly, but few quantitative data are available. Dowling and Booth[14] have shown an increase in the absorptive capacity of the jejunum for glucose after distal resections.

Disaccharidase activity is present throughout the entire small bowel mucosa;[15] therefore, disaccharides can be hydrolyzed into simple sugars for subsequent absorption at any level.

Impaired absorption of glucose, folic acid[16] and xylose[4] has been reported in patients with only 20 cm of jejunum remaining.

Fat and Nitrogen

Fat and protein are mixed with pancreatic and biliary secretions and are emulsified before they are absorbed. Lipids are absorbed in the proximal small intestine under normal physiologic circumstances.[17,18] When the lipid load is increased, the remaining lipid is absorbed by the ileum. Shortened exposure of lipid to a limited small bowel surface area, as in intestinal hurry, may contribute to steatorrhea, particularly in distal small bowel resections.

Studies in animals and in man identify the distal small bowel as the major site of bile salt absorption. The ileum has been shown to be the only intestinal site of active transport of both conjugated and unconjugated bile salts.[10]

Malabsorption of amino acids, accompanied by large losses of nitrogen in the feces, may occur in massive intestinal resection.[3] However, positive nitrogen balance can be maintained by a high-protein intake if some part of the jejunum is present. This may be partly the result of reduction in urinary nitrogen, an attempt by the body to conserve tissue nitrogen.

Calcium and Magnesium

Calcium may be lost in large quantities initially following resection, but tetany is an infrequent and usually a late complication. Serum and urine calcium levels may remain normal for long periods. Magnesium losses parallel calcium losses, since they share a similar transport system.[19] The effect of deficiency of this ion is discussed in Chapter 7, Section B.

Vitamins

Booth has shown that vitamin B_{12} is absorbed in the terminal ileum;[20] resection of that portion of the bowel will result in vitamin B_{12} malabsorption. Fat-soluble vitamins A, D and K are lost in large amounts in steatorrhea. The loss of vitamin D contributes to large calcium losses. Vitamin K losses may be reflected by a prolonged prothrombin time. Absorption of folic acid and other water-soluble vitamins is usually normal, providing 4 feet of proximal small bowel remains;[1] however, increased body needs may require supplements.

Electrolytes and Water

Excessive diarrhea leads to severe body potassium losses and to a lesser extent sodium, although serum values may be deceptively normal. Starvation leads to acidosis, and extensive water losses result in dehydration. Patients may show a delayed water absorption with nocturnal diuresis related to protein depletion.[21]

Plasma Protein

The small intestine is a site of catabolism of albumin.[22] It has been postulated that the albumin half-life should be prolonged in cases of massive bowel resection, and, indeed, studies in our laboratory showed a prolonged albumin survival in 2 patients with massive bowel resection.[23] The gut also plays an important role in the metabolism of immunoglobulins, both in synthesis and degradation.[24] If the gastrointestinal tract were the sole site of immunoglobulin synthesis, then reduction in bowel size by resection would tend to reduce the total body pool of these proteins. However, in 4 patients studied in this laboratory, Jabbari[25] found that IgG and IgA were high normal to elevated and IgM

was normal. The half-life of IgG was normal in 3 subjects tested. These observations suggested increased production rather than decreased catabolism. Accordingly, other important sites of production probably existed in these patients.

Gastric Secretion

Gastric hypersecretion has been observed in patients following extensive[3,26,27] bowel resection. Hypersecretion may worsen the patient's nutritional state by increasing the diarrhea and thereby interfere with absorption. The absorptive disturbance may be due in part to hypermotility and to alteration of gut intraluminal pH from that essential for optimal absorption. Vagotomy and pyloroplasty appear to improve the patient's clinical course following extensive intestinal resection.[26]

Clinical Course and Management

The clinical course of patients following massive resection may be divided into three phases: Phase 1 is the immediate postoperative period, when fluid and electrolyte losses, diarrhea and infection may overwhelm the patient. During phase 2 fluid and electrolyte problems decrease, diarrhea starts to diminish, wounds heal and the patient becomes more active and desires food. It is during this phase that the absorptive defects become apparent. The degree of malabsorption and general and specific nutrient deficiencies which depend on the amount and area of bowel resected may now be assessed. Phase 3 is the period during which the patient attains a balance with his disability, and his weight stabilizes at a level determined by the amount of nutrient absorbed by his remaining gut.

Metabolic balance studies indicate the loss of body nutrients. In general, the diet should contain 3,500 to 4,000 calories per day, provided largely by carbohydrate, since it is most easily absorbed, and by protein. Metabolic needs consume at least 50 gm per day of protein. If only 50 per cent of protein intake is absorbed, then at least 100 gm must be ingested. Provided caloric intake is adequate, this level of protein is consistent with positive nitrogen balance.

Since long-chain fatty acids are poorly absorbed, usual dietary fat is of limited usefulness in supplying absorbable calories. Fat intake should, therefore, be kept to the minimum needed to make the diet palatable. Medium-chain triglycerides (MCT) may be substituted for part of the dietary fat. Such supplements contribute to caloric intake and, together with adequate carbohydrate intake, prevent depletion of protein reserves.

For ordinary activity, 21 calories per pound of ideal body weight are necessary in order to maintain body weight. If the percentages of carbohydrate, protein and fat absorbed are known, then the caloric intake necessary to supply these requirements may be estimated. Initially, a deficit of 2,000 to 3,000 calories and later of 3,500 or more will cause 1-lb weight loss. Vitamin and mineral requirements can be estimated from tables in the Appendix and the chapters on individual nutrients.

Phase 1. During this postoperative period replacement of large volumes of fluids, salts, potassium, calcium, magnesium and amino acids or plasma protein will be required. Adequate caloric replacement can be provided intravenously (see Chapter 37). Oral or tube feeding should be initiated as soon as possible. Tube formulas may be necessary for variable periods. Generally, these feedings are composed of amino acid hydrolysates, simple sugars, electrolytes, calcium, magnesium and medium-chain triglycerides. Tube feeding can be given in a slow continuous 24-hour drip, which allows for more complete absorption and diminishes the diarrhea produced by ingestion of large amounts of formula at one time. During this time, if low gastric pH and large volumes suggest gastric hypersecretion, and if diarrhea is excessive and

wound healing delayed, vagotomy and pyloroplasty should be considered. If there is no evidence of gastric hypersecretion, but diarrhea is uncontrollable by usual measures, then insertion of an antiperistaltic bowel segment may become necessary. The segment is most helpful in patients in whom the ileocecal valve has been resected.[12]

Phase 2. Generally the patients prefer ordinary foods to prepared formulas and, if allowed "guided" selection, they will consume more calories. At first the feedings should be small and frequent, every 2 hours, during the course of the day. Later, as the patient improves, the amount may be increased and the interval between feedings lengthened. Caloric intake should be as high as the patient will accept and consist largely of carbohydrate. Simple sugars should be used. Particular attention should be given to the patient's tolerance for milk. Extensive resection of the bowel results in a reduction of lactase activity, whereupon ingestion of excessive lactose-containing foods may induce diarrhea. Decreased fluid intake will frequently decrease the volume of stool.

Restriction of fat intake to a minimum reduces steatorrhea and diminishes losses of fat-soluble vitamins, calcium and magnesium. It is difficult to maintain such restriction for long periods. Furthermore, the high caloric value of fat is desirable when it can be absorbed. Winawer et al.[3] reported a patient with massive intestinal resection who showed decreased steatorrhea, weight gain and improved calcium balance concomitant with MCT feeding.

Nitrogen balance improves during this phase. Calcium, magnesium and vitamin D losses parallel the degree of steatorrhea. Up to 3 gm of calcium per day may be required to maintain a positive calcium balance. Magnesium should be supplemented also, either in small oral doses or by parenteral routes. Since they are absorbed similarly, administration of calcium or magnesium alone may enhance the loss of the other. A "cocktail" of the following may be given twice daily: 1 gm calcium, 20 mEq magnesium, 5,000 U vitamin A, 500 U vitamin D and 30 mg of vitamin E. If the prothrombin time is prolonged, 10 to 20 mg vitamin K should be given by either the oral or the parenteral route, daily or as needed, to assure adequate blood coagulation. If malabsorption of vitamin B_{12} has been shown by the Schilling test, vitamin B_{12} (200 μg) may be given parenterally every month to prevent combined system disease and anemia. Replacement of other water-soluble vitamins, folic acid and iron is necessary only in extensive proximal resections. Use of pancreatic enzymes and bile salts should be avoided as they are of little benefit; in fact, they may be harmful. Complications in gastrointestinal function in under-nourished patients may require total or supplementary parenteral feeding. This is discussed in Chapters 36 and 37.

Phase 3. Most patients succumb during the second phase. Those few who reach this stage usually have less extensive resections. They can be sustained more easily by the program worked out in the previous stage and require less management.

Complications and Prognosis

Postoperative wound infections, breakdown of anastomoses, gastric hypersecretion, fluid and electrolyte losses have been discussed. Calcium and magnesium imbalance may lead to tetany. Deficiencies of folic acid, iron or vitamin B_{12}, if not replaced, will lead to anemia. Recurrent abdominal distention and occasional renal stone formation occur. Food rejection and emotional problems are common. Tuberculosis is common.

JEJUNOILEAL BYPASS FOR OBESITY

Consequences of morbid obesity include increased morbidity and mortality rates accompanied by numerous psychosocial problems. Conservative management with the most promising techniques available today—supervised dietotherapy, coupled with behavior modification—affords these patients only a 13 per cent success rate in achieving a 40-pound or greater weight loss.[1] The success rate of maintaining this weight loss over an extended period of time is obviously no better and, presumably, will be worse. Consequently, a more vigorous approach to the management of these patients, jejunoileal bypass surgery, has enjoyed a national upsurge with an experience to date of approximately 10,000 patients.[2] In general, this procedure has been restricted to those individuals who are more than 110 pounds overweight, who have a history of serious attempt(s) at weight reduction in the past and who are less than 50 years old. Qualifications are modified for those patients who do not meet these criteria but in whom a weight loss would ameliorate the sequelae of underlying disease, i.e. patients with complications of diabetes mellitus, hypertension, serious orthopedic problems, pulmonary alveolar hypoventilation (Pickwickian syndrome). A detailed discussion of indications and contraindications for intestinal bypass surgery for obesity may be found in the excellent text by Bray.[3]

Since its introduction in 1963, by Payne,[4] intestinal bypass surgery has undergone a number of modifications from the initial jejunocolic anastomosis to jejunoileal anastomosis, end to end, or end to side, with the remaining blind loop segment anastomosed to the ileum or to various locations in the colon. Advocates of each of the various procedures claim certain benefits, particularly reductions in the rates of various complications.

Physiologic Consequences

Weight loss is most rapid during the first 6 to 9 months. Losses recorded in over 100 patients averaged between 25 to 35 per cent of their initial weights, and, by the 30th month postoperatively, approached

30 to 40 per cent of their initial weights.[5] In a series of patients reported by Bray and his associates,[6] although the reduced intestinal absorbing surface contributed to weight loss, the major factor was a reduced caloric intake. Following intestinal bypass, caloric consumption declined from a mean of 6,300 kcal per day preoperatively to 1,300 kcal per day over the first 6 months postoperatively. Caloric consumption progressively increased over the next 18 months after operation. Additionally, the patients demonstrated a decrease in taste for sweetened solutions but not for salty solutions following surgery, which suggested that altered taste patterns may be an important consequence of intestinal bypass procedure.

Malabsorptive problems associated with jejunoilial bypass are similar to those encountered in massive small bowel resection, i.e. fat, protein, carbohydrate, fat and water-soluble vitamins, calcium, magnesium, potassium (see above). Intestinal adaptation following jejunoilial bypass was studied in 12 female patients under 30 years of age by Barry et al.[7] A series of events they reported was similar to that noted following massive small bowel resection. Morphologically, there was a hyperplasia of the small bowel epithelium and an elongation of the crypts 6 months postoperatively. Glucose absorption rates, measured over a 30-cm segment of a multilumen perfusion tube, were assessed prior to and following bypass procedure. Results obtained 6 months postoperatively indicated a mean reduction in glucose absorption in 9 of 10 patients of approximately 25 per cent compared to their preoperative status. Schilling tests for vitamin B_{12} absorption performed in individuals with end-to-end jejunoileal bypass were markedly decreased 2 weeks postoperatively, but approached normal levels 6 months postoperatively. In contrast, individuals with end-to-side bypass exhibited mean values on Schilling tests of approximately one-third of the preoperative values

2 weeks following surgery. At 6 months after operation, values for the Schilling test remained at this low level.

Fasting serum gastrin remained unchanged 6 months postoperatively. However, the serum gastrin response to a standard meal increased significantly following surgery.[7] The possibility suggested by this finding is that impaired glucose absorption may be related, in part, to increased gastrin release.[8] Basal gastric acid was increased 6 months postoperatively but peak gastric output remained unchanged.[7]

Bile in duodenal fluid showed an increased lithogenicity index in all patients 2 to 3 weeks postoperatively. By 6 months, however, an initial 30 per cent increase in cholesterol concentration was reduced to preoperative levels, with return of the lithogenic index to baseline values.[7] Decreased fecal bile acid concentration, and increased bile salt deconjugation have also been observed and have been suggested to be related to bacterial colonization of the functional remaining small bowel.[9]

Complications

Persistent Diarrhea. In studies carried out in over 100 morbidly obese patients in whom a jejunoileal bypass was performed, Dean et al.[11] reported that the duration of postoperative diarrhea was related to length of functional ileum. In patients in whom 30 cm of jejunum was anastomosed end to end with 30 cm of ileum, diarrhea ceased 3 months postoperatively. In individuals with 30 cm of jejunum, anastomosed to 20 cm, end to end, of ileum, persistent diarrhea was a problem for 17 per cent and, in those individuals with 30 cm of jejunum anastomosed to 15 cm of ileum, for 45 per cent.

Malabsorption of both exogenous and endogenous substrates results from the reduced intestinal absorbing surface and increased intestinal transit. At least two major factors contribute to the diarrhea observed in these patients:[12] The first is an inability to reabsorb bile salts in the enterohepatic circulation. This failure is accompanied by a compensatory increase in hepatic bile salt synthesis to maintain the bile salt pool. Thus both bile salt malabsorption and increased hepatic bile salt synthesis contribute to the increased levels of bile salts entering the colon. Dihydroxy bile acids, which reach high levels in the colons of these patients,[13] may inhibit absorption and promote secretion of water, sodium and chloride and thus contribute to diarrhea.

A second factor relates to the fat lost to the colon, which may serve as substrate for bacterial conversion to hydroxy fatty acids. It has been suggested, but not substantiated, that this may exert a cathartic effect.[14] Short-chain organic acids produced by bacteria from fat substrates may also exert an irritative effect on the bowel mucosa. The occurrence of "fatty acid" diarrhea generally precludes the occurrence of "bile acid" diarrhea. Bacterial modification of bile acids to less soluble species in the colon by 7-α-dehydroxylation is favored in the presence of a high fatty acid concentration. Consequently, bile acid precipitation occurs, diminishing bile salt diarrhea; in patients with intestinal bypass, the shorter the total length of functional small bowel, the greater is the likelihood of the development of "fatty acid" rather than "bile acid" diarrhea.[13]

Renal Calculi. Recurrent renal calculi were found in 6 to 32 per cent of patients who had undergone jejunoileal bypass[15,16] and their formation appears to be independent of the type of surgical bypass procedure used, i.e. end-to-end or end-to-side anastomosis. Generally, stones are calcium oxalate and are the consequence of hyperabsorption of dietary oxalate.[17] Impaired absorption of bile salts and dietary fat in these patients may result in alterations of colonic mucosal permeability and nonspecifically favor oxalate absorption.[18] Stauffer[19] suggested that, additionally, the increased intraluminal concentration of free fatty acids in these patients, as in

patients with inflammatory bowel disease, promotes the sequestration of calcium. Consequently, oxalate, which under normal circumstances would precipitate with intraluminal calcium, readily undergoes passive diffusion across the colonic mucosa.

Progressive Liver Disease. Progressive liver disease following jejunoileal bypass occurs in 1 to 17 per cent of patients,[20] among whom the fatality rate, although variable in different series, is no less than 17 per cent. In general, morbidly obese patients exhibit fatty infiltration of the liver prior to bypass[21] with a distribution pattern different from that seen in alcoholic patients. Degrees of hepatic dysfunction and associated hepatic morphology varying from steatosis and cellular necrosis to frank cirrhosis have been described.[22] Of interest are findings that, in 6 of 151 patients with jejunoileal bypass reviewed by Kern et al.,[21] 3 exhibited Laennec's cirrhosis and 3 had fibrosis, but presumably none was alcoholic. The mechanism(s) for these effects is (are) unknown although a number of possibilities have been suggested: (1) protein calorie malnutrition, (2) absorption of bacterial endotoxin or other toxic components derived from the flora colonizing the bypassed loop and (3) absorption of increased levels of the hepatotoxin lithocholic acid.[23] Recent evidence, however, suggests that lithocholic acid is not an important etiologic factor.[24]

Colonic Pseudo-obstruction. Abdominal distention and fluid levels, fever and toxic symptoms[25,26] have been noticed in a number of patients within 4 weeks following jejunoileal bypass. Presumably, bacterial overgrowth in the defunctionalized bowel contributes in some manner, since symptomatic improvement following antibiotic therapy has been shown.[27]

Arthritis and Arthralgia. In a small number of patients in whom colonic pseudo-obstruction occurred following jejunoileal bypass, symptoms of arthritis and arthralgias were manifest.[28] It has been suggested that systemically absorbed bacterial antigens may contribute to cryoprotein complexes. The latter have been associated with complement components and antibody against E. coli and Bacillus fragilis and may be important in the pathogenesis of the arthritis. Tetracycline administration has provided symptomatic improvement.[29]

Nutritional Management

Protein-calorie malnutrition is a common sequela in most, if not all, patients following jejunoileal bypass;[30] its severity is variable and, for the most part, the condition is permanent. Presumably, it contributes to the development of transient or permanent hepatic steatosis in these patients. Attempts at oral amino acid supplementation show a modest effect on protein-calorie malnutrition and no effect on progressive liver disease. Oral oligopeptide administration, with amino acid supplementation parenterally, appears to be of some benefit.[20]

Prevention of renal calculi is best accomplished by inhibiting the absorption of dietary oxalate. Dietary oxalate intake should be restricted to 50 mg per day by excluding high-oxalate-containing foods.[17] Calcium restriction is contraindicated in these patients since the excessive fecal fat loss contributes to calcium deficit. Furthermore, deficit of calcium prevents precipitation of insoluble calcium oxalate in the gut lumen. Consequently, therapy is aimed at maintaining a high level of intraluminal calcium. As an adjunct to calcium supplementation, 6 to 12 gm daily,[31] aluminum hydroxide antacid, providing 3.5 gm of elemental aluminum, has been found to be effective in inhibiting oxalate absorption.[32] Restricting saturated fats and thereby preventing sequestration of calcium by unabsorbed fat appears to be beneficial.[33] Additionally, medium-chain triglyceride substituted for saturated fat has been effective in reducing urinary oxalate excretion.[34] Hypocalcemia and hypomagnesemia resulting from the shortened absorptive surface, increased intestinal motility and sequestration by dietary fat lost to the stool are problems requiring constant surveillance. Iron deficiency anemia is an occasional complication of jejunoileal bypass surgery and is readily corrected by iron supplementation. Vitamin B_{12} malabsorption generally results from an inadequate length of terminal ileum compounded by bacterial overgrowth in the nonfunctional loop of small bowel and is corrected by parenteral B_{12}. Transient deficiencies in fat-soluble vitamins, as well as folate and vitamin C, have been noted and are correctable by oral supplementation.

Management of diarrhea in these patients is similar to the management of that of massive small bowel resection. High intakes of dietary fat and lactose have been frequent factors in refractory diarrhea.[11] Hypokalemia may be corrected by oral supplementation with 45 to 60 mg potassium daily.

MALABSORPTIVE SYNDROMES

The *diffuse disorders* of the small intestinal mucosa, such as are seen in the flat bowel mucosa syndromes (Tables 31B–1 and 2), are variously termed primary or idiopathic steatorrhea, nontropical sprue, adult celiac disease, celiac sprue and childhood celiac disease. The less severe disorders thereof are termed subacute atrophy. Creamer[1] concluded that the flat jejunal biopsy was not specific for adult celiac disease, since this may be seen in a variety of other diseases (Table 31B–1). Others have ascribed some degree of specificity to this group of disorders (Table 31B–2).

Determination of the extent, severity and type of nutritional deficiency seen in any and all of these disorders requires investigation by a wide variety of absorption tests and tests for specific nutrients, as described elsewhere in this text.

Diagnosis dependent upon roentgeno-

Table 31B–1. Diseases Associated with Flat Jejunal Mucosa (Primary and Secondary Celiac Syndromes)*

Primary celiac syndrome
  Gluten-sensitive enteropathy (celiac disease of children, adult celiac disease, idiopathic steatorrhea)
Secondary celiac syndrome
(May or may not respond to gluten-free diet)
  Carcinoma and lymphoma within and without the gut
  Lactose toxicity in infants
  Diabetes mellitus
  Sarcoidosis
  Sjögren's syndrome
  Infectious hepatitis
  Ulcerative colitis
  Regional enteritis
  Postgastrectomy states
  Pancreatic disease
  Giardia lamblia
  Ancylostoma duodenale
  Strongyloidiasis
  Coccidiosis
  Widespread dermatitis
  Acne rosacea
  Kwashiorkor
  Rigid dieting in obesity
  Experimental malnutrition in animals
  Excessive ingestion of cathartics
  Accompanying oral contraceptive agents
  Tropical sprue
  Hypo- and agammaglobulinemias
  IgA deficiency

*From Creamer.[1]

Table 31B–2. Diagnostic Usefulness of Peroral Biopsy of the Small Intestine*

Diagnosable Lesions
  Celiac sprue
  Acanthocytosis (A-beta-lipoproteinemia)
  Whipple's disease
  Lymphangiectasia
Controversial Areas
  Amyloidosis
  Carcinoma (small bowel)
  Cholera
  Cirrhosis
  Cystic fibrosis
  Diabetes mellitus
  Disaccharidase deficiency
  Diverticulosis
  Hepatitis and other viral illnesses
  Hypogammaglobulinemia
  Iron deficiency anemia
  Lymphoma
  Parasitic diseases
  Peptic ulcer
  Scleroderma
  Tropical sprue
Alleged Abnormalities
  Neomycin malabsorption
  Gastrectomy
  Regional enteritis
  Ulcerative colitis
Miscellaneous—no significant mucosal pathology within proximal jejunum
  Pancreatic insufficiency
  Pernicious anemia
  Chronic gastritis
  Chronic idiopathic diarrhea
  Severe malnutrition
  Folate deficiency
  Systemic mast cell disease

*From Rubin and Dobbins.

gram is often nonspecific. The introduction of the peroral biopsy techniques[2] made possible the prompt pathologic diagnosis of small bowel disease, and provided a morphologic basis for evaluation of therapy.[3–5]

GLUTEN-SENSITIVE ENTEROPATHY

Gluten-sensitive enteropathy is also called primary idiopathic steatorrhea, nontropical sprue, and adult celiac disease.

Although the cause of celiac disease is unknown, dietary elimination of wheat, oats, barley and rye has been used with dramatic relief since Dicke[1] first reported the relationship of wheat products to celiac disease. Subsequently, it was shown that the offending agent in wheat is confined to the protein moiety, gluten.[2] Precipitation of gluten with 70 per cent alcohol yields an alcohol insoluble portion—glutenin, which is nontoxic—and an alcohol-soluble fraction—gliadin, which is toxic to the sensitive individual. As little as 3 gm per day of this latter fraction, fed to celiac patients in remission, produces diarrhea and steatorrhea. Attempts to further fractionate this portion enzymatically and to purify the toxic component chemically are still the subject of considerable debate.

Kowlessar, Warren and Bronstein[3] summarized these reports as well as studies concerned with mucosal cell enzymic defect, histochemical findings and immunologic phenomena in celiac disease. They offered the following hypothesis: The enzymic defect in celiac patients is one in which N-pyrrolidone peptides derived from intraluminal digestion of wheat protein enter the mucosal epithelial cell but cannot be further degraded. Increased intracellular levels of N-pyrrolidone peptides interfere with metabolism in such a way as to transform normal columnar to stratified squamous cells. The damaged mucosal epithelium is rendered permeable to wheat glycopeptides and other soluble wheat and milk proteins, which may be antigenic. Participation of these proteins in antigen-antibody reactions might thus account for high antibody titers to food proteins in the sera of celiac patients.[4] Transmucosal passage of food antigens across a damaged small bowel mucosa has also been suggested[5] to account for high titers of antibodies to milk proteins and gluten fractions in the serum found in a patient with systemic mast cell disease studied in this laboratory.

In adult celiac disease there may be diffuse involvement of the entire intestinal mucosa with more severe involvement of the upper small bowel than of the more distal small bowel.[6,7] The diminution of absorptive area may result in impaired absorption of all nutrients, principally fat, although sugar, protein, vitamin and mineral malabsorption may be present in varying degrees.[8]

The average age of onset is 35 to 40 years,[9-13] although sometimes the history of diarrhea may date to childhood. The disease is characterized by exacerbations and remissions. Pregnancy, infection and other stresses may precede the onset of symptoms initially or precipitate exacerbations.[8,9] The presenting symptoms in over 75 per cent of the cases are weight loss, malaise and weakness and diarrhea.[10-12,14,15] Stools characteristically are bulky, light in color and foul smelling. Occasionally, however, a patient will complain of constipation. Physical examination reveals evidence of weight loss and malnutrition. Some patients may exhibit pallor, peripheral edema, hyperpigmentation, bleeding tendencies, clubbing and hypotension.[16] It is not uncommon to find evidence of hypofunction of all the endocrine glands.

Roentgenograms of the small bowel show hypomotility, dilatation, coarsening of the mucosal folds, puddling, segmentation and flocculation of the barium.[14,17-19] This nonspecific pattern is the result of a variety of causes and is described more fully in Chapter 21.

Peroral biopsy of the small intestinal mucosa has confirmed the early observations of Sakula and Shiner[20] and Rubin and co-workers.[21] They reported varying degrees of villus change, abnormalities of the epithelial cells and inflammatory infiltration of the lamina propria. These changes, no longer considered specific for celiac disease, have been seen in many disease states (Table 31B-1).[22]

Marked histologic improvement of mucosal specimens usually occurs within the first few weeks of therapy, but months to years may be needed for return to the normal state. Improvement in clinical parameters of absorption precedes histologic improvement.[2,6,23-26]

Fecal fat and xylose tests, almost always abnormal in the untreated patient, are helpful in assessing the improvement in bowel function. In general, improvement parallels strictness of adherence to the gluten-free diet.[27,28] Disaccharide intolerance, particularly for lactose, is common in this disease, and milk ingestion may contribute to diarrhea. Oral tolerance tests of lactose, sucrose and starch may be normal or they may give a flat blood sugar response. Disaccharidase levels in the small intestinal mucosa are usually low. Disaccharide hydrolysis and subsequent monosaccharide absorption are usually diminished.[29-33]

Fat malabsorption is often accompanied by deficiency of fat-soluble vitamins. Fatty acids released by bacterial action can contribute to influx of fluid into the gut lumen. Pancreatic and biliary secretions may be normal in celiac disease, and thus lipolysis of dietary fat to triglycerides and free fatty acids may be normal.[8] Subsequent micelle formation takes place but these lipids and bile salts are lost in the stool.

Hypocalcemia and hypomagnesemia lead to tetany, paresthesias and bone fractures.[34-36] Serum alkaline phosphatase[37] may be elevated. Electrolyte deficiencies from excessive loss of potassium and sodium into the stool may occur in severe diarrhea.

Since the greatest morphologic and absorptive defects occur in the proximal intestine, folate deficiency may occur.[40] Depending upon the degree of injury to the terminal ileum, vitamin B_{12} absorption may or may not be adequate. Macrocytic red blood cells, hypersegmented polymorphonuclear leukocytes and a megaloblastic bone marrow may result from deficiency of folic acid alone or from a combination of both deficiencies. In cases of severe disease it may be reasonably assumed that the water-soluble vitamins are inadequately absorbed.

When the diagnosis is made, gluten is withdrawn from the diet. The successful treatment of this disease depends heavily on the dietitian's ability to teach the patient how to select foods free of gluten-containing products and the patient's willingness to abide by this diet (see Appendix Table A–25). The diet should contain as many calories as the patient can tolerate. A 3,000- to 3,500-calorie diet is recommended, high in carbohydrate and protein if the patient is underweight. Initially, fat intake should be restricted to approximately 40 to 60 gm per day. Fat intake can

be increased as bowel function improves. Milk and products containing lactose should be limited initially if lactose intolerance is suspected.

Potassium supplements may be given in oral liquid form and continued as long as necessary if potassium depletion exists.

Initially, folic acid or folinic acid, 5 mg per day, may be given parenterally. Oral folic acid (15 mg per day) will suffice in many instances. The distal bowel is less severely affected in this disease than the proximal. Since the distal bowel heals first, vitamin B_{12} deficiency may not be a continuing problem. If the Schilling test demonstrates deficient absorption, vitamin B_{12}, 100 μg per month, should be given parenterally. Folic acid should not be given without vitamin B_{12} unless adequate vitamin B_{12} absorption is assured, for fear of obscuring the development of combined system disease. Some degree of iron deficiency usually exists.[8] Parenteral iron preparations may be given when oral preparations are not tolerated. Iron is absorbed primarily in the duodenum[38,39] where the low pH of gastric acid converts ferrous iron to the ferric state. The addition of ascorbic acid either in the form of food, e.g. orange juice, or in tablet form at the time of iron ingestion facilitates its absorption. (See Chapter 7C for discussion of iron absorption.)

Water-soluble vitamins, ascorbic acid, 100 gm per day, and B complex, may be given freely. If the patient is unable to eat, initial intravenous fluid therapy should contain vitamin supplements. As the condition improves these vitamins can be given by the oral route, preferably in liquid form. Many multivitamin preparations contain added minerals also. The quantity present, however, is not sufficient for adequate mineral replacement in the celiac patient. Calcium, 8 to 12 gm per day orally, is often required, given in 3 to 4 divided daily doses. When there is evidence of bone fracture or bone pain, the dose may be increased to 20 gm per day. One gram, given as a solution of calcium gluconate, may be administered slowly intravenously when tetany supervenes. As noted in Chapter 7 Section B, magnesium depletion should be suspected when serum calcium is depressed in a malabsorptive state. This should be checked and the deficiency, if present, treated with intravenous or intramuscular magnesium sulfate (2 to 4 gm daily) until normal serum levels are achieved and maintained on a normal diet. Vitamin D, 50,000 I.U. per day orally, is usually adequate where there is evidence of a pathologic bone condition.[41] When continued vitamin D therapy is required, or larger dosages are deemed necessary, careful monitoring of serum calcium levels is essential.

The principal therapeutic goal is the establishment of an effective gluten-free diet. Nutritional management usually becomes less demanding once the gluten-free diet is achieved. Although a gluten-free diet is usually effective in children, 15 to 25 per cent of adults will not respond satisfactorily.

When further evaluation fails to reveal other causes for the disorder, corticosteroid therapy may be used.[42-44] The usual dosage is 40 to 60 mg of prednisolone per day in divided oral doses.[45] Parenteral preparations may also be used. Less is known about the effectiveness of ACTH in this disease. Within the first week of therapy the patient should show increased appetite, decreased diarrhea and improved sense of well-being. The usual risks of corticosteroid therapy obtain; adequate potassium, magnesium, calcium and vitamin D should be provided. Osteoporosis and osteomalacia already present may be enhanced. Infection, handled poorly by the deficient patient, may be masked by this therapy.

Diuretics should be used cautiously, if at all, for the hypoproteinemic edema. The edema is usually not severe and responds to diet as the body protein stores are replenished. Diuretics tend to augment the potassium deficit already present and can precipitate hypokalemia and its consequences.

Testosterone or estrogen therapy may be useful in some children whose growth is retarded. Anabolic steroids may lend temporary support to some patients.

Patients should be observed closely for infections or bone fractures and treated promptly. Specific treatment for the decreased function of the pituitary, adrenal and thyroid glands is usually not necessary as these functions improve as metabolic deficits are replenished.

Tropical Sprue

Tropical sprue is a chronic recurrent afebrile disease of uncertain cause(s), occurring most commonly in the tropical and subtropical area such as Puerto Rico, Cuba, Hong Kong and India.[1] It is manifested clinically by diarrhea, steatorrhea, malnutrition and usually macrocytic anemia resulting from the malabsorption of folic acid and/or vitamin B_{12}. Bacteria, viruses[4] and parasites[5] have been implicated, but to date isolation and identification of a single causative agent have not been successful. Findings that well-nourished individuals arriving in the tropics from a temperate climate may acquire the disease within days or weeks of arrival,[6,7] the occurrence of epidemics in India and Burma[8-10] and the response to broad-spectrum antibiotics provide circumstantial evidence of an infectious component in the etiology.

Dammin[11] and Bayless and associates[12] studied the viral and bacteriologic flora in patients with tropical sprue, but their findings were inconclusive. Using newer techniques, Gorbach et al.[13] established that the small bowel of untreated patients with tropical sprue is generally colonized with coliform organisms. Klipstein et al.[14,15] isolated 3 serotypes of Klebsiella pneumoniae and a strain of Enterobacter cloacae from the small bowel of Puerto Rican patients. All isolates were toxigenic when assessed in the in vivo rabbit intestinal loop. The investigators suggested that enterotoxin elaborated by these organisms was capable of producing functional and structural abnormalities of the small bowel mucosa similar to those observed in tropical sprue. They also isolated similar enterotoxin-producing organisms from Haitian patients with tropical sprue, but not from patients with mild intestinal abnormalities.[16]

Protein deficiency is chronic in the tropics and parasitic infestations of the intestinal tract are common; both conditions may be associated with altered gut morphology.[17] It is apparent that the small bowel reflects the numerous factors acting on it, i.e. nutritional deficiencies, parasites, bacteria, viruses, etc., which alter gut morphology and further influence the absorption of available nutrients. This leads to an interacting cycle which is variously manifested clinically. Klipstein and Baker[18] editorialized that the syndrome of tropical sprue primarily involved impaired absorptive function of the gastrointestinal tract. Vitamin and mineral deficiencies and megaloblastic anemia were considered secondary to the malabsorptive state. Ghitis and co-workers[19] suggested that protein-calorie malnutrition may lead also to malabsorption, but these individuals can be differentiated from tropical sprue patients by relatively normal values of serum folate and vitamin B_{12}. This distinction is not clear-cut since other workers[20] noted considerable overlap between the two groups.

Gorbach and associates,[20] in studies of the small bowel microflora, observed that bacterial overgrowth was a frequent finding in tropical sprue and far less frequent in protein-calorie malnutrition. They documented bacterial interference with absorption in 80 per cent of the sprue cases but not in malnourished individuals. An additional point of differentiation was offered by Banwell et al.[21] who demonstrated that fluid secretion from the small intestinal mucosa was the usual event in tropical sprue but rarely occurred in protein-calorie malnutrition. In this regard the small bowel in tropical sprue patients has secretory characteristics similar to those observed in other chronic diarrheal diseases such as nontropical sprue,[22] scleroderma[23] and in the acute infectious diarrhea associated with Vibrio cholera[24] and E. coli.[25]

Physical examination reveals varying degrees of malnutrition: pallor, weight loss, submucosal and subepidermal hemorrhages, cheilosis, glossitis, hyperpigmentation of pressure points, generalized loss of muscle tone and occasionally signs of posterolateral column involvement of the nervous system.

Intestinal structure may be normal or show flattening of the villi, increase in the crypt/villus ratio and varying degrees of inflammatory reaction within the lamina propria.[2,3] The small bowel mucosa may differ histologically from that of celiac disease, primarily in severity of lesion and in location. In tropical sprue the lesion is usually milder, but the mucosa is more uniformly involved than is that of celiac disease, in which the proximal bowel is more severely damaged and frequently markedly atrophic.

In tropical sprue the villi are frequently "leaf" shaped. Some villi which appear normal under the dissecting microscope may be found under light microscopy to contain a dense inflammatory infiltrate in the lamina propria, and the epithelial cells may be abnormal. Klipstein et al. attempted to distinguish tropical sprue from celiac disease on the basis of the location and distribution of lipid droplets in basement membrane and lacteals.[26] Swanson et al.[27] showed that with folate and with vitamin B_{12} repletion the villus structure improved.

Laboratory studies may reveal a macrocytic anemia and megaloblastic bone marrow, reduction in serum proteins, calcium, magnesium, phosphorus and potassium.[28] Quantitative stool fat analysis frequently demonstrates steatorrhea of a mild degree. Xylose absorption is impaired.[26] Hypoacidity or anacidity following gastric analysis has been demonstrated in 50 per cent of the cases.[29] The absorption of vitamin B_{12} with intrinsic factor is usually impaired.[30] Absorption of folic acid and tissue stores[30] are decreased.[31] Smears of buccal and gastric epithelial cells reveal changes similar to those seen in untreated pernicious anemia.[32]

Jeejeebhoy found lowered serum vitamin B_{12} levels in 30 per cent of sprue patients studied, lowered folate levels in 70 per cent and combined vitamin B_{12} and folate deficiency in 20 per cent. These deficiencies may occur in the presence or absence of steatorrhea. In the majority of persons with tropical sprue B_{12} malabsorption results from ileal malabsorption.[33] Herbert and associates[34] demonstrated a lack of receptors for intrinsic factor B_{12} complex in morphologically normal ileal tissue obtained from several Puerto Rican expatriates in New York City. In others, reduced secretion of intrinsic factor has also been implicated in the vitamin B_{12} deficiency seen in these patients.[35] Development of folate deficiency in persons with tropical sprue may be related to two separate physiologic abnormalities of folate absorption: malabsorption of folate monoglutamate which appears to be related to the severity of the mucosal abnormality[36-38] and malabsorption of folate polyglutamate which may occur in patients with normal absorption of folic acid.[38]

Hypoalbuminemia and edema occur in approximately 25 per cent of patients with tropical sprue[39-41] because of an inadequate dietary intake, impaired albumin synthesis in the liver[42] and excessive protein leakage into the gastrointestinal tract.[43]

Hypocalcemia, a frequent finding in tropical sprue, has been considered a consequence of malabsorption and deficiency of vitamin D.[44] More likely, hypocalcemia may be induced by magnesium depletion rather than being secondary to vitamin D deficiency.[45] The presence of steatorrhea depends primarily upon the severity of the mucosal lesion.[46] Disaccharidase activity may be diminished in proportion to the severity of the gut mucosal lesion.[47,48] Oral absorption tests of disaccharides, especially lactose, give flat responses. Sucrosuria has been reported as a persistent finding. Steatorrhea is present more often in patients with severe malabsorption of vitamin B_{12}, suggesting involvement of distal bowel or a more diffuse lesion than that seen in patients with malabsorption of folic acid and d-xylose alone.

A nutritious diet—consisting of 2,400 to 3,000 calories, 100 to 150 gm of protein and an adequate supply of folate—is the primary requisite. If steatorrhea is a problem, the amount of fat may be reduced to 50 to 60 gm per day initially. Ingestion of lactose-containing foods in the presence of a relative lactase deficiency may augment diarrhea. Such substances should be deleted from the diet until improvement has occurred following therapy.

Intravenous electrolyte and fluid replacement is necessary in extremely ill patients; however, oral supplements of potassium, calcium and vitamin D usually suffice. Occasionally, there will be an indication for parenteral magnesium. Multivitamin supplements may be given.

Clinical remission has been reported when the tropical sprue patient is treated with oral sulfonamides or broad-spectrum antibiotics.[26,44,49-51] Tetracycline and oxytetracycline (1 gm per day) in divided doses are commonly prescribed. Hematologic remission and symptomatic improvement have occurred with folic acid and/or vitamin B_{12} alone, although Sheehy reported that vague gastrointestinal symptoms and steatorrhea persisted in 60 per cent of patients treated with vitamins alone.[52] Klipstein[26] reported folate repletion occurring in some patients treated with tetracycline alone, and noted further clinical and histologic improvement with the addition of folic acid. At the present time, many prefer to treat with all three.

Crystalline folic acid, 15 mg per day orally, and 100 μg IM of vitamin B_{12} at monthly intervals are the usual doses. These may be continued until the respective serum levels and all absorption parameters return to normal. Guerra et al.[49] advocate continuing therapy until patients are at least morphologically stabilized. They also reported effective long-term results following treatment with 300 to 500 mg of oxytetracycline for 6 months.

Whipple's Disease (Intestinal Lipodystrophy)

This previously fatal, chronic disorder is characterized by episodic fever, arthritis and polyserositis, diarrhea progressing to steatorrhea, marked weight loss, anemia, hyperpigmentation, lymphadenopathy and, occasionally, splenomegaly.

The usual laboratory tests give evidence of malabsorption of fat, xylose, and vitamin B_{12}.[1] Loss of fat-soluble vitamins and hypocalcemia, hypomagnesemia and hypokalemia may result from excessive steatorrhea and diarrhea. Serum proteins, particularly albumin,[2] may be diminished. Radiologic changes in the small bowel are compatible with a malabsorption pattern. Stools are intermittently positive for blood, the actual mechanism for which has not been elucidated. The diagnosis of Whipple's disease is made histologically by peroral biopsy of the intestinal mucosa.[3] Macrophages of the lamina propria of the small intestinal mucosa contain PAS-positive staining material. Light and electron microscopy has shown this material to consist of bacilli.[3-5] Other tissues, especially lymph nodes, may also be involved. Following treatment with antibiotics or steroids the bacilli disappear from the lamina propria and to a large extent from the macrophages, only to reappear with clinical relapses. The lacteals may be distended with fat globules, which are present in the lamina propria also. This derange-ment returns toward normal following therapy.[3,4] Vitale et al.[6] produced gastrointestinal lesions in primates similar to those observed in humans with Whipple's disease.

Numerous attempts have been made to culture the rod-like organisms present in the lamina propria of the bowel and in the lymph nodes. In one study[7] more than 30 identifiable strains were obtained from 8 biopsies in the same patient. The interpretation of this and other studies is rendered difficult because of the problems of gut luminal contamination. Charache[8] circumvented the problem by studying blood and lymph nodes obtained aseptically. Initial isolation revealed atypical bacterial forms—pleomorphic and rod-like gram-negative organisms—that reverted to β hemolytic, Lancefield group D enterococcus on repeated subcultures. High serum antibody titer against this organism, 1:128, but a low titer against a variety of other organisms were noted. Drug sensitivity correlated with the clinical response to therapy. The relationship of this or other organisms isolated from the blood to the pathogenesis of Whipple's disease is still to be ascertained. A 30 per cent incidence of endocarditis in these patients at autopsy complicates the interpretation of blood cultures, since these may represent an extension of the primary offender or represent secondary bacterial invasion. It is not known if patients with Whipple's disease have impaired bacterial resistance or if only one or more than one organism produces the clinical syndrome.[9]

Diet and replacement therapy are the same as those employed for other malabsorptive states and are based upon nutritional deficits, on-going needs and the specific absorptive defects.

Antibiotic therapy may bring about dramatic improvement.[1,3-5,10,11] Ruffin et al.[10] used procaine penicillin and streptomycin for a 10- to 14-day period, followed by long-term (10 to 12 months) broad-spectrum antibiotics such as tetracycline or oxytetracycline, with success. Serial peroral intestinal mucosal biopsies have shown the gradual disappearance of the PAS-positive staining material.[1,3–5,10,11] Therapy should be continued as long as this material is detectable. Clinical recovery may antedate the histologic reversion to normal by months to years. Relapse does occur and responds to the reintroduction of antibiotic therapy.[4]

Adrenocorticotropin and adrenocorticosteroid therapy are also reported to reverse the course of the disease in some patients.[12] Reasons for this effect are obscure and Pirola et al.[13] suggested that the use of corticosteroids be restricted to the critically ill patient unresponsive to antibiotics.

Malabsorption from Bacterial Contamination of the Gut (including Small Intestinal Diverticulosis, Blind Loop Syndrome and Scleroderma)

Anatomic derangements of the small bowel resulting in stasis or inadequate propulsion of the bolus with subsequent bacterial proliferation may lead to a malabsorption of fat and vitamin B_{12} deficiency. Among these conditions are the long afferent loop of duodenum following gastric surgery (blind loop), strictures or fistulization of the bowel and small bowel diverticulosis. Small duodenal diverticula commonly seen on roentgen examination have not been shown to cause significant disease. Occasionally, a single very large diverticulum may result in malabsorptive problems. Since bacterial overgrowth is common to these conditions, they will be considered together.

Symptoms associated with a *blind loop syndrome* or with *small bowel diverticulosis* vary; they include vague abdominal pains, particularly after meals, flatulence, colicky pain postprandially, weight loss, diarrhea, constipation, nausea and vomiting. Physical examination may be normal or show varying degrees of malnutrition and evidence of vitamin B_{12} deficiency.

Clinical studies by Doig and Girdwood[1] and experimental studies by Donaldson[2–4] show that the intraluminal bacteria compete with the host for vitamin B_{12}. A wide variety of enteric microorganisms, both gram-positive and gram-negative, aerobic and anaerobic, which may or may not require exogenous vitamin B_{12} for growth, can bind vitamin B_{12}.[5] Competitive binding and/or utilization by the bacterial flora explain the vitamin B_{12} deficit leading to the macrocytic anemia. Antibiotic therapy interrupts this process; the exact mechanism, be it suppression or alteration of the flora or alteration of the host defense, is not yet clear.[6]

While competitive uptake by the luminal flora may deprive the host of vitamin B_{12}, a less direct mechanism appears to be involved in steatorrhea associated with conditions of stasis. Dawson and Isselbacher[7] first suggested that bacterial hydrolysis of conjugated bile salts may play a role in the pathogenesis of steatorrhea in the blind loop syndrome.

Conjugated bile salts promote fat absorption by aiding the emulsion of the fat in the intestine, by activating pancreatic lipase, by incorporating the products of lipolysis into micelles[8] and by stimulating reesterification within the epithelial cells. Free or unconjugated bile salts are either inactive or inhibitory to these processes under in vitro conditions simulating those in the intestine. Although current evidence points to a deficiency of conjugated bile salts as the explanation for steatorrhea in the blind loop syndrome, the toxic or inhibitory effects of unconjugated bile salts may be contributory. Deconjugation of bile salts by bacteria colonizing the small bowel yields free bile acids, which are somewhat less effective than conjugated bile salts for micelle formation. More important is the fact that at a luminal pH below 7.0 (small bowel luminal pH 5.5 to 7.0) bile acids, unlike bile salts, are protonated, unionized and relatively insoluble in an aqueous environment. Consequently, precipitation of bile acids contributes to the bile salt deficiency noted in these patients.[6,9] Furthermore, the precipitation of bile acids under these conditions may provide an explanation for the occurrence of bile acid enteroliths occasionally noted in areas of stasis in the small bowel.

Dietary treatment consists of a diet abundant in calories (2,500 to 3,500), high in protein and reduced in fat and in bulk, i.e. a bland diet. Frequent small feedings are recommended. If lactose intolerance is noted, milk products should be excluded. Medical treatment is adequate in many patients. Surgical removal may be accomplished when the diverticula are confined to a short segment of gut, when they are large and empty slowly radiographically or when perforation, ulceration or hemorrhage occurs.

Iron supplements may be necessary if the duodenum is involved. Parenteral replacement, 200 μg of vitamin B_{12}, should be given each month. Therapy with a broad-spectrum antibiotic such as tetracycline or chlortetracycline in divided doses has been used successfully.[10] Intermittent therapy is desirable to minimize development of resistant organisms or overgrowth by yeasts. Whether folic acid therapy is necessary or whether it is synthesized in adequate amounts by the gut flora is not known.[11,12] Serum determinations should be performed when deficiency is suspected.

Scleroderma may involve the entire gastrointestinal tract. Histologically, atrophy and fragmentation of the muscular coat of the gastrointestinal tract with increased deposition of collagen and a largely intact mucosa are characteristic of this lesion.[13,14] Marked impairment of motility and development of dilated, static segments further contribute to bowel malfunction. The chief absorptive defect appears to be that of fat; vitamin B_{12} and xylose absorption are not consistently impaired.[14,15]

Impaired motility and stagnation within the small bowel favor abundant bacterial growth in the proximal small intestine. Salen et al.[16] suggested that the malabsorption pattern resulting from this bacterial overgrowth is similar to that seen in blind loop or intestinal diverticula.

Oral treatment with broad-spectrum antibiotics has been effective clinically. Maintenance of nutrition is hampered by the relentless course of this disease. However, reduction of fat in the diet will reduce the amount of diarrhea when steatorrhea is a problem. The patient should receive parenteral vitamin B_{12} therapy, 100 μg per month, oral supplements of water-soluble vitamins and minerals. Corticosteroid therapy or vitamins alone have been ineffective. When an isolated segment of the bowel is involved, surgical resection of that portion of the gut may lead to prolonged improvement.[15]

Mastocytosis

The skin lesions of systemic mastocytosis appear initially, but the disease may ultimately progress to involve many other organs including the intestine. Bank and Marks[1] reported one patient with systemic mastocytosis and malabsorption of carbohydrates, fat and vitamin B_{12}. Partial villous atrophy, with a prominent eosinophilic infiltrate of the lamina propria, was noted on surgical small bowel biopsy, as was the lack of mast cells. Rubin and Dobbins reported similar findings.[2] Jarnum and Zacharie,[3] however, noted a prominent increase in mast cells in the small bowel lamina propria, muscularis mucosae and submucosa. Malabsorptive defects in association with systemic mastocytosis were studied by Broitman and associates[4] in a 61-year-old woman. Malabsorption of carbohydrates, fat and vitamin B_{12} indicated involvement of the entire small bowel. Surgical small bowel biopsy disclosed abnormal numbers of mast cells beneath the muscularis; a rectal biopsy disclosed abnormal numbers of mast cells in the lamina propria and submucosa. Peroral small bowel biopsy showed intense mucosal and submucosal round cell infiltrates containing large numbers of eosinophils. High titers of antibodies to gluten (fraction III), alpha-lactalbumin and beta-lactoglobulin indicated transmucosal passage of incompletely degraded food antigens. Sensitivity to gluten was demonstrated by a favorable response to a gluten-free diet and prompt exacerbation of steatorrhea and diarrhea following gluten challenge. This was considered to be secondary to mast cell invasion of the gastrointestinal tract rather than to primary adult celiac disease unmasked by systemic mastocytosis. On a daily fat intake of 100 gm incorporated into a gluten-containing diet, the attacks of facial flushing, abdominal pain, tachycardia and explosive diarrhea ceased. This occurred coincident with a decrease in serum magnesium; restoration of magnesium levels to normal was followed by a recurrence of attacks. It was speculated that hypomagnesemia may promote degranulation and/or prevent regranulation of mast cells in man.

Although the symptoms were similar to those observed in other patients with mastocytosis, urinary histamine levels were normal. Histidine loading did not enhance symptoms or increase histaminuria above that of control subjects.

PROTEIN-LOSING ENTEROPATHIES

The gastrointestinal tract plays a prominent role in the metabolism and homeostasis of plasma proteins in normal and in pathologic states. Intact gamma globulin is absorbed in newborn animals; the gut synthesizes serum proteins, including immunoglobulins and lipoproteins, and degrades the plasma proteins. Serum proteins are normally lost into the gastrointestinal tract where they are degraded rapidly into their constituent amino acids for reabsorption and resynthesis of protein. Hypoproteinemia, therefore, develops when the rate of loss by excretion and catabolism exceeds the rate of nitrogen reabsorption and serum protein resynthesis.

Thus, diseases manifesting protein-losing enteropathy have no single common etiology and pathogenesis. Regardless of cause, patients exhibit a reduced circulating and total body pool of albumin, a normal or slightly increased rate of albumin synthesis and a markedly shortened albumin survival, determined by testing with radioactive labeled substances.[1]

Excessive protein loss into the bowel may result from numerous causes: (1) obstructed outflow of the gastrointestinal lymphatics, with consequent loss of lymph and protein into the gut lumen (lymphangiectasia, intestinal lipodystrophy, lymphoma, carcinoma, constrictive pericarditis), (2) exudation through an inflamed or ulcerated mucosa (regional enteritis, ulcerative colitis, celiac sprue), (3) excessive secretion of mucus (atrophic gastritis, Menetrier's disease—hypertrophic gastritis—and gastrointestinal cancer) or (4) excessive loss in other disorders (nephrosis, defective gamma globulin synthesis and some of the aminoacidurias).

Mineral losses—iron,[2] copper,[3] calcium[4]—and lipid loss[5] may accompany gastrointestinal protein loss. The constant finding of lymphocytopenia in patients with lymphatic channel abnormalities is suggestive of the loss of lymphocytes via the gastrointestinal tract.[1]

Clinically, the patient with protein-losing enteropathy may exhibit only edema and hypoproteinemia. In some, gastrointestinal complaints or symptoms of hypocalcemic tetany may prevail. Others may exhibit growth retardation. Occasionally, iron deficiency anemia, lymphocytopenia, eosinophilia or aminoacidurias may be noted as well. A comprehensive review of this subject is provided by Waldmann.[1]

"Allergic Gastroenteropathy"

Six infants were described by Waldmann[6] and Bookstein[7] with rhinitis, asthma, eczema, growth retardation, periorbital edema, anemia, hypoalbuminemia, hypogammaglobulinemia and eosinophilia. The patients had precipitating antibodies to milk and Charcot-Leyden crystals in their stools. They exhibited a normal to increased rate of albumin synthesis, but a shortened albumin survival and increased fecal excretion of protein. Absorption tests showed no steatorrhea and minimal xylose malabsorption. Roentgenograms showed evidence of mucosal edema in 5 of the 6 patients, only one of whom showed segmentation and puddling of barium.

Biopsies performed on 5 patients revealed increased infiltration of the lamina propria with some eosinophilia. Two were normal. Serum levels of albumin and IgA and IgG were reduced. Elimination of milk from the diet of 3 patients ameliorated their symptoms and the disordered protein metabolism. Reintroduction of milk caused recurrence of symptoms and increased the protein losses. Corticosteroid therapy in 3 other patients reversed the protein loss. Eosinophilia and response to steroids support the suggestion of an allergic or hyperimmune state.[8]

Hypogammaglobulinemia

This condition, with multiple granulomatous ulcers in the terminal ileum and cecum associated with an increased gastrointestinal protein loss, was described by Holman[9] in a patient with repeated infections. Intestinal resection ameliorated the intestinal protein loss, but gamma globulin concentration continued to decrease. Another report[10] indicates that in some patients IgA and IgM may be decreased more than IgG. Biopsies of the jejunal mucosa have shown considerable variability, ranging from normal[11,12] to nodular lymphoid hyperplasia with a normal intervening mucosa and villus architecture[10,11,13] to partial or total villus atrophy.[11,14] The malabsorptive defect in these patients does not appear to have a single cause. In some patients giardial infestation in association with hypogammaglobulinemia was observed.[10,15] Elimination of the parasite was accompanied by

cessation of diarrhea and steatorrhea in some.[10,11]

In the absence of detectable pathogens in the stool, antibiotic therapy has been unsuccessful in alleviating steatorrhea.[14] Patients with total atrophy of the jejunal mucosa have been treated with a gluten-free diet with variable results.[11,14] Corticosteroids may be of some benefit in the management of patients with localized granulomatous disease.[11] While the enteric loss of protein may be ameliorated and albuminemia may be corrected with the various therapeutic regimens listed above, gamma globulin synthesis remains unaffected. Waldmann[1] states that the primary disorder in these patients is defective gamma globulin synthesis, leading secondarily to gastrointestinal tract lesions and consequent loss of serum proteins via the gastrointestinal tract.

Cardiomyopathies

Excessive enteric protein loss occurs in congestive heart failure, especially in constrictive pericarditis,[16,17] in familial cardiomyopathies and in association with valvular and septal defects. Hypoproteinemia and edema are the chief presenting findings. Diarrhea and steatorrhea occur occasionally. In addition to the serum albumin decrease, the gamma globulins are also lowered. The total body protein pool is reduced, albumin survival time is markedly shortened and fecal protein losses are excessive. Xylose tolerance tests have been reported to be normal.[18] Microscopically, dilatation of the submucosal lacteals and lymphatics in the small bowel have been described in two cases.[18,19]

A functional disorder of the intestine secondary to an increase in the central venous pressure has been suggested as the mechanism of protein losses into the gut associated with congestive heart failure.[20] Increased thoracic duct pressure and flow rate have been demonstrated in patients with constrictive pericarditis.[18,21]

Treatment is aimed at the cause. In congestive heart failure the usual measures are employed: digitalis, diuretics and low salt diet. Recovery from hypoproteinemia with disappearance of lymphatic dilatation has been reported following pericardectomy.[18,20,22-24]

Intestinal Lymphangiectasia

This syndrome in children or young adults is characterized by generally mild gastrointestinal symptoms, but occasionally by severe diarrhea and steatorrhea, nausea, vomiting, and abdominal pain, asymmetric edema, chylous effusions, hypoalbuminemia, hypogammaglobulinemia and lymphocytopenia.[1,9,25-28] Waldmann showed a decreased serum half-life of albumin and stated that this was the result of gastrointestinal protein loss. Subsequent studies by Herskovic et al. showed that trapping of ^{131}I labeled albumin in the edematous extremities contributes to the reduced circulating albumin.[29] Malabsorption of nutrients other than fat is uncommon.[25] The diagnosis is made by the demonstration of increased albumin loss and by the morphologic changes observed in small bowel biopsy, namely, markedly dilated and telangiectatic lacteals and lymphatics in the lamina propria of the mucosa, submucosa or serosa.[25]

Treatment has been unsatisfactory. Steroids and antibiotics have been unsuccessful.[30] Satisfactory resection of a lesion confined to a short segment of bowel has been reported in two studies[1,26] but poor results were obtained in another.[1] Dietary fat restriction decreases the "load" on the lacteals and reduces intestinal lymph flow and pressure, thereby diminishing retrograde enteric "leakage." This effect is further enhanced by substituting medium-chain triglycerides for part of the dietary fat.[30-32]

CARBOHYDRATE INTOLERANCE

Carbohydrate "intolerance" or "dyspepsia" has been recognized for a number of years. Bloating, abdominal discomfort, nausea, vomiting and explosive acidic diarrhea occur following ingestion of the offending sugar.[1]

At least 50 per cent of man's daily caloric intake is provided by carbohydrate. Dietary starch and glycogen are hydrolyzed by alpha-amylase in the intestinal lumen to maltose (glucose-α-1-4 glucose) and isomaltose (glucose-α-1-6 glucose). Sucrose (glucose-fructose) from cane or beet sugar and lactose (galactose-glucose), milk sugar, are the major free dietary disaccharides. Further hydrolysis of disaccharide to monosaccharides is mediated by enzymes located in the brush border membrane of the intestinal villus.[2] Human jejunal mucosa contains up to 5 maltases, 1 or 2 sucrases and an alpha-dextrinase (an isomaltase). Of the two lactases described, only one has the properties of a digestive enzyme. It is specific for lactose, has a pH of 6.0 optimal and is missing in patients unable to tolerate lactose. The second β-galactosidase can utilize substrates in addition to lactose, persists at normal levels in lactose-intolerant individuals and may not play a significant role in lactose digestion.[3]

Intolerance may occur to disaccharides or monosaccharides. Monosaccharide intolerance, a rare condition, is manifested at birth and requires prompt diagnosis for infant survival.[4] It appears to result from an alteration of the transport mechanism for glucose and galactose. Treatment consists of elimination of glucose and galactose and replacement with fructose.[5-7]

More commonly, intolerance may occur to any of the four disaccharides lactose, sucrose, maltose or isomaltose, either singly or in combination.[7] Disaccharide intolerance occurs in infants and adults as a primary, inherited enzyme defect[8-10] or as an acquired defect secondary to other diseases of the small intestine (see Table 31B-3). Combined disaccharidase deficiencies may occur in any disorder of the small bowel epithelium such as celiac disease, sprue,[11-13] giardiasis,[1] acute enteric infections,[14] cystic fibrosis[15] and kwashiorkor.[16,17]

Table 31B–3. Classification of Disaccharide Intolerance.*

Lactose Intolerance
  Congenital physiologic lactase deficiency in premature infants
  Congenital lactase deficiency, presumably genetically determined (1) Some cases associated with lactosuria
  (? related to acute gastroenteritis in infants)
  Acquired lactase deficiency in children and adults, probably genetically determined
  Acquired: part of generalized disaccharidase deficiency and secondary to diffuse mucosal damage resulting
  from:
    Celiac disease, tropical sprue, Whipple's disease, intestinal lymphangiectaseia, etc.
    Acute gastroenteritis (especially in infants)
    Kwashiorkor
    Administration of neomycin or PAS
    Giardia lamblia infestation (presumed mucosal damage)
    Postbowel surgery in infants (presumed mucosal damage)
  Acquired: secondary to alteration in intestinal transit resulting from:
    Small bowel resection (may decrease lactase level also)
    Postgastrectomy or pyloroplasty (may unmask a preexisting deficiency)
    Lactose intolerance without lactase deficiency
  Suggested disease associations
    Cystic fibrosis
    Osteoporosis
Sucrose Intolerance
  Congenital sucrase-isomaltase deficiencies; rare, genetically determined (63 cases as of 1965)
  Seemingly acquired sucrose intolerance, sucrase-isomaltase deficiency in adults, presumably also genetically
  determined and similar to the congenital deficiencies
  Acquired: secondary to diffuse mucosal damage
Glucose-galactose Malabsorption
  Congenital, inherited inability to absorb these monosaccharides
  Acquired: secondary to diffuse mucosal damage in infants

*From Bayless and Christopher.[31]

Lactose ingestion most frequently causes clinical symptoms. According to Haemmerli and associates,[11] this may result from the lesser amount of lactase activity normally found per gram of mucosal tissue compared to other disaccharidases. Deficiency of lactase is the most frequently reported isolated enzyme deficiency.[18] Isolated sucrose and combined sucrose-isomaltose intolerances have been reported in infants and children.[19,20] Apparently these intolerances are lost with age, since only an occasional case has been reported in adults.[10] We have found no reports of isolated maltase deficiency. Among the congenital forms of disaccharide intolerance in infants, however, lactose intolerance seems to be the most common. Clinically symptomatic intolerance to lactose is seen even more frequently in the adult. Therefore, it must be either an inherited enzyme deficiency with delayed manifestation or an acquired deficiency. Cuatrecasas et al.[21] suggested that prolonged abstinence from milk and milk products results in lowered enzymatic activity. However, there is no evidence to date that such a deficiency, clinically symptomatic, can be induced in man. Starvation causes an equal lowering of activity of all the disaccharidases and all are raised equally by refeeding glucose alone. Knudsen suggests that this response is a result of the caloric effect.[22]

Adaptive changes in rat gut mucosal disaccharidase activity in response to disaccharide feeding have been studied by Deren and associates.[23,24] Despite increases in lactase activity on lactose feeding, absorption was unchanged.[23] Diminished activity of this enzyme following weaning occurs commonly in many animals.[25] Sunshine and Kretchmer[26] have demonstrated complete absence of this enzyme in the sea lion pup, which from birth requires no milk.

Lactase deficiency in the North American adult population is reported to vary from 16 to 55 per cent, with the higher incidence in blacks.[27,28] The incidence in children between the ages of 11 months to 11 years with similar eating habits and socioeconomic status varies from 10 per cent in Caucasians to 35 per cent in blacks.[29] The increasing frequency of lactose-induced symptoms in black children with advancing age suggests a gradual decline in enzymatic activity. Cook and Kajubi[30] reported significant variances in the tribal incidences of lactase deficiency in Uganda, despite apparently similar diets.

Frequently, gut lactase activity may be the only abnormally low disaccharidase in an otherwise normal adult. While Scandinavians and west Europeans show the lowest incidence (2 to 8 per cent are lactose intolerant), Greek Cypriots, Arabs and Ashkenazic Jews have an incidence of lactose intolerance of 60 to 80 per cent. Approximately 70 per cent of American Negroes and greater than 90 per cent of African Bantus, Japanese, Thais, Formosans and Filipinos are intolerant to lactose.[31,32] In general, the majority of adults the world over exhibit low gut lactase activity, implying that this may indeed be the "normal" situation. Recently, the variations in gut lactase activity in different populations have been the subject of anthropologic studies.[33] The question posed by these findings is whether the inherited tendency is the result of low consumption of milk over many generations or whether low consumption of milk is the result of low gut lactase in these populations.

Lactose intolerance following gastric operation for peptic ulcer disease[11,34] has been attributed to preexisting lowered lactase activity made symptomatic by the altered intestinal anatomy and physiology.[10]

Milk allergy, rapid delivery of a hyperosmotic load to the upper small bowel and inadequate lactose hydrolysis[35] may be contributing factors.

Intolerance to lactose and hypolactasia have also been reported in "irritable bowel syndrome,"[36] dermatitides,[37] ulcerative colitis[38] and regional ileitis.[39]

When disaccharides are not hydrolyzed and absorbed, they remain within the gut lumen where they exert a hyperosmolar effect. As large volumes of water are drawn into the gut lumen, distention and discomfort develop. The flora of the lower small bowel and colon metabolize the sugar, forming lactic, butyric and other irritant volatile acids and causing cramps and diarrhea.[1]

Following ingestion of 100 gm of lactose, the nondeficient individual shows a rise of at least 20 mg per 100 ml glucose in serum.[40] In the presence of lactase deficiency, however, the blood glucose curve is "flat" and the patient develops clinical symptoms. If the patient is given equimolar amounts of glucose and galactose, however, the expected rise of at least 20 mg occurs. The stool of the lactase-deficient patient contains large amounts of lactic acid. The pH of the stool may not fall below 6 in the adult, but in children it may go as low as 4.5 in a matter of 1 to 2 hours. Peroral biopsy of the small intestine is usually normal; however, a flat mucosa on biopsy, which reverted to normal on withdrawal of the sugar, has been reported by Burke et al. in intolerant infants fed lactose.[41] In this instance lactose appeared to be toxic to the mucosa in a manner similar to gluten in celiac disease. Kern and associates reported steatorrhea in association with lactose intolerance in a woman.[42] A similar finding was noted by Welch in a small percentage of 100 patients with isolated deficiency.[43] Assay of the small bowel mucosa for enzymatic activity by the method of Dahlqvist[44] in intolerant individuals revealed low or absent values for lactase and normal activity for the other disaccharidases. Welch suggested that the best single method of defining this group was on the basis of an increase in the sucrase/lactase ratio.[43]

Because intestinal biopsy presents some difficulty in infants, various indirect tests for detecting lactase deficiency have been tried.[45,46] ^{14}C-Lactose has been utilized and the quantity of [14]CO_2 activity in the breath following an oral load permits the detection of a reasonable number of lactase deficient subjects. Analysis of breath hydrogen following an oral lactose load appears to be an even more sensitive test for detecting lactase-deficient patients than either direct or other indirect tests. In this test, unabsorbed lactose provides a substrate for hydrogen production by colonic bacteria. This is measured in the breath of test subjects over a 4-hour period after lactose ingestion.

Treatment in the infant is simple once the offending sugar is identified. Numerous formula preparations contain sucrose and dextrins which can easily be substituted for lactose-containing preparations without losing calories. In sucrose-isomaltose malabsorption lactose is substituted. The older child or adult with sucrose-isomaltose intolerance requires thorough dietary education and diligent management. In the lactose-intolerant adult, elimination of lactose-containing foods results in prompt relief; for those who have had symptoms for many years without correct diagnosis this relief may be gratifying indeed.

METABOLIC DISORDERS
Diabetes

"Diabetic diarrhea" is associated with peripheral or autonomic neuropathy.[1,2] Steatorrhea, when present, is variable.

Abetalipoproteinemia (Acanthocytosis)

A syndrome of severe hypolipidemia, progressive neuromuscular ataxia, atypical retinitis pigmentosa and acanthocytosis in which there is a hereditary absence or deficiency of β-lipoprotein has been described.[1-3] Steatorrhea is usually present and serum cholesterol, carotene and vitamin A are markedly reduced. Monosaccharide absorption is normal; however, lactose absorption and lactase activity within the intestinal mucosa are decreased, as reported by Isselbacher. Peroral biopsy of the jejunal mucosa has revealed large amounts of intraepithelial fat globules.[2]

During the process of fat absorption, reesterification of triglycerides occurs within the mucosal epithelium (see Chapter 5). Triglycerides are then incorporated along with β-lipoprotein into the chylomicron. Isselbacher[4] suggested that this latter step may limit the rate of lipid movement across the mucosa into the lymphatic system. The impairment of protein synthesis by agents such as puromycin, acetoxycycloheximide or ethionine reduces the absorption of long-chain fatty acids.[5,6] Consequently, in experimental animals so treated and given an oral load of fat, plasma triglycerides did not reach a normal elevation. Further, plasma β-lipoproteins decreased while α-lipoproteins were unaffected. Morphologically, the intestinal mucosal epithelium was engorged with triglyceride droplets.[5] The close parallel between these findings and those in congenital β-lipoprotein deficiency implicates defective β-lipoprotein synthesis in chylomicron formation.[2,7] Normally about 75 per cent of the total circulating lipid consists of β-lipoprotein.[8] Van Buchem and associates[9] suggested that in abetalipoproteinemia steatorrhea develops when the accumulation of intracellular fat reaches a threshold value.

A convenient screening test for this disease, based upon autohemolysis of acanthocytic red blood cells, appears to be useful in assessing therapy.[10,11]

Isselbacher and associates[2] demonstrated weight gain and reduction in steatorrhea following replacement of dietary fat with 30 to 45 gm of medium-chain triglycerides.

Amino Acid Anomalies

Steatorrhea is sometimes associated with congenital abnormalities of active transport of amino acids, initially described in the renal tubule and subsequently shown in the small bowel.[1]

PARASITIC INFESTATION

Diarrhea is a frequent symptom of parasitic infestation of the intestine. Absorptive defects for one or more nutrients may accompany excessive fluid and electrolyte loss. Knowledge of the life cycle of the parasite in the human host is a prerequisite for understanding the several mechanisms of malabsorption: (1) Competition with the host for a particular nutrient, e.g. Diphyllobothrium latum,[1] the fish tapeworm, which consumes vitamin B_{12} within the gut lumen, deprives the host of this vitamin. (2) Invasion of the gut mucosa, e.g. Strongyloides stercoralis[2-4] attaches to the mucosa of the duodenum and upper jejunum where it reduplicates. Mucosal disruption and inflammation may prevent optimal absorption.[2,5] In hookworm infestation the worm Necator americanus attaches to the tips of the intestinal villi, deriving nutrients from the host.[2] The resultant bleeding causes microcytic, hypochromic anemia which responds promptly to iron.[6] (3) Interference with absorption can be caused by large numbers of organisms such as Giardia lamblia.[7,8] Although there is some controversy as to the invasiveness of Giardia, mechanical interference with absorption by enormous numbers of parasites appears to occur. The parasite may also competitively deprive the host of nutrients and provoke inflammatory reaction in some individuals, which accentuates absorptive defects.[7] Symptomatic infestation occurs most frequently in undernourished individuals and in those with impaired immune mechanisms. Some patients with symptomatic giardiasis have reduced immunoglobulin levels.[7,9]

Treatment of parasitic infestations has been reviewed by Marsden et al.[10,11] Diets high in calories, carbohydrates and protein and low in fats are used in patients with steatorrhea. Specific or multiple vitamin supplements are given as indicated. Iron preparations are given for iron deficiency anemia. During acute diarrhea, oral feedings may be withheld completely or clear liquids may be given.

ACUTE INFECTIOUS DIARRHEAS

An adequate discussion of this problem within the limited confines of this chapter is not possible. The reader is referred to extensive treatises on the subject, both general and specific.[1-3] Nutritional status influences susceptibility to and the consequences of bacterial infections.

Acute infectious diarrheas include, among others, salmonellosis, shigellosis, typhoid and paratyphoid fever, cholera, infantile diarrhea, E. coli diarrhea in adults, viral gastroenteritis, staphylococcal "food poisoning," and "traveler's diarrhea." In their more fulminant form these conditions are characterized by explosive diarrhea with immediate loss of fluid and electrolytes. Usually, however, they are self-limiting.

In general, therapy of infectious diarrheas is aimed at maintaining nutritional, fluid and electrolyte balance, while eliminating the causative microorganism. Eisenberg, Palazzola and Flippin[4] reported that as many as 74 per cent of adults with salmonellosis or shigellosis are afflicted with another or "primary" illness. Therapy, then, must be directed toward the primary illness as well as to the bacterial infection. Lindenbaum et al. showed evidence of malabsorption during and after recovery from acute intestinal infection in patients with acute enteritis, including cholera.[5,6] In infants with infectious enteritis Torres-Pinedo and associates[7] indicated that the volume and composition of diarrheal stools were partially determined by defective intestinal absorption of sugars. Following oral administration of glucose, fructose, lactose or sucrose, stool acidity markedly increased owing to an increase in organic acids. Presumably the latter was the result of bacterial fermentation. Additionally the accumulation of organic ions in the colon resulted in a cation-entrapment effect leading to increased losses of cations in the diarrheic stool.

Salmonellosis and Shigellosis

Salmonellosis, a major public health problem, is probably the most common cause of infectious gastroenteritis in the United States. During 1964, over 21,000 laboratory-confirmed human infections were reported.[1] Undoubtedly this represents but a small percentage of the total number of cases. In spite of its usual benign course in most adults, there may be serious manifestations, such as peritonitis, endocarditis, pneumonia, osteomyelitis, urinary tract infection and meningitis.[2-4] The incidence of infection and the fatality rate with food salmonellae are highest in infancy and decline with age.[5] The prime vehicle of salmonella transmission is food prepared from infected animals or contaminated during preparation. Virtually all types of food may be sources, especially those lightly cooked and subject to repeated handling.[6]

Duration and severity of the diarrhea appear in some cases to be related to the acid secretory status of the host. Patients with salmonellosis and impaired gastric acid secretion exhibit a cholera-like diarrhea as compared to patients with normal gastric acid secretion, who have mild diarrhea.[7,8] Salmonellae invade the small bowel mucosa, gain access to the general circulation via the small intestinal lymphatics and may ultimately favor sites such as joint spaces, kidney and bone marrow. Small bowel mucosal changes may vary from minimal inflammation and petechial hemorrhage, to frank ulceration and necrosis. These changes generally are most pronounced in the terminal ileum.

Shigellosis is localized to the gut, occasionally involving the terminal ileum but mainly affecting the colon, with lesions ranging from congestion and erythema to extravasation of blood and pus and, occasionally, ulceration and perforation. Chronic ulcerative colitis was considered to be a consequence of unusually severe shigellosis in approximately 15 per cent of cases by Felsen,[9] although the data were not conclusive.

Cholera

Cholera, caused by Vibrio cholerae, exemplifies a fulminant form of infectious diarrhea prevalent in malnourished populations. The major symptom is profuse watery diarrhea—isotonic with plasma. In the untreated case, vomiting and skeletal muscle cramping are early manifestations, probably secondary to marked electrolyte imbalance followed eventually by dehydration and circulatory collapse. The patient is afebrile and the disease has an average duration of 4.2 days.[1] The mortality rate is as high as 60 to 80 per cent[1,2] in untreated cases. Adequate treatment reduces the mortality rate to essentially zero.[1]

The relationship of malnutrition to cholera is not clear. Unquestionably the highest incidence is found among the poor living under primitive conditions. There appears to be a selective affinity for individual members in a family,[3] more frequently the young. Cruickshank has suggested that malnutrition may similarly affect the course of cholera.[3] Rosenberg, however, found no evidence of specific vitamin deficiencies.[4]

Fluid loss during the 3- to 6-day illness may exceed 30 liters. The average electrolyte composition of the stool in severe adult cholera is as follows, in mEq/L: Na^+ 140, K^+ 10, Cl^- 110 and HCO_3^- 40. Severe dehydration is evidenced by plasma protein concentrations as high as 14 gm per 100 ml. Diarrhea appears to be related to the production of an enterotoxin by V. cholerae, which increases small bowel intracellular cyclic AMP, or to be stimulated directly by enterotoxin or via adenyl cyclase.[5-7] Associated with increased cyclic AMP is a reversal of chloride transport, resulting in the net secretion of chloride. Sodium flux is also reduced to zero, but the net absorptive flux of sodium can be increased again by the addition of an actively transported sugar or amino acid. Realization of these phenomena has provided a major adjunct to the therapy of acute cholera.[7] Glucose (56 mM), along with bicarbonate, potassium, sodium and chloride (in concentrations equal to those found in the stool), administered orally, stimulates absorption of intestinal fluid and results in a prompt decrease in the volume of stools.

In severe cases, however, vomiting and other symptoms resembling the dumping syndrome occur when fluids are given orally. In such cases, fluid replacement must be administered intravenously.

Phillips' method of treating cholera is well suited for use in epidemics and may be applied by unskilled technicians in uncomplicated cases.[9] It relies on the measurement of plasma specific gravity by a copper sulfate method.[10] Four ml of fluid replacement per kg body weight are given for each increase of 0.001 plasma specific gravity above normal (1.025). Children and infants require relatively more fluid replacement.

The standard intravenous fluid regimen consists of 2 parts isotonic saline to 1 part isotonic sodium lactate or bicarbonate.[8] After determining the state of hydration by determination of plasma specific gravity, rapid rehydration is accomplished by administering 100 ml per minute; infusions are continued thereafter at a rate equal to the measured gastrointestinal fluid losses.

Tetracycline, 1 gm per day in divided doses, halves the duration of the disease and decreases the fluid requirements.[1]

Traveler's Diarrhea

This condition is usually far less severe than the acute bacterial diarrhea. Until recently, the search for conventional pathogens, bacterial, viral and protozoan, as etiologic agents has been unrewarding. Evidence newly available[1] has incriminated an organism indistinguishable by conventional techniques from Escherichia coli which comprises part of the normal fecal flora. It differs, however, in its ability to colonize the upper small bowel and elaborate an enterotoxin. Enterotoxigenic strains produce either a heat-labile and/or a heat-stable toxin; both result in fluid accumulation when instilled in the rabbit small bowel loop in vivo. Isolation of toxigenic E. coli has been reported from patients with traveler's diarrhea throughout the world. These are antigenically different from those known E. coli serotypes responsible for infant diarrhea.

It has been suggested that infection may be acquired conventionally by ingestion or may occur endogenously. In the latter instance, an individual may harbor enterotoxigenic E. coli in the colon with little consequence, since the enterotoxin appears specific for the small bowel. Under conditions which may result in transient small bowel stasis (presumably environmental changes, dietary variations, viral agents, etc.), the organisms may colonize the small bowel via retrograde spread from the colon and elaborate enterotoxin, resulting in a severe watery diarrhea. Fortunately it is self-limiting and responds to simple preventive or therapeutic aids.

CHRONIC INFLAMMATORY BOWEL DISEASE

Granulomatous Inflammatory Diseases—Regional Enteritis, Granulomatous Ileocolitis, and Granulomatous Colitis

Regional enteritis is an inflammatory disease of unknown etiology usually affecting the terminal ileum, but occasionally extending throughout the small intestine.[1] Acute and/or chronic inflammation of the lamina propria with granuloma formation accompanies obstruction of the lymphatics. Regional enteritis occurs less frequently than ulcerative colitis, but the two diseases have certain similarities.[2,3] As does ulcerative colitis, regional enteritis occurs most frequently in young adults, usually between ages 16 and 30. It appears to be more common in patients of Jewish origin and it is relatively uncommon among Negroes.[4]

Regional enteritis is characterized by bouts of abdominal pain, fever and diarrhea. Weight loss, anorexia, anemia and steatorrhea may be present in the chronic state. Rectal bleeding is usually less prominent than in ulcerative colitis. Physical examination frequently reveals wasting and a right lower quadrant tender mass.

Complications may consist of internal and external fistulization, scarring with obstruction, perforation with abscess formation and hemorrhage. Abscesses, uveitis, iritis, arthritis, selective or diffuse malabsorption, osteoporosis and liver disease may accompany regional enteritis as well as ulcerative colitis.[5] Systemic amyloidosis is a rare complication[6] and development of carcinoma at the site of involvement has been reported in only a few instances.[7-10]

The nutritional deficit depends upon the extent, severity, and location of the diseased bowel. Because of the frequency of involvement of the terminal ileum, vitamin B_{12} uptake and bile salt reabsorption may be impaired and steatorrhea and macrocytic anemia may occur. Fistulization may take place with formation of a blind loop in which excessive bacterial proliferation occurs. Anemia may be enhanced by decreased iron intake, malabsorption of iron and chronic blood loss into the gut. Hypoproteinemia and edema result from inadequate dietary intake of protein, increased tissue catabolism, increased enteric protein loss and malabsorption of amino acids. The net absorption of water and sodium may be diminished in the affected bowel.[11] Electrolyte losses, dehydration, folic acid deficiency and mineral and fat-

soluble vitamin losses parallel the severity of steatorrhea.

Maintenance of nutrition, allaying diarrhea, restoration of blood and fluid loss and control of infection are the aims of therapy.[12] Zetzel[3] recommended a high-calorie, high-protein, low-residue, low-fat, nonirritating diet, with elimination of milk and milk products, particularly if there is any suggestion of milk intolerance. High-residue foods can cause obstruction in a narrowed ileum and must be avoided; one of Brown's patients had four episodes of obstruction, all precipitated by corn and all relieved by medical treatment.[13] In the case of bacterial overgrowth from fistulization and stasis in patients unable to undergo further surgery, treatment is similar to that outlined for blind loop syndrome and includes intermittent antibiotic therapy, parenteral replacement of vitamin B_{12}, supplemental vitamin and mineral therapy and reduction of dietary fat.

Medication includes replenishment of vitamins, especially the vitamin B group, vitamin K and folic acid, and calcium, magnesium, iron and potassium, sedatives, tranquilizers, antispasmodic-anticholinergic drugs, salicylazosulfapyridine and, when needed, broad-spectrum antibiotics. Adrenocorticotropic hormone and adrenocorticosteroids have been used in acute as well as long-term management with some success. Sparberg and Kirsner reported apparent beneficial suppression of symptoms in 217 cases treated on a long-term basis with 30 mg or more daily of prednisone or prednisolone.[14] Perforation, abscess and sepsis, however, may be sequelae to such therapy and may further complicate management.

Patients with granulomatous disease may require surgical resection for palliation and control of obstruction, perforation and fistulization, and, rarely, cancer.

In recent years, largely because of combined efforts of English and American workers, granulomatous colitis has been recognized as a separate entity, clinically and pathologically, from nonspecific ulcerative colitis.[15-21] With regional ileitis, it shares a tendency to form palpable masses, fistulas and strictures and obstructions. It less commonly involves the rectum, differing thereby from nonspecific ulcerative colitis. In contrast to nonspecific ulcerative colitis, malignancy is rare, toxic megacolon has not been reported and bleeding and chronic anemia are less frequent. The clinical course, not surprisingly, resembles that of severe regional ileitis. Two types of clinical course have been recognized: (1) The disease is low-grade and indolent, obstructive symptoms are often the indication for surgery and patients generally do well after operation. (2) The clinical course is more severe, resembling severe regional ileitis and sharing its complications and surgical consequences.

The nutritional manifestations and treatment are similar to those described above.

With regard to the use of sulfonamides and corticosteroids Zetzel[22] commented that, although these are less effective in patients with granulomatous disease of the bowel than in those with ulcerative colitis, they afford sufficient benefit during the initial medical treatment to warrant their usage—unless, of course, this is contraindicated by complications.

Ulcerative Colitis

Nonspecific idiopathic ulcerative colitis is an acute and chronic febrile inflammatory and ulcerative disease of the colon and rectum[1] of unknown etiology. It is characterized by exacerbations and remissions and, occasionally, spontaneous recovery. Symptoms consist of abdominal pain, diarrhea, rectal bleeding, weight loss and debilitation. There is an increased incidence of allergic manifestations, e.g. asthma, hay fever and drug sensitivity. An allergic basis for the disease is further suggested by relief of symptoms after the elimination of certain foods such as milk, wheat, eggs and tomatoes in some patients and exacerbations during the "pollen season" in others.

The concurrence of ulcerative colitis with (1) conditions associated with hypersensitivity states, such as purpura, erythema nodosum, uveitis and arthritis, (2) the frequency of drug reactions, (3) the occasional elevation of serum alpha and gamma globulin and (4) the favorable response to corticotropin and corticosteroid therapy lends support to the hypothesis that ulcerative colitis has, as an immunologic basis, the so-called delayed allergy or tuberculin type of hypersensitivity. It is associated with a number of other diseases, including pyoderma gangrenosa, cirrhosis, nephrolithiasis, infections, osteoporosis and colonic carcinoma.[1-5]

Malnutrition is common, because of increased tissue catabolism, decreased food intake and excessive losses of nutrients, fluid and electrolytes. During exacerbations, loss of blood and plasma proteins occurs. Severe diarrhea leads to varying degrees of dehydration and losses of sodium, potassium and chloride. Steatorrhea and its sequelae (see above) may occur when the terminal ileum is involved. Anemia from iron deficiency is frequent.

Nonspecific jejunitis and jejunal villous atrophy have been reported by Salem and Truelove.[6] Flat curves following oral lactose tolerance tests and reduction in small bowel mucosal disaccharidase activity have been reported. After carbohydrate feeding, increased lactic acid and fatty acids occur in the stool[7] (see Carbohydrate Intolerance).

Nutritional management of ulcerative colitis is primarily supportive, symptomatic and nonspecific. Elimination diets are employed widely, but despite occasional dramatic responses there is no controlled evidence that they are actually beneficial. The frequent failure of a specific food allergy regimen is attributed by some to structural bowel changes complicated by secondary infection. The "low-residue" or "bland" diet is universally prescribed, but Kramer has pointed out the wide variation in these regimens.[8]

Kirsner[9] and Zetzel[10,11] have advocated the use of a diet devoid of the physical and chemical irritants contained in fruits, vegetables, fruit juices, condiments, alcoholic beverages and excessively hot or cold foods. A diet containing meat and potatoes but without fruits and vegetables is used initially. Cooked vegetables and canned fruits may then be added when stools are consistently formed and free of blood.[9] Diet may be further liberalized as the patient improves. For the acutely ill patient Kirsner has recommended a limited diet consisting of toast, butter, soft boiled eggs, clear broth, tea, rice, Jell-O, Cream of Wheat and custards.

Milk "allergy" has long been considered a factor in ulcerative colitis.[12,13] Hemagglutinins to the constituent milk proteins (lactalbumin) have been found in the serum of patients with ulcerative colitis by Taylor and Truelove,[14] but their origin and significance have not been satisfactorily explained. These same authors have observed that both the relapse rate and appearance of serial rectal biopsies were better when patients were on a milk-free diet than when they were fed gluten-free and milk-free or normal control diets. The histologic findings closely paralleled the clinical states. After maintenance on a milk-free diet many patients found that diarrhea ceased and that fruits and vegetables, which had previous been avoided, could again be eaten without symptoms. This response was noted particularly with the first attack of ulcerative colitis. Lactose has been suggested as the substance harmful in milk.[7] Lactase deficiency occurs more frequently in patients with ulcerative colitis than in the general population.[15]

Unreasonable restriction of diets can impose needless psychologic burdens on the patient. Success in overcoming the patient's disinterest in food requires patience in selecting attractive nutritious meals. Frequent small feedings are generally better tolerated than three regular ones. Not only is the patient less likely to consume as many calories when fed less frequently but

ingestion of larger volumes may stimulate bowel evacuation.

An intake of at least 2,400 to 3,600 calories containing at least 125 to 150 mg of protein may be needed to restore positive nitrogen balance. Protein supplements in the form of prepared formulas may be added to the diet; however, good-quality foods are preferred.

In patients with steatorrhea, restriction of dietary fat may be necessary to prevent further loss of nutrients and minerals. Reduction in the total pool of circulating bile salts may be one factor contributing to the steatorrhea. Substitution of a portion of the dietary fat with medium-chain triglycerides may be useful in the absence of adequate bile salts.[16] Kirsner[9] has emphasized that complete nutritional restoration may require at least 3 months or longer in the patient who has been acutely ill for a period of time.

Oral replacement of iron may cause gastrointestinal disturbances, even when taken with meals, and in such instances iron may be given by the parenteral route. If there is evidence of vitamin B_{12} malabsorption, then parenteral replacement in the amount of 100 to 200 μg per month should be given.

Potassium supplements are required only in exacerbations when excessive loss occurs. Anabolic steroid agents such as testosterone propionate have been prescribed to increase retention of nitrogen in tissue.

The goal is control rather than cure. Bed rest, sedation, tranquilizers, anticholinergics, antidiarrheal agents and occasionally short-term narcotics are used for control of symptoms.[9,10,17] Hospitalization frequently is necessary during acute exacerbations in order to remove the patient from stress in his environment, either known or unrecognized. As in any chronic disease state, tranquilizing drugs and, particularly, antidepressive preparations may be effective in alleviating depression and anxiety. Antispasmodic and anticholinergic medications such as tincture of belladonna help suppress the gastrocolic reflex and sphincter spasm. Antidiarrheal agents, e.g. diphenoxylate hydrochloride and paregoric, are useful in reducing bowel activity. Abdominal pain and tenesmus occasionally necessitate opiates but these should be avoided except for short-term usage, since they may mask perforations and lead to addiction.

Antibiotic agents should be used in presence of fever, evidence of sepsis, etc. Long-term therapy with sulfonamide preparations has been found to be particularly beneficial. The most commonly used preparation in the United States is salicylazosulfapyridine.

While not curative, ACTH and corticosteroid therapy have decreased morbidity and mortality.[18] The efficacy of short-term treatment with corticosteroid therapy, as opposed to long-term therapy, has been amply borne out by Truelove and Witts.[19] In a well-controlled double-blind study, cortisone (25 mg b.i.d.) did not decrease the relapse rate. During the initial acute attack the results of treatment with cortisone, 50 mg q.i.d. PO or ACTH, 80 U per day IM, were essentially the same. In subsequent acute exacerbations, however, ACTH was superior to cortisone in bringing about complete clinical remission in the course of 6 weeks' treatment. The chance of subsequent relapse was greater following ACTH therapy, as was the risk of complications, therby somewhat offsetting the beneficial results. It would seem that ACTH should be held in reserve. An occasional patient will need long-term therapy. Prednisone, 10 to 15 mg PO, is most frequently used. Hydrocortisone enemas have been employed with success not only during an acute episode but also on a long-term basis. Corticosteroid therapy is not without risk. When used for prolonged periods, calcium depletion with osteoporosis and ready fractures must be watched for. Perforations of diseased bowel may be masked.

In acute fulminant ulcerative colitis, general supportive measures may prove inadequate and operation may be required to control hemorrhage. Excessive fecal water, potassium and sodium losses lead to hypotension, prostration, renal impairment and oliguria, muscle flaccidity and cardiac arrhythmias.

"Toxic dilatation" of the colon is a state of rapid deterioration manifested by high fever, anorexia, nausea, vomiting and increasing prostration accompanied by colonic distention and tenderness. The diarrhea may decrease and bowel sounds cease. Radiographically, the transverse colon shows progressive distention. Perforation and sepsis may supervene. The exact mechanism is not known. The treatment recommended is cessation of all oral feeding, continuous gastric aspiration, restoration of blood, plasma, fluids and electrolytes, and parenteral antibiotics. A continuous intravenous drip of ACTH is recommended. If the patient does not show prompt response, surgery may be warranted.

The incidence of colonic carcinoma has been reported to be increased up to 20 times in ulcerative colitis. The appearance of cancer parallels the duration of the disease rather than its severity.[5]

Based on the hypothesis that ulcerative colitis is an autoimmune disease, a few preliminary reports suggested that the use of immunosuppressants such as azathioprine may be beneficial.[20] The efficacy of this therapy awaits further investigation. In the interim, Kraft and Kirsner[21] cautioned on the indiscriminate use of immunosuppressive treatment in inflammatory bowel disease. They emphasized the hazards of suppressing host defenses in patients who are vulnerable to many local and systemic risks, including infection and the possibility of development of primary neoplasms such as lymphoma and reticulum cell sarcoma, as noted in a small number of individuals given azathioprine therapy along with renal transplants. Additionally immunosuppressive drugs may enhance oncogenic viruses and alter host immunologic homeostasis, repressing immunologic mechanisms for the normal surveillance and rejection of malignant cells.[22]

OTHER COLONIC DISEASES

Colonic Diverticulum

A new concept has emerged in the treatment of diverticular disease of the colon, based on a better understanding of the pathophysiology.[1] Development of pulsion diverticula has been attributed to increased intraluminal pressure. The hypertrophied musculature of the sigmoid bowel wall exhibits motor activity to various stimuli in excess of that seen in normal controls.[2-4] With simultaneous intraluminal pressure recordings and cineradiography, Painter and Truelove[2] demonstrated that contraction of the thickened sigmoid muscle leads to narrowing and "blocking" of very short segments of the colon, which causes high intracolonic pressures. These high pressures contribute to the formation of diverticula. Almy[1] suggested that a large fecal mass in the sigmoid would prevent the close approximation of the colonic walls; hence, he recommended that the traditional low-residue diet be supplanted by one with large amounts of bulk and supplemented with hydrophilic colloids. Since morphine sulfate increases intraluminal pressures whereas meperidine does not, the latter drug is recommended for relief of pain in episodes of exacerbation of diverticular disease. Antibiotics are used when there is evidence of systemic infection manifested by fever and elevation of the white blood count.

Diverticulosis of the large bowel does not usually present nutritional complications until it is complicated by inflammation, formation of abscesses or fistulas, perforation or obstruction.

Villous Adenoma

Garis in 1941 reported a case of prerenal azotemia caused by fluid and electrolyte loss[1] accompanying a villous adenoma, but the relationship was not fully recognized until 1954 when McKittrick and Wheelock described the electrolyte depletion, dehydration, hypotension and azotemia.[2] Additional reports have appeared subsequently.[3,4]

In the normal colon there is a continuous exchange of water and electrolytes across the mucosa, the result being the efflux of water, sodium and chloride from the lumen and a net transfer of potassium and bicarbonate into the lumen to maintain isotonicity.[5] The normal fecal sodium output approximates 3.1 mEq per 24 hours and the potassium output 9.0 mEq per 24 hours.[6] In patients with villous tumors, large volumes of protein-rich mucosal fluid (3 to 4 L per 24 hours) may be passed, containing up to 160 mEq sodium and 70 mEq potassium. Such losses lead to lowered serum electrolyte concentrations.[7] Salem suggested that the sodium losses in this condition are quantitatively greater than potassium losses, but, because potassium balance is more precarious than sodium balance, the symptoms of hypokalemia are encountered more frequently than those of hyponatremia. The fecal potassium losses result from the increase in stool volume rather than from increased fecal potassium concentration. Therapy consists of colloid, fluid and electrolyte replacement. Sufficient bleeding may occur to warrant transfusion and protein losses may result in the lowering of serum protein values.[8]

This uncommon lesion, usually found in the rectum of older patients, may occur anywhere in the colon. Malignant change occurs in 30 to 74 per cent of the cases.[9,10] Surgical extirpation is the only definite therapy, but villous adenomas tend to recur.

USE OF MEDIUM-CHAIN TRIGLYCERIDES IN MALABSORPTION

Fat digestion and absorption entail (1) hydrolysis by pancreatic lipase catalyzed by bile salts, (2) micelle formation of the fatty acids and monoglycerides and bile salts, (3) passage into the epithelial cell by an as-yet-undefined mechanism, (4) reesterification of fatty acids of 10 or more carbon atoms to triglycerides within the intestinal mucosa; with shorter chain fatty acids, esterification is not obligatory, (5) subsequent incorporation of the reesterified triglycerides with phospholipids, cholesterol and protein into a beta-lipoprotein moiety, the chylomicron, and (6) continued movement of the lipid so packaged across the mucosa into the lymphatic system.[1]

In contrast, medium-chain triglycerides (MCT) and short-chain fatty acids appear to be absorbed about four times as efficiently as long-chain triglycerides (LCT) in experimental animals.[2] Although the rate of intraluminal lipolysis of MCT occurs faster than that of LCT,[3] a portion of the MCT enters the mucosal cell intact and undergoes intracellular hydrolysis.[4] Medium-chain fatty acids derived in this manner, as well as medium-chain fatty acids liberated within the intestinal lumen and absorbed, are transported without esterification to the liver via the portal vein.[1] Thus, diversion of pancreatic enzymes does not prevent hydrolysis of MCT[5] since extensive mucosal hydrolysis occurs. In conditions in which there are diminished concentrations of bile salts, less impairment of absorption of MCT occurs than of absorption of long-chain triglyceride, since bile salts are not required for dispersion of MCT in water. Clinically, in patients with pancreatic disease and biliary atresia, MCT is absorbed[6] more efficiently than LCT. Additional evidence that MCT are relatively well absorbed, despite low bile salt concentrations, was provided in normal individuals with cholestyramine-induced steatorrhea. Substitution of MCT for LCT abolished steatorrhea and no interference with cholestyramine sequestration of bile salts by MCT could be demonstrated.[7]

Both short-chain[8] and medium-chain triglycerides may be absorbed in part from the colon.[9] In the dog colon, Pihl, Glotzer and Patterson[10] demonstrated the absorption of 6-, 8- and 10-carbon fatty acids.

The differences between LCT (in which form most dietary fat occurs) and MCT (fractionated from coconut oil) make the latter useful in disorders of fat absorption. Commercial MCT is a bland oil composed primarily of the triglycerides of C_8 and C_{10} fatty acids.

Recent clinical observations have indicated that MCT are useful in treating patients with cystic fibrosis of the pancreas,[11,12] pancreatic insufficiency,[13-15] carcinoma of the pancreas,[12] extrahepatic biliary tract obstruction,[14] biliary atresia, bile fistula,[6] gastrectomy steatorrhea,[12,15-17] massive small bowel resection,[18,19] regional enteritis,[16] intestinal lymphangiectasia,[20,21] abetalipoproteinemia,[15,22] cholestyramine-induced steatorrhea[23] and cirrhosis.[16,24]

Senior[6] pointed out that MCT may play an important supplementary role in accelerating recovery from malabsorption treated by other therapies, including (1) gluten-free diets in celiac disease, (2) antibiotics in bacterial overgrowth of proximal gastrointestinal tract and (3) Whipple's disease on long-term antibiotic therapy, (4) pancreatic insufficiency responding partially to enzyme and bicarbonate replacement, but still fat intolerant, (5) tropical sprue during treatment with folic acid and antibiotics, (6) intestinal parasitism under specific therapy, (7) "bile salt diarrhea" with cholestyramine-produced steatorrhea.

In most cases diarrhea and steatorrhea decrease in patients responsive to MCT. To date, weight gain in patients given MCT supplements has been variable.[18] In this regard, it is interesting that the early clinical use of MCT was in the control of obesity.[26]

Saunders[27] called attention to the fact that the widely used van de Kamer[28] assay method does not completely extract MCT from stools. Indeed, the initial disillusionment during the clinical studies could be traced to the use of inappropriate methodology for quantitating the degree of steatorrhea following MCT-containing diets.[6] Less than 60 per cent of fatty acids such as octanoic can be recovered using the van de Kamer method. Braddock et al.[29] modified this by altering the ratio of ether and ethanol used in saponification and extraction of MCT and observed reliable results. Senior,[30] however, pointed out that the conventional van de Kamer method may give a reasonable estimation of fecal fat in patients given MCT, since the error of underestimation (owing to incomplete extraction of octanoic acid) is compensated for by an error of overestimation, when the fatty acid equivalent of 284 is used instead of 144 in the van de Kamer formula. The latter would be appropriate for such MCT fatty acids as octanoic. To circumvent these difficulties, Broitman et al. in this laboratory[31] urged the use of a fecal fat assay based on the principle of electrical capacitance.[32]

Despite evidence of clinical improvement in patients, long-term MCT feeding has not been entirely successful. Crampy abdominal pain and increased diarrhea have been reported with its use.[16] Increased steatorrhea has also been observed following the use of the oil preparation of MCT in one patient with short bowel syndrome.[16]

MCT is available as the purified oil or as the major fat constituent in commercially available powdered diets. Recipes are available for its use in cooking.[30] It may be substituted for long-chain fats in oral or tube formulas fed to patients with serious fat malabsorption.

It has been suggested[16] that MCT should not be used in patients with decompensated cirrhosis, because short-chain fatty acids inhibit oxidative phosphorylation[33] and may exert a narcotic effect on the central nervous system.[34] In cirrhotics, particularly those with hepatic encephalopathy, blood levels of short- and medium-chain fatty acids are increased.[35,36] MCT feeding may accentuate these effects. MCT are indicated in patients exhibiting continual nutritional caloric deterioration where all therapy has been unsuccessful in reversing the course of the malabsorptive disease, particularly in those instances where increased time for recovery and gain in body weight may result in spontaneous or therapeutic reversal of the initial problem. This is particularly relevant in infants, in whom nutritional considerations are critical.[6]

For additional information concerning biochemical and physiologic considerations and the clinical applications of MCT, the interested reader is referred to several excellent reviews.[25,30,37,38]

DIET AND THE CLINICIAN

The "diet" recommended by a physician is usually influenced by personal prejudice, mores and local dietary habits, many of which are carried over from times when little was known about the causes of gastrointestinal disorders and even less about specific medical therapy.

Weinstein et al.[1] and Donaldson[2] noted the need for more scientific information on the effect of diet in gastrointestinal diseases. The importance of using diets of proven usefulness is stressed. Such diets provide for: (1) avoidance of gluten in gluten-sensitive enteropathy,[3] (2) omission of disaccharides, e.g. lactose, in lactase-deficient patients,[4] (3) substitution of fructose in infants unable to actively transport glucose and galactose,[5] (4) substitution of artificially prepared medium-chain triglycerides for long-chain dietary lipids in patients with diminution or absence of pancreatic enzymes or bile salts[6] and with other malabsorptive disorders and (5) restriction of dietary fat in patients with steatorrhea in order to prevent further aggravation of steatorrhea with consequent loss of nutrients and minerals.

Diet therapy otherwise should be concerned with maintenance of nutrition or replacement of patient's losses. This is not an easy task and involves patience, imagination, time and much manipulation of foods. Perusal of diet manuals reveals great preoccupation with and wide variation in foods constituting so-called bland, high- and low-residue diets. Kramer[7] has pointed out the disparities in descriptions of high- and low-residue diets, which allegedly alter the intestinal contents or excreta. He advocates eliminating the word "residue," preferring "roughage" or "bulk" when referring to foods containing material resistant to chemical digestion. Cereals such as bran, vegetables, fruits and nuts contain the largest amount of roughage. Foods which increase the moisture content of excreta should be referred to as "laxative" foods or "juices," e.g. prune juice. Foods containing significant proportions of hemicellulose and/or cellulose, e.g. fruits and vegetables, would, therefore, be included in both categories.

The presence of large amounts of undigestible material or bulk within the intestinal lumen presumably acts as a mechanical stimulant in aiding evacuation. Bacterial action forming volatile acids within the colon also results in a laxative effect.[8]

Kramer studied the effect of foods commonly incriminated as causing alteration of bowel habits in otherwise healthy patients with ileostomies.[9] Excreta were checked for water content, wet and dry weights and electrolyte concentration following diets containing baked beans, cabbage, corn, prune juice, orange juice, pepper, milk and fried foods in amounts normally ingested. Cabbage increased the volume and weight in two-thirds of cases and baked beans increased dry weight only. The only substance he found consistently to increase stool weight and water content was prune juice, which contains diphenylisatin, a chemical laxative.[10] Water loading in this same group of patients by 6 to 8 glasses of water per day above the control intake did not appreciably alter the volume of ileal excreta, which remained at about 500 ml per day.[9] This apparently contradicts the common practice of prescribing increased water ingestion for the treatment of constipation. Whether his data are equally valid for the patient with a diseased colon or ileum remains to be studied.

BIBLIOGRAPHY

1. Zamcheck: Fed. Proc., *19*, 855, 1960.
2. Dubos, Shaedler and Costello: Fed. Proc., *22*, 1322, 1963.
3. Donaldson: N. Engl. J. Med., *270*, 938, 1964.
4. Sprinz: Fed. Proc., *21*, 57, 1962.
5. Spencer and Knox: Fed. Proc., *19*, 886, 1960.
6. Deren, Broitman and Zamcheck: J. Clin. Invest., *46*, 186, 1967.

Massive Resection of the Small Bowel

1. Booth: Postgrad Med. J., *37*, 725, 1961.
2. Kinney, Goldwyn, Barr and Moore: J.A.M.A., *179*, 529, 1962.
3. Winawer, et al.: N. Engl. J. Med., *274*, 72, 1966.
4. Jarnum, Schwartz, Thing and Thorsoe: Acta Chir. Scand., *122*, 428, 1961.
5. Cox, Meynell, Cooke and Gaddie: Gastroenterology, *35*, 390, 1958.
6. Shay, Gershon-Cohen and Fels: Am. J. Dig. Dis., *6*, 335, 1939.
7. Harrison and Harrison: J. Biol. Chem., *188*, 83, 1951.
8. Nicolaysen: Acta Physiol. Scand., *22*, 260, 1951.
9. Scheiner, Shils and Vanamee: Am. J. Clin. Nutr., *17*, 64, 1965.
10. Lack and Weiner: Am. J. Physiol., *200*, 313, 1961.
11. Hardison and Rosenberg: N. Engl. J. Med., *277*, 337, 1967.
12. Gazet and Kopp: Surgery, *56*, 565, 1964.
13. Fordtran, Clodi, Soergel and Ingelfinger: Ann. Intern. Med., *57*, 883, 1962.
14. Dowling and Booth: Lancet, *2*, 146, 1966.
15. Dahlqvist and Borgstrom: Biochem. J., *81*, 411, 1961.
16. Harrison and Booth: Gut, *1*, 237, 1960.
17. Booth, Read and Jones: Gut, *2*, 23, 1961.
18. Borgstrom, Dahlqvist, Lundh and Sjovall: J. Clin. Invest., *36*, 1521, 1957.
19. Alcock and MacIntyre: Biochem. J., *76*, 19P, 1960.
20. Booth and Mollin: Lancet, *1*, 18, 1959.
21. Klahr, et al.: Am. J. Med., *43*, 84, 1967.
22. Waldmann: Gastroenterology, *50*, 422, 1966.
23. Winawer, et al.: Am. J. Dig. Dis., *12*, 753, 1967.
24. Taylor: Gastroenterology, *51*, 1058, 1966.
25. Jabbari, Winawer and Zamcheck: Unpublished observations.
26. Frederick, Sizer and Osborne: N. Engl. J. Med., *272*, 509, 1965.
27. Osborne, Sizer, Frederick and Zamcheck: Am. J. Surg., *114*, 393, 1967.

Jejunoileal Bypass for Obesity

1. Penick, Filion, Fox and Stunkard: Psychosom. Med., *33*, 49, 1971.

2. Iber and Cooper: Am. J. Clin. Nutr., *30*, 4, 1977.
3. Bray: *The Obese Patient*. Philadelphia, W.B. Saunders, 1976.
4. Payne: Am. J. Surg., *106*, 273, 1963.
5. Scott, Brill and Price: Ann. Surg., *182*, 395, 1975.
6. Bray, Barry, Benfield, Castel-Nuovotedsco and Rodin: In *Hunger: Basic Mechanisms and Clinical Implications* (Wyrwyckee and Bray, Eds.). New York, Raven Press, 1976.
7. Barry, Barish, Bray, Sperling, Morin and Benfield: Am. J. Clin. Nutr., *30*, 32, 1977.
8. Moshal, Broitman and Zamcheck: Am. J. Clin. Nutr., *23*, 336, 1970.
9. Danö, Lenz and Justesen: Scand. J. Gastroenterol., *9*, 767, 1974.
10. Faloon, Rubulis, Knipp, Sherman and Flood: Am. J. Clin. Nutr., *30*, 21, 1977.
11. Dean, Scott, Shull and Gluck: Am. J. Clin. Nutr., *30*, 90, 1977.
12. Pi Sunyer: Am. J. Clin. Nutr., *29*, 409, 1976.
13. Hoffmann and Poley: Gastroenterology, *62*, 918, 1972.
14. Kim and Spritz: N. Engl. J. Med., *279*, 1424, 1968.
15. Dickstein and Frame: Surg. Gynecol. Obstet., *136*, 257, 1973.
16. O'Leary, Thomas and Woodward: Am. J. Surg., *127*, 142, 1974.
17. Gregory, Starkloff, Miyai and Schoenberg: J. Urol., *113*, 521, 1975.
18. Dobbins and Binder: Gastroenterology, *70*, 1096, 1976.
19. Stauffer: Am. J. Clin. Nutr., *30*, 64, 1977.
20. Peters: Am. J. Clin. Nutr., *30*, 53, 1977.
21. Kern, Heger, Payne and DeWind: Arch. Pathol., *96*, 342, 1973.
22. Drenick, Simmons and Murphy: N. Engl. J. Med., *282*, 829, 1970.
23. Moxley, Pozefsky and Lockwood: N. Engl. J. Med., *290*, 921, 1974.
24. Lockwood, Amatruda, Moxley, Pozefsky and Boitnott: Am. J. Clin. Nutr., *30*, 58, 1977.
25. Barry, Benfield, Nicell and Bray: Gut, *16*, 903, 1975.
26. Drenick, Ament, Fingold and Passaro: Am. J. Clin. Nutr., *30*, 76, 1977.
27. Barry, Chow, Billesdon and Benfield: Gut, *16*, 825, 1975.
28. Wands, LaMont, Mann and Isselbacher: N. Engl. J. Med., *294*, 121, 1976.
29. Shagrin, Frame and Duncan: Ann. Intern. Med., *75*, 377, 1971.
30. Holzbach: Am. J. Clin. Nutr., *30*, 43, 1977.
31. Buchwald, Varco, Moore and Schwartz: Curr. Probl. Surg., April, 1975.
32. Earnest: Am. J. Clin. Nutr., *30*, 72, 1977.
33. Anderson and Jagenburg: Gut, *15*, 360, 1974.
34. Earnest, Williams and Admirand: Clin. Res., *23*, 130, 1975 (abstract).

Malabsorptive Syndromes

1. Creamer: Gut, 7, 569, 1966.
2. Sakula and Shiner: Lancet, 2, 876, 1957.
3. Yardley, Bayless, Norton and Hendrix: N. Engl. J. Med., *267*, 1173, 1962.
4. Rubin, et al.: Gastroenterology, *43*, 621, 1962.

5. Bayless, Yardley and Hendrix: Arch. Intern. Med., *111*, 83, 1963.
6. Rubin and Dobbins: Gastroenterology, *49*, 676, 1965.

Gluten-sensitive Enteropathy

1. Dicke: *Investigation of the Harmful Effects of Certain Types of Cereal on Patients with Celiac Disease.* Utrecht, Thesis, 1950.
2. Dicke, Weijers and van de Kamer: Acta Paediatr., *42*, 34, 1953.
3. Kowlessar, Warren and Bronstein: In *Progress in Gastroenterology*, Vol. II (Glass, Ed.). New York, Grune & Stratton, 1970.
4. Kivel, Kearns and Liebowitz: N. Engl. J. Med., *271*, 769, 1964.
5. Broitman, et al.: Am. J. Med., *48*, 382, 1970.
6. Rubin, et al.: *Intestinal Biopsy* (Wolstenholme and Cameron, Eds.). Boston, Little, Brown & Co., 1962, pp. 67–83.
7. MacDonald, et al.: Gastroenterology, *47*, 573, 1964.
8. Adlersberg: *The Malabsorption Syndrome*. New York, Grune & Stratton, 1957.
9. Green and Wollaeger: Gastroenterology, *38*, 399, 1960.
10. Cooke, Peeney and Hawkins: Q. J. Med., *22*, 59, 1953.
11. Snell: Ann. Intern. Med., *12*, 1632, 1939.
12. Adlersberg and Schein: J.A.M.A., *134*, 1459, 1947.
13. Suarez: Ann. Intern. Med., *12*, 529, 1938.
14. Thaysen: *Non-tropical Sprue. A Study in Idiopathic Steatorrhea.* London, Humphrey Milford, 1932.
15. Manson-Bahr: *The Dysenteric Disorders.* 2nd ed. Baltimore, Williams & Wilkins, 1943.
16. Bossaak, Wong and Adlersberg: In *The Malabsorption Syndrome* (Adlersberg, Ed.). New York, Grune & Stratton, 1957.
17. Adlersberg, et al.: Gastroenterology, *26*, 548, 1954.
18. Laws, Booth, Shawdon and Stewart: Br. Med. J., *1*, 1311, 1963.
19. Marshak, Wolfe and Eliasoph: In *The Malabsorption Syndrome* (Adlersberg, Ed.). New York, Grune & Stratton, 1957.
20. Sakula and Shiner: Lancet, *2*, 876, 1957.
21. Rubin, Brandborg, Phelps and Taylor: Gastroenterology, *38*, 28, 1960.
22. Creamer: Gut, *7*, 569, 1966.
23. Rubin, et al.: Gastroenterology, *43*, 621, 1962.
24. McCarthy, Borland, Kurtz and Ruffin: Am. J. Pathol., *44*, 585, 1964.
25. McDonald, et al.: Gastroenterology, *47*, 573, 1964.
26. Yardley, Bayless, Norton and Hendrix: N. Engl. J. Med., *267*, 1173, 1962.
27. Benson, Kowlessar and Sleisenger: Medicine, *43*, 1, 1964.
28. Sleisenger: N. Engl. J. Med., *265*, 49, 1961.
29. Plotkin and Isselbacher: N. Engl. J. Med., *271*, 1033, 1964.
30. Shmerling, et al.: Helv. Paediatr. Acta, *19*, 507, 1964.
31. Nordio, Lamedica, Vignok and Berrio: Ann. Paediatr., *204*, 3, 1965.

32. Lifshitz, Klotz and Holman: Am. J. Dig. Dis., *10*, 47, 1965.
33. Arthur: Arch. Dis. Child., *41*, 519, 1966.
34. Astley and French: Br. J. Radiol., *24*, 321, 1951.
35. Anderson, Astley, French and Gerrard: Br. J. Radiol., *25*, 526, 1952.
36. Balint and Hirschowitz: N. Engl. J. Med., *265*, 631, 1961.
37. Cooke, et al.: Gut, *4*, 279, 1963.
38. Granick: J. Biol. Chem., *164*, 737, 1946.
39. Stewart, et al.: J. Exp. Med., 92, 375, 1950.
40. Cox, Maynell, Cooke and Gaddie: Gastroenterology, *35*, 390, 1958.
41. Hartley: In *The Malabsorption Syndrome* (Adlersberg, Ed.). New York, Grune & Stratton, 1957, p. 172.
42. Badenoch and Callender: Lancet, *1*, 192, 1960.
43. Kelley, Logan and Christ: N. Engl. J. Med., *252*, 658, 1955.
44. Taylor, Wollaeger, Comfort and Power: Gastroenterology, *20*, 203, 1952.
45. Colcher: In *The Malabsorption Syndrome* (Adlersberg, Ed.). New York, Grune & Stratton, 1957.

Tropical Sprue

1. Frazer: In *Proceedings World Congress on Gastroenterology,* Vol. 1. Baltimore, Williams & Wilkins, 1959, p. 619.
2. Swanson and Thomassen: Am. J. Pathol., *46*, 511, 1965.
3. Butterworth and Perez-Santiago: Ann. Intern. Med., *48*, 8, 1958.
4. Bayless, Guardiola-Rotger and Wheby: Gastroenterology, *51*, 32, 1966.
5. Milanes, et al.: Gastroenterology, 7, 306, 1946.
6. Bayless, Wheby and Swanson: Am. J. Clin. Nutr., *21*, 1030, 1968.
7. O'Brien and England: Br. Med. J., *2*, 1157, 1966.
8. Ayrey: Trans. R. Soc. Trop. Med. Hyg., *41*, 377, 1948.
9. Keele and Bound: Br. Med. J., *1*, 77, 1946.
10. Mathan and Baker: Am. J. Clin. Nutr., *21*, 1077, 1968.
11. Dammin: Fed. Proc., *24*, 35, 1965.
12. Bayless, Guardiola-Rotger and Wheby: Gastroenterology, *51*, 32, 1966.
13. Gorbach, et al.: Lancet, *1*, 74, 1969.
14. Klipstein, et al.: Ann. Intern. Med., *79*, 632, 1973.
15. Klipstein and Schenk: Gastroenterology, *68*, 642, 1975.
16. Klipstein, et al.: Gastroenterology, *70*, 1035, 1976.
17. Creamer: Gut, 7, 569, 1966.
18. Klipstein and Baker: Gastroenterology, *58*, 717, 1970.
19. Ghitis, Tripathy and Mayoral: Am. J. Clin. Nutr., *20*, 1206, 1967.
20. Gorbach, et al.: Am. J. Clin. Nutr., *23*, 1545, 1970.
21. Banwell, et al.: Am. J. Clin. Nutr., *23*, 1559, 1970.
22. Fordtran, Rector, Locklear and Ewton: J. Clin. Invest., *46*, 287, 1967.
23. Phillips and Schmid: Gut, *10*, 990, 1969.
24. Banwell, et al.: J. Clin. Invest., *49*, 183, 1970.
25. Banwell, Gorbach, Mitra and Pierce: Gastroenterology, *58*, 925, 1970 (abstract).
26. Klipstein, Schenk and Samloff: Gastroenterology, *51*, 317, 1966.
27. Swanson, Wheby and Bayless: In Proceedings 63rd Annual Meeting American Association Pathology and Bacteriology, Cleveland, 1966.
28. Haddock, Vega de Rodriguez, Floch and Cintron-Rivera: Am. J. Dig. Dis., 7, 967, 1962.
29. Rodriguez-Olleros and Hernandez-Morales: Puerto Rico J. Public Health Trop. Med., *15*, 274, 1940.
30. Meyer, et al.: Proc. Soc. Exp. Biol. Med., *83*, 681, 1953.
31. Girdwood: Lancet, *2*, 53, 1953.
32. Graham and Rheault: J. Lab. Clin. Med., *43*, 235, 1954.
33. Klipstein: Scand. J. Gastroenterol., *6* (Suppl.), 93, 1970.
34. Herbert: Am. J. Clin. Nutr., *21*, 1115, 1968.
35. Wheby and Bayless: Blood, *31*, 817, 1968.
36. Anderson, Belcher, Chanarin and Mollin: Br. J. Haematol., *6*, 439, 1960.
37. Klipstein: Blood, *21*, 626, 1963.
38. Hoffbrand, Necheles, Maldonado, Horta and Santini: Br. Med. J., *2*, 543, 1969.
39. Baker and Mathan: In *Tropical Sprue.* London, Churchill and Sons, 1970.
40. Jeejeebhoy, Desai, Borkar, Deshpande and Pathare: Am. J. Clin. Nutr., *21*, 994, 1968.
41. Tandon, Iyenger, Deo and Saraya: J. Assoc. Physicians India, *14*, 197, 1966.
42. Jeejeebhoy, et al.: Gastroenterology, *56*, 252, 1969.
43. Rubini, Sheehy, Meroney and Louro: J. Lab. Clin. Med., *58*, 902, 1961.
44. Haddock and Vasquez: J. Clin. Endocrinol., *26*, 859, 1966.
45. Shils, M. E.: Personal communication, 1972.
46. Jeejeebhoy, et al.: Gastroenterology, *51*, 333, 1966.
47. Bayless, Walter and Barber: Clin. Res., *12*, 445, 1964 (abstract).
48. Desai and Jeejeebhoy: Indian J. Pathol. Bacteriol., *10*, 107, 1967.
49. Guerra, Wheby and Bayless: Ann. Intern. Med., *63*, 619, 1965.
50. Klipstein: Ann. Intern. Med., *61*, 721, 1964.
51. French, Gaddie and Smith: Q. J. Med., *25*, 333, 1956.
52. Sheehy, Baggs, Perez-Santiago and Floch: Ann. Intern. Med., *57*, 892, 1962.

Whipple's Disease

1. Bobruff, DiBianco, Loebel and Groisser: Gastroenterology, *45*, 108, 1963.
2. Laster, Waldmann and Fester: Proceedings American Gastroenterological Association, New York, April 27, 1962.
3. Sugarman, Bigman and Jarkowski: J.A.M.A., *174*, 2192, 1960.
4. Trier, Phelps, Eidelman and Rubin: Gastroenterology, *48*, 684, 1965.

5. Yardley and Hendrix: Bull. Johns Hopkins Hosp., *109*, 80, 1961.
6. Vitale et al.: Personal communication.
7. Kok, Dybkaer and Rostgaard: Acta Pathol. Microbiol. Scand., *60*, 431, 1964.
8. Charache, Bayless, Shelley and Hendrix: Trans. Assoc. Am. Physicians, *79*, 399, 1966.
9. Bayless: Adv. Intern. Med., *16*, 171, 1970.
10. Ruffin, Kurtz and Roufail: J.A.M.A., *195*, 476, 1966.
11. England, French and Rawson: Gastroenterology, *39*, 219, 1960.
12. Holt, Isselbacher and Jones: N. Engl. J. Med., *264*, 1335, 1961.
13. Pirola, Mishkel and MacDonald: Med. J. Aust., *2*, 985, 1967.

Malabsorption Due to Bacterial Contamination of the Gut

1. Doig and Girdwood: Q. J. Med., *29*, 333, 1960.
2. Donaldson, Corrigan and Natsios: Gastroenterology, *43*, 282, 1962.
3. Strauss, Donaldson and Gardner: Lancet, *2*, 736, 1961.
4. Donaldson: Gastroenterology, *43*, 271, 1962.
5. Giannella, Broitman and Zamcheck: J. Clin. Invest., *50*, 1100, 1971.
6. Donaldson: Ann. Intern. Med., *64*, 948, 1966.
7. Dawson and Isselbacher: J. Clin. Invest., *39*, 730, 1960.
8. Hofmann and Borgström: J. Clin. Invest., *43*, 247, 1964.
9. Dowling and Small: Gastroenterology, *54*, 1291, 1968 (abstract).
10. Tabaqchali and Booth: Lancet, *2*, 12, 1966.
11. Klipstein and Samloff: Am. J. Clin. Nutr., *19*, 237, 1966.
12. Hoffbrand, Tabaqchali and Mollin: Lancet, *1*, 1339, 1966.
13. Heinz, Steinberg and Sackner: Ann. Intern. Med., *59*, 822, 1963.
14. Hoskins, Norris, Gottlieb and Zamcheck: Am. J. Med., *33*, 459, 1962.
15. McBrien and Lockhart-Mummery: Br. Med. J., *2*, 1653, 1962.
16. Salen, Goldstein and Wirts: Ann. Intern. Med., *64*, 834, 1966.

Mastocytosis

1. Bank and Marks: Gastroenterology, *45*, 535, 1963.
2. Rubin and Dobbins: Gastroenterology, *49*, 676, 1965.
3. Jarnum and Zacharie: Gut, *8*, 64, 1967.
4. Broitman, et al.: Am. J. Med., *48*, 382, 1970.

Protein-losing Enteropathies

1. Waldmann: Gastroenterology, *50*, 422, 1967.
2. Ulstrom and Krivit: Am. J. Dis. Child., *100*, 509, 1960.
3. Waldmann, Morell, Wochner and Sternlieb: J. Clin. Invest., *44*, 1107, 1965 (abstract).
4. Milhaud and Vesin: Nature, *191*, 872, 1961.
5. Mistilis, Skyring and Stephen: Lancet, *1*, 77, 1965.

6. Waldmann, Gordon, Dutcher and Wertlake: In *Plasma Proteins and Gastrointestinal Tract in Health and Disease.* Copenhagen, Ejnar Munksgaards Forlag, 1962.
7. Bookstein, French and Pollard: Am. J. Dig. Dis., *10*, 573, 1965.
8. Waldmann, Wochner, Laster and Gordon: N. Engl. J. Med., *276*, 761, 1967.
9. Holman, Nickel and Sleisenger: Am. J. Med., *27*, 963, 1959.
10. Hermans, et al.: Am. J. Med., *40*, 78, 1966.
11. Waldmann and Laster: J. Clin. Invest., *43*, 1025, 1964.
12. McCarthy, Austad and Read: Am. J. Dig. Dis., *10*, 945, 1965.
13. Allen and Hadden: Br. Med. J., *2*, 486, 1964.
14. Collins and Ellis: Am. J. Med., *39*, 476, 1965.
15. Hoskins, et al.: Gastroenterology, *53*, 265, 1967.
16. Paul, Castleman and White: Am. J. Med. Sci., *216*, 361, 1948.
17. Gimlette: Br. Heart J., *21*, 9, 1959.
18. Petersen and Hastrup: Acta Med. Scand., *173*, 401, 1963.
19. Kaihara, et al.: Jpn. Heart J., *4*, 386, 1963.
20. Davidson, Waldmann, Goodman and Gordon: Lancet, *1*, 899, 1961.
21. Petersen and Ottosen: Acta Med. Scand., *176*, 335, 1964.
22. Díaz, Linazasoro, López-Garcia and Guedes: Rev. Clin. Esp., *77*, 252, 1960.
23. Oeff and Lerche: Klin. Wochenschr., *39*, 100, 1961.
24. Plauth, Waldmann, Wochner and Braunwald: Pediatrics, *34*, 636, 1964.
25. Waldmann, et al.: Gastroenterology, *41*, 197, 1961.
26. Jeejeebhoy: Lancet, *1*, 343, 1962.
27. Marshak, Wolf, Cohen and Janowitz: Radiology, *77*, 893, 1961.
28. Schwartz and Jarnum: Lancet, *1*, 327, 1959.
29. Herskovic, et al.: Pediatrics, *40*, 345, 1967.
30. Steinfeld, Davidson, Gordon and Green: Am. J. Med., *29*, 405, 1960.
31. Jeffries, Chapman and Sleisenger: N. Engl. J. Med., *270*, 761, 1964.
32. Holt: Pediatrics, *34*, 629, 1964.

Carbohydrate Intolerance

1. Durand: *Disorders Due to Intestinal Defective Carbohydrate Digestion and Absorption.* Rome, Il Pensiero Scientifico, 1964.
2. Miller and Crane: Biochim. Biophys. Acta, *52*, 293, 1961.
3. Gray: Gastroenterology, *58*, 96, 1970.
4. Laplane, et al.: Arch. Fr. Pediatr., *19*, 895, 1962.
5. Schneider, Kinter and Stirling: N. Engl. J. Med., *274*, 305, 1966.
6. Lindquist and Meluwisse: Acta Paediatr., *51*, 674, 1962.
7. Abraham, Levin, Oberholzer and Russell: Arch. Dis. Child., *42*, 592, 1967.
8. Littman and Hammond: Gastroenterology, *48*, 237, 1965.
9. Ferguson and Maxwell: Lancet, *2*, 188, 1967.
10. Sonntag, et al.: Gastroenterology, *47*, 18, 1964.

11. Haemmerli, et al.: Am. J. Med., *38*, 7, 1965.
12. Welsh, et al.: Arch. Intern. Med., *117*, 495, 1966.
13. Weser and Sleisenger: Gastroenterology, *48*, 571, 1965.
14. Welsh, May, Drewry and Walker: Clin. Res., *13*, 32, 1965 (abstract).
15. Sunshine and Kretchmer: Pediatrics, *34*, 38, 1964.
16. Cozzetto: Pediatrics, *32*, 228, 1963.
17. Bowie, Brinkman and Hansen: Lancet, *2*, 550, 1963.
18. Dahlqvist: J. Clin. Invest., *41*, 463, 1962.
19. Weijers and van de Kamer: Acta Paediatr., *51*, 371, 1962.
20. Auricchio, Dahlqvist, Murset and Parker: J. Pediatr., *62*, 165, 1963.
21. Cuatrecasas, Lockwood and Caldwell: Lancet, *1*, 14, 1965.
22. Knudsen, et al.: Clin. Res., *14*, 300, 1966 (abstract).
23. Broitman, Thalenfeld and Zamcheck: Clin. Res., *15*, 229, 1967 (abstract).
24. Deren, Broitman and Zamcheck: J. Clin. Invest., *46*, 186, 1967.
25. Heilskov: Acta Physiol. Scand., *24*, 84, 1951.
26. Sunshine and Kretchmer: Science, *144*, 850, 1964.
27. Bayless and Rosensweig: J.A.M.A., *197*, 968, 1966.
28. Littman and Hammond: Gastroenterology, *48*, 237, 1965.
29. Huang and Bayless: N. Engl. J. Med., *276*, 1283, 1967.
30. Cook and Kajubi: Lancet, *1*, 725, 1966.
31. Bayless and Christopher: Am. J. Clin. Nutr., *22*, 181, 1969.
32. Gilat, Kuhn, Gelman and Mizrahy: Am. J. Dig. Dis., *15*, 895, 1970.
33. Simoons: Am. J. Dig. Dis., *15*, 695, 1970.
34. Welsh, Shaw and Walker: Ann. Intern. Med., *64*, 1252, 1966.
35. Hellemans: Acta Med. Scand., *148*, 367, 1954.
36. Weser, Rubin, Ross and Sleisenger: N. Engl. J. Med., *273*, 1070, 1965.
37. Paton, Murray and Watson: Br. Med. J., *1*, 459, 1966.
38. Frazer, et al.: Lancet, *1*, 503, 1966.
39. Struthers, Singleton and Kern: Ann. Intern. Med., *63*, 221, 1965.
40. Dunphy, et al.: Gastroenterology, *49*, 12, 1965.
41. Burke, et al.: Paediatr. J., *1*, 147, 1965.
42. Kern, Struthers and Attwood: Gastroenterology, *45*, 477, 1963.
43. Welsh: Medicine, *49*, 257, 1970.
44. Dahlqvist: Anal. Biochem., *7*, 18, 1964.
45. Isokoski, Jussilia and Sarna: Gastroenterology, *62*, 28, 1972.
46. Newcomer, et al.: N. Engl. J. Med., *293*, 1232, 1975.

Metabolic Disorders

Diabetes

1. Rundles: Medicine, *24*, 111, 1945.
2. Wruble and Kalser: Am. J. Med., *37*, 118, 1964.

Abetalipoproteinemia

1. Salt, et al.: Lancet, *2*, 325, 1960.
2. Isselbacher, Scheig, Plotkin and Caulfield: Medicine, *43*, 347, 1964.
3. Sobrevilla, Goodman and Kane: Am. J. Med., *37*, 821, 1964.
4. Isselbacher: Gastroenterology, *50*, 78, 1966.
5. Sabesin and Isselbacher: Science, *147*, 1149, 1965.
6. Hyams, Sabesin and Isselbacher: Fed. Proc., *24*, 671, 1965 (abstract).
7. Gotto, Levy, John and Fredrickson: N. Engl. J. Med., *284*, 813, 1971.
8. Eder: Am. J. Med., *23*, 269, 1957.
9. van Buchem, et al.: Am. J. Med., *40*, 794, 1966.
10. Simon and Ways: J. Clin. Invest., *43*, 1311, 1964.
11. Ways and Simon: J. Clin. Invest., *43*, 1322, 1964.

Amino Acid Anomalies

1. Milne: Br. Med. J., *1*, 327, 1964.

Parasitic Infestation

1. Von Bornsdarff: Parasitol. Rev., *5*, 207, 1956.
2. Faust, Russell and Jung (Eds.): *Craig and Faust's Clinical Parasitology*, 8th ed. Philadelphia, Lea & Febiger, 1970.
3. Amir-Ahmadi, et al.: Am. J. Dig. Dis., *13*, 959, 1968.
4. Milner, et al.: Gut, *6*, 574, 1965.
5. Stemmermann: Gastroenterology, *53*, 59, 1967.
6. Sheehy, Meroney, Cox and Soler: Gastroenterology, *42*, 148, 1962.
7. Hoskins, et al.: Gastroenterology, *53*, 265, 1967.
8. Yardley, Takano and Hendrix: Bull. Johns Hopkins Hosp., *115*, 389, 1964.
9. Hermans, et al.: Am. J. Med., *40*, 78–89, 1966.
10. Marsden and Hoskins: Gastroenterology, *51*, 701, 1966.
11. Marsden and Schultz: Gastroenterology, *57*, 724, 1969.

Acute Infectious Diarrheas

1. Morgan: In *Bacterial and Mycotic Infections in Man* (Dubos and Hirsch, Eds.). Philadelphia, J. B. Lippincott, 1965, p. 610.
2. Watt: In *Preventive Medicine and Public Health*, 9th ed. (Sartwell, Ed.). New York, Appleton-Century-Crofts, 1965.
3. Raffensperger: *Gastroenterology 2* (Bockus, Ed.). Philadelphia, W. B. Saunders, 1964.
4. Eisenberg, Palazzola and Flippin: N. Engl. J. Med., *253*, 90, 1955.
5. Lindenbaum, Alam and Kent: Br. Med. J., *2*, 1616, 1966.
6. Lindenbaum: Br. Med. J., *2*, 326, 1965.
7. Torres-Pinedo, Rivera and Rodriguez: Ann. N.Y. Acad. Sci., *176*, 284, 1971.

Salmonellosis and Shigellosis

1. Communicable Disease Center: Morbidity and Mortality Weekly Report, *14*, 393, 1965.
2. Saphra and Winter: N. Engl. J. Med., *256*, 1128, 1957.
3. Esenberg: Am. J. Med. Sci., *235*, 497, 1958.

4. Black, Kunz and Swartz: N. Engl. J. Med., 262, 811, 1960.
5. Cruickshank: Med. Clin. North Am., 51, 643, 1967.
6. Bowmer: J. Milk Food Technol., 28, 74, 1965.
7. Giannella, Broitman and Zamcheck: Am. J. Dig. Dis., 16, 1000, 1971.
8. Giannella, Broitman and Zamcheck: Am. J. Dig. Dis., 16, 1007, 1971.
9. Felsen: In Current Therapy (Conn, Ed.). Philadelphia, W. B. Saunders, 1945.

Cholera

1. Phillips: Ann. Intern. Med., 65, 922, 1966.
2. Gordon, et al.: Ann. Intern. Med., 64, 1328, 1966.
3. Cruickshank: Med. Clin. North Am., 51, 643, 1967.
4. Rosenberg, Greenough, Lindenbaum and Gordon: Am. J. Clin. Nutr., 19, 384, 1966.
5. Carpenter: Am. J. Med., 50, 1, 1971.
6. Field: N. Engl. J. Med., 284, 1137, 1971.
7. Greenough, et al.: In Progress in Gastroenterology II (Glass, Ed.). New York, Grune & Stratton, 1970.
8. Taylor, Hirschhorn and Phillips: Fed. Proc., 26, 384, 1967 (abstract).
9. Phillips: In Current Therapy (Conn, Ed.). Philadelphia, W. B. Saunders, 1964.
10. Phillips, et al.: J. Biol. Chem., 183, 305, 1950.

Traveler's Diarrhea

1. Gorbach, et al.: N. Engl. J. Med., 292, 933, 1975.
2. Nalin, et al.: Lancet, 2, 1116, 1975.
3. Merson, et al.: N. Engl. J. Med., 294, 1299, 1976.

Chronic Inflammatory Bowel Disease

Granulomatous Inflammatory Diseases

1. Crohn, Ginzburg and Oppenheimer: J.A.M.A., 99, 1323, 1932.
2. Zetzel: N. Engl. J. Med., 254, 990, 1956.
3. Zetzel: In Cecil-Loeb Textbook of Medicine, 11th ed. Philadelphia, W. B. Saunders, 1963.
4. Mendeloff, Monk, Siegel and Lilienfeld: Gastroenterology, 51, 748, 1966.
5. Soren: Arch. Intern. Med., 117, 78, 1966.
6. Werther, Schapira, Rubinstein and Janowitz: Am. J. Med., 29, 416, 1960.
7. Weingarten, Parker, Chazen and Jacobson: Arch. Surg., 78, 483, 1959.
8. Ginzburg, Schneider, Dreizen and Levinson: Surgery, 39, 347, 1956.
9. Atwell, Duthie and Goligher: Br. J. Surg., 52, 966, 1965.
10. Berman and Prior: J. Mt. Sinai Hosp., 31, 30, 1964.
11. Atwell and Duthie: Gastroenterology, 46, 16, 1964.
12. Kirsner: J.A.M.A., 169, 433, 1959.
13. Brown and Daffner: Ann. Intern. Med., 49, 595, 1958.
14. Sparberg and Kirsner: Am. J. Dig. Dis., 11, 865, 1966.
15. Lockhart-Mummery and Morson: Gut, 1, 87, 1960.

16. Lindner, Marshak, Wolf and Janowitz: N. Engl. J. Med., 269, 379, 1963.
17. Crohn and Yarnis: J. Mt. Sinai Hosp., 33, 503, 1966.
18. Marshak, Lindner and Janowitz: Gut, 7, 258, 1966.
19. Lockhart-Mummery and Morson: Gut, 5, 493, 1965.
20. Jones, Lennard-Jones and Lockhart-Mummery: Gut, 7, 448, 1966.
21. Morson: Proc. R. Soc. Med., 61, 79, 1968.
22. Zetzel: N. Engl. J. Med., 282, 600, 1970.

Ulcerative Colitis

1. Kirsner: Postgrad. Med., 22, 132, 1957.
2. Korelitz and Coles: Gastroenterology, 52, 78, 1967.
3. Wright, et al.: Q. J. Med., 34, 229, 1965.
4. Deren, Porush, Levitt and Khilnani: Ann. Intern. Med., 56, 843, 1962.
5. Goldgraber and Kirsner: Cancer, 17, 657, 1964.
6. Salem and Truelove: Br. Med. J., 1, 827, 1965.
7. Frazer, et al.: Lancet, 1, 503, 1966.
8. Kramer: Gastroenterology, 47, 649, 1964.
9. Kirsner: J.A.M.A., 169, 433, 1959.
10. Zetzel: N. Engl. J. Med., 271, 891, 1964.
11. Zetzel: In Cecil-Loeb Textbook of Medicine, 11th ed. Philadelphia, W. B. Saunders, 1963.
12. Wright and Truelove: Br. Med. J., 2, 142, 1965.
13. Dudek, Spiro and Thayer: Gastroenterology, 49, 544, 1965.
14. Taylor and Truelove: Br. Med. J., 2, 924, 1961.
15. Struthers, Singleton and Kern: Ann. Intern. Med., 63, 221, 1965.
16. Iber, Hardoon and Sangree: Clin. Res., 11, 185, 1963 (abstract).
17. Wright and Truelove: Br. Med. J., 2, 138, 1965.
18. Korelitz and Lindner: Gastroenterology, 46, 671, 1964.
19. Truelove and Witts: Br. Med. J., 2, 1041, 1955.
20. Wright: Gastroenterology, 58, 875, 1970.
21. Kraft and Kirsner: Gastroenterology, 60, 922, 1971.
22. Kirsner: Scand. J. Gastroenterol., 6 (Suppl.), 63, 1970.

Other Colonic Diseases

Colonic Diverticulum

1. Almy: Gastroenterology, 49, 109, 1965.
2. Painter, Truelove, Ardran and Tuckey: Gastroenterology, 49, 169, 1965.
3. Painter and Truelove: Gut, 5, 201, 1964.
4. Arfwidsson: Acta Chir. Scand., Supplement, 342, 1964.

Villous Adenoma

1. Garis: Ann. Intern. Med., 15, 916, 1941.
2. McKittrick and Wheelock: Carcinoma of Colon. Springfield, Charles C Thomas, 1954.
3. Goldgraber and Kirsner: Gastroenterology, 35, 36, 1958.
4. Davis, Seavey and Sessions: Ann. Surg., 155, 806, 1962.

5. Levitan, Fordtran, Burrows and Ingelfinger: Clin. Invest., *41*, 1754, 1962.
6. Dempsey, Caroll, Albright and Henneman: Metabolism, 7, 108, 1958.
7. Salem, Prokipchuk and Hendrix: Bull. Johns Hopkins Hosp., *117*, 69, 1965.
8. Masson, Heremons and Dive: Gastroenterologia, *105*, 270, 1966.
9. Scarborough and Klein: Am. J. Surg., *76*, 723, 1948.
10. Wheat and Ackerman: Ann. Surg., *147*, 476, 1958.

Medium-chain Triglycerides in Malabsorption

1. Isselbacher: Gastroenterology, *50*, 78, 1966.
2. Bennett: Q. J. Exp. Physiol., *49*, 210, 1964.
3. Greenberger, Rodgers and Isselbacher: J. Clin. Invest., *45*, 217, 1966.
4. Playoust and Isselbacher: J. Clin. Invest., *43*, 878, 1964.
5. Bennett and Holt: Clin. Res., *13*, 535, 1965 (abstract).
6. Senior: Am. J. Med. Sci., *257*, 75, 1969.
7. Zurier, Hashim and Van Itallie: In *Recent Advances in Gastroenterology,* Vol. 2. Tokyo, Third World Congress of Gastroenterology, 1967.
8. Dawson, Holdsworth and Webb: Proc. Soc. Exp. Biol. Med., *117*, 97, 1964.
9. Linscheer, et al.: J. Clin. Invest., *43*, 1280, 1964 (abstract).
10. Pihl, Glotzer and Patterson: J. Appl. Physiol., *21*, 1059, 1966.
11. Kuo and Huang: J. Clin. Invest., *44*, 1924, 1965.
12. Holt, Hashim and Van Itallie: Am. J. Gastroenterol., *43*, 549, 1965.
13. Hashim, Roholt and Van Itallie: Clin. Res., *10*, 394, 1962 (abstract).
14. Iber, Hardoon and Sangree: Clin. Res., *11*, 185, 1963 (abstract).
15. Law: Clin. Res., *14*, 48, 1966 (abstract).
16. Greenberger, Ruppert and Tzagournis: Ann. Intern. Med., *66*, 727, 1967.
17. Pinter, McCracken, Lamar and Goldsmith: Am. J. Clin. Nutr., *15*, 293, 1964.
18. Winawer, et al.: N. Engl. J. Med., *274*, 72, 1966.
19. Zurier, Cambell, Hashim and Van Itallie: N. Engl. J. Med., *274*, 490, 1966.
20. Holt: Pediatrics, *34*, 629, 1964.
21. Herskovic, et al.: Pediatrics, *40*, 345, 1967.

22. Isselbacher, Scheig, Plotkin and Caulfield: Medicine, *43*, 347, 1964.
23. Zurier, Hashim and Van Itallie: Gastroenterology, *49*, 490, 1965.
24. Linscheer, et al.: J. Clin. Invest., *45*, 1317, 1966.
25. Tantibhedyangkul and Hashim: Bull. N.Y. Acad. Med., *47*, 17, 1971.
26. Kaunitz, et al.: J. Nutr., *64*, 513, 1958.
27. Saunders: Gastroenterology, *52*, 135, 1967.
28. van de Kamer, ten Bokkel Huinink and Weyers: J. Biol. Chem., *177*, 347, 1949.
29. Braddock, Fleisher and Barbero: Gastroenterology, *55*, 165, 1968.
30. *Medium Chain Triglycerides* (Senior, Van Itallie and Greenberger, Eds.). Philadelphia, University of Pennsylvania Press, 1968.
31. Broitman, Pizzolante and Zamcheck: Unpublished observations.
32. Wolochow, Broitman, Williams and Zamcheck: J. Lab. Clin. Med., *65*, 334, 1965.
33. Samson, Dahl and Dahl: J. Clin. Invest., *35*, 1291, 1956.
34. Hird and Weidemann: Biochem. J., *98*, 378, 1966.
35. Muto and Takahaski: Postgrad. Med., *37*, A158, 1965.
36. Zieve: Arch. Intern. Med., *118*, 211, 1966.
37. Holt: In *Progress in Gastroenterology* (Glass, Ed.). New York, Grune & Stratton, 1968, pp. 277–298.
38. Greenberger and Skillman: N. Engl. J. Med., *280*, 1045, 1969.

Diet and the Clinician

1. Weinstein, et al.: J.A.M.A., *176*, 935, 1961.
2. Donaldson: Gastroenterology, *52*, 897, 1967.
3. Dicke, Weijers and van de Kamer: Acta Paediatr., *42*, 34, 1953.
4. Littman and Hammond: Gastroenterology, *48*, 237, 1965.
5. Lindquist and Meenwisse: Acta Paediatr., *51*, 674, 1962.
6. Iber, Hardoon and Sangree: Clin. Res., *11*, 185, 1963 (abstract).
7. Kramer: Gastroenterology, *47*, 649, 1964.
8. Williams and Olmsted: Ann. Intern. Med., *10*, 717, 1936.
9. Kramer, Kearney and Ingelfinger: Gastroenterology, *42*, 535, 1962.
10. Baum, Sanders and Straub: J. Am. Pharm. Assoc., *40*, 348, 1951.

C. Nutrition in Diseases of the Pancreas

Phani Dhar,
Norman Zamcheck
and
Selwyn A. Broitman

Advanced chronic pancreatitis or, less commonly, neoplastic obstruction of the pancreatic duct may result in a syndrome characterized by steatorrhea and weight loss with or without diabetes mellitus and/or pancreatic calcification.[1-5] When chronic inflammation is the underlying cause, the pancreatic parenchyma shows atrophy and fibrous replacement, the ducts show areas of dilatation and obstruction ("chain-of-lakes" appearance) and deposits of calcium may be found both in the parenchyma and within the ductal system. Malabsorption results from impaired secretion of pancreatic juice. When the underlying disease is a tumor, malabsorption results largely from obstruction to the outflow of pancreatic juice even though the acini are intact. Digestion is impaired to the extent to which availability of pancreatic juice is compromised. The spectrum of insufficiency ranges from subclinical abnormalities detectable only by secretory tests to overt steatorrhea characterized by pale, bulky, malodorous stools and marked wasting and emaciation. Diabetes mellitus accompanies the above syndrome when the islands of Langerhans are destroyed and is one of the common clinical manifestations of pancreatic insufficiency.[2,4,6-8]

Inadequate digestion may be accompanied by malabsorption of the lipid-soluble vitamins A, D, E and K. Steatorrhea may thus be complicated by manifestations of hypovitaminosis. Functional integrity of the pancreas is also necessary for the absorption of vitamin B_{12}.[9-11] Toskes et al. have reported that deficiency of this vitamin is reversible on pancreatic substitution therapy, both in pancreatectomized rats and in patients with exocrine pancreatic insufficiency.[12,13] Low duodenal pH in the absence of pancreatic bicarbonate may encourage excessive iron absorption and lead to hemosiderosis.[14-16] A clinically significant defect in iron metabolism, however, does not occur frequently in patients with pancreatic insufficiency.[17]

Other, less frequent causes of pancreatic insufficiency are surgical resection of the pancreas, gastrectomy, cystic fibrosis, protein-calorie malnutrition and Zollinger-Ellison syndrome.[18-20]

ROLE OF PANCREAS IN NORMAL NUTRITION

The human pancreas secretes 1,500 to 4,000 ml of juice per day with a pH between 7.5 and 8.5 and containing 6 to 12 gm of enzymes necessary for the digestion of protein, fat and carbohydrate. Secretion of this juice is initiated by vagal stimulus and subsequently maintained by the hormones secretin and pancreozymin. Secretin is released from the duodenal mucosa following contact with the acid contents of the stomach; it stimulates the secretion of water and electrolytes, mainly bicarbonate.Pancreozymin, released from the small bowel mucosa in response to contact with peptones and other products of gastric digestion, stimulates the secretion of enzymes. Secretion of both the aqueous and the enzymatic components of the pancreatic juice is stimulated by gastrin, released from the antrum in response to distention. Of the dietary stimuli for pancreatic secretion, protein and fat are most potent.

There are three main classes of pancreatic enzymes:

1. The proteolytic enzymes consist of trypsinogen, chymotrypsin, procarboxypeptidases A and B and proelastase. In addition, there are two nucleolytic enzymes, ribonuclease and deoxyribonuclease. Produced in the ribosomes of the acinar cells, the proteases are encased in lipid membranes by the Golgi apparatus and secreted into the pancreatic ductules as inactive precursors. In the duodenum trypsinogen is activated to trypsin by enterokinase in the presence of calcium. Trypsin, in turn, initiates the hydrolysis of ingested proteins, activates other proteolytic enzymes and autocatalyzes the conversion of inactive trypsinogen into trypsin. The proteases, thus released, hydrolyze the ingested proteins to dipeptides and amino acids. Hydrolysis of dipeptides to amino acids is completed by dipeptidases of the intestinal mucosal cells. Approximately 70 to 80 per cent of dietary proteins are digested and absorbed by the time they reach the ileum.

2. The pancreatic lipolytic enzymes consist of lipase, phospholipases A and B and cholesterol esterase. Emulsification of dietary fat, ingested mainly as water-insoluble triglycerides, is achieved by bile salts aided by lysolecithin; the latter is derived from the action of pancreatic lecithinase-A on the dietary and biliary lecithins. Pancreatic lipase, working at the water-lipid interfaces, hydrolyzes triglycerides to diglycerides and fatty acids with liberation of glycerol. Monoglycerides, which constitute 70 to 75 per cent of the hydrolyzed fat, are then incorporated into the bile salt micelles and transported across the mucosa by mechanisms incompletely understood. Chey et al. suggest that, in addition to causing lipolysis, pancreatic secretions may also assist in the absorption of fatty acids.[21] Digestion and absorption of specific dietary lipids are discussed in Chapter 5.

3. The amylolytic component of pancreatic juice, alpha amylase, hydrolyzes starch to oligosaccharides, disaccharides and small amounts of monosaccharides. Further hydrolysis of disaccharides is accomplished by the disaccharidases of the intestinal mucosal cells.

COMPENSATORY DIGESTIVE MECHANISMS IN PANCREATIC INSUFFICIENCY

The reserve potential of the digestive system is well appreciated. Davenport has made the point that fat malabsorption is clinically recognized in only 15 per cent of subjects with impaired pancreatic secretions and that pancreatic trypsin may be reduced by 90 per cent or more before malabsorption becomes apparent.[18] Kalser et al. found completely normal fat assimilation in a patient with 75 per cent pancreatectomy.[22] Several other workers have observed that frank steatorrhea occurs only occasionally even in patients with long-standing pancreatic disease.[2,4,23] In the absence of pancreatic enzymes, a number of alternative digestive mechanisms may contribute to normal digestion. Digestion of dietary starch may be carried out by the salivary and the intestinal mucosal amylases. Limited lipolysis may be accomplished by the human gastric juice independent of the influence of acid or regurgitated duodenal contents.[24] Lipase is also present in desquamated mucosal cells but its physiologic role is not understood. One class of dietary fats, the medium-chain triglycerides (MCT), can be absorbed without prior lipolysis.[25]

Of the dietary proteins, 10 to 15 per cent may be hydrolyzed to amino acids in the stomach. In dogs 22 to 85 per cent of ingested proteins can be absorbed in the total absence of pancreatic secretions. Following total pancreatectomy, 46 and 62 per cent of 75 gm of proteins fed daily were absorbed by a patient described by Davenport.[18] Thus overt malabsorption in patients with chronic pancreatic disease is relatively infrequent because of an impressive reserve capacity of the pancreas and the presence of a number of compensatory digestive mechanisms.

DIAGNOSIS OF PANCREATIC INSUFFICIENCY

Patients with pancreatic insufficiency may present themselves with either the symptoms of pancreatic inflammation or those of the consequent digestive disturbances. Symptoms suggestive of both may coexist, but it is uncommon for pain, steatorrhea, diabetes and pancreatic calcification to be present all in the same patient.[2] Maldigestion must thus be demonstrated in patients with obvious pancreatic disease (characteristic pain and hyperamylasemia with a background of alcoholism, biliary calculi or other predisposing causes) or, conversely, the presence of pancreatic disease must be established in patients with obvious malabsorption (weight loss, diarrhea, steatorrhea, etc). Steatorrhea, however, may not be obvious even when pancreatic lipolysis is impaired;[26] it is completely obscured in patients who avoid dietary fat for relief from diarrhea and flatulence. Nutritional deficiency in such patients may be attributed erroneously to alcoholism, undernutrition, occult neoplasm or other unrelated causes.

Error can also be made in assuming that malabsorption in patients with pancreatic disease is always exclusively the consequence of pancreatic dysfunction. Indeed, in the alcoholic patient defect in absorption may frequently result from subclinical protein malnutrition,[27,28] from bile salt abnormalities[29-31] or from the other digestive disturbances that often accompany alcoholism.[32,33] Consideration must also be given to other diagnostic possibilities, such as defects of the small bowel, metabolic and endocrine disorders and postoperative states, all of which can impair absorption with or without pancreatic disease.[20,26,34] Thus, lactase deficiency may complicate pancreatic dysfunction in cystic fibrosis[35] and render patients refractory to usual therapy. Steatorrhea in diabetics may suggest pancreatic insufficiency in patients who, in fact, have celiac disease or bacterial overgrowth resulting from reduced intestinal motility.[34] Special laboratory tests are invaluable for defining the pathophysiology and for objective assessment of therapy.

The tests listed in Table 31C-1 are available at most hospitals and are well standardized and therefore readily interpretable. They do not measure the secretory capacity of the pancreas; instead they help to demonstrate the pancreatic pathologic condition indirectly by characterizing the digestive disturbance. In pancreatic disease, both fat and nitrogen contents of the stool increase since isolated enzyme deficiency is rare. This finding serves to distinguish pancreatic disease from bile salt abnormalities, in which only fat is malabsorbed.[20] Fecal fat determination quantitates the degree of fat malabsorption, while the D-xylose test and upper

Table 31C-1. Tests Commonly Used for Differential Diagnosis of Malabsorption

Test	Findings in Pancreatic Insufficiency
Stool examination[36]	Gross: pale bulky, loose and greasy Microscopic: >10 meat fibers per coverslip >6 fat globules per low power field (>8 globules after acid and heating)
Chemical analysis[37-39]	>2.5 gm nitrogen per day >5-7 gm fat per day
Serum carotene	<50 μg/100 ml (<20 μg/100 ml usually in small bowel malabsorption)[40]
Fasting blood sugar and glucose tolerance test	Diabetic curve in about 66% of patients[41]
D-xylose test (with 25 gm oral D-xylose)	>4.5 gm excretion of D-xylose in 5-hour urine collection (decreased in small bowel diseases and bacterial overgrowth syndromes)
Upper gastrointestinal roentgen examination with small bowel follow-through	Normal small bowel pattern. (Pancreatic calcification and extrinsic duodenal abnormalities in relation to the head of the pancreas may sometimes be present)

gastrointestinal radiography with or without small bowel biopsy help to exclude lesions of the small bowel. Serum carotene measurement is a relatively insensitive test but continues to be used primarily because of the ease with which it can be performed. Simple microscopic examination of the stool with the patient on a diet containing 75 to 100 gm of fat per day is still useful in screening for steatorrhea. Drummey et al. found definite microscopic evidence of increased fecal fat in 75 per cent of patients with 6 to 10 per cent and in 94 per cent of patients with 11 to 15 per cent fecal excretion of the dietary fat.[42] Moore et al., using a slightly different technique, found a lower percentage of positive results, but concluded that this method compared favorably with other screening techniques.[36]

In addition to the above, a number of other techniques are sometimes employed for evaluating pancreatic function (Table 31C–2). Their routine use is limited at present.[43,44]

Other tests which do not measure digestive disturbance but help indirectly by establishing or excluding the presence of pancreatic disease include measurement of sweat electrolytes (increased in cystic fibrosis), operative or duodenoscopic pancreatography, selective arteriography, scintiscanning and serum carcinoembryonic antigen determination (positive results are found in 85 per cent of patients with pancreatic cancer).[59,60]

NUTRITION AND PANCREATIC INSUFFICIENCY

Nutrition in Acute Pancreatitis

Proper alimentation of patients with acute pancreatitis is essential and often difficult. This is specially so when the inflammation is prolonged or is complicated by pseudocyst or abscess formation. Preexisting nutritional deficiencies, attendant nausea and vomiting and massive loss of fluid, electrolytes and albumin in

Table 31C–2.   Other Tests for Malabsorption and Pancreatic Dysfunction

Test	Findings in Pancreatic Insufficiency
Stool enzymes	—Trypsin: <20 μg/gm of stool[45] —Chymotrypsin: <74 μg/gm of stool[45] or <165 units/kg body weight/ 24 hrs.[46] *Note:* Positive results more frequent in cystic fibrosis.[43] Enzymes get partially bound to insoluble debris in ileum.[47]
Serum enzymes[23] (evocative test)	—Peak serum amylase value of >159 units or a rise in serum amylase by >72 units following secretin/pancreozymin stimulation. *Note:* Positivity reflects ductal obstruction. Percent positivity varies widely from series to series.[48]
Analysis of duodenal contents following secretin (1 unit/kg body weight, IV) stimulations.[49]	—Total volume: <2 ml/kg body weight —Bicarbonate concentration: <90 mEq/liter —Total amylase: <6 units/kg body weight. *Note:* The only test directly measuring pancreatic exocrine function. —Reagents vary in potency requiring extensive standardization possible only at specialized laboratories.[43] —Various modifications include "augmented secretin test,"[50,51] use of pancreozymin[52] with determination of total protein output,[44,53] use of test meal instead of hormones,[54,55] use of inert markers to assess accuracy of collection[51] and cytologic studies on the aspirate.
Tests using labeled fats (administered orally) ^{131}I triolein and ^{131}I oleic acid	—Normal serum radioactivity with oleic acid but low with triolein —High stool radioactivity after triolein. (5–5.6% of ingested dose).[36,56] *Note:* Measurement of fecal radioactivity is considered better than that of blood. However, studies comparing this method with the chemical fat determination show widely variable correlations.[36, 57, 58]

the inflammatory exudate constitute a heavy metabolic load. Nasogastric suction further compounds the nutritional problem.

Attempts to meet this metabolic demand must be made through the parenteral route and replacements made in proportion to the losses incurred.[61,62] Rehydration is monitored by skin turgor, moistness of tongue, urine output, hematocrit and occasionally central venous pressures. Sodium and potassium lost in vomiting and calcium lost by precipitation as soaps of fatty acids and by other mechanisms[62,63] have to be replaced according to the clinical and electrocardiographic signs and the serum levels. Initial hematocrit is usually high as a result of hemoconcentration. If on rehydration it falls to anemic levels, as in acute hemorrhagic pancreatitis or in pancreatitis complicated by gastrointestinal hemorrhage, whole blood should be transfused.[64] Infusion of colloids, e.g. albumin or plasma, may be indicated if the hematocrit is adequate but the attack is severe, prolonged or complicated by exudative ascites or drop in the level of serum albumin. Elliott et al. have shown that prompt and adequate replacement of colloid losses may be lifesaving during a fulminant attack of pancreatitis.[65] The use of systemic protease inhibitors, e.g. Trasylol, however, continues to be disputed.[66,67] It has not been shown to change the course of disease once the necroinflammatory activity is established. Rosenberg et al. suggest that Trasylol in a dosage of 150,000 to 320,000 units per day, given by the intravenous route early in the course of disease, may be useful.[68]

Impairment of carbohydrate metabolism is encountered in almost all patients with acute pancreatitis but it is transient and only rarely requires treatment with insulin.[69]

Nutrition in the Phase of Recovery

The average patient with uncomplicated pancreatitis is free from pain, nausea and vomiting usually within 2 to 3 days on a regimen consisting of intravenous alimentation and nasogastric suction with or without anticholinergics and/or antibiotics.[1] By this time normal bowel sounds return and serum amylase declines to normal range. The nasogastric tube is clamped now for about 12 hours and gastric acids are neutralized by hourly administration of an antacid. If the patient continues to be asymptomatic the tube may be removed and an "ulcer type" of diet started. Diets rich in protein and fat which stimulate pancreatic secretion should be avoided in preference to carbohydrates.[70] By the end of the first week most patients are able to tolerate a 6-meal bland diet.

Nutrition in Patients with Acute Complications

When acute illness persists longer than a few days with persistent or recurrent elevation in serum amylase, continued abdominal pain and ileus, or when cessation of nasogastric suction is followed by return of symptoms, the presence of a complication such as pancreatic abscess, pseudocyst or obstruction to main pancreatic ducts is suspected. Oral feeding has then to be curtailed for longer periods of time and nutrition has to be maintained by the intravenous route; total parenteral nutrition may be necessary (Chapter 37).

Nutrition in Chronic Pancreatic Insufficiency

The object of therapy in such patients is to prevent further damage to the pancreas, forestall further attacks of acute inflammation, alleviate pain, treat steatorrhea and correct malnutrition. Large meals must be avoided; the frequency of attacks may be reduced by substituting for these frequent small feedings of a low-fat diet. All gastric stimulants such as coffee, tea, spices and condiments should be avoided. Specific treatment of pancreatic maldigestion consists of manipulation of the diet and enzyme replacement therapy. A number of complete and supplementary synthetic diets and formulas are available (see Appendix Tables 26, 31, 32). They may substitute for regular diet in the subacute phase of the disease or supplement the restricted diet recommended for patients with chronic pancreatitis. MCT-containing diets low in lactose may be particularly useful in patients with cystic fibrosis complicated by lactase deficiency.

Protein absorption can be readily increased by increasing protein intake. The same, however, is not true for dietary fat which, when undigested, causes flatulence and diarrhea. Fat intake must be restricted to 50 to 70 gm a day or less and protein and carbohydrate correspondingly increased to as much as 120 and 450 gm respectively.[5] Appropriate dietary patterns are given in the Appendix Table 26.

To improve fat absorption, two approaches may be used:

Enzyme Replacement Therapy. Desiccated extracts of porcine and bovine pancreas (pancreatin, pancrelipase) are commercially available as tablets, powder or capsules.[71] The active ingredients are contained either in the core of enteric coated tablets or in the form of acid-resistant granules. Giulian et al. tested the in vitro lipolytic activity of 15 commercial preparations, and found greatest activity in Cotazym (Organon), Lipan (Spirt & Co.), Panteric (Parke, Davis and Co.) and Viokase (VioBin Corp.).[72] The usual daily dose of 10 to 20 gm may be given in 3 divided doses with or immediately after meals.[73] Jordan and Grossman found better therapeutic results by administering 0.66 gm of Viokase every hour for 12 hours every day.[74] Kalser et al., however, did not find any advantage of hourly doses over conventional thrice-daily doses.[22] Schneider et al. recommended that the powder be sprinkled directly on the food immediately before eating.[75]

Therapeutic results can sometimes be improved by the addition of antacids, e.g. bicarbonate or aluminum hydroxide gel, to the regimen. The antacids prevent gastric inactivation of pancreatic supplements[76] and, in the absence of pancreatic bicarbonate, restore optimum pH in the duodenum for the action of pancreatic enzymes. Knill-Jones et al. found that fat absorption could be significantly improved by the addition of proteolytic enzymes from pineapple stem (bromelains) to the pancreatic extract.[77] However, bromelains given alone did not improve fat absorption in patients with pancreatic insufficiency.

Varying opinions regarding the ideal enzyme preparation, dose requirements and administration schedule presumably arise from both differences in methods of assessment and variability among the patients. The studies of Kalser and Warren and their colleagues[22,73] provide ample justification for initiating therapy in all patients with 1 to 2 gm of pancreatic extract administered thrice daily with meals. The regimen may then be modified according to the individual patient's response.

Use of Medium-chain Triglycerides. Medium-chain triglycerides (MCT) are neutral lipids which contain fatty acid molecules with chain lengths varying from 6 to 12 carbon atoms. Substantial quantities of such lipids may be hydrolyzed in the stomach and the intestine in the absence of pancreatic lipase. Small quantities of MCT enter the mucosal cells without prior hydrolysis.[25] Substitution of dietary fat by MCT in patients with pancreatic insufficiency may relieve steatorrhea and lead to gain in weight.[25,78] References regarding preparations and administration of MCT can be found in Chapter 31, Section B, on diseases of the intestines. To avoid monotony fish, chicken and lean meat may be included in the menu several times a week within the limits of toleration for long-chain triglycerides. Inclusion of other low-fat foods, such as apples, bananas, lettuce, celery and rice, may further improve the palatability of the diet.[79]

The usual side effects of MCT, namely, nausea, vomiting, abdominal distention, cramps and diarrhea, seen in about 10 per cent of the patients, can be avoided by initiating therapy with small supplements of a palatable preparation. Use of MCT is contraindicated in patients with cirrhosis of the liver, especially when complicated by encephalopathy.[25,79]

Diabetes Mellitus in Association with Pancreatic Disease[69]

Almost all patients with acute pancreatitis have impaired glucose tolerance with glycosuria in about 11 per cent. This abnormality is transient and may represent the combined effect of several factors, including (1) increased glycogenolysis resulting from increased serum amylase activity, (2) increased insulin degradation and (3) general reaction of the body to stress. Specific treatment in the acute phase is seldom necessary. In patients with chronic pancreatitis the incidence of diabetes mellitus varies from 13 per cent in those without calcification to 45 per cent in those with. It is usually mild and labile and is only rarely complicated by retinopathy or glomerulosclerosis.

Mild carbohydrate intolerance may be controlled by low-carbohydrate diet. If the above fails, therapy with insulin is indicated. Strict precautions against insulin overdose are necessary, especially in the alcoholic patient, for death from irreversible hypoglycemia is well documented in such individuals.[41]

MANAGEMENT OF SPECIFIC CONDITIONS

Alcohol-induced Pancreatitis

Chronic pancreatitis is usually associated with excessive consumption of alcohol.[1,3-5, 80,81] A number of pathogenetic mechanisms have been postulated, including (1) stimulation of pancreatic secretion with obstruction to the outflow,[82,83] (2) direct toxicity of ethanol to pancreatic paren-

chyma,[84-86] (3) regurgitation of infected duodenal contents[87] and (4) malnutrition.[23,27] Strict avoidance of alcohol is recommended, since this alone may reduce the frequency of painful attacks in such patients. However, the damage caused by alcoholic pancreatitis is irreversible and "no degree of repentance" can "resolve the original sin" (Spiro).[81] Diet and enzyme therapy for chronic pancreatic insufficiency have been described above. In addition, supplements of folic acid and thiamin, which are poorly absorbed in alcoholic patients,[88,89] and of other B vitamins and ascorbic acid, which may be deficient on account of reduced dietary intake, should be prescribed. Other alcohol-related problems[32,33] that may contribute to nutritional depletion should be simultaneously diagnosed and treated.

Protein-calorie Malnutrition. There is convincing evidence in the literature that both exocrine and endocrine pancreatic insufficiency may occur in association with protein-calorie malnutrition (Chapter 24). Pancreas of rats fed ethionine (thus functionally methionine deficient) develop marked acinar atrophy and fibrosis, and secrete diminished amounts of trypsin, chymotrypsin and lipase.[90] Tandon et al. have reported reversible impairment of pancreatic exocrine functions in patients taking protein-deficient diets.[91] Clinical examples of "trophopathic pancreopathy"[92] are also seen in children with kwashiorkor[93] and in adults with alcoholism.[27] Shaper has suggested that if malnutrition is prolonged the reversible functional changes may be followed by extensive fibrosis and calcification within the pancreas.[7] Pancreatic calcification has indeed been reported in 6 to 13.3 per cent of young diabetic patients from areas of the world where chronic protein-calorie malnutrition is common.[94]

Therapy is directed to correction of nutritional deficiencies. Complete clinical recovery may be achieved in a period of 12 to 14 weeks by feeding the patient a diet providing 50 calories per kg body weight, containing 1.5 gm per kg of protein, 80 gm of fat and the remainder of carbohydrates.[91] Supplements of iron and vitamins may be given as needed. Specific therapy with enzymes and/or insulin is indicated only in patients with irreversible pancreatic damage. Infections, especially tuberculosis and malaria, parasitic infestations and cirrhosis, where present, must also be treated.

Pancreatitis with Biliary Calculi

The dramatic onset of pancreatitis resulting from biliary calculi leads to its prompt diagnosis and management; this probably accounts for the low incidence of associated chronic pancreatic insufficiency.[81,95] Careful exclusion of biliary tract disease is mandatory in all patients with acute pancreatitis. Contrast studies should best be done 4 to 6 weeks after the acute attack, after pancreatic edema and transient liver function abnormalities have subsided.

Cystic Fibrosis

Pancreatic insufficiency is a common consequence of cystic fibrosis, seen mostly in children and sometimes in young adults. There is widespread involvement of the exocrine glands but the principal manifestations occur in the respiratory and the digestive systems.[35] Diagnosis is established by demonstration of increased chloride in sweat. Meticulous therapy for bronchiolar abnormalities with aerosols, mucolytic agents and antibiotics is essential to prevent morbidity and mortality from recurrent infections.[99] The nutritional abnormalities are mainly secondary to pancreatic insufficiency but may sometimes be complicated by small bowel malabsorption and hepatic abnormalities. Treatment with high-protein, low-fat diet with adequate supplements of fat-soluble vitamins and enzyme preparations often helps. The dose requirement of pancreatic enzymes is relatively high, in the range of 0.1 to 0.3 gm pancreatin per kg body weight per day.[71] Disaccharidase (mainly lactase) deficiency may coexist, requiring elimination of milk products from the diet.[35] Good results have been reported with the use of MCT preparations.

Surgical Conditions

Postgastrectomy (Chapter 31–A). Surgery of the upper gastrointestinal tract occasionally results in the uncovering of latent defects in absorption or in the de novo appearance of malabsorption.[20,34] This may be a consequence either of inadequate mixing of chyme with the enzymes or of diminished secretion of the enzymes because of interruption of normal physiologic stimuli, e.g. low acid, resected antrum, bypass of duodenum, etc.[96] Diagnostic possibilities are multiple, and in addition to pancreatic insufficiency include undernutrition resulting from small stomach, dumping syndrome, afferent loop dysfunction,[97] inadvertent gastroileostomy and unmasked gluten enteropathy. Pancreatic dysfunction, when suspected, must be confirmed by laboratory tests. Conservative therapy for pancreatic insufficiency often fails,[98] necessitating surgical procedures to restore normal digestive anatomy and physiology.

Pancreatic Resection. Patients with massive pancreatic resection frequently develop both exocrine and endocrine insufficiencies and thus require treatment for maldigestion as well as for diabetes mellitus.[22,73] Requirements of patients vary according to the proportion of pancreas resected, the state of the remaining pancreas and associated conditions. Therapy should thus be individualized using glucose tolerance and fat absorption as guidelines.

Zollinger-Ellison Syndrome. Malabsorption in Z-E syndrome probably results from a number of factors:[20,100] (1) The increased acidity may cause an irreversible denaturation of the pancreatic enzymes in the proximal small bowel. (2) Low duodenal pH may deconjugate the bile acids and thus impair micellar solubilization of fat. (3) Structural and functional changes of the intestinal mucosa itself may depress absorption. Daily fecal excretion of fat averages 26 ± 3.6 per cent of the dietary intake. Xylose absorption is only slightly depressed and vitamin B_{12} absorption is usually normal.

In addition to maldigestion and malabsorption, diarrhea and hypokalemia may result from hypermotility secondary to increased intestinal fluid volumes and increased vagal activity.[34] Alkalinization of duodenal contents may prevent inactivation of pancreatic enzymes[101] but uncontrolled gastrin release by the tumor defeats this effort. Continuous nasogastric suction with vigorous intravenous alimentation and replacement of fluid and electrolyte losses is necessary to maintain life in the seriously ill patient. Definitive therapy consists of total gastrectomy, or rarely, resection of an isolated pancreatic adenoma.

Pancreatic Cancer. Maldigestion in patients with cancer of the pancreas, specially of the head, generally results from interruption of the flow of pancreatic juice to the duodenum. Steatorrhea seldom occurs, presumably because of reduced food intake. Therapy with sufficient dosage of pancreatic enzymes may improve digestion in the pre- and postoperative patient.

BIBLIOGRAPHY

1. Comfort, Gambill and Baggenstoss: Gastroenterology, 6, 239, 376, 1946.
2. Gambill, Baggenstoss and Priestley: Gastroenterology, 39, 404, 1960.
3. Dreiling, Janowitz and Perrier: Pancreatic Inflammatory Disease. A Physiologic Approach. New York, Harper & Row, 1964.
4. Marks, Bank and Louw: In Progress in Gastroenterology, (Glass, Ed.). New York, Grune & Stratton, 1968, p. 412.
5. Berk and Guth: Med. Clin. North Am., 54, 479, 1970.
6. Zuidema: Trop. Geogr. Med., 11, 70, 1959.
7. Shaper: Lancet, 1, 1223, 1960.
8. Gee Verghese, Pillai, Joseph and Pitchumoni: J. Assoc. Physicians India, 10, 173, 1962.
9. Veeger, Abels, Hellmans and Niewig: N. Engl. J. Med., 267, 1341, 1962.
10. Editorial: N. Engl. J. Med., 268, 955, 1963.
11. Jeffries: N. Engl. J. Med., 284, 666, 1971.
12. Toskes, Hansell, Cerda and Deren: N. Engl. J. Med., 284, 627, 1971.
13. Toskes and Deren: J. Clin. Invest., 51, 216, 1972.
14. Davis: Lancet, 2, 749, 1961.
15. Biggs and Davis: Lancet, 2, 814, 1963.
16. Benjamin, Cortell and Conrad: Gastroenterology, 53, 389, 1967.
17. Balcerzak, Peternel and Heinle: Gastroenterology, 53, 257, 1967.
18. Davenport: Physiology of the Digestive Tract. An Introductory Text, 2nd ed. Chicago, Year Book Medical Publishers, 1966.
19. Isselbacher and Senior: Gastroenterology, 46, 287, 1964.
20. Wilson and Dietschy: Gastroenterology, 61, 911, 1971.
21. Chey, Shay and O'Leary: Gastroenterology, 45, 196, 1963.
22. Kalser, Leite and Warren: N. Engl. J. Med., 279, 570, 1968.
23. Fitzgerald, Fitzgerald, Fennelly, McMullin and Boland: Gut, 4, 193, 1963.
24. Cohen, Morgan and Hofman: Gastroenterology, 60, 1, 1971.
25. Greenberger and Skillman: N. Engl. J. Med., 280, 1045, 1969.
26. Kirsner: Med. Clin. North Am., 53, 1169, 1969.
27. Mezey, Jow, Slavin and Tobon: Gastroenterology, 59, 657, 1970.
28. Adibi and Allen: Gastroenterology, 59, 404, 1970.
29. Kalant: Gastroenterology, 56, 380, 1969.
30. Rosenberg, Hardison and Bull: N. Engl. J. Med., 276, 1391, 1967.
31. Gracey, Burke, Oshin, Barker and Glasgow: Gut, 12, 683, 1971.
32. Small, Longarini and Zamcheck: Am. J. Med., 27, 575, 1959.
33. Dinoso, Chey, Padow, Rosen, Ottenberg and Lorber: Am. J. Gastroenterol., 56, 209, 1971.
34. Jeffries, Weser and Sleisenger: Gastroenterology, 46, 434, 1964.
35. di Sant' Agnese: In The Exocrine Pancreas (Beck and Sinclair, Eds.). London, J. & A. Churchill, 1971, p. 227.
36. Moore, Englert, Bigler and Clark: Am. J. Dig. Dis., 16, 97, 1971.
37. Wallaeger, Comfort and Osterberg: Gastroenterology, 9, 272, 1947.
38. Van De Kamer, Huinink, Ten and Weyers: J. Biol. Chem., 177, 347, 1949.
39. Wolochow, Broitman, Williams and Zamcheck: J. Lab. Clin. Med., 65, 334, 1965.
40. Ingelfinger: In Year Book of Medicine, 1967–1968 Series. Chicago, Year Book Medical Publishers. 1967, p. 466.
41. Marks and Bank: S. Afr. Med. J., 37, 1039, 1963.
42. Drummey, Benson and Jones: N. Engl. J. Med., 264, 85, 1961.
43. Brooks: N. Engl. J. Med., 286, 300, 1972.
44. Hanscom: Med. Clin. North Am., 52, 1483, 1968.
45. Haverback, Dyce, Gutentag and Montgomery: Gastroenterology, 44, 588, 1963.
46. Muller, Wisniewski and Hansky: Aust. Ann. Med., 1, 47, 1970.
47. Roy, Campbell and Goldberg: Gastroenterology, 53, 584, 1967.

48. Shay, Sun, Chey and O'Leary: Am. J. Dig. Dis., 6, 142, 1961.
49. Dreiling: In *The Exocrine Pancreas* (Berk and Sinclair, Eds.). London, J. & A. Churchill, 1971, p. 154.
50. Hartley, Gambill and Summerskill: Gastroenterology, 48, 312, 1965.
51. Lagerlof, Schutz and Holmer: Gastroenterology, 52, 67, 1967.
52. Sun: Gastroenterology, 45, 203, 1963.
53. Hanscom and Littman: Gastroenterology, 45, 209, 1963.
54. Lundh: Gastroenterology, 42, 275, 1962.
55. Thaysen, Mullertz, Worning and Bang: Gastroenterology, 46, 23, 1964.
56. Wormsley: Gut, 4, 261, 1963.
57. Cox: Gastroenterology, 44, 275, 1963.
58. Rufin, Blahd, Nordyke and Grossman: Gastroenterology, 41, 220, 1961.
59. Ona, Dhar, Moore, Kupchik and Zamcheck: Clin. Res., 20, 463, 1972 (abstract).
60. Moore, Kupchik, Marcon and Zamcheck: Am. J. Dig. Dis., 16, 1, 1971.
61. Nugent: Med. Clin. North Am., 53, 431, 1969.
62. Banks: Gastroenterology, 61, 382, 1971.
63. Turner-Warwick: Lancet, 2, 546, 1956.
64. Elliott: Arch. Surg., 75, 573, 1957.
65. Elliott, Zollinger, Moore and Ellison: Gastroenterology, 28, 563, 1955.
66. Beck, Mekenna, Zylberszac, Solymar and Eisenstein: Gastroenterology, 48, 478, 1965.
67. Grozinger, Hollis and Artz: J.A.M.A., 178, 652, 1964.
68. Rosenberg and Janowitz: Gastroenterology, 48, 350, 1965.
69. Williams: *Textbook of Endocrinology*, 4th ed. Philadelphia, W. B. Saunders, 1968.
70. Snodgrass: In *Harrison's Principles of Internal Medicine*. New York, McGraw-Hill Book Co., 1970.
71. Editorial. Br. Med. J., 2, 161, 1970.
72. Giulian, Singh, Mansfield, Pairent and Howard: Ann. Surg., 165, 564, 1967.
73. Warren, Poulantzas and Kune: Ann. Surg., 164, 830, 1966.
74. Jordan and Grossman: Gastroenterology, 36, 447, 1959.
75. Schneider, Sammons and Beale: Br. Med. J., 2, 735, 1970.
76. Heizer, Cleveland and Iber: Bull. Hopkins Hosp., 116, 261, 1965.
77. Knill-Jones, Pearce, Batten and Williams: Br. Med. J., 4, 21, 1970.
78. Iber, Hardoon and Sangree: Clin. Res., 11, 185, 1963, (abstract).
79. Holt: Gastroenterology, 53, 961, 1967.
80. Mayday and Pheils: Med. J. Aust., 1, 1142, 1970.
81. Spiro: In *The Exocrine Pancreas* (Beck and Sinclair, Eds.). London. J. & A. Churchill, 1971, p. 212.
82. Gross and Hallenbeck: Gastroenterology, 38, 919, 1960.
83. Pirola and Davis: Aust. Ann. Med., 1, 24, 1970.
84. Janowitz and Bayer: Ann. Intern. Med., 74, 444, 1971.
85. Darle, Ekholm and Edlund: Gastroenterology, 58, 62, 1970.
86. Sarles, Lebreuil, Tasso, Figarella, Clemente, Devaux, Fagonde and Payan: Gut, 12, 377, 1971.
87. McCutcheon: Gut, 9, 296, 1968.
88. Halsted, Griggs and Harris: J. Lab. Clin. Med., 69, 116, 1967.
89. Tomasulo, Kater and Iber: Am. J. Clin. Nutr., 21, 1341, 1968.
90. Libre and McFarland: Proc. Soc. Exp. Biol. Med., 8, 452, 1964.
91. Tandon, Banks, George, Sama, Ramachandran and Gandhi: Gastroenterology, 58, 358, 1970.
92. Coppo and Cavazzuti: Gastroenterology, 99, 145, 1963.
93. Davies: Lancet, 1, 317, 1948.
94. Ramalingaswami: Lancet, 2, 733, 1969.
95. Sarles, Sarles, Camatte, Muratore, Gaini, Guien, Pastor and LeRoy: Gut, 6, 545, 1965.
96. Lundh: Gastroenterology, 42, 637, 1962.
97. Wirts and Goldstein: Ann. Intern. Med., 58, 25, 1963.
98. Marks, Bank and Airth: Gut, 41, 217, 1963.
99. Lobeck: In *The Metabolic Basis of Inherited Disease*, 3rd ed. (Stanbury, Wyngaarden and Fredrickson, Eds.). New York, McGraw-Hill Book Co., 1972, p. 1605.
100. Moshal, Broitman and Zamcheck: Am. J. Clin. Nutr., 23, 336, 1970.
101. Vogel, Weinstein, Herskovic and Spiro: Ann. Intern Med. 67, 816, 1967.

D.   *Diseases of the Liver*

Charles S. Davidson

Diet therapy is generally accepted as an important, if not the most important, factor in the management of patients ill with diseases of the liver.[1,2] When the scientific evidence for this conclusion is examined, many data are found to be still wanting but, until proven otherwise, this form of therapy is advised, as it has stood the test of time and may, in fact, turn out to be as important as it seems. In certain specific instances, alterations of the diet have a proved relationship to some of the complications of liver disease, specifically to ascites formation and to hepatic coma.

The part contributed by ill-balanced diets and secondary nutritional disorders in the pathogenesis of hepatic diseases in man is presently the center of controversy and experiment.

Everyone seems to agree that malnutrition can and does produce functional, structural and clinical alterations of the liver in kwashiorkor and other types of "fatty" liver. Many deny, however, that nutritional hepatic injury alone causes cirrhosis in man.

NUTRITIONAL FACTORS IN EXPERIMENTAL LIVER DISEASE IN ANIMALS[3,4]

Liver lesions in experimental animals resulting from abnormal diet are chiefly fatty change, massive necrosis and cirrhosis. Most of the studies have been done in rats, although more recently other animals, particularly nonhuman primates, have been studied.

In this latter connection, Lieber, Rubin and their colleagues have reproduced what they believe is classical fatty liver, hepatitis and cirrhosis of the alcoholic human in baboons by giving about half of the calories as alcohol and the remainder as a diet presumably furnishing ample quantities of all of the essential nutrients. These studies, although beautifully carried out and exciting, require extension and confirmation. Some authorities have been critical of the conclusions and others have pointed out that, in man, alcoholism is nearly always accompanied by a deficient diet which therefore must be taken into consideration in etiology and certainly in therapy (see Chapter 40).

Best and his colleagues, in their classical

experiments, found that fatty livers developed in pancreatectomized dogs maintained on insulin.[5] It was later shown that this effect was largely, if not entirely, a result of a deficiency of the external secretion of the pancreas which failed to promote the proper digestion and absorption of protein and thus of the essential amino acid methionine. Choline was likewise found to prevent and cure this fatty liver. Methionine was shown to act as a methyl donor, allowing the synthesis of the nutrient choline from ethanolamine.

A protein-deficient diet or, more particularly, one deficient in methionine and choline will regularly produce fatty liver in experimental animals (chiefly rats) and, if continued long enough, will lead to cirrhosis in some animals. Deficiency of other amino acids and, in some studies, of other substances will also lead to fatty liver, but the most severe fatty liver, and the one most likely to lead to cirrhosis, results from protein-choline-methionine deficiency. The place of vitamin B_{12} in fatty liver production is under investigation.

The massive necrosis observed in rats is produced by an entirely different dietary means. The diets usually have been high in protein, mostly furnished by Torula yeast, and deficient in sulfur-containing amino acids and vitamin E. In addition, a third factor is necessary to produce this lesion, trace quantities of organic selenium, an element which, in larger amounts in the diet, will *induce* liver disease.

These lesions have been considered the prototypes of hepatic disease in man, the former resembling the cirrhosis in alcoholics. The massive hepatic necrosis and postnecrotic scarring resemble somewhat, although distantly, the massive hepatic necrosis and so-called postnecrotic cirrhosis or postnecrotic scarring of man.

A note of caution is proper at this time to those eager to transfer concepts based on dietary hepatic disease in rats to the interpretation of hepatic disease in man. Elias has shown that the microscopic structure of the liver of the rat is different from that of man. Moreover, fatty liver in the rat has been produced in many circumstances apparently unrelated to nutritional disturbances. For example, fatty liver and other liver lesions resembling alcoholic liver disease have been produced in experimental animals[6] by alcohol ingestion in spite of a presumably adequate diet (see Chapter 40).

NUTRITIONAL ASPECTS OF LIVER DISEASE IN MAN[11]

In this chapter, we shall consider first the nutritional aspect of viral hepatitis, then of alcoholic liver disease and some miscellaneous liver diseases, including hemachromatosis, Wilson's disease and some others. Finally, the treatment of some of the complications of liver disease will be discussed. These will include the hepatic coma syndrome, ascites and edema and renal disease in particular.

Once the liver is severely damaged, there is no doubt that the general nutritional welfare of the body suffers and the majority of patients with chronic liver disease come to the physician nutritionally bankrupt. The disturbances may be multiple, in some cases because of deficient intake from anorexia or altered or impaired digestion and absorption of nutrients or, finally, because of abnormalities of intermediary metabolism which may occur in established liver disease.

The Fatty Liver

The association of fatty liver with pellagra, with starvation, with diseases of inanition—such as ulcerative colitis and tuberculosis—and with alcoholism is well known. Many believe that fatty liver is the forerunner of some forms of dietary cirrhosis, of tropical cirrhosis and of alcoholic Laennec's cirrhosis. The exact progression to cirrhosis from the fatty liver is still cloaked in mystery. Studies in Africa and elsewhere would seem to indicate that, in man, cirrhosis may not develop as a result of nutritional deficiency alone (see Kwashiorkor below). Should this be correct, it would seem that cirrhosis associated with alcoholism and other nutritional disturbances, such as ulcerative colitis, may not be the result simply of nutritional deficiency but of toxic factors which cause hepatic cellular necrosis, or, possibly, autoimmune responses which produce further damage.

Workers in several laboratories have explored the causes of the alcoholic fatty liver[6,9–11] (see Chapter 40). It has been assumed that the accumulation of fat was on the basis of the nutritional deficiency common among alcoholics. Probably deficiency of nutrients (protein, choline, methionine) contributes; perhaps it is most important. The metabolic effects of alcohol must, however, be considered. Large amounts, acutely given, appear to mobilize fat from adipose tissue to the liver as do some other stressful situations, operating through the pituitary and the adrenal glands. Lesser amounts, more in keeping with the usual alcoholic's drinking habits, exert an important effect upon the liver itself, increasing the synthesis of fat in this organ. It has been possible, in experimental animals and in man, to induce fatty change in the liver when alcohol is substituted for sucrose in an otherwise adequate diet.[10]

Kwashiorkor

Until recently, western physicians did not recognize that primary malnutrition—due to an unbalanced diet—produced fatty liver disease in man as it does in the laboratory animal. As a result of clinical studies in the past several decades, it has become clear that primary nutritional fatty liver disease is widespread in the tropics and is perhaps, after caloric deficiency, the most common nutritional disease of man.

Kwashiorkor is a disease of widespread tropical geographic distribution.[10] Patients with the disease have been found in Central and South America, Africa, India and Southeast Asia. Occasional instances have been reported from Europe during famines (Mehlnährschaden). It is rare in the United States. Many prefer the term "protein-calorie malnutrition," which is now often used for situations in the adult in which deficits of energy and protein are found. This syndrome is discussed more fully in Chapter 24.

Viral Hepatitis

The term "viral hepatitis" usually refers to the two diseases which were previously called "infectious hepatitis" and "serum hepatitis," and which are now called "virus A hepatitis" and "virus B hepatitis," respectively. There may be a "virus C" and perhaps more, now usually grouped as "non A, non B" virus(es). It is well to remember other viruses, for example, yellow fever, cytomegalovirus, Q fever, the virus of infectious mononucleosis, ECHO virus (type 9), Coxsackie virus (type B–3), occasionally the herpes virus, varicella and undoubtedly others, as hepatitis causes. Moreover, some bacteria (e.g. brucellosis), spirochetes (e.g. syphilis), some fungi (e.g. histoplasmosis), protozoa (e.g. amebae) and helminths (e.g. schistosomes) may cause liver disease.

Unfortunately, the nutritional aspects of most infectious diseases involving the liver have not been studied, except for infectious and serum hepatitis. These have been studied thoroughly because of their high incidence in military populations. Two broad questions need consideration with regard to these two kinds of hepatitis: (1) Are malnourished, nonimmune individuals more liable to infection with these viruses than well-nourished individuals? (2) Does diet therapy affect the course of these diseases?

Few critical studies have been done on rates of infection in malnourished populations infected with hepatitis. After World War II there were no reports of overwhelming epidemics in prisoner-of-war camps. During the war, the attack rate of infectious hepatitis in well-nourished, meat-eating Indian soldiers was no different from that observed in ill-nourished, vegetarian Indian soldiers who eschewed meat on religious grounds.

Capps[12] was the first to suggest that convalescence might be prolonged in soldiers with viral hepatitis if food intake was inadequate. The study was a particularly difficult one because wartime conditions made strict control impossible. A later study in which better control was possible indicated that optimal dietary intakes did shorten convalescence, but the effect was not a large one.[13] The food consumed daily by these soldiers provided approximately 40 calories per kg body weight. Protein was about 13 per cent of the calories and fat 30 to 35 per cent. This partition of nutrients is similar to that in the food consumed each day by healthy active soldiers studied by Johnson and Kark.[14]

Occasionally, the hepatitis viruses infect pregnant women but, in most developed countries, the disease does not seem to be much different from that in nonpregnant females of the same age group. Reports from some developing countries, however, suggest that both the frequency and the severity of hepatitis may be increased. Whether this is because of increased frequency of exposure, larger doses of virus, nutritional deficiency or even other factors is not yet known, but attention should certainly be paid to the possibility that nutritional deficiency may be an important contributing factor.

Dietary Management of Uncomplicated Infectious Hepatitis. Anorexia is a cardinal symptom of hepatitis, particularly in the early stages. During this time it may occasionally be necessary to feed patients with glucose intravenously pending return of appetite. As soon as appetite has begun to return, simple foods may be eaten as desired, with emphasis on a well-balanced normal diet.

Usually frequent small feedings of attractive meals at regular intervals are best tolerated. Three large meals a day may serve only to make the patient nauseated. Many patients say during this stage that they are hungry but as soon as they have eaten a little anorexia and even severe nausea may occur. For these patients, a tasty liquid formula in small quantities at frequent intervals is sometimes well tolerated.

During convalescence from acute hepatitis, a well-balanced, nutritious, mixed diet contains all the essential nutrients needed. This may be provided by attractive meals served at regular intervals, when the patient is most likely to be hungry, and by interval feedings of milk shakes or eggnogs.

If the above measures do not ensure an adequate intake of food, then food may be given by tube feedings (Appendix Tables 31, 32, 34). Intravenous feedings of glucose will rarely be needed if the patient is urged to eat.

An adequate protein intake of 1 gm per kg body weight or above is usually easily obtained from a well-planned, mixed diet. The protein should come from both animal and vegetable sources. Adequate supplies of protein, choline, inositol, methionine and other amino acids and vitamins are provided in mixed protein-containing foods such as meats, fish, eggs, dairy products, legumes and cereals. Amino acid supplements are unnecessary, as digestion and absorption of protein seem satisfactory in this disease. Moreover, supplements of vitamins, choline, inositol, methionine, etc., are also unnecessary unless food intake is drastically altered from normal, as adequate quantities are in a good mixed diet.

In a few susceptible individuals with severe hepatitis, usually those with massive necrosis, high or even normal protein intake may induce the syndrome of hepatic precoma or coma (see below). When protein in normal amounts is poorly tolerated and leads to this syndrome, it is an extremely poor prognostic sign. It is proba-ble that the protein ingested has not further damaged the liver, but only that, because of the severity of the liver disease, it is poorly tolerated by critically ill patients. In this circumstance, the regimen for hepatic coma given below should be carefully followed.

There is no need to restrict fat intake in patients ill with hepatitis, unless disturbances of digestion result, probably from diminished bile salts reaching the intestine from the liver. High-fat diets also are not necessary, but 30 to 40 per cent of the calories per day from fat certainly adds palatability to the diet, carries fat-soluble vitamins and is generally well tolerated, certainly during convalescence. In general, it is wiser to provide fat through dairy products and eggs rather than fried foods and fatty meats.

An adequate carbohydrate intake is readily obtained, provided that a well-balanced diet is consumed in accordance with the principles noted above. It has been the custom of many physicians to provide hard candy ad libitum to patients ill with hepatitis. This should usually not be done, as sweets, particularly between meals, disturb the appetite and provide an unbalanced source of calories.

In hepatitis the plasma prothrombin level is often reduced. This is usually the result of disturbed liver function. The damaged liver is unable to synthesize prothrombin and some other clotting factors. This is not corrected by vitamin K. However, intrahepatic biliary obstruction does occur in infective hepatitis, and occasionally the exclusion of bile from the gut will interfere with absorption of vitamin K. Under these conditions, parenteral vitamin K, or oral, water-soluble vitamin K, will raise prothrombin levels. In 1940, Kark and Souter showed that the degree of response of prothrombin levels to vitamin K therapy was a good index of hepatic function. This has been accepted as an excellent test of liver functional impairment.

Usually, gross sodium and water retention does not complicate hepatitis. Although it is true that recovery from hepatitis is often ushered in with a mild diuresis, it is only in the severely ill patient that sodium retention needs to be treated through strict dietary regulation of salt and sodium-containing foods. When this is necessary, the low-salt regimen prescribed for the treatment of cirrhosis should be followed.

Liquid Preparations for Complete or Between-meal Feedings. For supplementary or complete feeding, palatable liquid formulas may be useful (Appendix Tables 31–35).

It should be remembered that formulas high in milk products may be poorly tolerated by some patients, especially if intestinal lactase deficiency is present. When poorly tolerated the quantity given may be reduced or the mixture somewhat diluted until the patient is able to take the full mixture, or low-milk formulas may be used.

A number of powdered supplementary foods (easily reconstituted by adding water or milk) are marketed. Sustagen or various "instant breakfasts" are excellent in many respects. They are bland, "balanced" foods fortified with vitamins at a therapeutic level, and cost per gram of protein is not excessive.

The palatability of all these drinks depends to a great extent on the thoroughness of mixing of the preparation. Electric milk-shake mixers are ideal, but hand beaters are satisfactory if used with care and thoroughness. The milk shakes should be made up freshly each day and kept refrigerated from preparation until service.

When low-sodium supplementary or between-meal feedings are necessary, a low-sodium drink is suggested (Appendix Tables 13, 14).

Tube or Gavage Feeding. When anorexia, nausea or vomiting is severe enough to limit caloric intake, tube feeding should be instituted without delay. One of the most significant advances in therapeutics in the past years has been the recognition that thin polyethylene or nylon tubing can be used for gavage feeding of individual patients for weeks at a time without causing distress to the patient and without damage to the mucous membranes of the upper respiratory or gastrointestinal tract. When once passed, it can usually be left in place. The patient can eat his usual meals without discomfort during the day with the tube in position, and during the night, while he sleeps, a tube feeding can be run into his stomach or duodenum. In precoma or comatose patients, the danger of aspiration pneumonia as a result of regurgitation of stomach contents must be kept in mind.

Intravenous Feeding. The indication for intravenous feeding is vomiting. Intravenous feeding may also be used as a supplement to oral or gavage feeding, especially to supply low-sodium amino acid supplements to low-protein diets. Techniques and formulas for intravenous feeding are given in Chapter 37.

Complications. When the patient with hepatitis comes under medical care much of the damage within the liver is done, and diet therapy serves to allow or to hasten healing and regeneration of the hepatic cells. There are grave doubts that optimal diet therapy prevents the relentless march to cirrhosis which develops in occasional patients with hepatitis (less than 1 per cent); nor does it seem able to prevent the chronic form of the disease. In childhood, fortunately, infectious hepatitis nearly always runs a benign course.

When hepatitis develops in the third trimester of pregnancy, the prognosis for mother and child is less benign, while in the first trimester no ill effects usually ensue.

The complications of hepatitis require modifications of dietary management. The most common complications are nausea and vomiting, which may have to be managed with tube feedings or intravenous feedings. The other complication is progression toward severe hepatic insufficiency which requires separate consideration, as indicated under Hepatic Coma Syndrome. The dietary management of chronic hepatitis is no different from that of cirrhosis and is discussed below under this heading.

The Hepatic Coma Syndrome

Physicians from Galen's age to our own have recognized a connection between hepatic dysfunction and cerebral function. Kinnear Wilson was the first to describe pathologic lesions of the brain in patients ill with cirrhosis, and histologic abnormalities have been observed in the brains of patients who have died with hepatic coma.

The manifestations of precoma and coma have been clarified by various clinical observations.[15-24] Walshe[16] describes as part of the clinical picture of coma: confusion, apathy, personality changes, spasticity, muscle spasms, choreiform movements, athetoid postures, lead pipe and cogwheel rigidity of the arms, flexion withdrawal of the legs and cholemic crying. Ankle clonus with plantar flexor Babinski responses is rather characteristic.[17]

The neurologic findings are not uncommonly complicated in the alcoholic by delirium tremens, by hemorrhage into the brain as a result of prothrombin or other clotting factor deficiency, by other types of hemorrhagic disturbances such as scurvy, and by Wernicke's encephalopathy, the result of thiamin deficiency.

The neurologic signs and symptoms of hepatic coma and precoma have been observed in Eck-fistula dogs given meat, in patients with portacaval shunts, in patients with portal vein occlusion and in patients with a wide variety of hepatic disorders ranging from Chiari's syndrome to acute hepatitis. In many of these persons, attacks have been precipitated by oral feedings of meat, high-protein diets, casein hydrolysates, amino acid mixtures, amino acids, ammonium chloride, ammonium citrate, urea, cation-exchange resins containing ammonium and particularly after gastrointestinal bleeding.

It also appears that methionine or amino acid mixtures given by mouth will regularly precipitate neurologic signs in some patients ill with liver disease. It has been shown that the administration of oral, broad-spectrum antibiotics will inhibit the neurologic ill effects of protein feeding in patients in a state of impending coma. The observations and data on hand suggest that nitrogenous substances from the bowel—presumably the result of bacterial action on protein foods or nitrogenous chemicals—produce the neurologic and mental changes described above; the most studied has been ammonia, but other compounds such as amines may be active. These changes can occur when blood is shunted directly from the portal system into the systemic system. The healthy liver detoxifies or utilizes the toxic nitrogenous material as it passes up the portal vein. Thus, ammonia is quantitatively converted to urea. When the hepatic cells are damaged (anoxia, fatty infiltration, infection, etc.) or when vascular shunts develop within the liver, the toxic nitrogenous materials also pass into the systemic blood stream.

Abnormalities of amino acid metabolism have been postulated as contributing factors. Increases in blood aromatic amino acids and reduction of the 3 branched-chain amino acids may allow the former to enter the brain more easily; there they could alter neurotransmission.

Treatment of Hepatic Coma and Precoma. Consumption of an adequate diet with at least normal protein content is recognized as an essential part of the therapy of many forms of liver disease, but may precipitate hepatic precoma or coma. In the nutritional therapy of liver disease, the physician and the patient must walk a tightrope. Too much protein may induce hepatic coma, too little may prolong a patient's illness. A proper balance can usually be achieved by careful observation of the patient for the signs of impending coma. Treatment with broad-spectrum antibiotics, such as neomycin, should be instituted when the syndrome appears. If the syndrome progresses despite the antibiotic or the patient is first seen when in coma, protein administration should be omitted altogether.

At each visit to the sickroom the patient must be asked to cock up his hands; if the "flapping tremor" is noted or mental confusion is found, antibiotics should immediately be prescribed. At this stage it is usually not necessary to reduce the protein content of the diet—at least not below the recommended dietary allowance of approximately 1 gm per kg of body weight per day.

If the patient cannot eat, nutrition may be maintained as described above utilizing less protein.

Toxic Hepatitis and Cirrhosis

Opie and others have clearly indicated that the resistance to and repair of hepatic damage by toxic agents such as carbon tetrachloride is enhanced by diet therapy. Iatrogenic jaundice may be the result of endocrine therapy (methyltestosterone jaundice), some oral contraceptives, psychochemotherapy (chlorpromazine and iproniazid jaundice) and other drugs. Acute toxic hepatitis should be managed by regimens suitable for patients with other forms of hepatitis, and those ill with chronic toxic hepatitis or cirrhosis should be treated as are patients with Laennec's cirrhosis.

The development of toxic liver diseases other than those described above has also been related to nutritional factors. Senecio cirrhosis is seen in South Africa. It is the result of eating bread and other foods made from flour contaminated with the crushed seeds of species of Senecio, a plant which grows in the wheat fields of the Cape Province. In North America, Senecio poisoning is one cause of cirrhosis in cattle. Selzer[25] and her colleagues have shown that Senecio cirrhosis develops in rats only when the weed is added to an experimental diet poor in protein; an adequate protein intake protects the animals. These experiments may bear on the problem of infantile hepatic necrosis in Indians and on Jamaican infantile veno-occlusive hepatitis, which resembles Senecio cirrhosis and which occurs in weanlings living on low-protein diets and fed decoctions of local plants.

Cirrhosis and Fibrosis of the Liver.[26]

Cirrhosis is a disease common in the tropics and in alcoholics, and occurs occasionally in individuals who have had attacks of hepatitis. It also is part of the pathologic changes in patients suffering from disorders such as hemochromatosis, biliary cirrhosis, cholangiolitic jaundice and hepatolenticular degeneration. It may appear after infection with Brucella abortus, spirochetes and amoebae, after infestation with schistosomes, or as a result of metabolic or cardiac diseases. While diet therapy is used to treat the cirrhosis which develops in all these conditions, outstanding success is not attained in all instances. It is true that many alcoholics with Laennec's cirrhosis can be restored to and kept in good health by diet therapy, provided that they do not drink. Other patients with cirrhosis progress slowly or rapidly to death in hepatic failure, or as a result of rupture of esophageal varices.

Manipulations of diet have constituted a major advance in our attack on the problem, but diet therapy is only one part of the therapeutic regimen found to be of benefit. In essence, the regimen consists of bed rest during acute phases, absolute prohibition of all forms of alcohol, protection of the patient from hepatotoxic drugs and chemicals and provision of a diet rich in protein, calories and other nutrients. Sodium restriction is used when necessary. Particular attention is paid to actual daily dietary intake, to simple supportive psychotherapy and to the daily weight of the patient. When specific deficiencies coexist with cirrhosis, the patients should be treated immediately with a good diet and oral or parenteral water-soluble vitamins. After the lesions have gone away, extra vitamins are not necessary if a well-balanced diet is consumed each day.

Klatskin and Gabuzda have shown that marked improvement occurs in alcoholic cirrhotic patients even when they are given a minimal dietary regimen, provided alcohol intake is stopped, although this is not recommended therapy.

Intravenous albumin, methionine, choline, the B complex vitamins and liver extract do not seem to confer any special benefits and may sometimes be dangerous.

With regard to the treatment of cirrhosis in alcoholics, complete abstention must be the goal.

Dietary Treatment of Edema and Ascites in Cirrhosis. Hidden water retention, frank edema, and ascites are common complications of cirrhosis.[27] They are usually associated with nutritional, endocrinologic and secondary metabolic disorders. The signs of malnutrition commonly seen are loss of flesh and a raw, beefy tongue—both caused by protein wastage—scurvy, pellagra, cheilosis and other signs of B complex deficiency. Endocrinologic changes consist in the main of spider nevi, liver palms, loss of libido, testicular and prostatic atrophy, loss of hair on the chest, gynecomastia and amenorrhea or menorrhagia. These latter findings may be related to abnormal metabolism of hormones produced by malnutrition and also to the inability of the damaged liver to conjugate or otherwise dispose of normally circulating hormones. Metabolic defects are hypoalbuminemia, depressed levels of prothrombin and cholinesterase in the serum and electrolyte imbalance. The retention of sodium and water has been related to raised portal pressure, increased antidiuretic hormone, secondary aldosteronism, hypoalbuminemia and tissue permeability defects, among other factors. Restriction of dietary sodium to levels about equal to that lost by the body from the skin, stool and urine (200 mg per day) prevents further ascites accumulation. Repair of tissue mass is also associated with a slow, steady loss of excess water as the restoration of protein nutri-

tion moves the patient's tissue from depletion toward the normal state. With tissue repair, a long-term, slow, steady diuresis occurs, and eventually the kidney is once again able to handle the sodium load of a normal salt-containing diet.[27,28]

Restriction of Sodium. Restriction of sodium has been a most useful procedure in the delivery of ascitic and edema fluid, in preventing the reaccumulation of ascites following paracentesis and in restoration of tissue in malnourished cirrhotics. The difficulties encountered in therapy are mainly economic, for repair of tissue wasting and restoration of hepatic integrity may take many months or even several years. In addition, the diet is made up of expensive protein foods, some of which have to be processed commercially to remove sodium.

With the use of modern diuretics, particularly chlorothiazide and spironolactone, severe restriction may not be necessary at all times, and may in some instances, particularly when a good proportion of the ascites has gone, be harmful. Once the ascites and edema have gone, or are minimal, cautious removal of diuretics can be tried. If this is tolerated without gain in ascites (best measured by gain in weight) sodium can cautiously be added to the diet.

Hidden sources of sodium in intravenously administered plasma and whole blood (sodium citrate) transfusions, in the diet—as in bread or drinking water which has been artificially softened—or in some oral and parenteral drugs may cause an unexpected reaccumulation of fluid in patients who are "dry."

An instance of the effects of adding sodium to the diet is shown in the study of the cirrhosis patient J. D. (Fig. 31D–1), where 10 gm of salt (170 mEq of sodium) were added each day for 3 days to his low-sodium diet at a time when he was "dry" and when his weight was steady. As a result of this, he gained 5 pounds of weight in 4 days, and it took a week for him to lose this extra water bound in his body by the excess sodium. The rapid weight gain induced by deliberate salting during therapy with low-sodium diets and the length of time required to restore equilibrium are exceedingly useful methods for demonstrating to the individual patient the good effects of a low-sodium regimen and the ill effects of straying from the regimen. It may sometimes be wise for the physician to

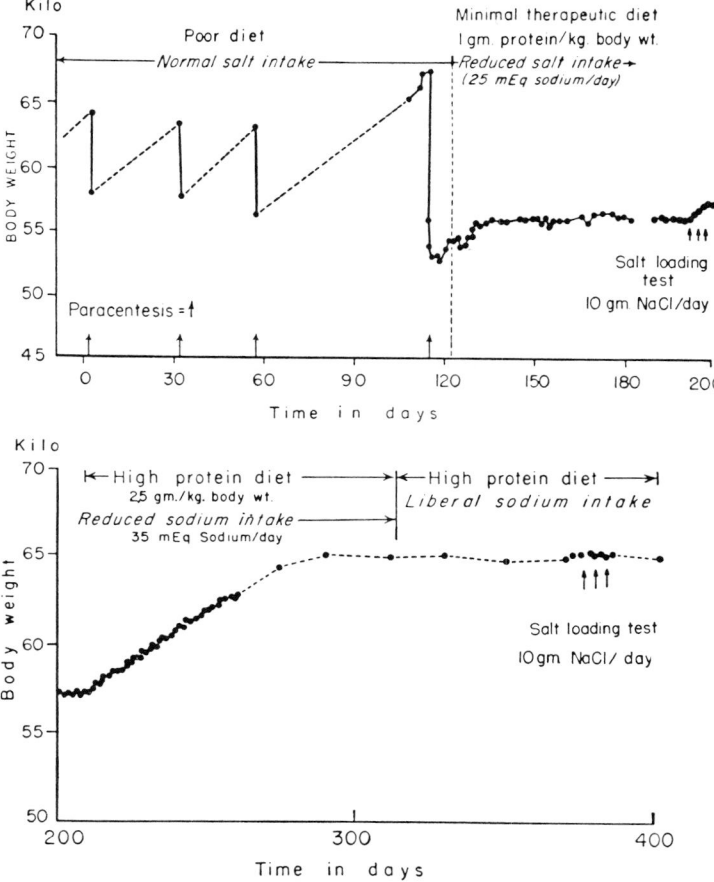

Fig. 31D–1. The effect of various diets on body weight and ascitic fluid accumulation in patient J. D., ill with alcoholism, cirrhosis and ascites.

From day 0 to 110 patient was treated at home by repeated paracenteses. At this time his diet was poor; he had a normal salt intake, and he reaccumulated fluid rapidly.

On day 111, a paracentesis was done, and he began to reaccumulate water. He was placed on a minimal therapeutic diet (1 gm of protein per kg body weight, and basal plus 150 per cent calories). Sodium was reduced to 25 mEq per day. On this regimen he stopped collecting fluid but did not gain weight. On day 190 a salt-loading test was started. He was unable to handle sodium, and reaccumulated water.

On day 200, the diet was changed by increasing the protein to 2.5 gm per kg body weight per day. This addition raised the sodium intake to 35 mEq per day. On this regimen there was a rapid restoration of body tissue, with reduction in liver size. Spider nevi disappeared. The steady gain in tissue was associated with a concomitant loss of water.

On day 310, the regimen was changed to a diet containing liberal amounts of salt. The patient did not gain water, and on day 376, when a salt-loading test was administered, there was no reaccumulation of water. Restoration of tissue mass and regeneration of liver tissue allowed the kidney to handle sodium normally.

demonstrate to the patient and his family the value of sodium restriction by deliberate salting of diets for short periods of time.

To control the level of sodium intake in the diet, it is necessary to weigh the patient *each day* or to have him weigh himself, preferably the first thing in the morning. These weights should be charted. Rapid gain in body weight means that water is accumulating because of sodium retention and too much sodium in the diet. On the other hand, a slow, steady gain of weight associated with clinical improvement is usually due to restoration of tissue mass. Rarely, rapid gain in body water and body weight is the result of "low-salt syndrome."

When patients have been on the low-sodium diet for some months and when clinical improvement is obvious, the daily output of sodium in urine begins to increase and eventually they can return to a diet containing moderate or normal quantities of salt. The decision to increase the amount of sodium in the diet should be implemented by a trial of salt feeding. This must be controlled by daily weighing. If, for example, 5 gm of salt are added each day to the diet and if the weight increases each day at a rapid rate, then the patient has not recovered his ability to excrete sodium and to handle the excess salt. Obviously, he must remain on his low-sodium diet for a further period of therapy until it is considered wise to attempt a second trial of salt feeding. Measurement of 24-hour urinary sodium excretion is worthwhile at this time.

Hazards of Sodium Restriction. Sodium restriction is not without hazard. A few patients with cirrhosis and ascites continue to demonstrate ascites and edema for a time even if sodium intake is controlled. They will thus develop hyponatremia. A moderately low serum sodium concentration is not unusual in cirrhotic patients (125 to 135 mEq per L). This degree of hyponatremia does not require drastic treatment, especially if it is chronic. Much

greater reductions in serum sodium concentration (e.g. below 120 mEq per L) may require treatment, especially when rapidly induced by overhydration, with or without excessive sodium loss from gastrointestinal bleeding, overuse of powerful diuretics, etc.

Fluid intake restriction must be carefully done. Overzealous limitation may be followed by oliguria which is sometimes not noted for several days. This alarming state of affairs can sometimes be prevented by gauging fluid intake to equal output (including insensible loss). Treatment of moderate oliguria may not be required, but if the condition is severe drastic therapy may be required. Adequate fluid intake is the basis for such therapy, which may include albumin infusions and other measures.

In view of the dangers of salt depletion, it is most important to test renal function before initiating low-sodium diet therapy in cirrhosis. When the dietary regimen is started, measurements of nonprotein nitrogen, plasma carbon dioxide-combining power and serum sodium and potassium should be made at least once a week for the first few weeks after treatment has been instituted. The physician should watch for the development of cramps, abdominal pain or unusual drowsiness.

If renal function is moderately disturbed salt restriction may be instituted, starting rather cautiously and allowing an initial intake of between 50 and 60 mEq of sodium per day, thereafter increasing or decreasing intake as indicated by changes in body weight, urine output, the clinical conditions of the patient and biochemical data.

Nutrient Intake with Low-sodium Diet.[26] Most patients ill with cirrhosis, and especially those who have ascites, show the ill effects of long-continued protein and caloric starvation. In them, part of the cellular protein has been replaced by water and possibly by electrolytes. This chronic cellular waterlogging may be clinically occult, but contributes to edema and ascites when they develop. With low-sodium and high-protein intakes even nonedematous patients deliver water and salt and lay down tissue protein. Moreover, patients ill with cirrhosis and ascites frequently improve on a diet which is "well balanced" by present concepts, and provides 1 gm of protein per kg of body weight. Sample low-sodium diets are given in Appendix Table 13.

When a nutritionally well-balanced, low-sodium, adequate protein diet is offered and consumed day after day by the cirrhotic patient, supplementation of the diet with choline, methionine and vitamins is not necessary. In our hands, intravenous injection of liver extracts has not been of value in the management of cirrhotic patients. Its exact usefulness awaits further evaluation. When patients with cirrhosis present themselves initially for examination, they are often ill with vitamin deficiency syndromes, but these are not as commonly seen now as formerly. When deficiency states are noted, treatment with water-soluble vitamins should be vigorous. It is our custom, when we diagnose vitamin deficiencies in our cirrhotic patients, to give a B complex vitamin mixture, or an intramuscular injection of a water-soluble B complex mixture, once a day for several days or until the patient is eating well.

Many alcoholics, especially those with liver disease, are deficient in folic acid, judging from the megaloblastic anemia which responds to folic acid[29] and the low blood levels of this vitamin which have been found.[30] Thus, folic acid should be given not only when it is proven to be deficient but should always be included in the vitamin B complex mixture used. It is important to note that many manufactured vitamin B complex mixtures do not contain folic acid because of its masking effect in pernicious anemia; it must then be given separately.

To replace the taste of the salt which is missing in the diet, patients may use a salt substitute. This may be sprinkled ad libitum over the food, as it contains no sodium. We have used two sodium-free glutamic acid flavoring agents, ammonium glutamate and calcium glutamate. These condiments certainly add zest to low-sodium diets. A few drops of lemon squeezed on meat add much to the flavor.

Biliary Tract Disease[31]

Onions and French-fried potatoes, and other cooked fatty foods, are anathema to most patients who are dyspeptic and who also suffer from chronic cholecystitis, biliary stones or other diseases involving the biliary tract. This is not surprising, since a number of nutrients affect the quality and quantity of bile, the motility of the gallbladder and the tone of the sphincter of Oddi. Moreover, the bile is essential for proper absorption of fats, fat-soluble vitamins and a number of hormones and metabolic substances which cycle through the enterohepatic circulation during consumption and digestion of food.[31] However, it is surprising to find that only 5 to 10 per cent of patients with gallstones are dyspeptic.

Effects of Diet on the Biliary Tract and Bile. High-protein diets and, to a lesser extent, high-fat diets increase bile production. Dehydration and high-carbohydrate diets decrease bile formation. Fatty food cholagogues—cream, egg yolk and olive oil—cause the sphincter of Oddi to relax and initiate contraction of the gallbladder. This process is thought to be initiated by food through the hormone cholecystokinin, which is released from the upper intestinal wall into the blood stream and is carried to the gallbladder and sphincter of Oddi. Thus, at mealtimes a store of gallbladder bile is released into the duodenum when it is most needed to help in the digestion and absorption of fats.

Many clinicians suspect that aberrations of this mechanism are responsible for initiating biliary or pancreatic disorders. It has been postulated that, following large meals high in fat and protein, the gallbladder may contract against an unrelaxed sphincter of Oddi (achalasia of the sphincter of Oddi) or against a spastic sphincter of Oddi (biliary dyskinesia). This may result in acute or recurrent biliary colic, and obstructive jaundice may develop. If an anomalous pancreatic duct opens directly into the biliary duct, then, when the situation described above develops, bile may regurgitate into the pancreas and acute or relapsing chronic pancreatitis may ensue.

Nutrition and the Development of Gallstones and Cholecystitis.[32-34] Recent studies have clearly demonstrated that neither bile nor gallstones nor gallbladder wall from patients with gallstones or cholecystitis is infected with organisms. This and other investigations strengthen the concept that cholecystitis is not an infectious disease but the result of a chemical inflammation of the wall of the gallbladder. Thus it seems that the genesis of cholecystitis and gallstones (except pigment stones resulting from hemolytic phenomena) must be sought in that rather vague but important field of medical endeavor which relates body build, race and other genetic factors to environmental, endocrinologic and nutritional abnormalities. Cholecystitis—and in particular gallstones—varies in incidence from country to country. It appears to be high in those who live on a high-calorie, high-fat diet, is rarely seen among the Japanese, is common in Jewish people, appears in families and in the obese and fair, becomes troublesome at the menopause and occurs more commonly in females than in males. The development of cholecystitis and gallstones appears to be related to cardiovascular disease, to familial hypercholesterolemia, to pancreatic disease and to diabetes.

While there is no proof that dietary habits are the prime cause of cholecystitis and gallstones, the data collected thus far are highly suggestive. Worldwide studies are needed on the incidence of gallbladder diseases in populations consuming different diets—studies which would be similar to those made in different parts of the world which relate degenerative heart disease with high-fat diets and high blood cholesterol levels.

Dietary Management of Patients with Dyspepsia, Gallstones and Cholecystitis.[35-37] A cholesterol-free diet cannot be regarded as a means of preventing gallstones. On the other hand, prescription of a low-fat diet is a time-honored dietary regimen for patients with chronic flatulent dyspepsia who have, in addition, physical or radiologic evidence of chronic cholecystitis or gallstones. Greasy or fried foods, eggs, mayonnaise, salad dressings, cheese and pork products and high-fat pastries rich in cream or suet should be avoided. Many patients recognize that they cannot tolerate onions, sauerkraut, cabbage, radishes, turnips, cucumbers and spicy foods such as chili con carne and curry. Vegetable fats, such as olive oil or corn oil which are rather unsaturated, seem to be beneficial when the gallbladder is functioning normally, as they stimulate bile flow. Their employment in the regimen must depend on the patient's ability to tolerate them.

When acute cholecystitis develops, no fried food should be fed, and the patient may need to be fed parenterally. Immediately after an acute attack, the diet should be limited to small amounts of carbohydrate foodstuffs such as fruit juices, pureed potatoes, rice and tapioca. Later, more solid cereals can be added, together with skim milk, broiled fish and lean broiled meats. Nonfat white chicken or turkey meat may also be employed.

Nutrition and Chronic Obstructive Jaundice. Chronic obstructive jaundice is most commonly seen as a result of postoperative traumatic stricture of the bile ducts, congenital lesions of the bile ducts, undetected calculi, carcinoma of the pancreas or hepatic ducts, cysts in the head of the pancreas, biliary cirrhosis and cholangiolitis.[37,38] In all these lesions, the nutrition and metabolism of the body are disturbed by acholia. In essence, the main pathophysiologic disturbance is steatorrhea with malnutrition resulting from loss of calories, fat-soluble vitamins and minerals.

Loss of dietary calories raises the demand for calories from protein sources, with resultant development of fatty liver and impaired production of plasma proteins. Medium-chain triglycerides permit better fat absorption and, hence, more calories. Failure to absorb vitamin K produces prothrombin deficiency, manifested by needle puncture hematomata, spontaneous bruising and a hemorrhagic tendency.

The loss of calcium and vitamin D produces osteomalacia, with demineralized bone, kyphosis, fractures, collapse of vertebrae and herniation of the intervertebral disc into the vertebral bodies (Schmorl's nodes). In addition, osteoporosis may be present, perhaps due to protein deficiency and reduced steroid output as a result of malnutrition. Vitamin A deficiency produces night blindness and hyperkeratosis, while failure of absorption of unsaturated fatty acids may result in eczematous-like skin lesions. Vitamin E deficiency may produce muscle weakness.[39] Loss of potassium may cause potassium nephropathy, atony of the bowel and typical muscle weakness.

Prevention of the ill effects of chronic obstructive jaundice consists of providing a regimen sufficient in calories and rich in protein. Fat is poorly tolerated and badly absorbed and should be limited.

The failure to absorb fat normally is due primarily to the lack of bile salts in the intestine. Bile salts are necessary for fat absorption, at least in part to form micelles with fat.

If prothrombin levels are low, vitamin K may have to be given by intramuscular injection each day until the deficiency is corrected. Bone lesions, if present, may have to be treated vigorously with vitamin D, usually vitamin D_3.[40] A maintenance dose of 6 gm of calcium gluconate per day should be taken in addition to skim milk, buttermilk and other high-calcium foods. If there is severe osteomalacia, the calcium should be increased to 2 to 3 times the maintenance dose per day.

There is some evidence that the anemia of chronic obstructive jaundice is the result of iron deficiency, and, if there is no response to vitamin B complex medication, ferrous sulfate grains, 7½ per day, may have to be continued indefinitely. Occasionally, intravenous iron therapy or transfusions may be necessary.

The development of cirrhosis in chronic obstructive jaundice needs special dietary attention, as described above.

BIBLIOGRAPHY

1. Patek and Post: J. Clin. Invest., 20, 481, 1941.
2. Symposium on Liver Disease. Am. J. Clin. Nutr., 21, 1325, 1968.
3. Alpers and Isselbacher: In Diseases of the Liver, 4th Ed. (Schiff, Ed.). Philadelphia, J. B. Lippincott, 1975.
4. Himsworth: Liver and Its Diseases. Cambridge, Harvard University Press, 1950.
5. Best and Ridout: Annu. Rev. Biochem., 8, 349, 1939.
6. Lieber (Ed.): Metabolic Aspects of Alcoholism. Baltimore, University Park Press, 1977.
7. Lieber and Davidson: Am. J. Med., 33, 319, 1962.
8. Lieber, Jones and DeCarli: J. Clin. Invest., 44, 1009, 1965.
9. Lieber: Gastroenterology, 65, 821, 1973.
10. Brock and Autret: WHO Monogr. Ser., 5, 1, 1952.
11. Davidson: Ann. N.Y. Acad. Sci., 104, 1026, 1963.
11a. Alter, Holland, Purcell and Popper: Lancet, 1, 459, 1978.
12. Capps and Barker: Ann. Intern. Med., 26, 405, 1947.
13. Chalmers: J. Clin. Invest., 34, 1163, 1965.
14. Johnson and Kark: Science, 105, 378, 1947.
14a. Bohrmanmanesh: In Problems in Liver Diseases, (Davidson, Ed.). New York, Stratton Intercontinental, 1979.
15. Walshe: Lancet, 1, 1075, 1953.
16. Walshe: Q. J. Med., 20, 421, 1951.
17. Adams and Foley: Trans. Am. Neurol. Assoc., 74, 271, 1949.
18. Davidson: In Gastroenterology, Vol. 3, (Bockus, Ed.). Philadelphia, W. B. Saunders, 1976.

19. Davidson and Gabuzda: N. Engl. J. Med., *243*, 779, 1950.
20. Phillips, Gabuzda and Davidson: J. Clin. Invest., *31*, 351, 1952.
21. Sherlock, Summerskill, White and Phear: Lancet, *2*, 453, 1954.
22. Murphy, Chalmers, Eckhardt and Davidson: N. Engl. J. Med., *239*, 605, 1948.
23. Gabuzda, Phillips and Davidson: N. Engl. J. Med., *246*, 124, 1952.
24. Phillips, Schwartz, Gabuzda and Davidson: N. Engl. J. Med., *247*, 239, 1952.
25. Selzer, Parker and Sapeicka: Br. J. Exp. Pathol., *32*, 14, 1951.
26. Davidson: *Liver Pathophysiology*. Boston, Little, Brown & Co., 1970.
27. Eisenmenger, Ahrens, Blondheim and Kunkel: J. Lab. Clin. Med., *34*, 1029, 1949.
28. Davidson: J. Am. Diet. Assoc., *62*, 515, 1973.
29. Jandl: J. Clin. Invest., *34*, 390, 1955.
30. Herbert, Zalusky and Davidson: Ann. Intern. Med., *58*, 977, 1963.
31. Warren and Tan: In *Diseases of the Liver,* 4th ed. (Schiff, Ed.). Philadelphia, J. B. Lippincott, 1975.
32. Small: N. Engl. J. Med., *279*, 588, 1968.
33. Small: In *Diseases of the Liver,* 4th ed. (Schiff, Ed.). Philadelphia, J. B. Lippincott, 1975.
34. Bennion, et al.: N. Engl. J. Med., *300*, 873, 1979.
35. McDermott: *Surgery of the Liver and Portal Circulation*. Philadelphia, Lea & Febiger, 1974.
36. Taylor (Ed.): *The Biliary System.* Philadelphia, F. A. Davis, 1965.
37. Editorial. Lancet, *1*, 805, 1978.
38. Ahrens, et al.: Medicine, *29*, 299, 1950.
39. Klatskin and Krehl: J. Clin. Invest., *29*, 1528, 1950.
40. Long, et al.: Br. Med. J., *1*, 75, 1978.

Chapter *32*

DIET IN THE TREATMENT OF DIABETES MELLITUS

Gerald J. Friedman

Recent studies on genetic and environmental factors influencing the development of diabetes mellitus have led to considerable advancement in the understanding of the disease, but the cause (causes?) of it remains a mystery.[1]

Diabetes mellitus is one of the most common maladies encountered in mankind. It has been estimated that it now affects 5 per cent of the population of the United States, having increased by more than 50 per cent between 1967 and 1973.[2] There are an estimated 10 million diabetics in the United States (9 million obesity induced).[3] An increase in diabetes has been noted also in the rest of the world.

Diabetes is the third-ranking cause of death in the United States, and remains one of the most crippling of all diseases because of its chronicity and complications (i.e. arteriosclerotic heart disease, hypertension and renal failure).[2] In addition to the long-term degenerative complications, diabetes causes blindness and is associated with acute infections. Until the roles of the multiple factors implicated in the pathogenesis are clearly defined, the treatment will probably remain palliative. The importance of research directed at the etiology of diabetes cannot be overemphasized since it may ultimately lead to the prevention and/or cure of the disease.[4]

DEFINITION OF DIABETES MELLITUS

Much of the difficulty in defining diabetes mellitus arises from the lack of a specific genetic marker, the evidence for genetic heterogeneity, the diversity of clinical manifestations and the multiple factors that influence the biochemical constituents (hyperglycemia, absolute or relative insulin deficiency and disturbances of intermediary metabolism).[5]

The disturbance might depend upon diet, primary or secondary failure of the beta cells of the islets of Langerhans through one or more hereditary defects, or any of the other factors that influence insulin synthesis, secretion, transport and action in responsive tissue.[6] Regardless of the mechanisms involved, diabetics, young and old, with mild or severe disease, suffer from a subnormal ability to utilize glucose in their systems.

From the clinical point of view, idiopathic or primary diabetes mellitus may be defined as an hereditary disease of metabolism in which there is an inadequate supply of effective insulin, characterized by disturbances of carbohydrate, fat and protein homeostasis and by macroangiopathic, microangiopathic and neuropathic changes.

Genetic factors are crucial in the development of diabetes mellitus. However, no known mechanism explains the frequency of the disease in the population.[7,8]

Some of the major intricacies that make the study of inheritance of diabetes a "geneticist's nightmare" include the complex presentations of the disease itself, i.e. a wide spectrum of subclinical and clinical profiles; the age of onset; diverse incidence rates in different ethnic and geographic groups with no definite relationship with phenotype, diet or habitat; and perhaps, most important of all, lack of availability of a genetic marker or an heritability index. In the present state of our ignorance, the mechanisms that probably best explain the manifestations of the diabetic potentiality include a combination of a polygenic or multifactorial inheritance and some, as yet, poorly understood environmental influences.[1]

In the human, two classical types of "idiopathic" diabetes mellitus are generally recognized—the insulin-dependent (juvenile-onset) and the noninsulin dependent (maturity-onset) types—depending upon the age of onset and the severity. Different modes of inheritance of these two forms have been speculated upon but not proven.[8,9] Recent studies suggest that there are definite differences in the genetic transmission of these two types as well as in the mechanisms underlying the clinical expression of the diabetic trait as well.

If diabetes were entirely determined by genetic factors we would expect to see a 100 per cent concordance rate for the disease in identical (monozygotic) twins. A concordance rate of 92 per cent was found when the diabetes occurred in the index twin after the age of 40, and only 50 per cent when the age of the index twin was less than 40.[10,11] The many years of continued discordance in younger twin-pairs underscores the influence of nongenetic (environmental) factors in such individuals.

The incidence of diabetes mellitus in offspring of conjugal diabetics is only 6 to 10 per cent. Twenty-five to 40 per cent of offspring of conjugal diabetic parents have "chemical" (latent) diabetes. On repeated testing 55 to 60 per cent of the offspring have nonprogressive chemical diabetes. It is estimated that only one-third of the offspring will eventually have "overt" diabetes—of which the majority will be the mild maturity-onset type—whereas 50 per cent of the offspring will have nonprogressive, chemical diabetes as determined by repetitive testing.[12-16]

The Insulin-dependent (Juvenile-onset) Type of Diabetes Mellitus

Insulin-dependent diabetes is unstable or labile. Juvenile diabetics account for 5 per cent of the total diabetic population; an additional 5 per cent are "brittle" adult diabetics.

Insulin-dependent diabetes usually, but not always, arises during childhood or puberty. It is abrupt in onset and symptomatic, occurs usually in undernourished patients, has wide variations in blood sugar values in response to small changes in insulin dose, exercise or infection, is difficult to control and is frequently associated with ketosis. While insulin production may be normal at the onset of the disease it usually becomes nonexistent within a few years.[17] The essential abnormalities in juvenile diabetes are related to absolute insulin deficiency. Vascular complications and degenerative changes are infrequent until the disease has been present for 5 years.

Insulin-dependent diabetes is probably the result of a genetic vulnerability of the islets of Langerhans to environmental insults (such as viruses) acutely, additively or with autoimmune sequelae.[5] An extensive search has been under way for associations between major-histocompatibility-complex antigens and specific diseases in man. It has been noted that certain human leukocyte antigens (HLA) are found with increased frequency in patients with certain diseases as compared with healthy controls.[18] Recent studies have revealed a two- to fourfold risk of insulin-dependent, juvenile-onset type diabetes in individuals possessing a relative excess of HLA B-8 and BW-15 antigens, both in the SD-2 (locus B) series.[19-21] Such an excess was not observed in those with maturity-onset type diabetes.[19] A new locus (D) has been found recently and two antigens in this series, Dw3 and Dw4, have an even stronger association with juvenile-onset diabetes than do the B-8 and BW-15.[22] One HLA antigen (B-7) appears to be associated with reduced risk for juvenile-onset diabetes.[23]

When one member of an identical twin-pair is affected by juvenile onset of diabetes mellitus, the other twin is affected in 50 per cent of the pairs, suggesting that there is 50 per cent penetrance of the genotype.[24] Rubinstein and his colleagues investigated the genetic predisposition to juvenile diabetes in the families of 31 index cases in relation to the inheritance of the HLA D system. They felt that the diabetes-predisposing gene was recessive because the diabetic sibs in index cases shared both their HLA genes with a significantly increased frequency. Rubinstein et al. prepared tables for the computation of risks to relatives based on the hypothesis of recessivity, HLA linkage and 50 per cent penetrance.[25] Neel feels there may be multiple genetic paths to the absence of insulin that characterizes the disease, each with a different penetrance and occurring with different frequencies in different populations.[26]

It has been postulated that the HLA-linked immune response genes might be involved in the interaction with certain viral agents capable of producing beta cell injury. In the past decade evidence has accumulated suggesting the importance of viral factors in the development of insulin-dependent diabetes—the seasonal and geographical trend, the occasional acute outbreaks in association with acute viral illnesses, the high frequency in young adults with congenital rubella, the association of juvenile diabetes with infectious mononucleosis, infectious hepatitis, mumps and Coxsackie B virus and the development of animal models of "viral diabetes."[27-30] Recent studies are suggestive of the ability of certain viruses to infect and damage the beta cells of the pancreas, causing diabetes in man.[132]

There is evidence for an *autoimmune component* in the etiology of insulin-dependent diabetes mellitus. A clinical association between it and other autoimmune diseases has been reported repeatedly (i.e. thyroid disorders, adrenal insufficiency, pernicious anemia, etc.).[31-35] In addition, some of the autoimmune diseases, such as Graves' disease, Addison's disease and myasthenia gravis, have a high incidence of HLA B-8.[18,36] Histologic "islitis" with lymphocytic infiltration has been described in immunized animals and in young untreated diabetics who died within a few months of diagnosis.[37,38] Several investigations have added evidence for an autoimmune component by the demonstration of circulating antibodies to pancreatic islet cells in insulin-dependent (juvenile-onset) diabetics.[39-41] Huang and MacLaren recently described insulin-dependent diabetes as a "disease of autoaggression." They demonstrated destruction of human pancreatic beta cells by the lymphocytes from young patients with juvenile diabetes.[42]

Insulin-dependent diabetes is probably caused by the interaction of environmental factors with the underlying genes. The diabetic has inherited a susceptible complex of immune-response genes, determined by their HLA determinants. The environmental insult (such as virus) may result in tolerance to a "foreign" antigen and a subsequent "autoimmune reaction." The concept of gene-virus interaction does not explain certain features of this type of diabetes (i.e. variation in insulin dependency in diabetics from different ethnic and geographic backgrounds, the "ketosis-resistance" of the disease in the tropics and certain American Indian and other tribes, despite relatively severe hyperglycemia). Dietary and other physical characteristics help explain some of the discrepancies, but other unknown factors may be functioning.

Noninsulin-dependent Type of Diabetes (Ketosis-resistant)

The obese noninsulin-dependent type of patient accounts for 80 per cent of the diabetic population, while the nonobese, stable, adult type makes up 10 per cent.

The ketosis-resistant diabetic has a gradual onset of the disorder usually after the age of 35 years, is usually overweight, may have minimal to no symptoms, may have narrow variations in blood sugar, may be relatively easy to control especially if he adheres to his diet, rarely develops ketosis except in the presence of unusual stress or severe infection and has a plasma-insulin response that, although delayed or diminished, is not absent. Vascular complications and degenerative changes are common.

This type of diabetes is a noninsulin-dependent disease, in which the genetic factors are dominant with a high family prevalence. Environmental factors (obesity, pregnancy and infection) may play a significant role in the pathogenesis of the disease. The primary defect may be in the islets of Langerhans or in the periphery. The islets may be deficient in number; there may be an insidious, variable premature senescence of the beta cells; there may be abnormalities in stimulus recognition, message propagation, insulin biosynthesis, storage and extrusion.

The defect in the periphery may result from generalized glucoreceptor deficiency, a possible faulty feedback with insulin antagonists (i.e. glucagon, STH), a possible cellular "impedance" to insulin action on an intracellular biochemical basis, a possible cellular resistance to insulin because of abnormalities in insulin receptors (i.e. receptor number, affinity of antibodies to insulin receptors) or a possible altered neurohumoral tone.

Noninsulin-dependent diabetes is probably caused by genetic limitations in some intrinsic aspect of islet function which may be expressed by environmental stress. It probably consists of multiple syndromes with multiple intrinsic etiologies and extrinsic factors.[5]

NATURAL HISTORY OF DIABETES MELLITUS

Primary or genetic diabetes may be classified into four stages.

Prediabetes

The first stage is prediabetes which exists prior to the onset of identifiable diabetes mellitus. It involves the period of time from conception until the development of impaired glucose tolerance in an individual predisposed to diabetes on genetic grounds. It can be suspected in an identical twin of a diabetic, in the offspring of two diabetic parents, in the presence of diabetes-like vascular lesions and in the woman with a history of large babies or frequent miscarriages.

The prediabetic state is characterized by normal glucose tolerance but delayed or decreased elevation in plasma insulin secretion following glucose or amino acid stimulation.[43-45] The latter also occurs in nondiabetic relatives of diabetic patients[46] and is similar to the defect present in clinical diabetes mellitus. The disappearance rate of intravenously administered glucose (k value) is significantly lower than in the control group, although still within the normal range. Cerasi and Luft[47] have postulated that a diminished insulin response to glucose is the basic pathogenic factor in the development of the different stages of the diabetic syndrome. The presence of low insulin response in healthy monozygotic twins of diabetic patients indicates that this insulin deficiency is inherited and antedates the appearance of decreased glucose tolerance.[48] The diagnosis of prediabetes can be made with assurance only in retrospect.

Subclinical Diabetes

The second stage is subclinical diabetes.[49] The fasting blood sugar and glucose tolerance tests are normal, but islet cell decompensation can be demonstrated by an abnormal cortisone-glucose tolerance test. The glucose tolerance test may be abnormal during pregnancy ("gestational diabetes") or stress.

Latent Diabetes

The third stage is latent (or chemical) diabetes. In this group the diagnosis is made by the presence of an abnormal glucose tolerance test or elevation of one fasting blood sugar in the absence of symptoms of diabetes.

Overt Diabetes

The fourth, and most advanced, stage of diabetes is overt (or clinical) diabetes. The classical symptoms of polyuria, polydipsia, polyphagia, pruritis and/or weight loss, as well as fasting hyperglycemia and glycosuria, are present.

Changes in Stage

In the natural history of diabetes, progression or regression from one stage to another may occur slowly over many years, may be rapid or may never occur.[50] Fluctuations in carbohydrate metabolism are common. Reversion from abnormal to normal glucose tolerance with regression from the latent stage to the prediabetes stage and even from overt, ketotic diabetes to prediabetes has been reported.[51–53] On the other hand, Fajans and Conn[50] have reported rapid progression from prediabetes to overt diabetes without going through the latent stage.

The carbohydrate intolerance of noninsulin-dependent diabetes may show no change in severity over the course of many years. Many have shown the nonprogressive course of carbohydrate intolerance of the maturity-onset type of diabetes, which may exist in asymptomatic states for years or decades in those middle-aged individuals in whom the occurrence of occlusive vascular disease or neuropathy is the presenting complication. Insulin-dependent diabetes was thought to be characterized by a rapid deterioration of insulin reserves. However, in 1960 Fajans and Conn reported latent (asymptomatic) diabetes in children and adolescents manifested only by an abnormal glucose tolerance test.[54]

DEFECTS IN METABOLISM IN DIABETES MELLITUS

Glucose homeostasis depends on a balance among absorption, production, storage and utilization of carbohydrate. In the fasted stage glucose uptake occurs primarily in the brain and, to a lesser extent, in the formed elements of the blood and muscle tissue.[55] In these sites glucose consumption is not insulin dependent. To meet the needs of these tissues, glucose is continuously released by the liver at rates of 2 to 3 mg per kg per min (a total of 150 to 250 gm per day).[56] Glycogenolysis accounts for 75 per cent of the glucose released, while gluconeogenesis (from lactate, alanine and glycerol) is responsible for the remaining 25 per cent.

Fuel allocation is managed by the islets of Langerhans which possess the functional requirements of a regulator of fuel distribution: (1) the ability to sense the availability and need for key fuels, (2) the ability to act bidirectionally and promote storage of fuels when they are abundant, or to promote their release from storage sites when they are needed and (3) the ability to vary the flux rates of an obligatory fuel such as glucose without allowing its concentration to change beyond a certain narrow range.[57]

The major factor regulating the production of glucose by the liver is the fall in circulating insulin levels from concentrations of 50 to 100 microunits (μU) per ml in the fed state to 10 to 20 microunits per ml in the fasted state.[58] Glucagon also is necessary (50 to 100 picograms (pg) per ml) for the maintenance of glucose production by the liver and the output of glucose into the extracellular space.[57]

In addition to the proper hormonal setting, it is essential that glucose precursors (especially alanine) be delivered to the liver in adequate concentrations, especially when hepatic glycogen stores have been depleted and when gluconeogenesis is responsible for an increased proportion of the total hepatic output of glucose.[55]

When glucose is absorbed from the intestine, plasma insulin levels increase two- to tenfold, and there is an efflux of glucose into the insulin-dependent tissues, most importantly in the liver, where it may be stored as glycogen or converted to fatty acids and triglyceride. The serum glucose concentration thus remains stable within a relatively narrow range despite the intermittent administration of mixed meals. The increase in plasma insulin also increases the uptake of amino acids (especially the branched-chain valine, leucine and isoleucine) by muscle tissue where they are used in protein synthesis.[59]

When protein is ingested, the hyperinsulinemia increases the uptake of glucose by the insulin-responsive tissues. This would result in hypoglycemia were it not for a concomitant increase in glucagon secretion.[60] The stimulatory effect of protein feeding on hepatic glucose production is probably a consequence of the rise in plasma glucagon, which in the diabetic is exaggerated and occurs in a setting of absolute insulin deficiency.[61,62] Felig has shown, however, that despite the persistent hyperglucagonemia the increase in glucose production does not persist. He feels that the hyperglycemia which accompanies protein feeding in the insulin-deficient diabetic is the result of failure to metabolize the increased glucose delivered to the periphery rather than of a glucagon-mediated stimulation of hepatic glucose production. "Regardless of the relative contributions of glucagon excess and/or insulin deficiency, the data indicate that protein feeding exaggerates the glucose overproduction and hyperglycemia of the diabetic state."[63]

DIETARY MANAGEMENT OF DIABETES MELLITUS

The principal objective in the treatment of a patient with diabetes mellitus is to permit him to lead a satisfactory life in good health in his normal environment. The treatment program should be designed to correct defects in metabolism, preserve pancreatic functions, prevent chronic diabetic complications and promote psychosocial adjustment.[64] The major objectives of dietary treatment are: (1) improvement in the overall health of the patient by attaining and maintaining optimum nutrition, (2) achievement and maintenance of weight that is close to "ideal body weight," (3) freedom from abnormal symptoms including hypoglycemic reactions and ketoacidosis, (4) maintenance of blood glucose at levels that prevent complications under stressful situations, (5) development of a diet which takes into account medical needs other than the diabetes and is consistent with the patient's ethnic background,[65,129] i.e. by providing for normal physical growth in the child, providing adequate nutrition for the pregnant woman and her fetus and providing adequate nutrition for lactation if she chooses to breast feed her infant, and (6) development and provision of a diet as attractive and realistic as possible.

The basic nutritional requirements for patients with diabetes mellitus are, in general, the same as those for all individuals and include adequate quality and quantity of all nutrients. Such a dietary program should be an integral component of general health care that includes periodic medical examinations, regular exercise, avoidance of cigarette smoking, attendance to personal hygiene and prevention of infection.

Long-term success in the treatment of diabetes correlates closely with the ability of the physician to educate patients and to keep them functioning in their normal environment. It is not possible to control diabetes unless diet therapy is optimal. If treatment with diet is to succeed, effective continuing communication is of critical importance, and patients must modify their behaviour as recommended by the physician, dietician and nurse. Professionals must be well informed and persistent. They must be persuasive and able to hold their patient's attention for the months or years that are necessary to change deeply ingrained, and usually inappropriate, eating habits.[66]

Total Calories

The majority (80 per cent) of diabetics are the obese, adult-onset type. About 90 per cent of the known diabetics are above ideal body weight at the time the diabetes is discovered. About 70 million Americans are 20 per cent or more above their ideal body weights and are, by definition, obese. As age increases, the incidence and degree of obesity increase. The incidence of diabetes increases from 0.1 per cent in those below 20 years of age to about 15 per cent in those above 60.[66] Epidemiologic data strongly support the hypothesis that most cases of noninsulin-dependent diabetes are precipitated by excessive caloric intake and resultant obesity.[67]

Caloric restriction and weight reduction are effective in lowering the blood sugar level in obese diabetics. Clinical studies[68] as well as studies on insulin receptors and obesity[69] have demonstrated the effectiveness of weight loss on tissue receptivity to insulin and improvement in carbohydrate tolerance.

In the obese patient the primary aim of diet therapy should be the provision of a diet restricted in calories that is nutritionally adequate. The caloric requirements of the diabetic will depend on the activity, age, sex, body weight and climate. Patients who are sedentary and overweight seldom need more than 20 kcal per kg of body weight per day. If they are overweight and perform moderate activity they require 30 kcal per kg per day. Those who are overweight and perform strenuous activity require 35 kcal per kg per day. Those who are of normal weight and do sedentary work require 30 kcal per kg per day; for moderate activity 35 kcal per kg per day are required, and for marked activity 40 kcal per kg per day. Underweight diabetics require 35 kcal per kg per day for sedentary work, 40 kcal per kg per day for moderate activity and 45 to 50 kcal per kg per day for strenuous activity. Active adolescent boys during their peak growth period need 3,100 to 3,600 kcal per day and adolescent girls from 2,400 to 2,700 kcal per day. In general, children require 1,000 kcal per day plus an additional 100 kcal for every year of age. "Achievement of this goal (of weight reduction) may be associated with the reduction or disappearance of the requirement for exogenous insulin, improvement or correction of fasting hyperglycemia and glucose intolerance, and reduction of known risk factors for atherosclerotic vascular disease such as obesity, hypertension, hyperlipidemia and hyperglycemia."[70]

The findings of an abnormal glucose tolerance in the presence of an elevated plasma insulin level suggests that the patient is insensitive to his own insulin. This situation is commonly seen in the obese, adult-onset type of diabetic and is corrected by weight reduction which will enhance sensitivity to endogenous insulin and will tend to normalize the glucose tolerance. Even in nondiabetics, the obese have a greater output of insulin after a carbohydrate meal than do thin nondiabetics. The increased output of insulin has been explained, in part, by the insulin-resistant state of the tissues, particularly the adipose tissues of the obese individual.[71] Obese individuals not only have hyperinsulinemia following a glucose load but also high basal levels of insulin. The combination of a high fasting insulin level and an exaggerated increase of insulin above baseline may result in a total insulin output that is markedly greater than that for a slender person.[72] Prolonged over-stimulation of impaired islet cell tissue by high blood glucose levels may cause progressive failure of insulin secretion. In part, this may be reversed. The diabetic state is aggravated by obesity in that higher plasma insulin levels are required to produce a given degree of glucose tolerance.

Restricted caloric diets presumably improve glucose tolerance in several ways. Weight reduction will result in a reduction of fat cell size, an increase in the glucose metabolism by insulin, an increased rate of fatty acid synthesis from glucose and a decrease in the intracellular nonesterified fatty acids. As the fat cell gets smaller there is an increase in its capacity for triglyceride storage. The fasting plasma free fatty acids, amino acid, glycerol, triglyceride, cholesterol and insulin decrease with weight loss. There is an increased glucose tolerance and a decreased insulin release in response to oral or intravenous glucose or intravenous arginine. There is an increased sensitivity of fat cells to insulin (in vivo) and an increased insulin-stimulated glucose uptake by the forearm muscles. The deficiency of insulin receptors on adipocytes, monocytes and liver cells in obesity is reversed by weight reduction. The rate of production of very-low-density lipoprotein triglycerides decreases and removal rate (by increased lipoprotein lipase activity in plasma) may increase.[3]

Observations such as those of Doar et al., that nearly all of their patients improved their glucose tolerance with dietary treatment and that most of them achieved satisfactory diabetic control,[73] imply that diet should remain the first line of management in newly diagnosed nonketotic diabetic patients. Hadden et al. assessed the effectiveness of intensive dietary management in the treatment of maturity-onset diabetics in their clinic and found that good control could be obtained by diet alone. The "poor dieters" had higher plasma insulin and triglyceride levels than those who were "good dieters."[74]

Populations characterized by obesity have a high incidence of abnormal glucose tolerance and clinical diabetes. Each 20 per cent increment of excess body weight doubles the prevalence of diabetes. Those characterized by slimness have a low incidence of diabetes. A worldwide diabetic survey demonstrated a decrease in glucose tolerance with increasing obesity, increasing sugar consumption, increasing dietary fat and protein and increasing economic status.[75]

In treating obesity-induced diabetes mellitus it is essential to devise an individualized diet designed to produce weight loss and attain ideal body weight. West noted that, in some ways, the problem of achieving weight reduction is the most important challenge in the therapy of diabetes.[76] Unfortunately this is a difficult goal to attain; less than 15 per cent reduce and stay reduced over the long range. Much of our present effort in diet counseling of obese patients is ineffective and wasteful. Many physicians, dietitians, nurses and patients have only modest incentive because they do not appreciate sufficiently the beneficial effects of weight reduction in maturity-onset diabetes.

Davidson[3] recommends short-term fasts (one week) in initiating diet therapy in individuals who are 50 or more pounds over the ideal body weight and in those above ideal body weight who are symptomatically hyperglycemic (if they are not pregnant). If the patient falls behind the planned rate of weight reduction, the fast may be repeated.

It is important to be aware of the metabolic effects of fasting when the intermittent fast regimen is used:

1. Hyperuricemia develops and gout or renal stones may be precipitated if fluid intake is insufficient.
2. Ten to 14 grams of nitrogen (60 to 84 gm of protein) are lost initially, decreasing to 3 to 4 gm of nitrogen (18 to 24 gm of protein) per day by the 30th day.
3. Sodium, potassium and water diuresis occurs and hypovolemia develops. Weakness, dizziness and faintness may result. Calcium

and magnesium are lost and the acidity of the phosphates, chlorides, sulfates and keto acids must be balanced by ammonium ion, titratable acid and some fixed base.

4. Plasma ketones rise and ketones appear in the urine on the third day. The ratio between beta-hydroxybutyrate and acetoacetate rises from 1:1 on the 1st day to 4:1 by the 8th day.

5. pH may fall to 7.30, with carbon dioxide dropping to 16 mEq/L by the 10th day.

6. Insulin decreases; glucagon increases.

7. Total fasting may cause nausea, vomiting, postural hypotension, weakness and faintness from plasma volume contraction. Hair growth may be arrested and dry, scaly skin may develop. The hematocrit may fall. Fatty infiltration of the liver may occur. Electrolyte imbalance, vitamin deficiency, neutropenia and death may occur.

8. Diuretics and all hypotensive drugs should be discontinued when a fast is started.

9. A water intake of 3,000 cc per day has been recommended as essential. Low-calorie protein supplements may be useful.

10. Fasting is contraindicated in patients who are pregnant, who have preexisting renal insufficiency or who have a psychosis in remission.

11. Drenick[77] reported an average loss of 65 pounds in 56 fast days in 137 patients whose mean initial body weight was 307 pounds.

The beneficial metabolic effects of weight loss in the treatment of the maturity-onset diabetic were:

1. Weight loss was successful in lowering blood sugar, cholesterol and triglycerides with a reversion to normal of the glucose tolerance test.

2. Insulin therapy could be discontinued in some patients after treatment with intermittent fasting and hypocaloric diets.

Bistrian[78] recommends a modified regimen using a protein-sparing modified fast instead of the absolute fast:

1. 1.3 to 1.5 gm protein per kg ideal weight per day as lean meat, fish or fowl (30 to 40 per cent fat—400–700 kcal per day).

2. RDA of vitamins and minerals.

3. Fluid ad libitum—1,500 cc per day.

4. 25 mEq potassium per day.

5. 300 to 500 mg calcium per day.

6. Low or absent carbohydrate.

7. Meal feeding 2 to 3 per day.

The modified fast does not result in an increase in bilirubin or BSP, a decrease in creatinine clearance, or the degree of hyperuricemia, the loss of tissue or the occasional dysphoria that occur with the total fasting regimen. The patient may be treated as an outpatient while on the modified protein-sparing fast.

If the rate of weight loss is less than predicted, additional intermittent short-term fasts (on an outpatient or inpatient basis) may be alternated with appropriate caloric restriction.[3]

Caloric restriction, with resultant weight reduction, is effective in lowering the blood sugar in obese diabetics. Attaining and maintaining ideal body weight and euglycemia can be achieved through diet therapy in about 80 per cent of patients who are intensively educated and continuously monitored by a well-informed, highly motivated team of physicians, dietitians and nurses.[66]

Genuth recently reported at The Second International Congress on Obesity in Washington (1978) on 1,200 patients treated with protein-supplemented fasting. His patients drink the protein (intact) supplement as their only source of food for an average of 6 months. In spite of the controversy over the smallest amount of protein needed to maintain nitrogen balance, similar results were obtained in three programs in which the protein supplement varied. Of 270 patients treated for one year, 12 per cent dropped out of the program after an initial weight loss while 21 per cent failed to lose weight. The major clinical benefit of the program was the improvement in hypertension. Most of the diabetic patients had a return of the fasting blood sugar to normal as a major benefit of protein-supplemented fasting.

Van Itallie at the same conference warned of the dangers of protein-supplemented fasting, noting that depletion of protein is a complex problem and better methods are needed to detect its effect. He warned that its study belonged in the hands of experienced physicians who are aware of the metabolic effects. Side effects of the protein-sparing fast were diarrhea (initially), fatigue, orthostatic dizziness, cold intolerance, skin dryness, hair loss and muscle cramps. Unusual occurrences were unilateral peroneal nerve palsy (which was reversible), cholecystitis, pancreatitis and distortion of self-image.

Four deaths occurred in the 1,200 patients treated by Genuth in four years. One patient aspirated gum; the other 3 presumably died from cardiac arrhythmias secondary to underlying coronary disease. None had a decreased potassium level or orthostatic hypotension, according to Dr. Genuth.

The occurrence of a number of deaths in individuals restricting their intake to a liquid protein hydrolysate indicates the need for extreme caution in the use of this form of weight reduction.

Prolonged total withdrawal from food does not change the appetite. Physicians, nurses, dietitians—forming a team—must continue to work with patients to maintain weight loss. Much of our present effort in counseling obese diabetics is ineffective. The programs require incentive, vigor and skill on the part of all involved, with an appreciation of the profoundly beneficial effects of weight reduction in the obese maturity-onset diabetic.

Carbohydrate Requirements

There has been, and continues to be, disagreement among workers in the field of diabetes as to the relative merits of a high-carbohydrate versus a low-carbohydrate diet in the treatment of diabetes.[79] Wood and Bierman have published an excellent review on the history of this subject.[80] The discovery of insulin in 1921 made it possible to liberalize carbohydrate intake. In 1923 Geyelin began to prescribe high-carbohydrate diets to diabetic patients treated with insulin. In 1935, after reviewing 10 years of his experience with the high-carbohydrate, low-fat diet, he concluded that the increased effectiveness of

insulin that consistently followed the institution of a high-carbohydrate diet was "chiefly dependent on the degree to which fat is curtailed."[81] Rabinowitch[82] was another advocate of the high-carbohydrate, low-fat diet. His goal was to keep his patients 5 to 10 pounds under their average body weights. He suggested that even less fat be included in the diet than previous observers had advocated (i.e. less than 50 gm a day) and believed that the restriction of dietary fat would help lower the incidence of cardiovascular-renal disease. He also observed that "potential diabetes can be activated and mild diabetes can be made severe by too rigid restriction of carbohydrate."[82]

Himsworth[83] demonstrated that diets high in carbohydrates improved glucose tolerance in normal persons when caloric intake was controlled. These observations of the effects of high-carbohydrate diet on oral glucose tolerance in normal subjects have been confirmed by others.[84-86]

A number of dietary surveys have been made in conjunction with studies of the prevalence of diabetes. The Zulus consume about 85 per cent of their calories as carbohydrate but they are thin and virtually free of diabetes. In the same area of the world, the Masai, who live on meat, milk and blood and eat only 20 per cent of their calories as carbohydrate, also remain thin and are spared from diabetes.[87] Various American Indian tribes who have remained relatively homogeneous have a high incidence of abnormal glucose tolerance and clinical diabetes.[88] Like those of other low-income Americans, their diets are high in carbohydrate and fat with the result that over half the population exceed 125 per cent of optimal weight. The diabetes is the maturity-onset type and is associated with a high incidence of large-vessel disease. On the other hand, Mouratoff et al.[89] found two other groups, the Eskimos and the Athabaskan Indians in Alaska, who have been spared from diabetes and atherosclerosis on a high-fat, low-carbohydrate diet (less than 50 gm per day). Both of these groups have a low incidence of obesity. The Indians in India have a low incidence of diabetes on a high-carbohydrate, low-calorie diet. However, those who migrated to South Africa and ate the same high-carbohydrate diet but at a higher caloric intake had a high incidence of maturity-onset diabetes and vascular disease. The Yemenite Jews who migrated to Israel and adopted the European diet high in calories and carbohydrates in place of their former diet (a high-fat, low-caloric diet) now have an increased incidence of diabetes and obesity.[87] Asians who consume high-carbohydrate, low-caloric diets have very low rates of diabetes.

Albrink and Davidson[65] feel that the most important fact that emerges from clinical and epidemiologic studies is the deleterious effect of *obesity* on diabetes. They indicate that the fewest vascular complications are found when the habitual dietary intake results in leanness, regardless of the proportion of carbohydrate or fat in the diet.

A difference of opinion exists as to the optimal proportion of carbohydrate and fat to be recommended to the diabetic who is of normal weight or underweight. At the present time most clinics permit 40 per cent of the total calories as carbohydrate, close to the normal average in the United States where 45 per cent of the calories ingested are in the form of carbohydrates. One group feels that carbohydrate intake should not be liberalized in either the insulin-dependent or insulin-independent diabetic on the grounds that a high-carbohydrate intake will accentuate postprandial hyperglycemic peaks, which should be avoided. Gabbay[90,91] has shown that, with decreased insulin activity and hyperglycemia, glucose is converted via the insulin-independent polyol pathway to sorbitol and fructose which accumulate in nervous tissue in experimental diabetic neuropathy. In addition to osmotic swelling, a number of other concomitant functional changes have been described in this situation. In human and experimental diabetic neuropathy the earliest clinical expression of demyelinization is a decrease in nerve-conduction velocity. Correction of hyperglycemia, by diet or hypoglycemic agents, in diabetic patients has resulted in improvement in the delayed nerve-conduction velocity.[92] Clinical studies have shown a greater effect of ingested glucose than of its equivalent as starch upon the rise of circulating glucose and insulin.[93] Yudkin has suggested that a high intake of refined carbohydrate results in an increased incidence of atherosclerosis and diabetes,[94] but this has been seriously challenged.[95,96]

Brunzell and his colleagues[97] reported an improved glucose tolerance with high-carbohydrate feedings in mild diabetes. Glucose and immunoreactive insulin levels were measured in normal persons and subjects with mild diabetes maintained on basal (45 per cent) carbohydrate and high (85 per cent) carbohydrate diets in order to evaluate the effect of increased dietary carbohydrate in diabetes mellitus. Fasting blood glucose levels fell in all subjects and oral glucose tolerance improved significantly after 10 days of high-carbohydrate feeding. Fasting insulin levels also were lower on the high-carbohydrate diet. However, insulin response to oral glucose testing did not change significantly. These data suggest that the high-carbohydrate diet increased the sensitivity of peripheral tissues to insulin. Preliminary data[98] suggest that patients with moderate and severe diabetes after treatment with oral drugs or insulin respond to the same carbohydrate diet in a manner similar to those with mild diabetes. Insulin, either endogenous or exogenous, must be available to obtain this effect. This short-term study is in agreement with the long-term effect of a high-carbohydrate diet noted by Stone and Connor.[99] These investigators are of the opinion that in mild diabetes, regardless of weight, a high-carbohydrate, low-fat diet improves glucose tolerance and decreases cholesterol levels and therefore should be used for diabetic management.

The Committee on Food and Nutrition of the American Diabetes Association in their 1971 dietary recommendations[70] for patients with diabetes mellitus stated:

> There no longer appears to be any need to restrict disproportionately the intake of carbohydrates in the diet of most diabetic patients. Increase of dietary carbohydrate, even to the extremes, *without increase of total calories*, does not appear to increase insulin requirement in the insulin treated diabetic patient. In the less severe, typically obese diabetic substitution of carbohydrate for fat does not appear to elevate blood glucose or worsen glucose tolerance. . . . The average proportion of calories consumed as carbohydrate in the U.S. population as a whole approximates 45 per cent; this proportion, or even higher, appears to be acceptable for the usual diabetic patient as well.

The Committee in its 1979 "current concepts" recommends that carbohydrate should account for 50 to 60 per cent of the total calories of the diabetic diet, preferably in the form of complex carbohydrate. For patients with hypertriglyceridemia, it is recommended that the diet should contain 35 per cent of its calories in the form of carbohydrate.

West,[76] in his excellent analysis of the failure of diet therapy in diabetes mellitus, stressed the need for regulation of carbohydrate intake "to assure appropriate consistency in the timing, division, amounts, and characteristics (sugar or starch) of the carbohydrates consumed and to assure that the total amounts do not increase caloric consumption above the optimal levels." Well-spaced, moderate-sized feedings are preferable to large ones and simple, concentrated carbohydrates such as sucrose should be avoided or limited. Diabetics who cannot handle rapid alterations in blood sugar should be protected from carbohydrates that produce rapid swings in blood sugar.

There is no doubt of the beneficial influence of a high-carbohydrate diet on the pancreas. Starvation, or a normal caloric diet in which carbohydrate is restricted, produces an impairment of the insulin production in response to a glucose challenge and may result in an abnormal glucose tolerance test. Preparing the patient with 300 gm of glucose for 3 days prior to the test may then result in a normal test. This is an excellent clinical example of the beta cell reserve which is present even in diabetic patients; such patients, when presented with sufficient carbohydrate for a period of time, are able to increase the amount of insulin produced following a subsequent carbohydrate challenge. Whether this will aid in the maintenance of beta cell integrity in the long run is not proven. Preventing the possible progression of the loss of the beta cell population and/or a decrease in the ability to secrete insulin is an important goal—especially in the many patients where the ability to secrete insulin seems to become more impaired with time. It would seem desirable to keep the carbohydrate intake in diabetic patients at that level where beta cell function is optimal.

The role of carbohydrate intake in the control of the plasma lipid levels was noted by Stone and Connor.[99] They increased the carbohydrate intake from 40 to 64 per cent, together with other manipulations of the diet, and noted improvement in the hyperglycemia, hypertriglyceridemia and hypercholesterolemia in their patients.

The effect of a high-carbohydrate diet on serum triglycerides seems to be a transitory one. There is an initial rise in triglycerides with an increase of lipogenesis and an increased production of very-low-density lipoproteins; with subsequent adaptation (even on an 85 per cent carbohydrate diet) there is a return of the triglycerides to normal. Bierman[72] has shown that during the adaptation phase, while the *fasting* triglycerides *are* higher, the triglyceride concentration integrated throughout the day is not higher. Thus, the carbohydrate induction of hypertriglyceridemia is, at most, a temporary phenomenon and cannot be used as a basis for prescribing a low-carbohydrate diet in the treatment of patients with diabetes, except in unusual cases.

Liberalization of the carbohydrate intake in the diet of patients with diabetes mellitus is warranted if the caloric intake is regulated. Restriction in carbohydrate intake has no short- or long-term advantage for the diabetic and often contributes to poor compliance and failure of diet therapy.

Dietary glucose and sucrose cause similar serum glucose and insulin responses. The complex carbohydrate starch causes flatter glucose and insulin responses. Different starches cause different responses. Crapo has shown that potato has the same effect on the blood sugar and insulin responses as dextrose, whereas rice results in a flatter response. This holds in those with normal glucose tolerance curves, chemical diabetes, or noninsulin-dependent diabetes. The difference between starches becomes more prominent with differences in carbohydrate tolerance. Since the responses to the starches differ they should be individualized rather than grouped together in standard diets.

Glucose and sucrose are more glucogenic than fructose in patients with a mild glucose intolerance, chemical diabetics and noninsulin-dependent diabetics. The same differences exist for the insulin response to the 3 sugars.

Where an insulin deficiency exists, fructose may have an advantage over the other sugars in diabetes mellitus.[130]

Fat Requirements

The epidemiologic and experimental evidence relating circulating lipids to atherosclerotic cardiovascular disease applies to diabetics as well as to nondiabetics (see Chapter 34).[100,101] Since diabetics are particularly susceptible to atherosclerosis and its complications, it seems prudent, on the basis of present information, for such patients to consume a diet that will favor the reduction of serum cholesterol and triglycerides. Limiting the saturated fat and cholesterol in the diet has been shown repeatedly to cause a fall in serum cholesterol even in the absence of weight loss.[99,102,103]

The level of triglycerides is controlled by multiple factors including the amount of carbohydrate, the proportion of saturated fat, the change in body weight and caloric intake and the initial serum triglyceride level.[104-110]

Wiensier et al.[104] studied the effect of high- and low-carbohydrate diets on diabetic control, insulin secretion and blood lipids. Despite an increased carbohydrate load from 40 to 60 per cent (with fat decreased from 45 to 25 per cent), control of diabetes and insulin secretory capacity were maintained, serum cholesterol was not altered by the change in dietary fat and the high-carbohydrate intake did not increase the mean level of serum triglycerides. Their data suggest a seasonal trend for both serum cholesterol and triglycerides. Stone and Connor, and others, have found no deleterious effect on the diabetes and no increase in the triglyceride level in nonobese, insulin-dependent diabetics on a low-fat (20 per cent of calories), low-cholesterol (100 mg per day) diet at the end of 12 months.

Diabetics who live in underprivileged areas have less macroangiopathy than those in the United States or Canada.[111,112] They usually live on a high-carbohydrate, low-saturated-fat diet which suggests that the major problem is the saturated fat. Sugar intake is also low in these areas, suggesting to some[94] but not to others[95,96] that sugar is an important factor in atherogenesis.

Diabetics with hyperlipidemia are exceedingly prone to atherosclerosis and must adhere to dietary regulations, i.e. decreased caloric intake, low saturated fat and low cholesterol. Since most diabetics are obese, their hypertriglyceridemia often responds to caloric restriction.

The low-saturated-fat diet used in the treatment of hypercholesterolemia may be prescribed in one of two ways: (1) The fat calories may be replaced by carbohydrate with a resultant lowering of the total intake of saturated fats. (2) The saturated fats may be replaced by polyunsaturated fats.

The use of a low-saturated-fat diet supplemented with large amounts of polyunsaturated fat results in an additional cholesterol-lowering effect. This supplementation makes the diet easier to follow and permits greater variety.

The dietary treatment of hyperlipidemia is essential in diabetes mellitus. However, it requires good planning and counseling. Gotto et al.[113] studied the effect of recommending therapeutic diets plus dietary counseling by a physician and dietitian as compared to the effect of similar diets but with little counseling. There was a marked decrease in the triglyceride level and better weight reduction in the group given counseling as compared to that not given such counseling.

"Control" of the diabetes will to some extent ameliorate hyperlipidemia. Controlled *hyper*triglyceridemic patients consumed greater amounts of sucrose, alcohol and total calories than controlled normotriglyceridemic patients.[114] In addition, the tendency to overweight and subtle increments of fasting blood glucose levels were shown to contribute to hypertriglyceridemia. Thus, it seems that the lipid disorder in controlled diabetics is multifactorial in origin and that well-conducted diet therapy and stricter regulation of the blood sugar are essential in the management of hyperlipdemia.

The Committee on Food and Nutrition of the American Diabetes Association in its 1979 special report of its dietary recommendations suggests that 30 to 38 per cent of the total calories be in the form of fat. The saturated fat should be reduced to less than 10 per cent of the total calories, and the polyunsaturated fatty acids should be increased to 10 per cent of the total calories. The remainder of ingested fat should be monounsaturated.[129]

Protein Requirements

The requirements for protein at different ages have been considered in Chapter 3 and the recommended allowances are set forth in the Appendix (Table A-1). Twelve to 20 per cent of the total calories of the diabetic diet should be from protein. The diabetic patient is likely to require extra protein to offset losses from the excessive gluconeogenesis and ketogenesis associated with impaired glucose utilization. The presence of infection, pregnancy and debilitating disease also requires additional protein. Patients with nephrosis or malabsorption may suffer appreciable losses of protein in the urine or feces and require replacement. Renal or hepatic failure usually dictates decreased amounts of protein depending on the extent of disease (Chapter 33). Thus, in diabetic patients whose hepatic and renal status permits, an additional allowance of protein ranging up to 0.5 gm per kg per day should be considered, depending upon the metabolic condition of the individual concerned.

Vitamin and Mineral Requirements

Diets for diabetic patients under good control usually contain the adequate amounts of vitamins recommended by the Food and Nutrition Board (Appendix Table A1). However, in those with poorly controlled diabetes, infection, malabsorption or other complications, vitamin supplementation may be necessary.

It had been taught that vitamin and mineral deficiencies are not present in the United States except in alcoholics and the chronically ill. Well-planned surveys by the Department of Agriculture and the Public Health Service within the past 10 years have shown that 40 to 50 per cent of the middle-class American population surveyed were not meeting the minimal requirements for one or more nutrients.

In the diabetic the conversion from carotene to vitamin A may be impaired. Adequate dietary sources of vitamin A should be available (i.e. liver, eggs, whole milk and cheese) or supplements may be required to meet this need.

In the study done by the Department of Agriculture it was found that the B vitamins were being taken in inadequate amounts. The need for B complex increases with the use of certain drugs (i.e. oral contraceptives) which increase the requirements for folic acid and B_6. The vitamins function as coenzymes in a great many vital reactions and they must not be limited in availability. Any diet that contains 1,000 calories or less requires supplementation with vitamins.

Calcium and iron are often suboptimal in our diets. Patients, especially teenagers, rarely drink enough milk to meet their needs. The equivalent of 3 glasses of milk (any form is acceptable) is required to satisfy calcium requirements (1 ounce of cheese is equivalent to 1 glass of milk). Neither cheese nor ice cream can be relied on to meet the calcium requirements. Skim milk and buttermilk are essentially free of fat and are the preferred sources of calcium. Cottage cheese is inadequate because much of the calcium and phosphorus are lost in processing. Iron was found to be grossly deficient in the surveys, and a recommendation was made that wheat bread be supplemented with iron. Eggs and red meat are the best sources in the diet.

Diabetic patients with poorly controlled disease usually develop deficits of water, sodium, potassium and chloride. This is especially true when diuresis or excessive sweating occurs. It is dramatically demonstrated in a patient in diabetic ketoacidosis. Deficiencies of certain electrolytes can also occur in prolonged diarrhea and renal disease with abnormalities of tubular absorption. Prolonged use of certain diuretics may produce electrolyte and acid-base

disturbances. Large doses of insulin, which cause hypoglycemia, will lower blood potassium. At times the diabetic patient must restrict sodium and/or potassium because of associated renal, hepatic or cardiovascular disease. During acute illnesses, especially when anorexia, vomiting or diarrhea occurs, the patient must be observed closely so that water and electrolyte balance may be maintained. Intravenous fluids may be necessary but patients should be returned to more normal diets as soon as possible. The control of fluid and electrolyte balance has been considered in Chapter 8.

The maintenance of adequate amounts of calcium, phosphorus, iron, copper, iodine, manganese, cobalt and zinc usually presents no problem to the well-controlled diabetic. Trivalent chromium, a glucose-tolerance factor for rats, may possibly be related to glucose tolerance for a small number of people with diabetes mellitus. In a preliminary and as yet unsubstantiated report Glinsmann and Mertz studied the effect of supplementing a diet with 60 to 1,000 μg of chromium ion, administered orally three times a day with meals for periods ranging from 15 to 133 days, and found that there was an improvement in the glucose tolerance in 3 out of 6 patients studied.[115,116] The chromium ion supplementation had no effect on the glucose tolerance of normal individuals. After chromium administration was stopped, glucose tolerance of the responsive diabetic patients reverted to the prechromium state.

Alcohol

Ethanol causes hypoglycemia in fasting subjects.[117] This effect has been attributed to inhibition of hepatic gluconeogenesis during ethanol oxidation. It does not seem to be mediated by an increased output of insulin. It is still unclear[118,119] whether ethanol increases or decreases[120,121] the rate of peripheral utilization of glucose. The insulin response to intravenous and oral glucose is potentiated by alcohol[118,122] but the mechanism is uncertain. Nikkila and Taskinen[123] found that ethanol accelerates the utilization of intravenous glucose and increases the early insulin response to glucose loading. It also causes an overstimulation of insulin output which accentuates the reactive hypoglycemia that follows glucose loading. Some individuals develop moderate to severe hypoglycemic symptoms in response to alcohol, with blood glucose falling to extremely low levels. Thus, heavy drinking of alcohol in combination with a carbohydrate-rich meal may cause postprandial hypoglycemia.

The effect of ethanol on the glucose-induced insulin response is much smaller in obese and diabetic subjects than in the normal. This suggests that the beta cells undergo qualitative changes in obesity. The obese also fail to develop postglucose hypoglycemia on administration of ethanol—possibly because of the increased insulin resistance of obesity.

Diabetics are even more resistant than obese nondiabetics to the actions of ethanol. Little or no increase in the glucose-mediated insulin response has been observed in diabetics upon administration of ethanol. This may be the result of the severe insulin deficiency in the diabetics. Ethanol may improve insulin secretion in those diabetics who still have an insulin reserve for prolonged release but not in those whose insulin pools have been depleted by the diabetes.

Glucose tolerance decreased in all subjects given alcohol to the extent of 25 per cent of their total caloric intake, even though none was a chronic alcoholic and none had liver disease. Since the plasma insulin response was not changed by the alcohol, the decreased glucose tolerance must have been caused by increased insulin resistance of the tissues.

Alcohol in moderation may be taken by the diabetic provided that the intake is really moderate and the calories provided are included within the daily limit. The problem with regular alcohol intake is that its use often leads to excess calories through disregard of caloric restriction advice.

Patients taking the sulfonylurea drugs may exhibit a peculiar idiosyncrasy to alcohol manifested by flushing, nausea and dizziness.

Fiber

There is evidence that fiber-depleted diets may be related to colon disturbances, coronary heart disease and diabetes mellitus.[129,131] High-fiber diets have been reported to lower postprandial blood sugar, decrease glycosuria, decrease insulin needs and increase tissue sensitivity to insulin. Whenever feasible, natural foods containing unrefined carbohydrate with fiber should be substituted for highly refined carbohydrates which are low in fiber.

CALCULATION OF THE DIABETIC DIET

Estimate the ideal body weight in pounds by referring to the standard height/weight table (Appendix Table A-4a). A rough approximation may be made by allowing 105 lb for the first 5 feet of height and 5 lb for each additional inch over 5 feet; for medium and heavy frames add 5 to 10 lb. For example, a patient with a normal frame who is 5'6" tall will have an ideal body weight of 135 lb.

Convert the ideal body weight from lb to kg by dividing the pounds by 2.2.

Calculate the total amount of kcal the patient needs per day for each kg of ideal body weight on the basis of body weight and activity as follows:

	Sedentary	Moderate Activity	Marked Activity
Overweight	20–25	30	35
Normal	30	35	40
Underweight	35	40	45–50

Composition: (1) Protein: Consider 1.5 gm per kg of ideal body weight as the protein requirement for the diabetic patient whose hepatic and renal status permits. (2) Carbohydrate: In the absence of carbohydrate-induced hypertriglyceridemia type IV the carbohydrate allowance may be 50 to 60 per cent of the total calories. In the presence of this type of hypertriglyceridemia the carbohydrate allowance may be between 125 and 150 gm per day. (3) Fat: The remaining calories should be given in the form of fat. The saturated fat intake should be limited to less than 10 per cent of the total calories and polyunsaturated fats increased to 10 per cent of the total calories. Most clinics recommend a limitation of total fat calories to 35 per cent or less of the total caloric intake, with a polyunsaturated/saturated fat ratio of 2.5.

Translate the calculated diet into food servings and distribute as desired among three meals plus extra feedings (examples of such diets are given in Appendix Table A-11). All patients receiving insulin must have a bedtime feeding. Children should have midmorning and midafternoon feedings as well.

The American Diabetes Association (A.D.A.) has revised its exchange lists with the emphasis on calories and decreasing the saturated fat intake.

According to Arky[124] the initial objectives of the exchange system are: (1) to group together foods of similar nutrient composition and caloric content, (2) to provide a system whereby meals can be planned to allow a variety of foods, (3) to develop a basic teaching tool that is applicable to most patients with diabetes as well as to others who require diet counseling and (4) to offer a basic instrument which dietitians and other counselors can modify or incorporate into teaching protocols for patients.

The recent A.D.A. revision attempts to bring its teaching into line with the diet philosophy of other organizations such as the American Heart Association, the American College of Cardiology and the National Institute of Heart and Lung Diseases, and to stress the importance of diet in the treatment of the majority of diabetic patients—the obese, adult-onset noninsulin-requiring diabetics. The use of low-fat milks, lean meats and starchy vegetables has been emphasized.

The dietitian can and does play a major counseling role and must have opportunity for thorough follow-up visits in addition to the initial consultation. The diet counselor should integrate ethnic dishes and those which are easy to prepare and convenient into the meal plan.

The exchange method is only one approach to diet therapy, with drawbacks as well as benefits. Other systems may be used with satisfactory results.

Individualization and Meal Spacing

The diabetic patient who requires insulin therapy must adjust not only his caloric intake but his eating habits as well. Food intake should be spaced in a fashion that takes into account administered insulin and physical activity in order to avoid intermittent hypoglycemia. Regularity of food intake and regularity of exercise are of paramount importance. Any dietary program, to be practical and effective, must be based on appropriate patient motivation coupled with diagnostic evaluation, dietary instruction and follow-up by the physician and dietitian.

Diet therapy must be adapted to the specific needs of individual patients. It is essential that the diet for the diabetic patient take into account his individual food preferences, background, economic status and the setting in which he eats his meals.[125] The rationale of the diet must be carefully explained in an effort to enlist the patient's full cooperation.

That this is a complex situation is emphasized by the results of surveys. Tunbridge and Wetherill[126] repeated a study in 1968 similar to that done in 1948 to determine whether patients were adhering to their prescribed diets. In both surveys less than one-third of the patients were keeping within 10 per cent of such diets. There was considerable fluctuation in intake from day to day, with no particular pattern discernible during the week; variability was noted even in patients who were adhering closely to the prescribed diet. The extreme example of such variation was in a patient with a caloric range of 1,265 to 2,850 kcal per day within a week. Based on single but searching interviews, Bloom[127] found that 17 of 111 insulin-dependent diabetics adhered strictly and regularly to their prescribed diets, 60 adhered in a "general" way and the other 34 were unable to follow regular diets.

It must be noted that half the diabetics in the United States have incomes of $4,000 or less per year. It has been pointed out that the cost of the diabetic diet may be much greater than the cost of normal diets for certain groups, and thus may contribute to the lack of dietary adherence.[116] The increased consumption of food as the symbol of success by persons who have recently escaped poverty also plays a factor in dietary adherence.

Between-meal snacks, including a small meal before bedtime, are often essential for the diabetic. They are particularly important to children, adolescents and certain adult patients who have a high daily requirement for calories. Short-term clinical studies have shown improved glucose tolerance with a schedule of 10 feedings compared to 3 meals or a single isocaloric feeding.[129] In epidemiologic surveys in which men were grouped according to habitual meal frequency, those who ate 3 meals or less per day showed significantly more obesity, higher serum cholesterol levels and diminished glucose tolerance. Multiple frequent feedings, avoiding large evening meals, are far less detrimental to the diabetic.

Insulin-dependent diabetics must eat multiple meals in order to avoid hypoglycemia. Their meals must be spaced according to the type of insulin they are taking and the period of peak action. The basic pattern of caloric intake must be individualized to promote maximum cooperation from the patient for day-to-day consistency. This consistency may result in greater safety from hypoglycemia and the avoidance of hyperglycemia.

Diet instructions should be as simple as possible while the monotony of diet can be avoided by teaching the patient to use suitable food exchanges. The patient must be taught the foods he must limit and those he can consume in unlimited quantities.

The diet must be tailored to the patient. For example, if he becomes physically ill when forced to eat breakfast, the insulin injections and midmorning snacks must be readjusted without upsetting the patient or the overall adequacy of the diet. Since diabetes is frequently associated with other medical disorders which may require special dietary treatment or restrictions, the basic diet must be altered accordingly. Sodium restriction may be necessary for those who have heart and kidney disease; the composition and consistency of the diet may be varied for patients with gastrointestinal disorders, e.g. peptic ulcer, gallbladder disease or colitis; the fat content may have to be reduced for those with gallbladder disease and protein restriction may be necessary in those with either renal or advanced hepatic insufficiency.

Adherence to Dietary Advice

It has been recognized by most diabetologists that adherence to diet in the treatment of diabetes has been a problem to date for the majority of patients and that compliance over long periods of time is minimal. Davidson[66] has reported excellent results with his patients in Georgia and has suggested some tactics that increase diet therapy success rates as well as some pitfalls that decrease success rates.

Factors That Lead to *Success* in Diet Therapy[66]

1. The team approach (physician-dietitian-nurse-patient).
2. Short-term fasts (one week) to initiate diet therapy in obese diabetics.

3. Individualized diet prescriptions, intensive education and continuous follow-up until patients attain ideal body weight; then a change to maintenance diet and continued follow-up.

4. Instruction of patients in the regular use of diet manual at home; they should be asked to bring it to the office at each visit.

5. Instruction of patients to measure food at frequent intervals and to keep a diary of diet, weight and urine glucose level (and acetone level if fasting).

6. Education of the family member who prepares the food (if someone other than patient), so that meals will be prepared, measured and served correctly.

7. Informing patients of anticipated rate of weight loss and of current weight and plasma glucose level at each visit. When patients adhere to the diet, praise them liberally; when they do not, find out why and encourage them to try harder. When low-calorie diets fail, intermittent outpatient or inpatient fasting often succeeds.

8. Encouraging patients to adapt to life-style of diabetes by: substituting water or non-caloric foods or drinks when hunger pangs create the urge to eat between meals or to eat excessively at meals, avoiding compulsive and socially induced eating and drinking (especially alcoholic beverages), avoiding "dietetic" and "health" foods, buying only prescribed types and amounts of food, eating the prescribed food on a regular schedule, slowly savoring each bite, and avoiding the preparation of food for others, if possible, until adequate weight loss has taken place.

9. Prescription of regular exercise if there are no contraindications; walking 5 miles a day is optimal.

Factors That Lead to *Failure* in Diet Therapy[66]

1. Failure to understand that hyperglycemia is frequently induced by obesity, and that one of the two primary objectives in treatment of diabetes is to attain and maintain ideal body weight. (The other is to attain and maintain normoglycemia.)

2. Failure to write a satisfactory dietary prescription.

3. Failure to utilize services of dietitians and nurses who can help to instruct patients on appropriately prescribed diet.

4. Use of outdated or incomplete diet publications that patients do not understand or that are alien to their life-styles.

5. Failure to modify patient behavior related to food intake because of insufficient education or follow-up.

6. Substitution of oral hypoglycemic agents or insulin for caloric restriction and weight loss in obese diabetics.

7. Substitution of appetite suppressants, diuretic agents, thyroid extract and occasionally even intestinal bypass surgery for caloric restriction and weight loss.

8. Failure to encourage patients to markedly restrict or discontinue alcohol intake.

9. Failure to challenge patients' statements such as "I don't overeat," "I can't afford the diet" or "I will be sick (or look bad, or be physically or sexually unattractive, or be unable to work) if I lose weight." (What we eat will determine what we weigh until the second law of themodynamics is repealed.)

SUMMARY OF GENERAL CONSIDERATIONS AND RECOMMENDATIONS

The noninsulin-dependent diabetic must be made aware that, in many instances, adequate weight reduction will convert his abnormal glucose tolerance to normal. It will also reduce his risk of developing certain serious complications of diabetes such as coronary heart disease. The most important objective in dietary management of the obese, noninsulin-dependent diabetic is to attain and maintain the optimum weight.

The physician and dietitian must be prepared to consult frequently with the patient and to make adjustments to fit the patient's needs and preferences. The planning of a diabetic diet for a child requires free communications among physician, dietitian, nurse, mother and child. The diet must be interesting, palatable and flexible. Education of the diabetic is essential.

It is not necessary to buy special foods. The diet should be selected from the same foods purchased for the rest of the family and should conform with the eating habits of the patient's family and his own tastes. Simplicity of dietary prescriptions is desirable. Fad diets should be avoided.

When a diabetic patient, especially an

insulin-dependent one, is unable to take his usual feedings, the carbohydrate content of the diet must be replaced with a sweetened beverage, e.g. ginger ale or orange juice, or with parenteral glucose in order to prevent insulin reactions. Timing of meals, diet composition, energy content and physical activity must be considered in planning a diet for insulin-dependent diabetics.

Caloric requirements depend upon age, weight, height, rate of growth, sex, exercise and general condition of the patient.

The diet must frequently be adjusted to the insulin dose.

Controlling the diabetic's diet requires persistence and caring on the part of the physician, nurse and dietitian.

BIBLIOGRAPHY

1. Ganda and Soeldner: Arch. Intern. Med., *137*, 461, 1977.
2. Report of The National Commission on Diabetes to The Congress of the United States, Vol. 1. DHEW Publication No. (N.I.H.) 76–1018.
3. Davidson: American Diabetes Association 25th Postgraduate Course—Diabetes in Review. 1978.
4. Felig: Postgrad. Med., *59*, 113, 1976.
5. Freinkel: American Diabetes Association 24th Postgraduate Course—Diabetes in Review. 1977.
6. Williams and Ensinck: Diabetes, *15*, 623, 1966.
7. Neel: Adv. Metab. Disord., Suppl. 1, 1970.
8. Rimoin: Med. Clin. North Am., *55*, 807, 1971.
9. Simpson: Ann. Hum. Genet., *32*, 283, 1969.
10. Gottlieb and Root: Diabetes, *17*, 693, 1968.
11. Tattersall and Pyke: Lancet, *2*, 1120, 1972.
12. Kahn, et al.: N. Engl. J. Med., *281*, 343, 1969.
13. Radder and Terpstra: Diabetologia, *11*, 135, 1975.
14. Tattersall and Fajans: Diabetes, *24*, 452, 1975.
15. Tattersall and Fajans: Diabetes, *24*, 44, 1975.
16. Fajans, Floyd and Tattersall: Arch. Intern. Med., *136*, 194, 1976.
17. Conn and Fajans: Am. J. Med., *37*, 839, 1961.
18. McDevitt and Bodmer: Lancet, *1*, 1269, 1974.
19. Nerup, et al.: Lancet, *2*, 864, 1974.
20. Cudworth and Woodrow: Diabetes, *24*, 345, 1975.
21. Carpenter: N. Engl. J. Med., *294*, 1005, 1976.
22. Thomsen, et al.: Transplant Rev., *22*, 125, 1975.
23. Creutzfeldt, Kobberling and Neel (Eds.): *Genetics of Diabetes Mellitus.* Berlin, Springer-Verlag, 1976.
24. Pyke and Nelson: In *Genetics of Diabetes Mellitus* (Creutzfeldt, Kobberling and Neel, Eds.). Berlin, Springer-Verlag, 1976, p. 194.
25. Rubinstein, Suciu-Foca and Nicholson: N. Engl. J. Med., *297*, 1036, 1977.
26. Neel: N. Engl. J. Med., *297*, 1062, 1977.
27. Craighead: Prog. Med. Virol., *19*, 161, 1975.
28. Steinke and Taylor: Diabetes, *23*, 631, 1974.
29. Forrest, Menser and Burgess: Lancet, *2*, 332, 1971.
30. Ross, et al.: Diabetes, *25*, 190, 1976.
31. Ganz and Kozak: Arch. Intern. Med., *134*, 430, 1974.
32. Irvine and Barnes: Clin. Endocrinol. Metab., *1*, 549, 1972.
33. Irvine, et al.: Lancet, *2*, 163, 1970.
34. Whittingham, et al.: Lancet, *1*, 763, 1971.
35. Bottazzo, Florin-Christensen and Doniach: Lancet, *2*, 1279, 1974.
36. Grumet, et al.: Clin. Res., *21*, 493, 1973.
37. Gepts: Diabetes, *14*, 619, 1965.
38. Nerup, et al.: Acta Allergol., *28*, 131, 1973.
39. MacCuish, et al.: Lancet, *2*, 1529, 1974.
40. Maclaren, Huang and Fogh: Lancet, *1*, 997, 1975.
41. Lendrum, Walker and Gamble: Lancet, *1*, 880, 1975.
42. Huang and Maclaren: Science, *192*, 64, 1976.
43. Cerasi and Luft: Diabetes, *21* (Suppl. 2), 685, 1972.
44. Colwell and Lein: Diabetes, *16*, 560, 1967.
45. Floyd, et al.: J. Clin. Endocrinol., *28*, 266, 1968.
46. Rull, Conn, Floyd and Fajans: Diabetes, *19*, 1, 1970.
47. Cerasi and Luft: Diabetes, *16*, 615, 1967.
48. Pyke, Cassar, Todd and Taylor: Br. Med. J., *4*, 649, 1970.
49. Conn and Fajans: Am. J. Med., *31*, 839, 1961.
50. Fajans and Conn: In *On The Nature and Treatment of Diabetes* (Leibel and Wrenshall, Eds.). New York, Excerpta Medica Foundation International Congress Series 84, 1965.
51. Kahn, et al.: N. Engl. J. Med., *281*, 343, 1969.
52. O'Sullivan and Hurwitz: Arch. Intern. Med., *117*, 769, 1966.
53. Peck, Kirtley and Peck: Diabetes, *17*, 93, 1968.
54. Fajans and Conn: Diabetes, *9*, 83, 1960.
55. Felig: Med. Clin. North Am., *61*, 43, 1977.
56. Felig: Am. J. Clin. Nutr., *26*, 998, 1973.
57. Unger and Orce: Arch. Intern. Med., *137*, 482, 1977.
58. Cahill, et al.: J. Clin. Invest., *45*, 1751, 1966.
59. Felig, Wahren and Hendler: Diabetes, *24*, 468, 1975.
60. Unger: Metabolism, *23*, 581, 1974.
61. Sherwin, et al.: N. Engl. J. Med., *294*, 455, 1976.
62. Felig, et al.: Diabetes, *25*, 1091, 1976.
63. Felig, Wahren, Sherwin and Palaiologos: Arch. Intern. Med., *137*, 507, 1977.
64. Knowles: In *Diabetes Mellitus: Diagnosis and Treatment*, Vol. II. New York, American Diabetes Association, 1967, p. 79.
65. Albrink and Davidson: Med. Clin. North Am., *55*, 877, 1971.
66. Davidson: Postgrad. Med., *59*, 114, 1976.
67. West and Kalbfleisch: Diabetes, *20*, 99, 1971.
68. Kalkhoff, Kim, Cerletty and Ferrov: Diabetes, *20*, 83, 1971.

69. Archer, et al.: J. Clin. Invest., *55*, 166, 1975.
70. Committee on Food and Nutrition, American Diabetes Association: Diabetes, *20*, 633, 1971.
71. Salans, Knittle and Hirsch: J. Clin. Invest., *47*, 153, 1968.
72. Bierman and Porte: Ann. Intern. Med., *68*, 929, 1968.
73. Doar, Wilde, Thompson and Sewell: Lancet, *1*, 79, 1263, 1975.
74. Hadden, et al.: Br. Med. J., *3*, 276, 1975.
75. West and Kalbfleisch: Diabetes, *19*, 656, 1970.
76. West: Ann. Intern. Med., *79*, 425, 1973.
77. Drenick: In *Obesity in Perspective* Vol. II, Part 2. Fogarty International Center Series on Preventive Medicine, 1974, p. 341.
78. Bistrian: American Diabetes Association 25th Postgraduate Course—Diabetes in Review, 1978.
79. Fajans: Diabetes, *21* (Suppl. 2), 678, 1972.
80. Wood and Bierman: Nutr. Today, *7*, 4, 1972.
81. Geyelin: J.A.M.A., *104*, 1203, 1935.
82. Rabinowitch: Can. Med. Assoc. J., *33*, 136, 1935.
83. Himsworth: Br. Med. J., *2*, 57, 1934.
84. Wales, Viktora and Wolff: Am. J. Med. Sci., *254*, 499, 1967.
85. Ford, Bozian and Knowles: Am. J. Clin. Nutr., *21*, 904, 1968.
86. Anderson, Herman and Zakin: Am. J. Clin. Nutr., *21*, 529, 1968.
87. Cleave, Campbell and Painter: *Diabetes, Coronary Thrombosis and the Saccharine Disease*, 2nd ed. Bristol, John Wright and Sons, 1969.
88. Henry, Burch, Bennett and Miller: Diabetes, *18*, 33, 1969.
89. Mouratoff, Carroll and Scott: Diabetes, *18*, 29, 1969.
90. Gabbay, Mierola and Field: Science, *151*, 209, 1966.
91. Gabbay: Diabetes, *18*, 336, 1969.
91a. Gabbay: Diabetes, *20*, 331, 1971.
92. Ward, et al.: Lancet, *1*, 428, 1971.
93. Swan, Davidson and Albrink: Lancet, *1*, 60, 1966.
94. Yudkin: Lancet, *2*, 4, 1964.
95. Burns-Cox, Doll and Ball: Br. Heart J., *31*, 485, 1969.
96. Howell and Wilson: Br. Med. J., *31*, 485, 1969.
97. Brunzell, et al.: N. Engl. J. Med., *284*, 521, 1971.
98. Brunzell, et al.: Diabetes, *19* (Suppl. 1), 379, 1970.
99. Stone and Conner: Diabetes, *12*, 127, 1963.
100. Cornfield and Mitchell: Arch. Environ. Health, *19*, 382, 1969.
101. Intersociety Commission for Heart Disease Resources: Circulation, *42*, A53, 1970.
102. Van Eck: Am. J. Med., *27*, 196, 1969.
103. Kempner, Peschel and Schlayer: Postgrad. Med., *24*, 359, 1958.
104. Weinsier, et al.: Ann. Intern. Med., *80*, 332, 1974.
105. Grande, Anderson and Keys: Am. J. Clin. Nutr., *25*, 53, 1972.
106. Lees and Frederickson: Clin. Res., *13*, 327, 1965.
107. Ahrens, Hirsch and Ouette: Trans. Assoc. Am. Physicians, *74*, 134, 1961.
108. Ernest, Hallgren and Svanborg: Metabolism, *11*, 912, 1962.
109. Horlick: Can. Med. Assoc. J., *85*, 1127, 1961.
110. Nestel, Carrol and Havenstein: Metabolism, *19*, 1, 1970.
111. West: *Nutrition and Diabetes Mellitus*, VI Capri Conference (Froesch and Yudkin, Eds.). Milano, Il Ponte, 1972, p. 405.
112. Tsuji and Wada: *Diabetes Mellitus in Asia, 1970*. Amsterdam, Excerpta Medica Foundation, 1971.
113. Gotto, et al.: J.A.M.A., *237*, 1212, 1977.
114. Maruhama, Abe, Okuguchi and Ohneda: Diabetes, *26*, 94, 1977.
115. Glinsmann and Mertz: Metabolism, *15*, 510, 1966.
116. Anon: Nutr. Rev., *25*, 49, 1967.
117. Freinkel, et al.: J. Clin. Invest., *42*, 1112, 1963.
118. Metz, Berger and Mako: Diabetes, *18*, 517, 1969.
119. Searles, et al.: Metabolism, *23*, 1023, 1974.
120. Lochmer, Wulff and Madison: Metabolism, *16*, 1, 1967.
121. Kreisberg, Siegal and Crawford: J. Clin. Invest., *50*, 175, 1971.
122. Dornhorst and Ouyang: Lancet, *2*, 957, 1971.
123. Nikkila and Taskinen: Diabetes, *24*, 933, 1975.
124. Arky: American Diabetes Association 24th Postgraduate Course—Diabetes in Review. 1977.
124a. Arky: Med. Clin. North Am., *62*, 655, 1978.
125. Van Itallie and Campbell: *Diabetes Mellitus: Diagnosis and Treatment*, Vol. 2. New York, American Diabetes Association, 1967, p. 91.
126. Tunbridge and Wetherill: Br. Med. J., *2*, 78, 1970.
127. Bloom: Proc. R. Soc. Med., *60*, 149, 1967.
128. Fabry and Tepperman: Am. J. Clin. Nutr., *23*, 1059, 1970.
129. American Diabetes Association: Special Report, Committee on Food and Nutrition. Diabetes Care, Nov.–Dec., 1979.
130. Crapo: 39th Annual Meeting, American Diabetes Association, Los Angeles, June 1979.
131. Anderson: 39th Annual Meeting, American Diabetes Association, Los Angeles, June 1979.
132. Yoon, Austin, Onodera and Notkins: N. Engl. J. Med., *300*, 1173, 1979.

Chapter *33*

NUTRITION, HYPERTENSION AND KIDNEY DISEASES

Robert M. Kark
and
Joseph H. Oyama

The kidneys, particularly the proximal convolutions of the nephrons, are the guardians of the nutritional wealth of the body. Each day, for example, nearly 2 kg of ascorbic acid are filtered through the walls of the glomerular tufts into the lumen of the renal tubules and all but a few milligrams are returned to the blood stream. The excretion of ascorbic acid in the urine, like that of many other water-soluble nutrients, is said to be determined by its plasma level, the rate of glomerular filtration and the maximum rate of tubular reabsorption; of these functions, the latter is crucial in preventing urinary wastage of the vitamin.[1] The extraordinary reabsorptive capacity of the proximal convolutions of the tubules in both health and disease is one reason why measurement of the urinary output of the water-soluble vitamins is of little value in the diagnosis of the classic deficiency diseases. The efficiency of the proximal convolutions in defending the body against loss of such water-soluble substances as ascorbic acid, glucose, amino acids and other nutrients is more than matched by the lower reaches of the nephron which act to conserve water and electrolytes. Even in chronic renal disease or in diabetes insipidus, when large amounts of dilute urine are passed each day, there is little or no excessive loss of ascorbic acid, and clinical deficiencies of ascorbic acid, or of other water-soluble vitamins, must be extremely uncommon on the basis of renal wastage. Nevertheless, renal wastage of other nutrients does occur. Excessive urinary loss of water, electrolytes, calcium and phosphorus, as well as protein and amino acids, is present in many renal disorders.

Prevention and treatment of renal wastage of nutrients are one side of the coin the physician has to deal with; on the other side, he finds renal *retention* of nutrients and their toxic metabolic products. Elimination and control of bodily excesses of water, of water and sodium (edema), of potassium, phosphorus, chloride and protons, and of the nitrogenous- and sulfur-containing metabolites of protein are necessary functions of the kidney. In the face of altered function, dietary modification and medications are often necessary to maintain homeostatic balance. The widespread availability of dialysis devices for those with end-stage kidney failure imposes additional factors which can disturb the nutritional economy of the body.

STRUCTURE, FUNCTION AND METABOLIC ACTIVITIES OF THE KIDNEYS

The anatomy of the kidney is extraordinarily complex, particularly the intertwining of tubules and blood vessels. In 184_ Bowman clearly related filtration of plasma and secretion of urine to the intimate relationship of blood-filled glomeru_ and the tubular capsule which envelops them. Since then, it has become more and more apparent that structure subserves function.

Function

Broadly, the kidney has three kinds of functions.* These are (1) the excretory functions, (2) their homeostatic and metabolic functions and (3) their endocrine activity. The first is concerned with expulsion of excess water, solutes, waste products of metabolism (including protons), dead and dying renal cells, minute amounts of proteins—particularly renal mucoproteins—and ingested poisons. The second function is related to the first. It deals with the maintenance of normal nutrition, acid-base and electrolyte balance and the water economy of the body. The third concerns hormones secreted by the organ. Among these are renin (see below) and erythropoietin, which balances hemoglobin and red cell production. A third hormone (or group of hormones, the prostaglandins) is present in the medulla. It may act to preserve normal blood pressure, and regulate sodium transport in man.[2] We now know that the kidney converts vitamin D into its active form and vitamin D can properly be termed a renal hormone (Chapter 6B).

Metabolic and Synthetic Activities

The metabolic and synthetic activities of the kidney are second only to those of the liver. The formation of ammonia in the renal tubules from glutamine and other amino acids is a well-known and well-studied function, but the kidney is also an active site of glucose formation. In addition, it synthesizes proteins, mucoproteins and fats, and uses energy and inorganic

---

*No comprehensive account of renal function can be given here. For those who need to refresh their memories, we suggest they browse in the following: R.F. Pitts: *Physiology of the Kidney and Body Fluid; An Introductory Text,* 4th ed. Chicago, Year Book Medical Publishers, 1974.

substances. The kidney has the highest oxygen consumption of any organ, save the minute carotid chemoreceptors. The oxygen consumption of the renal cortex is the highest of any tissue, while its respiratory quotient is one of the lowest. The studies of Lee et al.[3] indicate that the oxidation of fatty acids is the principal energy-yielding process in the cortex's highly aerobic metabolism, but the cortex is capable of utilizing a variety of substrates, including glucose, fructose, mannose, pyruvate and acetate. The oxygen consumption of the renal medulla is about one-sixth that of the cortex, and it is primarily dependent on glucose to supply energy for its predominantly anaerobic glycolytic metabolism.

Older investigators believed that three-fourths of the theoretical work of the kidney was involved in excreting urea and advised restriction of dietary protein intake to "rest" the kidney injured by disease. It is true that dietary protein is restricted in the treatment of certain renal disorders but not, as we shall see, to rest the kidney. Although we do not know exactly what the kidney does with most of the energy released by its metabolism, we now know that little is expended on the excretion of urea. Most of the energy released appears to be used in the active reabsorption of solutes and nutrients such as sodium in the proximal and distal (cortical) convolutions of the tubule.[4]

RENAL DISORDERS IN EXPERIMENTAL ANIMALS ON INADEQUATE DIETS

Disturbances of renal function and structure have been produced, with some difficulty, in experimental animals by dietary manipulations. Nocturia, hematuria, renal calculi and tubular abnormalities have developed as a result of inadequate food intake. Thus far, deficiencies of ascorbic acid, vitamin K, vitamin A, alpha tocopherol, linoleic acid, choline, potassium, magnesium and chloride have been shown to affect the kidneys of animals—usually the tubules.[5] The pathologic changes have not always been clear-cut, and this is, perhaps, because of present-day difficulties in interpreting structural abnormalities in tubular cells by available techniques.

The older literature—what little there is of it—deals mainly with the effects of high- or low-protein diets on renal hypertrophy and repair after nephrectomy, or with short-term effects of different diets on renal function, and has been completely reviewed by Smith.[6]

It has been known for some time that an excessive intake of vitamin D can produce hypercalcemia, hypercalciuria and metastatic calcification in the kidney, which may lead to either fatal or reversible renal failure. Dietary imbalance, with a high-calcium, low-phosphorus diet, has been shown to promote renal lithiasis.[7] In recent years, it has been suspected that an excessive intake of common salt was a factor in the production of essential hypertension. The relationships between sodium intake and the kidney have been explored by Meneely and his colleagues,[8] who produced renal lesions and hypertension in rats by diets containing large amounts of salt.

Best and Hartroft[9] have produced hypertension and renal disease in adult rats by an acute deprivation of choline during their infancy, the rats being fed at a luxus level during their life spans. Their observations, coupled with Hartroft's finding of glomerulosclerotic-like deposits in the kidneys of choline-deficient rats,[10] again raise the question of the origin of the vascular complications of diabetes, long suspected of being dietary in origin. It is interesting to recall the investigations of Burr and his associates[11,12] on linoleic acid deficiency and renal lesion in rats and to speculate that imbalances of fat intake may be a factor in producing hardening of the arteries in the kidney not only in diabetic patients but in many others.

RENAL FUNCTION, DIET AND DEFICIENCY DISORDERS IN MAN

Although the kidneys of man hardly ever suffer permanent damage as a result of dietary deficiency, function is affected by food and meals and on occasion manipulation of diet and water can produce functional disturbances which may be quite profound.

Maintenance of Normal Hydrogen Ion Concentration

In health, the renal tubules, together with the lungs, play a central role in maintaining the normal hydrogen ion concentration of plasma and extracellular fluids. Each day the nutritional and metabolic activity of the body produces an excess of acid metabolites. These consist mainly of 20 mol of carbonic acid, which is volatile and eliminated by the lungs, and 50 to 100 mEq of hydrogen ion as fixed acid (phosphate, sulfate, etc.), which must be excreted by the kidney. In the urine, the excess hydrogen ions are excreted as titratable acidity, present as acid phosphate (NaH_2PO_4 and KH_2PO_4) together with small amounts of organic acids such as citric acid. Normally this accounts for 20 to 30 mEq of hydrogen daily, while ammonium, which represents the larger part of the metabolic fixed acid excreted, amounts to 30 to 50 mEq daily.[13]

The net effect of both phosphate and ammonium excretion is to replenish the plasma bicarbonate level while excreting hydrogen ions. When acidosis occurs in individuals with healthy kidneys, acid phosphate excretion can increase relatively little but ammonium output may rise manyfold. The potential ability of the kidney to synthesize ammonium to take care of excess protons produced by severe exercise or disease is considerable. When patients become acidotic, for example during diabetic ketosis, the ammonium synthetic mechanism undergoes an adaptive stimulation and the tubular cells can produce and secrete many times the amount they normally present to the urine. This also occurs during consumption of the high-fat "ketogenic diet" and of culinary and other chemicals which produce acidosis (e.g. methanol, ammonium chloride).

Urinary pH

As with other renal functions, healthy kidneys can produce urine with a wide range of pH (between 4.5 and 8) but the pooled daily specimen is usually acid (pH 6). Immediately following a meal, the urine becomes less acid (the "alkaline tide") and a few hours later it becomes acid again. During sleep, decreased pulmonary ventilation causes respiratory acidosis and the urine becomes highly acid. Because of these physiologic facts, the urinary pH varies widely in health.

Ingestion of different foods, various diets and culinary chemicals (such as bicarbonate of soda) also affects the urinary pH. The usual diet of western man, rich in animal protein, produces an acid urine. Predominantly vegetable diets, such as commonly consumed in the east, in the tropics and by economically depressed individuals, produce an alkaline urine.

Effect of Diet on Renal Function

Studies on renal function with low-protein and high-protein diets on healthy individuals have been done using modern techniques, but no gross changes were observed.[14,16] With a high-protein intake a rise in filtration rate results from renal hyperemia. Dietary protein is important in the daily rhythm of glomerular filtration which parallels the rhythm of the metabolic processes of the body. The most exhaustive studies of the effects of diet on renal function of healthy young men have been made by Johnson and Sargent.[17-19] They showed that many alterations in function can be provoked by nutritional imbalance, caloric deficit, dehydration, physical work and extremes of temperature. In these investigations, the experiments involved all possible combinations of water deprivation, salt deprivation and protein deprivation, thus producing the three commonly recognized varieties of hydropenia, i.e. pure water depletion hydropenia, pure salt depletion hydropenia and mixed salt and water hydropenia. In the chronically and severely dehydrated subject, an ingested water load was retained only when the osmolar excretion exceeded 700 milliosmoles per day. Therefore, without knowledge of the rate of osmolar excretion, a subject cannot be considered well hydrated merely because he excretes a copious volume of dilute urine after a water load.

Ketonuria was easily produced by nutritional imbalance and aggravated by exposure to cold or hard work.[17] Transient albuminuria could be produced by an unbalanced diet or vigorous exercise, and exposure to cold accentuated this phenomenon. Microscopic hematuria and cylindruria could also be produced by starvation or unbalanced diet, especially one of pure carbohydrate. When a predisposition existed, moderate exercise could accentuate the microscopic hematuria and cylindruria. Further, a combination of chronic dehydration and a diet containing over 12 gm of nitrogen per day increased the concentrations of urea, creatinine and nonprotein nitrogen in the serum. Caloric deficiency decreased creatinine and urea clearances. Gross variations in diet could produce large alterations in the clearance values for sodium, chloride and total osmolar active substances.

Johnson and Sargent reviewed their findings in healthy men as they relate to the sick.[19] They stressed the need for the physician to recognize that abnormal urinalyses and tests of renal function might not be the result only of parenchymal renal disease but of dietary imbalance (oral or parenteral), dehydration or overhydration, fever or hypothermia, activity or rest, and these effects of illness or treatment must be taken into consideration when reviewing laboratory data on blood and urine. Teschan and his colleagues[20] have described increased excretion of white cells and cylindruria with exercise in young recruits. They have also described decreased osmolalities and decreased free-water clearance with severe exercise. Schedl and his colleagues[21] have shown the need for close dietary control when measuring the urinary creatinine clearance and osmolar clearance. In the former test, the 24-hour excretion of endogenous creatinine is influenced adversely by a low-protein diet. The latter test is of value only when solutes are available to the kidney for clearance, and erroneous results may be obtained when patients are tested while consuming a low-sodium or any other diet low in solutes.

It is evident that urinary sediment abnormalities and renal functional changes can be produced by dietary and environmental conditions and that additional studies are needed to determine the importance of dietary effects on commonly used renal function parameters.

Until the description of kaliopenic nephropathy, there had been no real evidence on hand to indicate that deficiencies of major nutrients seriously affected renal structure and function in man. This is surprising, since the kidneys must vigorously pursue the synthetic activities and other biochemical functions which serve the body. Despite their need for protein and nutrients to carry on their varied metabolic activities, they appear to be relatively resistant to the effects of nutritional deprivation. Their immunity to nutritional disease is probably related to their unique position in the nutritional economy of the body. They are small organs, but in an active man they receive over 1,700 liters of blood each day—one-fifth of the cardiac output and one-fifth of the circulating nutrients. Some of the alterations in renal function during nutritional deficiency are discussed below.

Protein-calorie Malnutrition. In severe chronic caloric malnutrition, renal function is disturbed and reduced. The most commonly described features have been polyuria, nocturia and hyposthenuria.[22] The pathophysiologic effects of starvation on the metabolic and excretory functions of the kidney recently have been greatly clarified by several investigators.

During prolonged starvation the body tends to protect its protein stores by decreasing protein catabolism and relies primarily upon utilization of fat stores for energy. Urea nitrogen, ordinarily the major nitrogenous end-product, rapidly diminishes to low basal excretion levels and ammonium nitrogen represents a greater proportion of total urinary nitrogen excretion. The reduction of urea nitrogen reflects the decreased gluconeogenesis from protein sources.

Owen et al.[23,24] have shown that the kidneys are very active metabolically during prolonged starvation. Oxygen consumption increases and CO_2 production increases. Various substrates, e.g. lactate, pyruvate, B-hydroxybutyrate, amino nitrogen, glycerol and fatty acids, are extracted across the renal bed. There is increased renal production of glucose and acetoacetate. Of the total amount of glucose synthesized daily during starvation, the kidney contributes 45 per cent and the liver the other 55 per cent. Analysis of individual amino acid concentration in arterial and venous renal blood has shown there is net uptake of glycine, alanine and proline with net release of serine during starvation.

The altered metabolic activity of the kidney during starvation is reflected in the constituents of the urine. Ketone bodies, principally β-hydroxybutyrate, are greatly increased; urea is diminished and ammonium is increased. Of the amino acids present in urine, glycine is excreted in greatest amounts. Ammonium production by the kidney has been shown to be closely tied to gluconeogenesis, and is promptly stimulated by conditions of acidosis.[25] During starvation the increased ammonium is needed to balance the increased excretion of B-hydroxybutyrate. The kidney thus reflects the change in metabolism of the body, i.e. the decrease in protein catabolism, the utilization of lipids for energy, and plays a major role in the daily production of glucose.

It has long been recognized that during starvation subjects excrete copious dilute urine. The structural and functional characteristics of the countercurrent multiplier system of the kidney have been well described.[26] Essential to the elaboration of a concentrated urine is the maintenance of an osmotic gradient in the deep medullary portion of the kidney. High-protein feedings increase the concentrative ability of the kidney. Studies by Klahr et al.[27] suggest that the mechanism of decreased concentrative ability in malnutrition is secondary to the failure to establish a hyperosmolar medullary gradient because of the diminished urea concentration in the medullary regions. The concentrative defect was restored in malnourished individuals by the intravenous administration of urea. Manitius et al.,[28] however, postulated that the enhanced concentrating ability on protein feeding was related to increased Na and K in the renal papilla.

The kidneys play a primary role in the regulation of electrolyte and hydrogen ion homeostasis. Acid loads are poorly handled by malnourished patients. Klahr et al.[29] found that the inability to excrete hydrogen ion loads was caused by a diminished titratable acid excretion. When malnourished patients were provided with phosphate ions by intravenous or oral supplementation, the ability to excrete acid loads and increase titratable acids in the urine was restored.

It has long been recognized that despite the virtual absence of sodium intake there is a continuing natriuresis associated with starvation.[30-32] This natriuresis can be abolished by feeding small amounts of carbohydrates, whereas fats do not have this sodium-sparing effect. Katz et al.[33] showed that protein or carbohydrate feedings, but not fat, would abolish the natriuresis of starvation. They postulate that the loss of sodium is the consequence of continuing breakdown of protein tissue with release of electrolytes and that this breakdown is diminished with protein and/or carbohydrate feedings.

Consolazio[34] and Keys[35] have studied urinary excretion of vitamins during prolonged starving. Vitamin excretion rapidly diminished during caloric restriction, but did not reach zero level during a 10-day period in the studies by Consolazio. Keys et al. had reported increased excretion of riboflavin during starvation.

When patients die of starvation, little is found in the kidney but atrophy. Gross structural changes are not often seen in kidneys of malnourished infants and children coming to autopsy. Some histologic alterations have been reported,[36] consisting of intense fatty metamorphosis of the convoluted tubules. Perhaps more detailed studies with electron microscopy and enzymatic analysis can shed further light.

Vitamin-deficient States. There are no characteristic renal structural or functional changes in pellagra and beriberi while scurvy and hemorrhagic hypoprothrombinemia are the only deficiency states known to produce hematuria. Eales[37] has described some changes in renal function in 14 patients with florid scurvy but these changes may have been results of the associated anemia and slight protein depletion. Thiamin and pyridoxine deficiencies have been implicated in the experimental production of renal stones, but their significance with regard to man is not clear.[38,39]

Mineral Deficiency States. The effects of deficiencies of sodium and potassium on renal function have been reviewed[40] and will not be extensively described here. The well-known effects of sodium deficit are reduction of plasma volume with consequent reduction of renal blood flow and glomerular filtration rate. Sodium-preserving homeostatic mechanisms come into play with reduction of urinary excretion of sodium and increased tubular reabsorption. No permanent structural alterations related to chronic hyponatremia have been described. Chronic hypokalemia can permanently alter the function and structure of the kidney[41] and is described in further detail below.

The effects of deficiencies of other minerals such as magnesium, calcium and phosphate on renal function have not yet been clearly defined, but there is some experimental evidence in animals to suggest that magnesium deficiency may alter renal function.[42]

THE COMMON NUTRIENTS AND RENAL DISORDERS

Because the kidneys are the guardian of the nutritional wealth of the body and are primary regulators of the balance between intake and excretion of nutrients and by-products, disturbances in various functions of the kidney can have important consequences to the nutritional well-being of the patient. Virtually every aspect of metabolism and nutrition can become altered in renal disorders. Water metabolism is altered, especially in disorders relating to the concentration and diluting ability of the kidney, e.g. diabetes insipidus where there is an absence of antidiuretic hormone (ADH), nephrogenic diabetes insipidus where the kidney is unresponsive to the hormone, in many cases of chronic renal failure and in acute renal failure. In addition, osmotic agents such as glucose, urea, mannitol and diuretic drugs can result in altered water metabolism. The above disorders will usually produce water loss and lead to dehydration with tragic consequences.

On the other hand, there are states of excessive water retention which produce the syndrome of water intoxication. Commonly, these are caused by injudicious administration of inappropriate solutions, particularly in circumstances where ADH activity prevents excretion of water loads. ADH activity is increased in many clinical settings, e.g. following surgery, with anxiety and with shock. Many drugs can increase secretion of ADH and many drugs are now known also to enhance the action of ADH on tubular cells. The syndrome of inappropriate ADH secretion and water intoxication has been well described.[43]

Calories

Caloric deficiency accompanies many renal disorders. Chronic renal failure is accompanied by loss of appetite, vomiting, altered gastrointestinal activity, so that caloric deficiency is often a major problem with uremia. Impaired growth has been particularly related to caloric deficiency in uremic children. Caloric deficiency is also a critical problem in instances of acute renal failure and in nephrosis. These are discussed in more detail below. On occasion, polycystic kidneys can be so large as to press on the stomach, mechanically interfering with eating and thus resulting in caloric deficiency.

Caloric excess and obesity are occasional problems in patients with renal diseases treated with corticosteroids. Obesity, per se, has also been implicated in causing nephrotic syndrome.[44]

Protein

Alterations in protein and amino acid metabolism are common in a variety of renal disorders. Protein deficiency and its manifold consequences are the primary problems in the nephrotic syndrome. Hypercatabolism of protein stores and consequent retention of toxic by-products are of major concern in acute renal failure. Chronic retention of protein products and alterations in protein metabolism are universal to any form of chronic renal failure.

In uremic poisoning, which is the common manifestation of renal failure, it is not clear which protein breakdown products are responsible for symptoms. Studies have implicated a wide variety of products to be responsible for the hematologic and neurologic disturbances associated with uremia.[45] Some substances, e.g. phenolic acids and guanidinosuccinic acids, have been identified as responsible, in part, for bleeding abnormalities.[46] Other substances, so-called middle molecule toxins, are being actively looked for to explain other clinical symptoms.[47] Suffice it to say that many by-products of normal and altered protein metabolism play an important role in uremia. Investigations are continuing in ways to alter diet or metabolic pathways to relieve symptoms and we await further information on this vital aspect of chronic renal failure.

Carbohydrate

Excessive consumption of certain fruits, such as plums, and vegetables, such as Jerusalem artichokes, allows escape in the urine of the uncommon carbohydrates the plants contain but produces no ill effects. Losses of carbohydrates also occur in genetic disorders. With renal tubular disorders, such as renal glycosuria of the Fanconi syndrome, sufficient glucose can be lost to produce symptoms of hypoglycemia. Glucose intolerance is a common feature of renal failure, even when those patients with diabetic nephropathy are excluded. Carbohydrate and insulin metabolism in renal failure has been reviewed.[48-50] There is a rough correlation of the intolerance with the retention of nitrogen. Glucose intolerance appears to be associated with a dialyzable antagonist, not yet identified, to the peripheral metabolic action of insulin, and improvement in tolerance occurs with repeated dialysis.[51] Other factors contributing to glucose intolerance in renal failure may include inadequate calorie intake, potassium depletion and chronic acidemia. Glucose intolerance is clearly undesirable and measures to improve correctable factors should be taken where possible. Occasionally, the hyperglycemia may require exogenous insulin for control. Tolerance of fructose, galactose and sorbitol is apparently normal in renal failure.[52]

Lipids

Clear-cut data are not available in man on the effects of fat consumption or disorders of lipids on the structure and function of the kidney and its vessels. Disorders of lipid metabolism have, however, been described in patients with chronic renal failure, particularly patients on chronic hemodialysis.[53-55] The observation of lactescent or milky blood flowing through tubing during hemodialysis suggested that abnormalities in triglyceride metabolism were present in chronic uremia. Most regularly dialyzed patients have elevated triglyceride levels. Many nondialyzed, nonnephrotic uremic patients were also found to have abnormal triglyceride levels. Hypertriglyceridemia, therefore, appears to be a feature of chronic renal failure itself, and is more marked in dialyzed patients.[56]

Since the work of Ahrens[57] and Dole[58] it has become obvious that carbohydrate and lipid metabolisms are very intimately related. As described above, uremic patients show glucose intolerance often associated with greater than normal basal insulin levels. Triglyceride and immunoreactive insulin levels have been found to be directly related, suggesting that increased synthesis of triglyceride-rich lipoprotein contributes to the triglyceride elevation in uremia.[54]

Triglyceride removal is believed to be mediated by the lipoprotein lipase enzyme system. Impaired removal may result in accumulation of both dietary and endogenous triglyceride. Postheparin lipolytic activity, an indirect measure of lipoprotein lipase activity, has been reported to be subnormal in both dialyzed and undialyzed uremic subjects.[55]

Lewis et al.[59] suggest that serum alpha-lipoprotein levels may be regulated by renal tissue. They found alpha-lipoprotein levels to be greatly decreased in anephric patients undergoing dialysis. Beta-lipoprotein levels were normal. After transplantation, alpha-lipoprotein levels became normal and remained normal as long as the kidney functioned well. If the kidney was rejected and removed, however, alpha-lipoprotein levels again decreased.

Hypercholesterolemia is, of course, a hallmark of the nephrotic syndrome and is further discussed below. Berlyne[60] has shown that ischemic heart disease is a complication of nephrotic syndrome that occurs with a frequency about 85 times that in the general population of the same age group. Every effort should be made to return plasma lipid values to normal in the nephrotic patient.

Sodium

Consumption of sodium in excess has been claimed to be related to the development of high blood pressure and is, perhaps, genetically mediated, as we shall see below. Retention of sodium with water as a result of functional or structural abnormalities of the kidney is common and is present in acute glomerulonephritis, in acute renal failure and in the nephrotic syndrome. Renal loss of sodium may be the result of functional disturbances of the tubule—Addison's disease is one example—but sodium wasting is more common with tubular damage, as in chronic renal failure and chronic pyelonephritis and in the diuretic phase of acute renal failure. Diets low in salt, diuretics and repeated paracenteses may produce serious deficits of salt and consequent reduction of plasma volume and thus interfere with renal function. The blood urea nitrogen may be spectacularly increased when this happens.

Potassium

Potassium retention is common in chronic and acute renal failure. Potassium deficiency is seen in functional or organic disorders such as renal tubular syndromes, chronic pyelonephritis or hyperaldosteronism. It develops commonly as a result of treatment with diuretic agents and steroid hormones and may follow self-induced diarrhea. Chronic deficiency results in kaliopenic nephropathy.

Calcium and Phosphorus

Small amounts of calcium are normally deposited in the kidney. Primary and secondary hyperparathyroidism, excess intake of vitamin D, neoplasms, immobilization, the milk-alkali syndrome, sarcoidosis and hyperthyroidism may all produce hypercalcemia, hypercalciuria, nephrocalcinosis and sometimes renal calculi. A low serum calcium is common in chronic renal failure; osteomalacia and deformities of bones may result from calcium wastage in renal tubular disorders (Fanconi syndrome). In the nephrotic syndrome, hypocalcemia is often related to the low serum protein levels. Phosphorus is retained in both acute and chronic renal disease and can be toxic. With renal tubular disorders, hyperparathyroidism and some other states of hypercalcemia, phosphaturia occurs and a low serum phosphorus can be noted.

Vitamin D

A great deal of recent research has uncovered much of the mechanism of vitamin D metabolism.[61] It is now known that vitamin D is converted in the body to metabolically active forms; these forms have greater activity than the parent compound in initiating intestinal calcium transport and bone mineral mobilization. One metabolite is 25-hydroxycholecalciferol. The liver appears to be the organ responsible for this step in hydroxylation. Another metabolite, 1,25-dihydroxycholecalciferol, appears to be the functionally active vitamin form, and is thought to be generated exclusively in kidney tissue. This observation explains much of the abnormality associated with decreased calcium absorption and vitamin D resistance in chronic renal failure. Moreover, Avioli[62] has shown that there are abnormalities in the metabolism and excretion of vitamin D in chronic renal failure.

Other Minerals

In Wilson's disease, which encompasses a tubular defect and excess tissue copper, renal wasting of copper and other nutrients may occur. Treatment with a copper-free diet has been used. Magnesium deficiency has been observed in aldosterone-producing tumors and in alcoholism. It is not clear whether deficiency of magnesium affects the kidney, although some animal work suggests that it does. Injection of magnesium has been used to treat eclampsia and also the muscle-twitching of uremia. This is a pharmacologic, not a nutritional, use of the element.

Occasionally, with gross hematuria from the urinary tract, as in Bilharzia, acute glomerulonephritis and tumors, iron-deficiency anemia may be seen. Anemia from lack of erythropoietin is much more common in chronic renal failure than is iron deficiency and does not respond to specific treatment with vitamins or iron; however, occasionally patients with chronic renal failure, particularly female patients, have associated iron-deficiency anemia, which responds to appropriate treatment.

HYPERTENSION, COMMON SALT AND POTASSIUM

High blood pressure, or hypertension, is not a disease. Rather, it is a symptom complex which may manifest itself in the course of many disorders, and the development of which may be based on one of several mechanisms. Guyton and his colleagues[63] have been the principal developers of the new systems approach to our as yet incomplete understanding of the complex physiologic and pathogenetic mechanisms which control arterial pressure in health and disease. Their work

expands on what was inferred 150 years ago, when in 1827 Richard Bright[64] hypothesized on the etiologies of the full pulse and hypertension of the heart in his patients with parenchymal renal involvement (Bright's disease).

Our modern pathophysiologic explanation is that hypertension and cardiac hypertrophy are the result of either or both increased peripheral resistance and effective blood volume expansion. This is also a gross oversimplification, and we do not have, as yet, adequate explanations of the intimate renal and other mechanisms which control the blood pressure in primary and secondary hypertension. Secondary hypertension is a symptom developing in the course of a number of renal, endocrinologic, vascular and nervous disorders. Among the renal and vascular causes are acute and chronic parenchymal renal disorders, congenital renal lesions, obstruction to the urinary conduit, eclampsia, renal artery stenosis and other forms of renovascular hypertension, coarctation of the aorta and ischemia of the kidneys. Pheochromocytoma, thyrotoxicosis, hyperparathyroidism, Cushing's syndrome and disease, acromegaly, adrenal virilism, adrenal hydroxylase deficiencies, primary hyperaldosteronism and utilization of oral contraceptives or excess mineralocorticoid medications are known hormonal causes of hypertension. Tumors of the brain, trauma to the head and intracranial hemorrhage are rarely associated with hypertension. All these conditions probably account for a very small percentage of hypertensive patients, at any one time. When hypertension occurs in the course of these conditions, management of the secondary hypertension is directed, for the most part, toward diagnosis and treatment of the underlying condition.

Primary or essential hypertension is a major, perhaps the major, health problem of modern man living in industrialized societies.[65-67] Nearly all who have studied the problem agree that it occurs as a result of environmental and genetic or familial factors.

Possible Etiologies

It is generally accepted that susceptibility to high blood pressure is genetic in nature, but the method of transmission is unclear. It has been suggested that inheritance is through a single incomplete dominant autosomal gene,[68,68a] but polygenic inheritance has also been postulated.[69] We believe that it is also possible that all men react normally to an environmental factor, such as abnormally high salt intake, by developing increasing blood pressure with age and that the small percentage of those who do not have inherited a genetic resistance to high blood pressure. Be that as it may, primary hypertension appears to have roots early in life.[70] Blood pressures in young children from families with history of hypertension are higher than those from families free of hypertension.

As industrialized populations grow older all but 15 to 20 per cent have increases in blood pressures. These latter may be genetically resistant to the development of hypertension. At some time or other in the life of each individual, an upward gradient of blood pressure may or may not eventually pass through those arbitrary levels defined by the World Health Organization and other medical organizations as "above normal." If it does and if it is maintained for a time, the individual will be declared "hypertensive." Rising blood pressure with age is typical of primary hypertension and differentiates it from the secondary forms of hypertension. Environmental factors considered to be acting in populations with high blood pressure are: the stresses of industrial life,[72] overcrowding,[73] air pollution,[74] psychosocial[75] and psychologic[76] perturbations and dietary disturbances. Among the latter, studies have incriminated "soft" drinking water,[77,78] high cadmium intake,[79] calcium consumption,[80] potassium/sodium ratio[81] and salt (sodium) intake.[82,83]

A great deal of evidence suggests that consumption of large amounts of salt and perhaps a simultaneous decreased intake of potassium are responsible for primary hypertension. Increased salt intake leads to expansion of extracellular fluid, increased cardiac output, overperfusion of the tissues; this by autoregulation leads to higher peripheral vascular resistance and high blood pressure with normalization of cardiac output. While there is no clear evidence of increased total body sodium or extracellular fluid sodium in primary hypertension, Tobian[84] has shown that arteries from hypertensives have an increased sodium content per unit of dry weight. This may add to the thickening of the artery wall, with a resulting increase in vascular resistance. It may also be related to enhanced vasoconstriction.

Because patients with Addison's disease are known to have low blood pressure and deplete their stores of sodium by excess loss through the dejecta, and because patients with Cushing's syndrome have hypertension and retain ingested sodium, attention has been focused on potential aberrant adrenal mechanisms as a cause of essential hypertension. Thirty or more years ago, adrenalectomy was a popular mode of treatment for uncontrollable high blood pressure. It appeared to be successful in about 20 per cent of patients with severe malignant or accelerated hypertension. At about that time, Goldblatt produced hypertension in dogs by clamping one renal artery.[85] He revived interest in the renal hormone renin as a cause of hypertension. In 1950, Conn described hypertension associated with aldosterone tumors of the adrenals.[86] From these and other studies developed our knowledge of the intricate interrelationships among aldosterone, renin, angiotensin I and II and their involvement with the sodium and potassium economy of the body as a mode of controlling effective blood volume and blood pressure in health, and in some diseases associated with hypertension. Thurston and Swales[87] and others have shown that the subdivision of primary hypertension into low, normal and high renin groups is arbitrary. Renin secretion is impaired in hypertensives and, while there may be prognostic or therapeutic value in selecting arbitrary "renin groups," this division has no demonstrated etiologic value.

Angiotensin II, a potent vasoconstrictor derived from the action of renin, is probably responsible for producing hypertension in renovascular disease. The best evidence for this is that saralasin, the competitive metabolic inhibitor of angiotensin II, usually causes a prompt decrease in blood pressure when infused into patients with renovascular hypertension. But saralasin and other angiotensin II inhibitors rarely lower blood pressure in other forms of hypertension, including primary hypertension.

Thus far, all attempts to find aberrant adrenal compounds which are responsible for primary hypertension have been unsuccessful. Nor have aberrations of the vasoactive compounds, such as the renal prostaglandins or kallikreins, been implicated as single causes of primary hypertension. Urinary kallikrein resembles renal kallikrein and differs from plasma kallikrein. The kallikreins release bradykinin or lasyl-bradykinin from an alpha-globulin substrate. Mills and his colleagues have shown that urinary kallikrein excretion in both normotensive and hypertensive persons is related to sodium excretion and therefore to salt intake.[88]

Many years ago, Morris[89] showed that the juxtaglomerular apparatus of the kidneys, which secrete renin, contains nerve endings. This led to studies demonstrating nervous control of renin secretion and has, recently, focused attention once again on central nervous system and carotid body (baroreceptor) disturbances as causes of hypertension.

It is also known that transplanting a healthy kidney from a normotensive patient into a patient with chronic renal failure and hypertension will usually reduce the blood pressure;[90] the same is true for rats.[90a] This has called attention to studies of renal perfusion pressures in relation to sodium excretion and blood flow in the kidney. Tobian[91-93] has found low renal papillary plasma flow in both Dahl-inbred sodium-sensitive rats and in Kyoto Wistar rats with spontaneous hypertension. In studying these isolated hypertensive rats' kidneys, it was found that they excrete subnormal amounts of sodium when perfused at "normal" pressures but will excrete normal amounts of sodium *only* when perfused at hypertensive pressures.

While there are "spontaneous" hypertensive inbred laboratory strains of rats,[94] man is the only animal living in its natural habitat in which hypertension is found. There are also many laboratory methods of producing hypertension in animals, from surgical operations on dogs to feeding turkeys aflatoxin. None of the animal models mimic the natural history of primary hypertension in man, but salt toxicity in rats comes close and illuminates its pathophysiology and pathogenesis.[95]

In Meneely's classic studies,[95,96] various diets containing salt in very small or very large amounts and with various intermediate levels were fed to laboratory rats over a 9-month period. It was seen that each increment in salt intake brought a concomitant increase in blood pressure. The rats eating 10 per cent salt in the dry diet developed gross hypertension. At 2 to 5 per cent salt in the diet, borderline or mild hypertension was observed. At the higher levels of blood pressure, there was obvious arteriolonephrosclerosis with severe renal damage.

Dahl showed that nearly 80 per cent of laboratory rats would develop high blood pressure when given large amounts of salt in their chow.[97] By inbreeding those most sensitive and least sensitive to salt intake, he developed two genetic strains of rats,[98,99] the "salt-sensitive" strain and the "salt-resistant" strain.

The salt-sensitive strain responds readily to any maneuver which usually produces hypertension in an unselected group of laboratory rats, such as renal artery stenosis, ingestion of mineralocorticoid hormones or consumption of sodium salts. With regard to high sodium consumption, the effect is not seen immediately; it is induced after some time has elapsed. The young animal is more susceptible to its effects than the adult rat, and once the blood pressure rise occurs it has a progressive upward trend. Salt restriction will modify the rate of climb but will not reverse it. Thus the genetic factor is permissive, not determinate. High blood pressure occurs only if the "sensitive" rat is exposed to the "environmental" stimulus—common salt.

Of course, there are many unanswered questions about the relationship of salt to primary hypertension. Why do the kidneys of those susceptible to hypertension handle sodium differently from those who have normal pressures? Why is peripheral resistance increased in those who are salt resistant? Perhaps the most important question is why does western man have a perverted and inappropriate taste for salt? One answer may be the presence of abnormal receptor sites for mineralocorticoid hormones in the cells of the arterioles.[99a]

"A Perverted and Inappropriate Taste for Salt"

Salt has been used for thousands of years, as a much sought after and precious condiment and as a safe preservative for food. In ancient times, it was a scarce commodity and to share salt was a sign of eternal friendship. To sit at the communal table "above the salt" was a mark of distinction, as those so honored could use as much salt as desired.

According to expert opinion,[100] salt was not available to primitive man in many parts of the world. The Odyssey (XI, 122 et seq.) speaks of inlanders who do not know the sea and use no salt in their food. Numidian nomads at the time of Sallust never ate salt with their foods. Among inland primitive people, a salt or brine spring was regarded as a special gift of the gods (Aristotle, Met. ii) and the ancient German tribes waged war for brine streams (Tacitus, Ann. XIII, 57). Salt was used as a part of religious activities in ancient times. Homer calls salt "divine," and Plato names it "a substance dear to the gods." The practice of using salt at sacrificial offerings, especially conjoined with cereals ("bread and salt") was prevalent among the Greek, Roman and Semitic peoples of the Mediterranean basin. The preservative qualities of salt were held to make it a peculiarly fitting symbol of an enduring compact, and a "covenant of salt" (Numbers XVIII, 19)* was used to seal an obligation to fidelity at the traditional meal which bound the parties. Even today, in some parts of the Orient, any meal that includes salt has a certain sacred character which creates a bond between the participants. The modern Persian phrase "unfaithful to salt" is used for those who are disloyal or ungrateful.

It appears that our habitual use and taste for salt is intimately connected with the advance from the nomadic life of the hunter-gatherer to the agricultural life, the use of cereals for food and the development of trade. The cereal foods used by the first agriculturists—parched wheat, flour pastes, porridge, unleavened bread, barley cakes, chapati, etc.—are so bland that sea salt was the obvious condiment to make them reasonably palatable.

In northern climes before the advent of the turnip and other advances in animal husbandry, it was not possible for farmers to feed all their stock over the winter; there was not enough feed nor any known satisfactory method to preserve it. A small number of breeding animals were culled from the herds to replenish the stock in the spring, and were kept alive with difficulty. The rest were slaughtered in the early

---

*"This is a perpetual covenant of salt before the Lord with you and your descendants also."

winter and the meat was salted down in barrels. Similarly, herrings caught in the fall were salted for winter use.

At one time almost the whole of salt in commerce was produced from the evaporation of sea water and, indeed, salt so made still forms a staple commodity, especially in countries possessing a seaboard where the climate is dry and the summers of long duration. Some of the oldest trade routes were created for traffic in salt. Such was the *Via Salaria* up which the produce of the salt pans of Ostia were carried into the hills of Rome, even before it was a city. Heroditus describes the caravan routes to the salt oases in the Libyan desert, which are still in use. Very early caravan routes were opened up in Asia, in the Middle East and in Africa to exchange salt from the sea for incense, slaves and gold. Blocks of salt were used as money. The Romans paid their soldiers partly in salt, the *salarium* from which stems our word *salary*. The vast salt mines of northern India were worked before the time of Alexander (Strabo, V 2 and 6) and were centers of the widespread trade in that subcontinent. The economic importance of salt is also indicated by the almost universal prevalence of taxes on salt, as well as by government monopolies on its sale. In the distant past, once trade routes were opened up by land and especially by sea, salt was required (and in demand) to preserve provisions for the journey. Thus, "bread" and "trade," stemming from early technologic advances of man, are at the roots of hypertension.

"Low-salt" and "Low-blood-pressure" Societies

Among mammals, the penchant for salt is peculiar to man and, as indicated above, seems to be a taste associated with passage from uncultivated and primitive society to agricultural or sophisticated industrial life. However, even when abundant salt is available, primitive people do not necessarily succumb to the human taste for it.[101,102] For example, the primitive fishermen living on the tiny Olong Java atoll, which is surrounded by the sea, consume 50 mg per day. The Olong Java people have blood pressures in the range of 110/65 all their lives. Their plasma renin activity levels are 2.5 times those of a population sample in the United States studied under similar conditions of posture and activity.[103]

Similar "high" plasma renin and "high" urinary aldosterone values were reported in highland Yanomatio Indians by Oliver et al.[104,105] These high hormone levels reflect the "low" sodium intake of these people. They excrete less than 1.0 mEq of sodium daily, an habitual intake of 0.5 gm of salt. They lead extraordinarily active physical lives in the tropical rain forests of northern Brazil without symptoms of sodium depletion. Their blood pressures are "low" by our standards and stay "low" all their lives. They do not have any increase in blood pressure with aging, as do all but 15 to 20 per cent of people in industrial societies.

Since the early reports of Thomas in 1927[106] and of Morse and Beh in 1937,[107] there have been more than thirty studies on a variety of populations with low salt intakes who do not have primary hypertension among their ills. These have been reviewed by Page,[103,108] Meneeley,[109] Tobian[91] and others. These low-salt, low-blood-pressure societies are generally groups of people who have not yet become acculturated into an industrial, western type of civilization. They represent the different races of man, they live in different climates, they have different customs and thrive on a variety of diets.

Among such populations are Greenland Eskimos,[110] African Nigerians, West Chinese in Szechwen Province,[107] Naga Hill tribesmen,[111] Polynesians,[112] East African Nomadic Semburu,[113,114] Congo Pygmies,[115] Kalahari-Kang bushmen[116] and the famous Masai warriors.[117] These low-salt populations are of great interest because they have escaped all mechanisms known to elevate blood pressure. They are *not* genetically protected from developing high blood pressures with age. A large number of studies, such as those of Cruz-Coke,[118] Prior[119] and Shaper[120] have demonstrated that when these low-blood-pressure people migrate into towns or acculturate into western ways of living upward trends in blood pressure soon appear and hypertension eventually follows. For example, Prior noted that natives in small villages in New Guinea had virtually no hypertension and that the blood pressures in old men were no higher than those in young men. This indicated for the first time that blood pressure is not necessarily compelled to rise with advancing age. Moreover, Prior found that these New Guinea natives nearly always developed their hypertension when they moved to "modern" coastal cities. The salt in the citified diet was suspected as a cause of the emergence of hypertension. Shaper reported that East African Sembura farmers greatly increased their salt intake, to 18 gm per day, when they were drafted into the army and ate army rations. Their blood pressure did not begin to rise immediately but, rather, during the second year of army service.

The migration of low-blood-pressure preindustrial people to cities and the change of environment may be responsible for the changes in blood pressure. With acculturation, they experience the stresses of modern life and "cultural shock," as well as changes in diets. Acculturation is a highly complex process and its effects are difficult to analyze. Several years ago, Lot Page and an expedition of expert anthropologists from the Peabody Museum at Harvard initiated a study of tribal groups in the Solomon Islands[103] which were beginning to change to a western culture. They selected eight populations which were all either unacculturated or at very low levels of acculturation. These eight groups were racially fairly homogeneous, but different in habitat, way of life and subsistence. All lived in rural tribal areas, away from roads, towns and other western influences. Although all were at very low levels of acculturation, important differences in degree of western influence occurred among them. Using eight separate criteria, Page and his colleagues ranked the degrees of acculturation. They found blood pressures to be rising with age in the five most acculturated groups. This upward trend, when it occurred, was more pronounced in females than in males. In looking for specific correlates for these trends, urban and psychosocial stresses were found to be virtually absent in all eight groups. Measures of general health and nutrition did not vary significantly among the eight and, unlike more advanced societies, body weight decreased with age in all. Diet varied widely among them, depending on habitat. Some lived entirely on root crops and leafy vegetables, others on fish, canned meat, canned fish, wheat flour and rice. Analysis of the data indicated that salt intake correlated with blood pressure more strongly than did other dietary items or the acculturation index—or indeed any of its components singly or together.

"High-salt" and "High-blood-pressure" Societies

If the low salt intake of preindustrial societies protects them from the rise of blood pressure with age and from development of hypertension, does primitive life of itself protect against hypertension even when there is a high consumption of common salt? Once again, Page has provided some information. He has recently studied Gashgai nomads living in the deserts of southern Iran. "Although the data are not fully analyzed, it is evident that these people, who use large amounts of salt but whose way of life has remained largely unchanged for hundreds of years, have strikingly high blood pressure."[121]

Meneely and Dahl[82,122,123] have reported on acculturated populations where the daily intake of common salt is very high, e.g. farmers in Honshu in northern Japan[124-126] and coastal fishermen in Newfoundland.[127] In these two populations, there is an extraordinarily high incidence of hypertension, stroke and ischemic heart disease. Meneely and Dahl plotted population sodium intake against the incidence of "hypertensives" in five societies (Fig. 33–1). They reported that in the United States the average intake of salt at the time the data were published was 10 gm per day. Data from the Framingham study collected many years ago (Table 33–1) also show that at age 45 most people consumed 10 or more gm of salt per day and indicated that hypertension increased with increasing salt intake.

Table 33–1. Framingham Study: Sodium Intake and Hypertension*

Sodium Chloride				
Consumed in gms	8	10	13	13
Average Age	44	44	44	45
% Hypertensive	20	24	27	36

*From Stamler, Stamler and Pullman.[73]

Potassium Intake

Although these epidemiologic data on low-salt and high-salt populations provide a most convincing association between salt intake and development of high blood pressure, studies of individuals with high blood pressure often do not show sig-

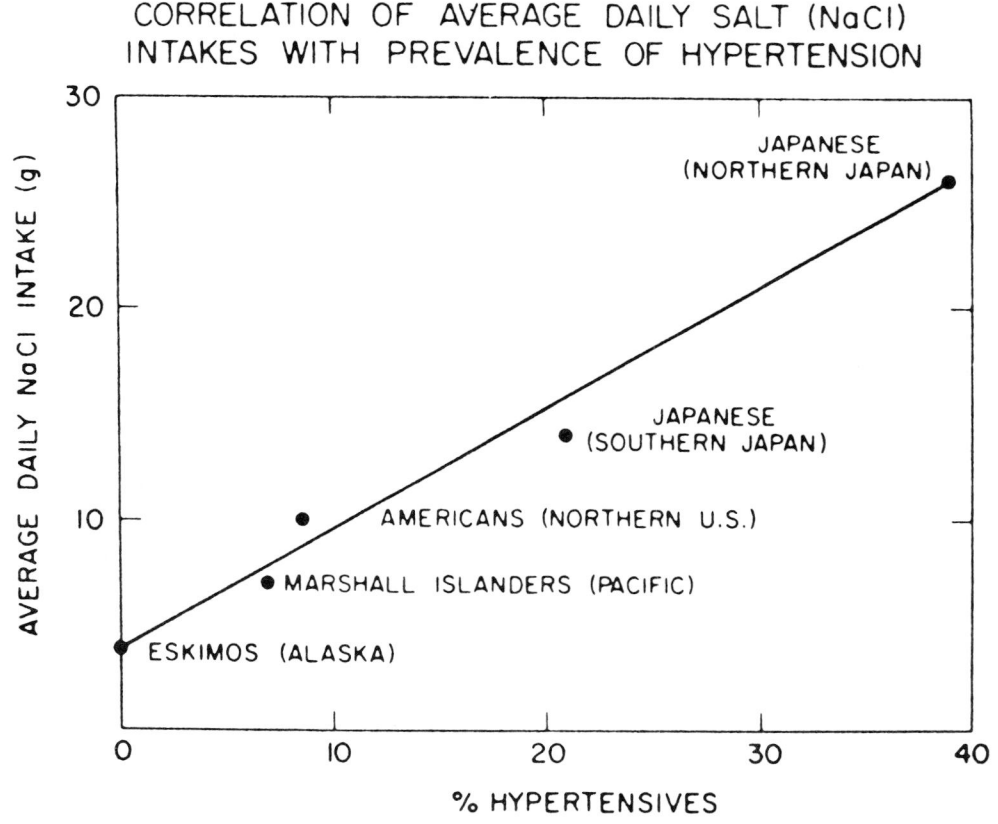

CORRELATION OF AVERAGE DAILY SALT (NaCl) INTAKES WITH PREVALENCE OF HYPERTENSION

Fig. 33-1. Salt intake and prevalence of high blood pressure in different populations. (Adapted from Meneely and Dahl[82] and Dahl.[122])

nificant correlations between hypertension or systolic or diastolic pressures and sodium intake measured over a short period of time. Of course, there are many problems to contend with in individual studies, including the fact that a person may be responding maximally at a lower level of intake than his habitual level of sodium consumption. Be that as it may, when we compare primeval dietary intake of man or the diets of low-salt, low-blood-pressure societies, there is a significant difference in potassium as well as in sodium intake. Primitive man and man in preindustrial or underdeveloped societies consume a "high-potassium, low-salt intake" by our standards.[128]

Meneely and his colleagues[97,129] fed high-salt hypertensive rats large amounts of potassium and in very well controlled studies demonstrated that large amounts of potassium added to the hypertensive diet dramatically enhanced survival with prolongation of median duration of life by 2 to 8 months. Dahl et al.[130] found that their salt-sensitive rats had higher blood pressures the higher the sodium/potassium ratio of their food when they kept sodium constant and varied potassium.

Addison in 1928[131] reported that potassium chloride regularly produced a drop in blood pressure while sodium chloride regularly produced a rise, and in 1962 Priddle confirmed these studies[132] and Sasaki showed that hypertension was not a problem in a Japanese group eating very large amounts of potassium while consuming a diet high in salt.[129] McQuarrie[133,134] reported metabolic studies on diabetics whose blood pressure increased when fed sodium chloride. When potassium was added, the blood pressure returned to normal. More recently, Langford, Schoenberger and their colleagues[135] have shown that, while most studies of western persons fail to show a direct correlation between sodium excretion and blood pressure, this is not true for Na/K urinary ratios. Na/K ratios were correlated with systolic and diastolic pressures, weight and other parameters. There was a significant correlation between Na/K ratio and diastolic blood pressure (p = 0.347 and t = 0.02), but other correlations were not significant. They also reported that when potassium intake was increased from 50 to 200 mEq each day there was a natriuresis of over 200 mEq sodium, and they indicated that the protective influence of potassium in preventing hypertension may be by this action.

Sources of Sodium Consumed by Man in the United States

Common salt is the major chemical used by the food industry to prevent spoilage of food. It is inexpensive, readily available and effective. Salt brines are used to pickle vegetables, fruits such as olives, meats and fish. Common salt has been layered in barrels between slabs of meat or fish ever since man used ships to ply long voyages. Salt is used to preserve cheese, caviar, sausages and bacon.

Many other chemicals are employed in the food industry to prolong shelf life, enhance texture, improve color, ensure uniformity and strengthen or change flavors during processing. When manufacturers purify or synthesize food or pharmaceutical chemicals they nearly always end by making sodium salts of the compounds they distribute or sell, such as sodium benzoate, sodium nitrate, sodium citrate, sodium phosphate and sodium monoglutamate. There are also many medicines, both oral and parenteral, such as "elemental" diets, amino acids and antibiotics, which can and do add a daily burden of sodium to the bodies of those who are ill. It is unusual for manufacturers deliberately to make calcium or potassium salts of the common chemicals added to foods, beverages and medications. They are not accustomed to doing this, as there seems to them to be no commercial advantage or reason to prepare, synthesize or use nonsodium salts.

Manufacturers do, however, respond to reason. When cyclamate sweeteners were first synthesized, many years ago, the manufacturers were informed that a potential market existed among diabetic and obese persons with congestive heart failure who should not consume the sodium salt of cyclamate. They made calcium cyclamate for sale. Manufacturers were also persuaded by the Academy of Pediatrics[136] to stop adding common salt to processed baby foods,[137] because Dahl's studies had indicated that salt-sensitive strain *infant* rats were susceptible to its toxic effects.[138]

Salt is commonly added to canned foods in large amounts (Table 33–2). In general, frozen foods contain less salt than canned foods, but foods such as frozen fish fillets are rich in salt from the sea brine in which they are frozen. (See Appendix for sodium content of other foods.)

Sodium hydroxide or other sodium salts are used to precipitate vegetable proteins from soy beans, algae and other sources of vegetable protein concentrates before extruding or spinning the vegetable protein fibers into palatable textured protein foods. Removing such added sodium salts is a problem which needs to be solved. In most of our metropolitan areas, exchange ions are used commonly to "soften" water. They are also used to remove the potassium bitartrate from red wines to prevent sediment formation. The ion exchangers act by removing calcium or potassium in exchange for sodium and thereby degrade the nutritional value of water and wine.

Some of the common foods we eat are dusted with salt (potato chips) or covered with salt crystals (pretzels) to increase our thirst and fluid requirement when consuming beer or other alcoholic beverages. Cocktail parties are notorious for the salty foods provided which also invoke thirst.

In the United States chefs, cooks and housewives use salt liberally. They cater to their own tastes and to those of the persons they feed who have acquired a taste for salt from infancy or childhood. Depending on the recipe, they add a pinch or a handful of salt to food during preparation. They rub handsful of salt into roasts before putting them into the oven—they apply salt to salads. They also use flavored salts (garlic salt or onion salt) and add salty olives, bacon, cheese and anchovies to some salads. They drop salted crackers into salty fish or clam chowders. Once food is on the table, consumers shake on salt (Table 33–3) and frequently ketchup, pickles or other salted condiments are added to spice up the fare.

In the past few decades, coincident with the development and growth of television, food companies have been developing, manufacturing and distributing more and more convenience foods (e.g. T.V. dinners) and more and more food snacks. Moreover, social change has increased the consumption of sodium and decreased the intake of potassium. Many women are working outside the home and have less time for planning and preparing meals.

Table 33–2. Effects of Canning and Preparation on Sodium and Potassium Content of Green Peas (per 100 gm)*

	Na Content mg/mEq	K Content mg/mEq
Fresh Green Peas	0.9/0.04	380/9.7
Canned Peas (Liquid Removed)	230/10	180/4.6
Canned Peas (Salt and Butter added)	643/28	180/4.6

*From Kark: Unpublished data.

Table 33–3. Salt Added to Food*

	NaCl mg/mEq
"A pinch of salt"	= 206/3.5
Lightly salted food	= 813/13.8
Heavily salted food	= 2252/38
"A handful of salt"	= 4768/81

*From Kark: Unpublished data.

This means that more convenience foods and manufactured foods are purchased for use in the home than fresh food and fresh produce, which were what we ate at family meals in the past. The highly varied and mobile life of many people means that each day's nutrition is the total of various meals and snacks consumed at different times and places rather than 2 or 3 planned meals at home. There is little thought about the nutritional contribution of convenience foods. Restaurants, cafeterias, and delicatessens are doing a thriving business. They use more and more convenience foods to feed their customers instead of fresh produce as in the past. Sixty per cent of the foods now served in restaurants are convenience

Table 33–4.   Sodium Content of Servings of Prepared Foods*

Frozen Entrées in One Estimated Serving of:

Salisbury steaks: Sodium content averaged 1472 mg Na (range 623 to 2381 mg Na)

Sliced beef: Average 1415 mg Na (range 794 to 2087 mg Na)

Sliced turkey: Average 2199 mg Na (range 955 to 3107 mg Na)

Banquet Foods:

Fried chicken: 16 ozs. 3.2 gm Na; meat loaf, turkey, salisbury steak (19-oz portion) 3.6 to 3.7 gm Na

Dessert pies: 1.6 gm to 2.5 gm Na per 20-oz portion

Variety entrées: 1.4 gm to 2.5 gm Na per serving

Buffet supper entrées: 32 oz, 4981 mg to 6599 mg Na per serving

Weight Watchers: Turbot: 8.5 oz, 516 mg; turkey dinner: 19.0 oz, 2279 mg; eggplant parmigiana: 13 oz, 1049 mg Na (per serving)

Morton: Turkey pot pie: 514 mg Na per 100 gm; spaghetti and meatballs: 413 mg Na per 100 gm

USDA: Frozen pancake and link sausage: 677 mg/100 gm; chicken chow mein and rice: 515 mg per 100 gm; meat loaf and whipped potatoes: 442 mg per 100 gm

MacDonald: Hamburger (99.3 gm) Na 530 mg; cheeseburger (114.2 gm) Na 752 mg; Big Mac (186.7 gm) Na 960 mg

*Sodium content of servings of prepared foods collected from commercial publications of manufacturers; see Consumer Reports, May 1977.

foods. These nearly all contain large quantities of common salt (Table 33–4).

Many hospitals are now using convenience foods from caterers for both "regular" and special diets. In one hospital near Chicago, the regular diet from such a caterer supplied 23 gm of sodium each day. All of the above facts underline the increasing consumption of salt and sodium in the United States.

Diet and the Prevention of Hypertension

All antihypertensive drugs have adverse effects some of which may be fatal. Some, such as the diuretics, may, on occasion, seriously deplete the body stores of potassium and then may produce chronic interstitial nephritis in some patients or digitalis intoxication in those on this drug.

Irving Page's[139] statement of 1966 about antihypertensive drugs is still germane to the problem of both prevention and treatment of hypertension. "Then began the era of drug treatment of hypertension. This era is quite fascinating because each drug we used produced a new disease of its own. There was hexomethomium lung disease; hydralazine disease, which is like lupus erythematosus. Reserpine depression or Parkinsonism. While intriguing to us, this type of treatment is a little rough on the patient."

As a result of the VA Cooperative Study on Hypertension[140-142] reported by Fries[143] vigorous programs are being developed for detecting all individuals with high blood pressure with the aim of treating them with antihypertensive drugs. This approach is fraught with danger. The iatrogenic diseases which would develop in that enormous population of hypertensives would be worse for many than no treatment at all. It is important to add that, at the fourth Nephrological Symposium held in Hanover in June 1976, Fries warned against excessive enthusiasm and also indicated the dangers of potential toxicity of antihypertensive drugs. Side effects and incompatibility limit the usefulness of antihypertensive drugs. The chances of success of antihypertensive treatment with respect to life expectancy decrease quite substantially with the presence of additional risk factors such as arteriosclerosis, diabetes mellitus, obesity or hyperlipemia. The decision as to whether a patient should be treated with drugs should not be made on the basis of the absolute blood pressure levels alone but, rather, with adequate consideration of the presence of additional risk factors. Because the usefulness of drug treatment cannot yet be demonstrated as clearly in mild hypertension as in severe hypertension, the decision as to whether the patient should be treated must be an individual one, in which case the sex and age, the presence or absence of risk factors, evidence or absence of organ damage typical of hypertension and family history must be taken into consideration.

While there is danger from iatrogenic disease in the drug treatment of hypertension, reverting to a diet low in salt and high in potassium can do no harm to the population as a whole. There is much direct evidence to support the concept that sodium "restriction" in man is well tolerated. Metabolic studies have shown that sodium balance can be maintained for indefinite periods in healthy western adults on an intake of 200 mg Na per day or even less.[144] Although the data on the electrolyte consumption (or excretion) in various segments of the population are remarkably scanty, and although more data are required, it is apparent that we consume at least 5 to 20 times the amount of sodium eaten by healthy primitive people—vastly above physiologic needs. For all the reasons cited above, we have for some time embarked on preventive action for our patients, which we feel is harmless, prudent and effective.

When a patient is seen for the first time in our office and there is a clear-cut family history of hypertension, we feel it is important to inform the individual about the probabilities of developing hypertension and the possibility of prevention with a low-sodium, high-potassium diet. In our experience this is best done in the setting of a family conference, at which time the patient and spouse are informed of risk factors (such as smoking and obesity) for stroke, cardiac hypertrophy, cardiac arrest and coronary artery disease; the hedonistic inappropriate taste for salt we have acquired; facts on low-salt, low-blood-pressure societies and particularly the abundance of sodium in the foods and beverages we eat (including ionized soft water). At that time, personal and family eating habits, food preferences, and food purchases and preparation are reviewed. Instruction is given on how to reduce sodium consumption at home and when eating out. Emphasis is placed on the need for low-sodium, high-potassium intake for infants and children as indicated. The patient and spouse are asked to purchase and review Ruth Leverton's small paperback book, *Food Becomes You,* to give them an adequate background in nutrition. Diet sheets listing high-salt or sodium foods and beverages and high-potassium foods and beverages (if not inappropriate) are reviewed. Thereafter, the burden of changing family food habits is turned over to a dietitian. At return visits to the physician's office, the changes in eating patterns are reviewed by us, sometimes jointly with the dietitian.

The same preventive action is suggested to those individuals *without a family history of hypertension* when, after multiple visits over the years, it becomes apparent that blood pressure is climbing toward hypertensive levels and there is no evidence of secondary hypertension. The patient and, if desired, the spouse are informed that, while there is no family history of high blood pressure, they may desire to make a prudent family dietary change which can do no harm.

In the public domain, the Food and Drug Administration is moving to ensure labeling of all packaged foods with their sodium and potassium content.[145] It is time that other public health authorities and influential medical bodies move to inform the food industry, restaurant owners, directors of schools for chefs and cooks and the chefs and cooks in the United States of the need for a sharp reduction in the use of common salt (and sodium) in the preparation of foods and food items for purchase. Moreover, the public needs to be informed of the ill effects produced on the blood pressure by the unnecessary inappropriate hedonistic consumption of salt. Salt substitutes are not satisfactory as yet and new ones which are fully acceptable need to be developed as quickly as possible to allow behavioral scientists time to determine how to turn off man's culturally induced salt appetite and perception.

Diet and the Treatment of Primary Hypertension

Caloric Restriction. Although there is no direct etiologic relationship, obesity is common in patients who have essential hypertension.[146] In fat hypertensives, the heart labors under the double load of high blood pressure and obesity, and for this reason the total caloric intake should be restricted. Total food consumption at any meal should be limited, as great fluctuations in blood pressure often occur after the ingestion of large meals because of decreased efficiency of vasomotor regulation in patients who have essential hypertension. Furthermore, it is known from experience that overfilling the stomach with food may result in embarrassment to the ischemic heart during digestion.

For information with regard to calorically restricted diets applicable to hypertensive patients who are obese, the reader is referred to Appendix Table A–12. As a general rule, a diet restricted to 1,000 to 1,200 calories daily will bring about desired results without harm to the patient. In most cases reduction of excessive weight is not accompanied by more than a mild decrease in blood pressure, but, in some cases, the drop in blood pressure is notable or even striking. Even when blood pressure is not lowered, improvement in subjective symptoms, such as fatigue and dyspnea, may be noted in a degree concomitant with the loss in weight.

Although reduction of caloric intake and regular moderate daily exercise (a brisk walk for 30 minutes per day) are indicated in the treatment of obese patients who have uncomplicated hypertension, dietary restriction should not be too severe on patients suffering from uncomplicated early hypertension, as this is frequently productive of more harm than good.

Less frequently, hypertensive patients are greatly underweight and undernourished. No evidence exists to support the thesis that hypertension is benefited by undernutrition; hence, in these patients it is important to restore weight and nutrition to as nearly normal levels as possible. However, reduced intake of food with due consideration for a properly balanced diet may have beneficial effects in hypertensive patients entirely apart from blood pressure level, e.g. in the latent diabetic and in subjects with elevated blood lipid levels or hyperuricemia.

In summary, the best interest of either the overweight or underweight patient is served by the adjustment of caloric intake to bring the weight of the patient to a normal level.

Protein. For years, belief in the effectiveness of sharp restriction of protein was widely accepted in the treatment of essential hypertension by some members of the medical profession and laity alike. This belief was inculcated so firmly in the minds of the laity that many patients who had hypertension literally had a phobia concerning meat and its supposedly harmful effects. There is no evidence to show that ingestion of protein plays any role in the production or aggravation of hypertension. Therefore, there is no justification for rigid restriction of protein in the diet of hypertensive patients as long as the ability of the kidneys to excrete nitrogen remains adequate. Protein restriction in chronic renal failure is discussed below.

Fluid Intake. In the absence of symptoms and signs of cardiac or renal insufficiency, the hypertensive patient should be allowed a normal intake of fluids of the usual variety. No hard evidence exists that alcohol, as such, plays any part in the causation or aggravation of hypertension, despite a recent study[146a] in which no investigation of salt or potassium intake or excretion was reported. Consequently, the temperate use of alcoholic beverages by patients who have uncomplicated hypertension is not contraindicated. However, because of the other effects of alcohol, the use of these beverages in other than moderate quantities should be discouraged. If hyperlipidemia, liver disease or other contraindications coexist, alcohol should not be used. The use of coffee or tea in moderation is probably harmless to most patients who have essential hypertension. However, their use in patients who suffer from nervousness, irritability or insomnia should be restricted.

Restriction of Salt. The evidence that restriction of salt intake is beneficial to patients who have essential hypertension, as well as other forms of cardiovascular renal disease, is not new and appears to have arisen as the result of the report of Ambard and Beaujard[147] in 1904. In 1922, Allen and Sherrill[148] found that diets sharply restricted in salt were effective in lowering the blood pressure of some hypertensive patients. As were Ambard and Beaujard and others, Allen and Sherrill were initially of the opinion that restriction of chloride rather than sodium was the effective feature of a low-salt regimen.

The introduction by Kempner in 1944[149] of the rice-fruit diet constituted one of the major and heroic attempts at control of essential hypertension by dietary means. This diet, made up solely of rice, fruit and fruit juice, provides approximately 20 gm of protein per day; it contains no protein

of animal origin and approximately 0.2 gm of sodium per day. Kempner[150,151] observed objective improvement in almost two-thirds of 500 patients; this improvement was evidence of significant decrease in blood pressure, reduction in cardiac size, reversal of abnormal electrocardiographic patterns, return to normal or near normal values for urea and other retained metabolites in the blood and regression of characteristic hypertensive changes in the ocular fundi. The clinical trial of the British Medical Research Council in 1950 completely confirmed Kempner's studies,[152] but indicated that it was the sodium content of the diet which was effective.

Grollman and his associates[153] observed a striking decrease in the blood pressure of six patients who had essential hypertension and who were treated with a diet more liberal than the rice-fruit diet which provided less than 0.5 gm of sodium (1.3 gm of sodium chloride) daily. They considered the basis for the success of this form of treatment to be the drastic restriction of sodium chloride in the diet and stated that moderate rather than drastic restriction of sodium in the diet may account for many of the therapeutic failures reported. This point of view has been generally accepted and has led to avoidance of the severe protein restriction of the Kempner diet. However, reduction of sodium in the diet to 0.5 gm per day has been difficult and expensive to achieve in the individual patient living in industrialized societies.

The development of potent antihypertensive drugs and particularly natriuretic diuretic agents has revolutionized the treatment of established severe hypertension. Rigid dietary sodium restriction (less than 0.2 gm per day) is hardly ever used. It is essential to remember, nevertheless, that the effectiveness of these drugs is considerably enhanced by moderate restriction of sodium while chronic depletion of potassium (which the diuretic natriuretic agents produce) is likely to be aggravated by consuming modern diets high in salt. Therefore, in most hypertensive patients and in the absence of heart failure, the amount of sodium chloride permitted in the diet should range from 2.0 to 3.5 gm daily (see Appendix Tables A–13, A–14). The appearance of hypotensive reactions is an indication for reduction in the dosage of one or more of the drugs rather than for an increase in the salt intake. Foods high in potassium (Appendix Table A–16) should be prescribed. Potassium supplements are often necessary as part of the regimen when diuretic drugs are used continuously, particularly if the baseline potassium (pretreatment serum K) cannot be maintained. A drop in serum potassium is evidence of depletion of total body potassium. However, a high-potassium intake is dangerous when a potassium-sparing diuretic (e.g. triamterene) is used.

When a decision is made to use diets low in salt, the same advice and the same mode of education and control should be provided for those patients with established hypertension, be it mild, moderate or severe, as for those on the preventive dietary regimens described above.

Appropriate sodium restriction assists greatly in control of blood pressure in renal disease and hypertension. However, when patients have renal failure, particular care must be given to avoid sodium restriction so severe as to cause gross depletion of extracellular volume. It is critical that blood pressure not be decreased too severely as this can cause further renal insufficiency. In advanced renal failure, control of blood pressure may need to be sacrificed in favor of expansion of plasma volume to increase glomerular filtration and avoid damage to target organs. Such hypertension should be permitted only long enough to establish dialysis or transplantation if the patient is a candidate for such a program. A number of patients with advanced renal disease and hypertension may require bilateral nephrectomy and

maintenance on chronic dialysis. In such nephrectomized patients, significant correlation between total exchangeable body salt and blood pressure in the renoprival state has been reported. Salt intake is important in maintenance of acceptable blood pressures.

PREECLAMPSIA OF PREGNANCY

The toxemias of pregnancy (which include preeclampsia and eclampsia) continue to be controversial.[154a,154b] Their causes and mechanisms are obscure. Prevention and treatment are largely empiric and etiologies are uncertain. They continue to be diseases of theories. Hypertension, proteinuria and edema are the cardinal clinical features of preeclampsia of pregnancy in which the glomeruli are enlarged, swollen and ischemic. Edema of the cells of the glomerular tufts is the most prominent pathologic feature, and the glomerular change is widespread through the kidney, all glomeruli being equally affected.

The presence of fibrin, IgM, C_3 and other plasma components can be found by immunofluorescence in the glomerular tufts of some patients with preeclampsia-eclampsia. Exactly what this means is controversial.[154b] It is probably an epiphenomenon. In some cases, the pathogenetic consequences may be clinically and histologically irreversible. One the other hand, the uncomplicated glomerular lesions of preeclampsia-eclampsia are reversible.

Clinically, the unusual spasm of the retinal arteries and the increase in the level of the serum uric acid are valuable criteria for distinguishing preeclampsia from hypertensive vascular disease in pregnancy.

The clinical pattern and the geographic distribution of preeclampsia are similar to primary nutritional disorders, particularly pellagra. Epidemic outbreaks occur in various parts of the world. The disease is endemic in some areas, and the sporadic cases which we see in large cities tend to appear in the poor and the ignorant and in those whose nutrition has been disturbed by food fads or for other reasons. Theobald[154c] was among the first to draw attention to its peculiar geographic distribution and to relate its appearance to nutritional factors. He recalls that when he was in charge of the largest obstetric service in Bangkok, Thailand, he saw only 8 cases of eclampsia from 1926 to 1929. When he moved to Ceylon, the situation was quite different. The incidence there was 28 per thousand live births, probably the highest in the world. On returning to Great Britain, he found that the mortality rates were higher in Scotland than in Wales. He also noted that the incidence of eclampsia doubled in Hong Kong during 1941 when gross malnutrition was rife as a result of the war. On the other hand, preeclampsia increased in Belgium and Holland after their liberation from German occupation, at a time when food became more plentiful.

There is a marked variation in the incidence of preeclampsia in different areas of South Africa.[155] In Cape Town, where four groups of people live under distinct social and economic conditions, eclampsia is common in the Cape Malays and less common among Bantu, Cape colored and European population groups.[156] The Cape Malays are Moslems, artisans and fishermen. They are descendants of slaves brought to South Africa from Java and Malaya in the 18th century, and they have an unusual pattern of food intake[157] and characteristic methods of preparing their diet.[158]

Wachstein and others have suggested that the metabolism of vitamin B_6 is altered in pregnancy,[159] but it does not appear that a simple deficiency of this vitamin is responsible for the specific lesion of the kidney in preeclampsia. It seems more likely that the lesion may be the result of a complex metabolic disturbance involving abnormal hormone activity and an unbalanced dietary intake.

Although most investigators have felt that the disease is precipitated by excess salt consumption, this concept has not been documented. Recent reports cast grave doubt on this concept and there is a real question of efficacy, and safety, of strenuous salt restriction or diuretic therapy. Salres[160] has found that, after a control period of 10 to 12 days on a 120-mEq sodium diet, the excretion of a 25-gm sodium chloride load was identical in normal pregnant patients and preeclamptics. Schewitz[161] suggests that preeclamptics on low-salt diets are salt depleted and retain it avidly when given, accounting for the often reported decreased sodium excretion after an acute load of sodium. In normal pregnancy, renin levels are found to be very high, as are aldosterone secretion rates, suggesting to some that there is a physiologic need for sodium retention in normal pregnancy.[162] A thorough dietary investigation of salt intake early in pregnancy by Robinson[163] demonstrated a high incidence of preeclampsia in women taking small amounts of salt compared to those taking large amounts. A series of detailed studies on salt intake in pregnant rats by Pike and her colleagues[164] indicates that the physiologic disturbances in the animals on low-salt intake parallel those in pregnant women with preeclampsia. These studies strengthen the concept of chronic water intoxication as the pathophysiologic change in preeclampsia. All of these studies indicate that much work is still required to clarify the nutritional aspects of preeclampsia.

Where the disorder has appeared, the traditional therapy has been a low-salt diet, antihypertensive drugs and natriuretic agents. The evidence cited above calls into question this traditional approach. Schewitz[161] has recommended high-protein, high-vitamin and a high or, at least, unrestricted salt intake. Thiazide diuretics are not recommended. Hypertension is treated if blood pressure is above 180/120 mm Hg. Sedation and bed rest are the most important measures.

Rigid salt restriction has been associated with vascular collapse during labor or immediately after delivery. When thiazide diuretics are used, it is imperative to see that adequate amounts of potassium are given to prevent hypokalemia (3 gm of potassium chloride or its equivalent). Of great interest is the report by Perey and his colleagues[165] who have induced multiple cysts in the kidneys of fetal rabbits by producing potassium deficiency in the pregnant does. If this work is confirmed, it may well have fundamental bearing on the problem of congenital renal disease in man.

There is no deficiency of magnesium in preeclamptic women. Parenteral magnesium sulfate is commonly used by obstetricians to treat preeclampsia and eclampsia. This is a pharmacologic not a nutritional usage.

ACUTE GLOMERULONEPHRITIS

Many disorders produce the classical clinical picture of acute glomerulonephritis—hematuria, edema, hypertension—and the histologic picture of proliferation of cells in the glomerulus. Among these disorders are lupus nephritis, periarteritis, Goodpasture's syndrome and many unknown causes. Most cases and most studies, however, have involved the relatively common and usually benign disease of childhood poststreptococcal glomerulonephritis. The troubling problems in hospitalized patients are usually edema, hypertension and azotemia. Massive proteinuria, acute renal failure and progression to chronic renal failure are other potential complications, but these aspects are dealt with later under separate headings.

Based on erroneous concepts of the work involved in urea excretion,[166,167] a low-protein diet had been advocated in treatment of this disease. We now know that limiting protein is of no value. Illingsworth[168] treated patients by allocating

them at random to two dietary regimens: strict protein restriction and the ordinary diet. Children were observed for a year. No advantage was detected by restricting protein. Mortensen[169] treated 44 patients with either high- or low-protein diets and evaluation after two years indicated that those on high protein did better. There is, therefore, no rationale for protein restriction in the usual care of poststreptococcal nephritis unless oliguria or renal failure develops.

Hypertension and edema are usually related to an increased body pool of sodium secondary to diminished excretion. When sodium balance is restored to normal by judicious use of diuretics or dietary restriction, hypertension and edema are much improved. While sodium restriction is not necessary in every case, those patients with problem hypertension or edema can be benefited by sodium restriction.

THE NEPHROTIC SYNDROME

The metabolic, nutritional and clinical consequences of continued massive albuminuria constitute the nephrotic syndrome. Florid cases are readily recognized from infancy to extreme old age, and the diagnosis can be confirmed rapidly in the laboratory by urinalysis and simple biochemical studies of the blood.

Biochemical Changes

The well-known metabolic hallmarks of the nephrotic syndrome are proteinuria, hypoalbuminemia and hypercholesterolemia,[170] but the full-blown picture presents many more biochemical aberrations than this. Albumin is the major protein lost in the urine, accounting for approximately 70 per cent of the total. As can be seen from Table 33–5, other nutritionally important plasma proteins, such as ceruloplasmin, also run to waste in the urine. The continued drain of proteins in the urine compromises the tissue and cellular stores of protein, and the clinical consequences of this impoverishment are tis-

Table 33–5. Some Biochemical Changes in the Urine of Patients with the Nephrotic Syndrome

Increased	Decreased	Variable
Albumin	Sodium	Glucose
Alpha globulin	Chloride	Potassium
Beta globulin		Amino acids
Gamma globulin		Nitrogen
Protein-bound iodine		
Ceruloplasmin		
Siderophilin		
Antidiuretic substance		
Complement		
Prothrombin		
Antithrombin		
Proconvertin		

Table 34–6. Some Biochemical Changes in the Blood of Patients with the Nephrotic Syndrome

Increased	Decreased	Variable
Total lipid	Albumin	Alpha globulin
Triglycerides	Protein-bound iodine	Gamma globulin
Phospholipids	Siderophilin	Alpha lipoprotein
Free cholesterol	Ceruloplasmin	Sodium
Cholesterol esters	Complement	Chloride
Beta lipoprotein	Osmotic pressure	Calcium
Alpha globulin	Plasma volume	
Beta globulin		
Fibrinogen		
Cholinesterase		
Aldosterone		

sue wastage, malnutrition, fatty metamorphosis of the liver, sodium retention, decreased resistance to infections and edema.[171] Depletion of complement and immunoglobulins makes the nephrotic patient particularly susceptible to infection, and loss of specialized proteins, such as those which bind thyroid hormone and iron, explains the apparent hypothyroidism and tendency to anemia. More difficult to explain is the marked increase in circulating serum lipids and relatively large plasma proteins such as cholinesterase and fibrinogen[172] (Table 33–6).

These changes may develop as a result of disturbance in the transport of fats, or they may be the result of some as yet unidentified mechanism. The metabolic changes seen in the nephrotic syndrome appear to be the result of increased hepatic synthesis of protein and fats,[173] called forth by depletion of hepatic albumin and made evident by the retention of large protein molecules in the blood stream and the loss of the small ones in the urine. Studies on nephrotic rats and man have clearly demonstrated that infusion of large amounts of serum albumin can restore both the protein and the lipid abnormalities in the plasma to normal.[174] Massive loss of albumin in the urine is not invariably accompanied by all the clinical or biochemical stigmata of the nephrotic syndrome. The loss of protein may not be sufficient to overwhelm the body's homeostatic mechanisms and clinical edema may never appear. These patients with subclinical forms feel well and rarely appear in the clinic unless proteinuria is detected on routine examination. In other formes frustes the serum lipid levels are normal or decreased in amount.

Treatment

The causes of nephrotic syndrome are legion. In some cases specific therapy can be directed at a specific etiologic course. In many instances, there may be no known specific treatment. Nevertheless, general principles of treatment, especially dietotherapy, are available and essential to the well-being of the patient. There is much that can be done to alleviate the conditions of edema, protein malnutrition and hyperlipidemia.

Sodium Intake. Salt restriction is one of the most important of the measures designed to prevent edema and to initiate diuresis; while low-salt diets are widely prescribed, little attention is paid by many clinicians to ensuring that these are sufficiently low in sodium. An intake of less than 10 mEq per day (580 mg sodium chloride) almost always prevents the accumulation of edema and will often start a diuresis, even without other forms of therapy. Limitation of salt intake to this level is now relatively easy with low-sodium milk powders or low-sodium fresh milk. Sodium retention and positive sodium balance are evidenced by the very low urinary excretion of sodium—in the untreated nephrotic, it will often be less than 10 to 20 mEq daily. The mechanism of this avid sodium retention is multifactorial but disturbed renal hemodynamics and hormonal changes play a prominent role. Massive loss of albumin diminishes plasma oncotic pressure and will lead to interstitial fluid accumulation. Intravascular plasma volume may fall with reduction in renal blood flow. Alterations in renal hemodynamics lead to increased renal renin production and inevitably to increased adrenal aldosterone production. The end-results are enhanced tubular reabsorption of sodium and eventually clinically apparent edema.

Low-sodium diets are essential to prevent the continuing accumulation of salt and water. Diuretics are useful in promoting a natriuresis to restore sodium balance to normal. A variety of diuretic agents are now available which differ in mode of action and efficiency. Since most nephrotics exhibit hyperaldosteronism, spironolactone (an aldosterone blocking agent) is frequently effective in maintaining a natriuresis. Other groups of diuretics will enhance potassium loss and potassium deficiency and must be guarded against.

Once patients have responded to diuretics, the patient is edema free and sodium balance is achieved, modest amounts of sodium (20 to 60 mEq per day) may be added to diets to make meals more palatable. Adjustments in dosage of diuretics may be necessary to prevent recurrence of edema. It should be noted that the use of low-sodium diets and diuretics to relieve or prevent edema does not affect the underlying kidney abnormality per se. As mentioned previously, the renal disturbance may not be amenable to specific therapy. Where it is not, adherence to measures outlined above is essential to keep the nephrotic free of salt and water abnormalities.

Protein Intake. The level of protein intake required by these patients has been the cause of much argument. High-protein diets of 150 gm per day or more have been employed with considerable success to maintain serum albumin levels. A rise in the urinary protein loss has been observed on such diets and some have interpreted this as deterioration in the renal condition. On the basis of animal studies, it was also argued that high-protein diets were undesirable as the prognosis in nephrotoxic serum nephritis was worse when high-protein diets were given. Also, the kidney was said to be required to do more "work" in excreting the additional urea load. Neither of these hypotheses is tenable, as it has been shown that increased proteinuria is to be expected with small rises of serum proteins and, as discussed previously, the work load caused by the excretion of urea is a very small fraction of that required by other tubular secretory processes in the kidney either normally or in the nephrotic syndrome.

The demonstration on high-protein diets of prolonged positive nitrogen balances, at times amounting to 500 gm nitrogen in some patients with proteinuria of many months' duration, suggests the presence of a severe body deficit of protein, of which the reduced serum proteins are only one manifestation. In adult patients, no maximal level of protein intake could be observed other than that set by the patient's appetite, and positive nitrogen balances were recorded with protein intakes ranging from 65 to 200 gm, higher intakes leading to higher positive balances. Since this body nitrogen deficit seems of fundamental importance in the patient with prolonged proteinuria, it would appear advisable to replace protein as rapidly as possible; in practice, it had been found that intakes of 120 gm per day for the average adult, with high-calorie intakes (50 to 60 kcal per kg), have provided satisfactory repletion without unpalatable diets. Higher levels may be obtained on occasion with tube feeding, and there seems to be no contraindication to their use (see Appendix). A variety of high-protein supplements are available commercially. In selected cases, these supplements are more easily tolerated than high-protein diets. It is, of course, essential to ensure that patients actually take such diets; too often, high-protein, high-caloric diets are advised but not consumed. The poor appetite of the edematous patient requires constant supervision and coaxing to ensure that adequate intakes are obtained. Where

renal impairment restricts excretion of urea and other nitrogenous products, appropriate limitation of protein and a balance between protein nutrition and nitrogen retention must be consistent with the patient's clinical state.

Mineral Intake. In some patients with severe and prolonged nephrotic syndrome deficiencies of calcium and potassium may appear as clinical symptoms. Bone pain and bone rarefaction may occur; myopathy and myalgias may reflect potassium depletion. Kaliopenic nephropathy (discussed below) may complicate the kidney problem. Avioli[62] has demonstrated the urinary loss of vitamin D metabolites in proteinuric states. What role this plays in calcium deficiency is not, as yet, certain. Fortunately, these complications are uncommon and diets with adequate calcium and potassium prevent them.

Hyperlipidemia

The nephrotic syndrome is characterized by high serum cholesterol levels, as well as phospholipids and triglycerides. Although the pathophysiologic mechanisms of hyperlipidemia are not completely understood, increased synthesis of lipoproteins by the liver is considered to be the source. There is, however, evidence that suggests abnormalities in lipoprotein lipase activity as well. Decreased postheparin lipoprotein lipase activity has been reported in nephrotic children.[175]

In a study of 96 adult nephrotic patients, Newmark et al.[176] studied lipoproteins and lipoprotein profiles. Ratios of serum cholesterol to serum albumin, serum triglycerides to serum albumin and 24-hour urinary protein loss to serum albumin were all significantly inversely correlated. All lipoprotein types except type 1 were found. The profiles fell into three nearly equal groups—11a, 11b and V. Type IV abnormality, the most common abnormality in uremia, was uncommon.

Berlyne[60] has observed that nephrotics have an increased incidence of coronary artery disease and deaths. This increased incidence suggests that the lipid abnormalities play a role in accelerated atherosclerosis in these patients. Measures to decrease hyperlipidemia are advised.

ACUTE RENAL FAILURE

The causes of oliguria or anuria are legion. Acute obstruction of the urinary tract, dehydration and various types of water and electrolyte disturbance may disturb urine formation and urine flow. Insults to the body remote from the kidney, such as an acute myocardial infarct, may reduce glomerular filtration to such low levels that little or no urine is formed. Finally, nephrotoxins, parenchymatous renal disease, endotoxins, hemolytic crises, renal vascular damage and acute allergic or immunologic reactions may disturb the function of the kidney, damage its cells and produce acute renal failure.

When acute renal failure occurs the body's ability to regulate fluid and nutritional balance is profoundly disturbed, leading to disastrous effects on normal organ functions. The course of acute renal failure may be short or long and can be divided into four phases: onset, oliguric or anuric phase, diuretic phase and late recovery phase. The disorder may be mild or severe and, while the course may be predicted initially from the type of disorder which has precipitated the failure (e.g. nephrotoxins, shock, glomerulonephritis, etc.) in at least 30 per cent of cases, no clear etiology is found.[177] The slope of the daily rise in blood urea is one good index of tissue breakdown and a measure of mildness or severity of catabolism and renal failure.

The aims of treatment are to discover the cause and deal with it (if possible), to maintain fluid, mineral and acid-base balance, to prevent uremia and, increasingly important, to maintain adequate nutritional status. The latter will promote tissue healing, resistance to infections, a sense of general well-being and general strength.

Treatment may be conservative, consisting primarily of agents to enhance renal function and urine output and dietary modifications to prevent uremia, or in more prolonged and severe cases treatment will require dialysis and intravenous or enteral alimentation.

Conservative Management

Mannitol and other diuretics may be used and can be effective in promoting adequate urine flow and function to prevent continuing rises in urea or fluid accumulation. If it is expected that the course will be a short one and uncomplicated by infection, hypercatabolism, etc., the dietary treatment is to provide adequate calories to maintain body weight and to keep endogenous protein catabolism to a minimum.[178] Minerals and fluid are given to replace continuing losses. This is done by measuring and charting, each day, the total fluid output from dejecta (urine, stool, drains, fistulas, vomitus, etc.). The next day, the patient is given the amount of fluid and minerals contained in those fluids (these can be measured or found in a standard reference). An additional 300 to 500 ml of water are allowed, which with the water of metabolism and release of tissue water from some endogenous protein catabolism will balance insensible water loss. Adjustments for fever must be taken into consideration. As a further control, the patient can be weighed daily and he should lose 0.25 to 0.5 kg per day. Greater weight losses suggest inadequate fluid administration or hypercatabolism. An increasing weight indicates overhydration.

Adequate calorie intake is primarily aimed to minimize endogenous protein breakdown (and consequent uremia) while the kidney repairs itself. There are clearcut data that intakes of at least 100 gm carbohydrate must be consumed to achieve some protection. There is, in addition, data that suggests that increased intakes up to 3,000 calories from carbohydrate sources may even further prevent nitrogen wastage.[179]

The main problem in conservative therapy is delivering enough calories with a limited fluid volume. In times past, patients have been given oral mixtures of oil, glucose and vitamins but these were often poorly tolerated and caused increased nausea and vomiting. Dietitians now, with the availability of high-calorie nonprotein supplements and with creative imaginations, can usually deliver 600 to 2500 calories in a palatable form. In difficult cases, it is preferable to go to parenteral or enteral feedings than to allow a patient to become malnourished. The emergence of crystalline amino acid solutions, elemental diets and intravenous fat emulsions has greatly benefited nutritional care of many patients, including those in acute renal failure.

Abel et al.[180,182] have demonstrated the efficiency of essential amino acid and hypertonic glucose solutions (delivered via central venous catheter) in maintaining adequate nutritional status in acute renal failure. Balance studies have shown that patients can be maintained in positive nitrogen balance without increasing urea nitrogen levels. In addition, utilization of nutrients and promotion of anabolism are associated with intracellular potassium and phosphorus shift, reducing hazards of hyperkalemia and calcium/phosphorus imbalances. Dialytic intervention can be reduced by such techniques. There is even the suggestion, which needs further confirmation, that recovery of renal function may be enhanced by such nutritive therapy. The ability to provide adequate calories by peripheral intravenous lipid emulsions in small volumes is beneficial in reducing the risk involved with central venous catheter feedings. Enteral feedings with amino acid and calorie sources are equally useful when adequate gastrointestinal function is assured.

The field of parenteral and enteral nutrition is expanding with new formulas and widening of applications. As discussed in more detail under chronic renal failure, the use of enteral or parenteral keto-analogs of essential amino acids may permit maintenance by protein and nitrogen balance with a virtually nitrogen-free diet in renal failure. When the requirements for fluid and nutritional support exceed the kidney's ability to maintain the patient free of overhydration or uremia, dialytic measures (hemodialysis or peritoneal dialysis) should be instituted before the patient deteriorates.

Potassium

A special note of caution is necessary regarding potassium intoxication in acute renal failure. Potassium is released into the blood stream from pus, pockets of blood, hemolysis, dead and dying tissue and, unfortunately, from inadvertent administration. The effects of hyperkalemia on the myocardium are aggravated in acute renal failure by other factors such as hypocalcemia, acidosis and hyponatremia. The net effect of hyperkalemia may be a life-threatening—indeed fatal—cardiac catastrophe. It is also vital to recall that the electrocardiogram does not always reflect the level of hyperkalemia. Serial measurements of serum potassium and vigilant monitoring of cardiac function are essential to avoiding an unnecessary death. The emergency treatment of severe hyperkalemia can be found in many references.

CHRONIC RENAL FAILURE

In patients with chronic renal failure, few functioning nephrons remain. These are usually hypertrophied and functioning at the upper limits of their activity. They have little reserve left to deal efficiently with new catabolic loads which may appear as a result of infection, trauma and overenthusiastic treatment with diets and drugs. Moreover, during the slow development of chronic renal failure, the cells of the body are bathed in an abnormal fluid and, in many cases, appear to have come into a new homeostatic equilibrium with the altered humoral environment. It is important to recognize that changing personally established patterns of fluid intake and diet (which often occur when these patients are admitted to the hospital for any cause) may do more harm than good. Under these circumstances, establishing new dietary regimens—if this is what the physician wants to do—must be done cautiously and with circumspection.

The interests of nutrition and chronic renal failure conflict. Good nutrition requires a liberal intake of calories, proteins, minerals and vitamins. Renal failure, however, prevents the excretion of excesses or by-products of such a nutritious diet. In addition, chronic renal failure may alter the normal handling of elements in the diet or, parodoxically, may even result in excess loss of some elements. In essence, however, uremia is the poisoning of the body by retention of its own nutritional excesses or metabolites. The blood with elements not kept within reasonable limits by the kidneys is "spoiled," therefore, of its purpose of nutrition.

Chronic renal failure patients are, as a group, malnourished. To what extent poor nutrition is secondary to retention of toxins or to what extent to inadequate diet is not fully resolved. Disturbances in metabolism of all major nutrient groups are found in chronic renal failure. We shall consider these in more detail below.

Metabolism in Renal Failure

Protein. Urea is a major end-product of protein metabolism and has for decades been the principally measured index of renal failure. The accumulation of urea, which of itself may not be toxic, is accompanied by other toxic by-products of altered protein metabolism. Guanidine derivatives interfere with platelet function and contribute to bleeding disorders in uremia. Phenolic acids and other organic acids accumulate and are reported to disturb hematologic functions. Much research is currently under way into identification of so-called middle molecules—some of which appear to be small peptide groups—which are felt to contribute to neurologic, hematologic and cardiac abnormalities in uremia.

Early treatment methods concerned themselves principally with restriction of protein intake in efforts to diminish retention of toxic products. The absolute minimal protein requirement for normal man is about 0.23 gm per kg per day of high-quality protein in order to maintain nitrogen balance.[183] Kempner was able to maintain nitrogen balance in hypertension patients with a rice diet containing 0.25 gm of protein per kg per day. It was from such studies that the impression was obtained that the optimum intake of protein for renal failure patients should be about 20 gm per day (0.28 gm per kg per day for a 70-kg man). Giordano,[184,185] Giovannetti[186] and others[187-189] popularized the concept of providing minimum requirements with protein of high biologic value and adequate calories. In this way, daily requirements of essential amino acids were provided with a minimum of nonessential nitrogen. Nitrogen balance could be maintained and urea accumulation (and inferentially other toxic products) would be minimized. Such diet therapy was successful in alleviating symptoms and prolonging life. These results, however, were overshadowed in many instances by the resultant malnutrition which occurred with stringent minimal protein diets.

It has been shown that chronic renal failure patients need more protein to maintain nitrogen balance. The results of many studies show that a total protein intake of less than 0.4 gm per kg per day is associated with an initial negative nitrogen balance which remains negative for many months.[190]

The efficiency of low-protein diets rests on the ability of the body to synthesize nonessential amino acids from endogenous carbon and nitrogen sources. Urea had for many years been considered an inert end-product of protein metabolism. Hydrolysis of urea to ammonia and carbon dioxide by rumen bacteria is a well-known physiologic fact. We now know urea is metabolized by nonruminants as well, that the hydrolysis takes place in the gut (principally the colon) and that bacterial ureases are responsible for splitting urea. This potential mechanism for reutilization of urea nitrogen exists in man. Many investigators have demonstrated the mechanisms which regulate hydrolysis, reabsorption and reutilization of the urea-derived nitrogen.[191,192] Richards et al.[193] have clearly demonstrated the utilization of gut-absorbed urea-derived nitrogen for synthesis of body protein.

The basic mechanism for synthesis of nonessential amino acids is through transamination of a keto acid precursor of the amino acid: the keto acid loses its oxygen and picks up an amino group (NH_2) and thus becomes an amino acid (e.g. alpha-ketoglutarate + $NH_3 \longrightarrow$ glutamic acid). The carbon precursors of the *nonessential* amino acids are abundant and widely available from carbohydrate metabolic pathways in man. The transaminases capable of the conversion of the precursors into their analog amino acids are present in liver, kidney and muscle.[194,195] The carbon skeletons of *essential* amino acids are more complicated structures and are not available from endogenous carbohydrate metabolic pathways. Rose[196] speculated forty years ago that the carbon skeletons were the essential parts of essential amino acids. This implied that, given the appropriate precursor, the human ought to be able to manufacture the essential amino acid by transamination reactions.

It has been clearly demonstrated[197–201] that all precursor keto acids and amino acids (except lysine and threonine) can participate in this type of recycling, called transamination, whereby a keto acid becomes an amino acid. The process is reversible so that amino acids can become donors of the amino group as well. The process by which amino groups can be passed back and forth appears to have evolved as a way of adjusting the proportions of free amino acids to the body's needs; amino acids in demand are manufactured preferentially to those that are not. Several nonessential amino acids, notably glutamine, alanine and glutamic acid, tend to participate in transamination reactions as amino group donors. By contrast, essential amino acids are more likely to be amino group receivers, although in certain instances they can also function as amino group donors. These transamination reactions and the utilization of urea-derived nitrogen are enhanced when dietary protein intake is restricted.

These observations implied that a uremic patient given the appropriate precursor such as the keto acid or alpha-hydroxy acid analog, ought to be able to manufacture essential amino acids. That this is so has been demonstrated for all the essential amino acids (except lysine and threonine) in uremic man.[202,203] The uremic patient can be maintained in nitrogen balance with stable urea levels on keto acid diets, given orally or intravenously. The use of keto acid precursors meets the protein requirements of the body with essentially nitrogen-free compounds. Since proteins are in essence nitrogenous compounds, this appears, at first sight, a contradiction. As we have seen, however, the essentiality of the amino acids is related to the carbon skeletons and not to the amino groups. These recent discoveries raise the future possibilities of maintaining adequate protein nutrition in the renal failure patient with essentially nitrogen-free diets or supplements. Since many renal failure patients may not be amenable to dialysis or transplantation and since improved dietary management can offer large numbers of patients important benefits at less expense and discomfort, the applications of these principles have tremendous potential.[204–207]

Plasma amino acid levels and patterns are abnormal in renal failure. The metabolism of phenylalanine and histidine is altered. Phenylalanine hydroxylase activity is deficient and less phenylalanine is converted to tyrosine. Interference with histidine metabolism results in low histidine levels so that histidine becomes an essential amino acid in uremia. Indeed, recent studies have suggested that histidine may, in fact, be an essential amino acid for the normal as well as the uremic man. Supplementation of histidine to uremics has been associated with increased hemoglobin production and improved nitrogen balances. There is thus accumulating evidence that amino acid metabolism and protein synthesis are altered in renal failure. We do not yet know the mechanisms (e.g. toxin inhibition, lack of precursors or vital coelements, etc.) which are responsible for these alterations. There is little question that much yet must be learned about protein metabolism in uremia.

On a practical note, some basic rules must be remembered. Dietary restriction too soon and too drastic will inevitably lead to a protein-malnourished renal failure patient who has little tolerance to the complications which can beset him. Once it is necessary to restrict a patient's diet to 40 or 50 gm protein to prevent clinical uremia, other long-term programs, i.e. dialysis and transplantation, must be considered.

Carbohydrate. Abnormal carbohydrate metabolism in uremia has been recognized for many years and has been recently reviewed.[49] Fasting blood sugars may be elevated but the abnormality is more evident on oral glucose tolerance testing. There are elevated peak glucose levels with delay in return to normal or fasting levels. The presence of peripheral insulin antagonism in uremia appears well founded. Although precise mechanisms are not yet elucidated, dialysis appears to improve peripheral insulin responsiveness, suggesting a dialyzable antagonist. Plasma insulin response to

oral and intravenous glucose varies widely in uremia; investigators have found normal, decreased and increased insulin response to glucose loads. Most studies agree that fasting and late insulin levels are elevated along with elevated glucose levels in many cases, again indicating a resistance to the peripheral action of insulin. Other hormonal factors (e.g. glucagon, growth hormone) and potassium metabolism also play roles in glucose metabolism in the uremic.

The kidneys also play a major role in the disordered insulin metabolism in uremia.[48] The normal kidney extracts and degrades 30 to 40 per cent of the insulin carried to it. Severe kidney disease markedly reduces renal insulin extraction, prolongs its half-life and decreases its metabolic clearance rate. These abnormalities, in part, explain the hyperinsulinemia in uremic patients and the decreased insulin requirements of diabetics who develop renal failure.

In summary, glucose intolerance occurs in well over 50 per cent of chronic renal failure patients. Many factors contribute to this abnormality; chronic dialysis can partially correct the glucose intolerance. Abnormally high insulin levels are commonly found and may contribute to hyperlipidemia, another frequently observed abnormality in uremics.

Lipid. The hyperlipidemia that accompanies renal disease without the nephrotic syndrome has been well documented.[53,54] In contrast to the hypercholesterolemia commonly observed in nephrotic syndrome, renal failure is characterized by elevated plasma triglyceride levels and only infrequently by high cholesterol. Lipoprotein electrophoresis usually shows high plasma levels of very-low-density lipoproteins, characteristic of type IV hyperlipidemia.[56] Lipid abnormalities are present in at least 50 per cent of uremic patients and appears to be exaggerated with chronic dialysis.

Two mechanisms appear to be responsible for the phenomenon.[56] Excessive hepatic triglyceride synthesis has been found and appears correlated to the hyperinsulinemia. Other studies have supported the thesis of deficient lipolysis in uremics. Diminished post-heparin plasma lipolytic activity and reduced adipose tissue lipoprotein lipase activity and triglyceride turnover have been described. The lipid abnormalities of uremics may play a significant role in the accelerated atherosclerosis which occurs in patients on maintenance dialysis.[208] Cardiovascular disease causes at least 50 per cent of deaths in these patients and is a critical determinant of the long-term prognosis of dialyzed patients. Since many other risk factors are also involved (e.g. hypertension, glucose intolerance, hyperuricemia, etc.), the role of lipid abnormalities is difficult to determine and additional studies are needed. Dietary modifications may be important in improving these abnormalities, as has recently been reported.[209]

Vitamins. Deficiencies of water-soluble vitamins may occur in uremic patients because limitations on protein and minerals result in consumption of a vitamin-deficient diet. The uremic state may also alter the excretion or metabolism of vitamins, resulting in functional deficiencies. In addition, the use of dialysis will increase losses of many vitamins, as discussed further below. Folic acid deficiency has been found in undialyzed uremic patients.[210] Although low vitamin C levels have been found in dialyzed patients,[211] no data concerning nondialyzed patients are available. No clinical deficiency of thiamin, riboflavin, nicotinic acid, pantothenic acid or biotin have been reported in the nondialyzed uremic.

Pyridoxine deficiency has been found with regularity in both dialyzed and nondialyzed uremics.[212,213] Based on erythrocyte glutamine oxaloacetic transaminase (SGOT) determinations, as many as 70 per cent of uremics may have B_6 deficiency. Inhibition of pyridoxal kinase activity by uremic toxins, rather than insufficient supply, appears to be the primary factor. Many of the symptoms common to uremia are those found in severe B_6 deficiency. Since B_6 impairs cellular and humoral immune responses, it may play a significant role in altered host resistance in uremia. Daily pyridoxine supplements can prevent the reduction of erythrocyte SGOT activity.

Recent advances in understanding of the metabolism of vitamin D and the discovery that the kidney is responsible for conversion of vitamin D to its biologically active metabolite, 1,25 dihydroxycholecalciferol, has greatly clarified the role of vitamin D in renal failure.[61] The primary physiologic action of vitamin D is maintenance of normal blood calcium levels. This is accomplished by stimulating intestinal absorption of calcium and potentiating the action of parathyroid hormone on calcium mobilization from bone. Deficiency of the active form of vitamin D in uremia is now well documented and explains the long-recognized findings of decreased calcium absorption and osteomalacia of uremia. We now also know that PTH is intricately involved in the renal conversion of 25-hydroxycholecalciferol into active or inactive metabolites. Trials with active vitamin D metabolites have demonstrated their efficacy in increasing calcium absorption and in repairing osteodystrophy.[214-216] The prospects for commercially available active vitamin D metabolites are promising and will do much to improve the abnormalities in uremia.

No abnormalities of vitamin E or K in uremia have been reported.

Sodium. With regard to nutrition, at present, the major error perpetrated by the practitioner in dietary care of the uremic patient is to prescribe a diet too low in sodium. Many patients with chronic renal failure do not retain sodium and, in fact, some waste salt excessively in the urine. This occurs particularly in cystic disease of the medulla and in chronic pyelonephritis, but is not uncommon in any form of chronic renal failure. There-fore, a common dietary complication seen in hospital is a low-salt syndrome from diets, diuretics, diarrhea, vomiting and the misguided use of intravenous fluids which are low in sodium or, perhaps, contain no electrolytes. Most of these patients need 80 to 100 mEq of sodium each day, and some may require massive amounts. This re-quirement can be determined by mea-surement of 24-hour urinary electrolyte output.

Potassium. Potassium retention is not an early problem in chronic renal failure. Only in severe end-stage failure is excre-tion of potassium unable to prevent hyperkalemia. When hyperkalemia exists before this stage, the likely causes are ex-cesses of potassium-containing foods or potassium-containing drugs (including salt substitutes which are mainly potassium salts) or potassium-retaining medications (e.g. spironolactone). Excessive potassium loss is a rare occurrence in renal failure.

When potassium retention is a problem, in addition to reduction in intake by re-striction of potassium-containing foods or-ally administered ion exchange resins are helpful. Such resins exchange one cation (typically sodium) for potassium and in certain instances the cation gained may be inappropriate and lead to further compli-cations, however.

Calcium/Phosphate. Calcium/phospho-rus abnormalities and bone disease are very common in chronic renal failure but the symptoms are not specific. As noted above, disturbed vitamin D metabolism plays an important role in the genesis of some of these abnormalities. We also have much data regarding the role of phosphate retention and PTH-related osteodystrophy (i.e. osteitis fibrosa cystica). Of central im-portance to this form of osteodystrophy are phosphate intake and phosphate reten-tion. Bricker[217] has described a "trade-off hypothesis" as the pathogenesis of second-ary hyperparathyroidism in the uremic pa-tient. As nephron damage occurs,

glomerular filtration rate falls. Phosphate is retained with elevation of serum phos-phate. A reciprocal fall in serum calcium occurs which stimulates secretion of PTH which causes renal tubular cells to promote excretion of phosphate and to normalize serum phosphate and calcium. Phosphate and calcium are maintained at normal levels as a trade-off for continued high PTH levels. Each time GFR falls, there is repetition of this sequence of events. Thus, the level of PTH rises progressively throughout the history of chronic renal disease if the phosphate intake is not di-minished.

As the disease advances, a point is reached (usually when the GFR has fallen to 20 to 30 per cent of normal) where maximal phosphate excretion is not sufficient to maintain normal serum phos-phate levels. Persistent hyperphos-phatemia and hypocalcemia result. PTH secretion may be further stimulated and extremely high levels, with resultant os-teitis fibrosa cystica, may occur. Increased PTH levels have been found in early renal failure and extremely high levels have been reported in severe renal failure.[218,219] Human and animal investigations have shown that, if phosphate intake is reduced commensurately with reduction in GFR, hyperphosphatemia does not occur and PTH levels do not increase.[220,221] Of course, at whatever stage in the disease, if vitamin D resistance occurs, with reduced intestinal absorption of calcium this will also contribute to the genesis of osteodys-trophy. Chronic metabolic acidosis is asso-ciated with demineralization of bone and can be an additional factor.[222]

Treatment of Osteodystrophy

Prevention and management of uremic bone disease can be successful only with full knowledge of the clinical condition, metabolic balances and bone pathology. Calcium, phosphorus and alkaline phos-phatase levels and x-ray films of bones are used as guides. The goal is to try to maintain levels of calcium and phosphate as near normal as possible, while maintaining acid-base balance and clinical well-being, thereby preserving the skeleton and preventing extraosseous calcification. Hyperphosphatemia can be prevented by reducing phosphate in diets or by reduction of absorption of phosphate with phosphate-binding antacids. Calcium intake should be generous (at least 500 mg per day) and, since many foods contain phosphate as well as calcium, calcium may be supplied as the carbonate, lactate or gluconate.

Vitamin D therapy should be restricted to patients with proven osteomalacic features. In such patients, the dosage required may vary widely. The initial dose may be 10,000 to 50,000 units daily and slowly increased if no response is apparent in a month; occasionally 10 to 50 times the usual doses are required. Careful monitoring of calcium, phosphate and alkaline phosphatase is required. It may take a year or more before healing occurs. The action of vitamin D is prolonged, and, to prevent vitamin D intoxication, reduction of dosage should be considered when improvement appears. Active vitamin D metabolites, particularly 1 α hydroxy cholecalciferol and the 1,25 dihydroxy form, are available and offer great promise for the future.

When osteitis fibrosa is present and the serum calcium $\times$ phosphorus product is above 75, vitamin D should not be used. Such patients may require subtotal parathyroidectomy for control of symptoms. The exact indications are yet unsettled, but, with newer techniques of directly measuring PTH levels and the response to dietary and drug therapy, it may soon be possible to select patients on a rational basis.

Dialysis and Nutrition

Dialytic therapy, peritoneal or hemodialysis, acute or chronic, has now become commonplace in the treatment of severe renal failure. Thousands of patients now undergo regular hemodialysis on a long-term basis. The intervention of such techniques has resulted in the discovery of nutritional complications consequent to the method of therapy itself in addition to the abnormalities consequent to renal failure as discussed above. Dialysis, per se, has required modification in dietotherapy of the renal failure patient. This is so particularly because of the potential for deficiency syndromes related to nutrient losses via dialysis. If we consider that virtually all of the essential nutrients filtered through the glomerulus are normally reabsorbed by the renal tubules, while there is little effective reabsorptive capability of a dialysis machine, it is little wonder that significant amounts of water-soluble low-molecular-weight substances can be readily lost. In addition, an artificial kidney machine has no metabolic, hormonal or synthetic capability, as does a normal kidney. Thus, while dialysis, especially long-term hemodialysis, has revolutionized the care of the terminal renal failure patient, it is yet at best limited in its ability to restore or maintain ideal health and nutritional status.

Peritoneal Dialysis. The technique, indications and hazards of peritoneal dialysis are covered elsewhere[223] and will not be discussed here. Peritoneal dialysis is associated with significant loss of protein, chiefly as albumin, IgG and amino acids. The loss of protein may be as great as 20 to 60 gm, depending on the duration of dialysis.[224] In addition, Berlyne[225] has reported losses of 5 to 10 gm of amino acids during peritoneal dialysis. In the undernourished uremic patients, these losses of albumin and amino acids can result in persistent hypoproteinemia, wasting and increased susceptibility to infections. Detailed studies of plasma amino acids in such patients indicate a pattern similar to that found in patients known to have chronic protein deficiency.[226,227] The losses of proteins and amino acids should be replaced with increased dietary proteins or by parenteral plasma or amino acid solutions. It has been shown that addition of amino acids to the dialysate can reduce the loss of amino acids as well.[228]

All the B vitamins are water soluble and have molecular weights which render them dialyzable. Folic acid is also lost during peritoneal dialysis, but there is no significant loss of vitamin B_{12}, perhaps because of its tight protein binding.[229] Deficiency states attributable to loss of B complex vitamins and folic acid during peritoneal dialysis have been reported.[230] It is suggested that daily vitamin and folic acid supplements be given to patients who regularly undergo peritoneal dialysis.

Hemodialysis. Contrasted to peritoneal dialysis, very small amounts of protein are lost during hemodialysis since the large protein molecules do not pass through the dialyzer membrane. However, smaller molecules, electrolytes, vitamins, folate and amino acids pass readily through the membrane. The loss varies with type of dialyzer, various flow characteristics and other factors, but losses of free amino acids of 1.1 gm per hr and total amino acids of 3 gm per hr of dialysis have been found by Giordano.[231] Comparable or greater losses have been reported by others.[232,233]

If patients are not given supplements of high-quality protein, the nitrogen losses are not made up and patients can become progressively malnourished. Indeed, when plasma aminograms were studied in a group of chronically dialyzed, undernourished patients, a pattern similar to that found in kwashiorkor was found.[234] A number of studies have commented on the need for increased dietary nitrogen in chronically dialyzed patients.[190,233] Approximately 0.75 gm per kg per day of high-biologic-value protein is necessary to maintain nitrogen balance in anephric patients who undergo twice-weekly dialyses.

Schaeffer et al.[227] have found signs of protein malnutrition in dialysis patients who were ingesting 0.97 gm protein per kg body weight. Mean concentrations of total protein, transferrin, valine and the ratio of

essential amino acids to nonessential amino acids were significantly lower than in normal subjects. A possible reason may be that protein requirements are higher for patients on long-term dialysis. Additionally, dietary intake was variable in dialysis patients. Some patients were stable with less than 20 per cent variation in daily intake. Another group showed significantly lower intakes on dialysis days and yet another significantly higher dietary intakes on dialysis days. Signs of malnutrition occurred more frequently in the latter groups.

Intravenous supplementation of essential amino acids and histidine at the end of each hemodialysis treatment has been shown to improve serum concentrations of total protein, transferrin and components of the complement system.[233-237] The patterns of essential amino acids used were according to the data of Rose, plus histidine which has been found to be essential in uremia. Further studies are needed to determine whether such supplementation is beneficial and particularly the pattern of amino acids which is of greatest benefit.

Megaloblastic anemia with low folate levels, presumably secondary to loss of folate in the dialysate, has been reported.[238] Low B vitamin levels and ascorbic acid depletion have also been reported in dialysis patients.[239] Regular supplementation of vitamins is recommended.[240]

The loss of electrolytes is prevented by dialysis against a bath with added electrolytes. Similarly, the addition of amino acids to the bath fluid can reduce the loss of amino acids. This hardly seems practicable, however, when additional dietary protein or intravenous supplementation will do just as well.

Impairment of fat metabolism has been found in dialysis patients. Hyperlipidemias, especially hypertriglyceridemia, perhaps caused by impaired lipoprotein lipase activity, have been described. Chronic dialysis patients have been found to have higher basal insulin levels which correlate strongly with high triglyderide levels.

Bone disease is a frequent and often serious complication of chronic renal failure; it appears to be of even greater importance in patients undergoing long-term hemodialysis. Since essentially all patients receiving hemodialysis have progressed beyond the end-stage renal failure phase of their disease, the severity and duration of their uremia are, on the whole, much more severe and much longer than those with chronic renal failure who are manageable without dialysis.

The need for greater amounts of protein results in greater amounts of phsophate, and serum phosphate levels can be extremely elevated in dialysis patients. The hyperphosphatemia may be resistant to dietary measures, dialysis and phosphate-binding gels. Secondary hyperparathyroidism and manifestations of bone disease may appear and seem to increase as duration of dialysis is extended. The treatment for bone disease in dialysis patients is similar to that outlined above for chronic renal failure.

There are very little data concerning trace mineral metabolism in chronic renal failure and in dialysis patients. The data available,[241] however, suggest disturbances of magnesium, fluoride, tin, copper, cadmium, molybdenum and rubidium. The clinical importance of trace element disturbances has not yet been defined, but it is known that these elements can produce profound alterations in normal metabolic and physiologic processes.

Zinc deficiency has been suggested to exist in uremia.[241] However, since zinc is dependent in part upon the kidney for its excretion, levels may be elevated, particularly if given parenterally to azotemic patients. Zinc may play a role in taste perception and may be an important element in the altered taste threshold and anorexia common in uremia. Additional studies in mineral metabolism in uremia are needed.

Transplantation

The complete excretory, metabolic, synthetic activities of a kidney can be recovered only with an adequately functioning kidney. Successful transplantation can lead ultimately to restoration of a normal state of health if no permanent sequelae of renal failure have occurred in other organs. With an adequately functioning transplanted kidney, diet and therapy will be governed by considerations other than nitrogen retention, e.g. obesity, underweight, etc. Many transplanted kidneys, however, will suffer episodes of rejection which may sufficiently compromise the function so that restrictions of protein, salt and other minerals may again be necessary.

NUTRITION AND RENAL CALCULI

Renal calculi are a common and serious malady. They were well known to Hippocrates and Galen and the ancient Arabic physicians described instruments for breaking up stones. Nutritional factors have long been suspected in their pathogenesis and throughout the centuries various strange and expensive diets have been advised. It has been, however, only since the latter half of the 19th century, when the chemical composition of the stones became known, that serious research and a rational approach to the nature and treatment of calculus disease have been undertaken.

Renal lithiasis is not a single entity. Stones are found under a variety of conditions with many factors contributing to their formation. Extensive reviews of renal stones are available.[242,243] Three major theories of stone formation have been proposed. The precipitation-crystallization theory implies that supersaturation of urine with crystalloids leads to precipitation and crystal growth. Such a mechanism seems well supported in the formation of stones composed of uric acid and xanthine. The matrix-nucleation theory implies that some matrix substance forms an initial nucleus upon which further stone growth occurs. Matrix substance A, a urinary microprotein, has been extensively studied by Boyce,[244] but its role in stone formation is not yet clear. Since normal urine can hold larger amounts of crystalloid in solution than simple aqueous solutions, the inhibitor-absence theory has been proposed to explain stone disease, especially in patients with normal concentrations of urinary crystalloids. Despite the arguments surrounding each of these theories, the care of most patients involves a search for and treatment of increased excretion of specific urinary crystalloids.

In the United States, two-thirds of all renal stones are composed of either calcium oxalate or calcium oxalate mixed with calcium phosphate in the form of hydroxyapatite.[245] Stones composed of magnesium ammonium phosphate (struvite) account for about 15 per cent and occur almost exclusively in patients with recurrent infections. Uric acid and cystine stones together account for another 10 per cent. Approximately 10 per cent are made up of other substances or mixtures. Accumulating evidence suggests that two disorders, idiopathic hypercalciuria and hyperuricosuria, account for about 65 per cent of calcium stones.[246] These disorders and hyperoxaluria have nutritional interrelations and are discussed below.

Idiopathic Hypercalciuria

Hypercalciuria is the most frequently found metabolic abnormality in nephrolithiases. The study of renal excretion of calcium is a complex problem and involves consideration of protein binding, inhibitors, chelations, hormonal influence, relationship to other electrolytes and as yet undefined conditions. Hypercalciuria is often related to hyperparathyroidism, bone disease, ingestion of milk and alkali, sarcoidosis and renal tubular acidosis. However, the most common abnormality is idiopathic hypercalciuria, present in about 42 per cent of a series of stone-forming patients.[247]

The underlying pathogenesis of idiopathic hypercalciuria is not yet known, but most investigators attribute it to disordered renal tubular cell handling of calcium. Some alteration in handling of dietary calcium in these patients, however, has also been found. Normally, about one-third of dietary calcium is absorbed and subsequently excreted in the urine, with two-thirds excreted in fecal material. These ratios are reversed in the idiopathic hypercalciuric patient: two-thirds of dietary calcium may be absorbed and subsequently excreted in urine.[248] Urinary calcium varies over a fairly wide range on normal diets, with values of 250 mg daily for women and 300 mg daily for men considered upper normal. Values in excess of 400 mg daily are often found in idiopathic hypercalciuria. This disorder is largely confined to males. There were only 24 females in a total of 186 patients with idiopathic hypercalciuria in one series.[247]

Elevated levels of PTH in serum have been found in patients with idiopathic hypercalciuria.[249] Reversal of hypercalciuria by thiazide diuretic caused a progressive decline in PTH toward normal. Hypercalciuria is induced by furosemide, a drug known to depress calcium reabsorption. These observations support defective renal tubular calcium reabsorption as the major factor in idiopathic hypercalciuria. Increased intestinal calcium absorption is, however, also present in virtually all patients with idiopathic hypercalciuria. A primary renal tubular defect may cause an elevated PTH level that increases gastrointestinal calcium absorption either on its own or through stimulation of vitamin D activation. Intestinal hyperabsorption, however, has been documented with normal serum PTH levels.[250] Coe[246] has raised an interesting theory proposing that hypophosphatemia, which can itself stimulate renal activation of vitamin D, may be of prime importance in the generation of increased calcium absorption and hypercalciuria. Hypophosphatemia is found in idiopathic hypercalciuria and phosphate depletion causes hypercalciuria in animals and humans by reducing renal tubular calcium absorption.[251] Continued research should clarify these areas.

Clinically many patients with idiopathic hypercalciuria will normalize urinary calcium with low calcium intakes. Restriction to 250 to 400 mg calcium daily is easily achieved and usually well tolerated. When reduction of dietary calcium is not sufficient, further reduction in urinary calcium can be achieved through use of thiazide diuretics.[247] Such therapy has had great success in reducing stone episodes.

Hyperuricosuria

Hyperuricemic conditions associated with increased production of uric acid are frequently complicated by hyperuricosuria and uric acid stone disease. Approximately 25 per cent of patients with primary overproduction gouty disease have stone episodes. About 40 per cent of patients with hyperuricemia secondary to lymphoproliferative or myeloproliferative disease have uric acid stones.[243]

Other mechanisms contribute to uric acid stones. Many patients with recurrent uric acid stones have persistent acid urine which favors precipitation of uric acid.[252] An abnormality in renal tubular ammonia production has been documented in some patients. A small group of patients have neither hyperuricosuria nor any abnormality in urine acidification and continue to have stone episodes. In some patients restriction of purine-rich foods will contribute significantly to reducing hyperuricosuria. In these patients, continued restriction is advised. All patients with uric acid stone disease will benefit from raising urine pH to the range of 7.0. This is easily accomplished by regular doses of alkalinizing agents, e.g. bicarbonates or citrates.

Coe[246] has found that calcium stone formers often have concomitant hyperuricosuria; the prevalence was much greater than was hyperuricosuria in a normal population. His studies indicate that hyperuricosuria with recurrent calcium stone disease seems mainly related to diet, although overproduction may have a role in as many as 30 per cent of cases. Data suggest that sodium urate and uric acid could promote growth of calcium oxalate crystals because of certain shared interatomic dimensions. Reduction of hyperuricosuria, primarily by use of allopurinol, was associated with significant decrease in calcium stone episodes. Since most hyperuricosuric patients with calcium stones may be purine gluttons, substitution of fish, meat and poultry with starches and grains may be beneficial.

Hyperoxaluria

Oxalate is a major component of two-thirds of all kidney stones. Hyperoxaluria as a cause of renal stones is a rare event except in patients with ileal resection or bypass. Major causes of hyperoxaluria are (1) increased ingestion of oxalate or its precursor, (2) pyridoxine deficiency, (3) primary hyperoxaluria—a hereditary enzyme deficiency that exists in two forms and (4) hyperoxaluria from small bowel dysfunction.

Oxalic acid is commonly found in many green leafy vegetables, being especially high in rhubarb, spinach and asparagus. In normal persons, it is usually poorly absorbed and endogenous production of oxalate from glyoxylate metabolism is the usual source of the body pool.

Hyperoxaluria has been said to occur with ingestion of diets extremely rich in oxalates (rhubarb poisoning) but data are not well documented. Ascorbic acid in massive doses (greater that 4 gm daily) may lead to hyperoxaluria, but an instance of stone disease has not yet been reported.

Pyridoxine is an important cofactor in the metabolism of glycine-glyoxylate. Deficiencies of this vitamin have been shown, experimentally, to result in increased oxalate production and hyperoxaluria.[253] Thiamin deficiency and magnesium deficiency have also been found to be associated with hyperoxaluria.[253]

The hyperoxaluria associated with small bowel disease appears to be the most common in man. Hyperoxaluria seems to be related to specific hyperabsorption of dietary oxalates. Hyperoxaluria and stones have been reported with diseases such as regional ileitis,[254] ileal resection for a variety of reasons[255] and ileal bypass procedures for obesity.[256] The exact mechanism for enteric-related hyperoxaluria is not yet determined but recent data indicate the colon is the site of and required for increased oxalate reabsorption.[257] The degree of steatorrhea has also appeared to be related to hyperreabsorption.[258] Regardless of the mechanism, reduction of dietary oxalates appears to be of prime importance in this intriguing hyperoxaluric syndrome.

In summary, nephrolithiasis is usually a chronic condition and patients may have many recurrences throughout life. Careful evaluation will uncover a specific cause or associated metabolic abnormality in most cases. Therapeutic measures and dietary modifications as discussed above, where appropriate, are therefore part of a long-time program. Since most studies show that saturation of urine with crystalloids favors stone formation, the simple expediency of drinking copious amounts of fluid (3000 ml daily) to dilute the urine is an important aspect of all therapeutic programs. Since deficiencies of pyridoxine, magnesium and thiamin have been shown to be associated with stone formation, it is equally obvious that a well-balanced nutritionally complete diet is important.

RENAL TUBULAR DEFECTS

In 1956, Dent and his colleagues[259] described, in the Hartnup family, a hereditary pellagra-like skin rash with unusual aminoaciduria and bizarre biochemical features. They speculated that the findings might be the result of abnormal metabolism or requirements for niacin. In addition, a renal tubular defect was found which is of particular interest to us because tubular defects fail to conserve filtered nutrients and are a prime renal cause of deficiency diseases.

Fanconi first proposed the concept that a defect in the function of the tubular cells could account for the clinical syndrome which bears his name.[260] Children afflicted with this disease have a genetically inherited abnormality in which a histologic defect in the proximal tubule is associated with defective tubular reabsorption and wastage of glucose, amino acids and phosphates. The latter disturbance leads to rickets or osteomalacia (Milkman's syndrome), depending on the age of the patient.[261,262] Fanconi's name has become generally used as an eponym to describe the various types of "tubular failure," such as "the adult Fanconi syndrome" and "the secondary Fanconi syndrome" which occur in patients ill with renal disorders such as pyelonephritis or multiple myeloma. A wide variety of clinical syndromes have been described as a result of failure of the tubules to reabsorb nutrients (Table 33-7)

Table 33-7. Proximal Tubular Syndromes*

Tubular Syndromes due to Congenital Disorders

Inborn errors of metabolism with secondary tubular involvement
  Cystinosis
  Wilson's disease
  Galactosemia
  Lowe syndrome
  Hartnup syndrome
  Glycogen storage disease
Syndromes of possibly primary tubular origin
  Idiopathic de Toni-Debre-Fanconi syndrome
  Incomplete tubular syndromes
Malformation of the urinary tract associated with tubular dysfunctions

Tubular Syndromes due to Acquired Disorders

Syndromes caused by poisons and toxins (accidental and experimental)
Kidney diseases associated with tubular syndromes
Idiopathic renal tubular acidosis
  Infantile form (Lightwood)
  Late form (Butler-Albright)

*After Bickel: In *Renal Disease* (Black, ed.). Oxford, Blackwell Scientific Publications, 1962.

and further additions to the list may be anticipated. It is possible that the whole spectrum of primary nutritional diseases could be mimicked by renal wastage of specific nutrients, and it is possible that, in some instances, the inherited genes may be lethal. Proximal renal tubular defects can be classified in many ways. Often they present multiple biochemical and structural defects or a single substance (renal glycosuria; renal phosphaturia) or related substances (aminoaciduria) may be involved.

Treatment of these disorders is not satisfactory at this time and consists of attempts to restore blood levels of involved nutrients by diet or pills. For example, phosphate or potassium supplements are given if either of these nutrients is at a low level in the blood. Frequent carbohydrate feedings may be necessary in occasional patients with gross hypoglycemia and symptoms. Some patients, particularly those with phosphate diabetes, are throught to have vitamin D resistance and may respond to treatment with massive doses of the vitamin. No satisfactory dietary treatment exists for most of the genetic or hereditary forms of tubular disorders and, as yet, treatment of the secondary forms of tubular defect, such as Wilson's disease, is experimental and described elsewhere in this volume.

KALIOPENIC NEPHROPATHY

Potassium depletion produces functional and structural derangements in the kidneys of man and animals.[236,264] If the deficiency is severe in degree and prolonged in nature, the kidneys are liable to be permanently damaged. What is distressing, however, is the development of renal disease in a number of people depleted of potassium for a relatively short period of time. These individuals, as are most patients we see with potassium deficiency and healthy kidneys, are, in the main, brought to this state by the injudicious use of powerful hormones or diuretic agents. These useful and life-saving drugs produce

kaliopenia unless the physician employing them takes pains to see that the potassium lost in the urine is replaced each day by potassium-containing medicines. It is not enough to prescribe foods rich in potassium. Patients unfortunately are more impressed with drugs than diets.

Since the advent of steroid hormones such as prednisone and particularly the thiazide diuretics, kaliopenic nephropathy has become a common disorder. Previously, it was rarely seen. In fact, the relationship of renal disease to potassium depletion was not clearly recognized until 1950 when Perkins, Peterson and Riley[265] first described renal lesions in patients with potassium deficiency owing to chronic diarrhea (Table 33–8). We now recognize that potassium depletion may develop as a result of many disorders, producing either a renal or a gastrointestinal loss of the element. Pure dietary deficiency in man has been produced only experimentally,[266] but loss of appetite and other causes of

Table 33–8. Causes of Kaliopenia and Kaliopenic Nephropathy in Man

Dietary Deficiency

Experimental

Gastrointestinal Loss

Diarrhea: particularly ulcerative colitis, regional colitis and ileitis, dysentery, malabsorption syndrome, acute infectious diarrhea
Purgatives: usually self-induced
Enemas or colonic lavage: often self-induced
Uterosigmoidostomy
Fistulas: particularly small bowel drainage
Vomiting
Combinations of above

Urinary Loss

Endocrine disturbances: aldosterone tumors, primary hyperaldosteronism, Cushing's syndrome, primary and secondary hypertrophy of the juxtaglomerular apparatus, diabetic coma
Renal diseases: renal tubular dysfunction, chronic pyelonephritis, interstitial nephritis, chronic renal failure, diuretic phase of acute renal failure

Iatrogenic

Diuretic drugs
Steroid hormones

inadequate intake of dietary potassium such as anorexia nervosa contribute to depletion in many instances. Of course, potassium loss is common in wasting disorders such as cirrhosis, but these losses occur pari passu with nitrogen wasting which has different effects from loss of potassium alone. The best-known effects of potassium depletion—aside from its potentiation of digitalis action and its effects on the electrocardiogram—are nocturia, muscle weakness or paralysis, vasopressin-resistant failure to concentrate the urine and inability to acidify the urine. Table 33–9 outlines some of the effects of potassium depletion on the kidney. In

Table 33–9.   Effects of Potassium Depletion on the Kidney

Biochemical Changes in Renal Tubules

Intracellular acidosis
Decreased capacity to accumulate para-aminohippurate
Increased glutaminase, D-amino oxidase and carbonic anhydrase activity
Increased lactic dehydrogenase activity in the collecting tubules
Decreased lactic dehydrogenase activity in the loop of Henle

Functional Changes of Renal Tubules

Vasopressin-resistant hyposthenuria or isosthenuria
Impaired para-aminohippurate extraction and excretion
Inability to establish minimal urinary pH; relative increase in urinary ammonia
Decreased urinary citric acid and other organic acids
Impaired capacity to conserve sodium when consuming a low dietary sodium intake
Phosphaturia

Structural Changes in Renal Tubules

Vacuolar (hydropic) nephropathy of proximal tubules
Granular degeneration and atrophy of cells in distal and collecting tubules
Increased intercalated cells in the collecting tubules
Alterations in mitochondria of the collecting tubules

Structural Changes in Interstitial Tissues

Edema
Fibrosis

most instances, these changes appear quite rapidly and are easily reversible with ingestion of adequate amounts of potassium by mouth (3 gm of potassium chloride or its equivalent per day). Infusion of potassium ions is necessary at times but may be fraught with danger as levels in the blood can pile up rapidly and cause cardiac arrest.

Muehrcke and McMillan[267] have reviewed cases from our clinic and from the world literature. They point out that the patients with gastrointestinal loss of potassium usually seek medical advice because of diarrhea, dehydration or other symptoms. Their electrolyte disorders are diagnosed and effectively treated early in the course of the potassium depletion. Consequently, irreversible histologic changes are less frequent in patients with gastrointestinal disorders than in patients with renal loss of potassium who may have had hypokalemia for many years without symptoms. Moreover, in these patients the renal tubular cells are the actual site of potassium loss and suffer greater functional and structural damage than when they are actively conserving potassium, which is what they do when the gastrointestinal tract is the site of potassium loss.

It is a curious fact that, once the irreversible destructive process of interstitial nephritis or pyelonephritis has developed in potassium-depleted patients, their kidneys are peculiarly prone to continue to lose potassium, notwithstanding the original site of loss. These studies, as do others, indicate that the renal tubular cell needs adequate supplies of potassium to preserve its integrity. The physician using agents such as steroids and diuretics which deplete the body of this electrolyte must be aware of the possibilities of damaging the kidney by his actions and of involving the organ in a secondary permanently harmful renal infection. Moreover, the physician must be on the lookout for clues to the diagnosis of potassium deficiency (nocturnal frequency, fatigue, weakness of the limbs and early changes in the electrocardiogram). Exact diagnosis comes with measurement of serum potassium, but the degree of depletion is often difficult to assess and may require metabolism studies for exact knowledge.

For prevention and treatment, enteric-coated tablets of potassium chloride were commonly used. Because patients may get abdominal cramps from the hypertonic solution formed during fragmentation of the tablet in the gut or, as sometimes happens, because the tablets may cause dangerous bowel disease including bowel performance, we prefer a liquid formula.

BIBLIOGRAPHY

1. Selkurt: Am. J. Physiol., 142, 182, 1944.
2. Heinemann and Lee: Am. J. Med., 61, 681, 1976.
3. Lee, Vance and Cahill: Am. J. Physiol., 206, 27, 1962.
4. Lassen, Mauck and Thaysen: Acta Physiol. Scand., 51, 37, 1961.
5. Follis: The Pathology of Nutritional Disease. Springfield, Charles C Thomas, 1948.
6. Smith: The Kidney: Structure and Function in Health and Disease. New York, Oxford University Press, 1951, p. 472.
7. McCarrison: Br. Med. J., 1, 1009, 1931.
8. Meneely, Tucker, Darby and Auerbach: Ann. Intern. Med., 39, 991, 1953.
9. Best and Hartroft: Fed. Proc., 8, 610, 1949.
10. Hartroft: Am. J. Pathol., 31, 381, 1955.
11. Burr and Burr: J. Biol. Chem., 82, 345, 1929.
12. Burr and Burr: J. Biol. Chem., 86, 587, 1930.
13. Simpson: Medicine, 50, 503, 1971.
14. Pullman, Alving, Devor and Landowne: J. Lab. Clin. Med., 44, 320, 1954.
15. Nielsen and Bang: Acta Med. Scand., 130, 382, 1948.
16. Nielsen and Bang: Scand. J. Clin. Lab. Med., 1, 295, 1949.
17. Sargent and Johnson: Am. J. Clin. Nutr., 4, 466, 1956.
18. Kachadorican and Johnson: J. Appl. Physiol., 28, 748, 1970.
19. Sargent and Johnson: Arch. Intern. Med., 99, 190, 1957.
20. Schrier, et al.: Am. J. Clin. Nutr., 4, 466, 1956.
21. Bleiler and Schedl: J. Lab. Clin. Med., 50, 945, 1962.
22. McCance: Medical Research Council Special Report Serial Number 275. London, His Majesty's Stationery Office, 1951.
23. Owen, et al.: J. Clin. Invest., 48, 574, 1969.
24. Felig, Owen, Wahren and Cahill: J. Clin. Invest., 48, 584, 1969.
25. Alleyene: Rush-Presly. St. Luke Hosp. Bull., 9, 84, 1970.
26. Berliner and Bennett: Am. J. Med., 42, 777, 1967.
27. Klahr, et al.: Am. J. Med., 43, 84, 1967.
28. Manitius, Pigeon and Epstein: Am. J. Physiol., 205, 101, 1963.
29. Klahr, Tripathy and Lotero: Am. J. Med., 48, 325, 1970.
30. Bloom: Arch. Intern. Med., 106, 321, 1960.
31. Gamble: Harvey Lect., 42, 247, 1947.
32. Hervey and McCance: Proc. R. Soc. Lond. Ser. B, 130, 527, 1952.
33. Katz, Holingsworth and Epstein: J. Lab. Clin. Med., 72, 93, 1968.
34. Consolazio, et al.: Am. J. Clin. Nutr., 20, 672, 1967.
35. Keys, et al.: Human Starvation. Minneapolis, University of Minnesota Press, 1951.
36. Davies: Am. J. Clin. Nutr., 4, 539, 1956.
37. Eales: Am. J. Clin. Nutr., 4, 529, 1956.
38. Gershoff, Faragalla, Nelson and Andrus: Am. J. Med., 27, 72, 1959.
39. Liang: Biochem. J., 82, 429, 1962.
40. Schwartz and Relman: N. Engl. J. Med., 276, 383, 452, 1967.
41. Conn and Johnson: Am. J. Clin. Nutr., 4, 523, 1966.
42. Conn and Johnson: Nutr. Rev., 28, 72, 1960.
43. Bartters and Schwartz: Am. J. Med., 42, 790, 1967.
44. Weisinger, Kempson, Eldridge and Swenson: Ann. Intern. Med., 81, 440, 1974.
45. Symposium on Uremic Toxins. Arch. Intern. Med., 126, 773, 1970.
46. Shaikin, Giatt and Berlyne: Kidney Int., 7, S302, 1975.
47. Scribner and Babb: Kidney Int., 7, S349, 1975.
48. Rubenstein and Sptiz: Diabetes, 17, 161, 1968.
49. DeFronzo, Andres, Edgar and Walker: Medicine, 52, 469, 1973.
50. Feldman and Singer: Medicine, 54, 345, 1975.
51. Hampers, Soeldner, Doak and Merrill: J. Clin. Invest., 45, 1719, 1966.
52. Luke, Briggs, McKiddie and Kennedy: In Nutrition in Renal Disease (Berlyne, Ed.). Baltimore, Williams & Williams, 1968, p. 170.
53. Bagdade, Porte and Bierman: N. Engl. J. Med., 279, 181, 1968.
54. Bagdade: J. Clin. Nutr., 21, 426, 1968.
55. Tsaltas and Friedman: Am. J. Clin. Nutr., 21, 430, 1968.
56. Wochos, Anderson and Mitchell: Mayo Clin. Proc., 51, 660, 1976.
57. Ahrens, Tsaltas, Hersch and Intull: J. Clin. Invest., 34, 918, 1955.
58. Dole: J. Clin. Invest., 35, 150, 1956.
59. Lewis, et al.: N. Engl. J. Med., 275, 1097, 1966.
60. Berlyne and Malliek: Lancet, 2, 399, 1969.
61. DeLuca: Ann. Intern. Med., 85, 367, 1976.
62. Avioli, Birge, Lee and Slatopolsky: J. Clin. Invest., 47, 2239, 1968.
63. Guyton, et al.: Circ. Res., 35, 159, 1974.
64. Bright: Guys Hosp. Rep., 1, 338, 1836.

65. Pickering: *High Blood Pressure*. New York, Grune & Stratton, 1955.
66. Nat. Center Health Statistics. USDHEW: Vital and Health Statistics Series II, No. 13, 1976.
67. U.S. DHEW: Statistics Series II, No. 4, 1976, p. 9.
68. Hamilton, Pickering, Roberts and Sowry: Clin. Sci., *13*, 11, 1954.
68a. Thomas: In *Hypertension, Mechanisms and Management* (Onesti, et al. Eds.). New York, Grune & Stratton, 1973, p. 66.
69. McKusick: Circulation, *22*, 857, 1960.
70. Medical News: J.A.M.A., *235*, 785, 1976.
71. Buck: J. Chronic Dis., *26*, 101, 1973.
71a. Kass, et al.: In *Epidemiology and Control of Hypertension* (Paul, Ed.). New York, Stratton Intercontinental Medical Book Co., 1975, p. 360.
72. Lee and Schneider: J.A.M.A., *167*, 1447, 1958.
73. Stamler, Stamler and Pullman: In *The Epidemiology of Hypertension*. New York, Grune & Stratton, 1967.
74. Dawber, et al.: In *The Epidemiology of Hypertension*. New York, Grune & Stratton, 1967, pp. 255–288.
75. Scotch and Geiger: J. Chronic Dis., *16*, 1183, 1963.
76. Henry and Cassel: Am. J. Epidemiol., *90*, 171, 1969.
77. Morris, Crawford and Healy: Lancet, *1*, 860, 1961.
78. Biorck, Bostrom and Widstrom: Acta Med. Scand., *178*, 239, 1965.
79. Schroeder: J.A.M.A., *172*, 1902, 1960.
80. Langford and Watson: Trans. Am. Clin. Climatol. Assoc., *83*, 125, 1922.
81. Priddle: Can. Med. Assoc. J., *86*, 1, 1962.
82. Meneely and Dahl: Med. Clin. North Am., *45*, 271, 1961.
83. Dahl and Love: J.A.M.A., *164*, 397, 1957.
84. Tobian and Binion: Circulation, 5, 754, 1952.
85. Goldblatt: J. Exp. Med., *59*, 347, 1934.
86. Conn: Ann. Intern. Med., *44*, 1, 1956.
87. Thurston and Swale: Lancet, *2*, 930, 1976.
88. Adetuyibi and Mills: Lancet, *2*, 203, 1972.
89. Morris, Robinson and Scheck: Can. Med. Assoc. J., *90*, 272, 1964.
90. Kolf, et al.: Circulation, *30* (Suppl. 2), 23, 1964.
90a. Bianchi, et al.: Clin. Sci. Mol. Med., *47*, 435, 1974.
91. Tobian: In *Epidemiology and Control of Hypertension*. New York. Stratton Intercontinental Medical Book Corp., 1975, pp. 131–146.
92. Tobian, et al.: Circ. Res., *36, 37* (Suppl.), 1, 1975.
93. Tobian, et al.: Circ. Res., *39*, 337, 1976.
94. Smirk: In *The Epidemiology of Hypertension*. New York, Grune & Stratton, 1967, pp. 39–55.
95. Meneely, Ball and Youmans: Ann. Intern. Med., *47*, 263, 1957.
96. Meneely, et al.: Circulation, *12*, 401, 1955.
97. Dahl and Schackow: Can. Med. Assoc. J., *90*, 155, 1964.
98. Dahl, Heine and Tassinari: J. Exp. Med., *118*, 605, 1963.
99. Dahl, et al.: J. Exp. Med., *126*, 687, 1967.
99a. Kornel: Personal communication, 1977.
100. *Encyclopedia Britannica* (11th ed.), New York, 1911.
101. Denton: Nutr. Abstr. Rev., *39*, 1043, 1969.
102. Wotman, et al.: J. Chronic Dis., *20*, 833, 1967.
103. Page, Damon and Moellering: Circulation, *49*, 1132, 1974.
104. Oliver, Cohen and Neel: Circulation, *52*, 146, 1975.
105. Chagnon: National Geographic, August 1976, pp. 211–222.
106. Thomas: J.A.M.A., *88*, 1559, 1927.
107. Morse and Beh: Lancet, *1*, 966, 1937.
108. Page: Am. Heart J., *91*, 527, 1976.
109. Meneely and Batterlee: Am. J. Cardiol., *38*, 768, 1976.
110. Thomas: J.A.M.A., *88*, 1559, 1927.
111. Kark: Unpublished observations, 1945.
112. Maddocks: Lancet, *2*, 396, 1961.
113. Shaper: Am. Heart J., *63*, 437, 1962.
114. Shaper, Wright and Kyobe: East Afr. Med. J., *46*, 273, 1969.
115. Mann, et al.: J. Chronic Dis., *15*, 341, 1962.
116. Truswell, et al.: Am. Heart J., *84*, 5, 1972.
117. Mann, et al.: J. Atheroscler. Res., *4*, 289, 1964.
118. Cruz-Coke, Etchevery and Nagel: Lancet, *1*, 697, 1964.
119. Prior, et al.: Int. J. Epidemiol., *3*, 225, 1974.
120. Shaper, et al.: East Afr. Med. J., *46*, 282, 1969.
121. Page: Personal Communication, 1977.
122. Dahl: N. Engl. J. Med., *258*, 1152, 1958.
123. Dahl: Am. J. Clin. Nutr., *25*, 231, 1972.
124. Takahashi, et al.: Hum. Biol., *29*, 139, 1957.
125. Sasaki: Jpn. Heart J., *3*, 313, 1962.
126. Sasaki: Geriatrics, *19*, 735, 1964.
127. Fodor, Abbott and Rusted: Can. Med. Assoc. J., *108*, 1365, 1973.
127a. Stamler: In *The Epidemiology of Hypertension* (Stamler and Pullman, Eds.). New York, Grune & Stratton, 1967.
128. Meneely and Battarbee: *Present Knowledge of Nutrition*. Washington, The Nutrition Foundation, 1976.
129. Meneely and Ball: Am. J. Med., *25*, 713, 1958.
129a. Lemley-Stone, Darby and Meneely: Am. J. Cardiol., *8*, 527, 1961.
130. Dahl, Leitl and Heine: J. Exp. Med., *136*, 318, 1972.
131. Addison: Can. Med. Assoc. J., *18*, 281, 1928.
132. Priddle: Can. Med. Assoc. J., *25*, 5, 1931.
133. Thompson and McQuarrie: Proc. Soc. Exp. Biol. Med., *31*, 907, 1934.
134. McQuarrie, Thompson and Anderson: J. Nutr., *11*, 77, 1936.
135. Langford, Watson, Marino and Schoenberger: J. Clin. Res., *25*, 512A, 1977.
136. Committee on Nutrition, American Academy of Pediatrics: Pediatrics, *53*, 115, 1974.
137. Dahl: Am. J. Clin. Nutr., *21*, 787, 1968.
138. Dahl, et al.: Proc. Soc. Exp. Biol. Med., *133*, 1405, 1970.
139. Page: *In* Pickering, G. (Reference 65).
140. Veterans Administration Cooperative Study: Arch. Intern. Med., *106*, 81, 1970.
141. Veterans Administration Cooperative Study: J.A.M.A., *213*, 1143, 1970.

142. Veterans Administration Cooperative Study: Circ. Res., *38*, 362, 1976.
143. Fries: Arch. Intern. Med., *133*, 982, 1974.
144. Brown, et al.: Circulation, *43*, 508, 1971.
145. Forbes: Personal communication, 1977.
146. Mann: N. Engl. J. Med., *291*, 178, 1975.
146a.Klatsky: N. Engl. J. Med., *297*, 450, 1977.
147. Ambard and Beaujord: Arch. Gin Med., *1*, 520, 1904.
148. Allen: *Treatment of Kidney Diseases and High Blood Pressure.* Morristown, The Physiatric Institute, 1925.
149. Kempner: N.C. Med. J., *5*, 125, 1944.
150. Kempner: N.C. Med. J., *6*, 61, 1945.
151. Kempner: Am. J. Med., *4*, 545, 1948.
152. Medical Research Council: Lancet, *2*, 509, 1950.
153. Grollman, et al.: J.A.M.A., *129*, 533, 1945.
154a.*Maternal Nutrition and the Course of Pregnancy.* Washington, National Academy of Science, 1970.
154b.Lindheimer, Katz and Zuspan: *Hypertension in Pregnancy.* International Symposium University of Chicago. New York, John Wiley, 1976.
154c.Theobald: In *Ciba Foundation Symposium.* Philadelphia, The Blakiston Company, 1950, p. 23.
155. Chrichton: Transactions International Congress Obstetricians and Gynaecologists, Dublin, 1947.
156. Brock: Personal communication, 1956.
157. duPlessis: *The Cape Malays.* Cape Town, Maskew Miller, 1944.
158. Gerber: *Traditional Cookery of the Cape Malays.* Cape Town, A.A. Balkema, 1957.
159. Wachstein and Gudaitis: Am. J. Clin. Pathol., *22*, 652, 1952.
160. Sarles, et al.: Am. J. Obstet. Gynec., *102*, 1, 1968.
161. Schewitz: Med. Clin. North Am., *55*, 47, 1971.
162. Brown, et al.: Lancet, *2*, 900, 1963.
163. Robinson: Lancet, *1*, 78, 1958.
164. Kirksey and Pike: J. Nutr., *77*, 34, 43, 1962; *78*, 325, 1962; *80*, 421, 1963.
165. Perey, Herdman, Vernier and Good: J. Lab. Clin. Med., *70*, 881, 1967.
166. Camera, Reimer and Newburgh: Univ. Mich. Med. Bull., *18*, 285, 1952.
167. Von Rohrer: Arch. Ges. Physiol., *109*, 375, 1905.
168. Illingsworth, Philpott and Rendle-Short: Arch. Dis. Child., *29*, 551, 1954.
169. Mortensen: Acta Med. Scand., *129*, 321, 1947.
170. Kark, et al.: Ann. Intern. Med., *49*, 751, 1958.
171. Squire: Am. J. Clin. Nutr., *4*, 509, 1956.
172. Baxter: Arch. Intern. Med., *109*, 742, 1962.
173. Marsh and Drabkin: Metabolism, *9*, 946, 1960.
174. Baxter, Goodman and Allen: J. Clin. Invest., *40*, 490, 1961.
175. Hyman, Wong and Grossman: Pediatrics, *44*, 1021, 1969.
176. Newmark, Anderson, Donadio and Ellefson: Mayo Clin. Proc., *50*, 359, 1975.
177. Cattell: In *Recent Advances: Renal Diseases* (Jones, Ed.). London, Churchill Livingstone, 1975.
178. Chapman, et al.: Adv. Nephrol., *6*, 321, 1976.
179. Sargent, Sargent, Johnson and Stolpe: WADC Technical Report 53–484, Part II, Vols. I and II. Dayton, Wright Air Development Center, 1955.
180. Abel, Abbott and Fischer: Arch. Surg., *103*, 513, 1971.
181. Abel, Abbott and Fischer: Am. J. Surg., *123*, 632, 1972.
182. Abel, et al.: N. Engl. J. Med., *288*, 695, 1973.
183. Hegsted, Tsongas, Abbott and Stare: J. Lab. Clin. Med., *31*, 261, 1946.
184. Giordano: J. Lab. Clin. Med., *62*, 231, 1947.
185. Giordano, et al.: Am. J. Clin. Nutr., *21*, 394, 1968.
186. Giovannetti and Maggiore: Lancet, *1*, 1000, 1964.
187. Berlyne, Gaan and Ginks: Am. J. Clin. Nutr., *21*, 547, 1968.
188. Robson, Kerr and Ashcroft: In *Nutrition in Renal Disease* (Berlyne, Ed.). Baltimore, Williams and Wilkins, 1968, p. 93.
189. Furst, Josephson and Vinars: In *Nutrition in Renal Disease* (Berlyne, Ed.). Baltimore, Williams and Wilkins, 1968, p. 99.
190. Ford, Phillips, Toye, Luck and DeWardener: Br. Med. J., *1*, 735, 1969.
191. Walser: J. Clin. Invest., *53*, 1385, 1974.
192. Richards, et al.: In *Nutrition in Renal Disease* (Berlyne, Ed.). Baltimore, Williams and Wilkins, 1968, p. 93.
193. Richards, Brown, Houghton and Wrong: Clin. Nephrol., *3*, 173, 1975.
194. Cammarata and Cohen: J. Biol. Chem., *187*, 439, 1950.
195. Awapara and Seale: J. Biol. Chem., *194*, 497, 1952.
196. Rose: Science, *86*, 298, 1937.
197. Richards, Houghton and Brown: Lancet, *2*, 128, 1971.
198. Richards, Brown and Lowe: J. Nutr., *102*, 1547, 1972.
199. Giordano, Phillips and DePascale: Lancet, *1*, 178, 1972.
200. Rudman: J. Clin. Invest., *50*, 90, 1971.
201. Sapir, Owen, Pozefsky and Walser: J. Clin. Invest., *54*, 974, 1974.
202. Walser: Clin. Nephrol., *3*, 180, 1975.
203. Walser, Coulter, Dighe and Crantz: J. Clin. Invest., *52*, 678, 1973.
204. Gulyassy and DeTorrente: Kidney Int., *7*, S311, 1975.
205. Simenhoff: Kidney Int., *7*, S314, 1975.
206. Tam, Kopple, Wang and Sevendeid: Kidney Int., *7*, S328, 1975.
207. Giordano, et al.: Br. Med. J., *4*, 714, 1973.
208. Bagdade: Kidney Int., *7*, S370, 1975.
209. Sanfelippo, Swenson and Reaven: Kidney Int., *11*, 54, 1977.
210. Hampers, et al.: N. Engl. J. Med., *276*, 551, 1967.
211. Sullivan and Eirenstein: Am. J. Clin. Nutr., *23*, 1339, 1970.
212. Dobbelstein, et al.: Kidney Int., *5*, 233, 1974.
213. Stone, Warnock and Wagner: Am. J. Clin. Nutr., *28*, 950, 1975.

214. Brickman, Coburn, Norman and Massry: Am. J. Med., *57*, 28, 1974.
215. Brickman, Coburn and Massry: Ann. Intern. Med., *80*, 161, 1974.
216. Chan, Oldharn, Holick and DeLuca: J.A.M.A., *234*, 47, 1975.
217. Bricker: N. Engl. J. Med., *286*, 1093, 1972.
218. Reiss, Canterbury and Kanter: Arch. Intern. Med., *124*, 417, 1969.
219. Fornier, Arnoud and Johnson: J. Clin. Invest., *50*, 599, 1971.
220. Slatopolsky, Robson and Elkan: J. Clin. Invest., *47*, 1865, 1968.
221. Slatopolsky, Caglar and Pennell: J. Clin. Invest., *50*, 492, 1971.
222. Lennon: Arch. Intern. Med., *124*, 557, 1969.
223. Dunea: Med. Clin. North Am., *55*, 155, 1971.
224. Berlyne, Jones, Hewitt and Nitwarangkur: Lancet, *1*, 738, 1964.
225. Berlyne, et al.: Lancet, *1*, 1339, 1967.
226. Young and Parsons: Clin. Sci., *97*, 1, 1969.
227. Schaeffer, et al.: Clin. Nephrol., *3*, 228, 1975.
228. Glessing: Lancet, *2*, 812, 1968.
229. Sevit and Hoffbrand: Br. Med. J., *2*, 18, 1961.
230. Palmer, Newell, Gray and Quinton: N. Engl. J. Med., *274*, 248, 1966.
231. Giordano, et al.: In *Nutrition in Renal Disease* (Berlyne, Ed.). Baltimore, Williams and Wilkins, 1968, p. 23.
232. Young and Parson: Clin. Sci., *31*, 299, 1969.
233. Ginn, Frost and Lacy: Am. J. Clin. Nutr., *21*, 385, 1968.
234. Gulassy, Peters, Lin and Ryan: Am. J. Clin. Nutr., *21*, 565, 1968.
235. Bergstrom, Furst and Noree: Clin. Nephrol., *3*, 187, 1975.
236. Noree and Bergstrom: Clin. Nephrol., *3*, 195, 1975.
237. Heidland and Kult: Clin. Nephrol., *3*, 234, 1975.
238. Whitehead, Comty, Posen and Kaye: N. Engl. J. Med., *279*, 970, 1968.
239. Sullivan and Eisenstein: Am. J. Clin. Nutr., *23*, 1339, 1970.
240. Kopple and Swendseid: Kidney Int., *7*, S79, 1975.
241. Mansouri, Halsted and Gambos: Arch. Intern. Med., *125*, 88, 1970.
242. Symposium on Stones. Am. J. Med., *45*, 5, 1968.
243. Williams: N. Engl. J. Med., *290*, 33, 1974.
244. Boyce: Am. J. Med., *45*, 673, 1968.
245. Herring: J. Urol., *88*, 545, 1962.
246. Coe and Kavalach: N. Engl. J. Med., *291*, 1344, 1974.
247. Yendt: Can. Med. Assoc. J., *102*, 479, 1970.
248. Henneman, Benedict, Forbes and Dudley: N. Engl. J. Med., *259*, 802, 1958.
249. Coe, Canterbury, Firpo and Reiss: J. Clin. Invest., *52*, 134, 1972.
250. Wills, et al.: Clin. Sci., *39*, 95, 1970.
251. Coburn and Massry: J. Clin. Invest., *49*, 1073, 1970.
252. Gutman and Yu: Am. J. Med., *45*, 756, 1968.
253. Gershoff and Prien: Am. J. Clin. Nutr., *20*, 393, 1967.
254. Stauffer, Humphreys and Weir: Ann. Intern. Med., *79*, 389, 1973.
255. Smith, Fromm and Hofmann: N. Engl. J. Med., *286*, 1371, 1972.
256. Gilbert, Brewer, Fajardo and Weinstein: Arch. Intern. Med., *137*, 239, 1977.
257. Dobbins and Binder: N. Engl. J. Med., *296*, 298, 1977.
258. Chadwick, Modha and Dowling: N. Engl. J. Med., *289*, 172, 1973.
259. Baron, et al.: Lancet, *271*, 421, 1956.
260. Fanconi: Jahrb. Kinderheilkd., *147*, 299, 1936.
261. Milkman: Am. J. Roentgenol., *24*, 29, 1930.
262. Albright, et al.: Medicine, *28*, 399, 1946.
263. Schwartz: N. Engl. J. Med., *253*, 601, 1955.
264. Milne, Muehrcke and Heard: Br. Med. Bull., *13*, 15, 1957.
265. Perkins, Petersen and Riley: Am. J. Med., *8*, 115, 1950.
266. Black and Milne: Clin. Sci., *11*, 397, 1952.
267. Muehrcke and McMillan: Ann. Intern. Med., *59*, 427, 1963.

Chapter *34*

DIET, HYPERLIPIDEMIA AND ATHEROSCLEROSIS

Nancy Ernst
and
Robert I. Levy

Arteriosclerosis is a general term for the degeneration of the arteries, resulting in thickening and hardening of the arterial wall. Atherosclerosis, one type of arteriosclerosis, is characterized by accumulation of lipids (primarily cholesterol, but also phospholipid and triglycerides) in the walls of medium and large arteries. Atherosclerosis is a disorder that underlies most arteriosclerotic heart disease (coronary artery disease) and, in addition, plays a major role in cerebrovascular disease.[1,2]

Atherosclerosis has a devastating effect on the health of Americans and on the nation's economy. Virtually all Americans are to some degree affected with atherosclerosis, and 27 million suffer from hypertension. Each year there are over 850,000 cardiovascular deaths in the United States from atherosclerosis and its sequelae and about 200,000 of these deaths occur before age 65. In 1976 more than 1.25 million Americans suffered heart attacks, and of these 20 to 30 per cent died suddenly before they received any medical care. In addition to human suffering, these diseases cost the nation an estimated $45 billion in sickness, lost wages and benefits.[3]

The role of epidemiology in the study of the prevalence of coronary heart disease (CHD) began to emerge in the early part of the 20th century.[4,5] Findings of subsequent and numerous epidemiologic surveys have helped to define apparent biologic, demographic and social differences between normal and coronary-prone individuals—hence, the development of the term *risk factors*, i.e. habits or traits which appear to be associated with or promote *risk* for coronary heart disease. Among those factors felt to convey increased risk are elevated blood lipids (most specifically cholesterol), cigarette smoking, hypertension, hyperglycemia (diabetes), obesity, sedentary living, psychosocial tension and a positive history of premature atherosclerotic disease. At least 37 different variables have been correlated with atherosclerosis.[6] Hypercholesterolemia, hypertension and cigarette smoking have the strongest statistical correlation to premature coronary heart disease.[7]

Inherent to the risk factor approach is the concept of decreasing risk through appropriate medical intervention. This concept appears to be true for cessation of cigarette smoking and normalization of elevated blood pressure. Unfortunately, despite numerous studies it is not yet clear whether modifications of all risk factors will substantially reduce mortality from coronary heart disease. Intervention trials of better design, employing adequate numbers of patients, are clearly needed. Presumptive evidence at this time would suggest, however, *the clinical modification when possible of all detected risk factors.*

ENVIRONMENTAL FACTORS

It is theorized that environmental factors are responsible for the findings that the cardiovascular death rate for migrants, particularly men, is, in most cases, closer to the cardiovascular mortality in the United States than that of the country of birth.[8] Diet, cigarette smoking, stress and tension and patterns of physical activity are influential environmental factors and often confuse the interpretation of endogenous variables.

Diet

The 20th-century man has become more reluctant to accept deterioration of coronary arteries and subsequent development of atherosclerosis as a necessary accompaniment of the aging process or of his personal being or so-called constitution. In a search for associated factors from his mode of life, diet has become one of the focal points of inquiry.

Gradually, the question has become, not whether diet can be associated with coronary heart disease, but to what extent diet influences the development of coronary heart disease in man. Is diet a preventive measure? Can diet improve deteriorating coronary status? If intensive investigations can prove dietary change commendable, is it feasible to achieve and maintain long-term dietary change in those individuals at predictable risk for coronary heart disease?

Unfortunately, a review of the nutritional literature does not provide answers to these questions. It is apparent that diet and atherosclerosis, from early investigational days, have been marked by numerous conflicting observations and controversies.

Clinical and Laboratory Studies. In the early 1900s, investigators demonstrated that by feeding large amounts of cholesterol to rabbits it was possible to produce arterial lesions similar to those found in human atherosclerosis.[9] These observations were significant at the time and insti-

gated a closer look at the cholesterol picture. The role of diet—specifically the effect of cholesterol feeding on serum cholesterol—was demonstrated in other laboratory animals by several investigators. The accepted concept was that the level of plasma cholesterol was determined solely by the cholesterol in the diet.[10] However, the possibility of cholesterol synthesis by animal (and man) was soon considered and in 1925 evidence was presented that cholesterol is synthesized in the animal organism.[11] Supportive and clarifying data soon followed.[12,13]

Today, it is recognized that in most animals except primates the lipoprotein spectrum is different from that of man. Man has more low-density lipoprotein and less high-density lipoprotein (see below) than laboratory animals such as rats, rabbits, sheep and dogs, and there appear to be differences in lipid transport functions. Therefore, an important contribution is the well-controlled study of primates (Rhesus monkey) which revealed that atherosclerotic lesions developed during 17 months of high-cholesterol feeding and regressed after 40 months of cholesterol-free chow.[14]

Dietary Cholesterol. Dietary studies in man have produced much conflicting and often confusing evidence. In the early 1950s, many investigators believed that cholesterol synthesis controlled serum cholesterol levels and that diet was not an important factor. Keys, one of the early opponents of cholesterol restriction, stated that the blood cholesterol was independent of the cholesterol intake over a wide range. He argued that the plasma cholesterol concentration responded to a zero intake of cholesterol—such as the rice diet—but that administration of large doses of cholesterol produced only trivial changes in the plasma cholesterol of man.[15] In 1956, Keys reported "definitive" findings from dietary experiments and population surveys that cholesterol in the natural diet had no effect on blood cholesterol if the other elements in the diet are held constant.[16] At that time, Kinsell[17] and Ahrens[18] were in agreement with this theory.

Subsequent studies have shown that dietary cholesterol has an undeniable hypercholesterolemic effect.[19-21] Furthermore, the effect of a given intake of dietary cholesterol is independent of the fat or fatty acid composition of the diet.[22-24] Keys postulated that "other things being equal, the serum cholesterol appears to be a linear function of the square root of the cholesterol in the daily diet."[23] It is probable that some of the earlier conflicting data regarding dietary cholesterol were misinterpreted because cholesterol was not fed in a form suitable for absorption. Cholesterol must be dissolved in or closely associated with other fats in order to be absorbed.[23]

Furthermore, it was initially thought that man's maximum daily absorption of dietary cholesterol, despite dietary intake, could not exceed 300 to 500 mg per day.[25,26] It is now clear that cholesterol absorption is proportional to cholesterol ingestion at all levels of cholesterol intake.[25-28] Patients fed as much as 3 gm per day absorbed up to 1 gm of cholesterol.[28,29]

Total Dietary Fat. By the middle 1950s some investigators were labeling the intake of dietary fat—and not cholesterol—as the dietary factor related to coronary heart diseases.[30-34]

Polyunsaturated Fatty Acids. Subsequent studies refuted reports that a high-fat diet per se is always associated with an increase in serum cholesterol.[35-37] These studies showed that the polyunsaturated oils (safflower, corn, cottonseed, for example) produce decreases in serum cholesterol, while isocaloric amounts of the saturated fats (butter, coconut oil and palm oil) increase levels of serum cholesterol. Keys ultimately concluded that polyunsaturated fatty acids have half the effect per gram on decreasing serum cholesterol concentrations as do saturated fatty acids acting in the opposite direction.[38] The principal polyunsaturated fatty acids in the diet are linoleic (C_{18}:2) and linolenic (C_{18}:3) which are most abundant in oils of grains, seeds and nuts. Longer-chain highly unsaturated acids are present in fish oils.

Saturated Fatty Acids. Saturated fat is present in the diet in animal products such as meat, egg yolk, dairy products, and in certain vegetable products such as coconut oil and hydrogenated shortenings and margarines. Saturated fatty acids vary in the degree of cholesterol influence. For example, stearic acid (C_{18}) has little or no effect on serum cholesterol,[39-42] while the saturated acids lauric (C_{14}), and palmitic (C_{16}) dramatically increase cholesterol concentrations.[39,40] Since palmitic is more abundant in food than lauric or myristic, it may be the primary fatty acid affecting cholesterol concentrations.[39] Saturated fatty acids containing 10 carbons or less (MCT) have not been shown to have any effect on cholesterol levels.[43,44]

Monounsaturated Fatty Acids. The most abundant monounsaturated fatty acid in the diet is oleic acid (C_{18}:1) which is found in all food fats and is especially high in olive oil. Dietary studies have reported that monounsaturated acids have no effect on serum cholesterol concentrations.[45-47]

Hydrogenated Oils. Hydrogenated oils have been reported to produce higher serum cholesterols than the corresponding unhydrogenated oils.[42,46,47] Oils are treated with hydrogen to increase their stability and to produce the degree of hardness required for shortenings and margarines.

Dietary Carbohydrate. The influence of dietary carbohydrate on the pathogenesis of coronary heart disease has received considerable attention in recent years. It has been shown that carbohydrate influences serum lipids, particularly triglycerides.[48-50] The normal response to a high-carbohydrate diet is an increase in triglycerides by approximately 50 to 100 per cent. In some lipidemic subjects, a high-carbohydrate intake produces more intense lipemia with triglyceride levels increasing by 1,000 mg per 100 ml or more.[51]

The intake of sucrose has attracted particular interest. J. Yudkin[52,53] claims that there is significant positive correlation between the intake of refined sugars and the incidence of coronary heart disease among the populations of various countries. In support of this concept, Yudkin reported that patients with occlusive vascular disease consume more sugar than do men with normal cardiac status.[54,55] These results are disputed by other investigators.[56-61]

The possible relationship between the kind of dietary carbohydrate consumed and serum lipid levels has been reviewed by McGandy.[62] A more recent compendium on the role of dietary carbohydrates in lipid disorders has been prepared by Albrink.[63] It has been reported that substitution of the simple sugars for starch results in increased concentrations of serum triglycerides and often in increased serum cholesterol,[64-69] that at a moderate carbohydrate intake sucrose has only a slight effect, if any, on serum lipids[70] and that the effects of dietary carbohydrate on serum lipids are of much smaller magnitude than are the effects of dietary fat.[71] At this time the relationship between sugar intake and coronary heart disease has not advanced beyond the state of inadequate knowledge and controversy.[72] The previously cited studies suggest that there is a very individualistic variability in lipid response to carbohydrate feeding. It appears that interchanging different sugars for starch will produce significant change in triglyceride and cholesterol concentrations only in certain individuals.

Dietary Fiber. With regard to fiber, a lipid-lowering relationship has been hypothesized but thus far the evidence is conflicting. The reason for this confusion stems partly from the imprecise definition of dietary fiber and from the failure to distinguish its constituents in experimental studies. The lack of a precise definition of dietary fiber relates to deficiencies in the analytic method of Einhof that dates back to 1809 and determines only crude fiber. Crude fiber is defined as the indigestible, fibrous residue that remains after sequential extraction with solvent, dilute aqueous acid and dilute alkali. Fiber includes cellulose, hemicellulose, pectin and lignin. These specific components of fiber vary in cholesterol-lowering effectiveness, i.e. lignin and pectin have been shown to lower serum cholesterol whereas the effect of cellulose on serum cholesterol is debatable.[73-76]

This area has a number of problems to be considered and resolved, including conflicting concepts of what constitutes fiber, the definition of lignin, cellulose and hemicellulose, achieving separation of lignin, the isolation of indigestible fiber and its relation to the true fiber of food, and the failure of hemicellulose, cellulose and lignin to be chemically or biologically similar in different plant materials.[77] Hypothesis and controversies regarding dietary fiber were featured in the recent Marabou Symposium: Food and Fibre.[78]

Epidemiologic Findings. An extensive review and summary of 278 references relating to the world epidemiology of coronary heart disease, the frequency of the disease in various populations and postulations for intrapopulation differences are available.[61] Many of the epidemiologic studies have provoked in-depth studies of nutritional relationships with respect to the apparent differences in the prevalence and incidence of CHD among racial and geographically distinct population groups. Notable among these studies are those involving the Bantu,[79,80] the Masai,[81] groups in the Middle East[80-83] and Central America[86] and various Oriental or Oriental-American groups.[89-91] In general, the findings report parallels among dietary fat, serum cholesterol and CHD incidence. The populations with a low incidence of CHD had low serum cholesterol and ate low-fat diets (specifically low saturated fat). The Masai have been cited in attempts to refute the theory that development of CHD is affected by the intake of cholesterol and saturated fat. However, there are striking dietary differences and apparent metabolic aberrations which probably protect the Masai from developing hypercholesterolemia and atherosclerosis as a result of a diet high in saturated fat and a significant amount of cholesterol.[90,91]

The mammoth seven-countries study[92] is a landmark in providing evidence that development of coronary heart disease is associated with cholesterol and saturated fat in the habitual diet. However, it has been difficult to elicit an association of diet with blood lipids within populations. The Framingham Study[93] reported that no statistical relationship of any of the measured dietary components to serum cholesterol could be demonstrated. The Honolulu Heart Study[94] demonstrated a weak but positive correlation of total dietary fat and saturated fat with blood cholesterol levels and a negative correlation of total carbohydrate and complex carbohydrate intake with serum cholesterol. The Puerto Rico Study data reports similar correlations in the urban population.[95,96] Recent publications from the Tecumseh Study report that serum lipid levels could not be shown to correlate with dietary habits.[97,98] Hence, it can only be said with conviction that while it has been difficult to elicit an association of diet with blood lipids *within* populations it has also been found that no populations subsisting on low saturated fat diets have an appreciable amount of coronary disease.

Clinical Trials. Several studies have been conducted to determine whether changing the composition of the diet will affect the atherosclerotic process and the incidence and mortality from coronary heart disease. The diet trials of the late 1960s and early 1970s include those of Dayton,[99] Turpeinen[100] and Leren.[101,102] These studies all incorporated the basic principles of diet therapy necessary to

lower serum cholesterol levels: restricted intake of cholesterol and saturated fat, with polyunsaturated fats substituted for saturated fats. All three studies reported a decrease in the incidence of new coronary events as compared with other groups. Reviews summarizing some of the major studies designed to demonstrate the efficacy of cholesterol diets are available.[103,104]

A recent dietary test of the lipid hypothesis is the 4½ year Minnesota Coronary Survey—a double-blind trial of 9,500 men and women over 21 years of age in a closed population in seven mental institutions. There was no difference in the overall death rate or number of heart attacks for the group as a whole. There were fewer deaths in men under 50 on the cholesterol-lowering diet, but the results were not statistically significant because of insufficient numbers.[105] Exploration of the lipid hypothesis demands that lipid levels be lowered as much as possible by simultaneous dietary and drug interventions. The World Health Organization (WHO) Cooperative Trial[106] and the Lipid Research Clinics Primary Prevention Trial will supply additional data on the effects of lipid lowering both before and after myocardial infarction. These trials must demonstrate the acceptability of combined diet/drug regimens in order to achieve long-term coherence and obtain evidence of the lack of serious toxicity of such long-term interventions.

Many dietary trials, including the National Diet-Heart Feasibility Study 1960–1967,[107] have shown that cholesterol concentrations can be effectively lowered by 8 to 18 per cent with diet. None of the studies has conclusively proven, however, that this cholesterol lowering will prevent or delay coronary heart disease or coronary mortality. Most of the dietary studies can be criticized in terms of study design, observer bias or improper and often "soft" end-points.[108] The cost of carrying out an effective dietary trial in the United States today is enormous, requiring a large number of subjects (and paramedical personnel) and prolonged time intervals to gain statistically valid differences in coronary morbidity and mortality.[109] Without such studies, however, arguments for lowering cholesterol through diet in coronary-prone patients remain primarily circumstantial.

Cigarette Smoking

Cigarette smoking is one of the most important exogenous factors which tend to increase incidence of coronary heart disease. Indeed, it has been found that the incidence of myocardial infarction is three times greater and death from coronary heart disease is five times greater in smokers than in nonsmokers.[110] There are those, however, who feel that cigarette smoking has no cumulative or permanent effect on the development of coronary heart disease.[110-113] Other data indicate that cigarette smoking has a cumulative effect and that the coronary disease risk for ex-smokers does not revert as quickly to nonsmoker levels as was once emphasized.[114] There is general agreement in these studies that risk is proportionate to the number of cigarettes smoked and that pipe and cigar smokers (qualified by Kahn[114] to 4 per day) suffer no greater mortality than nonsmokers.

Psychologic and Social Findings

One review[115] cited findings from over 160 papers, the majority of which report a relationship between coronary heart disease and such psychologic or social variables as education, religion, income, occupation, social mobility, personality traits and the like.

There seems to be a clinical impression that stress is associated with sudden death and probably development of coronary heart disease.[116] However, the Framingham Study reported that some aspects of stressful living—extremes of family size, marital stress, degree of affluence and

heavy consumption of coffee and tea (indirect measurement of stress)—were not associated with increased risk of coronary heart disease.[113]

Physical activity is one of the variables which has been studied within occupational groups, thereby minimizing possible effects of socioeconomic variations. Data collected in these studies support the hypothesis that men in the more sedentary occupations have more fatalities from coronary heart disease than men in occupations requiring at least moderate activity.[117-119] The Framingham Study revealed that the more sedentary individuals developed an excess of lethal attacks, not, however, of angina pectoris (arm and chest pain produced by effort and secondary to insufficient coronary blood flow). Physical activity also was related to ability to survive an attack.[113] The thought has been expressed that activity improves collateral coronary circulation,[113] but it is also hypothesized that the sedentary individual may choose less exercise because of general poor health.[99]

Epidemiologists have pointed out that methodologic inadequacies of many psychosocial studies impair interpretation as to absolute correlation.[113]

ENDOGENOUS FACTORS

Endogenous factors, perhaps by being more readily stratified, have been extensively studied, and the presence of hypertension, hyperlipidemia, obesity and diabetes is generally accepted as an index for increased susceptibility to coronary heart disease. Other determinants such as age, electrocardiographic abnormalities, increased uric acid levels and a positive family history also have associations of varying significance with increased atherogenesis.

Hypertension

Hypertension has been correlated with both an increased rate of new myocardial infarction and sudden death.[120] A positive correlation has been established between coronary heart disease and elevations in both systolic and diastolic blood pressures.[113,121]

The Framingham Study reported a 2.6-fold increase in risk in hypertensive men, ages 40 to 59, and a 6-fold increase in hypertensive women of the same age.[120] Another study reported that hypertensives 60 to 70 years of age had an increased rate of angina pectoris.[123]

Seasonal variations in blood pressure have been documented and should be recognized in interpretation of long-term epidemiologic studies.[121]

Diabetes Mellitus

The association of diabetes mellitus and increased incidence of coronary heart disease has long been recognized. The person with diabetes is reported to have a coronary heart disease occurrence rate two times that found in normal persons,[120] and diabetics are noted to be more susceptible to a lethal outcome.[111] In a large industrial population the risk of myocardial infarction in diabetic men, ages 25 to 64, was 2.55 times higher than in nondiabetics.[124] For the individual with diabetes who survives the initial myocardial infarction, long-term prognosis after myocardial infarction is poor. Statistics relate survival rates 5 years after heart attack for diabetics that are significantly below those for non-diabetics.[125]

An impaired glucose tolerance, even in the absence of overt diabetes, has been associated with coronary heart disease.[126] Epstein[127] reviews data suggesting that hyperglycemia, expressed not only as diabetes mellitus but also in lesser degrees of glucose tolerance, should be recognized as a predictive indication of coronary heart disease. The Tecumseh Study[128-129] found a greater prevalence of coronary heart disease when hyperglycemia was present than when glucose tolerance was normal; this finding was independent of blood pressure and blood cholesterol levels.

Obesity

Morbidity and mortality are significantly higher in the overweight than in those of normal weight, with the death rate from heart and circulatory disorders at least 1.5 times that of nonoverweight subjects.[130] In the Framingham Study, obesity was associated with increased risk of angina pectoris and sudden death but not of myocardial infarction.[113] Data from the Tecumseh population support this evidence, concluding that relative weight has an effect on incidence of coronary heart disease that is independent of blood pressure and blood sugar levels.[128]

Obesity is often associated with diabetes, hyperlipidemia and hypertension. There is no doubt that obesity increases coronary heart disease risk in subjects with hypertension, diabetes or hypercholesterolemia. Certain data indicate that the relationship of coronary heart disease and obesity has no statistical significance when the association with the previously mentioned risk factors is discounted.[122,130,131]

Positive Family History

Serum lipid levels, blood pressure and blood sugar levels are under both genetic control and environmental influences. Coronary heart disease apparently occurs in families. The question is whether this is because of the genetic variables mentioned above or other possible genetic mutations. Disagreement on interpretation of data arises when exogenous factors such as diet, smoking and other family habits are not satisfactorily excluded.[132]

Although there is no cogent proof that coronary heart disease is itself familial, there is evidence that coronary heart disease tends to aggregate among blood relatives.[133] It has been reported that the coronary heart disease pattern is family clustered, but some studies report that this trend is largely confined to the younger age groups.[134] The Tecumseh Study did find familial occurrence of coronary heart disease. Fatal coronary heart disease occurred more frequently in those individuals whose parents died of coronary heart disease before age 65 than when parental death was due to other causes.[135] In the United States, Goldstein et al.[136,138] have provided the impetus for promising research into the genetics of familial hyperlipidemia. Current knowledge regarding the role of genetics and atherosclerotic disease and their risk factors has been summarized in the Report from the National Heart and Lung Institute's Task Force on Genetic Factors in Atherosclerotic Disease.[139]

Electrocardiographic Abnormalities

Certain electrocardiographic abnormalities, in particular left ventricular hypertrophy (LVH) and intraventricular block (LVB), have an association with increased morbidity to coronary heart disease.[113] A definite ECG-LVH finding is correlated with a threefold increase of coronary heart disease after adjustment for the effect of coexisting hypertension.[140]

Other Factors, Multiplicity of Risk Factors and Age

Other factors associated with increased risk of coronary heart disease, but yet in need of supportive data, are hemoglobin levels exceeding 17 gm,[131] elevated uric acid levels, rapid pulse at rest and low vital capacity.[113]

The effect of any given risk factor or combination of factors increases with age, signifying that *age* itself must be considered a factor of risk in the forecast of coronary heart disease. This trend is reflected in the study of eight periodic health examination programs[140] where the incidence rate per 1,000 man years was 2.1 at age 30 to 39, increased to 8.1 at age 40 to 49 and 17.4 at age 50 to 59. Furthermore, those individuals having multiple risk factors are especially prone to the development of coronary heart disease, the risk being proportional to the number of factors found. The additive effect of risk factors is evident in all the studies and

aptly summarized in the Framingham report.[113] The individual who had any one of three risk factors (hypercholesterolemia, hypertension or cigarette smoking) had a risk 1.5 times that of someone having none of these factors. The presence of two factors increased the risk to approximately three times normal and the combination of three factors was associated with an eight times greater risk than someone at the same age with no risk factors.[32,69]

Hyperlipidemia

When the concentration of one or more of the plasma lipids is abnormally elevated, the condition is called hyperlipidemia. Hyperlipidemia may exist as a secondary manifestation of another disease, e.g. diabetes or hypothyroidism, or may result from dietary extremes. It may also appear as a hereditary or primary disorder. The plasma lipids of the greatest clinical interest are cholesterol and triglyceride.

Hypercholesterolemia, the most extensively measured lipid, is strongly associated with coronary heart disease. The degree of risk rises in proportion to the concentration of cholesterol,[113,123] the effect of cholesterol being greatest at younger ages[131] and usually manifested by myocardial infarction rather than by angina pectoris,[122] with the risk gradient remaining even when adjustment is made for other factors related to coronary heart disease risk and to blood lipids.[139]

Hypertriglyceridemia has also been associated with increased prevalence of coronary heart disease.[142,143] The problems relating to accurate measurement of triglyceride levels and the frequent association of hypertriglyceridemia with hypercholesterolemia have presented difficulties in the clear identification of hypertriglyceridemia alone as an indication of susceptibility to premature coronary heart disease.

All of the major lipids of the blood (cholesterol, triglyceride, and phospholipid) circulate in association with specific proteins as lipid-protein complexes. Since lipids are not water soluble in an uncombined state, these proteins (lipoproteins) serve to solubilize and transport all lipids in plasma.[144] Almost all body fats circulate between points of origin and catabolism as lipid-protein complexes. Under normal metabolic functioning, this process accounts for more than 100 gm of triglyceride, phospholipid and cholesterol each day. In arteriosclerosis, the lipoproteins provide most of the cholesterol which accumulates in the arterial wall. Thus, they are instrumental in the pathogenesis of atherosclerosis, both in physiologic and in quantitative terms.

Cholesterol and triglyceride elevations can be localized to one or more of the specific groups of lipoproteins that transport the lipids in plasma. This translation of hyperlipidemia helps determine which of the fat transports is overloaded and makes management of the hyperlipidemia more rational and often more successful.

Classification of Lipoproteins. This is generally based either on mobility (on electrophoresis) or on density (by ultracen-

APPROXIMATE % COMPOSITION OF LIPOPROTEINS

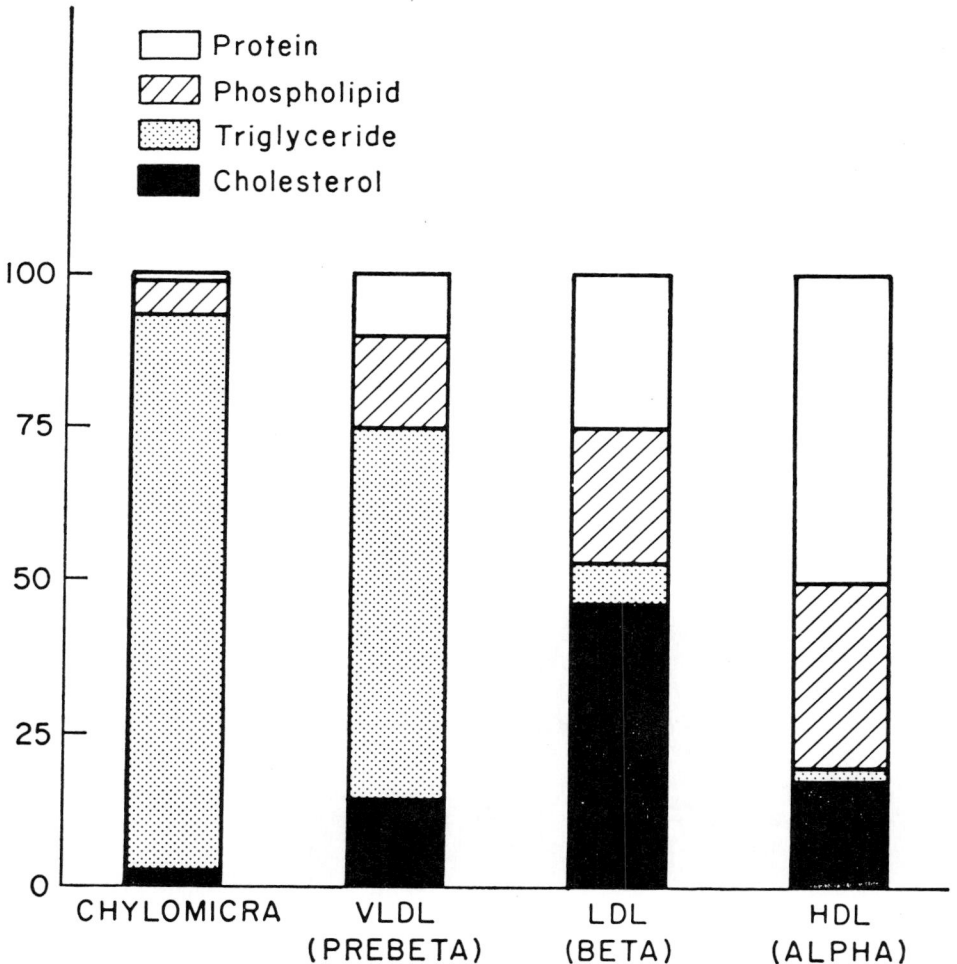

Fig. 34-1. Schematic representation of the four lipoprotein families as defined by paper electrophoresis and analytic ultracentrifugation. (From J. Am. Diet. Assoc., 58, 406, 1971.)

trifugal separation).[145] Each lipoprotein contains cholesterol, phospholipid, triglyceride and protein, but in different proportions (Fig. 34–1).

The designations for the lipoproteins separated with the ultracentrifuge are chylomicrons, very-low-density lipoproteins (VLDL), intermediate-density lipoproteins (IDL), low-density lipoproteins (LDL) and high-density lipoproteins (HDL). These can be correlated with electrophoretically defined chylomicrons, prebeta lipoproteins, broad beta lipoproteins, beta lipoproteins and alpha lipoproteins (Fig. 34–2).

Chylomicrons are the largest and lightest of the lipoproteins. Their principal component is triglyceride (80 to 95 per cent of the particle's weight), derived entirely from dietary (exogenous) fat (Fig. 34–2). The remaining components are cholesterol (2 to 7 per cent), phospholipid (3 to 6 per cent) and protein (1 to 2 per cent). These lipoproteins are synthesized in the intestine and serve to transport dietary (exogenous) glycerides from the intestinal mucosa via the thoracic duct to the tissues and are ultimately cleared by the liver and other cells (Fig. 34–3). Chylomicrons can be detected on agarose gel and paper electrophoresis. They adhere to the electrophoretic origin and are termed nonmigrating. They are also defined by their tendency as large particles to refract light and produce turbidity. Plasma appears turbid when chylomicrons are present. Furthermore, if plasma is allowed to stand at 4°C for 12 to 24 hours, the chylomicrons float to the top of the tube and form a layer. The presence of chylomicrons in the fasting state, 12 to 16 hours after the last meal, is abnormal and indicates a defective handling of dietary fat.

VLDL (very-low-density lipoproteins) are the next smallest and lightest of the lipid transport forms. The average triglyceride content is 55 to 65 per cent, cholesterol 10 to 15 per cent, phospholipid 15 to 20 per cent and protein 5 to 10 per cent. On agarose gel and paper electrophoresis they have a prebeta mobility and are sometimes called the prebeta lipoproteins. Their density is less than 1.006. Increased concentrations of VLDL produce turbid plasma.

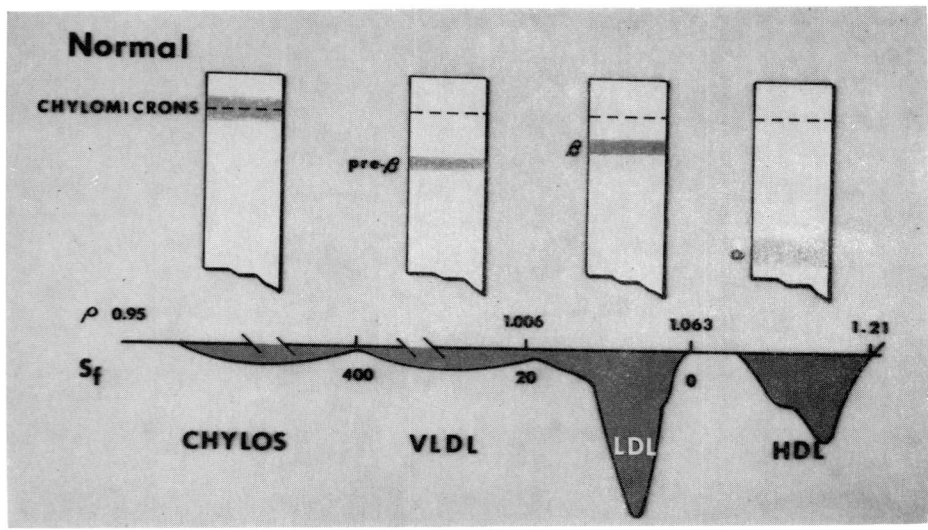

Fig. 34-2.   Representation of approximate percentage of lipoproteins. (From Prog. Cardiovasc. Dis., *14*, 341, 1972.)

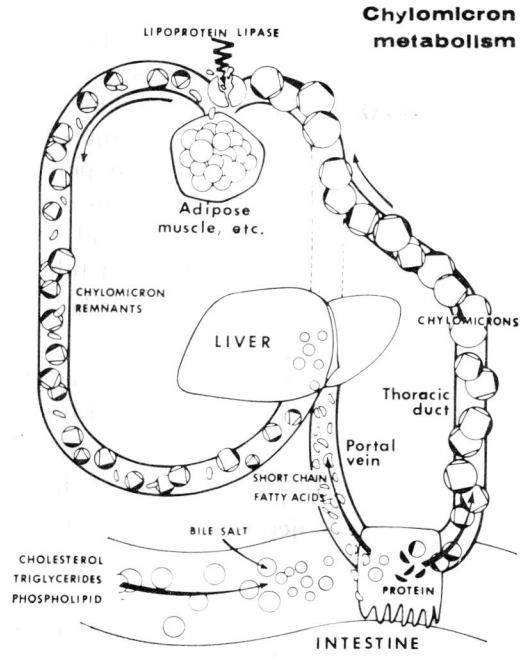

Chylomicron metabolism

Fig. 34-3. Schematic view of the metabolism and transport of chylomicrons (dietary fat). For explanation see text.

Intermediate-density lipoproteins (IDL) are not a separate species of lipoprotein, but an intermediate in the conversion of VLDL to LDL. Turnover occurs so rapidly (within 2 to 6 hours) that IDL are not normally identified, although they do define Type III hyperlipoproteinemia. The particles contain approximately 40 per cent triglyceride, 30 per cent cholesterol, 20 per cent phospholipid and 10 per cent protein. Elevated concentrations of IDL produce plasma turbidity. Clinical features associated with increased levels of IDL include premature atherosclerosis, glucose intolerance, hyperuricemia and tendinous tuberoeruptive and palmar planar xanthoma.

Low-density lipoproteins (LDL) may be defined by density range of separation (from 1.019 to 1.063) in the ultracentrifuge. On agarose gel and paper they have the electrophoretic mobility of the beta globulins and hence are often referred to as beta lipoproteins. By weight, LDL are approximately 45 per cent cholesterol, 22 per cent phospholipid, 10 per cent triglyceride and 25 per cent protein. It is suspected that LDL originate, at least in part, from VLDL degradation. The further pathway is unclear, although the liver appears to be primarily responsible for clearance. LDL elevation is associated with premature atherosclerosis, corneal arcus, tendinous and tuberous xanthoma.

High-density lipoproteins (HDL) are the fourth and smallest of the lipoprotein species. HDL contain approximately 45 to 50 per cent protein, 30 per cent phospholipid and 20 per cent cholesterol. In the ultracentrifuge, HDL floats between densities of 1.063 and 1.21 and on paper or agarose gel electrophoresis exhibit alpha mobility. HDL are normal constituents of fasting plasma and do not produce turbidity when present in increased amounts. HDL originate in the liver but are largely independent of VLDL production. Their precise function has not been elucidated.

The turbidity of VLDL, unlike that of chylomicrons, remains uniformly distributed throughout the sample after storage in the cold; layering out at the top does not occur. A small amount of VLDL is present in normal fasting plasma. In the absence of chylomicrons, an increase in VLDL can be directly correlated with plasma levels of triglyceride. VLDL consists primarily of triglyceride which is derived (endogenously) from the liver, synthesized from various precursors such as fatty acids and carbohydrates. It is presumed that these lipoproteins initiate a complex metabolic process whereby VLDL is eventually degraded into LDL via the short-lived intermediate lipoprotein. The precise workings of this mechanism have not yet been clarified. Increased levels of VLDL are generally associated with glucose intolerance, obesity, hyperuricemia, premature atherosclerosis and eruptive xanthoma.

HDL have invoked considerable interest of late. In contrast to the other lipoproteins, increased levels of HDL appear to be associated with a decreased risk of CHD. The appearance of HDL as a negative risk factor can be traced to Barr et al. in 1951.[146] The finding of *decreased* HDL in coronary heart disease has now been confirmed in several studies.[147–149] The mechanism for such a protective relationship is unexplained. Miller and Miller[150] hypothesize that HDL transport cholesterol from peripheral tissues to the liver for catabolism and excretion. The exact mechanism as well as the reported finding that physical activity and weight loss increase HDL are concepts inviting further exploration.[151–154]

Physiology of Lipid Transport.[144,155–157] Present-day concepts consider the lipoprotein moiety (protein, cholesterol and phospholipid) as the vehicle for the transport of glyceride, a neutral fat with a turnover rate of 100 to 150 gm per day. Kinetic studies demonstrate that the turnover of phospholipid and cholesterol is quite slow—both less than 1 to 2 gm a day. On a normal diet, from 70 to 150 gm of glyceride enter from the intestine each day and are cleared by the periphery; an additional 10 to 50 gm glyceride can enter each day from the liver. In any state in which too much triglyceride is mobilized from the liver or intestine or too little cleared, glyceride-rich lipoprotein accumulates in the plasma. Thus, a major determinant of plasma lipoprotein levels is the demand for glyceride transport.

Exogenous glyceride transport is depicted in Figure 34–3. The ingested fat is emulsified, hydrolyzed into smaller fragments by the pancreatic lipase in the intestine and these are solubilized in micelles by conjugated bile salts. (Chap. 5). Resynthesized fat is then associated with protein cholesterol and phospholipid in the cells of the intestine to form chylomicrons which enter the blood stream via the lymphatics. A small amount of fatty acids and the medium chain triglycerides enter the circulation directly via the portal system.

Exogenous hypertriglyceridemia can occur because of an increased intake of glyceride or because of inadequate peripheral clearance. Exogenous hyperlipemia is a daily phenomenon. Associated with each meal that we consume there is a tide of exogenous glyceride chylomicrons. Following a standard 100-gm fat meal in a normal person, chylomicrons will appear and reach a peak after approximately 4 hours. In the normal subject the chylomicrons will be cleared approximately 8 to 12 hours after the last meal. Awareness of this exogenous triglyceride is important in evaluating patients. In testing an individual for a lipid transport disorder the blood sample should be taken approximately 12 to 16 hours after the last meal, when the normal chylomicron tide will have cleared.

Endogenous hyperglyceridemia is more difficult to visualize. The liver synthesizes

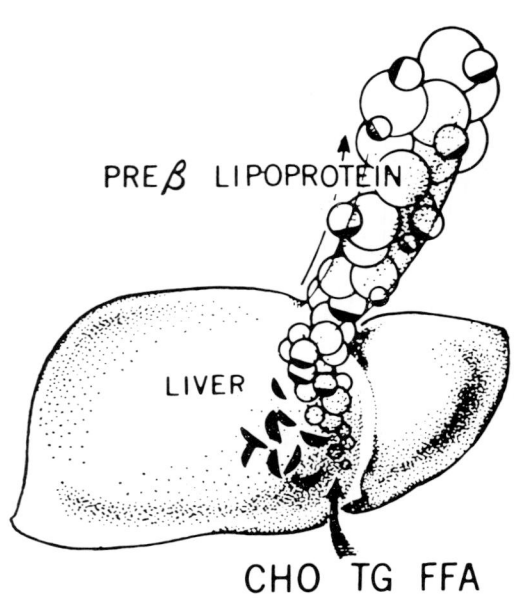

Fig. 34-4. Schematic view of endogenous glyceride production in the liver. (From J. Am. Diet. Assoc., 58, 406, 1971.)

glycerides de novo from absorbed carbohydrate, from fatty acid mobilized from adipose tissue, and from a number of different 2-carbon sources (Figure 34–4). If the liver is synthesizing glyceride at too rapid a rate, or if it is not being cleared, endogenous glyceride (prebeta lipoprotein, VLDL) will accumulate in the plasma. Endogenous hyperglyceridemia is a common phenomenon and can be produced in normal individuals with a high-carbohydrate diet. Although carbohydrate ingestion is accompanied by an increase in triglycerides as a normal phenomenon, some patients demonstrate increased sensitivity to carbohydrate which may result in higher and persistently elevated triglyceride levels.

Both exogenous and endogenous glycerides must be cleared from the plasma. This occurs predominantly in the liver, adipose tissue and muscle where the glycerides are stored or metabolized. At these sites of glyceride clearance, lipoprotein lipase is probably active in the break-down of the large glyceride-containing moieties into smaller more soluble lipoproteins and fatty acids. The adipose cell, the storage vat for fat, does not have the capacity for synthesizing lipoprotein. Therefore, glyceride cannot be released into the plasma. Rather, the only lipid leaving the adipose cell is fatty acid, which produces glyceridemia only secondarily; the fatty acid travels to the liver and stimulates endogenous glyceride release. Thus, hyperglyceridemia can occur because of too much glyceride entering from the intestine, too much glyceride production by the liver or too little glyceride clearance by the periphery.

A much less dynamic but important factor in controlling the plasma levels of lipoprotein is the state of cholesterol balance. There are two sources of plasma cholesterol—the exogenous cholesterol, i.e. the cholesterol in the diet, and the cholesterol made de novo predominantly in the liver and intestine.[158] Cholesterol entering from the intestine seems to exert

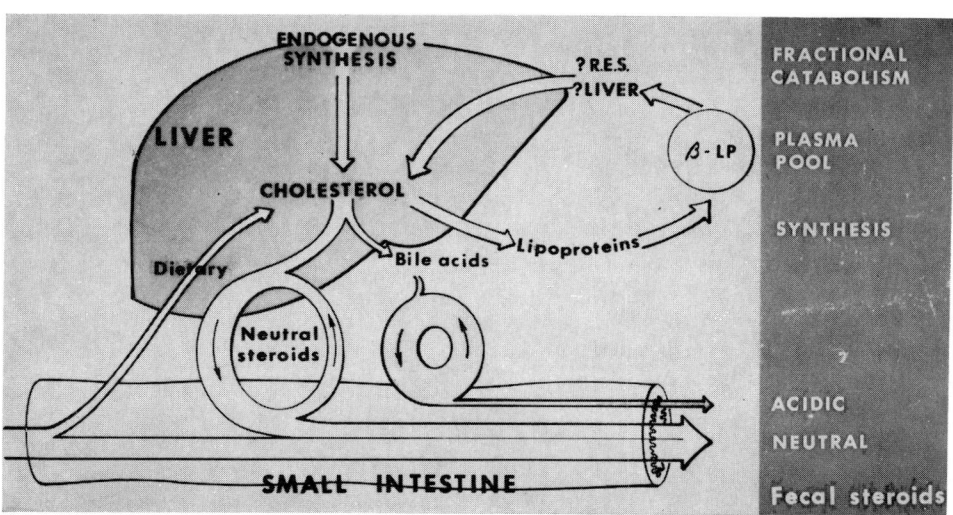

Fig. 34-5.   Schematic view of the dynamics of hepatic cholesterol metabolism. Liver cholesterol comes from three sources: endogenous synthesis, lipoprotein catabolism and the diet. Hepatic cholesterol leaves the liver via the blood stream on lipoproteins and via the biliary tree as neutral and acidic sterols. As shown here the acidic and neutral sterol constantly recirculates between the liver and intestine in what is known as "the enterohepatic cycle."

a negative feedback and inhibits the cholesterol production in the liver. If the exogenous load of cholesterol is decreased, the liver will synthesize more cholesterol. If less cholesterol is consumed (less than 300 mg per day), plasma cholesterol will fall considerably despite the increase in endogenous cholesterol synthesis. Bile acids are the major degradation products of cholesterol. Much of the bile acids are reabsorbed and constantly recycled in what is called the enterohepatic cycle (Fig. 34–5).

Other determinants, which are more difficult to measure but which play a significant role in controlling the concentration of lipoproteins in the plasma, include the availability of carbohydrates and proteins and the action of a number of hormones, including insulin, thyroxin, glucagon, epinephrine and adrenal and pituitary factors. These hormones act primarily by increasing or decreasing lipogenesis and/or lipolysis in the liver and adipose tissue. Insulin tends to maintain glyceride in the adipose tissue. Certain hormones, e.g. epinephrine, the catecholamines and glucagon, influence the breakdown of glyceride in adipose tissue, resulting in their release as fatty acids into the plasma, thereby giving rise to a secondary form of endogenous hyperlipemia. Age, weight change, emotion, stress, drugs and illness also affect lipoprotein concentrations.[159]

Lipoprotein Abnormalities. The hyperlipoproteinemias may be considered as a group of disorders characterized by excessive concentrations of one or more lipoproteins.[155] There are two general reasons for the accumulation: (1) inadequate clearance of the lipoprotein from the plasma and (2) increased production of a lipoprotein. The hyperlipoproteinemias may be simplistically categorized into six numbered types, according to the lipoprotein(s) present in excess[160] (Table 34–1). The numbering serves as a convenient code for rapid identification of the different phenotypes, both in the laboratory and in

Table 34–1.   Types of Hyperlipoproteinemia*

Type	Abnormality	Incidence
I	↑ Chylomicrons	Rare
IIa	↑ LDL	Common
IIb	↑ LDL & VLDL	Common
III	↑ IDL	Uncommon
IV	↑ VLDL	Common
V	↑ VLDL & Chylomicrons	Uncommon

*Curr. Probl. Cardiol. *1*, 3, 1976.

the clinic. Ideally, the definitive nomenclature should be based ultimately on the metabolic defect responsible for each lipoprotein abnormality. At present, although we can characterize the hyperlipoproteinemias by their respective lipoprotein patterns, we can only speculate as to the reasons for most of them. Clinical features of the six types of lipoprotein excess are summarized in Table 34–2.[155]

Classification of Hyperlipoproteinemia. *Type I.* In Type I or chylomicronemia, there is an enormous increase in the fasting concentration of chylomicrons which accumulate and streak at the origin on paper and agarose gel electrophoresis. The plasma will appear creamy and, after storage in the cold, often separates at the top into a distinct fatty layer. The ratio of triglyceride to cholesterol is greater than 5:1 and often greater than 10:1. The fasting plasma triglyceride usually is more than 2,000 mg per 100 ml when the patient is on a regular diet, while the cholesterol is either normal or elevated to a much lesser extent.

Primary Type I generally appears in infancy, often marked by chronic abdominal pain associated in some instances with pancreatitis. Other clinical features include eruptive xanthoma, hepatosplenomegaly and lipemia retinalis. In the familial form, the apparent defect involves the enzyme lipoprotein lipase. Clearance of dietary fat (chylomicrons) is inhibited because of either a deficiency or a decreased activity

Table 34–2. Distinguishing Features of the Primary Hyperlipoproteinemia

Features	Type I	Type II	Type III	Type IV	Type V
Incidence	Very rare	Common	Relatively uncommon	Common	Uncommon
Appearance of plasma	Cream layer over clear infranate on standing	Clear	Clear, cloudy or milky	Slightly turbid to cloudy, unchanged with standing	Cream layer over turbid infranate on standing
Cholesterol	Normal or elevated	Elevated	Elevated	Normal or elevated	Elevated or normal
Triglyceride	Markedly elevated	Normal or slightly elevated	Usually elevated	Elevated	Elevated to markedly elevated
Clinical presentation	Eruptive xanthomas, abdominal pain, lipemia retinalis	Xanthelasma, tendon and tuberous xanthomas, premature corneal arcus, premature atherosclerosis	Xanthoma planum; tuberoeruptive premature xanthomas; atherosclerosis of coronary and peripheral vessels	Premature coronary vessel disease, abnormal glucose tolerance, hyperuricemia	Eruptive xanthomas, hepatosplenomegaly, abdominal pain, hyperglycemia, hyperuricemia, lipemia retinalis
Origin; possible mechanism	Genetic recessive; deficiency in lipoprotein lipase	When genetic, dominant, sporadic; decreased catabolism of beta lipoprotein	Genetic mode of transmission unclear; sporadic	When genetic, dominant sporadic; excessive endogenous glyceride synthesis or deficient glyceride clearance?	Probably genetic, dominant, sporadic
Age of detection	Early childhood	Early childhood (in severe cases)	Adulthood (over age 20)	Adulthood	Early adulthood
Conditions to be excluded	Dysgammaglobulinemia, insulinopenic diabetes, lupus erythematosus	Dietary cholesterol excess, myxedema, nephrosis, porphyria, obstructive liver disease	Myxedema, dysgammaglobulinemia	Diabetes, glycogen storage disease, nephrosis pregnancy, stress, alcohol excess	Diabetic acidosis, nephrosis, alcoholism, pancreatitis, myeloma, dysproteinemias

of this enzyme. The deficiency can be detected electrophoretically following intravenous administration of heparin. Primary Type I has not been linked with the premature development of atherosclerosis. Secondary conditions which have been associated with Type I (chylomicron excess) include insulinopenic diabetes, dysglobulinemia and lupus erythematosus.

Type II. Type II is subdivided into two patterns: IIa (hypercholesterolemia) in which LDL alone is elevated, and IIb (hypercholesterolemia with endogenous hyperglyceridemia) in which both LDL and VLDL are increased. Cholesterol levels usually range from 300 to 600 mg per 100 ml. To distinguish this "mixed hyperlipidemia" from Types III and IV, it is necessary to quantify LDL levels. A visual check of the plasma after overnight storage at 4°C will show turbidity if VLDL is elevated; otherwise, the plasma remains clear.

Primary Type II hyperlipoproteinemia (familial hypercholesterolemia) is the most common of all the familial lipid disorders. It correlates positively with a high risk of developing premature ischemic heart disease.[160] Genetic forms of primary Type II may be present at birth and can be diagnosed in cord blood samples. The condition appears to be inherited as an autosomal dominant trait; therefore, there is a strong likelihood that one parent and approximately one-half of all first-degree relatives will be affected. Familial Type II is often accompanied by tendinous and tuberous xanthomas, xanthelasma and premature corneal arcus. These usually develop in adolescence or young adulthood in heterozygous forms of the disease. Patients with the most severe form, homozygous Type II, generally develop xanthomas in early childhood, and planar lesions are very common. Atherosclerotic heart disease usually develops early and progresses rapidly. The defect in primary familial Type II appears to be a decreased rate of LDL clearance, rather than in-

creased synthesis of those lipoproteins.[161] It may be related to a defect in binding (receptors) at cell surface, leading to faulty clearance of LDL.[162] The precise mechanism, however, is unknown.

In its milder forms, hypercholesterolemia may be caused by dietary excesses. Other secondary disorders to be excluded in the differential diagnosis of Type II are obstructive liver disease, hypothyroidism, nephrosis, porphyria, myxedema and multiple myeloma.

Familial Combined Hyperlipidemia. Familial combined hyperlipidemia is a genetic disorder most frequently associated with the Type IIb lipoprotein phenotype. However, in some individuals the phenotype may be Type IV or even Type IIa. This disorder has also been associated with an increased incidence of coronary heart disease. Xanthomas may occur. There is some evidence that the disorder is inherited as a monogenic, dominant trait. Perhaps the most distinct difference between familial combined hyperlipidemia and familial hypercholesterolemia is that the biochemical defect is present from birth in the latter but is not usually detected until adulthood in the former.[137]

Type III Hyperlipoproteinemia. Type III is defined biochemically by an increase in IDL levels. Both triglyceride and cholesterol concentrations are elevated in plasma, usually ranging from 350 to 1,000 mg per 100 ml. Often the ratio of triglyceride to cholesterol is close to 1:1. Chylomicrons may be seen in fasting plasma. The plasma may appear clear, cloudy or milky, depending on the extent of hypertriglyceridemia.

Type III has been alternately described as an increase in "VLDL of abnormal composition" or in "floating beta lipoprotein." In any case, it has a lipoprotein pattern quite distinct from Types II and IV but for which there is no absolute diagnostic test. Several definitions have been proposed in recent studies,[164] none of which is totally foolproof and all of which are based on techniques more complex than needed for routine clinical measurement.

The "floating beta" definition refers to a lipoprotein which has the flotation properties of VLDL, yet has beta mobility on electrophoresis. One drawback of relying solely on this definition is that the broad beta band does not always appear on electrophoresis. Other diagnostic tests for Type III involve the use of the preparative ultracentrifuge to determine the relative content of cholesterol and triglyceride in all lipoproteins of density less than 1.006 (so-called abnormal VLDL). A characteristic of Type III is a higher-than-normal cholesterol/triglyceride ratio, which is often accompanied by the presence of cholesterol-rich chylomicrons. None of these techniques alone, however, will furnish absolutely specific diagnoses of Type III. If there is reason to suspect the disorder, therefore, a combination of tests is desirable to confirm the diagnosis.

A distinguishing clinical feature which often is a basis for recognition of Type III is the presence of orange-yellow deposits along the palmar creases, referred to as palmar or plantar xanthomas. Palmar xanthomas may also be encountered in biliary cirrhosis. Tuberoeruptive xanthomas over the buttocks, knees and elbows are common but are not specific to Type III; they may occur in other hyperlipidemic disorders when the plasma triglyceride is greater than 2,000 mg per 100 ml.

Glucose tolerance is impaired in about 40 per cent of the subjects. There is an abnormal increase in the concentration of triglyceride when individuals with Type III are fed a high-carbohydrate diet—the phenomenon of carbohydrate induction.

Type III appears to be linked with a high incidence of premature peripheral vascular disease as well as with coronary artery disease, hence the importance of its recognition.[164] In contrast to other hyperlipoproteinemics, patients with this disorder respond rapidly to both dietary and drug therapy, particularly in combination. The condition is not at all as rare as had been supposed previously, nor is it as common as Type II. It is genetic in its primary form and usually appears in the second or third decade in men and 10 to 15 years later in women. The mode of inheritance is still unclear, although it has been reported both as an autosomal recessive and an autosomal dominant trait. It may also be secondary to myxedema, dysgammaglobulinemia and hypothyroidism. The suspected abnormality in Type III is unclear. It may be secondary to overproduction of VLDL or a blockage in the conversion of VLDL to LDL, both of which could cause accumulation of IDL and chylomicron remnants.

Type IV Hyperlipoproteinemia. This is a very common lipid disorder. Triglyceride levels usually range from 400 to 1,000. Plasma cholesterol levels may be normal. At higher levels of hypertriglyceridemia the plasma cholesterol may also be elevated since VLDL contains about 1 mg cholesterol per 5 mg of triglyceride. The severity of the hypertriglyceridemia is correlated with the appearance of the fasting plasma, which may vary from clear to very turbid.

Clinical features associated with primary Type IV include glucose intolerance in roughly 50 per cent of all cases, often coupled with hyperuricemia. Eruptive xanthomas can occur in patients with severely increased VLDL levels. Otherwise, external stigmata are rare. Obesity and excessive alcohol consumption will aggravate both primary and secondary forms of the disorder. Conversely, reduction to ideal body weight will invariably lower triglyceride concentrations. The disorder generally appears in the second decade, although there have been instances of its discovery in children. The pathophysiology of primary Type IV has been linked both to overproduction of VLDL and to an impaired rate of its clearance. The variability of the genetic and etiologic factors of the disorder certainly complicates the ascertainment of its metabolic defects.

Type IV is most frequently found in women aged 20 to 50 who are using oral contraceptives—the most common cause of Type IV in that age and sex group. Type IV can be secondary to diabetes, glycogen storage disease, the nephrotic syndrome, pregnancy, stress and alcoholism. Although there is still no conclusive proof that Type IV can lead to premature atherosclerosis, mounting evidence suggests that there may be an association between this disorder and an increased risk of developing CHD.

Type V Hyperlipoproteinemia. This is a mixed pattern in which the fasting plasma contains both chylomicrons (exogenous triglycerides) and an increased concentration of VLDL (endogenous triglycerides). Plasma triglyceride elevations are in the range of 1,000 to 6,000 mg per 100 ml. The plasma cholesterol is often elevated, but the ratio of triglyceride to cholesterol is about 5:1 or higher. The fasting plasma is creamy.

Clinical features of Type V are similar to those of Type I, except that they occur in adulthood rather than in infancy. The clinical finding of greatest concern is that of recurrent abdominal pain which may provoke an unneeded abdominal exploration. Acute pancreatitis sometimes accompanies the bouts of abdominal colic. Eruptive xanthoma and hepatosplenomegaly occur in about 30 per cent of affected subjects.

While Type V may be transmitted in certain families as a dominant trait with delayed penetrance, it more frequently is a secondary consequence of diabetic acidosis, alcoholism or nephrosis. Common biochemical findings are hyperuricemia and a diabetic glucose tolerance test. The Type V patient is often sensitive to increased dietary loads of both fat and carbohydrate. Plasma postheparin lipolytic activity is not severely depressed (in contrast to Type I) but is near the lower limit of the normal range.

Screening for Hyperlipoproteinemia. The suspicion of hyperlipidemia may be obtained from detailed personal and family history and a physical examination. One family history indicator is the occurrence of premature vascular disease (Types II, III, IV). Other important history and clinical findings are a history of turbid fasting plasma (Types I, IIb, III, IV and V), hyperuricemia (Types IV and V), diabetes (Types III, IV, V), premature corneal arcus (Type II) and xanthomata—tendinous (Types II and III), eruptive (Types I and V) or palmar (Type III).

The next step is to measure the plasma concentrations of both cholesterol and triglyceride. The sample should be obtained after an overnight fast and stored at 4°C. The measurement should reflect a steady state: (1) a regular diet for at least 2 weeks prior to sampling, (2) stable weight, (3) no acute illnesses within 4 to 6 weeks and (4) no medications, particularly hypolipidemic agents or hormones. Myocardial infarction, pregnancy, stress and other traumatic episodes can be expected to affect lipid levels. Measurements obtained during these periods should not be assumed to reflect baseline levels. Normal values of lipid and lipoprotein concentrations are listed in Table 34–3. Normal values are at best arbitrary. Lower values may be more desirable.

The underlying cause of hyperlipidemia may be metabolic, genetic or secondary to another disorder. If hyperlipidemia is secondary to another disease, then treatment of the underlying disease is undertaken. No further treatment of lipid elevation should be undertaken until the basic disorder is controlled. Potential causes of hyperlipidemia are dietary excess, diabetes mellitus, hypothyroidism, dysproteinemia, nephrosis, liver disease and alcoholism. Therefore, dietary assessment should be obtained as well as laboratory tests for blood sugar, thyroid, liver and renal function and a plasma protein electrophoresis.

Table 34–3.   Plasma Lipid Concentrations (mg/dl)*

| | Plasma Cholesterol Mean Values by Age Groups† | | | | | | Plasma Triglycerides Mean Values by Age Groups† | | | | | |
| | White Males | | | White Females Not on Hormones | | | White Males | | | White Females Not on Hormones | | |
Age (Years)	N	Mean	S.D.	N	Mean	S.D.	N	Mean	S.D.	N	Mean	S.D.
0–4	238	154.6	27.2	186	156.0	26.9	238	56.4	24.2	186	63.9	24.3
5–9	1253	159.9	25.3	1118	163.7	24.7	1253	55.7	22.7	1118	60.3	25.3
10–14	2278	157.6	25.6	2080	159.6	24.1	2278	65.6	30.6	2080	75.4	30.9
15–19	1980	149.9	26.5	1911	156.6	26.4	1980	78.0	38.1	1911	72.4	32.5
20–24	882	166.5	28.6	778	164.1	29.6	882	100.3	56.4	778	72.4	35.3
25–29	2042	182.2	35.0	1329	170.7	29.0	2042	115.8	104.3	1329	74.7	37.0
30–34	2444	192.2	36.8	1569	175.4	31.2	2444	128.3	121.2	1569	78.5	40.1
35–39	2320	201.3	36.8	1606	184.3	31.7	2320	144.9	120.8	1606	86.2	49.0
40–44	2428	206.5	36.5	1583	193.0	34.6	2428	151.4	148.8	1583	98.4	82.0
45–49	2296	212.2	36.0	1515	202.5	37.5	2296	151.7	115.8	1515	104.5	69.5
50–54	2138	212.7	37.0	1257	217.7	37.8	2138	151.8	117.8	1257	114.8	69.6
55–59	1621	213.9	38.3	1112	230.5	39.0	1621	141.4	88.1	1112	125.0	76.7
60–64	905	213.0	36.7	723	230.8	39.9	905	142.3	94.4	723	126.9	88.5
65–69	750	212.6	34.8	593	232.8	40.4	750	136.7	142.2	593	131.3	110.1
70–74	484	208.2	34.7	411	228.5	45.7	484	129.5	70.8	411	133.8	112.1
75–79	244	204.9	34.7	207	231.0	37.9	244	129.1	69.1	207	127.9	101.0
80+	122	206.6	42.9	130	222.1	37.3	122	132.1	120.6	130	135.2	103.8
All Ages	24428			18108			24428			18108		

*Data from Lipid Research Clinics North American Population Study.
†Mean levels are not necessarily safe or acceptable levels.

Since hypercholesterolemia or hyper-triglyceridemia indicates the elevation of one or more lipoproteins, the definition of the precise lipoprotein pattern is often obtained before beginning therapy. In addition to history and physical findings, two other simple procedures will usually suffice for identifying the types of hyper-lipoproteinemia: (1) Observation of the plasma which has been refrigerated overnight at 4°C is instructive. A floating "cream" layer identifies the presence of chylomicrons. This observation suggests either a nonfasting subject or an abnormality worthy of further investigation. A turbid infranate is caused by increased concentrations of VLDL. A clear infranate may contain elevated concentrations of LDL, since these molecules are small, completely soluble and do not refract light. Using these guidelines, a cream layer and a clear infranate suggest a Type I pattern. Turbid plasma without evidence of chylomicrons indicates Types IIb, III and IV. In Type III a scant cream layer of chylomicrons may be noticed. In Type IIa, the plasma may be clear or in Type IIb slightly turbid since VLDL is elevated in addition to LDL. (2) The cholesterol and triglyceride values indicate the type of hyperlipoproteinemia:[166,167]

High cholesterol, normal triglycerides usually indicate Type IIa. The plasma is clear with no chylomicron layer.

High cholesterol, triglycerides 150–400 usually identify Type IIb or Type IV but may occur in Type III. Plasma is turbid in all these types but Type III will show a slight cream supranate because of the chylomicrons. Lipid values which fluctuate widely from week to week are often an indication of Type III. If additional laboratory tests reveal the presence of the lipoprotein IDL, and the patient has palmar xanthoma, diabetes or premature vascular disease, the diagnosis will almost always be Type III.

High cholesterol, triglycerides 400–1,000 usually signify either Type IV or Type V.

A positive chylomicron test, in general, indicates Type V.

Normal cholesterol, high triglycerides almost invariably mean Type IV. It can also infrequently signify Type III.

In some instances quantification of the LDL fraction is necessary using either ultracentrifugal fractionation or electrophoretic analysis.

Management of Hyperlipoprotein-emia.[167] Treatment of hyperlipoproteinemia is undertaken primarily on the assumption that lowering lipids will reduce the risk of premature coronary heart disease. In some instances, therapy is undertaken to alleviate symptoms of severe hyperglyceridemia such as eruptive xanthomata and the abdominal pain sometimes associated with pancreatitis and hepatosplenomegaly.

Management of all hyperlipidemia (hyperlipoproteinemia) should begin with diet. Often no other treatment is needed. Mild hyperlipoproteinemia of Types IIa, IIb and IV can often be treated successfully with moderate diet therapy. For Types IIb and IV, management might begin with weight reduction, decreased intake of alcohol and perhaps carbohydrate. Types IIa, IIb and sometimes Type IV can begin with a prudent diet that restricts cholesterol intake to 300 mg and saturated fat to approximately 10 per cent of the calories from fat. More specifically tailored dietary guidelines for all types of hyperlipoproteinemia[168] continue to be effective tools of dietary management and are available upon request from the National Heart, Lung, and Blood Institute (see Summary, Table 34–4). The recommended diets for the treatment of primary hyperlipoproteinemia are outlined briefly below (Table 34–4).

Type I. At the present time, dietary modification is the only effective therapy for Type I. The high levels of chylomicrons which are present while the patient with this disorder is on a normal diet will disap-

Table 34–4. Therapy for Hyperlipoproteinemia*

	Type I	Type IIa	Type IIb & Type III	Type IV	Type V
Diet Prescription	Low fat 25–35 gm	Low cholesterol polyunsaturated fat increased	Low cholesterol approximately: 20% cal pro. 40% cal fat 40% cal CHO	Controlled CHO Approximately 45% of calories Moderately restricted cholesterol	Restricted fat 30% of calories Controlled CHO 50% of calories Moderately restricted cholesterol
Calories	Not restricted	Not restricted	Achieve and maintain "ideal" weight, i.e. reduction diet if necessary	Achieve and maintain "ideal" weight, i.e. reduction diet if necessary	Achieve and maintain "ideal" weight, i.e. reduction diet if necessary
Protein	Total protein intake is not limited	Total protein intake is not limited	High protein	Not limited other than control of patient's weight	High protein
Fat	Restricted to 25–35 gm Kind of fat not important	Saturated fat intake limited Polyunsaturated fat intake increased	Controlled to 40% calories (polyunsaturated fats recommended in preference to saturated fats)	Not limited other than control of patient's weight (polyunsaturated fats recommended in preference to saturated fats)	Restricted to 30% of calories (polyunsaturated fats recommended in preference to saturated fats)
Cholesterol	Not restricted	As low as possible; the only source of cholesterol is the meat in the diet	Less than 300 mg—the only source of cholesterol is the meat in the diet	Moderately restricted to 300–500 mg	Moderately restricted to 300–500 mg
Carbohydrate	Not limited	Not limited	Controlled—concentrated sweets are restricted	Controlled—concentrated sweets are restricted	Controlled—concentrated sweets are restricted
Alcohol	Not recommended	May be used with discretion	Limited to 2 servings (substituted for carbohydrate)	Limited to 2 servings (substituted for carbohydrate)	Not recommended

*From Fredrickson, Levy, Bonnell and Ernst.[168]

pear entirely on a fat-free regimen. Fat intake should be reduced to a level which will relieve symptoms and prevent abdominal pain. In general, this corresponds to 25 to 35 gm per day in adults and 10 to 15 gm per day in children. Fats, nuts, baked goods containing fat, all fatty meats and dairy products containing fat are eliminated. Although no other restrictions are necessary, the diet is difficult to follow because of its unpalatability and lack of satiety. Fat intake, however, generally brings on severe attacks of abdominal pain which will often stimulate adherence to the diet. Prescription of medium-chain triglyceride (MCT) adds variability and interest to meal preparation. MCT permits fat intake without chylomicron formation because the fatty acids are transported directly from the intestine to the liver via the portal system (Fig. 34–3).

Type IIa. The diet for management of Type II includes a cholesterol restriction to less than 300 mg per day, a decrease in saturated fats and an increase in the consumption of polyunsaturated fats. This plan is more restrictive than a prudent control. It eliminates egg yolks, limits the kinds and quantities of meat and allows only very-low-fat dairy products. Caloric and carbohydrate intake may be controlled in Type IIb in which reduction to ideal weight is recommended before starting the Type II maintenance diet. Weight loss alone, however, generally will not lower serum cholesterol to desired levels.

Dietary alteration may not lower serum cholesterol to desired levels in familial forms of Type IIa. Pharmacologic intervention is then a consideration.

Type IIb. In Type IIb, reduction to ideal weight may normalize triglyceride levels. Weight loss alone, however, will not normalize cholesterol levels. At ideal weight, the dietary principles applicable to the management of Type III—controlled calories, alcohol and carbohydrate—are sometimes needed to promote lower triglyceride concentrations. Cholesterol in-

take and saturated fat are also restricted. A drug supplement may be necessary to achieve optimum results.

Type III. Patients with Type III generally respond rapidly to dietary treatment. Even in the most severe cases, lipid values can return to normal through therapy, sometimes with the addition of drugs. Ideal weight should be sought and maintained. The Type III maintenance is similar to that prescribed for diabetics. Cholesterol is restricted to less than 300 mg. The distribution of total calories is 40 per cent each of carbohydrate and fat and 20 per cent protein. The dramatic response to therapy of patients with Type III is particularly gratifying because of the association of this disorder with xanthomas, premature vascular disease and, sometimes, coronary heart disease.

Type IV. The keystone of diet therapy in Type IV patients is weight control. It is suspected that Type IV is precipitated by weight gain in adults which, in turn, may be caused by a metabolic defect that manifests itself in adulthood. Weight loss will often reduce triglyceride concentrations to normal. Patients should be placed on a reducing diet to achieve ideal weight, which is then maintained by curtailing alcohol and carbohydrate intake. Cholesterol is moderately restricted (300 to 500 mg), but is not necessary for those few patients who manifest desired levels of serum cholesterol.

Type V. Because of the increase in VLDL and chylomicrons which characterizes the Type V disorder, patients generally manifest both fat and carbohydrate sensitivity. Both should be restricted in order to lower triglyceride levels, but fat intake should be controlled more rigidly since its ingestion often precipitates acute attacks of abdominal pain (as in Type I). Caloric restriction to achieve ideal weight is also important in Type V, as in other forms of endogenous hyperglyceridemia. Triglyceride levels in most patients will drop in response to weight loss, and tolerance of carbohydrates and fats also improves markedly. In lean patients, however, it may sometimes be necessary to add drugs.[159]

Drug Therapy. A variety of hypolipidemic agents are now available for the management of hyperlipoproteinemia (Table 34–5). However, no one drug is effective in all types of hyperlipoproteinemia and the longitudinal aspects of drug therapy are not available. It is crucial that drug therapy not be undertaken until the effectiveness of diet has been tested. Six weeks of diet therapy are desirable, during which time lipid values should be recorded at regular intervals. To establish a baseline, a minimum of three control values should be taken over a period of several days. If there is no appreciable change in lipid levels, and *only* then, should the addition of a drug be considered. Drug therapy should be a supplement to rather than a substitute for dietary control. Both forms of treatment should be continued concomitantly because their combined effects are cumulative. Drugs should be instituted one at a time. The effects of a particular drug should be fully established before another is introduced to supplement or replace it.

Long-term therapy with a drug should be contingent upon a marked reduction in plasma lipid levels. The yardstick for this decision should be an approximate 15 per cent decrease in lipid levels within 4 to 6 weeks. Another important criterion for continuation of a drug regimen is the absence of any serious side effects. Patients should also be carefully monitored for potential toxicity. Any complications will generally disappear soon after use of the drug is discontinued. Frequently, however, a simple adjustment in dosage will suffice to alleviate most abnormalities. Familial forms of hyperlipoproteinemia will generally require more intensive treatment than the environmentally induced disorders.

Conclusions and Prospects. Considerable progress has been made in the management of hyperlipoproteinemia in recent years. A vast amount of information has been acquired on lipid and lipoprotein metabolism, which has promoted a better understanding of the lipid transport disorders. It is now known that a high serum cholesterol level is simply the signal of an underlying lipoprotein abnormality and that attention should be focused on that abnormality rather than on its symptoms. Indeed, while the total plasma cholesterol as well as the cholesterol carried by the low-density lipoproteins (LDL) correlate quite positively with coronary artery disease, levels of high-density lipoprotein cholesterol (HDL) are inversely related to coronary artery disease. Moreover, each type of hyperlipoproteinemia represents distinct disorders which differ from one another in origin, clinical signs and response to therapy. It is precisely through the awareness of these disparities that a more pragmatic approach to management has evolved.

Identification of the specific lipoprotein phenotype (translating hyperlipidemia to

Table 34–5.   Preferred Drugs*

Type I	Type II	Type III	Types IV and V
None effective at present	Cholestyramine 16–32 gm/day	Clofibrate 2 gm/day *also* Nicotinic acid 3–6 gm/day D-Thyroxine 3–8 mg/day	Nicotinic acid 3–6 gm/day *sometimes* Clofibrate 2 gm/day

*From Levy, Morganroth and Rifkind.[167]

hyperlipoproteinemia) will help distinguish those patients who are at greatest risk and will also provide a more rational basis for the selection of therapy. Although many patients will respond well to dietary adjustment alone, in other cases supplemental medication may be needed. The prospects for successful lipid-lowering have been greatly improved by the development of highly effective hypolipidemic agents. Drug therapy, however, places an onus on the patient in terms of cost, long-term adherence and side effects. These drawbacks seem even harder to tolerate in the absence of any definitive justification for hypolipidemic therapy. Although the evidence associating hyperlipoproteinemia (except for excess HDL or chylomicrons) with CHD is overwhelming, it is nonetheless largely circumstantial and the ultimate benefits of lipid-lowering are still presumptive.

Diet is the cornerstone of therapy for each of the primary lipid transport disorders. Diet therapy should always be tried before any drug is used. Often dietary manipulations alone will allow normalization of plasma lipid levels. If the addition of drugs proves necessary, diet should be continued since the effects of diet and drugs are additive and more powerful than those of either alone. Though the evidence that dietary intervention in the coronary-prone patient will actually decrease coronary morbidity and mortality is still primarily presumptive, logic demands an active and aggressive approach to the high-risk patient.

The success of dietary management depends on the rapport of the doctor, dietitian and patient. The physician should explain the significance of the lipids to the patient. The dietitian should understand the patient's disease and dietary needs and counsel him on its practical aspects. Frequent return visits, teaching aids and family dietary counseling are all of benefit. The patient should be encouraged to call or write for additional information. The patient's motivation and understanding of the diet are essential in dietary management. Successful management of the high-risk patient with hyperlipoproteinemia depends on a close and enthusiastic working relationship among physician, dietitian and patient.

BIBLIOGRAPHY

1. Getz, Vesselinovitch and Wissler: Am. J. Med., 46, 657, 1969.
2. Fredrickson: In Harrison's Principles of Internal Medicine (Wintrobe, Thorn, Adams, Bennett, Braunwald, Isselbacher and Petersdorf, Eds.). New York, McGraw-Hill Book Company, 1970, pp. 1239–1252.
3. The National Heart, Lung, and Blood Institute's Fact Book for Fiscal Year 1976. DHEW Publication No. (NIH) 77–1172, Washington, U. S. Superintendent of Documents, October 1976.
4. De Langen: Geneeskd. Ned. Ind., 56, 1, 1916.
5. Snapper: Chinese Lessons to Western Medicine, New York, Interscience, 1941.
6. Strasser: WHO Chron., 26, 7, 1972.
7. Gordon and Kannel: J.A.M.A., 215, 1617, 1971.
8. Kreuger and Morijama: Am. J. Public Health, 57, 496, 1967.
9. Anitschkow: In Cowdry's Atherosclerosis–A Survey of the Problem, 2nd ed. (Blumenthal, Ed.). Springfield, Charles C Thomas, 1967, pp. 21–44.
10. Ahrens: Am. J. Med., 23, 928, 1957.
11. Randles and Knudson: J. Biol. Chem., 66, 459, 1925.
12. Schoenheimer and Breusch: J. Biol. Chem., 103, 439, 1933.
13. Rittenberg and Schoenheimer: J. Biol. Chem., 121, 235, 1937.
14. Armstrong, Warner and Connor: Circ. Res., 27, 59, 1970.
15. Keys, Michelsen, Miller and Chapman: Science, 112, 79, 1950.
16. Keys, Anderson, Mickelsen, Adelson and Flaminio: J. Nutr., 59, 39, 1956.
17. Kinsell, Partridge, Boling, Margen and Michaels: J. Clin. Endocrinol. Metab., 12, 909, 1952.
18. Ahrens, Tsaltas, Hirsch and Insull: J. Clin. Invest., 34, 918, 1955.
19. Steiner, Howard and Akgun: J.A.M.A., 181, 186, 1962.
20. Erickson, Coots, Mattson and Kligman: J. Clin. Invest., 43, 2017, 1964.
21. Connor, Hodges and Bleiler: J. Clin. Invest., 40, 894, 1961.
22. Connor, Stone and Hodges: J. Clin. Invest., 43, 1691, 1964.
23. Keys, Anderson and Grande: Metabolism., 14, 759, 1965.
24. Anderson, Grande and Keys: Am. J. Clin. Nutr., 29, 1184, 1976.

25. Kaplan, Cox and Taylor: Arch. Pathol., 76, 359, 1963.
26. Wilson and Lindsey: J. Lipid Res., 44, 1805, 1965.
27. Borgstrom: J. Lipid Res., 10, 331, 1969.
28. Quintao, Grundy and Ahrens: J. Lipid Res., 12, 221, 1971.
29. Quintao, Grundy and Ahrens: J. Lipid Res., 12, 233, 1971.
30. Keys: J. Chronic Dis., 4, 364, 1956.
31. Mayer, Connell, DeWolfe and Beveridge: Am. J. Clin. Nutr., 2, 316, 1954.
32. Wilmot and Swank: Am. J. Med. Sci., 223, 25, 1952.
33. Starke: Am. J. Med., 9, 494, 1950.
34. Hildreth, Mellinkoff, Blair and Hildreth: J. Clin. Invest., 30, 649, 1951.
35. Kinsell, Michaels, Partridge, Boling, Balch and Cochrane: J. Clin. Nutr., 1, 224, 1953.
36. Ahrens, Blankenhorn and Tsaltas: Proc. Soc. Exp. Biol. Med., 86, 872, 1954.
37. Beveridge, Connell, Mayer, Firstbrook and DeWolfe: Circulation, 10, 593, 1954.
38. Keys, Anderson and Grande: Lancet, 1, 787, 1957.
39. Keys, Anderson and Grande: Metabolism, 14, 776, 1965.
40. Hegsted, McGandy, Myers and Stare: Am. J. Clin. Nutr., 17, 281, 1965.
41. Horlick and Craig: Lancet, 2, 566, 1957.
42. Ahrens, Insull, Bloomstrand, Hirsch, Tsaltas and Peterson: Lancet, 1, 943, 1957.
43. Grande, Anderson and Keys: J. Nutr., 74, 420, 1961.
44. Hashim, Arteaga and Van Itallie: Lancet, 1, 1105, 1960.
45. Keys, Anderson and Grande: Proc. Soc. Exp. Biol. Med., 98, 387, 1958.
46. Keys, Anderson and Grande: Metabolism, 14, 747, 1965.
47. Anderson, Grande and Keys: J. Nutr., 75, 388, 1961.
48. Antonis and Bersohn: Lancet, 1, 3, 1961.
49. Antonis and Bersohn: Lancet, 1, 998, 1962.
50. Albrink: J. Am. Diet. Assoc., 62, 626, 1973.
51. Anderson: Am. J. Clin. Nutr., 20, 168, 1967.
52. Yudkin: Am. Heart J., 66, 835, 1963.
53. Yudkin: Lancet, 2, 4, 1964.
54. Yudkin and Roddy: Lancet, 2, 6, 1964.
55. Yudkin and Morland: J. Clin. Nutr., 20, 503, 1967.
56. Burns-Cox, Doll and Ball: Br. Heart J., 31, 485, 1969.
57. Howell and Wilson: Br. Med. J., 3, 145, 1969.
58. Keys: Atherosclerosis, 14, 193, 1971.
59. Keys: Atherosclerosis, 18, 352, 1973.
60. Walker: Atherosclerosis, 14, 137, 1971.
61. Keys: Atherosclerosis, 22, 149, 1975.
62. McGandy, Hegsted and Stare: N. Engl. J. Med., 277, 186, 245, 1967.
63. Albrink: Prog. Biochem. Pharmacol., 8, 242, 1973.
64. MacDonald and Braithwaite: Clin. Sci., 27, 23, 1964.
65. Groen, Balogh, Yaron and Cohen: Am. J. Clin. Nutr., 19, 46, 1966.
66. Antar and Ohlson: J. Nutr., 85, 329, 1965.
67. Kuo and Bassett: Ann. Intern. Med., 62, 1199, 1965.
68. Kuo: In Cardiac and Vascular Diseases (Conn and Horwitz, Eds.). Philadelphia, Lea & Febiger, 1971.
69. Kaufmann, Poznanski, Blondheim and Stein: Am. J. Clin. Nutr., 18, 261, 1966.
70. Dunnigan, Fyfe, McKiddie and Crosbie: Clin. Sci., 38, 1, 1970.
71. McGandy, Hegsted, Myers and Stare: Am. J. Clin. Nutr., 18, 237, 1966.
72. Walker: Am. J. Clin. Nutr., 28, 195, 1975.
73. Balmer and Zilversmit: J. Nutr., 104, 1319, 1974.
74. Kritchevsky and Story: J. Nutr., 104, 458, 1974.
75. Editorial: Lancet, 2, 353, 1975.
76. Trowell: Am. J. Clin. Nutr., 28, 798, 1975.
77. Van Soest and McQueen: Proc. Nutr. Soc., 32, 123, 1973.
78. Fifth Annual Marabou Symposium: Food and Fiber. Nutr. Rev., 35, 1977.
79. Becker: S. Afr. J. Med. Sci., 11, 97, 1946.
80. Higginson and Pepler: J. Clin. Invest., 33, 1366, 1954.
81. Mann, Shaffer, Anderson and Sandstead: J. Atheroscler. Res., 4, 289, 1964.
82. Toor, Katchalsky, Agmon and Allalouf: Circulation, 22, 265, 1960.
83. Keys, Fidanza, Scardi, Bergami, Keys and DiLorenzo: Arch. Intern. Med., 93, 328, 1954.
84. Keys, Vivanco, Minon, Keys and Mendoza: Metabolism, 3, 195, 1954.
85. Keys, Aravanis and Sdrin: Voeding, 27, 575, 1966.
86. Mann, Munos and Scrimshaw: Fed. Proc., 13, 467, 1954.
87. Keys, Kimura, Kusukawa, Bronte-Stewart, Larsen and Keys: Ann. Intern. Med., 48, 83, 1958.
88. Yano and Ueda: J. Biol. Med., 35, 504, 1963.
89. Lee: Am. J. Cardiol., 13, 30, 1964.
90. Mann: Cardiovascular Disease Epidemiology Conference. San Diego, March 4, 1974.
91. Biss, Ho, Mikkelsen, Lewis and Taylor: N. Engl. J. Med., 284, 694, 1971.
92. Keys: Circulation, 41 (Suppl. 1), 1, 1970.
93. Kannel and Gordon (Eds.): The Framingham Study: An Epidemiological Investigation of Cardiovascular Disease. Section 24. Diet and the Regulation of Serum Cholesterol. Bethesda, National Institutes of Health, 1969.
94. Kato, Tillotson, Nichaman, Rhoads and Hamilton: J. Epidemiol., 97, 372, 1973.
95. Garcia-Palmieri, Costas, Schiffman, Colon and Nazario: Circulation, 45, 829, 1972.
96. Garcia-Palmieri, et al.: Am. J. Clin. Nutr., in press.
97. Nichols, Ravenscroft, Lamphiear and Ostrander: J.A.M.A., 25, 1948, 1976.
98. Nichols, Ravenscroft, Lamphiear and Ostrander: Am. J. Clin. Nutr., 29, 1384, 1976.
99. Dayton, Pearce, Hashimoto, Dixon and Tomiyasu: Circulation, 39, 40, Suppl. 2, 1969.
100. Lehtosuo and Alivirta: Am. J. Clin. Nutr., 21, 255, 1968.
101. Leren: Acta Med. Scand., Suppl. 466, 1966.

102. Leren: Circulation, *42*, 935, 1970.
103. Anderson, Grande and Keys: J. Am. Diet. Assoc., *62*, 133, 1973.
104. Aherns: Ann. Intern. Med., *85*, 87, 1976.
105. Frantz, Dawson, Kuba, Brewer, Gatewood and Bartsch: Circulation, *52* (Suppl. 2), 4, 1975.
106. Heady: WHO Bull., *48*, 243, 1973.
107. The National Diet Heart Study Final Report: Circulation, *37* (Suppl. 1), 1, 1968.
108. Cornfield and Mitchell: Arch. Environ. Health, *19*, 382, 1969.
109. Report of the National Heart and Lung Institute, Task Force on Arteriosclerosis, Vol. I. DHEW Publication No. (NIH) 72–137. Washington, U.S. Superintendent of Documents, 1976.
110. Doyle, Dawber, Kannel, Heslin and Kahn: N. Engl. J. Med., *266*, 796, 1962.
111. Doyle, Dawber, Kannel, Kinch and Kahn: J.A.M.A., *190*, 886, 1964.
112. Shapiro, Weinblatt, Frank and Sager: J. Chronic Dis., *18*, 527, 1965.
113. Kannel, Castelli, and McNamara: J. Occup. Med., *9*, 611, 1967.
114. Kahn: NCI Monograph 19, 1, 1966.
115. Jenkins: N. Engl. J. Med., *284*, 307, 1971.
116. Doyle: Mod. Concepts Cardiovasc. Dis., *35*, 81, 1966.
117. Breslow and Bull: J. Chronic Dis., *11*, 421, 1960.
118. Kahn: Am. J. Public Health, *53*, 1058, 1963.
119. Taylor, Klepetor, Keys, Parlin, Blackburn and Puchner: Am. J. Public Health, *52*, 1697, 1962.
120. Stamler, Lindberg, Berkson, Shaffer, Miller and Poindexter: J. Chronic Dis., *11*, 405, 1960.
121. Paul, Lepper, Phelan, Dupertuis, McMillan, McKean and Park: Circulation, *28*, 20, 1963.
122. Kannel, Dawber, Kagan, Revotskie and Stoke: Ann. Intern. Med., *55*, 33, 1961.
123. Chapman and Massey: J. Chronic Dis., *17*, 933, 1964.
124. Pell and D'Alonzo: J.A.M.A., *185*, 831, 1963.
125. Partamian and Bradley: N. Engl. J. Med., *273*, 455, 1965.
126. Epstein, et al.: Am. J. Epidemiol., *81*, 307, 1965.
127. Epstein: Circulation, *36*, 609, 1967.
128. Epstein, Ostrander, Johnson, Payne, Hayner, Keller and Francis: Ann. Intern. Med., *62*, 1170, 1965.
129. Ostrander, Francis, Hayner, Kjelsberg and Epstein: Ann. Intern. Med., *62*, 1188, 1965.
130. Marks: Bull. N.Y. Acad. Med., *36*, 296, 1960.
131. Dunn, Ipsen, Elsom and Ohtani: Am. J. Med. Sci., *259*, 309, 1970.
132. Murphy: Can. Med. Assoc. J., *97*, 1181, 1967.
133. Bloor: Circulation, *39, 40* (Suppl. IV), 130, 1969.
134. Epstein: Isr. J. Med. Sci., *3*, 594, 1967.
135. Deutscher, Ostrander and Epstein: Am. J. Epidemiol., *91*, 233, 1970.
136. Goldstein, Hazzard, Schrott, Bierman and Motulsky: J. Clin. Invest., *52*, 1533, 1973.
137. Goldstein, Hazzard, Schrott, Bierman and Motulsky: J. Clin. Invest., *52*, 1544, 1973.
138. Goldstein, Hazzard, Schrott, Bierman and Motulsky: J. Clin. Invest., *52*, 1569, 1973.
139. National Heart and Lung Institute, Division of Heart and Vascular Diseases: Report by the Task Force on Genetic Factors in Atherosclerotic Diseases. DHEW Publication No. (NIH) 76–922, Washington, U.S. Superintendent of Documents, 1976.
140. Kannel, Gordon, Castelli and Margolis: Ann. Intern. Med., *72*, 813, 1970.
141. Kannel, Castelli, Gordon and McNamara: Ann. Intern. Med., *74*, 1, 1971.
142. Albrink, Meigs, Wister and Mann: Am. J. Med., *31*, 4, 1961.
143. Brown, Kinch and Doyle: N. Engl. J. Med., *273*, 947, 1965.
144. Fredrickson, Levy and Lees: N. Engl. J. Med., *276*, 32, 94, 148, 215, 273, 1967.
145. Eisenberg and Levy: In *Advances in Lipid Research*, 13th ed. New York, Academic Press, 1975, pp. 1–83.
146. Barr, Russ and Eder: Am. J. Med., *11*, 480, 1951.
147. Gofman, Young and Tandy: Circulation, *34*, 679, 1966.
148. Medalie, Kahn, Neufeld, Riss and Goldburt: J. Chronic Dis., *26*, 329, 1973.
149. Castelli, et al.: Circulation, *53* (Suppl. II), 97, 1975.
150. Miller and Miller: Lancet, *1*, 16, 1975.
151. Wood, Klein, Lewis and Haskell: Circulation, *50*, 111, 1974.
152. Lopez, Vial, Balart and Arroyare: Atherosclerosis, *20*, 1, 1974.
153. Wilson and Lees: J. Clin. Invest., *51*, 1051, 1972.
154. Hulley, Wilson, Burrows and Nichaman: Lancet, *2*, 551, 1972.
155. Fredrickson and Levy: In *The Metabolic Basis of Inherited Disease*, 3rd ed. (Stanbury, Wyngarden and Fredrickson, Eds.). New York, McGraw-Hill, 1972, pp. 545–611.
156. Fredrickson, Gotto and Levy: In *The Metabolic Basis of Inherited Disease*, 3rd ed. (Stanbury, Wyngarden and Fredrickson, Eds.). New York, McGraw-Hill, 1972, pp. 493–530.
157. Nikkila: Adv. Lipid Res., 7, 63, 1969.
158. Dietschy and Wilson: N. Engl. J. Med., *282*, 1128, 1179, 1241, 1970.
159. Fredrickson: Circulation, *39, 40* (Suppl. IV), 99, 1969.
160. WHO Memorandum: Circulation, *45*, 501, 1972.
161. Stone and Levy: Prog. Cardiovasc. Dis., *14*, 341, 1972.
162. Langer, Strober and Levy: J. Clin. Invest., *51*, 1528, 1972.
163. Brown and Goldstein: Science, *191*, 150, 1976.
164. Fredrickson, Morganroth and Levy: Ann. Intern. Med., *82*, 150, 1975.
165. Morganroth, Levy and Fredrickson: Ann. Intern. Med., *82*, 158, 1975.
166. Levy, et al.: Ann. Intern. Med., *77*, 267, 1972.
167. Levy, Morganroth and Rifkind: N. Engl. J. Med., *290*, 1295, 1974.
168. Fredrickson, Levy, Bonnell and Ernst: Dietary Management of Hyperlipoproteinemia. DHEW Publication No. (NIH) 76–110. Washington, U.S. Superintendent of Documents, 1975.

Chapter *35*

ALLERGY AND DIET

Vincent J. Fontana
and
Fernando Moreno-Pagan

THE IMMUNOLOGY OF FOOD ALLERGY

Rosenau and Anderson[1] were probably the first to demonstrate that sensitization could be produced through the digestive tract, by passage of proteins through the gastrointestinal mucous membranes. Walzer's experiments[2,3] showed that in 90 per cent of normal human beings undigested protein could be absorbed through the mucous membrane of the intestine and demonstrated in the blood.

In those cases in which allergic symptoms apparently occur on the first ingestion of a food, Zinsser[4] feels that active sensitization may have occurred in utero by passage of the exciting agent (antigen) from the mother through the placenta, and Ratner[5] suggests that pregnant and nursing mothers with allergic histories should refrain from using large quantities of foods with high sensitizing capacity, such as fish and eggs, and that milk should be thoroughly boiled. Infants are rarely born hypersensitive, for the skin sensitizing antibodies are unable to pass through the placenta and the fetus is never passively sensitized to an antigen.

The gamma E globulins exhibit all the properties of the reaginic antibody. They fix to human skin, they combine with allergens that can neutralize them and they are heat labile. The association between reaginic antibody and a unique immunoglobulin class IgE or gamma E is now firmly established.[5a] There is available evidence that histamine release from leukocytes by white cell-bound gamma E globulin upon antigen contact may make the mucosa of the shock organs of the allergic individual more vulnerable to antigenic stimulation.[5b]

Skin-sensitizing antibodies are found in the blood of a child of known allergic parentage before the child itself begins to exhibit allergic symptoms.[6] Thus, the clinical form of allergy would not seem to be determined by the mere presence in the blood of these antibodies. As a necessary attribute for clinical sensitization, some sensitized tissue area, or "shock organ," must exist.[7] There is conclusive evidence of the ability of normal persons to absorb proteins from the gastrointestinal tract apparently unaltered and in sufficient quantities to sensitize human beings.[8-12] The absorption of proteins through the intestinal wall occurs with greater regularity than is generally believed.[13] If normal guinea pigs are fed milk sensitization in these animals may be demonstrated by intravenous injection of milk.

Fink and Quinn[14] studied antibody production in inbred strains of mice and found that young mice produced much less antibody than more mature animals. Cannon and Longmire[62] showed that 5 to 10 per cent of skin grafts exchanged between pairs of newly hatched chicks of different breeds are tolerated and survive into adult life but the percentage of successes falls rapidly as the age at which the chicks are operated upon increases. It reaches zero if the operation is delayed to the end of the second week.

Even more striking results are obtained when antibody response is studied in the prenatal period. A group of English workers led by Medawar[63] found that mice never develop, or develop only to a limited degree, the power to become sensitized to foreign homologous tissue cells to which they have been exposed sufficiently in fetal life. Burnet[64] discusses the possibility that, during early embryonic life, an animal may accept foreign cells and develop a lasting tolerance to them; its ability to recognize the difference between "self" and "not-self" does not come until later, some time before birth. This would raise the question of whether it would not be advantageous, by means of a widely varied maternal diet, to expose the fetus at a very early age to as many foods as possible so that they be accepted as "self," no antibody formation being elicited upon later contact with them. This effect would depend, of course, upon the passage of sufficient food protein into the maternal circulation and through the placenta.

Glaser and Johnstone[15] suggested that a physiologic immunologic immaturity exists in the early months of postnatal life and that the absorption of unaltered proteins from the intestinal tract produces sensitization and clinical symptoms in potentially allergic children. They fed soybean from birth to infants whose antecedents included one parent or sibling with allergic disease. Only 14 (15 per cent) of this group showed major allergic diseases, compared with 42 (64 per cent) of the sibling control group and 91 (52 per cent) of a nonrelated control group of comparable ages. Their experiments showed that four times as many infants in the control groups developed major allergic conditions as in the experimental group where the foreign food (cow's milk) was withheld from the infant diet and a nonantigenic casein hydrolysate (soybean) substituted. Apparently, therefore, practically all individuals, nonallergic, allergic, and potentially allergic, are exposed to prolonged parenteral contact with undigested foreign protein.

That all individuals are not clinically sensitive to foods indicates, as Cooke[16] has suggested, that intimate exposure to the foreign protein is not of itself a sufficient cause. There must be some predisposing mechanism present, some capacity for sensitization mediated, at least in part, by a hereditary factor.[17,18] It would seem, therefore, prudent to expose the infant, especially if potentially allergic, to the least possible quantity of those food antigens notorious for their high sensitizing potential (such as milk, egg, fish and nuts), whether ingested directly or transmitted in the breast milk[19,20] of a nursing mother eating these foods, perhaps excessively.

THE CLINICAL MANIFESTATIONS OF ALLERGY

Allergic reactions may occur in any area of the body, since antibody is distributed throughout the various cells and tissue fluids. There are sites, however, characteristic for each clinical allergic malady, in which the tissues are thought to have a greater concentration of antibody, and which therefore show greater allergic activity upon exposure to the invading specific antigen. These sites may be the portals of entry where the primary invasion of antigen occurs. Often, however, the sites of the greatest allergic activity are distant from the portals of entry, the antigen being transported to them by the blood and lymph. For instance, in the individual asthmatic to horse dander, the symptoms result from allergic activity in the respiratory tissues, which are also the site of invasion of the airborne antigen. In the individual asthmatic to a food such as egg, symptoms also result from allergic activity in the respiratory tissues, but here the antigen has been transported from its portal of entry, the intestinal membrane.

The various clinical forms of allergy may be classified according to the major systems of the body in which the sensitized tissue areas chiefly involved in the allergic response are found: respiratory, alimentary, cutaneous, neural, cardiovascular, genitourinary and articular. Since tissue areas in several major systems may be sensitized to the same antigen, several manifestations of clinical allergy may result in an individual from a single type of invading antigen. In the individual sensitive to clams, for instance, the ingestion of his specific excitant may result simultaneously in coryza, bronchial asthma, pruritus, urticaria, tracheal edema, abdominal cramps and diarrhea, caused by activity in various sensitized areas of the respiratory, cutaneous and alimentary systems.

Cooke[21] pointed out that the allergic response may be of either an immediate reaction type, occurring within 4 hours after contact with the antigen, or a delayed type, requiring from 4 to 72 hours for the appearance of the symptoms. Both types may be present in a single patient, but to different excitants; a person may develop asthma immediately upon contact with horses, but urticaria only after a delay of 24 hours following the eating of egg. Furthermore, a food antigen may cause immediate symptoms in one patient, delayed in another. While the length of the reaction time may vary from person to person and from cause to cause, it is always a constant in any one individual to any given antigen. The immediate type is also termed the skin-sensitive, or wheal, type, since the immediately positive skin test, with typical wheal formation, may be obtained in sensitive individuals on application of the extract of the specific excitant by intracutaneous or scarification procedures. The delayed reaction type is also designated as the skin-negative, nonwheal type, because of its behavior upon skin test.

MANIFESTATIONS OF FOOD ALLERGY

Food allergy may produce any of the various manifestations of sensitivity previously enumerated, with the exception of pollenosis, which is always caused by plant pollens, bacterial allergy and physical allergy. It may be a sole or a contributing cause, producing symptoms of the immediate or delayed type, acute or chronic, mild or severe. Sensitivity to foods may manifest itself in the respiratory system as coryza, conjunctivitis, bronchitis, bronchial asthma and sinusitis; in the alimentary system as gastroenteritis with herpes, stomatitis, bad breath, "bilious" attacks, gingivitis, nausea, vomiting, flatus, abdominal distention and pain, colitis, diarrhea, constipation, pruritus ani; in the cutaneous system as pruritus, dermatitis, urticaria, angioedema, purpura; in the neural system as headache, peripheral neuritis, optic neuritis, vertigo, allergic labyrinthitis; in the cardiovascular system as tachycardia; in the genitourinary system as hematuria, pruritus vulvae; in the articular system as arthralgia; in the ocular system as conjunctivitis, corneal ulcers. It must be emphasized that food sensitivity is only an occasional or rare cause of many of these manifestations. The symptoms of food allergy may mimic those of many other clinical conditions. It is often difficult, even impossible, to demonstrate its presence and to prove its etiologic significance.

Psychosomatic factors may be important in activating and altering latent allergic symptoms. To the chore of collecting data on the incidence of food allergy by history or by trial-and-error methods may be added the difficulties of comparing the results of skin testing by different investigators, using food extracts of varying potencies and employing varying skills and methods of testing. Even when standardized extracts and techniques of skin testing are constant, as with a single investigator, the results may be unsatisfactory since approximately one-half of the authentic food allergic cases fail to give positive skin tests.

Most cases of food sensitivity occur in early life. From a study of 200 cases of bronchial asthma,[23] it was found by intracutaneous and clinical testing that only individuals 3 years or younger developed symptoms from foods alone. Inhalant substances (pollens, dusts and animal danders) gradually replace the food allergies so that by the age of 5 to 10 years the majority of patients were no longer clinically food-sensitive, although the skin test reaction often persisted. In only 5 per cent of adult asthmatic patients could a food allergy be demonstrated as the sole excitant.

It is generally agreed that the incidence of food allergy depends greatly on age. In the infant, sensitization to various foods is relatively high and ranks in importance with infection, while after the age of 5 years there is a tendency toward spontaneous disappearance of food allergy. Therefore, according to Chobot[23] the incidence of clinical food allergy is low in relation to that caused by inhalant substances and infection. On the other hand, Rinkel[24] feels that there is a higher incidence of food allergy in adults than in children, although it is less readily demonstrable. The comparative simplicity of the diet in childhood makes for easier diagnosis.

FOOD ALLERGY IN CHILDREN

It is not known why some infants develop a specific sensitization shortly after birth, although heredity may play a dominant role. Spain and Cooke[18] have shown that where both parents are allergic, as indicated by the occurrence of bronchial asthma and/or hay fever, approximately 70 per cent of the offspring will develop a clinical allergic condition by the age of 10 years. Where there is an antecedent unilateral history of bronchial asthma and/or hay fever, 50 per cent of the offspring will develop clinical allergic symptoms by the age of 30 years. It would seem, therefore, that both incidence and age of onset of

clinical allergic conditions are influenced by the strength of the inherited trait. Infections, focal or constitutional, and changes in the general health of the patient may play an important part in predisposing to the development or precipitation of allergic manifestations.

It is significant that Rowe and Rowe[25] and Stoesser[26] found allergy to food most important in asthma of early childhood, while inhalants were more significant in the latter part of the preschool period. Ratner and Untracht[27] found that 5 per cent of 500 allergic children were sensitive, clinically and by skin test, to a single food—egg. In the child, as in the adult, the allergic process can affect any of the body systems.

Milk and egg are usually the first foods to which the infant becomes sensitive, probably because they are among the initial foods comprising his diet. In Clein's series of 140 allergic infants,[28] 1 of every 15 was sensitive to cow's milk. Among the conditions they developed were eczema, pylorospasm and colic, while some felt "unhappy all the time." Less common symptoms were cough, choking and gasping, nose colds, constipation, asthma, anorexia, attacks of sneezing.

Heiner has reported a syndrome found in infants that includes intestinal blood loss and a hypochromic microcytic anemia thought to result from milk allergy.[29] Iron therapy and blood transfusions correct the anemia but do not alleviate the fetal blood loss thought to be milk induced. Ingestion of cow's milk, therefore, must cause the occult loss of significant quantities of blood in the gastrointestinal tract of some children with hypochromic microcytic anemia. This syndrome should be considered in any infant or child with occult fecal blood losses, especially with a family history of allergy.

The symptoms produced by a food allergy may involve any tissue of the body. The possibility of a food allergy should be considered in a child with constitutional or generalized signs of easy fatigability, irritability, insomnia, poor work in school or intermittent headaches and stomach aches. These children oftentimes find it difficult to get along with their siblings or peers. If the children have a positive family or personal history of allergy and are experiencing the constitutional tension-fatigue symptoms described, a thorough investigation for a food allergy should be undertaken.

Direct skin testing by either the scratch or intradermal methods is rarely employed in such cases because of the threat of a possible violent reaction to the use of an excitant of high potency. The diagnosis is usually established by the history, the indirect skin test method, the food diary and trial-and-error procedures.

Sensitization to milk presents a considerable though essential replacement problem. In the case of other foods, simple removal is sufficient, but where milk is to be avoided some substitute that fulfills the nutritional and mineral requirements must be given to the infant or young child. Such proprietary products as Mullsoy, Neo-Mullsoy, Pro-Sobee or Isomil are often satisfactory milk substitutes unless the infant is sensitive to soybean, in which case Nutramigen or a meat-base formula may be tried. In cases of disaccharide intolerance, a disease which may mimic milk allergy or soybean sensitivity, the use of a meat-base or carbohydrate-free formula will be helpful in making a diagnosis. After alleviation of the patient's symptoms, special formulas containing milk, soybean or disaccharide may be tried individually to elicit the true etiologic cause of the patient's symptoms. Specifications for their use are supplied by the makers of all these substances. Goat's milk, fresh or canned, often offers a highly satisfactory replacement, although an allergenic factor common to both cow's and goat's milk may prevent its use. A number of lactose-free nutritionally adequate formulas are also now available (see Appendix Table 31).

The infant or child highly allergic to egg must avoid all traces of it. In those with a more moderate degree of sensitization, the white of egg may be the excitant; the yolk is readily tolerated, as is poultry. Fortunately, most infants and children do not demonstrate an exquisite degree of food intolerance, and can satisfactorily follow a diet which need not be too restricted, provided heat-treated or cooked items are used.

ALLERGY AND NUTRITIONAL STATUS

Severe allergic conditions may have an adverse effect upon nutrition. The individual with uncontrolled bronchial asthma is frequently undernourished, since he has come to realize that the lightest of meals may cause embarrassed digestion and abdominal distention, with a consequent heightening of the asthmatic distress. Anorexia, nausea, flatus, diarrhea and constipation may result from apprehensions concerning health and from nervous tension caused by fear of precipitating an attack by the unwitting ingestion of some highly potent excitant, unidentifiable in some food preparation. Anemia, avitaminosis, underweight and, in the child, lack of proper growth, with a reduced vital capacity, are the evidences of impaired nutrition. The interruption of sleep, respiratory or intestinal symptoms or irritability and tension from antiasthmatic stimulating drugs such as ephedrine may intensify the problem. One of the first evidences of an improved allergic status and success in allergic management is a gain in weight.

In forms of severe food allergy, such as urticaria, dermatitis, gastroenteritis, colitis and headaches, evidence of malnutrition often result from self-inflicted, but usually unjustified, curtailment of the diet. The whims, fads and phobias regarding food allergy which plague many persons, both allergic and nonallergic, force upon the physician the added responsibility of attempting to reeducate the patient, to reassure him and to encourage him to adopt an adequate diet.

DIAGNOSIS AND TREATMENT

An immediate type of food allergy is often simple to identify, but the delayed type is often difficult to locate. The presence of food allergy may be established by (1) history, (2) cutaneous tests, (3) food diary and (4) clinical tests employing trial-and-error methods and restrictive diets.

History Taking. History taking is the most important of all diagnostic procedures, and should be completed first. It may provide information of great consequence, not only as to the specific food causes but also as to the degree to which they affect the patient. With such knowledge, the investigator is forewarned and may avert what might have been a hazardous exposure of the hypersensitive patient to the active food excitant by routine skin testing or clinical trial. In the immediate reaction type, where symptoms follow swiftly upon exposure to the exciting food, the patient is usually fully aware of at least the more obvious and more potent food factors and the extent of disturbance they produce. The individual who describes the prompt development of edema of the lips and tongue upon accidental contact with traces of egg, nut or fish, or who reports asthma from the inhalation of their odors, is not a candidate for further exposure to such foods by skin test or by ingestion experiments. Until the history and the degree of sensitivity can be verified, testing should be scrupulously avoided with those food excitants described as producing swift, severe symptoms; this is especially the case when the route of contact is by surface exposure of mucosa or skin or by inhalation of food odors. Patients with a history of such a high degree of sensitivity should be investigated by the passive transfer method.

A comprehensive investigation of the occurrence of allergic conditions in the patient and his family should be obtained, since the presence of bronchial asthma, allergic coryza or hay fever in the antecedent or collateral members of the family furnishes evidence of the inherited nature of sensitivity[17,18] and strongly suggests that cutaneous tests will be of value. An inherited capacity for vigorous allergic response is usually present in food-sensitive cases with an immediate reaction time. Sensitivity in any form may show itself in other members of the family, and at times the same specific food cause and the same pattern of symptoms may persist through many generations.

A point of diagnostic importance is the character of the symptoms. They may be acute, explosive in nature and even hazardous to life in the immediate reaction type, insidious and obscure, although severe, in the delayed reaction type. A description should be obtained of the frequency, intensity and duration of the symptoms, their paroxysmal or continuous character, their relation to meals and to the daily, weekly or monthly routine of the patient. Such correlations may usually be established through the maintenance of a food diary. Usually, the more acute the attack the briefer is the reaction time. The length of the symptom-free periods between attacks depends upon the frequency of exposure to the food excitant. The attacks may be of a cumulative nature, as when a food eaten regularly, usually daily, becomes irritating only when a limit of tolerance is reached.

A characteristic of food allergy of the immediate reaction type is the fact that symptoms of overwhelming intensity may result from exposure to minute amounts of the food factor; here the symptoms speedily reach a crucial stage, marked by almost instantaneous nausea, vomiting, diarrhea and asthma and by ominous attacks of urticaria and angioedema. Individuals subject to attacks of such great intensity live in a continual state of dread and apprehension, because of the threat of sudden diarrhea or of edema which may swiftly involve an area of such vital importance as the tongue or larynx. Such persons are usually quite aware of the inciting food cause, such as egg, nut or a seed, but may be unable to avoid it completely because of its presence in sauces, salads or in a multiplicity of commercially prepared food mixtures. An exquisite degree of sensitivity to egg has forced one patient to avoid all food and drink outside the home, and to use china and silverware kept constantly segregated from that employed in the household, for fear of contamination with egg in washing and handling. Such patients, fortunately rare, may have multiple abdominal scars, the results of repeated emergency operations necessitated by acute intestinal episodes usually caused by edema of the gut. In their abruptness and severity, the symptoms successfully mimic those of the acute "surgical abdomen" resulting from such varied causes as volvulus, intussusception, mesenteric thrombosis, biliary colic and acute appendicitis. The surgeon, even if he is aware that the symptoms *may* be caused by a food allergy, may be forced to operate in order to resolve the dilemma of whether the allergy or a surgically correctable crisis is responsible.

Both severity and periodicity of symptoms of food allergy may be influenced by other associated and intimately linked allergic conditions. Attacks of hay fever or bronchial asthma, for instance, may intensify the attacks of a food allergy or activate a latent food allergy. It is a frequent observation that hay fever patients are able to ingest without allergic discomfort such foods as peaches, melon, sweet corn, chocolate or seafood except during the hay fever season when they are contending with intense and disturbing symptoms of pollenosis. At these times, such food excitants may cause dermatitis, urticaria, bronchial asthma or increased coryza. The skin tests are often positive to the exciting foods not only during the pollen period but nonseasonally.

In food allergy, as in other types of sensitivity and, indeed, in many other en-tirely different maladies, the frequency and severity of symptoms may be influenced by worry, anxiety and states of physical stress. In searching for a diagnosis, the physician must be fully aware of the complexities produced by such psychosomatic factors. These are obviously operative in many individuals and may well prove an obstacle to improvement even where the physical factor, the offending food, is known. A young housewife whose urticarial attacks were identified by positive skin test as resulting from celery was able to eat it without ill effect once the problems of her household budget were solved. Occasional attacks occurred when celery was eaten at the first of the month, when the question of payment of bills was acute. Considerable time, effort and patience must be expended by both physician and patient in collecting data on the dietary habits and reactions to food of the patient being studied. No filling of blank history forms, no pattern of routine questioning is sufficient since problems in food allergy differ considerably among themselves. Questioning and cross-questioning are essential, especially in those cases with delayed reaction times and negative skin test results.[22] Such inquiry may offer the only clue to possible food factors. Foods notorious for their outstanding antigenic activity and for their high incidence as excitants should be particularly suspected. These are, in most instances, ingested uncooked, hence with their characteristic proteins unaltered by heat. They are: milk, eggs, seafood, nuts, seeds as mustard, chocolate, orange, tomato. However, not only these but the individual items in all food groups (meat, seafood, fruits, vegetables, cereals, beverages and spices) must be considered separately and in detail.

Foods Eaten to Excess. Patients may eat immoderate amounts of a food because of food fads, efforts to gain or lose weight on unbalanced diets or economic reasons. Milk, tomato juice, orange juice and chocolate are common offenders. A candidate for the football squad may drink several quarts of milk daily to gain weight; a dowager may consume excessive quantities of orange or tomato juice to lose weight; a stenographer may eat many chocolate bars to save lunch money. Such extremes may lead to food intolerance, where a moderate and less monotonous intake of the same foods would cause no discomfort.

Foods Eaten Though Disliked. Dislike of a food may be only a whim or a fancy, but it should be regarded as significant until proven otherwise. Aversion to egg or milk in children may be the result of nature's protective effort, often misinterpreted by parents.

Foods Eaten Though Causing Recognized Mildly Related Allergic Symptoms. A patient may be fully aware that a food such as chocolate may cause stomatitis, without realizing that it also produces his allergic headaches. Any food described as causing mildly associated effects should be placed on the suspect list.

Foods Eaten Though Known to Have Caused Earlier, Now Absent, Forms of Sensitivity. A patient may remember that in childhood a severe chronic dermatitis disappeared when a food such as egg was eliminated from the diet, although its return to the diet in recent years was not followed by a reappearance of the dermatitis. It is not realized that the present allergic manifestation, such as colitis, may be the result of a less obvious sensitization to the same food.

Foods Eaten Though Known to Cause Allergic Symptoms in Another Member of the Family. An allergy to a food such as egg or milk in an antecedent or collateral member of the family directs suspicion against this food as a cause of the patient's symptoms.

Such prolonged investigative procedures, applied to all types of foods, may often prove pleasurable and exciting to the patient who delights in discussing his diet, but they may prove wearisome to the physician; they are certainly not adaptable to mass production methods. Each patient is a separate and different problem, upon whom adequate information cannot be obtained in a few minutes or at a single visit. Only after the expenditure of considerable time and effort can satisfactory data be obtained.

Immediate Reaction

In this type of allergy, because of the brief interval between ingestion of the disturbing food and the occurrence of symptoms, the patient is able to inform the investigators at least partially of the exciting causes and of the degree to which they affect him. He may, however, be unaware of the importance of related but possibly less disturbing food substances, or that certain preparations may contain a food he knows to be an offender. Thus, an individual may be conscientiously avoiding egg as such while continuing to eat food mixes containing egg.

Upon skin test, definitely positive results are usually obtained with the extracts of these foods known to the patient for their immediate effect. As previously stated, such tests may be hazardous and should usually be avoided. Skin tests should be completed, however, with the extracts of other foods which may cause a definite but less obvious allergic disturbance.

Cutaneous Testing Procedures. *The Direct Method.* Whether the scarification or the intradermal technique be employed, the diagnostic skin testing procedure should not be attempted until the history has been completed. A full discussion of the methods of cutaneous testing of foods is not pertinent to this chapter and may be readily found in many textbooks on allergy. It should be mentioned, however, that frequently foods suspected and subsequently proven by clinical test to be authentic causes of immediate symptoms cannot be identified by skin test. Such negative effects are the result in many instances of the disparity between the food as eaten, often altered by cooking, and the extract of it which is prepared from unheated material. Then, too, it may well be that many food extracts are rendered ineffective by changes resulting from the chemical manipulations essential to their preparation and by changes occurring during storage. Also frequent are false-positive reactions due to nonspecific irritation of the cells of the skin.

The Indirect Method. Direct testing of the skin may be contraindicated because of wishes of the parents, the presence of eczematous or lichenified skin or the threat of an extreme degree of sensitization. The sera from allergic persons of the immediately reacting type usually contain skin-sensitizing antibodies responsible for the development of the wheal characteristic of the positive test.[30] Such antibodies may be shifted to the skin of a normal individual by intracutaneously injected deposits of the allergic serum, conferring temporary and local sensitization to the food excitants which are disturbing to the patient. This phenomenon can usually be shown by the positive results upon testing the serum sites with specifically offending antigens. This procedure has its limitations but is usually safe, although systemic reactions (vertigo, faintness, diarrhea and oppression of the chest) have been known to occur in normal recipients in whom sites made with serum from an exquisitely sensitive patient were tested with extracts or excessive high potency.

The Specifically Restricted Diet. Foods which give a positive reaction in direct or indirect skin tests (as indicated by an immediate wheal with pseudopods, itching and a surrounding zone of erythema) should be retested for verification; if the reaction is again positive, they should be removed from the diet on the assumption that they are at least partially the cause of the patient's symptoms. He should be supplied with a written list not only of the foods banned but of those permitted. A typed or printed form may be adjusted to each person's needs by crossing from the list all culpable foods that are to be avoided (see Appendix Table 27). In the adult

suffering from chronic bronchial asthma or chronic allergic enteritis or colitis, it is also advisable to have the patient avoid all flatulence-producing foods even though they are not incriminated as specific excitants.

Patients sensitive to milk, egg, wheat or nuts must be cautioned against the use of many of the preparations and food mixes supplied by manufacturers. Such processed substances may contain the specific food excitants in quantities sufficient to produce allergic symptoms, as in the case of egg and milk in pancake mixes for home use. Since the labels on packages of such products list all the ingredients, the patient should be urged to develop the habit of reading all such labels as a protective measure. Fish-sensitive patients must be warned against acquiring the habit of licking labels. While adhesives used on postage stamps and many envelopes are not of fish origin, fish collagen is used as adhesive upon some types of labels, stamps and stickers.

In the diet prepared for the patient, rigid restrictions against more than one or two food items are rarely permanent. Early changes are often desirable in an effort to enlarge and simplify the diet. Once the patient becomes symptom free, the banned foods are tried singly, at 3-day intervals, in a trial-and-error procedure as outlined subsequently. The problem of maintaining proper nutrition is simplified by providing the patient with data upon the mineral and vitamin content of important foods. Where added vitamin preparations are indicated, the synthetic varieties should be employed if possible.

Delayed Reaction

In those cases of food allergy where the interval is prolonged, 4 to 72 hours elapsing between contact with the food and appearance of symptoms, not only is the cause usually unknown to the patient but the allergic nature of the problem often is unknown, as well. Unfortunately in just these instances, where the skin testing procedure would be most helpful, it fails. In at least some instances, the negative results upon test are due to a lack of the proper antigen, which may not be the food itself but some digestive product requiring several hours for its appearance and its allergic effect upon the patient. This was true in Cooke's[31] case where allergic symptoms appeared several hours after the ingestion of milk. Skin tests were negative to milk itself but positive to the milk proteoses. Where neither history nor skin test affords information, but where there is reason to suspect an active food allergy, paroxysmal or continuous, an attempt at diagnosis should be made by food diary maintenance, dietary elimination and trial-and-error methods.

Food Diary. Entries should be made by the patient each day of the separate items of food, beverage and drugs ingested at each meal, between each meal and at bedtime. At the end of the day's entry, the patient should note any occurrence or continuance of his allergic symptoms. Once weekly the physician should attempt to correlate repetitive symptoms with repetitive ingested items, the interval of from 4 hours to 3 days being a constant for each suspected item. Should it be found, for instance, that headache occurred consistently on the third day following the ingestion of egg, that food should be suspected; if the interval proved to vary, being 24 hours at some entries and 3 days at others, the case against egg would be weakened, as, too, it would be if headache did not occur in most instances after egg was ingested. Foods suspected should be banned until subsequent verification of their allergenic importance can be attempted by trial-and-error procedure.

Simple Elimination Diets. The simplest attempt at elimination consists of removal from the diet of those foods most notorious as excitants: milk, egg (but not at the same time as milk), seafood, nuts, seeds, chocolate, orange, tomato. Care must be taken to explain to the patient the need for thorough avoidance, and he should be provided with a list of foods or food compounds in which the banned items may be present in disguised form, as shown in Appendix Table 27, in the milk-poor, egg-poor, seafood-poor, wheat-poor and nut-poor diets. Few patients object to abstinence from these food items for a 4-week period—usually sufficient for a proper evaluation. Occasionally, the chronic nature of the symptoms requires a longer period for evaluation. If promising results have been obtained from the restricted diet, the patient becoming symptom free, the diet should be continued and, at intervals of 31 days, the several banned items should be tried separately; those showing negative results, usually the majority, should be returned to the diet.

Trial-and-error Procedure. If the patient is fortunate enough to become symptom-free as a result either of this relatively simple dietary procedure or of restrictions based on positive findings in the clinical history or skin test, an attempt should be made to verify the fact that the excluded foods were offenders. Each banned item, obtained from the original source and prepared as identically as possible, should be separately and cautiously introduced into the diet by feeding a small portion on an empty stomach, preferably 1 hour before the midday meal. It is helpful in eliminating the personal equation if the food can be given in a disguised form, so that the patient is unaware of its identity; however, this is often impossible. If no symptoms are induced, the food is tried again after an interval of three days, in double quantity. If no symptoms occur from the first and second attempt, it may be concluded that the food under study may be eaten without discomfort, at least in moderate amounts and infrequently, although it must be remembered that a cumulative effect is always possible. If symptoms appear, the suspected food is eliminated, to be tried again once the patient is symptom free. The same or even a lesser amount of the food is to be eaten, depending upon the severity of the condition previously produced. The eliciting of symptoms typical of the patient's allergic complaint upon both first and second trials is presumptive evidence of a positive food cause if the patient was aware of the item under study; it may be considered positive proof if the food was fed in a disguised form. If either the first or second test alone is positive, further study is necessary.

The Rigidly Restricted Diet. When a relatively simple procedure is not successful, more austere methods may be necessary. The rigidly restricted diet is justified only in patients with severe, presumably allergic problems—recurrent headaches, urticaria, edema or colitis—and should not be employed in children or in the severely ill. The choice of foods is limited to the specific items, but the quantities ingested are not curtailed. With symptoms occurring frequently, at daily or weekly intervals, the patient's preferences may be consulted in the selection, after the first day, of the three vegetables, the meat and the three fruits to be studied. Beef or chicken may thus be substituted for lamb and other vegetables and fruits for those listed for the first five days of the diet. If improvement in symptoms has occurred at the end of the week, additional food items may be attempted singly and at intervals of three days, by trial-and-error procedures, until the daily menu meets the nutritional requirements of the normal diet. If at the end of two weeks no improvement has occurred, the diet should be replaced with a similar one with entirely different food constituents. If this should prove unsuccessful, the presence of a food allergy is doubtful.

Where the symptoms ordinarily occur at intervals of 7 to 14 days or longer, symptom-free periods of 2 to 4 weeks are usually required to determine whether offending foods have been removed from the diet. To the urban dweller, dependent upon restaurants for his meals, the use of these and all other types of restrictive diets poses a formidable problem.

Where foods are eliminated for test or therapeutic purposes, it is essential that the physician or dietitian review the diets in advance and at intervals to ensure that they are nutritionally adequate.

BIBLIOGRAPHY

1. Rosenau and Anderson: Hygiene Laboratory Bulletin No. 29, 1906. U.S. Government Printing Office.
2. Walzer: J. Immunol., *14*, 143, 1927.
3. Walzer and Walzer: Am. J. Med. Sci., *173*, 279, 1927.
4. Zinsser: *Resistance to Infectious Diseases.* New York, Macmillan, 1931.
5. Ratner, Jackson and Gruehl: J. Immunol., *14*, 249, 1927.
5a. Ishizaka and Ishizaka: J. Immunol., *99*, 1187, 1967.
5b. Ishizaka, et al.: J. Immunol., *102*, 884, 1969.
6. Baldwin: J. Immunol., *13*, 345, 1927.
7. Coca, Walzer and Thommen: *Asthma and Hay Fever.* London, Bailliere, Tindall & Cox, 1931.
8. Anderson and Schloss: Am. J. Dis. Child., *26*, 451, 1923.
9. Gillette: J.A.M.A., *50*, 40, 1908.
10. Weaver: Arch. Intern. Med., *3*, 485, 513, 1909.
11. Billard: C. R. Soc. Biol., *73*, 462, 1912.
12. Bernard, Debre and Porak: J. Physiol. Pathol., *14*, 971, 1912.
13. Ratner and Gruehl: J. Clin. Invest., *13*, 517, 1934.
14. Fink and Quinn: J. Immunol., *70*, 61, 1953.
15. Glaser and Johnstone: J.A.M.A., *153*, 620, 1953.
16. Cooke: *Allergy in Theory and Practice.* Philadelphia, W. B. Saunders, 1947.
17. Cooke and VanderVeer: J. Immunol., *1*, 201, 1916.
18. Spain and Cooke: J. Immunol., *9*, 521, 1924.
19. O'Keefe: Boston Med. Surg. J., *185*, 194, 1921.
20. Donnally: J. Immunol., *9*, 15, 1930.
21. Cooke: Am. J. Med., *3*, 523, 1947.
22. Spain: Proc. Conn. Med. Soc., *141*, 105, 1933.
23. Chobot: *Pediatric Allergy.* New York, McGraw-Hill, 1951.
24. Rinkel, *Food Allergy.* Springfield, Charles C Thomas, 1951.
25. Rowe and Rowe: Calif. Med., *69*, 261, 1948.
26. Stoesser: Minn. Med., *23*, 412, 1943.
27. Ratner and Untracht: Am. J. Dis. Child., *63*, 309, 1952.
28. Clein: Ann. Allergy, *9*, 195, 1951.
29. Heiner, Wilson and Lahey: J.A.M.A., *189*, 568, 1964.
30. Prausnitz and Küstner: Zentralbl. Bakterial., *86*, 160, 1921.
31. Cooke: Ann. Intern. Med. *16*, 71, 1942.

Chapter *36*

DIET AND NUTRITION IN THE CARE OF THE SURGICAL PATIENT

Maurice E. Shils
and
H. T. Randall

There is increasing recognition of an unacceptably high incidence of malnutrition in hospitals. While physicians and dietitians are becoming more aware of this problem, optimal prevention and treatment are far from satisfactory in many institutions. The problem and methods of approach have been reviewed in Chapter 22. However a few statistics related to surgical patients are instructive.

In a series of surgical patients in a large American hospital nearly 50 per cent had some evidence of protein-calorie malnutrition.[7] Similar general findings have been made in general surgical wards in an English hospital; approximately one-half of the patients remaining in hospital more than a week after major surgery had anemia, vitamin deficiency, weight loss, loss of muscle mass and/or low plasma values of transferrin and albumin.[8] Patients with inflammatory bowel disease who were candidates for urgent surgery had a significant lowering of a number of the nutritional parameters mentioned above.[9] Seven of the 9 patients who developed major complications after surgery had been admitted earlier for urgent surgery and none had received any specific nutritional therapy.[9] Similar findings of significant malnutrition have been made in patients with inflammatory bowel disease referred to an American surgical service;[10]

more than 82 per cent of 74 patients had lost more than 10 per cent of their usual weight, and serum albumin and transferrin levels were low.

Depressed cellular immunity has been established as having a correlation with malnutrition and can be reversed by nutritional repletion in approximately 2 to 3 weeks.[11] The status of delayed hypersensitivity by means of skin testing was used as an indicator of risk for morbidity and mortality in a large number of patients admitted to surgical wards and intensive care units.[12] Of 322 patients tested preoperatively, 21 (6.5 per cent) were anergic; a similar percentage were relatively anergic and 280 (87 per cent) were normal. The sepsis rates in these three groups were 19.0, 23.8 and 4.6 per cent, respectively. Mortality in the anergic and relatively anergic groups was 33.3 per cent in each, as contrasted to 4.3 per cent in those that were normal. Sequential testing of individual patients throughout the hospital course was of even greater prognostic value. Of 83 patients who remained normal throughout there was a 10.8 per cent sepsis rate and a 1.2 per cent mortality rate. Fifty-four abnormal responders who remained abnormal had a 53.5 per cent sepsis rate and a 75.9 per cent mortality rate. Of the 91 patients who were initially anergic or relatively anergic and *converted to normal,* 38.3 per cent had sepsis and 4.3 per cent died. All 5 patients who were initially normal and became and remained abnormal developed sepsis and died. Anergy and relative anergy were found to be associated with malnutrition, sepsis, shock and trauma. Effective treatment of these associated conditions, especially the maintenance of body cell mass by nutritional means, was associated with reversal of the anergic state and an improved prognosis.

In an effort to develop preoperatively a reliable assessment of potential operative morbidity and mortality based on nutritional parameters, Mullen et al. assessed the nutritional status of 161 elective surgical patients preoperatively using a battery of tests and monitored them for complications until death or discharge.[13] They developed the following equation:

Predicted risk (%) = 158 − 16.6 (alb) − 0.78 (TSF) − 0.2 (TFN) − 5.8 (DH)

where alb = gm per dl serum albumin, TSF = mm of triceps skinfold thickness, TFN = mg per dl serum transferrin and DH = delayed hypersensitivity reactivity.

When this equation was applied to the pertinent observations in 121 surgical patients, 51 patients at low risk (< 30 per cent) had a complication rate of 11.7 per cent, major sepsis rate of 7.8 per cent and death rate of 2.0 per cent, whereas a group of 32 deemed at high risk (> 59 per cent) had a complication rate of 81 per cent, major sepsis rate of 46.5 per cent and death rate of 59.4 per cent. An intermediate risk group (30 to 59 per cent) had a complication rate of 36.8 per cent, major sepsis rate of 5.3 per cent and a death rate of 7.9 per cent.

A significant number of surgical patients require that their nutritional program be planned as carefully as their operative procedure. These patients are of two general types: those who preoperatively are debilitated and malnourished as the result of chronic or subacute disease, and those who for prolonged periods of time may be unwilling or unable to eat adequately as the result of obstruction, high bowel fistulas, severe trauma, sepsis or complications of surgery. Examples of patients with major preoperative debility include those with severe inflammatory disease of large or small bowel, carcinoma of the esophagus, stomach or colon, chronic pancreatitis, chronic infection, particularly of lung or bone, and some forms of liver, kidney or heart disease. All of these patients have substantial weight loss with severe reduction of their skeletal muscle mass and total body protein. Most patients have an increase in relative proportion of extracellular fluid and total sodium, despite quite common hyponatremia. Two examples of the changes in body composition produced by chronic illness are shown in Figure 36–1.[14] In both cases there has been loss of body weight and relative expansion of extracellular fluid. In the patient with congestive heart failure, the body cell mass remains at normal levels while body fat has been substantially reduced and the extracellular fluid increased. In the patient with regional enteritis substantial loss of body weight is reflected by the fact that the skeleton is more than twice its normal proportion of total body weight; body cell mass is substantially reduced even on a percentage basis of the depleted body and the extracellular fluid compartment is markedly expanded. Patients with these derangements of body composition resulting from malnutrition and disease represent severe operative risks and require major attention to nutritional management in the preoperative as well as the postoperative period.

More acute problems include patients with acute or subacute pancreatitis, unresolved peritonitis, high-output fistulas from the gastrointestinal tract to skin, abdominal trauma, major wound sepsis, retroperitoneal hematomas and, most particularly, patients with major burns or multiple injury including femoral and pelvic

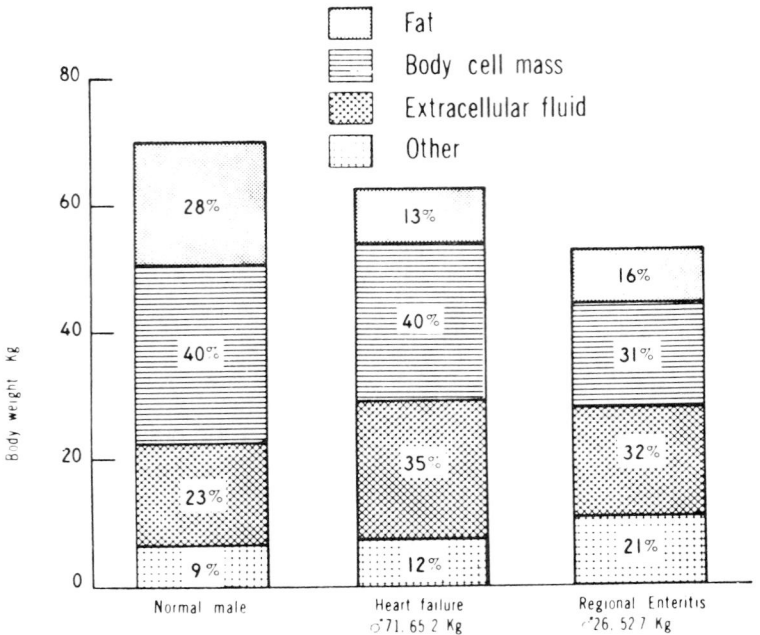

Fig. 36–1. Alteration in body composition in subacute and chronic illness. Body fat is reduced and extracellular fluid (ECF) increased with moderate weight loss as seen in heart failure. Major loss of weight in chronic illness results in both a proportional reduction of body cell mass with expansion of the ECF, and an absolute reduction of even greater magnitude, as shown by the high proportion of body weight represented by the skeleton and other extracellular nonfluid tissues. (Data from Moore et al.[14])

fractures. Most of these patients were healthy and well nourished before the onset of the acute problem; however, because of major catabolic response to trauma and sepsis and simultaneous partial starvation, the demands on fat and especially protein are so great that expendable protein may be exhausted from within 2 to 4 weeks. Death will occur from muscle weakness resulting in pulmonary infection and respiratory failure, unless food is provided in sufficient quantity and proper qualities to spare essential body cell mass. A loss of one-third of total body protein within 30 days appears to be lethal in man as well as in experimental animals.[15]

ENERGY, PROTEIN AND AMINO ACID INTERRELATIONS

Trauma

The trauma necessitated by a surgical procedure is the first of the four major clinical factors affecting nutritional status. Those who have operations which, for one or another reason, induce the second factor (namely, interference with normal ingestion, digestion and absorption of food) face the third factor, namely, partial or total starvation. All are at risk for the fourth factor, sepsis. Aspects of partial or total starvation have been reviewed in Chapters 1, 3 and 24 and in the General References with consideration of the adaptive mechanisms which occur in the nonhypermetabolic individual. Trauma and sepsis result in accelerated catabolism and these are considered below.

In 1930 Cuthbertson[16] published data to validate and in part to explain the well-recognized clinical observation that there is an extraordinary wasting of skeletal muscle and a decrease in strength following severe skeletal trauma; such changes occur often despite a seemingly adequate oral intake of both calories and protein. Cuthbertson reported that immobilization of normal male volunteers who were on a regular diet caused only a small negative nitrogen balance (1 to 2 gm a day) which occurred within 1 to 2 days. Subsequent surgery increased the rate of nitrogen loss in these patients greater than that produced by immobilization alone despite maintenance of the same diet.

Cuthbertson's observations were confirmed and extended by Howard and his associates[17,18] who compared the nitrogen balance of patients in convalescence following long bone fractures to that of patients undergoing operation on the skeleton. All the patients with long bone fractures showed nitrogen losses of considerable magnitude following injury, i.e. the equivalent of an average loss of 6.6 kg of lean body mass in a 70-kg man. The peak nitrogen loss in fracture cases occurred on the sixth day after injury; the patients undergoing operations on the skeleton sustained a much smaller total nitrogen loss with an earlier peak and a much more rapid repletion.

The marked rise in urinary nitrogen following moderate to severe trauma in previously healthy individuals is attributable primarily to an increase in urea, which comprises 80 to 90 per cent of the total urinary nitrogen. This is associated with increased urinary losses of potassium, phosphorus, magnesium, zinc and creatine. Cuthbertson's early work indicated that these losses came from soft tissue (even though the subjects had suf-

fered major long bone fractures) inasmuch as the losses of nitrogen, sulfur and phosphorus in the first 10 to 12 days after trauma were excreted in proportions similar to those found in muscle. This conclusion has been confirmed by subsequent investigators using various techniques.

Previously debilitated or malnourished individuals or experimental animals who are injured have markedly attenuated or no increased output of nitrogen in the urine. Rats which had been fed a protein-free, calorically sufficient diet for some time prior to injury had no increase in urine nitrogen following fracture of the femur.[19] Similarly, the quantity of protein in the diet before injury, but not after injury, affected the response to trauma. These findings demonstrate the importance of a dietary-dependent endogenous protein pool. Similar differences have been noted between well-nourished or poorly nourished patients undergoing surgery.[20,21]

Unless diarrhea occurs, stool losses following trauma are low and dependent on the level of protein ingestion, i.e. usually less than 10 per cent of ingested nitrogen. Protein losses may be significant when it comes from draining open wounds or from burn wounds prior to closure.[22]

In previously well-nourished individuals the extent of nitrogen loss is related to the size of the injury, the severity of any accompanying infection and the time interval (Fig. 36–2). This figure also reveals that heat production is also related to the degree of trauma and recovery. Cumulative nitrogen losses that may occur in the first ten days in a patient on ad libitum feeding may be 170 gm for a major burn, 150 gm for multiple injury, 136 gm for peritonitis, 115 gm for a simple fracture, 50 gm for major surgery and 24 gm for minor surgery.

This positive correlation between nitrogen losses and energy expenditure should not be taken to mean that the primary source of fuel from the body tissues

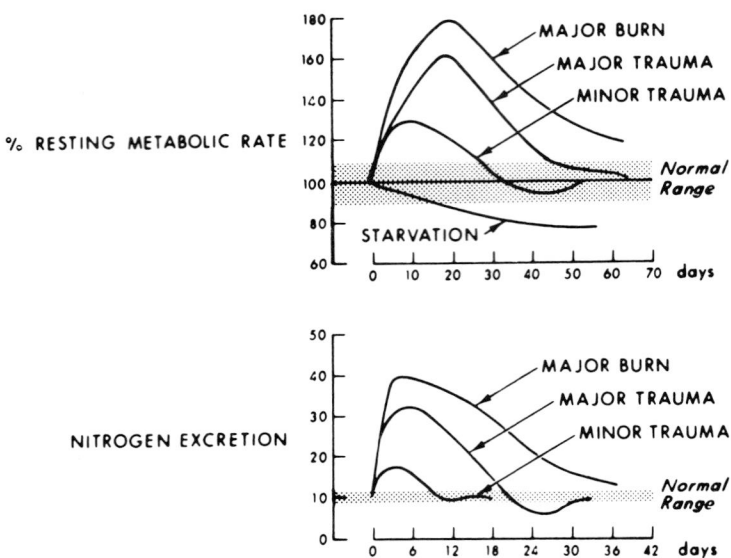

Fig. 36–2. The degree of increased energy metabolism and nitrogen excretion is related to the extent of trauma and stress. Note that, unlike trauma, starvation alone results in a decreased metabolic rate. (Adapted from Kinney by Wilmore.[5])

metabolized to meet the increased need is protein. Duke et al. found that the average contribution of protein to resting metabolic expenditure was 16.5 ± 4.3 per cent in preoperative patients destined for elective surgery.[23] The maximum figure for protein contribution to energy expenditure was 20.4 ± 7.7 per cent in traumatized individuals. In the starving, injured or septic patient body fat is the only other major source of fuel to meet the increased demands for energy. Additional factors augmenting protein losses are immobilization in bed,[24] poor caloric intake and a low ambient temperature.[25] As noted above the post-traumatic and sepsis-related nitrogen losses appear to derive from a combination of increased protein breakdown from muscle (as evidenced by increased creatine, creatinine and 3-methylhistidine excretion) together with decreased synthesis rates.[26]

When inadequate amino acids are available as in semistarvation in post-traumatic man[27] or in rats,[28] protein synthesis rates are decreased and this contributes to nitrogen losses. However, if adequate amino acids are provided, most protein synthesis rates are increased.[28]

As Figure 36–2 indicates, trauma and sepsis differ from starvation alone in that they are associated with an increased metabolic rate (ergo, the "hypermetabolic state") and with appreciably larger nitrogen losses. The mechanisms of the hypermetabolic response have been the objective of much research in the past but well-substantiated factors are only recently being elucidated, with active research in this field continuing. The increased nitrogen excretion and metabolic rate and hepatic gluconeogenesis noted in injured patients are associated with endocrine changes. Figure 36–3 summarizes the time sequence and relationships of the hormonal and metabolic changes. Although insulin levels may be normal in the early period, insulin effect is dampened[29,30] but becomes more normal following burn shock resuscitation.[30] In the early period

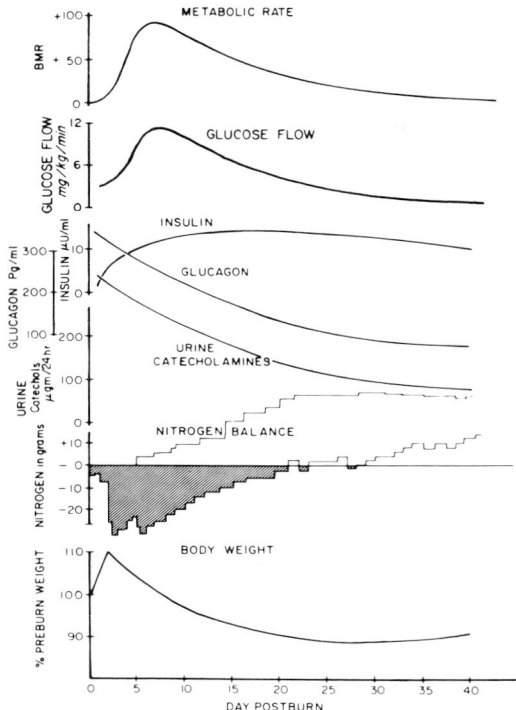

Fig. 36-3. Hormonal and metabolic changes following thermal injury. The increased rate of hepatic glucose production (glucose flow) parallels the hypermetabolic response and these are associated, in turn, with negative nitrogen balance and high levels of glucagon and catecholamines relative to insulin. As these hormonal mediators return to normal, oxygen consumption and hepatic glucose production fall and nitrogen balance becomes positive. (From Wilmore.[5])

following thermal injury when alpha receptor inhibition is apparent, diabetic tolerance curves are manifest. Increased glucagon and catecholamine levels stimulate hepatic glucose production. Beta-adrenergic receptor stimulatory effects become apparent in the second week with increases in glucose production, hypermetabolism and negative nitrogen balance. As adrenergic activity recedes, metabolic rate and muscle catabolism slow and positive nitrogen balance occurs as the patient improves clinically.[30]

Sepsis

The occurrence of sepsis also accentuates nitrogen losses in the urine and oxygen consumption. Figure 36-4 correlates nitrogen balance with caloric intake in burn patients with and without bacteremia. Nitrogen losses were increased by approximately one-third in patients with bacteremia as compared to those without it across a wide range of administered calories. However, both groups responded in a proportional manner to increasing calories.[31]

With the onset of acute infectious disease a complex and progressive variety of interrelated nutritional and metabolic responses are initiated within the host. Many of these have been documented and discussed by Beisel and his associates.[32–34] Figure 36-5 indicates the metabolic and nutritional responses and their time sequence in the course of a systemic febrile illness. Although the exact series of events depicted in the figure does not necessarily emerge in every acute infection, many host metabolic-nutritional responses do seem to follow predictable patterns. Variations may occur in relation to the type of infecting microorganism, severity of infection, the occurrence of complications or predominant involvement of one organ system e.g. intestine, kidney or central nervous system. Beisel emphasizes the fact that alterations in patterns of host protein metabolism are the most important general nutritional consequence of infection.[33] Defense mechanisms employed by the host to combat infections all ultimately depend upon the ability of host tissues or single cells to manufacture specific key proteins in sufficient quantity. Protein is being synthesized at increased rates in the form of phagocytic cells, cells of the lymphoid series, immunoglobulins and acute-phase reactant glycoproteins and others; albumin, on the other hand, is decreased in virtually all infections.[33,35]

Detailed balance data for nitrogen and other nutrients have been published for

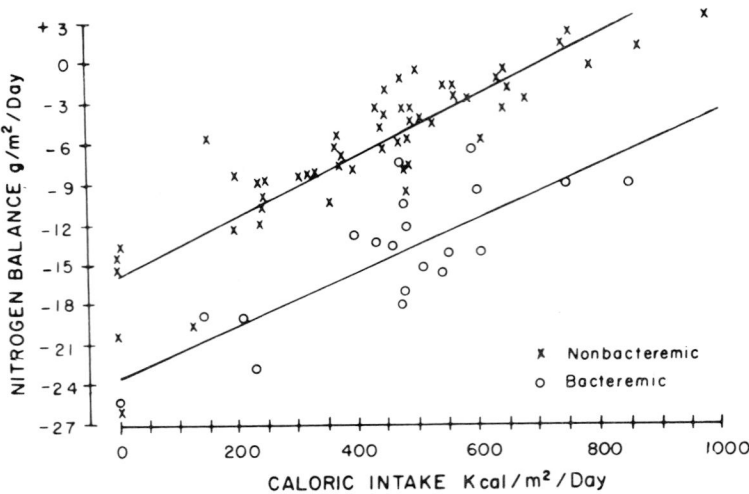

Fig. 36–4. Nitrogen balance per square meter of body surface (M^2) in relation to caloric intake per M^2 from glucose and amino acids in patients with thermal injuries. The bacteremic patients had significantly greater nitrogen losses at any given caloric intake. The slopes of the regression lines are not significantly different but each line represents a significantly different population of points. (From McDougal et al.[31])

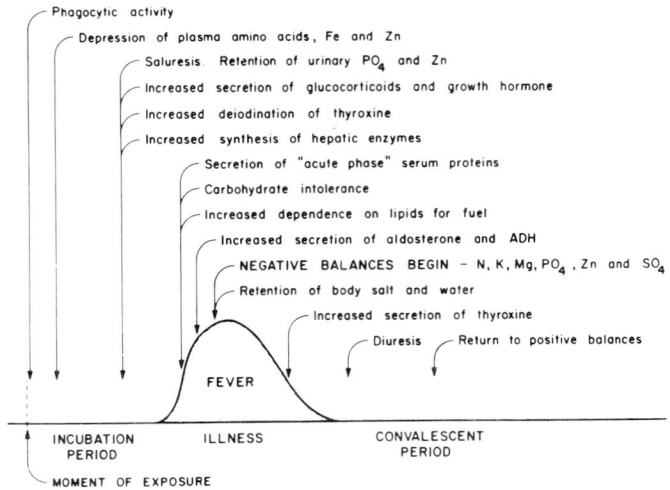

Fig. 36–5. Schematic representation of the sequence of nutritional responses that evolves during the course of a "typical febrile infectious illness." (From Beisel.[33])

various acute infections.[32] During infection and trauma the changes occurring in the rates of intake and of excretory loss of nitrogen contribute to the negative balances. Anorexia is usually present and may result in a marked reduction in food intake. To ascertain the extent to which semistarvation per se contributes to negative nitrogen balance, balance data were obtained on individuals with tularemia and on pair-fed nonexposed controls. The latter lost only about one-third as much nitrogen as the infected individuals in approximately two weeks; further, at that time the controls had essentially made up for their nitrogen losses while the infected subjects were still in serious negative nitrogen deficit.[32,33]

Hormonal Influences in Sepsis. The pathophysiologic mechanisms which account for the observed responses to sepsis —similar to the effects of trauma—include endocrine alterations in association with substrate availability.

Several decades ago, there was a strong assumption that an increased output of adrenal glucocorticoid hormones could account almost entirely for the metabolic consequences of an acute infection. However, Beisel and associates have demonstrated that the magnitude of the adrenal glucocorticoid response to infectious stress was relatively small and short-lived.[33,36] They estimate that production of such hormones is increased only two to fivefold above normal during the first several days of an acute febrile infection, then declines to normal values after several days of continuing infection and may become subnormal if the infection becomes subacute or chronic. Plasma cortisol loses its typical circadian rhythm early in the infection and levels are generally maintained over the day at values normally reached at the morning peak. Where increased concentrations occur in overwhelming sepsis, it is probable that the rise is explained by failure of hepatic enzymes to conjugate the steroids to glucuronide products. Negative

nitrogen balance was not produced when normal subjects were administered corticosteroids in daily doses that equaled or exceeded the glucocorticoid response measured during acute tularemia.[33,36] Hence, in nonlethal acute infections adrenal glucocorticoid activity does not explain the observed complex of metabolic and nutritional changes.

An interplay of various endocrine responses is involved in such patients. Adrenal mineralocorticoids increase in infection and contribute to the renal retention of salt and water.[36] All hormones that regulate carbohydrate metabolism appear to participate in the host responses to infection. A number of groups have documented an increased fasting concentration of both glucagon and insulin in the serum.[5,33] If a glucose tolerance test is performed in patients with an early febrile infection, the resultant insulin secretion appears to be exaggerated both in magnitude and duration, the elevated fasting concentrations of plasma glucagon decline in an appropriate manner and a paradoxical oversecretion of growth hormone becomes evident.[37] The catecholamines help to stimulate gluconeogenesis during infections, especially those caused by gram-negative microorganisms.[38] Although gluconeogenesis is initially stimulated during febrile infections and is abetted by the contribution of substrate amino acids derived from muscle protein, the body may eventually become severely hypoglycemic. In patients with serious trauma, glucose flow and hepatic gluconeogenesis increase, but if gram-negative sepsis occurs these decrease toward normal during the infection. In such patients, alanine administration fails to cause a rise in serum glucose.[39] Glucagon infusion but not insulin administration will increase hepatic production, indicating that the liver is the primary site of decreased gluconeogenesis in infection.

The thyroid hormones do not appear to play a primary role in initiating or sustaining the hypermetabolic response to fever.

However, thyroxine and 3,5,3'-triiodo-thyronine (T_3) are both metabolized at a somewhat accelerated rate during a variety of infections studied in man and experimental animals.[40,41] Despite the more rapid deiodination of its hormones in peripheral tissues, the thyroid gland response, as estimated by secretion rate measurements for thyroidal hormones, seems to be sluggish during early periods of an infection. Later and in early convalescence, the thyroid gland seems to catch up and may for a period of time overshoot its requirements. This sequence of responses may cause an early decline in thyroid hormone concentrations in plasma with a late rebound to somewhat elevated values. Serum concentrations of "reverse" 3,3',5'-triiodothyronine (rT_3), become elevated during febrile illnesses[42] as well as in starvation in man.

Metabolic Consequences of Phagocytic Activity and Inflammation. Metabolic, nutritional and biochemical responses during infection are also influenced importantly by biologically active substances released from host cells. After their encounter with invading microorganisms or their participation in a localized inflammatory reaction, host cells may liberate substances such as serotonin, histamine and prostaglandins, as well as a large variety of lysosomal enzymes. These biologically active substances can initiate localized effects at the anatomic site of invading bacteria; they can also affect more distant tissues or lead to generalized intravascular phenomena such as activation of the kinin and complement systems or the clotting cascade.[33-35] Activated phagocytic cells also release endogenous pyrogen into the blood stream and exert their specific effects on cells in distant anatomic locations. Endogenous pyrogens released by various types of body cells stimulate neuronal centers in the hypothalamus to initiate the febrile response. Similar substances stimulate the release of granulocytes from the bone marrow, accelerate uptake of iron, zinc and plasma amino acids by the liver and increase hepatocellular synthesis of nucleic acids and various acute-phase reactant glycoproteins.[33-35]

Energy Substrates in Trauma Sepsis. Major insights into the effects of injury and sepsis have been derived by measuring the metabolism of the various substrate sources in these conditions. Modification of overall nitrogen metabolism has been considered above. Hyperglycemia is known to occur commonly following injury and sepsis with the rise in blood sugar above normal being generally correlated with the degree of stress. This is associated with an increase in the size of the glucose pool (i.e. serum glucose × extracellular fluid compartment)[43,44] and an increased rate of hepatic gluconeogenesis.[45]

In a series of patients with acute severe gram-negative sepsis, most of whom had peritonitis, O'Donnell et al. have studied the levels and uptake or production of a number of energy substrates.[46] These were obtained by comparing concentrations of these substrates in femoral arterial and venous blood and applying flow measurement data to the arteriovenous (A-V) differences. The data obtained in 7 patients with "high-flow" sepsis (cardiac index (C.I.) > 2.8 L/M²/min) and 9 with "low-flow" sepsis (C.I. < 2.8 L/M²/min) are compared with those obtained in previous studies in 6 fasting normal subjects and in 10 patients with major injury without sepsis, primary multiple fractures and soft tissue wounds (Tables 36–1, 36–2). The latter group had been on dextrose-free solutions for 72 hours whereas the septic patients had been given 100 gm of glucose per 24 hours for at least 72 hours prior to the study. The elevated arterial glucose levels mentioned above were present in the injured and septic patients but A-V differences were increased in only the patients with decreased cardiac output. However, because of the increased flow rate in the high-flow sepsis patients, glucose uptake was similar to that of the low-flow group

Table 36–1. Comparison of Arterial Substrate Profile and Leg Exchange Data in Fasting, Major Injury and Sepsis*Φ

		Fasting Normals—72 Hr. (n = 6)	Noninfected Major Injury—72 Hr. (n = 10)	High-flow Sepsis—72 Hr. (n = 7)	Low-flow Sepsis (n = 9)
Glucose (mM)	Arterial	3.7 ± 0.3	5.0 ± 0.6	7.6 ± 0.59	7.15 ± 0.71
	ΔArteriovenous	0.17 ± 0.02	0.18 ± 0.03	0.15 ± 0.01	0.52 ± 0.09
Lactate (mM)	Arterial	0.6 ± 0.04	0.8 ± 0.1	1.73 ± 0.2	3.14 ± 0.74
	ΔArteriovenous	-0.07 ± 0.02	-0.17 ± 0.04	-0.16 ± 0.02	-0.68 ± 0.17
Glycerol (mM)	Arterial	0.17 ± 0.05	0.13 ± 0.05	0.08 ± 0.01	0.10 ± 0.02
	ΔArteriovenous	-0.08 ± 0.01	-0.12 ± 0.03	-0.035 ± 0.016	-0.092 ± 0.02
Alanine (mM)	Arterial	0.18 ± 0.02	0.28 ± 0.04	0.29 ± 0.031	0.43 ± 0.05
	ΔArteriovenous	-0.04 ± 0.02	-0.08 ± 0.03	-0.13 ± 0.01	-0.33 ± 0.12
Free fatty acid (μEq)	Arterial	1.2 ± 0.4	0.84 ± 0.42	0.701 ± 0.12	0.95 ± 0.15
	ΔArteriovenous	0.64 ± 0.2	0.32 ± 0.01	-0.059 ± 0.021	-0.17 ± 0.05
Ketone (mM)	Arterial	2.0 ± 0.5	0.8 ± 0.02	0.014 ± 0.003	0.035 ± 0.007
	ΔArteriovenous	0.1 ± 0.02	0.06 ± 0.02	—	—
Insulin (μU/ml)	Arterial	10 ± 8	30 ± 9	42 ± 4	6 ± 1
Nitrogen balance (gm/24)		9 ± 2	14 ± 2	16 ± 3	18 ± 4
Cardiac index (L/M²/min)		2.8	3.21 ± 0.43	4.38 ± 0.33	1.66 ± 0.41

*Mean ± S.E.M.
ΦFrom O'Donnell et al.[46]

Table 36–2. Comparison of Uptake or Production of Substrate Fuels in Sepsis and Fasting*[Φ]

	Fasting (n = 6)	High-flow[†] Sepsis (n = 7)	Low-flow[‡] Sepsis (n = 9)
Glucose uptake (+)	+0.17	+0.28	+0.29
Lactate production (−)	−0.07	−0.33	−0.40
Glycerol production (−)	−0.08	−0.05	−0.06
Alanine production (−)	−0.04	−0.16	−0.18
Free fatty acid uptake (+) or production (−)	+0.6	−0.06	−0.10
Ketone uptake (+)	+0.1	0	0

* mM/M^2/min or mEq/M^2/min

$$[†] \; AV \cdot \frac{CI\ sepsis}{CI\ fasting} \cdot 1.2.$$

$$[‡] \; AV \cdot \frac{CI\ sepsis}{CI\ fasting} \cdot 1.$$

[Φ] From O'Donnell et al.[46]

(Table 36–2). Despite the increased glucose uptake (compared to fasting subjects), the insulin levels were very different in the two groups of septic patients, suggesting insulin insensitivity in the high-flow patients and a noninsulin-dependent method of glucose transport in the low-flow group. Glycerol production was about the same in all groups. Major differences occurred with respect to free fatty acid A-V differences; these were appreciably higher in the fasting subjects with the expected uptake whereas the septic patient had negative A-V differences indicating that they were producing fatty acids in the periphery. Ketone body levels were very low in the septic patients, particularly in the high-flow group, and ketogenesis was apparently suppressed; injury without sepsis was associated with a less depressed fatty acid and ketone body utilization.

The markedly elevated lactate production in the low-flow group and its mild increase in high-flow sepsis are indicative of a decreased entry of pyruvate into the Krebs tricarboxylic acid cycle. Increased alanine production (as well as lactate production) may signify both increased production and decreased hepatic utilization. Lactate and alanine serve as glucose precursors.

In summary, sepsis and, to a lesser degree, trauma without sepsis are associated with increased gluconeogenesis, decreased fat catabolism and ketogenesis and mobilization of alanine from peripheral tissues. The metabolic pathways of the alanine-glucose cycle have been discussed in Chapter 4. Production of alanine permits the complete oxidation of the branched-chain amino acids leucine, isoleucine and valine, yielding 42, 43 and 32 ATP per mole, respectively, and thus providing up to 25 times more ATP than the Cori cycle and filling the energy deficit in muscle.[46,47] Recent data indicate increased glucose turnover (i.e. ref. 43) in sepsis and trauma.

Plasma Amino Acids in Trauma and Sepsis

There has been increasing interest in the patterns of plasma amino acids in various disease states. Of relevance to amino acid patterns in sepsis have been the observations on the changes resulting from hepatic dysfunction secondary to cirrhosis and portacaval shunting. A number of investigators have demonstrated that the amino acid pattern in the latter situation is altered from normal. The aromatic amino acids (AAA) phenylalanine, tyrosine and tryptophan and the neutral amino acids methionine and threonine tend to be elevated, whereas the branched-chain amino acids (BCAA) tend to be low.[48] Fischer et al. have demonstrated in dogs and then in men[48] that the plasma amino acid pattern may be normalized by infusing an amino acid solution high in BCAA and low in AAA. The restoration of the pattern toward normal has been associated with improvement in symptoms of hepatic encephalopathy.

Evidence from other sources indicated that sepsis, hemorrhage and surgery were associated with increased levels of AAA and changes in other amino acids.[49–52] More recent studies of septic patients have revealed plasma amino acid patterns characterized by an elevation in total amino acids mainly because of high levels of the AAA phenylalanine and tyrosine and of the sulfur-containing amino acids, cystine, methionine and taurine.[53] Alanine, aspartic acid, glutamic acid and proline were also elevated, but to a lesser degree. The BCAA were within normal limits, as were glycine, serine threonine, lysine, histidine and tryptophan. Those patients who did not survive sepsis had higher levels of aromatic and sulfur-containing amino acids than did those who survived. The latter had higher levels of alanine and BCAA (Fig. 36–6).

Infusion into septic patients of a crystalline amino acid solution enriched with BCAA, together with 23 per cent dextrose

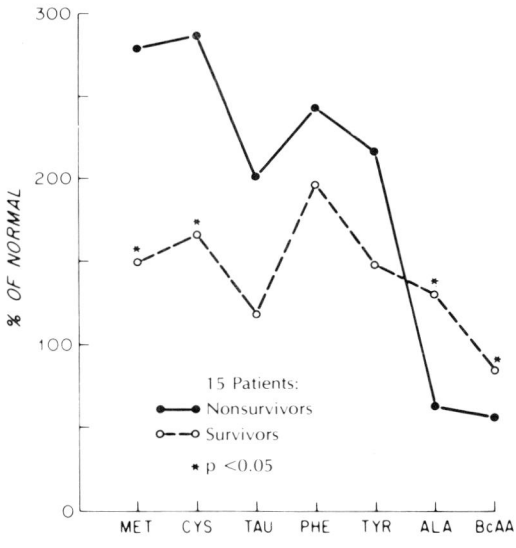

Fig. 36–6. Plasma amino acid patterns as per cent of normal values in septic patients who ultimately survived as compared to those who did not survive the episode of sepsis. The survivors had higher (more normal) levels of alanine and branched-chain amino acids and lower (more nearly normal) plasma concentrations of the aromatic amino acids (phenylalanine and tyrosine) and sulfur-containing amino acids (methionine, cysteine and taurine). (From Freund et al.[53])

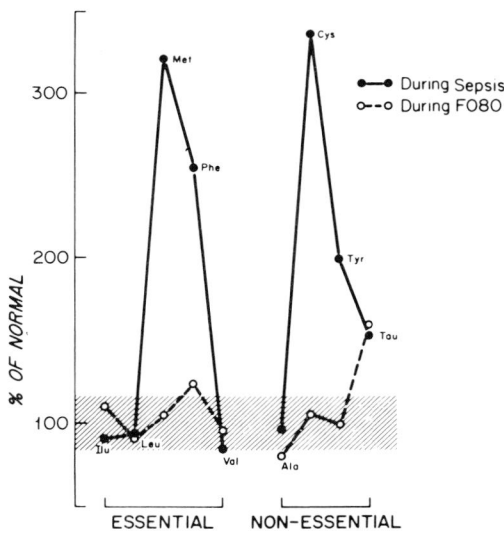

Fig. 36–7. Mean plasma levels (as per cent of normal) of aromatic, sulfur-containing, branched-chain amino acid (BCAA) and alanine in five patients during acute sepsis and during treatment with a BCAA-rich solution (FO80). The normalization of the amino acid pattern during infusion of FO80 also coincides in all five patients with reversal of metabolic encephalopathy. (From Freund et al.[53])

and other nutrients, normalized the plasma amino acids and reversed an existing encephalopathy (Fig. 36–7).[53] The authors postulate the following sequence to account for their observations and those of other investigators: (1) The septic patient develops insulin resistance in peripheral tissues, primarily muscle (in a situation, it should be added, of increased caloric need). (2) Insulin resistance and the inability to utilize fat lead to increased muscle proteolysis, which results in the release into the blood of large amounts of various amino acids. (3) The muscle is able to oxidize BCAA which meets the muscle's own energy requirements as well as supplying alanine for gluconeogenesis. (4) Extensive muscle proteolysis coupled with relative hepatic insufficiency—which is often present in sepsis—results in the elevation of the plasma levels of most of the amino acids present in muscle, particularly the AAA and sulfur-containing amino acids.

MEETING CALORIC AND NITROGEN NEEDS

Gamble's studies emphasized that ingestion of approximately 100 gm of glucose per day markedly decreased (but did not prevent) negative nitrogen balance in fasting men and also spared sodium and water by preventing starvation ketoacidosis.[54] Administration of glucose alone above 600 to 700 kcal per day does not further minimize nitrogen losses.[55] Additional studies performed during World War II as part of military ration research in rats, dogs and healthy men indicated that nitrogen equilibrium could not be achieved despite the presence of protein in a mixed orally ingested diet until total caloric intake was raised to a major percentage of caloric needs.[55–58] In healthy young men ingesting a daily caloric intake of somewhat less than 900 kcal, dietary protein was utilized as an energy source. At 900 kcal, 6.3 gm of dietary nitrogen partially decreased the negative balance; increasing the nitrogen did not improve the situation.[55] However,

further increases in non-nitrogen caloric sources improved nitrogen retention.

The intimate relation between nitrogen retention and caloric intake was further demonstrated in studies wherein increasing caloric intake by mouth improved nitrogen balance at any level of nitrogen intake and, conversely, at any level of caloric intake increasing nitrogen intake also improves nitrogen balance. These relationships have been reexplored and found to hold under various dietary conditions in healthy individuals and in traumatized and septic patients fed either enterally or parenterally.[31,59–62]

An example of this relationship is given in Figure 36–8 for burn patients at three different intakes of glucose and a wide range of nitrogen intakes.

A frequent problem encountered in surgical patients is their need for adequate nutritional support during periods when voluntary intake is impaired or not possible. Much effort has been expended over the years to solve the technologic, nutritional and metabolic problems posed by this situation.

During World War II Elman[63] and Brunschwig et al.[64] studied the effectiveness of parenteral solutions of casein hydrolysates in altering postoperative nitrogen loss in surgical patients. While there was an increased excretion of total nitrogen with the use of these preparations, there was also a reduction in the amount of patient-derived nitrogen. Neither group was able to achieve nitrogen equilibrium in any patient after major surgery when preoperative nutrition had been normal. Reigel and associates[65] and CoTui et al.[66] found that nitrogen equilibrium could be achieved in many patients postoperatively if elevated levels of protein intake and substantial additional calories were administered. The latter group was able to achieve positive nitrogen balance in patients within a very short period following surgery for duodenal ulcer by administering pureed beef into the gastrointestinal

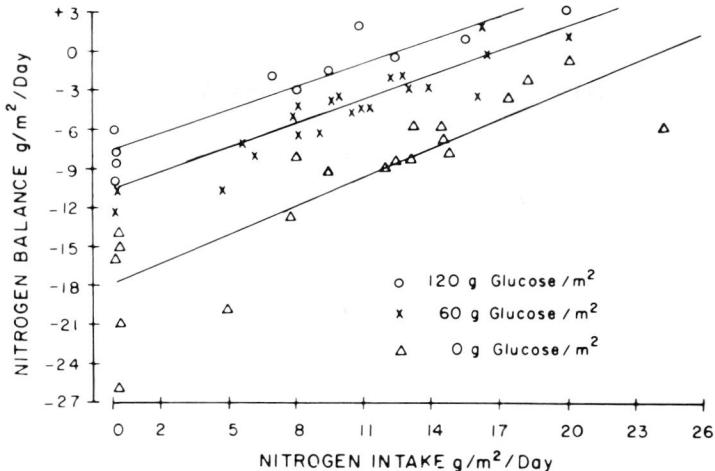

Fig. 36–8.   Nitrogen balance per square meter (M²) (corrected for alterations in BUN) expressed as a function of nitrogen intake at three different levels of glucose intake in nonbacteremic patients with thermal injuries. The slopes of the linear regression lines are not significantly different, but each line represents a distinct population of points significantly different from each of the other two with p > 0.001. (From McDougal et al.[31])

tract. However, most of the patients were relatively debilitated preoperatively, which undoubtedly enhanced their ability to retain nitrogen.

Separation of the effects of starvation from the effects of trauma of surgery was further elaborated by the studies of Werner[67] and Werner et al.[68] using purified amino acids. They showed that patients undergoing surgery and given parenteral nutrition (consisting of 18 to 24 kcal per kg per day of a 10 per cent solution of glucose with 12.5 to 14.4 gm of nitrogen as amino acids), had nitrogen losses considerably less than those noted in another group of patients maintained postoperatively on routine parenteral fluids consisting of 5 per cent dextrose with some sodium and potassium chlorides. They concluded that starvation played the major role in postoperative nitrogen loss under the conditions of their studies.

By the end of the 1940s and early 1950s the relationships among caloric intake, nitrogen intake and nitrogen utilization were recognized by clinicians knowledgeable in the field.[63–70] The technical problem with parenteral feeding involved supplying adequate calories via peripheral vein. This obstacle appeared to be overcome with the development of a stable commercial fat emulsion (IV Lipomul) and a number of studies indicated attainment of nitrogen balance in postoperative patients.[71] Unfortunately, the toxicity of this emulsion in long-term use led to its withdrawal. Credit for the development of a lipid emulsion (Intralipid) which was safe with continued use goes to Wretlind and associates.[72] Although Intralipid was approved for clinical use in most European countries by 1963, it did not receive official sanction until 1973 in Canada and 1977 in the United States.

The infusion of very hypertonic glucose solutions by a central venous catheter to provide adequate calories in conjunction with other nutrients gained wide popularity following the animal and human studies of Dudrick and associates.[73] These intravenous forms of total nutritional therapy have important applications in a number of surgical patients and are discussed in detail in Chapter 37.

Although there is good evidence that healthy individuals can utilize fat as the major source of calories to permit amino acids to be utilized for protein synthesis and positive nitrogen balance, there is presently some controversy on this point in traumatized or septic patients. This is discussed in Chapter 37.

"Protein-sparing" Infusion

Reference has been made above to publications indicating an inefficient utilization of dietary protein during ingestion of diets of mixed composition and insufficient calories to meet energy needs, particularly at very low caloric intakes. There has been general acceptance of this conclusion, which has served as the basis for the widespread use of 5 or 10 per cent dextrose in water with electrolytes and vitamins in immediate postoperative patients who do not require nutritional repletion or more adequate nutrition support.

This position has been challenged as the result of the studies of Blackburn and associates who reported that infusion of an isotonic 3 per cent amino acid solution (90 gm) into fasting surgical patients with moderate protein catabolism and into other subjects greatly minimized the negative nitrogen balance when compared to those given 100 gm of glucose.[74,75] The studies were short term (5 to 15 days). In some patients positive nitrogen balance with amino acids alone was achieved. In the group infused with amino acids alone, serum insulin levels fell and fatty acids and ketone bodies increased. The explanation offered for the reported superiority of the amino acids over that of glucose was that insulin production was stimulated by the glucose which, in turn, reduced fatty acid mobilization and their energy contribution; hence, protein catabolism was greater with the glucose.

These reports have stimulated much investigation because of the theoretic and clinical interest in the potential for sparing body protein in situations of caloric deficiency.

Studies have been performed in postoperative,[74-80] in nonoperated malnourished individuals,[81] in normal[82-84] patients with chronic duodenal ulcers,[85] in obese subjects[81,86] and in burn patients.[31] The experiments varied, not only in the types of subjects but also in the amounts of amino acids and glucose given and with respect to the contributions of administered fat. In these experiments essential and nonessential amino acids were given as commercial mixtures or as intact protein. Certain generalizations appear warranted: (1) Amino acid mixtures by themselves spared protein significantly in most studies but to varying degrees; generally, the subjects remained in some degree of negative nitrogen balance. (2) The urea excretion increased markedly over the levels occurring in fasting controls or glucose-fed subjects as the major portion of the administered amino acids was catabolized. (3) Hypocaloric amounts of glucose given with the amino acids increased nitrogen retention over that observed with amino acids in many (e.g. Fig. 36–8) but not all studies. It would appear, therefore, that the original hypothesis relating protein sparing to decreased insulin levels was not correct; the effect appears related to the amino acid supply directly. (4) Provision of amino acids alone is associated with maintenance of postabsorptive insulin and glucose concentrations, elevation of glucagon and free fatty acids and ketonemia. (5) Increased sparing seems to occur when amino acids are given to previously depleted individuals, probably reflecting the effects of exogenous supply, decreased catabolism and increased reutilization.

Glycerol as well as fat emulsion improves nitrogen retention when amino acids are given intravenously.[83] Glycerol is liberated from triglyceride hydrolysis (endogenous or exogenous) and is converted to glucose by way of pyruvate or lactate. The protein-sparing effect of Intralipid is attributable to the glycerol liberated from the triglycerides and to that added to the emulsion to make it isotonic.

Animal experiments have demonstrated that feeding protein alone conserved tissue and body nitrogen as long as sufficient adipose stores were maintained but, thereafter, had no advantage over lower protein intakes supplemented with carbohydrate.[87] Balance data do not give information on possible interorgan differences in protein economy. At a level of energy restriction with protein ingestion which permits positive nitrogen balance, liver nitrogen in dogs was as depressed as in a group on a protein-free diet. At less severe energy restriction, however, dietary protein was found to conserve liver nitrogen.[88]

Studies with ^{15}N-glycine have demonstrated that, when glucose was added to amino acid infusion in fasting man, there was increased whole-body protein synthesis while protein-breakdown rates remained unchanged.[84]

The protein-sparing effect of amino acids raises the practical question of its clinical usefulness as a replacement for peripheral infusion of isotonic glucose in routine postoperative care. While more comparative data on relative effectiveness would be useful, opinions have been expressed in the American[89] and British[85] literature that, for short-term use, the extent of the increase in nitrogen retention with amino acids over that of glucose does not warrant its routine use because of the extra cost. Where more prolonged use of intravenous feeding is required, and particularly when a significant degree of malnutrition has occurred or is expected to occur with routine glucose infusions, serious consideration should be given to total parenteral nutrition or at least to peripheral parenteral nutrition with amino acids, glucose 10 per cent and intravenous fat (Chapter 37).

Nitrogen-sparing Effect of Branched-chain Amino Acids (BCAA)

Interesting insights have developed into the effects of giving branched-chain amino acids during fasting or trauma. It has been demonstrated that the addition of BCAA to rat skeletal muscle in vitro promoted protein synthesis and decreased protein breakdown, indicating a regulatory role for these amino acids or their metabolic products.[90,91] Infusion of the three BCAA at their usual daily requirements into fasting guinea pigs resulted in significantly lower net nitrogen excretion when compared to animals infused with only the basal electrolyte solution or with glucose.[92] Injured rats given 3 per cent amino acids with varying proportions of BCAA (22, 35, 52 and 100 per cent of the total amino acids infused) had appreciably less nitrogen losses in short-term studies than controls given 5 per cent dextrose in water; the 35 and 100 per cent BCAA solutions appeared to be associated with minimum nitrogen losses and the 100 per cent BCAA group had essentially normal plasma and muscle total and individual amino acids.[93]

Infusion of the α-ketoanalogs of BCAA (4.7 gm per day) into fasting obese women for one week resulted in a significant lowering of urinary nitrogen as compared to that occurring in the same subjects during total fasting without the analogs. Furthermore, the decreased nitrogen persisted into the next week of fasting after the analogs had been discontinued.[94]

The mechanism for the protein sparing effect of BCAA is unclear but does not appear to be related to hormonal, ketone body or energy changes.

NUTRITIONAL PROBLEMS FOLLOWING SURGERY OF THE ALIMENTARY TRACT

Surgical resection at any point or alteration of the normal pathway of movement of food in the alimentary tract may result in the development of nutritional problems. These effects may be subtle and

Table 36–3. Surgical Modification of the Alimentary Tract Predisposing to Nutrition Problems

1. Radical resection of oropharyngeal area
   A. Chewing and swallowing difficulties
   B. Possible necessity for tube feeding
2. Esophagectomy and esophageal reconstruction
   A. Gastric stasis and hypochlorhydria secondary to vagotomy
   B. Steatorrhea
   C. Diarrhea
3. Gastrectomy (high subtotal or total)
   A. Dumping syndrome
   B. Malabsorption
   C. Achlorhydria and lack of intrinsic factor
   D. Hypoglycemia
4. Intestinal resection
   A. Jejunum
      (1) Decreased efficiency of absorption of many nutrients
   B. Ileum
      (1) Vitamin B_{12} deficiency
      (2) Bile salt losses with diarrhea
      (3) Hyperoxaluria
   C. Massive bowel resection
      (1) Life-threatening malabsorption
      (2) Malnutrition
      (3) Metabolic acidosis
   D. Ileostomy and colostomy
      (1) Complications of salt and water balance
5. Blind loop syndrome
6. Pancreatectomy
   A. Malabsorption
   B. Diabetes mellitus

insidious or acute and obvious. It is the responsibility of the surgeon to be aware of these potential problems and to institute the necessary preventive and therapeutic measures that will maintain optimum nutritional states in the patient.

A listing of some of the nutritional problems resulting from surgical intervention is given in Table 36–3. Modification of normal function may be further complicated by adjunctive treatments such as radiation and chemotherapy or by the development of complications such as fistulas.

Surgery of the Head and Neck

Radical surgery of the head and neck region, including partial or total glossectomy and/or mandibulectomy, often interferes with mastication and swallowing. With some training or with laryngectomy, which prevents aspiration of fluids and food, oral food intake is possible. In other cases, prolonged tube feeding may be required. Liquid diets are prepared by blending the types of food ordinarily consumed by the family, having made certain that the pattern is nutritious. Where the personal situation does not permit this, simple and inexpensive tube formulas may be used (see Appendix). Many elderly individuals do not tolerate large amounts of fluids. The composition of the formula should be modified as concomitant cardiovascular, renal or endocrine disease indicates. Attention should be paid to psychologic aspects of food with tube feedings, e.g. the aroma of a separate cup of coffee may be important. Patients can be taught to insert the nasopharyngeal tube themselves so that they avoid the psychologic trauma and throat irritation associated with an indwelling tube. For those unable to pass the tube, its insertion via an esophagostomy or gastrostomy is recommended.

Esophagectomy

Esophagectomy often induces significant malabsorption of fat.[95,96] The cause of this peculiar dysfunction appears to be the bilateral vagotomy inherent in the procedure; however, the precise intestinal mechanism causing the steatorrhea is unknown. The previously recognized sequelae of vagotomy—gastric stasis (necessitating a drainage procedure) and diarrhea—also occur in esophagectomized patients. Carbohydrate absorption is normal. The use of medium-chain triglycerides (MCT) as a major portion of fat intake diminishes the steatorrhea.[95] Cholestyramine has been reported to reduce postvagotomy diarrhea but support-ing evidence is awaited.

Gastrectomy

The physiologic and nutritional conse-quences of subtotal and total gastrectomy have been reviewed in Chapter 31A and elsewhere.[97] It suffices to state here that clinical problems increase proportionately to the extent of the resection. In addition to the well-known occurrences of dumping syndrome, hypoglycemia, steatorrhea, af-ferent loop syndrome and loss of intrinsic factor, emphasis is needed on the long-term consequences of loss of the stomach with the insidious development of various vitamin and mineral deficiencies.[98-101] Serious and persistent attention by the physician to prevent these nutritional problems is essential for long-term health when the underlying disease leading to the need for operation is benign or malig-nancy has been eradicated.

Intestinal Resection

Clinical studies in normal subjects and in those with ablation of varying portions of small intestine indicate that all nutrients studied, with the exception of vitamin B_{12}, are most efficiently and (in the usual di-etary amounts) rather completely absorbed in the proximal small bowel.[102,103] How-ever, following jejunal resection, the ileum, with its reserve absorptive capacity, can absorb these nutrients in good degree if adequate nutritional status is maintained.

When the terminal ileum has been re-moved there will be poor absorption of both vitamin B_{12} and conjugated bile salts since this is the site of their physiologic absorption. Provision of vitamin B_{12} in-tramuscularly in doses of 100 μg every month or two will prevent the develop-ment of B_{12} deficiency.

Failure to reabsorb conjugated bile salts will result in one of several problems. If the ileal resection is not extensive (usually less than 100 cm)[104] sufficient bile salts

enter the large bowel to induce a brown watery diarrhea which may be very distress-ing to the patient. Cholestyramine may be dramatically effective in controlling such a choleric diarrhea by its mechanism of bind-ing bile salts. The loss of bile salts as the result of ileal resection interrupts the nor-mal enterohepatic circulation which efficiently retains and recirculates conju-gated bile salts. The synthetic capacity of the liver to synthesize sufficient new bile salts is exceeded and the concentration of bile salts in the intestinal lumen becomes low, especially with successive meals. When the ileal resection is greater (usually more than 100 cm), the luminal content of bile salts will fall below the critical level for formation of micelles; consequently, fat absorption will be depressed and steator-rhea will ensue.[104,105] In such a situation, the patient will be helped by the feeding of a diet low in long-chain fats and use of medium-chain triglycerides which do not require bile salts for their absorption. The use of water-soluble forms of vitamin K and more of the other fat-soluble vitamins is indicated to prevent deficiency of these nutrients. Sufficient polyunsaturated fats should be fed to assure adequate essential fatty acids.

Another consequence of ileal resection is hyperoxaluria and renal oxalate stone formation. This is explainable on the fact that the normal precipitation of oxalate ion by intestinal calcium ions is prevented by a shortage of such free calcium ions because of binding to fatty acids present in in-creased amounts in the remaining small bowel and colon by the steatorrheic ileec-tomized patients. The soluble oxalate is then absorbed in the colon and appears in the urine in increased concentrations, with resultant probability of precipitation as calcium oxalate in the renal tubule.[106,107] On the basis of this explanation a reduced fat intake appears advisable, together with an increased intake of calcium salts.

Massive small bowel resection, with a

residual of three feet or less, presents serious and long-term problems in maintaining adequate nutrition, including water and electrolytes. If there is some radiation damage of remaining bowel or loss of the ileocecal valve and portions of the colon, the problems are intensified. However, the application of present knowledge with respect to care of these patients will often permit a successful outcome. These principles include:

1. The postoperative period is often a stormy one complicated by infection, ileus and weight loss. During this period, it is essential that all factors tending to weight loss and malnutrition be combatted vigorously. This includes preparation at operation for long-term parenteral nutrition with sterile insertion of an indwelling central venous catheter for institution of total parenteral nutrition (cf Chapter 37) and the formation of a feeding gastrostomy for future use.

2. Absorptive capacity of many of these patients improves with time, so that patience and a carefully developed nutritional program, designed to meet nutritional needs are essential.[108-111] As gastrointestinal function returns, special gastrostomy feedings can be initiated, utilizing round-the-clock feedings, if indicated, with hydrolyzed protein or amino acids and other nutrients capable of rapid absorption. This route is increasingly utilized as conditions improve, to the point where IV feedings are discontinued and eventually oral intake commences, supplemented by gastrostomy feedings when necessary. Protracted and meticulous follow-up care is essential with adequate provision at home—as in hospital—of all necessary nutrients including minerals and trace elements.

3. A marked reduction in the intake of long-chain fats reduces diarrhea and decreases fecal calcium, magnesium and other electrolyte losses.[112] The use of medium-chain triglycerides (MCT) in increasing amounts (as tolerated by the patient and consistent with an acceptable level of diarrhea) is often of value in increasing calories.[113] Given in significant amounts it causes some ketosis and acidosis which may require additional sodium bicarbonate.[114]

4. The acidosis associated with malabsorption and diarrhea will tend to increase calcium and potassium losses in urine and should be watched for and treated on a continuing basis.

5. Persistent gastric hypersecretion may occasionally occur[115,116] and this possibility should be investigated. In our experience, it is rare. When it does occur, without spontaneous improvement, the use of an H_2 antagonist is useful.

6. As noted above, vitamin B_{12} injections are to be given and dietary prescriptions made which minimize steatorrhea and hyperoxaluria.

7. The surgeon should retain the ileocecal valve whenever possible, since it appears to slow the exit of small bowel contents and, hence, improves absorption and perhaps acts to hinder retrograde movement of colonic bacteria. The use of an antiperistaltic segment of bowel as a replacement for the valve has been recommended with more or less enthusiasm.[117,118] The inherent dangers posed by the possibility of sacrificing further absorptive surface in a patient with massive bowel resection, together with the danger of obstruction, are, presumably, the reasons why this procedure is rarely reported as being performed now.

Ileostomy

This procedure is usually followed by large sodium and water losses but, within 7 to 10 days, these usually decrease to the range which will characterize the otherwise healthy individual on a stable diet. Generally, these stabilized individuals lose 300 to 600 ml of water daily, with 40 to 100 mEq of sodium and 2.5 to 10 mEq of potassium, emphasizing the physiologic role of the colon in absorbing water and sodium and in exchanging potassium for sodium. Gastroenteritis, partial intestinal obstruction and prolonged excessive sweating impose additional losses. Studies in man and in dogs during sodium depletion have demonstrated a reduction in sodium concentration of ileostomy material as depletion progressed, accompanied by increased potassium concentration.[119,120]

Pancreatectomy

The consequent loss of digestive enzymes leads to loss into the stool not only of fats and of protein but also of significant amounts of various vitamins and minerals. Since pancreatectomy necessitates partial gastrectomy, this is a complicating factor.

The situation is further complicated by the fact that even subtotal pancreatectomy with anastomosis of the remaining portion of the pancreatic duct to jejunum leads to exocrine insufficiency in a significant proportion of patients.[121] Total pancreatectomy, of course, induces diabetes mellitus. The diabetic state occurring in conjunction with impaired carbohydrate, protein and fat digestion further complicates the nutritional problems of such patients. The use of MCT and oligosaccharides may be beneficial.[121]

Pancreatic enzyme insufficiency may be effectively replaced by potent pancreatic extracts given with meals or at 2-hour intervals. Recent evaluations have been made of various pancreatic extracts,[122,123] dosage schedules[124,125] and ancillary treatment such as antacids and an H_2 receptor antagonist.[126] Important factors are adequate dosage with meals and use of antacids or H_2 receptor antagonist when gastric secretion is normal or high since the latter may inactivate the pancreatic enzymes. There may be impaired vitamin B_{12} absorption with pancreatectomy, improved by administration of pancreatic extract.[121,126] The diabetes mellitus following the resection is usually of the "brittle" type, requiring relatively small amounts of insulin, and is rather difficult to control with precision. Hence, tolerance of some glucosuria is safer than the hypoglycemic episodes which may occur with achievement of glucose-free urine.

Major Hepatic Resection

The liver has a remarkable ability to regenerate by cellular hypertrophy and hyperplasia following massive resection. Immediate postoperative problems are met by glucose and albumin infusions and adequate replacement of electrolytes including phosphate.[121]

Ureterosigmoidostomy

This procedure, which is now rarely performed, involved implantation of the ureters into the sigmoid colon following total cystectomy. It often led to significant disturbances in acid-base balance with development of a hyperchloremic acidosis, hypokalemia and hypophosphatemia.[127] These abnormalities occur much less commonly in patients with cutaneous *ureteroileostomy* (ileal conduit), which has replaced ureterosigmoidostomy.[128]

Management of External Gastrointestinal Fistulas

Major advances in the management of such fistulas have occurred as the result of the availability of effective antibiotics, more aggressive drainage of abscesses and recognition of the importance of nutritional support. There has been an increase in survival and rates of successful closures either spontaneously with improved nutrition or by surgical intervention following rehabilitation. The improvement in mortality over a span of years is shown in Table 36–4.

There were surgeons who were aware years ago of the importance of nutrition and took vigorous steps to ensure that their fistulized patients were aggressively treated. For example, Smith and Lee reported in 1956 the treatment of duodenal fistulas by intrajejunal administration of nutritional liquid formulas, with excellent results.[136] Tube and enterostomy feedings employed by Dunphy and his colleagues in the treatment of intestinal fistulas resulted in fistula closure of 89 per cent in patients receiving more than 1,600 kcal per day as compared to 37 per cent in those receiving less calories.[37] The widespread acceptance and application of total parenteral nutrition by surgeons has led to major improvements in spontaneous closure and survival where, apparently, nutritional support had previously not been adequate. A comparison has been made of experience with high-output small-bowel fistulas in the same hospital before and after institution of TPN.[138] In the period prior to institution of TPN when mean caloric intake was low (500 kcal per day[139]) in 66 patients, the nonoperative cure rate was 27

**Table 36–4. Surgical and Conservative Treatment of
External Gastrointestinal Fistulas†**

Ref/Yr	Number of Cases	Fistula Location (external fistulas)	Medical Management (% of cases)	Surgical Treatment (% of cases)	Overall Mortality (%)
129/1960	157	Gastroduodenal, small bowel, large bowel	22	78	44
130/1969	18	Small bowel	8.6	91.4	30
131/1971	21	Duodenal, small bowel	33.4	66.6	22
132/1971*	51	Gastroduodenal, small bowel, large bowel	36.3	64.7	12
133/1972	55	Small bowel	40	60	30
134/1973*	61	Gastroduodenal, small bowel, large bowel	73.7	18.3	9.8
135/1974*	38	Gastroduodenal, small bowel, large bowel	29.0	71.1	21
135a/1975*	71Φ	Esophagus to large bowel	43	67 ΦΦ	28
135b/1978*	25	Small bowel	60	40	20

† Taken in part from Aguirre et al.[135]
* Parenteral nutrition utilized.
Φ 66 with cancer; 39 with abdominal radiation.
ΦΦ In 35 per cent surgical closure either not attempted or failed.

per cent, surgical cure 32 per cent and one-third of the patients died. With TPN permitting administration of a mean of 2,500 kcal per day in 25 patients, nonoperative cure rate was 56 per cent, surgical cure was 36 per cent and only two patients died. The importance of nutrition support, regardless of whether it is by the enteral or parenteral route, has been emphasized.[140] Improved rates of closure with TPN alone or with TPN and surgery and marked decreases in mortality have been reported (Table 36–4). Similar observations have been made with defined formula diets as the sole[141] or major source following postoperative TPN.[142,143] The presence of malignancy in the abdomen, irradiated bowel or inflammatory bowel disease and other factors decreases the likelihood of spontaneous closure.[134,140] However, improved nutrition greatly increases surgical cure rates in such instances.

The period of time that should elapse before deciding on operative closure is a subjective decision. Dunphy advises wait-ing approximately one month after completely controlling infection and after nutrition is adequate.[144] MacFayden et al. reported 100 per cent spontaneous closure of duodenal fistulas in an average of 18.7 days, jejunal fistulas (88 per cent) in 33.8 days, colon fistulas (79 per cent) in 45.7 days. Only 40 per cent of ileal fistulas and 50 per cent of gastric fistulas closed; the average times to closure, spontaneous and operative, were 45.7 and 52.1 days, respectively.[134]

Pre- and Postoperative Feeding

It has been traditional to place patients who are to undergo abdominal surgery on a clear liquid diet for several days. Such a diet provides little in the way of nutrition and has been challenged as an unnecessary and undesirable withholding of potentially important nutritional support. The suggested alternative has been low-residue chemically defined formulas providing a complete diet in liquid form. One of the initial arguments favoring such formula diets was the belief that they would also decrease the types and concentration of bacterial flora,[145] but this has not proven to be the case.[146] There is merit, however, in providing more adequate nutrition in a form which permits a clean bowel, provided that the formula offered is palatable enough to be taken voluntarily in adequate amounts or fed by tube. Experience with such feedings have been published.[147,148]

There are few surgeons in the United States who believe that gastric decompression is unnecessary after abdominal surgery. Nasogastric suction, as advocated and popularized by Wangensteen,[149] is much more widely used than is temporary gastrostomy; decompression is usually continued from the stomach and upper intestine to prevent postoperative vomiting until functional activity becomes obvious.

There have been suggestions, especially in the British medical literature,[150,151] for considering earlier postoperative feeding, specifically intrajejunal. Such advocacy is based on postoperative audiographic, pressure and roentgen studies in normal and postoperative studies at various levels of the intestinal tract. Although surgery inhibits gastric and colonic motility, the small bowel appears to retain good activity.[150-152] Absorption of tritiated water given by the oral and colonic routes is retarded but that given intrajejunally is normally absorbed by man after abdominal surgery.[153] After small intestinal anastomosis and formation of a Stamm gastrostomy in dogs, intrajejunally administered glucose and ^{22}NaCl were absorbed normally.[154]

INTRAVENOUS WATER AND ELECTROLYTES

These requirements can be considered in three categories:

1. Baseline requirements: The calculation of baseline requirements disregards any preexisting dehydration or any abnormal losses, but baseline volumes may require modification in patients with extracellular fluid excess or dilutional hyponatremia.

2. Abnormal losses: What does the patient require in order to replace ongoing abnormal fluid and electrolyte losses resulting from the disease or its treatment, or both?

3. Deficits or excesses: What deficits (or excesses) does the patient have in water, electrolytes, blood volume, plasma proteins, and micronutrients? What should be done to correct these abnormalities, and at what rate should reconstitution be effected?

The orders written for parenteral fluid and electrolyte therapy should take into consideration these three major categories. The parenteral fluids required are the sum of baseline requirements and abnormal losses plus a part of or all the deficits existing at the time treatment is begun or minus a part or all of the excesses present when initiating treatment.

Baseline Requirements

Water. Normal water requirements have been discussed in Chapter 8. The usual surgical patient may not have the normal degree of renal efficiency; in addition he may be subjected to an increased solute load as the result of trauma and increased catabolism of body cell mass. Therefore, a urine volume of 1,200 to 1,500 ml per day is desirable in the average adult following operation. However, this goal for urine volume may be either excessive or inadequate with certain types of serious impairment of renal function; it may not be achievable in the early postoperative period when post-traumatic inhibition of renal free water clearance is to be expected with previously normal renal function. A patient with a normal body temperature, living in a comfortable environment of both temperature and humidity, will lose between 800 and 1,000 ml of water per day as insensible loss. The rate of loss is somewhat higher in men than in women and is proportionate to body surface area and to respiratory minute volume. There is a small insensible loss of sodium, potassium and chloride because of a combination of minimal sweating and electrolyte lost in desquamation of the epidermis. Balance studies have suggested an insensible loss of approximately 20 mEq of sodium per day, an equal amount of chloride and between 5 and 10 mEq of potassium.

The daily caloric requirement of the afebrile patient at bed rest will vary from 1,500 to 2,300 kcal. If the patient is receiving 400 to 500 kcal by the administration of glucose, the baseline production of endogenous water in this situation will be from 150 to 200 ml, or about 10 per cent of the total daily requirement. However, fever, trauma, infection and immobilization greatly increase endogenous water production, and the seriously ill patient suffering from extensive trauma or massive infection may provide as much as 1,000 ml of sodium-free, potassium-rich endogenous water a day. This must be taken into account in considering fluid balance.

Normal baseline parenteral water requirements vary from 1,250 to 3,000 ml per day depending on body cell mass size, age and sex. Table 36–5 illustrates two methods of estimating the baseline parenteral fluid requirements of surgical patients. Both these methods depend upon an estimation of the ideal body weight for height, sex and age in those patients who are obese, since excess fat has little metabolic activity or effect other than increasing somewhat the total body surface area.

Both methods should be considered rule-of-thumb guides for baseline fluid requirements to be modified as necessary in accordance with the needs of the individual patient.

Weights of patients on restricted parenteral fluid therapy of glucose, water and electrolytes should decrease with a loss of approximately 0.3 to 0.5 per cent of body weight per day until adequate nutrition is instituted. Exceptions occur with blood transfusions, with deliberate changes in hydration and during the first 24 to 48 hours following trauma or operation with local sequestration of fluid and increased parenteral therapy to compensate for it. The patient who otherwise gains weight while on this type of hypocaloric glucose parenteral therapy is almost certainly being overhydrated. The patient who loses weight rapidly, except during the normal post-traumatic diuresis, usually has abnormal fluid losses which are being underestimated and underreplaced.

Table 36–5.   Baseline Water Requirements

Computed per day for relatively normal semistarving patients without massive trauma, dehydration, or chronic illness.

Method 1: based on "ideal" body weight for height, sex and age for obese patients and on actual body weight for others:

   1. Children over 20 kg—1,500 ml + 30 ml/kg above 20 kg
   2. Previously vigorous young adults with large muscle mass—40 ml/kg/day
   3. Adults between 18 and 55 years—35 ml/kg/day
   4. Older patients with no major cardiac or renal disease—30 ml/kg/day

Method 2: for all patients except infants weighing less than 5 kg, based on "ideal" body weight for height, sex and age for obese patients and on actual body weight for others:*

	ml/kg/day
First 10 kg of body weight	100
Second 10 kg of body weight	50
All weight above 20 kg	20 if < 50 years old
	15 if > 50 years old

*Modified from recommendations of Kiesewetter.[155]

Daily (or more frequent) body weight measurements are the single most important method of controlling water balance.

Factors Which Increase Baseline Requirements. These are essentially ones which increase the insensible loss.

Fever. Fever increases the baseline water requirements largely through hyperventilation with increased water evaporation. A patient with a fever of 103° F (39.4° C) will require about 500 ml of additional baseline water per day. Endogenous water production is also increased.

Sweating. A rule of thumb with respect to sweat loss is to increase the average adult baseline water requirements by 500 ml per day for each 5° above 85° F of ambient temperature. This is dependent on the humidity. Sweat is about one-third isotonic sodium chloride in the summer and nearly two-thirds isotonic in winter, so that additional salt must be provided in baseline therapy to compensate. When the environmental temperature approaches body temperature, the seriously ill patient should be cooled, preferably by air conditioning, because insensible loss of water becomes very large when the ambient temperature exceeds body temperature.

Increased Metabolism. Hyperthyroidism increases the baseline water turnover substantially, as it does caloric requirements. Hyperthyroid patients in the semistarving state tend to consume massive amounts of lean body tissue and body fat, producing unusual amounts of endogenous water; simultaneously they lose water by both respiratory evaporation and skin sublimation as well as by sweating.

Factors Which Reduce Baseline Water Requirements. These include reduced metabolic activity, as seen in hypothyroidism, in the elderly and in situations in which there is an excessive amount of body water with overexpanded extracellular fluid space as in cardiac edema, in hypoproteinemia with starvation, in prolonged infection, in carcinoma of the gastrointestinal tract and in the special circumstance of acute renal failure.

Electrolytes. In the absence of abnormal losses or of dehydration and salt deficits, the baseline sodium requirements of the average previously healthy adult are easily met by a maximum of 500 ml of 0.9 per cent sodium chloride with 5 per cent dextrose. This provides 76 mEq each of sodium and chloride ion. In addition, 40 mEq of potassium chloride per day for all adults except those suffering from acute dehydration or renal insufficiency will provide sufficient baseline potassium to prevent many problems of potassium depletion. Potassium chloride should not be administered in concentrations in excess of 40 mEq/L of fluid (unless precautions are instituted to avoid accidental excessive rate of infusion), and therefore the baseline requirement should be dissolved in at least 1,000 ml of otherwise isotonic infusion fluid. Another approach to the administration of baseline electrolytes is to provide 3 mEq of sodium and 2 mEq of potassium per 100 ml of infusion fluid in the form of chloride salts. This method is particularly useful in pediatric surgical therapy but may result in an excessive electrolyte load for baseline fluids in the adult.

Magnesium (as $MgSO_4 \cdot 7H_2O$) should be given on a routine basis in parenteral solutions either daily at 8.5 mEq (= 2 ml 50 per cent solution) to 17 mEq or three times per week at double this amount in the stable adult patient without gastrointestinal losses or previous depletion.

In the presence of an overexpanded extracellular fluid space with excess total body sodium, the sodium chloride content of baseline fluids should be reduced or eliminated. In the presence of acute or chronic renal insufficiency or severe acidosis with elevation of the plasma potassium level, potassium should be reduced or withheld. Magnesium administration should also be reduced or withheld (as serum levels indicate) in patients with azotemia.

The remaining water requirement beyond that used to dissolve the electrolytes suggested is, of course, made up by the use of 5 or 10 per cent glucose in distilled water.

Administration of antibiotics such as sodium carbenicillin and/or amphotericin is often associated with significant urinary losses of potassium and magnesium. Serum levels should be determined daily (until the patient is stable) and additional amounts of these ions given; the amounts of potassium that may be necessary may be large (i.e. 150 to 250 mEq per day).

Abnormal Losses

These include both external abnormal losses of water, electrolytes and plasma protein, and internal fluid shifts with functional loss of fluids by sequestration within the body.

External abnormal loss may be in the form of excessive loss of water and electrolytes by normal routes of excretion or secretion, or losses may occur from intraluminal tubes, drains, fistulae or wounds. The most common of the sources of external abnormal losses in surgical patients is the gastrointestinal tract; next in frequency are losses from surgical wounds, increased evaporation from the skin and respiratory tract, and burns. Sequestration of extracellular fluids into areas of traumatized or infected tissue produces a decrease in the usual distribution of extracellular fluid without external loss or change in body weight.

Losses From the Gastrointestinal Tract. The normal daily volume of secretions into the gastrointestinal tract is not precisely known but has been estimated to be 8,000 to 10,000 ml, of which saliva constitutes 1 to 2 liters, gastric juice, including both acid and mucoid secretions, about 2,500 ml, bile 500 to 750 ml, and pancreatic juice more than 1,000 ml. In addition, secretion of the upper small bowel contributes between 2,000 and 3,000 ml. All but 100 to 200 ml is normally reabsorbed by the small bowel and the colon.

Abnormal losses from the gastrointestinal tract include water, electrolytes and varying amounts of protein. The electrolyte content of fluid from the gastrointestinal tract varies significantly with the level from which the bulk of the fluid is derived. Table 36–6 shows the average and the range of variation of sodium, potassium, chloride and bicarbonate in fluid from different levels of the intestine in patients with a variety of causes for drainage. It is important to note that of all the secretions of the gastrointestinal tract only bile and

Table 36–6. Electrolyte Concentration of Gastrointestinal Secretions*

Source of Fluid	Na, mEq/L	K, mEq/L	Cl, mEq/L	Effective HCO$_3$ mEq/L
Saliva, average of 3 pt (based on 1 ml/minute)	60	20	16	50
Gastric, average†	59	9.3	89	0–1
Range	30–90	4.3–12	52–155	
Upper small bowel, average	105	5.1	99	≅10
Range	72–128	3.5–6.8	69–127	
Ileum, average	117	5.0	106	15–20
Range	91–140	3.0–7.5	82–125	
Bile, average	145	5.2	100	≅50
Range	134–156	3.9–6.3	83–110	
Pancreatic fistula, average of 3 pt	141.6	4.6	76.6	≅70

*From Randall.[156]

† Range represents values for the middle two-thirds of a series of patients, except for gastric secretion, where a group of patients with high gastric acidity and a high Cl$^-$ concentration in gastric juice has been included at the upper limit.

pancreatic juice are approximately isotonic in their observed electrolyte content. The average calculated osmolarity of saliva is about 160 mO; of fasting gastric juice, in patients without duodenal ulcer, about 180 mO; of upper small bowel content, 220 mO; and of fluid from the distal ileum, about 240 mO. Other substances, including mucoproteins, other polysaccharides, urea, and calcium and phosphate, increase the total osmolality beyond these approximations.

The average values shown may be used for semiquantitative replacement of gastrointestinal tract losses. When volumes exceed 2,000 ml in 24 hours or when substantial losses (1 liter or more per day) continue for more than a few days, it is wise to send an aliquot of the 24-hr drainage to the laboratory for analysis for electrolytes and protein and to determine the pH of a freshly obtained specimen. With this information more precise replacement can be made.

A significant loss of protein may occur from distended and atonic small bowel. Losses of 20 to 30 gm of protein per liter of small bowel drainage have been observed. Larger losses of plasma protein, and substantial losses of whole blood, are seen in patients with severe diarrhea accompanying ulcerative colitis. A high percentage of this protein is serum albumin. Accordingly, when large volumes of bowel content are lost, replacement of lost plasma protein becomes necessary if a serious decrease in plasma protein concentration is to be avoided. If plasma, or preferably an albumin fraction, is used and the patient is otherwise adequately hydrated, the water and electrolyte content of the infusate must be considered.

Internal Fluid Shifts. If the intracellular and extracellular fluid spaces are considered as the two major body fluid compartments, an abnormal "third" fluid space is created when interstitial fluid, plasma and sometimes red blood cells are sequestered in abnormal amounts in an area of tissue injury. This sequestered fluid is in continuity with the remaining extracellular fluid from which it was derived, yet is unavailable for restoring diminished interstitial fluid and plasma volumes. It is apparent as edema in patients with burns; it also occurs in crush injuries, in peritonitis, in pulmonary infection, in soft tissue and wound infection and in areas distal to obstructed venous flow. Sequestered fluid is accumulated to some degree postoperatively in all surgical wounds and is substantial in retroperitoneal dissection or with visceral or muscle trauma.

A special type of internal fluid shift is seen with the development of transcellular pooling such as that which occurs within the gastrointestinal tract with intestinal obstruction or adynamic ileus; the volume of fluid involved may be quite large. These collections of transcellular fluid may become abnormal external losses if they are vomited or drained by intestinal intubation, or they may resolve by reabsorption as the patient recovers gastrointestinal function.

If the volume of sequestered fluid is significantly large, it must be replaced exactly as if an external loss had occurred. The major difference between development of a third space of sequestered fluid and an abnormal external fluid loss is that sequestered fluid remains within the body, so that there is no loss of weight. A gain in weight results from the necessary replacement of diminished plasma and interstitial fluid volumes of the rest of the body. Also, unlike an external loss, the sequestered fluid will eventually return to the circulation as normal function returns to the affected area—presenting a potential problem in water and electrolyte overloading.

Deficits or Excesses

The administration of water, electrolytes, calories, amino acids as such or as protein and vitamins as baseline therapy for replacement of abnormal external losses and for provision for internal fluid shifts is intended to help the patient to maintain normal functional volumes of body fluids, normal concentrations of electrolytes and a normal pH of plasma and interstitial fluid. However, patients may have deficits or excesses of some or all of the component body fluids at the time when they are first seen and treatment is begun. In other patients significant abnormalities of volume, concentration and pH may develop while the patient is under treatment. The replacement of deficits of water and electrolytes necessary to restore function when losses have occurred and the recognition and treatment of excessive fluid volumes or concentrations of electrolytes when present constitute the third major category for clinical consideration in fluid and electrolyte therapy.

Acute Dehydration. Acute change in the volume of total body water can occur either as the result of dehydration or through retention of an excessive amount of water, usually parenterally administered. There is, of course, a comparable change in body weights which, if known, greatly assists in diagnosis. Rapid weight loss through dehydration is almost entirely extracellular fluid. A loss of 2 per cent of body weight will produce thirst and some oliguria. A loss of 4 per cent of body weight (20 per cent of extracellular fluid) causes oliguria, tachycardia and often postural hypotension, and an acute extracellular fluid loss of 6 per cent of body weight is a life-threatening event, reducing interstitial fluid and plasma volumes by about 30 per cent and compromising both blood pressure and renal function.

Replacement of acute loss of extracellular fluid or its functional loss by sequestration or transcellular pooling is best accomplished by infusion of water containing the electrolytes of extracellular fluid. Balanced salt solutions such as Ringer's lactate or a solution of 2 parts of 0.9 per cent sodium chloride and 1 part M/6 sodium lactate are most effective. The rate of replacement can and usually should be rapid when the loss has occurred rapidly. If the loss causing the dehydration has been from vomiting, with an excess loss of hydrogen ion as hydrochloric acid, the plasma carbon dioxide content and pH will be elevated. Under these conditions the ideal fluid for rapid replacement is isotonic (0.9 per cent) sodium chloride. Where there is an indication for Na^+ restriction, N/10 hydrochloric acid solution may be infused as needed.[157,158] If a severe metabolic acidosis is present, with a low pH and carbon dioxide content of plasma, initial infusion of 88 mEq of sodium bicarbonate or 500 ml of M/6 sodium lactate solution should precede the use of a balanced salt solution. Close monitoring of serum potassium level is indicated with addition of KCl as indicated to prevent significant hypokalemia as potassium enters the cells with rising pH. Rapid infusion of glucose-containing solutions should be avoided to prevent a solute diuresis caused by glucose overloading. Glucose solutions should be introduced somewhat later, except in treatment of diabetic ketoacidosis where glucose will be required as administered insulin becomes effective.

Chronic Dehydration. A patient who has become chronically dehydrated over a period of several days to a week or more, as a result of inadequate intake of water and food, may well lose 10 per cent or more of body weight. The loss of body water in such instances is more evenly distributed between intracellular and extracellular fluids. The effects of combined fluid depletion are less severe than those with acute extracellular fluid dehydration; hypotension and hemoconcentration are less marked and the degree of oliguria is less.

Rehydration in such a patient requires replacement of the extracellular fluid deficit in sufficient volume to raise urine volume to 25 to 50 ml per hour and to reduce the hematocrit to normal levels. A period of days rather than hours is desirable for repletion of the intracellular water and potassium deficits. Emergency surgical measures, if required, can be performed after repletion of the extracellular fluid component. Complete rehydration should not result in return to predehydration weight because of the loss of protein and fat during the period of underhydration and semistarvation.

Dehydration by Primary Water Loss: Desiccation. This occurs as the result of excessive loss of water vapor or of very hypotonic solutions with the retention of extracellular fluid electrolytes and an increase in all the solutes of the plasma with a rise in plasma osmolality. The common clinical settings are those of excessive evaporation of water from the skin and respiratory tract, as seen with fever and hyperventilation caused by metabolic acidosis. Tracheostomy and the administration of insufficiently humidified oxygen by catheter are additional respiratory causes. A high volume of dilute urine, as seen with diabetes insipidus, use of osmotic diuretics and excessive sweating, all with inadequate water replacement, produce excessive water loss. The open treatment of burns with massive loss of water vapor from injured skin surfaces is particularly likely to produce desiccation dehydration. Oliguria, azotemia, fever, disorientation, coma, convulsions and death will follow. Hypotension is usually a late complication.

Laboratory findings in this setting demonstrate an increase in the concentration of all the solutes of plasma, with an increase in osmolality. Serum sodium concentration is the key, and values of 160 mEq/L or more may be found, denoting osmolality of more than 325 mO. The hematocrit will rise in proportion to loss of total body water when the process takes days to develop, as is usually the case; therefore it will not be as high as with acute extracellular fluid loss. Urine is highly concentrated and small in volume.

Treatment consists of the administration of water as 5 per cent glucose solution intravenously, or water by mouth in sufficient volumes to restore electrolyte concentrations and urine volume to normal. The rate of administration will depend somewhat on the rate at which water was initially lost; the more rapid the loss, the more rapid can be rehydration. Usually 1 or 2 days are required to bring the serum sodium level down to normal. Some salt may be required in the later stages of rehydration if significant amounts have been lost as the process has developed. An estimation of the volume of water required can be made from the loss of total body water necessary to raise the hematocrit and serum sodium to the levels observed. In patients who excrete large volumes of dilute urine while becoming dehydrated and hypertonic, a response to injected vasopressin tannate is both diagnostic of diabetes insipidus and therapeutic in promoting restoration of water balance.

Chronic Overexpansion of Extracellular Fluid. With chronic illnesses such as cancer, liver disease, chronic infection, starvation or cardiac decompensation, the patient often will exhibit an overexpansion of the extracellular fluid space with an excess of total body sodium despite hyponatremia. Such a patient will have a decrease in the normal intracellular water because of a diminished relative volume of body cell mass. Figure 36–1 illustrates abnormalities of distribution of body water and cell mass seen in chronic illness. With the characteristic fall in body cell mass, as per cent of weight, there is a relative expansion of the extracellular fluid space. Such patients are usually hyponatremic, with serum sodium concentrations in the low 130-mEq range. Usually total body potassium is markedly depleted although the plasma concentrations of potassium may be normal or even a little high. In addition, usually a considerable hypoproteinemia and a reduction in the normal osmolality of the plasma, with the osmolality in the range of 260 to 270 mO, are found.

Water and sodium retention are exaggerated postoperatively in such patients, and more marked hyponatremia and hyperkalemia often occur. There is poor tolerance for the administration of large volumes of extracellular fluid expander such as Ringer's lactate solution or saline solution. The expanded extracellular fluid space with hyponatremia is the most common pattern of water and electrolyte abnormality seen in surgical patients and is one of the most difficult to treat once it becomes established.

Treatment of this dilutional hyponatremia must *not* be by the administration of salt solutions on some formula based on unit deficit multiplied by a theoretical volume for extracellular fluid; rather it must be based on a combination of a restriction of water intake to less than that required by the normally hydrated individual and the restoration of the red cell mass and plasma volume to normal by the transfusion of blood or the infusion of plasma, or both. Since a large intracellular potassium deficit is usually present in such patients, the electrolyte need is usually for potassium rather than for sodium.

Hypertonicity Caused by Solute Loading. This is usually the result of inadequate intake of water in patients who are receiving *tube feedings of mixtures which are high in protein and salt* in relation to water content. The syndrome is likely to develop in patients who have had head and neck surgical treatment, those on gastrostomy feedings, unconscious patients being tube-fed and patients with brain stem injury. Hypertonicity resulting from solute loading can come from the exclusive use of an isotonic balanced salt solution such as Ringer's lactate solution given with the mistaken idea that such a solution will meet baseline requirements for patients receiving parenteral fluids. Unless renal function permits excretion of urine of very high specific gravity with elimination of excessive electrolyte, urea and other solutes in a volume of water smaller than that administered, both hypernatremia and azotemia will result.

Laboratory findings demonstrate an increased concentration of all plasma solutes, both electrolytes and crystalloids, which is out of proportion to changes in hematocrit. An elevated plasma sodium level in the presence of a moderate to large urine output is the key to diagnosis differentiating these patients from those with desiccation dehydration. The serum sodium may reach levels of 170 mEq/L or more in severe cases.

Treatment consists of administering large volumes of water orally or via the tube, or parenterally as 5 per cent glucose in water, while at the same time eliminating, or at least reducing, the osmolar load. Caution must be exercised in order to reduce the osmolality relatively slowly. The entire body, including the cerebrospinal fluid and brain, becomes hypertonic during the solute loading period; cerebral edema, convulsions or coma may result if the extracellular fluid osmolality is reduced too rapidly. Large volumes of urine will persist for several days during solute release, and the hematocrit will not change greatly unless dehydration has also been present in significant degree.

Overhydration, Hypotonicity and Water Intoxication. The opposite of solute overloading occurs with the excessive administration of water in the presence of antidiuresis. This condition exists in a chronic state in patients with wasting illnesses but may be seen acutely usually because of excessive and ill-advised parenteral administration of glucose and water.

Patients with cancer, heart disease, liver disease, renal insufficiency or chronic infection are likely to have an expanded extracellular fluid before surgical treatment. They are particularly prone, as previously noted, to retain water and electrolytes and further to expand and dilute extracellular fluid.

Water intoxication is an acute form of hypotonic dilution. Drowsiness, weakness, and a fall in urine volume are early symptoms, followed by convulsions and coma. A rapid weight gain will always occur. Peripheral and pulmonary edema may appear but are not always present. Water intoxication may result from excessive administration of parenteral glucose and water, from absorption of water from the colon as the result of enemas or colon irrigations given for distention or from water absorption from wounds and burns treated with hypotonic wet dressings. Water intoxication is a particular hazard of the dilute silver nitrate treatment of burns. It is particularly likely to occur in patients with inappropriate antidiuretic hormone release (see Chapter 8).

Laboratory findings include a low concentration of serum sodium, usually less than 120 mEq and often less than 110 mEq/L. The urine may contain a substantial concentration of sodium, 30 mEq/L or more despite the extremely low plasma value, because of an inappropriate sodium release in the presence of a very large extracellular fluid volume. Adrenal insufficiency and primary renal tubular disease may be excluded. The rapidity of fall of the plasma sodium concentration is apparently of greater significance than the absolute values. Cerebral edema from a shift of water into the cerebrospinal fluid resulting from the difference in osmolality is the probable cause of convulsions and coma.

Either total water restriction for a time or the very slow administration of a small volume of water as hypertonic glucose (20 per cent)—not more than 500 ml over 24 hours—is required. If the patient has good cardiovascular function and central venous pressure is within normal limits, small volumes (300 ml or less) of hypertonic sodium chloride solution (5 per cent) should be given slowly with monitoring of central venous pressure. This will begin restoration of extracellular fluid osmotic pressure and promote renal excretion of water. No attempt should be made to administer salt with a "formula" based on extracellular fluid deficit for severe overloading can

result. Time and patience will result in a rising urine volume and an increase in serum sodium concentration with recovery in most cases. In an emergency hemodialysis with ultrafiltration to remove water may be desirable.

VITAMINS

Several questions are relevant to the critically ill patient with respect to vitamins. They are: (1) Can acute depletion occur rapidly as the result of stress and trauma, even in previously adequately nourished individuals? (2) Does a depression of circulating vitamins impose additional risks for the critically ill? (3) Should additional amounts of vitamins be given to the critically ill and, if so, which vitamins should be given in extra dosage and what should that increment be?

During World War II and in the immediate postwar period there was a resurgence of concern about human nutrition with much interest centered on the need for vitamins, calories and protein of individuals who had suffered trauma, burns or major surgery. Although there was relatively little investigation into actual vitamin requirements, it was stated by various nutritional experts that there were significant increases in vitamin requirements for such patients. An authoritative review of this subject in 1952 for the National Research Council concluded that "little is known about changes from normal requirements for vitamins in disease and injury."[159] Nevertheless, despite this statement these and other authors recommended increased oral and parenteral dosages of many vitamins in therapeutic situations. These so-called therapeutic levels were appreciably higher than the recommended dietary allowances; furthermore, the suggestion was made that these be doubled or tripled in situations such as major fractures, burns or other marked "catabolic" situations. Specifically the dosage for ascorbic acid was recommended to be increased to as high as 1 gm or more. The reason for dwelling on this ancient history is the fact that such recommendations coming from an authoritative source served as a basis for the "therapeutic" vitamin formulations produced by many pharmaceutic companies. Such high-potency formulations have continued to the present time and a 1951 formulation appears in the Manual of Surgical Metabolism of the American College of Surgeons published in 1975.

In the intervening decades, considerable progress has been made in understanding the biochemical roles of vitamins and their metabolism. However, data concerning specific requirements for individuals with various diseases, infection or trauma have been meager. Furthermore, interpretation of the significance of changes in serum levels or urinary excretion is often difficult because of uncontrolled changes in intake, absorption or transport in complex clinical situations. This has been particularly true in reports of lowered levels of vitamin A, ascorbic acid and certain B vitamins in patients with acute infections.

Careful studies have been made of changes in certain vitamins in patients with severe burns, injury or infection.[161,162] Serum and urine levels of ascorbic acid and some B vitamins were appreciably lower than normal in such patients and proportionally large supplements of these vitamins were needed to raise the serum and urine levels. The data clearly indicated altered metabolism of these vitamins but did not per se rule in or rule out development of specific deficiency states at the biochemical level.

The complexity of the subject is shown by other observations on ascorbic acid. In an experimental approach to this problem Levenson et al. found that amounts of ascorbic acid that are adequate for wound healing in guinea pigs (2 mg per day) did not permit a normal rate of healing in the first 7 to 10 days following severe burns.[163] However, at 14 days there was no difference in healing between the burned and control animals. When 100 mg of the vitamin were given daily from the time of wounding, the burned animals healed their incisions at the same rate as unburned animals given 2 mg. These findings suggest that burns induce metabolic changes for a transient period during which small but normally adequate amounts of ascorbic acid are "unavailable" or rendered inadequate for wound healing. This observation raises the question of whether or not the catabolism of ascorbic acid is changed by stress. Salomon found that neither the rate constant for the catabolism of labeled ascorbic acid nor its biologic half-life was altered in guinea pigs which were stressed by diphtheria toxin.[164] Similarly, Hodges et al. noted that, when one of the human subjects on an experimental ascorbic acid depletion diet developed infection and fever on two occasions, there was no change in the apparent rate of catabolism of the vitamin.[165] Wound healing was not affected by ascorbic acid restriction in their experimental subjects.

Coon studied vitamin levels in patients undergoing major abdominal surgery. When riboflavin was withheld postoperatively for an average of 5.3 days, the urine excretion fell rapidly to very low levels; however the plasma riboflavin did not change consistently.[166] Complete omission of ascorbic acid resulted in a fall of blood levels only when initial values were 0.2 mg per 100 ml or above. When 75 mg per day were given, the blood level fell only when the preoperative level was above 0.5 mg per 100 ml; when it was below 0.5 mg per 100 ml, ascorbic acid levels increased.[167] In these studies with riboflavin and ascorbic acid, it was apparent that serum levels fell when the initial levels were high; when they were low they tended to rise with administration of moderate amounts of each vitamin. Coon also noted that urinary ascorbic acid excretion per unit time is strongly influenced by the rate of urine flow. This led him to abandon 24-hour excretion measurement of this vitamin as an index of ascorbic acid nutrition. No significant differences were noted between the requirements for ascorbic acid in those postoperative patients who have proven infections, those with fever without proven infection and those with no significant fever. He concluded that "the requirement for ascorbic acid in the usual patient undergoing a major operation is probably not much greater than that expected in comparable samples of normal population."

Acute generalized viral, bacterial and protozoan infections in man and other animals have been associated with decreased blood tissue levels of various vitamins,[168] undoubtedly caused in part by decreased intake. Acute infections in adults and children superimposed on a malnourished state have, on occasion, precipitated clinical signs of various vitamin deficiencies.[168]

What happens to previously well-nourished adults with the development of an acute infection when vitamin intake is continued at preillness levels? Artificially induced hyperthermia of 2 to 3° C in young adult males was associated with a reduction in serum vitamin A without appreciable changes in riboflavin or ascorbic acid.[169] Beisel et al.[170] have executed a carefully controlled study of vitamin levels in young men before and during infection with the sand fly virus. Vitamin intakes during the study were at or near those of the NRC Recommended Dietary Allowances. No changes attributable to the illness were detected in serum concentrations of vitamins A, C, folate or B_{12} or in the urinary excretions of thiamin, pyridoxine or niacin. Urinary riboflavin increased coincidentally with the fever and progressed during the early convalescent period. Others have documented such riboflavin losses during periods of negative nitrogen balance with or without fever and trauma.[171-173] The findings of Coon[167] and Beisel et al.[170] are at variance with earlier reports of Crandon et al.[174] and others implying very large ascorbic acid require-

ments for surgical and traumatized patients; such reports have led to the use of high vitamin dosages for such patients by many clinicians.

A number of reports relate a fall in serum vitamin A in various infections with a return to normal upon remission of the infectious disease,[168,169,173] but this was not observed by Beisel et al.[170] This vitamin is of major importance in the normal development of epithelial tissues and regulates membrane function. It stimulates the healing of wounds which has been retarded by cortisone, presumably with the antagonism occurring in the wound site.[175] Local application of vitamin A stimulates wound healing by a mechanism which is unclear but which may be related to the antagonism of endogenous cortisone.[176]

Under normal circumstances vitamin A is transported from the liver to the plasma bound to a specific retinol-binding protein (RBP). Plasma levels are normally highly controlled by the level of RBP. Hence abnormalities of these proteins may be associated with abnormalities in the levels of metabolism of plasma vitamin A. Liver dysfunction or protein malnutrition depresses RBP levels and retinol levels. In protein-calorie malnutrition retinol levels are low even though liver stores may be adequate.[178] It is quite possible that depressed levels of vitamin A in acute infection and trauma are related to decreased RBP concentrations and that liver stores are adequate in previously well-nourished individuals.

Giving large amounts of vitamin A does not lead to increased RBP and prealbumin; the increased plasma levels of the vitamin are in the form of the ester associated with lipoprotein. Apparently it is the latter form of the vitamin which, when presented to cell membranes, can cause the signs or symptoms of toxicity.[178] Excess vitamin A results in an increased lability of biologic membranes and has been shown to lead to increased synthesis and release of lysosomal enzymes. The total plasma vitamin A does not have to be markedly elevated to be associated with toxic effects; levels of 58 to 85 μg per 100 ml have been reported with toxicity. The critical factor appears to be the amount of retinyl esters. Hence, chronic administration of moderately large amounts to a patient with depressed RBP because of malnutrition and/or liver dysfunction may be potentially harmful. Studies in this area are urgently needed in view of the current use by a number of physicians of fairly large amounts of vitamin A in TPN or routine IV therapy.

Review of the literature is not helpful in answering the three questions which were posed above. Where the data indicate marked decreases in blood and urine levels, a metabolic effect other than increased excretion appears to be operative. Other studies with viral or artificial hyperthermia indicate isolated changes in vitamin levels.

Because it is often impossible to obtain rapid and adequate information on the vitamin status of critically ill patients, it appears prudent at the moment to provide levels for vitamin A and other fat-soluble vitamins at or near the RDA levels, and perhaps double the RDA for the water-soluble vitamins until the catabolic phase is terminated. Increased amounts of vitamins should be given to patients with a prior history of poor intake or poor absorption.

Attention should be given to the composition of vitamins prescribed for the critically ill whether they be given orally, intramuscularly or intravenously. A significant number of physicians appear to regard "vitamins" as a unitary concept with little regard for the actual composition of the vitamin formulation available from the pharmacy. Many oral preparations of the supplementary type are deficient or low in certain vitamins, especially folate. The therapeutic formulations tend to be high in many vitamins but may be deficient in a few.

At the present time there is no single all-inclusive parenteral vitamin preparation. In order to provide all of the vitamins known to be essential for man, it is necessary to use four or more different commercial preparations depending on the composition of each. Even in using such combinations some of the vitamins provided are still in relatively low amounts while others are at high levels. Because of this somewhat complex situation, it behooves each physician to review the vitamin formulations used in his or her hospital to be certain that complete and adequate coverage is being given. This problem has been discussed in Chapter 37.

IRON

The importance of iron in human nutrition has been discussed in Chapter 7C. However, mention should be made of the significance of the fall in serum iron with infection and the question of attempting to supplement the infected patient with iron. It is well established that both serum iron and zinc decrease significantly in a matter of hours in many acute infections in both man and experimental animals.[179-182] Similar changes are produced by injection of leukocyte-derived factors or in response to phagocytosis of killed organisms.[180] This decline in the iron has two phases: (1) a rapid change without concomitant fall in transferrin and (2) a delayed decrease in transferrin. Concomitant with their serum decline, iron and zinc accumulate primarily within the liver. It is known also that intestinal absorption of iron is suppressed with infection and that iron is sequestrated in the area of inflammation.[181-183] Studies by Cartwright and associates have indicated that the iron stored during infection is not utilized for hemoglobin synthesis as long as the infection persists. Iron given as therapy in this situation also enters into storage depots and not into hemoglobin.

Protein-calorie malnutrition leads to hypoferremia by decreased concentration of transferrin. To raise serum iron levels in this situation requires supplementation with protein and/or calories. In the presence of iron deficiency, iron supplementation is, of course, necessary.

The potential danger of iron administration to the infected individual rests on the arguments that microorganisms require iron for growth, that the tight binding of iron by serum and tissue proteins is a defense against such growth and that excess iron in serum or tissues neutralizes the antimicrobial activity of these proteins.[181] Since serious anemia in infected, critically ill patients is best treated with packed red cells, it seems prudent not to give iron as such unless there is good evidence for preexisting and significant iron deficiency.

ZINC

Inasmuch as zinc also leaves the serum in response to infection, it is logical to ask whether there is any value in administering this ion during infection. To my knowledge there is no evidence that giving zinc exacerbates infection in man. There is good reason for trying to assure normal zinc stores in view of its positive roles in protein synthesis, immune processes and phagocytic activity together with other minerals (e.g. phosphate and magnesium).

Serum copper and ceruloplasmin rise with infection as zinc and iron levels fall.[183]

Cuthbertson et al. studied excretion of zinc and other nutrients in patients following moderate to severe bone injuries or surgery.[184] Urine zinc excretion correlated significantly with nitrogen excretion with approximately two- to threefold increases above normal for zinc but usually not leading to more than an additional loss of 1 mg per day.

The needs for trace elements in parenteral feeding have been reviewed in Chapter 37. However, it is worth emphasizing here that hypozincemia is most likely to occur in patients with significant losses of gastrointestinal fluids because of the increased loss of this ion in such fluids.[185]

METHODS OF FEEDING

Oral

Where it is feasible, the optimal and preferred method is the oral route. Where there is significant anorexia this is often difficult to accomplish. The efforts of the physician should be directed to treating impaired appetite secondary to depression or oversedation. The efforts of the dietitian should be directed to ascertaining and meeting desires for special foods and, particularly, to providing foods based on ethnic patterns. Improvement in caloric and nutrient intake may be achieved by substituting palatable nutritious liquid formulas for low-calorie liquids. This is best accomplished by placing the liquids by the patient's bedside, in ice if desired, with instructions to sip repeatedly throughout the day. The formulas may range from milkshakes (if tolerated) to commercial formulas (see Appendix).

Tube

A significant number of patients are unable to ingest food orally in adequate amounts for a variety of reasons. In such circumstances, tube and IV feeding must be considered. Some of the factors that should enter into the final decision on the route to be used are listed in Table 36–7. Where the patient is well nourished and ingesting a significant proportion of his nutritional needs orally, or where depressed appetite or alimentary tract

Table 36–7. Alternatives to Oral Feeding: Factors Influencing a Decision

Degree and duration of failure in achieving adequate oral intake: the nutritional status of the patient
Contraindications to oral intake (partial or total)
Plans for patient treatment
Safety and potential complications of alternatives
Duration of need of alternatives
Acceptance of alternatives by patient and family
Medical capability in offering alternatives
Patient capacity to respond to alternatives
Costs to hospital and to patient

difficulty is likely to be of a few days' duration only, then no serious effort to meet total body needs by tube or parenteral means is indicated. Alternatives must be considered and appropriate action must be taken when a current situation causing depletion is likely to be extended without expectation of immediate significant improvement or where plans for further treatment are likely to preclude adequate oral intake and absorption for a significant time. The decision as to the alternative preferred will depend upon the variables in the list of factors. When either tube or IV routes are feasible, the factors of safety, potential complications, duration of treatment and cost to the hospital and to the patient must be considered.

A list of contraindications, either partial or total, to oral intake is given in Table 36–8. Complete bowel obstruction obviously leaves only one suitable alternative pending definitive treatment, namely, parenteral feeding. If the small intestine is patent, then feeding into the alimentary tract is an attractive alternative if aspiration is not a significant potential danger. These many qualifications indicate the need for careful consideration of the factors listed in Table 36–5 in conjunction with experience and competence in the necessary techniques.

Other situations in which tube feeding should be considered as an alternative to oral feeding include: (1) severe and persistent anorexia requiring a form of force

Table 36–8. Contraindications to Oral Feeding

Severe mucositis
Obstruction
Impairment of swallowing mechanisms
Ileus
Fistulas, especially of upper tract
Coma
Symptomatic exacerbation of disease with oral intake
Severe malabsorption and/or diarrhea, exacerbated
  by oral intake
Severe vomiting

feeding, (2) the treatment of a fistula in the upper alimentary tract where the feeding is given through a tube bypassing the fistula, (3) severe malabsorption requiring the administration of a formula that must be fed slowly and continuously to permit absorption or that is so unpalatable that the patient refuses to ingest adequate amounts on a prescribed schedule or (4) inflammatory bowel disease which may improve with very slow drip feedings of special formulas.

Entry Sites for Tubes. *Nasopharyngeal Tube.* It is preferable to have the tip of the tube in the lower esophagus rather than in the stomach since the latter may be associated with increased reflux, especially when the patient is supine. In most patients, it is easily and safely placed and replaced. Where required for long periods, some patients can be taught to remove and reinsert the tubes after a feeding.

Many patients have had prior experience with nasal tubes for aspiration following surgery and are often strongly opposed to further encounters with them when they remember sore throats and difficulty in swallowing with the tube in place. We have found that tubes of silicone elastomer or other special elastomers are tolerated much better than the same caliber polyethylene or rubber feeding tubes. A number of soft small-caliber (#5 to #8 French) feeding tubes are available;* some are mercury weighted.† Once induced to allow insertion of a fine tube, the patient is often willing to keep it. Small-bore tubes require a finely dispersed formula to prevent plugging.

---

*Very fine caliber tubes are available from Med-Pro, P.O. Box 144, Sun Prairie, Wisconsin 53590 and Argyle Co., St. Louis, Missouri 63103. Silastic tubes of different caliber may be purchased in 8-ft lengths and cut to size from Extracorporeal Medical Specialties, King of Prussia, Pa. 19406.

†Mercury-weighted tubes of various calibers are available from Hedco, 1 Pulgas Avenue, Palo Alto, California 94303 and Biosearch Med. Products Inc., 77 Tilman Street, Raritan, New Jersey 08869.

The potential for aspiration of formula must always be considered. This hazard is increased in debilitated patients having a depressed cough reflex, particularly when there is a preexisting pulmonary problem. It is our policy to restrict the use of nasopharyngeal feedings in such patients and, rather, to insert a long mercury-weighted tube which is allowed to pass into the upper small bowel prior to institution of feeding; when in place, the formula is given by drip. To minimize aspiration, it is essential that strict procedures be adhered to by the staff. These include preliminary testing with water and then dilute formula at slow infusion rates and progressive increases while monitoring the ability of the patient to tolerate the formula and while keeping the patient in a semisitting or sitting position during the feeding and for a period afterward. The potential for aspiration is decreased by slow-drip feeding from a bag or bottle. Feeding is not done when there is hiccoughing nor is it continued when the patient is sent off the floor for a test.

Esophagostomy Tube. A tube may be inserted into the pyriform sinus as recommended by Graham and Royster.[186] Where there is no contraindication, it is an alternative route to nasopharyngeal or gastrostomy tubes for long-term feeding. It is simpler than a gastrostomy and eliminates the psychologic and social problems faced by a patient who has to walk around with a tube protruding from his nose. Presumably, the large-caliber tubes have the same long-term potential disadvantages as do nasopharyngeal tubes of inducing esophagitis and stricture. Small-caliber tubes, especially those of Silastic, will reduce the esophagitis and are well tolerated even by patients with preexisting esophagitis. Esophagostomy is an alternative to jejunostomy for unobstructed patients needing long-term feeding who have had a prior subtotal gastrectomy or esophagogastrectomy with the stomach up in the chest.

Gastrostomy Tube. When surgically feasible, this is a highly desirable procedure for patients who are likely to need tube feedings for prolonged periods of time. When intestinal surgery is performed that is to result in significant malabsorption or the prolonged use of a feeding tube construction of a feeding gastrostomy should be included at that time. The usual gastrostomy closes spontaneously and fairly quickly where there is no longer need for it. Simple, adequate and reinforced directions to nursing staff, patient and family are necessary to prevent leakage and to ensure proper skin care at the entry site.

Jejunostomy Tube. Insertion of a feeding tube into the jejunum is indicated when there is obstruction at a higher level. The availability of soluble formulas that flow through fine-bore tubes has made feasible needle catheter jejunostomy.[187]

Rapid entry into the jejunum of hyperosmolar solutions may lead to the "dumping syndrome." This potential problem can be prevented by infusing the formula initially at reduced concentration and rate and increasing them as tolerance is demonstrated. Use is recommended of liquid formulas of relatively low osmolality incorporating polysaccharides or glucose oligosaccharides (in preference to mono- or disaccharides) and some fat. Intrajejunal feeding presents the possibility of inadequate mixing of the formula with bile and pancreatic juice with resultant depressed digestion. While usually not a significant problem, it can be overcome by various procedures such as the use of pancreatic extract, medium-chain triglyceride (which has less dependence on pancreatic lipase and bile salts for its digestion), oligosaccharides and protein hydrolysate or free amino acids which can be absorbed without pancreatric extract or bile. Such a formula is useful in patients with preexisting pancreatic insufficiency.

Formula Composition. For patients without digestive or absorptive disorders, a wide variety of foods in blenderized form may be used in tube feeding.

Knowledge of the widespread occurrence of lactase "deficiency" and lactose intolerance in various population groups and in those with small bowel disease has resulted in marked modification of the usual hospital tube formula that was once based primarily on milk and milk products. Hospital tube formulas with lower milk concentrations have been developed that have the added advantage that the concentrations of various nutrients such as fat, sodium and potassium can be easily modified (Appendix, Table A–33). Commercial formulas are available that are restricted in lactose content (Appendix Table A–31). Formulas of a more "purified" composition and with very little or no residue are also available and can be used for routine tube feedings (Appendix Table A–32). Many of these formulas are cheaper than liquid formulas made with natural foods such as eggs and meat. When these formulas are nutritionally complete and adequate for long-term feedings, there is no objection to their use. Some patients who are accustomed to regular bowel elimination are unhappy with low-residue formulas that cause them to be "constipated." There is inadequate information on the frequency of fecal impaction with prolonged use of such low-residue formulas.

Physicians and dietitians should give consideration to the costs of tube-feeding formulas for inpatients and for outpatients. For the latter, formulas made from regular family fare (with assistance from a dietitian to ensure overall nutritional adequacy) are appreciably cheaper than commercial formulas, as are those for which supplies are purchased in bulk and mixed at home. For hospitalized patients without absorptive disorders, there is no need for expensive "chemically defined" types of diet.

Defined-formula Diets for Medical Purposes. In recent years there has been an outpouring from the pharmaceutic industry of special liquid formulations.

These have been designated as "chemically defined" diets or "elemental" diets. Because most of these formulations are neither chemically defined nor elemental in a chemical sense, I have recommended that a more general term, *defined-formula diets*, be used to designate such formulations.[188] Their numbers and diversity in composition have created a field requiring special expertise on the part of the physician and dietitian who are faced with decisions on their use. Comparative analytic data on composition are now available (Appendix Tables A–31—A–33).

Being nutritionally complete, defined-formula diets are both a boon and a problem to the physician and dietitian. They are easy to store, order and administer. Serious problems, however, may arise from the very fact that formula compositions are "fixed." Patients having metabolic problems may be unable to tolerate the amounts of one or more nutrients in the formula given in the volumes necessary to meet overall nutritional requirements. Such a formulation may, in fact, be either potentially or actually hazardous for such patients because of the development of adverse effects. The physician must be aware of specific composition and possible contraindications. In these situations, the dietitian must modify the formula by either adding desired ingredients while diluting out those that are undesirable or, alternatively, devising a completely different preparation from specific nutrients.

Manufacturers could overcome the limitation of fixed formulations by preparing formula diets in "modular" form with certain critical items such as fat or sodium and potassium salts being made available in separate containers to be added or modified in amounts as indicated by a patient's need.

Other Precautions in Feeding. The total calories and nutritional composition of the formula supplied should be that needed by the individual at that particular time. There is a serious tendency on the part of many attending physicans, house staff and nurses to underfeed patients via a tube even though precise suggestion on the objectives have been made by the consultant. Continuing education and oversight are essential to ensure achievement of nutritional goals. When serious absorption problems exist, slow continuous feeding utilizing a pump is often essential. Inasmuch as large fluid, protein, carbohydrate and other nutrient loads may be involved in the use of some defined-formula diets, patients should be followed initially as closely as those on IV feeding. Formulas should be instituted in decreased concentration and at reduced volume per time period. Serial physical examinations, laboratory studies, urine fractional analyses and weighings should be standard practice with frequency dictated by the patient's response. Hyperosmolar nonketotic coma can occur in diabetic patients on high-carbohydrate tube-fed formulas when adequate precautions are not taken. There may be exacerbation of metabolic problems related to protein intake in patients with renal and hepatic disorders. Serious losses of water and electrolytes may result with tube feedings in patients with serious malabsorption secondary to bowel fistulas or damaged or resected small intestine.

Effects on Enteric Organisms. The intriguing possibility of markedly reducing the concentration and types of microorganisms in the large bowel through the use of defined-formula diets was presented by the report of Winitz et al.[189] in studies on normal volunteers. Since enteric organisms can conceivably enter the blood stream through mucosa damaged by chemotherapeutic agents or radiation with increased infection in patients with depressed bone marrow, this report had important clinical implications. Unfortunately, subsequent reports have been unable to duplicate these results.[190–194] These investigators uniformly found that the concentration of bacteria in the feces was unaffected by the test diet; however, since

the fecal volume was markedly decreased, the total number of organisms delivered from the large bowel also declined during the feedings. Nevertheless, the numbers of organisms in the large bowel were still enormous. Individual investigators found changes in certain constituents of the flora, but this could happen with certain individuals and not in others on the same diet and in the same study.

Pancreatic Secretion and Defined-formula Diets. Some of the best experimental work on defined-formula diets concerns their effects on pancreatic secretion and possible usefulness in the treatment of pancreatitis or pancreatic fistula. The data are applicable to those with massive bowel resection and large intestinal fluid losses where an attempt is made to minimize fluid losses. The studies of interest relative to pancreatic secretions are of four types: (1) Comparison of the effects of regular food versus defined formulas fed by mouth in dogs: In these the elemental diets appear to cause appreciably less volume of secretion without a change in enzyme concentration with a diet containing hydrolysate, or a delayed decrease in enzyme output requiring more than two weeks on Vivonex to manifest itself.[195] In this connection Rivilis et al.[196] showed that a diet with casein hydrolysate caused a markedly decreased gastric acid secretion when compared to regular dog food. (2) Comparison of defined-formula diet fed orally or intraduodenally: Administration of Vivonex intraduodenally prevented the response of water and bicarbonate secretion observed with its oral administration and decreased but did not prevent the protein response.[197] Hyperalimentation IV induced minor increases in pancreatic secretions when compared with the defined diet. (3) Intragastric versus jejunal loop administration: Vivonex instilled intragastrically into dogs markedly stimulated pancreatic secretion, whereas the formula infused into a Thiry-Vella jejunal loop did not stimulate secretion significantly.[198] (4)

Intrajejunal effects of regular and formula diets: The pancreatic secretory response to a diet with hydrolyzed protein was compared to that of a "blenderized ward diet" instilled into the proximal jejunum in dogs who had a stable 50 per cent maximum pancreatic secretory response to secretin and pancreazymin.[199] Both diets increased the volume and bicarbonate secretion, but there was a marked reduction in the protein (enzyme) concentration of the pancreatic juice with the "elemental" diet. The composition of the diets differed in terms of major nutrients as well as in the amino acid sources.

Diversion of pancreatic secretions has been reported to decrease the susceptibility of the intestinal mucosa to radiation damage.[200] If these findings are applicable to man the use of intrajejunally fed defined diets may be useful if they significantly decrease the pancreatic enzyme secretion while maintaining adequate nutrition during treatment with abdominal radiation.

Fistulas of the Alimentary Tract. Intrajejunal administration of a defined-formula diet was successfully utilized for the treatment of duodenal fistulas in 1956 by Smith and Lee.[201] With the advent of commercially available formulas, there have been additional reports of their use to achieve spontaneous fistula closure. In the treatment of high bowel fistulas, such as those in the esophagus, duodenum or upper jejunum, bypass of the fistula with a tube with the feedings entering distally is feasible. All of Smith and Lee's 11 duodenal fistulas closed; 64.8 per cent of 37 varied gastrointestinal-cutaneous fistulas of Rocchio et al.[202] and 75 per cent of those of Voitk et al.[202a] closed spontaneously using tube feedings. Eleven of the 37 patients of Rocchio et al.[202] had fistulas associated with cancer, 6 had spontaneous closure, 1 had an operative closure and 4 died; no data are given on the site of the fistula in the cancer patients and on

whether there had been radiation to the abdomen.

In the studies of Rocchio et al.[202] and of Kaminsky and Deitel,[203] feeding often preceded the use of the tube feedings. Feeding by the IV method is also a useful adjunct while tolerance of the tube and the volume of fistula drainage are evaluated as the formula is progressively increased to optimum amounts. When fluid and electrolyte losses are not serious, skin excoriation and pain are minimal and the tube is well tolerated, formula feedings may be continued without IV support. Otherwise parenteral feeding is indicated as the alternative.

Treatment of Malabsorption Syndromes. The requirement for and successful use of these formulations will depend upon the degree of malabsorption. At one end of the spectrum are adult patients who have such severe malabsorption (defined as a 5-hr xylose excretion in the adult of less than 0.8 gm following a 25-gm oral dose) that they cannot be successfully maintained even on an optimum tube formulation and administration rate and, hence, will require supplementary or total IV feeding until, hopefully, significant compensatory bowel hyperplasia occurs to permit maintenance on tube and/or oral feedings. At the other end of the spectrum are those with moderate malabsorption who do not require the highly purified formulations and do well with fairly normal types of diets taken frequently by mouth or by tube. The intermediate group can often be carried successfully with defined-formula diets of proper composition and rate of feeding. Tube feedings can be administered successfully in very young infants with malabsorption[204] as well as in children and adults.

The most difficult types of patients to maintain in good nutritional condition are those who have had severe radiation damage of the intestine combined with significant bowel resection. These patients often have significant malabsorption, since a significant portion of their remaining bowel is damaged by radiation, and they tend to have intermittent obstruction with fistulization and the need for further surgery. Careful attention to their nutritional needs using IV and tube feeding can have beneficial results.

The Route of Feeding and the Intestinal Epithelium

Short-term fasting leads to decreased weight, DNA, protein, glycolytic and disaccharidase concentrations of the small bowel.[205] Entry of food into the alimentary tract increased such parameters in the epithelium of intact[206] and postresection residual bowel[207] when compared with IV feeding only. Certain gastrointestinal hormones have trophic effects on individual organs of the alimentary tract, e.g. gastrin on gastric, duodenal and intestinal epithelium, and on the pancreas,[208] cholecystokinin on the pancreas[210] and insulin on the liver.[209] Pancreatic and biliary secretions also appear to have a stimulatory effect.[210] An important factor in maintaining organ mass and composition is the passage of food through the alimentary tract with its stimulus to endocrine and paracrine secretions and/or neural mechanisms and consequent trophic effects. Dworkin et al.[211] have presented further evidence indicating that intraluminal nutrition augments small intestinal mass both by direct contact with epithelial cells and by the indirect effects of hormonal or neurovascular stimuli. Intragastric infusion into rats of a complete formula with free amino acids had a significantly greater effect than IV infusion of the same solution in terms of gut and mucosal weight, DNA and protein content and sucrase activity. While these differences between the different routes of feeding were greater in bowel in continuity, there were consistent and significant differences in bypassed segments of small bowel that were not

exposed to food. When rats were fed a carbohydrate-free diet for 3 days, the normal proximal-distal small bowel gradient of the specific activities of 3 glycolytic enzymes disappeared. When glucose was infused directly into the ileum, the normal gradient of these enzymes was restored, suggesting a humoral and/or neural mechanism rather than a direct local luminal effect of the sugar itself.[212] The subject of intestinal adaptation following resection and other factors has been reviewed in detail.[213]

Treatment of Organ Failure

Because of depressed appetite and frequent nausea and lethargy seen in patients with serious renal dysfunction, oral intake of diets with restricted protein and electrolytes is often poor. Administration of formulas by tube may therefore be highly desirable. While special diets with essential amino acids including histidine (Amin-Aids, McGaw) are now available for those with advanced renal failure, diets containing restricted amounts of intact protein diets may do just as well providing adequate calories are ingested.[214] Formulas for tube feeding of nitrogen-free analogs of essential amino acids may prove useful in such patients in light of the studies of Walser.[215] The use of formulas with increased branched-chain amino acids in cirrhotic liver failure and sepsis which are under investigation in parenteral studies and which have been reviewed above may well be applicable to enteral feeding.

Weight, Dietary Intake and Output Records

Of importance in the care of seriously ill surgical patients are accurate records of weight and of intake and output. This should include not only fluid intake but also total caloric and protein intakes. When patients are on an oral and/or tube feeding intake a daily estimate of the calories and protein taken as food (actually eaten, not just served), together with a record of any supplemental calories and protein given, should be recorded in the chart by the dietitian. These data serve as an important guide to the surgeon in treating the patient.

Parenteral Feeding

When the contraindications to oral intake apply equally well to tube feeding, the only remaining alternative is parenteral feeding. Total parenteral nutrition, via a central venous catheter, and peripheral parenteral nutrition are discussed in detail in Chapter 37.

GENERAL REFERENCES

1. Moore: *Metabolic Care of the Surgical Patient.* Philadelphia, W. B. Saunders, 1959.
2. Clowes (Ed.): Symposium on response to infection and injury—II. Metabolism. Surg. Clin. North Am., *56*, 977, 1976.
3. Ballinger, et al. (Eds.): *Manual of Surgical Nutrition.* Philadelphia, W. B. Saunders, 1975.
4. Schwartz (Ed.): Principles of Surgery, 2nd ed. New York, McGraw Hill, 1974.
5. Wilmore: *The Metabolic Management of the Critically Ill.* New York, Plenum Press, 1977.
6. Brooks (Ed.): *Gastrointestinal Pathophysiology,* 2nd ed. New York, Oxford University Press, 1978.

REFERENCES CITED

7. Bristrian, Blackburn, Hollwell and Heddle: J.A.M.A., *230*, 858, 1974.
8. Hill, et al.: Lancet, *1*, 689, 1977.
9. Hill, Blackett, Pickford and Bradley: Br. J. Surg., *64*, 894, 1977.
10. Mullen, et al.: Ann. Surg., *187*, 523, 1978.
11. Law, Dudrick and Abdou: Ann. Intern. Med., *79*, 545, 1973.
12. Peitsch, Meakins and MacLean: Surgery, *82*, 349, 1977.
13. Mullen, et al.: Surg. Forum, *25*, 1979 (in press).
14. Moore, et al.: *The Body Cell Mass and Its Supporting Environment. Body Composition in Health and Disease.* Philadelphia, W. B. Saunders, 1963.
15. Morgan, Filler and Moore: Surgical nutrition. Med. Clin. North Am., *54*, 1367, 1970.
16. Cuthbertson: Biochem. J., *24*, 1244, 1939.
17. Howard, et al.: Bull. Johns Hopkins Hosp., *75*, 156, 1944.
18. Howard, et al.: Bull. Johns Hopkins Hosp., *78*, 282, 1946.
19. Munro and Chalmers: Br. J. Exp. Pathol., *26*, 396, 1945.
20. Abbott and Albertsen: Ann. N.Y. Acad. Sci., *110*, 941, 1963.
21. Johnson: Br. J. Surg., *54*, 438, 1967.
22. Soroff, Pearson and Artz: Surg. Gynecol. Obstet., *112*, 159, 1961.
23. Duke, et al.: Surgery, *68*, 168, 1970.
24. Birge and Whedon: In *Hypodynamics and Hypogravics.* (McCally, Ed.). New York, Academic Press, 1968.
25. Cuthbertson, Fell, Smith and Tilstone: Br. J. Surg., *59*, 925, 1972.
26. Wilmore: See Wilmore,[5] pp. 153–154.
27. O'Keefe and Sender: Lancet, *2*, 1035, 1974.
28. Stein, Leskiw, Wallace and Oram-Smith: Am. J. Physiol., *2*, E348, 1977.
29. Allison, Hinton and Chamberlain: Lancet, *2*, 1113, 1968.
30. Wilmore,[5] pp. 160–162.
31. McDougal, Wilmore and Pruitt: Surg. Gynecol. Obstet., *145*, 408, 1977.
32. Beisel, Sawyer, Ryll and Crozier: Ann. Intern. Med., *67*, 744, 1967.
33. Beisel: Am. J. Clin. Nutr., *30*, 1236, 1977.
34. Beisel: Am. J. Clin. Nutr., *30*, 1203, 1977.
35. Powanda: Am. J. Clin. Nutr., *30*, 1254, 1977.
36. Beisel, Bruton, Anderson and Sawyer: J. Clin. Endocrinol. Metab., *27*, 61, 1967.
37. Rayfield, Curnow, George and Beisel: N. Engl. J. Med., *289*, 618, 1973.
38. Groves, Griffiths, Leung and Meek: Ann. Surg., *178*, 102, 1973.
39. Wilmore, Mason and Pruitt: Surg. Gynecol. Obstet., *143*, 720, 1976.
40. Wartofsky, Martin and Earll: J. Clin. Invest., *51*, 2215, 1972.
41. Shambaugh and Beisel: J. Clin. Endocrinol. Metab., *27*, 1667, 1967.
42. Chopra, et al.: J. Clin. Endocrinol. Metab., *41*, 1043, 1975.
43. Long, Spencer, Kinney and Geiger; J. Appl. Physiol., *31*, 110, 1971.
44. Wilmore,[5] pp. 159–161.
45. Gump, Long, Killian and Kinney: J. Trauma, *14*, 378, 1974.
46. O'Donnell, et al.: Surgery, *80*, 192, 1976.
47. Odessey, Khairallah and Goldberg: J. Biol. Chem., *249*, 7623, 1974.
48. Fischer, et al.: Surgery, *80*, 77, 1976.
49. Wannemacher: Am. J. Clin. Nutr., *30*, 1269, 1977.
50. Marchuk, et al.: J. Surg. Res., *23*, 177, 1977.
51. Borders: In *Proceedings of Symposium on Metabolic Aspects of Critically Ill Patients.* Chicago, American Medical Association, 1979.
52. Clowes: In *Proceedings of Symposium on Metabolic Aspects of Critically Ill Patients.* Chicago, American Medical Association, 1979.
53. Freund, Ryan and Fischer: Ann. Surg., *188*, 423, 1978.
54. Gamble: Harvey Lect., *42*, 247, 1946.
55. Calloway and Spector: Am. J. Clin. Nutr., *2*, 405, 1954.
56. Swanson: Fed. Proc., *10*, 660, 1951.
57. Rosenthal and Allison: J. Nutr., *44*, 423, 1951.
58. Schwimmer and McGavack: N.Y. State J. Med., *48*, 1797, 1948.
59. Fitzpatrick, et al.: Surgery, *78*, 105, 1975.
60. Rudman, et al.: J. Clin. Invest., *55*, 94, 1975.

61. Jeejeebhoy, et al.: J. Clin. Invest., 57, 125, 1976.
62. Wilmore: In *Clinical Nutrition Update—Amino Acids*. Chicago, American Medical Association, 1977, pp. 47–57.
63. Elman: *Parenteral Alimentation in Surgery With Special Reference to Proteins and Amino Acids*. New York, Hoeber, 1947.
64. Brunschwig, Clark and Corbin: Ann. Surg., 115, 1091, 1942.
65. Reigel, et al.: J. Clin. Invest., 26, 18, 1947.
66. CoTui, et al.: Ann. Surg., 130, 688, 1949.
67. Werner: Ann. Surg., 126, 175, 1947.
68. Werner, Habif, Randall and Lockwood: Surg. Forum, 1, 458, 1951.
69. Ellison, McCleery, Zollinger and Case: Surgery, 26, 374, 1949.
70. Rice, Orr, Treloar and Strickler: Arch. Surg., 61, 977, 1950.
71. Symposium on Intravenous Fat Emulsions: Metabolism, 6, 591, 1957.
72. Schuberth and Wretlind: Acta Chir. Scand., 278(Suppl.):3, 1961.
73. Dudrick, et al.: Ann. Surg., 169, 974, 1969.
74. Blackburn, Flatt, Clowes and O'Donnell: Am. J. Surg., 125, 477, 1973.
75. Blackburn, et al.: Ann. Surg., 177, 588, 1973.
76. Hoover, Grant, Gorschboth and Ketcham: N. Engl. J. Med., 293, 172, 1975.
77. Greenberg, et al.: N. Engl. J. Med., 294, 1411, 1976.
78. Freeman, et al.: Arch. Surg., 110, 916, 1975.
79. Elwyn, et al.: Metabolism, 27, 325, 1978.
80. Schulte, Condon and Kraus: Arch. Surg., 110, 914, 1975.
81. Howard, et al.: Am. J. Clin. Nutr., 31, 226, 1978.
82. Freeman, et al.: Am. J. Clin. Nutr., 28, 477, 1975.
83. Wolfe, et al.: Ann. Surg., 186, 518, 1977.
84. Sim, et al.: Lancet, 1, 68, 1979.
85. Craig, Tweedle, Davidson and Johnston: Lancet, 2, 8, 1977.
86. Marliss, Murray and Nakhooda: J. Clin. Invest., 62, 468, 1978.
87. Nettleton and Hegsted: J. Nutr., 107, 1909, 1977.
88. Rosenthal and Allison: J. Agric. Food Chem., 4, 792, 1956.
89. Freeman, Stegink, Wittine and Thompson: Surg. Gynecol. Obstet., 144, 843, 1977.
90. Fulks, Li and Goldberg: J. Biol. Chem., 250, 290, 1975.
91. Buse and Reid: J. Clin. Invest., 58, 1251, 1975.
92. Kiene, Wolfe, Young and Burke: Life Sci., 23, 133, 1978.
93. Freund, Yoshimura, Lunetta and Fischer: Surgery, 83, 611, 1978.
94. Sapir and Walser: Metabolism, 26, 301, 1977.
95. Shils and Gilat: Gastroenterology, 50, 347, 1966.
96. Shils: Surg. Gynecol. Obstet., 132, 709, 1971.
97. Lawrence: Cancer Res., 37, 2379, 1977.
98. Hines, Hoffbrand and Mollin: Am. J. Med., 43, 555, 1967.
99. Deller, et al.: Gut, 5, 218, 1964.
100. Geokas and McKenna: Canad. Med. Assoc. J., 96, 411, 1967.
101. Eddy: Am. J. Med., 50, 442, 1971.
102. Booth: Postgrad. Med. J., 37, 725, 1961.
103. Stewart, et al.: Q. J. Med., 36, 425, 1967.
104. Hoffman and Poley: N. Engl. J. Med., 281, 397, 1969.
105. LeRusso, Korman, Hoffman and Hofmann: N. Engl. J. Med., 291, 689, 1974.
106. Saunder, Sillery and McDonald: Gut, 16, 543, 1975.
107. Dobbins and Binder: N. Engl. J. Med., 296, 298, 1977.
108. Dowling: Br. Med. Bull., 23, 275, 1967.
109. Wilmore, Dudrick, Daly and Vars: Surg. Gynecol. Obstet., 132, 673, 1971.
110. Weser: Gastroenterology, 71, 146, 1976.
111. Shils: Cancer Res., 37, 2432, 1977.
112. Booth, MacIntyre and Mollin: Q. J. Med., 33, 401, 1964.
113. Bochenek, Rogers and Balint: Ann. Intern. Med., 72, 205, 1970.
114. Bergen, Hashim and van Itallie: Diabetes, 15, 723, 1966.
115. Frederick, Sizer and Osborn: N. Engl. J. Med., 272, 509, 1965.
116. Hardison and Rosenberg: N. Engl. J. Med., 277, 337, 1967.
117. Wilmore and Johnson: Arch. Surg., 97, 784, 1968.
118. Winchester and Dorsey: Surg. Gynecol. Obstet., 132, 131, 1971.
119. Smiddy, et al.: Lancet, 1, 14, 1960.
120. Gallagher, Harrison and Skyring: Gut, 3, 219, 1962.
121. Shils: Cancer Res., 37, 2387, 1977.
122. Graham: N. Engl. J. Med., 296, 1314, 1977.
123. DiMagno, Malagelada, Go and Moertel: N. Engl. J. Med., 296, 1318, 1977.
124. Meyer: N. Engl. J. Med., 296, 1347, 1977 (editorial).
125. Regan, et al.: N. Engl. J. Med., 297, 854, 1977.
126. Morishita, et al.: Digestion, 11, 240, 1974.
127. Stamey: Surg. Gynecol. Obstet., 103, 736, 1956.
128. Bricker: Am. J. Surg., 135, 834, 1978.
129. Edmunds, Williams and Welch: Ann. Surg., 152, 455, 1960.
130. Lorenzo and Beal: Arch. Surg., 99, 394, 1969.
131. Nassos and Braasch: Surg. Clin. North Am., 51, 687, 1971.
132. Sheldon, Gardiner, Way and Dunphy: Surg. Gynecol. Obstet., 113, 490, 1971.
133. Roback and Nicoloff: Am. J. Surg., 123, 317, 1972.
134. McFayden, Dudrick and Ruberg: Surgery, 74, 100, 1973.
135. Aguirre, Fischer and Welch: Ann. Surg., 180, 393, 1974.
135a. Shils: Unpublished data.
135b. Blackett and Hill: Br. J. Surg., 65, 775, 1978.
136. Smith and Lee: Surg. Gynecol. Obstet., 103, 666, 1956.
137. Chapman, Foran and Dunphy: Am. J. Surg., 108, 157, 1964.
138. Himal, et al.: Br. J. Surg., 61, 724, 1974.

139. McLean: Discussion of,[140] p. 466.
140. Reber, Roberts, Way and Dunphy: Ann. Surg., *188*, 460, 1978.
141. Voitk, et al.: Surg. Gynecol. Obstet., *137*, 66, 1973.
142. Rocchio, Cha, Haas and Randall: Am. J. Surg., *127*, 148, 1974.
143. Kaminsky and Deitel: Br. J. Surg., *62*, 100, 1975.
144. Dunphy: Discussion of,[140] p. 467.
145. Winitz, et al.: Am. J. Clin. Nutr., *23*, 546, 1970.
146. Shils: Cancer Res., *37*, 2432, 1977.
147. Glotzer, Boyle and Silen: Surgery, *74*, 703, 1973.
148. Johnson: Arch. Surg., *108*, 32, 1974.
149. Wangensteen: West. J. Surg. Obstet. Gynecol., *40*, 1, 1932.
150. Baker and Dudley: Proc. R. Soc. Med., *57*, 391, 1964.
151. Wells, et al.: Lancet, *1*, 4, 1964.
152. Lancet, *2*, 1186, 1978 (editorial).
153. Tinckler and Kulke: Gut, *4*, 8, 1963.
154. Glucksman, Kalser and Warren: Surgery, *60*, 1020, 1966.
155. Kiesewetter: In *Manual of Preoperative and Postoperative Care*. Philadelphia, W. B. Saunders, 1967.
156. Randall: In *Modern Nutrition in Health and Disease* (Goodhart and Shils, Eds.), 5th ed. Philadelphia, Lea & Febiger, 1973, p. 956.
157. Abouna, Aldrete and Starzl: Surgery, *75*, 194, 1974.
158. Williams: Br. Med. J., *2*, 1189, 1976.
159. Pollack and Halpern: Therapeutic Nutrition. Publication No. 234. Washington, NAS/NRC, 1952.
160. Gann and Robinson: In *Manual of Surgical Nutrition*. Philadelphia, W. B. Saunders, 1975, p. 80.
161. Levenson, et al.: Ann. Surg., *124*, 840, 1946.
162. Lund, et al.: Arch. Surg., *55*, 537, 1947.
163. Levenson, et al.: Ann. Surg., *146*, 357, 1957.
164. Salomon: J. Biol. Chem., *228*, 163, 1957.
165. Hodges, et al.: Am. J. Clin. Nutr., *22*, 535, 1969.
166. Coon: Surg. Gynecol. Obstet., *120*, 1289, 1965.
167. Coon: Surg. Gynecol. Obstet., *114*, 522, 1962.
168. Scrimshaw, Taylor and Gordon: Interactions of Nutrition and Infection. WHO Monogr. Ser. 57, 1968.
169. Méndez. et al.: J. Appl. Physiol., *14*, 768, 1969.
170. Beisel, et al.: Am. J. Clin. Nutr., *25*, 1165, 1972.
171. Pollack and Bookman: J. Lab. Clin. Med., *38*, 561, 1951.
172. Consolazio, et al.: Am. J. Clin. Nutr., *24*, 1060, 1971.
173. Vitale: Am. J. Clin. Nutr., *30*, 1473, 1977.
174. Crandon, et al.: N. Engl. J. Med., *258*, 105, 1958.
175. Hunt, et al.: Ann. Surg., *170*, 633, 1969.
176. Seifter, et al.: Ann. Surg., *181*, 836, 1975.
177. Raz, Shiratori and Goodman: J. Biol. Chem., *245*, 1903, 1970.
178. Smith and Goodman: N. Engl. J. Med., *294*, 805, 1976.
179. Beisel: Am. J. Clin. Nutr., *30*, 1236, 1977.
180. Powanda: Am. J. Clin. Nutr., *30*, 1254, 1977.
181. Weinberg: Am. J. Clin. Nutr., *30*, 1485, 1977.
182. Cartwright, et al.: J. Clin. Invest., *25*, 65, 1946.
183. Gubler, Cartwright and Wintrobe: J. Biol. Chem., *184*, 563, 1950.
184. Cuthbertson, et al.: Br. J. Surg., *59*, 925, 1972.
185. Wolman, Anderson, Marliss and Jeejeebhoy: Gastroenterology, *76*, 458, 1979.
186. Graham and Royster: Surg. Gynecol. Obstet., *125*, 127, 1967.
187. Page, Ryan and Haff: Surg. Gynecol. Obstet., *142*, 184, 1976.
188. Shils: In *Proceedings of Conference on Defined Formula Diets for Medical Purposes* (Shils, Ed.). Chicago, American Medical Association, 1977.
189. Winitz, et al.: Am. J. Clin. Nutr., *23*, 546, 1970.
190. Attebery, Sutter and Finegold: Am. J. Clin. Nutr., *25*, 1391, 1972.
191. Bornside and Cohn: Ann. Surg., *181*, 58, 1975.
192. Bounous and Devroede: Gastroenterology, *66*, 210, 1975.
193. Crowther, et al.: Gut, *14*, 790, 1973.
194. Glotzer, Boyle and Silen: Surgery, *80*, 77, 1976.
195. McArdle, et al.: Am. J. Surg., *128*, 690, 1974.
196. Rivilis, McArdle, Waldek and Gurd: Ann. Surg., *179*, 226, 1974.
197. Kelly and Nahrwald: Surg. Gynecol. Obstet., *43*, 87, 1976.
198. Ragins, et al.: Am. J. Surg., *126*, 606, 1973.
199. Cassim and Allardyce: Ann. Surg., *180*, 228, 1974.
200. Morgenstern: Gastroenterology, *53*, 923, 1967.
201. Smith and Lee: Surg. Gynecol. Obstet., *103*, 666, 1956.
202. Rocchio, Cha, Haas and Randall: Am. J. Surg., *127*, 148, 1974.
202a. Voitk, et al.: Surg. Gynecol. Obstet., *137*, 68, 1973.
203. Kaminsky and Deitel: Br. J. Surg., *62*, 100, 1975.
204. Christie and Ament: J. Pediatr., *87*, 705, 1975.
205. Shils: Cancer Res., *37*, 2366, 1977.
206. Johnson, et al.: Gastroenterology, *68*, 1177, 1975.
207. Feldman, Dowling, McNaughton and Peters: Gastroenterology, *70*, 712, 1976.
208. Johnson: Gastroenterology, *70*, 278, 1976.
209. Starzl, Porter, Watanabe and Putnam: Lancet, *1*, 821, 1976.
210. Altman: Am. J. Anat., *132*, 167, 1971.
211. Dworkin, Levine, Farby and Spector: Gastroenterology, *71*, 626, 1976.
212. Espinoza, Clark, Hritz and Rosensweig: Gastroenterology, *71*, 295, 1976.
213. Williamson: N. Engl. J. Med., *298*, 1393; 1444, 1978.
214. Kopple and Swenseid: Am. J. Clin. Nutr., *27*, 806, 1974.
215. Walser: Life Sci., *17*, 1011, 1975.

Chapter *37*

PARENTERAL NUTRITION

Maurice E. Shils

Knowledge of human requirements, the availability of various essential nutrients and the means for their parenteral delivery over protracted periods are at a stage where nutritional status can be improved and maintained solely through intravenous feeding for prolonged periods.[2-6] This technique is termed *total parenteral nutrition* (TPN) or IV hyperalimentation. Achievement of this objective for a given patient requires expertise in formulating and preparing the solutions, in guaranteeing sterility, in safe administration and in patient monitoring. Programs have been developed in various hospitals which assist physicians and other staff to provide more easily this lifesaving but potentially hazardous procedure.

It is also feasible to provide parenteral caloric sources and various nutrients to meet total nutritional needs when intake of oral or tube-fed diets is inadequate. This is designated as *supplementary parenteral nutrition* (SPN). This chapter is directed primarily to a consideration of the nutritional and practical aspects of these forms of intravenous feedings.

The basic problem associated with conventional intravenous feeding of 5 or 10 per cent glucose solutions with electrolytes and vitamins is the inability to provide sufficient calories to meet the needs of undernourished or hypermetabolic patients and to permit efficient utilization of administered amino acids unless very large volumes of water are infused. Persistent negative caloric and nitrogen balances result in gradual loss of tissue and, if protracted, in debilitation with its multiple problems. Conventional parenteral feeding is, therefore, incapable of either maintaining the well-nourished for prolonged periods or of improving the already malnourished individual.

Aspects of the history of the development and rational use of fluids have been reviewed.[1,7,8] During and shortly after World War II much activity was directed toward achieving adequate nutrition by parenteral means; by the end of that decade the important relationships among caloric intake, nitrogen intake and nitrogen utilization were well recognized by clinicians knowledgeable in the field.[9-11] Provision of very hypertonic glucose solutions through catheters inserted in central veins became fairly common in managing severe renal failure in the period before the advent of simplified hemodialysis.[12] The combination of indwelling catheters, hypertonic glucose, protein hydrolysates and other nutrients was successfully utilized in the decade 1955–65 by a few clinicians on a limited basis, with or without the use of intravenous fat (IV Lipomul). This fat preparation could produce serious side effects with prolonged daily use;[7,13] it eventually was withdrawn from the market. The failure of this particular fat emulsion created a serious problem in the effort to provide adequate calories intravenously and delayed efforts at total parenteral nutritional therapy because of the need to provide calories as very hypertonic glucose.

Widespread interest and activity in parenteral nutrition developed following the reports of Dudrick and colleagues on the techniques and clinical value of this approach. They demonstrated in growing dogs and in malnourished infants and adults with various clinical problems that parenteral nutrition per se resulted in good growth, development of positive nitrogen balance and dramatic clinical rehabilitation.[14,15]

Dependence on glucose as the sole source of non-nitrogen calories has, fortunately, been terminated with approval in 1977 by the Food and Drug Administration of a 10 per cent soybean emulsion for intravenous use (Intralipid) (vide infra). Intralipid had been extensively used in most other countries before its approval in the United States.[16]

The persistent use of markedly hypertonic glucose (>10 per cent) solutions in parenteral nutrition requires their infusion via an indwelling catheter with its tip in a vessel with rapid and copious blood flow (e.g. superior vena cava). When fat calories are given with glucose at 5 or 10 per cent concentration, infusion of the nutrient solutions through a peripheral vein is feasible because the fat emulsion is isotonic. Hence total parenteral nutrition is possible with large amounts of fat emulsion through a peripheral line, provided that the infused amino acids can be efficiently utilized and the fat tolerated. Supplementary parenteral nutrition may be given through either a central or peripheral line, depending on the nutrient solution, the state of the patient's veins and his nutritional needs. The use of fat as the major source of calories presents important problems which must be considered by the physician in planning intravenous nutritional therapy.

The term *hyperalimentation* has appeared periodically in the clinical literature. In 1965 it described supplementary intravenous feeding of fat.[17] It has been used widely as a general term for total parenteral nutrition, reintroduced by the University of Pennsylvania group.[14,15]

"Hyperalimentation" may be mistakenly interpreted as meaning that all patients being maintained in adequate nutritional status solely by intravenous means require solutions providing calories, amino acids and other nutrients in amounts greater than those needed by patients on oral feeding. To the contrary, overweight patients dependent on parenteral nutrition will actually benefit by some caloric deficit in situations where wound healing is normal, other nutrient intakes are adequate and there is no hypermetabolic situation. Many other patients of acceptable weight will do quite well at maintenance caloric levels. Individuals with prior significant weight loss or with serious hypermetabolic problems will require increased calories, amino acids and certain other nutrients. The aim of parenteral nutrition, as is that of diet therapy by oral or tube-fed routes, is the provision of the calories and nutrients required by the specific patient. The phrases "total parenteral nutrition" and "total parenteral alimentation" appear more accurate and inclusive than does "hyperalimentation." The latter, if utilized, should refer to the administration of calories appreciably in excess of those usually required.

TOTAL PARENTERAL NUTRITION

Indications

The primary purpose of total parenteral nutrition is maintenance of an adequate nutritional state or its improvement in a previously undernourished individual when oral or tube feeding (nasopharyngeal, gastrostomy or jejunostomy) is contraindicated or is grossly inadequate, and when other parenteral support is no longer sufficient for his needs. With these indications and with the guidelines indicated below, this form of nutrition may be lifesaving in a variety of clinical situations, including obstructing lesions of the gastrointestinal tract where surgical intervention must be delayed, persistent ileus, "pseudo-obstruction," massive bowel resection prior to institution of tube or oral feeding, fistulas, hypermetabolic states associated with extensive burns, major trauma and severe infections where oral or tube feeding is not feasible or is inadequate, acute stages of inflammatory bowel disease, severe uncontrolled malabsorptive states, congenital anomalies in the neonate prior to surgery, intractable diarrhea, prolonged coma where hope for recovery is entertained and the danger of aspiration negates tube feeding, persistent nausea and/or vomiting secondary to cancer or other therapy or central nervous system lesions and metabolic disorders such as renal or hepatic failure where oral or tube feeding is inadvisable. In short, it is for "patients who cannot eat, should not eat, will not eat, or cannot eat enough."

The availability of total parenteral therapy should not be an excuse for procrastination in initiating more definitive therapy when this can be done without a significant increase in risk to the adequately nourished patient. Deficits of hemoglobin, water, electrolytes, vitamins and minerals can usually be replaced in a matter of days and operation can proceed in such cases.

The development of a pre- or postoperative or other complication precluding oral or tube feeding cannot be predicted. When such complications do occur, there is a tendency to hope for the best and to delay initiation of adequate parenteral feeding until serious weight loss or actual debilitation occurs. *Nutritional rehabilitation of the wasted patient is a slow affair.* Furthermore, the debilitated patient is prone to infection, skin breakdown, fluid and electrolyte problems and impaired wound healing—all of which complicate recovery.

There is persuasive evidence that malnutrition (manifested by serious loss of lean body mass—muscle and visceral—usually in association with depletion of body fat, low levels of albumin, depressed phagocytosis and cell-mediated immunity and electrolyte and fluid problems) is associated with marked increases in morbidity and mortality in patients with bowel fistulas[19] postoperatively or in traumatized septic patients[20,21] and children and adults with serious alimentary tract disorders.[14,22] As short a period as ten days with 5 per cent glucose as sole caloric intake can depress the response to hypoxia in previously well-nourished adults.[23] There is ample evidence that the occurrence of serious trauma, burns and sepsis markedly accelerates the metabolic rate and depletion of lean body tissues.[24-27] There may be a doubling or more of the rates occurring in a nonhypermetabolic starving individual. Failure to understand this fundamental fact and/or to act to meet the increased demand will result in rapid deterioration as the stress continues. This is the type of patient, who, when unable to be fed by other means, requires TPN early and in adequate amounts.

The decision to undertake total parenteral nutrition requires the weighing of a number of factors and due consideration for the patient's diagnosis and prognosis. When the clinical situation is such that prolonged maintenance or improvement in nutritional status will assist in recovery of the patient or will permit significant palliation of underlying disease, the TPN program has obvious merit and should be pursued vigorously. It has no place in prolonging life in the hopelessly ill or in routine short-term postoperative care.

Peripheral versus Central TPN. There is considerable experience in other countries and more recently in the United States with peripheral or central infusions where fat emulsion provides the major proportion of calories.[16,28-31] Peripheral infusion has the advantage of avoiding the insertion and maintenance of a central catheter. However, many patients requiring TPN have had numerous previous peripheral infusions and their peripheral veins are in a poor state for this or other reasons. As a result this route often becomes inadequate or unreliable before the need for TPN is fulfilled. Furthermore, for the sick patient one must have a reliable avenue for infusions around the clock.

Non-nitrogen Calories and Nitrogen Retention. There is solid evidence for the nitrogen-sparing effect of carbohydrate (including glycerol) in the absence of[32,33] and with[34] amino acids. In the absence of amino acids, fat appears not to spare nitrogen beyond its glycerol content released on metabolism.[33] There is disagreement on the nitrogen-sparing effect of fat in the presence of amino acids. Certainly on a mixed American type of diet positive nitrogen balance occurs with a considerable proportion of calories from fat, but there is an equal or greater proportion of calories from carbohydrate. The same has been observed in patients (children or adults) receiving parenteral feeding when a significant amount of fat was given but, again, where carbohydrate provided at least one-third and usually more of the calories.[29,35-37] Jeejeebhoy et al. alternated the same patients from high-glucose (91 per cent of calories) to high-fat infusions (75 per cent of calories as triglyceride); they noted that there was an adjustment period of 3 to 5 days after the patients were placed on the high-fat diets during which nitrogen excretion increased and then decreased to levels comparable to that observed with the high-carbohydrate diet.[28,29] In studies with stressed, burned or traumatized patients, Long et al. were unable to achieve nitrogen equilibrium or positive balance when fat was supplied as the non-nitrogen calories.[38] Calories from carbohydrate were required in an amount equal to the resting metabolic rate in order to achieve minimum nitrogen excretion. Long[39] has suggested that the data of Jeejeebhoy et al.[28,29] are interpretable as

resulting from a metabolic adaptation to a semistarvation state (i.e. ketosis) plus an effect of glycerol present in the fat. Wilmore has reviewed old data obtained in typhoid patients which also suggest that fat does not spare nitrogen in the hypermetabolic state.[27]

Intravenous fat emulsion is presently much more expensive on an equicaloric basis than 50 per cent dextrose in water.

Any objection to use of fat as the primary source of non-nitrogen calories in stressed patients does not negate its value as a portion of caloric contribution or as the source of essential fatty acids.

For the long-term patient or the individual with large caloric and other nutrient requirements, TPN via the central catheter is the procedure of choice, usually with glucose as the important contributor of calories.

Each patient requires decisions both on initiation of TPN and on the route, based on his specific needs. There are no clear-cut guidelines for deciding on the time of initiating the program for all patients. Assuming that the criteria mentioned in the preceding paragraphs have been met, certain generalizations can be made:

1. Prevent nutritional debilitation by initiating TPN early in patients who are obviously going to be unable to ingest food orally or by tube for some time regardless of cause. In particular, the presence of significant hypermetabolic factors such as infection and trauma dictate early and vigorous nutritional therapy.

2. Nontraumatized, noninfected, overweight or previously well-nourished individuals may be maintained on routine intravenous fluids with or without amino acids for periods of 7 to 10 days without serious debility. For longer periods more aggressive nutritional therapy is indicated by peripheral or central routes.

3. Children should not be permitted to lose weight and preferably should be fed intravenously early, so that weight gain continues in situations where oral or tube feeding is contraindicated.

4. Patients with more than 10 per cent weight loss below ideal weight or overweight pa-

tients who are hypermetabolic or with significant weight loss should be given adequate nutritional therapy.

Adherence to guidelines such as these will prevent the most common cause of malnutrition in patients unable to be fed orally or by tube, namely, physician procrastination in the vain hope that the patient's condition will improve and permit regular food intake to begin "within the next few days."

Infusion Routes. An indwelling central venous catheter is essential for infusion of very hypertonic solutions. This catheter, with its tip preferably in the superior vena cava, permits the prolonged administration of the nutrient solution directly into a region of high blood flow where rapid dilution occurs; this minimizes the occurrence of phlebitis and thrombosis.

The use of an indwelling central venous catheter imposes significant risks to the patient: the danger of microbial contamination and colonization of the catheter, pneumothorax or hemothorax or subclavian vein phlebitis or thrombosis with a subclavian catheter or carotid artery puncture and bleeding with a jugular vein insertion. These complications occur rarely when experienced personnel exercise strict precautions, which include aseptic techniques in catheter insertion and maintenance, insurance of proper placement (checked by x-ray study prior to use) and the delivery of sterile solutions. Insertion of the catheter should be treated as a serious surgical procedure. Techniques for catheterization of the superior vena cava by way of the subclavian or external jugular veins have been published.[15,40,41]

The catheter-related infection rates reported from various hospitals have varied greatly. In general, the infection rate varies inversely with the experience and utilization of trained personnel adhering to strict procedures. Because of potential hazards and the chance that a catheter inserted by a new venipuncture may not be properly placed, there is a tendency on the part of some physicians to maintain a preexisting catheter in place even though a patient becomes febrile. This is particularly true if a catheter has been burrowed under the skin in a subcutaneous tunnel, requiring a more elaborate procedure.

In general, sepsis should be seriously considered with the possibility of catheter colonization when the patient experiences sudden spiking fever and shaking chills. A sustained fever curve is more likely to be related to an abscess without catheter involvement. Other sources of infection should be sought, appropriate cultures taken and treatment (antibiotics and abscess drainage) instituted as indicated.

The use of a modified Seldinger technique is extremely valuable.[42,43] This involves rapid replacement of a central catheter over a flexible wire using appropriate sterile technique* but without another venipuncture. If the original catheter is in proper position, this procedure if properly performed assures that the new catheter will also be correctly positioned. Repeated x-ray study is indicated, nevertheless, before resuming infusion of the hypertonic glucose solutions. Blood cultures and culture of the tip of the removed catheter are mandatory, as is institution of antibiotic therapy if sepsis is suspected. The catheter may be replaced repeatedly if contamination of the skin or sinus tract is suspected. This technique greatly reduces the need for further venipunctures and possible complications.

Efforts to reduce infection along the insertion tract of central catheters have led some physicians to advocate subcutaneous tunnels of varying length for routine in-hospital use[44] and for outpatients.[45,46] No comparative data are available in controlled studies to allow an objective ap-

---

*A sterile wire stylet from a 24-inch central catheter or, preferably, a flexible guidewire may be used, e.g. U.S.C.I. #007004.

praisal of the value of this technique. Our experience and that of others indicate that, with aseptic technique and proper maintenance, indwelling catheters may remain safely in place for weeks, months or even years without infection.[2,40,41,43,45,46] The situation is less sanguine in patients with chronic infection, debility or diseases affecting immune mechanisms. However, even in such patients central catheters may be maintained for long periods without sepsis with care and with antibiotic coverage as indicated.

Internal or external arteriovenous (AV) shunts should be considered for long-term infusion of hypertonic solutions under special conditions. In the external technique, an AV shunt or the type used in hemodialysis is inserted and, after adequate flow is assured, a sidearm is placed between the arterial and venous arms to receive the infusion. The hypertonic solution is diluted with flowing blood in the shunt before it reaches the cannulated vein. High-flow shunts are desirable since they minimize clotting; long-term heparinization may be necessary to permit prolonged use of relatively low-flow shunts. Details of a delivery system utilizing external AV shunts have been published.[47,48] Infection and clotting have been the factors eventually causing removal. In nonuremic patients heparin may be required on a routine basis. In general, AV fistulas are useful only as a last resort. An internal fistula as the route for parenteral feeding has been proposed and a report of its long-term use has been published.[50] The author's experience with nonuremic patients indicates a very high incidence of clotting.[43]

A subcutaneous silicon elastomer chamber (Omaya shunt) connected to a subclavian vein has been used in a child.[51] Problems have been encountered by the author in an adult because of difficulty in penetrating the skin with a fine-bore needle.[43]

Delivery Systems

The nutrient solutions may be delivered from bottles or plastic bags by gravity flow, propulsion pump[52,53] or air pressure.[46,52] To assure an even flow rate, to overcome the increased resistance of filters of small porosity (especially with continued use) and to minimize the likelihood of clotting at the catheter tip, the utilization of a constant-flow propulsion pump is desirable. However, pumping of fluids—especially from bottles—presents the danger of air embolism; hence, this must be done only when there is constant supervision, or, preferably, when the pump has proven safeguards, e.g. a controlling photoelectric monitor attached to the drip chamber or a weight-sensing device.[52,53]

Although there is no uniformity of agreement on their value, in-line membrane filters have been used in an effort to provide greater assurance of sterile delivery of parenteral fluids and to prevent introduction of particulate matter.

The use of pliable plastic bags of various sizes eliminates the danger of breakage, simplifies transportation and storage and greatly reduces storage space requirements prior to and after filling, compared to glass or formed-plastic bottles. If the bags are free of albumin, lipids or blood, the usual water solutions of nutrients do not extract measurable amounts of the plasticizers or stabilizers used in their manufacture.[54]

Nutritional Considerations

General Requirements. Approximately 25 to 30 kilocalories (kcal) per kg of body weight per day should be sufficient to maintain weight for the adult patient who is in an acceptable weight range with restricted activity, little or no fever or other hypermetabolic condition.[55] (Appendix Table A-8) A nitrogen/calorie ratio of approximately 1:250 to 1:300 is appropriate.[56] Calories and amino acids should be increased to permit weight gain in individuals who are significantly underweight or who are stressed by trauma, burns or infection. In such adults the nitrogen/calorie ratio may have to be decreased to 1:150 to allow nitrogen equilibrium or positive balance.[27,55] The goals for infants and children are those of good pediatric practice: to allow growth and meet increased needs of trauma and infection.[22] All of the essential and sufficient nonessential amino acids should be provided in amounts needed for adequate protein synthesis. Essential fatty acids should be supplied regularly, particularly to malnourished adults and to all children. Mineral and vitamin intakes should meet individual requirements without excessive wastage or toxicity. These nutritional requirements are discussed in detail below. Water should be administered in volumes consistent with the renal and cardiovascular requirements of the patient and adequate to cover abnormal fluid losses.

Energy Sources and Requirements. Carbohydrate. Glucose is the most commonly used carbohydrate for caloric replacement and in the United States is the primary source of energy. It is readily available, relatively inexpensive and can be given in high concentrations and in large total amounts which are well tolerated by most patients after a period of adaptation. Glucose in parenteral fluids is glucose monohydrate; 1 gm provides 3.4 kcal. Infrequent but potentially serious complications may develop with hypertonic solutions. These include coma attributable to hyperosmolar nonketotic hyperglycemia[41,60] and osmotic diuresis with sodium loss and dehydration when glycosuria is pronounced. Fatty liver is noted fairly frequently when glucose is the non-nitrogen calorie source.[57-59] Accumulation of fat in liver with large amounts of glucose is more pronounced without amino acids[57] and may be related to failure to provide essential fatty acids.[59] Fructose offers no obvious advantage and is more expensive; when

administered rapidly, it has induced increased blood lactate levels and corresponding acidosis.[61] Fructose or xylitol infusions can decrease serum phosphate and raise lactate, urate and bilirubin. Fructose, xylitol and sorbitol are not recommended for parenteral use. Intravenous maltose is metabolized[62] but is not used in parenteral nutrition. Other disaccharides and the polysaccharides are not hydrolyzed significantly and, hence, are not available for metabolism.

Lipids. Intravenous fat is an obvious candidate as a source of calories and essential fatty acids. Following World War II much effort was expended in the development of a stable fat emulsion. A commercial product, IV Lipomul, was produced and used clinically;[63] however, because of undesirable side effects in patients who received it daily for some weeks, production ceased. A Swedish preparation, Intralipid, which was approved for sale there in 1961, has gradually appeared in many countries as 10 and 20 per cent emulsions. The 10 per cent emulsion was approved for use in the United States in 1977. This stable emulsion, which requires refrigeration, contains 10 per cent soybean oil, 1.2 per cent purified egg yolk, phospholipids, and 2.5 per cent glycerol. Other fat emulsions are available in Europe.[16] Experimental and clinical observations indicate that Intralipid is essentially free of the undesirable side effects of IV Lipomul. This experience has been summarized.[4] Intralipid 10 per cent provides 1.1 kcal per ml in an isotonic preparation which may be infused peripherally or centrally. Glucose H_2O is required in 32 per cent solution to provide an equal caloric concentration.

The triglycerides in the fat emulsion infused at 0.235 gm per kg per hr into adult man for 4 hours are cleared from serum within 4 hours of terminating the infusion; the rate of clearance is independent of a variation in concomitantly infused carbohydrate from 0.196 to 0.588

gm per kg per hr.[4] Serum free fatty acids are cleared more rapidly at the higher concentrations of simultaneously administered carbohydrate. Daily infusion of Intralipid over a 2-week period is associated with increased tolerance, as indicated by decreased preinfusion serum triglycerides.[64] Children[36,37] and malnourished or stressed adults[65] appear to tolerate increased amounts of intravenous fat very well.

The present upper limit standards (package insert) for intravenous fat as Intralipid are 2.5 gm per kg per day for adults and 4 gm per kg per day for children, although larger doses have been reported to be tolerated well.

After 7 days, infusion of Intralipid to provide 50 per cent of calories as lipid resulted in little or no elevation of triglycerides. There was a rise in serum cholesterol of some patients even though the fat emulsion has no cholesterol. Intralipid in amounts providing 83 per cent of calories caused a marked rise in cholesterol. In longer-term studies plasma phospholipid levels were markedly elevated at the end of the infusion period.[28] Long-term infusion (17 to 54 months) of 50 gm per day of Intralipid providing 20 to 25 per cent of total calories as lipid has been found to be safe and effective in a home TPN program with plasma lipoprotein profile, total triglyceride and cholesterol values within the normal range.[28]

As noted earlier, there is evidence that fat, per se, does not permit nitrogen retention in stressed patients unless the resting metabolic expenditure is met by carbohydrate, particularly in unadapted patients.[38] The glycerol of Intralipid is metabolized and some of the amino acids in the nutrient solution serve for gluconeogenesis, especially during an initial adaptation period. With lipid as the non-nitrogen source instead of glucose, plasma insulin level falls and glucagon level rises. There are increases in plasma free fatty acids and their metabolism increases.[28] This leads to sparing of body protein and reestablishment of nitrogen balance. Despite the cost of Intralipid, its utility in peripheral infusions has led to its clinical application by some clinicians as a major source of calories in TPN in hospitalized adults[16,28] and children.[16,36]

Intravenous fat is usually infused as a separate solution piggybacked into the tubing of a central or peripheral line with other solutions. In Europe several fat emulsions are mixed with amino acids, sorbitol or xylitol.[16] One home TPN system mixes Intralipid with other nutrients in a single reportedly stable suspension.[66]

Contraindications to daily administration of Intralipid include occasional minor acute reactions such as febrile response, chills, vomiting and chest pains. These are short term and do not contraindicate further administration. Occasional hematologic changes have been reported, primarily in young children.[16] There is contradictory evidence concerning transient decreases caused by Intralipid in pulmonary-diffusion capacity and membrane-diffusing capacity in normal subjects.[67-69] Low-birth-weight infants are at risk of developing bilirubin encephalopathy (kernicterus) at uncommonly low levels of bilirubin. Intralipid administration to such infants may result in very high plasma levels. The resulting high fatty acids can interfere with bilirubin-albumin binding, increasing the risk of development of free bilirubin. Hence, any jaundiced neonate receiving Intralipid should be monitored frequently to determine the status of bilirubin binding by albumin.[70]

Various fat emulsions given intravenously are known to result in deposition of a "ceroid" pigment in reticuloendothelial cells of the bone marrow, lymph nodes, spleen and the Kupffer cells and hepatocytes of the liver of man and laboratory animals.[71] Giant cells and microgranulomas may develop. To date no effect of these histologic changes on hepatic function has been discerned. Intralipid up to

100 gm of fat per day has been given to patients with moderate to severe liver damage without deleterious effect on liver function.[16]

Intralipid is contraindicated in patients with disorders leading to failure to clear lipids from blood. If in doubt, plasma should be examined before and 12 hours after conclusion of fat infusion.

Essential Fatty Acids. The nutritional and biochemical role of essential fatty acids (EFA) have been summarized in Chapter 5. Following discontinuation of IV Lipomul and prior to the availability of Intralipid there was no source of parenteral EFA. It is not surprising, therefore, that reports of biochemical and clinical evidence of EFA appeared of patients receiving TPN, particularly children, unable to ingest or absorb fat. A summary of various case reports indicates that biochemical changes were relatively common in children and adults, while dermatitis occurred more commonly and severely in children.[4] Hemolytic anemia has also been reported.[72]

The fatty acids of soybean oil in Intralipid consist for the major part of palmitic acid 9.1 per cent, oleic acid 26.3 per cent, linoleic acid 54.0 per cent and linolenic acid 7.7 per cent; there is no arachidonic acid. The biochemical and clinical manifestations of EFA deficiency have been corrected by giving this fat emulsion in an amount providing at least 4 per cent of the patient's calories as linoleic acid.[73,74] This amount of intravenous fat once or twice weekly (i.e. 500 or 1,000 ml) will prevent the development of the fatty acid changes.

Ethanol. Ethanol has been used as a source of calories in intravenous feedings. It cannot be given in large concentrations, and it has been my experience that older debilitated patients often do not tolerate even dilute solutions well. Its toxic-metabolic effects (Chapter 40) and the easy availability of other caloric sources make its use undesirable.

Amino Acids. Achievement of nitrogen equilibrium or positive nitrogen balance requires sufficient essential and nonessential amino acids (or a source of nitrogen for synthesis of the latter) together with adequate calories.[27,55,75]

Protein hydrolysates were the original sources of parenteral amino acids but are rapidly being replaced by solutions of free crystalline amino acids. Individual free amino acids are added to casein hydrolysate or beef fibrin hydrolysate to give a complete mixture. Approximately one-third of the amino acids in the hydrolysates are present as short-chain peptides, some of which may not be available for metabolism[76-79] and therefore make hydrolysates somewhat less efficient. However, in practice both types permit good nitrogen balance.[2,14,15,48,63,80]

Composition. The amino acid composition of a number of these commercially available solutions are given in Appendix Table A–29. L-Amino acids are added exclusively in most solutions, but one (FreAmine) has some D-methionine.

The original FreAmine has its basic amino acids as the hydrochloride without compensating acetate; its use resulted in development of metabolic acidosis, primarily in young children;[81] this was easily treated or prevented with sodium acetate or bicarbonate. Because of this the formula was changed to provide acetate instead of chloride (FreAmine II). The FreAmine I has use for patients with persistent metabolic alkalosis. All other free amino acid preparations have added acetate to prevent net anionic residue. Casein hydrolysate has a net cation residue when metabolized.[81]

The total amounts of amino acids vary among preparations, as do the amounts of individual amino acids. The eight essential amino acids are present in all, as are histidine and arginine. It will be noted that glycine and alanine are present in much greater concentration in the free amino acid preparations than in the hydrolysates; the former contain no aspartate and glutamate, whereas casein hydrolysate (Amigen) does. The ratio by weight of essential to total amino acids varies between 0.38 and 0.48 for crystalline mixtures, 0.72 for fibrin hydrolysate and 0.38 for casein hydrolysate.

Plasma or whole blood amino acid patterns (aminograms) have been utilized to assess the nutritional value of parenteral amino acid solutions and the effects of growth, malnutrition and disease states on specific amino acid requirements. Plasma amino acid concentrations are not a necessary reflection of various tissue levels, but increasing attention is being paid to them as an indication of metabolic defects and requirements. This was a topic considered at a recent conference on amino acids.[5] There is evidence for increased need of amino acids in sepsis.[77,82,83] Fasting or postprandial levels have been measured by various investigators. Plasma amino acids at the end of 4-day infusion paralleled the specific infusion concentrations. However, there were differences in certain amino acids depending on the amino acid formulation used, for example, with fibrin hydrolysate at 10 gm N per day in all subjects, subfasting levels of cystine, valine, phenylalanine and asparagine were noted, whereas subfasting levels were found only in the case of cystine, tyrosine and asparagine in subjects given the crystalline amino acid solution FreAmine. Sepsis resulted in altered levels of certain plasma amino acids (see Chapter 36).

Infusion of casein hydrolysate (Amigen) to malnourished adult patients with gastrointestinal diseases did not result in increases in whole blood levels of cystine plus methionine or phenylalanine plus tyrosine, in contrast to that observed with the crystalline amino acid solution Travasol 10 per cent. In the case of the latter, lysine and tryptophan did not increase.[79] Fasting and postprandial plasma aminograms have been obtained in a study of infants when infused with each of six different parenteral solutions.[84] Most of the essential amino acids were within or close to the postprandial ranges of normal infants; however, there were significant exceptions on either side of the normal range. Of the nonessential amino acids, glycine was high when the solutions were high in glycine. Arginine and its amino acid derivatives in the Krebs urea cycle were low following infusion of FreAmine and the hydrolysates.

All of the preparations, whether hydrolysate or crystalline amino acids, have been demonstrated to induce positive nitrogen balance in patients receiving TPN when given in adequate amounts and with adequate calories and other nutrients. The choice of a particular solution will depend on availability, cost per gram of nitrogen and the presence or absence of other nutrients, specifically minerals, in relation to the needs of patients with specific metabolic problems. Hyperammonemia has been reported in infants receiving hydrolysates[85] which contain appreciable amounts of preformed ammonium ion (and which should be used with caution in all patients with severe liver disease). Administration of FreAmine, which does not contain preformed ammoniun ion, has also been reported to cause symptomatic hyperammonemia postoperatively in some children after more than three weeks of use;[86] arginine and/or ornithine administration cured or prevented this condition. Hyperglycinemia has been reported in children receiving free amino acids containing relatively large amounts of glycine.[84]

The D-isomer of methionine is less well utilized by man than is the L-form; the administration of an amino acid mixture containing the D-form leads to elevated plasma levels and increased excretion in the urine.[84,87] Such preparations should probably not be given to patients with seriously compromised glomerular function.

Intravenous nutrition differs in two important aspects from normal oral food intake: (1) it is continuous for many or all hours of the day instead of being intermittent; (2) it bypasses the alimentary tract (with its hormonal, additive, mixing and metabolic activities and initial portal blood delivery to the liver) with infusion of the nutrients directly into the systemic circulation. The role of the gut and liver in regulating amino acid levels has been discussed in Chapter 3 and elsewhere.[88] Evidence is accumulating that modifications of certain plasma amino acids affect the transport of other amino acids into the brain and that certain disease states, such as sepsis, liver and renal dysfunction and genetic abnormalities, induce other changes in amino acid levels. These metabolic problems take on practical significance in view of existing differences in the amino acid composition of various commercial preparations.

Infants and children require an appreciably greater proportion of amino acid intake as essential amino acids than do adults; based on oral intakes, the ratio of essential to total amino acids for each of these age groups is 0.40, 0.36 and 0.19, respectively.[89] The ratios for parenteral feeding are not known with precision. Munro[89] has analyzed the data of Furst et al.[90] on healthy young women to indicate a ratio of not more than 0.25. It is probable that an optimum ratio for repletion of lean body mass in seriously debilitated adults is similar to that for older children.

Requirements. Assuming an adequate composition of the amino acid solution, the daily requirements for growth, maintenance or rehabilitation will depend upon age, nutritional status, metabolic needs and caloric contribution of non-nitrogen sources.

For infants the general range of amino acids is 2.5 to 4.0 gm per kg per day for either hydrolysate or crystalline mixtures. Heird et al. have found that the lower figure is preferable, since it permits positive nitrogen balance and weight gain equivalent to those with higher intakes but with less risk of azotemia.[22] This figure (2.5 gm per kg per day) is only slightly higher than that of 2.2 suggested for infants of less than 6 months in the recommended dietary allowances (Appendix Table A–1). For nonhypermetabolic older children of normal height and weight and for adults requiring TPN the RDA figures of 1.2 to 1.5 and 0.8 gm per kg respectively appear adequate. Since most patients on TPN, however, suffer from stressful conditions ranging from slight to major, the provision of amino acids should be appropriate to need.

Utilization of body nitrogen or retention of exogenous nitrogen bears a very close relation to energy requirements. During fasting fatty acids and their derivatives from adipose tissue provide a major source of energy but do not provide the glucose or carbohydrate intermediates necessary for the metabolism of certain cells. These must come from body protein (gluconeogenesis) and the glycerol from triglyceride hydrolysis. During infection and/or trauma, fatty acid catabolism is decreased despite adequate fat reserves. Despite the presence of hyperglycemia, the catabolism of lean body mass is accelerated.[38,55,82,91]

The energy requirements of the sick patient are those reflecting weight (often decreased), activity (also decreased) and a hypermetabolic state consonant with the status of disease or trauma. Kinney et al.[55,91] have noted that in surgical patients undergoing elective operations the postoperative energy expenditure will differ from the preoperative values by no more than 10 per cent in the absence of significant complications. The previously well-nourished patient who sustains multiple fractures will commonly demonstrate an increase in resting energy expenditure of 10 to 25 per cent over a period of 2 to 3 weeks. During the acute phase associated with major infections such as peritonitis, the energy expenditure is commonly increased from 20 to 50 per cent above predicted normal. A major thermal burn causes an increase from 50 to 125 per cent. Kinney has observed that the patient receiving parenteral feeding with a caloric intake exactly equal to his measured caloric expenditure will often not achieve weight or nitrogen equilibrium. Consequently, his practice is to provide a caloric intake which is 50 per cent above the estimated resting metabolic expenditure of a stressed patient (Table 37–1).

The ratio of total energy (kcal) to nitrogen (gm) in the daily diet of a healthy active adult usually falls between 180 and 280, i.e. 180 to 280 kcal per gm N. In the RDA the ratio for an infant is 322:1, in children 4 to 6 years 375:1, in males 23 to 50 years 301:1. Experience indicates that in the seriously hypermetabolic patient with reduced physical activity and increased protein breakdown a more effective ratio is 120 to 180:1.[55] The ratio of 150:1 is quoted as a practical guide for such patients;[27,82] however, it must be applied with due consideration of the metabolic status and the stage of the disease process.[92] Many clinicians routinely utilize a higher calorie/nitrogen ratio. Special care is indicated in the presence of renal and hepatic dysfunction.

It is of interest to consider the additional nitrogen and caloric requirements imposed by accretion of lean body mass in previously depleted adults and for growth of infants. There is good experimental evidence that previously protein-depleted laboratory animals[93] and man[27,94] utilize newly administered amino acids more efficiently than do repleted animals. When metabolic conditions are favorable for anabolism in adult patients, an average daily accretion rate for nitrogen (positive nitrogen balance) is approximately 4 gm, representing about 25 gm of protein or 125 gm of lean body mass.[15,95] For a 40-kg patient this represents a net retention of 0.10 gm nitrogen (derived from 0.63 gm amino acids) per kg per day. This, incidently, will require net retention of approximately 12 mEq of potassium and 2 mEq of magnesium per day.

Infants maintained by TPN postoperatively, receiving 110 to 120 kcal per kg per day (no fat) for a mean duration of 27 days, had an average weight gain of 11.8 gm per kg per day (range 7 to 18) and an average N balance of 0.19 gm per kg per day (range 0.10 to 0.28).[96] A group of 17 similar patients from another hospital who received Intralipid and glucose as equicalorie sources with an average of 88 kcal per kg per day had an average daily weight gain of 8.7 gm per kg (range 1 to 21.5). The differences were presumably related to caloric intake.

Physical therapy for the bedridden patient and mobilization whenever possible are essential for muscle renewal, bone mineral accretion and the prevention of

Table 37–1. Daily Caloric Intake of Average (70-kg) Man under Normal and Surgical Conditions*

Condition	Normal BMR	Measured Resting Expenditure		Caloric Intake (RME + 50%)
		ΔBMR(%)	Cal	
Normal	1,800			
Postoperative	1,800		1,800	2,700
Multiple fractures	1,800	+20	2,160	3,240
Major sepsis	1,800	+40	2,520	3,780
Major burn	1,800	+80	3,240	4,860

*From Kinney.[55]
RME = Resting metabolic expenditure.

undesirable consequences of prolonged bed rest.

Fat synthesis from carbohydrate is metabolically an expensive activity, resulting in high specific dynamic action and hypermetabolism.[97] Lipogenesis is an obviously desirable but limited objective in a patient who has little remaining subcutaneous fat, but prolonged excessive caloric feeding seems inappropriate in a patient with adequate fat stores where the basic nutrition problem is restoration or maintenance of lean body mass and repair of tissue damage.

Ionic Components of Amino Acid Solutions. It is essential that attention be given to the presence or lack of cations and anions in these solutions. They may be present either as additives, components of amino acids or contaminants. Some representative data from this and other laboratories are given in Table 37–2. Because casein is a phosphoprotein, the phosphate content is expected in solutions of casein hydrolysate and is often useful; approximately one-half of the phosphate is free and the other half is in bound form—both are available. FreAmine II has added phosphate, FreAmine I has none. Casein hydrolysate (Amigen) has significant amounts of sodium and potassium, some calcium and small amounts of magnesium. The crystalline amino acid solutions are low in electrolytes but certain manufacturers produce electrolyte-supplemented amino acid solutions. Anions as chloride or acetate are present. Evaluation of individual patient needs for electrolytes must take into account the contribution of the amino acid solution utilized in the final formulation.

In addition to the macrominerals, the amounts of trace elements also vary. Data on zinc, copper and chromium are available on a number of amino acid preparations (Table 37–3). Other large-volume parenterals provide insignificant amounts. It should be emphasized that the presence of trace elements is secondary to their occurrence in basic materials or water, i.e. they are contaminants. As such it is not surprising that their concentrations vary from lot to lot.

Vitamins. The presently available parenteral vitamin formulations have their origins in attitudes and suppositions about vitamin requirements for medical use stemming back to the 1940s and 1950s. At that time it was the opinion of the relatively few physicians active in clinical nutrition that there was a large requirement for parenteral vitamins in various disease states. The 1952 NRC review *Therapeutic Nutrition*[98] served as an authoritative source for this view and led to the commercial high-dosage "therapeutic" formulations which are still current.

The available parenteral multivitamin

Table 37–2. Electrolyte Composition of Amino Acid Solutions

A.A. Solution Name	%	Na mEq/L	K mEq/L	Cl mEq/L	Ca mg/L	P mg/L	Mg mEq/L
Hydrolysates							
Fibrin	5	3	16	10	20	10	2
Casein	10	66	38	34	230	460*	4
FreAmine II[Φ]	8.5	11	0	1	0	300	0
Travasol NE[Φ]	8.5	0	0	34	0	0	0
Travasol E[Φ]	8.5	70	60	70	200	930	10
Aminosyn[Φ]	10	0	5	0	0	0	0
Veinamine[Φ]	8	40	30	50	0	0	6

*Includes bound phosphate
Φ Added acetate

Table 37–3. Trace Elements in Parenteral Solutions (μg/L)

Solution	Zn	Cu	Cr	Mn	Fe	Ref.*
FreAmine I	70	0.2	0.01	—	—	1
	1260	0.6	—	—	—	5
FreAmine II	1700–3100	N.D.**	—	3.3	—	5
	820–4040	9–11	2.4	—	30–66	2
	1850	85	—	—	—	3
Aminosyn 5%	75	8	0.8	—	38	2
7%	120–140	N.D.	—	—	—	5
10%	30–60	N.D.	—	—	—	5
Veinamine 8%	130–150	13–15	8–24	—	—	2
Travasol 8.5%	140	N.D.	—	—	—	
Dextrose 50% (Mc)$^\Phi$	96–188	<10–12	1.8	—	<100	2
(C)	<25–96	<10	—	—	<100	2
(Mc)	N.D.	80	—	—	—	3
(C)	N.D.	80	—	—	—	3
(A)	30	N.D.	—	—	—	5
Dextrose 10% (C)	<25–158	<10	—	—	<100	2
(A)	N.D.	0.6	—	—	—	5
	N.D.–8	—	—	—	—	4
NaCl 0.9%	20–42	—	—	—	—	4
	108	16	—	—	—	5
Intralipid 10%	33–46	20–28	0.9	—	<100	2

*References:
1. Greene: *Zinc Metabolism*. New York, Liss, 1977.
2. Hauer and Kaminski: Am. J. Clin. Nutr., *31*, 264, 1978.
3. Hoffman and Ashby: Drug Intell., *10*, 74, 1976.
4. Jetton, Sullivan and Burch: Arch. Intern. Med., *136*, 782, 1976.
5. Shils and Alcock: Unpublished data.
$^\Phi$Mc = McGaw, C = Cutter, A = Abbott
**N.D. = not detectable

solutions have been used in various TPN formulations for infants, children and adults. The vitamins have usually been given in empirical fashion designed to meet established standards and with little published material on vitamin levels in serum or on tests of vitamin-related enzyme activity. Major concern has been in relation to dosages for infants and children. In the early days of TPN amounts of a solution containing vitamin A and D in fairly high concentration led to vitamin A and D toxicity in some infants and occasionally in adults.

The fasting plasma level of vitamin A depends on the concentration of retinol-binding protein (RBP). Vitamin A toxicity is related to amounts of vitamin A which exceed the capacity of the RBP.[99] Condi-

tions which depress the formation and circulating levels of RBP can lead to toxicity at plasma vitamin levels which are not extraordinarily high. In the presence of reduced RBP, a low fasting plasma A level does not necessarily mean tissue depletion. The observation that various vitamins circulate primarily in bound form has added complexity to our knowledge of vitamin requirements. A given level of a vitamin in plasma must be related to the level of its carrier in order to interpret plasma-tissue interrelations.

Parenteral vitamin preparations tend to have high concentrations of most water-soluble vitamins but also to be low or lacking in one or more. Given rapidly as a separate infusion, these vitamins may be quickly excreted. It is preferable to add the

Table 37–4. Parenteral Vitamin Schedule (Adults)*

	MVI (5 ml twice weekly)	Berocca C (2 ml twice weekly)	Total/Week	Avg/Day
Vitamin A (I.U.)	20,000	—	20,000	2,856
Vitamin D (I.U.)	2,000	—	2,000	286
Vitamin E (I.U.)	10	—	10	1.4
Thiamin (mg)	100	20	120	17
Riboflavin (mg)	20	20	40	5.7
Niacin (mg)	200	160	360	51
Pyridoxine (mg)	30	40	70	10
Pantothenate (mg)	50	40	90	13
Biotin (mg)	0	0.4	0.4	0.06
Ascorbate (mg)	1,000	200	1,200	171
Plus: Folate (mg)—1.5	twice weekly		3	0.43
B$_{12}$ (μg) 50	once weekly		100	14
Vitamin K$_1$ oxide (mg)	once weekly		5	0.7

*Children's dose: ¼ to ½ of adult dosage, depending on age.

vitamins to one or more TPN solutions and infuse them slowly over hours. The lack of one or more vitamins in various commercial preparations necessitates their addition from other sources on a daily or periodic basis.

It is essential that the physician and pharmacist involved in a TPN program review the composition of the parenteral vitamins in use in the hospital and take steps to assure proper and complete dosages with respect to age. Biotin, folic acid, vitamin B$_{12}$ and vitamin K are not present in many preparations and should be made available (unless contraindicated or modified, as for vitamin K in the patient taking Coumadin). Although biotin is normally synthesized by intestinal bacteria and absorbed, the patient receiving TPN who is not eating and who may be receiving antibiotics for long periods should have this vitamin added periodically to the formula.

The provision of all vitamins to a patient often requires the use of at least four different preparations over the course of a week. Several vitamin programs are given in Table 37–4 which have been found to provide normal blood levels for prolonged periods. Such formulations are not entirely satisfactory since the amounts of some

vitamins (particularly water-solubles) are quite high. Others, such as vitamin E, tend to be low; despite this, plasma E levels were in low normal limits, presumably because of the low intake of fat. Intralipid contains some tocopherol; if the fat is given frequently, this requires investigation.

The Food and Drug Administration has been involved with parenteral vitamin preparations as the result of the drug efficacy review conducted for it by the National Research Council–National Academy of Sciences in the late 1960s.[100] Following consultation and discussion with various pharmaceutical experts, physicians and biochemists, the Nutrition Advisory Group of the American Medical Association prepared a statement entitled Guidelines for Vitamin Preparations for Parenteral Use. This includes more rational parenteral vitamin formulations for daily administration as baseline maintenance of children and adults and recommendations for clinical testing of the formulations. A summary has been given.[101] The pediatric and adult formulations are given in Table 37–5. The pediatric formulation is designed to be given in amounts proportional to weight up to 10 kg.

Despite concern and various recom-

Table 37–5. Proposed Formulations for Intravenous Multivitamins for Daily Maintenance*

Vitamin	Units	Infants/ Children (under 11 yrs)	Adult
A (retinol)	I.U.	2300	3300
D	I.U.	400	200
E (α tocopherol)	I.U.	7.0	10.0
Vitamin K₁	mg	0.2	—
Thiamin	mg	1.2	3.0
Riboflavin	mg	1.4	3.6
Niacin	mg	17.0	40.0
Pyridoxine	mg	1.0	4.0
Pantothenic acid	mg	5.0	15.0
Folacin	μg	140	400
B₁₂	μg	1.0	5.0
Biotin	μg	20.0	60.0
Ascorbic acid	mg	80.0	100

*From Shils.[101]

Table 37–6. Minerals of Interest in TPN

Macro (>200 mg or 5 mM/day)	Micro (Trace) (<5 mg/day)
Sodium	Iron
Chloride	Zinc
Bicarbonate	Copper
Potassium	Iodide
Calcium	Fluoride
Magnesium	Chromium*
Phosphate	Cobalt***
Sulfate	Manganese*
	Molybdenum**
	Selenium**
	Vanadium**
	Nickel**
	Tin**

* Human requirements—tentative quantitative requirements proposed.
** Human requirement not established.
*** Cobalt in vitamin B₁₂ for man.

mendations for possible increased needs for vitamins as the result of trauma and infection, there are relatively few objective data on the subject which give reliable guidance; furthermore, published reports are conflicting. Even when the evidence indicates depressed urine excretion and plasma levels, the significance of the observations is unclear. The literature on this subject has been reviewed recently.[102]

Minerals. These ions may be divided into two broad groups on the basis of their quantitative requirements (Table 37–6).

Macronutrients. Probably the most critical aspect of total parenteral nutrition on a day-by-day basis concerns the requirements for electrolytes and for water. No matter how well constructed the overall formulation, it must be reviewed daily and sometimes more frequently when administered to patients with serious problems in fluid and electrolyte balance. Requirements for these ions will depend on the cardiovascular, renal, gastrointestinal and endocrine status of the patient. They have been discussed in detail in Chapters 7, 8 and 36. Ranges used in early TPN formu-

lations have been reviewed elsewhere.[103] Approximate daily requirements for patients without complications are given in Table 37–7.

Calcium and Phosphorus. Breast-feeding neonates ingest in the range of 34 to 44 mg of calcium and 21 to 24 mg of phosphorus per kg per day with absorptions of 55 and 89 per cent, respectively.[103] Suggested daily provision of these two ions for pediatric and adult use is given in Table 37–7. The desirable amount and frequency of calcium administration cannot be given categorically. The goal is maintenance of adequate bone mineralization without soft tissue calcification. Factors to be taken into account in deciding on calcium administration include parathyroid and renal status, age, state of bone mineralization, state of magnesium repletion and degree of mobilization. Unless there is a contraindication, such as hypercalcemia, a calcium salt such as calcium gluconate is routinely added to the basic formula to meet calcium need unless it is provided in adequate amounts in the form of casein hydrolysate.

Hypophosphatemia has been noted to

Table 37–7. Suggested Approximate Daily Intravenous Requirements for Minerals*

Ion	Units	Infants, Young Children (kg/day)	Adults (per day)
Sodium*	mEq	3–5	60 and up
Potassium*	mEq	3–5	60 and up
Magnesium*	mEq	0.3–0.5	8–10
Calcium	mg	20–40	200–400+
Phosphorus	mg	20–40	300–400
Sulfur		++	++
Iron	mg	1†	1-males and nm females** 2-m females**
Zinc	mg	0.10–0.25 (?)	2–4
Copper$^\Phi$	mg	0.01–0.02 (?)	0.5–1.0
Chromium (Cr+++)	μg	0.1–0.2 (?)	10–20 (?)
Fluoride	mg	0.001 (??)	1–2 (??)
Iodide	μg	3–5 (?)	1–2/kg
Manganese$^\Phi$	mg	0.005–0.01 (?)	0.15–0.25 (?)

* For patients without significant cardiovascular-renal dysfunction or intestinal or renal losses. The upper range is suggested for those with rapid growth rate. The upper ranges for sodium and potassium are variable and will depend on individual status.

 + Suitability of daily calcium administration in adult will depend on many factors, including those affecting bone resorption and soft tissue calcification.

++ Supplied as methionine.

 † May be given periodically as indicated after correcting deficiency.

** May be given periodically as indicated after correcting deficiency; nm = nonmenstruating females; m = menstruating females.

(?) Human requirements definite—range uncertain.

(??) Human requirement probable but not definite—range very uncertain.

$^\Phi$ Omit or give with close monitoring in patients with biliary obstruction.

develop in patients on high-glucose intravenous feeding in the absence of or with inadequate phosphate in the solution. The importance of phosphate in many stages of intermediary metabolism, in bone formation, and as a constituent of nucleic acids, phosphoproteins and phospholipids makes it desirable to maintain normal levels (2.5 to 4.5 mg per 100 ml for adults and up to 6.0 mg per 100 ml for infants) without waiting for hypophosphatemia to develop. Hypophosphatemia with levels of 1.0 mg or less may occur within 4 to 5 days after initiation of TPN with low or no phosphate supplements. Hypophosphatemic patients have reduced red cell glycolysis, decreased concentrations of 2, 3 diphosphoglycerate and ATP, increased hemoglobin-oxygen affinity,[105,106] revers-

ible hemolytic anemia and decreased phagocytosis.[107] Paresthesias, convulsions and coma have resulted from continued glucose infusion without phosphate repletion.[108]

The sudden infusions of large amounts of glucose (particularly into previously malnourished patients) can induce a rapid fall in serum phosphate even with daily provision of 225 to 450 mg of phosphorus as phosphate. These amounts are often adequate when repletion has occurred. Hence, progressive increase in glucose administration with larger amounts of phosphate and daily monitoring are indicated in such individuals. A major decrease or cessation of glucose administration causes a rise in serum phosphorus.

Magnesium. The importance of magnesium in human nutrition is well established (Chapter 7B). There is no known direct hormonal control of the serum level of this ion; the level will depend on a balance resulting from the amounts administered and released from tissue breakdown, renal excretion and gastrointestinal losses. The requirements for this ion by the IV route are not known with certainty. It is suggested[103] that 0.3 mEq per kg per day is adequate for infants and young children, although a wide range has been given in practice. Similarly, adult formulations vary widely from 4 to 25 mEq per 2,500 kcal;[103] 17 to 25 mEq (4 to 6 ml of 50 per cent $MgSO_4 \cdot 7H_2O$) are usually adequate.

Renal insufficiency in a patient requires careful monitoring of serum magnesium, potassium, phosphate and calcium. Antibiotics, particularly amphotericin and sodium carbenicillin, can lead to appreciable losses of potassium and magnesium in the urine; their use often requires persistent and relatively large supplementation with appropriate monitoring to ensure adequate but not excessive replacement. Serial determinations of serum and urine levels of these ions will afford a basis for evaluating the need for revision of dosages.

Sulfur. This element is present in tissues as methionine, cysteine, taurine, certain mucopolysaccharides and glycolipids, and sulfate esters of various metabolites. Adequate provision of methionine provides sufficient sulfur for formation of the other S-containing compounds. Sulfur enters into taurine along the metabolic pathway of cysteine and into sulfated compounds from inorganic sulfate derived from cysteine. Sulfate is incorporated into 3′-phosphoadenosine-5′-phosphosulfate which serves as a general agent for esterification of sulfate.

Microminerals (Trace Elements) *Iron.* Preexisting iron deficiency anemia should be corrected with intravenous or intramuscular iron. Maintenance iron may be given once weekly, biweekly or as indicated by periodic measurements of iron and transferrin and/or red cell indices. Suggested intravenous requirements are indicated in Table 37–7.

Other Trace Elements. The essentiality of zinc, copper and iodide for man is well established (Chapters 9A, 9B). Failure to recognize this need has led to the iatrogenic development of zinc and copper deficiencies in patients maintained by TPN without adequate replacement of these ions. Zinc depletion in such patients has been associated with dermatitis and possible alopecia,[109,110] and copper deficiency— primarily noted in children—with macrocytic anemia,[111] neutropenia[111] and fractures.[112] A recent report indicates that very prolonged (3½ years) TPN in a patient resulted in glucose intolerance, subjective ataxia and peripheral neuropathy which cleared with administration of chromium as chromic chloride.[113] Administration of various trace elements in TPN over prolonged periods has prevented deficiencies of the added ions. The use of plasma as a source of trace elements is inadvisable because of the danger of hepatitis, the cost and the inadequate amounts of zinc and copper that are supplied in the usual periodic infusions.

Recommended levels of trace elements are given in Table 37–8. It will be noted that the requirements given are for stable individuals without significant gastrointestinal or other losses. In the author's experience copper losses via small bowel contents are relatively small and probably do not require increased amounts once a patient is replete. Zinc losses from the small bowel, on the contrary, may be high and require an additional daily replacement of 1.0 to 4.0 mg per liter of intestinal losses in order to maintain normal serum levels. Serial determinations of trace elements are indicated in patients with large losses or previous depletion until daily needs are established and repletion occurs.

At the present time provision of zinc, copper, manganese and chromium appear indicated, either on a daily or regular

Table 37–8. Composition of Trace Element Solutions for Use in Parenteral Nutrition (per ml)

Form	Zinc	Copper	Manganese	Chromium
Ionic	2.0 mg	0.4 mg	0.1 mg	4 μg
Salt	8.8 mg	1.57 mg	0.31 mg	20.5 μg
	as	as	as	as
	$ZnSO_4 \cdot 7H_2O$	$CuSO_4 \cdot 5H_2O$	$MnSO_4 \cdot H_2O$	$CrCl_3 \cdot 6H_2O$

interval basis. Caution should be observed in the administration of copper and manganese to patients with biliary obstruction, since the primary route of excretion of these ions is in bile. Renal failure also requires caution and reduced dosage for those ions dependent on the urinary route.

Certain trace elements are present as contaminants in parenteral solutions (Table 37–3). The amounts in a given preparation should be taken into consideration in ordering trace element supplementation. Data are inadequate or lacking on the concentrations in parenteral fluids and additives of manganese, chromium, iodide, fluoride and the less-well-established trace minerals.

Individual or multitrace element solutions are easily prepared, sterilized and administered. Microbiologic sterility and absence of pyrogens must be assured before use.

Formulation and Preparation of Solutions

Formulation of the contents of parenteral solutions must be based on a combination of sound nutritional principles and the particular needs of the individual patient. Two approaches in general formulation are possible. One is the development of a basic unit solution providing a standard amount of kilocalories and nutrients per unit volume; the number of units supplied will depend upon individual needs. Adherence to a single unit preparation cannot possibly meet the needs of sick patients with differing nutritional and physiologic problems. Hence, most hospitals have a series of unit formulas prepared and issued on physicians' prescriptions.[114] The second approach is individual formulation, where specific patient requirements for water, calories, amino acids and electrolytes are estimated, prescribed and prepared in one or more containers.[115] The basic unit method is the one most widely used as a consequence of the publications of Dudrick et al.[14,15,18] Either method will work well with careful daily evaluation of the patient and flexibility in modifying the formulation as the clinical situation demands.

In the past, solutions were occasionally prepared in manufacturing pharmacies, utilizing bulk chemicals and large-volume filtering, sterilizing and bottling devices. However, with cessation of production of screw-cap containers for intravenous solutions this system is no longer used. The present method in general use is the mixing into unit containers of various commercially available sterile solutions and additives by open or, preferably, closed systems. Partially filled bottles with hypertonic glucose under vacuum are often used, and amino acids and other nutrients are added.[116] A partially filled bottle of 40 or 50 per cent glucose solution, together with a bottle of amino acid solution and a transfer set, is available in a kit for hospitals with minimum facilities and low demand for TPN. Sterile 1- or 2-liter empty bottles may be filled with the sterile solutions.[23,116] Flexible sterile plastic bags of 2+-liter capacity may be filled by gravity[115] or a 1-liter bag may be filled with a special vacuum apparatus.[116]

Strict and persevering adherence to sterile precautions with routine microbiologic monitoring is essential, regardless of method.

Examples of formulations based on a basic unit composition are given in Tables 37–9 and 37–10.

Table 37–9. Mixed Amino Acids (MAA) Solutions: Contents/Unit and Variations*

Ingredient (mEq unless otherwise indicated)	MAA Solution 900	MAA Solution 900 with Added Sodium	MAA Solution 900 with Insulin	MAA Solution 900 with Insulin and Added Sodium	MAA Solution 900 Low Potassium	MAA Solution 900 Low Potassium with Added Sodium
Protein equivalent (gm)	31.2	31.2	31.2	31.2	31.2	31.2
Nitrogen, utilizable (gm)	5.0	5.0	5.0	5.0	5.0	5.0
Dextrose (gm)	240.0	240.0	240.0	240.0	240.0	240.0
Total calories	959	959	959	959	959	959
Potassium	40	40	40	40	12	12
Sodium	20	50	20	50	20	50
Magnesium	6	6	6	6	6	6
Calcium	4.5	4.5	4.5	4.5	4.5	4.5
Calcium (mg)	90	90	90	90	90	90
Phosphate	26	26	26	26	12	12
Chloride	26	41	26	41	26	41
Acetate	30	45	30	45	16	30
Insulin (units)	None	None	15	15	None	None
Vitamins	B-group vitamins and ascorbic acid are added to each unit daily. Vitamins A, D,[a] and E[b] are added in addition to the B-group vitamins and ascorbic acid to each unit 1 day a week.					

*From Giovanoni: In Fischer,[3] p. 29.
[a] As ergocalciferol.
[b] As dl-alpha tocopheryl acetate.

Table 37–10. Selected Pediatric Solutions Available: Contents/Unit and Variations*

Ingredient (mEq unless otherwise indicated)	Solution 900		Solution 900 with Added Sodium		Solution 900 with Insulin		Solution 900 with Insulin and Added Sodium		Solution 900 Low Potassium		Solution 900 Low Potassium with Added Sodium	
	Hyd[a]	MAA[b]	Hyd	MAA	Hyd	MAA	Hyd	MAA	Hyd	MAA	Hyd	MAA
Protein equivalent (gm)	11.7	15.6	11.7	15.6	11.7	15.6	11.7	15.6	11.7	15.6	11.7	15.6
Nitrogen, utilizable (gm)	1.4	2.5	1.4	2.5	1.4	2.5	1.4	2.5	1.4	2.5	1.4	2.5
Dextrose (gm)	115	120	115	120	115	120	115	120	115	120	115	120
Total calories	447	480	447	480	447	480	447	480	447	480	447	480
Potassium	18	20	18	20	18	20	18	20	6	6	6	6
Sodium	16	10	31	25	16	10	31	25	31	10	31	25
Magnesium	3	3	3	3	3	3	3	3	3	3	3	3
Calcium	2.3	2.3	2.3	2.3	2.3	2.3	2.3	2.3	2.3	2.3	2.3	2.3
Calcium (mg)	45	45	45	45	45	45	45	45	45	45	45	45
Phosphate	13	13	13	13	13	13	13	13	13	13	13	13
Chloride	9.4	13	16.9	22	9.4	13	16.9	22	9.4	13	16.9	22
Acetate	7	15	19	23	7	15	19	23	4	8	12	15
Insulin (units)	0	0	0	0	15	15	15	15	0	0	0	0
Vitamins	0	0	0	0	0	0	0	0	0	0	0	0

One-half the adult amount of B-group vitamins and ascorbic acid is added to each unit (approximately 1,000 ml) daily. One-half the adult amount of vitamins A, D,[c] and E[d] is added in addition to the B-group vitamins and ascorbic acid to each unit 1 day a week.

*From Giovanoni: In Fischer,[3] p. 29.
[a] Hyd = Hydrolysate formula.
[b] MAA = Mixed amino acids formula.
[c] As ergocalciferol.
[d] As dl-alpha tocopheryl acetate.

Table 37–11.   Composition of Single-Formula TPN Solution*

Item		Volume (ml)	Kcal	Na (mEq)	K (mEq)	Cl (mEq)	Mg (mEq)	Ca (mg)	P (mg)
Crystalline amino acids	(8.5%)	750	255	8					225
Dextrose/water	(50%)	1000	1700						
Dextrose/saline	(10%)	250	85	39					
KCl (2 mEq/ml)		20			40	40			
NaCl (2.5 mEq/ml)		10		25		25			
Na acetate (2 mEq/ml)		10		20					
MgSO₄·7H₂O	(50%)	4					17		
Ca gluconate	(10%)	20						186	
K phosphate**		3			13				279
ZnCl₂***		1							
Total volume		2068	2040	92	53	65	17	186	504

IV supplements during week:
   Intralipid 10%—500 ml once weekly
   Vitamins^Φ—see below
   Trace elements^ΦΦ—1 ml twice weekly

* An example of an inpatient or home TPN formula for a stable 62-kg man with moderate gastrointestinal losses following bowel resection. It is prepared in a plastic bag of 2.8-L volume or in two 1-L bags connected by Y tubing.

^Φ Vitamins: MVI (conc) 5 ml twice/wk; Berocca C 2 ml twice/wk; vitamin K_1 oxide 5 mg/wk; folic acid 1.5 mg twice/wk; vitamin B_{12} 50 μg once/wk (see Table 37–4).

^ΦΦ Trace element solution (MH#3) containing $ZnCl_2$, $CuSO_4 \cdot 5H_2O$, $MnSO_4 \cdot H_2O$ and NaI in sterile saline. One ml provides 2.0 mg Zn++, 1.0 mg Cu++, 0.1 Mn++ and 0.056 mg I. This may be increased in volume as serial Zn, Cu and Mn levels indicate. For patients on TPN for more than 6 months, 1 ml of $CrCl_3 \cdot 6H_2O$ in sterile saline (= 38 μg of Cr+++) may be added once or twice weekly.

** If needed to supplement other phosphate sources.

*** $ZnCl_2$: 4 mg Zn++/ml: modify as periodic serum Zn++ levels indicate.

An example of a formulation based on an individual prescription is given in Table 37–11. If less fluid is desired in a given formulation without sacrificing caloric content, volume reduction is achieved by substituting 15 per cent sodium chloride for glucose/saline or 0.9 per cent salt solution in the formula. Further volume reduction can be achieved by using more concentrated amino acids and up to 70 per cent glucose solution (the latter is appreciably more expensive than 50 per cent glucose). When increased fluid volume is required without additional calories, this is achieved by diluting the formula with saline or sterile water as needed or, more simply, by running in sterile normal saline in piggyback fashion.

Additional calories may be given by replacing 10 per cent dextrose in saline with more concentrated glucose solutions. Less caloric intake is achieved by decreasing the volume of 50 per cent glucose.

Electrolytes may be increased or decreased by simple addition or omission from specified containers. Significant amounts of sodium chloride may be added in relatively small volume by using 15 per cent sodium chloride solution.

In the presence of metabolic acidosis, sodium acetate should be given in place of sodium bicarbonate, since the latter will precipitate any calcium present. When metabolic alkalosis is a problem, FreAmine I with its excess of H^+ and Cl^- is useful. Sterile N/10 HCl solution may be given slowly as needed with appropriate pump control into the tubing of the TPN solution.

TPN Use in Special Metabolic Situations

Renal Failure. As indicated in Chapter 33, serious renal dysfunction poses serious physiologic and nutritional problems to the patient. Giordano[117] and others[117,118] noted that a diet with a high percentage of essential amino acids, a low percentage of nonessentials and adequate calories could induce positive nitrogen balance in azotemic patients. This approach was applied via the parenteral route to groups of patients with acute and chronic renal failure by Dudrick et al.[120] and by Abel et al.[121,122] The latter compared the outcome and complication rates of two groups of patients with acute renal failure with prolonged ileus. One group received large amounts of parenteral hypertonic glucose and vitamins with electrolytes as needed and the other group 13.1 gm of eight essential amino acids in addition to the glucose, vitamins and minerals.[121] Although there were no differences in the requirement for dialysis between the two groups, a higher percentage of dialyzed patients receiving the amino acids survived. Their BUN and creatinine decreased to a greater extent, they withstood gastrointestinal hemorrhage better and showed an improved state of consciousness.

Histidine was not present in the amino acid formulation used in this study, nor was there a comparison with a group receiving both essential and nonessential amino acids. Furst had earlier given essential amino acids by mouth or intravenously to two uremic patients and had found that the patients in renal failure, unlike healthy or traumatized individuals, were unable to incorporate ^{15}N from urea into histidine.[123] Bergstrom et al. found that the addition of histidine or histidine and arginine enhanced positive nitrogen balance in patients with marked uremia maintained on a low-nitrogen diet orally and given essential amino acids intravenously.[124]

Comparison of the outcome of two groups in a nonrandomized, apparently retrospective study of patients in acute renal failure in an intensive care unit indicated a better survival rate in those given fibrin hydrolysate plus 100 or more grams of glucose than in those given glucose.[125]

Hepatic Failure. Abnormal plasma amino acid patterns associated with hepatic failure and encephalopathy have been noted by various workers over the past 20 years. In chronic liver disease (e.g. cirrhosis) with acute decompensation, neutral amino acids (phenylalanine, tyrosine, free tryptophan and methionine) are elevated and the branched-chain amino acids (leucine, isoleucine and valine) are decreased. Glutamate and aspartate are increased, which may reflect muscle catabolism. In patients with fulminant hepatitis the pattern is that of increase in almost all but the branched-chain amino acids. The changes noted in cirrhosis have suggested that there are resulting accumulations of false neurochemical transmitters and inhibition of normal norepinephrine synthesis or abnormal accumulations of other transmitters, e.g. serotonin.[126] These abnormalities are manifested by the development of hepatic coma in dogs with portacaval shunts or patients with cirrhosis.[127,128] The ratio of the plasma branched-chain amino acids to phenylalanine plus tyrosine in mammals is 3.0 to 3.5, but this decreases to 1.5 to 2.0 in patients with cirrhosis and in the presence of encephalopathy is often 0.6 to 1.0.[126] Correction can be accomplished by infusion of an amino acid solution (FO80) which has decreased amounts of methionine, phenylalanine and tryptophan and increased amounts of leucine, isoleucine, valine, threonine and arginine (as compared to FreAmine II). Infusion of FO80 has resulted in positive nitrogen balance in dogs in hepatic failure, resolution of coma and better survival than those on FreAmine.

Clearing of coma with this solution has also been noted in cirrhotic patients but not in those with fulminant hepatitis.[127,128]

The plasma amino acid pattern noted by various investigators in severe sepsis bears a remarkable similarity to that seen in hepatic insufficiency. This may be related to the fact that, in sepsis, fat metabolism and ketosis are inhibited, a relative hypoinsulinemic (and perhaps hyperglucagonemic) hyperglycemic state develops with resultant catabolism of protein and release of aromatic amino acids into the circulation and muscle metabolism of branched-chain amino acids to alanine and glutamate. Hepatic insufficiency, which is common in severe sepsis, depresses catabolism of the large amounts of the neutral amino acids presented to the liver. Disturbances in sensorium of such patients (not dissimilar to hepatic encephalopathy) may then ensue for the reasons postulated by Fischer et al.[129]

Administration

There are a number of precautions relating to administration. These should be incorporated in general instructions and specific medical orders by the physician for guidance of the house and nursing staffs. Reevaluation of nutrient and fluid need should be made daily on the basis of serial clinical and biochemical data until the patient is known to be stable; then laboratory tests may be made less frequently. Following insertion of the central venous catheter roentgenologic evidence of its correct position must be obtained *before* starting the solutions.

Testing the patient's ability to adjust to a large glucose load is essential. When glucose provides the major source of calories it is recommended that for the first 2 to 3 days the glucose content of the formula should be one-third or one-half of that desired. Fractional urines should be tested for glucose every 6 hours. Water balance data and daily weight should be obtained.

Since most patients develop a good tolerance to glucose, it is our policy to give insulin only for 3+ or 4+ glycosuria or ketonuria, or where glycosuria leads to an osmotic diuresis causing dehydration, or where blood glucose is persistently elevated despite minimal glycosuria. Except in diabetics with known insulin requirements, relatively small doses of insulin are given initially (4 units for 3+ and 8 units for 4+ without ketones) and modified as experience dictates. Monitoring blood glucose twice daily in the early days will help avoid potentially dangerous hyperosmolar nonketotic coma. When the patient manifests good tolerance or the insulin requirement is fairly well established with a given glucose load, increasing amounts of glucose may be given. Fractional urines continue to be monitored even though the patient is well stabilized and utilizing the glucose well, with or without exogenous insulin.

With previously known diabetics or those demonstrating persistent glucose intolerance as TPN progresses, Intralipid may be given daily to replace a significant proportion of glucose calories. It is the author's practice to add regular insulin to the containers in addition to the insulin given on the basis of fractional urine results. It has been demonstrated that approximately one-half of the added regular insulin, as determined by immunoassay, is absorbed to glass or plastic but the remainder is stable for at least 48 hours.[130] The patient's need for intravenous insulin in TPN with a given glucose load is determined by the serum glucose levels, and the requirement for subcutaneous insulin doses is indicated by fractional requirements on a 4- to 6-hour basis.

Physicians and nurses caring for the patient receiving insulin must be cautioned against (1) excessive insulin dosage and frequency and (2) discontinuation of hypertonic glucose solutions while endogenous or exogenous insulin levels are elevated. Hypertonic glucose infusions should be ended by gradual reduction of the infusion rate over 1 to 1½ hours.

Filters tend to clog with use and may impede or stop infusion rate by gravity flow or propulsion pump. They should be changed at intervals depending on pore size and experience with the solutions and additives in use.

A critical aspect of care involves sterile precautions when inserting tubing and filters, in making connections and in caring for the CV catheter and skin at its entry. Tubing from container to filter should be changed daily and preferably with each new container. When a filter is changed, the tubing connecting it to the catheter should be changed simultaneously; its reinsertion to the catheter should be made with antiseptic treatment of the joints and use of sterile gloves. A central catheter poses the possibility of an air embolus if accidentally detached. All joints must be firmly connected with sterile tape and direct tension on the catheter must be avoided.

Catheters must be sutured in place (unless there is subcutaneous tunneling with a cuff) to minimize to-and-fro movements at the skin opening and the danger of accidental dislodgment. Opinion differs on the value of antiseptic treatment and use of antibiotics at this entry site. The author uses a Betadine wash at the catheter insertion site, with fresh sterile dressings utilizing paper tape. An occlusive dressing is not essential unless the insertion site is likely to be contaminated by secretions, hair or other extraneous materials.

The Parenteral Nutrition Team

It is apparent from the preceding discussion that this potentially lifesaving and morbidity-reducing procedure is a complex one, posing multiple problems in patient care, nutrition, safety and equipment. It is constantly changing as new information and supplies become available. Experience indicates that the optimum care of the patient requiring TPN is most

adequately assured by a team approach. The smallest effective team should include a physician knowledgeable in clinical nutrition and physiology and technique, one or more nurses skilled in the various procedural aspects to supervise administration to the patient and to assist and educate floor nurses, and one or more pharmacists, nurses or other personnel trained in solution preparation. It is desirable for the team physician(s) either to insert the catheters or to take responsibility for ensuring that only those trained in catheter insertion are permitted to do so. It is advisable that the hospital medical board formally designate the team and issue a clear statement of its mission and responsibility.

Home Total Parenteral Nutrition

The experience with hospitalized patients on TPN led inevitably to the concept that this technique was applicable to certain individuals on an outpatient basis. In 1970 various centers began to utilize home TPN (HTPN), each utilizing its own procedures.[43,46,48,53] Criteria and patient population differ according to the types of disease encountered by those responsible for the in-hospital program. In general, the patients receiving HTPN are those with serious bowel dysfunction secondary to inflammatory bowel disease and massive bowel resection or radiation enteritis and bowel resection. They are usually in a stable clinical state by the time of discharge; were it not for HTPN they would be relegated to continuous institutional TPN or to death by malnutrition.

The final nutrient solutions may be prepared by the hospital pharmacists[131] or by the patient and/or family member.[43,53] They are infused at home using a gas pressure device[46,131] or one of several types of pump.[46,131] Patients have been successfully managed by this technique for more than five years and there is, theoretically, no limit to the duration of intravenous feeding, provided all required nutrients are given in adequate amounts and any systemic infection is quickly and adequately treated. The infusions are generally intermittent for 8 to 14 or more hours, with the patient free of solutions and connecting tubing during the remaining hours of the day by means of a "heparin lock." During the "free" period the patient can work and carry out usual activities as his basic medical status permits.

The estimated cost of HTPN for the original pump, equipment, and nutrient solutions and additives varies between $13,000 to $24,000 per year depending upon the composition of the solutions and where they are made. The exact number of patients who were discharged on this technique between 1970 and 1977 is unknown but was at least 400. An international registry of such patients is now in operation to assist in obtaining data on the numbers, procedures and follow-up of these unique individuals.

SUPPLEMENTARY PERIPHERAL OR CENTRAL PARENTERAL NUTRITION

In a large number of clinical situations oral intake or tube feeding is feasible but actual intake is inadequate in relation to overall requirements: e.g. with partial intermittent bowel obstruction and depressed appetite as the result of trauma, sepsis, renal or hepatic dysfunction, cancer, depression, serious malabsorption, cancer chemotherapy and other conditions. When food intake via the alimentary tract is 25 to 50 per cent of that required and when tube feeding is deemed inadvisable, supplementary intravenous nutrition via a peripheral or central line is useful in maintaining or improving nutritional status. The infusions may be continuous or intermittent with a heparin lock, daily or at intervals as the physiologic and nutritional status indicates. The intravenous nutritional requirements will vary from patient to patient and from time to time. A sample formula for supplementary peripheral infusion is given in Table 37–12. The daily administration of intravenous fat by peripheral vein makes this a relatively expensive procedure in comparison to that of 50 per cent glucose used in central TPN. The cost, however, is warranted when the technique permits a patient to be discharged more quickly from the hospital or allows outpatient maintenance of improved nutritional state and more normal physical activity during convalescence or further therapy.

Table 37–12. Sample Formulation for Supplementary Peripheral Parenteral Nutrition

Item		Volume (ml)	AA (gm)	Kcal	Na (mEq)	K (mEq)	Cl (mEq)	P (mg)	Mg (mEq)	Ca (mg)
Crystalline amino acids	(8.5%)Φ	500	42.5	170	5	—	—	150	—	—
Dextrose in water	(10%)Φ	1000	—	340	—	—	—	—	—	—
with additives:										
NaCl	(15%)	20	—	—	50	—	50	—	—	—
KCl (2 mEq/ml)		15	—	—	—	30	30	—	—	—
MgSO₄	(50%)	4	—	—	—	—	—	—	17	—
Ca gluconate	(10%)	20	—	—	—	—	—	—	—	186
Vitamins*										
Trace elements*										
Intralipid	(10%)Φ	500	—	550	—	—	—	—	—	—
Totals		2059	42.5	1060	55	30	80	150	17	186

Φ Each bottle infused piggyback simultaneously.
*Same formulations and frequency as in Table 37–11.

BIBLIOGRAPHY

General

1. Elman: *Parenteral Alimentation in Surgery.* New York, Paul Hoeber, 1947.
2. White and Nagy (Eds.): *Total Parenteral Nutrition.* Acton, Publishers Science Group, 1974.
3. Fischer (Ed.): *Total Parenteral Nutrition.* Boston, Little, Brown & Co., 1976.
4. Meng and Wilmore (Eds.): *Fat Emulsions in Parenteral Nutrition.* Chicago, American Medical Association, 1976.
5. Greene, Holliday and Munro (Eds.): *Amino Acids—Clinical Nutrition Update.* Chicago, American Medical Association, 1977.
6. Ballinger, et al. (Eds.): *Manual of Surgical Nutrition.* Philadelphia, W. B. Saunders, 1975.

Specific

7. Geyer: Physiol. Rev., *40*, 150, 1960.
8. Mengoli: Am. J. Surg., *121*, 311, 1971.
9. Ellison, McCleery, Zollinger and Case: Surgery, *26*, 374, 1949.
10. Rice, Orr, Treloar and Strickler: Arch. Surg., *61*, 977, 1950.
11. Levenson, et al.: Ann. Surg., *124*, 840, 1946.
12. Merrill: *The Treatment of Renal Failure.* New York, Grune & Stratton, 1955.
13. Shils: Postgrad. Med., *36*, A99, 1964.
14. Dudrick, Wilmore, Vars and Rhoads: Surgery, *64*, 134, 1968.
15. Dudrick, et al.: Ann. Surg., *169*, 589, 1969.
16. Wretlind: In Meng and Wilmore,[4] p. 109.
17. Watkin and Steinfeld: Am. J. Clin. Nutr., *16*, 182, 1965.
18. Dudrick and Ruberg: Gastroenterology, *61*, 901, 1971.
19. Dudrick and Long: Annu. Rev. Med., *28*, 517, 1977.
20. Pietsch, Meakins and MacLean: Surgery, *82*, 349, 1977.
21. Meakins, et al.: Ann. Surg., *186*, 241, 1977.
22. Heird, MacMillan and Winters: In Fischer,[3] p. 253.
23. Doekel, et al.: N. Engl. J. Med., *295*, 358, 1976.
24. Beisel: Am. J. Clin. Nutr., *30*, 1236, 1977.
25. Moore and Brennan: In Ballinger, et al.,[6] p. 169.
26. Brennan: Cancer Res., *37*, 2359, 1977.
27. Wilmore: In Greene, Holliday and Munro,[5] p. 47.
28. Jeejeebhoy, et al.: In Greene, Holliday and Munro,[5] p. 45.
29. Jeejeebhoy, et al.: J. Clin. Invest., *57*, 125, 1976.
30. Borreson, Coran and Knutrud: Ann. Surg., *172*, 291, 1970.
31. Wretlind: Nutr. Metab., *14* (Suppl. 1), 57, 1972.
32. Gamble: Harvey Lect., *42*, 247, 1947.
33. Brennan and Moore: J. Surg. Res., *14*, 250, 1973.
34. Wilmore: In Greene, Holliday and Munro,[5] p. 47.
35. Wretlind: In White and Nagy,[2] pp. 201–212.
36. Coran: In Meng and Wilmore,[4] p. 69.
37. O'Neill: In Meng and Wilmore,[4] p. 71.
38. Long, Wilmore, Mason and Pruitt: Ann. Surg., *185*, 417, 1977.
39. Long: In Meng and Wilmore,[4] p. 76.
40. Filler, et al.: N. Engl. J. Med., *281*, 589, 1969.
41. Ryan: In Fischer,[3] p. 55.
42. Blewett, Kyger and Patterson: Arch. Surg., *108*,, 241, 1974.
43. Shils: Am. J. Clin. Nutr., *28*, 1429, 1975.
44. Titone, Lefton and Sakwa: Surg. Gynecol. Obstet., *137*, 489, 1973.
45. Broviac, Cole and Scribner: Surg. Gynecol. Obstet., *136*, 602, 1973.
46. Langer, Michattie, Zohrab and Jeejeebhoy: J. Surg. Res., *15*, 226, 1973.
47. Scribner, et al.: J.A.M.A., *212*, 457, 1970.
48. Shils, Wright, Turnbull and Brescia: N. Engl. J. Med., *283*, 341, 1970.
49. Brescia, et al.: N. Engl. J. Med., *275*, 527, 1977.
50. Heizer and Orringer: Gastroenterology, *72*, 527, 1977.
51. Belin, Koster, Bryant and Griffen: Surg. Gynecol. Obstet., *134*, 491, 1972.
52. Shils: J.A.M.A., *220*, 1721, 1972.
53. Broviac and Scribner: Surg. Gynecol. Obstet., *139*, 24, 1974.
54. Rubin and Jaeger: In White and Nagy,[2] p. 359.
55. Kinney: In Fischer,[3] p. 135.
56. National Academy of Science: *Recommended Dietary Allowances,* 8th ed. Washington, 1974.
57. Daly, Steiger, Vars and Dudrick: Ann. Surg., *180*, 709, 1974.
58. MacDonald, Phillips and Jeejeebhoy: Gastroenterology, *64*, 885, 1973.
59. Jeejeebhoy, et al.: Gastroenterology, *65*, 811, 1973.
60. Wyrick, Rea and McClelland: J.A.M.A., *211*, 1697, 1970.
61. Bergstrom, Hultman and Roch-Norlund: Acta Med. Scand., *184*, 359, 1968.
62. Wretlind and Schumer: Colloquium—Carbohydrates. In White and Nagy,[2] pp. 186–196, 235–237.
63. Upjohn, Creditor and Levenson: Metabolism, *6*, 607, 1957.
64. MacFadyen, et al.: Surg. Gynecol. Obstet., *137*, 813, 1973.
65. Long: In Meng and Wilmore,[4] p. 76.
66. Solassol and Joyeux: In Fischer,[3] p. 285.
67. Greene: In White and Nagy,[2] p. 221; Meng and Wilmore,[4] p. 95.
68. Dimant and Shafrir: In Meng and Wilmore,[4] p. 99.
69. Wilmore: In White and Nagy,[2] p. 225.
70. Andrew, Chan and Schiff: In Meng and Wilmore,[4] p. 104.
71. Thompson: *The Pathology of Parenteral Nutritions with Lipids.* Springfield, Charles C Thomas, 1974.
72. Terry and Wixom: In Weng and Wilmore,[4] p. 18.
73. Collins, et al.: Nutr. Metab., *13*, 150, 1971.
74. Caldwell, Johnson and Othersen: J. Pediatr., *8*, 849, 1972.

75. Colloquium: In White and Nagy,[2] pp. 117–123.
76. Christensen, Lynch, Decker and Powers: J. Clin. Invest., 26, 849, 1947.
77. Long, Zikria, Kinney and Geiger: Am. J. Clin. Nutr., 27, 163, 1974.
78. Wretlind: In White and Nagy,[2] pp. 108, 114.
79. Anderson, Patel and Jeejeebhoy: J. Clin. Invest., 53, 904, 1974.
80. Patel, Anderson and Jeejeebhoy: Gastroenterology, 65, 427, 1973.
81. Heird, et al.: N. Engl. J. Med., 287, 943, 1972.
82. Long, Crosby, Geiger and Kinney: Am. J. Clin. Nutr., 29, 380, 1976.
83. Long: In Greene, Holliday and Munro,[5] p. 116.
84. Winters, Heird, Dell and Nicholson: In Greene, Holliday and Munro,[5] p. 147.
85. Johnson, Albritton and Sunshine: J. Pediatr., 81, 154, 1972.
86. Heird, et al.: J. Pediatr., 81, 162, 1972.
87. Steginkt: In Greene, Holliday and Munro,[5] p. 198.
88. Munro: In Greene, Holliday and Munro,[5] p. 141.
89. Munro: In White and Nagy,[2] p. 59.
90. Furst, Josephson and Vinnars: Scand. J. Lab. Clin. Med., 26, 319, 1970.
91. Kinney, Duke, Long and Gump: J. Clin. Pathol., 23 (Suppl. 4), 65, 1970.
92. Colloquium: In White and Nagy,[2] pp. 117–121.
93. Allison: Am. J. Med., 5, 419, 1948.
94. Werner: Ann. Surg., 126, 175, 1947.
95. Moore: Metabolic Care of The Surgical Patient. Philadelphia, W. B. Saunders, 1959.
96. Heird and Winters: J. Pediatr., 86, 2, 1975.
97. Blackburn: In Meng and Wilmore,[4] p. 65.
98. Pollack and Halpern: Therapeutic Nutrition. Publication 234, National Academy of Sciences/National Research Council. Washington, 1952.
99. Smith and Goodman: N. Engl. J. Med., 294, 805, 1976.
100. Federal Register 37, No. 241, 26626 Dec. 14, 1972.
101. Shils: Bull. Parenter. Drug Assoc., 30, 226, 1976.
102. Shils. In Nutrition in The Care of The Critically Ill (Long and Border, Eds.). Chicago, American Medical Association, 1979.
103. Shils: In White and Nagy,[2] p. 257.
104. Reference deleted.
105. Lichtman, Miller, Cohen and Waterhouse: Ann. Intern. Med., 74, 562, 1971.
106. Travis, et al.: N. Engl. J. Med., 285, 763, 1971.
107. Jacob and Amsden: N. Engl. J. Med., 285, 1446, 1971.
108. Knochel: Arch. Intern. Med., 137, 203, 1977.
109. Kay, et al.: Ann. Surg., 183, 331, 1976.
110. Arakawa, et al.: Am J. Clin. Nutr., 29, 197, 1976.
111. Karpel and Peden: J. Pediatr., 80, 32, 1972.
112. Vilter, et al.: N. Engl. J. Med., 291, 188, 1974.
113. Jeejeebhoy, Chu and Marliss: Am. J. Clin. Nutr., 30, 531, 1977.
114. Giovannoni: In Fischer,[3] p. 27.
115. Shils: J.A.M.A., 220, 1721, 1972.
116. Burke: In White and Nagy,[2] p. 329.
117. Giordano: J. Lab. Clin. Med., 62, 231, 1963.
118. Giovannetti and Maggiore: Lancet, 1, 1000, 1964.
119. Berlyne, et al.: Q. J. Med., 35, 59, 1967.
120. Dudrick, Steiger and Long: Surgery, 68, 180, 1970.
121. Abel, et al.: N. Engl. J. Med., 288, 695, 1973.
122. Abel: In Fischer,[3] p. 135.
123. Furst: Scand. J. Clin. Lab. Invest., 30, 307, 1972.
124. Bergstrom: Life Sci., 9, 787, 1970; Acta Med. Scand., 191, 359, 1972.
125. Back, et al.: Surg. Gynecol. Obstet., 141, 405, 1975.
126. Fischer and Baldessarini: In Progress in Liver Disease (Popper and Schaffner, Eds.). New York, Grune & Stratton, 1976.
127. Fischer, et al.: Surgery, 78, 276, 1975.
128. Fischer, et al.: Surgery, 80, 77, 1976.
129. Fischer: In Greene, Holliday and Munro,[5] p. 174.
130. Shils and Kurkus: Unpublished data.
131. Tsallas and Baun: Am. J. Hosp. Pharm., 29, 840, 1972.

Chapter *38*

NUTRITION AND NEOPLASIA

Maurice E. Shils

DIET AND NUTRITION AS MODIFYING FACTORS IN TUMOR GENESIS AND GROWTH

The major components of diet serve as the energy sources for the host and for the neoplasm which it may harbor. The amino acids from the diet provide the building blocks for the proteins and peptides of normal and tumor cells. Minerals have structural, metabolic and metallic coenzyme functions, and vitamins are coenzymes and regulators in many steps of intermediary metabolism in normal and malignant cells. It is, therefore, no surprise to find experimentally that manipulations of diet can affect tumor development and growth. However, the complexity, variability and unexpectedness of some of these relations and the potentiality for therapy impart considerable interest to this subject. Attention is directed in this section to dietary influences on tumor development and growth with brief attention to nutritional factors affecting carcinogenic action and immune responses.

Modification by Calories and Nutrients of Spontaneous Tumor Development in Experimental Animals

Various manipulations of dietary components have been utilized to test the effects of their intake. In some experiments, the diets have been adequate in all components but the major caloric contribution in the control diet, usually carbohydrate, has been partially withheld from the experimental group, leading to inadequate caloric intake; this technique is designated as "caloric restriction."[1] Another approach to calorie deficit has involved restricting all components of the control diet; this has been termed "underfeeding."[1] In most studies of these types the experimental animals were allowed to ingest only 50 to 70 per cent as much as their fully fed controls. The development of spontaneous tumors in mice and rats was inhibited by such restriction; however, the magnitude of inhibition was influenced by tumor type, the degree of restriction and the presence of carcinogenic agents.[1]

Several more recent long-term studies in rats confirm the older studies, but provide some exceptions and new data. When a commercial diet was compared to four purified diets varying in protein (casein), carbohydrate (sucrose) or in total calories in male rats, total tumor risk was found to be directly and exponentially related to caloric intake. Within each dietary group rats of heavier weight had greater tumor risk than lighter rats. Occurrence and malignancy of certain tumors correlated with the level of protein intake: malignant lymphomas were predominant in rats with high-protein intake, whereas fibromas and fibrosarcomas predominated in those with low-protein intake. Lowest incidence, greatest delay in time of occurrence, absence of malignant epithelial tumors and greatest life expectancy were observed when intakes of protein, carbohydrate and total calories were low.[2] In another study 10, 22 or 51 per cent casein in isocaloric diets was fed to male rats on an ad libitum or caloric-restricted basis. With ad libitum intake, the highest incidence of chromophobe adenomas of the anterior pituitary gland was found to be associated with the dietary group having the highest intake of protein. Under restricted conditions tumor incidence was directly related to the protein level in the diet. Restriction in both caloric and protein intakes depressed the incidence to the greatest extent. Among all six dietary groups, body weight of the rat early in life correlated directly with the tumor prevalence in later life.[3] Short-term (7-week) restriction of food intake by rats after weaning followed by an ad libitum regimen substantially reduced long-term growth and the incidence of neoplasms, particularly of benign tumors and endocrine adenomas. Animals restricted in their food intake throughout life had appreciably lower tumor incidence (benign and malignant) than did those on the short-term restriction or those fed ad libitum.[4]

Vitamin and Mineral Deficiencies and Tumor Development

There are important exceptions to the preceding evidence for decreased tumor incidence with restrictions of calories and major dietary components. Deficiencies of certain micronutrients have been associated with an increased incidence of spontaneous tumors in rats. Vitamin A deficiency has been related to the development of odontomas[5] and salivary gland tumors.[6] A cereal type of diet low in iodide has led to increased frequency of thyroid tumors and pituitary enlargement.[7] Magnesium deficiency in rats has been reported to induce an invasive thymoma;[8] other investigators, however, have not found the resulting enlarged thymus to be invasive although it does cause death.[9] Chronic myelogenous leukemia has also been reported in magnesium-deficient rats[10] but confirmation of this is not available. The development of cirrhosis and hepatoma which was noted to occur in rats

on choline-deficient diets[11] is now believed to be related to the concomitant exposure of aflatoxin, which was unknown at the time of the original experiments.[12]

NUTRIENT INTAKE AND ACTION OF CARCINOGENS

There is increasing evidence that chemical carcinogens play a significant role in the etiology in cancer in man. Hence, any maneuver is of potential value that will prevent exposure of susceptible cells, inhibit the interaction of a chemical carcinogen with a target cell or reverse such a reaction at an early phase. Carcinogens have a common reactive form, namely, a positively charged electrophilic species which binds to macromolecules; by one or more reactions, carcinogens are converted to this active form.[13] Various mechanisms for prevention of chemical carcinogenesis are known.[14] The information presently available comes from empirical studies, and the mechanism of action of many agents is still uncertain. Some of the protective mechanisms involve dietary components or food additives which modify the action of carcinogens. If inhibitors of chemical carcinogenesis are to have any practical value for man, they will have to be substances of little or no toxicity. Hence, there is a special interest in certain dietary or nutritional factors as possible protective mechanisms. Groups of compounds of interest which are considered here are those that: (1) alter (usually increase) the drug-metabolizing (microsomal oxidase) enzymes and which have maximum effectiveness when administered 24 to 48 hours prior to challenge by a carcinogen, (2) act as antioxidants which are inhibitory when administered shortly before the carcinogen, (3) prevent formation of the carcinogen and (4) reverse the early stages of carcinogenic activity.

Modification of Drug-metabolizing Enzymes

Endoplasmic reticulum (or its fragments, the microsomes) of various organs, especially the liver, contain enzyme systems which can convert many drugs and foreign chemicals into more polar compounds.[15] Administration to an animal of certain drugs or agents increases the capacity to metabolize a wide range of such drugs or chemicals by induction of these microsomal oxidase enzymes.[16] Among the wide variety of xenobiotic compounds which may be metabolized by these enzymes are many chemical carcinogens.[17] While drug and developmental factors play a role in the inducibility of these enzymes, such inducibility is also influenced by environmental factors, including diet and nutrition. The activities of these enzymes may be depressed by starvation, protein deficiency, fat and carbohydrate modification and certain mineral and vitamin deficiencies.[18]

The activities of microsomal oxidase enzymes in the small intestine and lung of experimental animals have been studied in relation to the effects of dietary factors. It has been suggested that the presence of these drug-metabolizing enzymes in the major portals of entry of food and air acts as an important protection against carcinogens entering by these routes.[19] Experiments with mice and rats have demonstrated that induction of these enzymes by various agents protects against a number of chemical carcinogens.[20] It has also been found that most, if not all, of the enzyme activity in these two organs resulted from exposure to exogenous inducing agents present in food and diets. Either starvation or the feeding of purified diets to the animals led to total loss of the ability to hydroxylate aromatic polycyclic hydrocarbons.

Efforts to identify the chemical natures of the inducers present in diets of natural foods disclosed that the most potent sources were vegetables of the Brassicaceae family, including brussels sprouts, cabbages and broccoli. Various indoles with inducing activity were isolated, namely, indole-3 acetonitrile, indole-3 carbinol and 3'-diinodolylmethane derived from hydrolysis of a parent compound.[21] Protection against a variety of chemical carcinogens has been afforded also by other inducers of microsomal enzymes; these include polycyclic hydrocarbons (which are toxic), flavones (which have little toxicity), barbiturates and phenothiazines.[14] While the increased activity of these enzymes is protective by virtue of their inactivation of primary carcinogens, it has been shown that they may also metabolize carcinogen precursors into active forms. Wattenberg has suggested that such activation of precarcinogens to proximate carcinogens is not likely to increase carcinogenesis.[14] In addition, he has pointed out that induction of the enzyme activity may be important in another manner: chemical carcinogens are subject to detoxification reactions as well as to activation or inactivation. For example, ring hydroxylation by enzymatic action results in detoxification whereas hydroxylation of the nitrogen causes activation. Hence, administration of inducers of the enzyme activity may cause a relatively larger portion of the carcinogen to be detoxified than to be activated.

Antioxidants

The use of antioxidants as possible inhibitors of chemical carcinogens has been based on the concept that the compounds may exert an inactivating effect on the reactive species of carcinogens. In early studies in which wheat germ oil and alpha-tocopherol were employed the published results are variable, so that their potential value is not clear. Wattenberg has not found alpha-tocopherol to be inhibitory.[22] Studies in the mouse and rat of phenolic antioxidants, in particular butylated hydroxyanisole (BHA) and butylated hydroxytoluene (BHT) and several nonphenolic antioxidants, have been shown to inhibit the expected carcinogenesis of a variety of compounds. The protective effect of BHA against benzpyrene appears to result from a decrease in epoxidation (which is an activation process) so that less carcinogen binds to DNA and, also, detoxification is increased.[14] Decreased binding to DNA of other carcinogens has been also shown with these antioxidants. BHA is of interest because of its extensive use as an additive in food for human consumption. Wattenberg estimates that the human consumption of this compound is of the order of several milligrams a day; on the basis of animal experiments, this amount may be important to man in inhibiting the effects of chronic exposure to low doses of carcinogens.[14]

An active nonphenolic antioxidant is ethoxyquin, which is used in commercial animal feed. Several organic isothiocyanates, which are naturally occurring constituents of edible plants, have been found to inhibit certain carcinogens. Similar effects have been found for coumarins which are also constituents of a wide variety of plants, including vegetables used for human consumption. Inhibition by selenium salts of experimental epidermal neoplasia induced by carcinogens has been reported by Shamberger.[23] An inverse relationship has been reported between the amount of selenium in soil and farm crops and human cancer death rates in the United States and Canada.[24]

The evidence to date is still inadequate to suggest that inhibitors of carcinogenesis should be deliberately added to food or ingested in other forms for this purpose. It is not too early to consider the criteria that would have to be met prior to such deliberate use, and such criteria have been suggested by Wattenberg.[14] He indicates the need for serious restraint in use, particularly for normal individuals, because of the possibility of toxicity and a need for long-term studies; however, population groups with elevated exposure to chemical carcinogens may well have less rigid restrictions in the use of certain inhibitors.

Certain compounds that prevent formation of carcinogens (e.g. the interaction of ascorbic acid with nitrite) and compounds that act to reverse early carcinogenic effects (e.g. retinoids) are considered below.

Specific Nutrient Modifications

One of the first and most intensively studied carcinogens the action of which is strongly influenced by nutritional factors is the azo dye p-dimethylaminoazobenzene (DMAB). In the 1930s, Japanese investigators observed that rats subsisting on rice developed liver cancer when given the dye. Addition of yeast or liver prevented the tumors. It was found by others that riboflavin and casein, together, markedly reduced tumor incidence when added to the rice diet. An ameliorating influence of nutritional factors has also been observed even after the initiating effect of the dye has been operating for some time; however, once adenomatous hyperplasia of the bile ducts, cholangioma or hepatoma was present, improvement in diet was without effect.[25] A biochemical basis for the effect of riboflavin was established by the finding that azo dye reductase (which splits DMAB) in liver requires riboflavin adenine nucleotide as a cofactor.[6] Demethylation of DMAB by drug-metabolizing enzymes results in loss of carcinogenicity.[26]

Protein, Fat and Lipotropes. Aflatoxins, a family of mycotoxins produced by certain strains of Aspergillus flavus, may contaminate peanuts, cereals and other foods.[27] These agents, particularly aflatoxin B_1, can induce both liver damage and hepatomas with marked species differences in susceptibility. Diets low in protein have had variable effects on aflatoxin toxicity and carcinogenicity.[28] Acute toxicity of aflatoxin B_1 is appreciably less in rats on a diet marginally low in lipotropes than in those on a controlled diet; however, following a carcinogenic dose, abnormal hepatocytes and hepatic carcinoma appeared much earlier in the experimental than in control rats.[29] Demethylating and hydroxylating enzymes were reduced in the livers of rats on the low lipotrope diet and the former were not induced by aflatoxin B_1.

A somewhat similar situation appears to occur with protein deficiency and dimethylnitrosoamine.[30] Protein deficiency protects rats against the acute lethal effects of the chemical but increases the later carcinogenic actions leading to kidney cancer. It is postulated that the metabolizing enzyme in liver is suppressed by a low-protein diet, thus decreasing the rate of metabolism of the toxic product and decreasing acute mortality but, at the same time, resulting in prolonged exposure of the kidney with increased methylation of DNA and increased carcinogenesis. Increased protein may increase carcinogenicity of other agents; for example, at levels of 15 and 22.5 per cent of total calories as protein the number and size of intestinal adenocarcinoma were greater than at the 7.5 per cent level in rats given dimethylhydrazine (DMH).[31] There was no difference in colon carcinogenesis between rats given beef or soybean as the protein sources when the diet contained 20 per cent fat from animal sources.[32] Consideration of the effects of specific amino acids depletion is given below.

The interest aroused by epidemiologic data suggesting a positive association between the prevalence of colon cancer in man and dietary fat intake (see below) has led, in recent years, to experimental studies on this subject.

Marginal deficiency of lipotropes (methionine, folate and choline) and a high level of fat in the diet increased or accelerated induction of hepatocarcinoma in rats, not only with aflatoxin B_1 but also with N-nitrosodiethylamine (NNDA), N-nitrosodibutylamine (DBN) and N-2-fluorenyl-acetamide; similarly, induction of colon tumors by this diet was enhanced by DMH.[33]

Carroll has reviewed data on spontaneous and carcinogen-induced tumors in relation to fat intake.[34] He concluded that dietary fat tends to promote tumorgenesis but only of certain types, such as mammary and colon tumors. Rats maintained for two generations on a 20 per cent fat diet were more susceptible than those on a 5 per cent fat intake to the induction of colon tumors by injections of DMH.[33]

The origin and degree of saturation of fat (corn oil versus lard) had no significant influence in some studies.[33,35] However, there is conflicting evidence to the claim that the type of fat has no influence on carcinogen-induced tumor growth. There are a series of papers from different laboratories indicating that dimethylbenzanthracene-induced tumor growth is enhanced in rats fed moderately large amounts of vegetable oils high in polyunsaturates as compared to those fed small amounts of corn oil or moderately large amounts of coconut oil or lard.[36-39] Inoculation of transplantable mammary adenocarcinoma cells into mice subsisting either on sunflower seed oil or on tallow-containing diets, each at 18.6 per cent, resulted in a greater incidence of tumors in those on the polyunsaturated-fat diet; this suggests that the effect of the fat was on the promotional stage of carcinogenesis.[40] It should be noted that the results in carcinogen-induced colon or liver tumors revealed no differences when the *type* of fat was varied, whereas studies related to carcinogen-induced mammary cancer indicated an enhancing effect of polyunsaturated fat. Further studies in this intriguing area are obviously necessary. The relationships among the amounts and types of fat and the influence of "fiber" are discussed further in considering human epidemiologic data on cancer incidence.

Fat intake stimulates bile secretion. Hill et al. have hypothesized and presented some evidence that bile salts are converted to carcinogens by certain bacteria.[41] Acting on this suggestion, bile salts have been fed, alone or with cholestyramine (a nonabsorbable resin which increases entry of bile salts into the colon); both increased the colon tumor-producing effect of certain carcinogens, as did the administration of cholestyramine alone.[39] Cholesterol added at 6 to 9 mg per day to a complete liquid cholesterol-free, low-fat formula markedly decreased the time to appearance of colon cancer in rats injected with DMH from that occurring when the formula was fed without cholesterol.[41a] A role for intestinal microflora in promoting or accelerating colon tumor production is indicated from experiments in which the induction of colon tumors by DMH was much greater in conventional rats than in germ-free rats.[35]

Vitamins. With the development of experimental animal models of carcinogen-induced neoplasia in various organ systems, there has been active interest in the effects of excesses or deficiencies of various vitamins on tumor genesis.

Vitamin A has been of particular interest because of its fundamental role in epithelial cell differentiation. A basic effect of its deficiency is increased DNA synthesis and mitotic activity with resultant hyperplasia of the basal cells of epithelium. Vitamin A-deficient rats have been found to be more susceptible than controls to induction of colon cancer by aflatoxin B_1;[33] contrariwise, vitamin A status did not appreciably affect DMH carcinogenesis[33] and vitamin A *deficiency* appeared protective against induction of colon cancer by N-methyl-N'-nitro-N-nitrosoguanidine.[35] Increased susceptibility to various carcinogens associated with vitamin A deficiency has been noted in rat respiratory tract[42] and bladder.[43]

Because the neoplastic process involves a dedifferentiation or an arrest of differentiation in epithelial tissue, the effect of topical or systemic administration of common forms of vitamin A has been tested by various investigators in an effort to inhibit the action of various carcinogens. Use of vitamin A has been associated with inhibition of development of carcinoma of the hamster forestomach and cervix,[44] tracheobronchial and bronchogenic epithelium,[45] skin[46] and breast. Other investigators have obtained conflicting results.[47]

Retinoids. The common retinyl esters have limitations as antitumor agents in pharmacologic doses because their met-abolic pathways limit availability at specific target sites (e.g. bladder epithelium) or because of their toxicity.[48] Accordingly, Sporn and associates have developed synthetic analogs (included in the general term *retinoids* which they introduced) which have lesser toxicity and different patterns of tissue distribution, metabolism and storage.[48]

Preliminary evidence is emerging of the value of specific retinoids in the prevention of development and growth of specific types of epithelial cancer. Several synthetic analogs have been found to be more effective against carcinogen-induced skin cancer in mice than *all-trans*-retinoic acid.[50] When fed for the life of hamsters following intratracheal benz [α] pyrene, 13-*cis*-retinoic acid has been shown to be protective.[49] The same analog decreased the incidence and extent of bladder papillomas and carcinomas in rats in which N-methyl-N-nitrosourea (MNU) had been instilled into their bladders.[51] Retinyl methylester and retinyl acetate greatly diminished the number of cancers per rat and delayed the onset of mammary cancer induced by MNU, whereas 13-*cis*-retinoic acid and another analog were ineffective.[52]

Ascorbic Acid. The potential role of nitrosoamines as carcinogenic, mutagenic and cytotoxic agents has focused attention on the nature and sources of their precursors. Nitrite ion reacts with naturally occurring and synthetic secondary and tertiary amines to form nitroso compounds. Nitrites and nitrates from food and water are of current concern and are discussed below. The findings that ascorbic acid reacts very rapidly with nitrite[53] and effectively competes with amines for nitrite in vitro[54] and in vivo[55] suggested that coadministration of ascorbic acid with potentially nitrosatable drugs and nitrite-containing foods may reduce the hazards associated with ingestion of these substances.[54,54a] Ascorbic acid has been reported to inhibit tumor induction in rats given nitrite with urea or amines or

N-nitroso compounds[56,57] and to decrease the formation of MNU in food incubated in vitro under simulated gastric conditions.[58] Other protective agents are gallic acid and thiocyanate.

Zinc. Dietary zinc deficiency increased the incidence and shortened the lag time for induction of esophageal tumors in rats given methylbenzylnitrosamine.[59] With high doses of this carcinogen, the incidence of invasive carcinomas was appreciably greater in the deficient animal than in the zinc-fed controls.

Examples of the opposite effect have been noted where increased amounts of nutrients augment carcinogens. Addition of tryptophan or other indoles to 2-acetyl-aminofluorene markedly increased the incidence of bladder tumors in rats.[60] Extra thiamin, given to rats on a grain diet with bracken fern (which contains a thiaminase), increased the incidence of bladder tumor without affecting the high incidence of intestinal tumors occurring in animals subsisting on the basic diet with the carcinogen.[61] A single injection of streptozotocin, a naturally occurring nitrosourea, when given with two injections of large doses of nicotinamide, resulted in the appearance of insulin-secreting pancreatic islet cell tumors in 92 per cent of male rats 226 to 547 days later. Streptozotocin by itself caused a 4 per cent tumor incidence; nicotinamide by itself had no effect.[62]

DIETARY DEFICIENCIES AND TUMOR GROWTH

The rationale for attempting inhibition or actual reversal of established neoplastic growth by induction of nutritional deficiencies is based on the possibility that certain tumor cells may be more sensitive to such depletion than are normal tissues. An increased sensitivity may reside in the presence of quantitative or even qualitative differences in the requirement for certain nutrients so that depletion by dietary means or the use of nutritional analogs (antimetabolites) which block metabolic pathways will adversely affect tumor cells to a greater degree than host cells.

It has been concluded that caloric intake can retard the establishment and growth of transplanted tumors only when the host weight diminishes.[1] Similarly, protein deprivation and other deficiencies are inhibitory only when associated with poor growth or weight loss.[1] An exception to this may occur with zinc deficiency in rats, where Walker 256 transplanted tumor growth was significantly reduced despite only small growth differences with weight-matched controls.[63] Variation in the proportion of dietary fat appears to have no consistent effect on transplant take and growth. When protein intakes of 0, 18 and 30 per cent were fed to rats for 2 weeks and Walker carcinosarcoma 256 was injected intraportally, it was noted that the greater the protein intake, the greater was the number of animals demonstrating hepatic metastases and the larger the tumors present.[64] The level of protein influenced the growth of metastases rather than the "take" of tumor cells. The incidence and size of metastases were no greater in fatty livers caused by a high-fat choline-free diet than in normal livers on choline-containing or low-fat diets.

Metabolic Advantages of Malignant Cells

One of the more interesting associations of tumor metabolism with nutrition concerns the ability of various experimental tumors to obtain their energy sources and amino acids from the host, especially in periods of deprivation.[65] There is also evidence that tumors in common with growing tissues are capable of taking up amino acids from the blood and concentrating them to a greater extent than do some other normal tissues. In rats fed ad libitum with transplanted tumors the host tissues begin to lose weight when the tumor begins to grow rapidly; anorexia is associated with this phase. Forced feeding by tube of such rats can prevent loss of host tissue in large part, but the tumor also grows; with continued feeding and no antitumor treatment undesirable metabolic reactions still occur and death ensues. Short-term intravenous feeding will also maintain host tissues; variable changes in tumor/host weight ratios have been reported.[66-68] The implications of forced feeding in the treatment of cancer in man are discussed below.

Amino Acids. Single omission of many but not all of the essential amino acids from the diets of rats with Walker 256 transplants[69] inhibited growth of the tumors but also resulted in loss of host body weight.

Experiments have also been conducted with mice where individual or several amino acids were restricted in amount below optimum requirement. Diets restricted in phenylalanine and tyrosine inhibited the growth of transplanted S91 melanoma in mice but not that of S37 sarcoma.[70] Rather similar restrictions of these amino acids had an insignificant effect on the growth of a hepatoma (BW7756) or mammary adenocarcinoma (C3HBA) in certain mouse strains.[71] Theuer has systematically studied the effects of restriction of each essential amino acid on the growth of transplanted BW10232 adenocarcinoma in female C57BL/J6 mice.[72] Dietary levels of tryptophan, threonine, leucine or methionine which significantly inhibited tumor growth also depressed host weight. However, reduced dietary levels of phenylalanine, valine or isoleucine significantly inhibited tumor weight without affecting host weight. Lysine restriction had no effect on either weight gain or tumor growth.

A different result was obtained by others in induction experiments in which groups of mice were fed diets restricted to 25 per cent of the control diet for phenylalanine-tyrosine, isoleucine or leucine.[72a] Although isoleucine deficiency caused obvious hair changes and weight inhibition as compared to controls, deficiencies of the other two caused little change in weight or appearance. Subcutaneous implantation of cellulose-paraffin discs impregnated with 5 per cent 3-methylcholanthrene (which leads to virtually 100 per cent tumor induction in susceptible strains) into the various dietary groups resulted in more rapid development of tumors and death in the phenylalanine-tyrosine depleted group. Deficiencies of the other two amino acids resulted in no significant differences in tumor incidence as compared to controls. The isoleucine-deficient animals had proportionately greater tumor weight to body weight than the other groups.

These conflicting results with phenylalanine-tyrosine and other restrictions in mice with transplanted or induced tumors emphasize again the fact that effective nutritional or other manipulation with one type of tumor or carcinogen may be ineffective with another.

There have been a small number of limited and unsatisfactory clinical trials with diets low in phenylalanine and tyrosine.[73] While not considered to be an essential amino acid, nutritional requirements have been found to exist for L-asparagine by certain neoplastic cells in tissue culture because of a deficiency of L-asparagine synthetase. A number of studies[74] have resulted in the finding that the enzyme L-asparaginase (which deaminates L-asparagine to aspartic acid) has antitumor action in neoplasms of the mouse, rat and dog. A wide variety of human neoplasms have been treated with L-asparaginase derived from E. coli; however, at this time, acute lymphocytic leukemia appears to be the most sensitive, with a high percentage of remissions which are not sustained.[74,75]

Amino acid analogs have been tested as inhibitors of tumor growth, but these have not been clinically useful.

Vitamins. Deficiencies of folic acid,[76] of pyridoxine[77] or of riboflavin[78] have each been found to result in significant inhibition of the growth of certain tumors beyond the effect of the vitamin deficiency per se.

Studies of the vitamin composition of various experimental tumors indicate that there is no specific qualitative difference from normal tissues. While a number of tumors tend to be low in certain vitamins, values as low or even lower are noted in some normal tissues.

Various vitamin antimetabolites have been tested against human neoplasms. At present, the only clinically useful analog is methotrexate, which plays an important role in the treatment of acute leukemias, metastatic choriocarcinoma and other malignancies. Large dosages are often given which are followed by leucovorin ("citrovorum rescue") to ameliorate damage to normal cells. Pyridoxine-low diets, combined in some cases with 4-deoxypyridoxine, had no definite antitumor effect in patients with advanced neoplastic diseases.[79] Possible approaches utilizing nutritional factors in cancer chemotherapy have been discussed.[73,80]

The inhibition of tumorgenesis and growth by dietary means involves a potentially complex and poorly understood problem. Dietary restriction or specific deficiency leads to many changes in the animal body. With endocrine-sensitive tumors, such as spontaneous mammary tumors, the principal effect may be related to reduced estrogen or other hormone production. A general phenomenon may be involved, such as that suggested by Bullough who postulated that inhibition is secondary to a decrease in the mean mitotic activity of the tissue.[81] Where a deficiency leads to tumor development the converse may occur, with increased mitotic activity of certain cells with neoplastic potential.

Nutritional Status and Immune Responses

The nature of immune responses has a number of facets of importance in relation to cancer. Depressed cellular immunity has been known to occur in cancer patients and, in the past, has frequently been attributed to the effects of cancer per se. As the result of studies done initially in children,[82] in adults[83] and then in cancer patients,[84] it has become obvious that altered immune responses can result from malnutrition. Malnutrition also induces altered phagocytosis, macrophage activity and depressed complement levels.[82] Efforts may be made to improve immunity either by improving nutritional status or, alternatively, by inducing certain deficiencies in an effort to slow tumor growth and enhance immune responses.[85] In 1949 Stoerk and Emerson found that induction of riboflavin deficiency in C3H mice at 6 to 14 days after implantation of lymphosarcoma 6C3H-CD resulted in marked to complete regression of the tumor within 10 days and in a 30 to 37 per cent cure rate; tumor reinoculated into "cured" mice with or without riboflavin in the diets failed to "take."[86] The authors believed that the deficiency slowed tumor growth and permitted immune defenses to become effective. Antibody directed against tumor antigens may increase tumor immunity as in antibody-dependent cellular cytotoxicity. On the other hand, production of other antibodies may diminish resistance.[87]

One possible explanation for the failure of host immune defenses to destroy malignant cells is the presence of serum inhibitors ("blocking antibody") which prevent their destruction by cell-mediated mechanisms. It has been suggested that certain deficiencies could inhibit formation of blocking antibody without depressing cellular immunity.[85] Protein-deficient mice showed increased responses to phytohemagglutinin and rejected skin allografts more rapidly than normally nourished controls, while showing decreases in splenic plaque-forming cells and antibody synthesis to sheep red cells.[88] Rats or mice fed a diet containing between 5 and 10 per cent casein showed depressed antibody responses but normal cellular immunity to tumor or transplantation antigens. Following immunization the normal animal developed specific antibody (blocking antibody) which partly or completely inhibited cell-mediated immunity in vitro. However, in the immunized animals with protein deficiency, the serum inhibitor was markedly reduced or absent. Consequently, cell-mediated immunity was more effective in this range of protein depletion. When the level of protein in the diet was reduced below 3 per cent of total calories, both humoral and cellular immunity were depressed and progressive weight loss and death followed.

The effects of modifying a single amino acid intake by mice have been observed in relation to humoral and cell-mediated immune responses to inoculation of allogenic tumor cells.[89] Moderate reduction of the amino acids phenylalanine-tyrosine, valine, threonine, methionine-cystine, isoleucine and tryptophan produced marked depression of hemagglutinating and blocking antibody responses without affecting cytotoxic cell-mediated immunity. Limitation of arginine, histidine and lysine gave rise to only slight depression of the immune responses. Moderate restriction of leucine resulted in a paradoxical depression of cytotoxicity with little effect on serum blocking antibody. The authors point out that these observations correlate with other reports on the effect or lack of effect of depletion of these amino acid deficiencies on tumor growth[72] and that deficiency or imbalance of essential amino acids may produce marked changes in the immune resistance of the host animal to tumors. Contrary evidence to this opinion has been presented recently. Worthington et al. have observed the effect of restriction of phenylalanine-tyrosine, isoleucine or leucine on the immune resistance of mice to a transplanted 3-methylcholanthrene (MCA)-induced tumor.[72a] There was rapid tumor development and 100 per cent incidence in nonimmune mice on the control

diet. Mice on the various deficient and control diets were immunized by inoculation of MCA tumor cells; when the tumor reached a certain size, it was totally excised. Three days later, the same animals were again inoculated with tumor cells. These reinoculated animals had a much slower tumor development and lower incidence than nonimmunized controls, but there was neither a protective nor deleterious influence of the various amino acid deficiencies as compared to controls receiving adequate amino acids.

It has been believed by a number of oncologists that the depressed cellular immunity often seen in cancer patients is the result of cancer per se. Copeland and associates have studied the effects of nutritional depletion and rehabilitation on immune competence, tumor growth and responsiveness to antitumor therapy.[84] Their data indicate that malnutrition leads to immunosuppression, as do surgery, radiation therapy and chemotherapy. The majority of patients who on initial testing gave a negative response to various intradermal antigens became positive (i.e. had increased cellular immunity) to skin testing following nutritional treatment with total parenteral nutrition despite chemotherapy and surgery. Radiation therapy prevented or reversed improved immune responses. Tumor-bearing rats with depressed cellular immunity induced by protein deficiency also responded to nutritional repletion with return of their immunity.[67] Provision of all amino acids administered as the only source of nutrition did not reverse the depressed immunity. In an uncontrolled study responses to chemotherapy occurred only in those patients who were or became skin-test positive.[84]

There is increasing clinical evidence that reestablishment of cellular immunity by nutritional means, together with control of infection, plays an important role in decreasing morbidity and mortality.[90] A number of nutritional deficiencies can adversely affect the various parameters of immune mechanisms (see Chapter 18). The importance of optimum defenses against infection in the cancer patient emphasizes the need for providing adequate nutrition.

HUMAN EPIDEMIOLOGIC DATA RELATING NEOPLASIA TO DIETARY PRACTICES

From the earliest medical records to the present, physicians and laymen have postulated an association (either protective or predisposing) between diet and the development of cancer.[91] This has proved a fertile area for a wide range of speculation extending from food faddists to epidemiologists.

There has been an upsurge in interest in this field as the result of epidemiologic surveys indicating: (1) marked differences in the prevalence of malignancies originating in different organ systems within a given population, (2) variations in the prevalence of malignancy in a specific organ among different populations which may or may not be geographically distant and (3) changes in prevalence of certain cancers associated with population migrations. Such data suggest that environmental factors are important even though they do not prove the identity of such factors. The role of diet as an important environmental variable has gained increasing attention as epidemiologic studies have associated differences in diet composition with regional differences in prevalence of types of cancer. The discovery that Aspergillus flavus grows on various foods under suitable conditions and produces the very potent liver carcinogen aflatoxin has focused attention on food contaminants as possible etiologic factors in human cancer.

The possible etiologic interrelations of a number of factors in cancer causation and their variations in various geographic areas have been emphasized.[92-94] Dietary factors of one type or another may induce changes in epithelial tissues, modify immune status or lead to formation of carcinogens in association with other factors such as viruses and alcohol.

Differences in the intake of a given dietary constituent, e.g. fat or carbohydrate, among population groups must be, by the nature of diet composition, associated with differences in intakes of other essential nutrients, caloric sources and food constituents so that the resulting differences, although ascribed to differences of a specific dietary constituent, may be, in fact, very complex. Such complexity should lead to caution and the development of more precise evidence before noncausative associations are mistakenly ascribed to "proven" etiologic factors.

Gastrointestinal neoplasms have been of special interest, since the incidence of malignancy in the upper and lower areas of the alimentary tract is often high in certain areas and the survival rate is often low. There is increasing evidence that the development and clinical expression of human alimentary tract carcinoma may run a course of many years. The initiating factors may not necessarily be present at the time of the epidemiologic survey, thereby creating difficulties in obtaining accurate retrospective individual data. Studies of migrant populations with those at the original site permit a more objective evaluation of environmental differences, including the effects of time, age and generation differences. Possible relations to diet are briefly discussed below by anatomic division of the alimentary tract.

Oropharyngeal and Esophageal Carcinoma

An association has been noted between the occurrence of Plummer-Vinson syndrome (sideropenic anemia with epithelial lesions) and cancer of the hypopharynx in Swedish women.[95] The syndrome is believed to be secondary to iron deficiency, but vitamin deficiencies are also involved. There is a decreasing trend in both the syndrome and the cancer in association with improved nutrition, health care and decreasing number of pregnancies.[96]

Esophageal carcinoma has a worldwide incidence which varies more than 100-fold.[97] There is an extremely high incidence in certain areas of various countries including France, India, the Soviet Union, Iran, Finland, China and Hong Kong, the West Indies and parts of Africa.[97] The disease is practically unknown in the west of Africa but is very common in east and south Africa. The high frequency in certain areas seems to be a development of the past 30 or 40 years.[98]

Increased use of alcohol and tobacco has been associated with occurrence of esophageal cancer in New York City and in parts of Brittany and Normandy.[97] In these areas the prevalence among males is much greater than among women. In the United States there has been a major increase among urban blacks of both sexes. In most of the world alcohol and tobacco do not appear to be factors of major importance. The poorer economic groups appear to be more affected by the malignancy. Further data are necessary to delineate basic factors.

Gastric Cancer

There are large demographic differences in the prevalence of this malignancy. Japan, Chile, Costa Rica, Finland and Iceland have rates (predominantly in males) five or more times those of U.S. Caucasians.[99] There appears to be a strong positive correlation between risk and mountainous living (e.g. Yugoslavia, Costa Rica, Guatemala and Colombia).[99] In the United States and in Europe, higher rates are

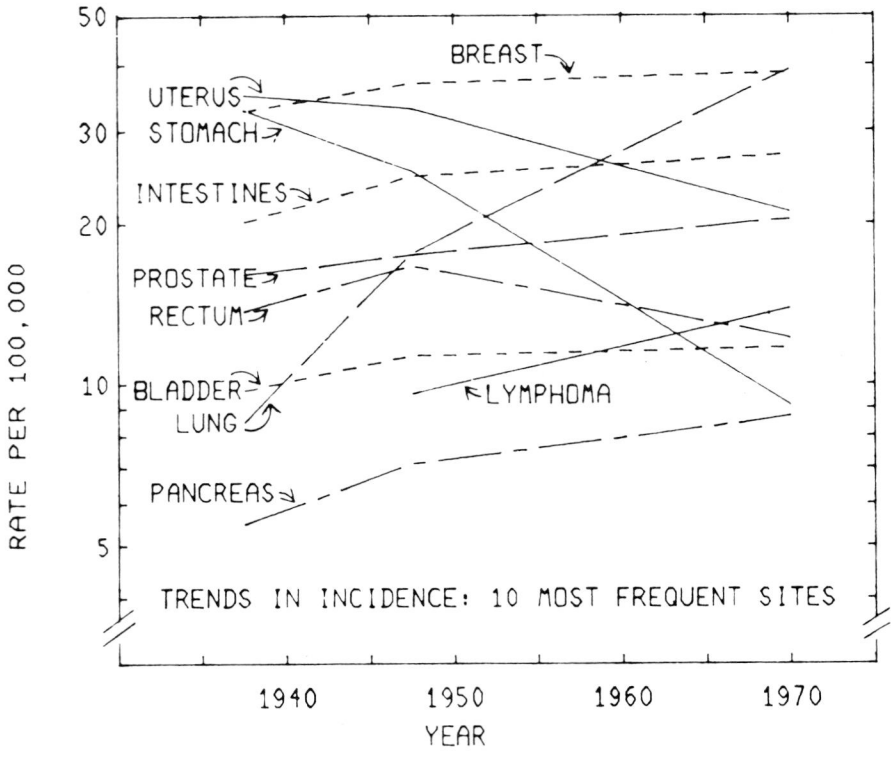

Fig. 38–1. Thirty-year incidence trends in the population of the United States for 10 most frequent sites of cancer. (From Devesa and Silverman.[101])

noted for gastric as well as esophageal cancer among low-income groups. Certain ethnic groups in this country appear to have increased risk, particularly the immigrant generation from countries with high risks for gastric cancer. Offspring born in the United States have a lower risk.[99,100] However, the most noteworthy trend has been the steady decline for more than 30 years, so that rates are now one-half to one-fifth their maximum since 1935[101] (Fig. 38–1). Similar downward trends became apparent later in western Europe and more recently in Japan, particularly in large city populations.[102]

There have been a number of studies of diet intake and practices in populations with varying prevalence of gastric cancer. While there are negative correlations between gastric cancer incidence and total fat consumption (and, hence, with living standard and meat consumption) and positive correlation with fish consumption, these relations are dependent on situations in specific countries[103] and hence are questionable. It has been concluded that no food can be identified that is common to all high-risk populations.[99] Some interview studies carried out among different populations in various cultures and geographic areas suggest positive risk association with high-starch diets in Tel Aviv, rice in Honolulu and potatoes in Buffalo.[104] Hirayama associates the declining trend in gastric cancer in Japan with increased intake of milk and milk products, meat, eggs and fruits and decreased intake of potatoes, especially sweet potatoes.[102]

Reference has been made above to the possible role of nitrites in cancer induction. Nitrite enters the food supply from nitrate in food or water and as preformed nitrite. Nitrate in considerable amounts was used in the United States as a food preservative, especially for fish and meat, prior to the widespread advent of refrigeration. With such refrigeration available there has been decreasing use of nitrate as a food additive and a tendency to its complete elimination from foods. Nitrates from fertilizer and soil offer a potential risk since they are ingested in agricultural products and well water. Approximately 86 per cent of ingested nitrate in the American diet derives from vegetables.[105] Such nitrate is reduced to nitrite by various microbial species during storage of foods at room temperature but not in the refrigerator.[58] Normal oral microbial flora in man can reduce nitrate to nitrite-producing levels as high as 6 to 10 ppm in the saliva of some individuals.[106] About 78.6 per cent of "ingested" nitrite arises from saliva as a result of this conversion and 21.2 per cent from cured meats in the American diet.[105] Increasing nitrate intake leads to marked increase in salivary nitrite within 90 minutes.[105a] Studies in Chile[107] and Colombia[108] show a strong positive correlation between the amount of nitrate fertilizer or intake of nitrate and gastric cancer incidence. It is well established that patients with pernicious anemia have an increased incidence of gastric cancer. It has been found that mean nitrite concentration in the gastric juice of such patients is nearly 50 times that of age-matched normal controls.[109] The number of bacteria in the gastric juice of patients with pernicious anemia was also greatly increased. In vitro studies suggest increased formation of nitrosamines under these conditions.

There is evidence that nitrite and nitrate are formed de novo in the human intestine.[109a] Absorbed nitrite is rapidly destroyed in the blood but nitrate is recycled into saliva, the stomach and the bladder.

Nitrite is used to preserve meats and fish in order to inhibit the spores of Clostridium botulinum with 150 to 200 ppm nitrite.[110] The levels of nitrite decline rapidly from the time of processing of meats until levels are no higher than 10 to 20 ppm at the time of food ingestion.[58,110] Nitrite in beans and cabbage products do not decline with storage.[58] There is recent evidence that nitrites added to food or water increase the incidence of lymphomas in rats.[54a] Thus, while the evidence for a causative effect of nitrites for cancer induction in man is circumstantial, the associations mentioned suggest that efforts be made to reduce nitrite and nitrate intake.

Foods are complex chemical mixtures with many, quantitatively minor, constituents, some of which may increase or decrease nitroso compound formation.[110] Ascorbate or erythorbate, phenolic compounds in curing smoke, gallic acid, cysteine and sodium sulfite block nitrosation.[110] The use of ascorbate and other agents in foods or diet to combine with nitrite, reduction of the amounts of nitrate and nitrite in foods and prevention of nitrate conversion to nitrite by refrigeration of food are practical measures which minimize nitrite intake and activity.[58]

Colon Cancer

Although older vital statistics included carcinoma of the sigmoid with that of the rectum and combined nonrectal colon cancer with that of the small intestine, it is now apparent that there is a heterogeneity in the frequency among populations of cancer in different parts of the colon.[111-113] More recent observations give specific data on occurrence in the cecum and ascending colon, transverse colon, descending colon, sigmoid colon (these sites are included in the term colon) and the rectum (up to 8 cm from the anus).[113] There is proportionately a greater incidence of left-sided colon (rectal) cancer in lower-risk population groups and an increase in the remainder of the colon in higher-risk groups. Carcinomas of the small intestine are relatively uncommon. When intestinal (e.g. colon) and rectal cancers are considered together, they are the most frequently diagnosed primary cancers in the United States.[101] Hence, there is increasing attention to these cancers in terms of early diagnosis and efforts at prevention. Colon cancer appears to be increasing slightly in white males, more so in nonwhite males, decreasing in white females and increasing in

nonwhite females, whereas rectal cancer is decreasing for all females and white males and increasing for nonwhite males.[101] The overall trend in the United States is shown in Figure 38–1. Death rates for cancer of the large bowel in a number of countries have a strong negative correlation with those of gastric cancer. However, there are a number of countries where there is a relatively low risk for both types.[112]

Colon cancer has an appreciably higher incidence in economically developed countries, with the outstanding exception of Japan and, to a lesser degree, Finland.[111,112] Despite this, no socioeconomic gradient has been found by *intra*population comparisons in the United States and western Europe. However, a study in Cali, Colombia, indicated a fourfold excess risk in upper classes in both sexes.[114] Colon cancer has been infrequent in Japan in the past but is now on the increase, with the ratio of incidence of colon to rectal cancer (C/R ratio) continuously increasing in males and females on logarithmic slopes similar to sex differences in the white population of the United States but with an estimated 60-year time difference.[102] The C/R ratio has an inverse association with the quantity of rice ingested per day.

The association of incidence with environment has been strengthened by observed changes following migration from a country of low risk to one of high risk. A striking example is the progressive increase in mortality from colon cancer in Japanese born and living in Japan, those migrating to Hawaii (Issei) and those of Japanese descent born in Hawaii (Nisei).[113] Figure 38–2 depicts differences in incidence rates for colon cancer in Japanese in Japan and Hawaii. Similar trends have been noted in Japanese in California and Puerto Ricans living in the island as compared to those in the continental United States. Contrary to the decline in gastric cancer, which does not express itself clearly until the first generation born to immigrants from high-risk areas, the in-

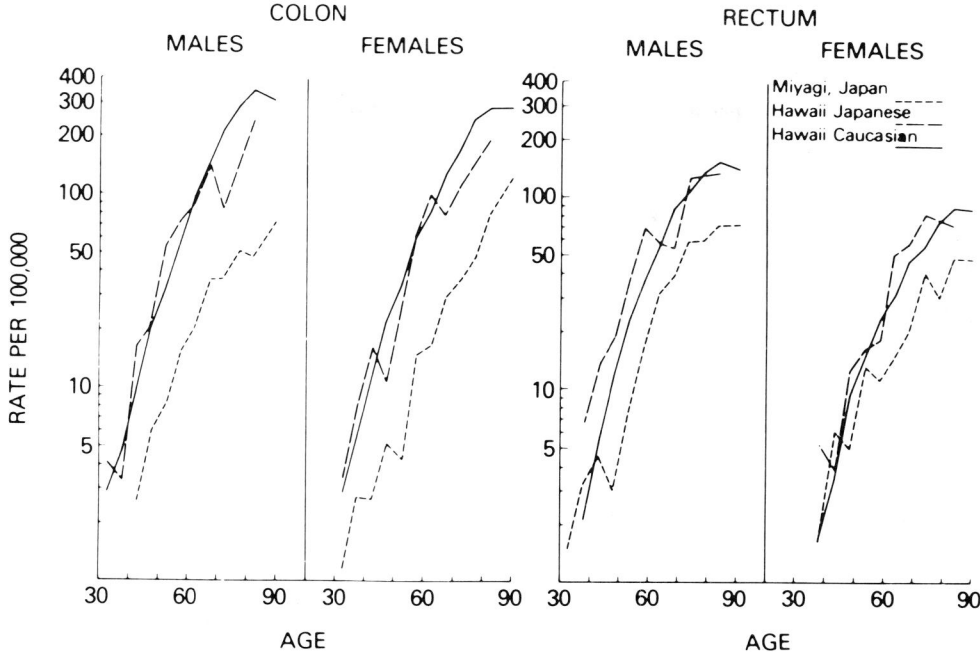

COLON

MALES   FEMALES

RECTUM

MALES   FEMALES

Miyagi, Japan
Hawaii Japanese
Hawaii Caucasian

RATE PER 100,000

AGE   AGE

Fig. 38–2. Incidence rates for cancer of the colon and rectum, by sex and age, for residents of Miyagi, Japan, 1968–1971 and for Japanese and Caucasians in Hawaii 1968–1972. (From Correa and Haenszel.[113])

crease in large-bowel cancer is seen in the immigrant generation. This indicates a strong environmental influence expressing itself clearly in a matter of about 10 years.

The strong environmental association has led to an increasing number of epidemiologic and experimental studies of dietary and nutritional influences. Wynder and associates have emphasized the worldwide correlation of colon cancer incidence, fat consumption and myocardial infarction.[111,115] Positive correlations with animal protein consumption[116] and with both animal fat and protein[117] have been reported. Armstrong and Doll found that the environmental variables most highly correlated with colon cancer rates are meat and animal protein consumption; the simple correlation coefficients were 0.85 and 0.89 for meat for male and female incidence, respectively, and 0.74 and 0.78 for total fat.[103] However, control of other vari-

ables reduced the correlation coefficient for total fat to 0.11 to 0.24, but no other variable reduced the correlation between meat consumption and incidence rate to less than 0.70. Similar strong epidemiologic correlations with meat, in particular beef, have been made.[118] Food consumption patterns are such, of course, that meat, animal protein and fat consumption are highly correlated with one another.

Data exist for regional differences in the United States for both sexes and among races. There is a striking north-south differential, with higher mortality rates throughout the northeast and lower rates in the south. High rates are associated with urbanization and the proportion of residents of Irish, German or Czech descent.[119] Although differential beef consumption between north and south has been noted,[118,120] it has been pointed out that the reported dietary differences were not large in 1966; however, they may have been greater in previous years.[118] Beef consumption is lower in the northeastern than in the central or western states where colon cancer rates are not especially high.[119] Although mortality from colon cancer is appreciably lower among both Mormons and non-Mormons in Utah than for the United States as a whole, a preliminary dietary survey found little difference in meat, fat and fiber consumption.[119a]

Enstrom has taken strong exception to the hypothesis that beef and fat consumption is involved in the etiology of colorectal cancer in the United States on the basis of his review of incidence and mortality trends in relation to socioeconomic, education, urban-rural and geographic differences in such consumption.[120] A similar exception has been taken to the claims for a positive correlation between the intake of animal fat and cancer with presentation of data indicating a negative or no correlation for animal fat but positive correlations with total fat and with vegetable fat.[121] The authors suggest that *trans* fatty acids may be exerting a metabolic role. The "fat hypothesis" will also need modification to take into account certain notable exceptions, e.g. the relatively low incidence of colon cancer in Finland despite the high fat intake.

It has been noted[103,121] that most of the epidemiologic studies which have compared cancer cases with controls have failed to demonstrate a clear association between colorectal cancer and meat or fat consumption, with the exception of the study indicating a positive association with beef (and bean) consumption in Hawaiian Japanese.[122] The latter are exceptional in having a considerable dietary heterogeneity based on previous practices and generation differences.

Assuming that fat is an etiologic factor, what is the metabolic action(s) which could induce malignancy? An hypothesis has been advanced to the effect that "western" types of diets have two complementary effects: (1) they increase bile secretion and (2) they induce a type of colon flora with an increase of anaerobes and the presence of certain strains of clostridia capable of converting bile acids by dehydrogenation into actual or potential carcinogens.[123-125] Significant differences have been reported in fecal flora between high- and low-risk groups subsisting on western or vegetarian types of diets[126-128] and the content of fecal sterols.[128,129] Similar changes have been noted in volunteers alternating from high-meat to low-meat diets.[130] Comparison of patients with colon cancer with controls indicated that the former had an increased amount of fecal bile acids[131,132] and dehydrogenating clostridia[131] and increased fecal bacterial 7-α-dehydroxylation of primary bile acids as compared to controls.[132] However, there are also reports which indicate only relatively few or no statistically significant differences in fecal flora in studies of individuals on Japanese and western diets,[133] between Seventh-Day Adventists (who abstain from smoking and drinking nor commonly use coffee, tea and certain condiments and 50 per cent of whom follow lacto-ovovegetarian diets[134]) who were strict vegetarians and those individuals on a usual American diet[135] or between vegetarian and nonvegetarian Seventh-Day Adventists.[136] Rotations of volunteers to normal-, low- and high-meat diets were associated with relatively minor changes in fecal flora.[137]

The fecal flora of man include a very large number of species, and a serious approach to quantitative analysis requires precise and sophisticated methods of collection and bacteriologic study. The most detailed studies of which the author is aware are those of Finegold and associates. In one study[136] approximately 150 different fecal bacterial species or subspecies were recovered. The authors compared four different diet groups and have reported several striking differences, e.g. fusobacterium and Clostridium perfringens counts were very low in the Adventists but lactobacillus counts were distinctly higher in that population. In comparing types of fecal flora between population groups at high or low risk for colon cancer, significant differences were found for 21 organisms or groups of organisms, 16 of which were obligate anaerobes. The clinical significance of these differences remains to be proven.

Decreased amounts of bile acids and their degradation products have been reported in Seventh-Day Adventists and recent Japanese migrants on Japanese types of diets as compared to individuals on typical American diets[128] and there are some data suggesting a positive association with past use of meat.[134] However, about one-fourth of the individuals on conventional American diets have been found to have a low conversion of cholesterol, with no differences observed between those with multiple adenomatous polyps and those who were polyp free.[138] No differences were noted in cancer mortality between Seventh-Day Adventist and non-Seventh-Day Adventist physicians, thus suggesting the role of selection factors.[134]

Regardless of changes in type of flora, it is possible that the potentially adverse metabolic activities of the flora are increased on western diets. It is also possible that certain bile acids, per se, present in increased amounts on such diets directly affect colonic mucosal function and lead to polypoid and malignant changes. Further research should clarify the etiologic pertinence of these many postulated factors.

"Fiber." Another hypothesis which has aroused interest and has led to active experimentation suggests an inverse relation between intake of nondigestible polysaccharides ("fiber") and large-bowel cancer.[139,140] As originally proposed the fiber theory postulated that a high-fiber diet results in a more rapid transit of food and other substances through the intestines and that the decreased transit time minimized opportunities for gut bacteria to produce carcinogens and also reduced

the chance for carcinogen-mucosal cell interaction; therefore populations living primarily on foods of vegetable origin with a relatively high fiber content should have a low incidence of colon cancer, while those ingesting foods which have a high content of refined or nonvegetable-derived foods should have a high incidence.

Fiber is not a single chemical substance but includes a variety of nonabsorbable polysaccharides and lignin entering the diet as part of cereals, fruits and vegetables; this aspect is discussed briefly in Chapter 4 and in detail by Southgate.[141] A western type of diet often includes a significant amount of fiber from vegetables and fruits; although the origins of the fiber are different, the amounts are not necessarily less than in a diet high in cereals and legumes. Glober et al. have noted that Japanese migrants in Hawaii who change to a western diet actually increase their total fiber intake.[141]

How do the postulates of the fiber hypothesis hold up in epidemiologic investigation? Contrary to the early claims[139,140] for a decreased transit time with increased fiber intake, others have found variable results depending on previous transit times of individuals,[143] no effect[144] or decreased transit times of individuals[145,146] when the same individuals acted as their controls. The transit time hypothesis is also challenged by the studies of Glober et al. who noted that Hawaiian-Japanese (both Issei and Nisei) had bowel transit times which were shorter than those of Caucasians of the same age.[142] On the basis of the original Burkitt hypothesis, the more traditional Issei should have had faster transit than the Nisei. In another study, Hawaiian-Japanese had transit times similar to Japanese in Japan although the risk of colon cancer is appreciably higher in the former. Both these groups had much shorter transit times than Caucasian-Hawaiians. Both Hawaiian groups had appreciably smaller stool weights than the Japanese in Japan.[147] There was no difference in mouth-anus transit time of food between population samples in Denmark and Finland despite a fourfold variation in colon cancer incidence. Although there were higher intakes of milk and fiber and lower consumption of meat in low-incidence areas of Finland, the data suggest that the etiology of colon cancer is not associated in a simple manner with dietary fat, neutral steroids, acid steroids or their bacterial metabolites.[148]

In the epidemiologic study of Armstrong and Doll,[103] the negative correlation of colon cancer with cereal consumption is accounted for by the positive association of the disease with meat. No relationship was observed between colon cancer and the total availability of crude fiber[117] but separation of fiber sources indicates a small (r = 0.30) but significant negative correlation.[149] In a case-controlled dietary study in Tel Aviv, Israel, of patients with cancer of the colon compared with neighbors and with hospitalized surgical patients (the latter without cancer), it was found that there was a significantly lower consumption of fiber-containing foods. However, the data reveal that in 80 of the patient-neighbor matched pairs the patient had a higher fiber intake, while in 114 pairs intake of the patient was less.[150] A case-controlled study in Japanese-Hawaiians revealed a positive association with the fiber-containing legumes, especially string beans.[122] As noted early, no correlation was found with fiber (and fat and meat) with decreased colon cancer of Utah residents despite a much lower colon incidence than that of the United States as a whole.[119a]

Certain fibrous materials, such as bagasse and bran, dilute fecal steroids and bagasse binds acid steroids. Increased fiber intake also increases fecal loss of acid steroids[124] and bile salts.[151] Thus, increased fiber intake may play a complementary role with a low-fat diet in reducing steroids in the colon available for modifica-tion. An extensive consideration of multiple aspects of dietary fiber has been published.[152]

The effects of fiber have been tested using rat models with dimethylhydrazine (DMH) as the carcinogen with some divergent results presumably due to differences in the fiber source, diets and levels of carcinogen. Ordinary wheat bran at high levels decreased the number of DMH-induced colon tumors in several studies[152a,152b] but not of duodenal tumors.[152b] At levels of 4.8 and 20 per cent dietary bran failed to modify colon cancer incidence or mortality as against no fiber in DMH-treated rats observed for one year.[152c] High levels of refined cellulose did not significantly decrease the numbers of DMH-induced colon tumors but did reduce the incidence of tumors of the small intestine.[152d]

A detailed list of the types of fiber products with their composition and suppliers has been published.[152e]

"Prudent" Diet. The reported epidemiologic correlations between fat and meat consumption and colon cancer have led to a recommendation for increased consumption of a "prudent diet" similar to that recommended many years ago by Jolliffe for prevention of atherosclerosis. Such a diet involves moderate restriction of calories and animal fat and a higher ratio of polyunsaturated to saturated fat.[111] One can justifiably take the position that the relation of specific dietary components to cancer of the colon is unsettled at present. However, the impressive progressive decline in deaths from myocardial infarction since 1963 provides a potent argument for the type of dietary recommendations incorporated in the prudent diet.[152f]

Hormone-dependent Cancers

These include malignancies of the breast, uterine corpus, testis, ovary, prostate and thyroid. The relation of cancer of the thyroid to iodide deficiency is well established and will not be discussed here. There is a fairly good correlation in many but not all areas between the incidence rates for bowel cancer and those for breast, uterine corpus, ovarian, testicular and prostatic cancers in declining order.[153] As with large-bowel cancer, a shift in breast cancer incidence to the pattern of the host country has been shown for Poles migrating to the United States[154] and Australia[155] and for Japanese resident in the United States.[156,157] As with the reverse trends in gastric cancer, these changes manifest themselves clearly in the children of the migrants, suggesting that environmental effects are playing a key role in relatively early life. In the case of breast cancer, this would be the time of puberty and breast development. There is increasing evidence of the importance of this period in influencing the risk of breast cancer.[153,158]

There is a high correlation between fat consumption and mortality data, not only for breast cancer[103,117,159,160] but also for those of the corpus uteri, ovary, prostate and testis.[103] The positive fat correlation for bowel- and endocrine-dependent tumors must be viewed in the context of socioeconomic factors, the type of fats consumed,[121] the adequacy of the dietary surveys, body stature and genetic differences. For example, up to the time of menopause age-specific rates for female breast cancer in American and Japanese women are fairly comparable—with some shift upward in age for the Japanese—despite marked differences in intakes of animal protein, fat and carbohydrates.[158] After menopause, differences appear with major increases occurring in American women and an abrupt leveling off in the Japanese. The Netherlands and Finland have a fairly similar per capita daily animal fat consumption but breast and colon cancer rates in the Netherlands are almost twice those of Finland. In addition to the animal fat consumed, the Dutch consume four times as much vegetable fats as the Finns (53 versus 13 gm).[121]

Weight and height differences among women 45 to 50 years and older with breast cancer in two Dutch cities and Aichi prefecture, Japan, suggest that approximately 50 per cent of the differences in incidence are attributable to differences in body weight and height.[161] Similar differences for postmenopausal women hold when cancer incidence is plotted against surface area. Overweight (excessive weight for a given height) was not deemed a risk factor in this study. This aspect of nutrition may explain the rise in breast cancer incidence noted in Japanese-Americans in the United States, which was also associated with increasing body weight and height following migration.[162] The association between breast cancer incidence and height and weight has not been noted in white women in North America.[158]

An area in which nutrition may play an important role in the development of breast cancer is in its modification of hormones. It is well established that thyroid, adrenal, ovarian and hypothalamopituitary activity can be altered by dietary modifications.[163] Can changes in the types of foods and percentages of major nutrients modify hormone profiles in various population groups? Evidence is accumulating that they can. Endocrine profiles of young Japanese women living in Hawaii have become more similar to those of Caucasian women than to those of women in Japan.[164] Premenopausal Japanese women have a higher level of estradiol than do Caucasian women; postmenopausal women have similar estradiol levels but the androstenedione and testosterone levels are significantly lower in the Japanese women.[158] Recent studies in prolactin levels indicate that volunteers on a western type of diet have higher levels than a similar group on a vegetarian diet, with the major difference occurring during deep sleep.[165]

Mention has been made of the role of fat in increasing susceptibility to carcinogen-induced colon cancer in experimental animals. Similar effects have been noted with respect to breast cancer.[34] As noted earlier, the enhancing effect appears to be related not only to the quantity of fat ingested but also to the type. The effect is greater when fat is given after carcinogen administration than before.[37]

Carcinoma of the corpus uteri is highly correlated with total fat consumption in statistics from 23 countries, being lowest in Japan and Nigeria and highest in the United States, Canada, New Zealand and western Europe.[103] A number of reports have associated obesity with this cancer.[103] There is also a relationship with infertility.[166] As with breast cancer, nutritional-endocrine interrelations are probably important but factual data are lacking.

Liver

Primary hepatic carcinoma is a major problem in certain population groups, especially males, in Africa, South China, Hawaii, Rumania and elsewhere.[98,167,168] In sub-Saharal Africa this is the most common of all forms of cancer, representing 10 to 30 per cent of all male tumors in most series.[98] In Bantu males in Laurenco Marques, Mozambique, it accounts for two-thirds of tumors in men (sex ratio about 3.4 to 1), with a rate approximately 500 times that observed in the United States in the 24- to 34-year age group.[169] In the United States the overall rate is about 2.4 per 100,000;[169] black males have a higher rate than white males but the rate in females of both races is about the same.[168] The variation in liver cancer is confined primarily to tumors of the hepatocytes, adenocarcinoma remaining constant except in areas in Asia where infection with Clonorchis sinesis is common.[169] It has been suggested that the high frequency in Africa and Asia is the result of a high proportion of cirrhotic livers developing neoplastic changes and that a similar trend is occurring elsewhere.[169] Although fatty liver is a common finding in protein-calorie malnutrition in children in areas where primary liver cancer is common, there is no good evidence suggesting a causal relation between the two occurrences.[169]

The carcinogenic properties of aflatoxins in many species—both accidentally and experimentally exposed—focused attention on those mycotoxins elaborated by the fungus Aspergillus flavus. Liver cancer has now been produced in a monkey after a number of years of exposure to aflatoxin B_1.[170] Various field studies have associated the incidence of liver cancer to the presence of aflatoxin in the food supply in African countries and Thailand.[171,172] There is as yet no direct evidence of a causative relation but the statistical associations are impressive. The aflatoxin studies do not explain satisfactorily the preponderance of male victims; however, males may convert aflatoxin to the ultimate carcinogen more efficiently than do females. Risk of exposure to aflatoxins is much less in technologically developed countries than in developing areas as the result of various procedures which reduce contamination of food at various stages of growth, storage and processing.

An additional factor in the development of liver cancer is viral hepatitis, inasmuch as large segments of the population in Asia and Africa are infected with hepatitis B virus. In these areas the infection is contracted at an early age, often at birth.[171] In a general population about 15 per cent of those infected develop chronic persistent hepatitis which appears to clear spontaneously, but about 5 per cent develop chronic active hepatitis and about one-half of these develop cirrhosis. The carrier state and infection affect males more frequently than females. As noted above, the incidence of primary liver cancer is generally much higher in cirrhotic individuals. The relation between hepatitis B infection and primary hepatocellular carcinoma has now been observed in a European-Caucasian (Greek) population with different racial, environmental and dietary circumstances than exist in Asia and Africa.[171a] This strengthens the belief in a significant influence of the viral infection.

NUTRITIONAL EFFECTS INDUCED BY CANCER

General Systemic Effects

A striking and presently unexplained effect of active neoplastic disease in a significant number of patients is the marked anorexia and wasting ("cancer cachexia") not directly attributable to obvious intestinal obstruction, sepsis, endocrine disorder or other causative anatomic lesions. Such observations have led to the belief that the disease process is capable of inducing profound alterations in the metabolism of the host.

Although anorexia is not unique to cancer, its high incidence, prolonged duration and deleterious effect make it of special concern. It is manifested most commonly and noticeably in patients with cancer in one or more areas of the alimentary tract, including the liver and pancreas,[173] and in those with widely disseminated disease. Its onset may be insidious and unaccompanied by manifestations of disease other than progressive weight loss. It is a dictum of medicine that a patient with an unexplained weight loss should undergo a thorough search for an occult neoplasm.

The degree of anorexia may range from mild to severe. Its etiology is uncertain although it and the weight loss seen in cancer have been the subject of many publications and conferences.[174-177] In many discussions anorexia and weight loss are linked. Obviously, impairment of food intake will lead to weight loss. However, as stated in the opening paragraph of this section, there is a common belief that other factors affect metabolism and accentuate weight loss. Anorexia and/or weight loss have been variably attributed to (1) development of a toxic factor by the tumor, although none has ever been identified, (2) abnormalities of hypothalamic control, although current and still fragmentary evidence is not positive,[177] (3) psychologic factors[178]—there is no question that fear of the disease and various accentuating diagnostic and intervention procedures often adversely affect appetite, although this does not explain initial anorexia and weight loss in undiagnosed patients nor their persistence with time as the patient's psychologic stress abates, (4) taste changes[176,179] and (5) metabolic changes.

The weight loss experienced by many cancer patients is for the most part attributable to inadequate food intake resulting from anorexia. It is common for such patients to ingest breakfast fairly well and then to eat progressively less of succeeding meals over the day. Often the anorexia is associated with alterations in taste and patients are prone to ascribe diminished appetite to the unpleasant taste of one or more foods. Efforts have been made to begin to dissect out the prevalence and types of taste alterations in cancer patients.[176,179] However, it is the opinion of this author that available data must be viewed as preliminary and variable to the point of being of questionable value. More precise studies are essential before we can establish the patterns (if any) that occur in relation to the type and stage of various malignancies. Efforts in this direction must take into account the complexities of neurophysiology and methodology inherent in this area.[180] Alterations in taste are probably not primary factors in anorexia but are associated with more basic changes initiated by tumors in association with psychosomatic factors.

It has been suggested by various investigators that cancer per se—apart from depressed food intake—alters energy metabolism so that requirements are increased beyond those of normal individuals of otherwise similar status. Possible mechanisms would be increased basal and resting metabolic rates as the result of modification of metabolism of fuel sources, the effects of variation in body organ size in relation to total body weight and changes in the rate of significant processes in energy expenditure (e.g. protein turnover and ion pumping).

More than a century ago Pettenkofer and Voit reported high energy production in a leukemic patient. Young[181] has reviewed eight reports published between 1922 and 1974 on the basal metabolic rate of cancer patients. The results were variable, the cases were relatively few and the available information was limited; however, the majority indicated a tendency toward elevation especially in patients with leukemia and Hodgkin's disease. Methodologic problems remain to be evaluated; for example, the reliability of the indirect method of Newburgh-Johnson used by some investigators for estimating caloric expenditure does not appear to have been tested for validity in cancer patients. A more recent study reported on 10 hospitalized afebrile cancer patients varying in the types of malignancy and degree of extension. Energy expenditure was calculated from continuous heart rate recordings and from oxygen consumption; the data were compared to the findings in control patients of similar age with nonmalignant diseases affecting physical activities to about the same extent.[182] The cancer patients were below normal in body weight and body cell mass. Although varying greatly, energy intake (mean 1,270 kcal per day) was not significantly different from that of the controls (mean 1,470 kcal per day). Both the daily energy expenditure (mean 2,020 kcal per 24 hr) and the resting metabolic rate (mean 1,630 kcal per 24 hr) were significantly greater in the cancer patients than in the controls (mean 1,420 and 1,170 kcal per 24 hr, respectively). Parallel to exacerbation of disease and reduced energy intake, energy expenditure and resting metabolic rate increased in relation to body cell mass in two patients. The variability of energy intake and expenditure of the cancer patients was great and there was a cluster of six cancer patients with expenditure similar to that of controls.

While more data are needed, there is reasonable evidence that some cancer patients do have increased resting metabolic expenditure occurring often in a setting of decreased energy intake. Obviously the anorexia is working against the nutritional interest of the patient by limiting caloric intake during a period of normal or increased expenditure. In the latter case, the patient is at increased risk of depletion during periods of impaired food intake.

Reports of energy expenditure in tumor-bearing animals are also variable, with some indicating increased expenditure[183,184] and another no consistent change in resting metabolism.[185]

A number of metabolic changes which may occur in cancer patients can modify energy expenditure. Fever, surgery and other causes of stress with increased corticosteroid and catecholamine production are not uncommon, and these increase protein catabolism with increased gluconeogenesis.[181] However, apart from such known stimulatory effects on energy requirements, consideration must be given to the effects of the malignancy, per se, on metabolic changes. It is well established that tumors have a high rate of anaerobic glycolysis with production of lactic acid. The metabolic cycle involving conversion of glucose to lactate and its resynthesis to glucose is termed the Cori cycle. It has been proposed that the increased rate of resynthesis of glucose in the liver from lactate produced by the tumor results in a significant energy drain on host tissues.[186] Cori cycle activity has been measured in a heterogeneous group of patients with metastatic carcinoma and found to be increased in those with progressive weight loss.[187] It has been pointed out, however, that increased Cori cycle activity does not appear to account for a significant fraction of daily energy expenditure.[181]

Under basal conditions the rates of glucose and free fatty acid oxidation and total CO_2 production in five patients with metastatic cancer did not differ appreciably from those of control subjects.[188] However, when a glucose load was given, oxidation of free fatty acids was suppressed to a lesser degree in cancer patients; in addition their rate of slow pool glucose oxidation was depressed, as was CO_2 production from nonglucose sources. If applicable to other cancer patients these findings would suggest increased energy cost as the result of increased conversion of glucose to fat before being metabolized.

Studies with isotopically labeled amino acids in experimental animals have demonstrated the marked capacity of tumor tissue for protein synthesis; the labeled amino acids tended to stay in the tumor, in contrast to their turnover in certain normal tissues.[189] It has also been demonstrated that various rapidly growing transplanted rodent tumors developed at the expense of host tissues; some obtained enough nitrogen for growth from the host tissues when the diet contained very little nitrogenous substance.[189,190]

Starvation in the tumor-bearing rat decreased total body and liver weight but tumor weight increased over that of pre-fasting controls.[192] During starvation a transplanted sarcoma increased its specific DNA activity, whereas the specific activity decreased in liver DNA in both tumor- and nontumor-bearing animals.[193] These and other observations have given rise to the concept of the tumor as a "nitrogen trap," i.e. incorporation of amino acids into tumor is essentially a one-way passage from metabolic pool to the tumor.[193]

However, experimental tumors are not entirely autonomous, and, depending on their type and growth phase, are influenced both nutritionally and metabolically by the host; furthermore, an interchange of nitrogen between tumor and host may occur. With certain tumors, improved nutrition in terms of protein and calories favors the host in terms of weight and nitrogen content, even though the experimental tumor may also grow larger (vide infra). Eventually, however, circumstances develop when even forced feeding is unable to prevent loss of normal host tissues.[194] Goodlad has summarized these and other relationships between protein metabolism and the growth of experimental tumors.[195]

With reference to the anorexia developing in tumor-bearing animals, it has been found that Walker tumor transplanted in rats previously made hyperphagic by lesions in the ventromedial hypothalamus resulted in depression of food intake, indicating that this tumor effect is not mediated by this center.[196]

In addition to the deleterious effects which may result from the systemic effects of cancer, nutritional problems may also develop as the result of "localized" effects of tumor and as a consequence of one or more treatment modalities (vide infra). The nutritional result of the combination of problems is evident from the following data: In 222 adult inpatients not resident in intensive care units, surveyed over a brief period in a large cancer center, 37 per cent were found to have lost more than 10 per cent and about 25 per cent had lost more than 20 per cent of their normal body weight; very few had gained weight.[197] In another series 24.3 per cent of 457 adult cancer patients studied at the time of admission had lost more than 10 per cent of their previous body weight and 17.3 per cent had lost more than 20 per cent.[198] Since a significant percentage of those losing weight had accumulated some edema which was included in the body weight, there was a tendency to underestimate body weight loss. These hospitalized patients presented a cross section of individuals at various stages of disease, before, during and after one or more forms of treatment. In a series of 1,112 patients initially appearing with gastric carcinoma, 84 per cent had already experienced weight loss.[173] In two series of patients appearing with pancreatic carcinoma, weight loss had occurred in 67 and 73 per cent, respectively. Approximately 40 per cent of 129 patients with limited bronchogenic carcinoma had lost at least 6 per cent of body weight.[199] The malnutrition most commonly seen in such patients is primarily that of calorie insufficiency. As anorexia and weight loss progress, secondary deficiencies of protein, minerals and vitamins may occur together with other manifestations of increasing debilitation.[197]

Creamer suggested that malignancies external to the gastrointestinal tract induced an abnormal small intestinal mucosa to which he attributed some of the ill health and loss of weight in malignancy.[200] A number of papers followed which claimed to support or deny these findings.[173] In a more definitive study Barry showed that malnourished patients with extra-alimentary tract malignancies often had abnormalities of mucosal histology, epithelial cell loss and lactose utilization; however, he found that similar changes occurred in seriously malnourished patients without cancer and suggested that such mucosal changes are the *result* of malnutrition rather than the direct cause of cachexia or the direct effect of malignancies outside of the gastrointestinal tract.[201] Once present, of course, impaired mucosal function can contribute further to malnutrition by depressed efficiency of absorption.

"Localized" Tumor Effects

In addition to the systemic effects of cancer, a number of more localized effects of various neoplasms lead to nutritional problems. Some of these are listed in Table 38–1.

By far the most common causes of malnutrition in this general category are interferences with food intake as a result of partial or complete obstruction of some portion of the gastrointestinal tract. Relief of obstruction by surgical or other treat-

Table 38–1. Some Effects of Neoplastic Diseases on Nutritional Status

1. Malnutrition secondary to persistent anorexia.
2. Malnutrition associated with impaired food intake secondary to obstruction.
3. Malabsorption associated with:
   A. Deficiency of pancreatic enzymes or bile salts.
   B. Infiltration of small bowel by neoplasms, such as lymphoma or carcinoma.
   C. Fistulous bypass of small bowel.
   D. Gastric hypersecretion inhibiting pancreatic enzymes (in Zollinger-Ellison syndrome).
   E. Blind loop secondary to partial upper small bowel obstruction.
   F. Malnutrition—induced villous hypoplasia.
4. Protein-losing enteropathy (e.g. in gastric carcinoma, lymphoma or with lymphatic obstruction).
5. Electrolyte and fluid balance disturbances associated with:
   A. Persistent vomiting in obstruction.
   B. Vomiting secondary to increased intracranial pressure from tumors.
   C. Small-bowel fluid losses from fistula.
   D. Diarrhea associated with hormone-secreting tumors (e.g. carcinoid syndrome, Zollinger-Ellison syndrome, Verner-Morrison syndrome) and villous adenoma of the colon.
   E. Inappropriate antidiuretic hormone secretion associated with certain tumors.
   F. Hyperadrenalism secondary to excessive corticotropin or corticosteroid production by tumors.

ment is necessary. Nutrition support by intravenous alimentation or tube feeding into a site distal to the obstruction may be very useful in sustaining such patients until normal oral feedings can be reinstituted following effective surgical or other therapy.

Involvement of the pancreas, pancreatic duct or common bile duct may lead to impaired digestion and absorption of fats and fat-soluble vitamins. Decreased fat absorption is associated with increased fecal losses of calcium and magnesium.[202] In addition, proteins may be much less efficiently absorbed with serious pancreatic insufficiency. The use of parenteral vitamin K and other fat-soluble vitamins is often helpful in restoring the patient to the best possible nutritional state for surgical procedure in such situations. Pancreatic insufficiency may be associated with impaired vitamin B_{12} absorption.[203]

Association of Carcinoma and Intestinal Mucosal Abnormalities. Bossak et al.[204] reviewed 94 patients with celiac disease (gluten enteropathy, nontropical sprue), 5 of whom had intestinal carcinomas. Harris et al.[205] reported 202 patients with adult celiac disease or sprue of whom 14 had carcinomas of the alimentary tract, 6 in the esophagus. Eighteen of 26 patients with such cancers were males. Various hypotheses have been suggested for the carcinomatous involvement in these patients, including possibilities that the abnormal small-bowel epithelium permits increased absorption of carcinogens, that the chronic inflammation of the lamina propria or lymphoid hyperactivity somehow plays a role or that environmental factors such as prolonged nutritional deficiency secondary to malabsorption or intestinal organisms may account for the malignant changes.

Celiac Syndrome and Intestinal Lymphomas. Prior to 1962 steatorrhea in lymphomatous patients was considered to be the consequence of mesenteric lymphoma causing obstruction of lymphatic flow or of diffuse lymphomatous infiltration of the small bowel. In 1962 Gough et al.[206] advanced the hypothesis that small-bowel reticulosis may develop as a complication in patients with celiac syndrome. Austed et al.[207] found a 10 per cent incidence of lymphoma in their celiac patients. Benson et al.[208] reported an incidence of 6.2 per cent, and Harris et al.[205] reported an incidence of 6.9 per cent (with a similar incidence of carcinoma in their series of 202 patients). Nine of the 14 patients of Harris et al.[205] had lymphoma involving the stomach, jejunum or ileum; 12 of the 14 had celiac disease diagnosed for more than 5 years (the average being 21 years for the group of 14). Of the 14, 4 had Hodgkin's disease without intestinal involvement. The others had reticulum cell sarcoma with the intestine involved in 8 patients. Many of the older studies had no histologic proof of villous atrophy by biopsy and the diagnosis of celiac syndrome was made by history or abnormal fat absorption and/or in response to gluten-free diets.

Lymphoma involving the small-bowel mesentery lymph nodes may appear as malabsorption.[209-211] Patients with abdominal lymphomas and malabsorption often exhibit abdominal pain, weight loss, anorexia and bulky stool suggestive of steatorrhea. They may have clubbing, glossitis, angular stomatitis and peripheral edema. Laboratory findings may include abnormal D-xylose absorption, flat glucose tolerance curves, hypoalbuminemia and fat and B_{12} malabsorption; megaloblastosis may be present. There may be deficits in fat-soluble vitamins. Folic acid deficiency may occur on occasion.[212] Because of this relationship lymphoma should be suspected with the onset of the celiac syndrome in middle age especially, but also in young people particularly with certain racial backgrounds.[210] Males above 40 years of age with long-standing celiac syndrome who are not eating a gluten-free diet are a major risk group.

Primary lymphomas originate in the intestinal tract in approximately 10 to 20 per cent of reported cases.[213] A majority of these tumors are lymphocytic lymphomas, with approximately 2[238] or 2.5 times as many[214] occurring in the stomach as in the small intestine. Disseminated lymphoma often secondarily involves one or more sites along the gastrointestinal tract; tumor, ulcerations, erosions and infection may occur with deleterious effects to the patient.[215]

The mechanisms for the development of malabsorption are several. The intestinal epithelium may be disrupted by the generalized villous atrophy found in association with lymphomatous involvement. Infiltration of the lamina propria and draining lymph nodes can lead to obstruction of mesenteric lymph channels and dilation of the lymphatics within the intestinal villi; this in turn can lead to development of a protein-losing enteropathy with hypoalbuminemia, hypoglobulinemia and lymphocytopenia.[215] Protein-losing enteropathy has also been described with cases of gastric carcinoma.[216]

The blind-loop syndrome in the upper small bowel secondary to partial obstruction with bacterial overgrowth may also result in steatorrhea and vitamin B_{12} deficiency. The blind-loop syndrome involves not only direct interaction of bacteria with certain nutrients but also the development of abnormalities of the intestinal epithelium to account for associated malabsorption.[217,217a]

Bypass of the small bowel as a result of gastrocolic and jejunocolic fistulas may also occur in the course of abdominal cancer, with significant malabsorption and electrolyte and fluid disturbances.

Nutritional replacement and support in such malabsorption syndromes are useful while direct antineoplastic treatment with surgery, radiation and chemotherapy are undertaken.

Ectopic Hormones. An area of expanding interest concerns the secretion by tumors of a variety of potent pharmacologic substances, including steroids, hormone polypeptides, kinins and prostaglandins.[218,219] A wide variety of nutritional-metabolic problems may develop in patients with such hormone-secreting neoplasia, some of which may produce more than one active agent. Diarrhea may occur with gastrin-secreting islet cell adenomas (Zollinger-Ellison syndrome),[220,220a] tumors, primarily of the pancreas (but also of bronchus and of the ganglia) which secrete vasoinhibitory peptide (VIP) and other hormones (Verner-Morrison syndrome or "pancreatic cholera"),[221,222] malignant carcinoma tumors of the intestine[223,224] and bronchus,[224] medullary carcinoma of the thyroid,[225] villous adenoma[225] and ganglioneuroma.[224] Losses of potassium and fluid with Verner-

Morrison syndrome and villous adenoma may be severe. Steatorrhea occurs in the Zollinger-Ellison syndrome; this has been attributed partly to inactivation of pancreatic lipase by excessive acid production in the stomach and partly to villous damage.[227] While the diarrhea of carcinoid is usually of the watery type, cases of steatorrhea have been reported.[228]

Hyponatremia, fluid retention and increased urinary sodium losses attributable to inappropriate antidiuretic hormone secretion have been described, most commonly in association with but not restricted to bronchogenic and oat cell carcinoma.[229] Medullary carcinoma of the thyroid gland (generally part of multiple endocrine adenomatosis, type III) secretes excessive amounts of calcitonin[230] as well as prostaglandins[225] and histamine[231] and may be associated with pheochromocytoma.[232] Calcitonin induces secretion of water and electrolytes by the jejunal mucosa, thereby explaining the diarrhea.[233] Calcitonin may result in hypocalcemia, but patients are usually normocalcemic probably because of stimulation of and increased secretion by the parathyroid gland.

There are reports of malabsorption and diarrhea occurring in patients with systemic mastocytosis, a disease associated with increased secretion of histamine from the mast cells.[234] Hypercalcemia resulting from parathormone excess or tumor-induced osteolysis induces anorexia in a significant percentage of patients. Hypercalcemia secondary to parathyroid-hormonelike substance occurs with a variety of tumors.[235] Electrolyte disturbances and increased nitrogen and calcium losses often occur in the hyperadrenal state, induced either by the secretion of adrenal cortical carcinoma or, less frequently, by corticotropin secreted by certain solid tumors, especially those in the lung.[236]

Fluid, Electrolyte and Other Changes. The major causes of fluid and electrolyte disturbances in cancer patients are vomiting and diarrhea secondary to partial or complete obstruction, and gastric and small-bowel fluid losses through a fistula. Losses of sodium, chloride, potassium, magnesium and zinc may be serious with large intestinal losses.

Fluid and electrolyte imbalances are often seen in patients with widespread hepatic metastases, ascites and liver failure, with cardiac metastases and failure, with metastatic ovarian carcinoma and ascites, with renal failure secondary to obstruction of the urinary tract by tumor, with obstruction of lymphatic or venous drainage in major areas and other situations listed in Table 38–1 and described above. Factitious hyperkalemia may be reported in patients with very high white counts as the result of cell breakdown in blood samples awaiting analysis.

Hypoalbuminemia and anemia are also frequently noted in advanced cancer cases. The depressed albumin levels are usually secondary to either (1) inability to produce sufficient albumin (as a result of serious protein-calorie deficiency, the metabolic effects of certain tumors or hepatic insufficiency secondary to parenchymal cell damage or replacement by tumor), (2) losses of albumin from the body in excess of synthetic capacity, e.g. protein-losing enteropathy or nephrotic syndrome and/or (3) dilution of albumin into abnormally large extracellular compartments (e.g. ascites and edema). Hypoalbuminemia will respond to appropriate nutritional therapy when malnutrition is the primary or an important contributory factor. Antitumor therapy is obviously indicated to treat the direct effects of neoplastic growth. The anemia may be secondary to insufficiency of hematopoietic nutritional factors and the etiology must be evaluated. A normochromic normocytic anemia is not infrequently associated with cancer and does not respond to nutritional factors. Radiation and chemotherapy may also be contributing factors.

Vitamins. Vitamin levels may be low in cancer patients. Undoubtedly, much of the depletion is secondary to poor intake, exacerbated in some by losses through abnormal alimentary tract and renal function.

Abnormalities in folate metabolism may occur in acute and chronic leukemias. Increased retention of this vitamin by such patients has been noted[237,238] in association with a tendency for increased vitamin content of leukocytes, especially in acute leukemias and chronic myeloid leukemia.[239] Patients with leukemias, disseminated lymphomas[240,241] and various metastatic carcinomas[242] tend to have low serum folate levels. It has been known for some time that serum vitamin B_{12} levels are elevated in certain leukemias[243,244] and in the presence of metastatic liver disease.[245] It is apparent that serum vitamin B_{12} as well as total and unsaturated B_{12} binding proteins tend to be increased in any situation with increased total body neutrophil pool with elevation in B_{12}-binding alpha-globulin. Furthermore, the dominant B_{12}-binding alpha-globulin in such myeloproliferative disorders does not release its bound vitamin to tissues, with the possibility of tissue depletion and biochemical abnormality.[246]

Abnormalities of vitamin B_6 and tryptophan metabolism in significant numbers of patients with Hodgkin's disease and in some with carcinoma of the breast and of the bladder have been reported,[247] with depressed plasma levels of pyridoxal phosphate in 8 of 14 untreated patients; 14 of 21 excreted increased quantities of at least one of the metabolic intermediates of tryptophan. The incidence of these abnormalities was correlated with the severity of the disease. The tests were normal in patients in remission after chemotherapy. All 8 patients with low pyridoxal phosphate were anergic. Pyridoxine administration raised the plasma pyridoxal phosphate but did not uniformly restore tryptophan metabolism to normal; this suggests that factors other than vitamin B_6 deficiency (perhaps increased secretion of corticosteroid) contribute to abnormal tryptophan metabolism.

Trace Elements. Increasing attention is being given to the trace-element status of cancer patients as the result of our improving understanding of their importance. The available data include serum and urinary levels and the tissue concentrations of various tumor types. The data are primarily those of the survey type, with little known of associated or etiologic factors. As with water-soluble vitamins, trace-element levels will reflect the intake, basic needs and losses. Impaired intake and/or increased excretion secondary to organ disease will lower serum values. Zinc losses are significant in small-bowel drainage and this is reflected in low serum levels. Failure to provide this and other essential trace elements in intravenous or tube feedings will exacerbate the problem. Since copper and manganese are dependent on bile secretion as a major avenue of elimination, increased levels of these elements occur with intrahepatic and extrahepatic biliary obstruction. Rapid tissue breakdown with chemotherapy or radiation will increase excretion and, in association with renal dysfunction, lead to rises in serum levels of those trace elements ordinarily excreted into the urine. Schwartz has reviewed the literature on serum, urine and tumor tissue trace element levels in various types of malignancies.[248]

Treatment

Reversal for any significant period of the undesirable metabolic and nutritional changes secondary to systemic and localized effects of cancer described depends primarily upon elimination of the malignancy entirely or in large part. The physician frequently faces the problem of having to correct significant malnutrition and fluid and electrolyte imbalances in patients requiring surgical procedures or in those who need to be maintained in the best possible state for as long as possible in order to permit a therapeutic trial of radia-

tion and/or chemotherapy. For such patients careful attention and a positive approach to correction of abnormalities are indicated. As with all chronic wasting diseases, one cannot and should not expect to restore significant amounts of tissue in a short period of time. Urgent surgical intervention cannot wait upon this goal of nutritional therapy. Correction of acute or chronic vitamin and mineral deficiencies, blood loss, and electrolyte and fluid imbalances can often be accomplished within a matter of days and this achievement improves the surgical risk. When operation is indicated for a debilitated patient and when there have been and are likely to be prolonged periods of little or no oral intake of food, an attempt to restore improved nutritional and metabolic status by adequate parenteral administration or tube feeding may be an aid to survival or to decreased morbidity and period of convalescence (cf Chapters 36 and 37).

NUTRITIONAL PROBLEMS ARISING FROM THE TREATMENT OF CANCER

Significant nutritional problems may arise as the result of the specific treatment given to control the neoplastic disease. This section discusses briefly some of the more common problems in this area (Table 38–2).

Radiation

A moving account by a physician relating her subjective reactions to the effects of destruction of the sense of taste following radiotherapy for cancer of the pharynx[249] serves to emphasize the need on the part of the attending physician to understand the profound psychologic, physiologic, and nutritional aftereffects which may occur with varied treatments.[250] The resulting loss of taste sensation ("mouth blindness") and xerostomia (dry mouth) consequent to decreased salivary secretion which makes chewing and swallowing difficult combine to create a potentially serious situation since "the patients are not hungry anyway,

Table 38–2. Consequences of Cancer Treatment Predisposing to Nutrition Problems

1. Radiation treatment.
    A. Radiation of oropharyngeal area.
        (1) Destruction of sense of taste; xerostomia and odynophagia; loss of teeth.
    B. Radiation to lower neck and mediastinum.
        (1) Esophagitis with dysphagia.
        (2) Fibrosis with esophageal stricture.
    C. Radiation of abdomen and pelvis.
        (1) Bowel damage, acute and chronic, with diarrhea, malabsorption, stenosis and obstruction, fistulization.
2. Surgical treatment.
    A. Radical resection of oropharyngeal area.
        (1) Chewing and swallowing difficulties.
        (2) Tube feeding possibly required.
    B. Esophagectomy and esophageal reconstruction.
        (1) Gastric stasis and hypochlorhydria secondary to vagotomy.
        (2) Steatorrhea.
        (3) Diarrhea.
    C. Gastrectomy (high subtotal or total)
        (1) Dumping syndrome.
        (2) Malabsorption.
        (3) Achlorhydria and lack of intrinsic factor.
        (4) Hypoglycemia.
    D. Intestinal resection.
        (1) Jejunum.
            (a) Decreased efficiency of absorption of many nutrients.
        (2) Ileum.
            (a) Vitamin B_{12} deficiency.
            (b) Bile salt losses with diarrhea.
            (c) Hyperoxaluria.
        (3) Massive bowel resection.
            (a) Life-threatening malabsorption.
            (b) Malnutrition.
            (c) Metabolic acidosis.
        (4) Ileostomy and colostomy.
            (a) Complications of salt and water balance.
    E. Blind-loop syndrome.
    F. Pancreatectomy.
        (1) Malabsorption.
        (2) Diabetes mellitus.
3. Chemotherapy treatment.
    A. Corticosteroids.
        (1) Fluid and electrolyte problems.
        (2) Nitrogen and calcium losses.
        (3) Hyperglycemia.
    B. Antimetabolites, alkylating agents and other drugs (see Table 38–3).

and it is easier to starve."[249] When all food becomes tasteless, appearance and aroma become much more important. Chewing and swallowing are assisted by use of gravies and salad dressings. Supplementary liquid formulas (see Appendix) improve total intake.

Radiation to the lower neck and the mediastinum may induce esophagitis after several weeks of therapy but this usually disappears following cessation of therapy. A delayed effect which may occur is fibrosis with esophageal stricture.

Radiation damage to small and large bowel occurs in a small but significant number of patients receiving external and/or internal radiation therapy.[250] The epithelium of the small bowel is second only to bone marrow in its sensitivity to radiation. Altered intestinal function may occur during therapy and usually disappears. In those in whom significant "late" radiation changes are developing, symptoms recur usually within the year, but sometimes not for 10 or more years. Flattening and ulceration of the mucosa, telangiectasis, fibrosis, endarteritis of small vessels and stenosis of the bowel develop and these changes are often progressive. Obstruction and fistula formation may occur and require bowel resection, which complicates preexisting diarrhea and malabsorption. While the damaged tissue may make operation more difficult, the obstructive symptoms are often remediable; consequently, exploratory laparotomy is recommended before malnutrition increases the risk. In our experience, patients with severe radiation damage and previous resection are more difficult to manage than patients with massive small-bowel resection alone. Intermittent obstruction, diarrhea, malabsorption and chronic intestinal and bladder blood loss create a multitude of problems in nutrition and electrolyte balance. However, with close follow-up and attention to nutritional requirements, these patients often do very well.

Surgery

The effects of ablative surgery may be varied and many. Most of these procedures and their sequelae are, of course, not peculiar to surgery for cancer. However, certain resections are much more common or limited almost entirely to patients with cancer (e.g. extensive resection of the head and neck, total esophagectomy or total gastrectomy).

Surgery of the Head and Neck. Radical surgery of the head and neck region, including partial or total glossectomy and/or mandibulectomy, often interferes with mastication and swallowing. With some training or with laryngectomy, which prevents aspiration of fluids and food, oral food intake is possible. In other cases, prolonged tube feeding may be required. Liquid diets are prepared by blending the types of food ordinarily consumed by the family, having made certain that the pattern is nutritious. Where the personal situation does not permit this, simple and inexpensive tube formulas may be used (see Appendix). Many elderly individuals do not tolerate large amounts of fluids. The composition of the formula should be modified as concomitant cardiovascular, renal or endocrine disease indicates. Attention should be paid to psychologic aspects of food with tube feedings, e.g. the aroma of a separate cup of coffee may be important. Patients can be taught to insert the nasopharyngeal tube themselves so that they avoid the psychologic trauma and throat irritation associated with an indwelling tube. For those unable to pass the tube, its insertion via an esophagostomy or gastrostomy is recommended (see Chapter 36).

Surgery of the Digestive Tract. Esophagectomy often induces significant malabsorption of fat.[251,252] The cause of this peculiar dysfunction appears to be the bilateral vagotomy inherent in the procedure; however, the precise intestinal mechanism causing the steatorrhea is unknown. The previously recognized sequelae of vagotomy—gastric stasis (necessitating a drainage procedure) and diarrhea—also occur in esophagectomized patients. Carbohydrate absorption is normal. The use of medium-chain triglycerides (MCT) as a major portion of fat intake diminishes the steatorrhea.[251] Cholestyramine has been reported to reduce postvagotomy diarrhea but supporting evidence is awaited.

Gastrectomy. The physiologic and nutritional consequences of subtotal and total gastrectomy have been reviewed in Chapter 31A and elsewhere.[253] It suffices to state here that clinical problems increase proportionately to the extent of the resection. In addition to the well-known occurrences of dumping syndrome, hypoglycemia, steatorrhea, afferent loop syndrome and loss of intrinsic factor, emphasis is needed on the long-term consequences of loss of the stomach with the insidious development of various vitamin and mineral deficiencies.[254-257] Serious and persistent attention by the physician to prevent these nutritional problems is essential for long-term health when the underlying disease leading to the need for operation is benign or malignancy has been eradicated.

Intestinal Resection. Clinical studies in normal subjects and in those with ablation of varying portions of small intestine indicate that all nutrients studied, with the exception of vitamin B_{12}, are most efficiently and (in the usual dietary amounts) rather completely absorbed in the proximal small bowel.[258,259] However, following jejunal resection, the ileum, with its reserve absorptive capacity, can absorb these nutrients in good degree if adequate nutritional status is maintained.

When the terminal ileum has been removed there will be poor absorption of both vitamin B_{12} and conjugated bile salts since this is the site of their physiologic absorption. Provision of vitamin B_{12} intramuscularly in doses of 100 μg every month or two will prevent the development of B_{12} deficiency.

Failure to reabsorb conjugated bile salts will result in one of several problems. If the ileal resection is not extensive (usually less than 100 cm[260]) sufficient bile salts enter the large bowel to induce a brown watery diarrhea which may be distressing to the patient. Cholestyramine may be dramatically effective in controlling such a choleric diarrhea by its mechanism of binding bile salts. The loss of bile salts as the result of ileal resection interrupts the normal enterohepatic circulation which efficiently retains and recirculates conjugated bile salts. The synthetic capacity of the liver to synthesize sufficient new bile salts is exceeded and the concentration of bile salts in the intestinal lumen becomes low, especially with successive meals. When the ileal resection is sufficiently greater (usually more than 100 cm), the luminal content of bile salts will fall below the critical level for formation of micelles; consequently, fat absorption will be depressed and steatorrhea will ensue.[260,261] In such a situation, the patient will be helped by the feeding of a diet low in long-chain fats and by the use of medium-chain triglycerides which do not require bile salts for their absorption. The use of water-soluble forms of vitamin K and more of the other fat-soluble vitamins is indicated to prevent deficiency of these nutrients. Sufficient polyunsaturated fats should be fed to assure adequate essential fatty acids.

Other consequences of ileal resection are hyperoxaluria and renal oxalate stone formation, explainable by the fact that the normal precipitation of oxalate ion by intestinal calcium ions is prevented by a shortage of such free calcium ions because of binding to fatty acids present in increased amounts in the remaining small bowel and colon by the steatorrheic ileectomized patients. The soluble oxalate is then absorbed in the colon and appears in the urine in increased concentrations, with resultant probability of precipitation as calcium oxalate in the renal tubule.[262,263] On the basis of this explanation a reduced fat intake appears advisable, together with an increased intake of calcium salts.

Massive small-bowel resection, with a residuum of three feet or less, presents serious and long-term problems in maintaining adequate nutrition, including water and electrolytes. If there is some radiation damage of remaining bowel or loss of the ileocecal valve and portions of the colon, the problems are intensified. However, the application of present knowledge with respect to care of these patients will often permit a successful outcome. These principles include the following:

1. The postoperative period is often a stormy one complicated by infection, ileus, and weight loss. During this period, it is essential that all factors tending to weight loss and malnutrition be combatted vigorously. This includes preparation at operation for long-term parenteral nutrition with sterile insertion of an indwelling central venous catheter for institution of total parenteral nutrition (cf Chapter 37) and the formation of a feeding gastrostomy for future use.

2. Absorptive capacity of many of these patients improves with time, so that patience and a carefully developed nutritional program designed to meet nutritional needs are essential.[264–267] As gastrointestinal function returns, special gastrostomy feedings can be initiated, utilizing round-the-clock feedings if indicated, with hydrolyzed protein or amino acids and other nutrients capable of rapid absorption. This route is increasingly utilized as conditions improve, to the point where IV feedings are discontinued and eventually oral intake, supplemented by gastrostomy feedings when necessary, commences. Protracted and meticulous follow-up care is essential with adequate provision at home—as in the hospital—of all necessary nutrients, including minerals and trace elements.

3. A marked reduction in the intake of long-chain fats reduces diarrhea and decreases fecal calcium, magnesium and other electrolyte losses.[268] The use of medium-chain triglycerides (MCT) in increasing amounts (as tolerated by the patient and consistent with an acceptable level of diarrhea) is often of value in increasing calories.[269] In significant amounts, this causes some ketosis and acidosis which may require additional sodium bicarbonate.[220]

4. The acidosis associated with malabsorption and diarrhea will tend to increase calcium and potassium losses in urine and should be watched for and treated on a continuing basis.

5. Persistent gastric hypersecretion may occasionally occur[271,272] and this possibility should be investigated. In our experience, it is rare. When it does occur, without spontaneous improvement, the use of an H_2 receptor antagonist is useful.

6. As noted above, vitamin B_{12} injections are to be given and dietary prescriptions made which minimize steatorrhea and hyperoxaluria.

7. The surgeon should retain the ileocecal valve whenever possible, since it appears to slow the exit of small-bowel contents and, hence, improves absorption and perhaps acts to hinder retrograde movement of colonic bacteria. The use of an antiperistaltic segment of bowel as a replacement for the valve has been recommended with varying enthusiasm.[272,273] The inherent danger posed by the possibility of sacrificing further absorptive surface in a patient with massive bowel resection and the danger of obstruction are, presumably, the reasons why this procedure is rarely reported as being performed now.

Ileostomy. This procedure is usually followed by large sodium and water losses but, within 7 to 10 days, these usually decrease to the range which will characterize the otherwise healthy individual on a stable diet. Generally, these stabilized individuals lose 300 to 600 ml of water daily, with 40 to 100 mEq of sodium and 2.5 to 10 mEq of potassium, emphasizing the physiologic role of the colon in absorbing water and sodium and in exchanging potassium for sodium. Gastroenteritis, partial intestinal obstruction and prolonged excessive sweating impose additional losses. Studies in man and in dogs during sodium depletion have demonstrated a reduction in sodium concentration of ileostomy material as depletion progressed, accompanied by increased potassium concentration.[274,275]

Pancreatectomy. This operation, with consequent loss of digestive enzymes, leads to loss into the stool not only of fats and protein but also of significant amounts of various vitamins and minerals. Pancreatectomy necessitates partial gastrectomy, a complicating factor. The situation is further complicated by the fact that despite subtotal pancreatectomy with anastomosis of the remaining portion of the pancreatic duct to the jejunum exocrine insufficiency occurs in a significant proportion of patients.[276] Total pancreatectomy, of course, induces diabetes mellitus in all. The diabetic state occurring in conjunction with impaired carbohydrate, protein and fat digestion further complicates the nutritional problems of such patients. The use of MCT and oligosaccharides may be beneficial.[276]

Pancreatic enzymes may be effectively replaced by potent pancreatic extracts given with meals or at 2-hr intervals. Recent evaluations have been made of various pancreatic extracts,[277,278] dosage schedules[279,280] and ancillary treatment such as antacids and an H_2 receptor antagonist.[281] Important factors are adequate dosage with meals and use of antacids or H_2 receptor antagonist when gastric secretion is normal or high, since the latter may inactivate the pancreatic enzymes. There may be impaired vitamin B_{12} absorption with pancreatectomy, improved by administration of pancreatic extract.[276,281] The diabetes mellitus following the resection is usually of the "brittle" type, requiring relatively small amounts of insulin, and is rather difficult to control with precision. Hence, tolerance of some glycosuria is safer than the hypoglycemic episodes which may occur with achievement of glucose-free urine.

Major Hepatic Resection. The liver has a remarkable ability to regenerate by cellular hypertrophy and hyperplasia following massive resection. Immediate postoperative problems are met by glucose and albumin infusions and adequate replacement of electrolytes including phosphate.[276]

Ureterosigmoidostomy. This procedure, which is now rarely performed, involved implantation of the ureters into the sigmoid colon following total cystectomy. It often led to significant disturbances in acid-base balance with development of a hyperchloremic acidosis, hypokalemia and hypophosphatemia.[282] These abnormalities occur much less commonly in patients with cutaneous *ureteroileostomy* (ileal conduit) which has replaced ureterosigmoidostomy.[283]

Chemotherapy

A relatively large number of antineoplastic agents have emerged in the last 30 years, the majority in the last 10 or so years. Although many of the current drugs were discovered empirically by animal testing against tumor models, more detailed biochemical study of their effects have yielded valuable information on the mechanisms by which many of these compounds affect cellular growth. This information has permitted a more rational therapeutic application of these agents singly and in combination. As a result of this new drug development and use, significant and, in some cases, dramatic improvement in the treatment of various forms of malignancy has occurred. Most of the present chemotherapeutic agents, aside from hormones, inhibit one or more key steps in the intermediary metabolism of cells—normal as well as neoplastic—particularly those reactions involving the synthesis of purines,

pyrimidines, DNA and RNA.[284] Since the epithelial cells of the small intestine have a relatively rapid turnover, it is to be expected that many of these drugs will adversely affect intestinal functions to a degree, depending upon the drug dosage, the duration of treatment, the rates of metabolism and individual susceptibility. The epithelium of the mouth and large bowel can also be affected, as can other organs.

Morphologic lesions and defective absorption have been described following treatment with a folic acid antagonist (e.g. methotrexate) of experimental animals[285,286] and man.[287] Pyrimidine analogs (e.g. 5-fluorouracil) exert a marked effect on the gastrointestinal mucosa of experimental animals[288] and similar effects may be seen in man at higher doses. The antibiotic actinomycin-D (Dactinomycin) also induces marked gastrointestinal changes; malabsorption of fat and other nutrients has been observed in rats following its administration.[289] Another antibiotic, bleomycin, may cause significant mucositis. The Vinca alkaloid vincistine has a neurologic effect which may lead to severe and obstructive constipation with prolonged administration. The enzyme asparaginase has relatively little effect on the mucosa of the intestines but may be toxic to liver, pancreas and kidneys. Many of these drugs induce anorexia, nausea and vomiting in clinical use. Table 38–3 summarizes the

Table 38–3. Alimentary Tract Effects of Cancer Chemotherapeutic Agents

Drug	Effect*	Drug	Effect*
Adriamycin	A,N,V,N	Daunorubicin	A,N,V,M
Asparaginase	A,N,V,	CDDP ("Cis-Pt")	A,N,V
BCNU	A,N,V	Hydroxyurea	N,V,M,D
Bleomycin	M	Methotrexate	A,N,U,P,M
Busulfan	N,V	Mithramycin	A,N,V,D
Cyclophosphamide	A,N,V,P	Procarbazine	A,N,U
Cytarbine	N,V,M,U	Vinblastine	N,V
Dactinomycin	A,N,V,D,M,P	Vincristine	P,O

*A = anorexia, N = nausea, D = diarrhea, M = mucositis, P = abdominal pain,
 O = obstipation, U = intestinal ulceration.

effects on the alimentary tract which may occur with these various agents. Adrenocorticosteroids, which are commonly used in treatment of certain types of cancer, have well-known metabolic and nutritional effects which include depletion of nitrogen from muscle and loss of calcium and potassium from the body; these may be significant depending on the type of steroid, dosage and duration of treatment.

There has been increasing use of multicombination high-dose cyclical chemotherapy as the result of (1) the frequent occurrence of resistance of malignant cells to a single drug, (2) the realization of the need to kill the entire population of neoplastic cells in order to obtain a "cure" and (3) improved understanding of the sites in DNA and RNA synthesis at which various chemotherapeutic agents have their effect. These treatment programs, while increasingly effective against various malignancies, also result in prolonged periods of anorexia and nausea as a result of their effects on the alimentary tract, with resultant impaired food intake. Since treatments may be prolonged, weight loss and progressive debility may be severe. These undesirable reactions are intensified when radiation therapy to the abdomen or operation on the intestinal tract further decreases appetite or impairs intestinal function.

NUTRITIONAL THERAPY IN A CANCER PATIENT

The systemic and localized manifestations of cancer combine with the effects of various treatments of the disease to adversely affect the nutritional status of a significant number of patients. This is demonstrated by the data in Figure 38–1, indicating weight changes in a large number of hospitalized adult cancer patients at various stages and treatments. Loss of more than 15 per cent of the preillness body weight in sick patients is certainly an indication of developing malnutrition. On this basis, 18 per cent of 457

patients were in this category on admission; the longer patients stayed in the hospital, the larger was the percentage in this category.

With the exception of certain leukemias, cancer has rarely been an acutely fatal disease. With more effective treatments it has become more and more a chronic or protracted illness and, consequently, a matter of concern for long periods for the patient and his physician. More successful palliation or potential "cure" of cancer is associated with the requirement for variably long-term chemotherapy treatment schedules. Years must elapse before the patient and physician are willing to admit that the disease may be "cured." Each is faced, in his own way, with the effects of the disease process, the psychologic impact of its presence and the long-term problems of treatment modalities and their side effects. These factors often combine to adversely affect the quality of life of the patient. When malnutrition is an additive factor the problems are accentuated and increased morbidity and mortality result. If the physician undertakes current treatment modalities, a sincere effort should be made to improve or maintain the quality of life which makes for a reasonably comfortable and functioning individual. This concern about patient status should begin with the planning for the initial treatment and continue to the hoped-for long-term survival.

Various principles of nutritional therapy in the cancer patient have been presented.[290] These may be summarized here as follows:

1. Malnutrition is not an obligatory response of the host to cancer. It is relatively uncommon to find a cancer patient who cannot be either maintained in good nutritional status or improved when previously malnourished by means of appropriate therapeutic nutritional modalities (i.e. oral, tube or intravenous feeding).
2. A rational nutritional therapeutic program for a patient requires analysis of the factors inducing depletion in that patient. Every

patient should have an early and then periodic assessments of nutritional status so that already malnourished patients or those at risk of developing malnutrition are detected early. Procedures for nutritional assessment have been outlined in Chapter 22 and elsewhere.[290,291] For the patient who is determined to be nutritionally depleted, procedures for the evaluation of the causes of depletion must be instituted (i.e. diet intake history, malabsorption workup, metabolic studies). As has been mentioned earlier, understanding of the complex interactions between cancer and its treatments and nutritional status is essential in order to correctly evaluate the cause(s) of depletion.

3. Nutritional therapy should be instituted early when the patient is deemed to be at risk for malnutrition, since it is much easier to maintain a reasonably good state of nutrition than it is to try to rehabilitate the already malnourished individual.

4. It is essential that the patient whose nutritional status has improved in the hospital be followed as an outpatient for assurance that the nutrition therapy program is not neglected after discharge. The application and evaluation of the effectiveness of the program must therefore become integral parts of good general clinical care for inpatients and outpatients and should be included in all medical audits.

5. Who is to be given aggressive nutritional therapy? If antitumor therapy of one type or another is to be undertaken, the patient deserves nutritional therapy so long as the treatment is applied and is being evaluated. If, on the other hand, the patient is not considered a suitable candidate for any further type of treatment, nutritional therapy is not to be stressed except in rare instances.

6. Nutritional therapy can be divided into: (a) supportive, (b) adjunctive and (c) definitive. *Supportive* therapy can be illustrated in the patient with bowel obstruction who is deemed a poor surgical risk because of malnutrition and who will be clinically improved by nutritional means to the point where surgery can be undertaken at appreciably lower risk. *Adjunctive* nutrition therapy is the type where nutrition becomes a part of the therapeutic program. Examples of this are: improving resistance to infection by improving immune status, permitting more rapid application and better adherence to a proposed antitumor therapeutic regimen by improved nutrition

or inducing spontaneous closure of an intestinal fistula as a result of nutritional therapy. *Definitive* nutrition therapy is defined as that where the therapy becomes the modality upon which the longer-term existence of the patient depends, i.e. when special oral, tube or intravenous nutritional programs permit the survival of a patient in good condition who has had a massive bowel resection or severe radiation enteritis or both and where debility or death will result without such therapy. This may be a short-term or long-term endeavor. The therapeutic modalities necessary to achieve these objectives should be available for inpatients and outpatients.

7. Nutritional status, tumor growth and antitumor treatment are intimately related. Many of the most potent cytotoxic agents used in antitumor therapy have optimum activity only against cells that are in the process of division. Hence, malignancies are most susceptible to chemotherapeutic measures where a high percentage of the cells are in that stage. Nutrition plays a role in the rate of cell growth and mitosis. As stated above, it is well established that experimental animals who have been deprived of food to the point of weight loss have a lower incidence of spontaneous tumors and a slower rate of growth of transplanted tumors. It is also well established that forced tube feeding[292,293] or parenteral nutrition[294-298] of experimental animals with transplanted tumors results in improved weight of the host. Repletion with a complete diet of previously protein-depleted tumor-bearing rats also appreciably increases the ratio of tumor weight to host tissue weight.[298] Recent observations of the effects of parenteral nutrition in tumor-bearing animals indicates some variability in results: In two or three reports total parenteral nutrition did not increase the relative tumor weight or size[295,296] while in one report the tumor growth was stimulated to a greater degree than was host weight.[294]

Clinical experience indicates it is a rare patient who has marked acceleration of growth of tumor during a period of improved nutrition. Increased growth of residual tumor would be expected in patients as a result of improved nutrition since tumor cells have a dependency on good nutrition, as do host cells. Furthermore, improved nutrition may be therapeutically useful since actively dividing tumor cells are more likely, as stated above, to be more sensitive to radiation therapy and chemotherapy than are slowly dividing cells. Preliminary studies in tumor-bearing experimental animals suggest that maintenance of better nutrition by intravenous[297] or oral[298] means improves the sensitivity of the tumor to chemotherapeutic agents. On the basis of such relatively preliminary data, it is the opinion of the author that it is not in the interest of the tumor-bearing patient who is a candidate for treatment to carry him on nutritional therapy without at the same time instituting adequate antitumor therapy.

BIBLIOGRAPHY

1. Tannenbaum: Nutrition and cancer. In *Physiopathology of Cancer*, 2nd ed. (Homberger, Ed.). New York, Hoeber-Harper, 1959, pp. 517–562.
2. Ross and Bras: J. Nutr., *87*, 245, 1965.
3. Ross, Bras and Ragbeer: J. Nutr., *100*, 177, 1970.
4. Ross and Bross: J. Nutr., *103*, 944, 1973.
5. Orten, Burn and Smith: Proc. Soc. Exp. Biol. Med., *36*, 82, 1937.
6. Rowe, Grammer, Watson and Nickerson: Cancer, *26*, 436, 1970.
7. Axelrad and Leblond: Cancer, *8*, 339, 1955.
8. Bois, Sandborn and Messier: Cancer Res., *29*, 763, 1969.
9. Alcock, Shils, Leiberman and Erlandson: Cancer Res., *33*, 2196, 1973.
10. Battifora, et al.: Arch. Pathol., *86*, 610, 1968.
11. Copeland and Salmon: Am. J. Pathol., *22*, 1059, 1946.
12. Butler and Newberne: Cancer Res., *29*, 236, 1969.
13. Miller and Miller: In *The Molecular Biology of Cancer* (Busch, Ed.). New York, Academic Press, 1973, pp. 377–402.
14. Wattenberg: J. Natl. Cancer Inst., *60*, 11, 1978; Adv. Cancer Res., *26*, 197, 1978.
15. Gillette: Adv. Pharmacol., *4*, 219, 1966.
16. Conney: Pharmacol. Rev., *19*, 317, 1967.
17. Conney and Burns: Science, *178*, 576, 1972.
18. Campbell and Hayes: Pharmacol. Rev., *26*, 171, 1974.
19. Wattenberg: Toxicol. Appl. Pharmacol., *23*, 741, 1972.
20. Wattenberg: Cancer Res., *35*, 3326, 1975.
21. Loub, Wattenberg and Davis: J. Natl. Cancer Inst., *54*, 985, 1975.
22. Wattenberg: J. Natl. Cancer Inst., *48*, 1425, 1972.
23. Shamberger: J. Natl. Cancer Inst., *44*, 931, 1970.
24. Shamberger and Willis: Clin. Lab. Sci., *2*, 211, 1971.
25. Sugiura: J. Nutr., *44*, 345, 1951.
26. Conney, Miller and Miller: Cancer Res., *16*, 450, 1956.
27. Wogan: Prog. Exp. Tumor Res., *11*, 134, 1969.
28. Newberne, Harrington and Wogan: Lab. Invest., *15*, 662, 1966.
29. Rogers and Newberne: Nature, *229*, 62, 1971.
30. McLean and Magee: Br. J. Exp. Pathol., *51*, 587, 1970.
31. Topping and Visek: J. Nutr., *106*, 1583, 1976.
32. Visek, et al.: Fed. Proc., *37*, 262, 1978.
33. Rogers and Newberne: Cancer Res., *35*, 3427, 1975.
34. Carroll: Cancer Res., *35*, 3374, 1975.
35. Reddy, et al.: Cancer Res., *35*, 3426, 1975.
36. Gammal, Carroll and Plunkett: Cancer Res., *27*, 1737, 1967.
37. Carroll and Khor: Lipids, *6*, 415, 1971.
38. Hopkins, West and Hard: Lipids, *11*, 328, 1976.
39. King, et al.: Fed. Proc., *36*, 1148, 1977.
40. Hopkins and West: J. Natl. Cancer Inst., *58*, 753, 1977.
41. Hill: Digestion, *11*, 289, 1974.
42. Nettesheim and Williams: Int. J. Cancer, *17*, 351, 1976.
43. Cohen, Willenberg and Bryan: Cancer Res., *36*, 2334, 1976.
44. Chu and Malmgren: Cancer Res., *25*, 884, 1965.
45. Saffiotti, et al.: Cancer, *20*, 857, 1967.
46. Shamberger: J. Natl. Cancer Inst., *47*, 667, 1971.
47. Smith, et al.: Cancer Res., *35*, 11, 1975.
48. Sporn: Nutr. Rev., *35*, 65, 1977.
49. Sporn, et al.: Fed. Proc., *35*, 1332, 1976.
50. Bollag: Eur. J. Cancer, *10*, 731, 1974.
51. Sporn, et al.: Science, *195*, 487, 1977.
52. Thompson, et al.: Fed. Proc., *37*, 261, 1978.
53. Dahn, Loewe and Bunton: Helv. Chim. Acta, *43*, 320, 1960.
54. Mirvish, et al.: Science, *177*, 65, 1972.
54a. Newberne: Science, *204*, 1079, 1979.
55. Ivancovic, et al.: Z. Krebsforsch., *79*, 145, 1973.
56. Mirvish: Toxicol. Appl. Pharmacol., *31*, 225, 1975.
57. Mirvish, et al.: J. Natl. Cancer Inst., *55*, 633, 1975.
58. Weisburger and Raineri: Cancer Res., *35*, 3469, 1975.
59. Fong, Sivak and Newberne: J. Natl. Cancer Inst., *61*, 145, 1978.
60. Dunning, Curtis and Mann: Cancer Res., *10*, 454, 1950.
61. Pamukcu, Yalciner, Price and Bryan: Cancer Res., *30*, 2671, 1970.
62. Rakieten, et al.: Proc. Soc. Exp. Biol. Med., *137*, 280, 1971.
63. DeWys, Pories, Richter and Strain: Proc. Soc. Exp. Biol. Med., *135*, 17, 1970.
64. Fisher and Fisher: Cancer, *14*, 547, 1961.
65. Mider: Annu. Rev. Med., *4*, 187, 1953.
66. Steiger, et al.: J. Surg. Res., *18*, 455, 1975.
67. Daly, Copeland, Quinn and Dudrick: Surg. Forum, *27*, 113, 1976.

68. Cameron and Pavlat: J. Natl. Cancer Inst., 56, 597, 1976.
69. Sugimura, Birnbaum, Winitz et al.: Arch. Biochem. Biophys., 81, 439, 1959.
70. Demopolous: J. Natl. Cancer Inst., 37, 185, 1966.
71. Ryan and Elliott: Arch. Biochem. Biophys., 125, 797, 1968.
72. Theuer: J. Nutr., 101, 223, 1971.
72a. Worthington, Syrotuck and Ahmed: J. Nutr., 108, 1402, 1978.
73. Bertino and Nixon: Cancer Res., 29, 2417, 1969.
74. Cooney and Handschumacher: Annu. Rev. Pharmacol., 10, 421, 1970.
75. Capizzi, Bertino and Handschumacher: Annu. Rev. Med., 21, 433, 1970.
76. Rosen, Sotobayashi and Nichol: Proc. Am. Assoc. Cancer Res., 5, 54, 1964.
77. Rosen, Mihich and Nicol: Vitam. Horm., 22, 609, 1964.
78. Morris and Robertson: J. Natl. Cancer Inst., 3, 479, 1943.
79. Gailani, Holland, Nussbaum and Olson: Cancer, 21, 975, 1968.
80. Nichol: Cancer Res., 29, 2422, 1969.
81. Bullough: Br. J. Cancer, 4, 329, 1950.
82. Suskind (Ed.): Malnutrition and the Immune Response. New York, Raven Press, 1977.
83. Law, Dudrick and Abdou: Ann. Surg., 179, 168, 1974.
84. Copeland, MacFadyen and Dudrick: Ann. Surg., 184, 60, 1976.
85. Jose, Cooper and Good: Nature, 231, 323, 1971.
86. Stoerk and Emerson: Proc. Soc. Exp. Biol. Med., 70, 703, 1949.
87. Bull: Cancer Res., 35, 3317, 1975.
88. Cooper, Mariani and Good: Fed. Proc., 29, 364, 1970.
89. Jose and Good: J. Exp. Med., 137, 1, 1973.
90. Meakins, et al.: Ann. Surg., 186, 241, 1977.
91. Hoffman: Cancer and Diet. Baltimore, Williams & Wilkins, 1937.
92. Nutrition in the Causation of Cancer (Conf. Proc.): Cancer Res., 35, 3321, 1975.
93. Doll: In Origin of Human Cancer (Hiatt, Watson and Winsten, Eds.). Cold Spring Harbor Laboratory, 1977, pp. 1–12.
94. Berg: In Origin of Human Cancer (Hiatt, Watson and Winsten, Eds.). Cold Spring Harbor Laboratory, 1977, pp. 15–19.
95. Ahlbom: Acta Radiol., 18, 163, 1937.
96. Larrson, Sandström and Westling: Cancer Res., 35, 3308, 1975.
97. Day: Cancer Res., 35, 3304, 1975.
98. Cooke and Burkitt: Br. Med. Bull., 27, 14, 1971.
99. Haenszel and Correa: Cancer Res., 35, 3452, 1975.
100. Haenszel, et al.: J. Natl. Cancer Inst., 49, 969, 1972.
101. Devesa and Silverman: J. Natl. Cancer Inst., 60, 545, 1978.
102. Hirayama: Cancer Res., 35, 3460, 1975.
103. Armstrong and Doll: Int. J. Cancer, 15, 617, 1975.
104. Graham: Cancer Res., 35, 3464, 1975.
105. White: J. Agric. Food Chem., 23, 886, 1975; cf Correction: J. Agric. Food Chem., 24, 202, 1976.
105a. Lowenfels, et al.: Gut, 19, 199, 1978.
106. Tannenbaum, et al.: J. Natl. Cancer Inst., 53, 79, 1974.
107. Zaldivar: Zentralbl. Bakteriol., 164, 193, 1977.
108. Nitrate and human cancer (editorial). Lancet, 2, 281, 1977.
109. Ruddell, et al.: Lancet, 1, 521, 1978.
109a. Tannenbaum, et al.: Science, 200, 1487, 1978.
110. Issenberg: Fed. Proc., 35, 1322, 1976.
111. Wynder: Cancer Res., 35, 3388, 1975.
112. Correa: Cancer Res., 35, 3395, 1975.
113. Correa and Haenszel: Adv. Cancer Res., 26, 1, 1978.
114. Haenszel and Correa: Cancer, 28, 14, 1971.
115. Wynder and Shigematsu: Cancer, 20, 1520, 1967.
116. Gregor, Toman and Prusova: Gut, 10, 1031, 1969.
117. Drasar and Irving: Br. J. Cancer, 27, 167, 1973.
118. Berg and Howell: Cancer, 34, 807, 1974.
119. Blot, et al.: In Origin of Human Cancer (Hiatt, Watson and Winsten, Eds.). Cold Spring Harbor Laboratory, 1977, pp. 25–26.
119a. Lyon and Sorenson: Am. J. Clin. Nutr., 31, S227, 1978.
120. Enstrom: Br. J. Cancer, 32, 432, 1975.
121. Enig, Munn and Keeney: Fed. Proc., 37, 2215, 1978.
122. Haenszel, et al.: J. Natl. Cancer Inst., 51, 1765, 1973.
123. Hill: Digestion, 11, 289, 1974.
124. Hill: Cancer Res., 35, 3398, 1975.
125. Hill: Am. J. Clin. Nutr., 27, 1475, 1974.
126. Aries, et al.: Gut, 10, 334, 1969.
127. Hill, et al.: Lancet, 1, 95, 1971.
128. Reddy and Wynder: J. Natl. Cancer Inst., 50, 1437, 1973.
129. Hill and Aries: J. Pathol., 104, 129, 1971.
130. Reddy, Weisburger and Wynder: J. Nutr., 105, 878, 1975.
131. Hill, et al.: Lancet, 2, 535, 1975.
132. Reddy and Wynder: Cancer, 39, 2533, 1977.
133. Finegold, Attebery and Sutter: Am. J. Clin. Nutr., 27, 1456, 1974.
134. Phillips: Cancer Res., 35, 3513, 1975.
135. Goldberg, Smith and Nichols: Ann. Surg., 186, 97, 1977.
136. Finegold, et al.: Am. J. Clin. Nutr., 30, 1781, 1977.
137. Maier, et al.: Am. J. Clin. Nutr., 27, 1470, 1974.
138. Hackman, et al.: Lancet, 1, 752, 1976.
139. Burkitt: Lancet, 2, 1229, 1969.
140. Burkitt, Walker and Painter: Lancet, 2, 1408, 1972.
141. Southgate: Am. J. Clin. Nutr., 31, S107, 1978.
142. Glober, et al.: Lancet, 2, 80, 1974.
143. Harvey, Pomare and Heaton: Lancet, 1, 1278, 1973.
144. Eastwood, et al.: Br. Med. J., 4, 392, 1973.

145. Walters, et al.: Br. Med. J., 2, 536, 1975.
146. Paylor: Lancet, 1, 1394, 1973.
147. Glober, et al.: Lancet, 2, 110, 1977.
148. International Agency for Research in Cancer: Lancet, 2, 207, 1977.
149. Irving and Drasar: Br. J. Cancer, 28, 462, 1973.
150. Modan, et al.: J. Natl. Cancer Inst., 55, 15, 1975.
151. Kern, Birkner and Ostrower: Am. J. Clin. Nutr., 31, 5175, 1978.
152. Symposium on Role of Dietary Fiber in Health. Am. J. Clin. Nutr., 31, S1, 1978.
152a.Wilson, Hutcheson and Wideman: Am. J. Clin. Nutr., 30, 176, 1977.
152b.Barbolt and Abraham: Proc. Soc. Exp. Biol. Med., 157, 656, 1978.
153c.Cruse, Lewin and Clark: Lancet, 2, 1278, 1978.
152d.Ward, Yamamoto and Weisburger: J. Natl. Cancer Inst., 51, 713, 1973.
152e.Crosby: Nutr. Cancer, 1, 15, 1978.
152f. Stamler: Circulation, 58, 3, 1978.
153. Berg: Cancer Res., 35, 3345, 1975.
154. Staszewski and Haenszel: J. Natl. Cancer Inst., 35, 291, 1965.
155. Staszewski, McCall and Stenhouse: Br. J. Cancer, 25, 559, 1971.
156. Haenszel and Kurihara: J. Natl. Cancer Inst., 40, 43, 1968.
157. Dunn: Cancer Res., 35, 3240, 1975.
158. Weisburger, Cohen and Wynder: In *Origin of Human Cancer* (Hiatt, Watson and Winsten, Eds.). Cold Spring Harbor Laboratory, 1977, pp. 584–594.
159. Lea: Lancet, 2, 323, 1966.
160. Carroll, Gammal and Plunkett: Can. Med. Assoc. J., 98, 590, 1968.
161. deWaard, et al.: Cancer, 40, 1269, 1977.
162. Buell: J. Natl. Cancer Inst., 51, 1479, 1973.
163. Gardner and Amacher (Eds.): *Endocrine Aspects of Malnutrition.* Santa Ynez, Kroc Foundation, 1973.
164. Dickinson, et al.: N. Engl. J. Med., 291, 1211, 1974.
165. Hill and Wynder: Lancet, 2, 806, 1976.
166. Dunn and Bradbury: Am. J. Obstet. Gynecol., 97, 465, 1967.
167. Doll: Natl. Cancer Inst. Monogr. No. 25, 1967, pp. 173–190.
168. Doll, Muir and Waterhouse (Eds.): *Cancer Incidence in Five Continents,* Vol. 2. New York, Springer, 1970.
169. Higginson: Gastroenterology, 57, 587, 1969.
170. Adamson, Correa and Dalgard: J. Natl. Cancer Inst., 50, 549, 1973.
171. Linsell and Peers: In *Origin of Human Cancer* (Hiatt, Watson and Winsten, Eds.). Cold Spring Harbor Laboratory, 1977, pp. 549–556.
171a. Trichopolous, et al.: Lancet, 2, 1217, 1978.
172. Wogan: Cancer Res., 35, 3499, 1975.
173. Shils: Cancer Res., 37, 2366, 1977.
174. DeWys: Cancer Res., 30, 2816, 1976.
175. Theologides: Ann. N. Y. Acad. Sci., 230, 14, 1974.
176. DeWys and Walters: Cancer, 36, 1888, 1975.
177. Morrison: Am. J. Clin. Nutr., 31, 1104, 1978.
178. Holland, Rowland and Plumb: Cancer Res., 37, 2452, 1977.
179. William and Cohen: Am. J. Clin. Nutr., 31, 122, 1978.
180. Pfaffman, et al.: Symposium on Sense of Taste and Nutrition. Am. J. Clin. Nutr., 31, 1057, 1978.
181. Young: Cancer Res., 37, 2336. 1977.
182. Warmold, Lundholm and Schirsten: Cancer Res., 38, 1801, 1978.
183. Kleiber and Chernikoff: J. Gerontol., 11, 140, 1956.
184. Pratt and Putney: J. Natl. Cancer Inst., 20, 173, 1958.
185. Morrison: Cancer Res., 31, 98, 1971.
186. Gold: Ann. N.Y. Acad. Med., 230, 103, 1974.
187. Holyroyde, et al.: Cancer Res., 35, 3710, 1975.
188. Waterhouse and Kemperman: Cancer Res., 31, 1273, 1971.
189. Henderson and LePage: Cancer Res., 19, 887, 1959.
190. White: J. Natl. Cancer Inst., 5, 265, 1945.
191. LePage, et al.: Cancer Res., 12, 153, 1952.
192. Brennan: Cancer Res., 37, 2359, 1977.
193. Mider: Cancer Res., 11, 281, 1951.
194. Stewart: Quoted by Fenninger and Mider: Adv. Cancer Res., 2, 229, 1954.
195. Goodlad: In *Mammalian Protein Metabolism,* Vol. 2 (Munro and Allison, Eds.). New York, Academic Press, 1964, pp. 415–444.
196. Baille, Millar and Pratt: Am. J. Physiol., 209, 296, 1965.
197. Shils: Cancer, 43, 2093, 1979.
198. Shils and Coiro: Unpublished data.
199. Lanzotti: Quoted by Costa: Cancer Res., 37, 2327, 1977.
200. Creamer: Br. Med. J., 2, 1435, 1964.
201. Barry: Gut, 15, 562, 1974.
202. Booth: Postgrad. Med. J., 37, 725, 1961.
203. Toskes, et al.: N. Engl. J. Med., 284, 627, 1971.
204. Bossak, Wang and Adlersberg: J. Mt. Sinai Hosp., 24, 286, 1957.
205. Harris, et al.: Am. J. Med., 42, 899, 1961.
206. Gough, Read and Naish: Gut, 3, 232, 1962.
207. Austed, et al.: Am. J. Dig. Dis., 12, 475, 1967.
208. Benson, Kowlessar and Sleisenger: Medicine, 43, 1, 1964.
209. Brunt, Sircus and MacLean: Lancet, 1, 180, 1969.
210. Eidelman, Parkins and Rubin: Medicine, 45, 111, 1966.
211. Novis, et al.: Q. J. Med., 40, 521, 1971.
212. Pitney, Joske and Mackinnon: J. Clin. Pathol., 13, 440, 1960.
213. Naqvi, Burrows and Kark: Ann. Surg., 170, 221, 1969.
214. Loehr, et al.: Ann. Surg., 170, 232, 1969.
215. Ehrlich, et al.: Gastroenterology, 54, 1115, 1968.
216. Waldman, Broder and Strober: Ann. N.Y. Acad. Sci., 230, 306, 1974.
217. Toskes, et al.: Gastroenterology, 68, 1193, 1975.
217a.Jonas, Krishnan and Forstner: Gastroenterology, 75, 791, 1978.

218. Thompson (Ed.): Gastrointestinal Hormones. Symposium. Austin, University of Texas Press, 1975.
219. Pearse, Polak and Bloom: Gastroenterology, 72, 746, 1977.
220. McGuigan and Trudeau: N. Engl. J. Med., 278, 1308, 1968.
220a. Deveney, Deveney and Way: Ann. Surg., 188, 384, 1978.
221. Verner and Morrison: Arch. Intern. Med., 133, 492, 1974.
222. Rambaud, et al.: Gastroenterology, 69, 122, 1975.
223. Sjoerdsma, Weissbach and Udenfriend: Am. J. Med., 20, 520, 1956.
224. Sandler, Karim and Williams: Lancet, 2, 1053, 1968.
225. Williams, Karim and Sandler: Lancet, 1, 22, 1968.
226. DaCruz, Gardner and Peskin: Am. J. Surg., 115, 203, 1968.
227. Shimoda, Saunders and Rubin: Gastroenterology, 55, 705, 1968.
228. Kowlessar, Law and Sleisinger: Am. J. Med., 27, 673, 1959.
229. Kleeman: Annu. Rev. Med., 21, 259, 1970.
230. Tashjian and Melvin: N. Engl. J. Med., 279, 279, 1968.
231. Baylin, Beaven, Engleman and Sjoerdsma: N. Engl. J. Med., 283, 1239, 1970.
232. Schimke, Hartmann, Prout and Rimoin: N. Engl. J. Med., 279, 1, 1968.
233. Gray, Bieberdorf, and Fordtran: J. Clin. Invest., 52, 3084, 1973.
234. Amman, Vetter and Deyhle: Gut, 17, 107, 1976.
235. Munson, Tashjian and Levine: Cancer Res., 25, 1062, 1965.
236. Liddle, Givens, Nicholson and Island: Cancer Res., 25, 1057, 1965.
237. Swendseid, Swanson, Meyers and Bethell: Blood, 7, 307, 1952.
238. Spray and Witts: Clin. Sci., 12, 385, 1953.
239. Swendseid, Bethell and Bird: Cancer Res., 11, 864, 1951.
240. Rao, Lagerlöf, Einhorn and Reizenstein: Lancet, 1, 1192, 1963.
241. Rose: J. Clin. Pathol., 19, 29, 1966.
242. Magnus: Cancer Res., 27, 490, 1967.
243. Beard, Pitney and Sanneman: Blood, 9, 789, 1954.
244. Hall and Finkler: Blood, 27, 611, 1966.
245. Klipstein and Smarth: Am. J. Dig. Dis., 14, 887, 1969.
246. Corcino, Zalinsky, Greenberg and Herbert: Blood, 20, 511, 1971.
247. Chalner, DeVita, Livingstone and Oliverio: N. Engl. J. Med., 282, 838, 1970.
248. Schwartz: Cancer Res., 35, 348, 1975.
249. MacCarthy-Leventhal: Lancet, 2, 1138, 1959.
250. Donaldson: Cancer Res., 37, 2407, 1977.
251. Shils and Gilat: Gastroenterology, 50, 347, 1966.
252. Shils: Surg. Gynecol. Obstet., 132, 709, 1971.
253. Lawrence: Cancer Res., 37, 2379, 1977.
254. Hines, Hoffbrand and Mollin: Am. J. Med., 43, 555, 1967.
255. Deller, et al.: Gut, 5, 218, 1964.
256. Geokas and McKenna: Can. Med. Assoc. J., 96, 411, 1967.
257. Eddy: Am. J. Med., 50, 442, 1971.
258. Booth: Postgrad. Med. J., 37, 725, 1961.
259. Stewart, et al.: Q. J. Med., 36, 425, 1967.
260. Hoffman and Poley: N. Engl. J. Med., 281, 397, 1969.
261. LeRusso, Korman, Hoffman and Hofmann: N. Engl. J. Med., 291, 689, 1974.
262. Saunder, Sillery and McDonald: Gut, 16, 543, 1975.
263. Dobbins and Binder: N. Engl. J. Med., 296, 298, 1977.
264. Dowling: Br. Med. Bull., 23, 275, 1967.
265. Wilmore, Dudrick, Daly and Vars: Surg. Gynecol. Obstet., 132, 673, 1971.
266. Weser: Gastroenterology, 71, 146, 1976.
267. Shils: Cancer Res., 37, 2432, 1977.
268. Booth, MacIntyre and Mollin: Q. J. Med., 33, 401, 1964.
269. Bochenek, Rogers and Balint: Ann. Intern. Med., 72, 205, 1970.
270. Bergen, Hashim and van Itallie: Diabetes, 15, 723, 1966.
271. Frederick, Sizer and Osborn: N. Engl. J. Med., 272, 509, 1965.
272. Hardison and Rosenberg: N. Engl. J. Med., 277, 337, 1967.
272a. Wilmore and Johnson: Arch. Surg., 97, 784, 1968.
273. Winchester and Dorsey: Surg. Gynecol. Obstet., 132, 131, 1971.
274. Smiddy, et al.: Lancet, 1, 14, 1960.
275. Gallagher, Harrison and Skyring: Gut, 3, 219, 1962.
276. Shils: Cancer Res., 37, 2387, 1977.
277. Graham: N. Engl. J. Med., 296, 1314, 1977.
278. DiMagno, Malagelada, Go and Moertel: N. Engl. J. Med., 296, 1318, 1977.
279. Meyer: Editorial. N. Engl. J. Med., 296, 1347, 1977.
280. Regan, et al.: N. Engl. J. Med., 297, 854, 1977.
281. Morishita, et al.: Digestion, 11, 240, 1974.
282. Stamey: Surg. Gynecol. Obstet., 103, 736, 1956.
283. Bricker: Am. J. Surg., 135, 834, 1978.
284. Calabresi and Parks: In The Pharmacological Basis of Therapeutics, 5th ed. (Goodman and Gilman, Eds.). New York, Macmillan, 1975, pp. 1248–1307.
285. Small, et al.: Am. J. Dig. Dis., 4, 700, 1959.
286. Baskerville and Batter-Hatton: Br. J. Exp. Pathol., 58, 663, 1977.
287. Trier: Gastroenterology, 43, 407, 1962.
288. Gardner, Sampson and Heading: Clin. Sci. Mol. Med., 54, 411, 1978.
289. Yeh and Shils: Fed. Proc., 25, 322, 1966.
290. Shils: Cancer, 43, 2095, 1979.
291. Butterworth and Blackburn: Nutr. Today, 10, 8, 1975.
292. Begg and Dickinson: Cancer Res., 11, 409, 1951.

293. Allison, et al.: J. Nutr., *54*, 593, 1954.
294. Cameron and Pavlet: J. Natl. Cancer Inst., *56*, 597, 1976.
295. Steiger, et al.: J. Surg. Res., *18*, 455, 1975.
296. Daly, Copeland and Dudrick: Surgery, *84*, 655, 1978.
297. Cameron and Rogers: J. Surg. Res., *23*, 279, 1977.
298. Reynolds, Daly, Copeland and Dudrick: Fed. Proc., *37*, 261, 1978.

Chapter 39

GENETIC ASPECTS OF HUMAN NUTRITION

Neil A. Holtzman,
Mark L. Batshaw and
David L. Valle

One species evolves from another as a result of mutations that increase adaptability to the environment. In a different environment those same mutations could have been detrimental and labelled "inborn errors of metabolism." Viewed in this context, inherited diseases represent only part of the spectrum of genetically determined adaptability. In this chapter we first consider the role that the nutritional environment plays in determining the value of a mutation and, consequently, the likelihood that those carrying the mutation will propagate. We will examine the extent of human variation, consider how gene function influences nutritional requirements, classify treatments for genetic diseases and conclude with consideration of a few specific metabolic defects.

EVOLUTION AND NUTRITION

The earliest forms of life were able to utilize energy for the synthesis of organic compounds from carbon dioxide, oxygen, water and nitrogen. Arising as a result of mutation, newer organisms were able to utilize the energy trapped in these organic compounds for the synthesis of more complex molecules. As long as their more primitive forebears were available for nutrition the new organisms could afford to lose the ability to synthesize the simpler organic compounds. Thus, evolutionary change involves both mutations that result in loss of function and others that gain new abilities for the organism.

Man's genetic endowment provides him with fewer nutritional capabilities than any other species. The energy and material that would have been used for nutrient synthesis can now be diverted to the acquisition of new functions. For instance, the loss by man and other primates of ascorbic acid synthesis frees glucose for other reactions.[1] In addition to his inability to synthesize most vitamins, man cannot synthesize some amino acids and cannot utilize cellulose, the most abundant energy-rich compounds in plants. He relies directly on plants for starches, some of the essential amino acids and vitamins and on them indirectly through foraging animals that convert cellulose to compounds that he can utilize. Not only do the bacteria in the rumen of cattle, sheep, goats and deer digest cellulose but they also synthesize the essential amino acids providing the animals themselves, and man, with another nutrient source.

Man's genetic endowment thus makes him markedly dependent on his environment. With the domestication of cereal grains, other plants and animals, man has diverted the high-energy compounds and nutrients synthesized by other species to his own benefit to a remarkable extent. On the evolutionary time scale, however, agriculture is a recent event. Even today, there are large segments of the earth's human population whose food supply is precarious. Thus, even after man evolved, mutations *within the species* that improved the ability to utilize nutrients from other species or to cope with the environment were, because of the selective advantage they offered, likely to spread. "Selective advantage" signifies only greater reproductive fitness: the probability that those with the advantage will live to propagate and will have more living offspring, some of whom will carry the advantageous mutation, is greater than in those who lack it. The hereditary persistence of lactase, diabetes mellitus and sickle-cell anemia provide possible examples.

Persistence of Intestinal Lactase

Milk is a ready source of protein and fat. Lactose, the carbohydrate of almost all mammalian milks, cannot, however, be absorbed. Unless hydrolyzed by lactase to glucose and galactose, sugars that are absorbed, lactose draws water into the gut osmotically; gastrointestinal motility increases, diarrhea ensues and absorption of fat and protein in the milk diminishes. Whereas intestinal lactase activity in most mammals and man declines at or soon after weaning, a mutation that resulted in its persistence into adulthood would benefit those to whom fresh animal milk was available for nutrition.[2] If a gene for persistence of lactase had a frequency of 5 per cent when dairying began, then, assuming that those who possessed it had 1 per cent more children per generation than intolerant individuals, in the ensuing 400 generations its frequency would have risen to 60 per cent. This approximates the gene frequency in modern milk-drinking populations. The hydrolysis of lactose also enhances calcium absorption; this may contribute to the high frequency of the adult lactase gene in northern Europe[3] where low sunlight increases the likelihood of calcium deficiency and, secondarily, of

bone deformities that diminish reproductive fitness.

Today, those with lactase deficiency live in milk-drinking cultures and, in addition, milk products are exported to adult populations deficient in lactase. Thus, lactose intolerance has emerged as a major cause of gastrointestinal discomfort in those in whom the enzyme does not persist, including blacks, Orientals and Jews.[4]

Diabetes Mellitus

Mutations that were advantageous when food was scarce may be disadvantageous when food becomes abundant. Because scarcity predominated until very recently, these mutations would still be present in high frequency. Although speculative, the high prevalence of diabetes mellitus today might result from a selective advantage of the diabetic genotype during the long period when famine, or alternating periods of famine and feast, characterized man's existence. There is no doubt that most forms of diabetes mellitus are inherited.

According to Neel,[5] increased insulin activity, which characterizes the common forms of diabetes, is closer to the primary defect than is resistance to its action which, he suggests, develops only in the presence of a persistently abundant food supply. Increased insulin activity, he speculates, could afford protection against future famine when food did present itself (or was captured) by stimulating greater hunger and, consequently, greater food intake. Hyperinsulinism could also result in greater glucose retention because the renal threshold for excretion of the sugar would be less likely to be exceeded. In either case, the margin of nutritional safety once famine supervened would be greater than in those without hyperinsulinism. The observations that symptomatic diabetes mellitus in western populations declines during modern periods of food scarcity and that it is more likely to develop in individuals from nutritionally marginal cultures who migrate to affluent ones than in those who remain behind[6] support the hypothesis that a large, steady supply of food is needed before the harmful aspects of the diabetic genotype become manifest.

The Sickle-cell Allele and Balanced Polymorphism

While Neel's explanation for the high frequency of diabetes mellitus remains conjectural, there is no doubt that the persistence of the sickle-cell gene results from the protection it affords the heterozygote against malaria.[7] Although the sickle-cell gene has little to do with nutrition, its discussion will enable us to introduce a number of terms and concepts useful later in the chapter.

Mutation, by definition, results in a new *allele* for the affected gene. The β hemoglobin chain that is coded by the sickle-cell allele differs from the chain coded by the usual or β^A allele by one amino acid. That difference has remarkable effects. Infants who inherit the sickle-cell allele (β^S) from both parents are, by definition, *homozygotes* for the β hemoglobin chain gene. In the absence of modern medical care they often die young from severe anemia or its complications. Thus the reproductive fitness of the homozygote is markedly impaired. *Heterozygotes,* who inherit the sickle-cell gene from only one parent, do not develop anemia (because of the presence of β^A hemoglobin). Moreover, they are resistant to the lethal effect of infection with Plasmodium falciparum malaria. Those who have inherited the β^A gene from both parents, and who are, therefore, homozygotes for the normal allele, do not have this protection against malaria. Thus the heterozygote has a selective advantage over the homozygous offspring. As the frequency of heterozygotes in the population increases, so too will the probability that heterozygotes will mate and produce homozygous offspring. Gene frequency will cease rising when the reproductive advantage of the heterozygote is offset by the loss of homozygotes. This is defined as balanced polymorphism.

The Extent of Human Variation

Thus far, we have described traits the relatively high frequency of which can be explained because of a selective advantage they offered in at least one stage of man's evolution, but such traits comprise only a small fraction of the genetic variation that exists within the human species. Examination of many different proteins obtained from hundreds of individuals indicates that for approximately one-third of all proteins a variant form occurs in at least 2 per cent of the population.[7] These variants, which do not convey any detectable advantage or disadvantage, are genetically determined, originating from mutation many generations ago. The explanation for their frequency is currently being debated. In the past, when man's environment differed from today's, some variant alleles may have been advantageous. Alternatively, they may have been neutral, in terms of reproductive fitness, becoming relatively frequent as a result of chance propagation or inbreeding.

Even genetic variants that produce disease may attain a relatively high frequency on the basis of random drift: (1) If the variant allele is harmful only when present in the homozygote, transmission of a single dose of the gene, from one heterozygote to another, would not be deleterious. (2) If the variant, in either the heterozygote or homozygote, causes disease *after* reproduction is completed, remaining silent or neutral until then, its transmission will not be affected by selective pressures. As the proportion of the population that lives beyond the age of reproduction increases, hitherto "silent" mutations will be expressed to a greater extent. This explains part of the high frequency today of heart disease associated with familial hypercholesterolemia (FH). Nutritional and other environmental changes have also altered the value of the FH mutation.

Familial Hypercholesterolemia. Coronary heart disease is the leading cause of death in the United States in all age groups over 35 years. Based on extensive family studies in Seattle, Goldstein and his colleagues established that patients who possess any one of three different mutant genes, including FH, account for about 20 per cent of all myocardial infarctions occurring before 60 years of age.[8] Another 5 per cent result from the simultaneous presence of several mutant genes. In FH, cellular receptors for the binding of low-density lipoprotein, which carries most of the cholesterol in the blood, are defective. As a consequence, the cell's synthesis of cholesterol is not inhibited.[9]

High concentrations of blood cholesterol can injure the endothelial lining of large arteries.[10] In heterozygotes for FH, the number of low-density lipoprotein receptor sites are reduced. This may result in higher levels of cholesterol in the blood stream and injury to the arterial wall. There may also be a greater propensity for cholesterol to accumulate at the site of injury.

About one in 500 persons in the general population is a heterozygote for FH. Until diets rich in saturated fats and cholesterol became widely available, the FH heterozygote may not have been at a disadvantage. Unless it reduces reproductive fitness, the FH gene may well persist. Survival to reproductive age is low in the FH homozygote but not necessarily in the heterozygote.

Variation in Nutritional Requirements. We have already described the extensive genetic variation within the human species. This creates a problem for those responsible for establishing nutritional requirements; the stipulated requirement may be inadequate for a significant proportion of the population[1,11] while for others it may be too high. In addition to the severe

inborn errors of metabolism, for which nutritional requirements are significantly altered,[12] there are less extreme genetic conditions in which nutritional requirements differ less profoundly from "normal." Many of these have only recently come to light, providing evidence for Williams' hypothesis that "whenever an extreme genetic character appears in an individual organism it should be taken as an indication ... that less extreme and graduated genetic characters of the same sort exist in other individual organisms."[13]

While the severe defects are rare, the less extreme forms occur with higher frequency. Often, they will manifest only when the supply of the nutrient in question deviates from the usual (Fig. 39–1). If the shift in supply is gradual, temporary and not excessive, individuals with these variant alleles may show neither permanent nor severe disease. For instance, infants who might have mild defects in copper absorption show signs of copper deficiency only when the intake of milk, which is low in copper, is prolonged and foods of higher copper content are withheld. This may happen with prematurity.[14] Let us now consider the genetically determined mechanisms that alter nutrient requirements.

GENETIC ALTERATIONS OF NUTRITIONAL REQUIREMENTS

Enzyme Defects

The utilization of nutrients depends on the presence of enzymes. The numbers of enzyme molecules available to catalyze a reaction, and the speed at which they do so, are both genetically determined. If the genes for the normal, or wild type, enzyme are altered by mutation either: (1) no enzyme is synthesized, (2) the amount of enzyme present is reduced by decreased enzyme synthesis or increased destruction, (3) a protein may be synthesized that is incapable of catalyzing the reaction or (4) the enzyme carries out the reaction at a

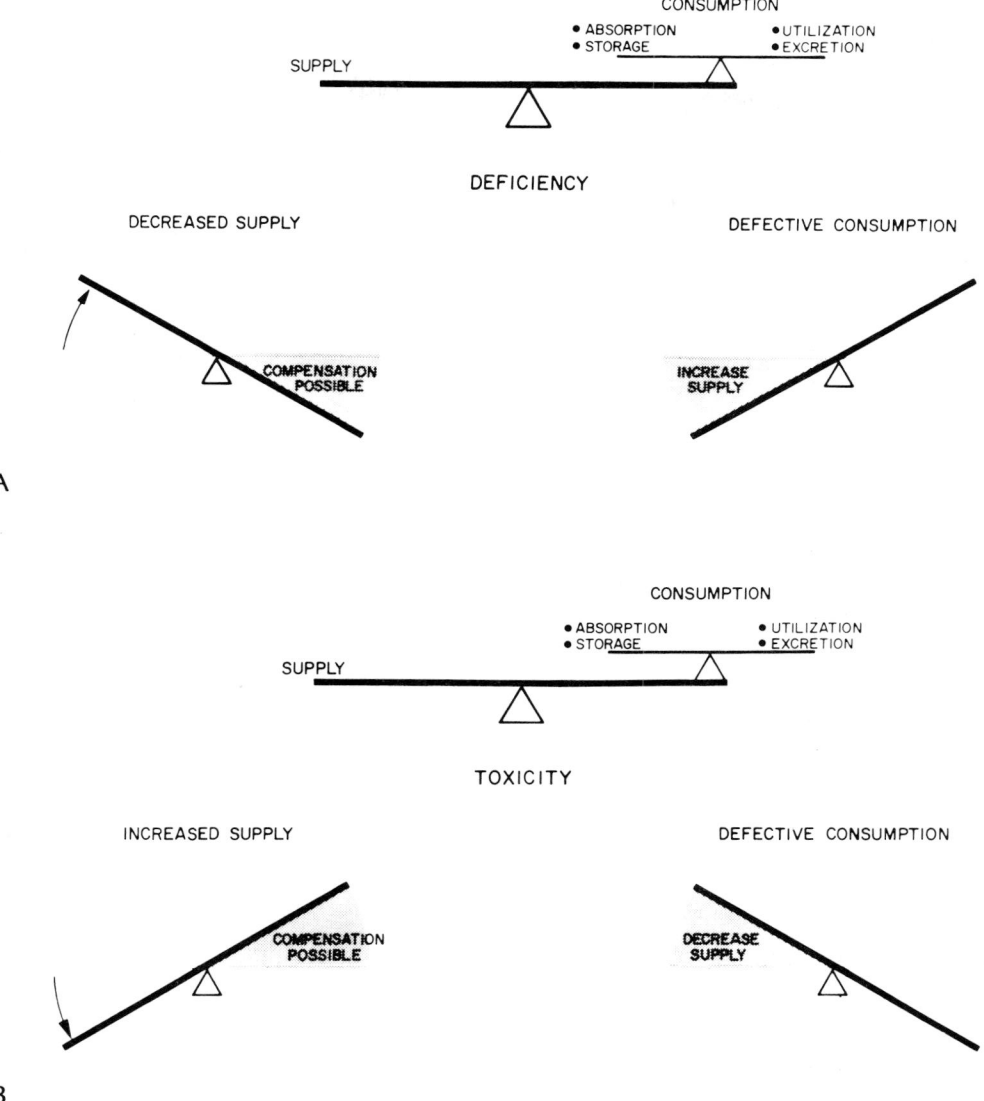

Fig. 39–1. **A:** Deficiency of a nutrient results from either decreased supply (left) or defective consumption (right). Confronted with diminished supply, the organism attempts to restore balance by increasing absorption, drawing on stored nutrient, improving utilization or diminishing excretion. These compensatory mechanisms are under genetic control and the magnitude of the nutrient deficiency for which compensation is possible, that is, for which balance can be restored, varies among individuals. When, on the other hand, an individual cannot maintain balance on a supply that is adequate for most others because of defective consumption (impairments of absorption, storage, utilization or excretion), his only recourse is to increase intake. **B:** Toxicity of a nutrient results from either increased supply (left) or defective consumption (right). The amount of excess nutrient that can be handled by the organism is under genetic control and varies among individuals. The mechanisms of compensation are as described in **A,** but in the opposite direction.

diminished rate. Enzymatic rates are also affected by mutations of genes for regulatory molecules.

As a result of such defects, the substance on which the enzyme acts, the substrate, will accumulate and, simultaneously, less product will be formed. Substrate may be diverted into other pathways and either it or some derivative, which is not ordinarily found in large amounts, may prove toxic. On the other hand, clinical disability may result from deficiency of the product.

Under ordinary circumstances, the rate at which most enzymes operate is considerably less than the maximum of which they are capable; otherwise, heterozygotes for absence of an enzyme, who have approximately one-half of the wild type activity, would encounter difficulty. However, for enzymes that normally operate at close to the maximum rate, or that are rate limiting for an entire pathway, any reduction in rate may be serious. Thus, heterozygotes for defects in the enzyme uroporphyrinogen I synthase suffer from acute intermittent porphyria.[15]

While the effect of moderately altered enzyme activity may be minimal *under ordinary circumstances,* departures from the usual can have profound consequences. Thus, if the environment ceases to supply a needed substance, individuals who have a diminished capability for synthesizing it, or cannot compensate for its loss in other ways, develop symptoms of disease, or perhaps even die, before those with greater capabilities (Fig. 39–1*A*). Similarly, if the environment suddenly presents large amounts of a potentially toxic material, those who have a diminished ability to detoxify it will suffer the most (Fig. 39–1*B*).

Transport Defects

The transport of many substances across cell membranes is an active process requiring energy. Frequently, a specific receptor on the cell surface recognizes the substance in question. Mutations that alter the number of these receptors, or their affinity for the substance, can result in intracellular deficiency or extracellular toxicity just as product deficiency or substrate toxicity results from enzyme defects. Again, in analogy with enzyme defects, if only some of the receptors are ordinarily involved in transport then disease might be manifest only when the defect is marked, as in homozygously affected individuals. If the transport system usually operates close to capacity, however, even heterozygotes might show signs of the deficiency. The reduction of low-density lipoprotein receptor in familial hypercholesterolemia, which we have already discussed, is one example of a transport defect in which heterozygotes suffer. One type of cystinuria, in which heterozygotes form kidney stones because of defects in the reabsorption of cystine, is another.[16]

Management of Genetic Disorders

Over one hundred genetic disorders have been reported in which harmful manifestations relate to toxicity or deficiency of nutrients or other environmental agents.[17] In some of them, modifications of the dietary supply alleviate the manifestations. In a large number, however, by the time symptoms and signs appear irreversible damage has already occurred. Successful management of these disorders will depend on identifying affected subjects while they are still presymptomatic. Because the disorders are genetic in origin, markers are theoretically present from the moment of conception. In practice, a number of disorders can be detected in the fetus in the 16th to 18th week of gestation by studies on amniotic fluid cells.[18] These and other disorders can be detected postnatally in the presymptomatic infant by analysis of blood serum, erythrocytes, leukocytes or fibroblasts cultured from skin biopsy. A search for presymptomatic genetic disease is most often undertaken only when there is a previous family history and the risk of recurrence is high. For a few disorders for which early treatment has proved effective, such as phenylketonuria, galactosemia or maple syrup urine disease, population-wide screening of newborns has been instituted so that a family need not have to suffer the disease once in order to manage it effectively in another child. In the future, population-wide presymptomatic detection will be extended to other disorders. Controlled trials to demonstrate the effectiveness of treatment must precede the initiation of routine screening programs. Table 39–1 lists genetic disorders in which modification of nutrient intake has been employed. Effectiveness has not been demonstrated for some of the therapies listed.

Table 39–1.   Genetic Disorders in Which Modifications of Nutrient Intake Play a Role in Management*

Disorder	*Nutrient Therapy*
Digestive Disorders	
Lactose intolerance	Lactose restriction
Sucrose-isomaltose malabsorption	Sucrose restriction
Intestinal Transport Disorders	
Abetalipoproteinemia	Medium-chain triglycerides, vitamins A, E
Acrodermatitis enteropathica	Zinc sulfate
Beta-sitosterolemia	Plant sterol restriction
Chloride diarrhea	Extra sodium chloride
Folic acid transport defect	Parenteral folate
Glucose-galactose malabsorption	Glucose, galactose restriction; fructose
Hartnup disease	Nicotinamide
Hypomagnesemia	Magnesium
Methionine malabsorption	Methionine restriction
Pernicious anemia	Vitamin B_{12} parenterally
Renal Transport Disorders	
Calcinosis, tumoral, with hyperphosphatemia	Low-phosphorus diet, aluminum hydroxide
Cystinosis and other causes of Fanconi's syndrome	Alkali, vitamin D, calcium
Diabetes insipidus	Water, low-solute diets (low protein)
Dibasic aminoaciduria	Protein restriction, arginine supplement
Glutamate-aspartate transport defect	Glutamine
Gout	Purine, protein restriction
Hypophosphatemia	Vitamin D, phosphorus
Oxalosis	Pyridoxine, magnesium, orthophosphate, water
Renal tubular acidosis	Alkali
Vitamin D-dependent rickets	Vitamin D_2 or D_3 or, preferably, their active forms
Internal Transport Disorders	
Hypercholesterolemia	Restriction of saturated fatty acids and cholesterol
Hyperlipoproteinemia I (familial hyperchylomicronemia)	Medium-chain triglycerides
Megaloblastic anemia due to transcobalamin II deficiency	Vitamin B_{12} parenterally
Metabolic Disorders	
Alkaptonuria	Ascorbic acid
Alpha-methylacetoacetic aciduria	Isoleucine restriction
Anemia, hypochromic, sideroblastic	Pyridoxine
Argininemia	Protein restriction
Argininosuccinic aciduria	Protein restriction
Ataxia with pellagra-like skin rash	Nicotinamide
Beta methylcrotonylglycinuria and beta hydroxyisovaleric aciduria	Biotin, leucine restriction

Table 39–1.   (Continued)

Disorder	Nutrient Therapy
Branched chain ketoaciduria	Branched-chain amino acid restriction; thiamin (in responsive form)
Chediak-Higashi	Ascorbic acid
Citrullinemia	Protein restriction
Combined hyperlipidemia	Caloric, carbohydrate, saturated fatty acid restriction
Cystathioninuria	Pyridoxine (in responsive form)
Ehlers-Danlos syndrome, lysyl hydroxylase defect	Ascorbic acid
Folic acid reductase deficiency	N^5-Formyltetrahydrofolic acid
Fructose intolerance	Fructose-free diet
Fructose-1,6-diphosphatase deficiency	Frequent glucose; folic acid
Galactokinase deficiency	Galactose-free diet
Galactosemia	Galactose-free diet; galactose restriction in pregnant heterozygotes
Galactose epimerase deficiency	Galactose
Glucose-6-phosphate dehydrogenase deficiency	Avoidance of fava beans and drugs that cause hemolysis
Glutaric acidemia	Protein restriction
Glycogen storage	
Type I (glucose-6-phosphatase defect)	Frequent feeding
Type III (amylo-1, 6-glucosidase defect)	Frequent feeding, high-protein diet
Type VI (phosphorylase defect)	Frequent feeding
Type VIII (phosphorylase kinase defect)	Avoid fasting; high-protein diet
Histidinemia	Histidine restriction
Homocystinuria	Pyridoxine (in responsive form)
Cystathionine synthase defect	Methionine restriction
N^5, N^{10}-methylenetetrahydrofolate reductase defect	Folic acid
Hydroxykynureninuria	Nicotinic acid
Hyperammonemia	
Ornithine transcarbamylase defect	Protein restriction; keto acids or essential amino acids
Carbamylphosphate synthetase defect	Protein restriction; keto acids or essential amino acids
Hyperbeta alaninemia	Pyridoxine
Hypertriglyceridemia	Weight reduction; carbohydrate restriction, high-protein diet
Isovaleric acidemia	Leucine restriction; protein restriction, glycine
Ketoacidosis of infancy	Glucose, alkali
Ketotic hyperglycinemia	Protein restriction, biotin (in responsive form)
Lactic acidosis, intermittent	High-fat, low-carbohydrate diet; thiamin (in responsive form)
Lysine intolerance (periodic hyperlysinemia with hyperammonemia)	Protein restriction
Megaloblastic anemia, thiamin responsive	Thiamin
Methylmalonic aciduria	
Methylmalonyl-CoA mutase defect	Protein restriction
Impaired synthesis of 5'-deoxyadenosylcobalamin	Vitamin B_{12}, parenterally
Methylmalonyl-CoA racemase defect	Protein restriction
Necrotizing encephalopathy, infantile, subacute, of Leigh	
Pyruvate carboxylase defect	Lipoic acid
Presence of an inhibitor of thiamin triphosphate synthesis	Thiamin tetrafurfuryl disulfide, thiamin propyldisulfide
Ornithinemia	Protein restriction
Orotic aciduria	Uridine
Periodic paralysis	
Hypokalemic	Carbohydrate restriction, potassium salts, sodium chloride

Table 39–1. **(Continued)**

Disorder	Nutrient Therapy
Hyperkalemic	Increased carbohydrates
Normokalemic	Sodium chloride
Phenylketonuria	Phenylalanine restriction
Porphyria, acute intermittent	Glucose, protein
Pyridoxine dependency with seizures	Pyridoxine, parenterally
Pyroglutamic aciduria	Alkali, protein restriction
Pyruvate carboxylase deficiency, partial	Thiamin
Refsum's disease	Phytanic acid restriction (diet low in dairy and ruminant fats)
Tryptophanuria with dwarfism	Nicotinic acid
Tyrosinemia	Phenylalanine, tyrosine restriction
Tyrosinemia with keratosis and corneal dystrophy	Protein restriction (phenylalanine and tyrosine)
Valinemia	Valine restriction
Vitamin A defect (beta-carotene 15,15'-dioxygenase)	Vitamin A
Vitamin B_{12} defect (conversion of B_{12} to precursor of 5'-deoxyadenosyl-B_{12} and methyl-B_{12})	Vitamin B_{12}
Vitamin K-dependent coagulation defect	Vitamin K
Xanthinuria	Purine restriction; allopurinol, fluids, alkali
Xanthurenic aciduria	Pyridoxine

*Other modes of therapy, including drugs, enzymes and transplantation, may be useful in the management of some of these conditions. See Bibliography for sources of additional information.[16,17,21,22]

Restriction of Harmful Substances. When a nutrient is toxic, restricting its supply may prove therapeutic. Excessive restriction may, however, prove harmful if the nutrient is essential. Thus, as we shall see, it is beneficial to restrict phenylalanine in phenylketonuria but enough must be provided to prevent deficiency.

Removal of Toxic Substances. When the dietary supply cannot be reduced below the toxic level, accumulations may, nevertheless, be prevented; e.g. the chelator, penicillamine, facilitates removal of copper in Wilson's disease, and allopurinol inhibits the synthesis of uric acid which is responsible for renal stone formation in gout. Later in this chapter we describe the use of keto acid analogs of amino acids that permit reduction in the intake of toxic substances and, at the same time, provide acceptors for ammonia, thereby reducing its toxicity.

Product Replacement. When deficiency causes symptoms, the substance may be provided exogenously either orally for low-molecular-weight, nondigestible and absorbable substances (such as uridine in hereditary orotic aciduria) or parenterally in the case of macromolecules (such as antihemophilic globulin in hemophilia or immunoglobulin in agammaglobulinemia).

Enhancement of Enzyme Activity. In a number of genetic disorders the affected enzyme retains some activity. For enzymes that depend on cofactor, the provision of greater-than-usual amounts of the vitamin that serves as cofactor, or as precursor of cofactor, boosts enzyme activity. In such cases, the defect involves either the utilization of the vitamin or the binding of the vitamin by the mutant enzyme.[16]

Synthesis of an increased number of partially defective enzyme molecules may also increase enzyme activity. For example, phenobarbitol may reduce bilirubin concentration in some inherited forms of hyperbilirubinemia by stimulating the synthesis of hepatic endoplasmic reticulum and the bilirubin conjugating enzymes associated with it.

In some disorders, increased enzyme activity causes harm. In familial hypercholesterolemia, intracellular cholesterol synthesis proceeds unchecked. The administration of substances that could reduce the activity of cholesterol-synthesizing enzymes might prove therapeutic.

Enzyme Replacement. Deficiencies of enzymes that act in the gut can be compensated for by predigesting the nutrient on which the enzyme acts. Examples include fermentation of lactose-containing milks in the case of lactase deficiency[4] or hydrolysis of protein in the case of trypsinogen deficiency. Digestive intestinal enzymes can also be provided directly, as is often done in children with cystic fibrosis.

Although the introduction of foreign proteins into the body when the native one is missing or defective presents enormous problems, a number of methods and a few actual human experiments have already been described.[19] Organ transplantation is another form of replacement therapy.[20]

INBORN ERRORS OF METABOLISM

We now turn to a number of inborn errors of metabolism that exemplify several points made thus far. We will describe variant forms of lesser severity for conditions with altered nutritional requirements and consider different modes of treatment, many of which involve dietary manipulation. The reader is referred elsewhere[12,16,21,22] for discussion of other disorders.

Phenylketonuria

Phenylketonuria (PKU) is a prototype of serious conditions that are detectable by neonatal screening and amenable to dietary therapy. In the classical form, activity of the enzyme phenylalanine hydroxylase, which is needed for the conversion of phenylalanine to tyrosine, is either absent or present in trace amounts.[23,24] As a result, phenylalanine accumulates and tyrosine becomes an essential amino acid (Fig. 39–2). We do not yet know the relative importance of phenylalanine toxicity, tyrosine deficiency or an elevated ratio of phenylalanine to tyrosine in causing retardation in the untreated patient. Diets that are low in phenylalanine and supplemented with tyrosine prevent mental retardation provided they are started in the first few months of life.[12,25,26] A slight reduction in I.Q. may still occur.[25]

As there are few, if any, signs of PKU in the first few months, early diagnosis depends on biochemical detection. To accomplish this newborns are screened for elevations of blood phenylalanine. Because some infants with PKU are missed by newborn screening,[27] phenylalanine should be determined in older infants with delayed development—particularly if associated with eczema, fair complexion, blonde hair and blue eyes.

Only a small proportion of infants with positive screening tests turn out to have PKU and to require treatment.[27] In the remainder of this section we discuss the evaluation of positive screening tests, the management of classical PKU, maternal phenylketonuria and variant forms of the disorder.

Evaluation of Positive Screening Tests. The risk of retardation is extremely high in infants with blood or serum phenylalanine concentrations of 20 mg per dl or greater. Not all infants with PKU will have yet attained such high concentrations when they are screened in the first few days of life. Consequently, the cutoff level must be set lower, usually between 2 and 6 mg per dl. As will be discussed further, the risk of retardation with elevations of less than 20 mg per dl is low. Before treatment is initiated two blood phenylalanine determinations of 20 mg per dl or higher with tyrosine concentrations of less than 5 mg per dl should be obtained.[28] Approximately 15 per cent of infants fulfilling these criteria develop the ability to convert phenylalanine to tyrosine during the first year of life. Consequently, every baby in whom the diet is started should be challenged with milk about three months after the start of dietary therapy. By the end of the first year of life most infants who have developed the ability to convert phenylalanine to tyrosine will require higher phenylalanine intakes to maintain their phenylalanine levels in the appropriate range than will those with the classical, persistent defect; a few may still require a challenge to make the distinction.[28]

Management of PKU. Once the diagnostic criteria are met, regular formula or breast feeding is discontinued and a casein hydrolysate from which most but not all of the phenylalanine has been removed is started instead. Such a formula, Lofenalac, is available in North America for infants with PKU. Hospitalization of the infant with newly discovered PKU provides an opportunity for health professionals to acquaint the parents with the management process and facilitates frequent monitoring of blood phenylalanine.

Phenylalanine is an essential amino acid and the amount needed per kilogram in newly diagnosed infant phenylketonurics to support adequate growth will be higher than at any subsequent age. Moreover, too-severe restriction can result in phenylalanine deficiency with growth failure and perhaps mental retardation.[12] A few ounces of regular cow's milk (or formula) will almost always have to be added to the special formula to prevent phenylalanine

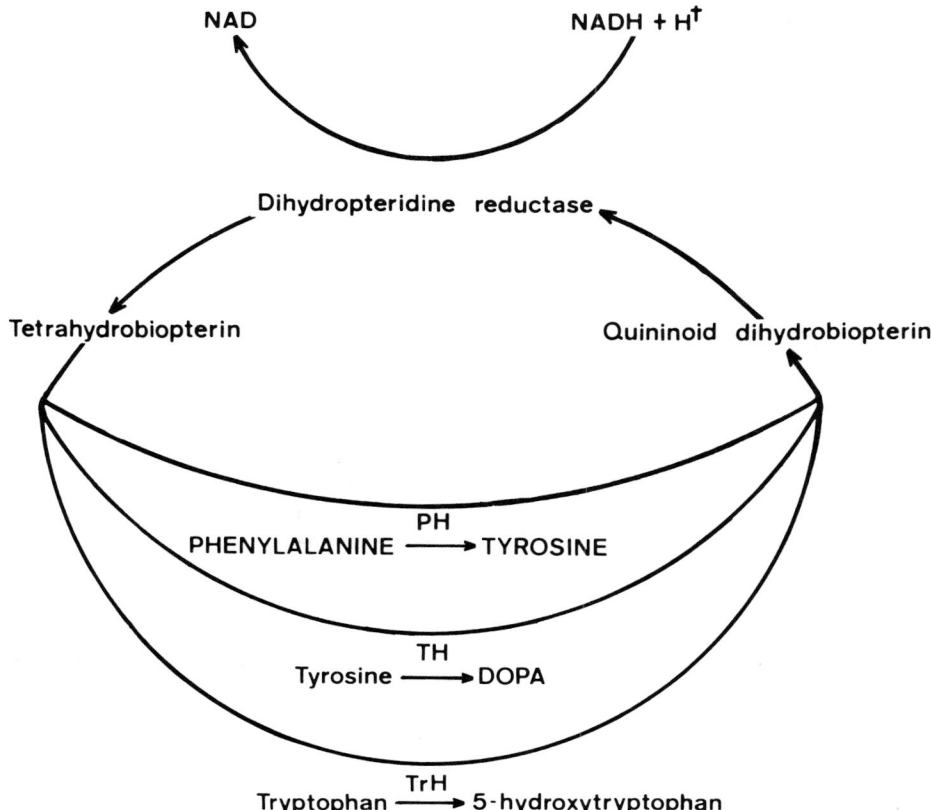

Fig. 39–2. Initial steps in phenylalanine, tyrosine and tryptophan metabolism. PH = phenylalanine hydroxylase, the enzyme that is defective in classical phenylketonuria, TH = tyrosine hydroxylase (central nervous system) or tyrosinase (melanocytes), TrH = tryptophan hydroxylase, NADH = nicotinamide dinucleotide, reduced, DOPA = dihydroxyphenylalanine.

deficiency. As the growth rate declines and as other foods are introduced, the serum phenylalanine level may rise. To assure that appropriate changes are made, blood phenylalanine should be measured once a week during the first year of life. Parents can be taught to collect the specimen themselves from a heel or finger prick. In some states a public health nurse and nutritionist visit the infant at home to collect the specimen and counsel the family.

The physical growth and mental development of PKU infants whose blood phenylalanine levels are maintained between 5.5 and 9.9 mg per dl are not significantly different at 4 years of age from those whose levels are maintained between 1.0 and 5.4 mg per dl.[25] Most physicians involved in PKU management aim to keep blood phenylalanine level between 3 and 8 mg per dl.

The PKU child will increasingly realize that many foods enjoyed by his peers are denied to him (or her). To allow the child somewhat greater latitude, an amino acid mixture from which phenylalanine is completely absent may be preferable to the low-phenylalanine formula used in infancy. Such a product is now available in the United States (Mead Johnson Phenyl-Free). Nevertheless, relatively small intakes of meat or dairy products will markedly raise the serum phenylalanine level. Efforts to maintain the serum phenylalanine within prescribed levels often meet with increased resistance from the child. Stealing and cheating ensue, threatening family stability. It is therefore important for investigators to determine how long the low-phenylalanine diet should be continued.

Although changes in behavior are noted when the blood phenylalanine concentration is raised abruptly, there is, as yet, little data to indicate the long-term effect that gradual termination of the low-phenylalanine diet after 4 years of age will have on either mental development or behavior. A clinical trial in which 4-year-old phenyl-

ketonurics were, with the consent of their parents, randomly assigned either to continue on the low-phenylalanine diet or to terminate it failed to reveal any significant difference in mental development between the two groups at 5 and 6 years of age.[29] Inasmuch as only 10 children were involved, the results cannot be considered conclusive. A randomized controlled trial of diet termination of approximately 100 6-year-old PKU children is currently in progress.

Maternal Phenylketonuria. Should diet termination in childhood prove safe, there will nonetheless be concern about completely stopping the diet in females. Off the diet, their blood phenylalanine will be high. When they become pregnant their fetuses will, regardless of the father's genotype, suffer from retardation, microcephaly and other congenital anomalies.[30]

Although a better outcome has been reported in a few infants whose PKU mothers were placed on low-phenylalanine diets during pregnancy, the duration of follow-up is too short, and the number of cases too small, to be confident that a low-phenylalanine diet instituted after conception will prevent damage to the fetus. As the concentration of phenylalanine in the amniotic fluid of the fetus from an untreated PKU mother was markedly elevated by the eighth week of gestation,[31] dietary restriction will probably have to be instituted early, perhaps even before conception, if a good outcome is to be obtained. Moreover, the restriction would have to be as complete as in the treatment of PKU in childhood; an infant born to a mother whose serum phenylalanine level was between 12 and 15 mg per dl during pregnancy was damaged.[32] The reinstitution of a low-phenylalanine diet is not easy; the formulas are not palatable to older subjects who have not been raised on them. Some physicians keep PKU girls on Lofenalac in small amounts to retain a taste for it should dietary restriction in pregnancy prove effective.

If damage to the infants of PKU mothers cannot be prevented by dietary treatment before and/or during pregnancy, the reduction in retardation from PKU which results from neonatal screening and early treatment may be offset by retardation in the offspring of PKU mothers.

Variant Forms. Approximately 20 infants in every 15,000 will have a positive screening test for PKU. Only 3, however, will have a positive follow-up test and only one, on the average, will prove to have phenylalanine levels before treatment of at least 20 mg per dl. Although all infants with such high elevations require therapy, they probably are a heterogeneous group.[33,34] The others will have moderate elevations between 6 and 20 mg per dl and in two-thirds of them serum phenylalanine will fall to normal within a few months. In the remaining one-third moderate elevation persists on a normal diet.[33] Phenylalanine hydroxylase activity, in those few in this category who have had liver biopsies, is approximately 10 per cent of normal.[24] This is much higher than in classical PKU[23,24] and is sufficient to prevent retardation even without dietary restriction.[35]

A rare variant has now been discovered that results from a deficiency of dihydropteridine reductase (DHPR), an enzyme needed to provide reduced biopterin cofactor not only for the conversion of phenylalanine to tyrosine but for the conversion of tyrosine to dihydroxyphenylalanine (DOPA) and of tryptophan to 5-hydroxytryptophan (Fig. 39–2). These, in turn, are converted to neurotransmitter substances in the brain; consequently, DHPR deficiency has profound effects on neuronal function. Seizures, mental deterioration and early death are observed despite dietary control of serum phenylalanine. Infants with this defect exhibit either marked or moderate phenylalanine elevation on screening.[36,37] As they do not respond to a low-phenylalanine diet alone but may respond to other therapy, the

diagnosis should be established early.[37] Recently, an infant discovered by newborn screening who failed to develop normally on a low-phenylalanine diet was found to have a deficiency of tetrahydrobiopterin (Fig. 39–2). His phenylalanine hydroxylase and DHPR activities were normal and he probably has a defect in biopterin synthesis. As biopterin does not enter the brain, the most appropriate therapy probably is DOPA and 5-hydroxytryptophan.[37a]

There is no conclusive evidence that heterozygotes for classical PKU suffer from carrying the gene. In fact, with a homozygote incidence of 1 in 15,000, the incidence of heterozygotes is approximately 1 in 60. Assuming that heterozygotes mate at random and that most classical phenylketonurics possess the same allele, such a high frequency suggests either a reproductive advantage for heterozygotes or random accumulation of the PKU gene. Ford reported that phenylalanine levels in heterozygotes, which are more likely to be slightly elevated than those in normal homozygotes, correlate positively with some aspects of intelligence and negatively with others.[38]

Bessman suggested that a pregnant PKU heterozygote will be less able than a normal homozygote to synthesize tyrosine for her fetus. The fetus then becomes dependent on the amino acids supplied in the mother's diet; when they are low, the fetus' needs may not be completely met. If the fetus is also a heterozygote, its inadequate tyrosine synthesis will be added to that of the mother. Mild physical or mental retardation, with frequencies higher than severe retardation due to homozygous PKU, could result.[39] Unless the mother is recognized as a heterozygote, which is unlikely, the etiology will remain obscure. Reproductive fitness would probably be affected if the mother's supply of tyrosine was low during pregnancy.

Much remains to be learned about the genes of PKU and the pathogenesis of the condition. Nevertheless, dietary restriction

Table 39–2. Other Congenital Defects Associated with Hyperammonemia

Disease	Defect	Biochemical Findings	Clinical Manifestations	Inheritance	Treatment
Ketotic hyperglycinemia Methylmalonic aciduria	Defect in degradation of branched-chain amino acids in fibroblasts	Ketoacidosis and accumulation of derivatives of branched-chain amino acid catabolism	Mental retardation Episodic coma	Autosomal recessive	Protein restriction B₁₂
Isovaleric acidemia Propionic acidemia					Glycine Biotin
Hyperornithinemia	?Ornithine amino transferase	Increased ornithine, homocitrullinuria	Feeding problems Mental retardation Seizures	Autosomal recessive	Protein restriction
Hyperdibasic amino aciduria	Defective intestinal absorption and renal tubular reabsorption of lysine	Increased lysine, arginine and glutamine-glutamate in urine. Plasma arginine and lysine low normal	Seizures Growth failure Mental retardation Hepatosplenomegaly	Unknown	
"Lysin-uric" protein intolerance	Increased renal clearance of arginine, lysine and ornithine. High-affinity transport system in renal tubular epithelium defective	Decreased plasma lysine, arginine and ornithine	Protein intolerance Growth failure Vomiting and diarrhea	Autosomal recessive Autosomal dominant	Administration of citrulline and lysine
Nonketotic hyperglycinemia	Glycine cleavage enzyme	Increased glycine in plasma and CSF	Seizures Mental retardation Coma	Autosomal recessive	Strychnine

of phenylalanine greatly improves the outcome. Care must be taken in establishing the diagnosis so that variants are not needlessly or dangerously treated.

Urea Cycle Enzyme Deficiencies

Hyperammonemia in early childhood commonly results from a deficiency of one of the five enzymes of the urea cycle. It may occasionally be associated with disorders of ornithine or lysine metabolism or inborn errors of branched chain amino acid catabolism (Table 39–2). Clinically, the disorders are marked by recurrent episodes of vomiting, lethargy and coma related to protein intake. Most children who survive are mentally retarded. The mainstay of therapy has been a protein-restricted diet. Although this may reduce the symptomatic episodes, it interferes with normal physical growth.

The Urea Cycle. Normally, ammonia is converted to urea in the liver through the Krebs-Henseleit cycle (Fig. 39–3). The first two enzymes of the cycle are mitochondrial. Carbamylphosphate synthetase I (CPSI) catalyzes the conversion of ammonia, ATP and bicarbonate to carbamylphosphate (cp). Ornithine transcarbamylase (OTC) carboxylates ornithine, forming citrulline. Citrulline is transported to the cytoplasm where it combines with aspartate to form argininosuccinic acid (ASA), a reaction catalyzed by argininosuccinic acid synthetase (ASA-S). Fumarate is cleaved by argininosuccinic acid lyase (ASA-L), yielding arginine. Urea is then formed by the action of arginase, regenerating ornithine which is transported back into the mitochondria.

Genetics. Congenital defects of each of the enzymes of the urea cycle have been described. Deficiencies of the cytosol enzymes, ASA-S, ASA-L and arginase, are thought to be inherited as autosomal recessives. The mode of inheritance of CPS deficiency is probably autosomal recessive although there have been few reported cases. There is evidence based on family

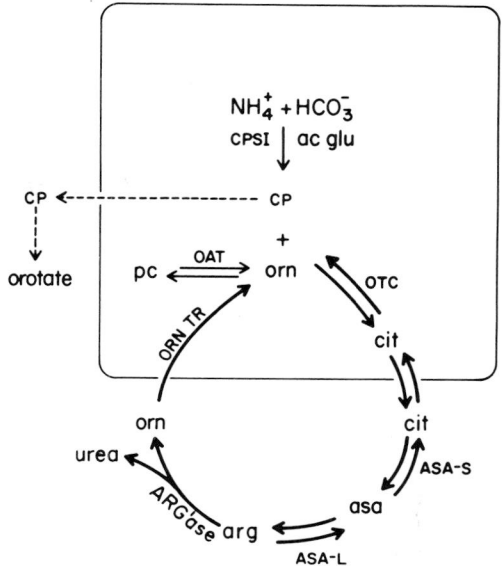

Fig. 39–3. The urea cycle. CPSI = carbamyl phosphate synthetase, OTC = ornithine transcarbamylase, ASA-S = argininosuccinic acid synthetase, ASA-L = ASA-lyase, Orn Tr = ornithine translocation, cp = carbamylphosphate, ac glu = N-acetyl-glutamate, OAT = ornithine aminotransferase, pc = Δ'pyrolline 5 carboxylate, ARG'ase = arginase. Boxed reactions are mitochondrial. Enzymes are denoted by capital letters and substrates by small letters.

studies that OTC deficiency is inherited as an X-linked trait.[40] The hemizygous males, with only the affected X chromosome, die in the neonatal period, while heterozygous females have milder and more variable symptoms ranging from a dislike of protein to episodes of lethargy and coma. Liver from a heterozygote female contains two distinct populations of hepatocytes: those with normal OTC activity and those with no activity.[41] This is compatible with the Lyon hypothesis that states that in any cell in a female only one X chromosome will be active.

Incidence. Although it is assumed that these disorders are rare, few studies of their frequency are available. Levy[42] reported an incidence of ASA-L deficiency of 1 in 70,000 newborn infants in Massachusetts between 1968 and 1973. The literature contains reports of more than 80 families with congenital urea cycle defects[43] (CPS deficiency 6, OTC deficiency 28, ASA-S deficiency 11, ASA-L deficiency 37, arginase deficiency 3). In response to a questionnaire, 109 genetic centers around the world identified 114 recently treated cases of congenital urea cycle defects, many of which have not been previously reported (Table 39–3).[44]

Rett[45] attempted to study the incidence of hyperammonemia in an institutionalized mentally retarded population. He found 30 female patients with a history of protein intolerance out of a population of 6,000. Of these patients, plasma ammonium values were reported for 21; 17 were abnormally high.

Laboratory Diagnosis. Diagnosis of urea cycle enzymopathies depends upon finding elevated plasma levels of ammonium and glutamine. Plasma ornithine concentration is normal and that of urea nitrogen is usually low normal.

The enzyme defect can be inferred from the specific metabolite that accumulates: orotic acid in the urine in OTC deficiency, citrulline, argininosuccinic acid and arginine in the plasma and urine in ASA-S, ASA-L and arginase deficiencies respectively. CPS deficiency is suggested by ex-

clusion of the other four enzymopathies and of hyperammonemia caused by acute or chronic liver diseases, Reye's syndrome, asparaginase treatment, propionic acidemia, hyperlysinemia, hyperornithinemia, isovaleric acidemia and methylmalonic aciduria. Definitive diagnosis[43] depends on enzyme assay in liver or a more accessible tissue (Table 39–3).

Urea Formation. Surprisingly, patients with urea cycle enzyme deficiencies usually have near-normal levels of blood urea nitrogen. One explanation has been that only a fraction of normal capacity is used to produce urea in the unaffected individual, so that partial enzyme deficiency still permits normal BUN concentrations.[46] It is also possible that the enzyme deficiency is not present in all organs.[47] Scott-Emuakpor et al.[48] proposed, in a case of citrullinemia, that an enzymatic path normally of little physiologic significance may be enhanced to compensate for the ASA-S defect and permit urea production. However, in a case of neonatal citrullinemia, whatever urea was formed came from dietary arginine via arginase. At the lowest level of arginine intake, 1.3 mM per kg per day, plasma urea nitrogen was only 0.7 mM, implying that at zero arginine intake urea synthesis would cease.[49]

Variability of Expression. Although hyperammonemia and its clinical sequelae of vomiting, lethargy and coma related to excessive protein intake are observed in all of the defects, the biochemical and phenotypic manifestations differ in the individual enzyme deficiencies. In ASA-L deficiency a specific hair abnormality, trichorrhexis nodosa, is evident. This may be related to arginine deficiency, although it is not a feature of the other urea cycle defects in which plasma arginine is low. While the clinical condition remains stable between hyperammonemic episodes in patients with defects of the first four enzymes, arginine deficiency has been associated with progressive degeneration of the central nervous system.[50]

Table 39–3. Distribution of Cases of Congenital Urea Cycle Enzyme Defects in 109 Genetic Centers

	CPS	OTC	ASA-S	ASA-L	Arginase
United States	3	18	6	16	3
Canada		5	1	4	
Japan		2	3		
Australia	1	5	1	1	
Belgium	3				3
England		1			
France	3	16	4	3	
Holland			1		5
Switzerland			2	2	
Germany		1	1		
TOTAL	10	48	19	26	11

Table 39–4. Demonstrated Presence of Urea Cycle Enzymes in Various Tissues

Enzyme	Liver	Jejunal Mucosa	RBC	WBC	Skin Fibroblasts
CPS	+	+	−	?	−
OTC	+	+	−	?	−
ASA-S	+	−	+	+	+
ASA-L	+	−	+	+	+
Arginase	+	−	+	+	−

Within each enzyme defect there is a spectrum of clinical manifestations ranging from death in the newborn period to cyclical vomiting and migraine in adolescence. For example, the typical male with OTC deficiency has less than 5 per cent activity and dies in the neonatal period. In a surviving male child with a variant form, the OTC enzyme shows decreased affinity for ornithine, a shift of pH optimum and 25 per cent of normal activity under physiologic conditions.[51]

Enzymatic evidence for genetic heterogeneity comes from kinetic studies in fibroblasts of three patients with ASA-S deficiency. All three showed decreased binding of citrulline and/or aspartate, but the residual ASA-S had a distinct and different curve of activity in each patient.[52] In a case of ASA-L deficiency, the enzyme was defective in the liver but not in the brain and kidney, suggesting that more than one gene may be responsible for ASA-L activity.[47]

Migraine as an Expression of the Heterozygous State. Russell[53] suggested that the heterozygous state of congenital hyperammonemia may be characterized by mild protein intolerance manifested clinically by migraine in adults and by cyclic vomiting in children. He noted that the grandmother and mother of two children with OTC deficiency suffered from migrainous attacks and voluntarily avoided high-protein foods. Ammonium chloride tolerance tests were done, and within 4 hours both women developed nausea and headache and their plasma ammonium levels rose to three times normal. Similar results were obtained when a protein tolerance test was done in two sibs and in the mother of a child with ASA-L deficiency.

When protein or ammonium chloride loads were administered to 15 children with migraine and cyclic vomiting, 9 had abnormally high baseline plasma ammonium levels. The tests produced marked hyperammonemia in 8; 6 developed migraine symptoms. Of 7 girls with cyclical vomiting subjected to enzyme assay, 3 were proven to have deficient activity of OTC.[53]

Treatment. The treatment of congenital urea cycle enzymopathies can be divided into acute and long-term therapy.

Acute Therapy. Peritoneal dialysis appears to be the most useful therapy in reducing plasma ammonium levels.[53a] Peritoneal dialysis for a period of seven days in a male neonate with OTC deficiency removed fifty times more ammonia than a single exchange transfusion.[54] However, peritoneal dialysis is not without difficulties and risks. Snyderman's patient developed Candida peritonitis. Recently sodium benzoate has been used successfully in reducing acute hyperammonemia in three patients.[54a] None of the many other maneuvers employed for acute management of congenital hyperammonemia has been very successful.[55]

Long-term Therapy. Because the goals of long-term therapy are adequate growth and maintenance of normal levels of the urea cycle precursors (ammonia, alanine and glutamine), all attempts at such therapy have included dietary restriction of protein supplemented with, or replaced by, amino acids. Severe protein restriction alone may be successful in ameliorating symptoms and reducing plasma ammonium and glutamine concentrations, but such dietary inadequacy prevents adequate growth. In order to promote growth, Buist[56] added arginine (a quasi-essential amino acid in all forms of congenital hyperammonemia except arginase deficiency) to a protein-restricted diet in a case of ASA-S deficiency. This corrected the imbalance caused by arginine deficiency, but the patient continued to maintain high plasma levels of ammonium and glutamine. However, in ASA-L deficiency, arginine supplements at a dose of 4 mM per kg per day have resulted in control of hyperammonemia and normal growth.[56a] Snyderman[54] managed a male with OTC deficiency with a mixture of the nine essential amino acids as well as arginine, cystine, tyrosine and aspartic acid; she used no additional dietary protein. This therapy resulted in a normal plasma ammonia level. Even though the patient died at age 45 days, the study demonstrated that limiting the nitrogen source to that which could be effectively utilized reduced the plasma ammonia levels.

Because they are readily transaminated to their corresponding amino acids, nitrogen-free analogs of essential amino acids could provide more effective therapy than the amino acids themselves. Not only do they share the beneficial effects of amino acids but, by virtue of their role as amino group acceptors, they lower labile nitrogen (glutamine, ammonia and alanine) levels more effectively. This capacity to accept amino groups would permit a greater and more varied protein intake. The greater palatability of the nitrogen-free analogs should also assure greater patient compliance than a regimen of amino acids with or without protein restriction. Furthermore, a fraction of these analogs is oxidized and, by an as yet undetermined mechanism, stimulates nitrogen sparing.[57]

The net result of addition of the nitrogen-free analogs to a protein-restricted diet would be to shunt the amino group of urea precursors into essential amino acids and thus reduce the requirement for urea synthesis as an outlet for ammonia.

The intravenous administration of nitrogen-free analogs of valine, leucine, isoleucine and phenylalanine to a 13-year-old girl with CPS deficiency resulted in a rise of the corresponding plasma amino acids, including tyrosine and alloisoleucine, and a fall in a component of the labile nitrogen pool, alanine.[58] A protein-restricted diet (0.75 gm per kg per day), together with oral supplements of the five nitrogen-free analogs plus the remaining essential amino acids and arginine, over an 18-month period led to increased growth (Fig. 39–4) and normal plasma amino acid and ammonia levels.[59] Clinically the child appeared more alert and had no further episodes of vomiting or lethargy. Following the initial six months of therapy the nutritional supplement was withdrawn. Fasting plasma ammonium, glutamine and alanine were normal during therapy, rose promptly to abnormal levels when therapy was stopped and then fell toward normal when therapy was resumed.

Determinations of nitrogen intake and urinary nitrogen output showed increased retention of nitrogen during therapy, suggesting a nitrogen-sparing effect. There is also some evidence that this regimen may have led to improved protein tolerance. Increasing the patient's nitrogen intake from 2.8 gm per day to 4.6 gm per day resulted in no change in the apparent nitrogen balance, nor did it precipitate hyperammonemia while she received the nitrogen-free analogs.

Therapy with a protein-restricted diet and mixtures of essential amino acids and their nitrogen-free analogs has been used in a 1-month-old male with zero activity of ASA-S who was in coma when treatment was begun.[60] Dramatic improvement oc-

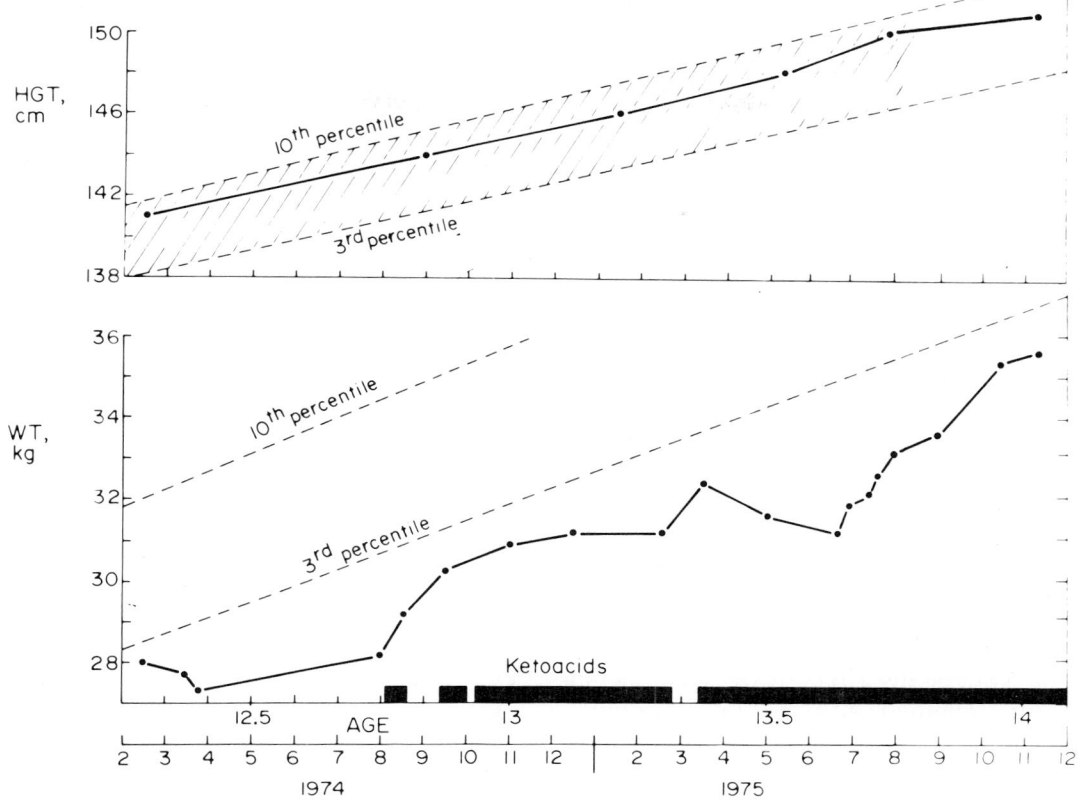

Fig. 39-4. The growth of the CPS-deficient patient before and during treatment with N-free amino acid analogs.

curred within 7 days with plasma ammonia levels falling from 620 μM to 180 μM and subsequently to normal. The child regained consciousness and seizure activity ceased. At 7 months of age, despite his stormy first few weeks, he was functioning developmentally at a 4-month level. On this mixture he was able to tolerate 1.3 gm protein per kg per day. His weight gain was satisfactory. Unfortunately the child became suddenly hyperammonemic at 8 months of age, probably as a result of a viral encephalitis, and expired.

The above results indicate that the long-term management of urea cycle enzymopathies should include: (1) sufficient arginine, except in the case of arginase deficiency, to meet the requirements for protein synthesis and to prevent ornithine supply from becoming rate limiting for citrulline synthesis, (2) provision of the remaining essential amino acids using the minimum quantities of nitrogen necessary for growth and (3) elimination of nitrogen accumulation by the use of nitrogen-free analogs of essential amino acids.

Genetic Disorders of Pyruvate Metabolism

Although inherited abnormalities of pyruvate metabolism are rare, study of their biochemistry is both interesting and informative as pyruvate metabolism is closely intertwined with carbohydrate, fat and amino acid metabolism.[16,61,62] The pathophysiologic mechanisms of these disorders include both precursor accumulation and product deficiency. Pyruvate accumulates and, since it is readily converted to lactate and alanine, these compounds

mits the oxidation of glyceraldehyde-3-phosphate, a glycolytic intermediate, thus ensuring continued glycolysis under anaerobic conditions.

The formation of lactate is summarized in Equation 1.

$$(1) \qquad CH_3 - \underset{\underset{O}{\|}}{C} - COOH + NADH_2 \rightleftharpoons CH_3 - \underset{\underset{OH}{|}}{CH} - COOH + NAD^+$$

are also present in plasma and urine in increased amounts.[61,62] The excessive accumulation of lactate may result in lactic acidosis,[63] which is a common feature of these conditions. Product deficiency also occurs with reduced production of either acetyl-coenzyme A (CoA) or of gluconeogenic intermediates, depending on the enzyme affected.

Early and exact biochemical diagnosis of the genetic disorders of pyruvate metabolism combined with an understanding of their pathophysiology has resulted in the development of rational nutritional therapy with some success.[61] A general consideration of the features of pyruvate metabolism is necessary before describing the clinical disorders.

Pyruvate Metabolism. Pyruvate occupies a central position in metabolism, and is product or precursor in at least six metabolic pathways (Fig. 39–5). The glycolytic pathway is a major source of pyruvate production, with 2 molecules of pyruvate being formed from each molecule of glucose. Phosphoenol pyruvate is the immediate precursor of pyruvate in this pathway and is converted to pyruvate by the enzyme pyruvate kinase in a reaction which also generates a molecule of ATP.

Reduction of pyruvate to lactate is the final reaction in anaerobic glycolysis. This reaction requires $NADH_2$ and is catalyzed by the cytoplasmic enzyme lactate dehydrogenase. The regeneration of NAD^+ by the conversion of pyruvate to lactate per-

The equilibrium constant for this reaction is described by Equation 2.

$$(2) \qquad K_{eq} = \frac{[lactate]\,[NADH_2]}{[pyruvate]\,[NAD^+]}$$

Solving for [lactate] we obtain Equation 3.

$$(3) \qquad [lactate] = [pyruvate] \times K_{eq}\,\frac{[NADH_2]}{[NAD^+]}$$

Accordingly, lactate concentration is dependent on two variables: (1) the pyruvate concentration and (2) the ratio of reduced to oxidized adenine dinucleotide. This adenine dinucleotide ratio is dependent upon the oxidation state of the particular tissue and thus the ratio of lactate to pyruvate concentration (L:P ratio) also reflects the state of tissue oxygenation. Under conditions of normal tissue oxygenation the L:P ratio is 10:1.[16]

All conditions with increased lactate concentrations can, therefore, be classified by the L:P ratio. Most commonly, lactate accumulations are the result of tissue anoxia secondary to some cardiopulmonary or hematologic abnormality.[63] Tissue anoxia results in decreased oxidation of $NADH_2$ by the reactions of oxidative phosphorylation. Thus the ratio $NADH_2:NAD^+$ increases, causing an increase of the L:P ratio to 20:1 or even higher. Stated another way, anoxia results in the accumulation of lactate in excess of pyruvate. Conversely, in the inherited disorders of pyruvate metabolism tissue

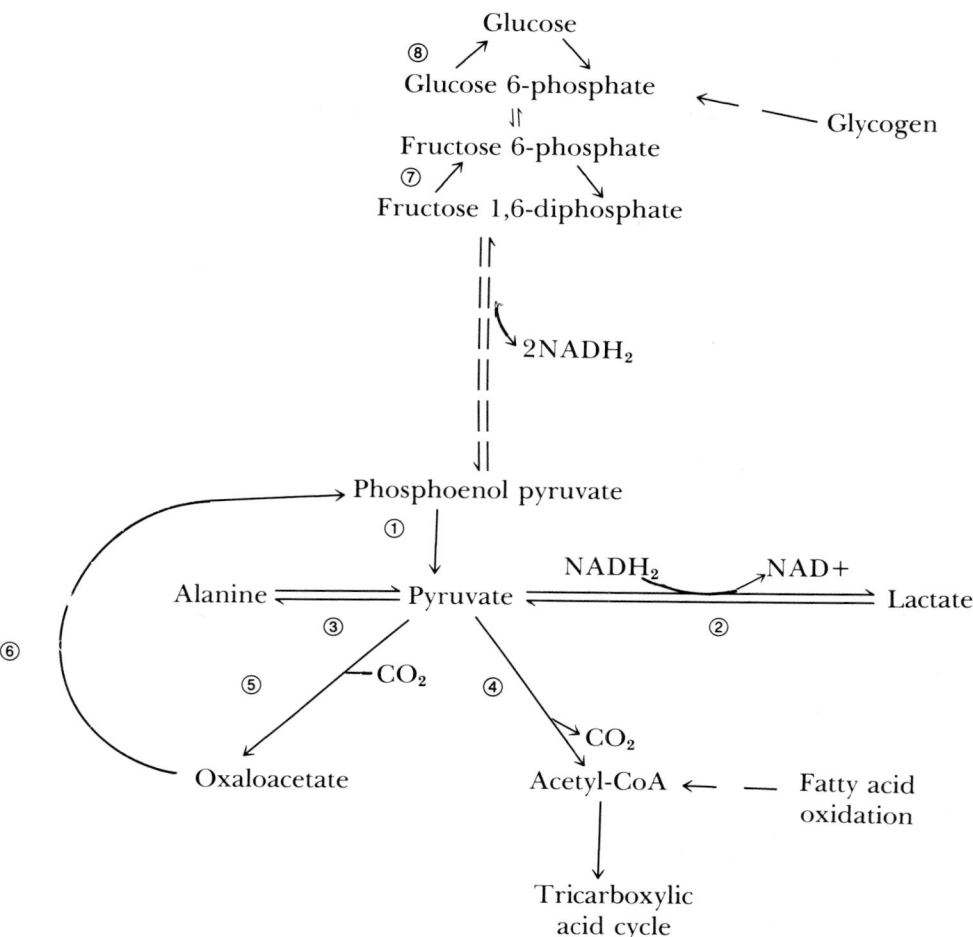

Fig. 39–5. Pyruvate metabolism. Key to enzymes: 1 = pyruvate kinase, 2 = lactate dehydrogenase, 3 = alanine aminotransferase, 4 = pyruvate dehydrogenase complex, 5 = pyruvate carboxylase, 6 = phosphoenol pyruvate carboxykinase, 7 = fructose 1,6-diphosphatase, 8 = glucose-6-phosphatase. Several of the intermediate steps in the glycolytic pathway have been deleted as indicated by the dashed arrows.

oxygenation is normal, the ratio of $NADH_2:NAD^+$ is normal, there is a concomitant increase in both lactate and pyruvate and the L:P ratio is normal.

Pyruvate is also converted to alanine in a readily reversible reaction catalyzed by alanine aminotransferase. The normal molar ratios of lactate:pyruvate:alanine are 10:1:3.[16] In the genetic disorders characterized by an accumulation of both pyruvate and lactate, alanine will also in-

crease, maintaining a normal 10:1:3 molar ratio. With hypoxia, however, lactate accumulates in excess of pyruvate, and alanine concentration remains low. Thus in evaluating conditions with lactate accumulation, the alanine concentration is of value in predicting the L:P ratio and can be used when pyruvate determinations are not available.[16]

A fourth major reaction for pyruvate is the conversion to acetyl-CoA catalyzed by the pyruvate dehydrogenase (PDH) complex located within the mitochondria. This reaction allows pyruvate formed from glucose, lactate or alanine to enter into the tricarboxylic acid cycle and be completely oxidized to CO_2 and water. The PDH complex consists of three catalytic and two regulatory enzymes.[62,64,65] As described below, there is good evidence for genetic defects of four of these five components.

Pyruvate decarboxylase, the first enzyme in the catalytic sequence (E_1), uses thiamin as a cofactor and functions to remove the C_1 carbon of pyruvate. The second enzyme in the sequence, lipoate acetyltransferase (E_2), uses lipoic acid as a cofactor and links the acetyl group formed by the C_2 and C_3 carbons of pyruvate to CoA to form acetyl CoA. The final enzyme of this complex, lipoamide dehydrogenase (E_3), uses NAD^+ and FAD^+ to reoxidize the reduced lipoate formed by E_2. On the basis of biochemical and genetic evidence (see below) E_3 is thought to be identical to the lipoamide dehydrogenase found in the α-ketoglutarate dehydrogenase enzyme complex.[66]

A further complexity of the PDH complex is the existence of E_1 in two forms: an inactive phosphorylated form ($E_1 - P$) and an active dephosphorylated form (E_1).[65,66] The ATP-dependent conversion of E_1 to $E_1 - P$ is catalyzed by PDH kinase, an enzyme inhibited by pyruvate and ADP. The activation of $E_1 - P$ is catalyzed by PDH phosphatase which, in turn, is activated by Ca^{++} and Mg^{++} and adenosine $3',5'$ cyclic phosphate (cAMP).[67] As the overall reaction catalyzed by the PDH complex is sequential, the phosphorylation-dephosphorylation of the E_1 component may regulate the overall reaction rate. Furthermore, the function of cAMP as an activator of PHD phosphatase suggests the possibility of hormonal regulation of the PDH complex.

In the postabsorptive state (i.e. following a 12- to 14-hour overnight fast) when inadequate amounts of glucose are available from dietary and glycogenolytic sources, the major flow of hepatic pyruvate metabolism is diverted from oxidation in the tricarboxylic acid cycle to the formation of glucose by the reactions of the gluconeogenic pathway.[68,69] The initial reaction of gluconeogenesis is the conversion of pyruvate to oxaloacetate by the mitochondrial enzyme pyruvate carboxylase. In the postabsorptive state acetyl CoA derived from fatty acid oxidation stimulates pyruvate carboxylase and diverts pyruvate to gluconeogenesis.[68] Oxaloacetate is then converted to phosphoenol pyruvate (PEP) in a GTP-dependent reaction catalyzed by PEP carboxykinase. The enzymes catalyzing the remainder of the gluconeogenetic pathway are the same as those used in glycolysis with the exception of fructose-1,6-diphosphatase and glucose-6-phosphatase. A defect in any one of the four enzymes (pyruvate carboxylase, PEP carboxykinase, fructose-1,6-diphosphatase and glucose-6-phosphatase) will result in decreased gluconeogenesis and accumulation of pyruvate and lactate.[61]

Clinical Syndromes. *General.* There are many inherited conditions which are associated with hyperpyruvic acidemia and lactic acidemia.[61] In most the accumulation of pyruvate results from its underutilization, but in others from its overproduction. Individuals affected with these disorders typically have intermittent or chronic elevation of plasma pyruvate (normal 0.03 to 0.1 mM) and plasma lactate (normal less than 1 mM) with normal L:P ratios of 10 or less.

Although pyruvate accumulation is the primary abnormality, patients with these conditions are usually discovered because of the secondary lactate accumulation; significant elevations of lactate cause metabolic acidosis and lactate determinations are available in most hospitals. Accumulation of lactate in excess of 2 mM associated with an acidic deviation of the blood pH is defined as lactic acidosis.[63] Lactic acidosis is documented by measuring the plasma lactate; it should be suspected in any patient with metabolic acidosis and an increase in the anion gap.[63,70] The anion gap is calculated by Equation 4.

$$(4) \quad ([Na^+] + [K^+]) - ([Cl^-] + [HCO_3^-]) = \text{Anion gap (mEq/liter)}$$

Normally, the anion gap is less than 16 mEq per liter and is made up of an unmeasured anion such as sulfate. In metabolic disorders in which there is an accumulation of an unmeasured anion such as lactate (or β-hydroxybutyrate or acetoacetate) the anion gap may increase to 20 to 30 mEq per liter. If the anion gap is excessive, lactate and, when possible, pyruvate concentrations should be measured and the L:P ratio determined. Plasma and urinary alanine determinations should be performed, especially if pyruvate determinations are not available.

An additional clue to pyruvate accumulation comes from the use of Acetest tablets.[71] Urine containing pyruvate in concentrations as low as 10^{-4}M causes a "dirty, grayish purple" reaction which is readily distinguished from the vivid purple color caused by ketone bodies.

PDH Complex Defects. Eighteen patients of both sexes have been described with decreased conversion of pyruvate to acetyl-CoA and associated chronic or intermittent elevations of plasma pyruvate and lactate concentrations. Eight children [62,65,72-76] have had abnormalities of the E_1 component (pyruvate decarboxylase). One infant[77] had a reduction in the E_1-activating enzyme PDH phosphatase. Three infants[78] had a reduction in both pyruvate dehydrogenase and in α-ketoglutarate dehydrogenase and therefore are thought to be defective in the E_3 component of PDH complex, which is also present in α-ketoglutarate dehydrogenase. Four other patients[62,71,80] had reduced PDH complex activity with normal E_1 activity and no abnormality of α-ketoglutarate dehydrogenase. Presumably these patients have a defect in the E_2 component. Two additional patients[80] have been reported with an uncharacterized reduction in PDH.

The clinical findings in these patients are variable, but in general two phenotypes have been described: a severe infantile form and a less severe, intermittent childhood form. Six patients have been reported with the infantile form in which severe lactic acidosis with normal L:P ratios developed in the first day(s) of life. Hypotonia, seizures, failure to thrive and a relentless downhill course usually result in death in the first weeks or months of life. The enzyme defects associated with this phenotype have included a severe reduction in E_1,[65,76] a partial reduction in PDH phosphatase[77] and a marked reduction in E_3.[78]

Long-term therapy for severely affected infants has in general been unsuccessful. Oral and intravenous bicarbonate and peritoneal dialysis with an *acetate-buffered* dialysis fluid temporarily corrects the acidosis. (Dialysis fluids buffered with lactate are probably contraindicated in these patients.) Vitamin therapy with pharmacologic doses of the known cofactors for PDH complex (thiamin, lipoic acid) has been unsuccessful but should probably be attempted.

Twelve patients with the childhood form of lactic acidosis associated with reduced PDH complex activity have been reported.[62] In these children the disorder is characterized by exacerbations of their biochemical and clinical abnormalities at times of physical or emotional stress. All of these children exhibited neurologic abnormalities with ataxia and choreoathetosis. Four of them had nystagmus or other oculomotor abnormalities. Seven of the 8 in which intellect is described were retarded and 5 have failed to grow normally.

The biochemical abnormalities in the patients with onset of symptoms in childhood are variable. Some of them have chronic mild elevations of lactate, pyruvate and alanine, while in others the concentrations of these compounds are increased only during an exacerbation of their disease. For example, a 9-year-old boy with intermittent ataxia and normal intelligence had mild but consistently increased urinary alanine and plasma pyruvate, but plasma lactate was increased only during ataxic episodes.[73] Biochemical characterization of the PDH in muscle homogenates and sonicates of cultured skin fibroblasts revealed an abnormality of the E_1 component resulting in a 70 per cent decrease in overall PDH complex activity. A similar patient was reported by Lonsdale et al.[72,74]

In a retarded 3-year-old female who had persistent lactic acidosis and "nystagmoid" eye movements[79] PDH complex activity in cultured fibroblasts was approximately 15 per cent of controls with normal activity of the E_1 component and a significant reduction of E_2.[62]

Cedarbaum et al.[71] reported an 8-year-old, severely retarded male with continuous choreoathetoid movements and a peculiar odor. Plasma pyruvate and lactate were normal on fasting specimens but were increased on 2-hour postprandial specimens, suggesting that postprandial samples may be a more sensitive screen for the disorder. Blood pyruvate concentrations were consistently abnormal during a standard glucose tolerance test. Profound lactic acidosis developed 48 hours after institution of a diet containing 65 per cent carbohydrate and 15 per cent fat. Biochemical studies on cultured fibroblasts demonstrated a reduction in PDH complex activity to 15 per cent of control values with evidence of normal function of the E_1 and E_3 component, suggesting a defect in the E_2 component.

Therapy for older children with PDH complex abnormalities has been primarily dietary. Vitamin therapy with thiamin has been ineffective but a therapeutic trial is worthwhile in each new case. Theoretically, diets low in carbohydrate (which would add to the pyruvate and lactate accumulations) and high in fat (which would bypass the metabolic block and supply energy substrates to the tricarboxylic acid cycle) would be beneficial in these patients. Some of the patients[80] have shown subjective improvement on a 65 per cent fat diet. It is hoped that in the future these patients will be identified earlier in life and prospective studies of high-fat diets will be performed.

In addition to these 18 infants and children with chronic or intermittent elevation of pyruvate and lactate caused by severe reductions in PDH complex activity, a recent report[81] suggests that Friedreich's ataxia may result from a moderate reduction in PDH complex activity. Friedreich's ataxia is an autosomal recessively inherited form of spinocerebellar degeneration characterized by progressive ataxia, dysarthria and peripheral neuropathy, with onset in late childhood. The PDH complex activity in fibroblasts cultured from 4 patients with the disease averaged 43 per cent of control values, although they had no accumulation of plasma pyruvate, lactate or alanine on high-carbohydrate diets.[81] The activity of α-ketoglutarate dehydrogenase was similarly reduced, suggesting a defect in the E_3 component. Further studies will be required before this modest reduction in PDH complex activity can be accepted as the primary abnormality in Friedreich's ataxia.

In summary, several clinical phenotypes have been reported in patients with reduced PDH complex activity. Severe reduction of PDH complex activity to less than 15 per cent of control values is associated with lactic acidosis, severe neurologic disease and death in infancy. Moderate reduction in PDH complex activity to values 15 to 30 per cent of control is associated with intermittent ataxia, choreoathetosis and lactic acidosis with onset in childhood. Moderate reductions of PDH complex activity to levels 40 to 50 per cent of control may result in spinocerebellar degeneration of the Friedreich's type with onset in late childhood or at puberty. Consideration of the metabolic role of the PDH complex and preliminary reports on a few patients suggest that dietary therapy with a high-fat intake may be of benefit in some of these patients.

We turn now to genetic defects of pyruvate metabolism in which gluconeogenesis is defective. As a result, hypoglycemia occurs in addition to increased concentrations of pyruvate, lactate and alanine.

Pyruvate Carboxylase Deficiency. Five patients have been reported with enzymatic evidence of decreased pyruvate carboxylase activity. In a 3-year-old female with profound psychomotor retardation, hyperpyruvic acidemia, hyperalaninemia, episodic lactic acidosis and hypoglycemia, biochemical investigation revealed reduced pyruvate carboxylase activity in liver homogenates.[82] Vitamin therapy with biotin, the cofactor for pyruvate carboxylase, was ineffective but therapy with thiamin seemed to improve the patient. The reasons for this are unclear but perhaps thiamin facilitated metabolism of pyruvate by the PDH complex.[16] The patient responded to a diet which provided adequate calories without excessive carbohydrate.

The other four patients[83,83a,83b] also exhibited mental retardation, lactic acidosis and hyperalaninemia. Pyruvate carboxylase activity was deficient in liver and/or fibroblasts. Extensive studies on the liver tissue of one of these patients suggested an important role for pyruvate carboxylase in modulating the concentration and intracellular distribution of hepatic acetyl-CoA.[83a]

In addition to these five patients, there have been over 100 children reported with Leigh's disease (subacute necrotizing encephalomyelopathy, SNE) a fatal neurodegenerative condition which may be caused by a deficiency of pyruvate carboxylase.[61,84] Children with SNE have focal areas of necrosis in the thalamus, pons and thoracic spinal cord; this results in somnolence, blindness, deafness and spasticity. Onset is usually within the first two years of life and inheritance appears to be autosomal recessive in nature. The biochemical evidence for a primary defect in pyruvate carboxylase in this disorder is inconclusive. However, some children with Leigh's disease have shown increases in plasma pyruvate, alanine and lactate. Four patients have been shown to have absent or reduced pyruvate carboxylase; however, this has not been a uniform finding.[61] An additional biochemical abnormality in SNE is the presence of a low-molecular-weight protein inhibitor of thiamin pyrophosphate phosphoryltransferase in the urine. The relationship of this inhibitor of an enzyme that catalyzes the formation of thiamin triphosphate to the abnormalities of pyruvate carboxylase is unclear. The interested reader is referred to recent reviews.[61,61a]

PEP Carboxykinase Deficiency. No patients have been reported with a deficiency of this enzyme.

Fructose-1,6-diphosphatase Deficiency. This defect manifests itself in early infancy with elevated plasma lactate, pyruvate and alanine concentrations and hypoglycemia.[61,85,86] Patients frequently have hepatomegaly and elevated serum transaminases. These findings are all similar to those in Type I glycogen storage disease. A glucagon tolerance test can distinguish these two disorders; patients deficient in fructose-1,6-diphosphatase have a hyperglycemic response whereas patients with Type I glycogen storage disease do not. Treatment of these children includes frequent carbohydrate feedings to avoid hypoglycemia and avoidance of fructose which may exacerbate the acidosis.[61]

Glucose-6-phosphatase Deficiency: Glycogen Storage Disease Type I. Hepatomegaly, profound hypoglycemia, ketosis and lactic acidosis in infancy are the presenting findings.[61,87] The lactate/pyruvate ratios are normal and the metabolic acidosis is usually compensated for. Hypoglycemia in these patients results in glucagon and epinephrine release which in turn stimulates liver glycogenolysis. Because of the absence of glucose-6-phosphatase, the end-products of glycogenolysis are pyruvate and lactate. Thus, pyruvate and lactate accumulate at least in part because of overproduction.[88] Additional regulatory factors may inhibit further metabolism of pyruvate and also contribute to the accumulation of these compounds.

Management of these patients is difficult; however, frequent carbohydrate feedings are helpful to prevent hypoglycemia and to promote positive nitrogen balance. In young children, continuous nasojejunal infusions of glucose are used when the patients are sleeping.[89] Chronic oral bicarbonate therapy has been useful in ameliorating the chronic lactic acidosis. Some authors have suggested avoidance of fructose and galactose, since these hexoses have been shown to exacerbate the lactic acidosis.[61]

Summary

Numerous genetic defects can elevate blood phenylalanine or interfere with the production of urea or the metabolism of pyruvate. The nutritional requirements of patients with severe defects in one of these three areas cannot be satisfied by usual diets. Frequently, knowledge of the precise defect is needed to manage the problem rationally.

In addition to the severe defects, we are now aware of variant forms for which nutritional requirements do not differ as-markedly from those of the "normal" population. The increased frequency with which these variants are being discovered suggests that "normality" has many shadings. As environments change and different adaptations are needed, normality itself becomes an elusive concept.

BIBLIOGRAPHY

1. Pauling: Science, *160*, 265, 1968.
2. McCracken: Curr. Anthropol., *12*, 479, 1971.
3. Flatz and Rotthaywe: Lancet, *2*, 76, 1973.
4. Simoons, et al.: Pediatrics, *59*, 98, 1977.
5. Neel: Am. J. Hum. Genet., *14*, 353, 1962.
6. Renold, et al.: In *The Metabolic Basis of Inherited Disease*, 3rd ed. (Stanbury, Wyngaarden and Fredrickson, Eds.). New York, McGraw-Hill, 1972, pp. 89–90.
7. Harris: *The Principles of Human Biochemical Genetics*, 3rd ed. Amsterdam, North Holland, 1975.
8. Goldstein, et al.: J. Clin. Invest., *52*, 1544, 1973.
9. Brown and Goldstein: N. Engl. J. Med., *294*, 1386, 1976.
10. Ross and Harker: Science, *193*, 1094, 1976.
11. Scrimshaw: N. Engl. J. Med., *294*, 136, 198, 1976.
12. Holtzman: Annu. Rev. Med., *21*, 335, 1970.
13. Williams: *Biochemical Individuality; The Basis for the Genetotrophic Concept.* New York, John Wiley and Sons, 1956.
14. Holtzman: Fed. Proc., *35*, 2276, 1976.
15. Meyer, et al.: N. Engl. J. Med., *286*, 1280, 1972.
16. Scriver and Rosenberg: *Amino Acid Metabolism and Its Disorders.* Philadelphia, W. B. Saunders, 1973.
17. Holtzman: In *Handbook of Nutrition* (Rechcigl, Ed.). Cleveland, CRC Press, in press.
18. Nadler: Adv. Pediatr., *22*, 1, 1976.
19. Desnick, et al.: Physiol. Rev., *56*, 57, 1976.
20. Advisory Committee to the Renal Transplant Registry: J.A.M.A, *232*, 148, 1975.
21. Stanbury, Wyngaarden, Fredrickson, Eds.: *The Metabolic Basis of Inherited Disease*, 3rd ed. New York, McGraw-Hill, 1972.
22. McKusick: *Mendelian Inheritance in Man: Catalogs of Autosomal Dominant, Autosomal Recessive, and X-linked Phenotypes.* Baltimore, Johns Hopkins, 1975.
23. Friedman, et al.: Proc. Natl. Acad. Sci., *70*, 552, 1973.
24. Bartholome, et al.: Pediatr. Res., *9*, 899, 1975.
25. Dobson, et al.: Pediatrics, *60*, 822, 1977.
26. Kang, et al.: Pediatrics, *46*, 881, 1970.
27. Holtzman, et al.: J.A.M.A., *229*, 667, 1974.
28. Shaw, et al.: *Management of Newborn Infants with Phenylketonuria.* Washington, Department of Health, Education and Welfare, DHEW Pub. No. (HSA) 78–5211, 1978.
29. Holtzman, et al.: N. Engl. J. Med., *293*, 1121, 1975.
30. Howell and Stevenson: Soc. Biol., *18*, S19, 1971.
31. Thomas, et al.: Am. J. Obstet. Gynecol., *111*, 38, 1971.
32. Levy and Shih: Pediatr. Res., *8*, 391, 1974.
33. Blaskovics, et al.: Arch. Dis. Child., *49*, 835, 1974.
34. Holtzman, et al.: Pediatrics, *53*, 353, 1974.
35. Berman, et al.: Am. J. Dis. Child., *117*, 54, 1969.
36. Kaufman, et al.: N. Engl. J. Med., *293*, 785, 1975.
37. Milstien, et al.: J. Pediatr., *89*, 763, 1976.
37a. Kaufman, et al.: N. Engl. J. Med., *299*, 673, 1978.
38. Ford and Bermon: Lancet, *1*, 767, 1977.
39. Bessman: J. Pediatr., *81*, 834, 1972.
40. Short, et al.: N. Engl. J. Med., *288*, 7, 1973.
41. Ricciuti, et al.: Am. J. Hum. Genet., *28*, 332, 1976.
42. Levy, et al.: Clin. Endocrinol. Metab., *3*, 153, 1974.
43. Shih: In *The Urea Cycle* (Grisolia, et al., Eds.). New York, John Wiley & Sons, 1976.
44. Batshaw: Unpublished observations.

45. Rett: Wien. Med. Wochenschr., *118*, 311, 1968.
46. Levin, et al.: Lancet, *2*, 170, 1969.
47. Glick, et al.: Am. J. Hum Genet., *28*, 22, 1976.
48. Scott-Emuakpor, et al.: Pediatr. Res., *6*, 626, 1972.
49. Walser, et al.: Clin. Sci. Mol. Med., *53*, 173, 1977.
50. Cederbaum, et al.: J. Pediatr., *90*, 569, 1977.
51. Levin, et al.: Arch. Dis. Child., *44*, 152, 1969.
52. Kennaway, et al.: Pediatr. Res., *9*, 554, 1975.
53. Russell: Mt. Sinai J. Med., *40*, 723, 1973.
53a. Batshaw, et al.: Pediatr. Res., *13*, 472, 1979.
54. Snyderman, et al.: Pediatrics, *56*, 65, 1975.
54a. Brusilow, et al.: Pediatr. Res., *13*, 417, 1979.
55. Hsia: Gastroenterology, *67*, 347, 1974.
56. Buist, et al.: J. Pediatr., *85*, 208, 1974.
56a. Brusilow, et al.: Lancet, *1*, 124, 1979.
57. Walser: Life Sci., *17*, 1011, 1975.
58. Batshaw, et al.: N. Engl. J. Med., *292*, 1085, 1975.
59. Batshaw, et al.: Pediatrics, *58*, 227, 1976.
60. Thoene, et al.: J. Pediatr., *90*, 218, 1977.
61. Israels, et al.: Adv. Pediatr., *22*, 267, 1976.
61a. Blass, et al.: Lancet, *1*, 1237, 1976.
62. Blass, et al.: In *Normal and Pathological Development of Energy Metabolism* (Hommes and Van dur Berg, Eds.). New York Academic Press, 1975, pp. 193–210.
63. Oliva: Am. J. Med., *48*, 209, 1970.
64. Reed, et al.: In *The Enzymes*, 3rd ed. (Boyer, Ed.). New York, Academic Press, 1970, pp. 213–240.
65. Farrell, et al.: Science, *187*, 1082, 1975.
66. Sakurai, et al.: J. Biol. Chem., *245*, 4453, 1970.
67. Wieland, et al.: Proc. Natl. Acad. Sci., *65*, 947, 1970.
68. Exton: Metabolism, *21*, 945, 1972.
69. Felig: Annu. Rev. Biochem., *44*, 933, 1975.
70. Anon: Lancet, *2*, 27, 1973.
71. Cederbaum, et al.: Pediatr. Res., *10*, 713, 1976.
72. Lonsdale, et al.: Pediatrics, *43*, 1025, 1969.
73. Blass, et al.: Arch. Neurol., *25*, 449, 1971.
74. Blass, et al.: Lancet, *1*, 1302, 1971.
75. Farmer, et al.: Neurology, *23*, 429, 1973.
76. Stromme, et al.: Pediatr. Res., *10*, 60, 1976.
77. Robinson, et al.: *9*, 935, 1975.
78. Haworth, et al.: Pediatrics, *58*, 564, 1976.
79. Blass, et al.: J. Clin. Invest., *51*, 1845, 1972.
80. Falk, et al.: Pediatr. Res., *9*, 350, 1975.
81. Blass, et al.: N. Engl. J. Med., *295*, 62, 1976.
82. Brunette, et al.: Pediatrics, *50*, 702, 1972.
83. Tada, et al.: Tohoku J. Exp. Med., *99*, 121, 1969.
83a. DeVivo, et al.: J. Clin. Endocrinol. Metab., *45*, 1281, 1977.
83b. Tada, et al.: Eur. J. Pediatr., *127*, 141, 1978.
84. Gruskin, et al.: Pediatr. Res., *7*, 832, 1973.
85. Baker, et al.: Lancet, *2*, 13, 1970.
86. Ragliara, et al.: J. Clin. Invest., *51*, 2115, 1972.
87. Howell: In *The Metabolic Basis of Inherited Disease*, 3rd Ed. (Stansbury, Wyngaarden and Fredrickson, Eds.). New York, McGraw-Hill, 1972, pp. 149–173.
88. Sadeghi-Nejad, et al.: J. Pediatr., *85, 49*, 1974.
89. Greene, et al.: N. Engl. J. Med., *294*, 423, 1976.

Chapter *40*

NUTRITION AND ALCOHOLISM

Spencer Shaw and
Charles S. Lieber

Nutrition and alcoholism interact at many levels. Alcoholic beverages are themselves nutrients, providing primarily caloric food value. However, they alter the balance of other nutrients in the diet and may displace them as well. Ethanol may affect the absorption and digestion of many nutrients and in some cases, e.g. the water-soluble vitamins, may alter dietary requirements. In turn, nutritional alterations may affect the metabolism of ethanol within the body. Chronic alcohol consumption may result in temporary or permanent damage to many organs—the liver, heart, brain and bone marrow—although these effects may be modified by nutritional factors such as dietary protein, fat and vitamins. Organ damage in turn may result in alterations in nutrient metabolism, most marked in the liver because of its central role in metabolism and its frequent alteration by alcohol. Permanent organ damage in the alcoholic can lead to marked alterations in pathophysiology that require complex nutritional therapy. Finally, the many effects of ethanol may collectively result in nutritional deficiencies requiring repletion.

THE NUTRITIONAL VALUE OF ALCOHOLIC BEVERAGES

Alcoholic beverages may contain varying amounts of carbohydrates, trace elements, B vitamins (such as niacin and thiamin) and other congeners.[1] However, aside from their ethanol content they provide little nutritive value. In unusual circumstances toxic amounts of lead, cobalt and iron may be present. While various metabolic effects of several congeners have been postulated, none has been definitely established.

Alcoholic beverages provide mainly caloric food value, derived from their ethanol content. Average national consumption figures indicate ethanol accounts for 4.5 per cent of calories in the average diet.[2] Ethanol liberates 7.1 kcal per gm when combusted, and sometimes may be an overlooked source of calories in the diet for those attempting weight reduction. However, ethanol does not provide caloric food value equivalent to carbohydrate.

Isocaloric replacement of carbohydrate calories by ethanol (50 per cent of total calories) in a balanced diet results in a decline in body weight[3] (Fig. 40–1). Furthermore, given as supplemental calories ethanol produces less weight gain than calorically equivalent food[3] (Figs. 40–2, 40–3). The mechanism by which this occurs is possibly related to an increase in the energy requirement of the body. Oxygen consumption is significantly higher in rats fed ethanol than in control animals fed isocaloric carbohydrate.[4] Furthermore, ethanol increases oxygen consumption in normal human subjects, and this effect is greater in alcoholics. Presumably, excess energy would be dissipated as heat. Evi-

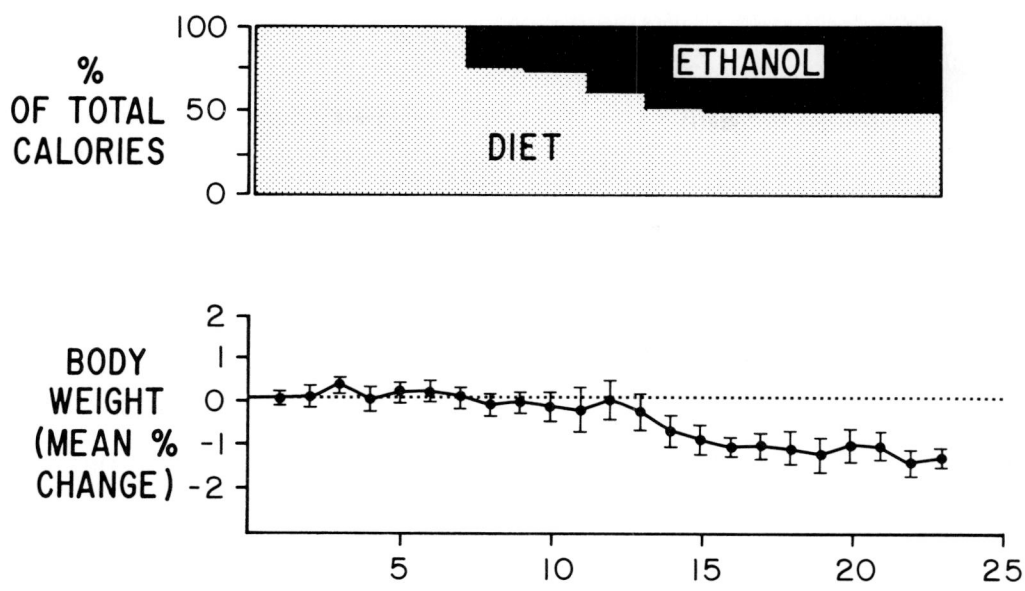

Fig. 40–1. Effect of the isocaloric substitution of ethanol for carbohydrate calories on body weight. Substitution of ethanol as 50 per cent of total calories results in a decline in body weight.[3]

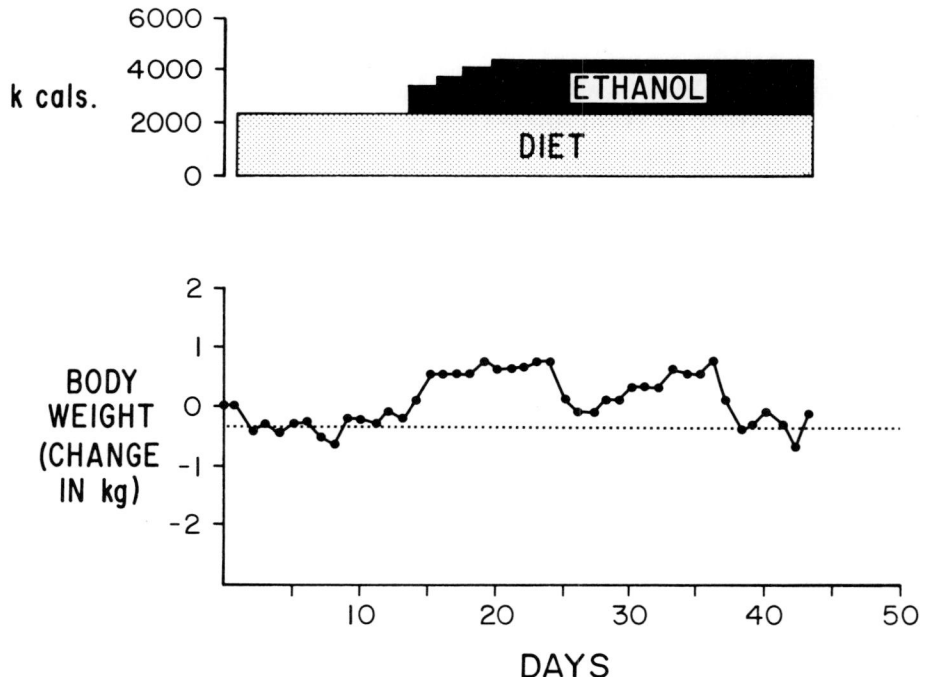

Fig. 40–2. Effect on body weight of the addition of alcohol-derived calories to the diet.

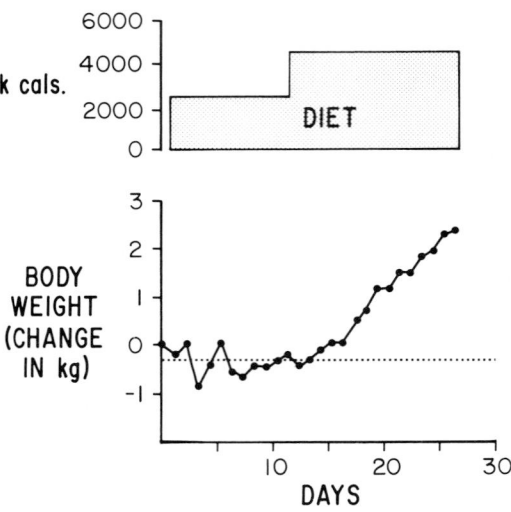

Fig. 40-3. Effect of nonalcohol-derived calories. Supplementary calories from ethanol produced less weight gain than calorically equivalent carbohydrate.[3]

dence for malabsorption or maldigestion as an explanation for ethanol-induced energy losses was lacking under conditions comparable to those pertaining to the studies depicted in Figures 40-1 to 40-3[4] although intake of ethanol in higher amounts for more prolonged periods of time may affect the gastrointestinal tract (vide infra).

EFFECTS OF ETHANOL ON DIGESTION AND ABSORPTION

Acute and chronic alcohol consumption may profoundly alter digestion and gastrointestinal absorption. The effects of ethanol, however, must often be differentiated from those of concurrent deficiency of nutrients such as folate. Many studies demonstrating acute effects of ethanol employ pharmacologic doses of ethanol in unphysiologic systems. The clinical relevance of such observatons to the nutritional status of human alcoholics is often not established. Nevertheless, alterations in digestion and absorption caused by alcohol may produce marginal deficiencies

or potentiate deficiencies arising from other causes.

The Gastrointestinal Tract

The stomach is exposed to higher concentrations of ethanol than the lower gastrointestinal tract, which may explain the vulnerability of the stomach to acute damage from alcohol. Ethanol disrupts the gastric musocal barrier[5] and is an accepted cause of acute gastritis. Its role in the production of gastric ulcer or chronic gastritis is controversial.[6] Acute gastritis may be accompanied by massive bleeding and thus result in iron deficiency. In addition to direct toxic effects, alcohol may impair gastric emptying[7] and may increase acid secretion although the latter effect is controversial.[8] The latter effect may secondarily enhance iron absorption[9] and may, in part, account for the tendency to increased iron retention noted in some alcoholics.

The duodenum, as is the stomach, is exposed to the highest concentrations of ethanol. Experimentally in the rat, ethanol-induced lesions in the intestine appear to be related directly to the concentration of ethanol, with the greatest damage resulting from those solutions with the highest concentrations of ethanol.[10] In man, the acute oral administration of ethanol (1 gm per kg) results in endoscopic and morphologic lesions in the duodenum.[11] These lesions are patchy in nature, a condition which may explain previous failures to observe them.[12]

The morphologic effects of ethanol on the small intestine are accompanied by functional changes. Alterations in mucosal enzymes and in absorption of many nutrients have been observed.[10,13,14] Oral and intravenous alcohol produces increased type III waves (propulsive waves) in the ileum and decreased type I waves (impeding waves) in the jejunum. These changes have been proposed as possible mechanisms to explain, at least in part, the diarrhea observed in binge drinkers.[15]

Chronic ethanol consumption is associated with many alterations in intestinal function. These effects, however, must be differentiated from those resulting from nutritional deficiencies. Indeed, malnutrition may lead to intestinal malabsorp-

tion,[16,17] and folate depletion, common in alcoholics, may be especially implicated in this regard.[18-21] Impaired absorption of folate, thiamin, B_{12}, fat and xylose has been described in alcoholics, with recovery after withdrawal and the institution of a nutritious diet.[19,22-25] By contrast, chronic ethanol administration with an adequate diet has been shown to result only in impairment of B_{12} absorption.[26] In well-nourished alcoholics, depressed levels of intestinal lactase and lactose intolerance have been observed,[27] with recovery following withdrawal from alcohol (Fig. 40–4). In this latter study blacks were more susceptible to this injurious effect of ethanol than were whites (Fig. 40–5). The functional significance of the reduced lactase values was revealed by the small blood glucose rise after a lactose load (Fig. 40–6). The subjects with low intestinal lactase and small blood glucose rises had a high frequency of intolerance (Fig. 40–6). The frequency of lactase deficiency, especially among black alcoholics, must be borne in

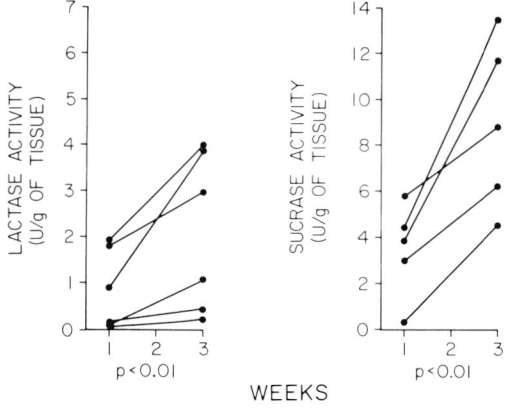

Fig. 40–4. Effect of withdrawal from alcohol upon intestinal lactase. A significant increase in intestinal lactase was observed following 1 to 3 weeks of withdrawal from alcohol. A similar effect was noted for intestinal sucrase activity.[27]

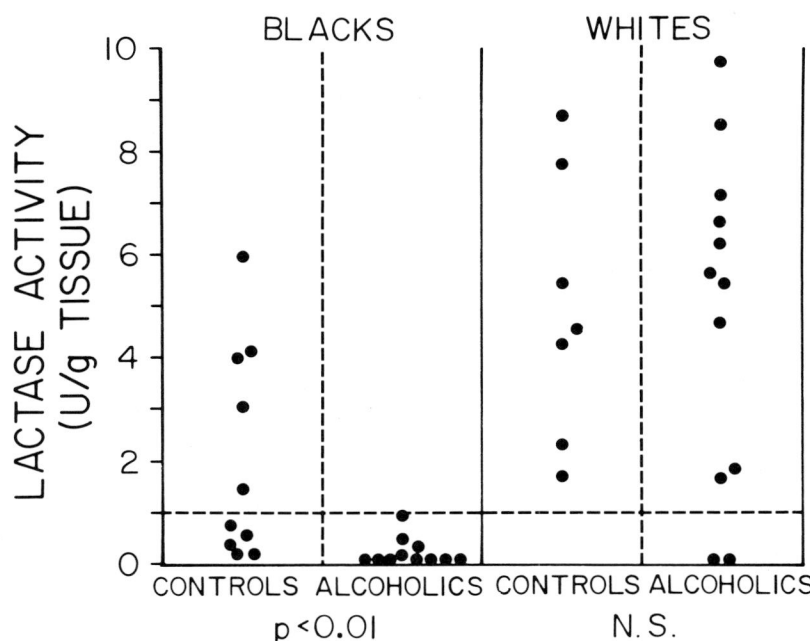

Fig. 40–5. The effects of chronic alcohol consumption on lowering intestinal lactase activity. Black alcoholics were found to be especially sensitive.[27]

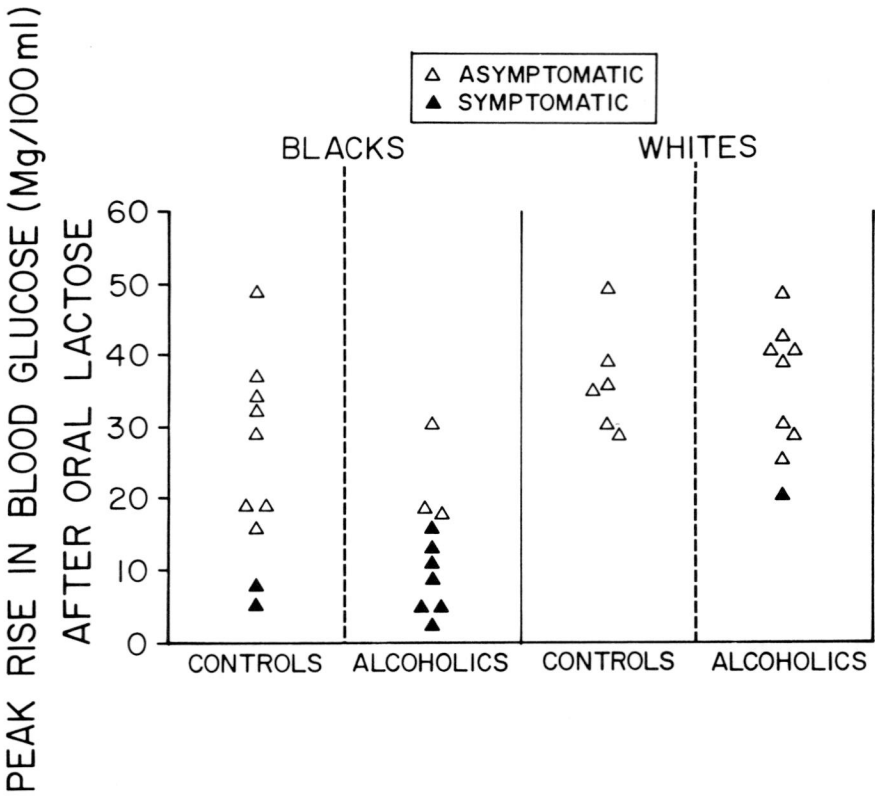

Fig. 40–6.   Effect of lactase deficiency on rise in serum glucose after oral lactose administration. Blood glucose rose the least in subjects with the most severe lactase deficiency. There was a good correlation between symptoms and the lack of rise in glucose.[27]

mind when diets are prescribed for alcoholics with gastritis or ulcer disease.

In alcoholics other factors may also contribute to intestinal dysfunction: portal hypertension,[28] therapeutic interventions as with neomycin,[29] pancreatic insufficiency, altered intestinal flora and altered bile salts.

Despite the many levels at which alcohol may alter the upper GI tract, the incidence of related nutritional deficiencies is relatively small. Even in patients with cirrhosis, the incidence of steatorrhea is uncommon and in one series was present in only 9 per cent of cases.[30]

Pancreas

Acutely, ethanol causes an increase in pancreatic secretion of water and bicarbonate when given orally; this may be mediated by release of secretin from the duodenum.[31-33] If gastric juice is prevented from reaching the duodenum, however, intravenous or intragastric ethanol results in a decrease in pancreatic secretion.[34-36] Increased tone at the sphincter of Oddi is observed after acute ethanol administration.[37] The physiologic significance of this effect, however, is not established.

Chronic alcohol consumption may result

in an increase in the protein content of pancreatic juice, with a concomitant decrease in water and electrolytes.[32] Precipitation of such protein within pancreatic ducts has been proposed as a key pathologic alteration in chronic calcific alcoholic pancreatitis. Both a high-fat, high-protein diet and, paradoxically, malnutrition have been implicated in the pathogenesis of this disorder.[38] Chronic pancreatitis may lead to pancreatic insufficiency and may contribute to steatorrhea and malabsorption. Acute pancreatitis may result in disturbances of fluid and electrolytes and diminished dietary intake. Both acute and chronic pancreatitis may cause alterations in glucose tolerance.

Bile Salts

Steatorrhea in an alcoholic may be potentiated by alterations in bile salt metabolism. Acutely, ethanol may decrease intraluminal bile salts.[36] Chronic ethanol feeding in rats prolongs the half-excretion time of cholic and chenodeoxycholic acid, increases the pool size slightly and decreases daily excretion.[39] In patients with alcoholic cirrhosis deoxycholate may be markedly diminished in the bile, possibly because of impaired conversion of cholate to deoxycholate by bacteria.[40] Decreased cholic acid synthesis, decreased total bile acid pools,[41] diminished concentrations of bile salts in intestinal juices and bacterial deconjugation of bile salts by altered intestinal flora[30] may all contribute to steatorrhea in patients with cirrhosis.

The incidence of pigmented gallstones is increased in patients with cirrhosis.[42]

ALTERATIONS OF NUTRIENT METABOLSIM

Water-soluble Vitamins

Overall Changes. The alterations of the metabolism of water-soluble vitamins in the alcoholic demonstrate the many levels at which ethanol, liver disease and other organ damage may affect nutrients. In addition to decreased intake and absorption the following have been noted: (1) decreased hepatic affinity for folate as measured by displacement studies,[43] (2) impaired activation or utilization of folate, thiamin and B_6,[44-48] (3) increased hepatic clearance of pyridoxal phosphate in cirrhosis.[49] The clinical significance of such alterations is not, however, clearly defined. Depressed circulating levels of vitamins may be found in 40 per cent of malnourished alcoholics, with folate and pyridoxine being most often lowered. Megaloblastic anemias related to folate or B_6 deficiency and neurologic syndromes related to thiamin deficiency are the most common clinical manifestations of vitamin deficiencies in the alcoholic. The effects of marginal deficiencies on such processes as recovery from liver injury is unknown.

The water-soluble vitamins have attracted special interest because they have been proposed as both a cure for alcoholism in high doses and a cause of alcoholism when deficient.[50] However, the human studies upon which these theories were based were uncontrolled and, similarly, the animal studies used as evidence are subject to many criticisms.[51]

Thiamin. Investigations of thiamin metabolism in alcoholism demonstrate how altered balance of other nutrients in the diet may affect vitamin metabolism. Administration of ethanol to rats using pair-feeding techniques may result in lowered tissue levels of thiamin or thiamin pyrophosphate (TPP) in liver, blood or brain, depending upon duration and conditions of feeding.[52-54] However, in some instances prolongation of ethanol feeding may result in an actual increase in tissue levels, for instance in the brain.[54] Furthermore, isocaloric substitution of ethanol for fat or carbohydrate in a thiamin-deficient diet delays the onset of opisthotonus and death in pigeons,[55] and isocaloric substitution for carbohydrate increases the urinary excretion of thiamin.[56] Thus, the effect of ethanol upon the dietary requirement for thiamin may depend on the balance of nutrient calories as well as on the duration of ethanol feeding.

In severe alcoholic liver injury such as cirrhosis the metabolism of thiamin may be altered. Normally, thiamin is activated within the liver to thiamin pyrophosphate, which is the active form of the vitamin. However, in patients with cirrhosis this conversion may be delayed.[46] In the latter case the clinical response of Wernicke's encephalopathy parallels the delayed activation of thiamin.[46]

Pyridoxine. Pyridoxine has been studied extensively with respect to the effects of ethanol metabolism. Veitch[57] found that, in rats fed alcohol as 36 per cent of total calories, there was a significant decrease in the hepatic content of pyridoxal phosphate both in the animals given a sufficient dietary amount of B_6 and in those rendered deficient. In isolated perfused livers, the addition of 18 mM ethanol lowered the pyridoxal phosphate content of livers and decreased the net synthesis of pyridoxal phosphate from pyridoxine in the B_6-deficient rats. Ethanol also diminished the rate of release of pyridoxal phosphate into the perfusate by the livers of B_6-deficient animals. These effects were abolished by 4-methylpyrazole, an inhibitor of alcohol dehydrogenase. Thus, the derangement in pyridoxal phosphate metabolism produced by ethanol is dependent upon its oxidation. One interpretation of these findings was that acetaldehyde may be the responsible agent, since in human erythrocytes it has been shown that acetaldehyde acts to enhance the enzymatic hydrolysis of pyridoxal-5-phosphate by cellular phosphatases.[58] Similar observations were made in isolated rat hepatocytes.[48] The latter study also reportedly showed that acetaldehyde can displace pyridoxal-5-phosphate from its binding protein and thereby promote its degradation.

Vitamin B_{12}. Vitamin B_{12} absorption has been shown to be impaired by chronic ethanol administration despite concomitant administration of pancreatin and intrinsic factor.[26] However, in the absence of other diseases, B_{12}-deficiency anemia is rare among alcoholics.

Folic Acid. The alcoholic may have decreased dietary intake, decreased absorption and decreased hepatic affinity for folate. The influence of these factors in the production of megaloblastic anemias is not clearly defined. The administration of alcohol, however, directly increases the dietary requirement for folate as assessed by hematologic parameters.[45]

Fat-soluble Vitamins

General Changes. The metabolism of fat-soluble vitamins may be altered in the alcoholic because of effects of alcohol, alcohol-induced tissue injury, steatorrhea, reduced dietary intake and concomitant nutritional alterations such as those related to calcium and zinc.

Vitamin A. Vitamin A is stored within the liver as retinol. Storage capacity, however, may be reduced with advanced liver disease. Activation of the vitamin occurs within target organs through oxidation by an alcohol dehydrogenase. Retinal, the active compound, is necessary for dark adaptation and spermatogenesis, both of which may be impaired in the alcoholic.[59,60] Ethanol may compete with retinol for alcohol dehydrogenase in the liver, retina[61] and testes.[62] Zinc deficiency, which may occur in the alcoholic, may exacerbate borderline deficiencies of vitamin A because zinc is a cofactor for alcohol dehydrogenase, needed for the activation of retinol to retinal.

Vitamin D. Vitamin D metabolism in the alcoholic has been of special interest because of the frequency of skeletal abnormalities—aseptic necrosis of the femoral head, osteomalacia and fractures. Vitamin D as well as other fat-soluble vitamins may be depleted through dietary insufficiency or steatorrhea. The liver is the first site of hydroxylation of vitamin D_3 (cholecalciferol); thus hepatocellular injury may result in deficient activation of dietary vitamin D and resistance to parenteral vitamin D therapy.[63] In alcoholic cirrhosis decreased clearance of cholecalciferol in the plasma and decreased urinary excretion of D_3 conjugates have been observed.[64]

Other postulated mechanisms of possible alterations in vitamin D metabolism include increased degradation of activated vitamin D by the cytochrome p-450 system (which is stimulated by chronic alcohol consumption) and decreased storage depots of fat and muscle in debilitated patients with chronic liver disease.[63] Ethanol-induced hypercorticism and parathyroid stimulation secondary to calcium-binding proteins in cirrhosis are other mechanisms by which bone metabolism may be altered. The extent to which altered vitamin D metabolism specifically contributes to clinical skeletal diseases in alcoholic populations and the sites of the abnormalities involved remain to be clarified.

Vitamin K. Vitamin K deficiency in the alcoholic may manifest itself as a bleeding diathesis related to failure to synthesize clotting factors in the liver. Dietary deficiency, decreased synthesis by intestinal bacteria and malabsorption may be contributory. Deficiency states are relatively uncommon, but marginal deficiencies may be potentiated by concomitant liver injury. Vitamin K may correct a prolonged prothrombin time in such instances;[65] failure to correct such an abnormality generally denotes severe parenchymal injury.

Minerals and Trace Elements

Minerals such as zinc, calcium and magnesium may be decreased in the plasma of alcoholics as the result of decreased dietary intake or ethanol-induced renal losses.[66-68] Calcium is of interest because of the skeletal abnormalities observed in alcoholics. Calcium absorption may be impaired when steatorrhea is present. Duodenal calcium transport is inhibited in rats by ethanol

ingestion. This defect is not reversed by the administration of vitamin D or 25-hydroxycholecalciferol[69] and cannot be related to intestinal calcium-binding activity. Thus, in addition to alterations of vitamin D metabolism, ethanol may directly inhibit calcium absorption through a vitamin D-independent pathway.

Hypomagnesemia has aroused considerable interest because of the similarity of the neuromuscular hyperexcitability seen in this condition and that observed following withdrawal from alcohol. However, as in the case of other trace elements, clinical correlations have not been significant and florid deficiency states remain exceedingly rare.[70] Similarly, abnormalities of other trace elements such as zinc, manganese and copper may be seen in chronic liver disease;[68] they are chiefly of investigational interest at present.

Iron

The question of the metabolism of iron is particularly relevant because of the association of hepatic injury with excess iron. Acute alcohol administration may increase iron absorption, possibly through stimulation of gastric acid secretion. This results in increased solubility of ferric ion in the small intestine.[9] Alcoholics may receive excessive dietary iron from the beverages they drink, such as certain wines, or through inadvertent treatment with iron-containing vitamin preparations. In addition, anemias unrelated to iron deficiency may be incorrectly treated with iron. Pancreatic insufficiency, folate deficiency, portosystemic shunting and cirrhosis may increase iron absorption.[71] By contrast, iron-deficiency anemia is uncommon in alcoholics unless factors such as gastrointestinal bleeding from varices, ulcers and gastritis, repeated phlebotomies, dietary extremes and chronic infections are present.[72] However, as mentioned, alcoholics have a propensity to develop increased iron stores which may potentiate tissue injury in the liver and other organs. Transfusions and iron therapy should be used with caution and only to the extent needed for correction of deficiencies. Routine iron supplements are not indicated.

Electrolytes

Alcoholics with chronic liver disease may have disorders of water and electrolyte metabolism, with sodium and water retention most common. Postulated mechanisms include portal hypertension, hypoalbuminemia, altered renal hemodynamics, endocrine abnormalities and changes in lymph flow.[73] Clinically, salt and water retention may be manifested as edema, ascites and pleural effusions.

Hypokalemia may occur and can be of special significance because of a secondary increase in renal vein ammonia and subsequent worsening of hepatic coma.[74] Low body potassium stores may result from vomiting, diarrhea, hyperaldosteronism, renal tubular acidosis, diuretic therapy and muscle wasting.

Carbohydrates

The absorption and digestion of carbohydrates are generally regarded as normal.[75] Experimentally, however, chronic alcohol administration impairs jejunal uptake and transport of carbohydrates.[76] Administration of alcohol has a priming effect on glucose-mediated insulin release[77] and causes glucose intolerance.[78] Chronic alcohol administration results in impaired glucose tolerance, elevated insulin levels and abnormal responses to glucagon.[79] These effects were noted in alcoholics with fatty liver as well as in those with cirrhosis. Alcohol-induced pancreatitis may result in a transient or permanent glucose intolerance, because of damage to pancreatic islet cells or the secondary release of steroids and catecholamines. Alcohol has many effects on the intermediary metabolism of carbohydrates[80] which may contribute to impaired gluconeogenesis and in part explain the symptomatic hypoglycemia seen in human alcoholics with prolonged fasting following heavy drinking. Other mechanisms which may contribute to hypoglycemia include glycogen depletion and autonomic dysfunction.[80]

Uric Acid

Hyperuricemia has been observed in patients following oral or intravenous administration of ethanol despite the absence of known disorders of uric acid metabolism or renal disease.[81] Following alcohol consumption hyperuricemia may persist for several days and thus be misdiagnosed as a primary rather than secondary disorder. NADH generation during ethanol metabolism by alcohol dehydrogenase may enhance lactate production or prevent the liver from completing the Cori cycle and utilizing lactate originating in peripheral tissues, especially lactate produced from muscle activity in alcoholic withdrawal.[82] Elevated serum lactate results in decreased urinary excretion of uric acid and is a major mechanism by which hyperuricemia occurs (Fig. 40–7). The effect of lactate is independent of alterations in urinary pH[81] and occurs despite the administration of probenecid.[83] Alcohol-induced hyperlipemia and ketogenesis, as well as starvation-induced ketosis, may also play a role in hyperuricemia. The changes in serum uric acid associated with alcohol administration are sufficient to precipitate acute gouty attacks;[83] the alterations in uric acid metabolism related to alcoholism may explain the clinical observation of the association between alcoholism and gout.

In advanced alcoholic liver disease serum uric acid may actually be decreased because of low xanthine oxidase activity in the damaged liver.

Lipids

The metabolism of lipids in alcoholics is of special interest because of the frequency of fatty liver and hyperlipidemias seen in these patients. Ethanol metabolism in the liver by alcohol dehydrogenase results in

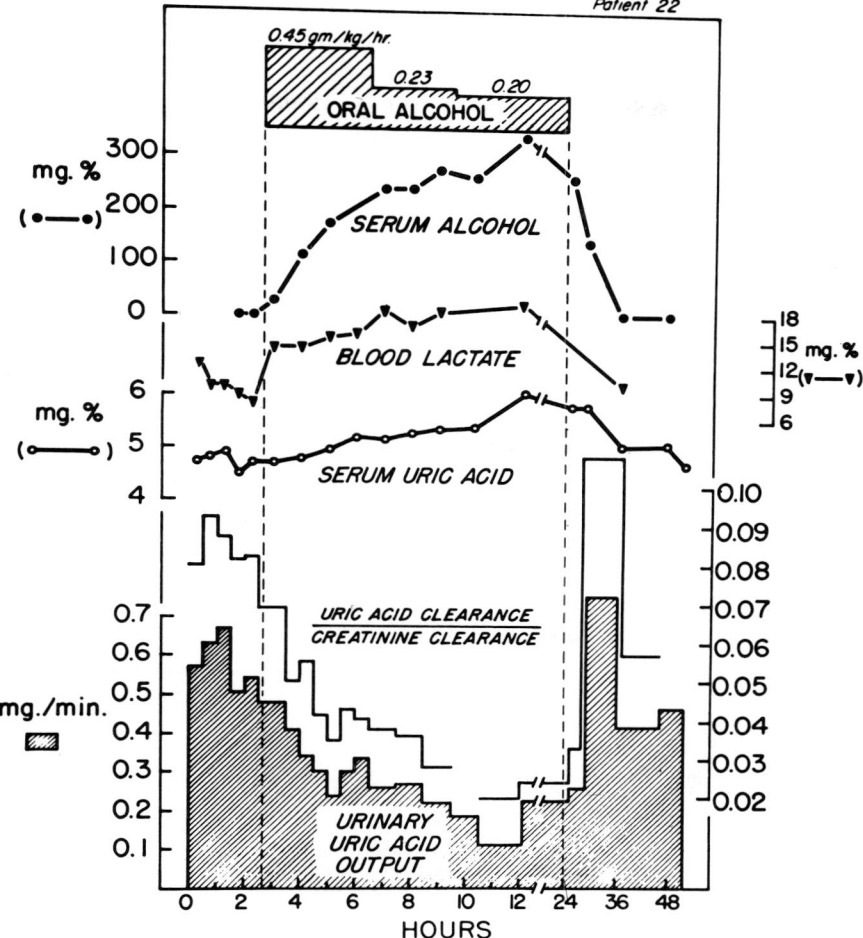

Fig. 40-7. Effect of ethanol administration on serum uric acid and uric acid excretion. Decreased excretion of uric acid and increased serum uric acid may in part be explained by the rise in blood lactate due to ethanol metabolism.[81]

excess hepatic production of NADH. Alcohol consumption also results in mitochondrial damage within the liver. These two effects may in large part account for the major alterations in lipid metabolism resulting from ethanol: decreased fatty acid oxidation, increased fatty acid synthesis and increased ketogenesis.[84,85] As a result of these alterations excess triglycerides may accumulate within the liver and produce steatosis or may be released into the blood as lipoproteins. Intestinal production of very-low-density lipoproteins has been observed,[86] although the contribution of this mechanism appears to be only minor.[87] The serum cholesterol may also be increased in alcoholism, a fact which may be related to an ethanol-induced increase in hepatic cholesterogenesis[39] and decreased bile salt secretion.[39]

The administration of ethanol to man results in hyperlipidemia, with the major elevation occurring in the serum triglycerides. This response may be greatly enhanced by a fat-containing meal.[88] Elevations in serum cholesterol and triglycerides have been directly attributed to chronic alcohol consumption.[89] A characteristic feature of alcohol-induced hyperlipemia is that all lipoprotein fractions are increased, albeit to a variable degree (Fig. 40–8). The major increase is in the very-low-density lipoproteins but a small percentage of alcoholics may have chylomicrons or chylomicron-like particles even in the fast-

ing state.[90] Furthermore, a similarly small percentage may have hypercholesterolemia due to hyperbetalipoproteinemia.

A marked sensitivity to the hyperlipidemic effects of alcohol may be observed in patients with Type IV familial or carbohydrate-induced hyperlipidemia,[91] patients with defective removal of lipids (decreased postheparin lipoprotein lipase),[92] diabetics and patients with pan-

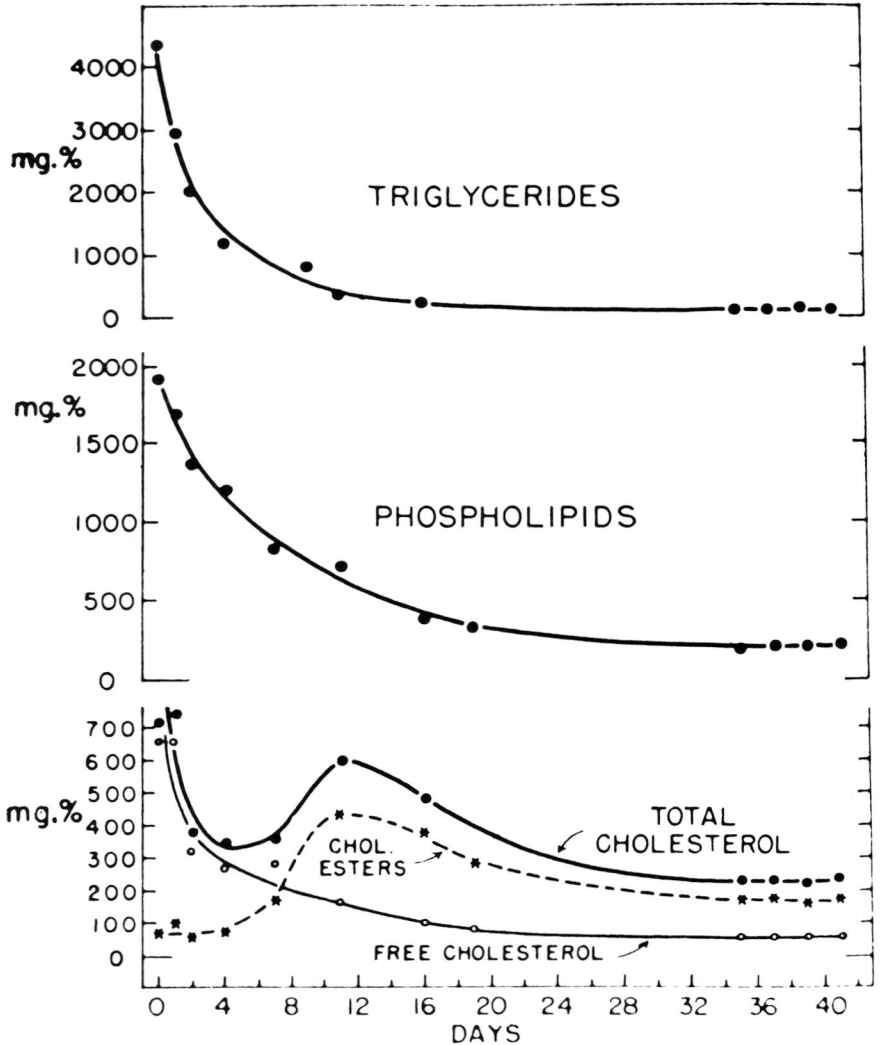

Fig. 40–8. Serum lipids in the alcoholic and effect of withdrawal from ethanol. Lipid fractions decrease at varying rates.[92]

creatitis. The latter condition has been associated with an inhibitor of lipoprotein lipase.[93] Ethanol may thus unmask a subclinical hyperlipidemia and should be excluded as a cause or contributor to observed hyperlipidemias. Marked hyperlipidemias may be associated with hemolysis,[94] which is transient and clears at the same time as the hyperlipidemia. Abdominal pain may occur with hyperlipidemia and differentiation of a primary effect from associated pancreatic, GI or hepatic pathology may be exceedingly difficult. The significance of alcohol-induced hyperlipidemia as a risk factor in coronary artery disease remains to be clarified. In patients with severe liver injury such as cirrhosis, hypolipemia usually prevails.[95,96]

Intrahepatic fat accumulation from alcohol may be affected by dietary lipids.[97] However, low-fat diets are not practical in a clinical setting because of their unpalatability.[98]

Protein

Acute ethanol administration has been observed to result in decreased hepatic synthesis of lipoproteins[99] and albumin.[100,101] By contrast, chronic alcohol feeding is associated with increased protein synthesis.[87] Furthermore, chronic feeding results in increased accumulation in the liver of transport protein such as albumin and transferrin[102] (Fig. 40–9). This effect may be mediated by the action of ethanol (or its metabolite acetaldehyde) on hepatic microtubules.[102] The accumulation of hepatic protein is comparable in magnitude, in terms of weight, to the accumulation of lipid.

Experimentally, alcohol has a complex effect on nitrogen balance, depending upon dietary conditions: given as supplementary calories ethanol may be nitrogen sparing but given as an isocaloric substitute for carbohydrate it increases urea excretion in the urine.[103,104]

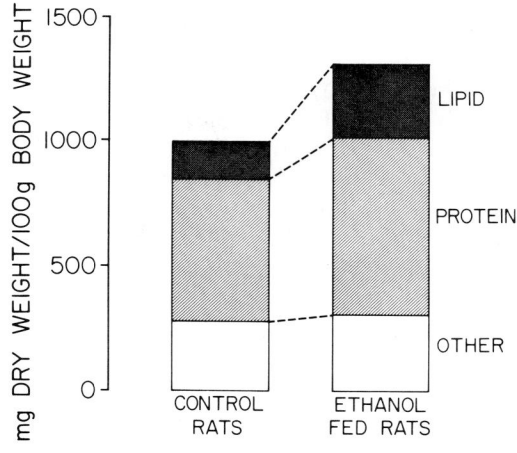

Fig. 40–9. Effect of ethanol feeding on hepatic dry weight, lipid and protein content. The increase in hepatic weight due to protein is comparable to that due to fat.[102]

Amino Acid Metabolism

General Changes. Amino acid metabolism in alcoholism is of special interest because of the relationship between amino acids and hepatic encephalopathy, the potential use of amino acids for parenteral feeding and the role of amino acids in the synthesis of central nervous system transmitters such as serotonin. Numerous alterations in amino acid metabolism have been observed,[105,106] but the clinical relevance of most observations remains to be established. This is especially true because of the failure of many studies to control the three main variables which may affect amino acid metabolism: alcohol, nutrition and liver injury.

Impairment of intestinal absorption of amino acids in the presence of alcohol has been noted;[13] however, increased nitrogen excretion in the stool is only rarely observed with chronic alcohol consumption. Ethanol impairs hepatic uptake of amino acids. This effect is mediated by the metabolism of ethanol.[107] However, hepatic protein and urea synthesis are increased after chronic alcohol feeding.[87,103] Therefore, the significance of the observed effects of alcohol on amino acid transport must be questioned.

Alterations of metabolism in the liver resulting from alcohol consumption and/or liver disease have been observed for almost every amino acid studied.[106] Several amino acids merit discussion in this regard.

Methionine. Chronic alcohol administration for 3 to 10 days to protein-deficient rats results in an increase in enzymes related to the degradation of methionine.[108] This is of interest because of the role of methionine as a lipotrope in rodents and because of the recent observation of increased alpha amino-n-butyric acid (a product of methionine catabolism) in the plasma following chronic alcohol consumption.[109]

Tryptophan. Tryptophan metabolism has aroused considerable interest because of its catabolism to the neurotransmitter serotonin as well as to nicotinic acid. Urinary excretion products have been measured but have yielded conflicting results regarding the effect of alcoholism on these competing pathways of catabolism.[106,110,111] This is not surprising in light of the many nutritional variables, such as pyridoxine availability, which are involved.

Branched-chain Amino Acids. Branched-chain amino acids (BCAA)— valine, leucine and isoleucine—have been observed to be decreased in the plasma of patients with alcoholism and/or liver injury.[112-114] In hepatic encephalopathy related primarily to Laennec's cirrhosis, patients have depressed BCAA and normal levels with disorders such as halothane hepatitis.[115] BCAA clearance from plasma is increased in patients with cirrhosis.[116] Recently, controlled studies conducted with animal models and patients have revealed that depressed BCAA observed in alcoholics result from dietary protein deficiency as well as advanced liver disease[109] (Figs. 40–10 and 40–11). Furthermore, chronic alcohol feeding results in a striking increase in BCAA if dietary protein intake is maintained[109] (Fig. 40–11). In addition to BCAA, chronic alcohol feeding also increases alpha amino-n-butyric acid in the plasma[109] (Fig. 40–11). This amino acid has recently proven useful as a biochemical marker of heavy drinking.[117]

Amino Acid Metabolism in Severe Liver

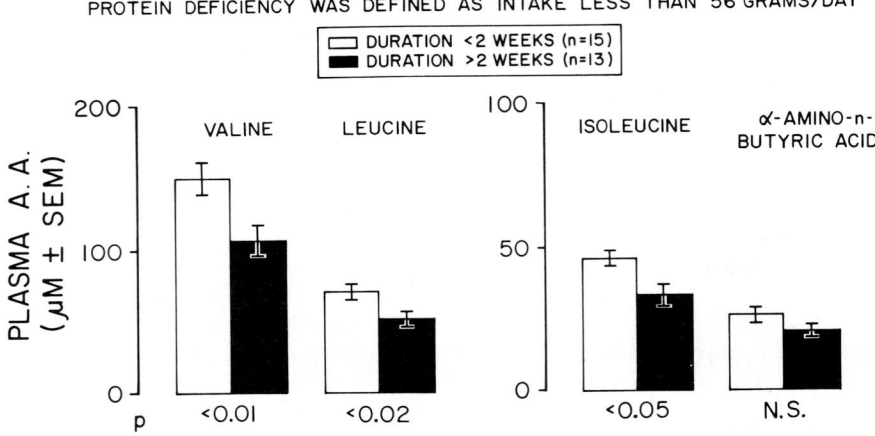

Fig. 40–10. Effects of dietary protein deficiency upon plasma amino acids in the alcoholic. Branched-chain amino acids valine, leucine and isoleucine as well as α-amino-n-butyric acid were depressed to a similar degree by dietary protein deficiency.[109]

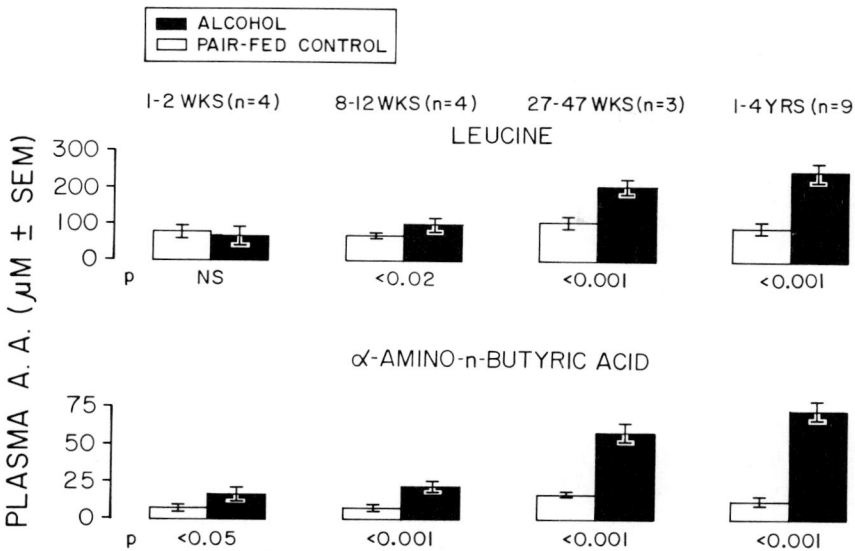

Fig. 40–11. Effect of chronic alcohol feeding on plasma amino acids in the presence of an adequate diet. Branched-chain amino acids and α-amino-n-butyric acid were increased by chronic feeding. A representative branched-chain amino acid, leucine, is shown, but similar results were observed for valine and isoleucine.[109]

Injury. Fulminant hepatic necrosis may result in a generalized nonspecific increase in plasma amino acids.[115,118] Cirrhotics have decreased conversion of phenylalanine to tyrosine, abnormal tyrosine tolerance test and elevated plasma levels of tyrosine, methionine, phenylalanine, tryptophan, glutamate and aspartate.[115,120–123] Elevated plasma levels of aromatic amino acids may be associated with elevated levels of their decarboxylation products because of metabolism in the GI tract. Recently, elevated levels of tyrosine and tyramine were reported in hepatic encephalopathy.[122] Tyrosine and other aromatic amino acid have been implicated in the pathogenesis of hepatic encephalopathy.[121,123]

THE EFFECTS OF DIETARY FACTORS ON ETHANOL METABOLISM

Alcohol dehydrogenase (ADH) is the enzyme which figures predominantly in ethanol metabolism. Under a variety of circumstances, it is the level of this enzyme which is rate limiting for the oxidation of ethanol.[124] The enzyme level may be affected by dietary factors which thus influence the rate of ethanol metabolism. Indeed, low-protein diets have been shown to reduce hepatic ADH levels in rats[125,126] and to considerably lower the rates of ethanol metabolism both in rats[126] and in man.[127]

Prolonged fasting markedly prolongs the metabolism of ethanol. In isolated rat liver cells the rate of ethanol oxidation is approximately twice as fast in the fed state than in the fasted state. The mechanism of this alteration in rate has been shown to result from decreased availability of metabolites to shuttle reducing equivalents into mitochondria needed for the metabolism of ethanol.[128]

The effects of dietary factors on the rate of ethanol metabolism may be of clinical significance. For a given alcohol intake, malnourished alcoholics may have higher and more sustained blood ethanol levels than do normal individuals; this results in increased brain effects of ethanol and decreased effects related to ethanol metabolism.

ALCOHOL, NUTRITION AND ORGAN DAMAGE IN THE ALCOHOLIC

Liver

Liver disease (fatty liver, hepatitis and cirrhosis) is the most significant medical complication in the alcoholic in terms of morbidity and mortality. The question of the respective roles of alcohol and malnutrition in the pathogenesis of alcoholic liver disease is significant both for the prevention and the treatment of the disease.

Malnutrition has been proposed as the predominant factor producing liver injury for several reasons: (1) poor nutritional status of alcoholics seen in some hospital populations, (2) poor dietary intake by history among patients with advanced liver disease (cirrhosis), (3) analogies between alcoholic fatty liver and the fatty liver present in kwashiorkor and following intestinal bypass for obesity. The nutritional status of alcoholics, however, is dependent upon the population studied; past stereotypes about the alcoholic may have stemmed from studies conducted primarily in skid-row alcoholics among city hospital populations. Dietary histories conducted in patients with cirrhosis[129] do not distinguish malnutrition and liver disease as cause and/or effect, since complications of cirrhosis such as ascites and encephalopathy may limit intakes. Furthermore, epidemiologic studies have failed to reveal relationships between malnutrition and cirrhosis in underdeveloped countries[130] and liver biopsies of severely malnourished prison camp victims of World War II revealed only minimal histologic abnormalities.[131]

The question of the role of lipotropes (such as methionine and choline) in the development of alcoholic liver disease is beset with confusion because of inappropriate extrapolation from animal models.

Primates are far less susceptible to lipotrope deficiency than are rodents[132] and, in fact, there is no evidence that a choline-deficient diet is deleterious to man. Treatment with choline of patients suffering from alcoholic liver injury has been found to be ineffective in the face of continued ethanol consumption;[133] experimentally, massive supplementation with choline failed to prevent fatty liver produced by alcohol in volunteer subjects.[134] Furthermore, the fatty liver of choline deficiency is biochemically distinct from that observed following ethanol administration: hepatic phospholipids are increased in alcoholic fatty liver[135] but decreased in fatty liver because of choline deficiency. Even in rodents, acute or chronic alcohol administration results in hepatic injury despite massive supplementation with choline.[136] Thus, hepatic injury induced by choline deficiency appears to be primarily an experimental disease of animals with little or no relevance to human alcoholic liver injury.

Some experimental studies in man and rats have revealed no adverse effects of alcohol in the face of adequate nutrition[137,138] and have been used to support the arguments against the importance of alcohol itself in the pathogenesis of alcoholic liver injury. However, such studies can be criticized because of the use of dosages of alcohol much below those of heavy drinkers. By contrast, much evidence supports the direct role of alcohol in the pathogenesis of alcoholic liver injury. Epidemiologically, a direct relationship has been demonstrated between the amount of alcohol consumed and the incidence of cirrhosis during Prohibition in the United States and during the rationing of alcoholic beverages in Europe during World War II.[139–140] Lelbach[141] has shown that the probability of developing cirrhosis is directly related to the amount and duration of ethanol consumed. Menghini[142] has observed that in sufficient quantity alcohol decreases the clearance of hepatic fat. Most significantly, alcohol has been shown to be directly toxic to the liver (morphologically and biochemically) in both alcoholics and nonalcoholics regardless of dietary variation in fat, protein, vitamins and lipotropes.[19,134,135,143,144] Recently, the full spectrum of alcoholic liver disease (fatty liver and cirrhosis) has been produced in a primate model given alcohol in conjunction with an adequate diet.[145-147]

The interaction of alcohol and malnutrition with respect to liver injury remains largely unexplored. Numerous experimental studies have demonstrated such interactions[97,148-151] but their clinical significance is unknown. In one recent clinical study of skid-row alcoholics with poor nutritional status the incidence of cirrhosis was surprisingly low.[152] Furthermore, experimentally, protein deficiency prevents the development of cirrhosis following CCl_4 administration in rats.[153] Thus, under some circumstances it is conceivable that malnutrition may even be protective with respect to some of the effects of ethanol on the liver.

Heart

Specific nutritional heart disease in the alcoholic may occur in the form of beriberi heart disease. Symptoms classically include those of congestive heart failure and hyperkinetic circulation. Low urinary thiamin and red cell transketolase confirm the diagnosis and other symptoms of thiamin deficiency may be present. In contrast to beriberi heart disease, alcoholic cardiomyopathy manifests itself with symptoms of congestive heart failure accompanied by a low cardiac output and peripheral vasoconstriction. The diagnosis is made essentially by exclusion.

Characteristic electron microscopic changes in alcoholic cardiomyopathy have been described[154] and compared to those produced experimentally in hypomagnesemic rats.[155] This has heightened interest in a possible nutritional etiology. However, alcoholics without evidence of heart disease or nutritional deficiency have been found to have abnormal left ventricular function when stressed.[156] Acute and chronic alcohol intake alters myocardial metabolism.[157] Acute alcohol administration sufficient to achieve blood levels of 150 mg per 100 ml causes a rise in end-diastolic pressure and decreases stroke output. Chronic alcohol administration in the face of a normal diet causes similar changes which persist for several weeks after withdrawal.[156] It is possible that alcohol and nutritional factors may, when combined, produce alcoholic cardiomyopathy. Such a case is illustrated by the cobalt-mediated cardiomyopathy in beer drinkers. The combination of small quantities of cobalt combined with large quantities of ethanol produces a fulminant cardiomyopathy in beer drinkers.[158] However, cobalt or ethanol alone taken in amounts comparable to those ingested by patients who developed cobalt beer-drinker's heart does not produce this disorder.

Blood and Bone Marrow

Deficiencies of pyridoxine and folate may result in hematologic abnormalities in alcoholics although the frequency and nature of the observed abnormalities are highly dependent upon the population selected. In one series of 65 patients admitted for alcoholism and not selected for hematologic problems, 40 per cent had megaloblastic erythropoiesis secondary to folate deficiency, 30 per cent had sideroblasts in the erythroid marrow and a small percentage had iron deficiency anemia. A total of 75 per cent had either anemia or bone marrow abnormalities. In middle- and upper-class alcoholics, folate levels are generally normal.[72] Small amounts of folic acid (250 μg intramuscularly and 150 μg by mouth) prevent megaloblastic changes and 1 mg of pyridoxine per day prevents sideroblastic changes during ethanol administration. However, pharmacologic doses of folic acid do not prevent vacuolization of erythroid elements in patients fed alcohol and eating an adequate diet.[159] Thus, alcohol has a direct toxic effect on the bone marrow despite adequate nutrition.

Thrombocytopenia and granulocytopenia have been described in alcoholics with varying frequency depending upon patient selection. Causes of thrombocytopenia include acute alcohol ingestion, folate deficiency, hypersplenism, infection and disseminated intravascular coagulation. Ethanol causes a depression in circulating platelets despite the concomitant administration of a nutritious diet and vitamin supplements, including large doses of folic acid.[159] In addition, chronic alcohol administration with an adequate diet and folate supplements impairs platelet function.[160] Granulocytopenia has been reported associated with alcohol intoxication in the absence of folate deficiency, hypersplenism or infection; there is rapid recovery after alcohol withdrawal.[161] However, in patients given alcohol chronically in the absence of nutritional deficiency, granulocytopenia does not develop.[159] Acute alcohol administration impairs leukocyte mobilization.[162]

Nervous System

A number of neurologic disorders seen in alcoholism have been traditionally attributed to nutritional deficiencies, especially those of the B vitamins. Recently, however, the nutritional etiology of some of these disorders, especially the Wernicke-Korsakoff syndrome, has been questioned.

Alcoholic polyneuropathy is characterized by generalized symmetrical involvement of peripheral nerves which spreads proximally. First symptoms include discomfort and fatigue in the anterior tibial muscles and paresthesias in the feet. This is usually followed by weakness in the toes and ankles, diminished ankle jerks and decreased fine movements and vibratory sense. Finally glove-and-stocking

hypalgesia and severe weakness may result.[163] Thiamin deficiency has been most strongly implicated in etiology, but other B vitamins are mentioned as well. B_{12}, pyridoxine, nicotinic acid and riboflavin deficiencies can be associated with peripheral neuropathy and pantothenic acid deficiency may produce symptoms of peripheral nerve disease.[163]

The Wernicke-Korsakoff syndrome is the most spectacular CNS-related neurologic problem in alcoholism. Wernicke's encephalopathy is characterized by weakness of eye movements, gait disturbance and confusion. Horizontal nystagmus, paralysis of external recti, paralysis of conjugate gaze and ataxia of gait and stance may be observed. Korsakoff's psychosis is characterized initially by anterograde amnesia, retrograde amnesia to a lesser extent, a disordered time sense and often confabulation in the acute stages. Cognitive deficits have also been observed.[164] Ophthalmoplegia in Wernicke's encephalopathy responds rapidly to thiamin administration, while the ataxia and confusion respond more slowly. The rapidity of response depends upon the conversion of thiamin to its active form in the liver; patients with advanced liver disease such as cirrhosis may therefore have a delayed response.[46]

The association of Korsakoff's psychosis with Wernicke's encephalopathy has led to their inclusion in one syndrome. However, while Wernicke's encephalopathy is a thiamin-responsive illness, the relationship of Korsakoff's psychosis to thiamin deficiency in terms of pathogenesis and treatment is less clearly delineated. Korsakoff's psychosis and Wernicke's encephalopathy are rarely if ever seen in clinical thiamin deficiency in the absence of alcoholism.[165] It has been postulated that this may be related to the impact of alcohol on the balance of dietary calories.[165] The Wernicke-Korsakoff syndrome is characterized by symmetrical CNS lesions in periaqueductal and perivestibular areas of the diencephalon, midbrain and cerebellum.[166] Symmetric and bilateral lesions are also observed in experimental thiamin deficiency in animals.[167] It is not surprising therefore that the psychosis and some aspects of the encephalopathy are only minimally or slowly responsive to thiamin treatment.[168] In addition to the structural similarity of lesions, the theory that Korsakoff's psychosis is related to thiamin deficiency, or at least nutritional deficiency, is supported by the observation that most alcoholics with memory and learning defects have a history of dietary deficiency.[169] Recently, an abnormality of a thiamin-requiring enzyme has been observed in patients with the Wernicke-Korsakoff syndrome.[170] Furthermore, clinical and pathologic evidence supports the concept that Wernicke's encephalopathy and the pathologic lesions associated with it are decreasing in association with improvement in nutrition in recent years.[166] However, a study from Holland has shown a recent increase in the Wernicke-Korsakoff syndrome[171] and experimentally it is difficult to demonstrate learning deficiencies related to thiamin deficiency alone in rats,[172] while alcohol in the absence of nutritional deficiencies readily produces such defects.[173] Thus, the precise interrelation of alcohol, thiamin and Korsakoff's psychosis awaits clarification.

Nutritional amblyopia is a disorder characterized by central or centrocecal scotomata. Vitamin B deficiency has been suggested as a cause although a specific etiology is not established.[164] Similarly, the influence of nutritional factors in the pathogenesis of central pontine myelinosis, Marchiafava-Bignami syndrome, alcoholic cerebellar degeneration and other rarer neurologic syndromes seen in alcoholics remains speculative. Cerebellar degeneration has, however, been reported as being responsive to thiamin.[174] Pellagra, although increasingly rare in alcoholics, may

be manifested by psychosis, dementia, neuropathy and posterior and lateral column disease. Skin changes and diarrhea may accompany the neurologic findings.

NUTRITIONAL THERAPY

Nutritional therapy must be viewed in terms of the nutritional deficiencies requiring repletion as well as the pathologic alterations induced by alcohol. Nutritional therapy may be limited by underlying organ damage. For example, repletion of dietary protein deficiency may be limited or restricted in the presence of concomitant encephalopathy.

Alcoholic Liver Injury

Fatty Liver and Alcoholic Hepatitis. Alcoholic fatty liver is the earliest and generally a completely reversible stage of alcoholic liver injury. The only specific requirement is abstinence from alcohol. Patients with fatty liver may have associated deficiencies or complications which require specific therapy. Similar measures are required for alcoholic hepatitis. However, alcoholic hepatitis may require specific supportive measures to ensure electrolyte balance, especially if pyrexia or nausea and vomiting are present.

Cirrhosis. Recovery from cirrhosis has been shown to be enhanced by a normal-protein, normal-fat, vitamin-enriched diet.[175-177] Thus diet remains the mainstay of the treatment of alcoholic liver disease. The components will be examined separately:

Fat. Low-fat diets are of theoretical interest in patients with alcoholic liver disease. However they are generally not advocated because of the lack of palatability of such regimens, especially for an already anorectic patient.[98]

Vitamins. Several times the daily requirements of water-soluble vitamins are generally given without known harmful effects or proven efficacy. An increased requirement for folic acid has been clearly demonstrated with clinically manifested hematologic abnormalities resulting from administration of the regular daily requirement with alcohol. Biochemical abnormalities of the metabolism of other vitamins have also been observed. Therefore, it seems prudent to prevent the possibility of marginal or subclinical deficiencies with supplementary vitamins.

Protein. Protein intake in patients with alcoholic liver injury must be adequate to prevent nitrogen wasting but not so great as to precipitate hepatic coma. Nitrogen balance studies have revealed essentially normal protein requirements in cirrhosis,[105] and some studies have even suggested increased nitrogen retention.[178] Dietary requirements for specific amino acids may be altered as evidenced by plasma levels and clearance rates. In general, patients with alcoholic liver disease have been found to have depressed plasma branched-chain amino acids[113,114,179,180] and increased clearance of these amino acids,[116] along with increased levels of aromatic amino acids[118-121] and decreased clearance of these amino acids.[119] Amino acids may differ with respect to their ability to produce ammonia and are tolerated to a different extent in hepatic encephalopathy[123] (see Hepatic Encephalopathy).

Calories. Caloric intake should be sufficient to prevent endogenous protein breakdown. The daily caloric requirement to achieve nitrogen sparing in the alcoholic or in the presence of alcoholic liver injury is unknown,[75] but it is a reasonable practice to give an amount of calories in excess of daily requirements if feasible.

Lipotropes. There is no evidence that lipotropes are useful in recovery from alcoholic liver injury and, in fact, they may prove harmful as an excess nitrogen load.[181]

Hepatic Encephalopathy

Hepatic encephalopathy represents a neuropsychiatric syndrome secondary to liver disease with a wide clinical spectrum ranging from personality changes to deep coma. Confusion, apathy, irritability and personality changes may represent the earliest findings. Clinical findings include constructive apraxia, hypothermia, asterixis and EEG changes. The etiology and pathogenesis of hepatic encephalopathy are complex. The major nutritional considerations include adjustment of exogenous and endogenous nitrogen loads, and potassium and acid-base balance.

Exogenous protein load must be minimized because of the adverse effects of the resultant nitrogen load on encephalopathy. Dietary protein may be eliminated initially in the treatment of hepatic encephalopathy but must be resumed after several days to prevent endogenous catabolism. Nitrogen sparing should be maintained through intravenous glucose if caloric intake is inadequate. Five per cent dextrose (as the monohydrate) contains only 170 kcal per 1000 ml and therefore it may be necessary to administer hypertonic glucose through a large-bore catheter, especially if fluid restriction is indicated. Hypercatabolic states such as infections with fever must be treated to prevent the adverse effects of protein catabolism. Patients with portacaval shunts may be especially sensitive to dietary protein.

Selective mixtures of essential amino acids (high in branched-chain amino acids, low in aromatic amino acids)[121] or keto analogs of amino acids[182] have been proposed for the treatment of hepatic insufficiency. The long-term efficacy of these therapies with respect to survival and nitrogen balance remains to be determined. Furthermore, they require special vigilance to avoid precipitation of hepatic coma or fluid and electrolyte disturbances. Dietary protein low in aromatic amino acids (generally vegetable as opposed to animal protein) has been advocated for patients with hepatic encephalopathy.[183-185] The long-term efficacy with respect to survival and nitrogen balance is, however, unknown.

Tolerance to dietary protein may be enhanced through concomitant administration of neomycin, lactulose and enemas. Neomycin inhibits the action of gastrointestinal flora which convert protein and urea to ammonia and other potentially toxic nitrogenous products within the gut. Decreased renal function (as with hepatorenal syndrome) may result in oto- and nephrotoxic blood levels of neomycin;[186] dosage must be markedly lowered or the drug discontinued under such circumstances. Recently, ampicillin has been found to prevent the conversion of urea to ammonia within the GI tract[187] and may prove to be a useful alternative to neomycin in these circumstances. Lactulose may also be used in place of neomycin and may be acting through acidification of bowel contents with resultant ammonia trapping (as ammonium) or through increased motility.[188]

Hypokalemia increases renal vein ammonia via a direct effect on renal ammonia production and possibly through increased back diffusion of ammonia from alkaline urine,[74] and may worsen encephalopathy. Parenteral or oral potassium may be given in dosages of approximately 100 to 200 mEq per day until deficits are corrected, provided that renal function is normal.

Ascites and Edema

Dietary regimen to combat ascites and edema is adjusted according to the severity of salt and water retention. Severe symptoms and refractory cases may require rigid sodium restriction (250 mg per day). Restriction at this level is advocated even if mild hyponatremia is present (serum sodium = 125 to 130 mEq per liter).[75] Symptomatic hyponatremia with serum sodium below this level may require intervention with hypertonic saline and rigid water restriction. Fluid restriction of 1500 to 2000 ml per day, including all liquids taken with medications, is recommended especially if hyponatremia is present. With less severe retention, sodium restriction of 500 to 2000 mg per day may be tried. Serum electrolytes and daily weights are necessary to guide therapy. Summerskill et al.[73] recommended that weight loss induced by dietary or diuretic therapy should not exceed 5 kg per week.

Renal Disorders

Oliguria, azotemia and elevated creatinine may indicate deteriorating renal function. Patients with alcoholic liver disease are especially susceptible to acute tubular necrosis through such complications as variceal bleeding. Spontaneous renal failure or the so-called hepatorenal syndrome may also occur. Rising serum urea caused by renal failure may present a special problem in the patient with alcoholic liver disease. Urea diffuses into the GI tract and is hydrolyzed to ammonia; thus, it acts as any nitrogenous compound. With increasing levels of urea the resultant ammonia becomes a significant problem and may worsen or precipitate hepatic coma.[189] In this case antibiotics (see Encephalopathy) may be given to prevent conversion of urea to ammonia, and enemas may be required.

Neurologic Disorders

Peripheral Neuropathy. In patients with peripheral neuropathy thiamin deficiency has been most strongly implicated in etiology, but other B vitamins have a place as well. B_{12}, pyridoxine, nicotinic acid and riboflavin deficiencies can be associated with peripheral neuropathy and pantothenic acid deficiency may produce symptoms of peripheral nerve disease.[163] Peripheral neuropathy, as with other neurologic disorders found in the alcoholic, is generally treated with abstinence and B-vitamin therapy. Empirically, B vitamins are given as a group rather than as a specific vitamin therapy. While the optimal therapeutic dosage has not been established, one recommendation is 10 × the normal daily requirement for 1 week and 5 × the daily requirement thereafter.[163]

Wernicke-Korsakoff Syndrome. In patients with the Wernicke-Korsakoff syndrome, the ophthalmoplegia responds rapidly to thiamin administration while the ataxia and confusion respond more slowly. Although 2 to 3 mg may be sufficient, usually larger doses (50 mg) are given. Rapidity of response depends upon the conversion of thiamin to its active form in the liver. Patients with advanced liver disease such as cirrhosis may therefore have a delayed response.[46]

Other Central Nervous System Disorders. Nutritional amblyopia, cerebellar degeneration, Marchiafava-Bignami syndrome and other rare central nervous system disorders seen in the alcoholic are prudently treated with abstinence and administration of B vitamins.

Hematologic Disorders

Iron deficiency, if present in the alcoholic, should be corrected cautiously because of the propensity of these patients, if liver disease is present, to retain iron and because of the potential injurious effects of iron excess upon the liver. Thrombocytopenia may respond simply to abstinence from alcohol or, if caused by vitamin deficiencies such as folate, to replacement therapy.

Anemias, low serum folate, megaloblastic marrow with or without sideroblasts may be used to diagnose folate- and pyridoxine-related hematologic abnormalities. Therapy includes abstinence and vitamin supplementation. While smaller doses may be adequate, many times the daily requirement of folate and pyridoxine are generally administered.

Cardiomyopathy

Thiamin repletion is the specific therapy for beriberi heart disease. Therapy of 5 to 10 mg per day is probably adequate, although generally larger amounts are administered. Empirically, however, in any alcoholic with cardiomyopathy, B vitamins are generally given as a group, with an adequate diet and abstinence from alcohol. Magnesium deficiency should be corrected if present although this is not a common clinical problem. Congestive heart failure from alcoholic cardiomyopathy is treated with conventional salt restriction and therapy used for heart disease of other etiologies.

THE NUTRITIONAL STATUS OF THE ALCOHOLIC

Alcoholism remains one of the few causes of florid nutritional deficiencies in our society. However, the stereotype of the malnourished alcoholic is probably unfounded as it applies to the millions of alcoholics in the United States. The spread of alcoholism to various socioeconomic classes, the greater availability and enrichment of foods and the investigation of broader populations of alcoholics have led to a modification of this view. Indeed, moderate alcohol consumption has been found to have little impact on nutritional status[190] and no significant differences have been found among alcoholics and nonalcoholics matched for socioeconomic and health history.[191] Nevertheless, alcohol may interact with nutrition at many levels to produce marginal if not clinically overt deficiencies. These interactions are summarized in Table 40–1. The clinical significance of such nutritional deficiencies by

**Table 40–1.	Alcohol-nutrition Interaction**

Primary Malnutrition (deficient intake)
  "Empty" calories
  Economic factors
  Impaired appetite secondary to GI-liver disorders
Secondary Malnutrition (deficient nutrient utilization)
  Ethanol-induced GI damage (maldigestion-malabsorption)
  Deficiency-induced intestinal dysfunction
  Energy wastage
  Decreased activation or increased inactivation of nutrients

themselves or in conjunction with alcohol with regard to organ damage remains an interesting area for further exploration.

BIBLIOGRAPHY

1. Leake and Silverman: In *Biology of Alcoholism* (Kissin and Begleiter, Eds.). New York, Plenum Press, 1974, p. 575.
2. Scheig: Am. J. Clin. Nutr., 23, 467, 1974.
3. Pirola and Lieber: Pharmacology, 7, 185, 1972.
4. Pirola and Lieber: Am. J. Clin. Nutr., 19, 90, 1976.
5. Davenport: Gastroenterology, 56, 439, 1969.
6. Lorber, Dinoso and Chey: In *Biology of Alcoholism* (Kissin and Begleiter, Eds.). New York, Plenum Press, 1974, p. 339.
7. Barboriak and Meade: Am. J. Clin. Nutr., 23, 1151, 1970.
8. Cooke: Gastroenterology, 62, 501, 1972.
9. Charlton, Jacobs, Seftel and Bothwell: Br. Med. J., 2, 1427, 1964.
10. Barona, Pirola and Lieber: Gastroenterology, 66, 226, 1974.
11. Gottfried, Korsten and Lieber: Am. J. Gastroenterol., 70, 587, 1978.
12. Pirola, Bolin and Davis: Am. J. Dig. Dis., 14, 239, 1969.
13. Israel, Valenzuela, Salazar and Ugarte: J. Nutr., 98, 222, 1969.
14. Hillman: In *Biology of Alcoholism* (Kissin and Begleiter, Eds.). New York, Plenum Press, 1974, p. 513.
15. Robles, Mezey, Halsted and Schuster: Johns Hopkins Med. J., 135, 17, 1974.
16. James: Lancet, 1, 333, 1968.
17. Mayoral, et al.: Am. J. Clin. Nutr., 20, 866, 1967.
18. Winawer, Sullivan, Herbert and Zamcheck: N. Engl. J. Med., 272, 892, 1965.
19. Halsted, Robles and Mezey: N. Engl. J. Med., 285, 701, 1971.
20. Hermos, et al.: Ann. Intern. Med., 76, 957, 1972.
21. Halsted, Robles and Mezey: Gastroenterology, 64, 526, 1973.
22. Tomasulo, Kater and Iber: Am. J. Clin. Nutr., 21, 1340, 1968.
23. Roggin, Iber, Kater and Tobon: Johns Hopkins Med. J., 125, 321, 1969.
24. Mezey, Jow, Slavin and Tobon: Gastroenterology, 59, 657, 1970.
25. Lindenbaum and Lieber: Nature, 224, 806, 1969.
26. Lindenbaum and Lieber: Ann. N.Y. Acad. Sci., 252, 228, 1975.
27. Perlow, Baraona and Lieber: Gastroenterology, 72, 680, 1977.
28. Losowsky and Walker: Gastroenterology, 56, 589, 1969.
29. Faloon: Am. J. Clin. Nutr., 23, 645, 1970.
30. Linscheer: Am. J. Clin. Nutr., 23, 488, 1970.
31. Walton, Schapiro and Woodward: Surg. Forum., 11, 365, 1960.
32. Sarles and Tiscornia: Med. Clin. North Am., 58, 1333, 1974.
33. Straus, Croach and Yalow: N. Engl. J. Med., 293, 1031, 1975.
34. Mott, Sarles, Tiscornia and Gullo: Dig. Dis., 17, 902, 1972.
35. Bayer, Rudick, Lieber and Janowitz: Gastroenterology, 63, 619, 1972.
36. Marin, Ward and Fischer: Dig. Dis., 18, 825, 1973.
37. Pirola and Davis: Gut, 9, 557, 1968.
38. Sarles: Gastroenterology, 66, 604, 1974.
39. Lefevre, DeCarli and Lieber: J. Lipid Res., 13, 48, 1972.
40. Knodell, Kinsey, Boedecker and Collins: Gastroenterology, 71, 196, 1976.
41. Vlahcevic, Juttijudata, Bell and Sewell: Gastroenterology, 62, 1174, 1972.
42. Nicholas, Rinaudo and Conn: Gastroenterology, 63, 112, 1972.
43. Cherrick, Baker, Frank and Leevy: J. Lab. Clin. Med., 66, 446, 1965.
44. Hines: J. Lab. Clin. Med., 74, 883, 1969.
45. Sullivan and Herbert: J. Clin. Invest., 43, 2048, 1964.
46. Cole, et al.: Am. J. Clin. Nutr., 22, 44, 1969.
47. Eichner and Hillman: Am. J. Med., 50, 218, 1971.
48. Veitch, Lumeng and Li: Gastroenterology, 66, 868, 1974.
49. Mitchell, et al.: Gastroenterology, 71, 1043, 1976.
50. Williams: *Alcoholism—The Nutritional Approach.* Austin, University of Texas Press, 1959
51. Mickelsen: J. Am. Diet. Assoc., 31, 570, 1955.
52. Kiessling and Tilander: Q. J. Study Alcohol, 22, 535, 1961.
53. Kontinnen, Oura and Suomalainen: Ann. Med. Exp. Pa., 45, 68, 1967.
54. Chan: Pharmacologist, 18, 237, 1976.
55. Westerfeld and Doisy: J. Nutr., 30, 127, 1945.
56. Butler and Saret: J. Nutr., 35, 539, 1948.
57. Veitch, Lumeng and Li: J. Clin. Invest., 55, 1026, 1975.
58. Lumeng and Li: J. Clin. Invest., 53, 693, 1974.
59. Patek and Haig: J. Clin. Invest., 18, 609, 1939.
60. Van Thiel and Lester: Gastroenterology, 71, 318, 1976.
61. Mezey and Holt: Exp. Mol. Pathol., 15, 148, 1971.
62. Van Thiel, Gavaler and Lester: Science, 196, 941, 1974.
63. Avioli and Haddad: Metabolism, 22, 507, 1973.
64. Avioli, et al.: J. Clin. Invest., 46, 983, 1967.
65. Roberts and Cederbaum: Gastroenterology, 63, 297, 1972.
66. McCollister, Flink and Lewis: Am. J. Clin. Nutr., 12, 415, 1963.
67. Markkanen and Nanto: Experientia, 22, 753, 1966.
68. Prasad, Oberleas and Rajasekaran: Am. J. Clin. Nutr., 23, 581, 1970.
69. Krawitt: J. Lab. Clin. Med., 85, 665, 1975.
70. Heaton, Pyrah, Beresford and Bryson: Lancet, 2, 802, 1962.

71. Grace and Powell: Gastroenterology, *67*, 1257, 1974.
72. Eichner, Buchanan, Smith and Hillman. Am. J. Med. Sci., *263*, 35, 1972.
73. Summerskill, Barnardo and Baldus: Am. J. Clin. Nutr., *23*, 499, 1970.
74. Shear and Gabuzda: Am. J. Clin. Nutr., *23*, 614, 1970.
75. Gabuzda: Med. Clin. North Am., *54*, 1455, 1970.
76. Lindenbaum, Shea, Saha and Lieber: Clin. Res., *20*, 459, 1972.
77. Metz, Berger and Mako: Diabetes, *8*, 517, 1969.
78. Phillips and Safrit: J.A.M.A., *217*, 1513, 1971.
79. Rehfeld, Juhl and Hilden: Gastroenterology, *64*, 445, 1973.
80. Arky: In *Biology of Alcoholism*. (Kissin and Begleiter, Eds.). New York, Plenum Press, 1974, p. 197.
81. Lieber, Jones, Losowsky and Davidson: J. Clin. Invest., *41*, 1863, 1962.
82. Newcombe: Metabolism, *21*, 1193, 1972.
83. MacLachlan and Rodan: Am. J. Med., *42*, 38, 1967.
84. Lieber: Lipids, *9*, 103, 1974.
85. Lieber: *Metabolic Aspects of Alcoholism*, Lancaster, England, MTP Press, 1977.
86. Mitstilis and Ockner: J. Lab. Clin. Med., *80*, 34, 1972.
87. Baraona, Pirola and Lieber: J. Clin. Invest., *52*, 296, 1973.
88. Wilson, Schreibman, Brewster and Arky: J. Lab. Clin. Med., *75*, 264, 1970.
89. Ostrander, et al.: Arch. Intern. Med., *134*, 451, 1974.
90. Chait, February, Mancini and Lewis: Lancet, *2*, 62, 1972.
91. Ginsberg, Olefsky, Farquhar and Raven: Ann. Intern. Med., *80*, 143, 1974.
92. Losowsky, Jones, Davidson and Lieber: Am. J. Med., *35*, 794, 1963.
93. Kessler, Kniffen and Janowitz: N. Engl. J. Med., *269*, 943, 1963.
94. Zieve: Ann. Intern. Med., *48*, 471, 1958.
95. Marzo, et al.: Klin. Wochenschr., *48*, 949, 1970.
96. Guisard, Gonand, Laurent and Debry: Nutr. Metab., *13*, 222, 1971.
97. Lieber and DeCarli: Am. J. Clin. Nutr., *23*, 474, 1970.
98. Crews and Faloon: J. Am. Med. Assoc., *181*, 754, 1962.
99. Schapiro, Drummey, Shimizu and Isselbacher: J. Clin. Invest., *43*, 1338, 1964.
100. Rothschild, Oratz, Mongelli and Schreiber: J. Clin. Invest., *50*, 1812, 1971.
101. Jeejeebhoy, et al.: Biochem.J., *126*, 1111, 1972.
102. Baraona, Leo, Borowsky and Lieber: Science, *190*, 794, 1975.
103. Klatskin: Yale J. Biol. Med., *34*, 124, 1961.
104. Rodrigo, Antezana and Baraona: J. Nutr., *101*, 1307, 1971.
105. Gabuzda and Shear: Am. J. Clin. Nutr., *23*, 479, 1970.
106. Orten and Sardesai: In *Biology of Alcoholism* (Kissin and Begleiter, Eds.). New York, Plenum Press, 1974, p. 229.
107. Piccirillo and Chambers: Res. Commun. Chem. Pathol. Pharmacol., *13*, 297, 1976.
108. Finkelstein, Cello and Kyle: Biochem. Biophys. Res. Commum., *61*, 525, 1974.
109. Shaw and Lieber: Gastroenterology, *74*, 677, 1978.
110. Pasquariello, Quadri and Tenconi: Pharmacology, *7*, 185, 1963.
111. Payne, Lu and Meyer: Am. J. Clin. Nutr., *27*, 572, 1974.
112. Siegel, Roach and Pomeroy: Proc. Natl. Acad. Sci., *51*, 605, 1964.
113. Iob, Coon and Sloan: J. Surg. Res., *7*, 41, 1967.
114. Zinneman, Seal and Doe: Am. J. Dig. Dis., *14*, 118, 1969.
115. Rosen, Yoshimura, Hodgman and Fischer: Gastroenterology, *72*, 483, 1977.
116. Iob, Coon and Sloan: J. Surg. Res., *6*, 233, 1966.
117. Shaw, Stimmel and Lieber: Science, *194*, 1057, 1976.
118. Wu, Bollman and Butt; J. Clin. Invest., *34*, 845, 1955.
119. Levine and Coon: J. Clin. Invest., *46*, 2012, 1967.
120. Iber, Rosen, Levenson and Chalmers: J. Lab. Clin. Med., *50*, 417, 1957.
121. Fischer, et al.: Surgery, *78*, 276, 1975.
122. Faraj, Bowen, Isaacs and Rudman: N. Engl. J. Med., *294*, 1360, 1976.
123. Fischer, et al.: Gastroenterology, *70*, 981, 1976.
124. Crow, Cornell and Veech: Alcoholism: Clin. Exp. Res., *1*, 43, 1977.
125. Horn and Manthei: Gastroenterology, *65*, 349, 1973.
126. Bode, Goebell and Stähler: Gesamte Exp. Med., *152*, 111, 1970.
127. Bode, Buchwald and Goebell: German Med. Mon., *1*, 149, 1971.
128. Meijer, Van Woerkom, Williamson and Tager: Biochem. J., *150*, 205, 1975.
129. Patek, et al.: Arch. Intern. Med., *135*, 1053, 1975.
130. Davidson: Am. J. Clin. Nutr., *23*, 427, 1970.
131. Sherlock and Walshe: Nature, *161*, 604, 1948.
132. Hoffbauer and Zaki: Arch. Pathol., *79*, 364, 1965.
133. Olson: In *Modern Nutrition in Health and Disease*, 5th ed. (Goodhart and Shils, Eds.). Philadelphia, Lea & Febiger, 1964.
134. Rubin and Lieber: N. Engl. J. Med., *178*, 869, 1968.
135. Lieber, Jones, and DeCarli: J. Clin. Invest., *44*, 1009, 1965.
136. Lieber and DeCarli: Gastroenterology, *50*, 316, 1966.
137. Hartroft and Porta: Can. J. Physiol. Pharmacol., *46*, 463, 1968.
138. Erenoglu, Edreira and Patek: Ann. Intern. Med., *60*, 814, 1964.
139. US Bureau of the Census: Vital Statistics Rates in the United States, 1900–1940, Government Printing Office, 1943.

140. Lederman: Alcohol, Alcoholisme, Alcoholisation. Institut National d'Etudes Demographiques, Travaux et Documents, Cahier No. 41, Paris, Presses Universitaires de France, 1964.
141. Lelbach: Acta Hepatosplenol., *14*, 9, 1967.
142. Menghini: Bull Schweiz. Akad. Med. Wiss., *16*, 36, 1960.
143. Rubin and Lieber: Fed. Proc., *26*, 1458, 1967.
144. Lieber and Rubin: Am. J. Med., *44*, 200, 1968.
145. Lieber and DeCarli: J. Med. Primatol., *3*, 153, 1974.
146. Rubin and Lieber: N. Engl. J. Med., *290*, 128, 1974.
147. Lieber, DeCarli and Rubin: Proc. Natl. Acad. Sci., *72*, 437, 1975.
148. Lieber and Spritz: J. Clin. Invest., *45*, 1400, 1966.
149. Klatskin, Krehl and Conn: J. Exp. Med., *100*, 605, 1954.
150. Lieber, Spritz and DeCarli: J. Clin. Invest., *45*, 51, 1966.
151. Lieber, Spritz, DeCarli: J. Lipid Res., *10*, 283, 1969.
152. Kyosola and Salorinne: Ann. Clin. Res., *7*, 80, 1975.
153. Bhuyan, Nayak, Deo and Ramalingaswami: Lab. Invest., *14*, 184, 1965.
154. Hibbs, et al.: Am. Heart J., *69*, 766, 1965.
155. Susin and Herdson: Arch. Pathol., *83*, 86, 1967.
156. Regan, et al.: Clin. Invest., *48*, 397, 1969.
157. Wendt, et al.: Ann. Intern. Med., *62*, 1068, 1965.
158. Morin and Daniel: Can. Med. Assoc. J., *97*, 926, 1967.
159. Lindenbaum and Lieber: N. Engl. J. Med., *281*, 333, 1969.
160. Haut and Cowan: Am. J. Med., *56*, 22, 1974.
161. Lindenbaum and Hargrove: Ann. Intern. Med., *68*, 526, 1968.
162. Brayton, Stokes, Schwartz and Louvian: N. Engl. J. Med., *282*, 123, 1970.
163. Hornabrook: Am. J. Clin. Nutr., *9*, 398, 1961.
164. Victor and Adams: Am. J. Clin. Nutr., *9*, 379, 1960.
165. Platt: In *Thiamine Deficiency: Biochemical Lesions and Their Clinical Significance* (Wolstenholme, Ed.). Boston, Little Brown and Co., 1967.
166. Neubueger: Arch. Pathol., *63*, 1, 1957.
167. Dreyfus and Victor: Am. J. Clin. Nutr., *9*, 414, 1961.
168. Phillips, Victor, Adams and Davidson: J. Clin. Invest., *31*, 859, 1952.
169. Victor and Adams: Am. J. Clin. Nutr., *9*, 379, 1961.
170. Blass and Gibson: N. Engl. J. Med., *297*, 1367, 1977.
171. Muller, Kobald and Endtz: Ned. Tijdschr. Geneeskd., *119*, 991, 1975.
172. Vorhees, Barrett and Schenker: Life Sci., *16*, 1187, 1975.
173. Walker and Freund: Science, *182*, 597, 1973.
174. Graham, Woodhouse and Read: Lancet, *2*, 107, 1971.
175. Morrison: Ann. Intern. Med., *24*, 465, 1946.
176. Patek and Post: J. Clin. Invest., *10*, 481, 1941.
177. Patek, et al.: J.A.M.A., *138*, 543, 1948.
178. Rudman, et al.: Am. J. Clin. Nutr., *23*, 1203, 1970.
179. Breuer and Breuer: Z. Klin. Chem. Klin. Biochem., *13*, 196, 1975.
180. Ning, Lowenstein and Davidson: J. Lab. Clin. Med., *70*, 554, 1967.
181. Phear, Ruebner, Sherlock and Summerskill: Clin. Sci., *15*, 93, 1956.
182. Maddrey, et al.: Gastroenterology, *71*, 190, 1976.
183. Bessman and Mirick: J. Clin. Invest., *37*, 990, 1958.
184. Fenton, Knight and Humperson: Lancet, *1*, 164, 1966.
185. Greenberger, et al.: Am. J. Dig. Dis., *22*, 845, 1977.
186. Kunin, et al.: N. Engl. J. Med., *262*, 380, 1960.
187. Meyers and Lieber: Gastroenterology, *70*, 244, 1976.
188. Huberl: Gastroenterology, *65*, 349, 1973.
189. Lieber and Davidson: Arch. Intern. Med., *106*, 749, 1960.
190. Bebb, et al.: Am. J. Clin. Nutr., *24*, 1042, 1971.
191. Westerfeld and Schulman: J.A.M.A., *170*, 197, 1959.

APPENDIX

Abby Stolper Bloch and Maurice E. Shils

The major portion of the Appendix provides information about diets and sup
plements to implement recommendations in the text for dietary management of specifi
disease entities. Because detailed and extensive tables of food composition are available
inclusion of this type of data has been limited. Dietary prescriptions may requir
modification in accordance with the clinical status and reactions of the individual patient

A major section on liquid formulas includes guidelines on use and detailed composi
tions of commercially available products and examples of special formulas for prepara
tion by hospitals or patients at home.

1244

Table A–1a. Food and Nutrition Board, National Academy of Sciences—National Research Council Recommended Daily Dietary Allowances,[a] Revised 1979 Designed for the Maintenance of Good Nutrition of Practically All Healthy People in the U.S.A.
Mean Heights and Weights and Recommended Energy Intake

Category	Age (Years)	Weight (kg)	Weight (lb)	Height (cm)	Height (in)	Energy Needs (with range) (kcal)	Energy Needs (with range) (MJ)
Infants	0.0–0.5	6	13	60	24	kg × 115 (95–145)	kg × .48
	0.5–1.0	9	20	71	28	kg × 105 (80–135)	kg × .44
Children	1–3	13	29	90	35	1300 (900–1800)	5.5
	4–6	20	44	112	44	1700 (1300–2300)	7.1
	7–10	28	62	132	52	2400 (1650–3300)	10.1
Males	11–14	45	99	157	62	2700 (2000–3700)	11.3
	15–18	66	145	176	69	2800 (2100–3900)	11.8
	19–22	70	154	177	70	2900 (2500–3300)	12.2
	23–50	70	154	178	70	2700 (2300–3100)	11.3
	51–75	70	154	178	70	2400 (2000–2800)	10.1
	76+	70	154	178	70	2050 (1650–2450)	8.6
Females	11–14	46	101	157	62	2200 (1500–3000)	9.2
	15–18	55	120	163	64	2100 (1200–3000)	8.8
	19–22	55	120	163	64	2100 (1700–2500)	8.8
	23–50	55	120	163	64	2000 (1600–2400)	8.4
	51–75	55	120	163	64	1800 (1400–2200)	7.6
	76+	55	120	163	64	1600 (1200–2000)	6.7
Pregnancy						+300	
Lactation						+500	

The data in this table have been assembled from the observed median heights and weights of children . . . together with desirable weights for adults . . . for the mean heights of men (178 cm) and women (163 cm) between the ages of 18 and 34 years as surveyed in the U.S. population (HEW/NCHS data).

The energy allowances for the young adults are for men and women doing light work. The allowances for the two older age groups represent mean energy needs over these age spans, allowing for a 2% decrease in basal (resting) metabolic rate per decade and a reduction in activity of 200 kcal/day for men and women between 51 and 75 years, 500 kcal for men over 75 years and 400 kcal for women over 75 (see original text). The customary range of daily energy output is shown for adults in parentheses, and is based on a variation in energy needs of ±400 kcal at any one age (see original text and Garrow, 1978), emphasizing the range of energy intakes appropriate for any group of people.

Energy allowances for children through age 18 are based on median energy intakes of children these ages followed in longitudinal growth studies. The values in parentheses are 10th and 90th percentiles of energy intake, to indicate the range of energy consumption among children of these ages (see original text).

From: Recommended Dietary Allowances, Revised 1979. Food and Nutrition Board, National Academy of Sciences—National Research Council, Washington, D.C.

Table A–1b.   Recommended Daily Dietary

	Age	Weight		Height		Protein	Fat-soluble Vitamins		
							Vita-min A (μg R.E.)[b]	Vita-min D (μg)[c]	Vita-min E (mg α T.E.)[d]
	(years)	(kg)	(lb)	(cm)	(in)	(g)			
Infants	0.0–0.5	6	13	60	24	kg × 2.2	420	10	3
	0.5–1.0	9	20	71	28	kg × 2.0	400	10	4
Children	1–3	13	29	90	35	23	400	10	5
	4–6	20	44	112	44	30	500	10	6
	7–10	28	62	132	52	34	700	10	7
Males	11–14	45	99	157	62	45	1000	10	8
	15–18	66	145	176	69	56	1000	10	10
	19–22	70	154	177	70	56	1000	7.5	10
	23–50	70	154	178	70	56	1000	5	10
	51+	70	154	178	70	56	1000	5	10
Females	11–14	46	101	157	62	46	800	10	8
	15–18	55	120	163	64	46	800	10	8
	19–22	55	120	163	64	44	800	7.5	8
	23–50	55	120	163	64	44	800	5	8
	51+	55	120	163	64	44	800	5	8
Pregnant						+30	+200	+5	+2
Lactating						+20	+400	+5	+3

[a] The allowances are intended to provide for individual variations among most normal persons living in the United States under usual environmental stresses. Diets should be based on a variety of common foods in order to provide other nutrients for which human requirements have been less well defined. See original text for detailed discussion of allowances and of nutrients not tabulated.

[b] Retinol equivalents. 1 Retinol equivalent = 1 μg retinol or 6 μg β parotene. See original text for calculation of vitamin A activity of diets as retinol equivalents.

[c] As cholecalciferol. 10 μg cholecalciferol = 400 I.U. vitamin D.

[d] α tocopherol equivalents (T.E.). 1 mg d-α-tocopherol = 1 α T.E. See original text for variation in allowances and calculation of vitamin E activity of the diet as α tocopherol equivalents.

[e] 1 NE (niacin equivalent) is equal to 1 mg of niacin or 60 mg of dietary tryptophan.

Table A–1c.   Estimated Safe and Adequate
Selected Vitamins

	Age (Years)	Vitamins			Trace Elements[b]	
		Vitamin K (μg)	Biotin (μg)	Pantothenic Acid (mg)	Copper (mg)	Manganese (mg)
Infants	0 – 0.5	12	35	2	0.5–0.7	0.5–0.7
	0.5– 1	10– 20	50	3	0.7–1.0	0.7–1.0
Children	1 – 3	15– 30	65	3	1.0–1.5	1.0–1.5
and	4 – 6	20– 40	85	3–4	1.5–2.0	1.5–2.0
Adolescents	7 –10	30– 60	120	4–5	2.0–2.5	2.0–3.0
	11+	50–100	100–200	4–7	2.0–3.0	2.5–5.0
Adults		70–140	100–200	4–7	2.0–3.0	2.5–5.0

[a] Because there is less information on which to base allowances, these figures are not given in the main table of the RDA and are provided here in the form of ranges of recommended intakes.

[b] Since the toxic levels for many trace elements may be only several times usual intakes, the upper levels for the trace elements given in this table should not be habitually exceeded.

Allowances,[a] Revised 1979

	Water-soluble Vitamins						Minerals					
Vitamin C (mg)	Thiamin (mg)	Riboflavin (mg)	Niacin (mg N.E.)[e]	Vitamin B₆ (mg)	Folacin[f] (µg)	Vitamin B₁₂ (µg)	Calcium (mg)	Phosphorus (mg)	Magnesium (mg)	Iron (mg)	Zinc (mg)	Iodine (µg)
35	0.3	0.4	6	0.3	30	0.5[g]	360	240	50	10	3	40
35	0.5	0.6	8	0.6	45	1.5	540	360	70	15	5	50
45	0.7	0.8	9	0.9	100	2.0	800	800	150	15	10	70
45	0.9	1.0	11	1.3	200	2.5	800	800	200	10	10	90
45	1.2	1.4	16	1.6	300	3.0	800	800	250	10	10	120
50	1.4	1.6	18	1.8	400	3.0	1200	1200	350	18	15	150
60	1.4	1.7	18	2.0	400	3.0	1200	1200	400	18	15	150
60	1.5	1.7	19	2.2	400	3.0	800	800	350	10	15	150
60	1.4	1.6	18	2.2	400	3.0	800	800	350	10	15	150
60	1.2	1.4	16	2.2	400	3.0	800	800	350	10	15	150
50	1.1	1.3	15	1.8	400	3.0	1200	1200	300	18	15	150
60	1.1	1.3	14	2.0	400	3.0	1200	1200	300	18	15	150
60	1.1	1.3	14	2.0	400	3.0	800	800	300	18	15	150
60	1.0	1.2	13	2.0	400	3.0	800	800	300	18	15	150
60	1.0	1.2	13	2.0	400	3.0	800	800	300	10	15	150
+20	+0.4	+0.3	+2	+0.6	+400	+1.0	+400	+400	+150	[h]	+ 5	+ 25
+40	+0.5	+0.5	+5	+0.5	+100	+1.0	+400	+400	+150	[h]	+10	+ 50

[f] The folacin allowances refer to dietary sources as determined by *Lactobacillus casei* assay after treatment with enzymes ("conjugases") to make polyglutamyl forms of the vitamin available to the test organism.

[g] The RDA for vitamin B₁₂ in infants is based on average concentration of the vitamin in human milk. The allowances after weaning are based on energy intake (as recommended by the American Academy of Pediatrics) and consideration of other factors such as intestinal absorption; see original text.

[h] The increased requirement during pregnancy cannot be met by the iron content of habitual American diets nor by the existing iron stores of many women; therefore the use of 30 to 60 mg of supplemental iron is recommended. Iron needs during lactation are not substantially different from those of nonpregnant women, but continued supplementation of the mother for two to three months after parturition is advisable in order to replenish stores depleted by pregnancy.

Daily Dietary Intakes of Additional and Minerals[a]

	Trace Elements[b]				Electrolytes		
Fluoride (mg)	Chromium (mg)	Selenium (mg)	Molybdenum (mg)		Sodium (mg)	Potassium (mg)	Chloride (mg)
0.1–0.5	0.01–0.04	0.01–0.04	0.03–0.06		115– 350	350– 925	275– 700
0.2–1.0	0.02–0.06	0.02–0.06	0.04–0.08		250– 750	425–1275	400–1200
0.5–1.5	0.02–0.08	0.02–0.08	0.05–0.1		325– 975	550–1650	500–1500
1.0–2.5	0.03–0.12	0.03–0.12	0.06–0.15		450–1350	775–2325	700–2100
1.5–2.5	0.05–0.2	0.05–0.2	0.1 –0.3		600–1800	1000–3000	925–2775
1.5–2.5	0.05–0.2	0.05–0.2	0.15–0.5		900–2700	1525–4575	1400–4200
1.5–4.0	0.05–0.2	0.05–0.2	0.15–0.5		1100–3300	1875–5625	1700–5100

From: Recommended Dietary Allowances, Revised 1979. Food and Nutrition Board, National Academy of Sciences—National Research Council, Washington, D.C.

Table A–2. Recommended Daily Nutrient

Age	Sex	Weight (kg)	Height (cm)	Energy[a] (kcal)	(MJ)[b]	Protein (gm)	Water-soluble Vitamins				
							Thiamin (mg)	Niacin (NE)[f]	Riboflavin (mg)	Vitamin B₆[g] (mg)	Folate[h] (μg)
0–6 mo	Both	6	—	kg × 117	kg × 0.49	kg × 2.2(2.0)[e]	0.3	5	0.4	0.3	40
7–11 mo	Both	9	—	kg × 108	kg × 0.45	kg × 1.4	0.5	6	0.6	0.4	60
1–3 yr	Both	13	90	1400	5.9	22	0.7	9	0.8	0.8	100
4–6 yr	Both	19	110	1800	7.5	27	0.9	12	1.1	1.3	100
7–9 yr	M	27	129	2200	9.2	33	1.1	14	1.3	1.6	100
	F	27	128	2000	8.4	33	1.0	13	1.2	1.4	100
10–12 yr	M	36	144	2500	10.5	41	1.2	17	1.5	1.8	100
	F	38	145	2300	9.6	40	1.1	15	1.4	1.5	100
13–15 yr	M	51	162	2800	11.7	52	1.4	19	1.7	2.0	200
	F	49	159	2200	9.2	43	1.1	15	1.4	1.5	200
16–18 yr	M	64	172	3200	13.4	54	1.6	21	2.0	2.0	200
	F	54	161	2100	8.8	43	1.1	14	1.3	1.5	200
19–35 yr	M	70	176	3000	12.6	56	1.5	20	1.8	2.0	200
	F	56	161	2100	8.8	41	1.1	14	1.3	1.5	200
36–50 yr	M	70	176	2700	11.3	56	1.4	18	1.7	2.0	200
	F	56	161	1900	7.9	41	1.0	13	1.2	1.5	200
51+ yr	M	70	176	2300[c]	9.6[c]	56	1.4	18	1.7	2.0	200
	F	56	161	1800[c]	7.5[c]	41	1.0	13	1.2	1.5	200
Pregnancy				+300[d]	1.3[d]	+20	+0.2	+2	+0.3	+0.5	+50
Lactation				+500	2.1	+24	+0.4	+7	+0.6	+0.6	+50

[a] Recommendations assume characteristic activity pattern for each age group.

[b] Megajoules (10^6 joules). Calculated from the relation 1 kilocalorie = 4.184 kilojoules and rounded to 1 decimal place.

[c] Recommended energy intake for age 66+ years reduced to 2000 kcal (8.4 MJ) for men and 1500 kcal (6.3 MJ) for women.

[d] Increased energy intake recommended during second and third trimesters. An increase of 100 kcal (418.4 kJ) per day is recommended during the first trimester.

[e] Recommended protein intake of 2.2 gm per kg body wt for infants age 0 to 2 mo and 2.0 gm per kg body wt for those age 3 to 5 mo. Protein recommendation for infants 0 to 11 mo assumes consumption of breast milk or protein of equivalent quality.

[f] 1NE (niacin equivalent) is equal to 1 mg of niacin or 60 mg of tryptophan.

[g] Recommendations are based on estimated average daily protein intake of Canadians.

[h] Recommendation given in terms of free folate.

[i] Considerably higher levels may be prudent for infants during the first week of life to guard against neonatal tyrosinemia.

Intake—Canada—Revised 1975*

| | | Fat-soluble Vitamins | | | | | Minerals | | | |
Vita-min B_{12} (μg)	Vita-min C (mg)	Vita-min A (RE)[j]	Vitamin D (μg cholecal-ciferol)[k]	Vitamin E (mg d-α-toco-pherol)	Calcium (mg)	Phosphorus (mg)	Magnesium (mg)	Iodine (μg)	Iron (mg)	Zinc (mg)
0.3	20[j]	400	10	3	500[m]	250[m]	50[m]	35[m]	7[m]	4[m]
0.3	20	400	10	3	500	400	50	50	7	5
0.9	20	400	10	4	500	500	75	70	8	5
1.5	20	500	5	5	500	500	100	90	9	6
1.5	30	700	2.5[l]	6	700	700	150	110	10	7
1.5	30	700	2.5[l]	6	700	700	150	100	10	7
3.0	30	800	2.5[l]	7	900	900	175	130	11	8
3.0	30	800	2.5[l]	7	1000	1000	200	120	11	9
3.0	30	1000	2.5[l]	9	1200	1200	250	140	13	10
3.0	30	800	2.5[l]	7	800	800	250	110	14	10
3.0	30	1000	2.5[l]	10	1000	1000	300	160	14	12
3.0	30	800	2.5[l]	6	700	700	250	110	14	11
3.0	30	1000	2.5[l]	9	800	800	300	150	10	10
3.0	30	800	2.5[l]	6	700	700	250	110	14	9
3.0	30	1000	2.5[l]	8	800	800	300	140	10	10
3.0	30	800	2.5[l]	6	700	700	250	100	14	9
3.0	30	1000	2.5[l]	8	800	800	300	140	10	10
3.0	30	800	2.5[l]	6	700	700	250	100	9	9
+1.0	+20	+100	+2.5[l]	+1	+500	+500	+25	+15	+1[n]	+3
+0.5	+30	+400	+2.5[l]	+2	+500	+500	+75	+25	+1[n]	+7

[j] 1RE (retinol equivalent) corresponds to a biologic activity in humans equal to 1 μg retinol (3.33 I.U.) or 6 μg ρ-carotene (10 I.U.).

[k] One μg cholecalciferol is equivalent to 1 μg ergocalciferol (40 I.U. vitamin D activity).

[l] Most older children and adults receive vitamin D from irradiation but 2.5 μg daily is recommended. This intake should be increased to 5.0 μg daily during pregnancy and lactation and for those confined indoors or otherwise deprived of sunlight for extended periods.

[m] The intake of breast-fed infants may be less than the recommendation but is considered to be adequate.

[n] A recommended total intake of 15 mg daily during pregnancy and lactation assumes the presence of adequate stores of iron. If stores are suspected of being inadequate, additional iron as a supplement is recommended.

*Reprinted by permission of the Minister of National Health and Welfare, Canada, from Dietary Standard for Canada, Table 13, rev. 1975, by Committee for Revision of the Canadian Dietary Standard, Bureau of Nutritional Sciences, Health and Welfare (Ottawa: Information Canada, 1975).

Table A–3.   Recommended Intakes of Nutrients—WHO—1974*

Age	Body Weight (kg)	Energy[1] (kcal)	(MJ)	Protein[1,2] (gm)	Vitamin A[3,4] (µg)	Vitamin D[5,6] (µg)	Thiamin[3] (mg)	Riboflavin[3] (mg)	Niacin[3] (mg)	Folic Acid[5] (µg)	Vitamin B_{12}[5] (µg)	Ascorbic Acid[5] (mg)	Calcium[7] (gm)	Iron[5,8] (mg)
Children														
<1	7.3	820	3.4	14	300	10.0	0.3	0.5	5.4	60	0.3	20	0.5–0.6	5–10
1–3	13.4	1360	5.7	16	250	10.0	0.5	0.8	9.0	100	0.9	20	0.4–0.5	5–10
4–6	20.2	1830	7.6	20	300	10.0	0.7	1.1	12.1	100	1.5	20	0.4–0.5	5–10
7–9	28.1	2190	9.2	25	400	2.5	0.9	1.3	14.5	100	1.5	20	0.4–0.5	5–10
Male adolescents														
10–12	36.9	2600	10.9	30	575	2.5	1.0	1.6	17.2	100	2.0	20	0.6–0.7	5–10
13–15	51.3	2900	12.1	37	725	2.5	1.2	1.7	19.1	200	2.0	30	0.6–0.7	9–18
16–19	62.9	3070	12.8	38	750	2.5	1.2	1.8	20.3	200	2.0	30	0.5–0.6	5–9
Female adolescents														
10–12	38.0	2350	9.8	29	575	2.5	0.9	1.4	15.5	100	2.0	20	0.6–0.7	5–10
13–15	49.9	2490	10.4	31	725	2.5	1.0	1.5	16.4	200	2.0	30	0.6–0.7	12–24
16–19	54.4	2310	9.7	30	750	2.5	0.9	1.4	15.2	200	2.0	30	0.5–0.6	14–28
Adult man (moderately active)	65.0	3000	12.6	37	750	2.5	1.2	1.8	19.8	200	2.0	30	0.4–0.5	5–9
Adult woman (moderately active)	55.0	2200	9.2	29	750	2.5	0.9	1.3	14.5	200	2.0	30	0.4–0.5	14–28
Pregnancy (later half)		+350	+1.5	38	750	10.0	+0.1	+0.2	+2.3	400	3.0	50	1.0–1.2	(9)
Lactation (first 6 months)		+550	+2.3	46	1200	10.0	+0.2	+0.4	+3.7	300	2.5	50	1.0–1.2	(9)

[1] Energy and Protein Requirements. Report of a Joint FAO/WHO Expert Group, FAO, Rome, 1972. [2] As egg or milk protein. [3] Requirements of vitamin A, thiamin, riboflavin and niacin. Report of a Joint FAO/WHO Expert Group, FAO, Rome, 1965. [4] As retinol. [5] Requirements of ascorbic acid, vitamin D, vitamin B_{12}, folate and iron. Report of a FAO/WHO Expert Group, FAO, Rome, 1970. [6] As cholecalciferol. [7] Calcium requirements. Report of a FAO/WHO Expert Group, FAO, Rome, 1961. [8] On each line the lower value applies when over 25 per cent of calories in the diet come from animal foods, and the higher value when animal foods represent less than 10 per cent of calories. [9] For women whose iron intake throughout life has been at the level recommended in this table, the daily intake of iron during pregnancy and lactation should be the same as that recommended for nonpregnant, nonlactating women of childbearing age. For women whose iron status is not satisfactory at the beginning of pregnancy, the requirement is increased, and in the extreme situation of women with no iron stores, the requirement can probably not be met without supplementation.

*From Passmore, Nicol and Rao: *Handbook on Human Nutritional Requirements*. Geneva, WHO Monogr. Ser. No. 61, 1974, Table 1.

ADDENDUM: Dietary allowances, official or unofficial for many European countries, as of 1976 or earlier, appear in the Proceedings of the Second European Nutrition Conference, Munich, 1976. (Nutr. Metab., 21:210, 1977.)

Table A–4a.   Desirable Weights for Men and Women, According to Height and Frame, Ages 25 and Over*

Height (in shoes)		Weight (in indoor clothing)					
		Small Frame		Medium Frame		Large Frame	
	(cm)	(lb)	(kg)	(lb)	(kg)	(lb)	(kg)
Men							
5 ft 2 in	158	112–120	51–55	118–129	54–59	126–141	57–64
5 ft 3 in	160	115–123	52–56	121–133	55–60	129–144	59–65
5 ft 4 in	163	118–126	54–57	124–136	56–62	132–148	60–67
5 ft 5 in	165	121–129	55–59	127–139	58–63	135–152	61–69
5 ft 6 in	168	124–133	56–60	130–143	59–65	138–156	63–71
5 ft 7 in	170	128–137	58–62	134–147	61–67	142–161	64–73
5 ft 8 in	173	132–141	60–64	138–152	63–69	147–166	67–75
5 ft 9 in	176	136–145	62–66	142–156	64–71	151–170	69–77
5 ft 10 in	178	140–150	64–68	146–160	66–73	155–174	70–79
5 ft 11 in	180	144–154	65–70	150–165	68–75	159–179	72–81
6 ft	183	148–158	67–72	154–170	70–77	164–184	74–84
6 ft 1 in	185	152–162	69–74	158–175	72–79	168–189	76–86
6 ft 2 in	188	156–167	71–76	162–180	74–82	173–194	79–88
6 ft 3 in	191	160–171	73–78	167–185	76–84	178–199	81–90
6 ft 4 in	193	164–175	74–79	172–190	78–86	182–204	83–93
Women							
4 ft 10 in	147	92–98	42–45	96–107	44–49	104–119	47–54
4 ft 11 in	150	94–101	43–46	98–110	45–50	106–122	48–55
5 ft	152	96–104	44–47	101–113	46–51	109–125	49–57
5 ft 1 in	155	99–107	45–49	104–116	47–53	112–128	51–58
5 ft 2 in	158	102–110	46–50	107–119	49–54	115–131	52–59
5 ft 3 in	160	105–113	48–51	110–122	50–55	118–134	54–61
5 ft 4 in	163	108–116	49–53	113–126	51–57	121–138	55–63
5 ft 5 in	165	111–119	50–54	116–130	53–59	125–142	57–64
5 ft 6 in	168	114–123	52–56	120–135	55–61	129–146	59–66
5 ft 7 in	170	118–127	54–58	124–139	56–63	133–150	60–68
5 ft 8 in	173	122–131	55–59	128–143	58–65	137–154	62–70
5 ft 9 in	175	126–135	57–61	132–147	60–67	141–158	64–72
5 ft 10 in	178	130–140	59–64	136–151	62–69	145–163	66–74
5 ft 11 in	180	134–144	61–65	140–155	64–70	149–168	68–76
6 ft	183	138–148	63–67	144–159	65–72	153–173	69–79

*Adapted from Overweight, its Prevention and Significance, a series of articles reprinted from *Statistical Bulletin*, Metropolitan Life Insurance Co., 1960, p. 5.

Table A–4b. Average Weight for Men and Women by Age and Height, United States, 1960–62*

Average Weight

Height[1]		18–24		25–34		35–44		45–54		55–64		65–74		75–79	
(in)	(cm)	(lb)	(kg)	(lb)	(kg)	(lb)	(kg)	(lb)	(kg)	(lb)	(kg)	(lb)	(kg)	(lb)	(kg)
									Years						
							Men								
62	158	140	63.6	139	63.2	150	68.2	142	64.6	145	65.9	161	73.2	140	63.6
63	160	150	68.2	143	65.0	154	70.0	150	68.2	155	70.5	152	69.1	135	61.4
64	163	139	63.2	147	66.8	154	70.0	159	72.3	158	71.8	154	70.0	136	61.8
65	165	149	67.7	156	70.9	169	76.8	163	74.1	152	69.1	159	72.3	153	69.6
66	168	160	72.7	161	73.2	166	75.5	164	74.6	163	74.1	159	72.3	153	69.6
67	170	153	69.6	167	75.9	165	75.0	168	76.4	168	76.4	155	70.5	169	76.8
68	173	157	71.4	165	75.0	170	77.3	174	79.1	172	74.6	164	74.6	182	82.7
69	175	166	75.5	173	78.6	174	79.1	172	78.2	173	78.6	164	74.6	158	71.8
70	178	165	75.0	180	81.8	179	81.4	183	83.2	173	78.6	174	79.1	173	78.6
71	180	166	75.5	181	82.3	190	86.4	191	86.8	178	80.9	179	81.4	[2]179	81.4
72	183	169	76.8	188	85.5	183	83.2	183	83.2	177	80.5	188	85.5	156	70.9
73	185	183	83.2	191	86.8	193	87.7	187	85.0	212	96.4	183	83.2	[2]189	85.9
74	188	185	84.1	182	82.7	204	92.7	203	92.3	216	98.2	185	84.1	[2]194	88.2

Women

57	145	117	53.2	128	58.2	122	55.5	144	65.5	132	60.0	136	61.8	132	60.0
58	147	121	55.0	121	55.0	117	53.2	117	53.2	136	61.8	140	63.6	124	56.4
59	150	121	55.0	118	53.6	138	62.7	135	61.4	141	64.1	143	65.0	133	60.5
60	152	122	55.5	124	56.4	138	62.7	137	62.3	148	67.3	142	64.6	148	67.3
61	155	124	56.4	127	57.7	137	62.3	150	68.2	147	66.8	146	66.4	146	66.4
62	158	128	58.2	133	60.5	143	65.0	143	65.0	159	72.3	154	70.0	133	60.5
63	160	126	57.3	135	61.4	146	66.4	146	66.4	160	72.7	145	65.9	145	65.9
64	163	126	57.3	140	63.6	147	66.8	155	70.5	156	70.9	158	71.8	156	70.9
65	165	135	61.4	142	64.6	140	63.6	156	70.9	161	73.2	145	65.9	144	65.5
66	168	142	64.6	139	63.2	148	67.3	157	71.4	145	65.9	154	70.0	[2]157	71.4
67	170	140	63.6	154	70.0	154	70.0	171	77.7	172	78.2	219	99.6	[2]160	72.7
68	173	131	59.6	150	68.2	160	72.7	169	76.8	158	71.8	200	90.9	162	73.6

[1] Height without shoes; weight partially clothed—clothing weight estimated as averaging two (2) pounds.

[2] Estimated values obtained from linear regression equations.

*From *Weight by Height and Age of Adults*. Vital Health Statistics Data. Washington, National Health Service, Pub. No. 1000, Series 11, No. 14, May 1966.

Table A–4c. Physical Growth NCHS Percentiles*
Girls: Birth to 36 Months

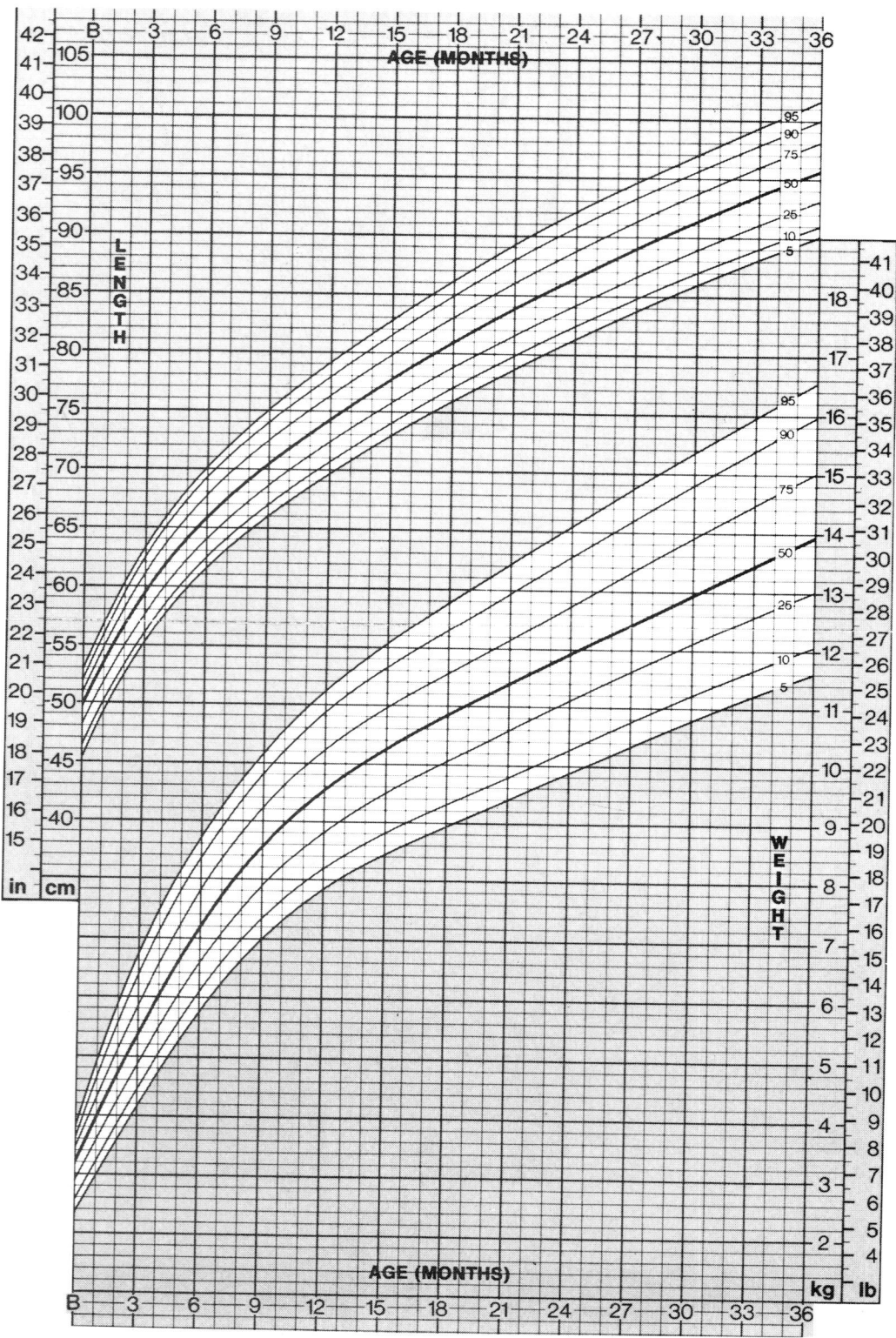

*These tables are used through the courtesy of Ross Laboratories who adapted the growth curves from the original data: National Center for Health Statistics, NCHS Growth Charts, 1976. Monthly Vital Statistics Report, Vol. 25, No. 3, Suppl. (HRA) 76–1120. Rockville, Health Resources Administration, June 1976. Data from The Fels Research Institute, Yellow Springs, Ohio.

Table A–4c. Boys: Birth to 36 Months

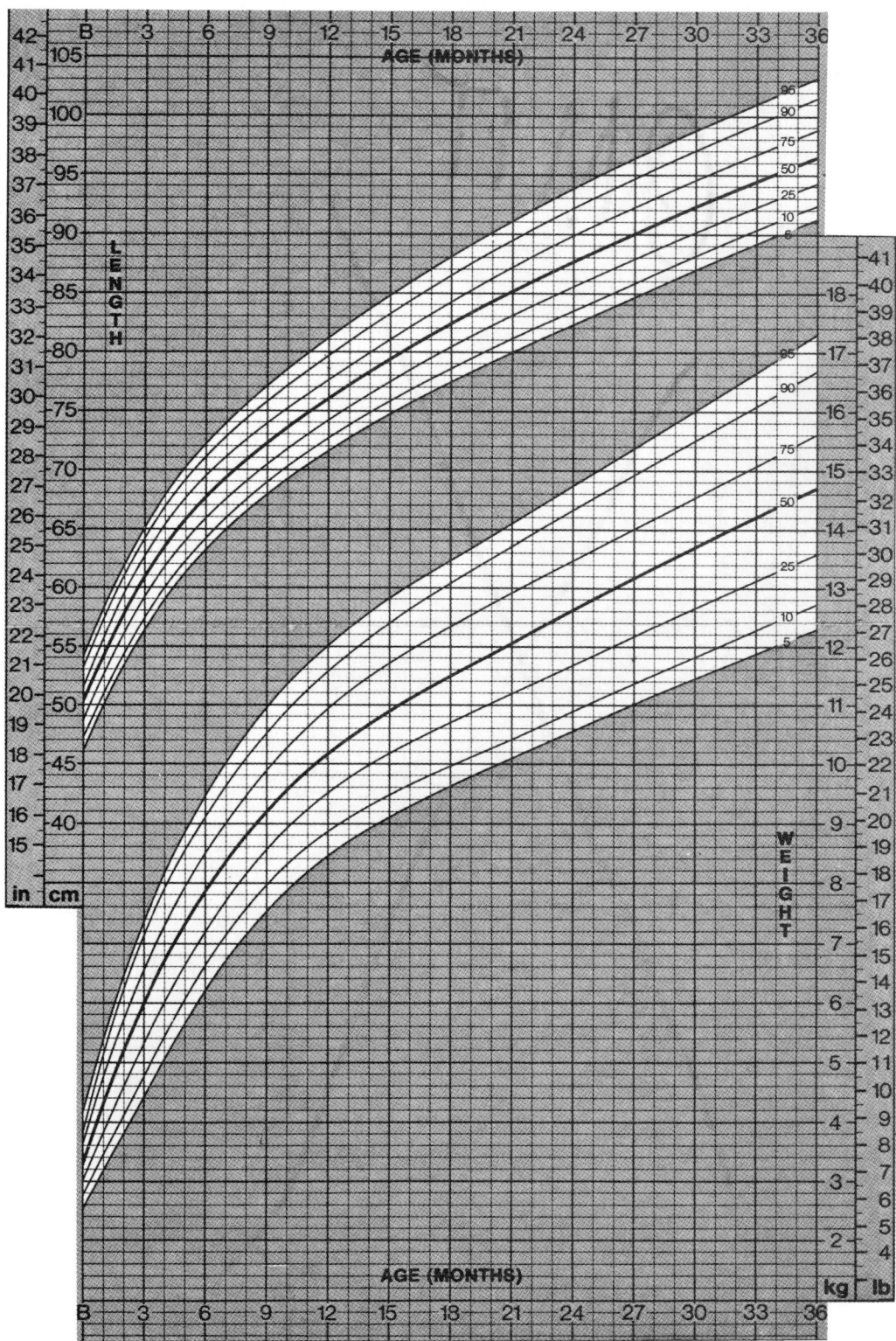

Table A–4c.   Girls: 2 to 18 Years

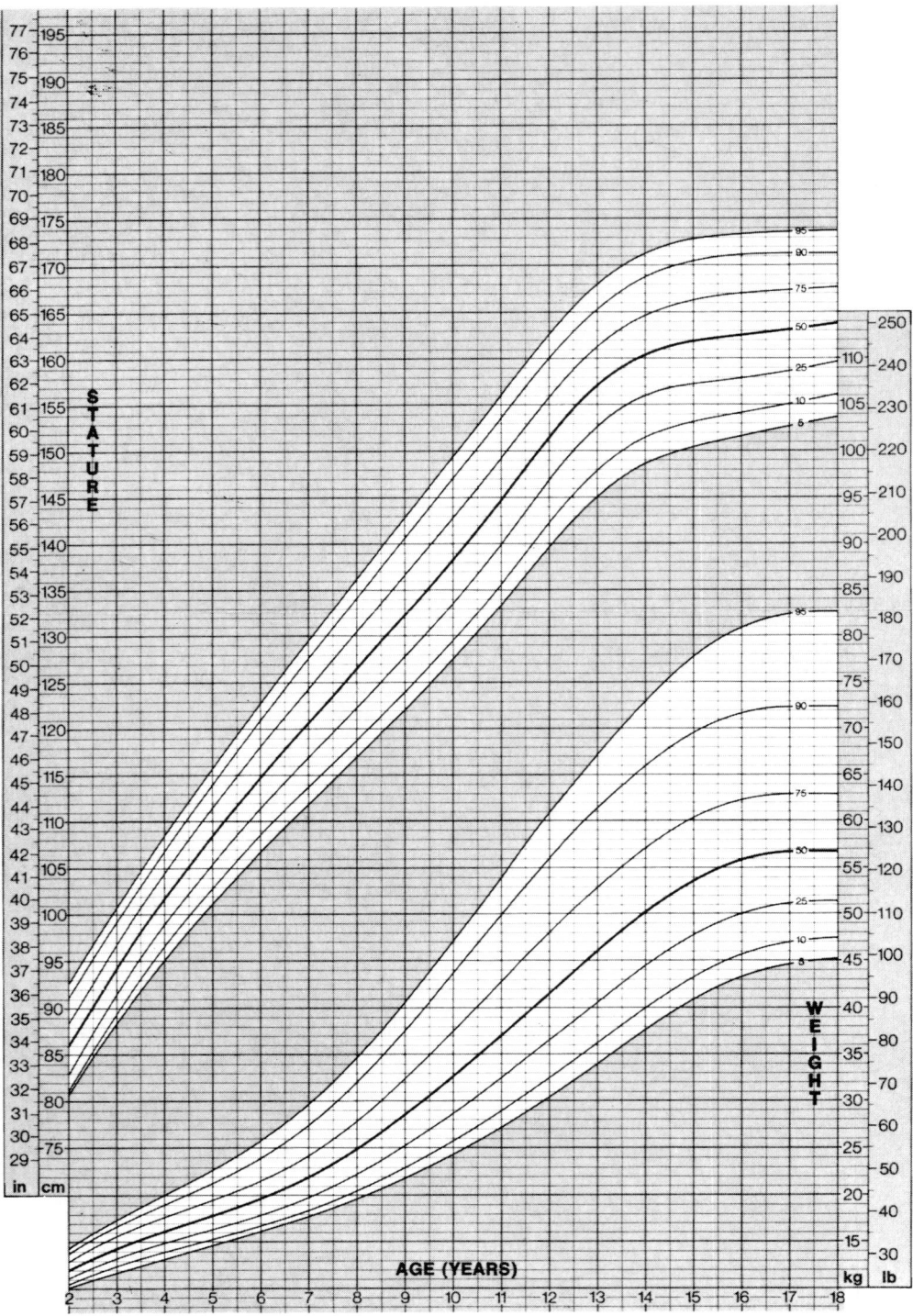

Table A–4c. Boys: 2 to 18 Years

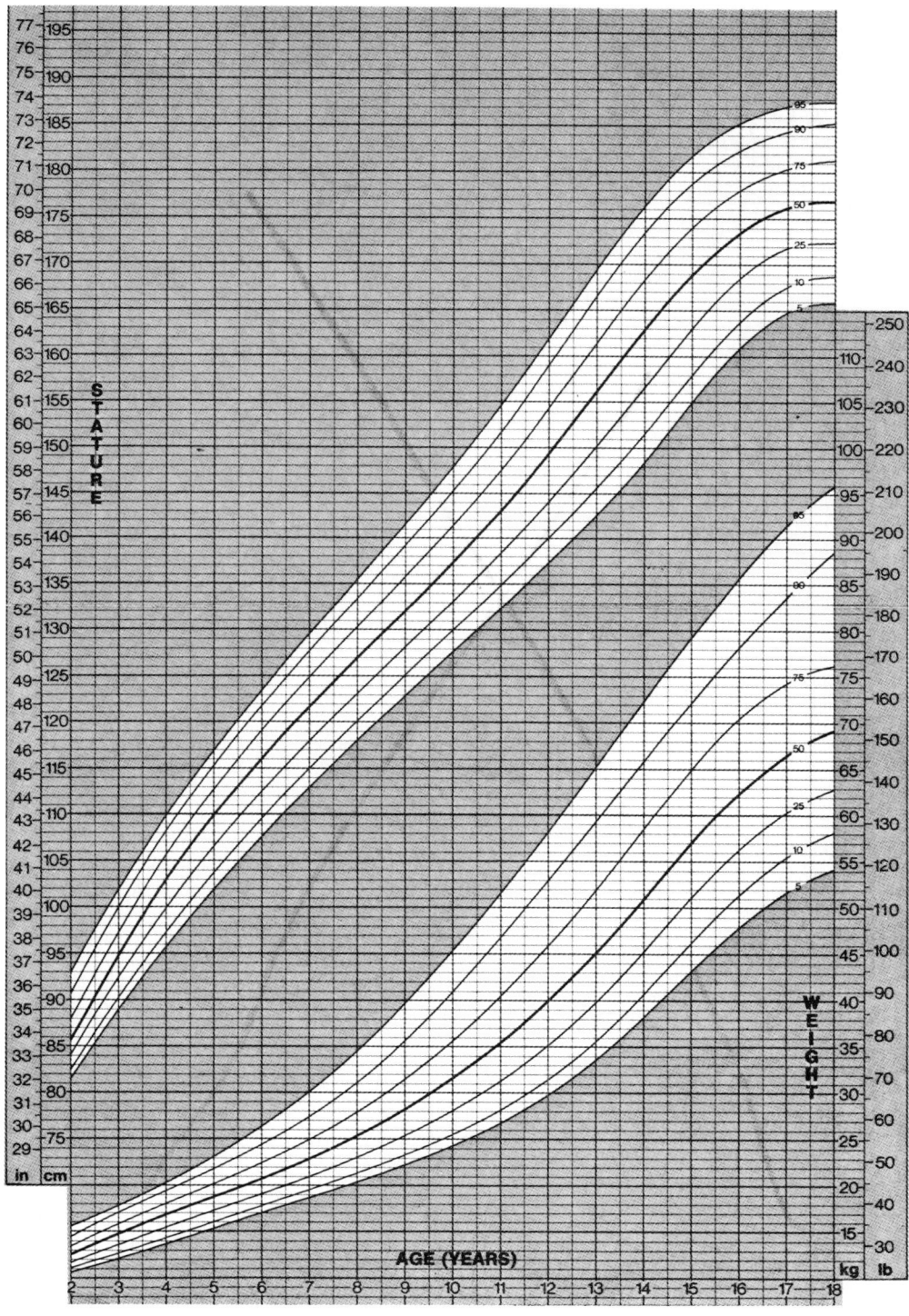

Table A–5.   Equivalent Weights and Measures

Volumes

Apothecaries' Measure		Metric	Household
1	fluid dram	4 milliliter (ml)	1 teaspoon (tsp)
2	fl dr	8 ml	1 dessert spoonful
½	fluid ounce (oz)	15 ml	1 tablespoon (tbsp) (3 tsp)
1	fl oz	30 ml	2 tbsp (⅛ cup)
1½	fl oz	45 ml	1 jigger
2	fl oz	59 ml	4 tbsp (¼ cup)
2⅔	fl oz	80 ml	5⅓ tbsp (⅓ cup)
4	fl oz	118 ml	8 tbsp (½ cup)
8	fl oz	237 ml	1 cup
16	fl oz	473 ml	1 pint (pt)
32	fl oz	947 ml	1 quart (qt)
128	fl oz	3,785 ml	1 gallon (gal)
1	minum	0.06 ml	
16.23	minum	1 ml	
3.38	fl oz	1 deciliter (dl) (100 ml)	
2.11	pints (pt)	1 liter (10^3 ml)	

Weights

Avoirdupois		Metric
1		picogram (pg) (10^{-12} gm)
1		nanogram (ng) (10^{-9} gm)
1		microgram (μg) (10^{-6} gm)
1	grain (gr)	0.065 gm (65 mg)
1	dram (dr) (27.3 gr)	1.77 gm
1	oz (16 dr)	28.35 gm
1	lb (16 oz)	453.59 gm
1	ton (2,000 lb)	0.91 metric tons
1.015	gr	1 milligram (mg) (10^{-3} gm)
15.4	gr (0.035 oz)	1 gram (gm)
2.2	lb	1 kilogram (kg) (10^3 gm)
220.5	lb	1 quintal (10^5 gm)
2,204.6	lb (1.1 tons)	1 metric ton (10^6 gm)

Length/Area

1	angstrom (Å)	10^{-7}	millimeter (mm)
1/2500	inch (in)	1	micron (μ) (10^{-3} mm)
0.039	in	1	mm
0.39	in	1	centimeter (cm)
1	in	2.54	cm
1	foot (ft) (12 in)	30.5	cm
39.4	in	1	meter (m)
1	yard (yd) (3 ft)	0.9	m
1093.6	yd (0.62 miles)	1	kilometer (km)
1	mile (mi) (5,280 ft)	1.61	km
1	acre	160	square rods (0.4 hectare)
1	hectare	2.47	acres

$$\text{Milliequivalents} = \frac{\text{Milligrams}}{\text{Atomic Weight}} \times \text{Valence}$$

Ion		Valence	Atomic Wt.	Equivalent Wt.
Bicarbonate	HCO_3^-	1	61.0	61.0
Calcium	Ca^{++}	2	40.1	20.0
Chloride	Cl^-	1	35.5	35.5
Magnesium	Mg^{++}	2	24.3	12.2
Phosphate*	HPO_4^{--}	2	96.0	48.0*
Potassium	K^+	1	39.1	39.1
Sodium	Na^+	1	23.0	23.0
Sulfate	SO_4^{--}	2	96.1	48.0

* At the normal pH of body fluids, 20 per cent of the phosphate radical is combined with one equivalent of base as BH_2PO_4 and 80 per cent with two equivalents of base as B_2HPO_4. Under these conditions, base equivalence per unit of HPO_4 is therefore $0.2 + (0.8 \times 2) = 1.8$ and the equivalent weight of 53.3 is obtained by dividing the ionic weight by 1.8 instead of by 2. Phosphorus content of phosphate solutions: 1 mEq provides approximately 15 mg. One mM provides approximately 31 mg.

Temperature conversions:
°F to °C: 5/9 (°F-32)
°C to °F: (9/5 × °C) + 32

Table A–6a. Daily Energy Expenditure in Various Activity Patterns*

Type of Activity[a]	Energy Expenditure (kcal/min)	(kJ/min)	Activity Pattern										
			A			B			C			D	
			Total No kcal	MJ	hr	Total No kcal	MJ	hr	Total No kcal	MJ	hr	Total No kcal	MJ
Men													
(1)	1.2	5.0	580	2.4	8	580	2.4	8	580	2.4	9	648	2.7
(2)	1.6	6.7	960	4.0	10	960	4.0	12	1152	4.8	13	1248	5.2
(3)	3.2	13.4	770	3.2	5	960	4.0	4	768	3.2	2	384	1.6
	(1.7–4.8)	(7.1–20.1)											
(4)	5.6	23.44	672	2.8	2	336	1.4	0	0	0	0	0	0
	(4.9–7.4)	(20.5–31.0)											
Totals			2982	12.4	24	2836	11.8	24	2500	10.4	24	2280	9.5
Women													
(1)	0.9	3.8	430	1.8	8	430	1.8	8	430	1.8	9	486	2.0
(2)	1.2	5.0	792	3.3	11	792	3.3	11	864	3.6	13	936	3.9
(3)	2.5	10.5	600	2.5	4	750	3.1	5	600	2.5	2	300	1.3
	(1.4–3.5)	(5.9–14.6)											
(4)	4.5	18.8	270	1.1	1	0	0	0	0	0	0	0	0
	(3.6–5.5)	(15.1–23.0)											
Totals			2092	8.7	24	1972	8.2	24	1894	7.9	24	1722	7.2

[a] The types of activities under (1), (2), (3) and (4) are described in Table A–6b.

*From Dietary Standard for Canada, p. 16, rev. 1975 (cf Table A–2).

Table A–6b. Breakdown of Activity Patterns*

	Types of Activity	Activity Pattern-Men				Activity Pattern-Women			
		A	B	C	D	A	B	C	D
		No. hours per day				No. hours per day			
(1)	Resting metabolism	8	8	8	9	8	8	8	9
(2)	Sitting or standing still	10	10	12	13	11	11	12	13
(3)	Walking slowly Light domestic work (e.g. ironing, sweeping floor, cooking, dishwashing, dusting) Light office or industrial work (e.g. typing, lab work, sewing, printing, machine-tool operating, garage mechanics) Sports involving light activity (e.g. bowling, golf, sailing)	4	5	4	2	4	5	4	2
(4)	Walking at moderate speed Moderate domestic work (e.g. scrubbing floor, window cleaning, furniture polishing) Moderate industrial work (e.g. painting, plastering, bricklaying, modern farming) Hobbies involving moderate activity (e.g. gardening, woodwork, dancing) Active sports (e.g. tennis, cycling, gymnastics, skiing, swimming)	2	1	0	0	1	0	0	0
	Total	24	24	24	24	24	24	24	24

*From Dietary Standard for Canada, p. 15, rev. 1975 (cf Table A–2).

Table A–7a. Energy Expenditure of a 65-kg Reference Man Distributed Over 24 Hours and Effect of Occupation*

Distribution of Activity	Light Activity		Moderately Active		Very Active		Exceptionally Active	
	(kcal)	(MJ)	(kcal)	(MJ)	(kcal)	(MJ)	(kcal)	(MJ)
In bed (8 hours)	500	2.1	500	2.1	500	2.1	500	2.1
At work (8 hours)	1 100	4.6	1 400	5.8	1 900	8.0	2 400	10.0
Nonoccupational activities (8 hours)	700– 1 500	3.0– 6.3	700– 1 500	3.0– 6.3	700– 1 500	3.0– 6.3	700– 1 500	3.0– 6.3
Range of energy expenditure (24 hours)	2 300– 3 100	9.7– 13.0	2 600– 3 400	10.9– 14.2	3 100– 3 900	13.0– 16.3	3 600– 4 400	15.1– 18.4
Mean (24 hours)	2 700	11.3	3 000	12.5	3 500	14.6	4 000	16.7
Mean (per kg of body weight)	42	0.17	46	0.19	54	0.23	62	0.26

Table A–7b. Energy Expenditure of a 55-kg Reference Woman Distributed Over 24 Hours and Effect of Occupation*

Distribution of Activity	Light Activity		Moderately Active		Very Active		Exceptionally Active	
	(kcal)	(MJ)	(kcal)	(MJ)	(kcal)	(MJ)	(kcal)	(MJ)
In bed (8 hours)	420	1.8	420	1.8	420	1.8	420	1.8
At work (8 hours)	800	3.3	1 000	4.2	1 400	5.9	1 800	7.5
Nonoccupational activities (8 hours)	580-980	2.4-4.1	580-980	2.4-4.1	580-980	2.4-4.1	580-980	2.4-4.1
Range of energy expenditure (24 hours)	1 800-2 200	7.5-9.2	2 000-2 400	8.4-10.1	2 400-2 700	10.1-11.8	2 800-3 200	11.7-13.4
Mean (24 hours)	2 000	8.4	2 200	9.2	2 600	10.9	3 000	12.5
Mean (per kg of body weight)	36	0.15	40	0.17	47	0.20	55	0.23

*From Passmore, Nicol and Rao: *Handbook on Human Nutritional Requirements*. Geneva, WHO Monogr. Ser. No. 61, 1974.

Table A–8. Weights for Heights[a] and Basal Metabolic Rates (BMR)[b] of Adults[c]*

Height		Men				Women			
		Median Weight		BMR		Median Weight		BMR	
(in)	(cm)	(lb)	(kg)	$\left(\dfrac{kcal}{day}\right)$	$\left(\dfrac{kcal}{kg}\right)$	(lb)	(kg)	$\left(\dfrac{kcal}{day}\right)$	$\left(\dfrac{kcal}{kg}\right)$
60	152					109 ± 9	50 ± 4	1399	28
62	158					115 ± 9	52 ± 4	1429	27
64	163	133 ± 11	60 ± 5	1630	27	122 ± 10	56 ± 5	1487	27
66	168	142 ± 12	64 ± 5	1690	26	129 ± 10	59 ± 5	1530	26
68	173	151 ± 14	69 ± 6	1775	26	136 ± 10	62 ± 5	1572	25
70	178	159 ± 14	72 ± 6	1815	25	144 ± 11	66 ± 5	1626	25
72	183	167 ± 15	76 ± 7	1870	25	152 ± 12	69 ± 5	1666	24
74	188	175 ± 15	80 ± 7	1933	24				
76	193	182 ± 16	83 ± 7	1983	24				

[a] Modified from Hathaway and Ford: Heights and Weights of Adults in the U.S. Home Economics Research Report No. 10, ARS. Washington, USDA, 1960, Table 80. Weights were based on those of college men and women. Measurements were made without shoes or other clothing. The ± refers to the weight range between the 25th and 75th percentile of each height category.

[b] Adapted from Talbot (FAO/WHO, 1973).

[c] To determine the daily energy need of an individual, allow for hours of sleep at 90 per cent of BMR and for time periods engaged in various activities as indicated below. Data are expressed as kcal per kg per hr.

Activity	Men	Women
Very light	1.5	1.3
Light	2.9	2.6
Moderate	4.3	4.1
Heavy	8.4	8.0

*Modified from *Recommended Dietary Allowances*, 8th ed. Washington, National Academy of Science, 1974.

Table A–9. Beverages and Alcoholic Drinks—Calories and Selected Electrolytes (per 100 ml)*

Beverage	Calories	Na (mg)	Na (mEq)	K (mg)	K (mEq)	Phosphorus (mg)
Pepsi	42	0.2	0.0	2.6	0.1	14.3
Diet Pepsi	—	17.6	0.8	3.4	0.1	16.9
Pepsi Light	19	2.5	0.1	3.3	0.1	13.2
Patio Grape or Orange	52	11.2	0.5	4.1ø	0.1	—
Mountain Dew	48	8.4	0.4	1.9	0.1	—
Teem	37	8.4	0.4	—	—	—
Root beer	45	1.0	0.1	3.9	0.1	—
Coca Cola	40	8.3	0.4	0.4	—	16.7
Sprite	40	17.5	0.8	0.4	—	—
Fanta, average	46	8.8	0.4	0.6	—	—
Fresca	1	23.8	1.0	0.7	—	—
Tab	—	12.5	0.5	0.5	—	12.5
Fanta Ginger Ale	35	12.5	0.5	—	—	—
Apricot nectar	57	trace	—	149.7	3.8	12.7
Apple juice	48	trace	—	100.0	2.6	9.7
Cranberry juice	67	trace	—	9.5	0.2	3.2
Grape juice, canned	67	3.16	0.1	117.1	3.0	12.7
Grapefruit juice, unsweetened	42	trace	—	116.8	4.2	12.9
Orange juice, unsweetened or fresh	49	1.1	0.1	202.1	5.2	17.1
Pear nectar	51	trace	—	38.5	1.0	6.4
Peach nectar	48	trace	—	77.2	2.0	9.6
Pineapple juice, unsweetened	54	trace	—	150.2	3.9	9.6
Tomato juice	20	200.7	8.7	227.0	5.8	16.5
Fruit-flavored beverages	45	—	—	—	—	—
Beer	43	6.7	0.3	26.7	0.7	30.0
Gin, rum, vodka, whiskey—86 proof	250	trace	—	3.6	0.1	—
Dessert wine, 18.5% alcohol/vol	137	3.3	0.1	76.7	2.0	—
Table wine, 12.2% alcohol/vol	86	3.5	0.1	93.1	2.4	10.3

ø Average.

*Brand name data supplied by the commercial producer of the product. Other data obtained from Nutritive Value of American Foods, in common units, Agriculture Handbook #456, Agriculture Research Service. Washington, USDA, 1975.

Note: According to one of the commercial soft drink companies, *approximate* average values of sodium and potassium in local drinking water supplied throughout the United States are as follows:

Sodium = 5 mg = 0.22 mEq/100 ml
Potassium = 0.5 mg = 0.01 mEq/100 ml

Alcoholic beverages are customarily served in special glassware, the size of which tends to standardize the alcoholic content:

1 cordial glass	= 20 ml	1 cocktail glass	= 90 ml	1 tumbler	= 240–360 ml
1 brandy glass	= 30 ml	1 burgundy glass	= 120 ml	1 mixing glass	= 360 ml
1 sherry glass	= 60 ml	1 champagne glass	= 150 ml	1 jigger	= 45 ml

Table A–10. Lipids and Polyunsaturates in Selected Foods, Fats and Oils*

100-gm Edible Serving	Total Fat (gm)	SFA (gm)	MFA (gm)	PFA (gm)	Oleic (gm)	Lin-Lin (gm)	P/S Ratio	Chol. (mg)
Beef approx. 6% fat, cooked	6.10	2.70	2.72	0.48	2.34	0.30	0.2	91.0
Beef approx. 30% fat, cooked	32.00	13.30	15.67	1.33	13.10	1.10	0.1	94.0
Lamb approx. 7% fat, cooked	7.00	2.95	2.69	0.42	2.50	0.33	0.1	100.0
Lamb approx. 30% fat, cooked	29.40	13.70	11.97	1.71	11.25	1.67	0.1	98.0
Veal approx. 6% fat, cooked	6.70	2.04	1.90	0.67	1.68	0.45	0.3	99.0
Veal approx. 25% fat, cooked	25.20	9.21	8.95	1.26	7.82	1.20	0.1	101.0
Chicken, turkey, Cornish hen, light meat without skin	3.40	0.88	0.76	0.76	0.62	0.56	0.9	78.0
Duck, goose (domestic) without skin	8.20	1.88	3.72	0.74	3.41	0.74	0.4	91.0
Beef, ground, fat unknown	32.00	13.30	15.67	1.33	13.10	1.10	0.1	94.0
Beef bologna	30.00	13.00	15.10	0.90	13.30	0.90	0.1	52.0
Pork, fresh, 30% fat, cooked	30.60	11.68	15.24	3.54	14.02	3.29	0.3	89.0
Frankfurter, all beef, cooked	30.00	12.70	14.80	1.20	13.00	1.20	0.1	51.0
Frankfurter, type unknown	27.20	10.06	13.52	3.17	12.33	3.17	0.3	62.0
Smoked pork, 25% fat, cooked	25.70	8.96	12.17	2.86	11.04	2.60	0.3	89.0
Bologna, salami, cold cuts, 25% fat	27.50	10.52	13.90	2.13	12.46	2.13	0.2	91.5
Bacon, regular, cooked	52.00	18.09	22.93	5.47	21.25	5.33	0.3	79.0
Cold cuts, variety unknown	27.50	10.52	13.90	2.13	12.46	2.13	0.2	91.5
Turkey frankfurters	23.76	5.72	9.92	5.78	7.06	5.61	1.0	98.5
Fish, 6% fat	4.00	1.08	1.07	1.55	0.70	0.18	1.4	66.0
Fish, 12% fat	13.40	2.28	3.17	4.56	1.55	0.77	2.0	84.0
Fish, 20% fat	0.90	0.21	0.17	0.37	0.09	0.02	1.8	66.0
Herring, canned, smoked, pickled	13.60	2.56	8.06	2.16	1.88	0.20	0.8	97.0
Salmon, pink, canned	5.90	0.98	1.75	2.66	1.02	0.30	2.3	35.0
Sardines, canned, drained	11.10	3.00	3.57	3.22	1.66	0.23	1.1	140.0
Tuna, canned, oil packed, drained	8.20	1.63	1.66	4.45	1.66	4.45	2.7	65.0
Tuna, canned, water packed	0.80	0.19	0.13	0.20	0.09	0.02	1.1	63.0
Clams, cooked	2.50	0.48	0.45	0.53	0.14	0.08	1.1	63.0
Crabmeat, cooked, canned	2.50	0.37	0.54	1.02	0.27	0.09	2.8	101.0
Crab, soft shell, steamed	2.50	0.25	0.34	0.55	0.18	0.05	2.2	100.0
Lobster, cooked	1.50	0.14	0.15	0.46	0.11	0.03	3.3	85.0
Oysters, cooked	2.20	0.75	0.42	0.84	0.16	0.09	1.1	45.0
Scallops, cooked	1.40	0.23	0.14	0.53	0.05	0.02	2.3	53.0
Shrimp, cooked	1.10	0.13	0.12	0.44	0.08	0.03	3.4	150.0
Caviar	15.00	3.71	4.65	6.29	3.51	0.03	1.7	300.0
Eggs, whole	11.50	3.40	4.54	1.38	4.16	1.29	0.4	504.0
Egg, yolk	30.60	10.10	13.42	4.11	12.30	3.83	0.4	1,480.0
Egg, white	—	—	—	—	—	—	—	0
Egg substitute, brand unknown	9.50	1.21	2.35	5.53	2.34	5.53	4.6	3.4
Creamer, imitation, liquid, frozen, saturated vegetable fat	11.00	8.50	0.10	0.00	0.10	0.00	—	0

Creamer—Poly Perx	10.00	1.50	4.60	3.90	3.10	3.30	2.6	0
Cream, light, sweet or sour, 20% fat	20.60	12.80	5.96	0.77	5.18	0.77	0.1	66.0
Buttermilk, 1% fat	0.80	0.50	0.23	0.03	0.20	0.03	0.1	2.3
Milk, 1% fat	1.00	0.60	0.28	0.03	0.25	0.03	0.1	2.9
Milk, 2% fat	2.00	1.20	0.58	0.08	0.50	0.08	0.1	5.8
Milk, whole	3.50	2.20	1.01	0.13	0.88	0.13	0.1	13.5
Cheese—grated, dry, creamed	26.50	16.80	7.71	0.58	6.83	0.58	0.0	95.0
cottage, low salt	2.00	1.24	0.58	0.07	0.50	0.07	0.1	8.3
cottage, creamed	4.20	2.60	1.09	0.12	0.91	0.12	0.1	14.7
cream, Neufchatel, 20% fat	21.18	13.17	6.12	0.78	5.32	0.78	0.1	76.0
cheddar, American, blue, feta, Liederkranz,	32.20	20.03	9.31	1.19	8.08	1.19	0.1	102.4
Camembert								
Yogurt—part skim, plain	1.70	1.00	0.41	0.04	0.34	0.04	0.0	7.0
part skim, all flavors	0.85	0.53	0.25	0.03	0.21	0.03	0.1	4.6
whole milk, all flavors	3.40	2.20	0.93	0.10	0.78	0.10	0.0	13.2
Ice cream, medium rich, 16% fat	16.10	10.01	4.65	0.60	4.04	0.60	0.1	57.0
Sherbet	1.20	0.75	0.35	0.04	0.30	0.04	0.1	3.5
Ice milk	5.10	3.20	1.42	0.19	1.28	0.19	0.1	14.4
Oil—corn	100.00	12.70	24.74	58.22	24.60	58.22	4.6	0
cottonseed	100.00	26.10	18.88	50.70	18.10	50.70	1.9	0
safflower	100.00	9.40	12.47	73.76	11.90	73.76	7.9	0
sesame	100.00	15.20	39.99	40.46	39.10	40.46	2.7	0
soybean, partially hydrogenated	100.00	13.00	47.00	40.00	31.00	33.00	3.1	0
olive	100.00	14.20	72.47	8.95	71.50	8.95	0.6	0
peanut	100.00	19.10	46.00	30.00	46.00	30.00	1.6	0
coconut	100.00	86.26	6.03	1.83	5.65	1.83	0.02	0
palm	100.00	47.90	38.30	9.30	37.90	9.30	0.2	0
Shortening, household, vegetable	100.00	32.03	42.06	19.60	26.77	16.73	0.6	0
Margarine—% fat unknown—tub	81.00	14.84	29.29	35.88	29.29	35.88	2.4	0
% fat unknown—stick	17.70	35.70	26.00	—	—	—	1.5	0
Mayonnaise, commercial or homemade	79.90	12.00	17.90	46.10	15.90	46.10	3.8	70.0
Peanut butter	50.60	9.66	23.28	15.18	23.28	15.18	1.6	0
Almonds	54.20	4.31	36.84	10.12	36.50	10.12	2.4	0
Cashews	45.70	9.20	26.44	7.42	26.20	7.42	0.8	0
Peanuts	48.70	9.30	22.40	14.61	22.40	14.61	1.6	0
Walnuts	64.00	6.94	9.90	41.81	9.70	41.81	6.0	0
Olives, black	13.80	1.96	10.01	1.24	9.87	1.24	0.6	0
Lard, rendered	100.00	39.60	44.34	11.77	40.90	11.40	0.3	95.0
Butter, sweet or salted	81.00	49.80	23.10	3.00	20.10	3.00	0.1	227.3
MCT oil	100.00	100.00				3.00		

*Data provided by The Nutrition Coding Center, University of Minnesota. Supported by Contract No. 1-HV-6-2941-L of the National Heart, Lung and Blood Institute.

øSFA = Saturated fatty acid, MFA = monounsaturated fatty acid, PFA = polyunsaturated fatty acid, Lin-Lin = linoleic-linolenic, P/S ratio = polyunsaturated/saturated fatty acids, Chol. = cholesterol.

Table A–11. Food Exchange Lists*

Milk Exchanges—List 1

One Exchange of Milk contains 12 gm of carbohydrate, 8 gm of protein, a trace of fat and 80 kcal.

Nonfat Fortified Milk

Skim or nonfat milk†	1 cup
Powdered (nonfat dry, before adding liquid)	⅓ cup
Canned, evaporated skim milk	½ cup
Buttermilk made from skim milk	1 cup
Yogurt made from skim milk (plain, unflavored)	1 cup

Low-fat Fortified Milk

1% fat fortified milk (omit ½ Fat Exchange)	1 cup
2% fat fortified milk (omit 1 Fat Exchange)	1 cup
Yogurt made from 2% fortified milk (plain, unflavored) (omit 1 Fat Exchange)	1 cup

Whole Milk (Omit 2 Fat Exchanges)

Whole milk	1 cup
Canned, evaporated whole milk	½ cup
Buttermilk made from whole milk	1 cup
Yogurt made from whole milk (plain, unflavored)	1 cup

Vegetable Exchanges—List 2

One Exchange of Vegetables contains about 5 gm of carbohydrate, 2 gm of protein and 25 kcal. The list shows the kinds of vegetables to use for one Vegetable Exchange. One Exchange is ½ cup.

Asparagus	**Beet Greens**	**Rutabaga**
Bean sprouts	**Chard Greens**	**Sauerkraut**
Beets	**Collard Greens**	**String beans, green/yellow**
Broccoli	**Dandelion Greens**	**Summer squash**
Brussels sprouts	**Kale Greens**	**Tomatoes**
Cabbage	**Mustard Greens**	**Tomato juice**
Carrots	**Spinach Greens**	**Turnips**
Cauliflower	**Turnip Greens**	**Vegetable juice cocktail**
Celery	**Mushrooms**	**Zucchini**
Cucumbers	**Okra**	
Eggplant	**Onions**	
Green pepper	**Rhubarb**	

The following raw vegetables may be used as desired:

Chicory	**Lettuce**
Chinese cabbage	**Parsley**
Endive	**Radishes**
Escarole	**Watercress**

Starchy vegetables are found in the Bread Exchange List.

---

*From American Diabetes Association, Inc. and The American Dietetic Association, Exchange Lists for Meal Planning, 1976.

†**Bold type indicates low-fat or nonfat item.** To plan a diet low in saturated fat and cholesterol, choose only those exchanges in **bold type.**

Fruit Exchanges—List 3

One Exchange of Fruit contains 10 gm of carbohydrate and 40 kcal.
The list shows the kinds and amounts of fruit to use for one Fruit Exchange.

Apple	1 small	**Mango**	½ small
Apple juice	⅓ cup	**Melon**	
Applesauce (unsweetened)	½ cup	**Cantaloupe**	¼ small
Apricots, fresh	2 medium	**Honeydew**	⅛ medium
Apricots, dried	4 halves	**Watermelon**	1 cup
Banana	½ small	**Nectarine**	1 small
Berries		**Orange**	1 small
Blackberries	½ cup	**Orange juice**	½ cup
Blueberries	½ cup	**Papaya**	¾ cup
Raspberries	½ cup	**Peach**	1 medium
Strawberries	¾ cup	**Pear**	1 small
Cherries	10 large	**Persimmon, native**	1 medium
Cider	⅓ cup	**Pineapple**	½ cup
Dates	2	**Pineapple juice**	⅓ cup
Figs, fresh	1	**Plums**	2 medium
Figs, dried	1	**Prunes**	2 medium
Grapefruit	½	**Prune juice**	¼ cup
Grapefruit juice	½ cup	**Raisins**	2 tbsp
Grapes	12	**Tangerine**	1 medium
Grape juice	¼ cup		

Cranberries may be used as desired if no sugar is added.

Bread Exchanges—List 4

One Exchange of Bread contains 15 gm of carbohydrate, 2 gm of protein and 70 kcal.
The list shows the kinds and amounts of breads, cereals, starchy vegetables and prepared foods to use for one Bread Exchange.

Bread

White (including French & Italian)	1 slice
Whole wheat	1 slice
Rye or pumpernickel	1 slice
Raisin	1 slice
Bagel, small	½
English muffin, small	½
Plain roll, bread	1
Frankfurter roll	½
Hamburger bun	½
Dried bread crumbs	3 tbsp
Tortilla, 6″	1

Bread Exchanges—List 4 (continued)

Cereal

Bran flakes	½ cup
Other ready-to-eat unsweetened cereal	¾ cup
Puffed cereal (unfrosted)	1 cup
Cereal (cooked)	½ cup
Grits (cooked)	½ cup
Rice or barley (cooked)	½ cup
Pasta (cooked)	½ cup
Spaghetti, noodles, macaroni	
Popcorn (popped, no fat added)	3 cups
Cornmeal (dry)	2 tbsp
Flour	2½ tbsp
Wheat germ	¼ cup

Crackers

Arrowroot	3
Graham, 2½″ sq.	2
Matzoth 4″ × 6″	½
Oyster	20
Pretzels, 3⅛″ long × ⅛″ dia	25
Rye wafers, 2″ × 3½″	3
Saltines	6
Soda, 2½″ sq	4

Dried Beans, Peas and Lentils

Beans, peas, lentils (dried and cooked)	½ cup
Baked beans, no pork (canned)	¼ cup

Starchy Vegetables

Corn	⅓ cup
Corn on cob	1 small
Lima beans	½ cup
Parsnips	⅔ cup
Peas, green (canned or frozen)	½ cup
Potato, white	1 small
Potato (mashed)	½ cup
Pumpkin	¾ cup
Winter squash, acorn or butternut	½ cup
Yam or sweet potato	¼ cup

PREPARED FOODS

Biscuit 2″ dia (omit 1 Fat Exchange)	1
Corn bread, 2″ × 2″ × 1″ (omit 1 Fat Exchange)	1
Corn muffin, 2″ dia (omit 1 Fat Exchange)	1
Crackers, round butter type (omit 1 Fat Exchange)	5
Muffin, plain small (omit 1 Fat Exchange)	1
Potatoes, French fried, length 2″ to 3½″	8
(omit 1 Fat Exchange)	
Potato or corn chips (omit 2 Fat Exchanges)	15
Pancake, 5″ × ½″ (omit 1 Fat Exchange)	1
Waffle, 5″ × ½″ (omit 1 Fat Exchange)	1

Meat Exchanges Lean Meat—List 5

One Exchange of Lean Meat (1 oz) contains 7 gm of protein, 3 gm of fat and 55 kcal.

This list shows the kinds and amounts of lean meat and other protein-rich foods to use for one low-fat Meat Exchange.

Beef:

> **Baby beef (very lean), chipped beef, chuck, flank**   1 oz
> **steak, tenderloin, plate ribs, plate skirt steak,**
> **round (bottom, top), all cuts rump, spare ribs,**
> **tripe**

Lamb:

> **Leg, rib, sirloin, loin (roast and chops), shank,**   1 oz
> **shoulder**

Pork:

> **Leg (whole rump, center shank), ham, smoked**   1 oz
> **(center slices)**

Veal:

> **Leg, loin, rib, shank, shoulder, cutlets**   1 oz

Poultry:

> **Meat without skin of chicken, turkey, Cornish**   1 oz
> **hen, guinea hen, pheasant**

Fish:

> **Any fresh or frozen**   1 oz
> **Canned salmon, tuna, mackerel, crab and lobster**   ¼ cup
> **Clams, oysters, scallops, shrimp**   5 or 1 oz
> **Sardines, drained**   3

Cheeses containing less than 5% butterfat   1 oz
Cottage cheese, dry and 2% butterfat   ¼ cup
Dried beans and peas (omit 1 Bread Exchange)   ½ cup

Meat Exchanges Medium-fat Meat

For each Exchange of Medium-fat Meat omit ½ Fat Exchange.

The list shows the kinds and amounts of medium-fat meat and other protein-rich foods to use for one medium-fat Meat Exchange.

Beef:

> Ground (15% fat), corned beef (canned), rib eye,   1 oz
> round (ground commercial)

Pork:

> Loin (all cuts tenderloin), shoulder arm (picnic),   1 oz
> shoulder blade, Boston butt, Canadian bacon,
> boiled ham

Liver, heart, kidney and sweetbreads (these are high in   1 oz
   cholesterol)

Cottage cheese, creamed   ¼ cup

Cheese:

> Mozzarella, ricotta, farmer's cheese, Neufchatel,   1 oz
> Parmesan   3 tbsp

Egg (high in cholesterol)   1

Peanut butter (omit 2 additional Fat Exchanges)   2 tbsp

For each Exchange of High-fat Meat omit 1 Fat Exchange.

This list shows the kinds and amounts of high-fat meat and other protein-rich foods to use for one High-fat Meat Exchange.

Beef:

Brisket, corned beef (brisket), ground beef (more than 20% fat), hamburger (commercial), chuck (ground commercial), roasts (rib), steaks (club and rib)   1 oz

Lamb:

Breast   1 oz

Pork:

Spare ribs, loin (back ribs), pork (ground), country-style ham, deviled ham   1 oz

Veal:

Breast   1 oz

Poultry:

Capon, duck (domestic), goose   1 oz

Cheese:

Cheddar types   1 oz

Cold Cuts:

4½″ × ⅛″ slice

Frankfurter:

1 small

Fat Exchanges—List 6 ‡

One Exchange of Fat contains 5 gm of fat and 45 kcal.

This list shows the kinds and amounts of fat-containing foods to use for one Fat Exchange.

Margarine, soft, tub or stick[a]	1 tsp
Avocado (4″ dia)	⅛
Oil, corn, cottonseed, safflower, soy, sunflower	1 tsp
Oil, olive[b]	1 tsp
Oil, peanut[b]	1 tsp
Olives[b]	5 small
Almonds[b]	10 whole
Pecans[b]	2 large whole
Peanuts[b]	
Spanish	20 whole
Virginia	10 whole
Walnuts	6 small
Nuts, other[b]	6 small
Margarine, regular stick	1 tsp
Butter	1 tsp
Bacon fat	1 tsp
Bacon, crisp	1 strip
Cream, light	2 tbsp
Cream, sour	2 tbsp
Cream, heavy	1 tbsp
Cream cheese	1 tbsp
French dressing[c]	1 tbsp
Italian dressing[c]	1 tbsp
Lard	1 tsp
Mayonnaise[c]	1 tsp
Salad dressing, mayonnaise type[c]	2 tsp
Salt pork	¾″ cube

[a] Made with corn, cottonseed, safflower, soy or sunflower oil only.

[b] Fat content is primarily monounsaturated.

[c] If made with corn, cottonseed, safflower, soy or sunflower oil can be used on fat-modified diet.

‡To plan a diet low in saturated fat select only those Exchanges which appear in **bold type;** they are polyunsaturated.

Table A–12. Diets for Weight Reduction, Diabetes and Reduced Soluble Carbohydrates (High-polyunsaturated-fat Diets)*

Total Daily Intake	kcal			
	800	1200	1800	2400
Carbohydrate (gm)	94	134	225	276
Protein (gm)	57	68	90	122
Fat (gm)	22	47	60	86
Total Exchanges for One Day (see Table A–11):				
Skim milk	2	2	2	3
Vegetable	2	2	2	4
Fruit	3	4	5	5
Bread	2	4	9	12
Meat†	5	6	8	10
Unsaturated fat	1	5	7	10
Sample Meal Pattern	Servings based on exchanges			
Breakfast				
Fruit	1	1	1	1 + 1 midmeal
Bread	1	1	3	3 + 1 midmeal
Meat†	0	0	2	2
Fat, unsaturated	1	1	2	3
Milk, skim	½	1	1	1 + 1 midmeal
Tea/coffee		as desired		
Lunch				
Meat†	2	2	3	3
Vegetable	0	1	1	2
Bread	½	1	3	3
Fat, unsaturated	0	2	2	3
Fruit	1	1	2	1
Milk, skim	1	½	0	1
Tea/coffee		as desired		
Dinner				
Meat†	3	3	3	3
Vegetable	2	1	1	2
Bread	½	1	2	3
Fat, unsaturated	0	1	2	3
Fruit	1	2	2	2
Milk, skim	½	0	0	0
Tea/coffee		as desired		
Evening				
Meat†	0	0	0	0
Bread	0	1	1	2
Milk, skim	0	½	1	0
Fat, unsaturated	0	0	2	1
Tea/coffee		as desired		

*This table, prepared by the authors, is based on the following dietary recommendations in *A Guide to Professionals: The Effective Application of Exchange Lists for Meal Planning,* American Diabetes Association, Inc., and The American Dietetic Association, 1977. Protein: 20 per cent of total calories for growing children and pregnant women, minimum of 0.5 gm per pound desirable body weight for other adults; carbohydrates: 50 to 70 per cent of nonprotein calories; fat: 30 to 50 per cent of nonprotein calories. An exception is the 800-kcal diet which has 29 per cent calories as protein. The percentage of fat in all the diets is in the low range, in keeping with the recently revised (1-24-78) *Dietary Goals for the United States,* 2nd ed. (Select Committee on Nutrition and Human Needs, U.S. Senate, Government Printing Office, 1978). Reduce fat consumption to 30 per cent of energy intake, providing equal proportions of saturated, monounsaturated and polyunsaturated fatty acids, reduce cholesterol to 300 mg per day, and increase complex carbohydrates and naturally occurring sugars to 48 per cent of energy intake, reduce consumption of refined and processed sugars to account for 10 per cent of total energy intake and reduce salt consumption to 5 gm per day.

†Eleven of 14 main meals per week should contain poultry (without skin), fish, lean veal, uncreamed cottage cheese or skim milk yogurt. Remaining meals may include servings of lean beef, lamb or pork. No more than 3 egg yolks (eating or cooking) should be taken per week.

Table A–13a. Sodium-restricted Diets*

Degree of Restriction:		Strict†	Moderate	Mild
Na in mg	=	500	1,000	2,400–4,500
Na in mEq	=	21.7	43.4	104.3–195.6
NaCl in gm	=	1.2	2.5	6.1–11.5

Approximate Composition	Unit			
Carbohydrate	gm	291	327	339
Protein	gm	84	147	111
Fat	gm	65	84	96.5
Calories		1,925	2,500	2,589.2
Calcium	mg	811	1,182	1,193
Phosphorus	mg	1,337	2,094	1,932
Iron	mg	12.7	19.5	15.8
Sodium	mg (mEq)	455 (20)	891 (44)	2,444 (106)
Potassium	mg (mEq)	3,840 (98)	4,765 (122)	4,267 (109)
Vitamin A	I.U.	6,178	7,222	7,358
Thiamin	mg	1.2	1.6	1.4
Riboflavin	mg	1.9	2.9	2.6
Niacin equivalents	mg	21.7	35.6	23.2
Ascorbic acid	mg	206	208	158

GENERAL RULES:

1. Avoid the use of all salt, baking soda and/or baking powder in cooking and for table use.
2. Avoid medicines, laxatives and salt substitutes unless prescribed by physician.
3. Read labels carefully for sodium or salt content of packaged foods.

Type of Food	Amount‡		Foods Included	Foods Excluded
Milk	Strict	‡2 cups	Evaporated, nonfat dry milk; skim milk; unsalted buttermilk and whole milk. ‡Additional milk must be low sodium, fluid or powdered.	Cultured buttermilk; condensed milk; all milk drinks prepared with malt, chocolate syrup and ice cream; yogurt; more than 2 cups of regular milk daily. (*Mild*—No restriction except limit to 3 cups)
	Moderate	3 cups		
	Mild			
	Mild			
Other beverages	Strict	2–3 cups	Cocoa prepared with milk allowance; coffee, instant and regular; Postum; Sanka; tea; fresh and frozen fruitades; carbonated beverages limit to one 8-oz bottle daily.	Ginger ale; commercial chocolate syrup, fountain beverages; instant cocoa and all powdered beverage mixes; all those not listed as allowed; alcoholic beverages allowed with physician's permission. (*Mild*—Only Dutch-process cocoa and alcoholic beverages without physician's permission.)
	Moderate	as desired		
	Mild			
	Mild	as desired		
Soup		1 cup (8 oz per cup)	Unsalted broth; unsalted vegetable soup made with allowed vegetables; unsalted cream soup made from butter and milk allowance; unsalted tomato bouillon.	All canned, dehydrated, and frozen soups containing salt; bouillon cubes; consomme and other commercial meat-extract soups.

Table A–13a.   Sodium-restricted Diets (continued)

Type of Food	Amount‡		Foods Included	Foods Excluded
Meat, poultry and fish	Strict Moderate Mild Mild	4 oz 10 oz 6 oz	Fresh, unsalted frozen or unsalted canned meats, fish and poultry such as beef, chicken, duck, lamb, liver (beef, calves or chicken liver allowed once every 2 weeks), pork, fresh tongue, turkey, veal; *use fresh fish only* such as bass, bluefish, cod, flounder, halibut, oysters, perch, salmon, snapper, sole, trout, tuna; sweetbreads and salt-free peanut butter. (*Mild*—Reg. tuna, salmon, shellfish)	All salted, koshered, smoked, corned, and canned (with salt) meats, fish and poultry; bacon, brains, kidneys, luncheon meats, chipped or corned beef, ham, frankfurters, anchovies, caviar, sardines, herring, regular canned tuna, salmon; shellfish: clams, crabs, lobsters, scallops, shrimps; regular peanut butter.
Cheese		1 svg. (1 oz)	Unsalted cottage cheese, unsalted cream cheese and unsalted American cheese. (*Mild*—American cheese, cheddar, Swiss, cottage, cream)	All other cheese not listed as allowed.
Eggs	Strict Moderate Mild	Limit to 1 a day 2 a day	Boiled, poached, scrambled or fried in unsalted butter.	None except in excess of amount allowed.
Potato or substitute		2 svgs. (½ cup per svg.)	Potatoes, white or sweet; macaroni; noodles; rice and spaghetti.	Potato chips and prepared potato products.
Bread	Strict Moderate Mild	4 svgs. 6 svgs. 4 svgs.	Unsalted bread and unsalted crackers such as melba toast and plain Passover or thin tea matzoth. (*Mild*—regular bread; graham crackers; biscuits; muffins)	Regular bread; rolls; biscuits; muffins and cereal products prepared with salt or baking soda; commercial mixes; graham crackers; saltines; soda crackers; salted matzoth and self-rising flour.
Cereals	Strict Moderate Mild	1 svg. (½ cup per svg.)	Unsalted slow-cooking unenriched cereals; barley; cornmeal; cornstarch; grits; tapioca; dry cereals; puffed rice; puffed and shredded wheat.	Quick-cooking and enriched cereals; dry cereals except those listed as allowed. (*Mild*—none)
Vegetables	Strict Moderate Mild	3 svgs. (½ cup per svg.) 4 svgs.	All fresh, frozen and unsalted canned vegetables except those listed under Foods Excluded; dried lima beans, lentils, split peas and soybeans. (*Mild*—all fresh, unsalted, canned and unsalted, frozen vegetables.)	Canned vegetables and vegetable juices to which salt has been added; artichokes; beets; beet greens; carrots; celery; collards; Swiss chard; dandelion greens; kale; mustard greens; sauerkraut; spinach; white turnips; frozen vegetables processed with salt such as lima beans, peas and mixed vegetables.

Table A–13a. Sodium-restricted Diets (continued)

Type of Food	Amount‡	Foods Included	Foods Excluded
Fruit and fruit juice	Strict ⎫ Moderate⎭ 3 svgs. (½ cup per svg.) Mild	Any fruit or fruit juice fresh, frozen or canned except those listed under Foods Excluded. Include one citrus fruit or juice daily.	Crystallized or glazed fruit; dried figs or raisins; tomato juice; all fruits to which sodium coloring, sodium flavoring or sodium benzoate has been added. (*Mild*—none)
Butter or fat	Strict 6 svgs. (1 tsp. per svg.) Moderate 6 svgs. Mild 5 svgs.	Unsalted butter; unsalted margarine; unsalted salad and cooking fats such as corn, cottonseed, Crisco, olive oil, Spry; unsalted French and mayonnaise dressings; unsalted gravy; sweet and sour cream, limit 2 tbsps per day. (*Mod.*—3 pats may be salted, 6 tsp sweet or sour cream) (*Mild*—3 oz butter; margarine; mayonnaise; French dressing; oil; plus 3 oz cream)	Salted butter and salted margarine; all commercial salad and mayonnaise dressings; bacon and pork fat; salted meat gravy. (*Mild*—bacon, bacon fat, excess of amount allowed)
Dessert	Strict ⎫ Moderate⎭ 1 svg. (1 svg. = ½ cup) Mild 3 svgs.	Fruit ice, gelatin made with fresh fruit juices; unsalted desserts made from milk and egg allowance such as custard, tapioca, cornstarch, and rice pudding; unsalted fruit crisps and unsalted fruit pies; junket except chocolate; unsalted sugar cookies. ‡Commercial ice cream and sherbet must be used as milk allowance. (*Mild*—cake, cookies and pies)	All commercial cakes; cookies; pies; puddings; Jell-O; chocolate junket; rennet tablets; all dessert made with baking powder, salt or soda; commercial ice cream and sherbet when not taken as milk allowance; gingersnaps; sandwich-type cookies; any dessert prepared with nuts.
Sweets	As desired	Sugar, white and brown; honey; jams; jellies made without the addition of sodium benzoate; hard candy; maple syrup and gum drops.	Commercial candies and syrups; chocolate syrups; molasses; saccharin and Sucaryl.
Spices	As desired	All except those listed in Foods Excluded.	Accent; dried or fresh celery leaves; celery salt; celery seed; garlic salt; horseradish prepared with salt; onion salt; salt substitutes unless recommended by physician; all seasonings with salt added.

Table A–13a.   Sodium-restricted Diets (continued)

Type of Food	Amount‡	Foods Included	Foods Excluded
Miscellaneous	As desired	Dietetic catsup, low-sodium dietetic meat extracts and tenderizers; cream of tartar; yeast; unsalted popcorn; unsalted nuts; sodium-free baking powders if allowed by physician.	Regular catsup; chili sauce; meat extracts; meat tenderizers; meat sauces; prepared mustard; olives; pickles; relishes; soy sauce; Worcestershire sauce; salted pretzels and popcorn; chips and all *snacks* containing salt; salted nuts.

*Modified from Diet Manual, Memorial Sloan-Kettering Cancer Center, rev. 1978.

Adequacy: This diet meets the 1979 Recommended Dietary Allowances of the National Research Council except for calories which may be low for an active individual and for iron for females. The calculations are based on the sample meal plan. Supplementation with iron and thiamin may be necessary in strict sodium regimens.

The use of water softeners may add significant amounts of sodium to the water supply.

†This strict diet can be modified to 250 mg sodium by eliminating regular milk and using only low-sodium milk and eliminating all commercial sherbets and ice cream.

‡Varying amounts of foods included relate to degrees of restriction.

Table A–13b.   Sample Meal Pattern for Strict Na Restriction (21.7 mEq)

Breakfast	*Serving Portion*	*Sample Menu*
Fruit	½ cup	Orange juice
Cereal	½ cup	Unsalted Wheatena
Egg	1	Soft-cooked egg
Bread	2 slices	Low-sodium toast
Fat	1 tsp	Unsalted butter
Milk	½ cup	Milk
Beverage	1 cup	Coffee
Sugar	1 tbsp	Sugar
Lunch		
Meat or substitute	2 oz	Unsalted broiled chicken
Potato	1	Baked potato
Vegetable	½ cup	Unsalted asparagus
Salad	½ cup	Sliced tomato
Dressing	1 tbsp	Unsalted French dressing
Dessert	½ cup	Lime ice
Bread	1 slice	Low-sodium bread
Fat	1 tsp	Unsalted butter
Milk	½ cup	Milk
Beverage	1 cup	Coffee or tea
Sugar	2 tsp	Sugar
Dinner		
Soup	1 cup	Unsalted broth
Meat	2 oz	Unsalted roast beef
Potato	1	Unsalted boiled potato
Vegetable	½ cup	Unsalted Brussels sprouts
Fruit	½ cup	Canned apricots
Bread	1 slice	Low-sodium bread
Fat	1 tsp	Unsalted butter
Beverage	1 cup	Coffee or tea
Sugar	2 tsp	Sugar
8:00 p.m.		
Milk	1 cup	Milk
Fruit	½ cup	Applesauce

Table A–14.   Sources of Information for Low-sodium Diet Management

1. American Heart Association:
   a. Your 500 Milligram Sodium Diet—Strict Sodium Restriction, New York, 1968.
   b. Your 1,000 Milligram Sodium Diet—Moderate Sodium Restriction, New York, 1969.
   c. Your Mild Sodium Restricted Diet, New York, 1969.
2. Payne, Alma Smith, and Callahan, Dorothy: *Low-Sodium-Fat Controlled Cookbook,* 3rd ed. Boston, Little, Brown and Company (34 Beacon Street, Boston, Mass.) 1966. Price $5.95.
3. *The Cookbook for Low Sodium Diets.* Boston, The Massachusetts Heart Association (85 Devonshire Street, Boston, Mass.) 1965. Price $0.25.
4. Conason and Metz: *The Salt-Free Diet Cookbook.* New York, Grosset and Dunlap, 1969. Price $1.45.
5. Margie and Hunt: *Living with High Blood Pressure, The Hypertension Diet Cookbook.* Bloomfield (N.J.), HLS Press, 1978. Appendix 7 contains names and addresses of companies supplying dietary products, pp 239–243.

Local Public Health Departments or Extension Services should be contacted for bulletins and brochures.

Individual food companies may be contacted for specific dietary information on their products.

Table A–15. Diet Information for Control of Renal Failure

Diet management of renal disease varies from patient to patient. References, lists of foods with specific nutrient values and basic dietary concepts are available for such dietary management (see references below). The USDA publication *Composition of Foods: Raw, Processed, Prepared*[3] gives a complete listing of foods commonly used with their protein, nitrogen and mineral values. A selected short list is given in Table A–16.

A widely practiced renal diet management program has been based on the Giordano-Giovanetti diet.[4] This is a two-part regimen for use when blood urea nitrogen is elevated above 100 mg per 100 ml on a normal protein diet. Initially, the diet includes 1800 to 3200 cals, low sodium, no protein of animal origin, 3 to 4 gm protein of vegetable origin. When the blood urea nitrogen falls, 12 to 40 gm animal and vegetable protein are given by using two eggs or the equivalent as milk, chicken or veal.

Less rigid dietary control based on equivalent lists is now the most acceptable approach for those patients currently being managed on dialysis programs (see references below).

Hospital manuals may also provide a good source of diet patterns for special regimens. Many food companies offer technical data about their dietary preparations.

Special products of interest for this purpose include:

Wheat products: Wheat starch, macaroni, baking mix, baking powder, Chicago Dietetic Supply, Inc.; Aproten low-protein flour, pastas, crisp bread, semolina, Dietetic Erba, Milan, Italy (U.S. distributor: General Mills Chemicals, Inc., Minneapolis, Minn.); Dietetic Paygel wheat starch, low-protein bread, baking mix, chocolate-flavored chip cookies, General Mills, Inc.; Precision Resource Baking Mix, Doyle Pharmaceutical Co., Minneapolis, Minn.; Amphogel Cookies, Phos-Lo Aluminum Hydroxide Wafers, Cobe Laboratories, Inc., Lakewood, Colo.; Jolly Joan Low-protein Bread Mix, Ener-G-Foods, Inc., Seattle, Wash.

Substitutes for light or whipped cream: Rich's Coffee Rich or Cafe-Lite, 0.8 per cent protein, 0.25 per cent sodium, trace potassium, ¼ cup = 88 kcal < 0.4 gm protein; Coffee Mate (Carnation), 3 gm = 16 kcal < 0.1 gm protein, 26.2 mg potassium, 3.6 mg sodium; Praise (Carnation) reconstituted, 1 fluid oz = 29 kcal < 0.13 gm protein, 3.6 mg potassium, 6.0 mg sodium; Praise (Carnation) whipped, ¼ cup = 50 kcal < 0.21 gm protein, 7.2 mg potassium, 12 mg sodium; Rich's, Whipped Topping = 0.00 per cent protein, 0.25 per cent sodium, trace potassium. Mocha Mix, RGB Laboratories, Kansas City, Missouri.

High-carbohydrate low-protein and electrolyte drinks: Hy-Cal, Beecham-Massengill Pharmaceuticals, Bristol, Tenn., 4 oz = 295 kcal < 0.03 per cent protein, 0.74 mg (0.02 mEq) potassium, 16.3 mg (0.71 mEq) sodium; Cal Power, General Mills, Minneapolis, Minn., 8-oz carton ≤ 0.3 gm protein, 30 mg (1.3 mEq)

sodium, 12 mg (0.31 mEq) potassium; Controlyte, low-protein, low-electrolyte, high-calorie dietary supplement, The Dolye Pharmaceutical Co., Minneapolis, Minn.; Amin-Aid, oral essential amino acids, fat, carbohydrate drink, McGaw Laboratories, Division of American Hospital Supply Corp., Irvine, Calif.

Supplements: Prono, a low-protein gelled dessert mix, General Mills Chemicals, Inc., Minneapolis, Minn.; dietetic portion-controlled salad dressings, condiments, jellies, William J. Elwood, New York, N.Y.; Polycose, low-protein pure-carbohydrate supplement, Ross Laboratories, Columbus, Ohio.

1. de St. Jeor, Carlston, Christensen, Maddock, and Tyler: *Low Protein Diets for the Treatment of Chronic Renal Failure.* Salt Lake City, University of Utah Press, 1970.
2. Margie, Anderson, Nelson, and Hunt: *The Mayo Clinic Renal Diet Cookbook.* New York, Western Publishing Co., 1974.
3. Watt and Merrill: Composition of Foods: Raw, Processed, Prepared, Agriculture Handbook No. 8. Washington, USDA, 1963.
4. Giovanetti and Maggiore: A low nitrogen diet with protein of high biological value for severe chronic uremia. Lancet, *1*, 1000, 1965.
5. Burton: Nutritional implications of renal disease. I. Current overview and general principles. J. Am. Diet. Assoc., *70*, 479, 1977.
6. Swendsied: Nutritional implications of renal disease. III. Nutritional needs of patients with renal disease. J. Am. Diet. Assoc., *70*, 488, 1977.
7. Anderson, Nelson, Margie, Johnson and Hunt: Nutritional therapy for adults with renal disease. J.A.M.A., *223*, 68, 1978.
8. Walser and Mitch: Dietary management of renal failure. *In* The Kidney, Vol. 10, #3. National Kidney Foundation, New York, 1977.
9. Stone: Vitamin supplementation of hemodialysis patients. Dial. Transplant., June, 51, 1977.
10. Mirahmadi, et al.: Serum ferritin level: Determinant of iron requirement in hemodialysis patients. J.A.M.A., *238,* 601, 1977.
11. Avioli: Renal osteodystrophy and vitamin D. Dial. Transplant., 7, 244, 1978.
12. A Guide to Protein Controlled Diets for Patients, A Guide to Protein Controlled Diets for Dietitians. Diet Therapy Committee, California Dietetic Association, Los Angeles District, 1609 Westwood Boulevard, Suite 101, Los Angeles, California 90024.
13. Liddle, et al.: Diet in transplantation. Dial. Transplant., May, 1977.
14. Symposium on Nutrition in Renal Disease, Proceeding of the First International Congress on Nutrition in Renal Disease, May 23–25, 1977, Würzburg, Germany (Kopple, Massry and Heidland, Eds). Part I—Am. J. Clin. Nutr., *31*, 1529, 1978; Part II—Am. J. Clin. Nutr., *31*, 1739, 1978.

Table A–16.   Protein, Sodium, Potassium, Phosphorus, and Zinc Contents of Selected Common Foods*

	Amount	Protein (gm)	Potassium (mEq)	Sodium (mEq)	Phosphorus (mg)	Zinc Φ (mg)
DAIRY PRODUCTS						
Eggs, large	1	6.1	1.67	3.00	90.0	0.72
Cottage cheese, salt-free, dry	1 oz.	4.9	0.24	0.15	29.5	0.13
Cream, light	1 tbsp	0.4	0.46	0.26	12.0	0.04
Cream, sour	1 tbsp	0.4	0.44	0.26	10.0	0.03
Milk, butter (fluid culture)	1 cup	8.1	9.51	11.17	219.0	1.03
Milk, regular	1 cup	8.0	9.49	5.22	228.0	0.93
Milk, skim	1 cup	8.3	10.41	5.48	247.0	0.98
Milk, low-sodium	1 cup	7.6	15.80	0.26	209.0	—
BUTTER OR FAT						
Butter, sweet	1 pat	0.03	0.03	0.02	1.0	4.6
Corn or olive oil	1 tsp	—	—	—	—	trace
Crisco	1 tsp	—	—	—	—	—
French dressing, low-calorie	1 tsp	0.04	0.11	1.83	0.67	trace
Margarine, salt-free	1 pat	—	0.03	0.02	1.0	trace
Mayonnaise	1 tsp	0.07	0.04	1.20	1.3	—
CEREAL						
Bran flakes, 40%	½ cup	1.8	1.75	4.50	68.5	0.62
Corn flakes	½ cup	1.0	0.38	5.40	4.5	0.05
Cream of rice, salt-free, cooked	1 cup	2.0	trace	trace	32.0	—
Cream of wheat, salt-free, quick-cooking	1 cup	4.9	trace	trace	145.0	1.23
Farina, salt-free, regular, cooked	1 cup	3.2	0.30	0.01	29.0	0.20
Oatmeal, cooked	1 cup	4.8	3.74	0.01	137.0	12.00
Puffed rice	½ cup	0.5	0.19	trace	7.0	0.25
Puffed and shredded wheat	½ cup	1.1	0.65	0.50	24.0	0.44
Rice Krispies	½ cup	0.9	0.37	6.15	14.0	0.25
Tapioca, salt-free, dry	1 tbsp	0.1	0.10	0.03	2.0	—

BREADS, COOKIES, CRACKERS

Food	Serving					
Bread, regular	1 slice	2.2	0.66	5.50	24.0	0.2
Bread, salt-free	1 slice	1.7	0.50	0.30	—	0.2
Bread, whole wheat	1 slice	2.6	1.74	5.73	57.0	0.5
Crackers, graham	2 squares	1.1	1.41	4.13	21.0	0.2
Crackers, salt-free	3 squares	3.1	0.30	0.04	—	0.3
Crackers, saltines	1 square	0.3	0.09	1.36	2.6	trace
English muffin, enriched	½	1.5	0.64	3.82	30.0	—
Italian bread, enriched	1 slice small	0.9	0.17	2.56	8.0	0.2
Roll, hard, enriched	½	2.5	0.60	6.80	23.0	1.13
Roll, soft, enriched	1	2.3	0.69	6.17	24.0	1.22
Vanilla wafers	5	1.1	0.37	2.20	25.0	—

MEAT, FISH

Food	Serving					
Boiled beef, cooked	1 oz	9.0	1.84	0.68	48.0	1.76
Chopped beef, lean, cooked	1 oz	8.2	2.35	0.87	68.9	1.27
Sirloin, cooked	1 oz	6.5	1.36	0.69	54.0	1.63
Chicken, dark, cooked	1 oz	7.9	2.30	1.10	64.8	0.46
Chicken, white, cooked	1 oz	8.9	3.00	0.80	74.9	0.25
Lamb, cooked	1 oz	6.1	1.76	0.65	48.6	1.23
Turkey, dark, cooked	1 oz	8.5	2.90	1.20	—	1.23
Turkey, white, cooked	1 oz	9.3	3.00	1.00	—	0.60
Veal, lean, cooked	1 oz	7.7	2.20	0.80	65.4	1.17
Bluefish, cooked	1 oz	7.4	—	1.26	81.0	—
Flat fish, raw	1 oz	4.7	2.47	0.95	55.2	—
Cod, cooked	1 oz	8.1	2.94	1.34	78.0	0.30
Halibut, cooked	1 oz	7.1	3.84	1.65	70.0	0.30
Shrimp, raw	1 oz	5.1	1.59	1.72	47.0	0.57
Tuna, regular, drained	1 oz	8.1	2.30	10.40	66.1	0.28
Tuna, salt-free	1 oz	7.9	2.02	0.50	53.7	0.28

Table A–16. Protein, Sodium, Potassium, Phosphorus, and Zinc Contents of Selected Common Foods* (continued)

	Amount	Protein (gm)	Potassium (mEq)	Sodium (mEq)	Phosphorus (mg)	Zinc Φ (mg)
SWEETS						
Candy, hard, sour balls	—	—	—	—	—	—
Honey	1 tbsp	0.1	0.28	0.04	1.0	0.02
Ice cream, regular	½ cup	3.0	3.10	1.80	76.5	0.30
Ice milk	½ cup	3.2	3.30	1.93	54.0	—
Jams, preserves	1 tbsp	0.1	0.50	0.40	2.0	0.07
Sherbet (fruit ice)	½ cup	0.9	0.50	0.20	12.5	—
Sugar, brown, packed	½ cup	0.0	4.41	0.65	9.5	—
Sugar, white	1 tbsp	0.0	trace	trace	0.0	0.06
JUICES						
Apple	3½ oz	0.1	2.59	0.03	8.87	—
Apricot nectar	3½ oz	0.3	3.90	trace	11.95	—
Cranberry	3½ oz	0.1	0.25	0.10	3.16	—
Grape	3½ oz	0.2	2.96	0.08	11.85	—
Grapefruit	3½ oz	0.5	4.14	0.03	14.17	—
Lemon, canned	3½ oz	0.4	3.61	0.03	9.83	—
Orange, canned	3½ oz	0.8	4.90	0.03	18.14	0.08
Orange, fresh	3½ oz	0.7	5.12	0.03	16.93	0.21
Pear nectar	3½ oz	0.3	1.00	0.05	5.20	—
Pineapple	3½ oz	0.4	3.82	0.05	9.20	0.01
Prune	3½ oz	0.4	6.00	0.09	19.92	—
Tomato	3½ oz	0.9	5.82	8.70	18.10	—
Tomato, salt-free	3½ oz	0.8	5.82	0.12	18.18	—

VEGETABLES

Asparagus, cut, canned	2.5	4.21	12.06	48.0	—
Asparagus, low-sodium	2.3	4.21	0.19	48.0	—
Beans, green, canned	1.0	1.64	6.93	17.0	0.2
Beans, green, low-sodium	1.0	1.64	0.06	17.0	0.2
Beans, wax, canned	0.9	1.64	6.93	16.5	—
Beets, canned	0.8	3.64	8.71	15.5	—
Beets, low-sodium	0.8	3.64	1.69	15.5	—
Broccoli, cooked, no added salt	2.4	5.30	0.34	48.0	0.1
Cabbage, cooked, no added salt	0.8	3.02	0.43	15.0	0.3
Carrots, canned	0.6	2.38	7.95	17.0	0.25
Carrots, low-sodium	0.6	2.38	1.30	17.0	0.25
Carrots, raw	0.8	6.30	1.47	26.0	0.3
Cauliflower, cooked, no salt	1.5	3.30	0.23	26.5	—
Celery, raw	0.4	3.48	2.17	11.0	—
Corn, canned	2.1	2.05	8.45	40.5	0.35
Corn, low-sodium	2.1	2.05	0.06	40.5	0.35
Cucumber, pared, raw	0.4	2.87	0.17	12.5	—
Peas, sweet, canned	4.0	2.08	8.71	57.0	1.0
Peas, low-sodium	3.8	2.08	0.11	57.0	1.0
Tomato, raw	1.4	7.69	0.17	33.0	0.2
Tomato, canned	1.2	6.70	6.80	23.0	0.25
Tomato, low-sodium	1.2	6.70	0.15	23.0	0.25
Potato, boiled	1.5	5.66	0.06	32.5	0.15
Noodles, egg, enriched, cooked, with no salt	3.3	0.89	0.06	47.0	0.35
Rice, enriched, no added salt	2.1	0.73	trace	28.5	0.40

Each row also bears the serving-size notation "½ cup drained" except: Carrots, raw — "1 medium"; Celery, raw — "1 stalk"; Tomato, raw — "1 medium".

Table A–16. Protein, Sodium, Potassium, Phosphorus, and Zinc Contents of Selected Common Foods* (continued)

	Amount	Protein (gm)	Potassium (mEq)	Sodium (mEq)	Phosphorus (mg)	Zinc Φ (mg)
FRUITS						
Apple, pared	1 medium	0.3	4.35	0.08	15.0	0.08
Applesauce, unsweetened	½ cup	0.25	2.43	0.10	6.0	0.15
Apricots, canned	3 halves	0.5	5.10	0.04	13.0	—
Banana	1 medium	1.3	11.28	0.04	31.0	0.30
Blueberries, fresh	½ cup	0.5	1.50	0.02	10.0	—
Cherries, canned, pitted	½ cup	1.2	4.15	0.06	16.5	—
Grapefruit, fresh	½ cup	0.45	3.02	0.04	14.0	—
Orange, fresh	1 medium	1.3	6.74	0.04	26.0	0.2
Peach, fresh, pared	1 medium	0.8	6.89	0.04	25.0	0.2
Peach, canned, in syrup	½ cup	0.5	4.26	0.10	15.5	0.15
Pear, raw	1 medium	1.1	5.46	0.13	18.0	—
Pear, canned, syrup	½ cup	0.25	2.74	0.06	9.0	—
Pineapple, canned	½ cup	0.4	3.14	0.06	6.5	—
Strawberries, raw	½ cup	0.5	3.12	0.02	15.5	—

*Data taken from Watt and Merrill: *Composition of Foods, Dairy and Egg Products, Raw-Processed-Prepared*, U.S. Department of Agriculture Handbook No. 8-1. Washington, USDA, 1976. *Nutritive Value of American Foods in Common Units*, U.S. Department of Agriculture Handbook No. 456. Washington, USDA, 1975. Watt and Merrill: *Composition of Foods, Raw-Processed-Prepared*, U.S. Department of Agriculture Handbook No. 8. Washington, USDA, 1963.

—Data are inadequate or variable.

Φ Murphy, et al.: Provisional tables on the zinc content of foods. J. Am. Diet. Assoc., 66, 345, 1975. Freeland and Cousins: Zinc content of selected foods. J. Am. Diet. Assoc., 68, 526, 1976.

Table A–17. Restricted Protein, Sodium and Potassium Diet
(30 gm protein, 20 mEq potassium, 35 mEq sodium)*

Purpose: This diet is designed for use in the feeding of patients with advanced renal disease where control of elevated blood urea and plasma sodium, potassium and other minerals by dietary means is indicated. Patients needing this diet are frequently anorectic or nauseated and the diet has been formulated to be palatable.

Approximate Composition	Unit	Amount
Carbohydrate	gm	236
Protein	gm	30
Fat	gm	50
Calories		1,437
Calcium	mg	217
Phosphorus	mg	460
Iron	mg	7.9
Sodium	mg (mEq)	896 (35)
Potassium	mg (mEq)	80 (20)
Vitamin A	I.U.	12,794
Thiamin	mg	.55
Riboflavin	mg	.57
Niacin equivalents	mg	6.3
Ascorbic acid	mg	25

Adequacy: This diet does not meet the 1979 RDA in any category and this inadequacy must be remedied when prescribed for more than a few days by addition of (1) more carbohydrate and fat calories given orally, by tube or intravenously, (2) a supplementary multivitamin and (3) by supplementation with a low mineral-low protein liquid formula such as the R-#3 formula (Table A–18).

Type of Food	Amount	Food Included	Food Excluded
Milk	None	None	Whole milk, skim milk, buttermilk, malted milk.
Other beverages‡	2 cups	Ginger ale, root beer, Seven-up, Kool-aid (unrestricted amounts).	Cola drinks, cocoa, tea, coffee,† Postum, Sanka.
Soup	None	None	All soups
Meat, poultry, fish	1½ oz	Beef, chicken, lamb, pork, liver, beef heart, beef kidney, sweetbreads. Salt-free canned salmon and tuna. Codfish, clams, lobster, haddock, perch, oysters, shad, shrimp, red snapper, whitefish, whiting. Canned crabmeat.	Meat extracts. Halibut, scallops, veal. Canned sardines. All others not listed as allowed.
Cheese	½ cup or ½ oz	Unsalted cottage cheese. Unsalted American cheese.	All others not listed as allowed.
Eggs	1	Any type prepared without milk (may be used as cheese substitute).	None
Potato substitute	1 svg. 1 cup	Enriched white rice, macaroni, noodles, spaghetti.	All potatoes (white or sweet). Canned potatoes, potato chips. Brown rice.
Bread	3 slices	Enriched white bread, saltines (5 only).	Rye bread, whole wheat bread, all those not listed as allowed.
Cereal	1 svg.	Cream of wheat, hominy grits, farina; all served without milk.	All others not listed as allowed.

Table A–17. Restricted Protein, Sodium and Potassium Diet
(30 gm protein, 20 mEq potassium, 35 mEq sodium)* (continued)

Type of Food	Amount	Food Included	Food Excluded
Vegetables	2 svg. ½ cup	Cooked or raw cabbage; fresh, frozen or salt-free canned green beans, salt-free canned carrots, cucumbers (6 slices), lettuce (2 leaves), salt-free canned peas, fresh or salt-free canned wax beans.	All others not listed as allowed.
Fruit	2 svg. ½ cup	Canned or fresh applesauce, blueberries, Royal Anne cherries, peaches, pears, pineapple, grapefruit sections; fresh blackberries, raspberries, strawberries, pineapple, grapes, apple, cherries; frozen raspberries, strawberries, cranberry sauce.	All dried fruits; all others not listed as allowed.
Fruit juice	2 svg.	Cranberry juice; frozen lemonade; frozen limeade.	All others not listed as allowed.
Butter or fat	3 tsp	Butter, margarine, corn oil (unrestricted amounts); mayonnaise or commercial salad dressing; cream cheese.	Cream gravies; all others not listed as allowed.
Desserts	1 serving	Gelatin made with Kool-aid and sugar; dietetic gelatin (D'Zerta); lime ice.	Commercial Jell-O: all others not listed as allowed.
Sweets	In moderation	Gum drops, hard candy, marshmallows; white sugar syrup—1 tsp.; jellies or jams.	Brown sugar, maple syrup, chocolate, molasses; all others not listed as allowed.
Spices	As desired	White pepper; vanilla; vinegar; peppermint extract; nutmeg; cinnamon; mace.	All others not listed as allowed.
Miscellaneous			Nuts; olives; pickles; catsup; coconut; peanut butter; bakers' yeast.

Sample Meal Pattern

Breakfast	Serving Portion	Sample Menu
Fruit	½ cup	Cranberry juice
Cereal	½ cup cooked	Farina
Bread	1 slice	Enriched white bread
Fat	1 tsp	Butter or margarine
Jelly	1 tbsp	Jelly
Sugar	1 tbsp	Sugar
Beverage	1 cup	Coffee†

Lunch		
Meat substitute	1 medium	Soft-cooked egg
Potato substitute	½ cup cooked	Unsalted white rice
Vegetable	½ cup	Salt-free green beans
Dessert	½ cup	Royal Anne cherries
Bread	1 slice	Enriched white bread
Fat	1 tsp	Butter or margarine
Beverage	1 cup	Ginger ale

Table A–17. Restricted Protein, Sodium and Potassium Diet
(30 gm protein, 20 mEq potassium, 35 mEq sodium)* (continued)

Type of Food	Amount	Food Included	Food Excluded
Dinner			
Meat	1½ oz	Salt-free roast beef
Vegetable	½ cup	Salt-free canned carrots
Fruit	½ cup	Applesauce
Bread	1 slice	Enriched white bread
Fat	1 tsp	Butter or margarine
Dessert	½ cup	Lime ice
8:00 p.m.			
Fruit juice	½ cup	Frozen lemonade

*Modified from Diet Manual, Memorial Sloan-Kettering Cancer Center, rev., 1978.
†May be ordered at the discretion of the physician.
‡Soft drinks vary in potassium and phosphate content. See Table A–9.

Table A–18. High-calorie, Low-protein and Low-mineral Liquid Supplement
(R-#3)*† (2000 ml volume)

	Gm	Household Measure
Dextrose (sugar)	240	1⅓ cup
Egg	250	5 eggs
Cornstarch	120	1 cup
Water	1284	5⅓ cups
Heavy cream	200	Skimpy cup
Chocolate syrup	90	4 tbsp (to taste)
Corn oil	30	1 oz

Preparation

Dissolve in saucepan dextrose, egg, cornstarch and about ½ measured water. Mix until no lumps are visible and nothing is stuck to the bottom of the pan.

Begin to cook on low to medium heat. Do not boil. When mixture just begins to thicken, remove from the heat.

Pour cooked mixture in blender. Turn on low speed and add remaining ingredients. Place top on blender and turn to high speed for 1 to 2 minutes (until well blended).

Pour into container. Use remaining water to rinse blender. Pour into container. Mix everything thoroughly. Refrigerate.

3 to 4 glasses (3 to 4 oz each) to be taken each day. Total volume should give a 3-day supply.

*100 ml (3½ oz) provides the following:

Calories	151	Mg (mg)	3
CH_2O (gm)	21	K (mEq)	1
Protein (gm)	2	Na (mEq)	1
Fat (gm)	7		
Ca (mg)	15		

†From Nutrition Support Kitchen, Memorial Sloan-Kettering Cancer Center, New York.

Table A–19.   Restricted Residue Diet*

Purpose: This diet is low in fibrous materials and is designed for patients with active diverticulitis, intermittent partial bowel obstruction or where a low-residue diet is desirable for other reasons. In fat-malabsorption cases, the fat in this diet should be reduced or one of the fat-restricted regimens should be ordered. When a milk restriction is prescribed, calcium should be given in the form of calcium salts by physician's order.

Approximate Composition	Unit	Amount
Carbohydrate	gm	221
Protein	gm	79
Fat	gm	112
Calories		2,200
Calcium	mg	801
Phosphorus	mg	1,226
Iron	mg	11.1
Sodium	mg (mEq)	1,904 (81)
Potassium	mg (mEq)	2,726 (70)
Vitamin A	I.U.	17,298
Thiamin	mg	1.2
Riboflavin	mg	1.8
Niacin equivalents	mg	19.5
Ascorbic acid	mg	120

Adequacy: This diet meets the 1979 Recommended Dietary Allowances of the National Research Council for men but may be low in iron for women. The calculations are based on the sample meal plan.

Physicians may order a diet decreasing the animal fat over a prolonged period. This order will imply the use of skim milk, margarine and vegetable oil. Limit lean broiled meat to one (1) serving per day and increase the use of fish and poultry.

Where lactose intolerance is evidenced, milk should be limited initially to 1 pint per day and may be increased as patient's tolerance improves.

Type of Food	Amount	Food Included	Food Excluded
Milk	1 pt (initially)	Whole milk, skim milk, buttermilk (including that used in cooking).	All in excess of 1 pt. (Ability of patient to increase quantity depends on tolerance.)
Other beverages	As desired	Coffee, tea, carbonated beverages.	Alcoholic beverages (unless ordered by physician).
Soup	1 cup	Bland broth. Cream soups made from strained vegetables allowed (limit of 2 cups milk daily in any form).	Spicy meat soups, highly seasoned soups. Bouillon cubes, canned soups, barley soups.
Meat, poultry, fish	6 oz	Tender or ground beef, pork, veal, lamb, chicken, turkey, chicken liver, beef liver, sweetbreads. Crisp bacon. Lean boneless fish. Canned salmon or tuna. Meats and fish should be baked, boiled, broiled, roasted or used in cream mixtures. Serve meat and fish without spicy gravy.	Pork mixtures, frankfurters, bologna, sausage, luncheon meats. Smoked, cured, canned, preserved meat or fish. Clams, oysters, shrimp, lobster. Processed smoked meats. Fried meats, fish or fowl. Shellfish.
Cheese	1–2 oz	Cottage, cream cheese, mild American cheese. Small amounts of mild flavored cheese may be used in cooking e.g. cream sauces or in combination with macaroni, noodles, rice, spaghetti or bread.	Cheese with added spices and herbs. Sharp cheese.

Table A–19. Restricted Residue Diet* (continued)

Type of Food	Amount	Food Included	Food Excluded
Egg	1	Soft, baked or hard cooked. Scrambled in double boiler without oil. Poached, creamed. Plain omelet or souffle.	Fried eggs.
Potato or substitute	2 svg.	White potato (no skin), boiled, baked, creamed, mashed, escalloped, au gratin. Pureed sweet potato. Plain macaroni, noodles, spaghetti, white rice (prepared with cream or mild cheese sauces or butter).	Fried potatoes, potatoes with skin. Potato chips. Whole-grain rice.
Bread	4 svg.	Fresh or toasted enriched white, light rye bread or rolls (without seeds). Saltines, soda crackers, melba toast, rusk, zweiback, milk toast.	Whole wheat, cracked wheat, dark rye bread. Whole wheat crackers, graham crackers, pretzels. Pancakes, waffles, muffins, corn bread, quickbreads. All others not listed as allowed.
Cereal	1 svg.	Cooked refined corn, rice and wheat cereals. Hominy grits, farina, strained oatmeal, rolled wheat, cornflakes, Rice Krispies, puffed rice.	Whole-grain cereals. Bran flakes, Ralston, Maltex, Wheatena, shredded wheat, Grapenut flakes, Wheat Chex. All other cereals not listed as allowed.
Vegetables	2 svg.	Well-cooked asparagus tips, carrots, beets. Cooked and pureed green beans, green peas. Acorn or yellow squash. Pumpkin. Pureed spinach, corn, lima beans. Baby foods with allowed vegetables.	Lentils, dried peas. Raw and seeded vegetables. All those not listed as allowed.
Fruit	3 svg.	Cooked, canned, baked or stewed fruits without skin or seeds. Apples, applesauce, Royal Anne cherries. Peeled apricots, peaches, pears. Fresh, ripe banana.	Raw fruits except those listed as allowed. Fruits with seeds or skin. Raisins, dates, figs. Canned plums, berries, fruit cocktail, pineapple and strawberries.
Fruit juice	2 svg.	Apple, apricot, pear, peach nectar. Strained fruit juice.	Fruit juices with pulp.
Butter or fat	3 svg.	Butter. Fortified margarine. Smooth peanut butter. Vegetable oils or shortenings may be used in moderation as seasonings or spreads. No more than ½ cup cream or half milk and half cream daily. Crisp bacon. Bland gravy made only of meat juice, flour and salt.	Spicy salad dressings. Crunchy peanut butter. Nuts. Spicy gravies.
Dessert	1 svg.	Cookies, e.g. arrowroot, plain sugar, vanilla wafers. Plain custard, ice cream, flavored gelatin (plain, whipped or with allowed fruit). Rennet dessert. Plain puddings. Fruit juice sponges. Snows, whips. Spanish cream, Bavarian cream. Sherbet. Cakes, e.g. angel food, sponge, plain white or yellow, plain pound, ladyfingers.	Tarts, pies, pastries, cakes, puddings that contain spices, nuts, fruits, raisins, seeds, frosting or coconut. Any others not listed as allowed.

Table A–19.   Restricted Residue Diet* (continued)

Type of Food	Amount	Food Included	Food Excluded
Sweets	In moderation	White sugar, brown sugar. Clear jelly. Honey, syrup, molasses. Clear sweet dessert sauces. Hard candy, gumdrops. Chocolate syrup.	Candy containing fruit or nuts. Jam, marmalade, sugar and candy in excess.
Spices		Salt (in moderation). Cinnamon, paprika, lemon, vanilla, vinegar.	All other spices, herbs and condiments not listed as allowed.
Miscellaneous		White sauce (within daily milk allowance).	Olives, pickles, popcorn, relishes. Excessive hot or cold foods.

BLAND RESTRICTED RESIDUE DIET

In addition to the above restricted residue, if the physician feels that the patient should be on a bland restricted diet the following foods are to be excluded:

All spices (except salt)	Pepper
Alcohol	Carbonated Beverages
Coffee	

Sample Meal Pattern

Breakfast	Serving Portion	Sample Menu
Fruit	½ cup	Strained orange juice
Cereal	½ cup	Farina
Egg	1	Soft-cooked egg
Bread	1 slice	Enriched white toast
Milk	½ cup	Whole milk
Fat	2 tsp	Butter
Sugar	1 tbsp	Sugar
Beverage	1 cup	Coffee or tea

Lunch		
Meat or substitute	3 oz	Broiled chicken
Potato or substitute	½ cup	Cooked rice
Vegetable	½ cup	Asparagus tips
Bread	1 slice	White enriched bread
Fat	2 tsp	Butter
Fruit	½ cup	Applesauce
Milk	½ cup	Whole milk
Sugar	2 tsp	Sugar
Beverage	1 cup	Coffee or tea

Dinner		
Meat or substitute	3 oz	Roast beef
Potato or substitute	1	Baked potato (no skin)
Vegetable	½ cup	Carrots
Bread	1 slice	White enriched bread
Milk	1 cup	Whole milk
Fat	2 tsp	Butter
Dessert	½ cup	Whole peeled apricots
Sugar	2 tsp	Sugar
Beverage	1 cup	Coffee or tea

9:00 p.m.		
Fruit	½ cup	Canned peaches

*Modified from Diet Manual, Memorial Sloan-Kettering Cancer Center, rev. 1978.

Table A–20. High-residue Diet*

Purpose: This diet is high in fibrous material and is designed for patients with asymptomatic diverticulosis or where a high-"fiber" diet is desired.

Approximate Composition	Unit	Amount
Carbohydrate	gm	324
Protein	gm	95
Fat	gm	130
Calories		2,747
Calcium	mg	997
Phosphorus	mg	1,872
Iron	mg	13.6
Sodium	mg (mEq)	2,551 (109)
Potassium	mg (mEq)	3,495 (90)
Vitamin A	I.U.	10,622
Thiamin	mg	1.2
Riboflavin	mg	2.0
Niacin equivalents	mg	26
Ascorbic acid	mg	69

Adequacy: This diet meets the 1979 Recommended Daily Allowance of the National Research Council for men but may be low in iron for women. The calculations are based on the sample meal plan.

Foods to be Emphasized on Regular Diet

Cereals	Oatmeal, whole wheat cereals, bran-type cereals.
Fruits	Three servings daily, one or more of which should be raw. All kinds, especially apples, dates, figs, grapes, raisins and prunes.
Fruit juices	All kinds, especially orange and prune.
Vegetables	Three servings daily. All kinds, especially cabbage, celery, corn, string beans, spinach, beet greens, lettuce, escarole, mixed vegetables; with inclusion of fresh raw vegetables.
Breads	Whole wheat, rye, cracked wheat, rusk, melba, zwieback, bran bread and bran muffins.
Beverages	Whole milk, buttermilk, skim milk.
Miscellaneous	Jams; molasses; salad dressing; nuts.

Sample Meal Pattern

Breakfast	Serving Portion	Sample Menu
Fruit	½ cup	Stewed prunes
Egg	1	Soft-cooked egg
Cereal	½ cup	All bran
Bread	1 slice	Rye bread
Fat	2 tsp	Butter
Milk	1 cup	Whole milk
Jam	1 tsp	Jam
Sugar	2 tsp	Sugar
Beverage	1 cup	Coffee or tea

Table A–20.   High-residue Diet* (continued)

Lunch

Meat or substitute	3 oz	Broiled chicken
Potato or substitute	½ cup	Wild rice
Vegetable	½ cup	Mixed vegetables
Salad	1 slice	Lettuce and tomato
Dressing	1 tbsp	Russian dressing
Bread	1 slice	Whole wheat bread
Fat	1 tsp	Butter
Milk	½ cup	Whole milk
Dessert	1 piece	Cherry pie
Sugar	2 tsp	Sugar
Beverage	1 cup	Coffee or tea

Dinner

Meat or substitute	3 oz	Roast beef
Potato or substitute	1	Baked potato
Vegetable	½ cup	Peas
Fruit	½ cup	Canned fruit cup
Bread	1 slice	Whole wheat bread
Fat	1 tsp	Butter
Salad		Tossed greens
Dressing	1 tbsp	Thousand Island dressing
Milk	1 cup	Whole milk
Sugar	2 tsp	Sugar
Beverage	1 cup	Coffee or tea

9:00 p.m.

Fruit	1	Fresh apple

*Modified from Diet Manual, Memorial Sloan-Kettering Cancer Center, rev. 1978.

Table A–21.   Soft-textured Diet*

Purpose: This diet is designed to provide an adequate nutritional intake for edentulous patients, for occasional postoperative patients not yet able to take a regular diet and for patients with mechanical or pathologic impairment of chewing and/or swallowing.

The diet is a modification of the regular diet and consists of food made soft enough to be mashed easily in the mouth and swallowed. The physiologic problems of patients to be placed on this diet should be given individual consideration and the diet varied where indicated.

Approximate Composition	Unit	Amount	
Carbohydrate	gm	246	
Protein	gm	84	
Fat	gm	128	
Calories		2,441	
Calcium	mg	728	
Phosphorus	mg	1,343	
Iron	mg	11	
Sodium	mg (mEq)	2,630	(112)
Potassium	mg (mEq)	2,900	(74.3)
Vitamin A	I.U.	17,372	
Thiamin	mg	1.2	
Riboflavin	mg	2.0	
Niacin equivalents	mg	20	
Ascorbic acid	mg	120	

Adequacy: This diet meets all the 1979 Recommended Dietary Allowances of the National Research Council for men but may be low in iron for women. The calculations are based on the sample meal plan.

Table A–21. Soft-textured Diet* (continued)

Type of Food	Amount	Food Included	Food Excluded
Milk	2 cups daily	Milk, buttermilk, skim milk; cocoa.	None
Other beverages	As desired	Tea, coffee, coffee substitutes; carbonated beverages.	None
Soups	As desired	Broths; strained or regular cream, vegetable, frozen or canned soups.	None
Meat, poultry, fish	6 oz or more daily	Any tender meat, fish, poultry, pureed or ground food if necessary.	Tough, fibrous meat
Cheese**		Ricotta, cottage cheese, cream cheese, American cheese, processed cheese.	Hard cheese; all others not listed as allowed.
Eggs	1 or more daily	Soft, medium, hard-cooked, poached, soft scrambled, chopped, fried.	
Potatoes and substitute	2 or more svg. daily	Pureed, mashed, baked potato (without skin); macaroni, rice, noodles, spaghetti.	All not listed as allowed.
Bread	3 svg. or more daily	Enriched white, whole wheat, rye (all without seeds); soft rolls; crackers; plain muffins.	Coarse bread or rolls with seeds, raisins or nuts; hard rolls.
Cereal	1 svg. daily	Any cooked cereal; dry cereal if tolerated.	None
Vegetables	2 svg. or more daily	Pureed; baby or tender whole cooked vegetables such as: asparagus tips, carrots, beets, squash (fresh, frozen or canned) if tolerated. Include at least 1 svg. of green or yellow cooked vegetables daily; sliced tomatoes if tolerated.	All others not listed.
Fruit	2 svg. or more daily	Pureed, baby or whole cooked fruits (fresh, canned or frozen); avocado; ripe tender raw fruits such as: banana, peaches, pears, melon, plums.	All raw fruits patient cannot tolerate.
Fruit juice	1 svg. or more daily	All—include 1 svg. daily of citrus fruit juice: orange, grapefruit, blended. If throat is sore, apricot, apple, pear, peach and grape are the mildest juices.	None
Butter or fat	6 or more tsp. daily	Butter, margarine; cream; salad dressing; vegetable fats and oils; gravies.	None
Desserts	As desired	Custards, junket, gelatin, puddings, fruit whips, ice cream, sherbet, soft cakes—all without nuts; soft fruit or cream pies; pureed or soft fruits.	Any dessert containing nuts, coconut or raisins.

Table A–21.   Soft-textured Diet* (continued)

Type of Food	Amount	Food Included	Food Excluded
Spices	As desired	Any that are tolerated by the patient, i.e. salt, pepper, garlic, paprika, cinnamon.	Any patient finds irritating.
Miscellaneous		White sauces; vinegar; salad dressing if tolerated.	Nuts; olives; pickles; popcorn; those foods which are chemically, mechanically or thermally irritating to the mouth and/or throat.
Sweets	As desired	Hard candy; honey; jellies; jams; sugar; syrups; molasses; soft chocolates without nuts.	All others not listed as allowed.

Sample Meal Pattern

Breakfast	Serving Portion	Sample Menu
Fruit	½ cup	Orange juice
Cereal	½ cup	Farina
Egg	1	Soft-cooked egg
Bread	1 slice	Enriched white toast
Fat	2 tsp	Butter or margarine
Milk	½ cup	Whole milk
Beverage	1 cup	Coffee
Sugar	1 tbsp	Sugar

Lunch		
Meat or substitute	3 oz	Ground chicken
Potato or substitute	½ cup cooked	Rice
Vegetable	½ cup	Asparagus
Fruit	½ cup	Canned cherries
Bread	1	Soft roll
Fat	2½ tsp	Butter or margarine
Milk	1 cup	Whole milk
Beverage	1 cup	Tea
Sugar	2 tsp	Sugar

Dinner		
Soup	½ cup	Cream of mushroom
Meat or substitute	3 oz	Ground beef
Potato or substitute	1	Baked potato (no skin)
Vegetable	½ cup	Diced carrots
Dessert	½ cup	Whole peeled apricots
Bread	1 slice	Light rye bread (no seeds)
Fat	2½ tsp	Butter or margarine
Milk	½ cup	Whole milk
Beverage	1 cup	Coffee
Sugar	2 tsp	Sugar

8:00 p.m.		
Fruit	½ cup	Applesauce

*Modified from Diet Manual, Memorial Sloan-Kettering Cancer Center, rev. 1978.
**Cheese is considered part of the protein allotment, e.g. a substitute for meat, poultry, fish.

Table A-22. Diet I for Peptic Ulcer Therapy

Purpose: In the past physicians have tended to administer this diet with antacids to patients admitted with acute ulcer symptoms. In recent years, gastroenterologists and other physicians have tended to depart from this procedure using antacids, *bland* diets, H_2 receptor antagonists and, where necessary, a diet low in lactose for the lactose-intolerant patient. For the more traditional physician, Diet I and Diet II may be used provided the patient is not lactose intolerant.

Approximate Composition	Unit	Gastric I (skim milk) 1,400 ml	Gastric I (milk) 1,400 ml	Gastric I (milk and cream) 700 ml and 700 ml
Carbohydrate	gm	71	69	64
Protein	gm	50	49	45
Fat	gm	1.4	49	169
Calories		500	911	1,958
Calcium	mg	1,694	1,652	1,540
Phosphorus	mg	1,330	1,302	1,211
Iron	mg	trace	trace	trace
Sodium	mg (mEq)	708 (31)	702(31)	6,408 (28)
Potassium	mg (mEq)	2,074 (53)	2,020(52)	1,856 (48)
Magnesium	mg (mEq)	196 (16)	182(15)	168 (14)
Vitamin A	I.U.	trace	1,960	6,860
Thiamin	mg	.5	.4	.4
Riboflavin	mg	2.6	2.4	2.3
Niacin equivalents	mg	1.4	1.4	1.4
Ascorbic acid	mg	14	14	14

Adequacy: These diets do not meet the 1979 Recommended Dietary Allowances of the National Research Council for any of the nutrients except calcium and riboflavin and for vitamin A when whole milk or cream is used.

Diet I (with milk, skim or whole): This routine consists solely of milk. When this routine is ordered 90 ml of milk are served on the hour from 7 a.m. to 10 p.m., inclusive, totaling 1,400 ml daily.

Diet I (with milk and cream): This routine consists solely of milk and light cream (half and half). When this routine is ordered 45 ml of milk and 45 ml light cream are served on the hour from 7 a.m. to 10 p.m., inclusive, totaling 1,400 ml daily.

Table A–23. Diet II for Peptic Ulcer Therapy

Purpose: To advance the symptomatic peptic ulcer patient to a more nutritious diet for a *limited* period. When hyperlipidemia or pyloric obstruction with gastric retention is of concern, skim milk is recommended (see Statement of Purpose for Diet I).

This routine consists of 120 ml milk or 60 ml milk and 60 ml light cream given hourly from 7 a.m. to 10 p.m. inclusive, plus 1, 3 or 6 supplements as ordered by the physician. Sugar and salt are permitted in moderation.

When 1 or 3 supplements are ordered they are served at mealtime and are selected from the following list:

Eggs—poached or soft cooked
Cream of wheat, farina, strained oatmeal
Milk toast
Junket, custard and gelatin desserts without fruit
Strained cream soup, prepared without meat stock

When 6 supplements are ordered they are served at meal hours as well as at 10 a.m., 3 and 8 p.m. Additional foods are selected from the following list:

Cottage cheese
White toast and butter
Vanilla ice cream, blanc mange, rice, tapioca, bread and cream puddings, except chocolate
Vanilla wafers
Plain soda crackers
Steamed rice with butter

Table A–24. Antidumping Diet

Purpose: Following partial or total gastrectomy, symptoms of dumping may occur, but patients vary greatly in the severity and duration of symptoms. The following approach is recommended regarding diets for partially gastrectomized patients:

1. Each patient must be evaluated individually regarding the diet that he can tolerate. While there are wide variations, the great majority are able to consume regular diets. Milk should be increased gradually as tolerance is proven.

2. To test and to prevent a dumping episode, a diet consists of six (6) equally spaced meals (restricted carbohydrate will be ordered). The carbohydrate should be in the form of starches, which are equally distributed among the six (6) meals. Sucrose and other soluble carbohydrates are to be avoided. All fluids must be consumed 45 to 60 minutes after ingestion of solid food. Fluids should be 4 oz or less per serving.

3. Patients with high subtotal gastrectomies may need stricter diet control. Consult your dietitian for the appropriate fat modification.

4. Increased food tolerance will encourage the patient to begin including those foods which currently appear in the excluded list of this diet. If the patient continues to be asymptomatic, a normal diet will be permitted.

5. Because patients may have a malabsorption for fat, minerals and vitamins, attention should be focused on the adequate intake of calories, protein, calcium, iron and vitamins. If a large fat intake is associated with frequent bulky stools, the fat should be restricted.

Approximate Composition	*Unit*	*Amount*
Carbohydrate	gm	153
Protein	gm	150
Fat	gm	121
Calories	—	2,328
Calcium	mg	819
Phosphorus	mg	1,944
Iron	mg	19
Sodium	mg (mEq)	1,977 (84)
Potassium	mg (mEq)	2,860 (73)
Vitamin A	I.U.	15,764
Thiamin	mg	1.2
Riboflavin	mg	2.1
Niacin equivalents	mg	44
Ascorbic acid	mg	123

Adequacy: This diet meets the 1979 Recommended Dietary Allowances of the National Research Council for all nutrients. The calculations are based on the sample meal plan.

Type of Food	Amount	Food Included	Food Excluded
Milk	1½ pt	Whole milk, buttermilk; plain yogurt (not chilled). Tolerance to milk and milk products should be tested.	All sweetened milk beverages; milk in all forms if not allowed by physician or if not tolerated.
Other beverages	See general instructions	Tea, coffee, Postum, Sanka; lemonade (without sugar or syrup—use saccharine).	Sweetened fruit beverages; cocoa, chocolate; alcoholic beverages including beer; carbonated beverages.
Soup	1 svg. ¾ cup per svg.	Broth, bouillon; cream soup (if milk is allowed).	All soups not listed as allowed.

Table A–24. Antidumping Diet* (continued)

Type of Food	Amount	Food Included	Food Excluded
Meat, poultry, fish	16 oz	All that are tolerated by patient.	None if tolerated by patient.
Cheese	1–2 oz	All cheeses, but preferably cream cheese.	None
Eggs	2–3	May be prepared in any way.	None
Potato, bread or substitute	6	All except those excluded.	Hot breads, waffles, muffins, pancakes; bread or its equivalent in excess of specified amount; whole grain and rye bread if not tolerated by patient.
Cereal	1 svg. ½ cup 4 oz	All kinds.	None except whole grain if not tolerated by patient.
Vegetable	2 svg. ½ cup per svg. Include 1 green or yellow vegetable.	All except those excluded.	Raw vegetables if not tolerated by patient; corn and lima beans (unless substituted for bread).
Fruit and fruit juice	2 svg. Include 1 citrus or 4 oz citrus juice	Unsweetened cooked, fresh or canned. All except those excluded.	Frozen and dried fruit; fruit cooked or canned with sugar; sweetened fruit juice; banana and prune juice (unless substituted for bread). Raw fruit if not tolerated by patient.
Butter or fat	10 tbsp 2–3 strips	Butter, cream, margarine, oils, fats, mayonnaise, French dressing. Crisp bacon	
Dessert	1 svg	Junket, custard. Gelatin (made without sugar—use saccharin or Sucaryl).	Cake, cookies, pastries, pies, puddings; sherbet, ice cream, sweetened sauces, gelatin candy.
Miscellaneous	In moderation	Nuts, smooth peanut butter; condiments including salt, saccharin and Sucaryl.	Sugar, jam, marmalade, jelly, honey, syrups, molasses, chocolate, marshmallows; snacks such as Fritos, popcorn, pretzels, potato chips; spices, condiments, pepper, catsup, chili sauce, mustard, vinegar.

Sample Meal Pattern

8:00 a.m.—Breakfast	Serving Portion	Sample Menu
Fruit	½ cup	Unsweetened applesauce
Eggs	2 each	Scrambled with
Butter	2 tsp	Butter
Cereal (calcium enriched)	½ cup	Farina

Table A–24.   Antidumping Diet* (continued)

9:00 a.m.

Milk		Milk
Beverage		Coffee

10:00 a.m.—Midmorning Nourishment

Crackers	4 each	Saltines
Cheese	1 oz	American cheese

12:00 p.m.—Lunch

Meat	5 oz	Roast chicken
Potato	½ cup	Rice
Vegetable	½ cup	Peas
Butter	2 tsp	Butter
Fruit	½ cup	Unsweetened apricots (drained)

1:00 p.m.

Beverage		Tea with lemon

3:00 p.m.—Midafternoon Nourishment

Bread	1 slice	White bread
Cheese	1 oz	Cream cheese

6:00 p.m.—Dinner

Meat	5 oz	Roast beef
Potato	1 medium	Baked potato
Butter or oil	2 tsp	Butter
Vegetable	½ cup	Carrots
Dessert	½ cup	Unsweetened peaches (drained)

7:00 p.m.

Beverage		Tea with lemon

8:00 p.m.—Evening Nourishment

Bread	1 slice	White bread
Meat	3 oz	Tuna
Butter	2 tsp	Mayonnaise

9:00 p.m.

Beverage	½ cup	Milk

General Instructions to the Patient

1. Eat regularly. Do not omit meals.
2. Eat small meals (6 per day).
3. The major amount of fluids should be taken 45 to 60 minutes (or later) after each meal.
4. Avoid excessively hot or cold foods.
5. Eat slowly; relax before and after meals.
6. As your tolerance for the diet improves, your physician will order the necessary modifications.
7. Some patients are not tolerant to milk and milk products following partial or total gastrectomies. Patient should test his tolerance by taking small amounts initially. Amounts may be increased gradually up to limit of acceptance by patient.

*Modified from Diet Manual, Memorial Sloan-Kettering Cancer Center, rev. 1978.

Table A–25.   Gluten-free Diet (Wheat, Rye, Oats, Barley and Buckwheat)*

Purpose: This diet is designed for the treatment of patients with gluten enteropathy (i.e. nontropical sprue, celiac disease), a malabsorption syndrome caused by sensitivity to gliadin or its products. Gliadin is a protein fraction of gluten found in all grains other than rice and corn. Therefore, gluten-containing cereals are eliminated in this diet. Since wheat, rye, oats, barley and buckwheat products are used in the manufacture of a variety of foods, beverages and confections, deviation from this diet is permitted only with the approval of the physician.

Approximate Composition	Unit	Amount
Carbohydrate	gm	297
Protein	gm	98
Fat	gm	107
Calories		2,505
Calcium	mg	823
Phosphorus	mg	1,371
Iron	mg	18.1
Sodium	mg (mEq)	2,757 (120)
Potassium	mg (mEq)	2,886 (74)
Vitamin A	I.U.	9,631
Thiamin	mg	1.7
Riboflavin	mg	2.7
Niacin equivalents	mg	26.8
Ascorbic acid	mg	219

Adequacy: This diet meets the 1979 Recommended Dietary Allowances of the National Research Council. The calculations are based on the sample menu.

Guidelines for Gluten-free Diets

This menu pattern is designed to provide adequate nutrition while eliminating wheat, rye, oats and barley from the diet. The fraction of gluten protein which injures the intestine of susceptible individuals is gliadin. When all sources of gliadin are removed from the diet, however, the intestine is able to regenerate and function normally.

Gluten may be present in foods either as a basic ingredient (that is, listed as wheat, rye, oats or barley), or added as a derivative when a food is processed or prepared. Thus, *reading labels carefully is very important.*

Since flour and cereal products are quite often used in the preparation of foods, it is important to be aware of the methods of preparation used as well as the foods themselves. This is especially true when dining out.

Type of Food	Amount	Foods Allowed	Foods to Avoid
Milk	2 or more cups	Fresh, dry, evaporated or condensed milk; cream, sour cream,† whipping cream; yogurt.†	Malted milk; some commercial chocolate drinks; some nondairy creamers.‡
Meat, fish, poultry	2 or more svg. 6 oz	All kinds of fresh meats, fish, other seafood, poultry; fish canned in oil or brine; some prepared meat products, such as hot dogs and lunch meats.‡	Prepared meats which contain wheat, rye, oats or barley, such as: some sausages,‡ hot dogs,‡ bologna,‡ luncheon meats,‡ chili con carne,‡ sandwich spreads.‡ Bread-containing products such as: Swiss steak, croquets, meat loaf. Some tuna canned in vegetable broth. Self-basting turkeys with HVP added.
Cheeses Can be used for meat and milk groups		All aged cheeses, such as: cheddar, Swiss, Edam, Parmesan. Cottage cheese,† cream cheese,† pasteurized processed cheese.†	Any cheese product containing oat gum as an ingredient.

Table A–25. Gluten-free Diet (Wheat, Rye, Oats, Barley and Buckwheat)* (continued)

Type of Food	Amount	Foods Allowed	Foods to Avoid
Eggs	1 or 2	Plain or in cooking.	Eggs in sauce made from gluten-containing ingredients (such as a regular, wheat-based white sauce)
Potato or other starch	1 or more svg.	White and sweet potatoes, yams; hominy; rice, wild rice; special gluten-free noodles (Aproten) made by General Mills; some Oriental rice and bean noodles.	Regular noodles, spaghetti, macaroni, some packaged rice mixes.‡
Vegetables	4 svg.	All plain, fresh, frozen or canned vegetables. Dried peas and beans, lentils; some commercially prepared vegetables.‡	Creamed vegetables,‡ vegetables canned in sauce,‡ canned baked beans,‡ commercially prepared vegetables and salads.‡
Fruits	2 to 3 svg.	All fresh, frozen, canned or dried fruits; all fruit juices; some canned pie fillings.	Thickened or prepared fruits; some pie fillings.‡
Breads	2–3 svg.	Specially prepared breads using only allowed flours. Examples of commercially available brands: Guisto's Lima-Soya Bread; Lima-Potato Bread; Rice Bread. Ener-G Foods' Rice Bread	All others containing wheat, rye, oat and/or barley flours.
Cereals	1 or more svg. enriched cereal	Hot cereals such as: corn meal, Cream of Rice, hominy, rice; cold cereals as follows: puffed rice, Kellogg's Sugar Pops, Post's Fruity and Chocolate Pebbles.	All others containing wheat, rye, oats and/or barley; bran; graham; wheat germ; malt; kasha; bulgur; buckwheat,†† millet.††

Flours and thickening agents		Arrowroot starch (A)
		Corn flour (B,C,D)
		Corn meal (B,C,D)
		Corn starch (A)
		Potato flour (B,C,E)
		Potato starch flour (B,C,E)
		Rice bran
		Rice flours:
		  Plain; brown (B,C,D)
		  sweet (B,C,D,F)
		Rice polish (B,C,G)
		Soy flour (B,C,G)
		Tapioca starch (A)
			Wheat starch (manufacturer states it contains residual protein—probably gluten). All flours containing wheat, rye, oats and/or barley.

(A) Good thickening agent
(B) Good combined with other flours
(C) Best combined with milk and eggs in baked product
(D) Grainy-textured products
(E) Drier product than with other flours
(F) Moister product than with other flours
(G) Adds distinct flavor to product—use with moderation

Crackers and snack foods		Rice wafers;‡ pure corn meal tortillas; popcorn; some crackers and chips.‡	All others containing wheat, rye, oats and/or barley.

Table A–25.   Gluten-free Diet (Wheat, Rye, Oats, Barley and Buckwheat)* (continued)

Type of Food	Amount	Foods Allowed	Foods to Avoid
Fats		Butter, margarine, vegetable oil; nuts, peanut butters; hydrogenated vegetable oils; some salad dressings,‡ mayonnaise.‡	Some commercial salad dressings.‡
Soups		Homemade broth and soups made with allowed ingredients; some commercially canned soups.‡	Most canned soups‡ and soup mixes;‡ bouillon.
Desserts		Cakes, quickbreads, pastries, puddings prepared with allowed ingredients. Cornstarch, tapioca and rice puddings; gelatin desserts; custard. Vanilla-flavored ice cream from: Arden, Carnation, Darigold, Foremost, Lucerne;‡ some pudding mixes.‡	Commercial cakes, cookies, pies, etc., made with wheat, rye, oats and/or barley; prepared mixes;‡ ice cream cones; puddings.‡
Beverages		Instant and ground coffee, instant tea, tea, carbonated beverages;‡ pure cocoa powder; unfortified wines, rums; some root beer.‡	Ovaltine, malted milk; ale, beer, gin, whiskies,# vodka; some root beer.‡
Sweets		Jelly, jam, honey; brown and white sugar; molasses; most syrups;‡ some candy;‡ chocolate, pure cocoa; coconut.	Some commercial candies.‡
Miscellaneous		Salt, pepper, herbs, extracts; food coloring; cloves, ginger, nutmeg, cinnamon, chili powder; tomato puree and paste; olives, pickles; cider and wine vinegar; yeast; bicarbonate of soda, baking powder,‡ cream of tartar, dry mustard; some other condiments;‡ monosodium glutamate (MSG).	Some curry powders,‡ some dry seasoning mixes,‡ some gravy extracts,‡ some meat sauces;‡ some catsup,‡ some mustard,‡ horseradish,‡ some soy sauce;‡ chip dips;‡ some chewing gum;‡ distilled white vinegar.#

Always check the source of the following ingredients before eating any product containing them.

Ingredient (as appears on product label)	Include	Avoid
Hydrolyzed vegetable protein (hvp)	Soy, corn	Mixtures of wheat, corn and soya
Flour or cereal products	Rice flour, corn flour, corn meal, potato flour, soy flour	Wheat, rye, oats, barley
Vegetable protein	Soy, corn	Wheat, rye, oats, barley
Malt or malt flavoring	Those derived from corn	Those derived from barley or barley malt syrup
Starch	Arrowroot, corn, potato, tapioca, waxy maize, maize	Wheat starch
Vegetable gum	Carob bean, locust bean, cellulose gum, guar gum, gum Arabic, gum acacia, gum tragacanth	Oat gum
Soy sauce, soy sauce solids	Those which do not contain wheat	Those which contain wheat

Table A–25. Gluten-free Diet (Wheat, Rye, Oats, Barley and Buckwheat)* (continued)

Sample Meal Pattern

Breakfast	Serving Portion	Sample Menu
Fruit	½ cup	Orange juice
Cereal	1 cup	Cream of rice
Egg	1	Soft-cooked egg
Bread	1 slice	Rice bread
Fat	2 tsps	Butter or margarine
Milk	1 cup	Milk
Beverage	1 cup	Coffee
Sugar	1 tbsp	Sugar

Lunch		
Meat or substitute	3 oz	Broiled chicken
Potato or substitute	1	Rice
Vegetable	½ cup	Asparagus
Salad		Sliced tomato
Dessert	½ cup	Custard
Bread	1 slice	Rice bread
Fat	2 tsp	Butter or margarine
Milk	½ cup	Milk
Beverage	1 cup	Coffee
Sugar	2 tsp	Sugar

Dinner		
Soup	1 cup	Bouillon, homemade
Meat or substitute	3 oz	Roast beef
Potato or substitute	1	Baked potato
Vegetable	½ cup	Brussels sprouts
Salad	½ carrot	Carrot sticks
Fruit	½ cup	Canned apricots
Fat	1 tsp	Butter or margarine
Beverage	1 cup	Coffee
Sugar	2 tsp	Sugar
	½ cup	Milk

8 p.m.		
Fruit	½ cup	Applesauce

*Approximate composition and sample meal pattern are modified from Diet Manual, Memorial Sloan-Kettering Cancer Center, rev. 1978. The Guidelines for Gluten-Free Diets were prepared by Elaine I. Hartsook, R.D., RC-14, Clinical Research Center, University Hospital, Seattle, Washington 98195. A gluten-free product list and newsletters are available from Ms. Hartsook.

†Check vegetable gum used

‡Contact manufacturer for clarification.

††Although botanically different from other gluten-containing grains, additional information is needed before this can be cleared.

#Distilled white vinegar uses grain as a starting material. Whiskies, including "corn whisky," use wheat, rye, oats or barley in the mash. According to chemistry professors consulted, in large-scale distillation processes it is possible that a very small amount of protein may be carried over into the distillate. The presence of such a small amount of gluten must be tested via immunoassay, an expensive and complex technique using laboratory animals to produce a gluten antibody. Currently, we are advising gluten-intolerant persons to use cider and wine vinegar in food preparation (salad dressings, pickles, and in cooking). Avoid all whiskies.

Commercially prepared pickles, ketchup, mustard, mayonnaise, steak sauce, and other condiments are usually made with distilled grain vinegar; however, the maximum amount of gluten which would be present in such products via the vinegar would be insignificant. Thus, moderate use of the above commercial condiments is recommended.

Table A–26. Fat-restricted Diets, 20 and 40 gm*†

Purpose: These diets are designed for patients with serious diseases of the biliary tract or pancreas or with malabsorption syndromes other than that caused by gluten sensitivity where a reduced fat intake may decrease diarrhea and nutrient losses. Medium-chain-length triglycerides (MCT) may be added to this diet in various recipes.** Pancreatic extract should be given where indicated.

Approximate Composition	Unit	20 gm		40 gm	
Carbohydrate	gm	391		369	
Protein	gm	91		98	
Fat	gm	21		42	
Saturated fatty acid	gm	6		14	
Unsaturated fatty acid	gm	7		19	
Calories		2,057		2,198	
Calcium	mg	979		925	
Phosphorus	mg	1,370		1,490	
Iron	mg	14		16	
Sodium	mg (mEq)	2,744	(115)	2,740	(115)
Potassium	mg (mEq)	3,272	(84)	3,422	(88)
Vitamin A	I.U.	12,000		13,000	
Thiamin	mg	1.5		1.5	
Riboflavin	mg	2.2		2.4	
Niacin equivalents	mg	19		23	
Ascorbic acid	mg	122		123	

Adequacy: These diets meet the 1979 Recommended Dietary Allowances for adult men of the National Research Council but may be low in iron for women. The calculations are based on the sample menu with an average weekly figure used for protein foods.

Type of Food	Amount	Food Included	Food Excluded
Milk	1 pt	Skim milk, fat-free buttermilk	Whole milk, cultured buttermilk, chocolate milk; yogurt
Other beverages	As desired	Coffee, tea, Sanka, Postum; carbonated beverages	All alcoholic beverages; Ovaltine, chocolate-flavored drinks, cocoa
Soup	As desired	Fat-free bouillon or broth, tomato bouillon; vegetable soup; skim milk soup	Any soup containing cream, fat or whole milk
Meat, poultry, or fish	6 oz cooked weights for 40-gm diet; 2 oz for 20-gm diet	All broiled, boiled, baked or cooked without fat in a Teflon pan. All visible fat must be removed. Meat and fish may be wrapped in foil before broiling or baking in order to retain juices. Lean cuts of beef, Canadian bacon, lamb, liver, veal, white meat of chicken and turkey—remove skin before cooking; organ meats. All fish, including canned pink salmon and sardines in tomato sauce, except those listed as not allowed.	Pork, ham, bacon, duck, goose, salami, pastrami, bologna, frankfurter, sausages, luncheon meats; frozen or canned meat dishes. Fish canned in oil (sardines, tuna); frozen fish sticks; fresh or frozen salmon.
Cheese	40-gm diet: as desired; 20-gm diet: additional 4 oz to replace meat portion	Fat-free cottage cheese, pot cheese, other skim-milk cheeseΦ	All others

Table A–26.   Fat-restricted Diets, 20 and 40 gm*† (continued)

Type of Food	Amount	Food Included	Food Excluded
Eggs	40-gm diet: 1 daily; omit on 20-gm diet	Medium or hard cooked, poached, scrambled in double boiler, cooked without fat in a Teflon pan, egg whites as desired.	More than 1 daily; eggs fried in fat
Potato or substitute	2–3 svg.	Baked, boiled, mashed without whole milk or fat; rice, spaghetti, macaroni; hominy	Escalloped or creamed potatoes, fried potatoes, potato chips, oven-browned potatoes; egg noodles
Bread	5 svg.	White, whole wheat, rye, French, hard rolls, soft rolls, matzoth, rye crisp, saltines, Uneeda biscuits, melba toast	All other breads and rolls; quickbreads, biscuits, popovers, muffins; egg matzoth; butter crackers
Cereals	1 svg.	All cooked and dry cereals	None
Vegetables	3 or more svg. including 1 green or yellow	All fresh; frozen or canned vegetables prepared without cream sauce, fats or oils	Creamed vegetables or vegetables prepared with fat or oil
Fruit and fruit juice	4 or more svg. including citrus or tomato	All fresh; frozen; canned and stewed except avocado and coconut; all fruit juices	Avocado and coconut
Butter or Fats	40-gm diet, 1 tsp if tolerated; 20-gm diet, omit	One of the following may be substituted for 1 tsp of butter or margarine: light cream 2 tbsp heavy cream 1 tbsp French dressing 1 tbsp mayonnaise 1 tsp oil 1 tsp	More than 1 tsp of butter or margarine; no gravies
Dessert	In moderation	Plain angel food cake, vanilla wafers, ladyfingers, arrowroot cookies, graham crackers, meringues, Jell-O, junket, cornstarch, rice and tapioca pudding made with skim milk and egg whites. Water ices, fruit whips made with gelatin or egg whites	All other cakes, pies, doughnuts, cookies, puddings, pastry, ice cream, puddings made with whole milk and egg yolks, or eggs
Sweets	In moderation	Sugar, honey, jelly, jam, marmalade, molasses, maple syrup and sugar, sour balls, gumdrops, jelly beans, marshmallows, hard candy and fondant	Chocolate, chocolate candy, chocolate syrup, candy made with cream, cocoa fats and nuts
Spices		Salt, paprika, herbs, mustard, nutmeg	Pepper
Miscellaneous		Catsup, chili sauce, vinegar, pickles, garlic, unbuttered popcorn, white sauce made with skim milk, vanilla	Olives, nuts, peanut butter, apple butter; cream sauces, gravies; buttered popcorn, waffles, pancakes, fritters

Table A–26.   Fat-restricted Diets, 20 and 40 gm*† (continued)

Sample Meal Pattern for 20-gm Fat Diet

Breakfast	*Serving Portion*	*Sample Menu*
Fruit	½ cup	Orange juice
Cereal	½ cup	Farina
Bread	2 slices	White enriched toast
Jelly	2 tsp	Jelly
Milk	½ cup	Skim milk
Sugar	1 tbsp	Sugar
Beverage	1 cup	Coffee or tea

Lunch		
Meat or substitute	3 oz	Broiled chicken (no skin)
Potato or substitute	½ cup	Rice
Vegetable	½ cup	Asparagus
Salad	1 svg.	Lettuce and tomato
Dressing		Vinegar
Fruit	½ cup	Canned cherries
Bread	1	Hard roll
Jelly	2 tsp	Jelly
Sugar	2 tsp	Sugar
Milk	½ cup	Skim milk
Beverage	1 cup	Coffee or tea

Dinner		
Soup	1 cup	Bouillon (fat-free)
Meat or substitute	3 oz	Baked flounder
Potato or substitute	1	Baked sweet potato
Vegetable	½ cup	Brussels sprouts
	½ cup	Carrot sticks
Fruit	½ cup	Apricots
Bread	1 slice	Rye bread
Milk	1 cup	Skim milk
Jelly	2 tsp	Jelly
Sugar	2 tsp	Sugar
Beverage	1 cup	Coffee or tea

8:00 p.m.		
Fruit	1	Apple

Table A–26.   Fat-restricted Diets, 20 and 40 gm*† (continued)

Sample Meal Pattern for 40-gm Fat Diet

Breakfast	Serving Portion	Sample Menu
Fruit	½ cup	Orange juice
Cereal	½ cup	Wheatena
Egg	1	Soft boiled
Bread	2 slices	White bread
Jelly	1 tbsp	Jelly
Milk, skim	1 cup	Skim milk
Beverage	As desired	Coffee
Sugar	1 tbsp	Sugar
Lunch		
Meat	3 oz	Sliced white chicken
Potato substitute	1 cup	Rice
Vegetable	1 svg.	Carrots
Salad	1 svg.	Sliced tomato
Bread	2 slices	White bread
Fat	1 tsp	Mayonnaise
Skim milk	½ cup	Skim milk
Beverage	1 cup	Tea
Sugar	1 tbsp	Sugar
Dessert	1 svg.	Canned peaches
Dinner		
Soup	½ cup	Bouillon
Meat	3 oz	Broiled steak
Potato	1 svg.	Baked potato
Vegetable	1 svg.	Steamed green beans
Salad	1 svg.	Celery hearts
Bread	1 svg.	Hard roll
Jelly	1 tbsp	Honey or jelly
Skim milk	½ cup	Skim milk
Beverage	1 cup	Coffee
Sugar	1 tbsp	Sugar
Dessert	1 svg.	Raspberry Jell-O
9 p.m.		
Fruit	1	Raw apple

*Modified from Diet Manual, Memorial Sloan-Kettering Cancer Center, rev. 1978.

†The 20-gm restricted fat diet contains approximately 6 gm saturated fatty acids or 27.9 per cent of the total fat, 7 gm polyunsaturated fatty acids or 34 per cent of the total fat. The 40-gm restricted diet contains 14 gm saturated fatty acids or 33 per cent of the total fat, 19 gm polyunsaturated fatty acids or 44.8 per cent of the total fat.

   The 40 gm will be decreased to 20 gm by omitting the egg and 1 tsp fat, reducing the meat allowance from 6 oz to 3 oz and adding 4 oz fat-free cottage cheese.

**MCT oil may be added to this diet to increase calories as potentially absorbable fat. For information and recipes on MCT see: *Medium-Chain-Triglycerides* (Senior: Ed.). Philadelphia, University of Pennsylvania Press, 1968.

ΦThe following is a partial list of some available low-fat cheeses: Caerphilly (70 per cent fat free), Gaperon (80 per cent fat free), Nökkelost (70 per cent fat free), Lorraine Swiss (85 per cent fat free), Swiss Chris (85 per cent fat free), Margarinost (100 per cent cholesterol free).

   The following are part skimmed or low fat: Jarlsberg, Fontina, Crem Havarti, Typo, Monterey Jack, pure goat cheeses.

Table A–27. Diet List to be Given Allergic Patient

This diet is not to be continued indefinitely without supervision. (Report for a possible revision at the end of 4 weeks.)

Avoid those foods which have been crossed out by your physician. Use all other foods.

Dairy Products

Milk, cream, ice cream, sherbets, milk soups and other milk-containing foods (see Milk-poor Diet below).

Butter, cheese, except cream cheese and cottage cheese.

Egg, unless hard boiled for 10 minutes, and egg-containing foods, as griddle cakes, waffles, egg sauce, etc. (see Egg-poor Diet below).

Meat and Fish

Chicken, duck, goose, turkey.
Bacon, crisp; smoked ham.
Fresh pork and pork sausage, lard.
Lamb (roast, chops, kidneys).
Beef (roast, steak, calves liver, chipped beef); all beef products.

Veal (roast, chops, kidneys).
Shellfish, except oyster.
Fish (see Seafood-free Diet below).

Cereals or Breadstuffs

Wheat and wheat products, as macaroni, noodles, spaghetti, Cream of Wheat, Wheatena, Shredded Wheat, bran flakes, cookies, cakes, etc. (see Wheat-poor Diet below).
Rye (pure rye bread, Ry-Krisp).
Corn (cornmeal muffins, corn flakes, farina, hominy).

Rice (also rice flakes, Cream of Rice cereal).
Oats, oatmeal
Barley
Soybean flour
Arrowroot
Tapioca

Vegetables

Artichokes	Eggplant	Pumpkin
Asparagus	Endive	Radish, horseradish
Beans, all types	Green pea	Spinach
Beets	Green pepper	Squash
Broccoli	Lentils	String beans
Brussels sprouts	Lettuce	Sweet corn
Cabbage, sauerkraut	Mushroom	Sweet potato
Carrots	Mustard	Tomato
Cauliflower	Okra	Turnip
Celery	Onion (baked or boiled)	Watercress
Chicory	Parsley	White potato (baked)
Cucumber	Parsnip	

Fruits

Apples	Grapefruit	Plums
Apricots	Grapes	Prunes
Avocado	Honeydew melon	Raisins
Banana	Lemon	Rhubarb
Berries	Lime	Strawberry
Cantaloupe	Orange	Tangerine
Cherries	Peaches	Watermelon
Cranberries	Pears	
Date	Pineapple	
Fig		

Table A-27. Diet List to be Given Allergic Patient (continued)

Beverages

All alcoholic drinks, including beer, ale, wine. Chocolate, cocoa.

Coffee, tea, cola drinks.

Miscellaneous

Nuts, peanut butter (see Nut-poor Diet below). Condiments, highly spiced foods. Foods fried in vegetable oils such as cottonseed, peanut and corn oils.

Excessively sweet foods. Intensely cold foods or drinks. Olives, pure olive oil. Gelatin.

Permitted foods should not be used constantly, but, whenever possible, in rotation.

Milk-poor Diet

Avoid:

Milk, buttermilk, cream, as such and in prepared foods, as ice cream, sodas, milk sherbet, Bavarian cream mousses, custards, gravies, cream sauces, soups, chowders.
Prepared flour mixes for home cooking.
Malted milk, hot chocolate or cocoa prepared with milk.

Cheese.
Evaporated, powdered, condensed milk (bakery products, as pies, breads and cakes containing small amounts of cooked milk can often be tolerated).

Butter and oleomargarine can usually be permitted in modest amounts.
Study the label on packaged foods for evidence of milk or milk products content.

Egg-poor Diet

Avoid:

Eggs: Fresh, frozen, powdered, cooked in any form.
Egg-containing foods, such as:
  Soups, broths made with egg.
  Prepared flour mixes for home cooking.
  Waffles, doughnuts, pretzels.
  Pancakes, griddle cakes, pastries, French toast.
  Macaroons, meringues, frostings.
  Cakes, cookies, unless known to be egg-free.
  Breads with glazed crust.
  Foods breaded with egg mixture.
  Sausages, croquettes, meat cakes, containing egg as binder.

Poultry, especially chicken, if fricasseed or in broth.
Salad dressings, unless known to be egg-free; Hollandaise, mayonnaise, and egg sauces.
Ice cream and sherbets, unless known to be egg-free.
Custards, cream candies, fondants, Bavarian cream.
Marshmallows.
Baking powder containing egg white.
Prepared drinks containing egg or egg powder for insomnia or underweight.

Study the labels on packaged foods for evidence of egg in any form.
Avoid vaccine made in egg, as for influenza, spotted fever, yellow fever.

Table A–27. Diet List to be Given Allergic Patient (continued)

Seafood-free Diet

Avoid:

Fish, shellfish, fresh, canned, smoked, pickled; fish liver oils and concentrates in vitamin preparations.

Fish and shellfish stews, bisques, broths, soups, salad, hors d'oeuvres, caviar.

Avoid licking labels, which may contain a fish glue adhesive.
Avoid injections of fish origin in the treatment of varicose veins.

Wheat-poor Diet

Avoid:

White, whole wheat, cracked wheat flour in breads, waffles, griddle cakes, doughnuts, muffins, pastries, pies, cakes, crackers, spaghetti, macaroni, dumplings, pretzels, zwieback, noodles.
Corn bread, unless known to be wheat-free.
Soy bread, unless known to be wheat-free.
Rye bread, unless known to be wheat-free.
Gluten bread.
Breakfast cereals, dry or cooked, containing wheat, whole wheat, cream soups, farina or bran.

Custards, gravies, sauces containing wheat.
Breaded foods prepared with wheat.
Coffee substitutes containing wheat; beer; ale.
Prepared meats, as sausages, frankfurters, meat loaf, croquettes made with wheat.
Prepared mixes for biscuits, muffins, pastries, pie crusts, cookies.

Study the label on prepared foods for evidence of wheat or wheat product content.

Nut-poor Diet

Avoid:

Nuts of all types, also peanuts (although a member of the bean family), cottonseed meal in health and laxative breads, soybean bread.
Nut crumbs on cookies, cake icings, ice cream.

Candies containing nuts.
Salad oils, lard substitutes, margarines made of coconut, soybean, cottonseed or peanut oils (many are so made). (Olive oil permitted.)

Individuals highly sensitive to nuts are often allergic to seeds, such as cottonseed, flaxseed, mustard (by external application in poultices, as well as when ingested as foods), beans, peas. Legumes, such as peas, beans, lentils, are often allergenic factors in the patient sensitive to nuts, but some patients tolerate legumes, such as peanuts, despite high degrees of nut sensitivity.

Table A–28.   Diet Exchanges for a Vegetarian Diet*

List 1—*Milk Exchanges*
   Kefir   1 cup (omit 2 Fat Exchanges)
   Soy milk (fortified)   1 cup (add ½ Bread Exchange)

List 2—*Vegetable Exchanges*
   Bamboo shoots   ¾ cup
   Bean sprouts: raw or cooked
      Alfalfa   1 cup
      Mung   1 cup
      Soy   1 cup
   Water chestnuts   4

List 3—*Fruit Exchanges*
   Carrot juice   ½ cup

List 4—*Bread Exchanges*
   Brown rice (cooked)   ⅓ cup
   Buckwheat flour (dark)   3 tbsp
   Bulgur wheat   2 tbsp
   Millet (cooked)   ½ cup
   Miso   3 tbsp
   Oats, dry   ¼ cup
   Pita (Syrian) bread   ½ of a 2½-oz loaf
   Rye flour   3 tbsp
   Wheat berries (cooked)   ⅓ cup
   Wild rice (cooked)   ½ cup

List 5—*"Lean Meat" Exchanges*Φ
   Dried beans and peas   ½ cup cooked
      Black-eyed peas   (omit 1 Bread Exchange)
      Broad beans   (omit 1 Bread Exchange)
      Garbanzo   (omit 1 Bread Exchange)
      Kidney   (omit 1 Bread Exchange)
      Lentils   (omit 1 Bread Exchange)
      Lima   (omit 1 Bread Exchange)
      Mung   (omit 1 Bread Exchange)
      Navy   (omit 1 Bread Exchange)
      Pinto   (omit 1 Bread Exchange)
   Soy flour   ¼ cup (omit ½ Bread Exchange)

      *"Medium-fat Meat" Exchanges*Φ
   Cheeses:
      Camembert   1 oz
      Edam   1 oz
      Liederkranz   1 oz
   Soybeans   ⅓ cup
   Tofu   2½" × 2¾" × 1"

      *"High-fat Meat" Exchanges*Φ
   Cheeses:
      Blue, Roquefort   1 oz
      Brick   1 oz
      Gorgonzola   1 oz
      Gouda   1 oz
      Gruyere   1 oz
      Limburger   1 oz
      Muenster   1 oz
      Parmesan   1 oz
      Swiss   1 oz

Table A-28. Diet Exchanges for a Vegetarian Diet (continued)

Hummus	4 tbsp (omit 1 Bread Exchange)
Peanuts #	4 tbsp (omit ½ Bread and 2 Fat Exchanges)
Pignolia nuts#	6 tbsp (omit ½ Vegetable and 1 Fat Exchanges)
Pumpkin seeds#	4 tbsp (omit ½ Bread and 1½ Fat Exchanges)
Sesame seeds#	4 tbsp (omit ½ Bread and 2 Fat Exchanges)
Sunflower seeds#	4 tbsp (omit ½ Bread and 2 Fat Exchanges)

List 6—*Fat Exchanges*

Tahini	1 tsp

Foods containing complementary proteins may be eaten together, thereby increasing protein quality. Examples of foods that may be complemented to yield high-quality protein are listed below.

Food	*Complementary Protein*
Grains	Combine rice with: cheese, legumes, sesame
	Combine wheat with: legumes, peanuts and milk, sesame and soybean
	Combine corn with: legumes
Legumes	Combine beans with: wheat, corn
	Combine soybeans with: rice and wheat, corn and milk, wheat and sesame, peanuts and sesame, peanuts and wheat and rice
Nuts and Seeds	Combine sesame with: beans, peanuts and soybeans, soybeans and wheat
	Combine peanuts with: sunflower seeds

Diet Patterns

LACTO-OVOVEGETARIAN
Calories: 1500
CH_2O—190 gm 50%
Pro—75 gm 20%
Fat—47 gm 30%

Daily Food Allowance
3 Skim Milk Exchanges
2 Vegetable Exchanges
4 Fruit Exchanges
7 Bread Exchanges
4 "Lean-meat" Exchanges
1 "Medium-fat Meat" Exchange
6 Fat Exchanges

Meal Pattern

Breakfast
1 Fruit Exchange
2 Bread Exchanges
1 "Medium-fat Meat" Exchange
2 Fat Exchanges
1 Skim Milk Exchange

Lunch
2 "Lean-meat" Exchanges
2 Bread Exchanges
1 Vegetable Exchange
2 Fruit Exchanges
2 Fat Exchanges

STRICT VEGETARIAN
Calories: 1500
CH_2O—190 gm 50%
Pro—75 gm 20%
Fat—47 gm 30%

Daily Food Allowance
3 Soybean Milk Exchanges (Note: Add ½ bread for each cup)
2 Vegetable Exchanges
4 Fruit Exchanges
7 Bread Exchanges
4 "Lean-meat" Exchanges
1 "Medium-fat Meat" Exchange
6 Fat Exchanges

Meal Pattern

Breakfast
1 Fruit Exchange
2 Bread Exchanges
1 "Medium-fat Meat" Exchange
2 Fat Exchanges
1 Milk Exchange

Lunch
2 "Lean-meat" Exchanges
2 Bread Exchanges
1 Vegetable Exchange
2 Fruit Exchanges
2 Fat Exchanges

Table A–28.   Diet Exchanges for a Vegetarian Diet (continued)

Dinner	*Dinner*
2 "Lean-meat" Exchanges	2 "Lean-meat" Exchanges
2 Bread Exchanges	2 Bread Exchanges
1 Vegetable Exchange	1 Vegetable Exchange
1 Fruit Exchange	1 Fruit Exchange
2 Fat Exchanges	2 Fat Exchanges
1 Skim Milk Exchange	1 Milk Exchange
Bedtime Snack	*Bedtime Snack*
1 Skim Milk Exchange	1 Milk Exchange
1 Bread Exchange	1 Bread Exchange

Guidelines for the Professional

You may want to revise the patient's meal plan to allow more calories from carbohydrate (50 to 60 per cent) because of the high consumption of complex carbohydrates by vegetarians.

Many vegetarians use butter instead of margarine because it is considered a natural food.

The commercial meat analogs are very high in sodium, ranging in values from 300 mg to 3000 mg per 100 gm edible portion. Nutritional analyses of these products are available upon request from Loma Linda Foods, Riverside, California 92505, and Worthington Foods, Miles Laboratories, Worthington, Ohio 43085.

Some vegetarians use diet supplements such as wheat germ and brewer's yeast. Include these in the diet as follows:

Brewer's yeast, powder: 1 level tbsp = ½ "Lean-meat" Exchange
Wheat germ: ¼ cup = 1 Bread Exchange

Vegetarian diets, unless fortified, could be deficient in iron. Iron absorption is enhanced by the inclusion of a vitamin C-rich food at each meal.

Vegetarian diets excluding dairy products may be inadequate in riboflavin and calcium. Two cups daily of fortified soybean milk or appropriate supplements should prevent deficiency.

For the strict vegetarian, vitamin B_{12} is also required as a vitamin supplement if 2 cups of fortified soybean milk are not consumed daily.

Suggested Reading for Vegetarians

1. Lappe: *Diet for a Small Planet.* New York, Ballantine Books, 1975.
2. Robertson, Flinders and Godfrey: *Laurel's Kitchen, A Handbook for Vegetarian Cookery and Nutrition.* Berkeley, Nilgiri Press, 1976.
3. National Academy of Sciences, National Research Council, Food and Nutrition Board. Committee on Nutritional Misinformation, Vegetarian Diets. J. Am. Diet. Assoc., 65, 121, 1974.
4. Williams: Making vegetarian diets nutritious. Am. J. Nurs., 75, 12, 1975.
5. Erhard: The new vegetarians, Part 1. Vegetarianism and its medical consequences. Nutr. Today, 8, 4, 1973. Part 2. The Zen macrobiotic movement and other cults based on vegetarianism. Nutr. Today, 9, 20, 1974.
6. Beckner, et al.: *Diet Manual Utilizing a Vegetarian Diet Plan.* Loma Linda, The Seventh Day Adventist Dietetic Association, 1975.
7. Smith: A guide to good eating the vegetarian way. J. Nutr. Educ., 7, 109, 1975.

---

*Supplement to Exchange Lists for Meal Planning Vegetarian Cookery. American Diabetes Association, Washington, D.C. Area Affiliate, Inc., Food and Nutrition Committee, 1978. See Table A–11 for Standard Exchange lists.

ΦMeat analogs: Vegetable protein foods which closely duplicate the flavor, texture and appearance of meat—"meatless" meats. See company information in the Guidelines for the Professional given below.

#Seeds and nuts can be considered a "High-fat Meat" exchange and a complete protein only when they are complemented.

Table A–29. Composition of Parenteral Amino Acid Solutions*

	Aminosyn Δ 10%	Freamine II 8.5%	Nephramine 5.1%	Veinamine 8%	Travasol** 8.5%	
Amino Acids: gm/100 ml						
Essential						
L-Isoleucine	0.720	0.590	0.560	0.493	0.406	
L-Leucine	0.940	0.770	0.880	0.347	0.526	
L-Lysine acetate	0.720	0.870	0.900	—	—	
L-Lysine hydrochloride	—	—	—	0.667	0.492	
[L-Lysine (free base)]§	[0.513]	[0.620]	[0.641]	[0.534]	[0.394]	
L-Methionine	0.400	0.450†	0.880	0.427	0.492	
L-Phenylalanine	0.440	0.480	0.880	0.400	0.526	
L-Threonine	0.520	0.340	0.400	0.160	0.356	
L-Tryptophan	0.160	0.130	0.200	0.080	0.152	
L-Valine	0.800	0.560	0.650	0.253	0.390	
Total gm per 100 ml	4.493Φ	3.940Φ	5.091Φ	2.694Φ	3.242Φ	
Nonessential						
L-Alanine	1.280	0.600	—	—	1.760	
Aminoacetic acid (glycine)	1.280	1.700	—	3.387	1.760	
L-Arginine	0.980	0.310	—	0.749	0.880	
Aspartic acid	—	—	—	0.400	—	
L-Cysteine : HCl : HOH	—	0.020	—	—	—	
Glutamic acid	—	—	—	0.426	—	
L-Histidine	0.300	0.240	—	0.237	0.372	
L-Proline	0.860	0.950	—	0.107	0.356	
L-Serine	0.420	0.500	—	—	—	
L-Tyrosine	0.044	—	—	—	0.034	
Total gm per 100 ml	5.164	4.320	0	5.306	5.162	
Per cent EAA per total AA	46.5%	47.7%	100%	33.7%	38.6%	
Electrolytes: mEq/liter					ME	EF
Acetate	30	42 (as lysine)	—	50	135	52
Chloride	—	—	—	50	70	34
Magnesium	—	—	—	6	10	—
Phosphate	—	20 (310 mg)	—	—	60 (930 mg)	—
Potassium	5.4	—	—	30	60	—
Sodium	—	10	6	40	70	—

*Table prepared through courtesy of L. Schloesser, M.S., R.Ph.

Δ Available also as 3.5%, 5% and 7% solutions with amino acid concentrations in proportion.

**Available also as 3.5% and 5% solutions with amino acid concentrations in proportion; available with (ME) and without (EF) added electrolytes.

§ Lysine (free base) calculated from salt forms and actually present in the solution.

† As D-L methionine.

Φ Calculated with lysine as free base.

INTRODUCTION TO SECTION ON LIQUID FORMULAS AND DEFINED FORMULA DIETS

When a physician or his surrogate places a patient on a liquid formula as the sole or major source of nutrients for periods longer than a few weeks, he or she assumes a serious responsibility. It is mandatory that the prescription be nutritionally adequate, that it meet special clinical requirements and that it is properly prepared and consumed. Reasonably close follow-up is required with the flexibility to modify the formula as clinical, nutritional and psychosocial needs of the patient dictate. It is suggested that the patient's tolerance for a specific complete formula be tested under close supervision with relatively slow administration initially, with some dilution with water; progression to the total undiluted formula should follow as rapidly as tolerance permits. Nutrient sources and milk, lactose and fiber contents should be noted. The fluid and salt content must always be evaluated in relation to individual need. A number of formulas contain very large amounts of certain minerals which may be excessive under certain conditions. Space does not permit statements of osmolality and vitamin content; these should be reviewed prior to prescription. Cost to the patient should also be considered in relation to nutritional content and clinical and nutritional requirements.

Attention to psychosocial and clinical needs of the patient restricted to formula feeding is very important. Such needs include prior explanation of the medical value of the formula, in-hospital use of insulated containers, in-hospital food service related temporally to that of other patients, mechanical assistance in holding funnels, education in avoidance of air entrapment in the feeding tube and separate serving of desired beverages such as coffee, tea, cocoa and alcoholic beverages.

Strict adherence to measures designed to avoid microbial contamination and growth is essential. A detailed compilation of many commercial formulations is included, together with indications for use.

LIQUID FORMULAS FOR ORAL AND TUBE FEEDING

An important aspect of clinical nutrition concerns liquid formulas designed to improve food intake by either oral or tube administration. In years past, the usual hospital tube-feeding formula was based on whole milk, skim milk and cream in various combinations. It is now known that most adult population groups have insufficient lactase concentrations in the intestinal brush border to permit adequate digestion of large amounts of milk and that milk intolerance occurs in individuals with gastric or intestinal resection, intestinal radiation damage and other diseases which adversely affect normal intestinal function. This has led to modifications in the composition of standard hospital formulas to ensure adequate nutrition without excessive lactose.

A recent development has been the commercial production of nutritionally complete liquid diets made with nutrients derived in purified form either from natural foods or ones that have been prepared synthetically. These have been given various designations such as "chemically defined" or "elemental" diets.† Their development was stimulated by predictions and subsequent claims that such formulations would be useful in treating patients with problems related to the ingestion, digestion or absorption of solid foods (Table A–30).

Very little basic work, however, has been done to date to establish the optimal nutri-

---

†Since these diets are usually not chemically defined, nor are they "elemental" in a chemical sense, it is suggested that they be designated "defined-formula diets for medical use."

Table A–30. Clinical Problems for Which Defined Formula Diets May Be Appropriate

Inborn Errors of Metabolism	*Hypermetabolic States*
	Severe trauma
Gastrointestinal Disease	Major burns
Ulcerative colitis	
Granulomatous bowel disease	*Incidental Uses*
Chronic partial obstruction	Preoperative bowel preparation
Malabsorption syndromes	Nonallergenic food source
Short-bowel syndrome	Food supplement
Infantile diarrhea	Toilet management problems
Fistulas	Protection of bowel mucosa against damaging
Pancreatitis	agents
	Feeding of premature infants
Renal Failure	Feeding of anorectic patients

tional requirements of these patients. Comparative studies assessing the effectiveness of the various preparations available also remain to be done.

Nutritional Preparations

A large number of commercially prepared liquid formulas are now on the market, varying greatly in composition and cost. They are summarized in terms of their composition in Tables A–31, A–32 and A–33. The data in these tables are presented on the basis of 1,000 kcal. The formulas are subdivided into categories on the basis of the following considerations.

Completeness of Nutritional Content. The formulas listed in Table A–31 (A through C) are adequate in composition as the sole source of nutrition, while those in Table A–32 are designed primarily either as dietary supplements or to meet special metabolic needs. Table A–33 lists formulas designed specifically for very special metabolic disorders.

Presence of "Fiber" or "Residue." Table A–31 (Sections B and C) lists formulas having no vegetable or animal fibrous products. Table A–31A includes several formulas with some nondigestible residue present in foods such as meat, vegetables and fruit.

Lactose Content. Formulas listed in Table A–31A have moderate to high lactose levels. Those in Tables A–31B and 31C have little or no lactose. The lactose content per 1,000 kcal is given.

Amino Acid Sources. Table A–31A includes formulas with intact protein derived from meat, milk products and/or eggs. The formulas in Table A–31B have intact protein as semipurified isolates from milk, soybean or egg. Table A–31C includes those with casein hydrolysate or fish protein concentrate supplemented with amino acids and those with free amino acids only.

Other Nutrients. The sources of fats and carbohydrates are given in quantitative terms where data are available. The amounts of minerals are listed. The osmolality of the formula, when prepared according to the manufacturer's directions, is given for most preparations. The volume of formula required to provide the amounts of vitamins necessary to meet the Recommended Dietary Allowances (RDA) for an adult (except for pediatric formulations) is indicated on the bottom line of Table A–31. The data on composition are derived from manufacturers' analyses.

Table A–32 lists some supplements for special nutritional needs including protein, carbohydrate and fat sources, formulas

Table A–31. Complete Defined Formula Diet

A. INTACT PROTEIN CONTAINING MILK. "COMPLEAT B," "FORMULA 2" AND

	Compleat B Doyle	Formula 2 Cutter	C.I.B.*† Carnation	Meritene Liquid* Doyle
PROTEIN, gm	40.0	37.5	55.2	60.0
Protein source	Beef Nonfat milk	Nonfat milk Beef	Nonfat milk Soy protein Na caseinate	Conc. skim milk Na caseinate
FAT, gm	40.0	40.0	27.6	33.3
Fat source	Corn oil	Corn oil Egg yolks	Milk fat	Corn oil Mono-diglycerides
CARBOHYDRATE, gm	120.0	122.5	124.1	115.0
Carbohydrate source	Hydrolyzed cereal solids 23.0 Maltodextrin ⎫ Vegetables ⎬ 73.4 Fruits ⎪ Orange juice ⎭	Sucrose Vegetables Orange juice Wheat flour	Sucrose Corn syrup solids Lactose	Corn syrup solids Sucrose
Lactose, gm	24.4	37.5	84.0	56.7
VOLUME TO GIVE 1,000 C, ml	1000 (can) 935 (bottle)	1000	880	1000
Minerals				
Calcium, mg	625.0	720.0	1206.9	1250.0
Phosphorus, mg	1250	560.0	972.4	1250.0
Magnesium, mg	250.0	100.0	403.5	333.3
Iron, mg	11.3	12.6	15.9	15.0
Iodine, μg	93.8	75.0	129.3	125.0
Copper, mg	1.3	1.0	2.0	1.7
Manganese, mg	2.5	0.2		3.3
Zinc, mg	9.4	7.5	13.7	12.5
Sodium, mEq	51.6	26.1	37.0	39.8
Potassium, mEq	33.6	45.1	63.3	42.7
Chloride, mEq	22.9	53.5		47.0
mOsm/kg	390 (can) 405 (bottle)	435–510		550–610
VOLUME NEEDED TO MEET 100% RDAs INCLUDING VITAMINS, ml	1600 (can) 1500 (bottle)	2000	1373	1200

*Vanilla flavor used.
†Whole milk added.
‡Infant formula. Volumes are modified to meet growing infant needs.
◇Unflavored.

Preparations (per 1,000 kcal)

VITANEED ARE *MODERATE RESIDUE;* ALL OTHERS ARE *LOW RESIDUE*

Meritene+Milk*† *Doyle*	*Nutri-1000** *Cutter*	*Sustacal Liquid** *Mead Johnson*	*Sustacal+Milk*†* *Mead Johnson*	*Sustagen+Water** *Mead Johnson*	*Vitaneed* *Organon*
65.1 Nonfat milk Whole milk	38.0 Skim milk Na caseinate	60.3 Na+Ca caseinate Soy protein	60.3 Nonfat milk Whole milk	60.0 Nonfat milk Whole milk Ca caseinate	34.3 Pureed beef Ca caseinate
32.5 Milk fat	52.0 Corn oil	23.0 Soy oil	24.4 Milk fat	8.6 Milk fat	39.2 Soy oil
112.0 Corn syrup solids 14.4	95.6 Sucrose 30.7 Corn syrup solids 14.8	137.8 Sucrose 97.2 Corn syrup solids 40.6	134.4 Sucrose 36.2 Corn syrup solids 11.8	171.4 Corn syrup solids 104.7 Glucose 9.3	127.4 Corn syrup solids Maltodextrins Green beans, peaches, carrots
97.5	50.1	0	85.8	57.3	0
940	946	1000		600	980
2168.6	1150.0	1000.0	1611.2	1828.6	563.5
1807.2	900.0	916.7	1333.4	1371.4	514.5
361.4	200.0	375.0	375.0	228.6	245.0
16.3	9.0	16.7	16.7	10.3	11.8
136.1	75.0	138.9	138.9	85.7	147.0
1.8	1.0	1.9	1.9	1.1	1.5
3.6	1.3	2.8	2.8	2.9	—
13.5	7.5	13.9	13.9	11.4	9.8
39.3	21.7	40.2	40.2	29.8	23.4
71.1	35.9	52.7	64.8	51.3	31.4
58.1	31.0	43.8	37.6		20.7
690	500	625	756	1334	400
1040	1920	1080		1050	1470

Table A–31 (Continued)

B. INTACT PROTEIN, PROTEIN ISOLATES

	Ensure* Ross	Ensure Plus* Ross	Isocal Mead Johnson	Isomil‡ Ross	Mull-Soy‡ Syntex	Neo Mull-Soy‡ Syntex
PROTEIN, gm	35.0	36.6	32.5	30.0	48.0	27.0
Protein source	Na+Ca caseinate Soy protein	Na+Ca caseinate Soy protein	Na caseinate Soy protein	Soy protein isolate L-methionine	Soy flour	Soy protein isolate L-methionine
FAT, gm	35.0	35.5	42.0	52.9	55.5	52.5
Fat source	Corn oil	Corn oil	Soy oil 33.6 MCT 8.4	Soy oil Coconut oil	Soy oil	Soy oil
CARBOHYDRATE, gm	136.7	133.2	125.0	100.0	79.5	96.0
Carbohydrate source	Corn syrup solids Sucrose	Corn syrup solids Sucrose	Glucose Oligo-saccharides	Corn syrup Sucrose	Sucrose Invert sucrose	Sucrose
Lactose, gm	0	0	0	0	0	0
VOLUME TO GIVE 1,000 C, ml	960	667	960	1470	1500	1500
Minerals						
Calcium, mg	500.0	420.0	600.0	1029.4	1875.0	1250.0
Phosphorus, mg	500.0	420.0	500.0	735.3	1250.0	950.0
Magnesium, mg	198.1	211.3	200.0	73.5	117.2	120.0
Iron, mg	9.0	9.5	9.0	17.6	15.6	15.6
Iodine, μg	74.5	70.7	75.0	220.6	234.4	234.4
Copper, mg	1.0	1.1	1.0	0.8	1.6	0.6
Manganese, mg	2.0	1.4	2.5	0.3	2.2	4.0
Zinc, mg	15.0	15.9	10.0	7.4	12.5	4.8
Sodium, mEq	30.4	30.7	21.7	19.2	28.1	26.2
Potassium, mEq	35.5	32.4	32.1	26.7	66.1	41.2
Chloride, mEq	28.2	29.9	28.2	14.9	24.0	14.1
mOsm/kg	450	600	300	250	252	275
VOLUME NEEDED TO MEET 100% RDAs INCLUDING VITAMINS, ml	1887	2000	1920			

*Vanilla flavor used.
†Whole milk added.
‡Infant formula. Volumes are modified to meet growing infant needs.
◇Unflavored.

Table A–31 (Continued)

—LOW LACTOSE, LOW RESIDUE

Precision HN Doyle	Precision Isotonic Doyle	Precision LR Doyle	Osmolite Ross	Portagen Mead Johnson	ProSobee‡ Mead Johnson	Nutri-1000 LF Cutter
41.7	30.0	23.7	36.7	35.0	37.5	37.8
Egg white solids	Egg white solids	Egg white solids	Na+Ca caseinate Soy protein isolate	Na caseinate	Soy protein isolate L-methionine	Ca+Na caseinate Soy protein
1.2	31.3	1.4	36.3	47.7	50.0	52.0
MCT, Soy oil Mono-diglycerides	Soy oil Mono-diglycerides	MCT, Soy oil Mono-diglycerides	MCT oil Corn oil Soy oil	MCT 41.0 Corn oil 5.5 Lecithin 1.3	Soy oil	Corn oil
205.7	150.0	223.2	136.8	115.0	100.0	95.4
Malto-dextrin 193.0 Sugar 12.7	Glucose oligo-saccharides Sugar	Malto-dextrin 208.4 Sugar 15.1	Corn syrup solids	Malto-dextrin 83.5 Sucrose 28.8 Other 2.5	Sucrose 62.0 Corn syrup solids 38.0	Corn syrup solids Sugar
0	0	0	0	<0.3	0	0
950	1040	900	943	1000	1500	946
333.3	667.0	526.3	500.0	937.8	1185.0	500.0
333.3	667.0	526.3	500.0	604.4	795.0	500.0
133.3	267.0	210.5	198.1	208.4	111.0	200.0
6.0	12.0	9.5	9.0	18.8	18.8	9.0
50.0	100.0	78.9	74.5	72.9	72.0	75.0
0.7	1.3	1.1	1.0	1.6	0.9	1.0
1.3	2.7	2.1	2.0	3.1	1.7	1.3
5.0	10.0	7.9	15.0	9.4	8.0	7.5
40.6	34.8	27.5	23.5	20.4	27.0	29.6
22.2	25.6	20.2	21.7	32.1	28.5	35.9
32.0	30.1	28.2	22.6	24.2	18.0	26.6
557	300	505–549	300	357	258	380
2850	1560	1710	1887	960		1920

Table A–31 (Continued)

C. HYDROLYZED PROTEIN, AMINO ACIDS—LOW LACTOSE, LOW RESIDUE

	Flexical Mead Johnson		Nutramigen‡ Mead Johnson		Vital Ross
PROTEIN, gm	22.4		32.5		41.7
Protein source	Hydrolyzed casein Amino acids		Hydrolyzed casein		Hydrolyzed Soy whey, meat, Amino acids
FAT, gm	34.0		39.0		10.3
Fat source	Soy oil MCT	27.4 6.6	Corn oil		Sunflower oil
CARBOHYDRATE, gm	154.0		130.0		185.0
Carbohydrate source	Sugar Dextrin Citrate	100.9 48.4 4.7	Sucrose Tapioca starch	93.6 36.4	Glucose oligo- and polysaccharides Sucrose Hydrolyzed corn starch
Lactose, gm	0		0		1.7
VOLUME TO GIVE 1,000 C, ml	1000		1500		1000
Minerals					
Calcium, mg	600.0		936.0		666.7
Phosphorus, mg	500.0		705.0		666.7
Magnesium, mg	200.0		109.2		267.0
Iron, mg	9.0		18.8		12.0
Iodine, μg	75.0		70.2		100.0
Copper, mg	1.0		0.9		1.3
Manganese, mg	2.5		1.6		1.3
Zinc, mg	10.0		6.3		10.0
Sodium, mEq	15.2		21.0		16.7
Potassium, mEq	32.0		25.5		29.8
Chloride, mEq	35.2		19.5		18.8
mOsm/kg	550		443		450
VOLUME NEEDED TO MEET 100% RDAs INCLUDING VITAMINS, ml	2000				1500

*Vanilla flavor used.
†Whole milk added.
‡Infant formula. Volumes are modified to meet growing infant needs.
◇Unflavored.

Table A–31 (Continued)

Vivonex◇ *Eaton*	*Vivonex HN* *Eaton*	*Vipep* *Cutter*	*Pregestimil‡* *Mead Johnson*	
20.4 Crystalline amino acids	43.3 Crystalline amino acids	25.0 Fish protein conc. Amino acids	28.5 Hydrolyzed casein Amino acids	
1.4 Safflower oil	0.9 Safflower oil	24.5 MCT oil Corn oil	41.0 Corn oil MCT oil	24.8 16.2
226.3 Glucose oligo- saccharides	211.0 Glucose oligo- saccharides	170.0 Corn syrup solids Sucrose Corn starch Tapioca flour	136.5 Corn syrup solids Tapioca starch	
0	0	0	0	
1000	1000	1000	1500	
555.0	333.0	600.0	936.0	
555.0	333.0	500.0	624.0	
222.0	133.0	200.0	109.2	
10.0	6.0	9.0	18.7	
83.0	50.0	75.0	70.2	
1.1	0 7	1.0	0.9	
1.6	0.9	1.3	0.3	
8.3	5.0	7.5	6.3	
37.4	33.5	32.6	20.4	
30.0	18.0	21.8	28.0	
51.8	52.4	47.9	24.2	
550	810	520	338	
1800	3000	2000		

Table A–32. Supplementary
(The number of new products is growing so rapidly that it was

	Cal-Power General Mills*	Casec Mead Johnson	Citrotein Doyle
PROTEIN, gm	0.6	237.6	60.5
FAT, gm	0	5.4	2.6
CARBOHYDRATE, gm	272.0	0	184.2
SODIUM, mEq	2.39	6.00	45.80
POTASSIUM, mEq	0.70	2.10	26.80
AMOUNT NEEDED TO GIVE 1,000 C	550 gm liquid	270.0 gm dry weight	263.4 gm dry weight
TYPE	Carbohydrate source	Protein source	Protein, vitamin supplement

*Dietary Specialty, General Mills Chemical, Inc.

Table A–32 (Continued)

	Pro Mix Beatrice Scientific	Lipomul-Oral Upjohn	Liprotein Upjohn	Lonalac Mead Johnson	Microlipid Organon	Lytren Mead Johnson
PROTEIN, gm	227.0	0.1	82.7	53.0	0	0
FAT, gm	0	111.1	64.3	54.7	111.1	0
CARBOHYDRATE, gm	22.7	1.1	22.1	74.2	0	253.0
SODIUM, mEq	18.52	2.90	8.00	1.70	0	100.00
POTASSIUM, mEq	116.51	0.09	42.46	48.08	0	83.30
AMOUNT NEEDED TO GIVE 1,000 C	284.0 gm dry weight	166.7 ml liquid	183.7 gm dry weight	1500 ml standard dilution or 196 gm dry weight	222 ml liquid	268 gm dry weight or 3333 ml standard dilution
TYPE	Protein source	Fat source	Calorie source	Low-sodium high-protein source	Fat source	Calorie and electrolyte source

Feedings (per 1,000 kcal).
impossible to include every known product now on the market.)

Controlyte Doyle	dp High p.e.r. Protein General Mills*	EMF Control Drugs	Gevral Lederle	Hy-Cal Beecham-Massengill
Trace	206.0	250.0	170.9	0.1
48.0	10.0	0	5.7	0.1
143.0	21.0	0	66.8	244.1
0.8	22.40	53.00	18.57	2.41
0.20	9.90	5.10	3.65	0.07
198.0 gm dry weight	258 gm dry weight	500 ml liquid	284.8 gm dry weight	407 ml liquid
Low-protein, low-electrolyte calorie source	Protein supplement and low electrolytes	Protein source	Protein-calorie supplement	Carbohydrate source

MCT Oil Mead Johnson	Pedialyte Ross	Polycose Ross	Probana Mead Johnson	Sumacal Organon	Sumacal Plus Organon	Sustacal Pudding Mead Johnson
0	0	0	60.0	0	0	28.3
120.5	0	0	32.0	0	0	39.5
0	250.0	250.0	118.0	250.0	312.5	133.1
0	150.00	12.00	40.50	4.34	4.60	21.70
0	100.00	2.5	46.50	2.94	4.20	30.95
120.5 gm liquid	5000 ml liquid	263 gm dry weight	1500 ml standard dilution	1000 ml liquid	400 ml liquid	625.0 gm
Medium-chain triglycerides	Calorie and electrolyte source	Oligo-saccharides	High protein banana powder formula for celiac condition and diarrhea	Carbohydrate source	Concentrated carbohydrate source	Nutritional supplement

Table A–33.   Defined Formula Diets for Special Metabolic Indications

Per 1000 kcal	Amin-Aid*	LofenalacΦ	Phenyl-FreeΨ	Hepatic Aid*
Protein, gm	9.72	32.5	50.0	25.9
Protein source	Ess. amino acids plus histidine	Casein hydrolysate, amino acids	Casein hydrolysates, amino acids	Amino acids (↑ BCAA ↓ AAA)
Fat, gm	35.2	39.8	16.75	22.0
Fat source	Partially hydrogenated soy oil	Corn oil	Corn oil	Partially hydrogenated soy oil, lecithin, mono-diglycerides
Carbohydrate, gm	162.0	129.2	162.5	174.5
Carbohydrate source	Maltodextrins	Corn syrup solids, tapioca starch	Corn syrup solids, tapioca starch	Maltodextrins, sucrose
Lactose, gm	0	0	0	0
VOLUME TO GIVE 1000 C, ml**	500	1500	1200	607
Minerals				
Calcium, mg	<60	936.0	1500.0	negligible
Phosphorus, mg	negligible	702.0	1125.0	"
Magnesium, mg	<36	109.2	175.0	"
Iron, mg	negligible	18.72	30.0	"
Iodine, mcg	"	70.2	112.5	"
Copper, mg	"	0.94	1.5	"
Manganese, mg	"	1.56	2.5	"
Zinc, mg	"	6.25	10.0	"
Sodium, mEq	<3	20.35	27.17	"
Potassium, mEq	<3	26.0	44.9	"
Chloride, mEq	negligible	19.8	35.2	"
mOsm/kg	1125		920.0	900/liter

Amin-Aid, Hepatic Aid by McGaw; Lofenalac, Phenyl-Free by Mead Johnson.
*Water for reconstituting will affect electrolyte concentration.
**When prepared according to package directions.
ΦBased on 20 kcal/fluid ounce.
Ψ16 oz (480 ml) is the suggested normal daily intake for the older PKU patient based on 25 kcal/fluid oz.
  BCAA = Branched-chain amino acids.
  AAA = Aromatic amino acids.

low or high in electrolytes, mixed calorie sources, and formulas for the treatment of renal failure.

Table A–33 lists defined formula diets for special metabolic indications. These are for patients with significant specific metabolic abnormalities which may be responsive to dietary modification.

Amin-Aid may be used for patients with severe renal disease who are eating poorly. It provides 8 essential amino acids together with histidine, carbohydrate and fat yielding approximately 2 kcal/ml. Amin-Aid contains no vitamins, no indigestible bulk or fibrous material and negligible electrolytes. It is to be supplemented with electrolytes and vitamins as indicated by the patient's metabolic status and frequency of dialysis. Amin-Aid is not palatable and may need to be given by tube.

Lofenalac is a low phenylalanine formula for use in special diets of infants and children with phenylketonuria. Casein hydrolysate is specially processed to remove most of the phenylalanine. Fat, carbohydrate, essential vitamins and minerals are included in appropriate amounts.

Phenyl-Free is a powder reconstituted for use as a beverage designed to permit greater flexibility in the diet of the PKU child previously receiving a Lofenalac-based diet as an infant. Phenyl-Free is not intended for use with infants. Phenyl-Free supplies all essential amino acids (except phenylalanine), vitamins and minerals, but fewer total calories than Lofenalac. The absence of phenylalanine allows a greater variety of other foods for the PKU child. This product should not be used as the sole diet at any time.

Hepatic Aid is a mixture of amino acids, carbohydrate, and fat which may be used as a nitrogen and calorie supplement to the diet of patients with serious hepatic insufficiency secondary to cirrhosis. Its special amino acid mixture contains a relatively high branch-chain amino acid content and a relatively low aromatic amino acid content. If the amino acids make the formula unpalatable to the patient, the preparation may be given by tube to assure adequate intake. It should be supplemented with vitamins and electrolytes based on the patient's metabolic status.

A variety of other formulas are available to meet the needs of children with other errors of metabolism. Among those available from Mead Johnson are:

1. MSUD (Maple Syrup Urine Diseases) Diet Powder, with an amino acid mixture free of branched-chain amino acids. The powder has fat, CH_2O, vitamins and minerals essential for infants.
2. Product 3200 AB, a powder low in tyrosine and phenylalanine designed for patients with hereditary tyrosinemia. Fat, CH_2O, vitamins and minerals are included in appropriate amounts to meet the infant's needs.
3. Product 3200 K, a soy protein powder containing no added methionine for use in the management of homocystinuric infants. Fat, CH_2O, vitamins,

minerals are supplied to meet the infant's needs. Plasma amino acid levels should be monitored.
4. Product 80056, a protein-free base for infants requiring the addition of specific mixtures of amino acids. This powder provides calories as CH_2O and fat in addition to all essential vitamins and minerals. Appropriate amino acid mixtures and adequate sodium must be supplied separately.

Two companies presently make a carbohydrate-free powder. Mead Johnson has Product 3232 A and Syntex has CHO-Free.‡ These formulas contain all essential vitamins and electrolytes but are free of carbohydrates. Calories are in the form of protein and fat. These formulas should be used, in our opinion, for two purposes: (1) as a test diet where carbohydrate intolerance of unknown types is being tested by systematically adding individual carbohydrates to the formula, (2) as a diet for patients with specific known carbohydrate intolerances which is supplemented with those carbohydrates demonstrated to be tolerated.

Indications for Use

Physicians, dietitians and nutritionists must evaluate the nutritional and clinical status of the patient in order to use defined-formula diets effectively, whether prepared commercially or by trained dietitians. Route of administration and flow rate must also be considered so that the nutritional and physiologic needs of the patient are met appropriately. For example, the composition of a specific formulation in terms of osmolality and the type and amounts of carbohydrates, amino acids and fats may be critical factors when fed rapidly to certain patients such as those with high subtotal gastrectomy or those on jejunostomy feedings. These same factors may pose little or no problem in the same

‡CHO-Free and Neo Mull Soy were removed from the market by the manufacturer at the time of this writing and presumably will be reformulated.

patient when a formulation is fed by slow drip over many hours. Hence, the technique of feeding will play a role in the choice of certain preparations.

Many other patients may require liquid feedings because of dysphagia or to supplement an inadequate intake of regular foods, even though they do not have maldigestion or malabsorption problems. Such individuals do not require defined-formula diets with hydrolysates or purified amino acids. Their need is for food dispersed in water. Too often, such patients are given relatively large amounts of "empty-calorie" fluids such as clear soups, tea or soft drinks instead of optimal nutritional supplementation in liquid form. Patients with maldigestion and malabsorption may need special formulas that are more readily absorbed than the usual hospital liquid formulas.

Palatability and acceptability become key factors when a formula is to be taken by mouth for many days, weeks or months. When there is no milk intolerance, varied formulations of milk products, eggs and fruit are useful. Where there is milk intolerance, defined-formula diets low in lactose and with intact protein are useful. Palatability is appreciably greater with preparations containing intact proteins than with those containing protein hydrolysates or free amino acids. Furthermore, those with free amino acids are more expensive than those with intact protein. Since a formula may be needed in fairly large amounts and over an extended period of time, it behooves the physician and dietitian to include the matter of cost when reviewing nutritional needs. Costs may be reduced for the patient at home by developing a diet which is prepared by the patient or family and which is relatively inexpensive because there is no charge for labor and the materials can be purchased in bulk. In considering costs, it is noteworthy that food technology and economics are such that many commercial defined-formula diets with intact proteins are now cheaper and have greater palatability than commercial liquid diets made of natural foods such as meat, eggs and fruit juices.

Formulations with protein hydrolysates or free amino acids are available with a variety of flavors for oral use. In our experience, they are not well accepted in large amounts by many of those patients most likely to benefit from their ingestion. The problem of palatability, of course, is not an issue when tube feeding is used.

Amino Acid Sources. These are derived either from: (1) intact protein in the form of puréed meat, eggs or milk, (2) protein isolates from milk (casein), soybean or egg white, (3) hydrolyzed protein with added amino acids to make a complete amino acid mix or (4) as purified free amino acids. It is well known that protein digestion in the normal intestinal tract proceeds fairly rapidly in the first 100 cm of the jejunum. There are relatively few data on the digestibility of processed proteins in various gastrointestinal disease states. When there is severe pancreatic insufficiency or malabsorption secondary to a short or damaged small bowel, it is postulated that amino acids are better absorbed from either hydrolyzed protein or free amino acids than from intact protein. There are increasing data indicating that the absorption of certain di- and tripeptides may be more efficient than that of individual free amino acids, but we are still lacking comparative data on the use of these peptides in malabsorptive states. Patients differ in the degree of their intestinal dysfunction; in some, a slow drip of a formula with intact protein may be just as well digested and absorbed as the amino acids from the hydrolysates or free amino acids.

Carbohydrates. These are the main source of calories in the formulations. The nature of the carbohydrate is of importance. Glucose or sucrose was used in early formulations which were also low in fat; the quantities required created a very high osmolality, with consequent problems of abdominal discomfort and diarrhea. These have been overcome by the use of starches, dextrins and glucose oligosaccharides. Oligosaccharides are soluble polymers of glucose containing 5 or more glucose molecules; these are hydrolyzed by enzymes in the intestinal mucosa without the need for pancreatic amylase. The preparation is useful for patients with severe pancreatic exocrine insufficiency. The low-osmolality formulas are useful when the "dumping syndrome" is of concern. Since oligosaccharides and longer-chain carbohydrates are not sweet, they can be included in relatively large amounts and be mixed with sucrose or glucose to meet individual taste preferences. In the commercial defined-formula diets, the percentage of calories derived from carbohydrates ranges from 40 to 90 per cent.

Fat. Fat may contribute from less than 1 to as much as 47 per cent of calories in commercial formulas, depending on the product. Most of the commercial formulas contain long-chain fats as corn oil, soy oil or safflower oil. Some products contain medium-chain triglycerides (MCT)# and those that do combine these in varying amounts with a long-chain triglyceride such as soy or corn oil. Fat contributes 9 kcal per gm and does not increase the osmolality of the formula; its presence often improves palatability.

When digestion or absorption is normal or is only slightly impaired, there is no reason to use a preparation containing free amino acids, particularly since they are expensive and tend to be low in fat. When significant maldigestion or malabsorption is present, a diet which is low in fat or which contains MCT oil may be useful. Fat can then be progressively added as tolerance is demonstrated. There are ample data indicating that MCT is absorbed better than long-chain fats when: (1) there is damage to the endothelium of the intestinal mucosa which inhibits the required resynthesis of long-chain fats, (2) the transport of fat from the epithelial cell into the lymphatic system is impaired by obstruction of lymphatic flow or (3) there is a decreased amount of conjugated bile salts or pancreatic enzymes in the upper small bowel. Ingestion and absorption of large amounts of MCT may be associated with increased ketone bodies and acidosis. MCT should be used with caution in patients with hepatic cirrhosis or portacaval shunts who have a tendency to hepatic encephalopathy.

Minerals and Vitamins. The commercial defined-formula diets contain all of the essential minerals, including trace elements, as well as vitamins in amounts which meet or exceed the National Research Council recommended dietary allowances. Give vitamin K as needed.

Trace Elements. For patients with severe malabsorption and/or marked gastrointestinal losses, trace elements supplied in commercial and hospital diets may not be sufficient. A rational approach to this problem requires initial and periodic monitoring of serum trace elements. Additional supplementation of those nutrients which have been identified as being deficient should be given when indicated.

We prepare trace element solutions both as a multiple or as individual solutions for oral or enteral use and the individual solutions have the following compositions:

Ferrous sulfate ($FeSO_4 \cdot 7H_2O$): 43.95 gm/L provides 8.83 mg/ml of Fe^{++}

Cupric sulfate ($CuSO_4 \cdot 5H_2O$): 3.26 gm/L provides 0.83 mg/ml of Cu^{++}

Zinc chloride ($ZnCl_2$): 10.35 gm/L provides 5.01 mg/ml of Zn^{++}

Manganese sulfate ($MnSO_4 \cdot H_2O$): 1.20 gm/L provides 0.38 mg/ml Mn^{++}

Sodium iodide (NaI): 0.05 gm/L provides 0.04 gm/ml I^-

Chromic chloride ($CrCl_3 \cdot 6H_2O$): 200 mg/L provides 38 μg/ml Cr^{+++}

#MCT is a bland oil derived from coconut oil. The fatty acids in the neutral fat vary from 6 to 10 carbons in length and have the unique physiologic property of being able to pass through the intestinal epithelium directly into the portal system as free fatty acids. One gram = 8 kcal.

Table A–34. Examples of Formulas Prepared for Hospital or Patient Preparation (per 1,000 kcal)

MSKCC Blenderized Tube Feeding. A general formula for patients with normal absorption. Sodium restriction to varying degrees is achieved by omission of salt and use of low-salt vegetables. Potassium restriction is achieved by modification of orange juice. Volume per 1000 kcal is 1000 ml.

Carrots, canned	45	gm
Chopped beefΦ	105	gm
Corn oil	30	gm
Dark Karo syrup	90	gm
Egg, cooked	68	gm
Farina, cooked	114	gm
Nonfat milk powder	20	gm
Orange juice	180	ml
Salt	1.5	gm
Water or vegetable juice	450	ml
Wax beans, canned	30	gm
Poly-Vi-Sol vitamins with iron	1	tablet/day

DeR Oral or Tube Formula. A palatable low-residue defined-formula as supplement. When used as only source of nutrition, magnesium oxide or chloride and trace elements are added. Modifications are easily made as needed. Volume per 1000 kcal is 800 ml.

Calcium caseinate	31	gm
Chocolate syrup	36	gm
Cornstarch, cooked	40	gm
Dextrose, anhydrous or oligosaccharides	80	gm
Egg, cooked	45	gm
Gevral protein	4.5	gm
Oil (corn or MCT)	27	gm
Potassium chloride	2.0	gm
Water	600	ml
Poly-Vi-Sol vitamins with iron**	1	tablet/day
Trace elements	2	ml

T-#23 Tube Formula. A formula with casein hydrolysate for use in patients with serious malabsorption, pancreatic insufficiency, inflammatory bowel disease or intestinal fistulas. Modifications are easily made. Volume per 1000 kcal is 900 ml.

Alcolec*	1.0	gm
Calcium lactate	0.9	gm
Calcium phosphate	0.9	gm
DL-methionine	0.23	gm
DL-tryptophan	0.23	gm
Egg, cooked	45	gm
Hy-Case, SF†	34	gm
Magnesium chloride	(as needed)	
Oil (corn or MCT) [initially low]	23	gm
Oligosaccharides (Polycose)	169	gm
Potassium gluconate and/or chloride	(as needed)	
Sodium chloride and/or bicarbonate	(as needed)	
Trace elements	2	ml
Water	690	ml
Poly-Vi-Sol vitamins with iron**	1	tablet/day

Φ Pureed beef is used for small-bore tubes to avoid clogging.
* Lecithin (emulsifying agent) if oil is used.
† Hydrolyzed casein.
** Add Vitamin K, 5 mg once weekly.

When preparing a multiple trace element solution containing all the above compounds, we add 5.0 ml 1 N hydrochloric acid to distilled water, then dissolve the salts and bring the final volume up to 1 liter. When zinc chloride is prepared individually, 1 to 2 drops of 1 N HCl is also added to 1 liter of solution to prevent formation of the hydroxide.

Ascorbic acid (50 to 100 mg) may be added to solutions containing ferrous sulfate to prevent oxidation to the ferric ion or to reverse the oxidation if it has occurred.

For our formulas (Table A–34) the multiple trace elements are added. Additional trace elements should be added as necessary. For general use 4 ml of the multiple trace element solution is prescribed per day.

These trace element solutions may be made by a trained dietitian or pharmacist or may be purchased commercially; they should be checked for proper content by analysis and for sterility by microbiologic testing prior to use.

Drawbacks With Commercial Formulations

Being nutritionally complete, defined-formula diets are both a boon and a problem to the physician and dietitian. They are easy to store, order and administer. Serious difficulties, however, may arise due to the very fact that formula compositions are "fixed." Patients having metabolic problems may be unable to tolerate the amounts of one or more nutrients provided by the formula in the volumes necessary to meet overall nutritional requirements. Such a formulation may, in fact, be either potentially or actually hazardous for such patients because of the development of adverse effects. This is true, for example, of patients with renal disease who cannot tolerate the levels of protein, sodium, potassium, phosphate or magnesium present in a given formulation, or of patients receiving corticosteroids who

are accumulating salt and water and cannot tolerate the amount of sodium present, or of those with hypercalcemia who should not be ingesting the amount of calcium present. The physician must be aware in each such instance of specific composition and possible contraindications. In these situations, the dietitian must modify the formula by either adding desired ingredients while diluting out those that are undesirable or, alternatively, devising a completely different preparation from specific nutrients.

Individual ingredients are available and can be combined with the proper medical prescription and the services of a dietitian trained in this field. Three examples of formulations which can be prepared in the hospital are given in Table A–34. The first is a general tube-feeding formula, the second is a palatable defined-formula for oral or tube feeding, and the third is designed for tube feeding in patients with pancreatic insufficiency, severe malabsorption or related problems. Modifications of major nutrients and electrolytes are easily executed.

Manufacturers could overcome the limitation of "fixed" formulations by preparing formula diets in "modular" form, with certain critical items such as fat or sodium and potassium salts being made available in separate containers to be added or modified in amounts as indicated by a patient's need.

Procedures in Tube Feeding

The preferred method of feeding anorectic patients is by the oral route when the alimentary tract is functioning normally. In practice, this is often difficult to accomplish. A palatable, high-calorie, nutritious liquid formula may contribute toward achieving an adequate intake. If this fails, an alternative method is tube feeding, using nasopharyngeal, esophagostomy, gastrostomy or jejunostomy tubes. In theory, such feeding should work very well; in practice, however, numerous problems may arise. Many patients who have had prior experience with nasogastric tubes are strongly opposed to further encounters with them. A medium- or fine-bore tube is tolerated much better than is the usual plastic or rubber feeding tube. However the small tube requires a finely dispersed formula to prevent clogging. Blenderized formulas of regular food usually do not flow well, whereas the highly dispersed defined-formula diets of low viscosity flow easily.

The potential hazard of formulas being aspirated must always be considered. This can be minimized by slow feeding to prevent accumulation in the stomach and by having the patient's head and chest kept at a 30-degree angle or higher while being fed. As a general policy, avoid tube feedings when the potential for aspiration is

significant, particularly when there is a preexisting pulmonary problem unless the tip of the tube can be placed in the duodenum or upper jejunum.

Small-caliber feeding tubes—which are usually well tolerated for prolonged periods because of their small diameter and flexibility—include long central venous catheters of 14 to 16 gauge, pediatric feeding tubes French 5 to 8, and tubes of silicone or polyurethane elastomers weighted with encapsulated mercury at the tip. Few patients require continuous round-the-clock feedings. Intermittent feedings for a variable number of hours are suitable for most formula patients. Consideration should be given to training the patient or a family member in the technique of passing the nasopharyngeal tube for each feeding when there is no contraindication. Some

Table A–35.   Modifications of MSKCC Blenderized Tube-feeding Formula (A-34) for Special Clinical Conditions

MCT oil: Eliminate 60 gm corn oil. Substitute 67 gm MCT oil (to maintain 2,000 kcal). Various proportions of both oils may be added as indicated by patient's condition.

Low fat: Eliminate 60 gm corn oil. Add 135 gm sugar (to maintain 2,000 kcal). Meat must be very lean. Fat = 26 gm.

Low Na: Eliminate 3.0 gm salt (44 mEq Na). If a severely restricted Na intake is indicated substitute salt-free carrots, salt-free wax beans for regular. Na will be less than 10 mEq.

Low protein, potassium and sodium: The restrictions of this diet are substantial and require close clinical supervision. Modifications should be made as soon as the patient's condition permits. An example of such a diet follows:

Wt.	Ingredients	Household Measures	Nutritive Analysis: 2,287 kcal*		
240 gm	cooked enriched farina	1 cup	Protein	17	gm
45 gm	egg, boiled	1	Fat	95	gm
20 gm	skim milk powder	2 tbsp	CH_2O	339	gm
45 gm	carrots, salt free	¼ cup			
60 gm	wax beans, salt free	½ cup	Ca	363	mg
90 gm	corn oil	3 oz	P	329	mg
300 gm	sugar	2 cups	Na	176/8	mg/mEq
	Water up to 2,000 ml		K	533/14	mg/mEq
	volume or as indicated		Fe	2.8	mg ⎫ plus
			Vit A	7,347	I.U. ⎪ those
			B_1	0.24	mg ⎪ in
			B_2	0.97	mg ⎬ multivitamin
			Niacin	1.54	mg ⎪ mineral
			Vit C	17.9	mg ⎭ supplement

*Does not meet 1974 RDA except for vitamin A. When multivitamin and mineral prescriptions are given, vitamin and mineral allowances may be achieved.

patients may be fed at night by slow drip (preferably pump monitored) and freed of the tube during much of the day.

Despite the antipathy of many patients toward feeding tubes, a large number will allow a small-caliber tube to be passed on a trial basis, with the understanding that the tube will be removed if it proves uncomfortable when long-term tube feeding is indicated. Most patients will keep the tube in place, and more highly motivated individuals will learn to pass the tube themselves.

Slow continuous feeding may be indicated in patients with a potential problem with aspiration, serious malabsorption, bowel fistula or partial obstruction. In this situation use of a delivery system which will ensure a controlled, slow drip is helpful. Various types of containers are available.

Table A–36. Oral or Tube Formula of Nonperishable Foods*

Purpose: This formula is nutritionally complete, is composed of ingredients which require no prior refrigeration and is easily prepared. It may be used for oral or tube feeding and is especially useful for patients on formula feeding who must travel. It contains skim milk and may not be satisfactory for those with lactose or milk intolerance. It is very low in residue and tends to be constipating. The materials are easily available and relatively inexpensive. Fruit juices, coffee or other beverages may be taken separately. The water volume will depend on the fluid requirements of the patient. Changes in kcal are accomplished by modifying the amounts of Karo syrup and corn oil. Sweetness may be modified by varying the amounts of Karo syrup or omitting Gevral Protein.

Preparation: Mix well in a blender at low speed or shake in a jar. Refrigerate. For better chocolate flavor use one or two packages of chocolate with one package of vanilla.

Ingredients for 2,400 ml:		*Nutritive Analysis:*	
321 gm	(9 packages) of Instant Breakfast or equivalent	Kcal	2,073
		Protein	80 gm
90 gm	(¼ cup) Karo syrup, dark	Fat	72 gm
6 gm	(1 tbsp) Gevral Protein (Lederle Labs)	CH_2O	276 gm
		Ca	1,157 mg
70 gm	(3 oz) corn oil	P	1,277 mg
2,160 ml	(9 cups) water	Na	59 mEq
		K	94 mEq
		Mg	19 mEq
		Fe	2.5 mg

*Modified by Shils, M. E., and Bloch, A. S. from a formula suggested by Mr. John Dewitt Norton.

This formula may be further adapted to a less expensive but complete nutritional intake by using the following:

Powdered skim milk	2½ cups dry
Vegetable oil	3 ounces
Sugar (or Karo)	½ cup
Juice of choice (citrus 2 to 3 times weekly)	½ cup
Vitamin/mineral supplement	1 tablet
Water—enough to reconstitute milk and meet daily fluid needs	

When convenient or available, include one cooked egg in formula.

Supplemental trace elements, folic acid, vitamin K and iron may be required if vitamin mineral preparation is inadequate in these factors.

The formulation provides 2,000 kcal, 73 gm protein, 90 gm fat, 223 gm CH_2O.

If calories or any single nutrient need to be adjusted to meet individual requirements, the specific nutrient may be increased or decreased to achieve a suitable intake.

One type of plastic feeding bag has two compartments: one for the formula, the other for ice. This bag comes with a large bore tubing. We recommend that the tubing be cut several inches below the bag and a standard IV drip chamber and tubing be inserted in its place for better control. Another type of bag has tubing which contains a microdrop drip chamber. Use of this bag for formulas other than the one for which it is designed may lead to clogged tubing or inconsistent rate of flow. Bottles are available with a screw-on fitted cap with small bore tubing to permit regulation of drip rate. The bottle caps are standard size and will screw onto most commercial formulas manufactured in bottles.

The need for a surgical procedure to insert esophagostomy, gastrostomy or jejunostomy feeding tubes often discourages physicians unduly from using tube feeding as an alternative method for ensuring that their patients' nutritional requirements are met. With jejunostomy feedings, the formula should be given slowly, particularly if it contains significant amounts of soluble sugars, until it has been demonstrated that the patient can tolerate the formula and the rate without developing dumping symptoms. The lower the osmolality of the formula, the more rapidly the infusion may be given.

The large number of commercial preparations listed in the tables offers a complex array from which choices must be made. It is suggested that physicians and dietitians who prescribe and serve such formulations perform their own taste tests, review the compositions, select a limited number of different types and carefully observe patient reactions to them. By using this approach, a short list of liquid formulas can be developed to meet specific patient nutritional needs.

Suggested Reading

1. Gray: N. Engl. J. Med., *292*, 1225, 1975.
2. Greenberger and Skillman: N. Engl. J. Med., *208*, 1045, 1969.
3. Heymsfield, Bethel, Ansley, Nixon and Rudman: Ann. Intern. Med., *90*, 63, 1979.
4. Matthews and Adibi: Gastroenterology, *71*, 151, 1976.
5. Shils: Cancer Res., *37*, 2432, 1977.
6. Shils (Ed.): *Proceedings from Conference on Defined Formula Diets for Medical Purposes.* American Medical Association, Chicago, 1975.
7. Bethel et al.: Am. J. Clin. Nutr., *32*, 1112, 1979.

INDEX

Page numbers in *italics* refer to illustrations; page numbers followed by t refer to tables.